BRIEF CONTENTS

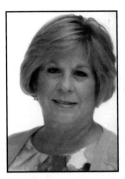

Linda Lane Lilley, RN, PhD

Linda Lilley received her diploma from Norfolk General School of Nursing, BSN from the University of Virginia, Master of Science (Nursing) from Old Dominion University, and PhD in Nursing from George Mason University. As an Associate Professor Emeritus and University Professor at Old Dominion University, her teaching experience in nursing education spans over 25 years, including almost 20 years at Old Dominion. Linda's teaching expertise includes drug therapy and the nursing process, adult nursing, physical assessment, fundamentals in nursing, oncology nursing, nursing theory, and trends in health care. The awarding of the University's most prestigious title of University Professor reflects her teaching excellence as a tenured faculty member. She has also been a two-time university nominee for the State Council of Higher Education in Virginia award for excellence in teaching, service, and scholarship. Linda received the 2012 Distinguished Nursing Alumni Award from Old Dominion University School of Nursing for her "continued work on the successful pharmacology textbook published by Elsevier" and to recognize her "extraordinary work and the impact [the book] has had on baccalaureate education." While at Old Dominion University, Linda mentored and taught undergraduate and graduate students as well as registered nurses returning for their BSN. Linda authored the MED ERRORS column for the *American Journal of Nursing* between 1994 and 1999 as well as numerous other peer-reviewed, published articles in professional nursing journals. After retiring in 2005, Linda continued to be active in nursing, serving as a member on dissertation committees with the College of Health Sciences and maintaining membership and involvement in numerous professional and academic organizations. Since January of 2014, Dr. Lilley continues to serves on the volunteer review panel for the monthly newsletter publication *Nurse Advise-ERR* (ISMP affiliated; the ISMP [Institute for Safe Medication Practices] is a nonprofit organization educating the healthcare community and consumers about safe medication practices). Linda has served as a consultant with school nurses in the city of Virginia Beach, a member on the City of Virginia Beach's Health Advisory Board, and a member of the City of Virginia Beach's Community Health Advisory Board and Youth Community Action Team (YCAT). Linda also served as an appointed member on the national advisory panel on medication errors prevention with the U.S. Pharmacopeia in Rockville, Maryland. She continues to educate nursing students and professional nurses about drug therapy and the nursing process and speaks on the topics of drug therapy, safe medication use, humor and healing, and grief and loss.

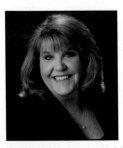

Shelly Rainforth Collins, PharmD

Shelly Rainforth Collins received her Doctor of Pharmacy degree from the University of Nebraska, College of Pharmacy in 1985, with High Distinction. She then completed a clinical pharmacy residency at Memorial Medical Center of Long Beach in Long Beach, California. She worked as a pediatric clinical pharmacist (neonatal specialist) at Memorial Medical Center before moving to Mobile, Alabama. She was the Assistant Director of Clinical Pharmacy Services at Mobile Infirmary Medical Center. After moving to Chesapeake, Virginia, she served as the Clinical Pharmacy Specialist/ Coordinator of Clinical Pharmacy Services at Chesapeake Regional Medical Center in Chesapeake, Virginia for 19 years. Her practice focused on developing and implementing clinical pharmacy services as well as medication safety and Joint Commission medication management standards and national patient safety goals. She is currently works as a clinical pharmacist for Sentara Obici Hospital. She is president of Drug Information Consultants, a business offering consultation and expert witness review for attorneys on medical malpractice cases. She holds certifications in Medication Therapy Management, Anticoagulation Management, and Immunizations. Shelly was awarded the Clinical Pharmacist of the Year Award in 2007 from the Virginia Society of Healthsystem Pharmacists. She led a multidisciplinary team that won the Clinical Achievement of the Year Award from George Mason University School of Public Health in 2007 for promoting safety with narcotics in patients with sleep apnea; this program has also received national recognition. She was awarded the Service Excellence Award from Chesapeake Regional Medical Center. Shelly's professional affiliations include the American Society of Healthsystem Pharmacists, the Virginia Society of Healthsystem Pharmacists, and the American Pharmacists Association.

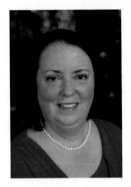

Julie S. Snyder, MSN, RN-BC

Julie Snyder received her diploma from Norfolk General Hospital School of Nursing and her BSN and MSN from Old Dominion University. After working in medical-surgical nursing, she worked in nursing staff development and community education. Later, she transferred to the academic setting and has since taught fundamentals of nursing, pharmacology, physical assessment, gerontologic nursing, and adult medical-surgical nursing. Julie is currently working as a Quality Initiative Coordinator at Chesapeake Regional Healthcare in Chesapeake, Virginia. She has been certified by the ANCC in Nursing Continuing Education and Staff Development and currently holds ANCC certification in Medical-Surgical Nursing. She is a member of Sigma Theta Tau International and was inducted into Phi Kappi Phi as Outstanding Alumni for Old Dominion University. She has worked for Elsevier as a reviewer, ancillary writer, and author since 1997. Julie's professional service has included serving on the Virginia Nurses' Association Continuing Education Committee, serving as Educational Development Committee chair for the Epsilon Chi chapter of Sigma Theta Tau, serving as an item writer for the ANCC, working with a regional hospital educators' group, and serving as a consultant on various projects for local hospital education departments. In addition, she has conducted NCLEX pharmacology review classes for recent nursing graduates.

PHARMACOLOGY
and the NURSING PROCESS
the

EIGHTH EDITION

Linda Lane Lilley, RN, PhD
University Professor and Associate Professor Emeritus (Retired)
School of Nursing
Old Dominion University
Norfolk, Virginia

Shelly Rainforth Collins, PharmD
Clinical Pharmacist
Sentara Obici Hospital
Suffolk, Virginia
President
Drug Information Consultants
Chesapeake, Virginia

Julie S. Snyder, MSN, RN-BC
Quality Initiative Coordinator
Chesapeake Regional Healthcare
Chesapeake, Virginia

ELSEVIER

ELSEVIER

3251 Riverport Lane
St. Louis, Missouri 63043

PHARMACOLOGY AND THE NURSING PROCESS   ISBN: 978-0-323-35828-6

Library of Congress Cataloging-in-Publication Data
Names: Lilley, Linda Lane, author. | Collins, Shelly Rainforth, author. | Snyder, Julie S., author.
Title: Pharmacology and the nursing process / Linda Lane Lilley, Shelly Rainforth Collins, Julie S. Snyder.
Description: 8th edition. | St. Louis, Missouri : Elsevier, [2017] | Includes index.
Identifiers: LCCN 2015040163 | ISBN 9780323358286 (pbk. : alk. paper)
Subjects: | MESH: Pharmacology—Nurses' Instruction. | Drug Therapy—Nurses' Instruction. | Pharmaceutical Preparations—administration & dosage—Nurses' Instruction.
Classification: LCC RM301 | NLM QV 4 | DDC 615/.1—dc23
LC record available at http://lccn.loc.gov/2015040163

Content Strategist: Jamie Randall
Content Development Manager: Billie Sharp
Publishing Services Manager: Catherine Jackson
Senior Project Manager: Clay S. Broeker
Design Direction: Margaret Reid

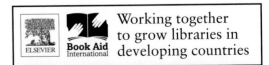

Printed in the United States of America

Last digit is the print number: 9 8 7 6 5 4 3 2

CONTRIBUTORS TO TEACHING/ LEARNING RESOURCES

Learning Strategies

Laura Jaroneski, MSN, RN, OCN, CNE
Adjunct Faculty
Macomb Community College
Warren, Michigan

Critical Thinking and Prioritization Questions

Julie S. Snyder, MSN, RN-BC
Quality Initiative Coordinator
Chesapeake Regional Healthcare
Chesapeake, Virginia

Key Points—Downloadable

Margaret Slota, DNP, RN, FAAN
Associate Professor and Director, DNP and Graduate Nursing
    Leadership Programs
Carlow University School of Nursing
Pittsburgh, Pennsylvania

PowerPoint® Slides

Valerie Baker, ACNS, BC
Assistant Professor
Villa Maria School of Nursing, Morosky College of Health
    Professions and Sciences
Gannon University
Erie, Pennsylvania

Review Questions for the NCLEX® Examination

Tara McMillan-Queen, RN, MSN, ANP, GNP
Cardiac Service Line Educator
Central Division, Carolinas HealthCare System
Charlotte, North Carolina

TEACH® for Nurses Lesson Plans

Deanne A. Blach, MSN, RN
DB Productions of NW Arkansas, Inc.
Green Forest, Arkansas

Linda Wendling, MA
Adult Learning Theory Consultant
Wordbench Educational
Fort Myers, Florida

Test Bank

Julie S. Snyder, MSN, RN-BC
Quality Initiative Coordinator
Chesapeake Regional Healthcare
Chesapeake, Virginia

Unfolding Case Studies

Jennifer D. Powers, MSN, FNP-BC, RN
Assistant Professor
National University Nevada
Henderson, Nevada

Kara Delaney, PharmD
St. Louis, Missouri

Nancy W. Ebersole, PhD, RN
Associate Professor of Nursing
Salem State University
Salem, Massachusetts

Margie L. Francisco, Ed. D, MSN, RN
Nursing Professor
Illinois Valley Community College
Oglesby, Illinois

Jennifer Hebert, MSN, RN-BC
Education Nurse Specialist
Chesapeake Regional Medical Center
Chesapeake, Virginia

Anne Marie Hood, RN
Nurse
Chesapeake, Virginia

Donna Walker Hubbard, RN, MSN, CNNE
Assistant Professor, Retired
University of Mary Hardin—Baylor
Bedford, Texas

Tiffany Jakubowski, BSN, RN, ONC
Nursing Faculty
Front Range Community College
Clinical Nurse II
Longmont United Hospital
Longmont, Colorado

Sarah Keeling, RN, BSN, MN
Associate Professor of Nursing
Georgia Perimeter College
Decatur, Georgia

Janis McMillan, RN, MSN, CNE
Nursing Instructor
Coconino Community College
Flagstaff, Arizona

Darla K. Shar, MSN, RN
Nursing Faculty
Hannah E. Mullins School of Practical Nursing
Salem, Ohio

Crystal R. Sherman, DNP, RN, APHN-BC
Assistant Professor
Shawnee State University
Portsmouth, Ohio

Lazette Nowicki, RN, MSN
Professor
American River College
Sacramento, California

Brian B. Walker, DNAP, MSNA, CRNA RN
Instructor
Texas State Technical College
Harlingen, Texas

Now in its eighth edition, *Pharmacology and the Nursing Process* provides the most current and clinically relevant nursing pharmacology content in a visually appealing, understandable, and practical format. The accessible size, clear writing style, and full-color design of *Pharmacology and the Nursing Process* are ideal for today's busy nursing student. The book not only presents drug information that nursing student needs to know but also provides information on what professional nurses may encounter during drug administration in a variety of health care settings, including accounts of real-life medication errors and tips for avoiding those errors. Edition after edition, the book has become increasingly inviting and engaging for the adult learner to read and study. Features that help set the book apart include:

- A focus on the role of prioritization in nursing care
- A strong focus on drug classes to help students acquire a better knowledge of how various drug classes work in the body, allowing them to apply this knowledge to individual drugs
- Ease of readability to make this difficult content more understandable
- Integrated learning strategies content that helps students understand and learn the particularly demanding subject of pharmacology while also equipping them with tools that they can use in other courses and as lifelong learners who are building an evidence-based practice.

The use of color has continued to complement the text by making the book more engaging for nursing students. Color is used throughout to:

- Highlight important content
- Illustrate how drugs work in the body in numerous anatomic and drug process color illustrations
- Improve the visual appearance of the content to make it more engaging and appealing to today's more visually sophisticated reader

We believe that the use of color and other visual engagement devices in these ways significantly improves students' involvement and understanding of pharmacology.

For this edition, the author team has continued to focus closely on providing the most "need-to-know" information, enhancing readability, and emphasizing the nursing process and prioritization throughout.

Sharing the goal of creating a nursing pharmacology textbook that is not only academically rigorous but also practical and easy to use, the authors bring together a unique combination of experience. The author team is comprised of an Associate Professor Emeritus with a PhD in nursing and more than 25 years of teaching experience, a clinical pharmacist with a PharmD and 28 years of experience in hospital pharmacy practice, and a nursing clinical instructor who holds a Master of Science in Nursing degree and has 25 years of teaching experience.

ORGANIZATION

This book includes 58 chapters presented in 10 parts, organized by body system. The 9 "concepts" chapters in Part 1 lay a solid foundation for the subsequent drug units and address the following topics:

- The nursing process and drug therapy
- Pharmacologic principles
- Lifespan considerations related to pharmacology
- Cultural, legal, and ethical considerations
- Preventing and responding to medication errors
- Patient education and drug therapy
- Over-the-counter drugs and herbal and dietary supplements
- Gene therapy and pharmacogenomics
- Drug administration techniques, including more than 100 drawings and photographs

Parts 2 through 10 present pharmacology and nursing management in a time-tested body systems/drug function framework. This approach facilitates learning by grouping functionally related drugs and drug groups. It provides an effective means of integrating the content into medical-surgical/adult health nursing courses or for teaching pharmacology in a separate course.

The 49 drug chapters in these 9 parts constitute the main portion of the book. Drugs are presented in a consistent format with an emphasis on drug classes and key similarities and differences among the drugs in each class. Each chapter is subdivided into two discussions, beginning with (1) a brief overview of anatomy, physiology, and pathophysiology and a complete discussion of pharmacology, followed by (2) a comprehensive yet succinct application of the nursing process.

Pharmacology is presented for each drug group in a consistent format:

- Mechanism of Action and Drug Effects
- Indications
- Contraindications
- Adverse Effects (often including Toxicity and Management of Overdose)
- Interactions
- Dosages

Drug class discussions conclude with specially highlighted Drug Profiles—brief narrative "capsules" of individual drugs in the class or group, including Pharmacokinetics tables for each drug. Key drugs (prototypical drugs within a class) are identified throughout with a ♦ symbol for easy identification. High-alert medications are identified with a ! symbol to increase awareness of high-alert medications.

The pharmacology section is followed by a Nursing Process discussion that relates to the entire drug group. This nursing content is covered in the following, familiar nursing process format:

- Assessment
- Nursing Diagnoses

- Planning (including Goals and Outcome Criteria)
- Implementation
- Evaluation

At the end of each Nursing Process section is a Patient-Centered Care: Patient Teaching box that summarizes key points for nursing students and/or practicing nurses to include in the education of patients about their medications. These boxes focus on teaching how the drugs work, possible interactions, adverse effects, and other information related to the safe and effective use of the drug(s). The role of the nurse as patient educator and advocate continues to grow in importance in professional practice, so there is emphasis on this key content in each chapter in this edition.

Additionally, each part begins with a Learning Strategies section that relates learning strategies to the unit being discussed. Topics include time management, note taking, studying, test taking, and others. This unique feature is intended to aid students who find pharmacology difficult and to provide a tool that may prove beneficial throughout their nursing school careers. This arrangement of content can be especially helpful to faculty who teach pharmacology through an integrated approach because it helps the student identify key content and concepts.

NEW TO THIS EDITION

To further improve the hallmark readability and user-friendliness of *Pharmacology and the Nursing Process*, each line of the text has been edited to improve readability.

The eighth edition of *Pharmacology and the Nursing Process* also features additional Quality and Safety Education for Nurses (QSEN) competencies by providing the following:

- Case studies with the relevant QSEN competency added to the case study title
- Selected case studies featuring collaboration and teamwork content
- New Safety: What Went Wrong? case studies
- Additional Safety and Quality Improvement: Medication Errors boxes
- New title for Patient Teaching Tips: Patient-Centered Care: Patient Teaching
- An explanation of the QSEN initiative as it relates to safety and quality of patient care included in the *Medication Errors* chapter

The QSEN initiative is also highlighted in this edition's *TEACH for Nurses* Lesson Plans (see Supplemental Resources).

The pharmacology and nursing content in each of the 58 chapters has been thoroughly revised and critically reviewed by nursing instructors, practicing nurses, and a PharmD to reflect the latest drug information and nursing content. Key updates include:

- New "Drugs in Action" illustrations show how specific drugs work in the body
- An icon indicating key drugs in the Dosages tables
- A red-flag icon to identify ISMP high-alert drugs
- Revised NCLEX® Examination Review Questions at the end of each chapter, including alternate-item format and new dosage calculation questions

ADDITIONAL TEACHING/LEARNING FEATURES

The book also includes a variety of innovative teaching/learning features that prepare the student for important content to be covered in each chapter and encourage review and reinforcement of that content. Chapter-opener features include the following:

- Learning Objectives
- Summary of Drug Profiles in the chapter, with page number references
- Key terms with definitions and page number references (key terms being in **bold blue** type throughout the narrative to emphasize this essential terminology)

The following features appear at the end of each chapter:

- Patient Teaching Tips related to drug therapy
- Key Points boxes summarizing important chapter content
- NCLEX® Examination Review Questions, with answers provided upside-down at the bottom of the section for quick and easy review
- Critical Thinking and Prioritization Questions, with answer guidelines provided on the Evolve website
- List of Evolve Resources available to students

In addition to the special boxes listed previously, other special features that appear throughout the text include:

- Case Studies, with answer guidelines provided on the Evolve website
- Dosages tables listing generic and trade names, pharmacologic class, usual dosage ranges, and indications for the drugs

For a more comprehensive listing of the special features, please see the inside back cover of the book.

SUPPLEMENTAL RESOURCES

A comprehensive ancillary package is available to instructors (and their students) who adopt *Pharmacology and the Nursing Process*. The following supplemental resources have been thoroughly revised for this edition and can significantly assist teaching and learning of pharmacology.

Study Guide

The carefully prepared student workbook includes the following:

- Student Study Tips that reinforce the Learning Strategies in the text and provide a "how to" guide to applying test-taking strategies
- Worksheets for each chapter, with NCLEX®-style questions (now with more application-based, alternate-item, and dosage calculation questions), critical thinking and application questions, and other activities
- Case Studies followed by related critical thinking questions
- An updated Overview of Dosage Calculations with helpful tips for calculating doses, sample drug labels, practice problems, and a quiz
- Answers to all questions (provided in the back of the book) to facilitate self-study

Evolve Website

Located at http://evolve.elsevier.com/Lilley/, the Evolve website for this book includes the following:

For students:

- More than 600 NCLEX® Examination Review Questions
- Printable, expanded Key Points for each chapter
- Content Updates
- Answers to Case Studies from the book
- Unfolding Case Studies

For instructors:

- *TEACH for Nurses* Lesson Plans that focus on the most important content from each chapter and provide innovative strategies for student engagement and learning. These new Lesson Plans include strategies for integrating nursing curriculum standards (QSEN, concept-based learning, and the BSN essentials), links to all relevant student and instructor resources, and an original instructor-only Case Study in each chapter.
- ExamView Test Bank that features more than 800 NCLEX® Examination–format test questions (including alternate-item questions) with text page references, rationales, and answers coded for NCLEX® Client Needs category, nursing process step, and cognitive level (new and old Bloom's taxonomy). The robust ExamView testing application, provided at no cost to faculty, allows instructors to create new tests; edit, add, and delete test questions; sort questions by NCLEX® Client Needs category, cognitive level, and nursing process step; and administer and grade tests online, with automated scoring and gradebook functionality.
- PowerPoint Lecture Slides consisting of more than 2100 customizable text slides for instructors to use in lectures. Audience Response System Questions (three or more discussion-oriented questions per chapter for use with i>Clicker and other systems) are folded into these presentations.
- An Image Collection with approximately 220 full-color images from the book for instructors to use in lectures
- Access to all student resources listed above

Pharmacology Online

Pharmacology Online for *Pharmacology and the Nursing Process*, eighth edition (ISBN: 978-0-323-37120-9), is a dynamic, unit-by-unit online course that includes interactive self-study modules, a collection of interactive learning activities, and a media-rich library of supplemental resources.

- *Self-Study Modules* go beyond the basic principles of pharmacology, with animations and NCLEX® Examination–style questions to help students assess their understanding of pharmacology concepts.
- *Interactive Case Studies* immerse students in true-to-life scenarios that require them to make important choices in patient care and patient teaching.
- "*Roadside Assistance*" video clips use humor and analogy in a uniquely fun and engaging way to teach key concepts.

- Interactive Learning Activities, Discussion Questions, Practice Quizzes for the NCLEX® Examination, and more are also included.

ACKNOWLEDGMENTS

This book truly has been a collaborative effort. We wish to thank the instructors who provided input on an ongoing basis throughout the development of the previous editions.

We thank Jamie Randall and Charlene Ketchum for helping make the eighth edition of the Lilley very successful. Jamie and Charlene's guidance, attention to detail, and support have been much appreciated, and suggestions for improving readability and organization of content helped to make the eighth edition better than ever. Thanks for their patience and nurturing manner! We thank Kristin Geen and Jamie Randall for their contributions and support throughout the fourth, fifth, and sixth editions. We are also extremely grateful to Clay Broeker for very capably guiding the project through to publication. Laura Jaroneski lent her study skills expertise and has updated the unique and appropriate Learning Strategies features for students; for her collaboration, we are most grateful. Finally, we thank Joe Albanese for his contributions to the first edition of the book, Bob Aucker for his contributions to the first three editions, and Scott Harrington for contributions through the sixth edition.

Linda thanks her daughter Karen for her unwavering and constant support. Long hours and time spent researching and writing has preempted time with family, but Karen has always understood. Linda wishes to dedicate this book to Karen Leanne Lilley Harris because she remains an inspiration and encouragement for all professional and personal endeavors and accomplishments. The memory of Linda's parents, John and Thelma Lane, who passed away during the fourth edition, and in-laws J.C. and Mary Anne Lilley, who passed away during the fifth and sixth editions, has continued to provide inspiration and a sense of pride in all her work. Students and graduates of Old Dominion University School of Nursing have been eager to provide feedback and support, beginning with the class of 1990 and continuing through the class of 2005. Without their participation, the book would not have been so user-friendly and helpful to students beginning the study of drug therapy. Linda attributes her successes and accomplishments to a strong sense of purpose, faith, and family and an appreciation for the light-hearted side of life. To Jibby Baucom, Linda offers many thanks, because without her recommendation to Mosby, Inc. back in the 1990s, the book would never have been developed. Robin Carter, Kristin Geen, Lee Henderson, Jamie Randall, and Jackie Twomey have been constant resources and more than just editors with Elsevier; they have been sources of strength and encouragement. Their excellent work ethic, positivity, and calming natures will be forever appreciated. The fifth through eighth editions have also involved Clay Broeker, who has been a tremendous resource in dealing with production issues; his contributions to all of these editions have been strong and forward-thinking. Elsevier has shared some of its best employees with Linda beginning with the first day of the first edition; for that, Linda is most thankful and extremely grateful.

Shelly wishes to dedicate this edition to her daughter Kristin Collins and to her father Charles Rainforth of Hastings, Nebraska, the two most important people in her life. You both have been an inspiration, a support system, and most importantly, a source of constant love. Kristin, it has been such a joy watching you grow into the wonderful woman you have become. You will make an amazing educator, and your students will be inspired by your passion, grace, and accomplishment. I am so very proud of you!! The memory of Shelly's mother, Rogene Rainforth, who passed away during the seventh edition, continues to provide a sense of pride and love. Shelly wishes to thank her brother, Randy Rainforth, for supporting their father when distance separates the family. Shelly would also like to thank Linda Lilley and Julie Snyder for giving her the opportunity to be affiliated with such a wonderful book. To the amazing editorial staff at Elsevier, thank you. To her dear friend, Anne Marie Hood, Shelly would like to thank you for all of your words of encouragement, support, and friendship. Finally, to the talented pharmacy department at Sentara Obici Hospital, Shelly thanks you for welcoming her to your family and is humbled to not only call you her colleagues but also her friends.

Julie wishes to dedicate this edition to her parents Willis and Jean Simmons for their unfailing love, support, and encouragement. She thanks Jonathan, her husband, for his patience during long hours of revision work, as well her daughter Emily Martin and son-in-law Randy Martin. She appreciates the support of the staff nurses who work alongside our nursing students in the clinical settings. Thanks also to Rick Brady and Chesapeake Regional Healthcare for their previous assistance with the photo shoot for the Photo Atlas of Drug Administration. The support and the encouragement of family, friends, and colleagues are vital to projects like this. Thanks to Jamie Randall and Charlene Ketchum for their assistance and guidance during this edition. Thanks also to Lee Henderson and Jackie Twomey at Elsevier for their assistance early on during this edition. A heartfelt thanks to Bridget Healy, who helped me to keep on track with deadlines. Thanks also to Shelly Rainforth Collins for her clinical insight and constant willingness to address questions. Julie is deeply grateful to Dr. Linda L. Lilley for her unwavering encouragement, mentoring, and friendship; her drive to make this book a success is inspiring. Thanks also to each student who has provided feedback during classes about the text and study aids. Most importantly, Julie gives thanks to God, our source of hope and strength. Finally, to those who teach, although your work may seem to go unnoticed or unappreciated, your impact will always be remembered through the accomplishments of your students. Thank you for teaching our future nurses.

WE WELCOME YOUR FEEDBACK

We always welcome comments from instructors and students who use this book so that we may continue to make improvements and be responsive to your needs in future editions. Please send any comments you may have for us to the attention of the publisher at j.randall@elsevier.com.

Linda Lane Lilley, RN, PhD
Shelly Rainforth Collins, PharmD
Julie S. Snyder, MSN, RN-BC

PHARMACOLOGY
and the NURSING PROCESS

Pharmacology Basics

Learning Strategies

INTRODUCTION

Opening your pharmacology textbook and glancing at the table of contents can seem overwhelming. You may wonder how you ever will be able remember so much information. You may wonder what the best approach is to tackling such a daunting topic. The good news is that there are many learning strategies available to help you not only learn about pharmacology but also apply the knowledge that you have learned.

As the title of the book implies, pharmacology is very important to the nursing process. As a nursing student, you will come to understand that learning in nursing is not about memorization but rather about application of that learning. While there will be many times when memorization is required to begin to understand a new field of knowledge, the ultimate goal will always be to take your learning to a higher level. In this introduction and in the following chapters, you will learn strategies that will guide you with techniques and suggestions on how you can shape the way you study and learn so it will become second nature to transform your thinking into deeper, long-term learning.

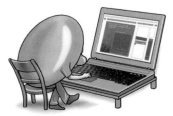

Continuing in your nursing education, you will soon realize that learning does not stop once you receive your degree and pass your state-licensing exam. As a professional nurse, you will come to understand that new information is always being added in the medical field. In the area of pharmacology, there are always new drugs being adopted for use by the Food and Drug Administration. So the strategies you learn here can be used again and again to assist you in staying on top of new discoveries and information in the nursing profession.

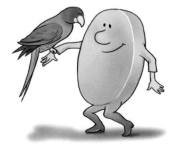

There is a new shift occurring in education today, which places the student in control of his or her own learning. You may have heard the terms "active" or "student-centered" learning. What this means is that the teacher is no longer standing in front of the class lecturing to impart all his or her knowledge on you, the student. Instead you are being asked to be an active participant in your learning. Your instructor acts more like a guide that assists you in attaining your fullest potential, allowing you to see the bigger picture or concept being taught. When students are taught this way, they gain more from their lessons because they are putting their learning into action. Also, that learning becomes embedded in their long-term memory because it is connected with a more complex thought process and has associated actions. In future chapters, you will see how this type of learning works well with your pharmacology textbook.

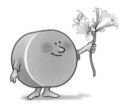

Another technique that you may have heard instructors are utilizing is "flipping the classroom." If your instructor uses this technique, you will be receiving some portion of your lesson outside of the classroom and participate in specific activities once you come to class. Again, this puts the responsibility of learning on the student and has the added benefit of the student being able to dig deeper into the content in class and leave with a greater understanding of the topic or content.

Both of these types of teaching strategies have proven beneficial to the student because they allow the students greater freedom in choosing how they learn best, while providing the instructors the ability to present the material through a variety of mediums like computer video streaming, YouTube presentations, case studies, human patient simulation, group presentations, chat rooms, and journaling. As a student, this may be a new way to learn, and some students may balk at the idea in the beginning. But once students are presented with the chance to participate in such a learning environment, they embrace it. Some students actually dislike it when their classes are strictly in lecture format.

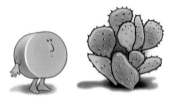

So you may ask yourself, "How does this affect me and how I learn pharmacology, if my instructor still lectures the 'old way'?" You will begin to see that, even if you are given an assigned reading from the textbook and receive a lecture on the material, it is still largely up to you to understand what you have read in the textbook and heard in the classroom. You will still need to be an active participant if you wish to fully comprehend and be able to apply pharmacology to your nursing knowledge/ practice. Nurses spend a large amount of their day giving medications to their patients. Anybody can open a pill packet, drop the pill in a cup, and give it to a person. However, safe

medication administration demands an enormous amount of knowledge and understanding about why a patient is receiving a medication, specific actions needed to take before you give the medication, expected outcomes anticipated from the dose of medication, and specific patient teaching needs. Other important things to know prior to giving medications are how to perform drug calculations for the correct dosage, and understanding the possible side effects or the contraindications of the medication. As you read your pharmacology textbook and listen to your instructors teaching on the subject, you will begin to understand why learning pharmacology is more than just memorizing drug facts.

Your textbook also contains terminology that is essential to your learning. You will be provided with techniques to help you learn the terminology that goes beyond rote memorization of the textbook definitions. The authors of the text have incorporated important boxes, tables, and case studies to help you understand the importance of patient safety and the prevention of errors. In future chapters, you will learn how to use the design and structure of the chapters to assist you in comprehending the content.

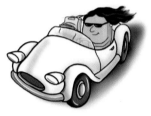

It is also suggested that students inherently understand the way they learn best. Are you a visual, auditory, or kinesthetic learner? Visual learners will benefit from seeing connections provided in maps and diagrams. They learn best through studying charts and watching demonstrations. Auditory learners gain the most learning through hearing the context or reciting aloud. These students benefit from audio flash cards, YouTube videos, and lectures. Kinesthetic learners learn through hands-on experience, but writing down information is also helpful to these students. Many students learn through more than just one type. Strategies for these different types of learning will also be addressed.

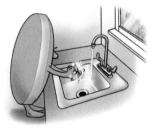

Various learning strategies are located throughout the textbook at the beginning of each major section. The strategies can be tailored to your specific need. In order to make the most of your learning, all learning strategies are listed here, so you can turn to those that will help you the most in the order that you need them. However, we suggest that you begin with the nursing process since it is a major component of understanding nursing and pharmacology.

Learning Strategies and their locations in this textbook are as follows:

- Introduction to Student Learning Strategies for Pharmacology—Part 1
- Nursing Process: Assessment, Nursing Diagnosis, Planning, Implementation, and Evaluation—Part 2
- Vocabulary, Text Notation, and Enhanced Typeface—Part 3
- Study Time: Learning Styles, Use of Apps, Mnemonics, and Flash Cards—Part 4
- Making the Most of Group Studying: Study Groups, Chat Rooms, and Discussion Groups—Part 5
- Time Management and Practice Questions—Part 6
- Active Questioning and NCLEX® Practice—Part 7
- Application of Pharmacology and Making Connections—Part 8
- Studying for Tests, Test-Taking Strategies, and Performance Evaluation—Part 9
- Future Application—Part 10

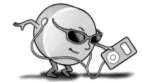

The Nursing Process and Drug Therapy

ⓔ http://evolve.elsevier.com/Lilley

OBJECTIVES

When you reach the end of this chapter, you will be able to do the following:

1. List the five phases of the nursing process.
2. Identify the components of the assessment process for patients receiving medications, including collection and analysis of subjective and objective data.
3. Discuss the process of formulating nursing diagnoses for patients receiving medications.
4. Identify the planning phase of the nursing process with outcome identification as related to patients receiving medications.

5. Discuss the evaluation process associated with the administration of medications and as reflected by outcome identification.
6. Develop a nursing care plan that is based on the nursing process and medication administration.
7. Briefly discuss the "Nine Rights" and other "Rights" associated with safe medication administration.
8. Discuss the professional responsibility and standards of practice for the professional nurse as related to the medication administration process.

KEY TERMS

Compliance Implementation or fulfillment of a prescriber's or caregiver's prescribed course of treatment or therapeutic plan by a patient. Use of *compliance* versus *adherence* in this textbook is supportive of the terms used in the current listing of NANDA-I nursing diagnoses. (p. 6)

Medication error Any preventable adverse drug event involving inappropriate medication use by a patient or health care professional; it may or may not cause the patient harm. (p. 13)

Noncompliance An informed decision on the part of the patient not to adhere to or follow a therapeutic plan or suggestion. Use of *noncompliance* versus *nonadherence* in this textbook is supportive of the terms used in the current listing of NANDA-I nursing diagnoses. (p. 7)

Nursing process An organizational framework for the practice of nursing. It encompasses all steps taken by the nurse in caring for a patient: assessment, nursing diagnoses, planning (with goals and outcome criteria), implementation of the plan (with patient teaching), and evaluation. (p. 4)

Outcomes Descriptions of specific patient behaviors or responses that demonstrate meeting of or achievement of behaviors related to each nursing diagnosis. These statements are specific while framed in behavioral terms and are measurable. (p. 5)

Prescriber Any health care professional licensed by the appropriate regulatory board to prescribe medications. (p. 7)

OVERVIEW OF THE NURSING PROCESS

The **nursing process** is a well-established, research-supported framework for professional nursing practice. The nursing process begins first with an understanding of underlying concepts associated with the art and science of nursing. It is a flexible, adaptable, and adjustable five-step process consisting of assessment, nursing diagnoses, planning with outcome identification, with implementation including patient education and evaluation. As such, the nursing process ensures the delivery of thorough, individualized, and quality nursing care to patients, regardless of age, gender, medical diagnosis, or setting. Through use of the nursing process combined with knowledge and skills,

the professional nurse will be able to develop effective solutions to meet patient's needs. The nursing process is usually discussed in nursing courses and/or textbooks that deal with the fundamentals of nursing practice, nursing theory, physical assessment, adult or pediatric nursing, and other nursing specialty areas. However, because of the importance of the nursing process in the care of patients, the process in all of its five phases is described in each chapter as it relates to specific drug groups or classifications.

Critical thinking is a major part of the nursing process and involves the use of thought processes to gather information and then develop conclusions, make decisions, draw inferences, and reflect upon all aspects of patient care. The elements of the nursing process address the physical, emotional, spiritual, sexual, financial, cultural, and cognitive aspects of a patient. Attention to these many aspects allows a more holistic approach to patient care. For example, a cardiologist may focus on cardiac functioning and pathology, a physical therapist on movement, and a chaplain on the spiritual aspects of patient care. However, it is the professional nurse who critically thinks and processes all points of information, incorporates this data about the patient, and then uses this information to develop and coordinate patient care. Therefore, the nursing process remains a central process and framework for nursing care. Box 1-1 provides guidelines for nursing care planning related to drug therapy and the nursing process.

Before further discussion of the phases of the nursing process, it is important to mention the trend of the implementation of QSEN initiatives in nursing education. The Quality and Safety Education for Nurses (QSEN) project was initiated in 2005. QSEN attempts to address the continued challenge of preparing future nurses with the knowledge, skills, and attitudes (called *KSAs*) needed to continuously improve the quality and safety of patient care within the health care system. These KSAs flow out of the QSEN initiatives and are being integrated into nursing education curricula and clinical outcomes. The six major initiatives include the following: patient-centered care, teamwork and collaboration, evidence-based practice (EBP), quality improvement (QI), safety, and informatics. Because of

---

BOX 1-1 Guidelines for Nursing Care Planning

This sample presents useful information for developing a nursing process–focused care plan for patients receiving medications. Brief listings and discussions of what must be contained in each phase of the nursing process are included. This sample may be used as a template for formatting nursing care plans in a variety of patient care situations/settings.

Assessment
Objective Data
Objective data include information available through the senses, such as what is seen, felt, heard, and smelled. Among the sources of data are the chart, laboratory test results, reports of diagnostic procedures, physical assessment, and examination findings. Examples of specific data are age, height, weight, allergies, medication profile, and health history.

Subjective Data
Subjective data include all spoken information shared by the patient, such as complaints, problems, or stated needs (e.g., patient complains of "dizziness, headache, vomiting, and feeling hot for 10 days").

Nursing Diagnoses
Once the assessment phase has been completed, the nurse analyzes objective and subjective data about the patient and the drug and formulates nursing diagnoses. The following is an example of a nursing diagnosis statement: "Knowledge, Deficient" written out as "Deficient knowledge related to lack of experience with medication regimen and second-grade reading level as an adult as evidenced by inability to perform a return demonstration and inability to state adverse effects to report to the prescriber." This statement of the nursing diagnosis can be broken down into three parts, as follows:
- Part 1—"Knowledge, Deficient" stated as Deficient Knowledge" This is the statement of the human response of the patient to illness, injury, medications, or significant change. This can be an actual response, an increased risk, or an opportunity to improve the patient's health status. The nursing diagnosis related to knowledge may be identified as either "Deficient" or "Readiness for Enhanced."
- Part 2—"Related to lack of experience with medication regimen and second-grade reading level as an adult." This portion of the statement identifies factors related to the response; it often includes multiple factors with some degree of connection between them. The nursing diagnosis statement does not necessarily claim that there is a cause-and-effect link between these factors and the response, only that there is a connection.

- Part 3—"As evidenced by inability to perform a return demonstration and inability to state adverse effects to report to the prescriber." This statement lists clues, cues, evidence, and/or data that support the nurse's claim that the nursing diagnosis is accurate.

Nursing diagnoses are prioritized in order of criticality based on patient needs or problems. The ABCs of care (airway, breathing, and circulation) are often used as a basis for prioritization. Prioritizing always begins with the most important, significant, or critical need of the patient. Nursing diagnoses that involve actual responses are always ranked above nursing diagnoses that involve only risks.

Planning: Outcome Identification
The planning phase includes the identification of outcomes that are patient oriented and provide time frames. Outcomes are objective, realistic, and measurable patient-centered statements with time frames.

Implementation
In the implementation phase, the nurse intervenes on behalf of the patient to address specific patient problems and needs. This is done through independent nursing actions; collaborative activities such as physical therapy, occupational therapy, and music therapy; and implementation of medical orders. Family, significant others, and caregivers assist in carrying out this phase of the nursing care plan. Specific interventions that relate to particular drugs (e.g., giving a particular cardiac drug only after monitoring the patient's pulse and blood pressure), nonpharmacologic interventions that enhance the therapeutic effects of medications, and patient education are major components of the implementation phase. See the previous text discussion of the nursing process for more information on nursing interventions.

Evaluation
Evaluation is the part of the nursing process that includes monitoring whether patient outcomes, as related to the nursing diagnoses, are met. Monitoring includes observing for therapeutic effects of drug treatment as well as for adverse effects and toxicity. Many indicators are used to monitor these aspects of drug therapy as well as the results of appropriately related nonpharmacologic interventions. If the outcomes are met, the nursing care plan may or may not be revised to include new nursing diagnoses; such changes are made only if appropriate. If outcomes are not met, revisions are made to the entire nursing care plan with further evaluation.

Modified from Herdman TH, Kamitsuru S (Eds): *NANDA-I: nursing diagnoses: definitions and classification 2015-2017*, ed 10, Oxford, 2014, Wiley Blackwell.

this growing trend for increasing core competencies of quality and safety within nursing education and practice, we have developed boxes of pertinent information related to pharmacology and the nursing process within some chapters of this edition.

ASSESSMENT

During the initial assessment phase of the nursing process, data are collected, reviewed, and analyzed from patient, family, group and/or community sources. Performing a comprehensive assessment allows you to organize the information collected and then place this information into meaningful categories of knowledge known as nursing diagnoses. Formulating a nursing diagnosis focuses on how the data collected signifies either a problem, strength, or vulnerability. For the purposes of this textbook, a nursing diagnoses will be related to drug therapy. Information about the patient may come from a variety of sources, including the patient; the patient's family, caregiver, or significant other; and the patient's chart. Methods of data collection revolve around interviewing, direct and indirect questioning, observation, medical records review, head-to-toe physical examination, and a nursing assessment. Data are categorized into objective and subjective data. Objective data may be defined as any information gathered through the senses or that which is seen, heard, felt, or smelled. Objective data may also be obtained from a nursing physical assessment; nursing history; past and present medical history; results of laboratory tests, diagnostic studies, or procedures; measurement of vital signs, weight, and height; and medication profile. A medication profile or a medication history review includes, but is not limited to, the following information: allergies of any type; any and all drug use; listing of all prescribed medications; use of home or folk remedies and herbal and/or homeopathic treatments, plant or animal extracts, and dietary supplements; intake of alcohol, tobacco, and caffeine; current or past history of illegal drug use; use of over-the-counter (OTC) medications (e.g., aspirin, acetaminophen, vitamins, laxatives, cold preparations, sinus medications, antacids, acid reducers, antidiarrheals, minerals, elements); use of hormonal drugs (e.g., testosterone, estrogens, progestins, oral contraceptives); past and present health history and associated drug regimen(s); family history and racial, ethnic, and/ or cultural attributes, with attention to specific or different responses to medications as well as any unusual individual responses; and growth and developmental stage (e.g., Erikson's developmental tasks) and issues related to the patient's age and medication regimen. A holistic nursing assessment includes gathering of data about the whole individual including physical/emotional realms, religious preference, health beliefs, sociocultural characteristics, race, ethnicity, lifestyle, stressors, socioeconomic status, educational level, motor skills, cognitive ability, support systems, lifestyle, and use of any alternative and complementary therapies. Subjective data include information shared through the spoken word by any reliable source, such as the patient, spouse, family member, significant other, and/or caregiver.

Assessment about the specific drug is also important and involves the collection of specific information about prescribed, OTC, and herbal/complementary/alternative therapeutic drug use, with attention to the drug's action; signs and symptoms of allergic reaction; adverse effects; dosages and routes of administration; contraindications; drug incompatibilities; drug-drug, drug-food, and drug–laboratory test interactions; and toxicities and available antidotes. Nursing pharmacology textbooks provide a more nursing-specific knowledge base regarding drug therapy as related to the nursing process. Use of current references or those dated within the last 3 years is highly recommended. Some examples of authoritative textbook sources include the *Physicians' Desk Reference, Mosby's Drug Consult,* drug manufacturers' inserts, drug handbooks, and/or licensed pharmacists. Authoritative journal references include professional journals within the last 3 to 5 years that are refereed. Refereed journals are professional journals or publications in which articles/papers are selected for publication by a panel of readers/referees who are experts in the field. Reliable online resources include, but are not limited to, the U.S. Pharmacopeia (USP) *(www.usp.org),* and the U.S. Food and Drug Administration *(www.fda.gov).* Other online resources are cited throughout this textbook.

Gather additional data about the patient and a given drug by asking these simple questions: What is the patient's oral intake? Tolerance of fluids? Swallowing ability for pills, tablets, capsules, and liquids? If there is difficulty swallowing, what is the degree of difficulty and are there solutions to the problem? Use of thickening agents with fluids or use of other dosage forms because of difficulty swallowing? What are the results of laboratory and other diagnostic tests related to organ functioning and drug therapy? What do renal function studies (e.g., blood urea nitrogen level, serum creatinine level) show? What are the results of hepatic function tests (e.g., total protein level, serum levels of bilirubin, alkaline phosphatase, creatinine phosphokinase, other liver enzymes)? What are the patient's white blood cell and red blood cell counts? Hemoglobin and hematocrit levels? Current as well as past health status and presence of illness? What are the patient's experiences with use of any drug regimen? What has been the patient's relationship with health care professionals and/or experiences with previous therapeutic regimens? What are current and past values for blood pressure, pulse rate, temperature, and respiratory rate? What medications is the patient currently taking, and how is the patient taking and tolerating them? Are there issues of **compliance**? Is there any use of folk medicines or folk remedies? What is the patient's understanding of the medication? Are there any age-related concerns? If patients are not reliable historians, family members, significant others, and/or caregivers may provide answers to these questions.

It is worth mentioning that there is often discussion about the difference between the terms *compliance* and *adherence.* Both of these terms, though not to be used interchangeably, are used to describe the extent to which patients take medications as prescribed. Often the term *adherence* is perceived as implying more collaboration and active role between patients and their providers (see Key Terms definition of *compliance*). Once assessment of the patient and the drug has been completed, the specific prescription or medication order (from any prescriber) must be checked for the following seven elements: (1) patient's name, (2) date the drug order was written, (3) name of drug(s), (4) drug dosage amount, (5) drug dosage frequency, (6) route of administration, and (7) prescriber's signature.

It is also important during assessment to consider the traditional, nontraditional, expanded, and collaborative roles of the nurse. Physicians and dentists are no longer the only practitioners legally able to prescribe and write medication orders. Nurse practitioners and physician assistants have gained the professional privilege of legally prescribing medications. Remain current on legal regulations as well as specific state nurse practice acts and standards of care.

Analysis of Data

Once data about the patient and drug have been collected and reviewed, critically analyze and synthesize the information. Clinical reasoning is the foundation of analyzing data and applying that to the development of nursing diagnoses. Verify all information and document appropriately. It is at this point that the sum of the information about the patient and drug are used in the development of nursing diagnoses.

CASE STUDY

Patient-Centered Care: The Nursing Process and Pharmacology

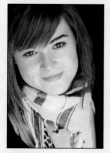 Dollie, a 27-year-old social worker, is visiting the clinic today for a physical examination. She states that she and her husband want to "start a family," but she has not had a physical for several years. She was told when she was 22 years of age that she had "anemia" and was given iron tablets, but Dollie states that she has not taken them for years. She said she "felt better" and did not think she needed them. She denies any use of tobacco and illegal drugs; she states that she may have a drink with dinner once or twice a month. She uses tea tree oil on her face twice a day to reduce acne breakouts. She denies using any other drugs.

1. What other questions does the nurse need to ask during this assessment phase?
2. After laboratory work is performed, Dollie is told that she is slightly anemic. The prescriber recommends that she resume taking iron supplements as well as folic acid. She is willing to try again and says that she is "all about doing what's right to stay healthy and become a mother." What nursing diagnoses would be appropriate at this time?
3. Dollie is given a prescription that reads as follows: "Ferrous sulfate 325 mg, PO for anemia." When she goes to the pharmacy, the pharmacist tells her that the prescription is incomplete. What is missing? What should be done?
4. After 4 weeks, Dollie's latest laboratory results indicate that she still has anemia. However, Dollie states, "I feel so much better that I'm planning to stop taking the iron tablets. I hate to take pills." How should the nurse handle this?

For answers, see *http://evolve.elsevier.com/Lilley.*

NURSING DIAGNOSES

Nursing diagnoses are developed by professional nurses and are used as a means of communicating and sharing information about the patient and the patient experience. Nursing diagnoses are the result of clinical judgement about a human response to health conditions and/or life processes, critical thinking, creativity, and accurate collection of data regarding the patient as well as the drug. Nursing diagnoses related to drug therapy will most likely grow out of data associated with the following: deficient knowledge; risk for injury; noncompliance; and various disturbances, deficits, excesses, impairments in bodily functions, and/or other problems or concerns as related to drug therapy. The development and classification of nursing diagnoses has been carried out by the North American Nursing Diagnosis Association International (NANDA-I) (formerly NANDA). NANDA-I is the formal organization recognized by professional nursing groups (e.g., the American Nurses Association [ANA]). NANDA-I is considered to be the major contributor to the development of nursing knowledge and the leading authority (on nursing diagnoses). The purpose of NANDA-I is to increase the visibility of nursing's contribution to the care of patients and to further develop, refine, and classify the information and phenomena related to nurses and professional nursing practice. In 2000, a classification system was adopted with a taxonomy including 13 domains divided into 106 classes and over 150 nursing diagnoses. Using this system, the nurse was able to choose a nursing diagnosis from the established list and individualize the nursing care plan. The 2009-2011 NANDA-approved nursing diagnoses included many changes with revisions, as well as several new diagnoses and a listing of retired nursing diagnoses. The newest list, the 2015-2017 NANDA-approved nursing diagnoses, includes 25 new and 13 revised nursing diagnoses, with each one based on the latest global evidence while also being approved by nurse experts in the areas of diagnostics, research and education. See Box 1-2 for more information about the 2015-2017 NANDA-I–approved nursing diagnoses.

Formulation of nursing diagnoses is usually a three-step process, with nursing diagnoses stated as follows: Part one of the statement is the human response of the patient to illness, injury, or significant change. This response may be an actual problem, an increased risk or vulnerability of developing a problem, or an opportunity/intent to improve the human response by the patient, family, group, or community. Part two of the nursing diagnosis statement is labeled as defining characteristics and identifies the factor(s) related to the response, with more than one factor often named. The nursing diagnosis statement does not necessarily claim a cause-and-effect link between these factors and the response; it indicates only that there is a connection between them. Part three of the nursing diagnosis statement contains a listing of clues, cues, evidence, signs, symptoms, or other data that support the nurse's claim that this diagnosis is accurate. Tips for writing nursing diagnoses include the following: Begin with a "statement" of a human response; connect the first part of the statement or the human response with the second part, the cause, using the phrase "related to"; be sure that the first two parts are not restatements

BOX 1-2 A Brief Look at NANDA-I and the Nursing Process

The North American Nursing Diagnosis Association International (NANDA-I) (formerly NANDA prior to 2002) fulfills the following roles: (1) increases the visibility of nursing's contribution to patient care; (2) develops, refines, and classifies information and phenomena related to professional nursing practice; (3) provides a working organization for the development of evidence-based nursing diagnoses; and (4) supports the improvement of quality nursing care through evidence-based practice and access to a global network of professional nurses. In 1987, NANDA and the American Nurses Association endorsed a framework for establishing nursing diagnoses, and in 1990 *Nursing Diagnoses* became the official journal of NANDA. In 2001 and 2003, NANDA modified and updated the listing of nursing diagnoses, but nursing diagnoses continued to be submitted for consideration by the Ad Hoc Research Committee of NANDA. This period resulted in changes such as replacement of the phrase *potential for* with *risk for*. The terms *impaired, deficient, ineffective, decreased, increased,* and *imbalanced* replaced the outdated terms *altered* and *alteration,* although the outdated terms may still be in use. In 2002, NANDA changed its name to NANDA-I ("I" for international) to reflect the organization's global reach. The official name of this organization is NANDA International, Inc. (no hyphenation), represented by the accepted abbreviation of NANDA-I with use of hyphenation. In 2007-2008, there were 188 nursing diagnoses (up from 172) with changes to defining characteristics and related or risk factors. There were also some 15 newly approved nursing diagnoses. More changes occurred in the 2009-2011 version of NANDA-I's *Nursing Diagnoses: Definitions and Classifications,* with 21 new, 9 revised, and 6 retired nursing diagnoses. More changes occurred with the listing of *2012-2014 NANDA-I Approved Nursing Diagnoses.* This list included 23 new, 33 revised, and 2 retired nursing diagnoses. The 2015-2017 edition of *Nursing Diagnoses: Definitions and Classification* includes 235 nursing diagnoses, with 25 new and 13 revised diagnoses, all appproved by a group of nurse experts, researchers, and educators. Visit *www.nanda.org/about-nanda-international.html* for further information.

NANDA-I, North American Nursing Diagnosis Association—International. From *Nursing Diagnoses: definitions and classification 2015-2017.* Copyright © 2014 Tenth Edition by NANDA International. Wiley-Blackwell Publishing, a company of John Wiley & Sons.

of one another; include several factors in the second part of the statement, such as associated factors, if appropriate; select a cause for the second part of the statement that can be changed by nursing interventions; avoid negative wording or language; and, finally, list clues or cues and/or more defininig characteristics that led to the nursing diagnosis in the third part of the statement or "as evidenced by." The common format when learning to formulate and write a nursing diagnosis looks like this: *nursing diagnosis or statement* of problem/strength/or risk _____ *related to etiologies, circumstances, facts, influences* that have a relationship such as a cause or contributing factor to the nursing diagnosis _____ *as evidenced by* defining characteristics/signs/symptoms. It is important to understand that "problem-focused" nursing diagnoses are not to be viewed as more important than "risk-related" statements because an at "risk" diagnosis may well be of highest prioirity for a patient. A listing of NANDA-I approved nursing diagnoses (2015-2017) most relevant to drug therapy is provided in Box 1-3. These nursing diagnoses, as well as all other phases of the nursing process, will be presented in the chapters that follow because the nursing process provides the framework of practice for all professional nurses and is also used to organize the nursing sections of this textbook.

PLANNING: OUTCOME IDENTIFICATION

After data are collected and nursing diagnoses are formulated, the planning phase begins; this includes identification of outcomes. The major purpose of the planning phase is to prioritize the nursing diagnoses and specify outcomes including the time frame for their achievement. The planning phase provides time to obtain special equipment for interventions, review the possible procedures or techniques to be used, and gather information for oneself (the nurse) or for the patient. This step leads to the provision of safe care if professional judgement is combined with the acquisition of knowledge about the patient and the medications to be given. In the 1990s, the American Nurses Association expanded the nursing process to include outcome identification as part of the planning phase. In past editions, we have included goals and outcomes as components of the planning phase of the nursing process. This edition has been changed in that goals are not identified or discussed. Instead, you will see the heading of **Planning: Outcome Identification** with outcomes further clarified.

Outcomes are objective, measurable, and realistic with an established time frame for their achievement. Patient outcomes reflect expected and measurable changes in behavior through nursing care and are developed in collaboration with the patient. Patient outcomes are behavior based and may be categorized into physiologic, psychological, spiritual, sexual, cognitive, motor, and/or other domains. They are patient focused, succinct, and well thought out. Outcomes also include expectations for behavior indicating something that can be changed and with a specific time frame or deadline. The ultimate aim of outcome identification is the safe and effective administration of medications. Outcomes need to reflect each nursing diagnosis and serve as a guide to the implementation phase of the nursing process. Formulation of outcomes begins with the analysis of the judgements made about patient data and subsequent nursing diagnoses and ends with the development of a nursing care plan. They also provide a standard for measuring movement toward goals. With regard to medication administration, these outcomes may address special storage and handling techniques, administration procedures, equipment needed, drug interactions, adverse effects, and contraindications. In this textbook, specific time frames are *not* provided in each chapter's nursing process section because patient care is individualized in each patient care situation.

IMPLEMENTATION

Implementation is guided by the preceding phases of the nursing process (i.e., assessment, nursing diagnoses, and planning). Implementation requires constant communication and collaboration with the patient and with members of the health care team involved in the patient's care, as well as with any family members, significant others, or other caregivers. Implementation consists of initiation and completion of specific nursing actions as defined by nursing diagnoses and outcome identification. Implementation of nursing actions may be independent, collaborative, or dependent upon a prescriber's

BOX 1-3	Current NANDA-I–Approved Nursing Diagnoses Most Relevant to Drug Therapy

Activity Intolerance (and, Risk for)	Insomnia
Airway Clearance, Ineffective	Knowledge (Deficient, Readiness for Enhanced)
Allergy Response, Risk for Aspiration, Risk for	Latex Allergy Response, (Risk for)
Bleeding, Risk for	Lifestyle, Sedentary
Body Image, Disturbed	Liver Function, Risk for Impaired
Body Temperature, Risk for Imbalanced†	Loneliness, Risk for
Breathing Pattern, Ineffective	Memory, Impaired
Cardiac Output, Decreased	Mobility (Impaired Bed, Impaired Physical†, Impaired Wheelchair)
Cardiovascular Function, Risk for Impaired*	Nausea
Comfort, Impaired (and Readiness for Enhanced)	Noncompliance
Communication, Readiness for Enhanced	Nutrition, Imbalanced (and Less than Body Requirements, Readiness for Enhanced)
Confusion (Acute, Chronic, and/or Risk for Acute)	Nutrition, Imbalanced: More than Body Requirements†
Constipation (and Perceived and Risk For)	Nutrition, Risk for Imbalanced: More than Body Requirements‡
Coping (Defensive, Ineffective, and Readiness for Enhanced)	Oral Mucous Membrane, Impaired (and Risk for Impaired*)
Death Anxiety†	Pain (Acute, Chronic)†
Decision-Making, Readiness for Enhanced	Peripheral Neurovascular Dysfunction, Risk for
Diarrhea	Poisoning, Risk for
Electrolyte Imbalance, Risk for	Powerlessness (and Risk for)
Energy Field, Disturbed‡	Self-Care Deficit (Bathing, Dressing, Feeding, Toileting)
Falls, Risk for	Self-Esteem, Chronic Low (and Risk for Chronic Low)
Fatigue	Self-Esteem, Low (Situational Low, Risk for Situational Low)
Fear	Sexual Dysfunction
Fluid Volume, Deficient	Sexuality Pattern, Ineffective
Fluid Volume, Excess†	Skin Integrity, Impaired (and Risk for Impaired)
Fluid Volume, Risk for Deficient (and Risk for Imbalanced)	Sleep Deprivation
Gas eExchange, Impaired	Sleep Pattern, Disturbed
Growth, Risk for Disproportionate	Standing, Impaired*
Growth and Development, Delayed‡	Stress Overload
Health Maintenance, Ineffective	Suicide, risk for
Home Maintenance, Impaired	Surgical Recovery, Delayed† (and Risk for Delayed*)
Human Dignity, Risk for Compromised	Swallowing, Impaired
Hyperthermia, Risk for*	Tissue Integrity, Impaired† (and Risk for Impaired*)
Hypothermia, Risk for Perioperative*	Tissue Perfusion, Ineffective Peripheral (Risk for Decreased Cardiac, Risk for
Incontinence (Functional Urinary, Overflow Urinary, Reflex Urinary, Stress Urinary, Urge Urinary, Risk for Urge Urinary)	Ineffective Cerebral, Risk for Ineffective Peripheral)
Infection, Risk for	Urinary Retention
Injury, Risk for	Verbal Communication, Impaired
	Walking, Impaired

NANDA-I, North American Nursing Diagnosis Association—International.
From *Nursing Diagnoses: definitions and classification 2015-2017.* Copyright © 2014 Tenth Edition by NANDA International. Wiley-Blackwell Publishing, a company of John Wiley & Sons.
*New nursing diagnosis.
†Revised nursing diagnoses or diagnoses in which a key word has changed.
‡Retired nursing diagnoses.

order. Interventions are defined as any treatment based on clinical judgement and knowledge and performed by a nurse to enhance outcomes. Statements of interventions include frequency, specific instructions, and any other pertinent information. With medication administration, you need to know and understand all of the information about the patient and about each medication prescribed. In years past, nurses adhered to the "Five Rights" of medication administration: right drug, right dose, right time, right route, and right patient. Use of "Six Rights" in the previous edition of this textbook included "right documentation." However, continued support exists for referring to up to "Nine Rights" of medication administration inclusive of the basic "Six Rights." The Nine Rights are discussed in

detail in the next section. These "rights" of medication administration have been identified as additional standards of care as related to drug therapy. Even implementation of these "rights" does not reflect the complexity of the role of the professional nurse because they focus more on the individual/patient than on the system as a whole or the entire medication administration process beginning with the prescriber's order.

Nine Rights of Medication Administration
Right Drug

The "right drug" begins with the registered nurse's valid license to practice. Most states allow currently licensed practical nurses to administer medications with specific guidelines. The registered nurse is responsible for checking all medication orders and/or prescriptions. To ensure that the correct drug is given, the specific medication order must be checked against the medication label or profile three times before giving the medication. Conduct the first check of the right drug/drug name during your initial preparation of the medication for administration. At this time, consider whether the drug is appropriate for the patient and, if doubt exists or an error is deemed possible, contact the prescriber and/pharmacist immediately. It is also appropriate at this time to note the drug's indication and be aware that a drug may have multiple indications, including off-label use and non–FDA-approved indications. In this textbook, each particular drug is discussed in a specific chapter that deals with its main indication, but the drug may also be cross-referenced in other chapters if it has multiple uses.

All medication orders or prescriptions are required by law to be signed by the prescriber involved in the patient's care. If a verbal order is given, the prescriber must sign the order within 24 hours or as per guidelines within a health care setting. Verbal and/or telephone orders are often used in emergencies and time-sensitive patient care situations. To be sure that the right drug is given, information about the patient and drug (see previous discussion of the assessment phase) must be obtained to make certain that all variables and data have been considered. See previous discussion about authoritative sources/references.

Avoid relying upon the knowledge of peers because this is unsafe nursing practice. Remain current in your knowledge of generic (nonproprietary) drug names as well as trade names (proprietary name that is registered by a specific drug manufacturer); however, use of the drug's generic name is now preferred in clinical practice to reduce the risk for medication

QSEN EVIDENCE-BASED PRACTICE

Nurses' Clinical Reasoning: Processes and Practices of Medication Safety

Review
In one of the first quality reports about medication safety in the series *To Err is Human* (2000), Kohn, Corrigan, and Donaldson identified medication errors as the most common of errors occurring in health care. In 2007 in another quality series, Aspden and colleagues reported that a patient in a hospital could expect at least one medication error per hospital day. They also reported that as many as 7000 deaths might occur in hospitals each year because of medication errors, with a great variation among hospitals as to the number of events reported. It is important to note that in 1994 (Leape), research on medication errors changed from one of individual focus to one of a series of failures or breakdowns in the complexity of health care systems. Lacking in most of the medication error research is the critical role that professional nurses play in preventing medication errors from reaching the patient. Not only did a process need to be researched but especially the phenomenon behind the process of prevention of errors, which led to this particular qualitative research study. This study was designed to look at the nurse's clinical reasoning and actions preventing the medication error prior to even reaching the patient.

Type of Evidence
Grounded theory was used to identify the essence of medication safety. This qualitative method research design was used in an attempt to understand the world of preventing medication errors by the nurse and to gain an understanding of their knowledge. Qualitative research is important to use in the context of exploring study participants within their environment … looking at understanding human behavior and reasons for that behavior … the why and how of decision-making versus the empirical investigation through statistical analysis. Nurses were interviewed face-to-face about what they thought and did to prevent errors. Additionally, they were asked to identify factors that they thought increased the likelihood of a medication error occurring and how they made a difference in the interception of errors. A purposive sample of 50 medical-surgical nurses from 10 mid-Atlantic hospitals was used. Interviews, conducted in private settings on hospital units, included open-ended questions regarding their processes, and taped recordings were about 60 minutes in length.

Results of the Study
The analysis of data was one of the discovery (of grounded theory) beginning with a line-by-line analysis of the narratives, with coding of data reflecting

the nurses' thoughts and actions when they recognized something was wrong with the medication and/or patient. An iterative (repetitive) process was used until all categories appeared to be saturated and theoretically sound. Emerging ideas were also categorized during the interviews, and the nurses' dialogues, researcher observations, and analytical memos provided the data for analysis. The analysis of data revealed that nurses, to ensure patient safety, needed to interact with others. A majority of the nurses clearly acknowledged their role in the process of "Five Rights" of medication administration as well as the need to extend safe practice beyond these five tasks. Two safety processes were found within the clinical reasoning: The first process was maintaining medication safety with various medication practices including advocacy with pharmacy, educating patients, and conducting medication reconciliation. The second process was managing the clinical environment with four environmentally focused safety categories including coping with interruptions and documenting "near misses." These processes and practices demonstrated nurses' clinical reasoning that served as a foundation of the "safety net" protecting patients from medication errors. Out of all these narratives, there also emerged a model for the processes and practices of safe medication administration.

Link of Evidence to Nursing Practice
Nurses in this study clearly demonstrated how clinical reasoning was used to prevent potential medication errors from reaching the patient. This evidence is critical to further development of medication safety practices for implementation by professional nurses. All processes, practices, and reasoning related to safe medication administration demonstrated by nurses need to be acknowledged, valued, and respected by nurse/health care managers/leaders within the various health care settings. Additionally, more research is needed on development of models for safe medication practice that reaches further than just the "Five Rights" and emphasis on astute clinical reasoning. Systemic policies for safer medication administration may be developed out of these practice models. Results of this study may also be helpful in development of nursing curricula focused on patient safety as the very basis of quality patient care.

From Dickson GL, Flynn L: Nurses' clinical reasoning: processes and practices of medication safety. *Qual Health Res* 22(1):3-16, 2012.

errors. A single drug often has numerous trade names, and drugs in different classes may have similarly spelled names, increasing the possibility of medication errors. Therefore, when it comes to the "right drug" phase of the medication administration process, use of a drug's generic name is recommended to help avoid a medication error and enhance patient safety. (See Chapter 2 for more information on the naming of drugs).

If there are questions about the medication order at any time during the medication administration process, contact the prescriber for clarification. Never make any assumptions when it comes to drug administration, and, as previously emphasized in this chapter, confirm at least three times the right drug, right dose, right time, right route, right patient, and right documentation before giving the medication.

Right Dose

Whenever a medication is ordered, a dosage is identified from the prescriber's order. Always confirm that the dosage amount is appropriate for the patient's age and size. Use of a current, authoritative drug reference is encouraged. Also, check the prescribed dose against the available drug stocks and against the normal dosage range. Recheck all mathematical calculations, and pay careful attention to decimal points, the misplacement of which could lead to a tenfold or even greater overdose. Leading zeros, or zeros placed before a decimal point, are allowed, but trailing zeros, or zeros following the decimal point, are to be avoided. For example, 0.2 mg is allowed, but 2.0 mg is not acceptable, because it could easily be mistaken for 20 mg, especially with unclear penmanship. Patient variables (e.g., vital signs, age, gender, weight, height) require careful assessment because of the need for dosage adjustments in response to specific parameters. Pediatric and elderly patients are more sensitive to medications than younger and middle-age adult patients; thus, use extra caution with drug dosage amounts for these patients.

QSEN ⚡ **SAFETY AND QUALITY IMPROVEMENT: PREVENTING MEDICATION ERRORS**

Right Dose?

The nurse is reviewing the orders for a newly admitted patient. One order reads: "Tylenol, 2 tablets PO, every 4 hours as needed for pain or fever."

The pharmacist calls to clarify this order, saying, "The dose is not clear." What does the pharmacist mean by this? The order says "2 tablets." Isn't that the dose?

NO! If you look up Tylenol (acetaminophen) in a drug resource book, you will see that Tylenol tablets are available in strengths of both 325 mg and 500 mg. The order is missing the "right dose" and needs to be clarified. *Never assume the dose of a medication order!*

Right Time

Each health care setting or institution has a policy regarding routine medication administration times. These policies need to be checked and committed to memory! Include in your three checks the frequency of the ordered medication, the time to be administered, and when the last dose of medication was given.

However, when giving a medication at the prescribed time, you may be confronted with a conflict between the timing suggested by the prescriber and specific pharmacokinetic or pharmacodynamic drug properties, concurrent drug therapy, dietary influences, laboratory and/or diagnostic testing, and specific patient variables. For example, the prescribed right time for administration of antihypertensive drugs may be four times a day, but for an active, professional 42-year-old male patient working 14 hours a day, taking a medication four times daily may not be feasible, and this regimen may lead to noncompliance and subsequent complications. For patient safety, your appropriate actions would include contacting the prescriber and inquiring about the possibility of prescribing another drug with a different dosing frequency (e.g., once or twice daily).

For routine medication orders, the standard of care is to give the medications no more than $\frac{1}{2}$ hour before or after the actual time specified in the prescriber's order (e.g., if a medication is ordered to be given at 0900 every morning, you may give it at any time between 0830 and 0930); the exception includes medications designated to be given stat (immediately) that must be administered within $\frac{1}{2}$ hour of the time the order is written. Assess and follow the health care institution policy and procedure for any other specific information concerning the "$\frac{1}{2}$ hour before or after" rule. For medication orders with the annotation "prn" (*pro re nata*, or "as required"), the medication must be given at special times and under certain circumstances. For example, an analgesic is ordered every 4 to 6 hours *prn* for pain; after one dose of the medication, the patient complains of pain. After assessment, intervention with another dose of analgesic would occur, but only 4 to 6 hours after the previous dose. In addition, because of the increasing incidence of medication errors related to the use of abbreviations, many prescribers are using the wording "as required" or "as needed" instead of the abbreviation "prn." Military time is used when medication and other orders are written into a patient's chart (Table 1-1).

Nursing judgement may lead to some variations in timing, and you must document any change and the rationale for the change. If medications are ordered to be given once every day, twice daily, three times daily, or even four times daily, the times of administration may be changed if it is not harmful to the patient or if the medication or the patient's condition does not require adherence to an exact schedule, but only if the change is approved by the prescriber. For example, suppose that an antacid is ordered to be given three times daily at 0900, 1300, and 1700, but the nurse has misread the order and gives the first dose at 1100. Depending on the specific policy of a hospital or other health care setting, the medication, and the patient's condition, such an occurrence may not be considered an error, because the dosing may be changed once the prescriber is contacted, so that the drug is given at 1100, 1500, and 1900 without harm to the patient and without incident to the nurse. If this were an antihypertensive medication, the patient's condition and well-being could be greatly compromised by one missed or late dose. Thus, falling behind in dosing times is not to be taken lightly or ignored. Never underestimate the effect of a change in the dosing or timing of medication, because one missed dose of certain medications can be life threatening.

TABLE 1-1   Conversion of Standard Time to Military Time

Standard Time	Military Time
1 AM	0100
2 AM	0200
3 AM	0300
4 AM	0400
5 AM	0500
6 AM	0600
7 AM	0700
8 AM	0800
9 AM	0900
10 AM	1000
11 AM	1100
12 PM (noon)	1200
1 PM	1300
2 PM	1400
3 PM	1500
4 PM	1600
5 PM	1700
6 PM	1800
7 PM	1900
8 PM	2000
9 PM	2100
10 PM	2200
11 PM	2300
12 AM (midnight)	2400

Other factors must be considered in determining the right time, such as multiple-drug therapy, drug-drug or drug-food compatibility, scheduling of diagnostic studies, bioavailability of the drug (e.g., the need for consistent timing of doses around the clock to maintain blood levels), drug actions, and any biorhythm effects such as occur with steroids. It is also critical to patient safety to avoid using abbreviations for *any* component of a drug order (i.e., dose, time, route). Spell out *all* terms (e.g., *three times daily* instead of *tid*) in their entirety. Be careful to write out all words and abbreviations, because the possibility of miscommunication or misinterpretation poses a risk to the patient. The Joint Commission created a "do not use" list of abbreviations in 2010 and integrated the list into their Information Management standards. For accredited facilities, abbreviations are not to be used in internal communications, telephone/verbal prescriptions, computer-generator labels, labels for drug storage bins, medication administration records, as well as pharmacy and prescriber computer entry screens. Further discussion is included in Chapter 5.

Right Route and Form

As previously stated, you must know the particulars about each medication before administering it to ensure that the right drug, dose, route, and dosage form are being used. A complete medication order includes the route of administration. Confirm the appropriateness of the prescribed route while also making sure the patient can take/receive the medication by the prescribed route. If a medication order does not include the route, be sure to ask the prescriber to clarify it. Never *assume* the route of administration. Additionally, it is critical to patient safety to be aware of the right form of medication. For example, there are various dosage forms of a commonly used medication, acetaminophen. It is available in oral suspension, tablet, capsule, gelcap, and pediatric drops as well as rectal suppository dosage forms. Nurses need to give the right drug via the right route with use of the correct dosage form. Another example is the administration of a controlled-release dosage form of a medication. This dosage form is not to be crushed or altered due to the subsequent immediate release of the drug (versus the controlled release) which, in some cases, may be life threatening.

Right Patient

Checking the patient's identity before giving each medication dose is critical to the patient's safety. Confirm the name on the order and the patient, and be sure to use several identifiers. Ask the patient to state his or her name, and then check the patient's identification band to confirm the patient's name, identification number, age, and allergies. With pediatric patients, the parents and/or legal guardians are often the ones who identify the patient for the purpose of administration of prescribed medications. With newborns and in labor and delivery situations, the mother and baby have identification bracelets with matching numbers, which must be checked before giving medications. In older adult patients or those with altered sensorium or level of consciousness, asking the patient his or her name or having the patient state his or her name is neither realistic nor safe. Therefore, checking the identification band against the medication profile, medication order, or other treatment or service orders is crucial to avoid errors. When available, use technology such as scanning a bar code on the patient's identification band. In 2008, The Joint Commission released National Patient Safety Goals for patient care. These goals emphasize the use of two identifiers when providing care, treatment, or services to patients. To meet these goals, The Joint Commission recommends that the patient be identified "reliably" and also that the service or treatment (e.g., medication administration) be matched to that individual. The Joint Commission's statement of National Patient Safety Goals indicates that the two identifiers may be in the same location, such as on a wristband. In fact, it is patient-specific information that is the identifier. Acceptable identifiers include the patient's name, an assigned identification number, a telephone number, or other patient-specific identifier. Arm bands are commonly used in the acute care setting and may serve as one identifier, with the other one being date of birth, Social Security number, or home address.

Right Documentation

Documentation of information related to medication administration is crucial to patient safety. Recording patient observations and nursing actions has always been an important ethical responsibility, but now it is becoming a major medical-legal consideration as well. Because of its significance in professional nursing practice, correct documentation became known as the "sixth right" of medication administration adding to the previous use of "Five Rights." Always assess the prescribed order in the patient's chart for the presence of the following information: date and time of medication administration, name of medication, dose, route, and site of administration. Document administration only after the medication has been given including the time, route, and any laboratory values or vital signs (as appropriate). Documentation of drug action may also be made in the regularly scheduled assessments for changes in symptoms the patient is experiencing, adverse effects, toxicity, and any other drug-related physical and/or psychological symptoms. Documentation must also reflect any improvement in the patient's condition, symptoms, or disease process as well as no change or a lack of improvement. You must not only document these observations, but report them to the prescriber promptly in keeping with your critical thinking and judgement. Document any teaching, as well as an assessment of the degree of understanding exhibited by the patient. Other areas of information that need to be documented include the following: (1) if a drug is *not* administered with the reason why and any actions taken (e.g., contacting the prescriber and monitoring the patient), (2) actual time of drug administration; and (3) data regarding clinical observations and treatment of the patient if a medication error has occurred. If there is a medication error, complete an incident report with the entire event, surrounding circumstances, therapeutic response, adverse effects, and notification of the prescriber described in detail. However, do not record completion of an incident report in the medical chart.

"Right reason" refers to the appropriateness in use of the medication to the patient. Confirm the rationale for use through researching the patient's history while also asking the patient the reason he or she is taking the drug. Always revisit the rationale for long-term medication use.

"Right response" refers to the drug and its desired response. Continually assess and evaluate the achievement of the desired response as well as any undesired response. Examples of data gathering include, but are not limited to, monitoring vital signs, weight, edema, intake and output, nutritional intake, laboratory values, results of diagnostic testing, and auscultating heart and lung sounds. Document any assessment, intervention, and monitoring as deemed appropriate.

The ninth "right" to discuss is that of the right of the patient to refuse. Patients refuse medications for a variety of reasons. If refusal of a medication occurs, always respect the patient's right (to refuse), determine the reason, and take appropriate action including notifying the prescriber. Document the refusal and a brief, concise description of the reason for refusal. Document any further actions you take at this time, such as vital signs and/or system assessment. If of consequence to the patient's condition and/or as hospital policy dictates, contact the physician. Never return unwrapped medication to a container,

and discard medication dose according to agency policy. If the wrapper remains intact, return the medication to the automated medication-dispensing system. Revise the nursing care plan as needed.

This list is never-ending and ever-changing, and additional rights to be considered when administering medications include the following:

- Patient safety, ensured by use of the correct procedures, equipment, and techniques of medication administration and documentation
- Individualized, holistic, accurate, and complete patient education with appropriate instructions
- Double-checking and constant analysis of the system (i.e., the process of drug administration including all personnel involved, such as the prescriber, the nurse, the nursing unit, and the pharmacy department, as well as patient education)
- Proper drug storage
- Accurate calculation and preparation of the dose of medication and proper use of all types of medication delivery systems
- Careful checking of the transcription of medication orders
- Accurate use of the various routes of administration and awareness of the specific implications of their use
- Close consideration of special situations (e.g., patient difficulty in swallowing, use of a nasogastric tube, unconsciousness of the patient, advanced patient age)
- Implementation of all appropriate measures to prevent and report medication errors, and the use of non-expired medications

Medication Errors

When the Nine Rights (and other rights) of drug administration are discussed, medication errors must be considered. Medication errors are a major problem for all of health care, regardless of the setting. The National Coordinating Council for Medication Error Reporting and Prevention defines a **medication error** as any *preventable* event that may cause or lead to inappropriate medication use or patient harm while the medication is in the control of the health care professional, patient, or consumer. Such events may be related to professional practice, health care products, procedures, or systems, including prescribing; order communication; product labeling, packaging, and nomenclature; compounding; dispensing; distribution; administration; education; monitoring; and use *(www.nccmerp .org/about-medication-errors)*. Both patient-related and system-related factors must always be considered when examining the medication administration process and the prevention of medication errors. See Chapter 5 for further discussion of medication errors and their prevention.

EVALUATION

Evaluation occurs after the nursing care plan has been implemented but also needs to occur at each phase of the nursing process. It is systematic, ongoing, and a dynamic phase of the nursing process as related to drug therapy. It includes monitoring the fulfillment of outcomes, as well as monitoring the patient's therapeutic response to the drug and its adverse effects and toxic effects. Documentation is also a very important component of evaluation and consists of clear, concise, abbreviation-free charting that records information related to goals and outcome criteria as well as information related to any aspect of the medication administration process, including therapeutic effects versus adverse effects or toxic effects of medications (see the Teamwork and Collaboration: Legal and Ethical Principles box).

Evaluation also includes monitoring the implementation of standards of care. Several standards are in place to help in the evaluation of outcomes of care, such as those established by state nurse practice acts and by The Joint Commission.

Guidelines for nursing services policies and procedures are established by The Joint Commission. There are even specific standards regarding medication administration to protect both the patient and the nurse. The ANA *Code of Ethics* and Patient Rights statement are also used in establishing and evaluating standards of care.

In summary, the nursing process is an ongoing and constantly evolving process (see Box 1-1). The nursing process, as it relates to drug therapy, involves the way in which a nurse gathers, analyzes, organizes, provides, and acts upon data about the patient within the context of prudent nursing care and standards of care. The nurse's ability to make astute assessments, formulate sound nursing diagnoses, identify outcomes, implement safe and accurate drug administration, and continually evaluate patients' responses to drugs increases with additional experience and knowledge.

QSEN ▶ **TEAMWORK AND COLLABORATION: LEGAL AND ETHICAL PRINCIPLES**

Do's and Don'ts of Charting

Do's
- Do check to be sure you have the correct chart before documenting.
- Do chart only the facts.
- Do include the time you gave a medication, the route of administration and the patient's response.
- Do chart patient teaching.
- Do chart any precautions or preventative measures.
- Do record each phone call to a physician with exact time, message and response.
- Do give prescise descriptions.
- Do chart patient care at the time you provide it.
- Do chart a patient's refusal to allow a treatment or to take a medication and report to the patient's physician and charge nurse.

Don'ts
- Don't chart a symptom, such as "c/o pain", without charting what you did to intervene on the patient's behalf.

- Don't alter a patient's record.
- Don't give excuses, such as "medication not given because not available".
- Don't chart care ahead of time.
- Don't mention the term *incident report* in charting. These reports are confidential and filed separately. Chart only the facts of the medication error or incident and appropriate actions taken.
- Don't use the following terms: *by mistake, by accident, accidentally, unintentional,* or *miscalculated.*
- Don't chart casual conversations with peers, prescribers, or other members of the health care team.
- Don't use abbreviations. Some agencies or facilities may still keep a list of approved abbreviations, but overall their use is discouraged.
- Don't use negative language.

Modified from *Do's and don'ts of documentation.* 2013, Nurses Service Organization. Available at *www.nso.com.* Accessed March 27, 2015.

KEY POINTS

- The nursing process is an ongoing, constantly changing and evolving framework for professional nursing practice. It may be applied to all facets of nursing care, including medication administration.
- The five phases of the nursing process include assessment; development of nursing diagnoses; planning with outcome identification; implementation, including patient education; and evaluation.
- Nursing diagnoses are formulated based on objective and subjective data and help to drive the nursing care plan. Nursing diagnoses have been developed through a formal process conducted by NANDA-I and are constantly updated and revised. Safe, therapeutic, and effective medication

administration is a major responsibility of professional nurses as they apply the nursing process to the care of their patients.
- Nurses are responsible for safe and prudent decision-making in the nursing care of their patients, including the provision of drug therapy; in accomplishing this task, they attend to the Nine Rights and adhere to legal and ethical standards related to medication administration and documentation. There are additional rights related to drug administration. These rights deserve worthy consideration before initiation of the medication administration process. Observance of all of these rights enhances patient safety and helps avoid medication errors.

NCLEX® EXAMINATION REVIEW QUESTIONS

1. An 86-year-old patient is being discharged to home on digitalis therapy and has very little information regarding the medication. Which statement best reflects a realistic outcome of patient teaching activities?
   a. The patient and patient's daughter will state the proper way to take the drug.
   b. The nurse will provide teaching about the drug's adverse effects.
   c. The patient will state all the symptoms of digitalis toxicity.
   d. The patient will call the prescriber if adverse effects occur.

2. A patient has a new prescription for a blood pressure medication that may cause him to feel dizzy during the first few days of therapy. Which is the best nursing diagnosis for this situation?
   a. Activity intolerance
   b. Risk for injury
   c. Disturbed body image
   d. Self-care deficit

3. A patient's chart includes an order that reads as follows: "Atenolol 25 mg once daily at 0900." Which action by the nurse is correct?
   a. The nurse gives the drug via the transdermal route.
   b. The nurse gives the drug orally.
   c. The nurse gives the drug intravenously.
   d. The nurse contacts the prescriber to clarify the dosage route.

4. The nurse is compiling a drug history for a patient. Which question from the nurse will obtain the most information from the patient?
   a. "Do you depend on sleeping pills to get to sleep?"
   b. "Do you have a family history of heart disease?"
   c. "When you have pain, what do you do to relieve it?"
   d. "What childhood diseases did you have?"

5. A 77-year-old man who has been diagnosed with an upper respiratory tract infection tells the nurse that he is allergic to penicillin. Which is the most appropriate response by the nurse?
   a. "Many people are allergic to penicillin."
   b. "This allergy is not of major concern because the drug is given so often."
   c. "What type of reaction did you have when you took penicillin?"
   d. "Drug allergies don't usually occur in older individuals due to built-up resistance to allergic reactions."

6. The nurse is preparing a care plan for a patient who has been newly diagnosed with type 2 diabetes mellitus. Which of these reflect the correct order of the steps of the nursing process?
   a. Assessment, Planning, Nursing Diagnoses, Implementation, Evaluation
   b. Evaluation, Assessment, Nursing Diagnoses, Planning, Implementation
   c. Nursing Diagnoses, Assessment, Planning, Implementation, Evaluation
   d. Assessment, Nursing Diagnoses, Planning, Implementation, Evaluation

7. The nurse is reviewing new medication orders that have been written for a newly admitted patient. The nurse will need to clarify which orders? (Select all that apply.)
   a. Metformin (Glucophage) 1000 mg PO twice a day
   b. Sitagliptin (Januvia) 50 mg daily
   c. Simvastatin (Zocor) 20 mg PO every evening
   d. Irbesartan (Avapro) 300 mg PO once a day
   e. Docusate (Colace) as needed for constipation

8. The nurse is reviewing data collected from a medication history. Which of these data are considered objective data? (Select all that apply.)
   a. White blood cell count 22,000 mm^3
   b. Blood pressure 150/94 mm Hg
   c. Patient rates pain as an "8" on a 10-point scale
   d. Patient's wife reports that the patient has been very sleepy during the day
   e. Patient's weight is 68 kg

1. a, 2. b, 3. d, 4. c, 5. c, 6. d, 7. b, e, 8. a, b, e

CRITICAL THINKING AND PRIORITIZATION QUESTIONS

1. When medications were administered during the night shift, a patient refused to take his 0200 dose of an antibiotic, claiming that he had just taken it. What is the best action by the nurse to maintain patient safety?

2. During a busy shift, the nurse notes that the chart of a newly admitted patient has a few orders for various medications and diagnostic tests that were taken by telephone by another nurse. The nurse is on the way to the patient's room to do an assessment when the unit secretary tells the nurse that one of the orders reads as follows: "Lasix, 20 mg, stat." What is the priority action by the nurse? How does the nurse go about giving this drug? Explain the best action to take in this situation.

For answers, see *http://evolve.elsevier.com/Lilley*.

Pharmacologic Principles

ⓔ http://evolve.elsevier.com/Lilley

OBJECTIVES

When you reach the end of this chapter, you will be able to do the following:

1. Define the common terms used in pharmacology (see Key Terms).
2. Understand the general concepts such as pharmaceutics, pharmacokinetics, and pharmacodynamics and their application in drug therapy and the nursing process.
3. Demonstrate an understanding of the various drug dosage forms as related to drug therapy and the nursing process.
4. Discuss the relevance of the four aspects of pharmacokinetics (absorption, distribution, metabolism, excretion) to professional nursing practice as related to drug therapy for a variety of patients and health care settings.
5. Discuss the use of natural drug sources in the development of new drugs.
6. Develop a nursing care plan that takes into account general pharmacologic principles, specifically pharmacokinetic principles, as they relate to the nursing process.

KEY TERMS

Additive effects Drug interactions in which the effect of a combination of two or more drugs with similar actions is equivalent to the sum of the individual effects of the same drugs given alone. For example, $1 + 1 = 2$ (compare with synergistic effects). (p. 32)

Adverse drug event Any undesirable occurrence related to administering or failing to administer a prescribed medication. (p. 32)

Adverse drug reaction Any unexpected, unintended, undesired, or excessive response to a medication given at therapeutic dosages (as opposed to overdose). (p. 32)

Adverse effects A general term for any undesirable effects that are a direct response to one or more drugs. (p. 30)

Agonist A drug that binds to and stimulates the activity of one or more receptors in the body. (p. 29)

Allergic reaction An immunologic hypersensitivity reaction resulting from the unusual sensitivity of a patient to a particular medication; a type of adverse drug event. (p. 32)

Antagonist A drug that binds to and inhibits the activity of one or more receptors in the body. Antagonists are also called *inhibitors*. (p. 29)

Antagonistic effects Drug interactions in which the effect of a combination of two or more drugs is less than the sum of the individual effects of the same drugs given alone ($1 + 1$ equals less than 2); it is usually caused by an antagonizing (blocking or reducing) effect of one drug on another. (p. 32)

Bioavailability A measure of the extent of drug absorption for a given drug and route (from 0% to 100%). (p. 21)

Biotransformation One or more biochemical reactions involving a parent drug; occurs mainly in the liver and produces a metabolite that is either inactive or active. Also known as *metabolism*. (p. 25)

Blood-brain barrier The barrier system that restricts the passage of various chemicals and microscopic entities (e.g., bacteria, viruses) between the bloodstream and the central nervous system. It still allows for the passage of essential substances such as oxygen. (p. 25)

Chemical name The name that describes the chemical composition and molecular structure of a drug. (p. 18)

Contraindication Any condition, especially one related to a disease state or patient characteristic, including current or recent drug therapy, which renders a particular form of treatment improper or undesirable. (p. 30)

Cytochrome P-450 The general name for a large class of enzymes that play a significant role in drug metabolism and drug interactions. (p. 26)

Dependence A state in which there is a compulsive or chronic need, as for a drug. (p. 31)

Dissolution The process by which solid forms of drugs disintegrate in the gastrointestinal tract and become soluble before being absorbed into the circulation. (p. 19)

Drug Any chemical that affects the physiologic processes of a living organism. (p. 18)

Drug actions The processes involved in the interaction between a drug and body cells (e.g., the action of a drug on a receptor protein); also called *mechanism of action*. (p. 19)

Drug classification A method of grouping drugs; may be based on structure or therapeutic use. (p. 19)

Drug effects The physiologic reactions of the body to a drug. They can be therapeutic or toxic and describe how the body is affected as a whole by the drug. (p. 28)

KEY TERMS—cont'd

Drug-induced teratogenesis The development of congenital anomalies or defects in the developing fetus caused by the toxic effects of drugs. (p. 33)

Drug interaction Alteration in the pharmacologic or pharmacokinetic activity of a given drug caused by the presence of one or more additional drugs; it is usually related to effects on the enzymes required for metabolism of the involved drugs. (p. 31)

Duration of action The length of time the concentration of a drug in the blood or tissues is sufficient to elicit a response. (p. 28)

Enzymes Protein molecules that catalyze one or more of a variety of biochemical reactions, including those related to the body's physiologic processes as well as those related to drug metabolism. (p. 29)

First-pass effect The initial metabolism in the liver of a drug absorbed from the gastrointestinal tract before the drug reaches systemic circulation through the bloodstream. (p. 21)

Generic name The name given to a drug by the United States Adopted Names Council. Also called the *nonproprietary name*. The generic name is much shorter and simpler than the chemical name and is not protected by trademark. (p. 18)

Glucose-6-phosphate dehydrogenase (G6PD) deficiency A hereditary condition in which red blood cells break down when the body is exposed to certain drugs. (p. 33)

Half-life In pharmacokinetics, the time required for half of an administered dose of drug to be eliminated by the body, or the time it takes for the blood level of a drug to be reduced by 50% (also called *elimination half-life*). (p. 27)

Idiosyncratic reaction An abnormal and unexpected response to a medication, other than an allergic reaction, that is peculiar to an individual patient. (p. 33)

Incompatibility The characteristic that causes two parenteral drugs or solutions to undergo a reaction when mixed or given together that results in the chemical deterioration of at least one of the drugs. (p. 32)

Intraarterial Within an artery (e.g., intraarterial injection). (p. 22)

Intraarticular Within a joint (e.g., intraarticular injection). (p. 22)

Intrathecal Within a sheath (e.g., the theca of the spinal cord, as in an intrathecal injection into the subarachnoid space). (p. 22)

Medication error Any preventable adverse drug event (see above) involving inappropriate medication use by a patient or health care professional; it may or may not cause patient harm. (p. 32)

Medication use process The prescribing, dispensing, and administering of medications, and the monitoring of their effects. (p. 32)

Metabolite A chemical form of a drug that is the product of one or more biochemical (metabolic) reactions involving the parent drug (see later). Active metabolites are those that have pharmacologic activity of their own, even if the parent drug is inactive (see *prodrug*). Inactive metabolites lack pharmacologic activity and are simply drug waste products awaiting excretion from the body (e.g., via the urinary, gastrointestinal, or respiratory tract). (p. 32)

Onset of action The time required for a drug to elicit a therapeutic response after dosing. (p. 28)

P-glycoprotein a transporter protein that moves drugs out of cells and into the gut, urine, or bile. (p. 26)

Parent drug The chemical form of a drug that is administered before it is metabolized by the body into its active or inactive metabolites (see *metabolite*). A parent drug that is not pharmacologically active itself is called a *prodrug*. A prodrug is then metabolized to pharmacologically active metabolites. (p. 20)

Peak effect The time required for a drug to reach its maximum therapeutic response in the body. (p. 28)

Peak level The maximum concentration of a drug in the body after administration, usually measured in a blood sample for therapeutic drug monitoring. (p. 28)

Pharmaceutics The science of preparing and dispensing drugs, including dosage form design. (p. 19)

Pharmacodynamics The study of the biochemical and physiologic interactions of drugs at their sites of activity. It examines the physicochemical properties of drugs and their pharmacologic interactions with body receptors. (p. 19)

Pharmacoeconomics The study of economic factors impacting the cost of drug therapy. (p. 19)

Pharmacogenomics The study of the influence of genetic factors on drug response that result in the absence, overabundance, or insufficiency of drug-metabolizing enzymes (also called *pharmacogenomics;* see Chapter 8). (p. 33)

Pharmacognosy The study of drugs that are obtained from natural plant and animal sources. (p. 19)

Pharmacokinetics The study of what happens to a drug from the time it is put into the body until the parent drug and all metabolites have left the body. Pharmacokinetics represent the drug absorption into, distribution and metabolism within, and excretion from the body. (p. 19)

Pharmacology The broadest term for the study or science of drugs. (p. 18)

Pharmacotherapeutics The treatment of pathologic conditions through the use of drugs. (p. 19)

Prodrug An inactive drug dosage form that is converted to an active metabolite by various biochemical reactions once it is inside the body. (p. 26)

Receptor A molecular structure within or on the outer surface of a cell. Receptors bind specific substances (e.g., drug molecules), and one or more corresponding cellular effects (drug actions) occur as a result of this drug-receptor interaction. (p. 29)

KEY TERMS—cont'd

Steady state The physiologic state in which the amount of drug removed via elimination is equal to the amount of drug absorbed with each dose. (p. 28)

Substrates Substances (e.g., drugs or natural biochemicals in the body) on which an enzyme acts. (p. 26)

Synergistic effects Drug interactions in which the effect of a combination of two or more drugs with similar actions is greater than the sum of the individual effects of the same drugs given alone. For example, 1 + 1 is greater than 2 (compare with *additive effects*). (p. 32)

Therapeutic drug monitoring The process of measuring drug levels to identify a patient's drug exposure and to allow adjustment of dosages with the goals of maximizing therapeutic effects and minimizing toxicity. (p. 28)

Therapeutic effect The desired or intended effect of a particular medication. (p. 28)

Therapeutic index The ratio between the toxic and therapeutic concentrations of a drug. (p. 30)

Tolerance Reduced response to a drug after prolonged use. (p. 31)

Toxic The quality of being poisonous (i.e., injurious to health or dangerous to life). (p. 19)

Toxicity The condition of producing adverse bodily effects due to poisonous qualities. (p. 28)

Toxicology The study of poisons, including toxic drug effects, and applicable treatments. (p. 19)

Trade name The commercial name given to a drug product by its manufacturer; also called the *proprietary name.* (p. 18)

Trough level The lowest concentration of drug reached in the body after it falls from its peak level, usually measured in a blood sample for therapeutic drug monitoring. (p. 28)

OVERVIEW

Any chemical that affects the physiologic processes of a living organism can be defined as a **drug**. The study or science of drugs is known as **pharmacology**. Pharmacology encompasses a variety of topics, including the following:

- Absorption
- Biochemical effects
- Biotransformation (metabolism)
- Distribution
- Drug history
- Drug origin
- Excretion
- Mechanisms of action
- Physical and chemical properties
- Physical effects
- Drug receptor mechanisms
- Therapeutic (beneficial) effects
- Toxic (harmful) effects

Pharmacology includes the following several subspecialty areas: *pharmaceutics, pharmacokinetics, pharmacodynamics, pharmacogenomics (pharmacogenetics), pharmacoeconomics, pharmacotherapeutics, pharmacognosy,* and *toxicology.* Knowledge of pharmacology enables the nurse to better understand how drugs affect humans. Without understanding basic pharmacologic principles, the nurse cannot fully appreciate the therapeutic benefits and potential toxicity of drugs.

Throughout the process of its development, a drug will acquire at least three different names. The **chemical name** describes the drug's chemical composition and molecular structure. The generic name, or nonproprietary name, is often much shorter and simpler than the chemical name. The **generic name** is used in most official drug compendiums to list drugs. The **trade name**, or proprietary name, is the drug's registered trademark, and indicates that its commercial use is restricted to the owner of the patent for the drug (Figure 2-1). The patent owner is usually the manufacturer of the drug. Trade names are generally created by the manufacturer with marketability in mind. For this reason, they are usually shorter and easier to pronounce and remember than generic drug names. The *patent life* (the length of time from patent approval until patent expiration) of a newly discovered drug molecule is normally 17 years. The research processes for new drug development normally require about 10 years, and the manufacturer generally has the remaining 7 years for sales profits before patent expiration. A significant amount of these profits serves to offset the

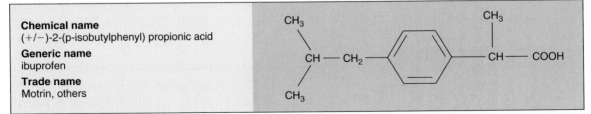

Chemical name
(+/−)-2-(p-isobutylphenyl) propionic acid

Generic name
ibuprofen

Trade name
Motrin, others

FIGURE 2-1 Chemical structure of the common analgesic ibuprofen and the chemical, generic, and trade names for the drug.

multimillion-dollar costs for research and development of the drug. A new category of the generic drug market is called *biosimilars*. Biosimilar, by definition, is a copy version of an already authorized biological product.

After the patent expires, other manufacturers may legally begin to manufacture *generic* drugs with the same active ingredient. At this point, the drug price usually decreases substantially. Due to the high cost of drugs, many institutions have implemented programs in which one drug in a class of several drugs is chosen as the preferred agent, even though the drugs do not have the same active ingredients. This is called *therapeutic equivalence*. Before one drug can be therapeutically substituted for another, the drugs must have been proven to have the same therapeutic effect on the body.

Drugs are grouped together based on their similar properties. This is known as a **drug classification**. Drugs can be classified by their structure (e.g., beta-adrenergic blockers) or by their therapeutic use (e.g., antibiotics, antihypertensives, antidepressants). Within the broad classification, each class may have subclasses; for example, penicillins are a subclass within the group of antibiotics, and beta-adrenergic blockers are a subclass within the group of antihypertensives.

Three basic areas of pharmacology—*pharmaceutics, pharmacokinetics,* and *pharmacodynamics*—describe the relationship between the dose of a drug and the activity of that drug in treating the disorder. **Pharmaceutics** is the study of how various dosage forms influence the way in which the drug affects the body. **Pharmacokinetics** is the study of what the body does to the drug. Pharmacokinetics involves the processes of absorption, distribution, metabolism, and excretion. **Pharmacodynamics** is the study of what the drug does to the body. Pharmacodynamics involves drug-receptor relationships. Figure 2-2 illustrates the three phases of drug activity, starting with the pharmaceutical phase, proceeding to the pharmacokinetic phase, and finishing with the pharmacodynamic phase.

Pharmacotherapeutics (also called *therapeutics*) focuses on the clinical use of drugs to prevent and treat diseases. It defines the principles of **drug actions**. Some drug mechanisms of action are more clearly understood than others. Drugs are also categorized into pharmacologic classes according to their physiologic functions (e.g., beta-adrenergic blockers) and primary disease states treated (e.g., anticonvulsants, antiinfectives). The U.S. Food and Drug Administration (FDA) regulates the approval and clinical use of all drugs in the United States, including the requirement of an expiration date on all drugs. This textbook focuses almost exclusively on current FDA-approved indications for the drugs discussed in each chapter and on drugs that are currently available in the United States at the time of this writing. Only FDA-approved indications are permitted to be described in the manufacturer's written information, or labeling, for a given drug product. At times, prescribers may choose to use drugs for non–FDA-approved indications. This is known as *off-label prescribing*. Evolving over time in clinical practice, previously off-label indications often become FDA-approved indications for a given drug.

The study of the adverse effects of drugs and other chemicals on living systems is known as **toxicology**. Toxic effects are often

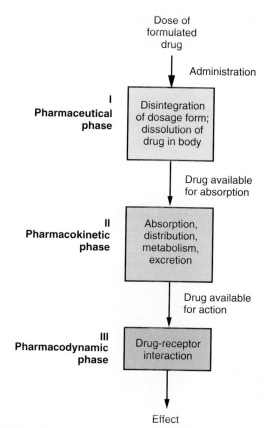

FIGURE 2-2 Phases of drug activity. (From McKenry LM, Tessier E, Hogan M: *Mosby's pharmacology in nursing*, ed 22, St Louis, 2006, Mosby.)

an extension of a drug's therapeutic action. Therefore, toxicology frequently involves overlapping principles of both pharmacotherapy and toxicology. The study of natural (versus synthetic) drug sources (i.e., plants, animals, minerals) is called **pharmacognosy**. **Pharmacoeconomics** focuses on the economic aspects of drug therapy.

In summary, pharmacology is a very dynamic science that incorporates several different disciplines, including chemistry, physiology, and biology.

PHARMACEUTICS

Different drug dosage forms have different pharmaceutical properties. Dosage form determines the rate at which drug **dissolution** (dissolving of solid dosage forms and their absorption, e.g., from gastrointestinal [GI] tract) occurs. A drug to be ingested orally may be in either a solid form (tablet, capsule, or powder) or a liquid form (solution or suspension). Table 2-1 lists various oral drug preparations and the relative rate at which they are absorbed. Oral drugs that are liquids (e.g., elixirs, syrups) are already dissolved and are usually absorbed more quickly than solid dosage forms. Enteric-coated tablets, on the other hand, have a coating that prevents them from being broken down in the acidic pH environment of the stomach and are not absorbed until they reach the higher (more alkaline) pH

TABLE 2-1	**Drug Absorption of Various Oral Preparations**
Oral disintegration, buccal tablets, and oral soluble wafers	Fastest
Liquids, elixirs, and syrups	
Suspension solutions	
Powders	
Capsules	
Tablets	
Coated tablets	
Enteric-coated tablets	Slowest

TABLE 2-2	**Dosage Forms**
Route	**Forms**
Enteral	Tablets, capsules, oral soluble wafers, pills, timed-release capsules, timed-release tablets, elixirs, suspensions, syrups, emulsions, solutions, lozenges or troches, rectal suppositories, sublingual or buccal tablets
Parenteral	Injectable forms, solutions, suspensions, emulsions, powders for reconstitution
Topical	Aerosols, ointments, creams, pastes, powders, solutions, foams, gels, transdermal patches, inhalers, rectal and vaginal suppositories

of the intestines. This pharmaceutical property results in slower dissolution and therefore slower absorption.

Particle size within a tablet or capsule can make different dosage forms of the same drug dissolve at different rates, become absorbed at different rates, and thus have different times to onset of action. An example is the difference between micronized glyburide and nonmicronized glyburide. Micronized glyburide reaches a maximum concentration peak faster than does the nonmicronized formulation.

Combination dosage forms contain multiple drugs in one dose, for example, the cholesterol and antihypertensive medications atorvastatin/amlodipine tablets called Caduet. There are large numbers of such combination dosage forms; key examples are cited in the various chapters of this textbook.

A variety of dosage forms exist to provide both accurate and convenient drug delivery systems (Table 2-2). These delivery systems are designed to achieve a desired therapeutic response with minimal adverse effects. Many dosage forms have been developed to encourage patient adherence with the medication regimen. Extended-release tablets and capsules release drug molecules in the patient's GI tract over a prolonged period. This ultimately prolongs drug absorption as well as duration of action. This is the opposite of immediate-release dosage forms, which release all of the active ingredient immediately upon dissolution in the GI tract. Extended-release dosage forms are normally easily identified by various capital letter abbreviations attached to their names. Examples of this nomenclature are SR (slow release or sustained release), SA (sustained action), CR (controlled release), XL (extended length), and XT (extended time). Convenience of administration correlates strongly with patient adherence, because these forms often require fewer daily doses. Extended-release oral dosage forms must not be crushed, as this could cause accelerated release of drug from the dosage form and possible toxicity. Enteric-coated tablets also are not recommended for crushing. This would cause disruption of the tablet coating designed to protect the stomach lining from the local effects of the drug and/or protect the drug from being prematurely disrupted by stomach acid. The ability to crush a tablet or open a capsule can facilitate drug administration when patients are unable or unwilling to swallow a tablet or capsule and also when medications need to be given through an enteral feeding tube. Capsules, powder, or liquid contents can often be added to soft foods such as applesauce or pudding, or dissolved in a beverage. Granules contained in capsules are usually for extended drug release and normally should not be crushed or chewed by the patient. However, they can often be swallowed when sprinkled on one of the soft foods. Consultation with a pharmacist or use of other suitable source is necessary if any question exists as to whether a drug can be crushed or mixed with a specific food or beverage.

An increasingly popular dosage form is one that dissolves in the mouth and is absorbed through the oral mucosa. These include orally disintegrating tablets as well as thin wafers. Depending on the specific drug product, the dosage form may dissolve on the tongue, under the tongue, or in the buccal (cheek) pocket.

The specific characteristics of the dosage form have a large impact on how and to what extent the drug is absorbed. For a drug to work at a specific site in the body, either it must be applied directly at the site in an active form or it must have a way of getting to that site. Oral dosage forms rely on gastric and intestinal enzymes and pH environments to break the medication down into particles that are small enough to be absorbed into the circulation. Once absorbed through the mucosa of the stomach or intestines, the drug is then transported to the site of action by blood or lymph.

Many topically applied dosage forms work directly on the surface of the skin. Once the drug is applied, it is in a form that allows it to act immediately. With other topical dosage forms, the skin acts as a barrier through which the drug must pass to get into the circulation; once there, the drug is then carried to its site of action (e.g., fentanyl transdermal patch for pain).

Dosage forms that are administered via injection are called *parenteral* forms. They must have certain characteristics to be safe and effective. The arteries and veins that carry drugs throughout the body can easily be damaged if the drug is too concentrated or corrosive. The pH of injections must be very similar to that of the blood for these drugs to be administered safely. Parenteral dosage forms that are injected intravenously are immediately placed into solution in the bloodstream and do not have to be dissolved in the body. Therefore, 100% absorption is assumed to occur immediately upon intravenous injection.

PHARMACOKINETICS

Pharmacokinetics is the study of what happens to a drug from the time it is put into the body until the **parent drug** and all metabolites have left the body. Specifically, drug absorption into, distribution and metabolism within, and excretion from the body represent the combined focus of pharmacokinetics.

Absorption

Absorption is the movement of a drug from its site of administration into the bloodstream for distribution to the tissues. Bioavailability is the term used to express the extent of drug absorption. A drug that is absorbed from the intestine must first pass through the liver before it reaches the systemic circulation. If a large proportion of a drug is chemically changed into inactive metabolites in the liver, then a much smaller amount of drug will pass into the circulation (i.e., will be bioavailable). Such a drug is said to have a high first-pass effect. First-pass effect reduces the bioavailability of the drug to less than 100%. Many drugs administered by mouth have a bioavailability of less than 100%, whereas drugs administered by the intravenous route are 100% bioavailable. If two drug products have the same bioavailability and same concentration of active ingredient, they are said to be bioequivalent (e.g., a brand-name drug and the same generic drug).

Various factors affect the rate of drug absorption. How a drug is administered, or its route of administration, affects the rate and extent of absorption of that drug. Although a number of dosage formulations are available for delivering medications, they can all be categorized into three basic routes of administration: enteral (GI tract), parenteral, and topical.

transported to the liver. Once the drug is in the liver, hepatic enzyme systems metabolize it, and the remaining active ingredients are passed into the general circulation. Many factors can alter the absorption of drugs, including acid changes within the stomach, absorption changes in the intestines, and the presence or absence of food and fluid. Various factors that affect the acidity of the stomach include the time of day; the age of the patient; and the presence and types of medications, foods, or beverages. Enteric coating is designed to protect the stomach by having drug dissolution and absorption occur in the intestines. Taking an enteric-coated medication with a large amount food may cause it to be dissolved by acidic stomach contents and thus reduce intestinal drug absorption and negate the coating's stomach-protective properties. Anticholinergic drugs slow GI transit time (or the time it takes for substances in the stomach to be dissolved for transport to and absorption from the intestines). This may reduce the amount of drug absorption for acid-susceptible drugs that become broken down by stomach acids. The presence of food may enhance the absorption of some fat-soluble drugs or of drugs that are more easily broken down in an acidic environment.

Drug absorption may be altered in patients who have had portions of the small intestine removed because of disease. This is known as *short bowel syndrome*. Similarly, bariatric weight loss surgery reduces the size of the stomach. As a result, medication absorption can be altered, because stomach contents are delivered to the intestines more rapidly than usual. This is called *gastric dumping*. Examples of drugs to be taken on an empty stomach and those to be taken with food are provided in Box 2-1. The stomach and small intestine are highly vascularized. When blood flow to this area is decreased, absorption may also be decreased. Sepsis and exercise are examples of circumstances under which blood flow to the GI tract is often reduced. In both cases, blood tends to be routed to the heart and other vital organs. In the case of exercise, it is also routed to the skeletal muscles.

Rectally administered drugs are often given for systemic effects (e.g., antinausea, analgesia, antipyretic effects), but they are also used to treat disease within the rectum or adjacent bowel (e.g., antiinflammatory ointment for hemorrhoids). In this case, rectal administration may also be thought of as a *topical* route of drug administration.

CASE STUDY

Patient-Centered Care: Pharmacokinetics

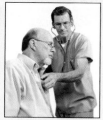

Four patients with angina are receiving a form of nitroglycerin, as follows:

Mrs. A. takes 9 mg PO twice a day to prevent angina.

Mr. B. takes a transdermal patch that delivers 0.2 mg/hr, also to prevent angina.

Mrs. C. takes 0.4 mg sublingually, only if needed for chest pain.

Mr. D. is in the hospital with severe, unstable angina and is receiving 20 mcg/hr via an intravenous infusion.

You may refer to the section on nitroglycerin in Chapter 23 or to a nursing drug handbook to answer these questions.

1. For each patient, state the rationale for the route or form of drug that was chosen. Which forms have immediate action? Why would this be important?
2. Which form or forms are most affected by the first-pass effect? Explain your answer.
3. What would happen if Mrs. A. chewed her nitroglycerin dose? If Mrs. C. chewed her nitroglycerin dose?

For answers, see *http://evolve.elsevier.com/Lilley.*

Enteral Route

In enteral drug administration, the drug is absorbed into the systemic circulation through the mucosa of the stomach and/or small or large intestine. Orally administered drugs are absorbed from the intestinal lumen into the blood system and

---

BOX 2-1   Drugs to Be Taken on an Empty Stomach and Drugs to Be Taken with Food

Many medications are taken on an empty stomach with at least 6 ounces of water. The nurse must give patients specific instructions regarding those medications that are not to be taken with food. Examples include alendronate sodium and risedronate sodium.

Medications that are generally taken with food include carbamazepine, iron and iron-containing products, hydralazine, lithium, propranolol, spironolactone, nonsteroidal antiinflammatory drugs, and theophylline.

Macrolides and oral opioids are often taken with food (even though they are specified to be taken with a full glass of water and on an empty stomach) to minimize the gastrointestinal irritation associated with these drugs. If doubt exists, consult a licensed pharmacist or a current authoritative drug resource. An Internet source to use is *www.usp.org.*

Sublingual and buccal routes. Drugs administered by the *sublingual* route are absorbed into the highly vascularized tissue under the tongue—the oral mucosa. Sublingual nitroglycerin is an example. Sublingually administered drugs are absorbed rapidly because the area under the tongue has a large blood supply. These drugs bypass the liver and yet are systemically bioavailable. The same applies for drugs administered by the *buccal route* (the oral mucosa between the cheek and the gum). Through these routes, drugs such as nitroglycerin are absorbed rapidly into the bloodstream and delivered to their site of action (e.g., coronary arteries).

Parenteral Route

The parenteral route is the fastest route by which a drug can be absorbed, followed by the enteral and topical routes. *Parenteral* is a general term meaning any route of administration other than the GI tract. It most commonly refers to injection. Intravenous injection delivers the drug directly into the circulation, where it is distributed with the blood throughout the body. Drugs given by intramuscular injection and subcutaneous injection are absorbed more slowly than those given intravenously. These drug formulations are usually absorbed over a period of several hours; however, some are specially formulated to be released over days, weeks, or months.

Drugs can be injected intradermally, subcutaneously, *intraarterially*, intramuscularly, *intrathecally*, intraarticularly, or intravenously. Physicians, or advanced practice nurses, usually give **intraarterial, intrathecal,** or **intraarticular** injections. Medications given by the parenteral route have the advantage of bypassing the first-pass effect of the liver. Parenteral administration offers an alternative route of delivery for medications that cannot be given orally. However, drugs that are administered by the parenteral route must still be absorbed into cells and tissues before they can exert their pharmacologic effect (Table 2-3).

⚡ SAFETY AND QUALITY IMPROVEMENT: PREVENTING MEDICATION ERRORS   QSEN

Does IV = PO?

The prescriber writes an order for "Lasix 80 mg IV STAT × 1 dose" for a patient who is short of breath with heart failure. When the nurse goes to give the drug, only the PO form is immediately available. Someone must go to the pharmacy to pick up the IV dose. Another nurse says, "Go ahead and give the pill. He needs it fast. It's all the same!" But is it?

Remember, the oral forms of medications must be processed through the gastrointestinal tract, absorbed through the small intestines, and undergo the first-pass effect in the liver before the drug can reach the intended site of action. However, IV forms are injected directly into the circulation and can act almost immediately because the first-pass effect is bypassed. The time until onset of action for the PO form is 30 to 60 minutes; for the IV form, this time is *5 minutes*. This patient is in respiratory distress, and the immediate effect of the diuretic is desired. In addition, because of the first-pass effect, the available amount of orally administered drug that actually reaches the site of action would be less than the available amount of intravenously administered drug. Therefore, IV does NOT equal PO! Never change the route of administration of a medication; if questions come up, always check with the prescriber.

TABLE 2-3   Routes of Administration and Related Nursing Considerations

Route	Advantages	Disadvantages	Nursing Considerations
Intravenous (IV)	Provides rapid onset (drug delivered immediately to bloodstream); allows more direct control of drug level in blood; gives option of larger fluid volume, therefore diluting irritating drugs; avoids first-pass metabolism	Higher cost; inconvenience (e.g., not self-administered); irreversibility of drug action in most cases and inability to retrieve medication; risk of fluid overload; greater likelihood of infection; possibility of embolism	Continuous intravenous infusions require frequent monitoring to be sure that the correct volume and amount are administered and that the drug reaches safe, therapeutic blood levels. Intravenous drugs and solutions must be checked for compatibilities. Intravenous sites are to be monitored for redness, swelling, heat, and drainage—all indicative of complications, such as thrombophlebitis and infection. If intermittent intravenous infusions are used, clearing or flushing of the line with normal saline before and after is generally indicated to keep the intravenous site patent and minimize incompatibilities.
Intramuscular (IM); subcutaneous	Intramuscular injections are good for poorly soluble drugs, which are often given in "depot" preparation form and are then absorbed over a prolonged period; onsets of action differ depending on route.	Discomfort of injection; inconvenience; bruising; slower onset of action compared to intravenous, although quicker than oral in most situations	Using landmarks to identify correct intramuscular and subcutaneous sites is always required and recommended as a nursing standard of care. For adults, the intramuscular site of choice is the ventral gluteal muscle with use of a 1½-inch (sometimes 1-inch in very thin or emaciated patients) and 20- to 25-gauge needle for aqueous solutions and 18- to 25-gauge needle for viscous or oil-based solutions. Subcutaneous injections are recommended to be given at a 90-degree angle with a proper size syringe and needle (½- to ⅝-inch); in emaciated or very thin patients, the subcutaneous angle is at 45 degrees. Subcutaneous injections require a 26- to 30-gauge, ½-inch needle inserted at a 90-degree angle. Selection of correct size of syringe and needle is key to safe administration by these routes and is based on thorough assessment of the patient as well as the characteristics of the drug.

TABLE 2-3 Routes of Administration and Related Nursing Considerations—cont'd

Route	Advantages	Disadvantages	Nursing Considerations
Oral	Usually easier, more convenient, and less expensive; safer than injection, dosing more likely to be reversible in cases of accidental ingestion (e.g., through induction of emesis, administration of activated charcoal)	Variable absorption; inactivation of some drugs by stomach acid and/or pH; problems with first-pass effect or presystemic metabolism; greater dependence of drug action on patient variables	Enteral routes include oral administration and involve a variety of dosage forms (e.g., liquids, solutions, tablets, and enteric-coated pills or tablets). Some medications are recommended to be taken with food, while others are recommended not to be taken with food; it is also suggested that oral dosage forms of drugs be taken with at least 6 to 8 ounces of fluid, such as water. Other factors to consider include other medicines being taken at the same time and concurrent use of dairy products or antacids. If oral forms are given via nasogastric tube or gastrostomy tube, tube placement in stomach must be assessed prior to giving the medication, and the patient's head is to remain elevated; flushing the nasogastric tube with at least 30 to 60 mL of water before and after the drug has been given is recommended to help maintain tube patency and prevent clogging.
Sublingual, buccal (subtypes of oral, but more parenteral than enteral)	Absorbed more rapidly from oral mucosa and leads to more rapid onset of action; avoids breakdown of drug by stomach acid; avoids first-pass metabolism because gastric absorption is bypassed	Patients may swallow pill instead of keeping under tongue until dissolved; pills often smaller to handle	Drugs given via the sublingual route are to be placed under the tongue; once dissolved, the drug may be swallowed. When using the buccal route, medication is placed between the cheek and gum. Both of these dosage forms are relatively nonirritating; the drug usually is without flavor and water-soluble.
Rectal	Provides relatively rapid absorption; good alternative when oral route not feasible; useful for local or systemic drug delivery; usually leads to mixed first-pass and non–first-pass metabolism	Possible discomfort and embarrassment to patient; often higher cost than oral route	Absorption via this route is erratic and unpredictable, but it provides a safe alternative when nausea or vomiting prevents oral dosing of drugs. The patient must be placed on his or her left side so that the normal anatomy of the colon allows safe and effective insertion of the rectal dosage form. Suppositories are inserted using a gloved hand and/or gloved index finger and water-soluble lubricant. The drug must be administered exactly as ordered.
Topical	Delivers medication directly to affected area; decreases likelihood of systemic drug effects	Sometimes awkward to self-administer (e.g., eyedrops); can be messy; usually higher cost than oral route	Most dermatologic drugs are given via topical route in form of a solution, ointment, spray, or drops. Maximal absorption of topical drugs is enhanced with skin that is clean and free of debris; if measurement of ointment is necessary—such as with topical nitroglycerin—application must be done carefully and per instructions (e.g., apply 1 inch of ointment). Gloves help minimize cross-contamination and prevent absorption of drug into the nurse's own skin. If the patient's skin is not intact, sterile technique is needed.
Transdermal (subtype of topical)	Provides relatively constant rate of drug absorption; one patch can last 1 to 7 days, depending on drug; avoids first-pass metabolism	Rate of absorption can be affected by excessive perspiration and body temperature; patch may peel off; cost is higher; used patches must be disposed of safely	Transdermal drugs are to be placed on alternating sites and on a clean, nonhairy, nonirritated area, and only after the previously applied patch has been removed and that area cleansed and dried. Transdermal drugs generally come in a single-dose, adhesive-backed drug application system.
Inhalational	Provides rapid absorption; drug delivered directly to lung tissues where most of these drugs exert their actions	Rate of absorption can be too rapid, increasing the risk for exaggerated drug effects; requires more patient education for self-administration; some patients may have difficulty with administration technique	Inhaled medications are to be used exactly as prescribed and with clean equipment. Instructions need to be given to the patient/family/caregiver regarding medications to be used as well as the proper use, storage, and safe-keeping of inhalers, spacers, and nebulizers. Chapter 9 describes how medications are inhaled and the various inhaled dosage forms.

NOTE: For more information on avoiding the use of abbreviations associated with dosage routes, dosage amounts, dosage frequency, and drug names, as well as the use of symbols, please visit *www.ismp.org*.

Subcutaneous, intradermal, and intramuscular routes. Injections into the fatty subcutaneous tissues under the dermal layer of skin are referred to as *subcutaneous* injections. Injections under the more superficial skin layers immediately underneath the epidermal layer of skin and into the dermal layer are known as *intradermal* injections. Injections given into the muscle beneath the subcutaneous fatty tissue are referred to as *intramuscular* injections. Muscles have a greater blood supply than does the skin; therefore, drugs injected intramuscularly are absorbed faster than drugs injected subcutaneously. Absorption from either of these sites may be increased by applying heat to the injection site or by massaging the site. In contrast, the presence of cold, hypotension, or poor peripheral blood flow compromises the circulation, reducing drug activity by reducing drug delivery to the tissues. Most intramuscularly injected drugs are absorbed over several hours. However, specially formulated long-acting intramuscular dosage forms called *depot drugs* have been designed for slow absorption over a period of several days to a few months or longer.

Topical Route

The topical route of drug administration involves application of medications to various body surfaces. Several topical drug delivery systems exist. Topically administered drugs can be applied to the skin, eyes, ears, nose, lungs, rectum, or vagina. Topical application delivers a uniform amount of drug over a longer period, but the effects of the drug are usually slower in their onset and more prolonged in their duration of action as compared to oral or parenteral administration. This can be a problem if the patient begins to experience adverse effects from the drug and a considerable amount of drug has already been absorbed. All topical routes of drug administration avoid first-pass effects of the liver, with the exception of rectal administration. Because the rectum is part of the GI tract, some drug will be absorbed into the capillaries that feed the portal vein to the liver. However, some drugs will also be absorbed locally into perirectal tissues. Therefore, rectally administered drugs are said to have a mixed first-pass and non–first-pass absorption and metabolism. Box 2-2 lists the various drug routes and indicates whether they are associated with first-pass effects in the liver.

BOX 2-2	**Drug Routes and First-Pass Effects**
First-Pass Routes	**Non–First-Pass Routes**
Hepatic arterial	Aural (instilled into the ear)
Oral	Buccal
Portal venous	Inhaled
Rectal*	Intraarterial
	Intramuscular
	Intranasal
	Intraocular
	Intravaginal
	Intravenous
	Subcutaneous
	Sublingual
	Transdermal

*Leads to both first-pass and non–first-pass effects.

Ointments, gels, and creams are common types of topically administered drugs. Examples include sunscreens, antibiotics, and nitroglycerin ointment. The drawback to their use is that their systemic absorption is often erratic and unreliable. Generally, these medications are used for local effects, but some are used for systemic effects (e.g., nitroglycerin ointment for maintenance treatment of angina). Topically applied drugs can also be used in the treatment of various illnesses of the eyes, ears, and sinuses. Eye, ear, and nose drops are administered primarily for local effects, whereas nasal sprays may be used for both systemic and local effects. Vaginal medications may be given for systemic effects (e.g., progestational hormone therapy with progesterone vaginal suppositories) but are more commonly used for local effects (e.g., treatment of vaginal yeast infection with miconazole [Monistat] vaginal cream).

Transdermal route. Transdermal drug delivery through adhesive patches is an elaborate topical route of drug administration that is commonly used for systemic drug effects. Transdermal patches are usually designed to deliver a constant amount of drug per unit of time for a specified time period. For example, a nitroglycerin patch may deliver 0.1 or 0.2 mg/hr over 24 hours, whereas a fentanyl patch may deliver 25 to 100 mcg/hr over a 72-hour period. This route is suitable for patients who cannot tolerate oral administration and provides a practical and convenient method for drug delivery.

Inhaled route. Inhalation is another type of topical drug administration. Inhaled drugs are delivered to the lungs as micrometer-sized drug particles. This small drug size is necessary for the drug to be transported to the small air sacs within the lungs (alveoli). Once the small particles of drug are in the alveoli, drug absorption is fairly rapid. Many pulmonary and other types of diseases can be treated with such topically applied (inhaled) drugs.

Distribution

Distribution refers to the transport of a drug by the bloodstream to its site of action (Figure 2-3). Drugs are distributed first to those areas with extensive blood supply. Areas of rapid distribution include the heart, liver, kidneys, and brain. Areas of slower distribution include muscle, skin, and fat. Once a drug enters the bloodstream (circulation), it is distributed throughout the body. At this point, it is also starting to be eliminated by the organs that metabolize and excrete drugs—primarily the liver and the kidneys. Only drug molecules that are not bound to plasma proteins can freely distribute to *extravascular* tissue (outside the blood vessels) to reach their site of action. If a drug is bound to plasma proteins, the drug-protein complex is generally too large to pass through the walls of blood capillaries into tissues (Figure 2-4). Albumin is the most common blood protein and carries the majority of protein-bound drug molecules. If a given drug binds to albumin, then there is only a limited amount of drug that is *not* bound. This unbound portion is pharmacologically active and is considered "free" drug, whereas "bound" drug is pharmacologically inactive. Certain conditions that cause low albumin levels, such as extensive burns and malnourished states, result in a larger fraction of free (unbound and active) drug. This can raise the risk for drug toxicity.

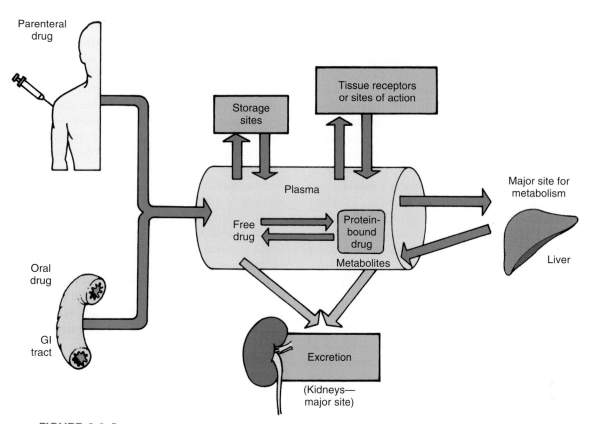

FIGURE 2-3 Drug transport in the body. *GI,* Gastrointestinal. (From McKenry LM, Tessier E, Hogan M: *Mosby's pharmacology in nursing,* ed 22, St Louis, 2006, Mosby.)

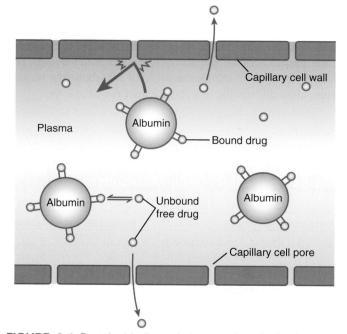

FIGURE 2-4 Protein binding of drugs. Albumin is the most prevalent protein in plasma and the most important of the proteins to which drugs bind. Only unbound (free) drug molecules can leave the vascular system. Bound molecules are too large to fit through the pores in the capillary wall.

When an individual is taking two medications that are highly protein bound, the medications may compete for binding sites on the albumin molecule. Because of this competition, there is more free, unbound drug. This can lead to an unpredictable drug response called a *drug-drug interaction.* A drug-drug interaction occurs when the presence of one drug decreases or increases the actions of another drug that is administered concurrently (i.e., given at the same time).

A theoretical volume, called the *volume of distribution,* is sometimes used to describe the various areas in which drugs may be distributed. These areas, or *compartments,* may be the blood *(intravascular space),* total body water, body fat, or other body tissues and organs. Typically a drug that is highly water-soluble (hydrophilic) will have a smaller volume of distribution and high blood concentrations. In contrast, fat-soluble drugs (lipophilic) have a larger volume of distribution and low blood concentrations. There are some sites in the body into which it may be very difficult to distribute a drug. These sites typically either have a poor blood supply (e.g., bone) or have physiologic barriers that make it difficult for drugs to pass through (e.g., the brain due to the **blood-brain barrier**).

Metabolism

Metabolism is also referred to as **biotransformation**. It involves the biochemical alteration of a drug into an inactive metabolite, a more soluble compound, a more potent active metabolite (as in the conversion of an inactive prodrug to its active form), or a less active metabolite. Metabolism is the next step after absorption and distribution. The organ most responsible for the metabolism of drugs is the liver. Other metabolic tissues include skeletal muscle, kidneys, lungs, plasma, and intestinal mucosa.

Hepatic metabolism involves the activity of a very large class of enzymes known as cytochrome P-450 enzymes (or simply P-450 enzymes), also known as *microsomal* enzymes. These enzymes control a variety of reactions that aid in the metabolism of medications. They target lipid-soluble (*nonpolar* [no charge]) drugs (also known as *lipophilic* ["fat loving"]), which are typically very difficult to eliminate. These include the majority of medications. Those medications with water-soluble (polar or *hydrophilic* ["water loving"]) molecules may be more easily metabolized by simpler chemical reactions such as hydrolysis. Some of the chemical reactions by which the liver can metabolize drugs are listed in Table 2-4. Drug molecules that are the metabolic targets of specific enzymes are said to be substrates for those enzymes. Specific P-450 enzymes are identified by standardized number and letter designations. Some of the most common P-450 enzymes and their corresponding drug substrates are listed in Table 2-5. The P-450 system is

one of the most important systems that influence drug-drug interactions. The list of drugs that are metabolized by the P-450 enzyme system is constantly changing as new drugs are introduced into the market. For further information, see websites such as *www.medicine.iupui.edu/clinpharm/ddis/* and *www.nursinglink.com/training/articles/320-clinically-significant-drug-interaction-with-the-cytochrome-p450-enzyme-system*. Another common drug interaction involves P-glycoprotein.

The metabolizing capabilities of the liver can vary considerably from patient to patient. Various factors that can alter the biotransformation include genetics, diseases, and the concurrent use of other medications (Table 2-6).

Many drugs can inhibit drug-metabolizing enzymes and are called *enzyme inhibitors*. Decreases in drug metabolism result in the accumulation of the drug and prolongation of the effects of the drug, which can lead to drug toxicity. In contrast, some drugs can stimulate drug metabolism and are called *enzyme inducers*. This can cause decreased pharmacologic effects. This often occurs with the repeated administration of certain drugs that stimulate the formation of new microsomal enzymes.

Excretion

Excretion is the elimination of drugs from the body. All drugs, whether they are parent compounds, active or inactive metabolites, must eventually be removed from the body. The primary organ responsible for this elimination is the kidney. Two other organs that play a role in the excretion of drugs are the liver and the bowel. Most drugs are metabolized in the liver by various mechanisms. Therefore, by the time most drugs reach the kidneys, they have undergone extensive biotransformation, and only a relatively small fraction of the original drug is excreted as the original compound. Other drugs may bypass hepatic metabolism and reach the kidneys in their original form. Drugs that have been metabolized by the liver become more polar and water-soluble. This makes their elimination by the kidneys much easier, because the urinary tract is water-based. The kidneys themselves are also capable of metabolizing various drugs, although usually to a lesser extent than the liver.

TABLE 2-4   Mechanisms of Biotransformation

Type of Biotransformation	Mechanism	Result
Oxidation Reduction Hydrolysis	Chemical reactions	Increase polarity of chemical, making it more water-soluble and more easily excreted. This often results in a loss of pharmacologic activity.
Conjugation (e.g., glucuronidation, glycination, sulfation, methylation, alkylation)	Combination with another substance (e.g., glucuronide, glycine, sulfate, methyl groups, alkyl groups)	Forms a less toxic product with less activity.

TABLE 2-5   Common Liver Cytochrome P-450 Enzymes and Corresponding Drug Substrates

Enzyme	Common Drug Substrates
1A2	acetaminophen, caffeine, theophylline, warfarin
2C9	ibuprofen, phenytoin
2C19	diazepam, naproxen, omeprazole, propranolol
2D6	codeine, fluoxetine, hydrocodone, metoprolol, oxycodone, paroxetine, risperidone, tricyclic antidepressants
2E1	acetaminophen, ethanol
3A4	acetaminophen, amiodarone, cyclosporine, diltiazem, ethinyl estradiol, indinavir, lidocaine, macrolides, progesterone, spironolactone, sulfamethoxazole, testosterone, verapamil

TABLE 2-6   Examples of Conditions and Drugs That Affect Drug Metabolism

Category	Example	DRUG METABOLISM Increased	DRUG METABOLISM Decreased
Diseases	Cardiovascular dysfunction		X
	Renal insufficiency		X
Conditions	Starvation		X
	Obstructive jaundice		X
	Genetic constitution		
	Fast acetylator	X	
	Slow acetylator		X
Drugs	Barbiturates	X	
	rifampin (P-450 inducer)	X	
	phenytoin (P-450 inducer)	X	
	ketoconazole (P-450 inhibitor)		X

The actual act of renal excretion is accomplished through *glomerular filtration, active tubular reabsorption,* and *active tubular secretion.* Free (unbound) water-soluble drugs and metabolites go through passive glomerular filtration. Many substances present in the nephrons go through active reabsorption and are taken back up into the systemic circulation and transported away from the kidney. This process is an attempt by the body to retain needed substances. Some substances may also be secreted into the nephron from the vasculature surrounding it. The processes of filtration, reabsorption, and secretion for urinary elimination are shown in Figure 2-5.

The excretion of drugs by the intestines is another route of elimination. This process is referred to as *biliary excretion.* Drugs that are eliminated by this route are taken up by the liver, released into the bile, and eliminated in the feces. Once certain drugs, such as fat-soluble drugs, are in the bile, they may be reabsorbed into the bloodstream, returned to the liver, and again secreted into the bile. This process is called *enterohepatic recirculation.* Enterohepatically recirculated drugs persist in the body for much longer periods. Less common routes of elimination are the lungs and the sweat, salivary, and mammary glands.

Half-Life

Another pharmacokinetic variable is the half-life of the drug. By definition, half-life is the time required for one-half (50%) of a given drug to be removed from the body. It is a measure of the rate at which the drug is eliminated from the body. For instance, if the peak level of a drug is 100 mg/L and the measured drug level in 8 hours is 50 mg/L, then the estimated half-life of that drug is 8 hours. The concept of drug half-life viewed from several different perspectives is shown in Table 2-7.

TABLE 2-7 Example of Drug Half-Life Viewed from Different Perspectives

Metric	Changing Values					
Hours after peak concentration	0	8	16	24	32	40
Drug concentration (mg/L)	100 (peak)	50	25	12.5	6.25	3.125 (trough)
Number of half-lives	0	1	2	3	4	5
Percentage of drug removed	0	50	75	88	94	97

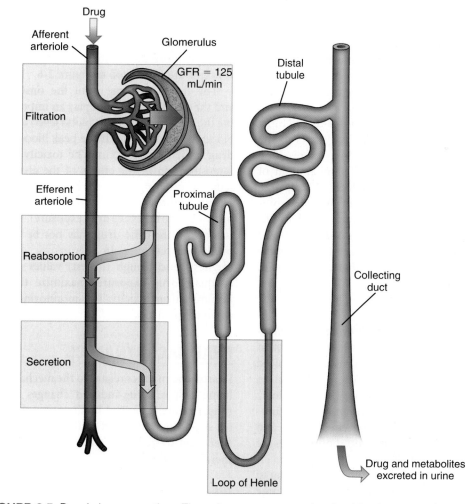

FIGURE 2-5 Renal drug excretion. The primary processes involved in drug excretion and the approximate location where these processes take place in the kidney are illustrated. *GFR,* Glomerular filtration rate.

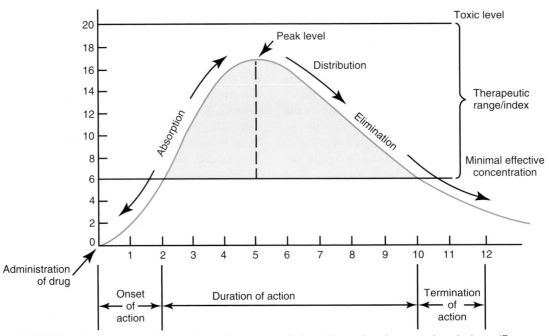

FIGURE 2-6 Characteristics of drug effect and relationship to the therapeutic window. (From McKenry LM, Tessier E, Hogan M: *Mosby's pharmacology in nursing,* ed 22, St Louis, 2006, Mosby.)

After about five half-lives, most drugs are considered to be effectively removed from the body. At that time approximately 97% of the drug has been eliminated, and what little amount remains is usually too small to have either therapeutic or toxic effects.

The concept of half-life is clinically useful for determining when steady state will be reached. **Steady state** refers to the physiologic state in which the amount of drug removed via elimination (e.g., renal clearance) is equal to the amount of drug absorbed with each dose. This physiologic plateau phenomenon typically occurs after four to five half-lives of administered drug. Therefore, if a drug has an extremely long half-life, it will take much longer for the drug to reach steady-state blood levels. Once steady-state blood levels have been reached, there are consistent levels of drug in the body that correlate with maximum therapeutic benefits.

Onset, Peak, and Duration

The pharmacokinetic terms *absorption, distribution, metabolism,* and *excretion* are all used to describe the movement of drugs through the body. Drug actions are the processes involved in the interaction between a drug and a cell (e.g., a drug's action on a receptor). In contrast, **drug effects** are the physiologic reactions of the body to the drug. The terms *onset, peak, duration,* and *trough* are used to describe drug effects. *Peak* and *trough* are also used to describe drug concentrations, which are usually measured from blood samples.

A drug's **onset of action** is the time required for the drug to elicit a therapeutic response. A drug's **peak effect** is the time required for a drug to reach its maximum therapeutic response. Physiologically, this corresponds to increasing drug concentrations at the site of action. The **duration of action** of a drug is the length of time that the drug concentration is sufficient (without more doses) to elicit a therapeutic response. These concepts are illustrated in Figure 2-6.

The length of time until the onset and peak of action and the duration of action play an important part in determining the **peak level** (highest blood level) and **trough level** (lowest blood level) of a drug. If the peak blood level is too high, then drug **toxicity** may occur. The toxicity may be mild, such as intensification of the effects of the given drug (e.g., excessive sedation resulting from overdose of a drug with sedative properties). However, it can also be severe (e.g., damage to vital organs due to excessive drug exposure). If the trough blood level is too low, then the drug may not be at therapeutic levels to produce a response. In **therapeutic drug monitoring**, peak (highest) and trough (lowest) values are measured to verify adequate drug exposure, maximize therapeutic effects, and minimize drug toxicity. This monitoring is often carried out by a clinical pharmacist.

PHARMACODYNAMICS

Pharmacodynamics relates to the mechanisms of drug action in living tissues. Drug-induced changes in normal physiologic functions are explained by the principles of pharmacodynamics. A positive change in a faulty physiologic system is called a **therapeutic effect** of a drug. Such an effect is the goal of drug therapy.

Mechanism of Action

Drugs can produce actions (therapeutic effects) in several ways. The effects of a particular drug depend on the characteristics of the cells or tissue targeted by the drug. Once the drug is at the

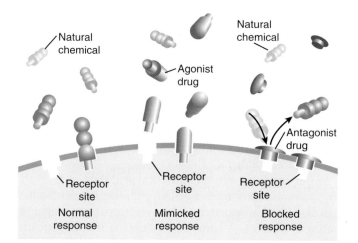

FIGURE 2-7 Drugs act by forming a chemical bond with specific receptor sites, similar to a key and lock. The better the "fit," the better the response. Drugs with complete attachment and response are called **agonists**. Drugs that attach but do not elicit a response are called **antagonists**.

TABLE 2-8	Drug-Receptor Interactions
Drug Type	**Action**
Agonist	Drug binds to the receptor; there is a response.
Partial agonist (agonist-antagonist)	Drug binds to the receptor; the response is diminished compared with that elicited by an agonist.
Antagonist	Drug binds to the receptor; there is no response. Drug prevents binding of agonists.
Competitive antagonist	Drug competes with the agonist for binding to the receptor. If it binds, there is no response.
Noncompetitive antagonist	Drug combines with different parts of the receptor and inactivates it; agonist then has no effect.

site of action, it can modify (increase or decrease) the rate at which that cell or tissue functions, or it can modify the strength of function of that cell or tissue. A drug cannot, however, cause a cell or tissue to perform a function that is not part of its natural physiology.

Drugs can exert their actions in three basic ways: through receptors, enzymes, and *nonselective interactions*. Not all mechanisms of action have been identified for all drugs. Thus, a drug may be said to have an unknown mechanism of action, even though it has observable therapeutic effects in the body.

Receptor Interactions

A **receptor** can be defined as a reactive site on the surface or inside of a cell. If the mechanism of action of a drug involves a receptor interaction, then the molecular structure of the drug is critical. Drug-receptor interaction is the joining of the drug molecule with a reactive site on the surface of a cell or tissue. Most commonly, this site is a protein structure within the cell membrane. Once a drug binds to and interacts with the receptor, a pharmacologic response is produced (Figure 2-7). The degree to which a drug attaches to and binds with a receptor is called its *affinity*. The drug with the best "fit" and strongest affinity for the receptor will elicit the greatest response. A drug becomes bound to the receptor through the formation of chemical bonds between the receptor on the cell and the active site on the drug molecule. Drugs interact with receptors in different ways either to elicit or to block a physiologic response. Table 2-8 describes the different types of drug-receptor interaction.

Enzyme Interactions

Enzymes are the substances that catalyze nearly every biochemical reaction in a cell. Drugs can produce effects by interacting with these enzyme systems. For a drug to alter a physiologic response in this way, it may either inhibit (more common) or enhance (less common) the action of a specific enzyme. This

process is called *selective interaction*. Drug-enzyme interaction occurs when the drug chemically binds to an enzyme molecule in such a way that it alters (inhibits or enhances) the enzyme's interaction with its normal target molecules in the body.

Nonselective Interactions

Drugs with nonspecific mechanisms of action do not interact with receptors or enzymes. Instead, their main targets are cell membranes and various cellular processes such as metabolic activities. These drugs can either physically interfere with or chemically alter cellular structures or processes. Some cancer drugs and antibiotics have this mechanism of action. By incorporating themselves into the normal metabolic process, they cause a defect in the final product or state. This defect may be an improperly formed cell wall that results in cell death through cell lysis, or it may be the lack of a necessary energy substrate, which leads to cell starvation and death.

PHARMACOTHERAPEUTICS

Before drug therapy is initiated, an end point or expected outcome of therapy needs to be established. This desired therapeutic outcome is patient-specific, established in collaboration with the patient, and, if appropriate, determined with other members of the health care team. Outcomes need to be clearly defined and must be either measurable or observable by monitoring. Outcome goals must be realistic and prioritized so that drug therapy begins with interventions that are essential to the patient's well-being. Examples include curing a disease, eliminating or reducing a preexisting symptom, arresting or slowing a disease process, preventing a disease or other unwanted condition, or otherwise improving quality of life. These goals and outcomes are not the same as nursing goals and outcomes. See Chapter 1 for a more specific discussion of the nursing process.

Patient therapy assessment is the process by which a practitioner integrates his or her knowledge of medical and drug-related facts with information about a specific patient's medical and social history. Items to be considered in the assessment are drugs currently used (prescription, over-the-counter, herbal, and illicit or street drugs), pregnancy and breastfeeding status, and concurrent illnesses that could contraindicate initiation of a given medication. A contraindication for a medication is any patient condition, especially a disease state that makes the use of the given medication dangerous for the patient. Careful attention to this assessment process helps to ensure an optimal therapeutic plan. The implementation of a treatment plan can involve several types and combinations of therapies. The type of therapy can be categorized as *acute, maintenance, supplemental* (or *replacement*), *palliative, supportive, prophylactic,* or *empiric.*

Acute Therapy

Acute therapy often involves more intensive drug treatment and is implemented in the acutely ill (those with rapid onset of illness) or the critically ill. It is often needed to sustain life or treat disease. Examples are the administration of vasopressors to maintain blood pressure, the use of volume expanders for a patient who is in shock, and intensive chemotherapy for a patient with newly diagnosed cancer.

Maintenance Therapy

Maintenance therapy does not eradicate pre-existing problems the patient may have, but will prevent progression of a disease or condition. It is used for the treatment of chronic illnesses such as hypertension. In this case, maintenance therapy maintains the patient's blood pressure within given limits, which prevents certain end-organ damage. Another example of maintenance therapy is the use of oral contraceptives for birth control.

Supplemental Therapy

Supplemental (or replacement) therapy supplies the body with a substance needed to maintain normal function. This substance may be needed either because it cannot be made by the body or because it is produced in insufficient quantity. Examples are the administration of insulin to diabetic patients and of iron to patients with iron-deficiency anemia.

Palliative Therapy

The goal of palliative therapy is to make the patient as comfortable as possible. Palliative therapy focuses on providing patients with relief from the symptoms, pain, and stress of a serious illness. The goal is to improve quality of life for both the patient and the family. It is typically used in the end stages of an illness when attempts at curative therapy have failed; however, it can be provided along with curative treatment. An example is the use of high-dose opioid analgesics to relieve pain in the final stages of cancer.

Supportive Therapy

Supportive therapy maintains the integrity of body functions while the patient is recovering from illness or trauma. Examples are provision of fluids and electrolytes to prevent dehydration in a patient who is vomiting and has diarrhea, administration of fluids, volume expanders, or blood products to a patient who has lost blood during surgery.

Prophylactic Therapy and Empiric Therapy

Prophylactic therapy is drug therapy provided to *prevent* illness or other undesirable outcome during *planned* events. A common example is the use of preoperative antibiotic therapy for surgical procedures. The antibiotic is given before the incision is made, so that the antibiotic can kill any potential pathogens. Another example is the administration of disease-specific vaccines to individuals traveling to geographic areas where a given disease is known to be endemic.

Empiric therapy is based on clinical probabilities. It involves drug administration when a certain pathologic condition has a high likelihood of occurrence based on the patient's initial presenting symptoms. A common example is use of antibiotics active against the organism most commonly associated with a specific infection before the results of the culture and sensitivity reports are available.

Monitoring

Once the appropriate therapy has been implemented, the effectiveness of the therapy—that is, the clinical response of the patient to the treatment—must be evaluated. Evaluating the clinical response requires familiarity with both the drug's intended therapeutic action (beneficial effects) and its unintended possible adverse effects (predictable adverse drug reactions). Examples of monitoring include observing for the therapeutic effect of reduced blood pressure following administration of antihypertensive drugs and observing for the toxic effect of leukopenia after administering antineoplastic (cancer chemotherapy) drugs. Another example is performing a pain assessment after giving pain medication. It should be noted that this textbook highlights only the most common adverse effects of a given drug; however, the drug may have many other less commonly reported adverse effects. Consult comprehensive references or a pharmacist when there is uncertainty regarding adverse effects that a patient may be experiencing.

All drugs are potentially toxic and can have cumulative effects. Recognizing these toxic effects and knowing their manifestations are integral components of the monitoring process. A drug can accumulate when it is absorbed more quickly than it is eliminated or when it is administered before the previous dose has been metabolized or cleared from the body. Knowledge of the organs responsible for metabolizing and eliminating a drug combined with knowledge of how a particular drug is metabolized and excreted enables the nurse to anticipate problems and treat them appropriately if they occur.

Therapeutic Index

The ratio of a drug's toxic level to the level that provides therapeutic benefits is referred to as the drug's therapeutic index. The safety of a particular drug therapy is determined by this index. A low therapeutic index means that the difference between a therapeutically active dose and a toxic dose is small. A drug with a low therapeutic index has a greater likelihood than other drugs of causing an adverse reaction, and therefore requires closer monitoring. Examples of such drugs are warfarin and digoxin. In contrast, a drug with a high therapeutic index, such as amoxicillin, is rarely associated with overdose events.

Drug Concentration

All drugs reach a certain concentration in the blood. Drug concentrations can be an important tool for evaluating the clinical response to drug therapy. Certain drug levels are associated with therapeutic responses, whereas other drug levels are associated with toxic effects. Toxic drug levels are typically seen when the body's normal mechanisms for metabolizing and excreting drugs are compromised. This commonly occurs when liver and kidney functions are impaired or when the liver or kidneys are immature (as in neonates). Dosage adjustments should be made in these patients to appropriately accommodate their impaired metabolism and excretion.

Patient's Condition

Another patient-specific factor to be considered is the patient's concurrent diseases or other medical conditions. A patient's response to a drug may vary greatly depending on physiologic and psychological demands. Disease of any kind, infection, cardiovascular function, and GI function can alter a patient's therapeutic response. Stress, depression, and anxiety can also be important psychological factors affecting response.

Tolerance and Dependence

To provide optimal drug therapy, it is important to understand and differentiate between tolerance and dependence. Tolerance is a decreasing response to repeated drug doses. Dependence is a physiologic or psychological need for a drug. *Physical dependence* is the physiologic need for a drug to avoid physical withdrawal symptoms (e.g., tachycardia in an opioid-addicted patient). *Psychological dependence* is also known as *addiction* and is the obsessive desire for the euphoric effects of a drug. Addiction typically involves the recreational use of various drugs such as benzodiazepines, opioids, and amphetamines. See Chapter 17 for further discussion of dependence and addiction.

Interactions

Drugs may interact with other drugs, with foods, or with agents administered as part of laboratory tests. Knowledge of drug interactions is vital for the appropriate monitoring of drug therapy. The more drugs a patient receives, the more likely that a drug interaction will occur. This is especially true in older adults, who typically have an increased sensitivity to drug effects and are receiving several medications. In addition, over-the-counter medications and herbal therapies and food can interact significantly with prescribed medications. See Table 2-9 for the most common food and drug interactions.

Alteration of the action of one drug by another is referred to as drug interaction. A drug interaction can either increase or decrease the actions of one or both of the involved drugs. Drug interactions can be either beneficial or harmful. Numerous drug interactions can occur and have been reported. Only those drug interactions that are considered to be significant with a good probability of occurring and/or those that require dosage/therapy adjustment are discussed in this textbook. An authoritative resource may be used as a means of exploring all possible drug interactions.

Concurrently administered drugs may interact with each other and alter the pharmacokinetics of one another during any of the four phases of pharmacokinetics: absorption, distribution, metabolism, or excretion. Table 2-10 provides examples of

TABLE 2-9   Common Food and Drug Interactions

Food	Drug (Category)	Result
Leafy green vegetables	warfarin (anticoagulant)	Decreased anticoagulant effect from warfarin
Dairy products	tetracycline, levofloxacin, ciprofloxacin, moxifloxacin (antibiotics)	Chemical binding of the drug leading to decreased effect and treatment failures
Grapefruit juice	amiodarone (antidysrhythmic), buspirone (antianxiety), carbamazepine (antiseizure), cyclosporine, tacrolimus (immunosuppressants), felodipine, nifedipine, nimodipine, nisoldipine (calcium channel blockers), simvastatin, atorvastatin (anticholesterol drugs)	Decreased metabolism of drugs and increased effects
Aged cheese, wine	Monoamine oxidase inhibitors	Hypertensive crisis

TABLE 2-10   Examples of Drug Interactions and Their Effects on Pharmacokinetics

Pharmacokinetic Phase	Drug Combination	Mechanism	Result
Absorption	antacid with levofloxacin	Antacids bind to the levofloxacin preventing adequate absorption.	Decreased effectiveness of levofloxacin, resulting from decreased blood levels (harmful)
Distribution	warfarin with amiodarone	Both drugs compete for protein-binding sites.	Higher levels of free (unbound) warfarin and amiodarone, which increases actions of both drugs (harmful)
Metabolism	erythromycin with cyclosporine	Both drugs compete for the same hepatic enzymes.	Decreased metabolism of cyclosporine, possibly resulting in toxic levels of cyclosporine (harmful)
Excretion	amoxicillin with probenecid	Inhibits the secretion of amoxicillin into the kidneys.	Elevation and prolongation of plasma levels of amoxicillin (can be beneficial)

drug interactions during each of these phases. Most commonly, drug interactions occur when there is competition between two drugs for metabolizing enzymes, such as the cytochrome P-450 enzymes listed in Table 2-5. As a result, the speed of metabolism of one or both drugs may be enhanced or reduced. This change in metabolism of one or both drugs can lead to subtherapeutic or toxic drug actions.

Many terms are used to categorize drug interactions. When two drugs with similar actions are given together, they can have additive effects (1 + 1 = 2). Often drugs are used together for their additive effects so that smaller doses of each drug can be given.

Synergistic effects occur when two drugs administered together interact in such a way that their combined effects are greater than the sum of the effects for each drug given alone (1 + 1 = greater than 2).

Antagonistic effects are said to occur when the combination of two drugs results in drug effects that are less than the sum of the effects for each drug given separately (1 + 1 = less than 2). Incompatibility is a term most commonly used to describe parenteral drugs. Drug incompatibility occurs when two parenteral drugs or solutions are mixed together and the result is a chemical deterioration of one or both of the drugs or the formation of a physical precipitate. The combination of two such drugs usually produces a precipitate, haziness, or color change in the solution. Before administering any intravenous medication, the nurse must always inspect the bag for precipitate. If the solution appears cloudy or if visible flecks are seen, the bag must be discarded.

Adverse Drug Events

The recognition of the potential hazards and detrimental effects of medication use is a topic that continues to receive much attention. This focus has contributed to an increasing body of knowledge regarding this topic as well as the development of new terminology.

Adverse drug event (ADE) is a broad term for any undesirable occurrence involving medications. A similarly broad term also seen in the literature is *drug misadventure.* Patient outcomes associated with adverse drug events vary from no effects to mild discomfort to life-threatening complications, permanent disability, disfigurement, or death. Adverse drug events can be preventable (see discussion of medication errors in Chapter 5) or nonpreventable. Fortunately, many adverse drug events result in no measurable patient harm. Adverse drug events can be both external and internal. The most common causes of adverse drug events *external* to the patient are errors by caregivers (both professional and nonprofessional) or malfunctioning of equipment (e.g., intravenous infusion pumps). An adverse drug event can be internal, or *patient induced,* such as when a patient fails to take medication as prescribed or drinks alcoholic beverages that he or she was advised not to consume while taking a given medication. An impending adverse drug event that is noticed before it actually occurs is considered a *potential* adverse drug event (and appropriate steps must be taken to avoid such a "near miss" in the future). A less common situation, but one still worth mentioning, is an *adverse drug withdrawal event.* This is an adverse outcome associated with discontinuation of drug therapy, such as hypertension caused by abruptly discontinuing blood pressure medication or return of infection caused by stopping antibiotic therapy too soon.

The two most common broad categories of adverse drug event are medication errors and adverse drug reactions. A medication error is a preventable situation in which there is a compromise in the "Six Rights" of medication use: *right drug, right dose, right time, right route, right patient,* and *right documentation.* Medication errors are more common than adverse drug reactions. Medication errors occur during the *prescribing, dispensing, administering,* or *monitoring* of drug therapy. These four phases are collectively known as the medication use process. See Chapter 5 for further discussion of medication errors.

An adverse drug reaction (ADR) (see Chapter 5) is any reaction to a drug that is unexpected and undesirable and occurs at therapeutic drug dosages. Adverse drug reactions may or may not be caused by medication errors. Adverse drug reactions may result in hospital admission, prolongation of hospital stay, change in drug therapy, initiation of supportive treatment, or complication of a patient's disease state. Adverse drug reactions are caused by processes inside the patient's body. They may or may not be preventable, depending on the situation. Mild adverse drug reactions usually do not require a change in the patient's drug therapy or other interventions. More severe adverse drug reactions, however, are likely to require changes to a patient's drug regimen. Severe adverse drug reactions can be permanently or significantly disabling, life threatening, or fatal. They may require or prolong hospitalization, lead to organ damage (e.g., to the liver, kidneys, bone marrow, skin), cause congenital anomalies, or require specific interventions to prevent permanent impairment or tissue damage.

Adverse drug reactions that are specific to particular drug groups are discussed in the corresponding drug chapters in this book. Four general categories are discussed here: pharmacologic reaction, hypersensitivity (allergic) reaction, idiosyncratic reaction, and drug interaction.

A pharmacologic reaction is an extension of the drug's normal effects in the body. For example, a drug that is used to lower blood pressure in a patient causes a pharmacologic adverse drug reaction when it lowers the blood pressure to the point at which the patient becomes unconscious.

Pharmacologic reactions that result in adverse effects are predictable, well-known, and result in minor or no changes in patient management. They are related to dose and usually resolve upon discontinuation of drug therapy.

An allergic reaction (also known as a *hypersensitivity reaction*) involves the patient's immune system. Immune system proteins known as *immunoglobulins* (see Chapters 48 and 49) recognize the drug molecule, its metabolite(s), or another ingredient in a drug formulation as a dangerous foreign substance. At this point, an *immune response* may occur in which immunoglobulin proteins bind to the drug substance in an attempt to neutralize the drug. Various chemical mediators, such as *histamine,* as well as *cytokines* and other inflammatory substances are released during this process.

This response can result in reactions ranging from mild reactions such as skin erythema or mild rash to severe, even life-threatening reactions such as constriction of bronchial airways and tachycardia.

It can be assumed throughout this textbook that use of any drug is contraindicated if the patient has a known allergy to that specific drug product. Allergy information may be reported by the patient as part of his or her history or may be observed by health care personnel during a patient encounter. In either case, every effort must be made to document as fully as possible the name of the drug product and the degree and details of the adverse reaction that occurred. For example: "Penicillin; skin rash, pruritus" or "Penicillin; urticaria and anaphylactic shock requiring emergency intervention."

In more extreme cases of disease or injury (e.g., cancer, snakebite), it may be reasonable to administer a given drug *in spite of* a reported allergic or other adverse reaction. In such cases, the patient will likely be premedicated with additional medications as an attempt to control any adverse reactions that may occur.

An **idiosyncratic reaction** is not the result of a known pharmacologic property of a drug or of a patient allergy, but instead occurs unexpectedly in a particular patient. Such a reaction is a genetically determined abnormal response to normal dosages of a drug. The study of such traits, which are solely revealed by drug administration, is called **pharmacogenomics** (see Chapter 8). Idiosyncratic drug reactions are usually caused by a deficiency or excess of drug-metabolizing enzymes. An example is **glucose-6-phosphate dehydrongenase (G6PD) deficiency** (see the Patient-Centered Care: Cultural Implications box).

The final type of adverse drug reaction is due to drug interactions. A drug interaction occurs when the presence of two (or more) drugs in the body produces an unwanted effect. This unwanted effect can result when one drug either enhances or reduces the effects of another drug. Some drug interactions are intentional and beneficial (see Table 2-10). However, most clinically significant drug interactions are harmful. Drug interactions specific to particular drugs are discussed in detail in the chapters dealing with those drugs.

BOX 2-3   Exogenous Causes of Cancer

Dietary customs	Environmental pollution
Drug abuse	Food-processing procedures
Carcinogenic drugs	Food production procedures
Workplace chemicals	Oncogenic viruses
Radiation	Smoking

Other Drug Effects

Other drug-related effects that must be considered during drug therapy are teratogenic, mutagenic, and carcinogenic effects. These can result in devastating patient outcomes and may be prevented in many instances by appropriate monitoring.

Teratogenic effects of drugs or other chemicals result in structural defects in the fetus. Compounds that produce such effects are called *teratogens*. Prenatal development involves a delicate program of interrelated embryologic events. Any significant disruption in this process of *embryogenesis* can have a teratogenic effect. Drugs that are capable of crossing the placenta can cause **drug-induced teratogenesis**. Drugs administered during pregnancy can produce different types of congenital anomalies. The period during which the fetus is most vulnerable to teratogenic effects begins with the third week of development and usually ends after the third month. Chapter 3 describes the FDA safety classification for drugs used by pregnant women.

Mutagenic effects are permanent changes in the genetic composition of living organisms and consist of alterations in chromosome structure, the number of chromosomes, or the genetic code of the deoxyribonucleic acid (DNA) molecule. Drugs that are capable of inducing mutations are called *mutagens*. Radiation, viruses, chemicals (e.g., industrial chemicals such as benzene), and drugs can all act as mutagenic agents in humans. Drugs that affect genetic processes are active primarily during cell reproduction (mitosis).

Carcinogenic effects are the cancer-causing effects of drugs, other chemicals, radiation, and viruses. Agents that produce such effects are called *carcinogens*. Some exogenous causes of cancer are listed in Box 2-3.

PHARMACOGNOSY

The source of all early drugs was nature, and the study of these natural drug sources (plants and animals) is called *pharmacognosy*. Although many drugs in current use are synthetically derived, most were first isolated in nature. The four main sources for drugs are plants, animals, minerals, and laboratory synthesis. Plants provide many weak acids and weak bases (alkaloids) that are useful and potent drugs. Animals are the source of many hormone drugs. Conjugated estrogens are derived from the urine of pregnant mares, hence the drug trade name Premarin. *Equine* is the term used for any horse-derived drug. Insulin comes from two sources: pigs (porcine) and humans. Human insulin is now far more commonly used than animal

QSEN ⊕ **PATIENT-CENTERED CARE: CULTURAL IMPLICATIONS**

Glucose-6-Phosphate Dehydrogenase Deficiency

Glucose-6-phosphate dehydrogenase (G6PD) is an enzyme found in abundant amounts in the tissues of most individuals. It reduces the risk for hemolysis of red blood cells when they are exposed to oxidizing drugs such as aspirin. Approximately 13% of African-American men and 20% of African-American women carry the gene that results in G6PD deficiency. Approximately 14% of Sardinians and more than 50% of the Kurdish Jewish population also show G6PD deficiencies. When exposed to drugs such as sulfonamides, antimalarials, and aspirin, patients with this deficiency may suffer life-threatening hemolysis of the red blood cells, whereas individuals with adequate quantities of the enzyme have no problems in taking these drugs.

insulins thanks to the use of recombinant DNA techniques. Heparin is another commonly used drug that is derived from pigs (porcine heparin). Some common mineral sources of currently used drugs are salicylic acid, aluminum hydroxide, and sodium chloride.

PHARMACOECONOMICS

Pharmacoeconomics is the study of the economic factors influencing the cost of drug therapy. One example is performing a *cost-benefit analysis* of one antibiotic versus another when competing drugs are considered for inclusion in a hospital formulary. Such studies typically examine treatment outcomes data (e.g., how many patients recovered and how soon) in relation to the comparative total costs of treatment with the drugs in question.

TOXICOLOGY

The study of poisons and unwanted responses to both drugs and other chemicals is known as *toxicology*. Toxicology is the science of the adverse effects of chemicals on living organisms. Clinical toxicology deals specifically with the care of the poisoned patient. Poisoning can result from a variety of causes, ranging from drug overdose to ingestion of household cleaning agents to snakebite. Poison control centers are health care institutions equipped with sufficient personnel and information resources to recommend appropriate treatment for the poisoned patient.

Effective treatment of the poisoned patient is based on a system of priorities, the first of which is to preserve the patient's vital functions by maintaining the airway, ventilation, and circulation. The second priority is to prevent absorption of the toxic substance and/or speed its elimination from the body

TABLE 2-11	Common Poisons and Their Antidotes*	
Substance	**Antidote**
Acetaminophen	Acetylcysteine
Organophosphates (e.g., insecticides)	Atropine
Tricyclic antidepressants, quinidine	Sodium bicarbonate
Calcium channel blockers	Intravenous calcium
Iron salts	Deferoxamine
Digoxin and other cardiac glycosides	Digoxin antibodies
Ethylene glycol (e.g., automotive antifreeze solution), methanol	Ethanol (same as alcohol used for drinking), given intravenously
Benzodiazepines	Flumazenil
Beta blockers	Glucagon
Opiates, opioid drugs	Naloxone
Carbon monoxide (by inhalation)	Oxygen (at high concentration), known as bariatric therapy

*These and other antidotes are discussed throughout this textbook where applicable.

using one or more of the variety of clinical methods available. Several common poisons and their specific antidotes are listed in Table 2-11.

SUMMARY

A thorough understanding of the pharmacologic principles of pharmacokinetics, pharmacodynamics, pharmacotherapeutics, and toxicology is essential in drug therapy and to safe, quality nursing practice. Application of pharmacologic principles enables the nurse to provide safe and effective drug therapy while always acting on behalf of the patient and respecting the patient's rights. Nursing considerations associated with various routes of drug administration are summarized in Table 2-3.

KEY POINTS

- The following definitions related to drug therapy are important to remember: *pharmacology*—the study or science of drugs; *pharmacokinetics*—the study of drug distribution among various body compartments after a drug has entered the body, including the phases of absorption, distribution, metabolism, and excretion; *pharmaceutics*—the science of dosage form design.
- The nurse's role in drug therapy and the nursing process is more than just the memorization of the names of drugs, their uses, and associated interventions. It involves a thorough comprehension of all aspects of pharmaceutics, pharmacokinetics, and pharmacodynamics and the sound

application of this drug knowledge to a variety of clinical situations. See Chapter 1 for further discussion of drug therapy as it relates to the nursing process.
- Drug actions are related to the pharmacologic, pharmaceutical, pharmacokinetic, and pharmacodynamic properties of a given medication, and each of these has a specific influence on the overall effects produced by the drug in a patient.
- Selection of the route of administration is based on patient variables and the specific characteristics of a drug.
- Nursing considerations vary depending on the drug as well as the route of administration.

NCLEX® EXAMINATION REVIEW QUESTIONS

1. An elderly woman took a prescription medicine to help her to sleep; however, she felt restless all night and did not sleep at all. The nurse recognizes that this woman has experienced which type of reaction or effect?
   a. Allergic reaction
   b. Idiosyncratic reaction
   c. Mutagenic effect
   d. Synergistic effect

2. While caring for a patient with cirrhosis or hepatitis, the nurse knows that abnormalities in which phase of pharmacokinetics may occur?
   a. Absorption
   b. Distribution
   c. Metabolism
   d. Excretion

3. A patient who had a thyroidectomy is now taking levothyroxine, a thyroid hormone, daily. Which term best describes this type of therapy?
   a. Palliative therapy
   b. Maintenance therapy
   c. Supportive therapy
   d. Supplemental therapy

4. The nurse is giving medications to a patient in heart failure. The intravenous route is chosen instead of the intramuscular route. What patient function does the nurse recognize as the most influential when deciding to use the intravenous route of drug administration?
   a. Altered biliary function
   b. Increased glomerular filtration
   c. Reduced liver metabolism
   d. Diminished circulation

5. A patient has just received a prescription for an enteric-coated stool softener. When teaching the patient, the nurse should include which statement?

   a. "Take the tablet with 2 to 3 ounces of orange juice."
   b. "Avoid taking all other medications with any enteric-coated tablet."
   c. "Crush the tablet before swallowing if you have problems with swallowing."
   d. "Be sure to swallow the tablet whole without chewing it."

6. Each statement describes a phase of pharmacokinetics. Put the statements in order, with 1 indicating the phase that occurs first and 4 indicating the phase that occurs last.
   a. Enzymes in the liver transform the drug into an inactive metabolite.
   b. Drug metabolites are secreted through passive glomerular filtration into the renal tubules.
   c. A drug binds to the plasma protein albumin and circulates through the body.
   d. A drug moves from the intestinal lumen into the mesenteric blood system.

7. A drug that delivers 300 mg has a half-life of 4 hours. How many milligrams of drug will remain in the body after 1 half-life?

8. The nurse is reviewing the various forms of topical medications. Which of these are considered topical medications? *(Select all that apply.)*
   a. Rectal ointment for hemorrhoids
   b. Eye drops for inflammation
   c. Sublingual tablet for chest pain
   d. Inhaled medication for asthma
   e. Intradermal injection for tuberculosis testing

1. b, 2. c, 3. b, 4. d, 5. d, 6. a = 3, b = 4, c = 2, d = 1, 7. 150 mg, 8. a, b, d

CRITICAL THINKING AND PRIORITIZATION QUESTIONS

1. Mr. L. is admitted to the trauma unit with multisystem injuries from an automobile accident. He arrived at the unit with multiple abnormal findings, including shock from blood loss, decreased cardiac output, and urinary output of less than 30 mL/hr. Which route of administration would you expect to be the best choice for this patient? Explain your answer.

2. You are administering medications to a patient who had an enteral tube inserted 2 days earlier for continuous feedings. As you review the medication list, you note that one drug is an enteric-coated tablet ordered to be given twice a day. What is the best action regarding giving this drug to this patient?

For answers, see *http://evolve.elsevier.com/Lilley*.

ⓔ EVOLVE WEBSITE

http://evolve.elsevier.com/Lilley
- Animations
- Answer Keys for Textbook Case Studies and Textbook Critical Thinking and Prioritization Questions

- Content Updates
- Key Points
- Review Questions
- Student Case Studies

3

Lifespan Considerations

OBJECTIVES

When you reach the end of this chapter, you will be able to do the following:

1. Discuss the influences of the patient's age on the effects of drugs and drug responses.
2. Identify drug-related concerns during pregnancy and lactation and provide an explanation of the physiologic basis for these concerns.
3. Summarize the impact of age-related physiologic changes on the pharmacokinetic aspects of drug therapy.
4. Explain how these age-related changes in pharmacokinetics influence various drug effects and drug responses across the lifespan.
5. Provide several examples of how age affects the absorption, distribution, metabolism, and excretion of drugs.
6. Calculate a drug dose for a pediatric patient using the various formulas available.
7. Develop a nursing care plan for drug therapy and the nursing process as related to the various lifespan considerations.

KEY TERMS

Active transport The active (energy-requiring) movement of a substance between different tissues via pumping mechanisms contained within cell membranes. (p. 36)

Diffusion The passive movement of a substance (e.g., a drug) between different tissues from areas of higher concentration to areas of lower concentration. (Compare with *active transport*.) (p. 36)

Neonate Pertaining to a person younger than 1 month of age; newborn infant. (p. 36)

Older adult Pertaining to a person who is 65 years of age or older. (NOTE: Some sources consider "older adult" to be 55 years of age or older.) (p. 40)

Pediatric Pertaining to a person who is 12 years of age or younger. (p. 38)

Polypharmacy The use of many different drugs concurrently in treating a patient, who often has several health problems. (p. 40)

OVERVIEW

From the beginning to the end of life, the human body changes in many ways. These changes have a dramatic effect on the four phases of pharmacokinetics—drug absorption, distribution, metabolism, and excretion. Newborn, pediatric, and older adult patients each have special needs. Drug therapy at both spectrums of life is more likely to result in adverse effects and toxicity. Fortunately, response to drug therapy changes in a predictable manner in younger and older patients. Knowing the effect that age has on the pharmacokinetic characteristics of drugs helps predict these changes.

Most experience with drugs and pharmacology has been gained from the adult population. The majority of drug studies have focused on the population between 13 and 65 years of age. It has been estimated that 75% of currently approved drugs lack U.S. Food and Drug Administration (FDA) approval for pediatric use and therefore lack specific dosage guidelines for neonates and children. Fortunately, many excellent pediatric drug dosage books are available. Most drugs are effective in younger and older patients, but drugs behave very differently in patients at the opposite ends of the age spectrum. It is vitally important from the standpoint of safe and effective drug administration to understand what these differences are and how to adjust for them.

DRUG THERAPY DURING PREGNANCY

A fetus is exposed to many of the same substances as the mother, including any drugs that she takes—prescription, nonprescription, or street drugs. The first trimester of pregnancy is generally the period of greatest danger of drug-induced developmental defects.

Transfer of both drugs and nutrients to the fetus occurs primarily by diffusion across the placenta, although not all drugs cross the placenta. Diffusion is a passive process based on differences in concentration between different tissues. Active transport requires the expenditure of energy and often involves some sort of cell-surface protein pump. The factors that contribute to the safety or potential harm of drug therapy

TABLE 3-1 Pregnancy Safety Categories

Category	Description
Category A	Studies indicate no risk to the human fetus.
Category B	Studies indicate no risk to the animal fetus; information for humans is not available.
Category C	Adverse effects reported in the animal fetus; information for humans is not available.
Category D	Possible fetal risk in humans has been reported; however, in selected cases consideration of the potential benefit versus risk may warrant use of these drugs in pregnant women.
Category X	Fetal abnormalities have been reported, and positive evidence of fetal risk in humans is available from animal and/or human studies. These drugs are not to be used in pregnant women.
New FDA rules, effective June 2015 for newly approved drugs: Drugs currently on the market are allowed to be phased in. This information will replace the A to X categories, but information is not completed at time of publication.	Three detailed subsections on "Pregnancy," "Lactation," and "Females and Males of Reproductive Potential"

during pregnancy can be broadly broken down into three areas: drug properties, fetal gestational age, and maternal factors.

Drug properties that impact drug transfer to the fetus include the drug's chemistry, dosage, and concurrently administered drugs. Examples of relevant chemical properties include molecular weight, protein binding, lipid solubility, and chemical structure. Important drug dosage variables include dose and duration of therapy.

Fetal gestational age is an important factor in determining the potential for harmful drug effects to the fetus. The fetus is at greatest risk for drug-induced developmental defects during the first trimester of pregnancy. During this period, the fetus undergoes rapid cell proliferation. Skeleton, muscles, limbs, and visceral organs are developing at their most rapid rate. Self-treatment of minor illness is strongly discouraged anytime during pregnancy, but especially during the first trimester. Gestational age is also important in determining when a drug can most easily cross the placenta to the fetus. During the last trimester, the greatest percentage of maternally absorbed drug gets to the fetus.

Maternal factors also play a role in determining drug effects on the fetus. Any change in the mother's physiology can affect the amount of drug to which the fetus may be exposed. Maternal kidney and liver function affect drug metabolism and excretion. Impairment in either kidney or liver function may result in higher drug levels and/or prolonged drug exposure, and thus increased fetal transfer. Maternal genotype may also affect how certain drugs are metabolized (pharmacogenomics). The lack of certain enzyme systems may result in adverse drug effects to the fetus when the mother is exposed to a drug that is normally metabolized by the given enzyme.

Although exposure of the fetus to drugs is most detrimental during the first trimester, drug transfer to the fetus is more likely during the last trimester. This is the result of enhanced blood flow to the fetus, increased fetal surface area, and increased amount of free drug in the mother's circulation.

It is important to use drugs judiciously during pregnancy; however, there are certain situations that require their use. Without drug therapy, maternal conditions such as hypertension, epilepsy, diabetes, and infection could seriously endanger both the mother and the fetus, and the potential for harm far outweighs the risks of appropriate drug therapy.

The FDA classifies drugs according to their safety for use during pregnancy. This system of drug classification is based primarily on animal studies and limited human studies. This is due in part to ethical dilemmas surrounding the study of potential adverse effects on fetuses. Traditionally, the most widely used index of potential fetal risk of drugs has been the FDA's pregnancy safety category system. The five safety categories are described in Table 3-1. It must be noted that in December 2014, the FDA issued its final rule on changes to pregnancy and lactation labeling for prescription drugs. This ruling takes effect on June 30, 2015 for newly approved drugs. The FDA is allowing all of the currently marketed drugs to be phased in gradually. It is anticipated that these new changes will not be fully in effect for several years. The student will likely encounter both the old categories (A to X) as well as the new rules throughout his or her career. The new rule requires the use of three subsections in the prescribing information titled "Pregnancy," "Lactation," and "Females and Males of Reproductive Potential." These subsections will include a summary of the risks of using a drug during pregnancy and breastfeeding, as well as data supporting the summary and information to help health care providers make prescribing decisions. The "Pregnancy" section will include information on dosing and potential risks to the developing fetus. The "Lactation" section will provide information regarding breastfeeding, such as the amount of drug in breast milk and the potential effect on the child. The "Females and Males of Reproductive Potential" section will include information about contraception, pregnancy testing, and infertility. The new information is not yet published for drugs included in this book at the time of publication. The information will be posted on *http://evolve.elsevier.com/Lilley* once it becomes available.

DRUG THERAPY DURING BREASTFEEDING

Breastfed infants are at risk for exposure to drugs consumed by the mother. A wide variety of drugs easily cross from the mother's circulation into the breast milk and subsequently to the breastfeeding infant. Drug properties similar to those discussed in the previous section influence the exposure of infants to drugs via breastfeeding. The primary drug characteristics that increase the likelihood of drug transfer via breastfeeding include fat solubility, low molecular weight, and high concentration.

Fortunately, breast milk is not the primary route for maternal drug excretion. Drug levels in breast milk are usually lower than those in the maternal circulation. The actual amount of exposure depends largely on the volume of milk consumed. The ultimate decision as to whether a breastfeeding mother takes a particular drug depends on the risk/benefit ratio. The risks of drug transfer to the infant in relation to the benefits of continuing breastfeeding and the therapeutic benefits to the mother must be considered on a case-by-case basis.

CONSIDERATIONS FOR NEONATAL AND PEDIATRIC PATIENTS

Pediatric patients are defined based on age. A *neonate* is defined as between birth and 1 month of age. An *infant* is between 1 and 12 months of age, and a *child* is between 1 and 12 years of age. The age ranges that correspond to the various terms applied to pediatric patients are shown in Table 3-2.

Physiology and Pharmacokinetics

Pediatric patients handle drugs much differently than adult patients, based primarily on the immaturity of vital organs. In both neonates and older pediatric patients, anatomic structures and physiologic systems and functions are still in the process of developing. The Patient-Centered Care: Lifespan Considerations for the Pediatric Patient box on this page lists those physiologic factors that alter the pharmacokinetic properties of drugs in young patients.

Pharmacodynamics

Drug actions (or pharmacodynamics) are altered in young patients, and the maturity of various organs determines how drugs act in the body. Certain drugs may be more toxic, whereas others may be less toxic. The sensitivity of receptor sites may also vary with age; thus, higher or lower dosages may be required depending on the drug. In addition, rapidly developing tissues may be more sensitive to certain drugs, and therefore smaller dosages may be required. Certain drugs are contraindicated during the growth years. For instance, tetracycline may permanently discolor a young person's teeth; corticosteroids may suppress growth when given systemically (but not when delivered

via asthma inhalers, for example); and quinolone antibiotics may damage cartilage.

PATIENT-CENTERED CARE: LIFESPAN CONSIDERATIONS FOR THE PEDIATRIC PATIENT

Pharmacokinetic Changes in the Neonate and Pediatric Patient

Absorption
- Gastric pH is less acidic because acid-producing cells in the stomach are immature until approximately 1 to 2 years of age.
- Gastric emptying is slowed because of slow or irregular peristalsis.
- First-pass elimination by the liver is reduced because of the immaturity of the liver and reduced levels of microsomal enzymes.
- Intramuscular absorption is faster and irregular.

Distribution
- Total body water is 70% to 80% in full-term infants, 85% in premature newborns, and 64% in children 1 to 12 years of age.
- Fat content is lower in young patients because of greater total body water.
- Protein binding is decreased because of decreased production of protein by the immature liver.
- More drugs enter the brain because of an immature blood-brain barrier.

Metabolism
- Levels of microsomal enzymes are decreased because the immature liver has not yet started producing enough.
- Older children may have increased metabolism and require higher dosages once hepatic enzymes are produced.
- Many variables affect metabolism in premature infants, infants, and children, including the status of liver enzyme production, genetic differences, and substances to which the mother was exposed during pregnancy.

Excretion
- Glomerular filtration rate and tubular secretion and resorption are all decreased in young patients because of kidney immaturity.
- Perfusion to the kidneys may be decreased, which results in reduced renal function, concentrating ability, and excretion of drugs.

Dosage Calculations for Pediatric Patients

Most drugs have not been sufficiently investigated to ensure their safety and effectiveness in children. In spite of this, there are numerous excellent pediatric dosage references. Because pediatric patients (especially premature infants and neonates) have small bodies and immature organs, they are very susceptible to drug interactions, toxicity, and unusual drug responses. Pediatric patients require different dosage calculations than do adults. Characteristics of pediatric patients that have a significant effect on dosage include the following:
- Skin is thinner and more permeable.
- Stomach lacks acid to kill bacteria.
- Lungs have weaker mucous barriers.
- Body temperature is less well regulated, and dehydration occurs easily.
- Liver and kidneys are immature, and, therefore, drug metabolism and excretion are impaired.

Many formulas for pediatric dosage calculation have been used throughout the years. Calculating the dosage according to

TABLE 3-2   Classification of Young Patients

Age Range	Classification
Younger than 38 weeks' gestation	Premature or preterm infant
Younger than 1 month	Neonate or newborn infant
1 month up to 1 year	Infant
1 year up to 12 years	Child

NOTE: The meaning of the term *pediatric* may vary with the individual drug and clinical situation. Often the maximum age for a pediatric patient may be identified as 16 years of age. Consult the manufacturer's guidelines for specific dosing information.

the body weight is the most commonly used method today. Most drug references recommend dosages based on milligrams per kilogram of body weight. The following information is needed to calculate the pediatric dosage:

- Drug order (as discussed previously)
- Pediatric patient's weight in kilograms (1 kilogram = 2.2 pounds) (For example, a 10-lb baby weighs 4.5 kg; divide the number of pounds by 2.2 to determine kilograms.)
- Pediatric dosage as per manufacturer or drug formulary guidelines
- Information regarding available dosage forms

When using either of the previous methods, the following must be done to ensure the correct pediatric dose:

- Determine the pediatric patient's weight in kilograms.
- Use a current drug reference to determine the usual dosage range per 24 hours in milligrams (mg) per kilogram (kg). It must be noted that some drugs are stated as mg/kg/dose.
- Determine the dose parameters by multiplying the weight by the minimum and maximum daily doses of the drug (the safe range).

- Determine the total amount of the drug to administer per dose and per day.
- Compare the drug dosage prescribed with the calculated safe range.
- If the drug dosage raises any concerns or varies from the safe range, contact the health care provider or prescriber immediately and do not give the drug!

A common source of medication error and potential toxicity is confusing pounds with kilograms. Unless otherwise noted, the child's weight is to be given in kilograms, not pounds. Take great care to ensure that the correct weight is reported to the prescriber. In calculating pediatric dosages, the factor of organ maturity must always be considered along with BSA, age, and weight. When all of these physical developmental factors are considered and doses are calculated correctly, the likelihood of safe and effective drug administration is increased. Emotional developmental considerations must also be a part of the decision-making process in drug therapy for pediatric patients (see the Patient-Centered Care: Lifespan Considerations for the Pediatric Patient box on this page).

QSEN PATIENT-CENTERED CARE: LIFESPAN CONSIDERATIONS FOR THE PEDIATRIC PATIENT

Age-Related Considerations for Safety in Medication Administration from Infancy to Adolescence

General Interventions

- Always come prepared for the procedure (e.g., prepare for injections with needleless syringe, and gather all needed equipment).
- Ask the parent and/or child (if age-appropriate) if the parent will remain for the procedure (for in-hospital administration).
- Assess for comfort methods that are appropriate before and after drug administration.

Infants

- While maintaining safe and secure positioning of the infant (e.g., with parent holding, rocking, cuddling, soothing), perform the procedure (e.g., injection) swiftly and safely.
- Allow self-comforting measures as age-appropriate (e.g., use of pacifier, fingers in mouth, self-movement).

Toddlers

- Offer a brief, concrete explanation of the procedure but with realistic expectations of the child's actual understanding of the information. Parents, caregivers, or other legal guardians must be part of the process. Hold the child securely while administering the medication.
- Accept aggressive behavior as a healthy response, but only within reasonable limits.
- Provide comfort measures immediately after the procedure (e.g., touching, holding).
- Help the child understand the treatment and his or her feelings through puppet play or play with stuffed animals or hospital equipment such as empty, needleless syringes.
- Provide for healthy ways to release aggression such as age-appropriate supervised playtime.

Preschoolers

- Offer a brief, concrete explanation of the procedure at the patient's level and with the parent or caregiver present.

- Provide comfort measures after the procedure (e.g., touching, holding).
- Identify and accept aggressive responses, and provide age-appropriate outlets.
- Make use of magical thinking (e.g., using ointments or "special medicines" to make discomfort go away).
- Note that the role of the parent in providing comfort and understanding is very important.

School-Age Children

- Explain the procedure, allowing for some control over body and situation.
- Provide comfort measures.
- Explore feelings and concepts through the use of therapeutic play. Art may be used to help the patient express fears. Use of age-appropriate books and realistic hospital equipment may also be helpful.
- Set age-appropriate behavior limits (e.g., okay to cry or scream, but not to bite).
- Provide age-appropriate activities for releasing aggression and anger.
- Use the opportunity to teach about the relationship between receiving medication and body function and structure (e.g., what a seizure is and how medication helps prevent the seizure).
- Offer the complete picture (e.g., need to take medication, relax with deep breaths; medication will help prevent pain).

Adolescents

- Prepare the patient in advance for the procedure but without scare tactics.
- Allow for expression in a way that does not cause losing face, such as giving the adolescent time alone after the procedure (e.g., once a seizure is controlled) and giving the adolescent time to discuss his or her feelings.
- Explore with the adolescent any current concepts of self, hospitalization, and illness, and correct any misconceptions.
- Encourage self-expression, individuality, and self-care.
- Encourage participation in procedures as appropriate.

Modified from McKenry LM, Salerno E: *Mosby's pharmacology in nursing,* ed 22. St Louis, 2006, Mosby; Hockenberry M, Wilson D: *Wong's essentials of pediatric nursing,* ed 9. St. Louis, 2013, Elsevier Mosby; and The Safer Health Care for Kids program. Available at www.aap.org/saferhealthcare. Accessed April 30, 2015.)

CONSIDERATIONS FOR OLDER ADULT PATIENTS

Due to the decline in organ function that occurs with advancing age, older adult patients handle drugs physiologically differently than adult patients. Drug therapy in the older adult is more likely to result in adverse effects and toxicity.

In this textbook, the word *older adult* is used instead of the word *geriatric* or *elderly*; however, these terms are synonymous. An **older adult** patient is defined as a person who is 65 years of age or older. This segment of the population is growing at a dramatic pace (see the Patient-Centered Care: Lifespan Considerations for the Older Adult Patient box on this page). At the beginning of the twentieth century, older adults constituted a mere 4% of the total population. At that time, more people died of infections than of chronic illnesses such as heart disease, cancer, and diabetes. As medical and health care technology has advanced, so has the ability to prolong life. This has resulted in a growing population of older adults. Today patients older than 65 years of age constitute 13.7% of the population. Life expectancy is currently approximately 81 years for females and 76 years for men. It is estimated that over 20% of the population will be 65 years of age or older by 2030. These trends are expected to continue as new disease prevention and treatment methods are developed.

QSEN **PATIENT-CENTERED CARE: LIFESPAN CONSIDERATIONS FOR THE OLDER ADULT PATIENT**

Percentage of Population Older Than Age 65

Year	Percentage Older Than Age 65
1900	4%
2000	12%
2020	20%

Issues in Clinical Drug Use in the Older Adult

The older adult population consumes a larger proportion of all medications than other population groups, taking 35% of all prescription drugs and over 42% of over-the-counter drugs. At any given time, the average older adult takes four or five prescription drugs as well as two over-the-counter medications, which can increase the risk for drug interactions. Commonly prescribed drugs for older adults include antihypertensives, beta blockers, diuretics, insulin, and potassium supplements. The most commonly used over-the-counter drugs are analgesics, laxatives, and nonsteroidal antiinflammatory drugs (NSAIDs). Older adults, especially those of certain ethnicities, may use various folk remedies of unknown composition that are unfamiliar to their health care providers.

Not only do older adult patients consume a greater proportion of prescription and over-the-counter medications, they commonly take multiple medications on a daily basis. About 1 in 3 older adults take more than 8 different drugs each day, with many taking 15 or more. One reason for the use of multiple medications is the more frequent occurrence of chronic diseases and the multiple drug options available for treatment. More than 80% of patients taking eight or more drugs have one or more chronic illnesses. More complicated medication regimens predispose older adults to self-medication errors, especially those with reduced visual acuity and manual dexterity. Such sensory and motor deficits can be particularly problematic when older adult patients split their own tablets. The practice of pill splitting occurs commonly for financial reasons, because lower- and higher-strength tablets often have similar costs. Furthermore, some insurance companies require tablet splitting for this reason. Other factors that may contribute to medication errors include lack of adequate patient education and understanding of their drug regimens, and use of multiple prescribers and multiple pharmacies. In this age of medical specialization, patients may see several prescribers for their many illnesses. Because of this, it is very important for the patient to use only one pharmacy so that monitoring for drug interactions and duplicate therapy can occur.

Older adult patients are hospitalized frequently due to adverse drug reactions. Many people use complementary and alternative medicines such as herbal remedies and dietary supplements, which can interact with prescription drugs. The simultaneous use of multiple medications is called **polypharmacy**. As the number of medications a person takes increases, so does the risk for drug interaction. For example, the chance of a drug interaction is approximately 6% for a patient receiving two medications. This risk rises dramatically as the number of drugs the patient is taking increases. For a patient taking five medications, the chance of a drug interaction is 50%, and for those taking 10 or more medications, the chance is 100%.

Some drugs may be given specifically to counteract the adverse effects of other drugs (e.g., a potassium supplement to counteract the potassium loss caused by certain diuretic medications), which is one example of what is known as the *prescribing cascade*. Sometimes it is difficult to distinguish adverse drug effects from disease symptoms. Although such prescribing is sometimes appropriate, it also increases the potential for more adverse drug events (including drug interactions, hospitalization or prolonged hospital stays, hip fractures secondary to drug-induced falls, addiction risk, anorexia, confusion, urinary retention, and fatigue). Recognizing polypharmacy and taking steps to reduce it whenever possible by decreasing the number and/or dosages of drugs taken can significantly reduce the incidence of adverse outcomes. Appropriate drug doses for older adults may sometimes be one-half to two-thirds of the standard adult dose. As a general rule, dosing for the older adult should follow the admonition, "Start low and go slow," which means to start with the lowest possible dose (often less than an average adult dose) and increase the dose slowly, based on patient response.

Another important issue is noncompliance, or nonadherence, with prescribed medication regimens. Drug nonadherence is reported to occur in roughly 40% of older adult patients and is associated with increased rates of hospitalization. Some patients want to adhere to their medication regimen but truly cannot afford the medicine. Patients in this situation need to be referred to a health care social worker or their prescriber.

Many drug companies offer patient assistance for expensive medications.

Physiologic Changes

Physiologic changes associated with aging affect the action of many drugs. As the body ages, the functioning of several organ systems slowly declines. The collective physiologic changes associated with the aging process have a major effect on the disposition and action of drugs. Table 3-3 lists some of the body systems most affected by the aging process.

The sensitivity of the older adult to many drugs requires careful monitoring and dosage adjustment. The criteria for drug dosages in older adults must include consideration of body weight and organ functioning, with emphasis on liver, renal, cardiovascular, and central nervous system function (similar to the criteria for pediatric dosages). With aging, there is a general decrease in body weight.

Changes in drug molecule receptors in the body can make a patient more or less sensitive to certain medications. For example, older adults commonly have increased sensitivity to central nervous system depressant medications (e.g., anxiolytics, tricyclic antidepressants) because of reduced integrity of the blood-brain barrier.

It is important to monitor the results of laboratory tests that have been ordered. These values serve as a gauge of organ function. The most important organs from the standpoint of the breakdown and elimination of drugs are the liver and the kidneys. Kidney function is assessed by measuring serum creatinine and blood urea nitrogen levels. Creatinine is a by-product of muscle metabolism. Because muscle mass declines with age, the serum creatinine level may provide a misleading index of renal function. For example, a frail older female may have a reported serum creatinine value that is lower than normal, and this may lead one to falsely think that her renal function is normal. In actuality, because this patient has limited muscle mass, she cannot produce creatinine. The seasoned clinician knows that renal function declines with age and that this value alone does not give an accurate estimate of renal function. The most accurate way to determine creatinine clearance is by collecting a patient's urine for 24 hours. This test is quite cumbersome, however, and is not used very often. Fortunately, several equations exist that allow pharmacists and prescribers to accurately assess renal function. Frequency of testing for renal function is often dictated by the degree of renal dysfunction and the type of medications being prescribed or used.

Liver function is assessed by testing the blood for liver enzymes such as aspartate aminotransferase (AST) and alanine aminotransferase (ALT). These laboratory values can help in assessing the ability to metabolize and eliminate medications and can aid in anticipating the risk for toxicity and/or drug accumulation. Laboratory assessments need to be conducted at least annually, both for preventive health monitoring and for screening for possible toxic effects of drug therapy. Such assessments may be indicated more frequently (e.g., every 1, 3, or 6 months) in those patients requiring higher-risk drug regimens.

Pharmacokinetics

The pharmacokinetic phases of absorption, distribution, metabolism, and excretion (see Chapter 2) may be different in the older adult than in the younger adult. Awareness of these differences helps ensure appropriate administration of drugs and monitoring. The Patient-Centered Care: Lifespan Considerations for the Older Adult Patient box on this page lists the four pharmacokinetic phases and summarizes how they are altered by the aging process.

PATIENT-CENTERED CARE: LIFESPAN CONSIDERATIONS FOR THE OLDER ADULT PATIENT

Pharmacokinetic Changes

Absorption
- Gastric pH is less acidic because of a gradual reduction in the production of hydrochloric acid in the stomach.
- Gastric emptying is slowed because of a decline in smooth muscle tone and motor activity.
- Movement throughout the gastrointestinal tract is slower because of decreased muscle tone and motor activity.
- Blood flow to the gastrointestinal tract is reduced by 40% to 50% because of decreased cardiac output and decreased perfusion.
- The absorptive surface area is decreased because the aging process blunts and flattens villi.

Distribution
- In adults 40 to 60 years of age, total body water is 55% in males and 47% in females; in those older than 60 years of age, total body water is 52% in males and 46% in females.
- Fat content is increased because of decreased lean body mass.
- Protein (albumin) binding sites are reduced because of decreased production of proteins by the aging liver and reduced protein intake.

Metabolism
- The levels of microsomal enzymes are decreased because the capacity of the aging liver to produce them is reduced.
- Liver blood flow is reduced by approximately 1.5% per year after 25 years of age, which decreases hepatic metabolism.

Excretion
- Glomerular filtration rate is decreased by 40% to 50%, primarily because of decreased blood flow.
- The number of intact nephrons is decreased.

TABLE 3-3 Physiologic Changes in the Older Adult Patient

System	Physiologic Change
Cardiovascular	↓ Cardiac output = ↓ absorption and distribution
	↓ Blood flow = ↓ absorption and distribution
Gastrointestinal	↑ pH (alkaline gastric secretions) = altered absorption
	↓ Peristalsis = delayed gastric emptying
Hepatic	↓ Enzyme production = ↓ metabolism
	↓ Blood flow = ↓ metabolism
Renal	↓ Blood flow = ↓ excretion
	↓ Function = ↓ excretion
	↓ Glomerular filtration rate = ↓ excretion

Absorption

Absorption in the older person can be altered by many mechanisms. Advancing age results in reduced absorption of both dietary nutrients and drugs. Several physiologic changes account for this reduction in absorption. Older adults have a gradual reduction in the ability of the stomach to produce hydrochloric acid, which results in a decrease in gastric acidity and may alter the absorption of some drugs. In addition, the combination of decreased cardiac output and advancing atherosclerosis results in a general reduction in the flow of blood to major organs, including the stomach. By 65 years of age, there is an approximately 50% reduction in blood flow to the gastrointestinal (GI) tract. Absorption, whether of nutrient or drug, is dependent on good blood supply to the stomach and intestines. The absorptive surface area of an older adult's GI tract is often reduced, thus decreasing drug absorption.

GI motility is important for moving substances out of the stomach and also for moving them throughout the GI tract. Muscle tone and motor activity in the GI tract are reduced in older adults. This often results in constipation, for which older adults frequently take laxatives. This use of laxatives may accelerate GI motility enough to actually reduce the absorption of drugs.

Distribution

The distribution of medications throughout the body is also different in older adults. There seems to be a gradual reduction in the total body water content with aging. Therefore, the concentrations of highly water-soluble (hydrophilic) drugs may be higher in the older adult because they have less body water in which the drugs can be diluted. The composition of the body also changes with aging, with a decrease in lean muscle mass and an increase in body fat. In both men and women, there is an approximately 20% reduction in muscle mass between 25 and 65 years of age and a corresponding 20% increase in body fat. Fat-soluble or lipophilic drugs, such as hypnotics and sedatives, are primarily distributed to fatty tissues and may result in prolonged drug actions and/or toxicity.

Older adults may have reduced protein concentrations, due in large part to reduced liver function. Reduced dietary intake and/or poor GI protein absorption can cause nutritional deficiencies and reduced blood protein levels. Regardless of the cause, the result is a reduced number of protein-binding sites for highly protein-bound drugs. This results in higher levels of unbound (active) drug in the blood. Remember that only drugs not bound to proteins are active. Therefore, the effects of highly protein-bound drugs may be enhanced if their dosages are not adjusted to accommodate any reduced serum albumin concentrations. Some highly protein-bound drugs include warfarin and phenytoin.

Metabolism

Metabolism declines with advancing age. The transformation of active drugs into inactive metabolites is primarily performed by the liver. The liver loses mass with age and slowly loses its ability to metabolize drugs effectively due to reduced production of microsomal (cytochrome P-450) enzymes. There is also a reduction in blood flow to the liver because of reduced cardiac output and atherosclerosis. A reduction in the hepatic blood flow of approximately 1.5% per year occurs after 25 years of age. All of these factors contribute to prolonging the half-life of many drugs (e.g., warfarin), which can potentially result in drug accumulation if serum drug levels are not closely monitored.

Excretion

Renal function declines in roughly two-thirds of older adults. A reduction in the glomerular filtration rate of 40% to 50%, combined with a reduction in cardiac output leading to reduced renal perfusion, can result in delayed drug excretion and therefore drug accumulation. This is especially true for drugs with a low therapeutic index such as digoxin. Renal function needs to be monitored frequently. Appropriate dose and interval adjustments may be determined based on the results of renal and liver function studies as well as the presence of therapeutic levels of the drug in the serum. If a decrease in renal and liver function is known, adjust the dosage so that drug accumulation and toxicity may be avoided or minimized.

Problematic Medications for the Older Adult

Certain classes of drugs are more likely to cause problems in older adults because of many of the physiologic alterations and pharmacokinetic changes already discussed. Table 3-4 lists some of the more common medications that are problematic. Some drugs to be avoided in the older adult have been identified by various professional organizations such as the American Nurses Association as well as by various other authoritative sources. Since the 1990s, a very effective tool, the Beers Criteria, has been used to identify drugs that may be inappropriately prescribed, ineffective, or cause adverse drug reactions in older adult patients (see the Evidence-Based Practice box). The Beers Criteria are very useful and help determine risk-associated situations for older adults and specific drugs that may be problematic.

NURSING PROCESS

ASSESSMENT

Before any medication is administered to a pediatric patient, obtain a health history and medication history with assistance from the parent, caregiver, or legal guardian. The following are some areas to be included:

- Age
- Age-related concerns about organ functioning
- Age-related fears
- Allergies to drugs and food
- Baseline values for vital signs
- Head-to-toe physical assessment findings
- Height in feet/inches and centimeters
- Weight in kilograms and pounds
- Level of growth and development and related developmental tasks

TABLE 3-4   Medications and Conditions Requiring Special Considerations in the Older Adult Patient

Medication	Common Complications
Analgesics	
Opioids	Confusion, constipation, urinary retention, nausea, vomiting, respiratory depression, falls
Nonsteroidal antiinflammatory drugs (NSAIDs)	Edema, nausea, gastric ulceration, bleeding, renal toxicity
Anticoagulants (heparin, warfarin)	Major and minor bleeding episodes, many drug interactions, dietary interactions
Anticholinergics	Blurred vision, dry mouth, constipation, confusion, urinary retention, tachycardia
Antidepressants	Sedation and strong anticholinergic adverse effects (see above)
Antihypertensives	Nausea, hypotension, diarrhea, bradycardia, heart failure, impotence
Cardiac glycosides (e.g., digoxin)	Visual disorders, nausea, diarrhea, dysrhythmias, hallucinations, decreased appetite, weight loss
Central nervous system (CNS) depressants (muscle relaxants, opioids)	Sedation, weakness, dry mouth, confusion, urinary retention, ataxia
Sedatives and hypnotics	Confusion, daytime sedation, ataxia, lethargy, increased risk for falls
Thiazide diuretics	Electrolyte imbalance, rashes, fatigue, leg cramps, dehydration

Condition	Drugs Requiring Special Caution and Monitoring
Bladder flow obstruction	Anticholinergics, antihistamines, decongestants, antidepressants
Clotting disorders	NSAIDs, aspirin, antiplatelet drugs
Chronic constipation	Calcium channel blockers, tricyclic antidepressants, anticholinergics
Chronic obstructive pulmonary disease	Long-acting sedatives or hypnotics, narcotics, beta blockers
Heart failure and hypertension	Sodium, decongestants, amphetamines, over-the-counter cold products
Insomnia	Decongestants, bronchodilators, monoamine oxidase inhibitors
Parkinson's disease	Antipsychotics, phenothiazines
Syncope, falls	Sedatives, hypnotics, opioids, CNS depressants, muscle relaxants, antidepressants, antihypertensives

QSEN EVIDENCE-BASED PRACTICE

Update on Application of the Beers Criteria for Prevention of Adverse Drug Events in Older Adults

Review

In 1991, a panel of experts led by Mark H. Beers, MD, identified a list of "potentially inappropriate medications" (PIM) for use in individuals 65 years of age and older. These criteria were intended for use with nursing home residents and then were expanded and revised to include all settings of geriatric care. The specific aim of the project was to predict adverse drug reactions (ADRs) in this age group. The Beers Criteria were updated in 1997 and 2002 and provided a listing of drugs and drug classes to be avoided in older adults. The criteria also identified disease states considered to be contraindications for some drugs. In 2005, research was conducted to confirm the relationship between PIM prescribing, as defined by Beers Criteria, and the occurrence of ADRs in older adult patients treated at outpatient clinics. In 2012, a list of medications was identified and classified into three categories: (1) potentially inappropriate medications and classes to avoid in older adults, (2) potentially inappropriate medications and classes to avoid in older adults with certain diseases and syndromes, and (3) medications to be used with caution in older adults.

Type of Evidence

The 2012 Beers Criteria were considered greatly improved because of the inclusion of important updates to the previous list of medications. Additionally, there was consideration of the challenges of assisting and guiding clinicians in avoiding certain drugs in older adults and/or the need for cautious use. The quality of the criteria was also improved by: (1) application of an evidence-based approach, (2) support of the American Geriatrics Society (AGS) in conjunction with an interdisciplinary panel of experts in geriatric care and pharmacotherapy, (3) use of a time-tested method for developing care guidelines while using the Institute of Medicine's standards for evidence/transparency as an important benchmark, and (4) an extensive review of more than 2000 high-quality research studies about prescription medications for this age group.

Results of the Study

Fifty-three medications/medication classes were included in the 2012 AGS Beers Criteria. There was a list of 34 medications and types of medications labeled as "potentially inappropriate," 14 common health problems with associated medications that were also potentially inappropriate, and 14 types of potentially inappropriate drugs to be used only with caution—all with older adults. Nineteen medications/medication classes were dropped from the 2003 list. The update allows thoughtful application of the Criteria for closer monitoring of drug use, application and interventions to decrease adverse drug events in older adults, and better patient outcomes.

Link of Evidence to Nursing Practice

These Criteria are improved and provide a much needed update for drugs to avoid and use with caution in older adults. They also increase awareness of inappropriate medication use in this age group and may also be integrated into electronic health records. With the support of the AGS, the Criteria will continue to develop over time and will continue to help improve the health of older adults.

Modified from American Geriatrics Society 2012 Beers Criteria Update Expert Panel. American Geriatrics Society updated Beers Critieria for potentially inappropriate medication use in older adults. *J Am Geriatri Soc* 60(4):616-631, 2012.

- Medical and medication history (including adverse drug reactions); current medications, related dosage forms, and routes; patient's tolerance of the forms and/or routes
- State of anxiety of the patient and/or family members or caregiver
- Use of prescription and over-the-counter medications in the home setting
- Usual method of medication administration, such as use of a calibrated spoon or needleless syringe
- Usual response to medications
- Motor and cognitive responses and their age-appropriateness
- Resources available to the patient and family

In addition, check and recheck the prescriber's orders because there is no room for error when administering medications to pediatric patients—or any patients for that matter. Carefully perform medication dosage calculations, and check several times for accuracy. Calculations for dosages take into account a variety of information and variables that may affect patient response, and use of body weight formulas (milligrams per kilogram) are recommended. In addition to an assessment of the patient, an assessment of the drug and related information is needed, focusing specifically on the drug's purpose, dosage ranges, routes of administration, cautions, and contraindications. The saying that pediatric patients are just "small adults" is incorrect, because in pediatric patients every organ is anatomically and physiologically immature and not fully functioning. As pediatric patients grow older, their weight is still lower, so extreme caution is continually needed when giving them medications. Immature organ and system development will influence pharmacokinetics and thus affect the way the pediatric patient responds to a drug. Organ function may be determined through laboratory testing. The prescriber may order the following studies before beginning drug therapy as well as during and after drug therapy: hepatic and renal function studies, red blood cell and white blood cell counts, and measurement of hemoglobin and hematocrit levels and serum protein levels.

Assessment data to be gathered for the older adult patient may include the following:
- Age
- Allergies to drugs and food
- Dietary habits
- Sensory, visual, hearing, cognitive, and motor-skill deficits
- Financial status and any limitations
- List of all health-related care providers, including physicians, dentists, optometrists and ophthalmologists, podiatrists, and alternative medicine health care practitioners such as osteopathic physicians, chiropractors, and nurse practitioners
- Past and present medical history
- Listing of medications, past and present, including prescription drugs, over-the-counter medications, herbals, nutritional supplements, vitamins, and home remedies
- Existence of polypharmacy (the use of more than one medication)
- Self-medication practices

- Laboratory test results, especially those indicative of renal and liver function
- History of smoking and use of alcohol with notation of amount, frequency, and years of use
- Risk situations related to drug therapy identified by the Beers Criteria (see the Evidence-Based Practice box on the previous page)

One way to collect data about the various medications or drugs being taken by the older adult is to obtain the information from the patient and/or caregiver using the brown-bag technique. This is an effective means of identifying various drugs the patient is taking, regardless of the patient's age and may be used in conjunction with a complete review of the patient's medical history or record. The brown-bag technique requires the patient/caregiver to place all medications used in a bag and bring them to the health care provider. All medications need to be brought in their original containers. A list of medications with generic names, dosages, routes of administration, and frequencies is then compiled. This list of medications is then compared with what is prescribed to what the patient states he or she is actually taking. Medication reconciliation procedures are performed in health care facilities when assessing and tracking medications taken by the patient (see Chapter 5). In addition, the patient's insight into his or her medical problems is a very beneficial piece of information in developing a plan of care. It is also important for the nurse to realize that although older adult patients may be able to provide the required information, many may be confused or poorly informed about their medications and/or health condition. In such cases, consult with a more reliable historian, such as a significant other, family member, or caregiver. Older adult patients may also have sensory deficits that require the nurse to speak slowly, loudly, and clearly while facing the patient.

With the older adult patient—as with a patient of any age—thoroughly assess support systems and the patient's ability to take medications safely. Whenever possible with the older adult, health care providers/prescribers need to opt for a nonpharmacologic approach to treatment first, if appropriate. Other data to collect include information about acute or chronic illnesses, nutritional problems, cardiac problems, respiratory illnesses, and GI tract disorders. Laboratory tests related to lifespan considerations that are often ordered include hemoglobin and hematocrit levels, red blood cell and white blood cell counts, blood urea nitrogen level, serum and urine creatinine levels, urine specific gravity, serum electrolyte levels, and protein and serum albumin levels.

NURSING DIAGNOSES

1. Imbalanced nutrition, less than body requirements, related to the impact of age and drug therapy and possible adverse effects
2. Deficient knowledge related to information about drugs and their adverse effects or about when to contact the prescriber

PATIENT-CENTERED CARE: LIFESPAN CONSIDERATIONS FOR THE OLDER ADULT PATIENT

A Brief Look at the Sixth Leading Cause of Death in the United States: Alzheimer's Disease

- Every 67 seconds, someone in the United States develops Alzhemier's disease.
- In 2015, an estimated 5.3 million Americans of all ages have Alzheimer's disease.
- In 2015, an estimated 700,000 people in the United States age 65 and older will die with Alzheimer's disease. Between 2000 and 2013, deaths attributed to Alzheimer's disease increased 71%, while deaths attributed to the number one of cause of death—heart disease—decreased by 14%.
- Alzheimer's disease is the sixth leading cause of death in the United States. It is the only cause of death among the top 10 causes in the United States that cannot be prevented, cured, or slowed.
- 1 in 3 seniors dies with Alzheimer's disease or another form of dementia.
- Almost two-thirds of Americans with Alzheimer's disease are women.
- Older African-Americans and Hispanics are more likely to have Alzheimer's disease and other dementias than older whites. In the United States, there are more non-Hispanic whites living with Alzheimer's disease and other dementias than any other racial or ethnic group.
- The cost of the disease is staggering at best. By 2050, these costs could rise as much as $1.1 trillion. In 2015, Alzhemier's disease and other dementias will cost the nation $226 billion.
- Ten warning signs of Alzheimer's disease include the following: memory loss that disrupts daily life; challenges in planning or solving problems; difficulty completing familiar tasks at home or work or at leisure; confusion with time or place; difficulty and trouble understanding visual images and spatial relationships; new problems with words while speaking and in writing; misplacing things and losing the ability to retrace steps; decreased or poor judgement; withdrawal from work or social activities; and changes in mood and personality. For a comparison to typical age-related changes, see www.alz.org.
- Alzheimer's disease is ultimately fatal. If one does not die from Alzheimer's disease, he or she dies with it. Survival with Alzheimer's disease may range from 4 to 20 years.
- Two abnormal structures in the brain of a person with Alzheimer's include plaques and tangles and are the prime suspects in damaging and killing nerve cells.

From *2015 Alzheimer's disease facts and figures.* Available at *www.alz.org.*

3. Risk for injury related to adverse effects of medications or to the method of drug administration
4. Risk for injury related to idiosyncratic reactions to drugs due to age-related drug sensitivity

PLANNING: OUTCOME IDENTIFICATION

1. Patient (caregiver, parent, or legal guardian) states measures to enhance nutritional status due to age- and drug-related factors with understanding of major food groups, as well as any adverse drug effects on everyday nutrition (e.g., nausea, vomiting, loss of appetite).

2. Patient (caregiver, parent, or legal guardian) states the importance of adhering to the prescribed drug therapy for its intended therapeutic effects (or takes medication as prescribed with assistance) as well as anticipated adverse effects.

3. Patient contacts the prescriber when appropriate, such as when unusual effects occur during drug therapy.

4. Patient (caregiver, parent, or legal guardian) identifies ways to minimize complications, adverse effects, reactions, and injury to self that are associated with the therapeutic medication regimen including drinking at least 4 to 6 ounces. of water with all oral medications, rotating of subcutaneous injection sites, and adherence to directions provided by the medication order/prescription.

IMPLEMENTATION

It is always important to emphasize and practice the Nine Rights of medication administration (see Chapter 1) and follow the prescriber's order and/or medication instructions. Each time *before* you administer a medication, it is the standard of care to systematically and conscientiously check your procedure three times against the following basic "Six Rights": right patient, right medication/drug, right dose, right route/form, right time, and right documentation. The other three "rights" are also considered at this time. This usually applies for acute care and long-term care inpatient and outpatient situations. For the *pediatric* patient, some specific nursing actions are as follows: (1) If needed, mix medications in a substance or fluid other than essential foods (e.g., milk, orange juice, or cereal) because the child may develop a dislike for the essential food item(s). Instead, find a liquid or food item that may be used to make the medication(s) taste better. Sherbet or flavored ice cream is often used. Only resort to this intervention if the patient cannot swallow the dosage form or if the taste needs to be made more palatable. (2) Do not add drug(s) to fluid in a cup or bottle because the amount of drug consumed would then be impossible to calculate if the entire amount of fluid is not consumed. (3) Always document special techniques of drug administration so that others involved in the patient's care may benefit from the suggestion. For example, if the child takes an unpleasant-tasting pill, liquid, or tablet after eating a frozen Popsicle, then this information would be valuable to another caregiver. (4) Unless contraindicated and if needed, add small amounts of water or fluids to elixirs to enhance the child's tolerance of the medication. Remember that it is essential for the child to take the entire volume, so remain cautious with this practice and only use an amount of fluid mixture that you know the child will tolerate. (5) Avoid using the word *candy* in place of the word *drug* or *medication*. Medications must be called *medicines* and their dangers made known to children. Taking medications is no game, and children must understand this for their own safety! (6) Keep all medications out of the reach of children of all ages. Be sure that parents and other family members in the same household understand this and request child-protective lids or tops for their medications. Childproof locks or closures may also be used on cabinets holding medications. (7) Inquire about how the child usually takes medication (e.g., preference of liquid versus pill or tablet dosage forms) and whether there are any helpful hints from the family/caregiver that may be helpful. See the Patient-Centered Care: Lifespan Considerations for the Pediatric Patient box for further information on medication administration beginning with infancy through adolescence. For more information about dosage calculations for medication administration in pediatric patients, an online site providing examples and programs to help with pediatric drug dosage calculations is available at *www.testandcalc .com* and *www.mapharm.com/dosage_calc.htm.*

Encourage *older adult* patients to take medications as directed and not to discontinue them or double up on doses unless recommended or ordered to do so by their health care provider/ prescriber. The patient or caregiver must understand the treatment- and/or medication-related instructions, especially those related to safety measures, such as keeping all medications out of the reach of children. Transdermal patches provide a different challenge in that if they fall off onto the floor or bedding, a child or infant in that environment may have accidental exposure to the effects of the medication. Serious adverse reactions have been reported concerning the accidental adhering of a transdermal patch to a child/infant while crawling or playing on the floor/carpet. Toxic and even fatal reactions may occur depending on the medication and dosage. Provide written and oral instructions concerning the drug name, action, purpose, dosage, time of administration, route, adverse effects, safety of administration, storage, interactions, and any cautions about or contraindications to its use. Remember that simple is always best! Always try to find ways to make the patient's therapeutic regimen easy to understand. Always be alert to polypharmacy. Be sure the patient or caregiver understands the dangers of multiple drug use. Patient education may prove to be helpful in preventing and/or minimizing problems associated with polypharmacy. If a nurse advocate or a nurse practitioner with prescription privileges has the opportunity to review the patient's chart, simplified written instructions must be provided with the purpose of the drug, how to best take the medication(s), and a list of drug interactions and adverse effects. Information must be provided in bold, large print. Among the specific interventions that have proved to be helpful in promoting medication safety in the older adult is the use of the Beers Criteria (see the Evidence-Based Practice box). These criteria provide a systematic way of identifying prescription medications that are potentially harmful to older adult patients. The prescriber and nurse must constantly remember that clinical judgment and knowledge base are important in making critical decisions about a patient's care and drug therapy. In addition, keeping abreast of evidence-based nursing, such as application of the Beers Criteria, is important for the nurse to remain current in clinical nursing practice. Specific guidelines for medication

administration by various routes are presented in detail in the photo atlas in Chapter 9.

In summary, drug therapy across the lifespan must be well thought out, with full consideration to the patient's age, gender, cultural background, ethnicity, medical history, and medication profile. When all phases of the nursing process and the specific lifespan considerations discussed in this chapter are included, there is a better chance of decreasing adverse effects, reducing risks to the patient, and increasing drug safety.

CASE STUDY

Safety: What Went Wrong? Polypharmacy and the Older Adult

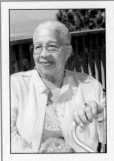 R.M., a 77-year-old retired librarian, sees several physician specialists for a variety of health problems. She uses the pharmacy at a large discount store but also has prescriptions filled at a nearby pharmacy, which she uses when she does not feel like going into the larger store. Her medication list is as follows:

Thiazide diuretic, prescribed for peripheral edema
Potassium tablets, prescribed to prevent hypokalemia
Beta blocker, prescribed for hypertension
Warfarin, taken every evening because of a history of deep vein thrombosis
Multivitamin tablet for seniors

1. What medications may cause problems for R.M.? Explain your answer.
2. What measures can be taken to reduce these problems?
    R.M. visits the pharmacy to pick up some medications for her "aches and pains." She has chosen a popular over-the-counter nonsteroidal anti-inflammatory drug. Two weeks later, she notices that she has increased bruising on her arms and legs, and that her gums bleed slightly when she brushes her teeth.
3. What went wrong? (Hint: check for potential drug interactions.) How could this problem have been prevented?

For answers, see *http://evolve.elsevier.com/Lilley.*

EVALUATION

When dealing with lifespan issues as related to drug therapy, observation and monitoring for therapeutic effects as well as adverse effects is critical to safe and effective therapy. You must know the patient's profile and history as well as information about the drug. The drug's purpose, specific use in the patient, simply stated actions, dose, frequency of dosing, adverse effects, cautions, and contraindications need to be listed and kept available at all times. This information will allow more comprehensive monitoring of drug therapy, regardless of the age of the patient.

KEY POINTS

- There are many age-related pharmacokinetic effects that lead to dramatic differences in drug absorption, distribution, metabolism, and excretion in the young and the older adult. At one end of the lifespan is the pediatric patient, and at the other end is the older adult patient, both of whom are very sensitive to the effects of drugs.

- Most common dosage calculations use the milligrams per kilogram formula related to age. Organ maturity may also be considered. It is important for the nurse to know that many elements besides the mathematical calculation itself contribute to safe dosage calculations. Safety must remain the first priority and concern with consideration of the Nine Rights of medication administration (see Chapter 1).

- The percentage of the population older than 65 years of age continues to grow, and polypharmacy remains a concern with the increasing number of older adult patients. A current list of all medications and drug allergies must be on their person or with their family/caregiver at all times.

- Your responsibility is to act as a patient advocate as well as to be informed about growth and developmental principles and the effects of various drugs during the lifespan and in various phases of illness.

NCLEX® EXAMINATION REVIEW QUESTIONS

1. The nurse is reviewing factors that influence pharmacokinetics in the neonatal patient. Which factor puts the neonatal patient at risk with regard to drug therapy?
   a. Immature renal system
   b. Increased peristalsis in the GI tract
   c. Irregular temperature regulation
   d. Smaller circulatory capacity

2. The physiologic differences in the pediatric patient compared with the adult patient affect the amount of drug needed to produce a therapeutic effect. The nurse is aware that one of the main differences is that infants have
   a. increased protein in circulation.
   b. fat composition lower than 0.001%.
   c. more muscular body composition.
   d. water composition of approximately 75%.

3. While teaching a 76-year-old patient about the adverse effects of his medications, the nurse encourages him to keep a journal of the adverse effects he experiences. This intervention is important for the older adult patient because of which alterations in pharmacokinetics?
   a. Increased renal excretion of protein-bound drugs
   b. More alkaline gastric pH, resulting in more adverse effects
   c. Decreased blood flow to the liver, resulting in altered metabolism
   d. Less adipose tissue to store fat-soluble drugs

4. When the nurse is reviewing a list of medications taken by an 88-year-old patient, the patient says, "I get dizzy when I stand up." She also states that she has nearly fainted "a time or two" in the afternoons. Her systolic blood pressure drops 15 points when she stands up. Which type of medication may be responsible for these effects?
   a. Nonsteroidal antiinflammatory drugs (NSAIDs)
   b. Cardiac glycosides
   c. Anticoagulants
   d. Antihypertensives

5. A pregnant patient who is at 32 weeks' gestation has a cold and calls the office to ask about taking an over-the-counter medication that is rated as pregnancy category A. Which answer by the nurse is correct?
   a. "This drug causes problems in the human fetus, so you should not take this medication."
   b. "This drug may cause problems in the human fetus, but nothing has been proven in clinical trials. It is best not to take this medication."
   c. "This drug has not caused problems in animals, but no testing has been done in humans. It is probably safe to take."
   d. "Studies indicate that there is no risk to the human fetus, so it is okay to take this medication as directed if you need it."

6. The nurse is preparing to administer an injection to a preschool-age child. Which approaches are appropriate for this age group? (Select all that apply.)
   a. Explain to the child in advance about the injection.
   b. Provide a brief, concrete explanation about the injection.
   c. Encourage participation in the procedure.
   d. Make use of magical thinking.
   e Provide comfort measures after the injection.

7. The nurse is preparing to give an oral dose of acetaminophen (Tylenol) to a child who weighs 12 kg. The dose is 15 mg/kg. How many milligrams will the nurse administer for this dose?

8. An 82 year-old patient is admitted to the hospital after an episode of confusion at home. The nurse is assessing the current medications he is taking at home. Which method is the best way to assess his home medications?
   a. Ask the patient what medications he takes at home.
   b. Ask the patient's wife what medications he takes at home.
   c. Ask the patient's wife to bring his medications to the hospital in their original containers.
   d. Contact the patient's pharmacy for a list of the patient's current medications.

1. a, 2. d, 3. c, 4. d, 5. d, 6. b, d, e, 7. 180 mg, 8. c

CRITICAL THINKING AND PRIORITIZATION QUESTIONS

1. A mother calls the clinic to ask how to give a tablet to her 4-year-old son. He is refusing to swallow it and won't chew it because it "tastes icky." The mother says she is ready to force her son to take this medication. What is the nurse's priority action?

2. A woman in her third trimester of pregnancy is having a checkup and asks for aspirin for a headache. What is the nurse's best response?

For answers, see *http://evolve.elsevier.com/Lilley.*

ⓔ EVOLVE WEBSITE

http://evolve.elsevier.com/Lilley
- Animations
- Answer Keys for Textbook Case Studies and Textbook Critical Thinking and Prioritization Questions

- Content Updates
- Key Points
- Review Questions
- Student Case Studies

Cultural, Legal, and Ethical Considerations

ℰ http://evolve.elsevier.com/Lilley

OBJECTIVES

When you reach the end of this chapter, you will be able to do the following:

1. Discuss the various cultural factors that may influence an individual's response to medications.
2. Identify various cultural phenomena affecting health care and use of medications.
3. List the drugs that are more commonly associated with variations in response due to cultural and racial/ethnic factors.
4. Briefly discuss the important components of drug legislation at the state and federal levels.
5. Provide examples of how drug legislation impacts drug therapy, professional nursing practice, and the nursing process.
6. Discuss the various categories of controlled substances, and give specific drug examples in each category.

7. Identify the process involved in the development of new drugs, including the investigational new drug application, the phases of investigational drug studies, and the process for obtaining informed consent.
8. Discuss the nurse's role in the development of new and investigational drugs and the informed consent process.
9. Discuss the ethical principles and how they apply to pharmacology and the nursing process.
10. Identify the ethical principles involved in making an ethical decision.
11. Develop a nursing care plan that addresses the cultural, legal, and ethical care of patients with a specific focus on drug therapy and the nursing process.

KEY TERMS

Bias Any systematic error in a measurement process. (p. 55)

Black box warning A type of warning that appears in a drug's prescribing information and is required by the U.S. Food and Drug Administration (FDA) to alert prescribers of serious adverse events that have occurred with the given drug. (p. 56)

Blinded investigational drug study A research design in which the subjects are purposely unaware of whether the substance they are administered is the drug under study or a placebo. This method serves to minimize bias on the part of research subjects in reporting their body's responses to investigational drugs. (p. 55)

Controlled substances Any drugs listed on one of the "schedules" of the Controlled Substance Act (also called *scheduled drugs*). (p. 53)

Culture The customary beliefs, social forms, and material traits of a racial, religious, or social group. (p. 50)

Double-blind investigational drug study A research design in which both the investigator(s) and the subjects are purposely unaware of whether the substance administered to a given subject is the drug under study or a placebo. This method minimizes bias on the part of both the investigator and the subject. (p. 55)

Drug polymorphism Variation in response to a drug because of a patient's age, gender, size, and/or body composition. (p. 51)

Ethics The rules of conduct recognized in respect to a particular class or group of human actions. (p. 58)

Ethnicity Relating to or characteristic of a human group having racial, religious, language, and other traits in common. (p. 50)

Ethnopharmacology The study of the effect of ethnicity on drug responses, specifically drug absorption, metabolism, distribution, and excretion as well as the study of genetic variations to drugs (i.e., pharmacogenetics). (p. 50)

Expedited drug approval Acceleration of the usual investigational new drug approval process by the FDA, usually for drugs used to treat life-threatening diseases. (p. 54)

Health Insurance Portability and Accountability Act (HIPAA) An act that protects health insurance coverage for workers and their families when they change jobs. It also protects patient information. If confidentiality of a patient is breached, severe fines may be imposed. (p. 53)

Informed consent Written permission obtained from a patient consenting to a specific procedure. (p. 55)

Investigational new drug (IND) A drug not yet approved for marketing by the FDA but available for use in experiments to determine its safety and efficacy. (p. 55)

Investigational new drug application An application that must be submitted to the FDA before a drug can be studied in humans. (p. 55)

Legend drugs Another name for prescription drugs. (p. 53)

Malpractice A special type of negligence or the failure of a professional and/or individual with specialized education and training to act in a reasonable and prudent way. (p. 57)

Narcotic A legal term established under the Harrison Narcotic Act of 1914. The term is currently used in clinical settings to refer to any medically administered controlled substance and in legal settings to refer to any illicit or "street" drug; also referred to as *opioid*. (p. 53)

Negligence The failure to act in a reasonable and prudent manner or failure of the nurse to give the care that a

reasonably prudent (cautious) nurse would render or use under similar circumstances. (p. 57)

Orphan drugs A special category of drugs that have been identified to help treat patients with rare diseases. (p. 53)

Over-the-counter drugs Drugs available to consumers without a prescription. Also called nonprescription drugs. (p. 52)

Pharmacogenomics The study of genetics in drug response. (p. 50)

Placebo An inactive (inert) substance (e.g., saline, distilled water, starch, sugar) that is not a drug but is formulated to resemble a drug for research purposes. (p. 55)

Race Descendants of a common ancestor; a tribe, family, or people believed to belong to the same lineage. (p. 50)

CULTURAL CONSIDERATIONS

The United States is a very culturally diverse nation as evidenced by its constantly and rapidly changing demographics. Based on the 2010 U.S. Census and official estimates through 2013, projections noted by Colby and Ortman (2015) reflect that between 2014 and 2060, the U.S. population is expected to increase from 319 million to 417 million, reaching close to 400 million in 2051. By 2044, more than half of all Americans are projected to belong to a minority group. Between the years 2014 and 2060, the native population is projected to increase by 62 million, and foreign-born people are expected to account for an increasing share of the total population, reaching some 19% in 2060. The African-American population is expected to increase by 14% by 2060. The Hispanic population is projected to be the third fastest growing group, with an increase from 55 million in 2014 to 119 million in 2060. The Asian population is projected to double to approximately 9.3% of the total population. The Native Hawaiian and Other Pacific Islander population is anticipated to increase by some 100% between 2014 and 2060. The U.S. Census Bureau has also identified the increase in the selection of "some other race" in the discussion of racial-ethnic groups. To address this, a combined race and ethnicity question is under consideration for 2020 within the U.S. Census Bureau data-collection process. The options to select would be identified as white, black, Hispanic/Latino/Spanish origin, American Indian/Alaska Native, Asian, Native Hawaiian/Other Pacific Islander, or some other race or origin. An additional line would be offered under each category for identification of more detail about one's origin, tribe, or race. Examples of this include German, African American, Mexican, Navajo, Asian Indian, and Samoan. However, worth mentioning is the fact that there are other racial-ethnic groups, not well-known, and are not included in the above listing but are increasing significantly in numbers. One such group, that is a cultural but not an ethnic group, includes the peoples of Appalachia. Of the some 300 plus million Americans in 2010, 25.2 million lived in the Appalachian region with a great variance in Appalachia's 420 counties. Their growth rate was nearly

7 percent higher as compared to the year 2000, which is slightly lower than the nearly 10 percent growth rate for the U.S. as a whole. The Appalachian regions include counties within Alabama, Georgia, Kentucky, Maryland, Mississippi, New York, North Carolina, Ohio, Pennsylvania, South Carolina, Tennessee, Virginia, and West Virginia (U.S. Census Bureau, 2000 and 2010 U.S. Census Bureau 2010 Decennial Census, *www.prb.org/pdf12/ appalachia-census-chartbook-2011.pdf*). The concern for these "newer" cultural, racial-ethnic groups is for their particular health care needs and barriers to health care. Appalachia is associated with being one of the unhealthiest areas in America, and so it is important to expose nursing students—and other students in the health care profession—to their cultural practices and health care beliefs. Resources providing current information about health care and cultural, racial-ethnic groups include the following: *www.ahrq.gov/nhqrdr10/nhqrdminority11.htm*, *www .cdc.gov/omhd/about/disparities.htm*, *www.commonwealthfund .org/usr_doc/mead_racialethnic*, and *www.cdc.gov/minorityhealth/ populations/REMP*.

The field of ethnopharmacology provides an expanding body of knowledge for understanding the specific impact of cultural factors on patient drug response. It is hampered by the lack of clarity in terms such as race, ethnicity, and culture. For example, although some researchers have used the term *Hispanic* to encompass geographic groups as diverse as Puerto Ricans, Mexicans, and Peruvians, others have used it to denote a specific racial group. Cultural assessment needs to be part of the assessment phase of the nursing process. Acknowledgment and acceptance of the influences of a patient's cultural beliefs, values, and customs is necessary to promote optimal health and wellness. Some relevant practices are discussed in the Patient-Centered Care: Cultural Implications box.

Influence of Ethnicity and Genetics on Drug Response

Pharmacogenomics is the study of how certain genetic traits affect drug response (see Chapter 8). The concept of polymorphism is critical to an understanding of how the same drug may

🌐 PATIENT-CENTERED CARE: CULTURAL IMPLICATIONS

A Brief Review of Common Practices among Selected Cultural Groups

Cultural Group	Common Health Beliefs and Alternative Healers	Verbal and Nonverbal Communication; Touch/Time	Family	Biologic Variations
African	Practice folk medicine; employ "root doctors" as healers, spiritualists Use herbs, oils, and roots	Asking personal questions of someone met for the first time seen as intrusive and not proper Direct eye contact seen as rude Present oriented	Have close extended family ties Women play important key role in making health care decisions	Keloid formation, sickle cell anemia, lactose intolerance, skin color
Asian	Believe in traditional medicine; hot and cold foods; herbs/teas/soups; use of acupuncturist, acupressurist, and herbalist; Tai Chi; QiGong	High respect for others, especially individuals in positions of authority Not usually comfortable with custom of shaking hands with those of opposite sex Present oriented	Have close extended family ties; family needs more important than individual needs	Many drug interactions, lactose intolerance, skin color, thalassemia
Hispanic	View health as a result of good luck and living right; see illness as a result of doing a bad deed Heat, cold, and herbs used as remedies; Use curandero, spiritualist	Expressing negative feelings seen as impolite Avoiding eye contact seen as respectful and attentive Touching acceptable between two persons in conversation	Have close extended family ties; all family members involved in health care decisions Past cultural experiences in the family with illness and healing practices holds significant value Strong adherence to cultural practices	Lactose intolerance, skin color
Native American	Believe in harmony with nature and ill spirits causing disease Use medicine man	Speak in low tone of voice Light touch of a person's hand is preferred versus a firm handshake as a greeting Present oriented	Have close extended family ties; emphasis on family	Lactose intolerance, skin color, cleft uvula problems

Giger JN. *Transcultural nursing: assessment & intervention*, ed 6. St Louis, 2013, Mosby.

result in very different responses in different individuals. For example, why does a Chinese patient require lower dosages of an antianxiety drug than a white patient? Why does an African-American patient respond differently to antihypertensives than a white patient? Drug polymorphism refers to the effect of a patient's age, gender, size, body composition, and other characteristics on the pharmacokinetics of specific drugs. Factors contributing to drug polymorphism may be categorized into environmental factors (e.g., diet and nutritional status), cultural factors, and genetic (inherited) factors.

Medication response depends greatly on the level of the patient's adherence with the therapy regimen. Yet adherence may vary depending on the patient's cultural beliefs, experiences with medications, personal expectations, family expectations and influence, and level of education. Prescribers must be aware that some patients use alternative therapies, such as herbal and homeopathic remedies, that can inhibit or accelerate drug metabolism and therefore alter a drug's response.

Environmental and economic factors (e.g., diet) can contribute to drug response. For example, a diet high in fat has been documented to increase the absorption of some drugs. Malnutrition with deficiencies in protein, vitamins, and minerals may modify the functioning of metabolic enzymes, which may alter the body's ability to absorb or eliminate a medication.

Historically, most clinical drug trials were conducted using white men, often college students, as research subjects. However, there are data that demonstrate the impact of genetic factors on drug *pharmacokinetics* and drug *pharmacodynamics* or drug response. Some individuals of European and African descent are known to be *slow acetylators*. This means that their bodies attach acetyl groups to drug molecules at a relatively slow rate, which results in elevated drug concentrations. This situation may warrant lower drug dosages. A classic example of a drug whose metabolism is affected by this characteristic is the antituberculosis drug isoniazid. In contrast, some patients of Japanese descent are more rapid acetylators and metabolize drugs more quickly, which predisposes the patient to subtherapeutic drug concentrations and may require higher drug dosages.

Levels of the cytochrome P-450 enzymes (see Chapter 2) are also known to vary between ethnic groups. This has effects on the ability to metabolize many drugs. This can affect plasma drug levels, and therefore the intensity of drug response, at different doses. Groups of Asian patients have been shown to be "poor metabolizers" of certain drugs and often require lower dosages to achieve desired therapeutic effects. In contrast, white patients are more likely to be classified as "ultrarapid metabolizers" and may require higher drug dosages.

Variations are also reported between ethnic groups in the occurrence of adverse effects. For example, African-American patients taking lithium may need to be monitored more closely for symptoms of drug toxicity, because serum drug levels may be higher than in white patients given the same dosage. Likewise, Japanese and Taiwanese patients may require lower dosages of lithium. For the treatment of hypertension, thiazide diuretics appear to be more effective in African Americans than in whites. Several additional examples of racial and ethnic differences in drug response are outlined in the Patient-Centered Care: Cultural Implications box.

⊕ PATIENT-CENTERED CARE: CULTURAL IMPLICATIONS

Examples of Varying Drug Responses in Different Racial or Ethnic Groups

Racial or Ethnic Group	Drug Classification	Response
African Americans	Antihypertensive drugs	African Americans respond... • Better to diuretics than to beta blockers and angiotensin-converting enzyme inhibitors. • Less effectively to beta blockers. • Best to calcium channel blockers, especially diltiazem. • Less effectively to single-drug therapy.
Asians and Hispanics	Antipsychotic and antianxiety drugs	Asians ... • Need lower dosages of certain drugs such as haloperidol. Asians and Hispanics... • Respond better to lower dosages of antidepressants. Chinese... • Require lower dosages of antipsychotics. Japanese... • Require lower dosages of antimanic drugs.

NOTE: The comparison group for all responses is whites.

Individuals throughout the world share common views and beliefs regarding health practices and medication use. However, specific cultural influences, beliefs, and practices do exist. Awareness of cultural differences is critical for the care of patients because of the constantly changing U.S. demographics. As a result of these changes, attending to each patient's cultural background helps to ensure quality nursing care, including medication administration.

For example, some African Americans have health beliefs and practices that include an emphasis on proper diet and rest; the use of herbal teas, laxatives, and folk medicine, prayer, and the "laying on of hands." Reliance on various home remedies can be an important component of their health practices. Some Asian-American patients, especially Chinese individuals, believe in the concepts of *yin* and *yang*. Yin and yang are opposing forces that lead to illness or health, depending on which force is dominant in the individual and whether the forces are balanced. Balance produces healthy states. Other common health practices of Asian Americans include use of acupuncture, herbal remedies, and heat. All such beliefs and practices need to be

considered—especially when the patient values their use more highly than the use of medications. Many of these beliefs are strongly grounded in religion. Some Native Americans believe in preserving harmony with nature or keeping a balance between the body and mind and the environment to maintain health. Ill spirits are seen as the cause of disease. Some individuals of Hispanic descent view health as a result of good luck and living right and illness as a result of bad luck or committing a bad deed. To restore health, these individuals seek a balance between the body and mind through the use of cold remedies or foods for "hot" illnesses (of blood or yellow bile) and hot remedies for "cold" illnesses (of phlegm or black bile). Hispanics may use a variety of religious rituals for healing (e.g., lighting of candles). It is important to remember that these beliefs vary from patient to patient; therefore, consult with the patient rather than assume that the patient holds certain beliefs because he or she belongs to a certain ethnic group.

Barriers to adequate health care for the culturally diverse U.S. patient population include language, poverty, access, pride, and beliefs regarding medical practices. Medications may have a different meaning to different cultures. Therefore, before any medication is administered, complete a thorough cultural assessment. This assessment includes questions regarding the following:

- Languages spoken, written, and understood; need for an interpreter
- Health beliefs and practices
- Past uses of medicine
- Use of herbal treatments, folk remedies, home remedies, or supplements
- Use of over-the-counter drugs
- Usual responses to illness
- Responsiveness to medical treatment
- Religious practices and beliefs (e.g., many Christian Scientists believe in taking no medications at all)
- Support from the patient's cultural community that may provide resources or assistance as needed, such as religious connections, leaders, family members, or friends
- Dietary habits

Cultural Nursing Considerations and Drug Therapy

It is important to be knowledgeable about drugs that may elicit varied responses in culturally diverse patients or those from different racial/ethnic groups. Varied responses may include differences in therapeutic dosages and adverse effects, so that some patients may have therapeutic responses at lower dosages than are typically recommended. For example, in Hispanic individuals taking traditional antipsychotics, symptoms may be managed effectively at lower dosages than the usual recommended dosage range (see the Patient-Centered Care: Cultural Implications box on this page).

Another aspect of cultural care as it relates to drug therapy is the recognition that patterns of communication may differ based on a patient's race or ethnicity. Communication also includes the use of language, tone, volume, as well as spatial distancing, touch, eye contact, greetings, and naming format. It is important to assess and apply these aspects of cultural and racial/ethnic variations to patient care and to drug therapy and the nursing process. One specific example of cultural diversity is the use of verb tense; some languages, such as the Chinese language, do not have numerous verb tenses as compared to the English language. Therefore, very precise instructions must be included in patient education about medication(s) and how to best and safely take them. Avoiding the use of contractions such as *can't, won't,* and *don't* is important with patients from other countries to prevent confusion. Instead, use of *cannot, will not,* and *do not* is recommended to improve understanding.

LEGAL CONSIDERATIONS

Prescription drug use is vital to treating and preventing illness. However, due to safety reasons, its use is regulated by several different agencies, including the Food and Drug Administration (FDA), The Drug Enforcement Agency (DEA), and individual state laws. Traditionally, only medical doctors (M.D.) and doctors of osteopathy (D.O.) had the privilege of prescribing medications. Dentists and podiatrists are also allowed to prescribe medications so long as it is within the scope of their practice. In some states, other health care professionals may also prescribe, including licensed physician's assistants (P.A.s) and advanced practice registered nurses (APRNs).

As the number and complexity of prescriptions continue to increase and technology continually changes, so do the laws regarding their use. Even more autonomy has been gained by the professional nurse over his or her nursing practice. With this increasing autonomy comes greater liability and legal accountability; therefore, the professional nurse must be aware and duly consider this responsibility as he or she practices. Specific laws

and regulations are discussed later and in the nursing process section of this chapter.

U.S. Drug and Related Legislation

Until the beginning of the twentieth century, there were no federal rules and regulations in the U.S. to protect consumers from the dangers of medications. The various legislative interventions that have occurred have often been prompted by large-scale serious adverse drug reactions (see Table 4-1). One example is the sulfanilamide tragedy of 1937. Over 100 deaths occurred in the United States when people ingested a diethylene glycol solution of sulfanilamide that had been marketed as a therapeutic drug. Diethylene glycol is a component of automobile antifreeze solution, and the drug was never tested for its toxicity. Another prominent example is the thalidomide tragedy that occurred in Europe between the 1940s and 1960s. Many pregnant women who took this sedative-hypnotic drug gave birth to seriously deformed infants.

A recent and significant piece of legislation is the Health Insurance Portability and Accountability Act (HIPAA) of 1996. HIPAA requires all health care providers, health and life insurance companies, public health authorities, employers, and schools to maintain patient privacy regarding protected health information. Protected health information includes any individually identifying information such as patients' health conditions, account numbers, prescription numbers, medications, and payment information. Table 4-1 provides a timeline summary of major U.S. drug legislation.

New Drug Development

Research into and development of new drugs is an ongoing process. The pharmaceutical manufacturing industry is a

TABLE 4-1 Summary of Major U.S. Drug and Related Legislation	
Name of Legislation (Year)	**Provisions/Comments**
Federal Food and Drugs Act (FFDA, 1906)	Required drug manufacturers to list on the drug product label the presence of dangerous and possibly addicting substances; recognized the *U.S. Pharmacopeia* and *National Formulary* as printed references standards for drugs
Sherley Amendment (1912) to FFDA	Prohibited fraudulent claims for drug products
Harrison Narcotic Act (1914)	Established the legal term narcotic and regulated the manufacture and sale of habit-forming drugs
Federal Food, Drug, and Cosmetic Act (FFDCA, 1938; amendment to FFDA)	Required drug manufacturers to provide data proving drug safety with FDA review; established the investigational new drug application process (prompted by sulfanilamide elixir tragedy)
Durham-Humphrey Amendment (1951) to FFDCA	Established legend drugs or prescription drugs; drug labels must carry the legend, "Caution—Federal law prohibits dispensing without a prescription"
Kefauver-Harris Amendments (1962) to FFDCA	Required manufacturers to demonstrate both therapeutic efficacy *and* safety of new drugs (prompted by thalidomide tragedy)
Controlled Substance Act (1970)	Established "schedules" for controlled substances (Tables 4-2 and 4-3); promoted drug addiction education, research, and treatment
Orphan Drug Act (1983)	Enabled the FDA to promote research and marketing of orphan drugs used to treat rare diseases
Accelerated Drug Review Regulations (1991)	Enabled faster approval by the FDA of drugs to treat life-threatening illnesses (prompted by HIV/AIDS epidemic)
Health Insurance Portability and Accountability Act (1996)	More commonly known by its acronym, *HIPAA*; officially required all health-related organizations as well as schools to maintain privacy of protected health information
Medicare Prescription Drug Improvement and Modernization Act (2003)	More commonly known as *Medicare Part D*; provides seniors and disabled persons with an insurance benefit program for prescription drugs; the cost of medications is shared by the patient and the federal government

AIDS, Acquired immunodeficiency syndrome; *FDA,* Food and Drug Administration; *HIV,* human immunodeficiency virus.

TABLE 4-2 Controlled Substances: Schedule Categories

Schedule	Abuse Potential	Medical Use	Dependency Potential
C-I	High	None	Severe physical and psychological
C-II	High	Accepted	Severe physical and psychological
C-III	Less than C-II	Accepted	Moderate to low physical or high psychological
C-IV	Less than C-III	Accepted	Limited physical or psychological
C-V	Less than C-IV	Accepted	Limited physical or psychological

TABLE 4-3 Controlled Substances: Categories, Dispensing Restrictions, and Examples

Schedule	Dispensing Restrictions	Examples
C-I	Only with approved protocol	Heroin, lysergic acid diethylamide (LSD), marijuana, mescaline, peyote, psilocybin, and methaqualone
C-II	Written prescription only* No prescription refills Container must have warning label	Codeine, cocaine, hydrocodone, hydromorphone, meperidine, morphine, methadone, secobarbital, pentobarbital, oxycodone, amphetamine, methylphenidate, and others
C-III	Written or oral prescription that expires in 6 months No more than five refills in a 6-month period Container must have warning label	Codeine with selected other medications (e.g., acetaminophen), pentobarbital rectal suppositories, and dihydrocodeine combination products
C-IV	Written or oral prescription that expires in 6 months No more than five refills in a 6-month period Container must have warning label	Phenobarbital, chloral hydrate, meprobamate, benzodiazepines (e.g., diazepam, temazepam, lorazepam), tramadol, and others
C-V	Written prescription or over the counter (varies with state law)	Medications generally for relief of coughs or diarrhea containing limited quantities of certain opioid controlled substances

*Legally permitted to be telephoned in for major emergencies only. If telephoned in, written prescription is required within 72 hours.

multibillion-dollar industry. Pharmaceutical companies must continuously develop new and better drugs to maintain a competitive edge. The research required for the development of these new drugs may take several years. Hundreds of substances are isolated that never make it to market. Once a potentially beneficial drug has been identified, the pharmaceutical company must follow a regulated, systematic process before the drug can be sold on the open market. This highly sophisticated process is regulated and carefully monitored by the FDA. The primary purpose of the FDA is to protect the patient and ensure drug effectiveness.

This U.S. system of drug research and development is one of the most stringent in the world. It was developed out of concern for patient safety and drug efficacy. Much time, funding, and documentation are required to ensure that these two very important objectives are met. Many drugs are marketed and used in foreign countries long before they receive approval for use in the United States. Drug-related calamities are more likely to be avoided by this more stringent drug approval system. The thalidomide tragedy mentioned earlier, which resulted from the use of a drug that was marketed in Europe but not in the United States, is an illustrative example. A balance must be achieved between making new lifesaving therapies available and protecting consumers from potential drug-induced adverse effects. Historically, the FDA has had less regulatory authority over vitamin, herbal, and homeopathic preparations because they are designated as dietary supplements rather than drugs. In 1994, Congress passed the Dietary Supplement Health and Education Act, which requires manufacturers of such products at least to ensure their safety (although not necessarily their efficacy) and prohibits them from making any unsubstantiated claims in the product labeling. For example, a product label may read "For depression" but cannot read "Known to cure depression." Reliable, objective information about these kinds of products is limited but is growing as more formal research studies are conducted. In 1998, Congress established the National Center for Complementary and Alternative Medicine as a new branch of the National Institutes of Health. The function of this center is to conduct rigorous scientific studies of alternative medical treatments and to publish the data from such studies. Consumer demand for alternative medicine products continues to drive this process. Patients must exercise caution in using such products and communicate regularly with their health care providers regarding their use.

U.S. Food and Drug Administration Drug Approval Process

The FDA is responsible for approving drugs for clinical safety and efficacy before they are brought to the market. There are stringent steps, each of which may take years, which must be completed before the drug can be approved. The FDA has made certain lifesaving investigational drug therapies available sooner than usual by offering an expedited drug approval process, also known as "fast track" approval. Acquired Immune Deficiency Syndrome (AIDS) was the first major public health crisis for which the FDA began granting expedited drug approval. This process allowed pharmaceutical manufacturers to shorten the approval process and allowed prescribers to give medications that showed promise during early phase I and phase II clinical trials to qualified patients with AIDS. In such cases, when a trial continues to show favorable results, the overall process of drug approval is hastened. The concept of expedited drug approval became controversial after the FDA-initiated manufacturer recall of the anti-inflammatory drug rofecoxib (Vioxx) in 2004. This recall followed multiple case reports of severe cardiovascular events, including fatalities, associated with the use of this drug. This unfortunate example has reduced the number of drugs approved via the expedited approval process. More information and specific drugs approved under this fast-track process can be found at *www.fda.gov*.

The drug approval process is quite complex and prolonged. It begins with *preclinical* testing phases, which include *in vitro* studies (using tissue samples and cell cultures) and animal studies. *Clinical* (human) studies follow the preclinical phase. There are four clinical phases. The drug is put on the market after phase III is completed if an **investigational new drug application** submitted by the manufacturer is approved by the FDA. The collective goal of these phases is to provide information on the safety, toxicity, efficacy, potency, bioavailability, and purity of the new drug.

Preclinical Investigational Drug Studies

Current medical ethics require that all new drugs undergo laboratory testing using both *in vitro* (cell or tissue) and animal studies before any testing in human subjects can be done. *In vitro* studies include testing of the response of various types of mammalian (including human) cells and tissues to different concentrations of the investigational drug. *In vitro* studies help researchers to determine early on if a substance might be too toxic for human patients. Many prospective new drugs are ruled out for human use during this preclinical phase of drug testing. However, a small percentage are referred for further clinical testing in human subjects.

Four Clinical Phases of Investigational Drug Studies

Before any testing on humans begins, subjects must provide informed consent, and it must be documented. **Informed consent** involves the careful explanation to the human test patient or *research subject* of the purpose of the study, the procedures to be used, the possible benefits, and the risks involved. This explanation is followed by written documentation on a *consent form*. The informed consent document, or consent form, must be written in a language understood by the patient and must be dated and signed by the patient and at least one witness. Informed consent is always voluntary. By law, informed consent must be obtained more than a given number of days or hours before certain procedures are performed and must always be obtained when the patient is fully mentally competent. The informed consent process may be carried out by a nurse or other health care professional, depending on how a given study is designed.

Medical ethics dictate that participants in experimental drug studies be informed volunteers and not be coerced to participate in any way. Therefore, informed consent must be obtained from all patients (or their legal guardians) before they can be enrolled in an **investigational new drug (IND)** study. Research subjects must be informed of all potential hazards as well as the possible benefits of the new therapy. It must be stressed to all patients that involvement in IND studies is voluntary and that any individual can either decline to participate or quit the study at any time without affecting the delivery of any previously agreed-upon health care services.

Phase I. Phase I studies usually involve small numbers of healthy subjects rather than those who have the disease that the new drug is intended to treat. The purpose of phase I studies is to determine the optimal dosage range and the pharmacokinetics of the drug and to ascertain if further testing is needed. Blood tests, urinalyses, assessments of vital signs, and specific monitoring tests are also performed.

Phase II. Phase II studies involve small numbers of volunteers who have the disease that the drug is designed to diagnose or treat. Study participants are closely monitored to determine the drug's effectiveness and identify any adverse effects. Therapeutic dosage ranges are refined during this phase. If no serious adverse effects occur, the study can progress to phase III.

Phase III. Phase III studies involve large numbers of patients who are followed by medical research centers and other types of health care entities. The purpose of this larger sample size is to provide information about infrequent or rare adverse effects that may not yet have been observed during previous smaller studies. Information obtained during this clinical phase helps identify any risks associated with the new drug. To enhance objectivity, many studies are designed to incorporate a placebo. A **placebo** is an inert substance that is not a drug. Placebos are given to a portion of the research subjects to separate out the real benefits of the investigational drug from the apparent benefits arising out of researcher or subject **bias** regarding expected or desired results of the drug therapy. A study that incorporates placebo is called a *placebo-controlled study*. If the study subject does not know if the drug he or she is administered is a placebo or the investigational drug, but the investigator does know, the study is referred to as a **blinded investigational drug study.** In most studies, neither the research staff nor the subjects being tested know which subjects are being given the real drug and which are receiving the placebo. This further enhances the objectivity of the study results and is known as a **double-blind investigational drug study** because both the researcher and the subject are "blinded" to the actual identity of the substance administered. Both drug and placebo dosage forms given to patients often look identical except for a secret code that appears on the medication itself and/or its container. At the completion of the study, this code is revealed to determine which study patients received the drug and which were given the placebo. The code can also be broken before study completion by the principle investigator in the event of a clinical emergency that requires a determination of what substance individual patients received.

The three objectives of phase III studies are to establish the drug's clinical effectiveness, safety, and dosage range. After phase III is completed, the FDA receives a report from the manufacturer, at which time the drug company submits a new drug application (NDA). The approval of the application paves the way for the pharmaceutical company to market the new drug exclusively until the patent for the drug molecule expires. This is normally 17 years after discovery of the molecule and includes the 10- to 12-year period generally required to complete drug research. Therefore, the manufacturer typically has 5 to 7 years after drug marketing to recoup research costs, which are usually in the hundreds of millions of dollars for a single drug.

Phase IV. Phase IV studies are postmarketing studies that are voluntarily conducted by pharmaceutical companies to obtain further proof of the therapeutic and adverse effects of the new drug. Data from these studies are gathered for at least 2 years after the drug's release. Often these studies compare the safety and efficacy of the new drug with that of another drug in the same therapeutic category. Some medications make it through all phases of clinical trials without causing any problems among study patients. However, when they are used in the larger general population, severe adverse effects may appear for the first time. If a pattern of severe reactions to a newly marketed drug begins to emerge, the FDA may request that the manufacturer of the drug issue a black box warning or a voluntary recall. A black box warning is the strictest warning from the FDA and indicates that serious adverse effects have been reported with the drug. The drug can still be prescribed; however, the prescriber must be aware of the potential risk and the patient must be warned. Black box warnings are included in the prescribing information of the drug, and the text of the warning has a solid black border, thus the name *black box*. The number of drugs with black box warnings is substantial, and it should be noted that not all black box warnings are presented in this textbook. For a list of all drugs with black box warnings, the student is directed to www.blackboxrx.com.

The FDA or the manufacturer may issue a drug recall anytime a problem with a drug is noted. There are three classes of recall that may be issued:

- **Class I:** The most serious type of recall—use of the drug product carries a reasonable probability of serious adverse health effects or death.
- **Class II:** Less severe—use of the drug product may result in temporary or medically reversible health effects, but the probability of lasting major adverse health effects is low.
- **Class III:** Least severe—use of the drug product is not likely to result in any significant health problems.

The FDA has a voluntary program called MedWatch in which professionals are encouraged to report any adverse events seen with newly approved drugs. Information can be found at www.fda.gov/medwatch. Drug information of this kind is continually evolving as new events are observed and reported. Recommended actions also change with time, thus it is imperative to utilize the most current information available along with sound clinical judgment.

The Controlled Substance Act requires the scheduling of every drug (see Tables 4-2 and 4-3). There are five classes of drugs, designated from C-I to CV-. Drugs in the C-I class are defined as drugs with no currently accepted medical use and a high potential for abuse. Drugs in Schedule II are defined as drugs with a medical use and a high potential for abuse. Schedule III drugs are defined as drugs with a moderate to low potential for physical and psychological dependence. Schedule IV drugs are defined as drugs with a low potential for abuse and low risk of dependence. Schedule V drugs are defined as drugs with lower potential for abuse than Schedule IV and consist of preparations containing limited quantities of certain narcotics.

Schedule V drugs are generally used for antidiarrheal, antitussive, and analgesic purposes. It should be noted that in 2014, the popular pain medicine hydrocodone (Vicodin, Lortab) was rescheduled from C-III to C-II, and tramadol (Ultram) was rescheduled to C-IV; prior to the change it was a schedule V.

Legal Nursing Considerations and Drug Therapy

State and federal legislation dictate the boundaries for professional nursing practice. Standards of care and nurse practice acts identify the definition of the scope and role of the professional nurse (Box 4-1). Nurse practice acts further define/identify: (1) the scope of nursing practice, (2) expanded nursing roles, (3) educational requirements for nurses, (4) standards of care, (5) minimally safe nursing practice, and (6) differences between nursing and medical practice. In addition, state boards of nursing define specific nursing practices such as rules concerning the administration of intravenous therapy. Additionally, guidelines from professional nursing groups (American Nurses Association), nursing specialty groups, institutional policies and procedures, and state/federal hospital licensing laws all help to identify the legal boundaries of nursing practice. There is also case law or common law consisting of prior court rulings that affect professional nursing practice.

The American Nurses Association (ANA) has developed standards for nursing practice, policy statements, and similar resolutions. The standards describe the scope, function, and role of the nurse and establish clinical practice standards. The ANA *Code for Nurses with Interpretive Statements* explains the goals, values, and ethical precepts that direct the nursing profession. The ANA believes that the *Code for Nurses* is nonnegotiable and to be upheld by each nurse (see *www.nursingworld. org*). The Joint Commission requires that accredited hospitals fulfill certain standards with regard to nursing practice. One such requirement is that these institutions must have written policies and procedures. These policies are usually quite specific and are contained in policy and procedures manuals found on most nursing units. For example, a policy and procedure will outline the steps to take when changing a dressing or administering a medication. The nurse must know the policies and

---

BOX 4-1   Nurse Practice Acts

Nurse Practice Acts (NPAs) are state laws that are instrumental in defining the scope of nursing practice and protect public health, safety, and welfare. In each state, the law directs entry into nursing practice, defines the scope of practices, and identifies disciplinary actions. State boards of nursing oversee this statutory law. NPAs are the most significant part of legislation as related to professional nursing practice. Together, it is NPAs and common law that define nursing practice. The National Council of State Boards of Nursing maintain an online database of each state's NPA, and each state has a website where the NPAs are defined and outlined. For example, if the nurse is practicing in Missouri, Virginia, or West Virginia, the websites are as follows:

Missouri: *http://pr.mo.gov/nursing-rules-statutes.asp*
Virginia: *www.dhp.virginia.gov/nursing/nursing_laws_regs.htm*
West Virginia: *www.wvrnboard.com/images/pdf/6707.pdf*

procedures of the employing institution, because if the nurse is involved in a lawsuit, these are one of the standards by which the nurse will be measured. Nursing specialty organizations also define standards of care for nurses who are certified in specialty areas, such as oncology, surgical care, or critical care. Standards of care help to determine whether a nurse is acting appropriately when performing professional duties. It is critical to safe nursing practice to remain up to date on the ever-changing obligations and standards of practice and care. If standards of care are not met, the nurse becomes liable for **negligence** and **malpractice** (Box 4-2). Current nursing literature remains an authoritative resource for information on new standards of care. State governments and/or state boards of nursing have websites that include links to specific nurse practice acts and standards of care.

TEAMWORK AND COLLABORATION: LEGAL AND ETHICAL PRINCIPLES

Ethical Terms Related to Nursing Practice

Autonomy: Self-determination and the ability to act on one's own; related nursing actions include promoting a patient's decision making, supporting informed consent, and assisting in decisions or making a decision when a patient is posing harm to himself or herself.

Beneficence: The ethical principle of doing or actively promoting good; related nursing actions include determining how the patient is best served.

Confidentiality: The duty to respect privileged information about a patient; related nursing actions include not talking about a patient in public or outside the context of the health care setting.

Justice: The ethical principle of being fair or equal in one's actions; related nursing actions include ensuring fairness in distributing resources for the care of patients and determining when to treat.

Nonmaleficence: The duty to do no harm to a patient; related nursing actions include avoiding doing any deliberate harm while rendering nursing care.

Veracity: The duty to tell the truth; related nursing actions include telling the truth with regard to placebos, investigational new drugs, and informed consent.

The legal-ethical dimensions of professional nursing care are also addressed in the legislation passed to amplify the guidelines contained in the HIPAA (1996). Under these federal regulations (see p. 53), the privacy of patient information is protected, and standards are included for the handling of electronic data about patients. HIPAA also defines the rights and privileges of patients in order to protect privacy without diminishing access to quality health care. The assurance of privacy—even prior to establishment of the HIPAA guidelines—was based on the principle of respect of an individual's right to determine when, to what extent, and under what circumstances private information can be shared or withheld from others, including family members. In addition, confidentiality must be preserved; that is, the individual identities of patients or research study participants are not to be linked to information they provide and cannot be publicly divulged. HIPAA addresses the issues of confidentiality and privacy by prohibiting prescribers, nurses, and other health care providers from sharing with others any

BOX 4-2   Areas of Potential Liability for Nurses

Area	Examples Related to Drug Therapy and the Nursing Process
Failure to assess/ evaluate	Failure to... • See significant changes in patient's condition after taking a medication • Report the changes in condition after medication • Take a complete medication history and nursing assessment/history • Monitor patient after medication administration
Failure to ensure safety	• Lack of adequate monitoring • Failure to identify patient allergies and other risk factors related to medication therapy • Inappropriate drug administration technique • Failure to implement appropriate nursing actions based on a lack of proper assessment of patient's condition
Medication errors	Failure to... • Clarify unclear medication order • Identify and react to adverse drug reactions • Be familiar with medication prior to its administration • Maintain level of professional nursing skills for current practice • Identify patient's identity prior to drug administration • Document drug administration in medication profile

patient health care information, including laboratory results, diagnoses, and prognoses, without the patient's consent. Conflicting obligations arise when a patient wants to keep information away from insurance companies, and matters remain complicated and challenging in the era of improving technology and computerization of medical records. Health care facilities continue to work diligently, however, to adhere to HIPAA guidelines and use special access codes to limit who can access information in computerized documents and charts.

In summary, federal and state legislation, standards of care, and nurse practice acts provide the legal framework for safe nursing practice, including drug therapy and medication administration. Further, as discussed in Chapter 1, the "Nine Rights" of medication administration with a specific emphasis on the basic "Six Rights" (right patient, drug, dose, time, route, and documentation) are yet another measure for ensuring safety and adherence to laws necessary for protecting the patient. Chapter 1 also discusses other patient rights that are part of the standards of practice of every licensed registered nurse and every student studying the art and science of nursing.

ETHICAL CONSIDERATIONS

Decisions in health care are seldom made independently of other people and are made with consideration of the patient, family, nurses, and other members of the health care team. All members of the health care team must make a concentrated effort to recognize and understand their own values and be considerate, nonjudgmental, and respectful of the values of others and ethics. The use of drug therapy has evolved from just administering whatever was prescribed to providing responsible drug therapy for the purpose of achieving defined outcomes that improve a patient's quality of life.

Ethical principles are useful strategies for members of the health care team (e.g., physician, pharmacist, nurse) and include standards or truths on which ethical actions are made. Some of the most useful principles in nursing and health care, specifically drug therapy, include autonomy, beneficence, nonmaleficence, and veracity (see the Teamwork and Collaboration: Legal and Ethical Principles box). However, day-to-day practice in nursing and health care pose many potential ethical conflicts. Each situation is different and requires compassionate and humane solutions. When answers to ethical dilemmas remain unclear and ethical conflict occurs, then the appropriate action must be based on ethical principles.

TEAMWORK AND COLLABORATION: LEGAL AND ETHICAL PRINCIPLES

Elements of Liability for Nursing Malpractice

Element	Example
Duty	Being responsible for accurate assessment of a patient's intravenous (IV) and site of IV during caustic drug infusion and the timely reporting of changes in the patient's condition
Breach of duty	Nurse does not notice that the IV site is swollen, red, painful, and warm to touch or that the IV has quit infusing properly
Causation	Nurse fails to note the signs and symptoms of extravasation at IV site (with a chemotherapy drug or other caustic drug) that results in the need for skin grafting
Damage	Extensive skin and nerve damage with several surgical skin grafts resulting in limited use of arm

Ethical Nursing Considerations and Drug Therapy

Ethical nursing practice is based on fundamental principles such as beneficence, autonomy, justice, veracity, and confidentiality. The American Nurses Association (ANA) *Code of Ethics for Nurses* (available at www.nursingworld.org/codeofethics) and the International Council of Nurses (ICN) *Code of Ethics for Nurses* serve as frameworks of practice for all nurses and as ethical guidelines for nursing care (see the Teamwork and Collaboration: Legal and Ethical Principles box on the next page). Adherence to these ethical principles and codes of ethics ensures that the nurse is acting on behalf of the patient and with the patient's best interest at heart. As a professional, the nurse has the responsibility to provide safe nursing care to patients regardless of the setting, person, group, community, or family

involved. Although it is not within the nurse's realm of ethical and professional responsibility to impose his or her own values or standards on the patient, it *is* within the nurse's realm to provide information and to assist the patient in making decisions regarding health care.

The nurse also has the right to refuse to participate in any treatment or aspect of a patient's care that violates the nurse's personal ethical principles. However, this must be done without deserting the patient, and in some facilities the nurse may be transferred to another patient care assignment only if the transfer is approved by the nurse manager or nurse supervisor. The nurse must always remember, however, that the ANA *Code of Ethics for Nurses* and professional responsibility and accountability require the nurse to provide nonjudgmental nursing care from the start of the patient's treatment until the time of the patient's discharge. If transferring to a different assignment is not an option because of institutional policy and because of the increase in the acuteness of patients' conditions and the high patient-to-nurse workload, the nurse must always act in the best interest of the patient while remaining an objective patient advocate. It is always the nurse's responsibility to provide the highest-quality nursing care and to practice within the professional standards of care. The ANA *Code of Ethics for Nurses,* the ICN *Code of Ethics for Nurses,* nurse practice acts, federal and state codes, ethical principles, and the previously mentioned legal principles and legislation are readily accessible and provide nurses with a sound, rational framework for professional nursing practice.

NURSING PROCESS

Only information on the cultural considerations related to drug therapy and the nursing process will be presented in the following sections. Legal issues and ethical principles are integrated into professional nursing practice, whereas there are specific racial-ethnic (cultural) factors that need to be addressed in each phase of the nursing process.

ASSESSMENT

A thorough cultural assessment is needed for the provision of culturally competent nursing care. A variety of assessment tools and resources to incorporate into nursing care are provided in Box 4-3. However, various factors must be assessed and then applied to nursing care, specifically drug therapy and the nursing process. Some of the specific questions about the patient's physical, mental, and spiritual health include the following:

MAINTAINING HEALTH

- *For physical health:* Where are special foods and clothing items purchased? What types of health education are of the patient's culture? Where does the patient usually obtain information about health and illness? Folklore? Where are health services obtained? Who are the health care providers (e.g., physicians, nurse practitioners, community services organizations, health departments, healers)?

TEAMWORK AND COLLABORATION: LEGAL AND ETHICAL PRINCIPLES

International Council of Nurses Code of Ethics for Nurses

The International Council of Nurses (ICN) first adopted the *Code of Ethics for Nurses* in 1953; the *Code* has been revised several times since then, most recently in 2012. The 2012 revision is available in English, French, Spanish, and German. The ICN *Code* serves as a guide for nursing actions and health care that is constantly changing in our world and based on social values and need. The Preamble identifies the four fundamental responsibilities of nurses—promoting health, preventing illness, restoring health, and alleviating suffering—and points out that the need for nursing is universal. The *Code* makes it clear that inherent in professional nursing practice is respect for human rights including the right to life, dignity, and the right to be treated with respect. Nursing care is rendered to the individual, family, and community and is respectful of gender, age, color, creed, culture, disability, illness, nationality, politics, race, and social status. Nurses render services to the individual, family, and community. The *Code* describes four principal elements that provide a framework for the standards of ethical conduct it defines: nurses and people, nurses and practice, nurses and the profession, and nurses and coworkers. For nurses to realize the purpose of this *Code*, it must be understood and used by nurses in their everyday professional nursing practice. The *Code* needs to be available to students and nurses throughout their academic program of study and professional work lives.

Another area of ethical consideration related to drug therapy and the nursing process is the use of placebos. A placebo is a drug dosage form (e.g., tablet, capsule) without any pharmacologic activity due to a lack of active ingredients. However, there may be reported therapeutic responses, and placebos have been found to be beneficial in certain patients, such as those being treated for anxiety. Placebos are also administered frequently in experimental studies of new drugs to evaluate and measure the pharmacologic effects of a new medicine compared with those of an inert placebo. Except in new drug studies, however, placebo use is often considered to be unethical and deceitful, possibly creating mistrust among the nurse, the prescriber, and the patient. In current clinical practice guidelines for pain management, the American Pain Society and the Agency for Health Care Policy and Research recommend the avoidance of placebos because their use is believed to be deceitful and to violate a patient's rights to the highest-quality care possible. Many health care agencies limit the use of placebos to research only to avoid the possible deceit and mistrust. If an order is received for a placebo for a patient, it is within the legal purview of a professional nurse to inquire about the order and to ask why a placebo is being prescribed; the order must never be taken lightly. If administration of the placebo is part of a research study or clinical trial, the informed consent process must be thorough and the patients must be informed of their right to (1) leave the study at any time without any pressure or coercion to stay, (2) leave the study without consequences to medical care, (3) receive full and complete information about the study, and (4) be aware of all alternative options and receive information on all treatments, including placebo therapy, being administered in the study.

BOX 4-3   Cultural Assessment Tools and Related Web Links

- Several cultural assessment tools have been developed over the last decade. Madeline Leininger's Sunrise Model focuses on seven major areas of cultural assessment, including educational, economic, familial and social, political, technologic, religious and philosophic, and cultural values, beliefs, and practices.
- Other comprehensive cultural assessment tools include those developed by Andrews and Bowls, 1999; Friedman, Bowden, and Jones, 2003; Giger and Davidhizar, 1999; and Purnell and Pcaulanka, 1998. Rani Srivastava's (2006), found in *The Healthcare Professional's Guide to Clinical Cultural Competence* (Healthcare Professional's Guides), contains further discussion on how populations are viewed by health care workers and not through the use of ethno-cultural/religious labels.

- *For mental health:* What are examples of culturally specific activities for the mind and for maintaining mental health, as well as beliefs about stress reduction, rest, and relaxation?
- *For spiritual health:* What are resources for meeting spiritual needs?

PROTECTING HEALTH

- *For physical health:* Where are special clothing and everyday essentials? What are examples of the patient's symbolic clothing, if any?
- *For mental health:* Who within the family and community teaches the roles in the patient's specific culture? Are there rules about avoiding certain persons or places? Are there special activities that must be performed?
- *For spiritual health:* Who teaches spiritual practices, and where can special protective symbolic objects such as crystals or amulets be purchased? Are they expensive, and how available are they for the patient when needed?

RESTORING HEALTH

- *For physical health:* Where are special remedies purchased? Can individuals produce or grow their own remedies, herbs, and so on? How often are traditional and nontraditional services obtained?
- *For mental health:* Who are the traditional and nontraditional resources for mental health? Are there culture-specific activities for coping with stress and illness?
- *For spiritual health:* How often and where are traditional and nontraditional spiritual leaders or healers accessed?

NURSING DIAGNOSES

1. Sleep deprivation related to a lack of adherence to cultural practices for encouraging stress release and sleep induction
2. Deficient knowledge (drug therapy) related to lack of experience and information about prescribed drug therapy
3. Risk for injury related to adverse and unpredictable reaction to drug therapy due to racial/ethnic or cultural factors

PLANNING AND OUTCOME IDENTIFICATION

1. Patient describes specific measures to enhance sleep patterns such as regular sleep habits, decrease in caffeine, meditation, relaxation therapy, journaling sleep patterns, and noting those measures that enhance or take away sleep.
2. Patient lists the various medication(s) with their therapeutic and adverse effects, dosage routes, and specific methods of

adequate self-administration, drug interactions, and any other special considerations.

3. Patient describes the impact of his or her racial/ethnic influences (e.g., metabolic enzyme differences) on specific medications and the resulting potential for increase in adverse effects, toxicity, and/or increased or decreased effectiveness (medication therapy).

IMPLEMENTATION

There are numerous interventions for implementation of culturally competent nursing care, but one very important requirement is that nurses maintain current knowledge about various cultures and related activities and practices of daily living, health beliefs, and emotional and spiritual health practices and beliefs. Specifically, knowledge about medications that may elicit varied responses due to racial/ethnic variations is most important with application of concepts of culturally competent care and ethnopharmacology to each patient care situation. Information of particular significance is the impact of cytochrome P-450 enzymes on certain phases of drug metabolism (see previous discussion on p. 26). Specific examples of differences in certain cytochrome P-450 enzymes can be found on p. 51. Consider additional factors, including the patient's verbal and nonverbal communication patterns; health belief systems; identification of health care provider and/or alternate healers; and interpretation of space, time, and touch. For example, with regard to adherence with the treatment regimen, Hispanics with hypertension have been found in some studies to be less likely than African Americans or whites to continue to take medication as prescribed, a finding that may reflect the patients' health belief systems. Other lifestyle decisions (e.g., use of tobacco or alcohol) may also affect responses to drugs and must be considered during drug administration. In addition, a patient's cultural background and associated socioeconomic status may create a situation that leads the patient to skip pills, split doses, and not obtain refills. This culture of poverty may be a causative factor in noncompliance and requires astute attention and individualized nursing actions.

EVALUATION

Culturally competent nursing care related to drug therapy may be evaluated through the actual compliance (or lack thereof) to the medication regimen(s). Safe, effective, and therapeutic self-administration of drugs with minimal to no adverse/toxic effects will be present only when the patient is treated as an individual and has a thorough understanding of the medication regimen.

CASE STUDY: TEAMWORK AND COLLABORATION

Clinical Drug Trial

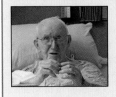

A patient on the cardiac telemetry unit has had a serious heart condition for years and has been through every known protocol for treatment. The cardiologist has admitted him to a telemetry unit for observation during a trial of a new investigational drug. The patient exclaims, "I have high hopes for this drug. I've read about it on the Internet and the reports are wonderful. I can't wait to get better!"

1. What is the best way for the research nurse to answer this statement?

The physician meets with the patient and the research nurse to explain the medication and how the double-blind experimental drug study will work. The purpose of the medication and potential hazards of the therapy are described, as well as the laboratory tests that will be performed to measure the drug's effectiveness. The physician then asks the research nurse to have the patient sign the consent form. When the nurse goes to get the patient's signature, the patient says, "I'll sign it, but I really didn't understand what that doctor told me about the placebo."

1. Should the research nurse continue with getting the consent form signed? Explain your answer.

2. The patient tells the research nurse, "How can I make sure I have the real drug and not the fake drug? I really want to see if it will help my situation." What is the nurse's best response?

3. After a week, the patient tells the research nurse, "I don't see that this drug is helping me. In fact, I feel worse. But I'm afraid to tell the doctor that I want to stop the medicine. What do I do?" What is the nurse's best response?

For answers, see *http://evolve.elsevier.com/Lilley.*

KEY POINTS

- A variety of culturally based assessment tools are available for use in patient care and drug therapy.
- Drug therapy and subsequent patient responses may be affected by racial and ethnic variations in levels of specific enzymes and metabolic pathways of drugs.
- Various pieces of federal legislation, as well as state law, state practice acts, and institutional policies, have been established to help ensure the safety and efficacy of drug therapy and the nursing process.
- HIPAA guidelines have increased awareness concerning patient confidentiality and privacy. It is important to understand this federal legislation as it relates to drug therapy and the nursing process.
- The Controlled Substance Act of 1970 provides nurses and other health care providers with information on drugs that

cause little to no dependence versus those associated with a high level of abuse and dependency.

- Always obtain informed consent as needed, with complete understanding of your role and responsibilities as patient advocate in obtaining such consent.
- In the IND research process, adhere to the study protocol while also acting as a patient advocate and honoring the patient's right to safe, quality nursing care.
- Adhere to legal guidelines, ethical principles, and the ANA *Code of Ethics for Nurses* so that your actions are based on a solid foundation.
- Placebo use remains controversial, and if a placebo is ordered, question the prescriber about the specific cause for its use.

NCLEX® EXAMINATION REVIEW QUESTIONS

1. A patient has been diagnosed with late-stage cancer. After consulting with his family, he tells the nurse, "I would like to try to live long enough to see my granddaughter graduate in 3 months, but after that I don't want any extra treatments." This patient is demonstrating which of these?
   a. Veracity
   b. Beneficence
   c. Maleficence
   d. Autonomy

2. When caring for an older adult Chinese patient, the nurse recognizes that which of these cultural issues may influence the care of this patient?
   a. Chest x-rays are seen as a break in the soul's integrity.
   b. Hospital diets are interpreted as being healing and healthful.
   c. The use of heat may be an important practice for this patient.
   d. Being hospitalized is a source of peace and socialization for this culture.

3. A patient is being counseled for possible participation in a clinical trial for a new medication. After the patient meets with the physician, the nurse is asked to obtain the patient's signature on the consent forms. The nurse knows that this "informed consent" indicates which of the following?
   a. Once therapy has begun, the patient cannot withdraw from the clinical trial.
   b. The patient has been informed of all potential hazards and benefits of the therapy.
   c. The patient has received only the information that will help to make the clinical trial a success.
   d. No matter what happens, the patient will not be able to sue the researchers for damages.

4. A new drug has been approved for use, and the drug manufacturer has made it available for sale. During the first 6 months, the FDA receives reports of severe adverse effects that were not discovered during the testing and considers withdrawing the drug. This illustrates which phase of investigational drug studies?
   a. Phase I
   b. Phase II
   c. Phase III
   d. Phase IV

5. A patient of Japanese descent describes a family trait that manifests frequently: She says that members of her family often have "strong reactions" after taking certain medications, but her white friends have no problems with the same dosages of the same drugs. The nurse recognizes that, because of this trait, which statement applies?

   a. She may need lower dosages of the medications prescribed.
   b. She may need higher dosages of the medications prescribed.
   c. She should not receive these medications because of potential problems with metabolism.
   d. These situations vary greatly, and her accounts may not indicate a valid cause for concern.

6. When evaluating polymorphism and medication administration, the nurse considers which factors? *(Select all that apply.)*
   a. Nutritional status
   b. Drug route
   c. Genetic factors
   d. Cultural beliefs
   e. Patient's age

7. The nurse is reviewing the four clinical phases of investigational drug studies. Place the four phases in the correct order of occurrence.
   4 a. Studies that are voluntarily conducted by pharmaceutical companies to obtain more information about the therapeutic and adverse effects of a drug.
   2 b. Studies that involve small numbers of volunteers who have the disease or ailment that the drug is designed to diagnose or treat.
   1 c. Studies that involve small numbers of healthy subjects who do not have the disease or ailment that the drug is intended to treat.
   3 d. Studies that involve large numbers of patients who have the disease that the drug is intended to treat; these studies establish the drug's clinical effectiveness, safety, and dosage range.

8. A patient shows the nurse an article in the newspaper about a new black box warning and states, "I take this drug! Is it safe for me to take now?" What is meant by a *black box warning*?
   a. The FDA is asking for a mandatory recall of this drug.
   b. Serious adverse effects have been reported with this drug, and he will not be able to take it again because the risks outweigh the benefits.
   c. Even though severe adverse effects have been reported, it can still be prescribed as long as the prescriber and patient are aware of the potential risks.
   d. Pharmacies will no longer be able to dispense this drug to patients.

1. d, 2. c, 3. b, 4. d, 5. a, 6. a, c, d, e, 7. a = 4, b = 2, c = 1, d = 3, 8. c

CRITICAL THINKING AND PRIORITIZATION QUESTIONS

1. During a busy shift, the nurse is called to the telephone to speak to a family member of Mrs. H., who was admitted with pneumonia. The caller states, "I'm her grandson, and I want to know if that pneumonia she has is that very contagious bug that's going around hospitals. Is she going to die?" The nurse will answer the family member by following which guidelines?

2. The nurse is assessing a newly admitted 85-year-old woman. During the assessment, the nurse finds that the patient is wearing a copper ring around her left ankle. The ankle is cool, pale, swollen with 3+ edema, and the copper ring is actually cutting into the skin. What is the nurse's priority action at this time?

For answers, see *http://evolve.elsevier.com/Lilley.*

ⓔ EVOLVE WEBSITE

http://evolve.elsevier.com/Lilley
- Animations
- Answer Keys for Textbook Case Studies and Textbook Critical Thinking and Prioritization Questions
- Content Updates
- Key Points
- Review Questions
- Student Case Studies

Medication Errors: Preventing and Responding

http://evolve.elsevier.com/Lilley

OBJECTIVES

When you reach the end of this chapter, you will be able to do the following:

1. Compare the following terms related to drug therapy in the context of professional nursing practice: adverse drug event, adverse drug reaction, allergic reaction, idiosyncratic reaction, medical error, and medication error.
2. Describe the most commonly encountered medication errors.
3. Develop a framework for professional nursing practice for prevention of medication errors.
4. Identify potential physical and emotional consequences of a medication error.
5. Discuss the impact of culture and age on the occurrence of medication errors.
6. Analyze the various ethical dilemmas related to professional nursing practice associated with medication errors.
7. Identify agencies concerned with prevention of and response to medication errors.
8. Discuss the possible consequences of medication errors for professional nurses and other members of the health care team.

KEY TERMS

Adverse drug event Any undesirable occurrence related to administration of or failure to administer a prescribed medication. (p. 64)

Adverse drug reactions Unexpected, unintended, or excessive responses to medications given at therapeutic dosages (as opposed to overdose); one type of adverse drug event. (p. 64)

Allergic reaction An immunologic reaction resulting from an unusual sensitivity of a patient to a certain medication; a type of adverse drug event and a subtype of adverse drug reactions. (p. 64)

Idiosyncratic reaction Any abnormal and unexpected response to a medication, other than an allergic reaction, that is peculiar to an individual patient. (p. 64)

Medical errors A broad term used to refer to any errors at any point in patient care that cause or have the potential to cause patient harm. (p. 63)

Medication errors Any preventable adverse drug events involving inappropriate medication use by a patient or health care professional; they may or may not cause the patient harm. (p. 64)

Medication reconciliation A procedure to maintain an accurate and up-to-date list of medications for all patients between all phases of health care delivery. (p. 70)

GENERAL IMPACT OF ERRORS ON PATIENTS

Medical errors and medication errors in particular have received much national attention. The Institute of Medicine (IOM) report "To Err is Human" brought medical errors to the public's attention. According to this report, the number of patient deaths from medical errors in U.S. hospitals ranged from 44,000 to 98,000 annually based on data from two large-scale studies. Preventable medication errors were responsible for 7000 deaths per year, and it is estimated that 3 to 6.9% of hospitalized patients experience a medication error. The IOM released a similar report in 2006 and found that medical errors harm at least 1.5 million people per year, including 117,000 hospitalizations at a cost of over $4 billion. A follow-up report in 2010 showed 25.1 "harms" per 100 admissions to the hospital. This report showed no significant change in rates of preventable errors since the IOM report. Health institutions have made prevention of medical errors a top priority. The key to preventing errors is to recognize that reporting of errors should not be punitive toward the reporter. In fact, all health care professionals are encouraged to report errors. It has been shown that reporting of errors can prevent errors from occurring. The IOM report brought forth the notion that most errors occur as a breakdown in the medication use system, as opposed to being the fault of the individual. This concept has been taken a step further and has created "Just Culture." Just Culture is an environment where, after a systematic review of an error, discipline is applied appropriately. Just Culture recognizes that competent professionals make mistakes but acknowledges that professionals may develop unhealthy habits (i.e., taking shortcuts). Staff is held accountable for their actions involving such habits. However, when the error is related to a system or process, staff are held blameless.

While the aforementioned IOM study has been instrumental in the discussion and prevention of medication errors within the system of health care, there are other ideas of thought regarding prevention and/or reduction of medication errors. One important new concept focusing on patient safety and error prevention/reduction emphasizes the way nursing students (and others in the health care professions) are educated. Some nursing leaders and health care experts believe that the education of all health professions needs a systemic change. Particular to mention is the 2003 report of the IOM, *Health Professions Education: A Bridge to Quality*, which built upon the IOM report in 2001, *Crossing the Quality Chasm: A New Health System for the 21st Century*. This study recommended a complete restructuring of clinical education across all health professions. A follow-up initial report came out of a multidisciplinary summit of health profession leaders (2002), and this high-level panel composed of 150 participants recommended the goal of "an outcome-based" education system. This outcome-based education system was recommended in the hopes of better preparation of clinicians to meet both the needs of patients and the requirements of a changing health system (IOM, 2003). With the 2003 IOM Report, *Health Professions Education: A Bridge to Quality*, all educators were challenged to alter the process of professional development so that health care professionals, including nurses, would graduate with an adequate understanding and acceptance that their jobs consist of caring for individual patients as well as continuously improving the quality, safety, and reliability of the health care systems within which they work. Nurse leaders supported and integrated these findings into the future of nursing education and developed specific competencies related to patient-centered care, interprofessional teamwork and collaboration, evidence-based practice, safety sciences, quality improvement methods, and informatics. These competencies were considered essential elements of future nursing curricula. "QSEN" (Quality and Safety Education for Nurses) was an initiative funded by the Robert Woods Johnson Foundation to support faculty development in order to support and accomplish this paradigm shift in nursing education. These initiatives will continue to be integrated into nursing curricula and are important to the assurance of the quality and safety in professional nursing practice. It is important to mention the IOM studies and QSEN initiatives in this chapter because of the impact they have on safety, including medication errors. It is important for nursing students to understand and recognize the significance of all these reports and be a constant changing force within their educational and work environments while constantly working toward high quality standards of professional nursing practice.

Medical errors can occur during all phases of health care delivery and involve all health professionals. Some of the more common types of error include misdiagnosis, patient misidentification, lack of patient monitoring, wrong-site surgery, and medication errors. Most studies have looked at medical errors occurring in hospitals; however, many serious medication errors occur in the home. Errors occurring in homes can be quite harmful, as potent drugs once used only in hospitals are now being prescribed for outpatients. The majority of fatal errors at home involve the mixing of prescription drugs with alcohol or other drugs. Intangible losses resulting from such adverse outcomes include patient dissatisfaction and loss of trust in the health care system. This, in turn, can lead to adverse health outcomes because patients are afraid to seek health services.

MEDICATION ERRORS

An **adverse drug event** is a general term that encompasses all types of clinical problems related to medication use, including **medication errors** and **adverse drug reactions**. The various subsets of adverse drug events and their interrelationships are illustrated in Figure 5-1. Adverse drug reactions are reactions that occur with the use of the particular drug. Two types of adverse drug reactions are **allergic reaction** (often predictable) and **idiosyncratic reaction** (usually unpredictable). Medication errors are a common cause of adverse health care outcomes and can range from having no significant effect to directly causing patient disability or death.

It is important to consider all of the steps involved in the medication use system when discussing medication errors. Identifying, responding to, and ultimately preventing medication errors require an examination of the entire medication use process. Attention must be focused on all persons and all steps involved in the medication use process. A systems approach takes the basic "Six Rights" one step further and examines the entire health care system, the health care professionals involved, and any other factor that has an impact on the error.

Drugs commonly involved in severe medication errors include central nervous system drugs, anticoagulants, and chemotherapeutic drugs. "High-alert" medications have been identified as those that, because of their potentially toxic nature, require special care when prescribing, dispensing, and/or administering.

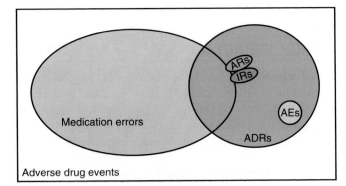

FIGURE 5-1 Diagram illustrating the various classes and subclasses of adverse drug events. *ADRs,* Adverse drug reactions; *AEs,* adverse (drug) effects; *ARs,* allergic reactions; *IRs,* idiosyncratic reactions.

High-alert medications are not necessarily involved in more errors than other drugs; however, the potential for patient harm is higher. Some high-alert medications are listed in Box 5-1. High-alert medications will be denoted with a red exclamation point throughout this textbook. Medication errors also result from the fact that there are drugs that have similarities in spelling and/or pronunciation (i.e., look-alike or sound-alike names). Several acronyms have been created to refer to these drugs, including SALAD (sound-alike, look-alike drugs) and LASA (look-alike, sound-alike). Mix-ups between such drugs are most dangerous when two drugs from different therapeutic classes have similar names. This can result in patient effects that are grossly different from those intended as part of the drug therapy. The Safety and Quality Improvement: Preventing Medication Errors box lists examples of commonly confused drug names. More information on high-alert medications and sound-alike, look-alike drugs can be found at the website of the Institute for Safe Medication Practices at *www.ismp.org.*

It is widely recognized that most medication errors result from weaknesses in the systems within health care organizations rather than from individual shortcomings. System weaknesses include failure to create a Just Culture environment, excessive workload, minimal time for preventive education, and lack of interdisciplinary communication and collaboration. All hospitals are required to analyze medication errors and implement ways to prevent them. Nurses must take the time to report errors, because without reporting, no changes can be made. When errors are reported, trends can be identified and processes can be changed to prevent the errors from occurring again. Nurses must rely on individual policies and procedures of the institution at which they are working.

ISSUES CONTRIBUTING TO ERRORS

Organizational Issues

Medication errors can occur at any step in the medication process: procuring, prescribing, transcribing, dispensing, administering, and monitoring. One study noted that half of all preventable adverse drug events begin with an error at the medication ordering (prescribing) stage. Administration is the next most common point in the process at which medication errors occur, followed by dispensing errors and transcription errors. It is very important for nurses to have good relationships with pharmacists, because the two professions, working together, can have a major impact in preventing medication errors. Hospital pharmacists are usually available 24/7 and serve as great resources when the nurse has any question regarding drug therapy.

⚡ SAFETY AND QUALITY IMPROVEMENT: PREVENTING MEDICATION ERRORS   QSEN

Institute for Safe Medication Practices: Examples of Look-Alike, Sound-Alike (LASA) Commonly Confused Drug Names

Names of Medications	Comments
carboplatin vs. cisplatin	Two different antineoplastic drugs
Celebrex vs. Celexa	Antiinflammatory drug vs. antidepressant drug
Depakote vs. Depakote ER	Same drug; immediate-release vs. extended-release dosage forms
dopamine vs. dobutamine	Vasopressor drugs of markedly different strengths; dobutamine is also a strong inotropic affecting the heart
glipizide vs. glyburide	Two different antidiabetic drugs
Humulin vs. Humalog	Short-acting vs. rapid-acting insulin
Lamictal vs. Lamisil	Anticonvulsant/mood stabilizer vs. antifungal drug
metronidazole vs. metformin	Antibiotic vs. antidiabetic drug
MiraLax vs. Mirapex	Laxative vs. antiparkinson drug
morphine vs. hydromorphone	Two different potency opioids
oxycodone vs. OxyContin	Immediate-release vs. long-acting oxycodone
Paxil vs. Plavix	Antidepressant vs. antiplatelet drug
trazodone vs. tramadol	Antidepressant vs. analgesic

Additional examples can be found at *http://www.ismp.org/Tools/ confuseddrugnames.pdf.* Accessed June 18, 2015.

The Joint Commission, the major accreditation body for many hospitals, began a patient public awareness campaign in 2006 called *Speak Up.* It encourages patients to take a more active role in their health care by "speaking up" and asking questions. The value of this program is twofold: patients learn

---

BOX 5-1   Examples of High-Alert Medications

Drug Classes/Categories

- Adrenergic agonists, IV (e.g., epinephrine, phenylephrine, norepinephrine)
- Adrenergic antagonists, IV (e.g., propranolol, metoprolol, labetalol)
- Anesthetic agents, general, inhaled, and IV (e.g., propofol, ketamine)
- Antidysrhythmics, IV (e.g., amiodarone)
- Antithrombotic agents, including warfarin, enoxaparin IV unfractionated heparin, factor Xa inhibitors (e.g., fondaparinux), direct thrombin inhibitors (e.g., argatroban, rivaroxaban), thrombolytics (e.g., alteplase), and glycoprotein IIb/IIIa inhibitors (e.g., eptifibatide)
- Cardioplegic solutions
- Chemotherapeutic agents, parenteral and oral
- Epidural or intrathecal medications
- Antidiabetic medications (e.g., insulin)
- Inotropic drugs, IV (e.g., digoxin, milrinone)
- Moderate sedation drugs, IV (e.g., midazolam)
- Narcotics/opiates, IV, transdermal, and oral neuromuscular blocking agents (e.g., succinylcholine, rocuronium, vecuronium)
- Total parenteral nutrition solutions

Specific Drugs

- Magnesium sulfate injection
- Methotrexate, oral, nononcologic use
- Concentrated electrolytes (potassium chloride for injection)
- Promethazine, IV
- Sodium chloride for injection, hypertonic (greater than 0.9% concentration)
- Sterile water for injection, inhalation, and irrigation (excluding pour bottles)

From Institute for Safe Medication Practices: ISMP's list of high-alert medications. Available at *www.ismp.org/Tools/highalertmedications.pdf.* Accessed June 18, 2015.

The World Health Organization (WHO) posts information on its website regarding initiatives to promote patient safety in medication administration. As the WHO notes, no adverse event should ever occur anywhere in the world if the knowledge exists to prevent it from happening. Knowledge is of little use, however, if it is not applied in practice. The WHO Collaborating Centre for Patient Safety Solutions has developed patient safety initiatives that can serve as a guide in redesigning the patient care process to prevent the inevitable errors from ever reaching patients. Information about the patient safety solutions approved by the WHO center is available at http://www.ccforpatientsafety.org. These patient safety concerns include avoiding confusion of medications with look-alike, sound-alike names; ensuring correct patient identification; enhancing communication during patient "hand-overs" between care units or care teams; ensuring performance of the correct procedure at the correct body site; maintaining control of concentrated electrolyte solutions; ensuring medication accuracy at transition points in care; avoiding catheter and tubing misconnections; and promoting single use of injection devices and improved hand hygiene to prevent health care–associated infections.

More information about patient safety and safety initiatives is also provided in a national campaign supported by The Joint Commission and the Centers for Medicare and Medicaid. These initiatives encourage patients to take a role in preventing health care errors by becoming more active, involved, and informed regarding all aspects of their health care. The *Speak Up* campaign features various brochures, posters, and buttons addressing a variety of patient safety issues and encourages the public to do the following: **S**peak up if you have any questions. **P**ay attention to your health care. **E**ducate yourself about medical diagnoses and be informed. **A**sk a family member or friend you trust to be your advocate. **K**now the medications you take and the reason for taking them. **U**se a hospital, ambulatory, or urgent care center or other type of health care institution. **P**articipate in all decisions about your treatment. For more information on the use of Speak Up and to look at the materials available, visit *http://www.jointcommission.org/speakup.aspx.*

coding of medications allows the nurse to use electronic devices for verification of correct medication at the patient's bedside. Computer programs are used in the pharmacy to screen for potential drug interactions. Despite all the benefits technology has to offer, workload issues (i.e., nursing staff shortage), inadequate education, or difficulties in using the complex technology can prevent the technology from eliminating errors as it was designed to do. A new set of medication errors have emerged from computerized order entry including overriding allergy or drug interaction alerts and the potential to choose the wrong drug during order entry. The nurse must never assume that technology eliminates potential medication errors and must always question any issue that does not seem correct.

Educational System Issues and Their Potential Impact on Medication Errors

All health professionals have an obligation to double-check any necessary information before proceeding. This includes stopping and checking medication orders and knowing about the drug *before* administering it Even the most capable health care provider cannot know everything or have immediate recall of every drug. Thankfully, there are numerous printed and on-line sources for drug information for health professionals. Patient safety begins in the educational process with nursing students and faculty members. Adopting the philosophy that "no question is a stupid question" allows students to begin their careers with greater confidence and with a healthy habit of self-monitoring. Commonly reported student nurse errors involve the following situations: unusual dosing times, medication administration record issues (unavailability of the record, failure to document doses given resulting in administration of extra doses, failure to review the record before medicating patients), administration of discontinued or "held" medications, failure to monitor vital signs or laboratory results, administration of oral liquids as injections, and preparation of medications for multiple patients at the same time.

Medication Errors and Related Sociologic Factors

Effective communication among all members of the health care team contributes to improved patient care. Disruptive physician behavior and lack of institutional response to it are significant factors affecting nurse job satisfaction and nursing staff retention. The majority of working nurses have witnessed or experienced disruptive behavior by a physician. This type of behavior may not only undermine patient care but also lead to staff dissatisfaction and turnover. Disruptive behavior, as defined by the American Medical Association (AMA), is personal verbal or physical conduct that affects or potentially may affect patient care in a negative fashion. These behaviors are classified into four types by the AMA: (1) intimidation and violence, (2) inappropriate language or comments, (3) sexual harassment, and (4) inappropriate responses to patient needs or staff requests.

Fortunately, communication between prescribers and other members of the health care team has improved over the years with newer generations of prescribers. This is due in large part to more progressive approaches in medical education that emphasize a team orientation.

more about their illnesses and the care provided, and they can advocate for their own safety at each health care encounter. The Institute for Safe Medication Practice (ISMP) is an excellent resource for medication safety errors and tips for prevention of such errors. The ISMP website is www.ISMP.org, and students are encouraged to utilize this throughout their careers. The World Health Organization also has error-reduction tips (Box 5-2).

Effective use of technologies such as computerized prescriber order entry and bar coding of medication packages has been shown to reduce medication errors. The U.S. Food and Drug Administration (FDA) requires bar codes for all prescription and over-the-counter medications. The cost of implementing current technology, including automated drug dispensing cabinets with electronic charting and computerized order entry, and bar code scanning may cost in excess of $20 million, which can be prohibitive for smaller hospitals. Nonetheless, these various technologic advances have been shown to reduce medication errors. For example, computerized order entry (also known as computerized physician order entry [CPOE]) eliminates handwriting and standardizes many prescribing functions. Bar

TEAMWORK AND COLLABORATION: LEGAL AND ETHICAL PRINCIPLES

Use of Abbreviations

Medication errors often occur as a result of misinterpretation of abbreviations. Therefore, the National Coordinating Council for Medication Error Reporting and Prevention recommends that the following abbreviations be written out in full and the abbreviations avoided. The U.S. Pharmacopeia and Institute of Safe Medication Practices endorse the avoidance of abbreviations whenever possible. NOTE: It is the philosophy of the authors of this textbook to *avoid* the use of any abbreviations whenever possible.

Abbreviation	Intended Meaning	Common Error
U	Units	Mistaken for a zero (0), a four (4), or cc.
μg	Micrograms	Mistaken for mg (milligrams).
Q.D.	Latin abbreviation for "every day"	The period after the "Q" can be mistaken for an "I" so that a medication is given "QID" (four times daily) instead of once daily.
Q.O.D.	Latin abbreviation for "every other day"	Misinterpreted as "QD" (daily) or QID. If "O" is poorly written, it may look like a period or "I."
D/C	Discharge or discontinue	Medications have been prematurely discontinued when D/C (intended to mean "discharge") was misinterpreted as "discontinue" because it was followed by a list of drugs. Use the word "Stop."
HS	Half strength	Misinterpreted as the Latin abbreviation "HS" (hour of sleep).
cc	Cubic centimeters	Mistaken for "U" (units) when written poorly.
AU, AS, AD	Both ears, left ear, right ear	Misinterpreted as the Latin abbreviation "OU" (both eyes), "OS" (left eye), "OD" (right eye). Also, some people forget which is right or left, or both, and which is eye or ear.

From Institute for Safe Medication Practices: ISMP's list of error-prone abbreviations, symbols, and dose designations. Available at *www.ismp.org/tools/errorproneabbreviations.pdf.* Accessed July 22, 2015.

PREVENTING, RESPONDING TO, REPORTING, AND DOCUMENTING MEDICATION ERRORS: A NURSING PERSPECTIVE

Preventing Medication Errors

Medication errors are considered to be any preventable event that could lead to inappropriate medication use or harm. The major categories of medication error are defined by the 2005 National Coordinating Council for Medication Error Reporting and Prevention as (1) no error, although circumstances or events occurred that could have led to an error; (2) medication error that causes no harm; (3) medication error that causes harm; and (4) medication error that results in death. Medication errors may be prevented through a variety of strategies, including: (1) Multiple systems of checks and balances should be implemented to prevent medication errors. (2) Prescribers must write legible orders that contain correct information, or orders entered electronically, if available (see Evidence Based Practice on computerized physician order entry [CPOE] on p. 68). (3) Authoritative resources, such as pharmacists or current (within the last three to five years) drug references/literature, must be consulted if there is any area of concern or lack of clarity, beginning with the medication order and continuing throughout the entire medication administration process. Do not use faculty members, nursing staff, or fellow nursing students as your authoritative source regarding medications and the safe practice of using appropriate resources. (4) Nurses need to always check the medication order three times before giving the drug and consult with authoritative resources (see earlier in the chapter) if any questions or concerns exist. (5) The basic "Six Rights" of medication administration should be used consistently and have been shown to substantially reduce the likelihood of a medication error. See the Patient-Centered Care: Lifespan Considerations for the Pediatric Patient box on the next page for a discussion of medication errors in pediatric patients and special considerations for this age group. See the Safety and Quality Improvement: Preventing Medication Errors box on p. 69 for a more concise and detailed listing of ways to help prevent medication errors.

Responding to, Reporting, and Documenting Medication Errors

Responding to and reporting medication errors are part of the professional responsibilities for which the nurse is accountable. If a medication error does occur, it must be reported, regardless of whether the error was made by a nursing student or a professional nurse. Follow health care institution policies and procedures for reporting and documenting the error closely and cautiously. Once the patient has been assessed and urgent safety issues have been addressed, report the error immediately to the appropriate prescriber and nursing management personnel, for example, the nurse manager or supervisor. If the patient cannot be left alone due to deterioration of the patient's condition or the need for close monitoring after the medication error, a fellow nurse or other qualified health care professional should remain with the patient and provide appropriate care while the prescriber is contacted. Follow-up procedures or tests may be ordered or an antidote prescribed. These orders should be implemented as indicated by the prescriber. Remember that the nurse's highest priority at all times during the medication administration process and during a medication error is the patient's physiologic status and safety.

When a medication error has occurred, complete all appropriate forms—including an incident report—as per the health care institution's policies and procedures, and provide appropriate documentation. Document the medication error, however, by providing only factual information about the error. Documentation should always be accurate, thorough, and objective. Avoid using judgmental words such as *error* in the documentation. Instead, chart factual information such as the medication that was administered, the actual dose given, and other details regarding the order (e.g., wrong patient, wrong route, and/or wrong time). Also note any observed changes in

QSEN **EVIDENCE-BASED PRACTICE**

Reduction in Medication Errors in Hospitals Due to Adoptions of Computerized Provider Order Entry Systems

Review

The occurrence of medication errors in hospitals is common, expensive, and sometimes harmful to patients. While medications are used to treat infectious diseases, manage symptoms of chronic disease, and help relieve pain and suffering, there are risks in taking any medication. Each year in the United States, adverse drug events, or injury resulting from the use of medication, result in over 700,000 visits to hospital emergency departments. This study's objective was to develop a national representative estimate of the reduction of medication errors in hospitals utilizing electronic prescribing through computerized provider order entry (CPOE) systems.

Type of Evidence

A systematic literature review was conducted and a random-effects meta-analytic technique used to establish a summary estimate of the effect of CPOE on medication errors. The pooled estimate was then combined with data collected from the 2006 American Society of Health-System Pharmacists Annual Survey, the 2007 American Hospital Association Annual Survey, and its 2008 Electronic Health Record Adoption Database supplement. These sources of data were used to estimate the percentage and absolute reduction in medication errors attributable to CPOE.

Results of the Study

The use of a CPOE system in the processing of a prescription drug order decreased the likelihood of a medication error on that order by 48%. With the

given effect size and the degree of CPOE adoption and use in hospitals in 2008, the researchers estimated a 12.5% reduction in medication errors, which equals approximately 17.4 million medication errors averted in the United States in 1 year. The findings of this study suggest that CPOE can substantially reduce the frequency of medication errors within inpatient acute-care settings. However, it is important to mention that these results translate into reduced harm for patients.

Link of Evidence to Nursing Practice

The Institute of Medicine estimates that there is an average of at least one medication error per day in hospitalized patients. They also estimate that at least $\frac{1}{4}$ of all mediation-related injuries are preventable and that CPOE may be one method to reduce medication errors and patient harm. Nurses deal directly with medication orders and the interpretation of handwriting and incorrect transcription. With computerized charting, the use of electronic entry of medication orders through CPOE may indeed reduce errors resulting from poor handwriting or incorrect transcription. Despite CPOE systems' effectiveness in preventing medication errors, their adoption and use in the United States remains modest, at best. Nurses can advocate for the use of CPOE and even conduct their own professional nursing research regarding the impact of this electronic order system and prevention of medication errors. Future research from various health care disciplines is needed to link the connection between CPOE and prevention of medication errors.

Centers for Disease Control (CDC) and Prevention: Medication Safety Program. Centers for Disease Control and Prevention, National Center for Emerging and Zoonotic Infectious Diseases (NCEZID) Division of Healthcare Quality Promotion (DHQP), 2013. Available at www.cdc.gov. Updated November 14, 2013. Accessed February 25, 2014.

QSEN **PATIENT-CENTERED CARE: LIFESPAN CONSIDERATIONS FOR THE PEDIATRIC PATIENT**

Medication Errors

Of all the ways a pediatric patient may be harmed during medical treatment, medication errors are the most common. As with older adult patients, when medication errors occur, there is a higher risk of death. The findings of several studies indicate that medication errors involving inpatient pediatric patients occur at a rate of 4.5 to 5.7 errors per 100 drugs used. The most common medication errors in pediatrics are dosing errors. Research has begun to identify some of the groups of pediatric patients who are at highest risk of medication errors. These include the following patients: (1) those younger than 2 years of age, (2) those in intensive care units (ICUs), specifically the neonatal ICU, (3) those in the emergency department between the hours of 4 AM and 8 AM or on the weekend and who are seriously ill, (4) those receiving intravenous and/or chemotherapeutic drugs, and (5) those whose weight has not been determined or recorded. Mathematical dosage calculations for pediatric patients are also problematic. In determination of the correct dosage once the drug has been ordered, the problems of most concern include the following: (1) inability of the nurse to understand/perform the correct calculation or dilution, (2) infrequent use of calculations, and (3) decimal point misplacement, with potential overdosing or underdosing.

The following are some of the actions that can be taken to prevent pediatric medication errors:

- Report all medication errors, because this information is part of the practice of professional nursing and helps in identifying causes of medication error.

- Know the drug thoroughly, including its on- and off-label uses, action, adverse effects, dosage ranges, routes of administration, high-alert drug status cautions (see Box 5-1), and contraindications (e.g., Is it recommended for use in pediatric patients?).
- Confirm information about the patient each and every time a dose is given, and check three times before giving the drug by comparing the drug order with the patient's medication profile and verifying for the right patient, right drug, right dose, right time, right route, and right documentation (see Chapter 1).
- Double-check and verify information in handwritten orders that may be incomplete, unclear, or illegible.
- Avoid verbal telephone orders in general. When they are unavoidable, always repeat them back to the prescriber over the telephone. Insist that the prescriber sign off any emergency in-person verbal orders before leaving the unit.
- Avoid distractions while giving medications.
- Communicate with everyone (e.g., parent, caregiver) involved in patient care.
- Make sure all orders are clear and understood with shift changes.
- Use authoritative resources such as drug handbooks, *Physicians' Desk Reference*, or information from the Food and Drug Administration website (http://www.fda.gov). For off-label use of drugs, see *www.fda.gov/Drugs/ResourcesForYou/Consumers/ucm143565.htm*.

QSEN ⚡ SAFETY AND QUALITY IMPROVEMENT: PREVENTING MEDICATION ERRORS

How to Prevent Medication Errors

- As the first step to defend against errors, assess information about drug allergies, vital signs, and laboratory test results.
- Use two patient identifiers before giving medications.
- Never give medications that have not been drawn up or prepared yourself or are prepared and properly labeled by the pharmacy.
- Minimize the use of verbal and telephone orders. If used, be sure to repeat the order to confirm with the prescriber. Speak slowly and clearly, and spell the drug name aloud.
- List the reason for use of each drug on the medication administration record and any educational materials.
- Avoid abbreviations, medical shorthand, and acronyms because they can lead to confusion, miscommunication, and risk of error (see the Teamwork and Collaboration: Legal and Ethical Principles box).
- Never assume anything about any drug order or prescription, including route. If a medication order is questioned for any reason (e.g., dose, drug, indication), never assume that the prescriber is correct. Always be the patient's advocate and investigate the matter until all ambiguities are resolved.
- Do not try to decipher illegibly written orders; instead, contact the prescriber for clarification. Illegible orders fall below applicable standards for quality medical care and endanger patient safety. If in doubt about any part of an order, always check with the prescriber. Compare the medication order against what is on hand by checking for the Right Drug, Right Dose, Right Time, Right Patient, and Right Route.
- Never use trailing zeros (e.g., 1.0 mg) in writing and/or transcribing medication orders. Use of trailing zeros is associated with increased occurrence of overdose. For example, "1.0 mg warfarin sodium" could be misread as "10 mg warfarin," a tenfold dose increase. Instead, use "1 mg" or even "one mg."
- Failure to use leading zeros can also lead to overdose. For example, .25 mg digoxin could be misread as 25 mg digoxin, a dose that is 100 times the dose ordered. Instead, write "0.25 mg."
- Carefully read all labels for accuracy, expiration dates, dilution requirements, and warnings (e.g., black box warnings).
- Remain current with new techniques of administration and new equipment.
- Encourage the use of generic names to avoid medication errors due to many sound-alike trade names.

- Listen to and honor any concerns expressed by patients. If the patient voices a concern about being allergic to a medication or states that a pill has already been taken or that the medication is not what he or she usually takes—then STOP, listen, and investigate.
- Strive to maintain your own health to remain alert, and never be too busy to stop, learn, and inquire. In addition, engage in ongoing continuing education.
- Become a member of professional nursing organizations to network with other nursing students or professional nurses to advocate for improved working conditions and to stand up for the rights of nurses and patients.
- Know where to find the latest information on which dosage forms can or should not be crushed or opened (e.g., capsules), and educate patients accordingly.
- Safeguard any medications that the patient had on admission or transfer so that additional doses are not given or taken by mistake. In such situations, safeguarding is accomplished by compiling a current medication history and resolving any discrepancies rather than ignoring them.
- If using paper medication administration records, always verify if they have been rewritten or reentered for any reason, and follow policies and procedures about this action.
- Make sure the weight of the patient is always recorded before carrying out a medication order to help decrease dosage errors.
- Provide for mandatory recalculation of every drug dosage for high-risk drugs (e.g., highly toxic drugs) or high-risk patients (e.g., pediatric or older adult patients) because there is a narrow margin between therapeutic serum drug levels and toxic levels (e.g., for chemotherapeutic or digitalis drugs, or in the presence of altered liver or kidney function in a patient).
- Always suspect an error whenever an adult dosage form is dispensed for a pediatric patient.
- Seek translators when appropriate—never guess what patients are trying to say.
- Educate patients to take an active role in medication error prevention, both in the hospital setting and at home.
- Involve yourself politically in advocating for legislation that improves patient safety.

the patient's physical and mental status. In addition, document the fact that the prescriber was notified and any follow-up actions or orders that were implemented. Patient monitoring should be ongoing.

Most facilities require additional documentation when a medication error occurs consisting of an incident report or unusual occurrence report. Always follow health care institution policies and procedures or protocols in completing an incident report. Documentation should include only factual information about the error as well as all corrective actions taken. Complete any additional sections of the form to help with the investigation of the incident. Because these forms are forwarded to the institution's risk management department, this complete and factual information may help prevent errors in the future. Do not document on the patient's chart that an incident report was filled out, and a copy of the incident report should not be kept. Incident reports are not to be placed in the patient's chart. The reporting of actual and suspected medication errors should offer the option of anonymity. This may help to foster improved error reporting and safe medication practices. Internal, institution-based systems of error tracking may generate data to help customize policy and procedure development. All institutional pharmacy departments are required to have an adverse drug event monitoring program.

Nurses as well as health care institutions may also be involved in external reporting of medication errors. There are nationwide confidential reporting programs that collect and disseminate safety information on a larger scale. One such program is the U.S. Pharmacopeia Medication Errors Reporting Program (USPMERP). The U.S. Pharmacopeia (USP) has created a nationwide database of medication errors and their causes, as well as potential errors. Any health care professional can report an error by contacting the USPMERP at 800-23-ERROR. Many important institutional changes have been made based on the data collected by this program. MedWatch is another useful error and adverse event reporting program provided by the FDA. Any member of the public can report problems with medications or medical devices via telephone or mail, or online at the FDA website. The Institute for Safe Medication Practices and the Joint Commission also provide useful information and reporting services to health care providers aimed at safety enhancement.

CASE STUDY

Safety: What Went Wrong? Preventing Medication Errors

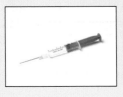

During your busy clinical day as a student nurse, the staff nurse assigned to your patient comes to you and says, "Would you like to give this injection? We have a 'now' order for Sandostatin (octreotide) 200 mcg subcutaneously. I've already drawn it up; 200 mcg equals 2 mL. It needs to be given as soon as possible, so I drew it up for you to save time." She hands you a syringe that has 2 mL of a clear fluid in it.

1. Should you give this medication "now," as ordered? Why or why not?

   You decide to check the order in the patient's electronic record. The physician ordered, "Octreotide, 200 mcg now, subcutaneously, then 100 mcg every 8 hours as needed." Before you have a chance to find your instructor, the nurse returns and says, "Your instructor probably won't let you give the injection unless you can show the medication ampules. Here are the ampules I used to draw up the octreotide. Be quick—your patient needs it now!"

   You show the two ampules and the syringe to your instructor. Together you read the electronic order and then check the ampules. Each ampule is marked "Sandostatin (octreotide) 500 mcg/mL."

2. If the nurse drew up 2 mL from these two ampules, how much octreotide is in the syringe? How does this amount compare with the amount on the order?

   The nurse is astonished when you point out that the ampules read "500 mcg/mL." She goes into the automated medication dispenser and sees two identical boxes of Sandostatin next to each other in the refrigerated section. One box is labeled "100 mcg/mL," and the other box is labeled "500 mcg/mL." She then realizes that she chose ampules of the wrong strength of drug and drew up an incorrect dose.

3. What would have happened if you had given the injection? (Consult a nursing drug handbook if needed.)

4. What needs to be done at this point? What contributed to this potential medication error, and how can it be prevented in the future?

For answers, see *http://evolve.elsevier.com/Lilley*.

Medication Reconciliation

Medication reconciliation is a process in which medications are "reconciled" at all points of entry and exit to/from a health care entity. Medication reconciliation requires patients to provide a list of all the medications they are currently taking (including herbals and over-the-counter drugs). The prescriber is then to assess those medications and decide if they are to be continued upon hospitalization. Medication reconciliation was designed to ensure that there are no discrepancies between what the patient was taking at home and in the hospital. Medication reconciliation is to occur at entry into the health care institution, upon transfer from surgery, upon transfer into or out of the intensive care unit, and at discharge.

Although this seems to be an easy process, numerous problems have been encountered since its inception in 2005. The first problem is that many times patients do not know exactly what medications they are taking and may report that they take a "blue pill for blood pressure." Sometimes the patient may have a list of medications but some of the medications were discontinued prior to admission, and they oftentimes fail to provide this vital piece of information. This can lead to the prescriber continuing a medicine based on faulty information. This particular problem has grown because many hospitals now use hospitalists (physicians that only take care of the patient in the hospital), and the primary care provider who has the most accurate list of medications is not involved. Medication reconciliation involves three steps:

1. Verification—Collection of the patient's medication information with a focus on medications currently used (including prescription drugs as well as over-the-counter medications and supplements)
2. Clarification—Professional review of this information to ensure that medications and dosages are appropriate for the patient
3. Reconciliation—Further investigation of any discrepancies and changes in medication orders

To ensure ongoing accuracy of medication use, the steps listed need to be repeated at each stage of health care delivery: *Admission, status change* (e.g., from critical to stable), *patient transfer* (within or between facilities or provider teams), and *discharge* (the latest medication list should be provided to the patient to take to his or her next health care provider visit.)

Some applicable assessment and education tips regarding medication reconciliation are as follows:

1. Ask the patient open-ended questions, and gradually move to yes-no questions to help determine specific medication information. (Details are important, maybe even critical!)
2. Avoid the use of medical jargon unless it is clear that the patient understands and is comfortable with such language.
3. Prompt the patient to try to remember all applicable medications (e.g., patches, creams, eyedrops, inhalers, professional samples, injections, dietary supplements). If the patient provides a medication list, make a copy for the patient's chart.
4. Clarify unclear information to the extent possible (e.g., by talking with the home caregiver or the outpatient pharmacy the patient uses).
5. Record the information in the patient's chart as the first step in the medication reconciliation process.
6. Emphasize to the patient the importance of always maintaining a current and complete medication list and bringing it to each health care encounter (e.g., as a wallet card or other list). Also encourage patients to learn the names and current dosages of their medications.

OTHER ETHICAL ISSUES

Notification of Patients Regarding Errors

A landmark article published in the *Journal of Clinical Outcomes Management* in 2001 recognized the obligation of institutions and health care providers to provide full disclosure to patients when errors have occurred in their care. The article not only emphasized the ethical basis for this practice but also addressed the legal implications and was a starting point for understanding the issue of notification of patients regarding medication errors. The point was made that patients who seek attorney services are often motivated primarily by a perceived imbalance in power between themselves and their health care providers and by fear of financial burden. Health care organizations can choose to proactively apologize and accept responsibility for obvious errors and even offer needed financial support (e.g., for travel expenses, temporary loss of wages). Research indicates that such actions help health care organizations to avoid litigation and potentially much larger financial settlements.

Possible Consequences of Medication Errors for Nurses

The possible effects of medication errors on patients range from no significant effect to permanent disability and even death in the most extreme cases. However, medication errors may also affect health care professionals, including nurses and student nurses, in a number of ways. An error that involves significant patient harm or death may take an extreme emotional toll on the nurse involved in the error. Nurses may be named as defendants in malpractice litigation, with possibly serious financial consequences. Many nurses choose to carry personal malpractice insurance for this reason, although nurses working in institutional settings are usually covered by the institution's liability insurance policy. Nurses should obtain clear written documentation of any institutional coverage provided before deciding whether to carry individual malpractice insurance.

Administrative responses to medication errors vary from institution to institution and depend on the severity of the error. One possible response is a directive to the nurse involved to obtain continuing education or refresher training. Disciplinary action, including suspension or termination of employment, may also occur depending on the specific incident. However, many hospitals have implemented a nonpunitive approach to medication errors. Nurses who have violated regulations of their state's nurse practice act may also be counseled or disciplined by their state nursing board, which may suspend or permanently revoke their nursing license. Student nurses, given their lack of clinical experience, must be especially careful to avoid medication errors, as well as errors in general. When in doubt about the correct course of action, students must consult with clinical instructors or more experienced staff nurses. Nonetheless, if a student nurse realizes that he or she has committed an error, the student is to notify the responsible clinical instructor immediately. The patient may require additional monitoring or medication, and the prescriber may also need to be notified. Although such events are preferably avoided, they can ultimately be useful, though stressful, learning experiences for the student nurse. However, student nurses who commit sufficiently serious errors or display a pattern of errors can expect more severe disciplinary action. This may range from a requirement for extra clinical time or repeating of a clinical course to suspension or expulsion from the nursing school program (see Educational System Issues and Their Potential Impact on Medication Errors earlier in the chapter).

SUMMARY

The increasing complexity of nursing practice also increases the risk for medication errors. Widely recognized and common causes of error include misunderstanding of abbreviations, illegibility of prescriber handwriting, miscommunication during verbal or telephone orders, and confusing drug nomenclature. The structure of various organizational, educational, and sociologic systems involved in health care delivery may also contribute directly or indirectly to the occurrence of medication errors. Understanding these influences can help the nurse take proactive steps to improve these systems. Such actions can range from fostering improved communication with other health care team members, including students, to advocating politically for safer conditions for both patients and staff. The first priority when an error does occur is to protect the patient from further harm whenever possible. All errors should serve as red flags that warrant further reflection, detailed analysis, and future preventive actions on the part of nurses, other health care professionals, and possibly even patients themselves.

KEY POINTS

- To prevent medication errors from misinterpretation of the prescriber's orders, avoid abbreviations. Medication errors include giving a drug to the wrong patient, confusing sound-alike and look-alike drugs, administering the wrong drug or wrong dose, giving the drug by the wrong route, and giving the drug at the wrong time.
- Measures to help prevent medication errors include being prepared and knowledgeable and taking time to always triple-check for the right patient, drug, dosage, time, and route. It is also important for nurses always to be aware of the entire medication administration process and to take a systems analysis approach to medication errors and their prevention.
- Encourage patients to ask questions about their medications and to question any concern about the drug or any component of the medication administration process.

- Encourage patients to always carry drug allergy information on their persons and to keep a current list of medications in their wallets or purses and on their refrigerators. This list should include the drug's name, reason the drug is being used, usual dosage range and dosage prescribed, expected adverse effects and possible toxicity of the drug, and the prescriber's name and contact information.
- Report medication errors. It is important to include in this documentation assessment of patient status before, during, and after the medication error, as well as specific orders carried out in response to the error.

NCLEX® EXAMINATION REVIEW QUESTIONS

1. The nurse keeps in mind that which measure is used to reduce the risk of medication errors?
   a. When questioning a drug order, keep in mind that the prescriber is correct.
   b. Be careful about questioning the drug order a board-certified physician has written for a patient.
   c. Always double-check the many drugs with sound-alike and look-alike names because of the high risk of error.
   d. If the drug route has not been specified, use the oral route.
2. During the medication administration process, it is important that the nurse remembers which guideline?
   a. When in doubt about a drug, ask a colleague about it before giving the drug.
   b. Ask what the patient knows about the drug before giving it.
   c. When giving a new drug, be sure to read about it after giving it.
   d. If a patient expresses a concern about a drug, stop, listen, and investigate the concerns.
3. If a student nurse realizes that he or she has made a drug error, the instructor should remind the student of which concept?
   a. The student bears no legal responsibility when giving medications.
   b. The major legal responsibility lies with the health care institution at which the student is placed for clinical experience.
   c. The major legal responsibility for drug errors lies with the faculty members.
   d. Once the student has committed a medication error, his or her responsibility is to the patient and to being honest and accountable.
4. The nurse is giving medications to a newly admitted patient who is to receive nothing by mouth (NPO status) and finds an order written as follows: "Digoxin, 250 mcg stat." Which action is appropriate?

   a. Give the medication immediately (stat) by mouth because the patient has no intravenous (IV) access at this time.
   b. Clarify the order with the prescribing physician before giving the drug.
   c. Ask the charge nurse what route the physician meant to use.
   d. Start an IV line, then give the medication IV so that it will work faster, because the patient's status is NPO at this time.
5. The nurse is reviewing medication orders. Which digoxin dose is written correctly?
   a. digoxin .25 mg
   b. digoxin .250 mg
   c. digoxin 0.250 mg
   d. digoxin 0.25 mg
6. The nurse is administering medications. Examples of high-alert medications include: *(Select all that apply.)*
   a. Chemotherapeutic agents
   b. Antibiotics
   c. Opiates
   d. Antithrombotics
   e. Potassium chloride for injection
7. Convert 250 micrograms to milligrams. Be sure to depict the number correctly according to the guidelines for decimals and zeroes.
8. The nurse is performing medication reconciliation during a patient's admission assessment. Which question by the nurse reflects medication reconciliation?
   a. "Do you have any medication allergies?"
   b. "Do you have a list of all the medications, including over-the-counter, you are currently taking?"
   c. "Do you need to take anything to help you to sleep at night?"
   d. "What pharmacies do you use when you fill your prescriptions?"

1. c, 2. d, 3. d, 4. b, 5. d, 6. a, c, d, e, 7. 0.25 mg, 8. b.

CRITICAL THINKING AND PRIORITIZATION QUESTIONS

1. Just after the nurse administers an oral antihypertensive drug, the patient asks, "Wasn't that supposed to be a half-tablet? I just took the whole tablet!" The nurse realizes that the patient was given twice the ordered amount. The order was for 25 mg, a half-tablet, and the entire 50-mg tablet was given. At this time, what would the nurse need to say to the patient? What are the nurse's priority actions?

2. The nurse is reviewing the orders on a newly admitted patient and reads this order: "Humalog insulin, 4 U q.d." What problems, if any, would the nurse identify in this order?

For answers, see *http://evolve.elsevier.com/Lilley*.

EVOLVE WEBSITE

http://evolve.elsevier.com/Lilley

- Animations
- Answer Keys for Textbook Case Studies and Textbook Critical Thinking and Prioritization Questions
- Content Updates
- Key Points
- Review Questions
- Student Case Studies

Patient Education and Drug Therapy

e http://evolve.elsevier.com/Lilley

OVERVIEW

Given the constant change in today's health care climate and increased consumer awareness, the role of the nurse as an educator continues to increase and remains a significant part of patient care, both in and out of the hospital environment. Patient education is essential in any health care setting and is a critical component of quality and safe health care. Without patient education, the highest quality and safest of care cannot be provided. Patient education is also very crucial in assisting patients, family, significant others, and caregivers to adapt to illness, prevent illness, maintain health and wellness, and provide self-care. Patient education is a process, much like the nursing process; it provides patients with a framework of knowledge that assists in the learning of healthy behaviors and assimilation of these behaviors into a lifestyle. The patient education process begins with assessment of the learner, development of appropriate nursing diagnoses, planning, implementation, and evaluation. Patient education may be one of the more satisfying aspects of nursing care because it is essential to improved health outcomes and can be easily measured. In fact, in the current era of increasing acuteness of patient conditions and the need to decrease length of stays in hospitals, patient education and family teaching become even more essential to effectively and efficiently meet outcome criteria. Patient education has also been identified as a valued and satisfying activity for the professional nurse. Additionally, patient education is a qualifier found in professional and accreditation standards. Health teaching is not only included in the American Nurses Association document *Nursing: Scope and Standards of Practice* (2004) but is also one of the grading criteria used by The Joint Commission (2011), which was formerly known as the Joint Commission on Accreditation of Healthcare Organizations (JCAHO). Visit http://www.thejointcommission.org for more information on accreditation, certification, standards, measurement, and related topics.

Contributing to the effectiveness of patient education is an understanding of and attention to the three domains of learning: the cognitive, affective, and psychomotor domains. It is recommended that one or a combination of these domains be addressed in any patient educational session. The cognitive domain refers to the level at which basic knowledge is learned and stored. It is the thinking portion of the learning process and incorporates an individual's previous experiences and perceptions. Previous experiences with health and wellness influence the learning of new materials, and prior knowledge and experience can serve as the foundation for adding new concepts. Thus, the learning process begins with the identification of what experiences the person has had with the subject matter or content. However, it is important to remember that thinking involves more than the delivery of new information because a patient must build relationships between prior and new experiences to formulate new meanings. At a higher level in the thinking process, the new information is used to question something that is uncertain, to recognize when to seek additional information, and to make decisions during real-life situations. For example, you would ask the patient if he or she had ever taken pain medication and, if so, how was the experience? Did the patient understand how often to take the pain medication? What did he or she remember about the risks of the medication? The answers to these questions would then help you, the nurse, determine the patient's understanding of the prescribed pain medication and further refine the teaching plan.

The affective domain is the most intangible component of the learning process. Affective behavior is conduct that expresses feelings, needs, beliefs, values, and opinions. It is well known that individuals view events from different perspectives and often choose to internalize feelings rather than express them. You must be willing to approach patients in a nonjudgmental manner, listen to their concerns, recognize the nonverbal messages being given, and assess patient needs with an open mind. If you are successful in gaining the trust and confidence of patients and family members, it may have a powerful effect on their attitudes and thus on the learning process. An example would include questions about how effective the pain medication was and how long the patient took it. The patient explains that she only took one dose of the pain medicine because a family member said it was addicting, and so she was in significant pain. Once the situation is assessed further and it is determined that the opinion about the pain medication being addictive was incorrect, you can provide accurate information with proper instructions so that the pain is controlled.

The psychomotor domain involves the learning of a new procedure or skill and is often called the *doing domain*. Learning is generally accomplished by demonstration of the procedure or task using a step-by-step approach with return demonstrations by the learner to verify whether the procedure or skill has been mastered. An example would be the use of return demonstration with an individual who is a newly diagnosed diabetic and has a prescription for insulin injections at home. Using a teaching approach that engages these domains—whether one, two, or a combination of all three—will certainly add to the quality and effectiveness of patient education sessions and subsequent learning.

The result of effective patient education is learning. Learning is defined as a change in behavior, and teaching as a sharing of knowledge. Although you may never be certain that patients will take medications as prescribed, you may carefully assess, plan, implement, and evaluate the teaching you provide to help maximize outcome criteria. Just like the nursing process, the medication administration process and the teaching-learning process provide systematic frameworks for professional nursing practice. The remainder of this chapter provides a brief look at patient education as related to the nursing process and drug therapy.

ASSESSMENT OF LEARNING NEEDS RELATED TO DRUG THERAPY

As previously mentioned, the patient education process is similar to the nursing process. A very important facet of the patient education process, like the nursing process, is a thorough assessment of learning needs. This may be incorporated as part of the health assessment interview. Complete this assessment before patients begin any form of drug therapy. As related to patient education and drug therapy, assessment includes gathering subjective and objective data about the following:

- Adaptation to any illnesses
- Age
- Barriers to learning (Box 6-1)
- Cognitive abilities
- Coping mechanisms
- Cultural background
- Developmental status for age group with attention to cognitive and mental processing abilities
- Education received including highest grade level completed and literacy level
- Educational resources
- Emotional status
- Environment at home and at work
- Folk medicine, home remedies, or use of alternative/complementary therapies (e.g., physical therapy, chiropractic therapy, osteopathic medicine, meditation, yoga, aromatherapy)
- Family relationships
- Generational differences; for example, Generation Y individuals are technologically dependent and need immediate feedback
- Health literacy (Box 6-2)
- Hierarchy of needs
- Motivation level and/or interest in health maintenance
- Psychosocial growth and development level according to Erikson's stages (Box 6-3)
- Health beliefs, including beliefs about health, wellness, and/or illness
- Information the patient understands about past and present medical conditions, medical therapy, and medications
- Language(s) spoken
- Level of knowledge about any medication(s) being taken
- Limitations (physical, psychological, cognitive, and motor)
- Medications currently taken (including over-the-counter drugs, prescription drugs, and herbal products)

BOX 6-1 Strategies to Enhance Patient Education and Reduce Barriers to Learning

- Work with available educational resources in nursing and pharmacy to collect or order and distribute materials about drug therapy. Make sure that written materials are available to all individuals and are prepared on a reading level that is most representative of the geographical area, such as an eighth-grade reading level. Most acute care and other health care facilities have electronic resources, so that printing educational materials is easy. Some examples of electronic or computerized programs are Micromedex and Lexi-PALS; these offer patient pamphlets that are in different languages and at appropriate reading levels.
- Be sure that written and verbal instructions are available in the language most commonly spoken, such as Spanish. Identify resources within the health care institution and in the community that can provide assistance with translation, such as nurses or other health care providers who are proficient in Spanish and other languages. Have the information available so that education is carried out in a timely and effective manner.
- Perform a cultural assessment that includes questions about level of education, learning experiences, past and present successes of therapies and medication regimens, language spoken, core beliefs, value system, meaning of health and illness, perceived cause of illness, family roles, social organization, and health practices or lack thereof.
- Make sure that written materials are available on the most commonly used medications and that all materials are updated annually to ensure that information is current.
- Have available information for patients on how they can prevent medication errors. The Institute for Safe Medication Practices offers informative pamphlets on the patient's role in preventing medication errors as well as web-based resources such as alerts for consumers with the proper citation.
- Work collaboratively in the health care setting, inpatient and outpatient, to develop a listing of medications that may be considered error prone, such as cardiac drugs, chemotherapeutic drugs, low–molecular-weight heparin, digoxin, metered-dose inhaled drugs, and acetaminophen. Lack of time for patient education is often a concern for nurses, but efforts should be undertaken to make materials available and to review these with patients and those involved in their care. Use all available resources, such as videotapes, verbal instructions, pictures, and other health care providers.
- For the adolescent, be sure to provide clear and simple directions for each medication, including clarification of information that may well be misinterpreted. For example, teenage girls may have the false idea that oral contraceptives prevent them from contracting sexually transmitted diseases.
- Use readability tools in the development of patient education materials if you are involved in this process. Several tools are available, such as the SMOG (Simple Measure of Gobbledygook) readability measure and the Fry readability formula. It is important to know that evidenced-based measures such as these are available to help in the creation of written materials and verbal instructions for patients. Online resources include http://www.readabilityformulas.com/smog-readability-formula.php and http://www.readabilityformulas.com/fry-graph-readability-formula.php.
- Never wait until discharge to teach patients. Include family or caregivers whenever possible, so that they become contributors to patient education and not barriers!

BOX 6-2 A Brief Look at Health Literacy

- According to the National Assessment of Adult Literacy, only 12% of adults have proficient health literacy, meaning that 9 out of 10 adults lack the basic skills needed to manage their health and prevent disease. It further states that 14% of adults have below basic health literacy and are more likely to report their health as poor and to lack health insurance than those adults with proficient health literacy.
- As related to patient education, assessing and addressing health literacy is only one aspect, but a very important aspect, of health communication and the cognitive domain of learning.
- If there is health illiteracy, studies have shown that issues of noncompliance to treatment regimens and disease complications as well as difficulty accessing health care are problematic, contributing to poor health as well as higher health care costs.
- Health illiteracy has been associated with less education, lower socioeconomic status, decrease in sensorial abilities, and multiple disease processes, so assessment of these factors is important to individualized patient education.
- Other areas to assess related to health literacy include reading level, ability to follow directions/instructions, as well as ability to manage everyday living activities such as self-care, grocery shopping, and meal preparation.
- Assessment of health literacy must be done with much sensitivity and not only relates to education but also to levels of stress/inability to cope with a new diagnosis/process and with new and complex information (e.g., patients with a higher level of education who are stressed and unable to process due to a disturbing diagnosis).

BOX 6-3 Erikson's Stages of Development

Infancy (birth to 1 year of age): Trust versus mistrust. Infant learns to trust himself or herself, others, and the environment; learns to love and be loved.

Toddlerhood (1 to 3 years of age): Autonomy versus shame and doubt. Toddler learns independence; learns to master the physical environment and maintain self-esteem.

Preschool age (3 to 6 years of age): Initiative versus guilt. Preschooler learns basic problem solving; develops conscience and sexual identity; initiates activities as well as imitates.

School age (6 to 12 years of age): Industry versus inferiority. School-age child learns to do things well; develops a sense of self-worth.

Adolescence (12 to 18 years of age): Identity versus role confusion. Adolescent integrates many roles into self-identity through imitation of role models and peer pressure.

Young adulthood (18 to 45 years of age): Intimacy versus isolation. Young adult establishes deep and lasting relationships; learns to make commitment as a spouse, parent, and/or partner.

Middle adulthood (45 to 65 years of age): Generativity versus stagnation. Adult learns commitment to the community and world; is productive in career, family, and civic interests.

Older adulthood (over 65 years of age): Integrity versus despair. Older adult appreciates life role and status; deals with loss and prepares for death.

- Misinformation about drug therapy
- Mobility and motor skills
- Motivation
- Nutritional status
- Past and present health behaviors
- Past and present experience with drug regimens and other forms of therapy, including levels of compliance

- Patient resources such as social support and financial resources
- Psychosocial development levels based on Erikson's Theory of Development and learning differences based on different developmental stages
- Race and/or ethnicity
- Readiness to learn

- Religion or religious beliefs
- Self-care ability
- Sensory status

During the assessment of learning needs, be astutely aware of the patient's verbal and nonverbal communication. Often a patient will not tell you how he or she truly feels. A seeming discrepancy is an indication that the patient's emotional or physical state may need to be further assessed in relation to his or her actual readiness and motivation for learning. Use of open-ended questions is encouraged, because they stimulate more discussion and greater clarification from the patient than closed-ended questions that require only a "yes" or "no" answer. Assess level of anxiety, because mild levels of anxiety have been identified as being motivating, whereas moderate to severe levels may be obstacles. In addition, if there are physical needs that are not being met, such as relief from pain, vomiting, or other physical distress, these needs become obstacles to learning. These physical issues must be managed appropriately before any patient teaching occurs.

NURSING DIAGNOSES RELATED TO LEARNING NEEDS AND DRUG THERAPY

Some of the most commonly used and currently approved NANDA-I (2015 to 2017) nursing diagnoses related to patient education and drug therapy are as follows (see Chapter 1 for a more complete listing):

- Falls, Risk for
- Health Maintenance, Ineffective
- Health Management, Ineffective
- Health Management, Readiness for Enhanced
- Injury, Risk for
- Knowledge, Deficient
- Knowledge, Readiness for Enhanced
- Memory, Impaired
- Noncompliance
- Powerlessness
- Sleep Deprivation
- Sleep Pattern, Disturbed

As an example of how nursing diagnoses related to patient education are derived, the nursing diagnosis of *deficient knowledge* refers to a situation in which the patient, caregiver, or significant other has a limited knowledge base or skills with regard to the medication or medication regimen. A nursing diagnosis of *deficient knowledge* develops out of objective and/or subjective data showing that there is limited understanding, no understanding, or misunderstanding of the medication and its action, indications, adverse reactions, toxic effects, drug-drug and/or drug-food interactions, cautions, and contraindications. This diagnosis may also reflect decreased cognitive ability or impaired motor skill needed to perform self-medication. Deficient knowledge differs from noncompliance in that the latter occurs when the patient does not take the medication as prescribed or at all; in other words, the patient does not comply with or adhere to the instructions given about the medication. Noncompliance is usually a patient's choice. A nursing diagnosis of *noncompliance* is made when data collected from the patient show that the condition or symptoms for which the patient is taking the medication have recurred or were never resolved because the patient did not take the medication per the prescriber's orders or did not take the medication at all. Although noncompliance is usually a patient decision, other factors need to be assessed to determine the cause of the noncompliance (e.g., lack of ability of the parent, family, or caregiver to administer the medication; other physical, emotional, or socioeconomic factors). These factors are associated with the nursing diagnosis of ineffective health maintenance and provide a patient-centered approach to the plan of care.

PLANNING: OUTCOME IDENTIFICATION AS RELATED TO LEARNING NEEDS AND DRUG THERAPY

The planning phase of the teaching-learning process occurs as soon as a learning need has been assessed and then identified in the patient, family, or caregiver. With mutual understanding, the nurse and patient identify outcome criteria that are associated with the identified nursing diagnosis and are able to relate them to the specific medication the patient is taking. Planning will identify the methods to be used that will meet the patient's educational needs. Outcome identification will include if an outcome is a cognitive (knowledge) change, a psychomotor (performance of a skill) change, or an affective (attitude or feeling/emotion) change. The following is an example of outcome identification related to a nursing diagnosis of *deficient knowledge* for a patient who is self-administering an oral antidiabetic drug and has many questions about the medication therapy. *Sample outcomes identification:* "Patient safely self-administers the prescribed oral antidiabetic drug within a given time frame" and "Patient remains without signs and symptoms of overmedication while taking an oral antidiabetic drug, such as hypoglycemia with tachycardia, palpitations, diaphoresis, hunger, and fatigue." When drug therapy outcomes are identified, appropriate time frames for meeting outcome criteria must be identified (see Chapter 1 for more information on the nursing process). In addition, outcomes need to be realistic, based on patient needs, stated in patient terms, and include behaviors that are measurable, such as *list, identify, demonstrate, self-administer, state, describe,* and *discuss*.

IMPLEMENTATION RELATED TO PATIENT EDUCATION AND DRUG THERAPY

After you have completed the assessment phase, identified nursing diagnoses, and created a plan of care, the implementation phase of the teaching-learning process begins. This phase includes conveying specific information about the medication to the patient, family, or caregiver. The domain of learning (see previous discussion) must match the specific teaching method. Teaching methods/sessions must always accommodate the priorities of the patient. Teaching-learning sessions must incorporate clear, simple, concise written instructions (Box 6-4); oral instructions; and written pamphlets, pictures, videos, or any

BOX 6-4 General Teaching and Learning Principles

- Make learning patient-centered and individualized to each patient's needs, including his or her learning needs. This includes assessment of the patient's cultural beliefs, educational level, previous experience with medications, level of growth and development (to best select a teaching-learning strategy), age, gender, family support system, resources, preferred learning style, and level of sophistication with health care and health care treatment.
- Adult learning principles include the following: learning is related to a need/deficit; is person centered; and is reinforced by application and prompt feedback with the nature of learning changing frequently.
- New information will draw on past experiences.
- Your role as patient educator is that of facilitation.
- Assess the patient's motivation and readiness to learn.
- Assess the patient's ability to use and interpret label information on medication containers.
- Some studies have shown that as much as 20% of the U.S. population is functionally illiterate. Therefore, ensure that educational strategies and materials are at a level that the patient is able to understand, while taking care to not embarrass the patient.
- If a patient is illiterate, he or she still needs to be instructed on safe medication administration. Use pictures, demonstrations, and return demonstrations to emphasize instructions.
- Consider, assess, and appreciate language and ethnicity during patient teaching. Make every effort to educate non–English-speaking patients in their native language. Ideally the patient needs to be instructed by a health professional familiar with the patient's clinical situation who also speaks the patient's native language. At the very least, provide the patient detailed written instructions in his or her native language.
- Assess the family support system for adequate patient teaching. Family living arrangements, financial status, resources, communication patterns, the roles of family members, and the power and authority of different family members must always be considered.
- Make the teaching-learning session simple, easy, fun, thorough, effective, and not monotonous. Make it applicable to daily life, and schedule it at a time when the patient is ready to learn. Avoid providing extraneous information that may be confusing or overwhelming to the patient.
- Remember that learning occurs best with repetition and periods of demonstration and with the use of audiovisuals and other educational aids.
- Patient teaching must focus on the various processes in the cognitive, affective, and/or psychomotor domains (see earlier discussion).
- Consult online resources for help in obtaining the most up-to-date and accurate patient teaching materials and information.

other learning aids that will help ensure patient learning. You may have to conduct several brief teaching-learning sessions with multiple strategies, depending on the needs of the patient. Several changes related to the growth and aging of patients affect teaching-learning, and Table 6-1 lists educational strategies for accommodating these changes in a plan of care. You may also need to identify aids to help the patient in the safe administration of medications at home, such as the use of medication day or time calendars, pill reminder stickers, daily medication containers with alarms, weekly pill containers with separate compartments for different dosing times for each day for the week, and/or a method of documenting doses taken to avoid overdosage or omission of doses.

As the United States experiences increasing diversity and growth in minority populations, our nursing and health care system will continue to see a staggering increase in the percentage of non-English speaking patients. With an estimated U.S. population of 319 million in 2014, it is projected that the total population will be close to 400 million in 2051 and 417 million in 2060. It is also anticipated that when the 2020 census is conduted, more than half the nation's children are expected to be part of of a minority race or ethnic group. By 2044, it is projected that more than half of all Americans will belong to a minority group. The African-American population is expected to increase by 14% by 2060, and the Hispanic population is estimated to increase from 55 million in 2014 to 119 million in 2060. Other minority groups are also expected to increase; the Asian population is expected to double to about 9.3% of the total population, and the Native Hawaiian and Other Pacific Islander population is expected to increase by some 100% between 2014 and 2060 (Colby and Ortman, 2015).

This increasing diversity leads to more complex issues with communication, especially when the patient speaks limited or no English. Communicate with the patient in the patient's native language, if you are proficient in that language. Joint Commission standards on language access have been instituted, and individuals with limited English proficiency have the right to what an English-speaking individual has when seeking health care services and/or health care information. Regardless of the situation, a credentialed professional needs to be an essential part of the health care team for the nurse and other members of the health care team to gain accurate and efficient insight into a patient's condition and needs. For the protection of patients and for health care providers, the individuals who are called upon need to be educated and certified in the languages so that the appropriate message is conveyed. Interpreting is a profession with standards of practice, codes of ethics, and competency criteria. Just like with nursing and with every member of the health care team, interpreters must be properly trained, educated, and certified by an accredited body so that they can be trusted to communicate a patient's needs in order to achieve quality outcomes. In these types of patient scenarios, a qualified health care team includes the certified medical interpreter to facilitate the exchange between nurse/provider and patient. Family members need to be an active part of patient care, but in the situations of non–English-speaking patients, it is best for the patient and for quality outcomes to avoid the use of family members, laypersons, and nonprofessionals as interpreters. Certified medical interpreters are essential to avoiding problems with bias, misinterpretation, and potential confidentiality concerns. A well-trained, certified medical interpreter is an asset to the health care team and ensures quality patient outcomes in our non–English-speaking population. For more information, visit the following websites: National Board for Certification of Medical Interpreters at *www.certifiedinterpreters.org;* The Certification Commission for Healthcare Interpreter Certification at *www.healthcareinterpretercertifcation.org;* and the National Board for Certification of Medical Interpreters at *www.certified medicalinterpreters.org.*

TABLE 6-1   Educational Strategies to Address Common Changes Related to Aging That May Influence Learning

Change Related to Aging	Educational Strategy
Cognitive and Memory Impairment	
Slowed cognitive functioning	Slow the pace of the presentation, and attend to verbal and nonverbal patient cues to verify understanding. New learning must relate to what the individual already knows; concrete and practical information presented with sensitivity and patience. Whenever possible, the readability and language used should be below the eighth-grade level—preferably at the fifth-grade level of English.
Decreased short-term memory	Limit content to one or two objectives. Provide smaller amounts of information at one time. Repeat information frequently. Provide written instructions for home use. Ask them to do, write, say or show something to confirm their understanding.
Decreased ability to think abstractly	Use examples to illustrate information. Use a variety of methods, such as audiovisuals, props, videotapes, large-print materials, materials with vivid color, return demonstrations, and practice sessions.
Decreased ability to concentrate	Decrease external stimuli as much as possible. Keep communication short, and use simple sentences without complex grammar. Keep handouts to one page, if at all possible.
Increased reaction time (slower to respond)	Always allow sufficient time, and be patient. Allow more time for feedback.
Disturbed Sensory Perception	
Hearing Impairment	
Diminished hearing	Perform a baseline hearing assessment. Use tone- and volume-controlled teaching aids; use bright, large-print material to reinforce.
Decreased ability to distinguish sounds (e.g., differentiate words beginning with *S, Z, T, D, F,* and *G*)	Speak distinctly and slowly, and articulate carefully.
Decreased conduction of sound	Sit on the side of the patient's best ear.
Loss of ability to hear high-frequency sounds	Do not shout; speak in a normal voice but a lower voice pitch.
Partial to complete loss of hearing	Face the patient so that lip reading is possible. Use visual aids to reinforce verbal instruction. Reinforce teaching with easy-to-read materials. Decrease extraneous noise. Use community resources for the hearing impaired.
Visual Impairment	
Decreased visual acuity	Ensure that the patient's glasses are clean and in place and that the prescription is current.
Decreased ability to read fine detail	Use printed materials with large print that is brightly and clearly colored. Print size needs to be fairly large (at least 14 points) if the older adult patient is using the materials at home.
Decreased ability to discriminate among blue, violet, and green; tendency for all colors to fade, with red fading the least	Use high-contrast materials, such as black on white. Avoid the use of blue, violet, and green in type or graphics; use red instead.
Thickening and yellowing of the lenses of the eyes, with decreased accommodation	Use nonglare lighting, and avoid contrasts of light (e.g., a darkened room with a single light).
Decreased depth perception	Adjust teaching to allow for the use of touch to gauge depth.
Decreased peripheral vision	Keep all teaching materials within the patient's visual field.
Touch and Vibration Impairment	
Decreased sense of touch	Increase the time allowed for the teaching of psychomotor skills, the number of repetitions, and the number of return demonstrations.
Decreased sense of vibration	Teach the patient to palpate more prominent pulse sites (e.g., carotid and radial arteries).

Modified from Touhy T, Jett K: *Ebersole and Hess gerontological nursing and healthy aging,* ed 4, St Louis, 2014, Mosby.

Publications provided for non–English-speaking patients may enable you to convey a sufficient amount of information in the patient's language to help effectively educate the patient while also allowing you to share materials with family members and caregivers for their use. Companies now also publish a variety of patient education materials for the discharge teaching process in both English and Spanish. Providing resources to a non–English-speaking patient in his or her native language is important in making the patient feel safe in the environment and helps to establish a therapeutic relationship, but this is not the same as interpreting.

The teaching of manual skills for specific medication administration is also part of the teaching-learning session. Sufficient time must be allowed for the patient to become familiar with any equipment and to perform several return demonstrations to you or another health care provider. Teaching-learning needs will vary from patient to patient. Make every effort to include family members, significant others, or caregivers in the teaching

QSEN **EVIDENCE-BASED PRACTICE**

A Drug by Any Other Name: Patients' Ability to Identify Medication Regimens and Its Association with Adherence and Health Outcomes

Review

Understanding and organizing medication regimens are challenging to patients as well as to members of the health care team. With the increase in use of prescription as well as over-the-counter medications, preventing errors and enhancing patient safety with medication administration is a task that needs to be aggressively and consistently addressed. Many patients struggle daily to properly and safely self-administer prescribed medications. This struggle often leads to less effective treatment, more adverse effects, and/or patient harm. Additionally, there are numerous generic prescription medications that sound alike and look alike. Generic prescriptions are prescribed more commonly due to economic reasons, thus adding further complexity to the picture. Patients often depend upon the familiarity of their "pill" or other dosage form and often rely upon the shape and/or color of their "pill" to ensure accurate dosing. This form of medication identification combined with the variables of age, diversity, language barriers, and lack of proper education about the medication's characteristics, name, dosage, action, and indication leads to an increased potential for adverse drug events and poor health outcomes. These issues with medication regimen may be the result of patients spending inadequate time discussing their medication regimen(s) or reconciling their medication with their health care providers.

Type of Evidence

This study looked at the familiarity that patients diagnosed with hypertension possessed about their prescribed medication regimen. Specifically, they compared a group of patients and related knowledge about the names and dosages of their prescribed medications as compared to patients who relied upon only the physical characteristics of the medication(s) such as size, shape, and color. In particular, the association between patients' self-reported regimen adherence, blood pressure control, and ability to identify their medications by name as compared to identification by visual characteristics was specifically explored. Other variables evaluated included specific patient attributes such as age, literacy skills, and comorbidity. Specific outcomes also evaluated included medication nonadherence, poor blood pressure control, and number of emergency room department visits and hospitalizations over the past year. Descriptive statistics with reporting of percentages, means, and standard deviation were calculated for demographic variables compared to how participants identified their medications (use of a one-way analysis of variance and chi-square). The outcomes of interest were also analyzed (see journal article for more specific information) as well as the risk ratio for each outcome of those identifying medications by physical appearance (or not at all) compared to those identifying the name of the medication while also controlling for age, gender, race, health literacy, number of antihypertensive drugs taken, and comorbid conditions.

Results of the Study

It was found that those patients who were dependent upon physical (visual) characteristic identification of prescription medicine reported worse adherence.

This group also had significantly lower rates of blood pressure control and greater risk for hospitalization.

The ability to identify prescribed medicines by name may be helpful for screening and responding to patients at greater risk for making medication errors or being less engaged with their regimen for adherence purposes. Those participants unable to identify their hypertension medications either by name or by appearance (44.8%) were more likely to miss taking a medication in the past week as compared to those who were able to identify by either name (22.5%) or appearance (21.8%). Participants identifying all medications by name tended to be less likely to have uncontrolled blood pressure, visit an emergency department, or be hospitalized in the past year as compared with participants who were unable to identify by name. Those who were able to identify (medicine) by appearance were more likely to have uncontrolled blood pressure and report being hospitalized in the past year compared with those who identified medications by name. Those who were unable to identify medications were also more likely to be hospitalized and were more likely to miss a medication in the past week. It was also found that those patients with the ability to properly name medications was associated with health literacy.

Link of Evidence to Nursing Practice

The findings of this study suggest that if a patient is unable to identify his or her antihypertensive medications by name, but only by physical characteristics, concerns are raised for patient outcomes of blood pressure control and health care utilization. These data also emphasize the need for attention during the medication reconciliation process to the accuracy of the medication list but also to the patient's understanding of his or her medications. The results of this study, in particular, emphasize the need for more intensive efforts toward increased education with understanding and comprehension of medication regimens with attention to indications and safe use. Nursing can continue with more research on patients' medical outcomes with their ability, or lack thereof, to identify their medications by name or physical characteristics. Additionally, research on measures for increasing medication adherence and safety or a combination of measures may lead to better patient outcomes. Predictors of safety in medication self-management in all levels of health literacy are another important area of research. These data underscore the continued need for attention to the issue of the medication reconciliation process to not only the accuracy of the medication list, but also to patients' understanding of their medications. Patients will only benefit from more intensive efforts to improve their identification, understanding, and comprehension of their medication regimens. As nurses, we need to inquire about all medications the patient is taking, and even if they do know the name of the medication(s), knowing the correct dose and frequency is also critical to medication safety.

Reference: Lenahan JL, McCarthy DM, Davis TC, et al: A drug by any other name: patients' ability to identify medication regimens and its association with adherence and health outcomes. *Journal of Health Communication: International Perspectives* 18(1):31-39, 2013.

session(s) for reinforcement purposes. Audiovisual aids may be incorporated and based on findings from the learning needs and nursing assessment. Resources for information about medications include *USP Drug Information* volume II, *Advice for the Patient,* which is published annually (along with the *Health Care Professional* volume) by Thomson Micromedex; this information is appropriate to share with the patient. This type of resource may be helpful to the patient when he or she seeks information about a medication (e.g., purpose, adverse effects, method of administration, drug interactions) and helpful to you in developing a patient teaching plan. Create a safe, nonthreatening, nondistracting environment for learning needs, and be open and receptive to the patient's questions. The following strategies may help ensure an effective teaching-learning session:

- Begin the teaching-learning process upon the patient's admission to the health care setting (see the Teamwork and Collaboration: Legal and Ethical Principles box).
- Individualize the teaching session to the patient.
- Provide positive rewards or reinforcement (verbal affirmation) after accurate return demonstration of a procedure, technique, and/or skill during the teaching session.
- Complete a medication calendar that includes the names of the drugs to be taken along with the dosage and frequency.

- Use audiovisual aids.
- Involve family members, significant others, or caregivers in the teaching session, as deemed appropriate.

Keep the teaching on a level that is most meaningful to the given patient. Research has shown that 20% of the population reads at or below a fifth-grade level, with most health care materials written at a tenth-grade level. Materials written at a sixth-grade or lower reading level are recommended preferably with pictures, diagrams, and/or illustrations. Box 6-4 lists some general teaching and learning principles to consider in providing patient education.

QSEN ⊕ PATIENT-CENTERED CARE: CULTURAL IMPLICATIONS

Patient Education

Research various cultures to enhance an individualized approach to nursing care. For example, with Mexican-American patients, aspects of nursing care must be approached in a sensitive manner with strong consideration for the family, communication needs, and religion. Approximately 90% of native Mexicans are Roman Catholic. To help meet the needs of these patients more effectively, consider speaking with them about their desire for clergy visits while in the hospital. Family members are generally involved, and Mexican Americans often have large extended families; therefore, take the time to include family members in the patient's care and when providing discharge instructions and medication instructions.

Health care professionals who work in a geographic area where a variety of non-English languages are widely spoken need to make an effort to learn one or more of these languages. Adult foreign language education is available in most U.S. cities, often at 2- and 4-year colleges or universities. Many classes are designed for working professionals and are scheduled at a variety of convenient times during the day and evening to accommodate demanding work schedules. Community colleges often offer quality courses that meet as little as 1 day or evening per week. Many employers will pay for job-related courses, and some courses may qualify for professional continuing education credits. Language

courses provide a means of networking and developing quality friendships with other highly motivated, empathic individuals both within and outside of the health care profession. A variety of self-study materials are also available. However, interpreting is a profession with standards of practice, competency criteria, and codes of ethics. For a non–English-speaking patient, make sure you know the resources available to you in that particular health care setting. An interpreter is needed any time the patient and nurse do not speak the same language.

Some of the common characteristics recommended for best-practice interpreter services systems include the following: (1) 24-hour access to oral language assistance for all limited–English-proficient patients or non–English-speaking patients, (2) timely delivery of interpreter services for all languages, and (3) systematic and uniform assessment, training, and evaluation of competency across the various type of oral language assistance utilized. One option for provision of services is to have available trained medical interpreters or translators. Another option is the use of remote interpreting services, and many hospital settings have proven these services to be successful. Being culturally competent and sensitive is critical to quality patient care; however, effective communication for non–English-speaking patients is their right.

Modified from Giger JN: *Transcultural nursing: Assessment and intervention*, ed 6, St. Louis, 2013, Mosby.

QSEN ⧐ TEAMWORK AND COLLABORATION: LEGAL AND ETHICAL PRINCIPLES

Discharge Teaching

The safest practices for discharge teaching are as follows:
- Always follow the health care institution's policy on discharge teaching with regard to how much information to impart to the patient.
- Do not assume that any patient has received adequate teaching before interacting with you.
- Always begin discharge teaching as soon as possible when the patient is ready.
- Minimize any distractions during the teaching session.
- Evaluate any teaching of the patient and/or significant others by having the individuals repeat the instructions you have given them.
- Contact the health care institution's social services department or the discharge planner if there are any concerns regarding the learning capacity of the patient.
- Written and/or verbal instructions for discharge medications should include information about the purpose of the drug(s), dosages and best timing for taking the medication(s), and side effects to report.

- Utilize all resources available, such as interpreters, for patients speaking a different language from yourself.
- Use the "teach back" method of teaching to ensure that the patient/family/significant others understand the at-home care plan and answer any questions.
- Assist the patient in arranging appointments for follow-up and post-discharge testing with input from the patient, family, and/or significant others.
- Document teaching-learning strategies used, such as videotapes and pamphlets.
- Document what you taught, who was present with the patient during the teaching, what specific written instructions were given, what the responses of the patient and significant others or caregivers were, and what your own nursing actions were, such as specific demonstrations or referrals to community resources. Any follow-up teaching encounter also needs to be documented, with attention to reinforcement of information.

Modified from *RARE (Reducing Avoidable Readmissions Effectively)*, 2015. Available at http://www.rareadmissions.org. Accessed March 30, 2015.

Upon completion of any teaching-learning process or patient education session, documentation needs to include notes about the learner assessment, outcomes, content provided, strategies used, patient response to the teaching session, and an overall evaluation of learning. Because of the significance of patient education related to drug therapy and the nursing process, this textbook integrates patient education into each chapter in the implementation phase of the nursing process. In addition, a Patient-Centered Care: Patient Teaching section is included at the end of most chapters.

EVALUATION OF PATIENT LEARNING RELATED TO DRUG THERAPY

Evaluation of learning outcomes needs to also be consistent with the identified domain of learning. Evaluation of patient learning is a critical component of safe and effective drug administration. To verify the success—or lack of success—of patient education, ask specific questions related to patient outcomes, and request that the patient repeat information or give a return demonstration of skills, if appropriate. The patient's behavior—such as adherence to the schedule for medication administration with few or no complications—is one key to determining whether or not teaching was successful and learning occurred. If a patient's behavior is characteristic of noncompliance or an inadequate level of learning, develop, implement, and evaluate a new plan of teaching.

CASE STUDY

Patient-Centered Care: Patient Education and Anticoagulant Therapy

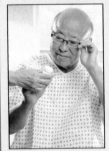

M.S., an 82-year-old retired librarian, has developed atrial fibrillation. As part of his medical therapy, he is started on the oral anticoagulant warfarin (Coumadin). His wife reports that he has some trouble hearing yet refuses to consider getting hearing aids. In addition, this is his first illness, and his wife states that he has "always hated taking medications. He's read about herbs and folk healing and would rather try natural therapy." The nurse is planning education about oral anticoagulant therapy, and M.S. says that he'll "give it a try" for now, but he "knows nothing about this drug."

1. What will the nurse assess, including possible barriers to learning, before teaching?
2. Formulate an education-related nursing diagnosis for this patient based on the information given above. In addition, provide at least three examples of outcome criteria for the nursing diagnosis.
3. What education strategies will the nurse plan to use, considering any age-related changes the patient may have?

For answers, see *http://evolve.elsevier.com/Lilley.*

SUMMARY

Patient education is a critical part of patient care, and patient education about medication administration, therapies, or regimens is no exception. From the time of initial contact with the patient throughout the time you work with the patient, the patient is entitled to all information about medications prescribed as well as other aspects of his or her care. Evaluation of patient learning and compliance with the medication regimen remains a continuous process; be willing to listen to the patient about any aspect of his or her drug therapy. Professional nurses are teachers and serve as patient advocates and thus have a responsibility to facilitate learning for patients, families, significant others, and caregivers. Accurate assessment of learning needs and readiness to learn always requires a look at the whole patient, including cultural values, health practices, and literacy issues. Every effort needs to be made to see that the patient receives effective learning to ensure successful outcomes with regard to drug therapy—and all parts of the patient's health care.

It is important to consult the resources mentioned earlier, as well as the U.S. Pharmacopeia (at http://www.usp.org), which serves as an advocate for patient safety and establishes standards for medications. This organization is a tremendous resource for the health care professional in obtaining information for the patient so that quality patient education can be provided. The U.S. Pharmacopeia values patient education as a means of enhancing patient safety as well as a means of decreasing medication errors in the hospital setting or at home. In addition, the Institute for Safe Medication Practices (at *www.ismp.org*) provides nurses with a wealth of information related to patient education, safety, and prevention of medication errors. As a nonprofit organization, this institute works closely with nurses, prescribers, regulatory agencies, and professional organizations to provide education about medication errors and their prevention, and is a premier resource in all matters pertaining to safe medication practices in health care organizations.

Another resource is the National Council on Patient Information and Education (NCPIE), which may be accessed at www.talkaboutrx.org. This site was developed with the purpose of stimulating and improving communication of information on the appropriate use of medications to consumers and health care professionals (Box 6-5). Centerwatch.com is a site providing information and views on the clinical trials industry. A PDF reprint can be obtained from this online resource. In summary, it is professional nurses who usually have the most contact with patients and see patients in a variety of settings. Because of this, nurses need to continue to be patient advocates and take the initiative to plan, design, create, and present educational materials for teaching about drug therapy.

BOX 6-5 National Council on Patient Information and Education (NCPIE): A Brief Review

- NCPIE, founded in 1982, is a non-profit multi-stakeholder coalition working toward improving communication and information on appropriate medication use to consumers and health care professionals.
- It is the leading authority for informing the general public and health care professionals on safe medication use through utilization of more effective communication leading to better health outcomes and quality of life.
- NCPIE works diligently to address critical medicine safe-use issues, including adherence improvent, prescription drug overuse prevention, medication error reduction and quality improvements in health care provider–patient medicine communication, and the safe storage or and disposal of medicines.
- It develops and provides valuable patient educational programs and educational resources.

- Some of NCPIE's public-facing websites include the following: *www.talkaboutrx.org; www.bemedicinesmart.org, www.bemedwise.org, www.mustforseniors.org,* and *www.recoveryopensdoors.org.*
- NCPIE's website, available at *www.talkaboutrx.org,* helps consumers make sound decisions about the use of medicines. Other resources available on NCPIE's website are Educate Before You Medicate: Knowledge Is the Best Medicine; Communicate Before You Medicate, Team Up and Talk, and Mustforseniors.org.
- Some of the programs that have been launched include Talk About Your Medicines and Align My Refills, targeted towards the safe use/preventing abuse and medication safety.

Data from National Council on Patient Information and Education: National Council on Patient Information and Education website, 2015. Available at *www.talkaboutrx.org.* Accessed March 31, 2015.

PATIENT-CENTERED CARE: PATIENT TEACHING

- Teaching needs to focus on either the cognitive, affective, or psychomotor domain or a combination of all three. The cognitive domain may involve recall for synthesis of facts, with the affective domain involving behaviors such as responding, valuing, and organizing. The psychomotor domain includes teaching someone how to perform a procedure.
- Realistic patient teaching outcomes must be identified and established with the involvement of the patient, caregiver, or significant other.
- Keep patient teaching on a level that is most meaningful to the individual. Most research indicates that reading materials need to be written at a sixth-grade reading level or lower but may be adjusted accordingly to patient assessment.
- Follow teaching and learning principles when developing and implementing patient education.
- Emphasize the name of the medication(s), dosage, and frequency. Encourage patients to update a listing of all medications and allergies and keep it on their person at all times.
- Be sure to control the environmental factors, such as lighting, noise, privacy, and odors. Provide dignified care while preparing the patient for teaching, and respect personal space. If there are distractions, such as television, radio, cell phone, or computer, work with the patient/family members to safely and appropriately quiet these items during teaching sessions.
- Make sure that all patient education materials are organized and at hand. If the patient wears eyeglasses or hearing aids, be sure they are made available prior to education.

KEY POINTS

- The effectiveness of patient education relies on an understanding of and attention to the cognitive, affective, and psychomotor domains of learning. After you have completed the assessment phase, identified nursing diagnoses, and created a plan of care, the implementation phase of the teaching-learning process begins; reevaluation of the teaching plan must occur frequently and as needed. The growth in cultural diversity, in particular the increase in the Hispanic population, demands that nursing and related health care professions provide patient education materials in both English and Spanish.
- In educational sessions, patients need to receive information through as many senses as possible, such as verbally and visually (e.g., through pamphlets, videotapes, and diagrams), to maximize learning. Information must be presented at the patient's reading level (in the patient's native language, if possible) and suitable for the patient's level of cognitive development (see Erikson's stages in Box 6-3).
- Teaching and learning principles also must be integrated into patient education plans. Evaluation of patient learning is a critical component of safe and effective drug administration.
- To verify the success—or lack of success—of patient education, nurses need to be very specific in their questions related to patient outcomes and request that the patient repeat information or perform a return demonstration of skills, if appropriate.
- Be knowledgeable about all available resources for non–English-speaking patients including the use of certified medical interpreters.

NCLEX® EXAMINATION REVIEW QUESTIONS

1. A 47-year-old patient with diabetes is being discharged to home and must take insulin injections twice a day. The nurse keeps in mind which concepts when considering patient teaching?
   a. Teaching needs to begin at the time of diagnosis or admission and is individualized to the patient's reading level.
   b. The nurse can assume that because the patient is in his forties he will be able to read any written or printed documents provided.
   c. The majority of teaching can be done with pamphlets that the patient can share with family members.
   d. A thorough and comprehensive teaching plan designed for an eleventh-grade reading level needs to be developed.

2. The nurse is developing a discharge plan regarding a patient's medication. Which of these statements about the discharge plan is true?
   a. It will be developed right before the patient leaves the hospital.
   b. It will be developed only after the patient is comfortable or after pain medications are administered.
   c. It will include videos, demonstrations, and instructions written at least at the fifth-grade level.
   d. It will be individualized and based on the patient's level of cognitive development.

3. The nurse is responsible for preoperative teaching for a patient who is mildly anxious about receiving pain medications postoperatively. The nurse recognizes that this level of anxiety may
   a. impede learning because anxiety is always a barrier to learning.
   b. lead to major emotional unsteadiness.
   c. result in learning by increasing the patient's motivation to learn.
   d. reorganize the patient's thoughts and lead to inadequate potential for learning.

4. What action by the nurse is the best way to assess a patient's learning needs?
   a. Quiz the patient daily on all medications.
   b. Begin with validation of the patient's present level of knowledge.
   c. Assess family members' knowledge of the prescribed medication even if they are not involved in the patient's care.
   d. Ask the caregivers what the patient knows about the medications.

5. Which technique would be most appropriate to use when the nurse is teaching a patient with a language barrier?
   a. Obtain an interpreter who can speak in the patient's native tongue for teaching sessions.
   b. Use detailed explanations, speaking slowly and clearly.
   c. Assume that the patient understands the information presented if the patient has no questions.
   d. Provide only written instructions.

6. A nursing student is identifying situations that involve the psychomotor domain of learning as part of a class project. Which are examples of learning activities that involve the psychomotor domain? *(Select all that apply.)*
   a. Teaching a patient how to self-administer eyedrops
   b. Having a patient list the adverse effects of an antihypertensive drug
   c. Discussing what foods to avoid while taking antilipemic drugs
   d. Teaching a patient how to measure the pulse before taking a beta blocker
   e. Teaching a family member how to give an injection
   f. Teaching a patient the rationale for checking a drug's blood level

7. The nurse is instructing an older adult patient on how to use his walker. Which education strategies are appropriate? *(Select all that apply.)*
   a. Speak slowly and loudly.
   b. Ensure a quiet environment for learning.
   c. Repeat information frequently.
   d. Allow for an increased number of return demonstrations.
   e. Provide all the information in one teaching session.

8. You are reviewing newly prescribed medications with the wife of a patient who will be discharged today on a liquid diet after jaw surgery. She will be giving the patient his medications. There is a prescription for liquid metoclopramide (Reglan), 10 mg PO before breakfast and dinner. The medication is available in a strength of 5 mg/mL. How many mL will she need to give for each dose?

1. a, 2. d, 3. c, 4. b, 5. a, 6. a, d, e, 7. b, c, d, 8. 10 mL.

CRITICAL THINKING AND PRIORITIZATION QUESTIONS

1. A nurse has been trying to communicate with a patient who does not speak English, but so far none of the communication techniques has been successful. What are the best strategies the nurse can use to develop a plan of care that addresses the patient's need for medication information on the cardiac drug digoxin and also focuses on the potential for toxicity? (Note: You may need to look up the drug in the textbook if you are not familiar with it.)

2. A patient has had hip replacement surgery and will be going home in a few days. The surgeon has requested that the nurses teach the patient and a family member how to give subcutaneous injections of the low–molecular-weight heparin that will be prescribed for him after his discharge. What is the priority regarding this patient's education? Explain your answer.

For answers see *http://evolve.elsevier.com/Lilley.*

EVOLVE WEBSITE

http://evolve.elsevier.com/Lilley
- Animations
- Answer Keys for Textbook Case Studies and Textbook Critical Thinking and Prioritization Questions
- Content Updates
- Key Points
- Review Questions
- Student Case Studies

Over-the-Counter Drugs and Herbal and Dietary Supplements

ⓔ http://evolve.elsevier.com/Lilley

OBJECTIVES

When you reach the end of this chapter, you will be able to do the following:

1. Discuss the differences between prescription drugs, over-the-counter (OTC) drugs, herbals, and dietary supplements.
2. Briefly discuss the differences between the federal legislation governing the promotion and sale of prescription drugs and the legislation governing OTC drugs, herbals, and dietary supplements.
3. Describe the advantages and disadvantages of the use of OTC drugs, herbals, and dietary supplements.
4. Discuss the role of nonprescription drugs, specifically herbals and dietary supplements, in the integrative (often called *alternative* or *complementary*) approach to nursing and health care.
5. Discuss the potential dangers associated with the use of OTC drugs, herbals, and dietary supplements.
6. Develop a nursing care plan related to OTC, herbal, and dietary supplement drug therapy and the nursing process.

KEY TERMS

Alternative medicine Herbal medicine, chiropractic, acupuncture, massage, reflexology, and any other therapies traditionally not emphasized in Western medical schools. (p. 89)

Complementary medicine Alternative medicine when used simultaneously with, rather than instead of, standard Western medicine. (p. 89)

Conventional medicine The practice of medicine as taught in Western medical schools. (p. 89)

Dietary supplement A product that contains an ingredient intended to supplement the diet, including vitamins, minerals, herbs, or other botanicals. (p. 88)

Herbal medicine The practice of using herbs to heal. (p. 89)

Herbs Plant components including bark, roots, leaves, seeds, flowers, fruit of trees, and extracts of these plants that are valued for their savory, aromatic, or medicinal qualities. (p. 89)

Iatrogenic effects Unintentional adverse effects that are caused by the actions of a prescriber, other health care professional, or by a specific treatment. (p. 89)

Integrative medicine Simultaneous use of both traditional and alternative medicine. (p. 89)

Legend drugs Medications that are not legally available without a prescription from a prescriber; also called *prescription drugs).* (p. 89)

Over-the-counter (OTC) drugs Medications that are legally available without a prescription. (p. 86)

Phytochemicals The pharmacologically active ingredients in herbal remedies. (p. 91)

OVER-THE-COUNTER DRUGS

Health care consumers are becoming increasingly involved in the diagnosis and treatment of common ailments. This has led to a great increase in the use of nonprescription or **over-the-counter (OTC) drugs.** More than 80 classes of OTC drugs are marketed to treat a variety of illnesses ranging from acne to cough and cold, pain relief, and weight control. There are currently more than 300,000 OTC products containing over 800 major active ingredients. OTC medications now account for about 60% of all medications used in the United States. Health care consumers use OTC drugs to treat or cure more than 400 different ailments. Over 40 medications that formerly required a prescription are now available OTC. Large numbers of older adults (40% to 87%) use one OTC product regularly, and 5.7% take five or more OTC or dietary supplements daily. Some of the most commonly used OTC products include acetaminophen (see Chapter 10), aspirin (see Chapter 44), ibuprofen (see Chapter 44), famotidine, omeprazole and antacids (see Chapter 50), loperamide (see Chapter 51), and cough and cold products (see Chapter 18).

In 1972, the FDA initiated an OTC Drug Review to ensure the safety and effectiveness of the OTC products available, as well as to establish appropriate labeling standards. As a result of this review, approximately one-third of the OTC products were determined to be safe and effective for their intended uses, and one-third were found to be ineffective. A small number were considered to be unsafe, and the remainder required submission of additional data. Products determined to be unsafe were removed from the market. Some established products that were found to be ineffective but not unsafe were "grandfathered" in and allowed to remain on the market. Many of these have gradually slipped into obscurity and are no longer sold. The FDA now requires new stricter "drug facts" labeling for OTC products that includes information on the following: purpose and uses of the product; specific warnings, including when the product should not be used under any circumstances; and when it is appropriate to consult a doctor or pharmacist. This labeling also describes side effects that could occur; substances or activities to avoid; dosage instructions; and active ingredients, warnings, storage information, and inactive ingredients.

Over 40 medications that were previously available by prescription only have been reclassified to OTC status. A drug must meet the criteria listed in Box 7-1 to be considered for reclassification. The required information is obtained from clinical trials and postmarketing safety surveillance data, which are submitted to the FDA by the manufacturer. Although this reclassification procedure has been criticized as overly time-consuming, it is structured to ensure that products reclassified to OTC status are safe and effective when used by the average consumer.

OTC status has many advantages over prescription status. Patients can conveniently and effectively self-treat many minor ailments. Some professionals argue that allowing patients to self-treat minor illnesses enables prescribers to spend more time caring for patients with serious health problems. Others argue that it delays patients from seeking medical care until they are very ill. Reclassification of a prescription drug as an OTC drug may increase out-of-pocket costs for many patients because third-party health insurance payers usually do not cover OTC products. However, overall health care costs tend to decrease when products are reclassified as OTC due to a direct reduction in drug costs, elimination of prescriber office visits, and avoidance of pharmacy dispensing fees. Some examples of drugs that have recently been reclassified as OTC products appear in Box 7-2.

The importance of patient education cannot be overstated. Many patients are inexperienced in the interpretation of medication labels (Figure 7-1), which results in misuse of the products. This lack of experience and possibly a lack of knowledge may lead to adverse events or drug interactions with prescription medications or other OTC medications. Small print on OTC package labels often complicates the situation, especially for older adults. According to a report by the Institute for Safe Medication Practices, parents gave children incorrect doses

---

BOX 7-1 Criteria for Over-the-Counter Status

Indication for Use
Consumer must be able to easily:
- Diagnose condition
- Monitor effectiveness
- Benefits of correct usage must outweigh risks.

Safety Profile
Drugs must have:
- Favorable adverse event profile
- Limited interaction with other drugs
- Low potential for abuse
- High therapeutic index*

Practicality for Over-the-Counter Use
Drugs must be:
- Easy to use
- Easy to monitor

*Ratio of toxic to therapeutic dosage.

BOX 7-2 Selected Reclassified Over-the-Counter Products

Analgesics
ibuprofen (Advil, Motrin)
naproxen sodium (Aleve, Naprosyn)

Histamine Blockers
H₁ Receptors
chlorpheniramine maleate (Chlor-Trimeton)
diphenhydramine hydrochloride (Benadryl)
fexofenadine (Allegra)
loratadine (Claritin)
cetirizine (Zyrtec)

H₂ Receptors
cimetidine (Tagamet HB)
famotidine (Pepcid AC)
nizatidine (Axid AR)
ranitidine (Zantac)

Nasal Steroids
Flonase Allergy Relief (fluticasone propionate)
Nasacort Allergy 24 HR (triamcinolone acetonide)

Proton Pump Inhibitors
Esomeprazole (Nexium-24)
lansoprazole (Prevacid-24)
omeprazole (Prilosec-OTC)

Smoking Deterrents
nicotine polacrilex gum (Nicorette)
nicotine transdermal patches (Nicoderm) (other dosage forms available)

Topical Medications
clotrimazole (Lotrimin)
butoconazole (Femstat)
miconazole (Monistat)
minoxidil solution and hydrocortisone acetate 1% cream (Rogaine)
terbinafine (Lamisil AT)

Weight Loss Products
orlistat (Alli)

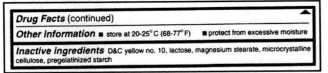

Drug Facts

Active ingredient (in each tablet)	Purpose
Chlorpheniramine maleate 2 mg..	............Antihistamine

Uses temporarily relieves these symptoms due to hay fever or other upper respiratory allergies: ■ sneezing ■ runny nose ■ itchy, watery eyes ■ itchy throat

Warnings
Ask a doctor before use if you have
■ glaucoma ■ a breathing problem such as emphysema or chronic bronchitis
■ trouble urinating due to an enlarged prostate gland

Ask a doctor or pharmacist before use if you are taking tranquilizers or sedatives

When using this product
■ drowsiness may occur ■ avoid alcoholic drinks
■ alcohol, sedatives, and tranquilizers may increase drowsiness
■ be careful when driving a motor vehicle or operating machinery
■ excitability may occur, especially in children

If pregnant or breast-feeding, ask a health professional before use.
Keep out of reach of children. In case of overdose, get medical help or contact a Poison Control Center right away.

Directions

adults and children 12 years and over	take 2 tablets every 4 to 6 hours; not more than 12 tablets in 24 hours
children 6 years to under 12 years	take 1 tablet every 4 to 6 hours; not more than 6 tablets in 24 hours
children under 6 years	ask a doctor

Drug Facts (continued)

Other information ■ store at 20-25°C (68-77°F) ■ protect from excessive moisture

Inactive ingredients D&C yellow no. 10, lactose, magnesium stearate, microcrystalline cellulose, pregelatinized starch

FIGURE 7-1 Example of an over-the-counter drug label. (From U.S. Food and Drug Administration: The new over-the-counter medicine label: take a look, 2011. Available at *www.fda.gov/ Drugs/EmergencyPreparedness/BioterrorismandDrug Preparedness/ucm133411.htm#.TnP-oVxzZyo.email.* Accessed July 7, 2014.)

of OTC fever medications more than 50% of the time. Use of OTC medications can be hazardous for patients with various chronic illnesses, including diabetes, hypertension, cardiovascular disease, and glaucoma. Patients are encouraged to read labels carefully and consult a qualified health care professional when in doubt.

OTC medications may relieve symptoms without necessarily addressing the cause of the disorder; this can cause delay in the effective management of chronic disease states or treatment of serious and/or life-threatening disorders.

OTC medications also have their own toxicity profiles. In 2008, the FDA issued recommendations that OTC cough and cold products not be used in children younger than 2 years of age. This followed numerous case reports of symptoms such as oversedation, seizures, tachycardia, and even death in toddlers medicated with such products. There is also evidence that such medications are simply not efficacious in small children. A follow-up study showed a dramatic decrease in young children's emergency department visits since the FDA recommendation (Shehab et al., 2010). Parents are advised to be mindful of how much medication they give and to be careful not to give two products that contain the same active ingredient(s).

Two other examples of OTC drug hazards include products containing acetaminophen (e.g., Tylenol) and nonsteroidal antiinflammatory drugs (NSAIDs) such as ibuprofen (e.g., Advil, Motrin) and naproxen (e.g., Aleve). Liver toxicity is associated with excessive doses of acetaminophen and is a leading cause of liver failure. Acetaminophen doses are not to exceed a total of 3 to 4 g/day. The use of NSAIDs is associated with gastrointestinal ulceration, myocardial infarction, and stroke. Patients may take excessive dosages of these and other OTC medications. In 2009, the FDA began requiring specific labeling for acetaminophen, aspirin, and NSAIDS to enhance consumer awareness of these risks.

Abuse can also be a potential hazard with the use of OTC drug products. Pseudoephedrine is found in a variety of cough and cold products (see Chapter 17); however, this drug is also used to manufacture the widely abused street drug methamphetamine. Because of the potential for abuse, products containing pseudoephedrine must be sold from behind the pharmacy counter. Many patients become addicted to OTC nasal sprays because they can cause rebound congestion and dependency. Dextromethorphan (used as a cough suppressant) is also commonly abused. It is known by the brand name of Robitussin, and abusing it is called *Robotripping*.

Several other OTC products can cause specific problems. The use of sympathomimetics (see Chapter 18) can cause problems in patients with type 1 diabetes and patients with hypertension or angina. Aspirin is not to be used in children as it can cause a rare condition called Reye's syndrome (see Chapter 44). Long-term use of antacids can result in constipation or impaction (see Chapter 50).

Normally, OTC medications are used only for short-term treatment of common minor illnesses. An appropriate medical evaluation is recommended for all chronic health conditions, even if the final decision is to prescribe OTC medications. Patient assessment includes questions regarding OTC drug use, including what conditions are being treated. Such questions may help uncover more serious ongoing medical problems. Inform patients that OTC drugs, including herbal products, are still medications. Their use may have associated risks depending on the specific OTC drugs used, concurrent prescription medications, and the patient's overall health status and disease states.

Health care professionals have an excellent opportunity to prevent common problems associated with the use of OTC drugs. Up to 60% of patients consult a health care professional when selecting an OTC product. Provide patients with information about choice of an appropriate product, correct dosing, common adverse effects, and drug interactions.

For specific information on various OTC drugs, see the appropriate drug chapters later in this text. (Table 7-1 provides cross-references to these chapters.)

HERBALS AND DIETARY SUPPLEMENTS

History

Dietary supplement is a broad term for orally administered alternative medicines and includes the category of herbal supplements. Dietary supplements are products that are intended to augment the diet and include vitamins, minerals, herbs or other botanicals, amino acids, and enzymes. Dietary supplements may be produced in many forms, such as tablets, capsules, liquids, and powders. These supplements may also be found in nutritional, breakfast, snack, or health food bars; drinks; and shakes.

TABLE 7-1	Common Over-the-Counter (OTC) Drugs	
Type of OTC Drug	**Examples**	**Where Discussed in this Book**
Acid-controlling drugs (H_2 blockers), antacids, and proton pump inhibitors	famotidine (Pepcid AC), ranitidine (Zantac); aluminum- and magnesium-containing products (Maalox, Mylanta); calcium-containing products (Tums), esomeprazole (Nexium 24), lansoprazole (Prevacid-24), omeprazole (Prilosec-OTC)	Chapter 50: Acid-Controlling Drugs
Antifungal drugs (topical)	clotrimazole (Lotrimin), miconazole (Monistat), terbinafine (Lamisil AT)	Chapter 56: Dermatologic Drugs
Antihistamines and decongestants	brompheniramine (Dimetapp), cetirizine (Zyrtec), chlorpheniramine (Theraflu), diphenhydramine (Benadryl), fexofenadine (Allegra), guaifenesin (Robitussin), loratadine (Claritin), pseudoephedrine (Sudafed)	Chapter 36: Antihistamines, Decongestants, Antitussives, and Expectorants
Eyedrops	artificial tears (Moisture Eyes)	Chapter 57: Ophthalmic Drugs
Hair growth drugs (topical)	minoxidil (Rogaine)	Chapter 56: Dermatologic Drugs
Pain-relieving drugs		
Analgesics	acetaminophen (Tylenol)	Chapter 10: Analgesic Drugs
Nonsteroidal antiinflammatory drugs	aspirin, ibuprofen (Advil, Motrin), naproxen sodium (Aleve)	Chapter 44: Antiinflammatory and Antigout Drugs
Nasal steroids	fluticasone (Flonase), triamcinolone (Nasacort)	Chapter 33: Adrenal Drugs

TABLE 7-2	Conventional Medicines Derived from Plants
Medicine*	**Plant**
atropine	*Atropa belladonna*
capsaicin	*Capsicum frutescens*
cocaine	*Erythroxylon coca*
codeine	*Papaver somniferum*
digoxin	*Digitalis lanata*
paclitaxel	*Taxis brevifolia*
scopolamine	*Datura fastuosa*
senna	*Cassia acutifolia*
vincristine	*Catharanthus roseus*

*Includes both over-the-counter and prescription drugs.

Herbs come from nature and have been used for thousands of years to help maintain good health. About 30% of all modern drugs are derived from plants (Table 7-2). In the early nineteenth century, scientific methods became more advanced and became the preferred means of healing. At this time, the practice of botanical healing was dismissed as quackery. **Herbal medicine** lost ground to new synthetic medicines during the early part of the twentieth century. In the 1960s, concerns were expressed over the **iatrogenic effects** of **conventional medicine.** These concerns, along with a desire for more self-reliance, led to a renewed interest in "natural health," and, as a result, the use of herbal products increased. In 1974, the World Health Organization encouraged developing countries to use traditional plant medicines. In 1978, the German equivalent of the FDA published a series of herbal recommendations known as the *Commission E monographs.* These monographs focus on herbs whose effectiveness for specific indications is supported by the research literature. Recognition of the increasing use of herbal products and **alternative medicine** led to the establishment of the Office of Alternative Medicine by the National Institutes of Health in 1992. This office was later renamed the National

Center for Complementary and Alternative Medicine (NCCAM). **Complementary medicine** refers to the simultaneous use of both traditional and alternative medicine. This practice is also referred to as **integrative medicine.** NCCAM classifies complementary and alternative medicine into the following five categories: (1) alternative medical systems, (2) mind-body interventions, (3) biologically based therapies, (4) manipulative and body-based methods, and (5) energy therapies.

Many controversies remain about the safety and control of herbals and dietary supplements. Their uses and touted advantages are widely publicized. As a result, these products are sold in grocery stores, pharmacies, health food stores, and fitness gyms and can even be ordered through television, radio, and the Internet. Adverse effects are considered to be minimal by the public as well as by the companies that sell these supplements. However, a false sense of security has been created because the view of the public tends to be that if a product is "natural," then it is safe. The information listed in this textbook regarding herbal products does not imply author or publisher endorsement of such products.

For many years, neither federal legislation nor the FDA provided any safeguards surrounding dietary supplements. Instead, manufacturers were responsible only for ensuring product safety. In 1993, the FDA threatened to remove dietary supplements from the market. The American public reacted with a massive letter-writing campaign to Congress, and the 103rd Congress responded by passing the Dietary Supplement and Health Education Act (DSHEA) of 1994. The DSHEA defined dietary supplements and provided a regulatory framework. In 2002, the U.S. Pharmacopeia, an independent organization that is the government's official standard-setting authority for dietary supplements, began certifying products that it had independently tested as part of its Dietary Supplement Verification Program.

A major difference between **legend drugs** (prescription drugs) and OTC products and dietary supplements is that the DSHEA requires no proof of efficacy and sets no standards

TABLE 7-3	Selected Herbs and Dietary Supplements and Their Possible Drug Interactions
Herb or Dietary Supplement	**Possible Drug Interaction**
Chamomile	Increased risk for bleeding with anticoagulants
Cranberry	Decreased elimination of many drugs that are renally excreted
Echinacea	Possible interference with or counteraction to immunosuppressant drugs and antivirals
Evening primrose	Possible interaction with antipsychotic drugs
Garlic	Possible interference with hypoglycemic therapy and the anticoagulant warfarin (Coumadin)
Gingko	May increase risk for bleeding with anticoagulants (warfarin, heparin) and antiplatelets (aspirin, clopidogrel)
Ginger root	At high dosages, possible interference with cardiac, antidiabetic, or anticoagulant drugs
Grapefruit	Decreases metabolism of drugs used for erectile dysfunction, estrogens, and some psychotherapeutic drugs. Increases risk for toxicity of immunosuppressants, HMG-CoA reductase inhibitors, and some psychotherapeutic drugs. Increases intensity and duration of effects of caffeine
Hawthorn	May lead to toxic levels of cardiac glycosides (e.g., digitalis)
Kava	May increase the effect of barbiturates and alcohol
Saw palmetto	May change the effects of hormones in oral contraceptive drugs, patches, or hormonal replacement therapies
St. John's wort	May lead to serotonin syndrome if used with other serotonergic drugs (e.g., selective serotonin reuptake inhibitors [see Chapter 16]). May interact with many drugs, including antidepressants, antihistamines, digoxin, immunosuppressants, theophylline, and warfarin.
Valerian	Increases central nervous system depression if used with sedatives

for quality control for supplements. In contrast, the FDA has specific and stringent requirements for manufacturers of legend drugs. However, in June 2007, the FDA announced that all manufacturers of dietary supplements would be required to comply with the same good manufacturing practices as prescription manufacturers. Under these new requirements, manufacturers must provide data that demonstrate product identity, composition, quality, purity, and strength of active ingredients. They must also demonstrate that products are free from contaminants such as microbes, pesticides, and heavy metals. Manufacturers of supplements may currently claim an effect but cannot promise a specific cure on the product label. Dietary supplements do not need approval from the FDA before they are marketed. The FDA posts warnings on herbal products on its website (http://www.fda.gov). Regulating agencies in Germany, France, the United Kingdom, and Canada require manufacturers to meet standards of herbal quality and safety.

Consumer Use of Dietary Supplements

Consumer use of dietary supplements is growing, with an estimated 50% of U.S. adults using some form of alternative medicine, despite the fact that one-fourth of the individuals who use them experience adverse reactions. Consumers use dietary supplements for the treatment and prevention of diseases and proactively to preserve health and wellness and boost the immune system. In addition, herbs may be used as adjunct therapy to support conventional pharmaceutical therapies.

Some herbal products may be used to treat minor conditions and illnesses (e.g., coughs, colds, stomach upset) in much the same way that conventional FDA-approved, OTC nonprescription drugs are used.

Safety

Dietary supplements, and especially herbal medicines, are often perceived as being natural and therefore harmless; however, this

is not the case. Many examples exist of allergic reactions, toxic reactions, and adverse effects caused by herbs. Some herbs have been shown to have possible mutagenic effects and to interact with drugs (Table 7-3). It is estimated that 70% of patients using dietary supplements do not disclose this to their health care providers. In addition, one study identified a relatively low level of knowledge of these products and their risks, even among regular users. This demonstrates the need for health care providers to develop a clinical knowledge base regarding these products and know where to find key information as the need arises. Because of underreporting, present knowledge may represent but a small fraction of potential safety concerns. Also, the FDA has limited oversight of how dietary supplements are prepared, whether herbal or not.

There are few published scientific data regarding the safety of dietary supplements. Two recent examples indicating some of the growing concerns about herbal remedies include the FDA warnings about possible liver toxicity with the use of kava and possible cardiovascular and stroke risks with the use of ephedra. The sale of ephedra was officially banned by the FDA in April 2004. Kava remains on the market despite a 2002 FDA consumer-warning letter regarding the risk for liver toxicity. Also, a state-of-the-art paper published in the *Journal of the American College of Cardiology* in 2010 suggests that many herbal products are best avoided in patients with cardiovascular diseases (Tachjian et al., 2010). Herbal products can increase bleeding risk with warfarin (see Chapter 26), potentiate digoxin toxicity (see Chapter 24), increase the effects of antihypertensive agents (see Chapter 22), and cause heart block or dysrhythmias (see Chapter 25).

Consumers are encouraged to report adverse effects to the FDA's MedWatch (800-332-1088). Other authoritative references that can be utilized for herbal information include Pharmacist's Letter/Prescriber's Letter Natural Medicines Comprehensive Database and Natural Standard, available at www.naturalstandard.com.

Level of Use

The FDA estimates that over 29,000 different dietary supplements are currently used in the United States, with approximately 1000 new products introduced annually. Estimates of the prevalence of dietary supplement use differ greatly. The wide disparity in these estimates is most likely due to the use of varying terminology (e.g., "herbs" versus "dietary supplements"). One recent estimate of the amount spent on dietary supplements was in excess of $20 billion annually in the United States. The use of botanical medicines is greater in other parts of the world than in the United States.

Herbal medicine is based on the premise that plants contain natural substances that can promote health and alleviate illness. The many different herbs in these preparations contain a wide variety of active phytochemicals (plant compounds). Some of the more common ailments and conditions treated with herbs are anxiety, arthritis, colds, constipation, cough, depression, fever, headache, infection, insomnia, intestinal disorders, premenstrual syndrome, menopausal symptoms, stress, ulcers, and weakness.

Herbal products constitute the largest growth area in retail pharmacy. Their use is increasing at a rate of 20% to 25% per year, which far exceeds the growth in the use of conventional drugs. Insurance plans and managed care organizations are beginning to offer reimbursement for alternative treatments. Some of the most commonly used herbal remedies are aloe, black cohosh, chamomile, echinacea, feverfew, garlic, ginger, ginkgo biloba, ginseng, goldenseal, hawthorn, St. John's wort, saw palmetto, and valerian. These products are covered in more detail in the Safety: Herbal Therapies and Dietary Supplements boxes that appear in the various drug chapters (see the inside back cover for a complete listing of these boxes with page numbers throughout the textbook).

NURSING PROCESS

ASSESSMENT

OVER-THE-COUNTER DRUGS

Nursing assessments are always important to perform, but they are especially important when a patient is self-medicating. Previous use of *OTC drugs* and the patient's response are important to note. Successes versus failures with drug therapies and self-medication, reading level, cognitive and developmental level, and motor abilities are other variables to be assessed.

Other assessment data include questioning about allergies to any of the ingredients of the drug. Include a list of all medications and substances used by the patient, including OTC drugs, prescription drugs, herbal products, vitamins, and minerals in the medication history. Also note use of alcohol, tobacco, and caffeine. Assess past and present medical history so that possible drug interactions, contraindications, and cautions are identified. Screen patients carefully before recommending an OTC drug because patients often assume that if a drug is sold OTC it is completely safe to take and without negative consequences. This is not true—OTC drugs can be just as lethal or problematic

---

⊕ PATIENT-CENTERED CARE: CULTURAL IMPLICATIONS   QSEN

Drug Responses and Cultural Factors

Responses to drugs—including over-the-counter (OTC) drugs, herbals, and dietary supplements—may be affected by beliefs, values, and genetics as well as by culture, race, and ethnicity (see Chapter 4 for more discussion of cultural considerations). As one example of the impact of culture on drug response and use, if patients who are Japanese experience nausea, vomiting, or bowel changes as adverse effects of OTC drugs, herbals, and/or dietary supplements, these often are not mentioned. The reason is that this culture finds it unacceptable to complain about gastrointestinal symptoms, and so they may go unreported to the point of causing risk to the patient.

Herbal and alternative therapies may also be used more extensively in some cultures than in others. Wide acceptance of herbal use without major concern for the effects on other therapies may be very problematic because of the many interactions of conventional drugs with herbals and dietary supplements. For example, the Chinese herb ginseng may inhibit or accelerate the metabolism of a specific medication and significantly affect the drug's absorption or elimination.

One genetic factor that has an influence on drug response is acetylation polymorphism; that is, prescription drugs, OTC drugs, herbals, and dietary supplements may be metabolized in different ways that are genetically determined and vary with race or ethnicity. For example, populations of European or African descent contain approximately equal numbers of individuals showing rapid and slow acetylation (which affects drug metabolism), whereas Japanese and Inuit populations may contain more rapid acetylators. See Chapter 4 for a more in-depth discussion of these specific genetic attributes.

From Yasuda SU, Zhang L, Huang SM: The role of ethnicity in variability in response to drugs: focus on clinical pharmacology studies. *Clinical Pharmacology and Therapeutics* 84(3):417-423, 2008.

⚡ SAFETY AND QUALITY IMPROVEMENT: PREVENTING MEDICATION ERRORS   QSEN

Measuring Over-the-Counter Liquid Medications Safely

The Institute for Safe Medication Practices (ISMP) sponsors ConsumerMedSafety. org, a website with the purpose of helping to protect consumers from medication errors. One safety focus is the measuring of over-the-counter liquid medications. Many people will use household measuring devices, such as teaspoons or tablespoons, to measure liquid medications. However, these devices are not calibrated for medicines and may deliver inaccurate doses. The website suggests these tips for accurate and safe measuring of liquid medications at home:

- Use the measuring device (cup or oral syringe) that comes with the OTC liquid medicine, not household measuring devices.
- If the medication does not come with a measuring device, ask the pharmacist to recommend one.
- If giving OTC liquid medications to a child, know the child's current weight. Many medications for children are dosed by weight, not by age.
- Wash the dosing device thoroughly after each dose, and store the medicine and the dosing device together.
- Do not use a dosing cup or syringe that was supplied for one medication for a different medication as this may lead to dosing errors.

For more information, see *www.consumermedsafety.org/tools-and-resources/medication-safety-tools-and-resources/consumer-medsafety-lists/item/601-ten-tips-for-measuring-over-the-counter-liquid-medications-safely.* Accessed April 12, 2015.

---

as prescription drugs if they are not taken properly or are taken in high dosages and without regard to directions (see discussion earlier in the chapter).

Assessment of the patient's knowledge about the components of self-medication, including the positive or negative consequences of the use of a given OTC drug, must be included. Assessment of the patient's (or caregiver's or family member's) level of knowledge and experience with OTC self-medication is critical to the patient's safety, as is assessment of attitudes toward and beliefs about their use, especially a too-casual attitude or a lack of respect for and concern about the use of OTC drugs. This is especially true if a casual attitude is combined with a lack of knowledge. Obviously this could result in overuse, overdosage, and potential complications. See Chapter 6 for more information on patient education.

Generally speaking, laboratory tests are not ordered before the use of OTC drugs, because they are self-administered and self-monitored. However, there are situations in which patients may be taking certain medications that react adversely with these drugs, and laboratory testing may be needed. Some patient groups are also at higher risk for adverse reactions to OTC drugs (as to most drugs in general), including pediatric and older adult patients; patients with single and/or multiple acute and chronic illnesses; those who are frail or in poor health, debilitated, or nutritionally deficient; and those with suppressed immune systems. OTC drugs must also be used with caution and may be contraindicated in patients with a history of renal, hepatic, cardiac, or vascular dysfunction. More assessment information for OTC drugs, herbals, and dietary supplements can be found in other chapters in this textbook when relevant (see Table 7-1). It is important to remember that consumer/patient safety and quality of care related to drug therapy of any kind begins with education. Thus, the best way for patients to help themselves is for them to learn how to assess each situation, weigh all the factors, and find out all they can about the OTC drug they wish to take *before* taking it!

HERBAL PRODUCTS AND DIETARY SUPPLEMENTS

Many *herbal products* and *dietary supplements* are readily available in drug, health food, and grocery stores as well as in home gardens, kitchens, and medicine cabinets. As noted earlier in the chapter, among the more commonly used herbals are aloe, black cohosh, chamomile, echinacea, feverfew, garlic, ginger, ginkgo biloba, ginseng, goldenseal, hawthorn, St. John's wort, saw palmetto, and valerian. Although patients generally self-administer these products and do not perform an assessment, in various settings you may be able to assess the patient through a head-to-toe physical examination, medical and nursing history, and medication history. Share assessment data and factors and variables to consider with the patient for the patient's safety. This sharing of assessment information allows you to be sure that the patient is taking the herbal product in as safe a manner as possible.

Many herbals and dietary supplements may lead to a variety of adverse effects. For example, some may cause dermatitis when used topically, whereas some taken systemically may be associated with kidney disorders such as nephritis. Therefore, for example, patients with existing skin problems or kidney dysfunction must seek medical advice before using certain herbals. It is also crucial to patient safety to consider any other contraindications, cautions, and potential drug-drug and drug-food interactions. See Table 7-3 for more information on drug interactions.

CASE STUDY

Safety: What Went Wrong? Over-the-Counter Drugs and Herbal Products

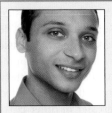 J.V., a 28-year-old graduate student, is at the student health clinic for a physical examination that is required before he goes on a research trip out of the country. As he completes the paperwork, he asks the nurse, "The form is asking about my medications. I don't have any prescribed medicines, but I take several herbal products and over-the-counter medicines. Do you need to know about these?"

1. How should the nurse answer J.V.?

   On the form, J.V. lists the following items:

   1 baby aspirin each day to prevent blood clots

   Sleep-Well herbal product with valerian at night if needed

   Benadryl as needed for allergies, especially at night

   Stress-Away herbal product with ginseng as needed

   Generic ibuprofen, 3 or 4 tablets three times a day for muscle aches from working out

   Memory Boost herbal product with ginkgo every morning

2. J.V. tells you that he has been wondering why he bruises so easily, and shows you some bruises on his arms and his knees. Examine the products on J.V.'s list, and state whether there are any concerns with interactions or adverse effects. You may need to refer to descriptions of the individual herbal products (see the inside back cover for a complete listing of Safety: Herbal Therapies and Dietary Supplements boxes located throughout the textbook) or to the appropriate drug chapters for more information. What do you think has happened?

3. Upon further questioning, J.V. remembers that he has had problems with "acid stomach" for about a year and takes Prilosec-OTC for that as needed. What concerns, if any, are there about this?

For answers, see *http://evolve.elsevier.com/Lilley*.

NURSING DIAGNOSES

Nursing diagnoses appropriate for the patient taking *OTC drugs, herbals,* and/or *dietary supplements* include the following (without related causes, because these are too numerous to include):

1. Activity intolerance
2. Acute pain
3. Chronic pain
4. Fatigue
5. Impaired memory
6. Impaired physical mobility
7. Ineffective health maintenance
8. Insomnia
9. Risk for injury
10. Urinary retention

PLANNING: OUTCOME IDENTIFICATION

1. Patient states that the actions of the OTC drug, herbal, and/or dietary supplement have been beneficial with relief of symptoms and increased physical mobility.
   - Patient experiences improving overall well-being and health status with minimal adverse effects or complications.

2. Patient experiences increased alertness and improved short-term and long-term memory with continued use of the herbal product and/or dietary supplement and reports any changes in orientation and/or memory.

3. Patient identifies measures to enhance urinary elimination patterns and minimize discomfort such as increasing fluid intake to 6 to 8 glasses of water per day, unless contraindicated, and taking time to void at regular intervals.

4. Patient describes nonpharmacologic approaches to the treatment of acute and chronic pain such as the use of hot or cold packs, physical therapy, massage, relaxation therapy, biofeedback, imagery, and hypnosis.

5. Patient takes measures to maximize energy levels through use of herbal and dietary supplements, sleeping 6 to 8 hours per night, increasing fluid intake, and intake of recommended daily amounts of food/caloric/protein.

6. Patient states that the actions of the OTC drug, herbal, and/or dietary supplement have been beneficial with relief of symptoms and subsequent increased ability to participate in activities of daily living (ADLs) as well as increase in other physical activities.

7. Patient states improved sleep patterns with increased hours of sleep (i.e., 6 to 8 hours of sleep) and less difficulty with onset of sleep while using OTC, herbal, and/or dietary supplement.

8. Patient experiences improved health maintenance with healthier behaviors as related to health maintenance by being more knowledgeable about self-medication administration with OTC drugs, herbals, and/or dietary supplements.
   - Patient inquires of pharmacist or health care provider about the safe daily healthy maintenance behavior of taking herbals and/or dietary supplements and deciphers information appropriately.

9. Patient remains free from injury and states the importance of taking drugs as directed and of immediately reporting any severe adverse effects or complications associated with the use of an OTC drug, herbal, and/or dietary supplement to the health care provider and pharmacist and to contact the poison control center, if needed.

IMPLEMENTATION

With *OTC drugs, herbals,* and *dietary supplements,* patient education is an important strategy to enhance patient safety. Patients need to receive as much information as possible about the safe

use of these products and to be informed that, even though these are not prescription drugs, they are *not* completely safe and are not without toxicity. Include information about safe use, frequency of dosing and dose, specifics of how to take the medication (e.g., with food or at bedtime), as well as strategies to prevent adverse effects, drug interactions, and toxicity in the patient instructions. Another consideration is the dosage form, because a variety are available such as liquids, tablets, enteric-coated tablets, transdermal patches, gum, and quick-dissolve tablets or strips. For transdermal patches (e.g., for smoking cessation), it is important to emphasize proper use and application. Make sure the patient is aware that the FDA does not regulate these products unless there is sufficient data to support a recall of the product. The companies that manufacture OTC drugs, herbals, and/or dietary supplements are not required to provide evidence of safety and effectiveness. As previously mentioned, many consumers believe that no risks exist if a medication is available OTC or is an herbal or a "natural" substance. See Box 7-1 for more information about the criteria for moving a drug from prescription to OTC status. The fact that a drug is an herbal or a dietary supplement does not mean that it can be safely administered to children, infants, pregnant or lactating women, or patients with certain health conditions that put them at risk.

EVALUATION

Patients taking *OTC drugs, herbals,* and/or *dietary supplements* need to carefully monitor themselves for unusual or adverse reactions and therapeutic responses to the medication to prevent overuse and overdosing. The range of therapeutic responses will vary, depending on the specific drug and the indication for which it is used. Therapeutic responses also vary depending on the drug's action; a few examples are decreased pain; decreased stiffness and swelling in joints; decreased fever; increased activity or mobility, as in increased ease of carrying out ADLs; increased hair growth; increased ease in breathing; decrease in constipation, diarrhea, bowel irritability, or gastrointestinal reflux or hyperacidity; resolution of allergic symptoms; decreased vaginal itching and discharge; increased healing; increased sleep; and decreased fatigue or improved energy. For more specific information about nursing diagnoses, planning with goals and outcome criteria, implementation, and evaluation related to various OTC drugs, herbals, and/or dietary supplements, see the appropriate chapters later in the book. Table 7-1 provides cross-references to these chapters.

QSEN   PATIENT-CENTERED CARE: PATIENT TEACHING

- Provide verbal and written information about how to choose an appropriate OTC drug or herbal or dietary supplement as well as information about correct dosing, common adverse effects, and possible interactions with other medications.
- Many patients believe that no risks exist if a medication is herbal and "natural" or if it is sold OTC, so provide adequate education about the drug or product as well as all the advantages and disadvantages of its use, because this is crucial to patient safety.

- Provide instructions on how to read OTC drug, herbal, and dietary supplement labels and directions. Encourage the reading of ingredients if using more than one product, as the ingredient/chemical may occur in both products. For example, a multivitamin supplement may contain ginseng, and taking additional ginseng supplements may lead to toxicity. Another example is with products containing acetaminophen (Tylenol). If the patient is taking acetaminophen and then also takes a cold/flu product, there may also be acetaminophen in that product, and consequently the risk of adverse effects and toxicity increases.

- Emphasize the importance of taking all OTC drugs, herbals, and dietary supplements with extreme caution, and being aware of all the possible interactions and/or concerns associated with the use of these products.
- Instruct the patient that all health care providers (e.g., nurses, dentists, osteopathic and chiropractic physicians) need to be aware about the use of any OTC drugs, herbals, and dietary supplements (and, of course, any prescription drug use).
- Encourage journaling of any improvement of symptoms noted with the use of a specific OTC drug, herbal, and/or dietary supplement.
- Encourage the use of appropriate and authoritative resources for patient information, such as a registered pharmacist,

literature provided from the drug company and pharmacist, and web-based information from reliable sites at an appropriate reading level for the patient (e.g., www.Webmd.com).

- Instruct the patient that all medications, whether an OTC drug, herbal, and/or dietary supplement, must be kept out of the reach of children and pets.
- Provide thorough instructions regarding the various dosage forms of OTC drugs, herbals, and dietary supplements. Provide specific instructions such as how to mix powders and how to properly use transdermal patches, inhalers, ointments, lotions, nose drops, ophthalmic drops, elixirs, suppositories, vaginal suppositories or creams, and all other dosage forms (see Chapter 9); also provide information about proper storage and cleansing of any equipment.

KEY POINTS

- Consumers use herbal products therapeutically for the treatment of diseases and pathologic conditions, prophylactically for long-term prevention of disease, and proactively for the maintenance of health and wellness.
- The FDA has established the MedWatch program to track adverse events and/or problems related to drug therapy. The toll-free number for reporting adverse effects of prescription drugs, OTC drugs, herbals, and dietary supplements is 800-332-1088. Nurses may report adverse events anonymously and without consequence via telephone. Adverse event reporting is also available inside of medical reference applications such as Epocrates or Medscape.

- Herbal products are not FDA-approved drugs, and therefore their labeling cannot be relied on to provide consumers and patients with adequate instructions for use or even information about warnings.
- The fact that a drug is an herbal product, dietary supplement, or OTC medication is no guarantee that it can be safely administered to children, infants, pregnant or lactating women, or patients with certain health conditions that may put them at risk.

NCLEX® EXAMINATION REVIEW QUESTIONS

1. The nurse is reviewing dietary supplements and recalls that the FDA requires manufacturers of dietary supplements to
   a. follow FDA standards for quality control.
   b. prove efficacy and safety of dietary supplements.
   c. identify the active ingredients on the label.
   d. obtain FDA approval before the products are marketed.
2. When educating patients about the safe use of herbal products, the nurse remembers to include which concept?
   a. Herbal and over-the-counter products are approved by the FDA and under strict regulation.
   b. Herbal products are tested for safety by the FDA and the U.S. Pharmacopeia.
   c. No adverse effects are associated with these products because they are natural and may be purchased without a prescription.
   d. Take the product with caution because labels may not contain reliable information.
3. When taking a patient's drug history, the nurse asks about use of over-the-counter drugs. The patient responds by saying, "Oh, I frequently take aspirin for my headaches, but I didn't mention it because aspirin is nonprescription." What is the nurse's best response?
   a. "That's true; over-the-counter drugs are generally not harmful."

   b. "Aspirin is one of the safest drugs out there."
   c. "Although aspirin is over the counter, it's still important to know why you take it, how much you take, and how often."
   d. "We need you to be honest about the drugs you are taking. Are there any others that you haven't told us about?"
4. When making a home visit to a patient who was recently discharged from the hospital, the nurse notes that she has a small pack over her chest and that the pack has a strong odor. She also is drinking herbal tea. When asked about the pack and the tea, the patient says, "Oh, my grandmother never used medicines from the doctor. She told me that this plaster and tea were all I would need to fix things." Which response by the nurse is most appropriate?
   a. "You really should listen to what the doctor told you if you want to get better."
   b. "What's in the plaster and the tea? When do you usually use them?"
   c. "These herbal remedies rarely work, but if you want to use them, then it is your choice."
   d. "It's fine if you want to use this home remedy, as long as you use it with your prescription medicines."

5. A patient tells the nurse that he has been using an herbal supplement that contains kava for several years to help him to relax in the evening. However, the nurse notes that he has a yellow tinge to his skin and sclera, and is concerned about liver toxicity. The nurse advises the patient to stop taking the kava and to see his health care provider for an examination. What else, if anything, should the nurse do at this time?
   a. Report this incident to MedWatch.
   b. Notify the state's pharmaceutical board.
   c. Contact the supplement manufacturer.
   d. No other action is needed.
6. The nurse is reviewing the drug history of a patient, and during the interview the patient asks, "Why are some drugs over-the-counter and others are not?" The nurse keeps in mind that criteria for over-the-counter status include: *(Select all that apply.)*
   a. The condition must be diagnosed by a health care provider.
   b. The benefits of correct usage of the drug outweigh the risks.

c. The drug has limited interaction with other drugs.
d. The drug is easy to use.
e. The drug company sells OTC drugs at lower prices.
7. A patient comes to the clinic complaining of elbow pain after an injury. He states that he has been taking two pain pills, eight times a day, for the past few days. The medication bottle contains acetaminophen, 325-mg tablets. Calculate how much medication he has been taking per day. Is this a safe dose of this medication?
8. The nurse is reviewing definitions for a pharmacology review class. Which of these products would be categorized as "legend drugs?" *(Select all that apply.)*
   a. acetaminophen (Tylenol)
   b. warfarin (Coumadin)
   c. gingko biloba
   d. morphine sulfate
   e. diphenhydramine (Benadryl)

1. c, 2. d, 3. c, 4. b, 5. a, 6. b, c, d, 7. 5200 mg/day, No, 8. b, d

CRITICAL THINKING AND PRIORITIZATION QUESTIONS

1. The nurse is discussing over-the-counter drugs and herbal products with neighbors. One neighbor comments, "Oh, the over-the-counter drugs and herbals are safe. As long as you use the recommended amounts, there won't be any bad side effects." What is the nurse's best response?
2. A patient tells the clinic nurse that he has been taking a "blood thinner" for several months and wants to ask about taking garlic capsules to reduce his blood pressure. He says

his sister uses it and it "works wonders." He also says, "I think it would be safe because I can buy it at the drug store. They wouldn't sell harmful drugs." What is the nurse's best response? (You may need to look up the drug warfarin and the herbal product elsewhere in the textbook.)

For answers see *http://evolve.elsevier.com/Lilley.*

ⓔ EVOLVE WEBSITE

http://evolve.elsevier.com/Lilley
- Animations
- Answer Keys for Textbook Case Studies and Textbook Critical Thinking and Prioritization Questions

- Content Updates
- Key Points
- Review Questions
- Student Case Studies

Gene Therapy and Pharmacogenomics

http://evolve.elsevier.com/Lilley

OBJECTIVES

When you reach the end of this chapter, you will be able to do the following:

1. Understand the basic terms related to genetics and drug therapy.
2. Briefly discuss the major concepts of genetics as an evolving segment of health care, such as principles of genetic inheritance; deoxyribonucleic acid (DNA), ribonucleic acid (RNA), and their functioning; the relationship of DNA to protein synthesis; and the importance of amino acids.
3. Describe the basis of the Human Genome Project and its impact on the role of genetics in health care.
4. Discuss the different gene therapies currently available.
5. Differentiate between direct and indirect forms of gene therapy.
6. Identify the regulatory and ethical issues related to gene therapy as related to nursing and health care professionals.
7. Briefly discuss pharmacogenomics and pharmacogenetics.
8. Discuss the evolving role of professional nurses as related to gene therapy.

KEY TERMS

Acquired disease Any disease triggered by external factors and not *directly* caused by a person's genes (e.g., an infectious disease, noncongenital cardiovascular diseases). (p. 97)

Alleles The two or more alternative forms of a gene. (p. 97)

Chromosomes Structures in the nuclei of cells that contain threads of deoxyribonucleic acid (DNA), which transmit genetic information, and are associated with ribonucleic acid (RNA) molecules and synthesis of protein molecules. (p. 97)

Gene The biologic unit of heredity; a segment of a DNA molecule that contains all of the molecular information required for the synthesis of a biologic product such as an RNA molecule or an amino acid chain (protein molecule). (p. 97)

Gene therapy New therapeutic technologies that directly target human genes in the treatment or prevention of illness. (p. 98)

Genetic disease Any disorder caused directly by a genetic mechanism. (p. 97)

Genetic material DNA or RNA molecules or portions thereof. (p. 97)

Genetic polymorphisms (PMs) Variants that occur in the chromosomes of 1% or more of the general population. (p. 99)

Genetic predisposition The presence of certain factors in a person's genetic makeup, or *genome* that increase the individual's likelihood of developing one or more diseases. (p. 97)

Genetics The study of the structure, function, and inheritance of genes. (p. 97)

Genome The complete set of genetic material of any organism. (p. 98)

Genomics The study of the structure and function of the genome, and the way genes and their products work in both health and disease. (p. 98)

Genotype The particular alleles present at a given site on the chromosomes that determine a specific genetic trait for that organism (compare *phenotype*). (p. 97)

Heredity The characteristics and qualities that are genetically passed from one generation to the next through reproduction. (p. 97)

Human Genome Project (HGP) A scientific project of the U.S. Department of Energy and National Institutes of Health to describe in detail the entire genome of a human being. (p. 98)

Inherited disease Genetic disease that results from defective alleles passed from parents to offspring. (p. 97)

Nucleic acids Molecules of DNA and RNA in the nucleus of every cell. DNA makes up the chromosomes and encodes the genes. (p. 97)

Personalized medicine The use of molecular and genetic characterizations of both the disease process and the patient for the customization of drug therapy. (p. 99)

Pharmacogenetics A general term for the study of the genetic basis for variations in the body's response to drugs, with a focus on variations related to a single gene. (p. 99)

Pharmacogenomics A branch of *pharmacogenetics* (see earlier) that involves the survey of the entire genome to detect multigenic (multiple-gene) determinants of drug response. (p. 99)

Phenotype The expression in the body of a genetic trait that results from a person's particular *genotype* (see earlier) for that trait. (p. 97)

Recombinant DNA (rDNA) DNA molecules that have been artificially synthesized or modified in a laboratory setting. (p. 98)

OVERVIEW

Genetic processes are a highly complex part of physiology and are far from completely understood. Genetic research is one of the most active branches of science today. Expected outcomes of this research include a deeper knowledge of the genetic influences on disease, along with the development of gene-based therapies. In 1996, the National Coalition for Health Professional Education in Genetics (NCHPEG) was founded as a joint project of the American Medical Association, the American Nurses Association, and the National Human Genome Research Institute *(www.nchpeg.org)*. The purpose of NCHPEG is to promote the education of health professionals and the public regarding advances in applied genetics.

Since the 1960s, published literature has described the role of nursing in genetics and genetic research. The Genetics Nursing Network was formed in 1984 and later became the International Society of Nurses in Genetics (ISONG). In 1997, the American Nurses Association designated genetics nursing as an official nursing specialty. In 2001, ISONG approved formation of the Genetic Nursing Credentialing Commission (GNCC). The growing understanding of genetics is creating demand for clinicians in all fields who can educate patients and provide clinical care that tailors health care services to each patient's inherent genetic makeup. This reality also calls for increasing the level of genetics education in nursing school curricula as well as continuing nursing education.

BASIC PRINCIPLES OF GENETIC INHERITANCE

Nucleic acids are biochemical compounds consisting of two types of molecules: deoxyribonucleic acid (DNA) and ribonucleic acid (RNA). DNA molecules make up the **genetic material** that is passed between all types of organisms during reproduction. A chromosome is a long strand of DNA that is contained in the nuclei of cells. DNA molecules, in turn, act as the template for the formation of RNA molecules, from which proteins are made. Humans normally have 23 pairs of **chromosomes**. **Alleles** are the alternative forms of a **gene** that can vary with regard to a specific genetic trait. Genetic traits can be desirable (e.g., lack of allergies) or undesirable (e.g., predisposition toward a specific disease). An allele may be dominant or recessive for a given genetic trait. A person's **genotype** for a given trait determines whether or not a person manifests that trait, or the person's **phenotype**. Genetic traits that are passed on differently to male and female offspring are said to be sex-linked traits because they are carried on either the X or Y chromosome. For example, hemophilia genes are carried by females but manifest as a bleeding disorder only in males. Hemophilia is an example of an **inherited disease**, that is, a disease caused by

passage of a genetic defect from parents to offspring. A more general term is **genetic disease**, which is any disease caused by a genetic mechanism. Not all genetic diseases are inherited. Chromosomal abnormalities (aberrations) can also occur spontaneously during embryonic development. In contrast, an **acquired disease** is any disease that develops in response to external factors and is not directly related to a person's genetic makeup. Genetics can play an indirect role in acquired disease, however. For example, atherosclerotic heart disease is often acquired in middle or later life. Many people have certain genes in their cells that increase the likelihood of this condition. This is known as a **genetic predisposition**. In some cases, a person may be able to offset his or her genetic predisposition by lifestyle choices, such as consuming a healthy diet and exercising to avoid developing heart disease.

Current literature differentiates "old genetics," which focused on single-gene inherited diseases such as hemophilia, from the "new genetics." The new genetic perspective recognizes that common diseases, including Alzheimer's disease, cancer, and heart disease, are the product of complex relationships between genetic and environmental factors. Environmental factors, such as diet or toxic exposures, can initiate or worsen disease processes. Research into disease treatment is beginning to look at genetically tailored therapy.

DISCOVERY, STRUCTURE, AND FUNCTION OF DNA

Genetics is the study of the structure, function, and inheritance of genes. **Heredity** refers to the qualities that are genetically transferred from one generation to the next during reproduction. A major turning point in the understanding of genetics came in 1953, when Drs. James Watson and Francis Crick first reported the chemical structures of human genetic material and named the primary biochemical compound deoxyribonucleic acid (DNA). They later received a Nobel Prize for their discovery.

It is now recognized that DNA is the primary molecule in the body that serves to transfer genes from parents to offspring. DNA molecules contain four different organic bases, which are linked to a type of sugar molecule known as deoxyribose. In turn, these sugar molecules are linked to a "backbone" chain of phosphate molecules, which results in the classic double-helix structure of two side-by-side spiral macromolecular chains. An important related biomolecule is ribonucleic acid (RNA). RNA has a chemical structure similar to that of DNA. RNA most commonly occurs as a single-stranded molecule. Certain new drug therapies involve synthetic analogues of both nucleosides and nucleotides (see Chapters 40, 45, 46, and 47). A related field is targeted drug therapy. Targeted drug therapy focuses on modifying the function of immune system cells (T cells and B cells) and biochemical mediators of immune response (cytokines). Current examples of targeted drug therapy are presented in Chapters 45, 46 and 48.

An organism's entire DNA structure is its **genome**, and refers to all the genes in an organism taken together. **Genomics** is the relatively new science of determining the location (mapping), structure (DNA base sequencing), identification (genotyping), and expression (phenotyping) of individual genes along the entire genome, and determining their function in both health and disease processes.

Protein Synthesis

Protein molecules drive the functioning of all biochemical reactions. Protein synthesis is the primary function of DNA in human cells. Mutations, undesired changes in DNA sequence, can affect the shape of protein molecules and impair or destroy their functioning.

In the cell nuclei, the double strands of DNA uncoil and separate, and a strand of mRNA forms on each separate DNA strand. This process is called *transcription* of the DNA. These mRNA molecules then detach from their corresponding DNA strands, leave the cell nucleus, and enter the cytoplasm, where they are then "read," or translated, by the ribosomes. Ribosomes are composed of a second type of RNA known as *ribosomal* RNA (rRNA). This translation process involves molecules of a third type of RNA, *transfer* RNA (tRNA). This whole process results in the creation of chains of multiple amino acids (polypeptide chains), which are known as protein molecules. Proteins include hormones, enzymes, immunoglobulins, and numerous other biochemical molecules that regulate processes throughout the body. They are involved in both healthy physiologic processes and the pathophysiologic processes of many diseases. Manipulation of genetic material, as in gene therapy, can theoretically modify the synthesis of these proteins and therefore aid in the treatment of disease.

Genetic testing and counseling are important for patients. Genetic counseling allows patients who are at risk for an inherited disorder to be advised of the consequences and nature of the disorder, the probability of developing or transmitting it, and the options open to them. One of the most common genetic testing is for the *BRCA* gene for breast cancer. Other common examples of genetic testing are prenatal testing to determine if a future child may have cystic fibrosis or Down syndrome.

Human Genome Project

In 1990, an unprecedented genetic research project began in the United States, the **Human Genome Project (HGP)**, and was coordinated by the U.S. Department of Energy and the National Institutes of Health (NIH). The project was completed in 2003, two years ahead of schedule. The goals of this project were to identify the estimated 30,000 genes and 3 billion base pairs in the DNA of an entire human genome. Additional goals included developing new tools for genetic data analysis and storage, transferring newly developed technologies to the private sector, and addressing the inherent ethical, legal, and social issues involved in genetic research and clinical practice.

GENE THERAPY

Background

Gene therapy is an experimental technique that uses genes to treat or prevent disease. It allows doctors to treat a disorder by inserting a gene into a patient's cells instead of using drugs or surgery. Researchers are testing several approaches to gene therapy, including:

- Replacing a mutated gene with a healthy copy of the gene
- Introducing a new gene into the body to help fight a disease
- Inactivating a mutated gene that is functioning improperly

Although hundreds of gene therapy clinical trials have been approved by the U.S. Food and Drug Administration (FDA), no gene therapy to date has been approved for routine treatment of disease in the United States. The goal of gene therapy is to transfer exogenous genes that will either provide a temporary substitute for, or initiate permanent changes in, the patient's own genetic functioning to treat a given disease. Originally projected to provide treatment primarily for inherited genetic diseases, gene therapy techniques are now being researched for treatment of acquired illnesses such as cancer, cardiovascular diseases, diabetes, infectious diseases, and substance abuse. In the future, *in utero* gene therapy may be used to prevent the development of serious diseases as part of prenatal care for the unborn infant. During gene therapy, segments of DNA are injected into the patient's body in a process called *gene transfer*. These artificially produced DNA splices are also known as **recombinant DNA (rDNA)**.

There are limitations to gene therapy, and the determination of an ideal gene transfer method remains a major challenge for gene therapy researchers. Viruses used for gene transfer can induce viral disease and can be immunogenic in the human host. The proteins produced by artificial methods can be immunogenic. Figure 8-1 provides a clinical example of the potential use of gene therapy.

Current Application

One indirect form of gene therapy is well established and is called *rDNA technology*. It involves the use of rDNA vectors in the laboratory to make recombinant forms of drugs, especially biologic drugs such as hormones, vaccines, antitoxins, and monoclonal antibodies. The most common example is the use of the *Escherichia coli* bacterial genome to manufacture a recombinant form of human insulin. When the human insulin gene is inserted into the genome of the bacterial cells, the resulting culture artificially generates human insulin on a large scale. Although this insulin must be isolated and purified from its bacterial culture source, the majority of the world's medical insulin supply has been produced by this method for well over a decade.

Regulatory and Ethical Issues Regarding Gene Therapy

Gene therapy research is inherently complex and can also carry great risks for its recipients. Thus, the issue of patient safety becomes significant. Research subjects who receive gene therapy often have a life-threatening illness, such as cancer, which may

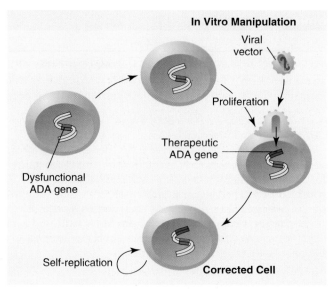

In Vitro Manipulation

Viral vector

Proliferation

Therapeutic ADA gene

Dysfunctional ADA gene

Self-replication

Corrected Cell

FIGURE 8-1 Gene therapy for adenosine deaminase (ADA) deficiency attempts to correct this immunodeficiency state. The viral vector containing the therapeutic gene is inserted into the patient's lymphocytes. These cells can then make the ADA enzyme. (From Lewis SL, Dirksen SR, Heitkemper MM, et al: Medical-surgical nursing: assessment and management of clinical problems, ed 8, St Louis, 2011, Elsevier.)

justify the risks involved. The FDA must review and approve all human clinical gene therapy trials, as it does for any type of drug therapy.

Any institution that conducts any type of research involving human subjects must have an institutional review board, whose purpose is to protect research subjects from unnecessary risks. Also required for institutions engaging in gene therapy research is an institutional biosafety committee. The role of this committee is to ensure compliance with the *NIH Guidelines for Research Involving Recombinant DNA Molecules.*

A major ethical issue related to gene therapy is that of eugenics. Eugenics is the intentional selection before birth of genotypes that are considered more desirable than others. For similar reasons, the prospect of being able to manipulate genes in human germ cells (sperm and eggs) is also a potential ethical hazard of gene therapy. Because of ethical concerns such as these, gene therapy research in the United States is limited to somatic cells only. Gene therapy in germ-line (reproductive) cells is currently not approved for funding by the National Institutes of Health. This limitation remains despite arguments from those who believe that human germ-cell research could potentially yield cures for many serious chronic illnesses and disabilities, such as Parkinson's disease and spinal paralysis.

PHARMACOGENETICS AND PHARMACOGENOMICS

Pharmacogenetics is a general term for the study of genetic variations in drug response and focuses on single-gene variations. A related science that pertains more directly to the HGP is **pharmacogenomics**. Pharmacogenomics is the combination of two scientific disciplines: pharmacology and genomics. Pharmacogenomics involves how genetics (genome) affect the body's response to drugs. Pharmacogenomics offer physicians the opportunity to individualize drug therapy based on a patient's genetic makeup. The ultimate goal is to predict patient drug response and proactively tailor drug selection and dosages for optimal treatment outcomes. Warfarin is an anticoagulant drug that is used to prevent blood clots (see Chapter 26). Research has shown that people with certain genetic variations (*CYP2C9*2* or *CYP2C9*3* alleles) are at increased risk for bleeding and require lower doses than those without the variation. In addition, variations in the gene that encodes *VKORC1* may make a patient more or less sensitive to warfarin. This genetic variation occurs most frequently in the Asian population. Several new drugs have been approved recently that target certain genes, including Ivacaftor (Kalydeco) for the treatment of cystic fibrosis and dabrafenib (Tafinlar) for the treatment of melanoma.

Individual differences in alleles that occur in at least 1% of a population are known as **genetic polymorphisms (PMs)**. The word *polymorphism* literally means "many forms." Polymorphisms are considered to be too frequent to result from random genetic mutations. Polymorphisms that alter the amount or actions of drug-metabolizing enzymes can alter the reactions to medications. Known examples include those PMs that affect the metabolism of certain antimalarial drugs, the antituberculosis drug isoniazid, and the variety of drugs that are metabolized by the subtypes of cytochrome (CYP) enzymes. Differences in CYP enzymes (see Chapter 2) are the best-studied PM effects thus far. Depending on their existing genes for these enzymes, patients can be genetically classified as "poor" or "rapid" metabolizers of CYP-metabolized drugs such as warfarin, phenytoin, codeine, and quinidine. With warfarin and phenytoin, a rapid metabolizer may need a higher dose of medication for the same effect, whereas a lower dose may be best for a poor metabolizer. With codeine, a poor metabolizer may actually need a higher dose to get the same analgesic effect that occurs when codeine is metabolized to morphine. In contrast, a rapid metabolizer may convert codeine to morphine too quickly, resulting in oversedation, and a lower dose may be sufficient. Because CYP enzymes are known to vary among racial and ethnic groups, the principle of "cultural safety" becomes one of the imperatives for routine gene-based drug dosing.

Studying both the genome of the patient and the genetic features of the pathology (e.g., tumor cells, infectious organisms) before treatment could allow for customized drug selection and dosing. Such analysis could permit the avoidance of drugs not likely to be effective as well as optimization of drug dosages to minimize the risk for adverse drug effects. These applications of pharmacogenomics are examples of **personalized medicine**.

Table 8-1 lists several examples of current clinical applications of pharmacogenomics.

APPLICATION OF THE NURSING PROCESS AS RELATED TO GENETIC PRINCIPLES

As noted previously, the recognition that genetic factors contribute, at some level, to most diseases continues to grow. Thus,

TABLE 8-1   Clinical Applications of Pharmacogenomics

Genetic Technique	Application
Genotyping for the presence of the CYP2D6 isoenzyme and for *CYP2D6* alleles determining whether patients are poor, intermediate, extensive, or ultra-rapid metabolizers related to these enzymes (under study)	*Psychiatry* and *general medicine:* Helps guide the prescribing of selected medications such as anticoagulants, immunosuppressants, antidepressants, antipsychotics, mood stabilizers, anticonvulsants, beta blockers, and antidysrhythmics
Genotyping for the presence of the *p-glycoprotein* drug transport protein (under study)	*Cardiology, infectious diseases, oncology, and other practice areas:* Assists in drug selection and dosing for drugs such as digoxin, antiretrovirals, and antineoplastics
Genotyping for variations in beta-adrenergic receptors (under study)	*Pulmonology:* Determines which asthma patients are more or less responsive to beta-agonist therapy (e.g., albuterol) and which patients might benefit from other types of drug therapy
Genotyping for the presence of the *HER2/neu* protooncogene	*Oncology:* Identifies a subset of breast cancer patients whose tumors express this gene, which indicates their suitability for treatment with the cancer drug trastuzumab (Herceptin)
Viral genotyping of hepatitis C viruses (under study)	*Infectious diseases:* Can determine whether a particular infection warrants 26 versus 48 weeks of drug therapy (thereby reducing both costs and adverse drug effects)
Genotyping for the presence of factor V gene mutation	*Women's health:* Identifies women with a 7 to 100 times greater risk of thrombosis with oral contraceptive use compared to women without the mutation
Genotyping for the presence of sodium channels associated with renin-angiotensin receptors and adrenal gland receptors	*Cardiology:* Allows refined antihypertensive drug selection
Race-based drug selection	*Cardiology:* Indicates use of the drug isosorbide dinitrate/hydralazine (BiDil) for treatment of hypertension in African-American patients due ultimately to genotypic variations in this patient population

CYP2D6, Cytochrome P-450 enzyme subtype 2D6; *HER2/neu,* human epidermal growth factor receptor 2.

genetic influences on health, including the interaction of genetic and environmental (non-genetic) factors, will routinely affect nursing care delivery. In general, it is expected that in the next few years genetic research will move from the laboratory to more clinical practice settings.

Nurses in general practice settings will not be expected to perform in-depth genetic testing or counseling. Nurses—or other health care providers—with specialty certification in the field of genetics will conduct genetic testing and counseling. However, all nurses will need to have a working knowledge of relevant genetic principles. In this era of the "new genetics" paradigm, nurses are fully aware of the fact that nearly all diseases have a genetic component. Conditions such as myocardial infarction, cancer, mental illness, diabetes, and Alzheimer's disease are now viewed in a different light because of the known complex interactions between a number of factors, including the influence of one or more genes and a variety of environmental exposures for patients. For more information about the need for more genetic content within undergraduate nursing education curriculum, see the Evidence-Based Practice box.

There are several other applicable skills regarding genetics as related to the nursing process. It is during the assessment phase of patient care that the nurse may uncover factors that may point to a risk for genetic disorders. Also, during the initial assessment, the nurse needs to obtain the patient's personal and family history. The family history is most effective if it covers at least three generations and includes the current and past health status of each family member. Assessment of factors possibly indicating an increased risk for genetic disorders is also important. A few examples of such factors include a higher incidence of a particular disease or disorder in the patient's family than in the general population; diagnosis of a disease in family members at an unusually young age; or diagnosis of a family member with an unusual form of cancer or with more than one type of cancer.

It is also important to inquire about any unusual reactions to a drug—on the part of either the patient, family members, significant others, and/or caregivers. An unusual or other than expected reaction to a drug in family members may point to a difference in the patient's ability to metabolize certain drugs. As indicated earlier in the chapter (as well as in Chapter 2), genetic factors may alter a patient's metabolism of a particular drug, resulting in either increased or decreased drug action. Each and every time a medication is administered, the patient's response to that drug must be assessed. Any unusual medication responses in a patient may point to a need for further investigation. Once a genetic variation is known, drug therapy may be adjusted accordingly.

As DNA chip technology becomes more affordable and accessible, it will be possible for patients to know in advance their relative risks for different diseases in later life. Genotype testing to identify a patient's drug-metabolizing enzymes will help prescribers better predict a patient's response to drug therapy.

Teaching about genetic testing and counseling may be another responsibility expected of the nurse. Patients will have questions and concerns about genetic testing and other issues. Nurses in general practice are not experts in genetic issues. However, the nurse may help with suggestions about genetic counseling, if appropriate. If genetic testing is ordered, the nurse may be a part of the testing process and will need to ensure that the informed decision-making and consent procedure has been carried out correctly.

Maintaining privacy and confidentiality is of utmost importance during genetic testing and counseling. The patient is the one who decides whether to include or exclude any family members from the discussion and from knowledge of the results of genetic testing. The patient needs to be reminded that he or she is not required to undergo the genetic test and that the patient has the right to disclose or withhold test results from anyone. Nurses must protect against improper disclosure of information to other family members, friends of the family, other health care providers, and insurance providers. Nurses share the responsibility with other health care providers to protect patients and their families against the misuse of the patients' genetic information. Other responsibilities of the professional nurse may include development of clinical and social policy such as genetic nondiscrimination and prenatal testing policies, testing of genetic products for reliability, and tasks in genetic informatics to meet the challenge of sifting through a continually expanding body of knowledge.

SUMMARY

Increasing scientific understanding of genetic processes is expected to revolutionize modern health care in many ways. The artificial manipulation and transfer of genetic material, although not yet a standard treatment for disease, is the focus of over 300 current human clinical gene therapy trials. The spectrum of diseases that may eventually be treatable by

QSEN EVIDENCE-BASED PRACTICE

Integrating Genomics into Undergraduate Nursing Education

Review

Scientists continue to make discoveries that contribute to the knowledge base and understanding of how human health and disease are impacted by genomics. No matter the setting of health care delivery, genomics will continue to change the approach to many aspects of medicine. The nursing profession, in order to keep up with these changes, needs to emphasize the importance and significance of genomics in their approaches to education and practice. Genomics is integral in the diagnosis, treatment, and prevention of disease. The purpose of this review of research and literature was to show the significance for the need to prepare the next generation of nurses. Additionally, faculty are now confronted with the challenge of integrating and incorporating genomics into nursing curriculum. This article and review presents a discussion on meeting of this challenge.

Type of Evidence

The organizing construct of this review includes steps to initiate curricular changes on how to include genomics into nursing curriculum. The question is whether it is more effective to create a genomic curriculum thread versus a stand-alone course (on genomics). The evidence presented is based on information gathered from a review of the literature as well as curriculum changes by the authors.

Results of the Study

Some of the models for integrating genomics into undergraduate nursing curriculum include the following: integration with faculty-initiated change; creating a curriculum thread focused on genomics; developing a stand-alone required or elective course; clinical practicums and/or simulation, and incorporating printed materials (bulletin boards) and/or technology (clickers, Web Quests, blogs). In recognition of the advances in genomics, there must be an increasing emphasis on the integration of this content into professional nursing practice, and more importantly, nursing education. Information must be included within didactic courses and then reinforced in the context of clinical settings while also using current technological advances/resources.

Link of Evidence to Nursing Practice

There is an undeniable need to prepare our next generation of nurse clinicians in the world of genomics. This need begins with the change in undergraduate nursing curriculum with faculty participation from the beginning of all planning and change. With application of the nursing process to nursing research and nursing education, assessment of faculty knowledge must be followed by implementation of a plan for integrating genetics and genomics into nursing courses and clinical experiences. Further research of a multifaceted approach with use of didactic courses, clinical practicum with various delivery elements, and current platforms is needed for delineating the most effective ways of presenting this crucial content in undergraduate nursing programs.

Daack-Hirsch S, Dieter C, Quinn Griffin MT: Integrating genomics into undergraduate nursing education, *J Nurs Scholarsh* 43(3):223-230, 2011.

CASE STUDY

Patient-Centered Care: Genetic Counseling

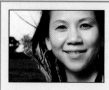

During the nurse's assessment of a newly admitted 38-year-old patient, the patient tells the nurse, "I'm allergic to codeine. Whenever I take it, it just knocks me out!" The patient tells the nurse that codeine does the same thing to all of her sisters. She insists that she's been allergic to codeine all of her life.

1. Does the patient have an actual allergy to codeine? What else could be happening?

   The next day, the patient's oncologist comes in and explains the results of a genetic test that was performed on an outpatient basis. The patient agrees to allow the nurse to sit in on the conversation. The physician tells

the patient that she has a type of gene that indicates a strong chance of developing breast cancer within the next 5 years. The oncologist recommends that she undergo a bilateral mastectomy soon to avoid the possibility of developing breast cancer and suggests that she share this information with her sisters and her daughter, who is 18 years old. After the physician leaves, the patient tells the nurse, "I don't know what to do. I haven't talked to one of my sisters for years and I just know she won't believe me. I also don't want to worry my daughter. She is so young, and I'm sure she's too young to get cancer."

2. Should the nurse tell the patient's sister and daughter? Explain your answer.

3. What is the best way for the nurse to handle this situation?

gene therapy includes inherited diseases that are present from birth, disabilities such as paralysis from spinal cord injuries, and life-threatening illnesses such as cancer. The science of pharmacogenomics has already identified some of the genetic nuances in how different individuals' bodies metabolize drugs to their benefit or harm. Continued study in this area is expected to result in proactive customization of drug therapy to promote therapeutic benefits while minimizing or eliminating toxic effects. Genetic procedures and therapeutic techniques will likely become an increasing part of nursing practice as well as of health care delivery in general.

KEY POINTS

- Genetic processes are a highly complex facet of human physiology, and genetics is becoming an integral part of health care that holds much promise in the form of new treatments for alterations in health.
- The Human Genome Project (HGP), spearheaded by the U.S. Department of Energy and the NIH, describes in detail the entire genome of a human individual.
- Basic genetic inheritance is carried by 23 pairs of chromosomes in each of the somatic cells; one pair of chromosomes in each cell is the *sex chromosomes*, identified as XX for females and XY for males.
- Applicable skills for general nurses include taking thorough patient, family, and drug histories, recognizing situations that may warrant further investigation through genetic testing, identifying resources for patients, maintaining confidentiality and privacy, and ensuring that informed consent is obtained for genetic testing and counseling.

NCLEX® EXAMINATION REVIEW QUESTIONS

1. Which is the most appropriate example of a product formed by an indirect form of gene therapy?
   a. Stem cells
   b. Vaccines
   c. Antigen substitution
   d. Platelet inhibitors
2. The nurse is explaining the general goal of gene therapy to a patient. With gene therapy, the general goal is to transfer exogenous genes to a patient for which result?
   a. To change the patient's own genetic functioning to treat a given disease
   b. To improve drug metabolism
   c. To prevent genetic disorders in the patient's future children
   d. To stimulate the growth of stem cells
3. The nurse is reviewing genetic concepts. Which is considered the biologic unit of heredity?
   a. Gene
   b. Allele
   c. Chromosome
   d. Nucleic acid
4. The presence of certain factors in a person's genetic makeup that increase the likelihood of eventually developing one or more diseases is known as a
   a. genetic mutation.
   b. genetic polymorphism.
   c. genetic predisposition.
   d. genotype.
5. The nurse is reviewing gene therapy. Which is the primary molecule in the body that serves to transfer genes from parents to offspring?
   a. RNA
   b. DNA
   c. Allele
   d. Chromosome

6. General responsibilities of the nurse regarding genetics may include which of these activities? (*Select all that apply.*)
   a. Assessing the patient's personal and family history
   b. Referring the patient to a genetic counselor or other genetics specialist
   c. Communicating the results of genetic tests to the patient and patient's family
   d. Maintaining privacy and confidentiality during the testing process
   e. Answering questions about genetic test results
7. The nurse is assessing a patient for a possible increased risk for genetic disorders. Which of these, if present, may indicate an increased risk for a genetic disorder? (*Select all that apply.*)
   a. Having a brother who died of a myocardial infarction at age 29
   b. Having a family member who has been diagnosed with more than one type of cancer
   c. Having an uncle who was diagnosed with prostate cancer at age 73
   d. A history of allergy to shellfish and iodine
   e. Having a maternal grandmother, two maternal aunts, and a sister who were diagnosed with colon cancer
8. Liquid potassium chloride is ordered as follows: Give 16 mEq per PEG tube twice a day. The dose on hand contains 20 mEq/15 mL. How much will the nurse give per dose?

1. b, 2. a, 3. a, 4. c, 5. b, 6. a, b, d, 7. a, b, e, 8. 12 mL.

CRITICAL THINKING AND PRIORITIZATION QUESTIONS

1. You are working on a medical-surgical unit and performing an assessment on a newly admitted patient. During the assessment, your patient states, "My doctor told me that I need to have genetic testing. I just don't understand. If they change my genes, then it will change the way I look!" What is the priority as you, the nurse, answer the patient's concerns?

2. An indirect form of gene therapy is already seen in contemporary health care practice. Explain this statement, and provide examples.

For answers, see *http://evolve.elsevier.com/Lilley*.

ⓔ EVOLVE WEBSITE

http://evolve.elsevier.com/Lilley
- Animations
- Answer Keys for Textbook Case Studies and Textbook Critical Thinking and Prioritization Questions
- Content Updates
- Key Points
- Review Questions
- Student Case Studies

Photo Atlas of Drug Administration

PREPARING FOR DRUG ADMINISTRATION

NOTE: This photo atlas is designed to illustrate general aspects of drug administration. For detailed instructions, please refer to a nursing fundamentals or nursing skills book.

When giving medications, remember safety measures and correct administration techniques to avoid errors and to ensure optimal drug actions. Keep in mind the "Nine Rights"—Right: right drug, right dose, right time, right route, right patient (using two identifiers), right documentation, right reason, right response to the medication, and the patient's right to refuse.

Refer to Chapter 1 for additional rights regarding drug administration. Other things to keep in mind when preparing to give medications are as follows:

- Remember to perform hand hygiene before preparing or giving medications (see Box 9-1, p. 108).
- If you are unsure about a drug or dosage calculation, do not hesitate to double-check with a drug reference or with a pharmacist. **DO NOT** administer a medication if you are unsure about it!
- Be punctual when giving drugs. Some medications must be given at regular intervals to maintain therapeutic blood levels.
- Figure 9-1 shows an example of a computer-controlled drug-dispensing system. To prevent errors, obtain the drugs for one patient at a time.
- Remember to check the drug at least three times before giving it. The nurse is responsible for checking original medication labels against the transcribed medication order. In Figure 9-2, the nurse is checking the drug against the electronic medication administration record. The drug must then be checked before opening it and again after opening it but before giving it to the patient. Some high-alert drugs (i.e., insulin and intravenous heparin) must be checked by two licensed nurses.
- Health care institutions have various means of checking the medication record when a new medication order is received, so be sure that you are giving medications from a medication profile that has been checked or verified before giving the medication. If the patient's medication record has a new drug order on it, the best rule of practice is to double-check that order against the original medication order on the patient's medical record.

- Check the expiration date of all medications. Medications used past the expiration date may be less potent or even harmful.
- Make sure that drugs that are given together are compatible. For example, bile acid sequestrants and antacids (see Chapters 27 and 50) must not be given with other drugs, because they will interfere with drug absorption and action. Check with a pharmacist if unsure. Before administering any medication, check the patient's identification bracelet. The Joint Commission's standards require two patient identifiers (name and birthday, or name and account number, according to the institution's policy). In many health care institutions, patient information is in a barcode system that is scanned (Figure 9-3). In addition, assess the patient's drug allergies before giving any medication.
- Be sure to take time to explain the purpose of each medication, its action, possible adverse effects, and any other pertinent information, especially drug-drug or drug-food interactions, to the patient and/or caregiver.

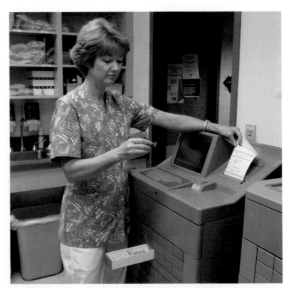

FIGURE 9-1 Using a computer-controlled drug-dispensing system to remove medication.

patient's hand
drugs with your
until you get to
ation and waste

be returned to the
e pharmacy if the
al policy. Discard
drugs that are not
ote on the patient's
patient's reason for

the floor or become

it takes the drugs. Do
le or the meal tray for

administering medica-
cation Administration).
n the medication record
ng to the next patient. Be
responses, adverse effects
nurse's notes. Many health
onic documentation, but
be used.

• Return to evaluate the patient's response to the drug. Remember that the expected response time will vary according to the drug route. For example, responses to sublingual nitroglycerin or intravenous (IV) push medications need to be evaluated within minutes, but it may take 1 hour or more for a response to be noted after an oral medication is given. Follow institutional policy for reassessment after pain medication is given.
• See Patient-Centered Care: Lifespan Considerations for the Pediatric Patient on p. 39 in Chapter 3 for age-related considerations for medication administration to infants and children.

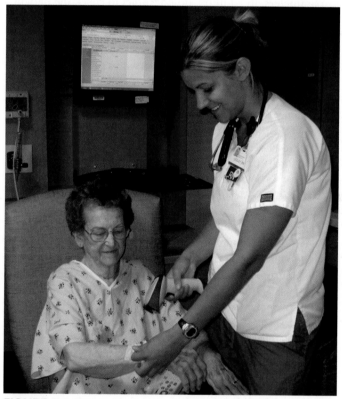

FIGURE 9-3 The nurse is using a bar-code scanner to identify the patient before medication administration. Always check the patient's identification, using two patient identifiers, and allergies before giving medications.

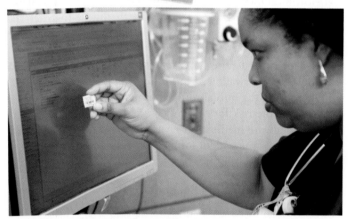

FIGURE 9-2 Checking the medication against the order on the electronic medication administration record.

ENTERAL DRUGS

Administering Oral Drugs

Always begin by performing hand hygiene and maintain Standard Precautions (see Box 9-1). When administering oral drugs, keep in mind the following points:

Oral Medications

- Administration of some oral medications (and medications by other routes) requires special assessments. For example, it is recommended that the apical pulse be auscultated for 1 full minute before any digitalis preparation is given (Figure 9-4). Administration of other oral medications may require blood pressure monitoring. Be sure to document all parameters. In addition, do not forget to check the patient's identification and allergies before giving any oral medication (or medication by any other route).
- If the patient is experiencing difficulty swallowing (dysphagia), some types of tablets can be crushed with a pill-crushing device (Figure 9-5) for easier administration. Crush one type of pill at a time, because if you mix together all of the medications before crushing (instead of crushing them one at a time) and then spill some, there is no way to know which drug has been wasted. Also, if all are mixed together, you cannot check the correct drug three times before giving the drug. Mix the crushed medication in a small amount of soft food, such as applesauce or pudding. Be sure that the pill-crushing device is clean before you use it, and clean it afterward. See Chapter 2 for more information on medications that are not to be crushed.
- **CAUTION:** Be sure to verify whether a medication can be crushed by consulting a drug reference book or a pharmacist. Some oral medications, such as capsules, enteric-coated tablets, and sustained-release or long-acting drugs, must *not* be crushed, broken, or chewed (Figure 9-6). These medications are formulated to protect the gastric lining from irritation or protect the drug from destruction by gastric acids, or are designed to break down gradually and slowly release the medication. If these drugs, designated with labels such as *sustained release* or *extended release*, are crushed or opened, then the intended action of the dosage form is destroyed. As a result, gastric irritation may occur, the drug may be inactivated by gastric acids, or the immediate availability of a drug that was supposed to be released slowly may cause *toxic* effects. Check with the prescriber to see if an alternate form of the drug is needed.
- Be sure to position the patient in a sitting or side-lying position to make it easier for him or her to swallow oral medications and to avoid the risk for aspiration (Figure 9-7). Always provide aspiration prevention measures as needed.
- Offer the patient a full glass of water; 4 to 6 ounces of water or other fluid is recommended for the best dissolution and absorption of oral medications. *Age-related considerations:* Young patients and older adults may not be able to drink a full glass of water but need to take enough fluid to ensure that the medication reaches the stomach. If the patient prefers another fluid, be sure to check for interactions between the medication and the fluid of choice. If fluid restriction is ordered, be sure to follow the guidelines.
- If the patient requests, you may place the pill or capsule in the patient's mouth with your gloved hand.
- Oral lozenges need to be dissolved slowly in the mouth, and are not be chewed unless specifically instructed/ordered.
- Effervescent powders and tablets need to be mixed with water and then given immediately after they are dissolved.
- Remain with the patient until all medication has been swallowed. If you are unsure whether a pill has been swallowed, ask the patient to open his or her mouth so that you can inspect to see if it is gone. Assist the patient to a comfortable position after the medication has been taken.
- Document the medication given on the medication record, and monitor the patient for a therapeutic response as well as for adverse reactions.

Sublingual and Buccal Medications

The sublingual and buccal routes prevent destruction of the drugs in the gastrointestinal tract and allow for rapid absorption into the bloodstream through the oral mucous membranes. These routes are not often used. Be sure to provide instruction to the patient before giving these medications.

- Sublingual tablets are placed under the tongue (Figure 9-8). Buccal tablets are placed between the upper or lower molar teeth and the cheek.
- Be sure to wear gloves if you are placing the tablet into the patient's mouth. Adhere to Standard Precautions (see Box 9-1).
- Instruct the patient to allow the drug to dissolve completely before swallowing.
- These drug forms are not taken with fluids. Instruct the patient not to drink anything until the tablet has dissolved completely.
- Be sure to instruct the patient not to swallow the tablet; saliva should not be swallowed until the drug is dissolved.
- When using the buccal route, alternate sides with each dose to reduce the risk for oral mucosa irritation.
- Document the medication given on the medication record, and monitor the patient for a therapeutic response as well as for adverse reactions.

Orally Disintegrating Medications

Orally disintegrating medications, either in tablet or medicated strip form, dissolve in the mouth without water within 60 seconds. These medications are placed *on* the tongue, not under the tongue, as in the sublingual route. The absorption through the oral mucosa is rapid with a faster onset of action than for drugs that are swallowed. The patient must be instructed to allow the medication to dissolve on the tongue and not to chew or swallow the medication.

- Be sure to wear gloves if you are placing the medication on the patient's tongue. Adhere to Standard Precautions (see Box 9-1).
- Make sure the patient has not eaten or had anything to drink for 5 minutes before and after taking these medications.
- Orally disintegrating medications are often packed in foil blister packs. Do not open the package until just before giving the medication. Carefully open *one* dose at a time. These medications are fragile and may break if they are

pushed through the blister pack. Once a blister or foil pack is opened, the tablet must either be taken or discarded; it cannot be stored for another time.

- Orally disintegrating medications cannot be split, broken, or torn.
- Instruct the patient to hold the medication on the tongue to allow it to dissolve, instead of chewing or swallowing it. This

usually takes about 1 minute. Warn the patient that there may be a sweet or even slightly bitter taste. Remind the patient not to drink water or to eat for 5 minutes after taking the medication.

- Document the medication given on the medication record, and monitor the patient for a therapeutic response as well as for adverse reactions.

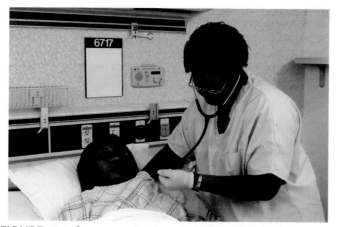

FIGURE 9-4 Some medications require special assessment before administration, such as taking an apical pulse.

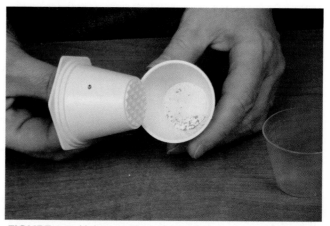

FIGURE 9-5 Using a pill-crushing device to crush a tablet.

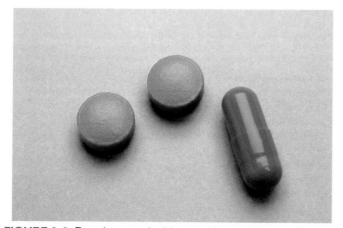

FIGURE 9-6 Enteric-coated tablets and long-acting medications are not to be crushed, broken, or chewed.

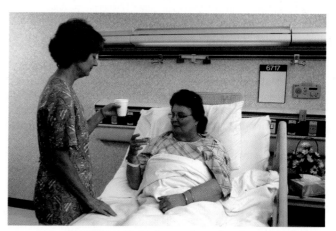

FIGURE 9-7 Giving oral medications.

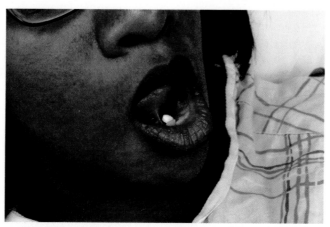

FIGURE 9-8 Proper placement of a sublingual tablet.

BOX 9-1 Standard Precautions

Always adhere to Standard Precautions, including the following:
- Wear clean gloves when exposed to or when there is potential exposure to blood, body fluids, secretions, excretions, and any items that may contain these substances. Always wash hands immediately when there is direct contact with these substances or any item contaminated with blood, body fluids, secretions, or excretions. Gloves must always be worn when giving injections and may be necessary during medication preparation. Be sure to assess the patient for latex allergy and use nonlatex gloves if indicated.
- Perform hand hygiene after removing gloves and between patient contacts. According to the Centers for Disease Control and Prevention, the preferred method of hand decontamination is with an alcohol-based hand rub, but washing with an antimicrobial soap and water is an alternative to the alcohol rub. Use soap and water to wash hands when hands are visibly dirty.
- Perform hand hygiene:
  - Before direct contact with patients
  - After contact with blood, body fluids, excretions, mucous membranes, wound dressings, or nonintact skin
  - After contact with a patient's skin (i.e., when taking a pulse or positioning a patient)
  - After removing gloves
- Wear a mask, eye protective gear, and face shield during any procedure or patient care activity with the potential for splashing or spraying of blood, body fluids, secretions, or excretions. Use of a gown may also be indicated for these situations.
- When administering medications, once the exposure or procedure is completed and exposure is no longer a danger, remove soiled protective garments or gear and perform hand hygiene.
- Never remove, recap, cap, bend, or break any used needle or needle system. Be sure to discard any disposable syringes and needles in the appropriate puncture-resistant container.

BOX 9-2 Safety and Medication Administration

- Always verify the patient's correct identity, using two patient identifiers.
- Always check for allergies to medications, foods, and other substances.
- Always know the reason for the drug as well as the correct dose and administration technique. Follow the manufacturer's guidelines for preparation and delivery.
- Always know the necessary assessments before giving the drug.
  - For antihypertensives, check the patient's blood pressure.
  - For insulin and other drugs that lower blood glucose levels, check the patient's blood glucose levels.
  - Know the patient's potassium levels before giving drugs that can change the level, such as oral supplements, corticosteroids, or ACE inhibitors.
  - Check the patient's apical pulse for one full minute before giving beta blockers, digoxin, or other drugs that cause bradycardia.
  - Assess the patient's CBC before administering chemotherapy.
  - Know the appropriate coagulation studies before administering anticoagulants.
- Double-check calculations with a second nurse or a pharmacist.
- Remove and then administer medications from the automated dispensing cabinet for one patient at a time.
- Follow the institution's protocol for verifying all medication orders (whether electronic or hand-written) before giving the medications.
- For oral medications, ensure that the patient is able to swallow and has an intact gag reflex. For those with difficulty swallowing, other routes may be necessary to avoid aspiration.
- Use appropriate personal protective equipment as indicated. Use the safety device on used needles, then dispose into the proper container. Never recap used needles.
- Administer medications via the prescribed route using correct technique.
- Do not bypass the safety features of electronic pumps used to deliver medications, such as infusion pumps, smart pumps, PCA pumps. Workarounds can lead to serious errors.
- Always verify correct placement of an enteral tube before giving medications. Watch the patient for signs of respiratory distress during medication administration through an enteral tube.
- Monitor the patient for adverse effects and signs of allergic reactions after medications are given.
- If a medication error or near miss incident occurs, report it per the institution's protocol.

Liquid Medications

- Liquid medications may come in a single-dose (unit-dose) package, may be poured into a medicine cup from a multi-dose bottle, or may be drawn up in an oral-dosing syringe (Figure 9-9).
- When pouring a liquid medication from a container, first shake the bottle gently to mix the contents if indicated. Remove the cap, and place it upside down on a paper towel on the counter. Hold the bottle with the label against the palm of your hand to keep any spilled medication from altering the label. Place the medicine cup at eye level, and fill to the proper level on the scale (Figure 9-10). Pour the liquid so that the base of the meniscus is even with the appropriate line measure on the medicine cup.
- If you overfill the medicine cup, discard the excess in the sink. Do not pour it back into the multidose bottle. Before replacing the cap, wipe the rim of the bottle with a paper towel.
- Doses of medications that are less than 5 mL cannot be measured accurately in a calibrated medicine cup. For small volumes, use a calibrated oral syringe. Do not use a hypodermic syringe or a syringe with a needle or syringe cap. If hypodermic syringes are used, the drug may be inadvertently given parenterally, or the syringe cap or needle, if not removed from the syringe, may become dislodged and accidentally aspirated by the patient when the syringe plunger is pressed.
- Document the medication given on the medication record, and monitor the patient for a therapeutic response as well as for adverse reactions.

Oral Medications for Infants and Children

- Liquids are usually ordered for infants and young children because they cannot swallow pills or capsules.
- A plastic disposable oral-dosing syringe is recommended for measuring small doses of liquid medications. Use of an oral-dosing syringe prevents the inadvertent parenteral administration of a drug once it is drawn up into the syringe.
- Position the infant so that the head is slightly elevated to prevent aspiration. Not all infants will be cooperative, and many need to be partially restrained (Figure 9-11).
- Place the plastic dropper or syringe inside the infant's mouth, beside the tongue, and administer the liquid in small amounts while allowing the infant to swallow each time.
- A clean empty nipple may be used to administer the medication. Place the liquid inside the empty nipple, and allow the infant to suck the nipple. Add a few milliliters of water to rinse any remaining medication into the infant's mouth, unless contraindicated.
- Take great care to prevent aspiration. A crying infant can easily aspirate medication. If the infant is crying, wait until the infant is calmer before trying again to give the medication.
- Do not add medication to a bottle of formula; the infant may refuse the feeding or may not drink all of it. Make sure that all of the oral medication has been taken, and then return the infant to a safe, comfortable position.
- A child will reject oral medications that taste bitter. The drug may be mixed with a teaspoon of a sweet-tasting food such as jelly, applesauce, ice cream, or sherbet. Using honey in infants is *not* recommended because of the risk for botulism. Do not mix the medication in an essential food item, such as formula, milk, or orange juice, because the child may reject that food later. After the medication is taken, offer the child juice, a flavored frozen ice pop, or water.

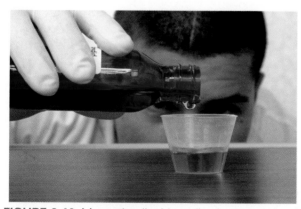

FIGURE 9-9 A, Liquid medication in a unit-dose package. **B,** Liquid measured into a medicine cup from a multidose container. **C,** Liquid medication in an oral-dosing syringe.

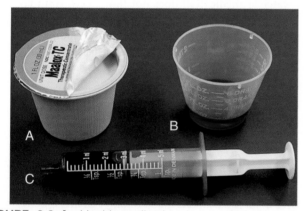

FIGURE 9-10 Measuring liquid medication at eye level.

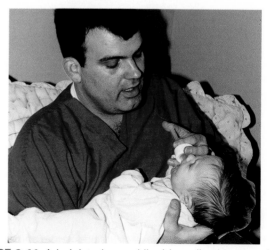

FIGURE 9-11 Administering oral liquid medication to an infant.

Administering Drugs through a Nasogastric or Gastrostomy Tube

Always begin by performing hand hygiene and maintain Standard Precautions (see Box 9-1). Gloves must be worn. When administering drugs via these routes, keep in mind the following points:

• Before giving drugs via these routes, position the patient in a semi-Fowler's or Fowler's position, and leave the head of the bed elevated for at least 30 minutes afterward to reduce the risk for aspiration (Figure 9-12).

• Assess whether fluid restriction or fluid overload is a concern. It will be necessary to give water along with the medications to flush the tubing.

• Check to see if it is recommended for the drug to be given on an empty or full stomach. In addition, some drugs are incompatible with enteral feedings. If the drug is to be given on an empty stomach or if incompatibility exists, the feeding may need to be stopped before and/or after giving the medication. Follow the guidelines for the specific drug if this is necessary. Examples of drugs that are not compatible with enteral feedings are phenytoin and carbidopa-levodopa.

• Whenever possible, give liquid forms of drugs to prevent clogging the tube.

• If tablets must be given, crush the tablets individually into a fine powder. Administer the drugs separately (Figure 9-13). Keeping the drugs separate allows for accurate identification if a dose is spilled. Be sure to check whether the medication can be crushed; enteric-coated and sustained-release tablets or capsules are not to be crushed (see Chapter 2). Check with a pharmacist if you are unsure.

• Before administering the drugs, follow institutional policy for verifying tube placement and checking gastric residual. Reinstill gastric residual per institutional policy, and then clamp the tube.

• Dilute a crushed tablet or liquid medication in 15 to 30 mL of warm water. Some capsules may be opened and dissolved in 30 mL of warm water; check with a pharmacist.

• Remove the piston from an adaptable-tip syringe, and attach the syringe to the end of the tube. Unclamp the tube, and pinch the tubing to close it again. Add 30 mL of warm water, and release the pinched tubing. Allow the water to flow in by gravity to flush the tube, and then pinch the tubing closed again before all the water is gone to prevent excessive air from entering the stomach. If a stopcock valve device is present on the enteral tube, then open and close the stopcock instead of pinching the tubing to clamp it.

• Pour the diluted medication into the syringe and release the tubing to allow it to flow in by gravity (Figure 9-14). Flush between each drug with 10 mL of warm water. Be careful not to spill the medication mixture. Adjust fluid amounts if fluid restrictions are ordered, but sufficient fluid must be used to dilute the medications and to flush the tubing.

• If water or medication does not flow freely, you may apply gentle pressure with the plunger or bulb of the syringe. Do not try to force the medicine through the tubing.

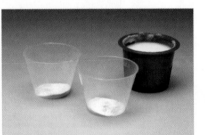

FIGURE 9-13 Medications given through gastric tubes need to be administered separately. Dilute crushed pills in 15 to 30 mL of water before administration.

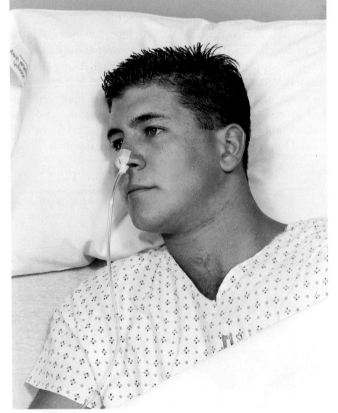

FIGURE 9-12 Elevate the head of the bed before administering medications through a nasogastric or other enteric tube.

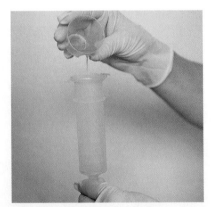

FIGURE 9-14 Pour liquid medication into the syringe, then unclamp the tubing and allow it to flow in by gravity.

- After the last drug dose, flush the tubing with 30 mL of warm water, and then clamp the tube. Resume the tube feeding when appropriate.
- Have the patient remain in a high Fowler's or slightly elevated right-side-lying position to reduce the risk for aspiration.
- Document the medications given on the medication record, the amount of fluid given on the patient's intake and output record, and the patient's response in the patient's record.

Administering Rectal Drugs

Always begin by performing hand hygiene and maintain Standard Precautions (see Box 9-1). Gloves must be worn. When administering rectal drugs, keep in mind the following points:

- Assess the patient for the presence of active rectal bleeding or diarrhea, which generally are contraindications for the use of rectal suppositories.
- Suppositories should not be divided to provide a smaller dose. The active drug may not be evenly distributed within the suppository base.
- Position the patient on his or her left side, unless contraindicated. The uppermost leg needs to be flexed toward the waist (Sims' position). Provide privacy and drape.
- Do not insert the suppository into stool. Gently palpate the rectal wall for the presence of feces. If possible, have the patient defecate. DO NOT palpate the patient's rectum if the patient has had rectal surgery.

- Remove the wrapping from the suppository, and lubricate the rounded tip with water-soluble gel (Figure 9-15).
- Insert the tip of the suppository into the rectum while having the patient take a deep breath and exhale through the mouth. With your gloved finger, quickly and gently insert the suppository into the rectum, alongside the rectal wall, at least 1 inch beyond the internal sphincter (Figure 9-16).
- Have the patient remain lying on his or her left side for 15 to 20 minutes to allow absorption of the medication.
- *Age-related considerations:* With children, it may be necessary to gently but firmly hold the buttocks in place for 5 to 10 minutes until the urge to expel the suppository has passed. Older adults with loss of sphincter control may not be able to retain the suppository.
- If the patient prefers to self-administer the suppository, give specific instructions on the purpose and correct procedure. Be sure to tell the patient to remove the wrapper.
- Use the same procedure for medications administered by a retention enema, such as sodium polystyrene sulfonate (see Chapter 29). Drugs given by enemas are diluted in the smallest amount of solution possible. Retention enemas need to be held for 30 minutes to 1 hour before expulsion, if possible, for maximum absorption.
- Document the medication given on the medication record, and monitor the patient for a therapeutic response as well as for adverse reactions.

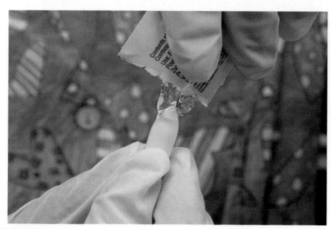

FIGURE 9-15 Lubricate the suppository with a water-soluble lubricant.

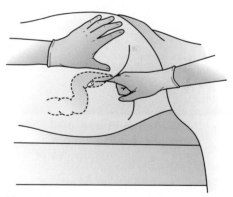

FIGURE 9-16 Inserting a rectal suppository.

PARENTERAL DRUGS

Preparing for Parenteral Drug Administration (Figures 9-17 through 9-28)

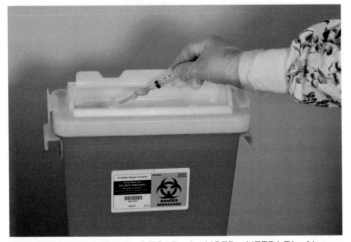

FIGURE 9-17 NEVER RECAP A USED NEEDLE! Always dispose of uncapped needles in the appropriate sharps container. See Box 9-1 for Standard Precautions.

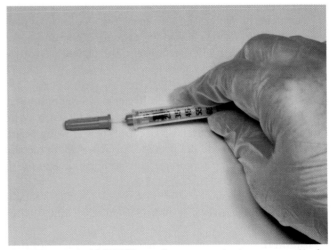

FIGURE 9-18 An UNUSED needle may need to be recapped before the medication is given to the patient, especially if the needle is fixed to the syringe, as with insulin syringes. The "scoop method" is one way to recap an unused needle safely. Be sure not to touch the needle to the countertop or to the outside of the needle cap.

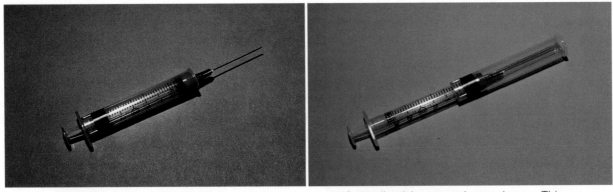

FIGURES 9-19 and 9-20 There are several types of needlestick prevention syringes. This example (Figure 9-19) has a guard over the unused syringe. After the injection, the nurse pulls the guard up over the needle until it locks into place (Figure 9-20).

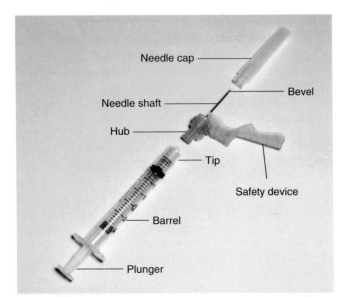

FIGURE 9-21 The parts of a syringe and hypodermic needle.

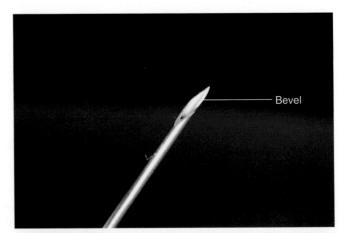

FIGURE 9-22 Close-up view of the bevel of a needle.

jections Overview

eedle Insertion Angles for Intramuscular, Subcutaneous, d Intradermal Injections

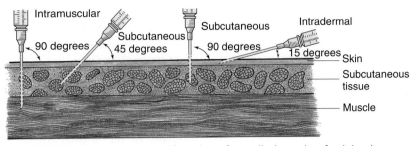

FIGURE 9-37 Comparison of angles of needle insertion for injections.

For any injection, if syringes are prepared at a medication cart or in a medication room, then each parenteral medication should be prepared separately and a label identifying the patient, the medication, the dose, and the route placed on the barrel of the syringe before the nurse leaves the preparation area.

For intramuscular (IM) injections, insert the needle at a 90-degree angle (Figure 9-37). Intramuscular injections deposit the drug deep into muscle tissue, where the drug is absorbed through blood vessels within the muscle. The rate of absorption of medications given by the intramuscular route is slower than that of medications given by the intravenous route but faster than that of medications given by the subcutaneous route. Intramuscular injections generally require a longer needle to reach the muscle tissue, but shorter needles may be needed for older patients, children, and adults who are malnourished. The site chosen will also determine the length of the needle needed. In general, aqueous medications can be given with a 22- to 27-gauge needle, but oil-based or more viscous (thick) medications are given with an 18- to 25-gauge needle. Average needle lengths for children range from ⅝ to 1 inch, and needles for adults range from 1 to 1½ inches. The nurse must choose the needle length based on the size of the muscle at the injection site, the age of the patient, and the type of medication used. For a normal, well-developed adult, 3 mL is the maximum amount used in a single injection. Follow institutional policy. If more than 3 mL is needed for the ordered dose, then the medication will need to be given in two separate injections. However, if the patient is an older adult or is thin, a smaller maximum volume, such as 2 mL, is recommended.

- For subcutaneous (subcut) injections, insert the needle at either a 45- or 90-degree angle (Figure 9-37). Subcutaneous injections deposit the drug into the loose connective tissue under the dermis. This tissue is not as well supplied with blood vessels as is the muscle tissue; as a result, drugs are absorbed more slowly than drugs given intramuscularly. Doses are usually 0.5 to 1 mL. In general, use a 25-gauge, ½- to ⅝-inch needle. A *90-degree angle* is used for an *average-sized* patient; a *45-degree angle* may be used for *thin, emaciated, and/or malnourished* adults and for children. To ensure

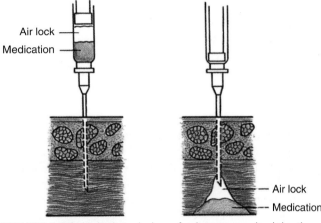

FIGURE 9-38 Air-lock technique for intramuscular injections.

correct needle length, grasp the skinfold with thumb and forefinger, and choose a needle that is approximately half the length of the skinfold from top to bottom.

- Intradermal (ID) injections are given into the outer layers of the dermis in very small amounts, usually 0.01 to 0.1 mL. These injections are used mostly for diagnostic purposes, such as testing for allergies or tuberculosis, and for local anesthesia. Very little of the drug is absorbed systemically. In general, choose a tuberculin or 1-mL syringe with a 25- or 27-gauge needle that is ⅜ to ⅝ inch long. The angle of injection is 5 to 15 degrees (Figure 9-37).
- For specific information about giving injections to children, see Box 9-3.

Air-Lock Technique

- Some health care institutions recommend administering intramuscular injections using the air-lock technique (Figure 9-38). Check institutional policy.
- After withdrawing the desired amount of medication into the syringe, withdraw an additional 0.2 mL of air. Be sure to inject using a 90-degree angle. The small air bubble that follows the medication during the injection may help prevent the medication from leaking through the needle track into the subcutaneous tissues.

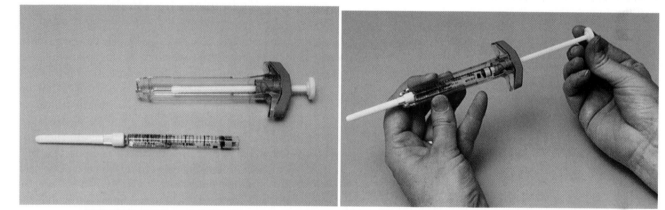

FIGURE 9-23 Be sure to choose the correct size and type of syringe for the drug ordered.

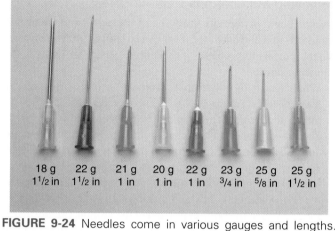

FIGURE 9-24 Needles come in various gauges and lengths. The larger the gauge number, the smaller the needle. Be sure to choose the correct needle—gauge and length—for the type of injection ordered.

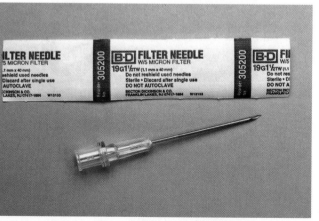

FIGURES 9-25 and 9-26 Some medications come in prefilled sterile medication cartridges. Figures 9-25 and 9-26 show the Carpuject prefilled cartridge and syringe system. Follow the manufacturer's instructions for assembling prefilled syringes. After use, dispose of the syringe in a sharps container; the cartridge is reusable. Some prefilled syringes come with an air bubble in the syringe; do not expel the bubble before administration.

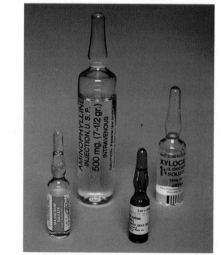

FIGURE 9-27 Ampules containing medications come in various sizes. The neck of the ampule must be broken carefully before the medication is withdrawn. (See Figures 9-30 and 9-31.)

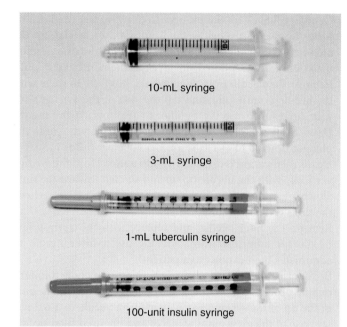

FIGURE 9-28 Use a filter needle when withdrawing medication from an ampule. Filter needles help to remove tiny glass particles that may result from the ampule breakage. DO NOT USE A FILTER NEEDLE FOR INJECTION INTO A PATIENT! Some health care institutions may also require the use of a filter needle to withdraw medications from a vial.

Removing Medications from Ampules

Always begin by performing hand hygiene and maintain Standard Precautions (see Box 9-1). Gloves may be worn. When performing these procedures, keep in mind the following points:

- When removing medication from an ampule, use a sterile filter needle (Figure 9-28). These needles are designed to filter out glass particles that may be present inside the ampule after it is broken. The filter needle IS NOT intended for administration of the drug to the patient and must be removed before the medication is given to the patient.
- Medication often rests in the top part of the ampule. Tap the top of the ampule lightly and quickly with your finger until all fluid moves to the bottom portion of the ampule (Figure 9-29).
- Place a small gauze pad or dry alcohol swab around the neck of the ampule to protect your hand. Snap the neck quickly and firmly, and break the ampule *away* from your body (Figures 9-30 and 9-31).
- To draw up the medication, either set the open ampule on a flat surface or hold the ampule upside down. Insert the filter needle (attached to a syringe) into the center of the ampule opening. Do not allow the needle tip or shaft to touch the rim of the ampule (Figure 9-32).

- Gently pull back on the plunger to draw up the medication. Keep the needle tip below the fluid within the vial; tip the ampule to bring all of the fluid within reach of the needle.
- If air bubbles are aspirated, do not expel them into the ampule. Remove the needle from the ampule, hold the syringe with the needle pointing up, and tap the side of the syringe with your finger to cause the bubbles to rise toward the needle. Draw back slightly on the plunger, and slowly push the plunger upward to eject the air. Do not eject fluid.
- Excess medication is disposed of into a sink. Hold the syringe vertically with the needle tip up and slanted toward the sink. Slowly eject the excess fluid into the sink, and then recheck the fluid level by holding the syringe vertically.
- Remove the filter needle, and replace with the appropriate needle for administration. NEVER use a filter needle to administer medications to a patient!
- Be sure to ensure the sterility of the injection needle throughout the process. Do not touch the open end of the needle hub, or the tip of the syringe, when attaching a needle to a syringe.
- Dispose of the glass ampule pieces and the used filter needle in the appropriate sharps container.

Removing Medications from Vials

Always begin by performing hand hygiene and maintain Standard Precautions (see Box 9-1). Gloves may be worn. When performing these procedures, keep in mind the following points:

- Vials can contain either a single dose or multiple doses of medication. Follow institutional policy for using opened multidose vials, such as vials of insulin. Mark multidose vials with the date and time of opening and the discard date (per institutional policy). If you are unsure about the age of an opened vial of medication, discard it and obtain a new one.
- Check institutional policy regarding which type of needle to use to withdraw fluid from a vial. With the exception of insulin, which must be withdrawn using an insulin syringe, fluid may be withdrawn from a vial using a blunt fill needle or a filter needle. Some health care institutions may use a needleless system to remove medications. Using a blunt fill needle or needleless system reduces the risk for injury with a sharp needle (Figure 9-33).

- If the vial is unused, remove the cap from the top of the vial.
- If the vial has been previously opened and used, wipe the top of the vial vigorously with an alcohol swab.
- Air must first be injected into a vial before fluid can be withdrawn. The amount of air injected into a vial needs to equal the amount of fluid that needs to be withdrawn.
- Determine the volume of fluid to be withdrawn from the vial. Pull back on the syringe's plunger to draw an amount of air into the syringe that is equivalent to the volume of medication to be removed from the vial. Insert the syringe into the vial, preferably using a needleless system. Figure 9-34 shows a needleless system for vial access. Inject the air into the vial.
- While holding onto the plunger, invert the vial and remove the desired amount of medication (Figure 9-35).
- Gently but firmly tap the syringe to remove air bubbles. Excess fluid, if present, must then be discarded into a sink.
- Some vials are not compatible with needleless systems and therefore require a needle for fluid withdrawal (Figure 9-36). Use a blunt fill needle if available (see Figure 9-33).

- When an injection requires two medications f___ ent vials, begin by injecting air into the first___ touching the fluid in the first vial), and then in___ second vial. Immediately remove the desir___ the second vial. Change needles (if possible), ar___ the exact prescribed dose of drug from the first___ care not to contaminate the drug in one vial___ from the other vial. Check with a pharmacist to___ two drugs are compatible for mixing in the san___
- For injections, if a needle has been used to rer___ tion from a vial, always change the needle befor___ ing the dose. Changing needles ensures that___ sharp needle is used for the injection. Me___ remains on the outside of the needle may cause___ the patient's tissues. In addition, the needle may___ if used to puncture a rubber stopper. However, so___ such as insulin syringes, have needles that are fi___ syringe and cannot be removed.
- Ensure the sterility of the injection needle___ the process. Do not touch the open end of the___ or the tip of the syringe, when attaching a needle___

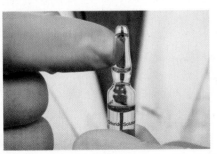

FIGURE 9-29 Tapping an ampule to move the fluid below the neck.

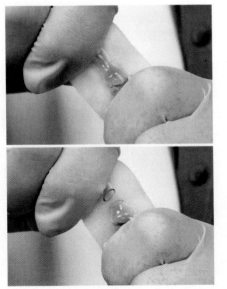

FIGURES 9-30 and 9-31 Breaking an ampule. Carefully break the neck of the ampule in a direction *away* from you and away from others near you.

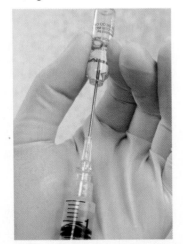

FIGURE 9-32 Using a filter needle to withdraw medication from an ampule.

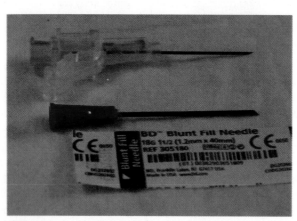

FIGURE 9-33 Comparison of the sharp tip of a needle for injection *(above)* with the blunt tip of a fill needle *(below)*, which is used to remove fluid from a vial.

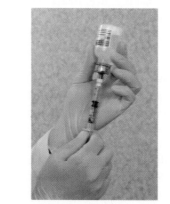

FIGURE 9-35 Withdrawing medication from a vial (needleless system shown).

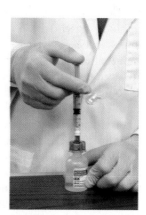

FIGURE 9-34 Insert air into a vial before withdrawing ___tion (needleless system shown).

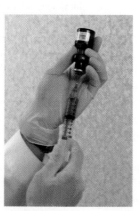

FIGURE 9-36 Using a needle and syringe to remove me___ tion from a vial.

Intradermal Injections

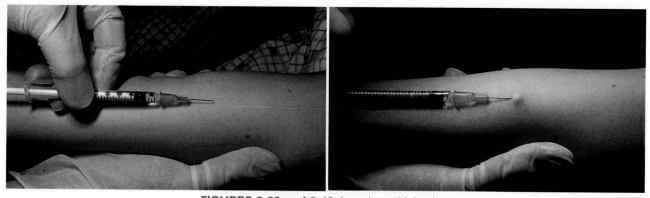

FIGURES 9-39 and 9-40 Intradermal injection.

Always begin by performing hand hygiene and maintain Standard Precautions (see Box 9-1). Gloves must be worn. When giving an intradermal injection, keep in mind the following points:

- Be sure to choose an appropriate site for the injection. Avoid areas of bruising, rashes, inflammation, edema, or skin discoloration.
- Help the patient to a comfortable position. Extend and support the elbow and forearm on a flat surface.
- In general, three to four finger widths below the antecubital space and one hand width above the wrist are the preferred locations on the forearm. Areas on the back that are also suitable for subcutaneous injection may be used if the forearm is not appropriate for the intradermal injection.
- Cleanse the site with an alcohol or antiseptic swab. Apply the swab at the center of the site, and cleanse outward in a circular direction for about 2 inches (5 cm) (see Figure 9-42); then let the skin dry.
- After cleansing the site, stretch the skin over the site with your nondominant hand.

- With the needle almost against the patient's skin, insert the needle, bevel UP, at a 5- to 15-degree angle until resistance is felt, and then advance the needle through the epidermis, approximately 3 mm (Figure 9-39). The needle tip should still be visible under the skin.
- Do not aspirate. This area under the skin contains very few blood vessels.
- Slowly inject the medication. It is normal to feel resistance, and a bleb that resembles a mosquito bite (about 6 mm in diameter) will form at the site if accurate technique is used (Figure 9-40).
- Withdraw the needle slowly while gently applying a gauze pad at the site, but do not massage the site.
- Dispose of the syringe and needle in the appropriate container. Use the safety device to cover the used needle. DO NOT RECAP the needle. Perform hand hygiene after removing gloves.
- Provide instructions to the patient as needed for a follow-up visit for reading the skin testing, if applicable.
- Document on the medication record the date of the skin testing and the date that results need to be read, if applicable.

Subcutaneous Injections

Always begin by performing hand hygiene and maintain Standard Precautions (see Box 9-1). Gloves must be worn. When giving a subcutaneous injection, keep in mind the following points:

- Be sure to choose an appropriate site for the injection (Figure 9-41). Avoid areas of bruising, rashes, inflammation, edema, or skin discoloration.
- Ensure that the needle size is correct. Grasp the skinfold between your thumb and forefinger, and measure from top to bottom. The needle must be approximately one-half this length.
- Cleanse the site with an alcohol or antiseptic swab. Apply the swab at the center of the site, and cleanse outward in a circular direction for about 2 inches (5 cm) (Figure 9-42); then let the skin dry.
- Tell the patient that he or she will feel a "stick" as you insert the needle.
- For an average-sized patient, pinch the skin with your nondominant hand and inject the needle quickly at a 45- or 90-degree angle (Figure 9-43).
- For an obese patient, pinch the skin and inject the needle at a 90-degree angle. Be sure the needle is long enough to reach the base of the skinfold.
- *Age-related considerations:* For a child or a thin patient, pinch the skin gently and be sure to use a 45-degree angle when injecting the needle.
- Injections given in the abdomen must be given at least 2 inches away from the umbilicus because of the surrounding vascular structure (Figure 9-44). The injection site must also be 2 inches away from any incisions, stomas, or open wounds, if present.
- After the needle enters the skin, grasp the lower end of the syringe with your nondominant hand. Move your dominant hand to the end of the plunger—be careful not to move the syringe.
- Aspiration of medication to check for blood return is not necessary for subcutaneous injections, but some institutions may require it. Check institutional policy. Heparin injections and insulin injections are NOT aspirated before injection.
- With your dominant hand, slowly inject the medication.
- Withdraw the needle quickly, and place a swab or sterile gauze pad over the site.
- Apply gentle pressure, but do not massage the site. If necessary, apply a bandage to the site.
- Use the safety device to cover the needle. Dispose of the syringe and needle in the appropriate container. DO NOT RECAP the needle. Perform hand hygiene after removing gloves.
- Document the medication given on the medication record, and monitor the patient for a therapeutic response as well as for adverse reactions.
- For injections of heparin or other subcutaneous anticoagulants, follow the manufacturer's instructions for injection technique as needed. Many manufacturers recommend the area of the abdomen known as the "love handles" for injection of anticoagulants. DO NOT ASPIRATE before injecting, and DO NOT MASSAGE the site after injection. These actions may cause a hematoma at the injection site.
- The air bubble should not be expelled from prefilled syringes, as this is designed to remain next to the plunger to ensure the whole dose is administered.
- Heparin doses are ordered in units, but it is important to note that units of heparin are not the same as units of insulin. Heparin is *never* measured with an insulin syringe.

Insulin Syringes

- *Always use an insulin syringe to measure and administer insulin.* When giving small doses of insulin, use an insulin syringe that is calibrated for smaller doses. Figure 9-45 shows insulin syringes with two different calibrations. Notice that in the 100-unit syringe (*A*), each line represents 2 units; in the 50-unit syringe (*B*), each line represents 1 unit. Note: A unit of insulin is NOT equivalent to a milliliter of insulin!
- Figure 9-46 shows examples of insulin pens used to help the patient self-administer insulin. These pens feature a multi-dose container of insulin and easy-to-read dials for choosing the correct dose. The needle is changed with each use. These devices are for single-patient use only and must never be used by more than one patient due to the risk for blood contamination of the medication reservoir.
- When two different types of insulin are drawn up into the same syringe, always draw up the rapid-acting or short-acting (clear) insulin into the syringe first (Figure 9-47). See p. 115 for information about mixing two different medications in one syringe.

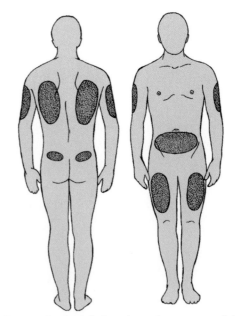

FIGURE 9-41 Potential sites for subcutaneous injections.

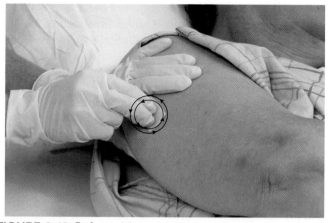

FIGURE 9-42 Before giving an injection, cleanse the skin with an alcohol or antiseptic swab using a circular motion.

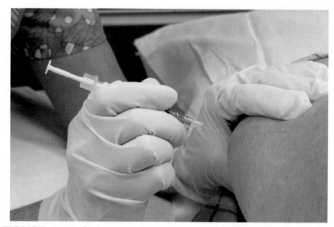

FIGURE 9-43 Giving a subcutaneous injection at a 90-degree angle.

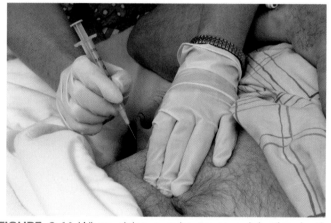

FIGURE 9-44 When giving a subcutaneous injection in the abdomen, be sure to choose a site at least 2 inches away from the umbilicus.

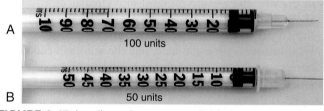

FIGURE 9-45 Insulin syringes are available in 100-unit **(A)** and 50-unit **(B)** calibrations.

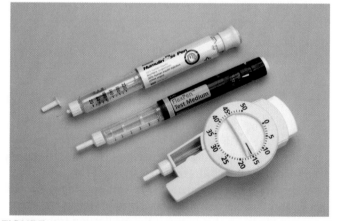

FIGURE 9-46 Examples of prefilled insulin pens for insulin injections.

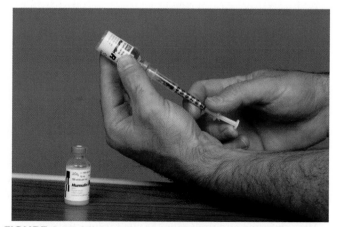

FIGURE 9-47 Mixing two types of insulin in the same syringe. NOTE: The rapid- or short-acting (clear) insulin is always drawn up into the syringe first.

Intramuscular Injections

Always begin by performing hand hygiene and maintain Standard Precautions (see Box 9-1). Gloves must be worn. When giving an intramuscular (IM) injection, keep in mind the following points:

- Choose the appropriate site for the injection by assessing not only the size and integrity of the muscle but the amount and type of injection. Palpate potential sites for areas of hardness or tenderness, and note the presence of bruising or infection.
- The dorsogluteal injection site is no longer recommended for injections because of the close proximity to the sciatic nerve and major blood vessels. Injury to the sciatic nerve from an injection may cause partial paralysis of the leg. The dorsogluteal site is not to be used for intramuscular injections; instead, the ventrogluteal site is the preferred intramuscular injection site for adults and children.
- Assist the patient to the proper position, and ensure his or her comfort.
- Locate the proper site for the injection. Cleanse the site with an alcohol or antiseptic swab. Apply the swab at the center of the site, and cleanse outward in a circular direction for about 2 inches (5 cm) (see Figure 9-42); then let the skin dry. Keep a sterile gauze pad nearby for use after the injection.
- With your nondominant hand, pull the skin taut. Follow the instructions for the Z-track method (see later) if appropriate.

- Grasp the syringe with your dominant hand as if holding a dart, and position the needle at a 90-degree angle to the skin. Tell the patient that he or she will feel a "stick" as you insert the needle.
- Insert the needle quickly and firmly into the muscle. Grasp the lower end of the syringe with the nondominant hand while still holding the skin back, to stabilize the syringe. With the dominant hand, pull back on the plunger for 5 to 10 seconds to check for blood return.
- If no blood appears in the syringe, inject the medication slowly, at the rate of 1 mL every 10 seconds. After injecting the drug, wait 10 seconds, and then withdraw the needle smoothly while releasing the skin.
- Apply gentle pressure at the site, and watch for bleeding. Apply a bandage if necessary.
- If blood does appear in the syringe, remove the needle, dispose of the medication and syringe, and prepare a new syringe with the medication.
- Use the safety device to cover the needle. Dispose of the syringe and needle in the appropriate container. DO NOT RECAP the needle. Perform hand hygiene after removing gloves.
- Document the medication given on the medication record, and monitor the patient for a therapeutic response as well as for adverse reactions.

Z-Track Method

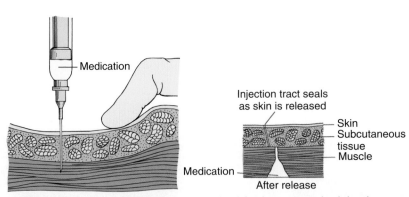

FIGURES 9-48 and 9-49 Z-track method for intramuscular injections.

- The Z-track method is used for injections of irritating substances such as iron dextran and hydroxyzine. The technique reduces pain, irritation, and staining at the injection site. Some health care institutions recommend this method for *all* intramuscular injections (Figures 9-48 and 9-49).
- After choosing and preparing the site for injection, use your nondominant hand to pull the skin laterally, and hold it in this position while giving the injection. Insert the needle at a 90-degree angle, aspirate for 5 to 10 seconds to check for

blood return, and then inject the medication slowly. After injecting the medication, wait 10 seconds before withdrawing the needle. Withdraw the needle slowly and smoothly, and maintain the 90-degree angle.
- Release the skin immediately after withdrawing the needle to seal off the injection site. This technique forms a Z-shaped track in the tissue that prevents the medication from leaking through the more sensitive subcutaneous tissue from the muscle site of injection. Apply gentle pressure to the site with a dry gauze pad.

Ventrogluteal Site

- The ventrogluteal site is the *preferred* site for adults and children. It is considered the safest of all sites because the muscle is deep and away from major blood vessels and nerves (Figure 9-50).
- Position the patient on his or her side, with knees bent and upper leg slightly ahead of the bottom leg. If necessary, the patient may remain in a supine position.
- Palpate the greater trochanter at the head of the femur and the anterosuperior iliac spine. As illustrated in Figure 9-51, use the left hand to find landmarks when injecting into the patient's right ventrogluteal site, and use the right hand to find landmarks when injecting into the patient's left ventrogluteal site. Place the palm of your hand over the greater trochanter and your index finger on the anterosuperior iliac spine. Point your thumb toward the patient's groin and fingers toward the patient's head. Spread the middle finger back along the iliac crest, toward the buttocks, as much as possible.

- The injection site is the center of the triangle formed by your middle and index fingers (see arrow in Figure 9-51).
- Before giving the injection, you may need to switch hands so that you can use your dominant hand to give the injection (Figure 9-52).
- Follow the general instructions for giving an intramuscular injection.

FIGURE 9-50 Finding landmarks for a ventrogluteal injection.

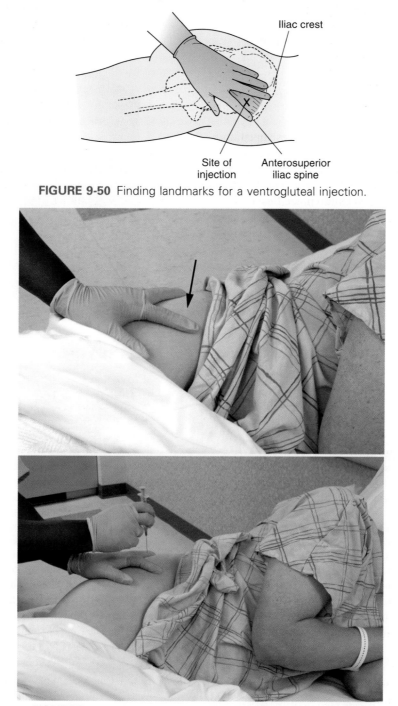

FIGURES 9-51 and 9-52 Ventrogluteal intramuscular injection.

Vastus Lateralis Site

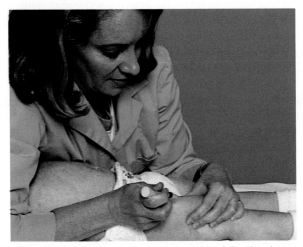

FIGURE 9-53 Vastus lateralis intramuscular injection in a small child. The nurse stabilizes the leg before giving the injection.

- Generally the vastus lateralis muscle is well developed and not located near major nerves or blood vessels. It is the preferred site of injection of drugs such as immunizations for infants and small children (Figure 9-53). For specific information about giving injections to children, see Box 9-3.
- The patient may be sitting or lying supine; if supine, have the patient bend the knee of the leg in which the injection will be given.
- To find the correct site of injection, place one hand above the knee and one hand below the greater trochanter of the femur. Locate the midline of the anterior thigh and the midline of the lateral side of the thigh. The injection site is located within the rectangular area (Figures 9-54, 9-55, and 9-56).

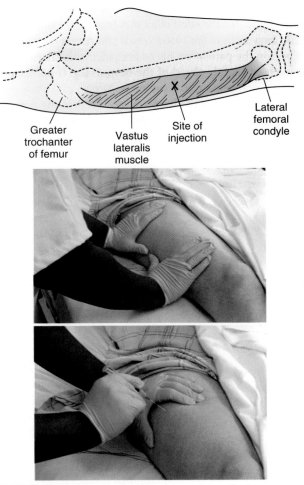

FIGURES 9-54, 9-55, and 9-56 Vastus lateralis intramuscular injection.

BOX 9-3   Pediatric Injections

Site selection is crucial for pediatric injections. Factors to consider are the age of the child, the size of the muscle at the injection site, the type of injection, the thickness of the solution, and the ease with which the child can be positioned properly. There is no universal agreement in the literature on the "best" intramuscular injection site for children. For infants, the preferred site is the vastus lateralis muscle. The ventrogluteal site may also be used in children of all ages. For immunizations in toddlers and older children, the deltoid muscle may be used *if* the muscle mass is well developed. Intramuscular injections for older infants and small children should not exceed 1 mL in a single injection. Refer to health care institutional policy.

Children are often extremely fearful of needles and injections. Even a child who appears calm may become upset and lose control during an injection procedure. For safety reasons, it is important to have another person available for positioning and holding the child.

Distraction techniques are helpful. Say to the child, "If you feel this, you can ask me to take it out, please." Be quick and efficient when giving the injection.

Have a small, colorful bandage on hand to apply after the injection. If the child is old enough, have the child hold the bandage and apply it after the injection. If possible, offer a reward sticker after the injection.

After the injection, allow the child to express his or her feelings. For young children, encourage parents to offer comfort with holding and cuddling. Older children respond better if they receive praise.

EMLA (lidocaine/prilocaine) cream or a vapocoolant spray, if available, may be used before the injection to reduce the pain from the needle insertion. However, because these agents do not absorb down into the muscle, the child may still experience pain when the medication enters the muscle. Apply EMLA cream to the site at least 1 hour and up to 3 hours before the injection. Vapocoolant spray is applied to the site immediately before the injection. Another option is to apply a wrapped ice cube to the injection site for 1 minute before the injection.

Deltoid Site

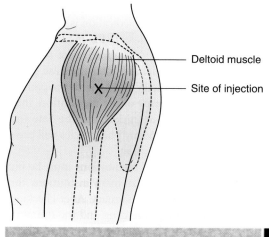

Deltoid muscle

Site of injection

FIGURES 9-57, 9-58, and 9-59 Deltoid intramuscular injection. The deltoid site is not considered a primary site for intramuscular injections but is used for immunizations for toddlers, older children, and adults. This site is not used for infants.

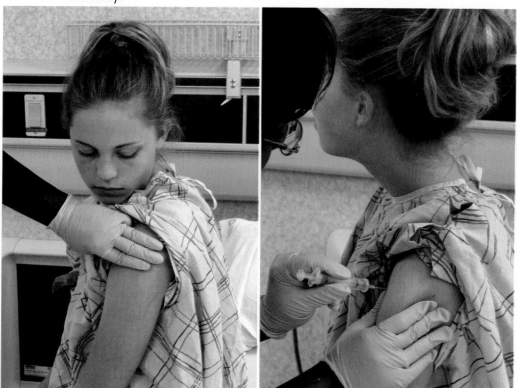

- Even though the deltoid site (Figure 9-57) is easily accessible, it is *not* the first choice for intramuscular injections because the muscle may not be well developed in some adults, and the site carries a risk for injury because the axillary nerve lies beneath the deltoid muscle. In addition, the brachial artery and radial, brachial, and ulnar nerves are also located in the upper arm. Always check medication administration policy, because some heath care institutions do not permit the use of the deltoid site for intramuscular injections. The deltoid site must only be used for administration of immunizations to toddlers, older children, and adults (not infants) and only for small volumes of medication (0.5 to 1 mL).
- The patient may be sitting or lying down. Remove clothing to expose the upper arm and shoulder; do not roll up

tight-fitting sleeves. Have the patient relax his or her arm and slightly bend the elbow.
- Palpate the lower edge of the acromion process. This edge becomes the base of an imaginary triangle (Figure 9-58).
- Place three fingers below this edge of the acromion process. Find the point on the lateral arm in line with the axilla. The injection site will be in the center of this triangle, three finger widths (1 to 2 inches) below the acromion process.
- *Age-related considerations:* In children and smaller adults, it may be necessary to bunch the underlying tissue together before giving the injection and/or use a shorter (⅝-inch) needle (Figure 9-59).
- To reduce patient anxiety, have the patient look away before giving the injection.

Preparing Intravenous Medications

Always begin by performing hand hygiene and maintain Standard Precautions (see Box 9-1). Gloves must be worn for most of these procedures. When administering intravenous (IV) drugs, keep in mind the following points:

- The intravenous route for medication administration provides for rapid onset and faster therapeutic drug levels in the blood than other routes. However, the intravenous route is also potentially more dangerous. Once an intravenous drug is given, it begins to act immediately and cannot be removed. The nurse must be aware of the drug's intended effects and possible adverse effects. In addition, hypersensitivity (allergic) reactions may occur quickly.
- Many institutions now use a needleless system for all infusion lines.
- Before giving an intravenous medication, assess the patient for drug allergies, assess the intravenous line for patency, and assess the site for signs of phlebitis or infiltration.
- When more than one intravenous medication is to be given, check with the pharmacy for compatibility if the medications are to be infused at the same time.
- Check the expiration date of both the medication and infusion bags.
- *Age-related considerations:* For children, infusion pumps *must* be used to prevent the risk for infusing the fluid and medication too fast.
- The Joint Commission requires that the pharmacy prepare intravenous solutions and intravenous piggyback (IVPB) admixtures under a special laminar airflow hood. On the rare occasion when you must dilute a drug for intravenous use, contact the pharmacist for instructions. Be sure to verify which type of fluid to use and the correct amount of solution for the dosage.
- Nurses must receive special training and certification before administering chemotherapy drugs.
- It is important to choose the correct solution for diluting intravenous medications. For example, phenytoin must be infused with normal saline, not dextrose solutions (see Chapter 14). Check with the pharmacist if necessary.
- Most IVPB medications come in vials that are added to the intravenous bag just before administration. This "add-a-vial" system allows the intravenous medication vial to be attached to a small-volume minibag for administration. Figure 9-60 shows two examples of IVPB medications attached to small-volume infusion bags.
- These IVPB medication setups allow for mixing of the drug and diluent immediately before the medication is given. Remember that if the seals are not broken and the medication is not mixed with the fluid in the infusion bag, then the medication stays in the vial! As a result, the patient does not receive the ordered drug dose; instead, the patient receives a small amount of plain intravenous fluid.
- One type of IVPB system that needs to be activated before administration is illustrated in Figure 9-61. To activate this type of IVPB system, snap the connection area between the intravenous infusion bag and the vial (Figure 9-62). Gently squeeze the fluid from the infusion bag into the vial, and allow the medication to dissolve (Figure 9-63). After a few minutes, rotate the vial gently to ensure that all of the powder is dissolved. When

the drug is fully dissolved, hold the IVPB apparatus by the vial and squeeze the bag; fluid will enter the bag from the vial. Make sure that all of the medication is returned to the IVPB bag.

- When hanging these IVPB medications, take care NOT to squeeze the bag. This may cause some of the fluid to leak back into the vial and alter the dose given.
- Always label the IVPB bag with the patient's name and room number, the name of the medication, the dose, the date and time mixed, your initials, and the date and time the medication was given. Many pharmacies will provide a printed label with this information.
- Some intravenous medications must be mixed using a needle and syringe. Again, in many institutions, this procedure will be performed in the pharmacy. After checking the order and the compatibility of the drug and the intravenous fluid, wipe the port of the intravenous bag with an alcohol swab (Figure 9-64).
- Carefully insert the needle into the center of the port, and inject the medication (Figures 9-65 and 9-66). Note how the medication remains in the lower part of the intravenous infusion bag. Turn the bag gently, end to end, to mix the fluid and added medication (Figure 9-67).
- Always add medication to a *new* bag of intravenous fluid, not to a bag that has partially infused. The concentration of the medication may be too strong if it is added to a partially full bag.
- Always label the intravenous infusion bag when a drug has been added (Figure 9-68). Label as per institutional policy, and include the patient's name and room number, the name of the medication, the date and time mixed, your initials, and the date and time the infusion was started. In addition, label all intravenous infusion tubing per institutional policy.

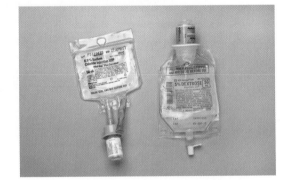

FIGURE 9-60 Two types of intravenous piggyback medication delivery systems. These intravenous systems must be activated before the drug is administered to the patient.

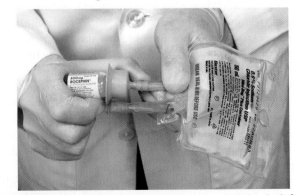

FIGURE 9-61 Activating an intravenous piggyback infusion bag (step 1).

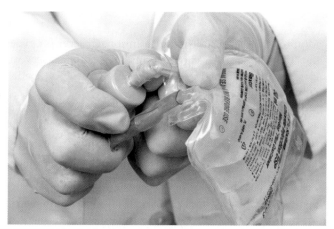

FIGURE 9-62 Activating an intravenous piggyback infusion bag (step 2).

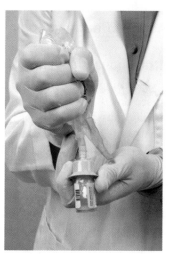

FIGURE 9-63 Activating an intravenous piggyback infusion bag (step 3).

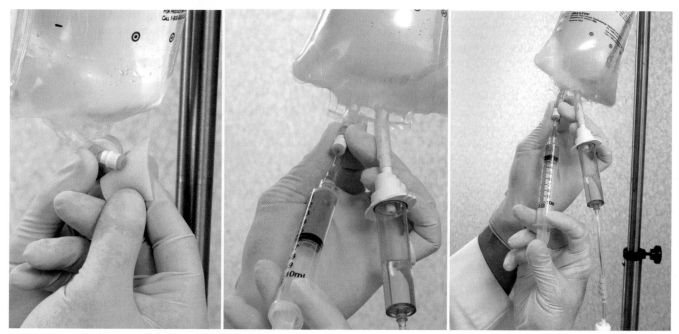

FIGURES 9-64, 9-65, and 9-66 Adding a medication to an intravenous infusion bag with a needle and syringe.

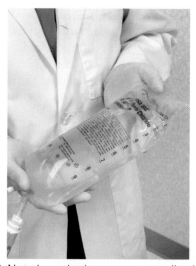

FIGURE 9-67 Note how the intravenous medication is concentrated at the bottom of the bag. Always mix the medication thoroughly before infusing by gently turning the bag end to end. Do not shake the bag.

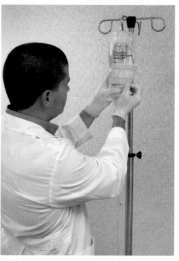

FIGURE 9-68 Label the intravenous infusion bag when medication has been added.

Infusions of Intravenous Piggyback Medications

Always begin by performing hand hygiene and maintain Standard Precautions (see Box 9-1). Gloves must be worn.

- Refrigerated medications may need to be left on the counter to warm to room temperature before administering. If you are infusing the IVPB medication for the first time, you will need to attach the medication bag to the appropriate tubing and "prime" the tubing by allowing just enough fluid through the tubing to flush out the air. Take care not to waste too much of the medication when flushing the tubing.
- If you are adding IVPB medication to an infusion that already has tubing, then use the technique of "backpriming" to flush the tubing. Backpriming allows for the administration of multiple intravenous medications without multiple disconnections, and thus reduces the risk for contamination of the intravenous tubing system.
- Backpriming also removes the old medication fluid that has remained in the IVPB tubing from the previous dose of intravenous medication. After ensuring that the medication in the primary infusion (if any) is compatible with the medication in the IVPB bag, close the roller clamp on the primary infusion if the intravenous fluid is infusing by gravity flow (not necessary if an infusion pump is used). Remove the empty IVPB container from the intravenous pole, lower it to below the level of the primary infusion bag, and open the clamp on the IVPB tubing (Figure 9-69). This will allow fluid to flow from the primary intravenous bag into the empty IVPB bag. Then close the clamp on the IVPB tubing, and squeeze the fluid that is in the drip chamber into the old IVPB bag to remove the old medication fluid. At this point, you may add the new dose of intravenous medication to the IVPB tubing.
- Backpriming will not be possible if the primary intravenous infusion contains heparin, aminophylline, a vasopressor, or multivitamins. Check with a pharmacist if unsure about compatibility.
- Stopping intravenous infusions of medications such as vasopressors for an IVPB medication may affect a patient's blood pressure; stopping intravenous heparin may affect the patient's coagulation levels. Be sure to assess carefully before adding an IVPB medication to an existing infusion. A separate intravenous line may be necessary so that the primary infusion is not stopped for the IVPB.
- Figure 9-70 shows an IVPB medication infusion (also known as the *secondary infusion*) with a primary gravity infusion. When the IVPB bag is hung higher than the primary intravenous infusion bag, the IVPB medication will infuse until empty, and then the primary infusion will take over again.
- When beginning the infusion, attach the IVPB tubing to the upper port on the primary intravenous tubing. A back-check valve above this port prevents the medication from infusing up into the primary intravenous infusion bag.
- Fully open the clamp of the IVPB tubing, and regulate the infusion rate with the roller clamp of the primary infusion tubing. Be sure to note the drip factor of the tubing, and calculate the drops per minute to set the correct infusion rate for the IVPB medication.

- Monitor the patient during the infusion. Observe for hypersensitivity and for adverse reactions. In addition, observe the intravenous infusion site for infiltration. Have the patient report if pain or burning occurs.
- Monitor the rate of infusion during the IVPB medication administration. Changes in arm position may alter the infusion rate.
- When the infusion is complete, clamp the IVPB tubing and check the primary intravenous infusion rate. If necessary, adjust the clamp to the correct infusion rate.
- Figure 9-71 shows an IVPB medication infusion with a primary infusion that is going through an electronic infusion pump.
- When giving IVPB drugs through an intravenous infusion controlled by a pump, attach the IVPB tubing to the port on the primary intravenous tubing above the pump. Open the roller clamp of the IVPB medication tubing. Make sure that the IVPB bag is higher than the primary intravenous infusion bag.
- Following the manufacturer's instructions, set the infusion pump to deliver the IVPB medication. Entering the volume of the IVPB bag and the desired time frame of the infusion (e.g., over a 60-minute period) will cause the pump to automatically calculate the flow rate for the IVPB medication. Start the IVPB infusion as instructed by the pump.
- Monitor the patient during the infusion, as described earlier.
- When the infusion is complete, the primary intravenous infusion will automatically resume.
- Document the medication given on the medication record, and monitor the patient for a therapeutic response as well as for adverse reactions.
- When giving intravenous medications through a saline lock, follow institutional policy for the flushing protocol before and after the medication is administered.
- Figure 9-72 illustrates a volume-controlled administration set that can be used to administer intravenous medications. The chamber is attached to the infusion between the intravenous infusion bag and the intravenous tubing. Fill the chamber with the desired amount of fluid, and then add the medication via the port above the chamber, as shown in the photo. Be sure to cleanse the port with an alcohol swab before inserting the needle in the port. Label the chamber with the medication's name, dose, and time added and your initials. Infuse the drug at the prescribed rate.
- In patient-controlled analgesia (PCA), a specialized pump is used to allow patients to self-administer pain medications, usually opiates (Figure 9-73). These pumps allow the patient to self-administer only as much medication as needed to control the pain by pushing a button for intravenous bolus doses. Safety features of the pump prevent accidental overdoses. A patient receiving PCA pump infusions must be monitored closely for his or her response to the drug, excessive sedation, respiratory depression, hypotension, and changes in mental status. Follow institutional policy for setup and use.

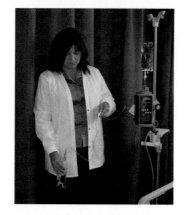

FIGURE 9-69 Flush the intravenous piggyback (secondary) tubing by using the backpriming method. Fluid is drained through the tubing into the old intravenous piggyback bag, which is then discarded. The new dose of medication is then attached to the primed secondary tubing.

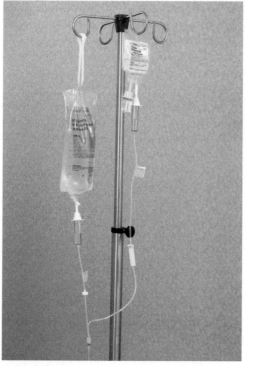

FIGURE 9-70 Infusing an intravenous piggyback medication with a primary gravity infusion. Note how the primary bag is lower than the IVPB.

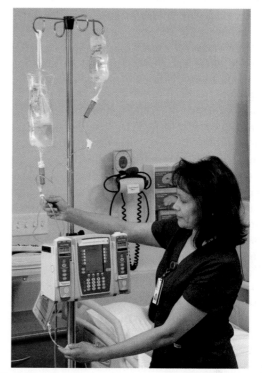

FIGURE 9-71 Infusing an intravenous piggyback medication with the primary infusion on an electronic (smart) infusion pump.

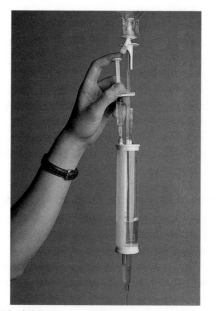

FIGURE 9-72 Adding a medication to a volume-controlled administration set.

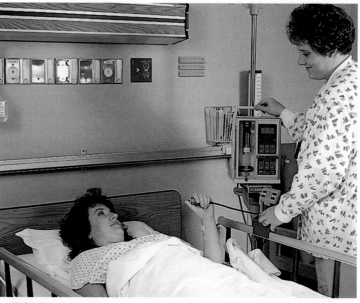

FIGURE 9-73 Instructing the patient on the use of a patient-controlled analgesia pump.

- Figure 9-74 displays a smart pump, an IV infusion safety system that has been designed to reduce IV medication errors. A smart pump contains built-in software that is programmed with institution-specific dosing profiles. The pump is able to "check" the dose-limits and other clinical guidelines, and when the pump is set up for patient use, it can warn the nurse if a potentially unsafe drug dose or therapy is entered.

Intravenous Push Medications

Always begin by performing hand hygiene and maintain Standard Precautions (see Box 9-1). When administering intravenous push (or bolus) medications, keep in mind the following points:

- Registered nurses are usually the only nursing staff members, besides a nurse anesthetist, allowed to give intravenous push medications. This may vary at different health care institutions.
- Intravenous push injections allow for rapid intravenous administration of a drug. The term *bolus* refers to a dose given all at once. Intravenous push injections may be given through an existing intravenous line, through an intravenous (saline) lock, or directly into a vein.
- Because the medication may have an immediate effect, monitor the patient closely for adverse reactions as well as for therapeutic effects.
- Follow the manufacturer's instructions carefully when preparing an intravenous push medication. Some drugs require careful dilution. Consult a pharmacist if you are unsure about the dilution procedure. Improper dilution may increase the risk for phlebitis and other complications.
- Some drugs are *never* given by intravenous push. Examples include dopamine, potassium chloride, and antibiotics such as vancomycin.
- Small amounts of medication, less than 1 mL, need to be diluted in 5 to 10 mL of normal saline or another compatible fluid to ensure that the medication does not collect in a "dead space" of the tubing (such as the Y-site port). Check institutional policy.
- Most drugs given by intravenous push injection are to be given over a period of 1 to 5 minutes to reduce local or systemic adverse effects. Always time the administration with your watch, because it is difficult to estimate the time accurately. Adenosine, however, must be given very rapidly, within 2 to 3 seconds, for optimal action (see Chapter 25). ALWAYS check packaging information for guidelines, because many errors and adverse effects have been associated with too-rapid intravenous drug administration.

Intravenous Push Medications through an Intravenous Lock

- Obtain two syringes of 0.9% normal saline (NS), often supplied in prefilled 10-mL syringes. Prepare medication for injection and follow institutional policy for intravenous lock flushes. If ordered, prepare a syringe with heparin flush solution.
- Cleanse the injection port of the intravenous lock vigorously with an antiseptic swab for 15 seconds (Figure 9-75).

- Insert the syringe of NS into the injection port (Figure 9-76). Open the clamp of the intravenous lock tubing, if present.
- Gently aspirate and observe for blood return. Absence of blood return does not mean that the intravenous line is occluded; further assessment may be required.
- Flush gently with saline while assessing for resistance. If resistance is felt, do not apply force. Stop and reassess the intravenous lock.
- Observe for signs of infiltration while injecting NS.
- Reclamp the tubing (if a clamp is present), and remove the NS syringe. Repeat cleansing of the port, and attach the medication syringe. Open the clamp again.
- Inject the medication over the prescribed length of time. Measure time with a watch or clock (Figure 9-77).
- When the medication is infused, clamp the intravenous lock tubing (if a clamp is present) and remove the syringe.
- Repeat cleansing of the port; attach an NS syringe and inject the contents into the intravenous lock slowly. If a heparin flush is ordered, attach the syringe containing heparin flush solution and inject slowly (per institutional policy).

Intravenous Push Medications through an Existing Infusion

Prepare the medication for injection. Check compatibility of the intravenous medication with the existing intravenous solution.

- Choose the injection port that is closest to the patient.
- Remove the cap, if present, and cleanse the injection port with an antiseptic swab.
- Occlude the intravenous line by pinching the tubing just above the injection port (Figure 9-78). Attach the syringe to the injection port.
- Gently aspirate for blood return.
- While keeping the intravenous tubing clamped, slowly inject the medication according to institutional policy. Be sure to time the injection with a watch or clock.
- After the injection, release the intravenous tubing, remove the syringe, and check the infusion rate of the intravenous fluid.

After Injection of Intravenous Push Medications

- Monitor the patient closely for adverse effects. Monitor the intravenous infusion site for signs of phlebitis and infiltration.
- Document medication given on the medication record, and monitor the patient for a therapeutic response as well as for adverse reactions.

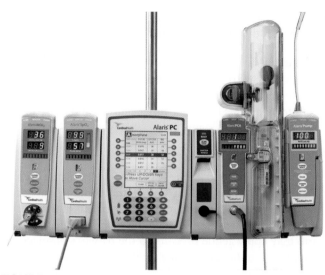

FIGURE 9-74 An electronic smart pump. The two components on the right side are a patient-controlled analgesia pump.

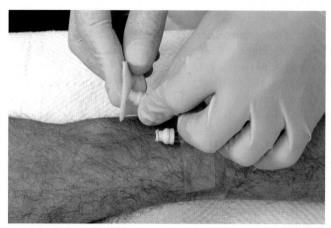

FIGURE 9-75 Cleanse the port vigorously for 15 seconds before attaching the syringe.

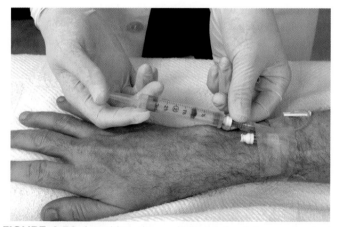

FIGURE 9-76 Attaching the syringe to the intravenous lock, using a needleless system.

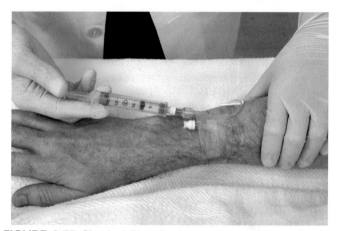

FIGURE 9-77 Slowly inject the intravenous push medication through the intravenous lock; use a watch to time the injection.

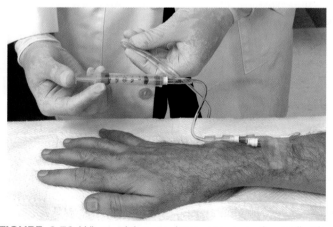

FIGURE 9-78 When giving an intravenous push medication through an intravenous line, pinch the tubing just above the injection port.

TOPICAL DRUGS

Administering Eye Medications

Always begin by performing hand hygiene and maintain Standard Precautions (see Box 9-1). Gloves must be worn. When administering eye preparations, keep in mind the following points:

- Make sure the patient is not wearing contact lenses. Assist the patient to a supine or sitting position. Tilt the patient's head back slightly.
- Remove any secretions with a sterile gauze pad; be sure to wipe from the inner to outer canthus (Figure 9-79).
- Have the patient tilt his or her head slightly back and look up. With your nondominant hand, gently pull the lower lid open to expose the conjunctival sac.

Eyedrops

- With your dominant hand resting on the patient's forehead, hold the eye medication dropper 1 to 2 cm above the conjunctival sac. Do not touch the tip of the dropper to the eye or with your fingers (Figure 9-80).
- Drop the prescribed number of drops into the conjunctival sac. Never apply eyedrops directly onto the cornea.
- If the drops land on the outer lid margins (if the patient moved or blinked), repeat the procedure.
- *Age-related considerations:* Infants often squeeze the eyes tightly shut to avoid eyedrops. To give drops to an uncooperative infant, restrain the head gently and place the drops at the corner near the nose where the eyelids meet. When the eye opens, the medication will flow into the eye.

Eye Ointment

- Gently squeeze the tube of medication to apply an even strip of medication (about 1 to 2 cm) along the border of the conjunctival sac. Start at the inner canthus and move toward the outer canthus (Figure 9-81).

After Instillation of Eye Medications

- Ask the patient to close the eye gently. Squeezing the eye shut may force the medication out of the conjunctival sac. A tissue may be used to blot liquid that runs out of the eye, but instruct the patient not to wipe the eye.
- You may apply gentle pressure to the patient's nasolacrimal duct for 30 to 60 seconds with a gloved finger wrapped in a tissue. This will help to reduce systemic absorption of the drug through the nasolacrimal duct and may also help to reduce the taste of the medication in the nasopharynx (Figure 9-82).
- If multiple eyedrops are due at the same time, then wait several minutes before administering the second medication. Check the instructions for the specific drug.
- Assist the patient to a comfortable position. Warn the patient that vision may be blurry for a few minutes.
- Document the medication given on the medication record, and monitor the patient for a therapeutic response as well as for adverse reactions.

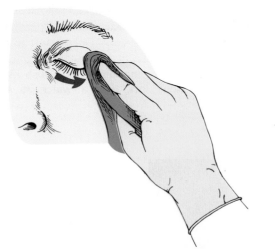

FIGURE 9-79 Cleanse the eye, washing from the inner to outer canthus, before giving eye medications.

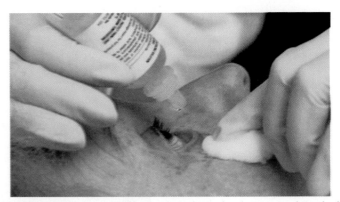

FIGURE 9-80 Insert the eyedrop into the lower conjunctival sac.

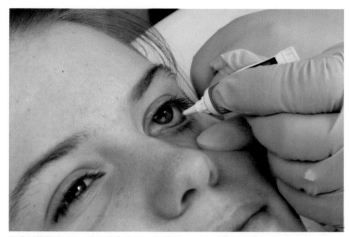

FIGURE 9-81 Applying eye ointment. Move from the inner to outer canthus, along the border of the conjunctival sac.

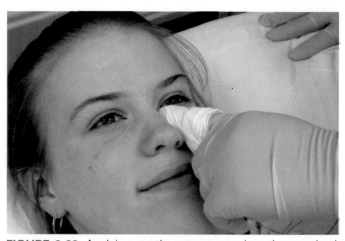

FIGURE 9-82 Applying gentle pressure against the nasolacrimal duct after giving eye medication.

Administering Eardrops

Always begin by performing hand hygiene and maintain Standard Precautions (see Box 9-1). Gloves may be worn. When administering ear preparations, keep in mind the following points:

- After explaining the procedure to the patient, assist the patient to a side-lying position with the affected ear facing up. If cerumen or drainage is noted in the outer ear canal, remove it carefully without pushing it back into the ear canal.
- Remove excessive amounts of cerumen before instillation of medication.
- If refrigerated, warm the ear medication by taking it out of refrigeration for at least 30 minutes before administration. Instillation of cold eardrops can cause nausea, dizziness, and pain.
- *Age-related considerations:* For an adult or a child older than 3 years of age, pull the pinna up and back (Figure 9-83). For an infant or a child younger than 3 years of age, pull the pinna down and back (Figure 9-84).

- Administer the prescribed number of drops. Direct the drops along the sides of the ear canal rather than directly onto the eardrum.
- Instruct the patient to lie on his or her side for 5 to 10 minutes. Gently massaging the tragus of the ear with a finger will help to distribute the medication down the ear canal.
- If ordered, a loose cotton pledget can be gently inserted into the ear canal to prevent the medication from flowing out. The cotton must remain somewhat loose to allow any discharge to drain out of the ear canal. To prevent the dry cotton from absorbing the eardrops that were instilled, moisten the cotton with a small amount of medication before inserting the pledget. Insertion of cotton too deeply may result in increased pressure within the ear canal and on the eardrum. Remove the cotton after about 15 minutes.
- If medication is needed in the other ear, wait 5 to 10 minutes after instillation of the first eardrops before administering.
- Document the medication given on the medication record, and monitor the patient for a therapeutic response as well as for adverse reactions.

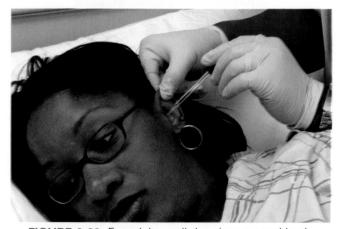

FIGURE 9-83 For adults, pull the pinna up and back.

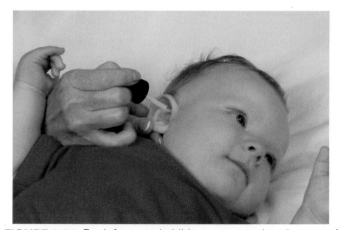

FIGURE 9-84 For infants and children younger than 3 years of age, pull the pinna down and back.

Administering Inhaled Drugs

Always begin by performing hand hygiene and maintain Standard Precautions (see Box 9-1). Gloves may be worn. Patients with asthma need to monitor their peak expiratory flow rates by using a peak flow meter. A variety of inhalers are available (Figure 9-85). Be sure to check for specific instructions from the manufacturer as needed. Improper use will result in inadequate dosing. When administering inhaled preparations, keep in mind the following points:

Metered-Dose Inhalers

- Shake the metered-dose inhaler (MDI) gently before using.
- Remove the cap and inspect the mouthpiece to ensure that there are no foreign objects in the mouthpiece. Inhalation of a foreign object could cause serious injury.
- Hold the inhaler upright and grasp it with the thumb and first two fingers.
- Tilt the patient's head back slightly.
- If the inhaler is used without a spacer, do the following:
  1. Have the patient open his or her mouth; position the inhaler 1 to 2 inches away from the patient's mouth (Figure 9-86). For self-administration, some patients may measure this distance as 1 to 2 finger widths.
  2. Have the patient exhale, then press down once on the inhaler to release the medication; have the patient breathe in slowly and deeply for 5 seconds.
  3. Have the patient hold his or her breath for approximately 10 seconds, then exhale slowly through pursed lips.
- *Age-related considerations:* Spacers can be used with children and adults who have difficulty coordinating inhalations with activation of metered-dose inhalers (see Chapter 37). If the inhaler is used with a spacer, do the following:
  1. Attach the spacer to the mouthpiece of the inhaler after removing the inhaler cap.
  2. Place the mouthpiece of the spacer in the patient's mouth.
  3. Have the patient exhale.
  4. Press down on the inhaler to release the medication, and have the patient inhale deeply and slowly through the spacer. The patient then needs to breathe in and out slowly for 2 to 3 seconds, and then hold his or her breath for 10 seconds (Figure 9-87).

- If a second puff of the same medication is ordered, wait 1 to 2 minutes between puffs.
- If a second type of inhaled medication is ordered, wait 2 to 5 minutes between medication inhalations or as prescribed.
- If both a bronchodilator and a corticosteroid inhaled medication are ordered, the bronchodilator needs to be administered first so that the passages will be more open for the second medication.
- Instruct the patient to replace the cap onto the mouthpiece of the inhaler.
- Instruct the patient to rinse his or her mouth after inhaling a corticosteroid medication to prevent the development of an oral fungal infection.
- Document the medication given on the medication record, and monitor the patient for a therapeutic response as well as for adverse reactions.
- It is important to teach the patient to be aware of the number of doses in the inhaler and to keep track of uses. Simply shaking the inhaler to "estimate" whether it is empty is not accurate and may result in its being used when it is empty. Many MDIs now come with devices that help to count the remaining doses. Dry powder inhalers have varied instructions, so follow the manufacturer's instructions closely. Instruct patients to cover the mouthpiece completely with their mouths. Capsules that are intended for use with these inhalers must NEVER be taken orally. Most dry powder inhalers also have convenient built-in dose counters.

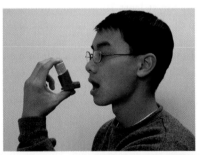

FIGURE 9-86 Using a metered-dose inhaler without a spacer.

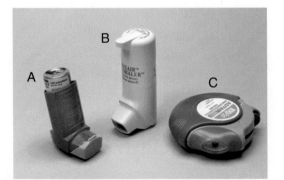

FIGURE 9-85 A, Metered-dose inhaler (MDI). **B,** Automated, or breath-activated, MDI. **C,** Dry powder inhaler that delivers powdered medication.

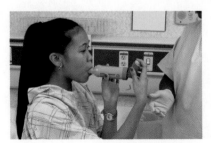

FIGURE 9-87 Using a spacer device with a metered-dose inhaler.

Small-Volume Nebulizers

- In some health care institutions, the air compressor is located in the wall unit of the room. A small portable air compressor is used at home and in areas where wall units are not available. Be sure to follow the manufacturer's instructions for use.
- Nebulizer treatments may be performed by a respiratory therapist or a nurse. Always closely monitor the patient before, during, and after the drug administration.
- Be sure to take the patient's baseline heart rate, especially if a beta-adrenergic drug is used. Some drugs may increase the heart rate.
- After gathering the equipment, add the prescribed medication to the nebulizer cup (Figure 9-88). Some medications will require a diluent; others are premixed with a diluent. Be sure to verify before adding a diluent.
- Have the patient hold the mouthpiece between his or her lips (Figure 9-89).
- *Age-related considerations:* Use a face mask for a child or an adult who is too fatigued to hold the mouthpiece. Special adaptors are available if the patient has a tracheostomy.
- Before starting the nebulizer treatment, have the patient take a slow, deep breath, hold it briefly, and then exhale slowly. Instruct patients who are short of breath to hold their breath every fourth or fifth breath.

- Turn on the small-volume nebulizer machine (or turn on the wall unit), and make sure that a sufficient mist is forming.
- Instruct the patient to repeat the breathing pattern mentioned previously during the treatment.
- Occasionally tap the nebulizer cup during the treatment and toward the end to move the fluid droplets back to the bottom of the cup.
- Monitor the patient throughout treatment to ensure that the nebulizer medication is properly administered.
- Monitor the patient's heart rate during and after the treatment.
- If inhaled steroids are given, instruct the patient to rinse his or her mouth afterward.
- After the procedure, clean and store the tubing per institutional policy.
- Document the medication given on the medication record, and monitor the patient for a therapeutic response as well as for adverse reactions.
- If the patient will be using a nebulizer at home, instruct the patient to rinse the nebulizer parts after each use with warm, clear water and to air-dry. Wash the parts daily with warm, soapy water and allowed to air-dry. Once a week, soak the nebulizer parts in a solution of vinegar and water (four parts water and one part white vinegar) for 30 minutes; rinse thoroughly with clear, warm water; and air-dry. Storing nebulizer parts that are still wet will encourage bacterial and mold growth.

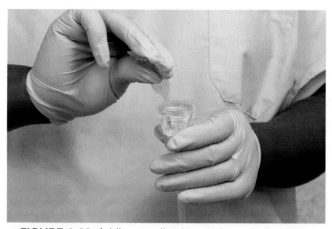

FIGURE 9-88 Adding medication to the nebulizer cup.

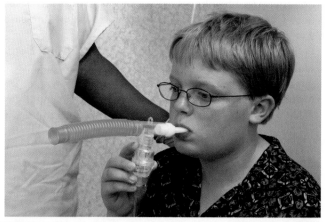

FIGURE 9-89 Administering a small-volume nebulizer treatment.

Administering Medications to the Skin

Always begin by performing hand hygiene and maintain Standard Precautions (see Box 9-1). Gloves must be worn. Avoid touching the preparations to your own skin. When administering skin preparations, keep in mind the following points:

Lotions, Creams, Ointments, and Powders

- Apply powder to clean, dry skin. Have the patient turn his or her head to the other side during application to avoid inhalation of powder particles.
- Apply lotion to clean, dry skin. Remove residual from previous applications with soap and water.
- Before administering any dose of a topical skin medication, ensure that the site is dry and free of irritation. Thoroughly remove previous applications using soap and water, if appropriate for the patient's condition, and dry the area thoroughly. Be sure to remove any debris, drainage, or pus if present.
- *Age-related considerations:* The skin of an older patient may be more fragile and easily bruised. Be sure to handle the skin gently when cleansing to prepare the site for medication and when applying medications.
- With lotion, cream, or gel, obtain the correct amount with your gloved hand (Figure 9-90). If the medication is in a jar, remove the dose with a sterile tongue depressor and apply to your gloved hand. Do not contaminate the medication in the jar.
- Apply the preparation with long, smooth, gentle strokes that follow the direction of hair growth (Figure 9-91). Avoid excessive pressure. Be especially careful with the skin of older adults, because age-related changes may result in increased capillary fragility and tendency to bruise.
- Some ointments and creams may soil the patient's clothes and linens. If ordered, cover the affected area with gauze or a transparent dressing.
- Nitroglycerin ointment in a tube is measured carefully on clean ruled application paper before it is applied to the skin (Figure 9-92). Unit-dose packages are not measured. Do not massage nitroglycerin ointment into the skin. Apply the measured amount onto a clean, dry site, and then secure the application paper with a transparent dressing or a strip of tape. Always remove the old medication before applying a new dose. Rotate application sites.

Transdermal Patches

- Be sure that the old patch is removed as ordered. Some patches may be removed before the next patch is due, so check the order. Clear patches may be difficult to find, and patches may be overlooked in obese patients with skinfolds. Cleanse the site of the old patch thoroughly. Observe for signs of skin irritation at the old patch site. Rotate sites of application with each dose.
- Transdermal patches need to be applied at the same time each day if ordered daily.
- The old patch can be pressed together and then wrapped in a glove as you remove the glove from your hand. Dispose of it in the proper container according to institutional policy.
- Select a new site for application and ensure that it is clean and without powder or lotion. For best absorption and fewest adverse effects, the site needs to be hairless and free from scratches or irritation. If it is necessary to remove hair, clip the hair instead of shaving to reduce irritation to the skin. Application sites may vary. Follow the drug manufacturer's specific instructions as to where to apply the patch.
- Remove the backing from the new patch (Figure 9-93). Take care not to touch the medication side of the patch with your fingers.
- Place the patch on the skin site, and press firmly (Figure 9-94). Press around the edges of the patch with one or two fingers to ensure that the patch is adequately secured to the skin. If an overlay is provided by the drug manufacturer, apply it over the patch.
- Instruct the patient not to cut transdermal patches. Cutting transdermal patches releases all of the medication at once and may result in a dangerous overdose.

After Administration of Topical Skin Preparations

- Document the medication given on the medication record, and monitor the patient for a therapeutic response as well as for adverse reactions.
- Provide instruction on administration to the patient and/or caregiver.

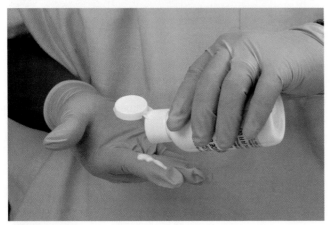

FIGURE 9-90 Use gloves to apply topical skin preparations.

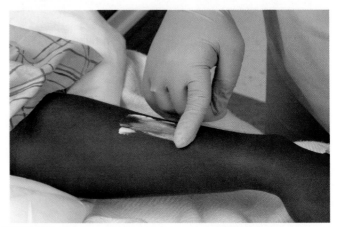

FIGURE 9-91 Spread the lotion on the skin with long, smooth, gentle strokes.

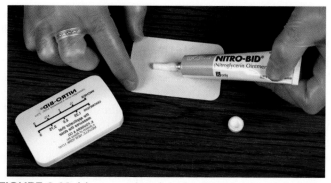

FIGURE 9-92 Measure nitroglycerin ointment carefully before application.

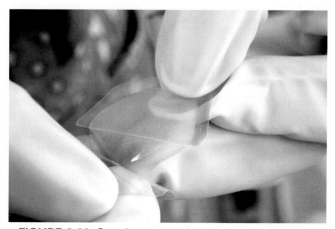

FIGURE 9-93 Opening a transdermal patch medication.

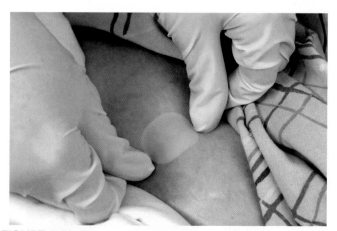

FIGURE 9-94 Ensure that the edges of the transdermal patch are secure after applying.

Administering Nasal Medications

Always begin by performing hand hygiene and maintain Standard Precautions (see Box 9-1). Patients may self-administer some of these drugs after proper instruction. Gloves must be worn. When administering nasal medications, keep in mind the following points:

- Before giving nasal medications, explain the procedure to the patient and tell him or her that temporary burning or stinging may occur. Instruct the patient that it is important to clear the nasal passages by blowing his or her nose, unless contraindicated (e.g., with increased intracranial pressure or nasal surgery), before administering the medication. Assess for deviated septum or a history of nasal fractures, because these may impede the patient's ability to inhale through the affected nostril.
- Figure 9-95 illustrates various delivery forms for nasal medications: sprays, drops, and metered-dose sprays.
- Assist the patient to a supine position. Support the patient's head as needed.
- If specific areas are targeted for the medication, position as follows:
  - For the posterior pharynx, position the head backward.
  - For the ethmoid or sphenoid sinuses, place the head gently over the top edge of the bed, or place a pillow under the shoulders and tilt the head back.
  - For the frontal or maxillary sinuses, place the head back and turned toward the side that is to receive the medication.

Nasal Drops

- Hold the nose dropper approximately $\frac{1}{2}$ inch above the nostril. Administer the prescribed number of drops toward the midline of the ethmoid bone (Figure 9-96).

- Repeat the procedure as ordered, instilling the indicated number of drops per nostril.
- Keep the patient in a supine position for 5 minutes.
- *Age-related considerations:* Infants are nose breathers, and the potential congestion caused by nasal medications may make it difficult for them to suck. If nose drops are ordered, administer them 20 to 30 minutes before a feeding.

Nasal Spray

- While the patient is sitting upright, occlude one nostril by pressing a finger against the outer nare. After gently shaking the nasal spray container, insert the tip into the other nostril. Squeeze the spray bottle into the nostril while the patient inhales through the open nostril (Figure 9-97).
- Repeat the procedure as ordered, instilling the indicated number of sprays per nostril.

After Administration of Nasal Medicines

- Offer the patient tissues for blotting any drainage, but instruct the patient to avoid blowing his or her nose for several minutes after instillation of the drops.
- Assist the patient to a comfortable position.
- Document the medication given on the medication record, and document drainage, if any. Monitor the patient for a therapeutic response as well as for adverse reactions.

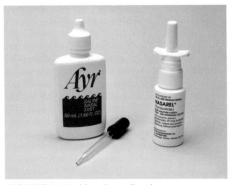

FIGURE 9-95 Nasal medications may come in various delivery forms.

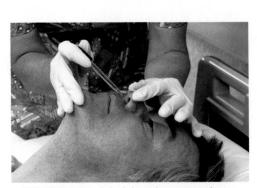

FIGURE 9-96 Administering nose drops.

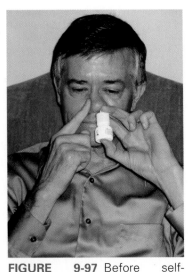

FIGURE 9-97 Before self-administering the nasal spray, the patient needs to occlude the other nostril.

Administering Vaginal Medications

Always begin by performing hand hygiene and maintain Standard Precautions (see Box 9-1). Gloves must be worn. When administering vaginal preparations, keep in mind the following points:

- Vaginal suppositories are larger and more oval than rectal suppositories (Figure 9-98).
- Figure 9-99 shows examples of a vaginal suppository in an applicator and vaginal cream in an applicator.
- Before giving these medications, explain the procedure to the patient and have her void the bladder.
- If possible, administer vaginal preparations at bedtime to allow the medications to remain in place as long as possible.
- Some patients may prefer to self-administer vaginal medications. Provide specific instructions if necessary.
- Position the patient in the lithotomy position and elevate the hips with a pillow, if tolerated. Be sure to drape the patient to provide privacy.

Creams, Foams, or Gels Applied with an Applicator

- Fit the applicator to the tube of the medication, and then gently squeeze the tube to fill the applicator with the correct amount of medication.
- Lubricate the tip of the applicator with a water-soluble lubricant.
- Use your nondominant hand to spread the labia and expose the vagina. Gently insert the applicator as far as possible into the vagina (Figure 9-100).
- Push the plunger to deposit the medication. Remove the applicator and wrap it in a paper towel for cleaning. Wash the applicator with soap and water, and store in a clean container for the next use.

Suppositories or Vaginal Tablets

- For suppositories or vaginal tablets, remove the wrapping and lubricate the suppository with a water-soluble lubricant. Be sure that the suppository is at room temperature.
- Using the applicator provided, insert the suppository or tablet into the vagina, and then push the plunger to deposit the suppository. Remove the applicator.
- If no applicator is available, use your dominant index finger to insert the suppository about 2 inches into the vagina (Figure 9-101).
- Have the patient remain in a supine position with hips elevated for 5 to 10 minutes to allow the suppository to melt and the medication to be absorbed.
- If the patient desires, apply a perineal pad.
- If the applicator is to be reused, wash it with soap and water and store in a clean container for the next use.
- Document the medication given on the medication record, and monitor the patient for a therapeutic response as well as for adverse reactions.

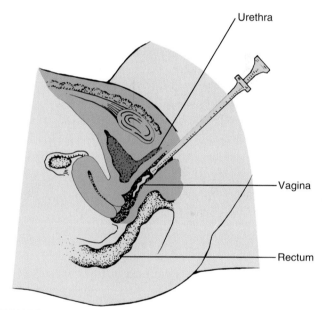

FIGURE 9-100 Administering vaginal cream with an applicator.

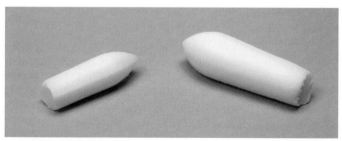

FIGURE 9-98 Vaginal suppositories *(right)* are larger and more oval than rectal suppositories *(left)*.

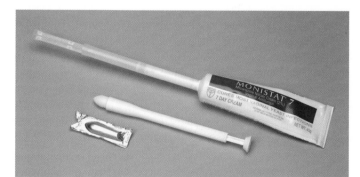

FIGURE 9-99 Vaginal cream and suppository, with applicators.

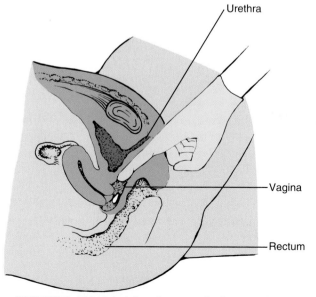

FIGURE 9-101 Administering a vaginal suppository.

ILLUSTRATION CREDITS

Figures 9-1, 9-4, 9-6, 9-7, 9-8, 9-10, 9-13, 9-15, 9-24, 9-28, 9-29, 9-30, 9-31, 9-32, 9-34, 9-35, 9-36, 9-42, 9-43, 9-44, 9-46, 9-51, 9-52, 9-55, 9-56, 9-58, 9-59, 9-60, 9-61, 9-62, 9-63, 9-64, 9-65, 9-66, 9-67, 9-68, 9-70, 9-75, 9-76, 9-77, 9-78, 9-81, 9-82, 9-83, 9-84, 9-85, 9-86, 9-88, 9-89, 9-90, 9-91, 9-92, 9-93, 9-94, 9-96, 9-97, 9-98, and 9-99 from Rick Brady, Riva, MD. Figures 9-2, 9-3, 9-5, 9-37, 9-41, 9-47, 9-48, 9-49, 9-74, and 9-79 from Perry AG, Potter PA: *Clinical nursing skills and techniques,* ed 8, St Louis, 2014, Mosby. Figure 9-9 from Perry AG, Potter PA, Elkin MK: *Nursing interventions and clinical skills,* ed 5, St Louis, 2012, Mosby. Figures 9-14, 9-38, 9-100, and 9-101 from Elkin MK, Perry AG, Potter PA: *Nursing interventions and clinical skills,* ed 3, St Louis, 2004, Mosby. Figure 9-11 courtesy Oscar H. Allison, Jr. In Clayton BD, Stock YN: *Basic pharmacology for nurses,* ed 15, St Louis, 2010, Mosby. Figure 9-16 modified from Perry AG, Potter PA: *Clinical nursing skills and techniques,* ed 8, St Louis, 2014, Mosby. Figures 9-19, 9-20, 9-22, 9-39, and 9-40 courtesy Chuck Dresner. Figures 9-25 and 9-26 from Potter PA, Perry AG: *Basic nursing: theory and practice,* ed 3, St Louis, 1995, Mosby. Figure 9-27 from Potter PA, Perry AG: *Fundamentals of nursing,* ed 5, St Louis, 2001, Mosby. Figure 9-45 from Mulholland J: *The Nurse, the math, the meds: using dimensional analysis,* ed 2, St Louis, 2011, Mosby. Figures 9-50, 9-54, and 9-57 modified from Potter PA, Perry AG: *Fundamentals of nursing: concepts, process, and practice,* ed 3, St Louis, 1993, Mosby. Figure 9-53 from Hockenberry MJ, Wilson D: *Wong's nursing care of infants and children,* ed 9, St Louis, 2011, Mosby. Figure 9-71 from Potter PA, Perry AG, Stockert PA, et al: *Fundamentals of nursing,* ed 8, St Louis, 2013, Mosby. Figure 9-72 from Potter PA, Perry AG: *Fundamentals of nursing,* ed 6, St Louis, 2005, Mosby. Figure 9-73 from Christensen BL, Kockrow EO: *Foundations and adult health nursing,* ed 6, St Louis, 2011, Mosby. Figure 9-80 from Potter PA, Perry AG, Stockert PA, et al: *Basic nursing,* ed 7, St Louis, 2011, Mosby. Figure 9-95 from Perry AG, Potter PA: *Clinical skills and techniques,* ed 6, St Louis, 2006, Mosby.

Drugs Affecting the Central Nervous System

Learning Strategies

NURSING PROCESS

In Chapter 1 you were introduced to the five phases of the nursing process. Throughout this textbook, you will see the Nursing Process applied to each category of drugs. This is a very important concept for you to understand. As you will recall, it was stated earlier in the introduction on learning strategies, that administering medications to patients involves more that the physical act of giving medications. The nurse needs to know the rationale and apply critical thinking with each patient encounter. The Nursing Process is a way to ensure that medications are administered accurately and safely. Nurses effortlessly use the nursing process every day. Students who are new to the nursing process learn best by using it frequently. One strategy to remember the different parts of the nursing process is to use the mnemonic ADPIE for assessment, diagnosis, planning, implementation, and evaluation.

ASSESSMENT

Every patient encounter starts with an Assessment. As you are learning pharmacology, the importance of the assessment will become clear. You will want to ask yourself some questions: Why is this drug being prescribed for this patient? What symptoms does the patient have? What assessments do I need to perform prior to administering the medication (e.g., checking the patient's blood pressure or laboratory values)? Does the patient have any allergies to this medication? Has the patient taken this medication before?

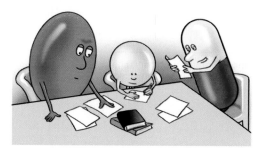

NURSING DIAGNOSIS

Each patient will receive a Nursing Diagnosis based on the assessment. There are nursing diagnoses that relate to the medical condition, such as Acute Pain related to hip surgery, and there are nursing diagnoses related to the actual medication the patient is receiving, such as Risk for Bleeding. In the first diagnosis, the medication administration will be part of the Implementation. The nurse will administer medication to relieve the pain from hip surgery. In the second diagnosis, the medication administration will be critically evaluated to watch for the adverse effect of bleeding that can be seen with anticoagulant drugs. In both of these examples, you can clearly see the relationship between pharmacology and the nursing process.

PLANNING

Once you have established the nursing diagnosis, you need to decide on a **Plan** of care for the patient. What is the outcome that you want the patient to achieve? For our first example, pain relief is a good outcome. It can further be defined by the pain level, less than 5 out of 10 on the pain scale. For the second example, the outcome would state that the patient not experience any bleeding episodes. As explained in Chapter 1, these outcomes will be patient specific and have a time frame associated with them.

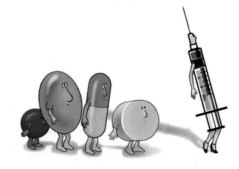

IMPLEMENTATION

The **Implementation** is where you devise the actions or interventions that you will provide to the patient to help him or her achieve the outcome you established. For our patient with Acute Pain, a good intervention is to provide pain medication. For our patient with a risk for bleeding, a good intervention would be teaching the patient to watch for signs and symptoms of unusual bleeding. So in these two examples you have seen that an Implementation can be something we do for the patient, and it can include something we teach the patient. Patient teaching is a very important component of nursing pharmacology.

EVALUATION

The last part of ADPIE is the **Evaluation**. This is where we look at our outcome and see whether or not our Implementation of the plan worked. Did the patient with hip pain obtain relief from the administration of the pain medication? Did the patient at risk for bleeding have any episode of bleeding, or did he or she understand the teaching we provided? If your outcome was not met, you will need to re-evaluate your outcome, the outcome time frame, or the interventions you implemented. Thus the nursing process is an ongoing and evolving process.

CONCEPT MAPPING

This entire **Nursing Process** can be learned and applied by using a method called a *concept map*. There are many forms of concept mapping. Many nursing schools use concept maps for planning the care of the patients. Here is a simplified concept map for our first example patient. Start with Assessment.

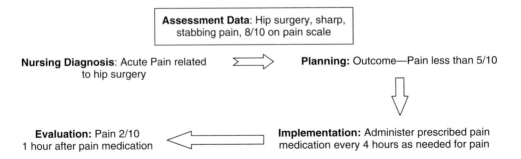

This concept map can be very simple or detailed depending on the patient's assessment. Several Nursing Diagnoses can be formulated on one patient. In the planning of care, more than one outcome can be written along with various implementations to achieve the outcome. Then each outcome should be evaluated to see if they were achieved. This concept map can help you better learn and understand the Nursing Process.

Looking at the second example, we can draw a concept map examining the medication more closely. It will still use the nursing process but from a different angle. We will start with the medication that the patient is prescribed.

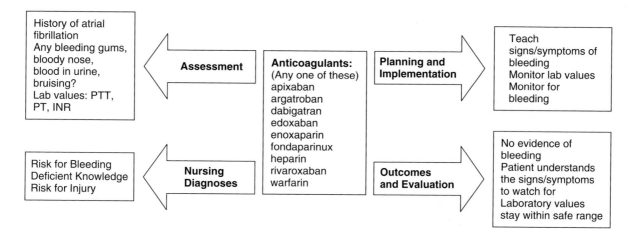

This concept map format can be used by students as a way to study the specific drug content in each of the chapters. If you look at the nursing process section in Chapter 26, you will notice that this concept map contains some of those key points from that chapter on anticoagulant drugs. Students can make this map as simple or as detailed as they need to learn the concepts.

When students find that a concept map is helpful to their learning, many times they will make a template on their computer. Then all they need to do is copy it and fill in the data. Writing the data into the boxes helps the brain make the connections and assists in remembering the information. Repeating an activity like concept mapping makes the nursing process easy as pie, ADPIE.

Analgesic Drugs

ⓔ http://evolve.elsevier.com/Lilley

OBJECTIVES

When you reach the end of this chapter, you will be able to do the following:

1. Define acute pain and chronic pain.
2. Contrast the signs, symptoms, and management of acute and chronic pain.
3. Discuss the pathophysiology and characteristics associated with cancer pain and other special pain situations.
4. Describe pharmacologic and nonpharmacologic approaches for the management of acute and chronic pain.
5. Discuss the use of nonopioids, nonsteroidal antiinflammatory drugs, opioids (opioid agonists, opioids with mixed actions, opioid agonists-antagonists and antagonists), and miscellaneous drugs in the management of pain, including acute and chronic pain, cancer pain, and special pain situations.
6. Identify examples of drugs classified as nonopioids, nonsteroidal antiinflammatory drugs, opioids (opioid agonists, opioids with mixed actions, opioid agonists-antagonists and antagonists), and miscellaneous drugs.
7. Briefly describe the mechanism of action, indications, dosages, routes of administration, adverse effects, toxicity, cautions, contraindications, and drug interactions of nonopioids, nonsteroidal antiinflammatory drugs (see Chapter 44), opioids (opioid agonists, opioids with mixed actions, opioid agonists-antagonists and antagonists), and miscellaneous drugs.
8. Contrast the pharmacologic and nonpharmacologic management of acute and chronic pain with the management of pain associated with cancer and pain experienced in terminal conditions.
9. Briefly describe the specific standards of pain management as defined by the World Health Organization and The Joint Commission.
10. Develop a nursing care plan based on the nursing process related to the use of nonopioid and opioid drug therapy for patients in pain.
11. Identify various resources, agencies, and professional groups that are involved in establishing standards for the management of all types of pain and for promotion of a holistic approach to the care of patients with acute or chronic pain and those in special pain situations.

DRUG PROFILES

♦acetaminophen, p. 158
!codeine sulfate, p. 155
!fentanyl, p. 155
♦!hydromorphone, p. 155
lidocaine, transdermal, p. 158

!meperidine hydrochloride, p. 155
♦!methadone hydrochloride, p. 156
♦!morphine sulfate, p. 156
♦naloxone hydrochloride, p. 156
naltrexone hydrochloride, p. 157

!oxycodone hydrochloride, p. 156
!tramadol hydrochloride, p. 158

_____
♦ = *Key drug*
! = *High-alert drug*

KEY TERMS

Acute pain Pain that is sudden in onset, usually subsides when treated, and typically occurs over less than a 6-week period. (p. 145)

Addiction A chronic, neurobiologic disease whose development is influenced by genetic, psychosocial, and environmental factors (same as *psychologic dependence*). (p. 147)

Adjuvant analgesic drugs Drugs that are added for combined therapy with a primary drug and may have additive or independent analgesic properties, or both. (p. 144)

Agonist A substance that binds to a receptor and causes a response. (p. 149)

Agonists-antagonists Substances that bind to a receptor and cause a partial response that is not as strong as that caused by an agonist (also known as a *partial agonist*). (p. 149)

Analgesic ceiling effect Occurs when a given pain drug no longer effectively controls pain despite the administration of the highest safe dosages. (p. 149)

Analgesics Medications that relieve pain without causing loss of consciousness (sometimes referred to as *painkillers*). (p. 144)

Antagonist A drug that binds to a receptor and prevents (blocks) a response. (p. 150)

Breakthrough pain Pain that occurs between doses of pain medication. (p. 147)

KEY TERMS—cont'd

Cancer pain Pain resulting from any of a variety of causes related to cancer and/or the metastasis of cancer. (p. 146)

Central pain Pain resulting from any disorder that causes central nervous system damage. (p. 146)

Chronic pain Persistent or recurring pain that is often difficult to treat. Includes any pain lasting longer than 3 to 6 months, pain lasting longer than 1 month after healing of an acute injury, or pain that accompanies a nonhealing tissue injury. (p. 145)

Deep pain Pain that occurs in tissues below skin level; opposite of *superficial pain.* (p. 146)

Gate theory The most well described theory of pain transmission and pain relief. It uses a gate model to explain how impulses from damaged tissues are sensed in the brain. (p. 146)

Narcotics A legal term that originally applied to drugs that produce insensibility or stupor, especially the opioids (e.g., morphine, heroin). Currently used to refer to any medically used controlled substance and to refer to any illicit or "street" drug. (NOTE: This term is falling out of use in favor of *opioid.*) (p. 149)

Neuropathic pain Pain that results from a disturbance of function in a nerve. (p. 146)

Nociception Processing of pain signals in the brain that gives rise to the feeling of pain. (p. 144)

Nociceptors A subclass of sensory nerves (A and C fibers) that transmit pain signals to the central nervous system from other body parts. (p. 144)

Nonopioid analgesics Analgesics that are not classified as opioids. (p. 146)

Nonsteroidal antiinflammatory drugs (NSAIDs) A large, chemically diverse group of drugs that are analgesics and also possess antiinflammatory and antipyretic activity. (p. 146)

Opioid analgesics Synthetic drugs that bind to opiate receptors to relieve pain. (p. 144)

Opioid naïve Describes patients who are receiving opioid analgesics for the first time and who therefore are not accustomed to their effects. (p. 165)

Opioid tolerance A normal physiologic condition that results from long-term opioid use, in which larger doses of opioids are required to maintain the same level of analgesia and in which abrupt discontinuation of the drug results in withdrawal symptoms (same as *physical dependence*). (p. 147)

Opioid tolerant The opposite of opioid naïve; describes patients who have been receiving opioid analgesics (legally or otherwise) for a period of time (1 week or longer). (p. 147)

Opioid withdrawal The signs and symptoms associated with abstinence from or withdrawal of an opioid analgesic when the body has become physically dependent on the substance. (p. 152)

Opioids A class of drugs used to treat pain. This term is often used interchangeably with the term *narcotic.* (p. 149)

Pain An unpleasant sensory and emotional experience associated with actual or potential tissue damage. (p. 144)

Pain threshold The level of a stimulus that results in the sensation of pain. (p. 144)

Pain tolerance The amount of pain a patient can endure without its interfering with normal function. (p. 145)

Partial agonist A drug that binds to a receptor and causes a response that is less than that caused by a full agonist (same as *agonist-antagonist*). (p. 150)

Phantom pain Pain experienced in the area of a body part that has been surgically or traumatically removed. (p. 146)

Physical dependence A condition in which a patient takes a drug over a period of time and unpleasant physical symptoms (withdrawal symptoms) occur if the drug is stopped abruptly or smaller doses are given. The physical adaptation of the body to the presence of an opioid or other addictive substance. (p. 145)

Psychologic dependence A pattern of compulsive use of opioids or any other addictive substance characterized by a continuous craving for the substance and the need to use it for effects other than pain relief (also called *addiction*). (p. 147)

Referred pain Pain occurring in an area away from the organ of origin. (p. 146)

Somatic pain Pain that originates from skeletal muscles, ligaments, or joints. (p. 145)

Special pain situations The general term for pain control situations that are complex and whose treatment typically involves multiple medications, and nonpharmacologic therapeutic modalities (e.g., massage, chiropractic care, surgery). (p. 166)

Superficial pain Pain that originates from the skin or mucous membranes; opposite of *deep pain.* (p. 146)

Synergistic effects Drug interactions in which the effect of a combination of two or more drugs with similar actions is greater than the sum of the individual effects of the same drugs given alone. For example, 1 + 1 is greater than 2. (p. 148)

Tolerance The general term for a state in which repetitive exposure to a given drug, over time, induces changes in drug receptors that reduce the drug's effects (same as *physical dependence*). (p. 145)

Vascular pain Pain that results from pathology of the vascular or perivascular tissues. (p. 146)

Visceral pain Pain that originates from organs or smooth muscles. (p. 146)

World Health Organization (WHO) An international body of health care professionals that studies and responds to health needs and trends worldwide. (p. 149)

OVERVIEW

The management of pain is a very important aspect of nursing care. Pain is the most common reason that patients seek health care, resulting in over 70 million office visits annually in the United States. Surgical and diagnostic procedures often require pain management, as do several diseases including arthritis, diabetes, multiple sclerosis, cancer, and acquired immunodeficiency syndrome (AIDS). Pain leads to much suffering and is a tremendous economic burden in terms of lost workplace productivity, workers' compensation payments, and other related health care costs.

To provide quality patient care, the nurse must be well informed about both pharmacologic and nonpharmacologic methods of pain management. This chapter focuses on pharmacologic methods of pain management. Nonpharmacologic methods are listed in Box 10-1.

Medications that relieve pain without causing loss of consciousness are classified as **analgesics**. There are various classes of analgesics, determined by their chemical structures and mechanisms of action. This chapter focuses primarily on the **opioid analgesics**, which are used to manage moderate to severe pain. Often drugs from other chemical categories are added to the opioid regimen as **adjuvant analgesic drugs** (or adjuvants) and are described later.

Pain is most commonly defined as an unpleasant sensory and emotional experience associated with either actual or potential tissue damage. It is a very personal and individual experience. Pain can be defined as whatever the patient says it is, and it exists whenever the patient says it does. Although the mechanisms of pain are becoming better understood, a patient's perception of pain is a complex process. Pain involves physical, psychologic, and even cultural factors (see the Patient-Centered Care: Cultural Implications box). Because pain intensity cannot be precisely quantified, health care providers must cultivate relationships of mutual trust with their patients to provide optimal care.

There is no single approach to effective pain management. Instead, pain management is tailored to each patient's needs. The cause of the pain, the existence of concurrent medical conditions; the characteristics of the pain; and the psychological and cultural characteristics of the patient need to be considered. It also requires ongoing reassessment of the pain and the effectiveness of treatment. The patient's emotional response to pain depends on his or her psychologic experiences of pain. Pain results from the stimulation of sensory nerve fibers known as **nociceptors**. These receptors transmit pain signals from various body regions to the spinal cord and brain, which leads to the sensation of pain, or **nociception** (Figure 10-1).

The physical impulses that signal pain activate various nerve pathways from the periphery to the spinal cord and to the brain. The level of stimulus needed to produce a painful sensation is referred to as the **pain threshold**. Because this is a measure of the physiologic response of the nervous system, it is similar for most individuals. However, variations in pain sensitivity may result from genetic factors.

There are three main receptors believed to be involved in pain. The mu receptors in the dorsal horn of the spinal cord appear to play the most crucial role. Less important but still involved in

BOX 10-1 Nonpharmacologic Treatment Options for Pain

- Acupressure
- Acupuncture
- Art therapy
- Behavioral therapy
- Biofeedback
- Comfort measures
- Counseling
- Distraction
- Hot or cold packs
- Hypnosis
- Imagery
- Massage
- Meditation
- Music therapy
- Pet therapy
- Physical therapy
- Reduction of fear
- Relaxation
- Surgery
- Therapeutic baths
- Therapeutic communication
- Therapeutic touch
- Transcutaneous electric nerve stimulation
- Yoga

⊕ PATIENT-CENTERED CARE: CULTURAL IMPLICATIONS   QSEN

The Patient Experiencing Pain

- Each culture has its own beliefs, thoughts, and ways of approaching, defining, and managing pain. Attitudes, meanings, and perceptions of pain vary with culture, race, and ethnicity.
- African Americans believe in the power of healers who rely strongly on the religious faith of people and often use prayer and the laying on of hands for relief of pain.
- Hispanic Americans believe in prayer, the wearing of amulets, and the use of herbs and spices to maintain health and wellness. Specific herbs are used in teas and therapies, often including religious practices, massage, and cleansings.
- Some traditional methods of healing for the Chinese include acupuncture, herbal remedies, yin and yang balancing, and cold treatment. *Moxibustion*, in which cones or cylinders of pulverized wormwood are burned on or near the skin over specific meridian points, is another form of healing.
- Asian and Pacific Islander patients are often reluctant to express their pain because they believe that the pain is God's will or is punishment for past sins.
- For many Native Americans, treatments for pain include massage, the application of heat, sweat baths, herbal remedies, and being in harmony with nature.
- In Arab culture, patients are expected to express their pain openly and anticipate immediate relief, preferably through injections or intravenous drugs.
- Remain aware of all cultural influences on health-related behaviors and on patients' attitudes toward medication therapy and thus, ultimately, on its effectiveness. A thorough assessment that includes questions about the patient's cultural background and practices is important to the effective and individualized delivery of nursing care.

pain sensations are the kappa and delta receptors. Pain receptors are located in both the central nervous system (CNS) and various body tissues. Pain perception is closely linked to the number of mu receptors. This number is controlled by a single gene, the mu opioid receptor gene. When the number of receptors is high, pain sensitivity is diminished. Conversely, when the receptors are reduced or missing altogether, relatively minor noxious stimuli may be perceived as painful.

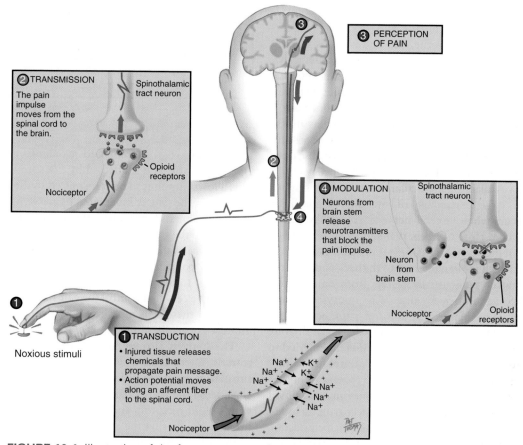

FIGURE 10-1 Illustration of the four processes of nociception. (From Jarvis C: *Physical examination and health assessment*, ed 6, St Louis, 2012, Saunders.)

The patient's emotional response to the pain is also molded by the patient's age, sex, culture, previous pain experience, and anxiety level. Whereas pain threshold is the physiologic element of pain, the psychologic element of pain is called **pain tolerance.** This is the amount of pain a patient can endure without its interfering with normal function. Because it is a subjective response, pain tolerance can vary from patient to patient. Pain tolerance can be modulated by the patient's personality, attitude, environment, culture, and ethnic background. Pain tolerance can even vary within the same person depending on the circumstances involved. Table 10-1 lists the various conditions that can alter one's pain tolerance.

Pain can also be further classified in terms of its onset and duration as either acute or chronic. **Acute pain** is sudden and usually subsides when treated. One example of acute pain is postoperative pain. **Chronic pain** is persistent or recurring, lasting 3 to 6 months. It is often more difficult to treat, because changes occur in the nervous system that often require increasing drug dosages. This situation is known by the general term **tolerance** or **physical dependence** (see Chapter 17). Acute pain and chronic pain differ in their onset and duration, their associated diseases or conditions, and the way they are treated. Table 10-2 lists the different characteristics of acute and chronic pain and various diseases and conditions associated with each.

Pain can be further classified according to its source. The two most common sources of pain are somatic and visceral. **Somatic**

TABLE 10-1	Conditions That Alter Pain Tolerance
Pain Threshold	**Conditions**
Lowered	Anger, anxiety, depression, discomfort, fear, isolation, chronic pain, sleeplessness, tiredness
Raised	Diversion, empathy, rest, sympathy, medications (analgesics, antianxiety drugs, antidepressants)

TABLE 10-2	Acute versus Chronic Pain		
Type of Pain	**Onset**	**Duration**	**Examples**
Acute	Sudden (minutes to hours); usually sharp, localized; physiologic response (SNS: tachycardia, sweating, pallor, increased blood pressure)	Limited (has an end)	Myocardial infarction, appendicitis, dental procedures, kidney stones, surgical procedures
Chronic	Slow (days to months); long duration; dull, persistent aching	Persistent or recurring (endless)	Arthritis, cancer, lower back pain, peripheral neuropathy

SNS, Sympathetic nervous system.

pain originates from skeletal muscles, ligaments, and joints. Visceral pain originates from organs and smooth muscles. Superficial pain originates from the skin and mucous membranes. Deep pain occurs in tissues below skin level. Pain may be appropriately treated when the source of the pain is known. For example, visceral and superficial pain usually require opioids for relief, whereas somatic pain (including bone pain) usually responds better to nonopioid analgesics such as nonsteroidal antiinflammatory drugs (NSAIDs) (see Chapter 44).

Pain may be further subclassified according to the diseases or other conditions that cause it. Vascular pain is believed to originate from the vascular or perivascular tissues and is thought to account for a large percentage of migraine headaches. Referred pain occurs when visceral nerve fibers synapse at a level in the spinal cord close to fibers that supply specific subcutaneous tissues in the body. An example is the pain associated with cholecystitis, which is often referred to the back and scapular areas. Neuropathic pain usually results from damage to peripheral or CNS nerve fibers by disease or injury but may also be idiopathic (unexplained). Phantom pain occurs in the area of a body part that has been removed—surgically or traumatically—and is often described as burning, itching, tingling, or stabbing. It can also occur in paralyzed limbs following spinal cord injury. Cancer pain can be acute or chronic or both. It most often results from pressure of the tumor mass against nerves, organs, or tissues. Other causes of cancer pain include hypoxia from blockage of blood supply to an organ, metastases, pathologic fractures, muscle spasms, and adverse effects of radiation, surgery, and chemotherapy. Central pain occurs with tumors, trauma, inflammation, or disease (e.g., cancer, diabetes, stroke, multiple sclerosis) affecting CNS tissues.

Several theories attempt to explain pain transmission and pain relief. The most common and well described is the gate theory. This theory, proposed by Melzack and Wall in 1965, uses the analogy of a gate to describe how impulses from damaged tissues are sensed in the brain. First, the tissue injury causes the release of several substances from injured cells, such as bradykinin, histamine, potassium, prostaglandins, and serotonin. Some current pain medications work by altering the actions and levels of these substances (e.g., NSAIDs → prostaglandins; antidepressants → serotonin). The release of these pain-mediating chemicals initiates action potentials (electrical nerve impulses) at the distal end of sensory nerve fibers through pain receptors known as *nociceptors*. These nerve impulses are conducted along sensory nerve fibers and activate pain receptors in the *dorsal horn* of the spinal cord. It is here that the so-called *gates* are located. These gates regulate the flow of sensory nerve impulses. If impulses are stopped by a gate at this junction, no impulses are transmitted to the higher centers of the brain. Conversely, if the gates permit a sufficient number and intensity of action potentials to be conducted from the spinal cord to the cerebral cortex, the sensation of pain is then felt. This is known as *nociception*. Figure 10-2 depicts the gate theory of pain transmission.

Both the opening and the closing of this gate are influenced by the activation of large-diameter A fibers and small-diameter C fibers (Table 10-3). Closing of the gate is affected by the activation of A fibers. This causes the inhibition of impulse

TABLE 10-3 A and C Nerve Fibers

Type of Fiber	Myelin Sheath	Fiber Size	Conduction Speed	Type of Pain
A	Yes	Large	Fast	Sharp and well localized
C	No	Small	Slow	Dull and nonlocalized

transmission to the brain and avoidance of pain sensation. Opening of the gate is affected by the stimulation of C fibers. This allows impulses to be transmitted to the brain and pain to be sensed. The gate is innervated by nerve fibers that originate in the brain and modulate the pain sensation by sending impulses to the gate in the spinal cord. These nerve fibers enable the brain to evaluate, identify, and localize the pain. Thus, the brain can control the gate, either keeping the gate closed or allowing it to open so that the brain is stimulated and pain is sensed. The cells that control the gate have a threshold. Impulses that reach these cells must rise above this threshold before an impulse is permitted to travel up to the brain.

The body is also equipped with certain endogenous neurotransmitters known as *enkephalins* and *endorphins*. These substances are produced within the body to fight pain and are considered the body's painkillers. Both are capable of bonding with opioid receptors and inhibiting the transmission of pain impulses by closing the spinal cord gates, in a manner similar to that of opioid analgesic drugs. The term *endorphin* is a condensed version of the term *endogenous morphine*. These endogenous analgesic substances are released whenever the body experiences pain or prolonged exertion. They are responsible for the phenomenon of "runner's high." Figure 10-1 depicts this entire process.

Another phenomenon of pain relief that may be explained by the gate theory is the fact that massaging a painful area often reduces the pain. When an area is rubbed or liniment is applied, large sensory A nerve fibers from peripheral receptors carry pain-modulating impulses to the spinal cord. Remember, the A fibers tend to close the gate, which reduces pain sensation in the brain.

TREATMENT OF PAIN IN SPECIAL SITUATIONS

It is estimated that one of every three Americans experiences ongoing pain. Pain is poorly understood and often undertreated. Patient-controlled analgesia (PCA) is commonly used in the hospital setting. In this situation, patients are able to self-medicate by pressing a button on a PCA infusion pump. This has been shown to be very effective and reduces the total opioid dose used. Morphine and hydromorphone are commonly given by PCA. Potential hazards of PCA include well-meaning family members' pressing the dosing button rather than letting able patients do so on their own. Numerous deaths have occurred when well-meaning family members have administered too much of the opioid drug. This is called *PCA by proxy*. The Institute for Safe Medication Practices (ISMP) advises against PCA by proxy. For patients who are unable to self-medicate using the PCA pump, a different method of pain control must be used.

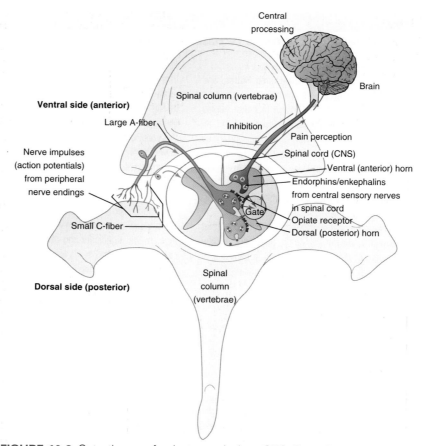

FIGURE 10-2 Gate theory of pain transmission. *CNS,* Central nervous system.

Patients with complex pain syndromes often benefit from a holistic or multimodal clinical approach that involves pharmacologic and/or nonpharmacologic treatment. Effective drug therapy may include use of opioid and/or nonopioid drugs. The main consideration in pain management for pain associated with cancer is patient comfort and not trying to prevent drug addiction (or psychologic dependence; see Chapter 17). Opioid tolerance is a state of adaptation in which exposure to a drug causes changes in drug receptors that result in reduced drug effects over time. This can occur in as little as 1 week. Because of increasing pathology (e.g., tumor burden), cancer patients usually require increasingly higher opioid doses and thus do become physically dependent on the drugs. Cancer patients are likely to experience withdrawal symptoms (see Chapter 17) if opioid doses are abruptly reduced or discontinued; however, actual psychologic dependence or addiction in such patients is unusual. For long-term pain control, oral, intravenous, subcutaneous, transdermal, and rectal dosing routes are favored over multiple intramuscular injections.

The treatment of acute pain in patients who are addicted to opioids is of great concern to health care professionals, who may be reluctant to prescribe opioid therapy. However, habitual street opioid users or patients with chronic pain are opioid tolerant and generally require high dosages. Effective management of acute-on-chronic pain requires patients to receive equivalent amounts of their chronic pain medication in addition to an extra 20% to 40% more opioids to treat the acute pain. Longer-acting opioids such as methadone or extended-release oxycodone are

usually better choices than shorter-acting immediate-release drug products for these patients. This is because the shorter-acting drugs are more likely to produce a psychologic "high" or euphoria, which only reinforces addictive tendencies. Genetic differences in cytochrome P-450 enzymes (see Chapters 2 and 8) can cause different patients, whether addicted or not, to respond more or less effectively to a given drug. For this reason, patients must not automatically be viewed with suspicion if they complain that a given drug does not work for them.

The label of "addict" can be used unfairly to justify refusal to prescribe pain medications, resulting in undertreatment of pain, even in patients who do not use street drugs. This is now regarded as an inappropriate and inhumane clinical practice. In these situations, control of the patient's pain takes ethical and clinical priority over concerns regarding drug addiction. Nonetheless, prescribers must contend with the reality of abuse of street and/or prescription drugs by patients without genuine pain conditions (see Chapter 17). Such patients often request excessive numbers of prescriptions and may use multiple prescribers and/or pharmacies.

For patients receiving long-acting opioids, breakthrough pain often occurs between doses of pain medications. This is because the analgesic effects wear off as the drug is metabolized and eliminated from the body. Treatment with "prn" (as needed) doses of immediate-release dosage forms (e.g., oxycodone IR) given between scheduled doses of extended-release dosage forms (e.g., oxycodone ER) is often helpful in these cases. Chewing or crushing of any extended-release opioid drug can

EVIDENCE-BASED PRACTICE

Pain Management Knowledge and Attitudes of Baccalaureate Nursing Students and Faculty

Review

Pain impacts approximately 76 million adults within the United States, and although it is a top priority in care and considered to be the fifth vital sign, pain continues to be inadequately addressed. It is a well-known fact that nurses spend more time with patients than any other health care professional and, as such, nurses are very aware of the patient's needs. One of the main priorities in nursing and health care is that of managing pain. Nurses need to be adequately prepared both in knowledge and clinical skills to assess, plan, implement, and evaluate the pain patients experience regardless of age and cultural diversity. Therefore, nurse educators/faculty members must offer didactic, clinical, and evidence-based knowledge about the complex issue of pain. The purpose of this research study was to examine the knowledge and attitudes that junior- and senior-level baccalaureate nursing students and their faculty members held about the management of pain toward patients in pain and to establish a systematic, comprehensive integration of pain in patients who were hospitalized.

Type of Evidence

This study was conducted at a university in Texas and utilized a convenience sample of both students and faculty. Participants were asked to complete a 36-item Knowledge and Attitudes Survey Regarding Pain (KASRP). This tool consists of two case studies, and respondents are asked to evaluate and manage the pain of the patients described (in the case study). Calculated scores were done as a percentage of correct responses with a minimum score of 80 out of 100%, which was required to earn a satisfactory rating.

Results of the Study

The final sample included 162 nursing students and 16 faculty members. The two case studies presented were identical in their pain complaints, but the first was described as grimacing and quiet and the second as smiling and conversing on the phone. 83% of the sample was white, female (87%), and younger than 30 years of age (81%). The scores on the KASRP varied from 28% to 86%. Statistically significant differences were found between the scores of the junior- and senior-level nursing students but not between the senior-level students and faculty (at 68% and 71%, respectively). Both scored in the unsatisfactory range. The survey items most frequently yet incorrectly answered were about pain medications. Those questions that were most frequently answered correctly were those about the assessment of pain. More specific information

about the case studies includes the following: Faculty accurately assessed pain in the second scenario as compared to the students; the students most accurately assessing pain in the second scenario were first-semester junior students (86%), whereas only 59.4% of second-semester students and 77% of first-semester senior nursing students made the correct assessment. In all cases, the nursing students who answered incorrectly were assessing the pain at a lower level than that of the patient's own pain assessment. Interestingly enough, students correctly assessing pain often chose incorrect pain management strategies with less than optimal doses of pain medication. In a few situations, no pain medication was selected at all. The findings of this research study must be interpreted with caution due to limitations, such as a small sample size and use of only a single academic institution. However, the findings are still significant and can assist in the care of patients with pain. Significant findings of this study (and consistent with other studies) offering us areas of direction for further education include the finding that knowledge deficits were found in the area of pain medications. Scores associated with pain assessment were found to be higher, as with other studies. Even if the student or faculty correctly assessed the patient's pain level, the selection of intervention was often incorrect.

Link of Evidence to Nursing Practice

The results of this study emphasize the fact that more needs to be done in regards to the adequate and thorough education of nursing students about pain and its assessment, management, and evaluation. Further research needs to be conducted using the same methodology, but in a larger sample and in a variety of educational programs for professional nurses. Emphasis also needs to be on specific levels of pain assessment and adequate dosing of pain medication, as prescribed. The significant findings of this study need to be replicated using a larger sample and across a variety of educational programs for future professional nurses. Areas of concentration need to be on the adequate assessment of pain and its effective management. Additionally, there needs to be assessment of specific knowledge deficits about pain medications in regard to their specific action, indication(s), and dosing. Nonpharmacologic pain management therapies need to also be researched. With pain being one of the top priorities in health care settings, more research needs to occur so that future professional nurses are adequately prepared both in their knowledge and clinical skills in the assessment, planning, implementation, and evaluation of all types of patient pain experiences.

Reference: Duke G, Haas BK, Yarborough S, Northam S: Pain management knowledge and attitudes of baccalaureate nursing students and faculty. *Pain Manag Nurs* 14:11-19, 2013.

cause oversedation, respiratory depression, and even death due to rapid drug absorption. If the patient is requiring larger doses for breakthrough pain, the dose of the scheduled extended-release opioid may need to be shortened or a more potent drug started.

Drugs from other chemical categories are often added to the opioid regimen as adjuvant drugs. These assist the primary drugs in relieving pain. Such adjuvant drug therapy may include NSAIDs (see Chapter 44), antidepressants (see Chapter 16), antiepileptic drugs (see Chapter 14), and corticosteroids (see Chapter 33). This approach allows the use of smaller dosages of opioids and reduces some of the adverse effects that are seen with higher dosages of opioids, such as respiratory depression, constipation, and urinary retention. It permits drugs with different mechanisms of action to produce synergistic effects.

Antiemetics (see Chapter 52) and laxatives (see Chapter 51) may also be needed to prevent or relieve associated constipation, nausea, and vomiting (Box 10-2). This multimodal approach has been shown to be very effective in treating pain.

Adjuvant drugs are commonly used in the treatment of neuropathic pain, where opioids are not completely effective. Neuropathic pain usually results from nerve damage secondary to disease (e.g., diabetic neuropathy, postherpetic neuralgia secondary to shingles, AIDS or injury, including nerve damage secondary to surgical procedures [e.g., post-thoracotomy pain syndrome occurring after cardiothoracic surgery]). Common symptoms include hypersensitivity or hyperalgesia to mild stimuli such as light touch or a pinprick, or the bed sheets on a person's feet. This is also known as *allodynia*. It can also manifest as hyperalgesia to uncomfortable stimuli, such as pressure

BOX 10-2   Potential Opioid Adverse Effects and Their Management

Constipation

Opioids decrease gastrointestinal (GI) tract peristalsis because of their central nervous system (CNS) depression, with subsequent constipation as an adverse effect. Stool becomes excessively dehydrated because it remains in the GI tract longer. **Preventative measures:** Constipation may be managed with increased intake of fluids, stool softeners such as docusate sodium, or the use of stimulants such as bisacodyl or senna. Agents such as lactulose, sorbitol, and polyethylene glycol (Miralax) have been proven effective. Bulk-forming laxatives, such as psyllium, may be used but do require an increase in fluid intake to avoid fecal impactions or bowel obstructions.

Nausea and Vomiting

Opioids decrease GI tract peristalsis, and some also stimulate the vomiting center in the CNS, so nausea and vomiting are often experienced. **Preventative measures:** Nausea and vomiting may be managed with the use of antiemetics such as phenothiazines.

Sedation and Mental Clouding

Any change in mental status must always be evaluated to ensure that causes other than drug-related CNS depression are ruled out. Respiratory depression is strongly associated with excessive sedation. **Preventative measures:** Safety precautions implemented. Persistent drug-related sedation may be managed with a decrease in the dosage of opioid or change in drug used. The prescriber may also order various CNS stimulants (see Chapter 13).

Respiratory Depression

Long-term opioid use is generally associated with tolerance to respiratory depression. **Preventative measures:** For severe respiratory depression, opioid antagonists (naloxone) may be needed.

Subacute Overdose

Subacute overdose may be more common than acute respiratory depression and may progress slowly (over hours to days), with somnolence and respiratory depression. Before analgesic dosages are changed or reduced, advancing disease must be considered, especially in the dying patient. **Preventative measures:** Often, holding one or two doses of an opioid analgesic is enough to judge if the mental and respiratory depression is associated with the opioid. If there is improvement with this measure, the opioid dosage is often decreased by 25%.

Other Opioid Adverse Effects

Dry mouth, urinary retention, pruritus, dysphoria, euphoria, sleep disturbances, or sexual dysfunction may occur but are less common than the aforementioned adverse effects. **Preventative measures:** Ongoing assessment is needed for each of the adverse effects so that appropriate measures may be implemented (e.g., sucking of sugar-free hard candy or use of artificial saliva drops or gum for dry mouth; use of diphenhydramine for pruritus).

---

from an inflated blood pressure cuff on a patient's limb. It may be described as heat, cold, numbness and tingling, burning, or electrical sensations. Examples of adjuvants commonly used in these cases are the antidepressant amitriptyline and the anticonvulsants gabapentin and pregabalin.

The three-step analgesic ladder defined by the World Health Organization (WHO) is often applied as the pain management standard. Step 1 is the use of nonopioids (with or without adjuvant medications) once the pain has been identified and assessed. If pain persists and/or increases, treatment moves to step 2, which is defined as the use of opioids with or without nonopioids and with or without adjuvants. If pain persists or increases, management then rises to step 3, which is the use of opioids indicated for moderate to severe pain, administered with or without nonopioids or adjuvant medications. Not all patients will be treated effectively using the ladder method, and some may need to seek an experienced pain management physician.

PHARMACOLOGY OVERVIEW

The terms opioids and narcotics are often used interchangeably. However, the appropriate term when discussing pharmacology is *opioid*. Opioids are classified as both mild agonists (codeine, hydrocodone) and strong agonists (morphine, hydromorphone, oxycodone, oxymorphone, meperidine, fentanyl, and methadone). Meperidine is not recommended for long-term use because of the accumulation of a neurotoxic metabolite, *normeperidine,* which can cause seizures. In 2010, the mild agonist propoxyphene (Darvocet) was withdrawn from the market due to adverse effects. The opiate agonists-antagonists

such as pentazocine and nalbuphine are associated with an analgesic ceiling effect. This means that the drug reaches a maximum analgesic effect, so that analgesia does not improve even with higher dosages. Such drugs are useful only in patients who have not been previously exposed to opioids and can be used for nonescalating moderate to severe pain. Finally, because of associated bruising and bleeding risks, as well as injection discomfort, there is now a strong trend away from intramuscular injections in favor of intravenous, oral, and transdermal routes of drug administration.

OPIOID DRUGS

The pain-relieving drugs currently known as *opioid analgesics* originated from the opium poppy plant. The word *opium* is a Greek word that means "juice." More than 20 different alkaloids are obtained from the unripe seed of the poppy.

Chemical Structure

Opioid analgesics are very strong pain relievers. They can be classified according to their chemical structure or their action at specific receptors. Of the 20 different natural alkaloids available from the opium poppy plant, only three are clinically useful: morphine, codeine, and papaverine. Of these, only morphine and codeine are pain relievers; papaverine is a smooth muscle relaxant. Relatively simple synthetic chemical modifications of these opium alkaloids have produced the three different chemical classes of opioids: morphine-like drugs, meperidine-like drugs, and methadone-like drugs (Table 10-4). Knowing the chemical structure of the different opioids can be important in determining the appropriate drug for patients who are

TABLE 10-4 **Chemical Classification of Opioids**	
Chemical Category	**Opioid Drugs**
Meperidine-like drugs	meperidine, fentanyl, remifentanil, sufentanil, alfentanil
Methadone-like drugs	methadone
Morphine-like drugs	morphine, heroin, hydromorphone, oxymorphone, codeine, hydrocodone, oxycodone
Other	tramadol, tapentadol

TABLE 10-5 **Opioid Receptors and Their Characteristics**		
Receptor Type	**Prototypical Agonist**	**Effects of Opioid Stimulation**
mu	morphine	Supraspinal analgesia, respiratory depression, euphoria, sedation
kappa	ketocyclazocine	Spinal analgesia, sedation, miosis
delta	Enkephalins	Analgesia

experience significant allergic reactions to a specific opioid. For example, if a patient experiences anaphylaxis from morphine, giving a drug with an unrelated structure such as fentanyl would be appropriate.

Mechanism of Action and Drug Effects

Opioid analgesics can also be characterized according to their mechanism of action. They are agonists, agonists-antagonists, or antagonists (nonanalgesic). An *agonist* binds to an opioid pain receptor in the brain and causes an analgesic response—the reduction of pain sensation. An *agonist-antagonist*, also called a partial agonist or a *mixed agonist,* binds to a pain receptor and causes a weaker pain response than does a full agonist. Different drugs in this class exert their agonist and/or antagonist effects by binding in different degrees to kappa and mu opioid receptors. Although not normally used as first-line analgesics, they are sometimes useful in pain management in obstetrical patients (because they avoid oversedation of the mother and/or fetus). An antagonist binds to a pain receptor but does not reduce pain signals. It functions as a *competitive antagonist* because it competes with and reverses the effects of agonist and agonist-antagonist drugs at the receptor sites.

The receptors to which opioids bind to relieve pain are listed in Table 10-5. The mu, kappa, and delta receptors are most responsive to drug activity, with the mu being the most important. Many of the characteristics of a particular opioid, such as its ability to sedate, its potency, and its ability to cause hallucinations, can be attributed to relative affinity for these various receptors.

Understanding the relative potencies of various drugs becomes important in clinical settings. *Equianalgesia* refers to the ability to provide equivalent pain relief by calculating dosages of different drugs and/or routes of administration that provide comparable analgesia. Box 10-3 lists equianalgesic doses for several common opioids and shows how to calculate dosage conversions for patients. For example, hydromorphone (Dilaudid) is seven times more potent than morphine. Deaths have been reported where a nurse gave the patient morphine and, not realizing the equialanagesic equivalency, gave the same patient hydromorphone a short time later. It is critical to understand that hydromorphone is seven times more potent than morphine.

Indications

The main use of opioids is to alleviate moderate to severe pain. The amount of pain control or unwanted adverse effects

depends on the specific drug, the receptors to which it binds, and its chemical structure.

Strong opioid analgesics such as fentanyl, sufentanil, and alfentanil are commonly used in combination with anesthetics during surgery. Use of fentanyl injection for management of postoperative and procedural pain has become popular due to its rapid onset and short duration. Transdermal fentanyl comes in a patch formulation for use in long-term pain management and is not to be used for postoperative or any other short-term pain control (see the Safety and Quality Improvement: Preventing Medication Errors box).

Strong opioids such as morphine, hydromorphone, and oxycodone are often used to control postoperative and other types of pain. Because morphine and hydromorphone are available in injectable forms, they are often first-line analgesics in the immediate postoperative setting. There is a trend away from using meperidine due to its greater risk for toxicity (see Drug Profile). All available oxycodone dosage forms are orally administered. The product OxyContin is a sustained-release form of oxycodone that is designed to last up to 12 hours. The "Contin" in the product name is a trademark of the original drug manufacturer, and refers to the "continuous-release" nature of the drug formulation. Recall that a continuous- or extended-release dosage form of a drug means that it has a prolonged duration of action, most often 8 to 24 hours (see Chapter 2). Similarly, the drug product MS Contin is a long-acting or sustained-release form of morphine. The "MS" stands for morphine sulfate. Both drugs are also available generically. In 2013, the FDA approved a risk evaluation and mitigation strategy (REMS) for long-acting opioids. The FDA requires prescriber and patient education to help combat prescription opioid misuse and deaths.

There are also immediate-release dosage forms of oxycodone and morphine in tablet, capsule, and liquid form. The analgesic effects of immediate-release oral dosage forms of all three drugs typically last for about 4 hours.

Opioids also suppress the medullary cough center, which results in cough suppression. The most commonly used opioid for this purpose is codeine (see Chapter 36). Hydrocodone is also used in many cough suppressants, either alone or in combination with other drugs. Constipation is often an unwanted side effect of opioids due to decreased gastrointestinal (GI) tract motility. It occurs because opioid drugs bind to intestinal opioid receptors. However, this effect is sometimes helpful in treating diarrhea. Some of the opioid-containing antidiarrheal preparations are camphorated opium tincture (paregoric) and diphenoxylate/atropine (Lomotil) tablets.

BOX 10-3 Calculating Dosage Conversions Between Commonly Used Opioids

EQUIANALGESIC DOSES

	Oral Dose (mg)	Parenteral Dose (mg)	Oral-to-Parenteral Dose Ratio	Dosing Interval (hr)
morphine	30	10	3:1	12 (continuous release) 4 (immediate release)
hydromorphone	7.5	1.5	5:1	4 (immediate release)
oxycodone	15	N/A	N/A	4 (immediate release)
hydrocodone	30	N/A	N/A	N/A

Basic Conversion Equation

$$\frac{\text{24-hour amount of current drug}}{x} = \frac{\text{EA dose of current drug}}{\text{EA dose of desired drug}}$$

Where x = the amount of desired opioid in 24 hours and EA = the equianalgesic dose obtained from the table above

For example: A patient with colon cancer is currently taking oral oxycodone 80 mg every 12 hours and needs to be converted to intravenous morphine due to a bowel obstruction. What is the equivalent IV morphine dose?

Step 1: **Determine the 24-hour amount of oxycodone taken by this patient:**
80 mg × 2 doses per 24 hours = 160 mg per 24 hours

Step 2: **Using the conversion table above, find the equianalgesic (EA) doses of oxycodone and parenteral morphine:**
15 mg oxycodone = 10 mg parenteral morphine

Step 3: Use the above equation and solve for x by cross-multiplying:

$$\frac{\text{24-hour amount of oxycodone (160 mg)}}{x} = \frac{\text{EA of current oxycodone (15 mg)}}{\text{EA dose of parenteral morphine (10 mg)}}$$

Where x = the amount of parenteral morphine in 24 hours (solve by cross-multiplying)

$$160\,\text{mg} \times 10\,\text{mg} = 15\,\text{mg}\, x \quad x = \frac{1600\,\text{mg}}{15\,\text{mg}}$$

$x = 107$ mg (approximately 100 mg of injectable morphine per 24 hours)

N/A, Not applicable.

OSEN ⚡ SAFETY AND QUALITY IMPROVEMENT: PREVENTING MEDICATION ERRORS

Fentanyl Transdermal Patches

When giving fentanyl transdermal patches, keep in mind several important points to avoid improper administration:

- These patches are recommended to be used *only* by patients who are considered opioid tolerant. To be considered opioid tolerant, a patient needs to have been taking, for a week or longer, morphine 60 mg daily, oral oxycodone 30 mg daily, or oral hydromorphone 8 mg daily (or an equianalgesic dose of another opioid). Giving fentanyl transdermal patches to non–opioid-tolerant patients may result in severe respiratory depression. Thorough assessment is important.
- Inform patients that heat, such as in the form of a heating pad/pack, must never be applied over a fentanyl transdermal patch. The increased circulation that results from the application of heat may result in increased absorption of medication, causing an overdose.
- Teach about the proper disposal of transdermal patches. The patch is customarily applied externally for 72 hours and then replaced with a new patch. Although a used patch may have been used for a 72-hour time period, it may still contain a significant amount of medication, which presents a tremendous health hazard/risk of accidental exposure (and even opportunity for diversion). Children have pulled used patches from the trash, which has resulted in death due to exposure to the drug. Additionally, there have been incidents of a patch becoming displaced and it becoming adhered to the skin of an infant, toddler, or child under a variety of means. For disposal at home, the product insert recommends that the patch be folded in half and disposed of by flushing down the toilet (see www.fda.org for the listing of medicines recommended for disposal by flushing). For the home setting and other facilities, when a drug contains instructions to flush it down the toilet it is because the FDA has been working with the manufacturer regarding the most appropriate method of disposal presenting the least risk to safety (see *www.fda.gov/ForConsumers/ConsumerUpdates*).
- Disposal practices in health care institutions may vary by area because of concerns for the water systems. Follow health care institution policy.
- Accidental drug poisoning with transdermal fentanyl has also occurred in health care settings where children accompany adults to visit patients. This includes long-term care institutions, so it is extremely important that used patches are disposed of very carefully and with the consideration of all institution drug-disposal policies.
- Keep patches, as well as all medications, away from children and pets. Do not store medications in warm, moist places such as medicine cabinets in the bathroom.
- Encourage patient education through printed and verbal instructions.
- The Institute for Safe Medication Practices has described examples of fatal patient incidents resulting from failure to follow the above points. It is essential for the patient's safety to read the product labeling and follow instructions precisely. For more information, visit www.ismp.org.

Contraindications

Contraindications to the use of opioid analgesics include known drug allergy and severe asthma. It is not uncommon for patients to state they are allergic to codeine, when in the overwhelming majority of these patients nausea was the "allergic" reaction. Many patients will claim to be allergic to morphine because it causes itching. Itching is a pharmacologic effect due to histamine release and not an allergic reaction. Thus, it is important to determine the exact nature of a patient's stated allergy. Although not absolute contraindications, extreme caution is to be used in cases of respiratory insufficiency, especially when resuscitative equipment is not available and in conditions involving elevated intracranial pressure (e.g., severe head injury); morbid obesity and/or sleep apnea; myasthenia gravis; paralytic ileus (bowel paralysis); and pregnancy, especially with long-term use or high dosages.

Adverse Effects

Many of the unwanted effects of opioid analgesics are related to their pharmacologic effects in areas other than the CNS. Some of these unwanted effects can be explained by the drug's selectivity for the receptors listed in Table 10-5. The various body systems that the opioids affect and their specific adverse effects are summarized in Table 10-6.

Opioids that have an affinity for mu receptors and have rapid onset of action produce marked euphoria, and are most likely to be abused. All opioid drugs have a strong abuse potential. They are common recreational drugs of abuse among the lay public and also among health care professionals, who often have relatively easy access. The person taking them to alter his or her mental status will soon become psychologically dependent (addicted; see Chapter 17).

In addition, opioids cause histamine release. It is thought that this histamine release is responsible for many of the drugs' unwanted adverse effects, such as itching or pruritus, rash, and hemodynamic changes. Histamine release causes peripheral arteries and veins to dilate, which leads to flushing and orthostatic hypotension. The amount of histamine release that an opioid analgesic causes is related to its chemical class. The naturally occurring opiates (e.g., morphine) elicit the most histamine release; the synthetic opioids (e.g., meperidine) elicit the least histamine release. (See Table 10-4 for a list of the various opioids and their respective chemical classes.)

TABLE 10-6	Opioid-Induced Adverse Effects by Body System
Body System	**Adverse Effects**
Cardiovascular	Hypotension, flushing, bradycardia
Central nervous	Sedation, disorientation, euphoria, lightheadedness, dysphoria
Gastrointestinal	Nausea, vomiting, constipation, biliary tract spasm
Genitourinary	Urinary retention
Integumentary	Itching, rash, wheal formation
Respiratory	Respiratory depression and possible aggravation of asthma

The most serious adverse effect of opioid use is CNS depression, which may lead to respiratory depression. When death occurs from opioid overdose, it is almost always due to respiratory depression. When opioids are given, care must be taken to titrate the dose so that the patient's pain is controlled without affecting respiratory function. Individual responses to opioids vary, and patients may occasionally experience respiratory compromise despite careful dose titration. Respiratory depression can be prevented in part by using drugs with very short duration of action and no active metabolites. Respiratory depression seems to be more common in patients with a preexisting condition causing respiratory compromise, such as asthma, chronic obstructive pulmonary disease, or sleep apnea. Respiratory depression is strongly related to the degree of sedation (see Toxicity and Management of Overdose later in the chapter).

GI tract adverse effects are common in patients receiving opioids due to stimulation of GI opioid receptors. Nausea, vomiting, and constipation are the most common adverse effects. Opioids can irritate the GI tract, stimulating the chemoreceptor trigger zone in the CNS, which in turn may cause nausea and vomiting. Opioids slow peristalsis and increase absorption of water from intestinal contents. These two actions combine to produce constipation. This is more pronounced in hospitalized patients who are nonambulatory. Patients may require laxatives (see Chapter 51) to help maintain normal bowel movements. Urinary retention, or the inability to void, is another unwanted adverse effect of opioids, caused by increasing bladder tone. Severe hypersensitivity or anaphylactic reaction to opioid analgesics is rare. Many patients will experience GI discomforts or histamine-mediated reactions to opioids and call these "allergic reactions." However, true anaphylaxis is rare, even with intravenously administered opioids. Some patients may complain of flushing, itching, or wheal formation at the injection site, but this is usually local and histamine mediated, and not a true allergy. See Box 10-2 for additional information on opioid adverse effects and their management.

Toxicity and Management of Overdose

Naloxone and naltrexone are opioid antagonists, and they bind to and occupy all of the receptor sites (mu, kappa, delta). They are competitive antagonists with a strong affinity for these binding sites. Through such binding, they can reverse the adverse effects induced by the opioid drug, such as respiratory depression. These drugs are used in the management of both opioid overdose and opioid addiction and can also be used in small doses to treat itching associated with opioid use. The commonly used opioid antagonists (reversal drugs) are listed in Table 10-7.

Some degree of physical dependence is expected in opioid-tolerant patients. The extent of opioid tolerance is most visible when an opioid drug is discontinued abruptly or when an opioid antagonist is administered. This usually leads to symptoms of **opioid withdrawal**, also known as *abstinence syndrome* (see Chapter 17). This can occur after as little as 2 weeks of opioid therapy in **opioid-naïve** patients. Gradual dosage reduction after chronic opioid use, when possible, helps to minimize the risk and severity of withdrawal symptoms.

TABLE 10-7   Opioid Antagonists (Reversal Drugs)

Generic Name	Trade Name	Adverse Effects
naloxone (IV)	Narcan	Raised or lowered blood pressure, dysrhythmias, pulmonary edema, withdrawal
naltrexone (PO)	ReVia	Nervousness, headache, nausea, vomiting, pulmonary edema, withdrawal

Respiratory depression is the most serious adverse effect associated with opioids. Stimulating the patient may be adequate to reverse mild hypoventilation. If this is unsuccessful, ventilatory assistance using a bag and mask or endotracheal intubation may be needed to support respiration. Administration of opioid antagonists (e.g., naloxone) may also be necessary to reverse severe respiratory depression. Careful titration of dose until the patient begins to breathe independently will prevent over-reversal. The effects of naloxone are short-lived and usually last about 1 hour. With long-acting opioids, respiratory depressant effects may reappear, and naloxone may need to be re-dosed.

The onset of withdrawal symptoms is directly related to the half-life of the opioid analgesic being used. Withdrawal symptoms resulting from the discontinuance or reversal of therapy with short-acting opioids (codeine, hydrocodone, morphine, and hydromorphone) will appear within 6 to 12 hours and peak at 24 to 72 hours. Withdrawal symptoms associated with the long half-life drugs (methadone, levorphanol, and transdermal fentanyl) may not appear for 24 hours or longer after drug discontinuation and may be milder.

Interactions

Potential drug interactions with opioids are significant. Co-administration of opioids with alcohol, antihistamines, barbiturates, benzodiazepines, phenothiazine, and other CNS depressants can result in additive respiratory depressant effects. The combined use of opioids, such as meperidine, with monoamine oxidase inhibitors, such as selegiline, can result in respiratory depression, seizures, and hypotension.

Laboratory Test Interactions

Opioids can cause an abnormal increase in the serum levels of amylase, alanine aminotransferase, alkaline phosphatase, bilirubin, lipase, creatinine kinase, and lactate dehydrogenase (see the Safety: Laboratory Values Related to Drug Therapy box). Other abnormal results include a decrease in urinary 17-ketosteroid levels and an increase in the urinary alkaloid and glucose concentrations.

Dosages

For the recommended initial dosages of selected analgesic drugs in opioid-naïve patients, see the Dosages table on p. 154.

QSEN SAFETY: LABORATORY VALUES RELATED TO DRUG THERAPY

Analgesics

Laboratory Test	Normal Ranges	Rationale for Assessment
Alkaline phosphatase (ALP)	30-120 units/L	ALP is found in many tissues but in highest concentrations in the liver, biliary tract, and bone. Detection of this enzyme is important for determining liver and bone disorders. Enzyme levels of ALP are increased in both extrahepatic and intrahepatic obstructive biliary disease and cirrhosis and/or other liver abnormalities.
Alanine aminotransferase (ALT); formerly serum glutamic-pyruvic transaminase (SGPT)	4-36 units/L Older adults may have slightly higher levels than the adult	ALT is found mainly in the liver and lesser amounts in the kidneys, heart, and skeletal muscle. If there is injury or disease to the liver parenchyma (cells), it will cause a release of this liver cellular enzyme into the bloodstream and thus elevate serum ALT levels. Most ALT elevations are from liver disease. Therefore, if medications are then metabolized by the liver, this metabolic process will be altered and possibly lead to toxic levels of drugs.
Gama-glutamyl transferase (GGT)	Male/female 45 years of age and older: 8-38 units/L	GGT is an enzyme that is present in liver tissue; when there is damage to the liver cells (hepatocytes) that manufacture bile, the enzyme will be released throughout the cell membranes and released into the blood. Individuals of African ancestry have normal values that are double the values of those who are white.
Aspartate aminotransferase (AST); formerly called serum glutamic-oxalocetic transaminase (SGOT)	0-35 units/L	AST is elevated with hepatocellular diseases. With disease or injury of liver cells, the cells lyse and the AST is released and picked up by the blood; the elevation of AST is directly related to the number of cells affected by disease or injury.
Lactic dehydrogenase (LDH)	100-190 units/L	LDH is found in cells of many body tissues including the heart, liver, red blood cells, kidneys, skeletal muscles, brain, and lungs. Because it is in so many tissues, the total LDH level is not a specific indicator of one disease. If there is disease or injury affecting cells containing LDH, the cells lyse and LDH is released from the cells into the bloodstream, thus increasing LDH levels. This enzyme is just part of the total picture of altered liver function, which, if present, will then decrease the breakdown/metabolism of drugs and other chemical compounds, resulting in elevated blood levels of drugs.

DOSAGES

Selected Analgesic Drugs and Related Drugs

Drug (Pregnancy Category)	Pharmacologic Class	Usual Adult Dosage Range	Indications/Uses
Opioids			
‼codeine sulfate (D)	Opiate analgesic; opium alkaloid	15-60 mg tid-qid 10-20 mg every 4-6 hr; do not exceed 120 mg/day	Opioid analgesia Relief of cough
‼fentanyl (Duragesic, Oralet, Actiq*) (D)	Opioid analgesic	All doses titrated to response, starting with lowest effective dose IV/IM: 50-100 mcg/dose titrated to response via continuous infusion. Duragesic (transdermal patch): 12.5-200 mcg/hr every 72 hr; Oralet, Actiq (buccal lozenges): begin with lowest dose (200 mcg) and titrate as needed NOTE: The FDA has placed restrictions on transmucosal fentanyl (only allowed for chronic pain)	Procedural sedation or adjunct to general anesthesia Relief of moderate to severe acute pain Relief of chronic pain, including cancer pain
◆‼hydromorphone (Dilaudid)	Opioid analgesic	IV/IM: 0.25-1 mg IV every 4-6 hr prn Oral: 2-4 mg PO every 6 hr prn	Seven times more potent than morphine. 1 mg hydromorphone = 7 mg morphine
‼meperidine HCl (Demerol) (D)	Opioid analgesic	PO/IV/IM/subcut: 50-150 mg every 3-4 hr prn	Meperidine use not recommended because of the unpredictable effects of neurometabolites at analgesic doses and risk for seizures
◆‼methadone HCl (Dolophine) (D)	Opioid analgesic	PO/IM/IV/subcut: 2.5-10 mg every 8-12 hr 40 mg or more once daily	Opioid analgesia, relief of chronic pain, opioid detoxification Opioid addiction maintenance
‼morphine sulfate (MSIR, Roxanol, others) (D)	Opiate analgesic; opium alkaloid	PO: 10-30 mg every 4 hr prn IV/IM/subcut: 2.5-10 mg every 2-6 hr prn	Opioid analgesia
◆‼morphine sulfate, continuous-release (MS Contin, Oramorph, Kadian) (D)	Opiate analgesic; opium alkaloid	PO: 15 mg every 8 hr to 200 mg every 8-12 hr	Relief of moderate to severe pain Cannot be crushed
‼oxycodone, immediate-release (OxyIR) (D)	Opioid, synthetic	PO: 5-20 mg every 4-6 hr prn	Relief of moderate to severe pain
‼oxycodone, continuous-release (OxyContin) (D)	Opioid, synthetic	PO: 10-160 mg every 8-12 hr	Relief of moderate to severe pain Cannot be crushed
Opioid Antagonists			
◆naloxone HCl (Narcan)	Opioid antagonist	IV: 0.4-2 mg IV; repeat in 2-8 min if needed IV: 0.1-0.2 mg IV; repeat at 2-3 min intervals	Treatment of opioid overdose Postoperative anesthesia reversal
naltrexone HCl	Opioid antagonist	PO: 50 mg every 24 hr or 100 mg every other day	Maintenance of opioid-free state
Nonopioids			
◆acetaminophen (Tylenol, others) (B)	Nonopioid analgesic, antipyretic	PO/PR: 325-650 mg every 4-6 hr not to exceed 3-4 g/day. In alcoholics, not to exceed 2 g/day	Relief of mild to moderate pain
‼tramadol (Ultram)	Nonopioid analgesic (with opioid-like activity)	PO: 50-100 mg every 4-6 hr not to exceed 400 mg/day	Relief of moderate to moderately severe pain

FDA, U.S. Food and Drug Administration; *HCl,* hydrochloride; *IM,* intramuscular; *IV,* intravenous; *IR,* immediate release; *MS,* morphine sulfate; *MSIR,* morphine sulfate immediate-release; *PCA,* patient-controlled analgesia; *PO,* oral; *PR,* rectal; *subcut,* subcutaneous.
*Actiq is not approved for use in patients younger than 16 years of age.
The maximum recommended daily dose of acetaminophen for a typical adult patient with normal liver function is 3000 mg/24 hr. For hepatically compromised patients, this dosage may be 2000 mg or even lower. If in doubt, check with a pharmacist or prescriber regarding a particular patient.

DRUG PROFILES

OPIOID AGONISTS

! codeine sulfate

Codeine sulfate is a natural opiate alkaloid (Schedule II) obtained from opium. It is similar to morphine in terms of its pharmacokinetic and pharmacodynamic properties. In fact, about 10% of a codeine dose is metabolized to morphine in the body. However, codeine is less effective as an analgesic and is the only agonist to possess a ceiling effect (meaning increasing the dose will not increase response). It is more commonly used as an antitussive drug in an array of cough preparations (see Chapter 36). Codeine combined with acetaminophen (tablets or elixir) is classified as a Schedule III controlled substance and is commonly used for control of mild to moderate pain as well as cough. When codeine is not combined with other drugs, it is classified as a Schedule II controlled substance, which implies a high abuse potential. Codeine causes GI tract upset, and many patients will say they are allergic to codeine, when in fact it just upsets their stomach. Codeine is no longer recommended for use in pediatric patients. For dosage information, see the table on the previous page.

Pharmacokinetics: Codeine

Route	Onset of Action	Peak Plasma Concentration	Elimination Half-life	Duration of Action
PO	15-30 min	34-45 min	2.5-4 hr	4-6 hr

! fentanyl

Fentanyl is a synthetic opioid (Schedule II) used to treat moderate to severe pain. Like other opioids, it also has a high abuse potential. It is available in several dosage forms: parenteral injections, transdermal patches (Duragesic), buccal lozenges (Fentora), and buccal lozenges on a stick (Actiq). The buccal dosage forms are absorbed through the oral mucosa. The injectable form is used most commonly in perioperative settings and in intensive care unit settings for sedation during mechanical ventilation. Fentanyl is a very potent analgesic. Fentanyl in a dose of 0.1 mg intravenously is roughly equivalent to 10 mg of morphine intravenously.

The transdermal delivery system (patch) has been shown to be highly effective in the treatment of various chronic pain syndromes such as cancer-induced pain, especially in patients who cannot take oral medications. This route is not to be used in opioid-naïve patients or for acute pain relief. Fentanyl patches are difficult to titrate and are best used for nonescalating pain.

Fentanyl patches take 6 to 12 hours to reach steady-state pain control after the first patch is applied, and supplemental short-acting therapy may be required. Most patients will experience adequate pain control for 72 hours with this method of fentanyl delivery. A new patch is to be applied every 72 hours. It is important to remove the old patch when applying a new one. It takes about 17 hours for the amount of fentanyl to reduce by 50% once the patch is removed.

The U.S. Food and Drug Administration (FDA) has issued many safety warnings about the use of fentanyl patches. Fentanyl patches are intended for management of chronic or cancer pain in opioid-tolerant patients whose pain is not adequately controlled by other types of medications. These patches are not to be used for acute pain situations such as postoperative pain. According to the FDA, patients who are considered opioid tolerant are those who have been taking at least 60 mg of oral morphine daily or at least 30 mg of oral oxycodone daily or at least 8 mg of oral hydromorphone daily or an equianalgesic dose of another opioid. Other hazards associated with the use of fentanyl patches are cutting the patch and exposing the patch to heat (e.g., via a heating pad or sauna), both of which accelerate the diffusion of the drug into the patient's body. Unused patches should be flushed down the toilet. Fentanyl patches are often cut into pieces and sold on the street as "chicklets." Patients should be warned to keep all fentanyl patches away from children, as deaths have occurred when toddlers inadvertently chewed fentanyl patches.

For dosage information, see the table on the previous page.

Pharmacokinetics: Fentanyl

Route	Onset of Action	Peak Plasma Concentration	Elimination Half-life	Duration of Action
IV	Rapid	Minutes	1.5-6 hr	30-60 min
Transdermal	12-24 hr	48-72 hr	Delayed	13-40 hr
PO	5-15 min	20-30 min	5-15 hr	Unknown

♦! hydromorphone (Dilaudid)

Hydromorphone (Dilaudid) is a very potent opioid analgesic and is a Schedule II drug. It is approximately seven times more potent than morphine. It is most often referred to as Diludid, because hydromorphone can be mistaken for morphine. One milligram of IV or IM hydromorphone is equivalent to 7 mg of morphine. Many nurses are unfamiliar with the potency difference, and because it is given in low doses (0.2-1 mg) some inadvertently assume low dose means low potency. Many medication errors and deaths have occurred because of lack of knowledge of this potency difference. Exalgo is the osmotic extended release oral delivery system of hydromorphone, which is difficult to crush or extract for injection, to help reduce the abuse potential. For dosage information, see the table on the previous page.

Pharmacokinetics: Hydromorphone (Dilaudid)

Route	Onset of Action	Peak Plasma Concentration	Elimination Half-life	Duration of Action
IV	Rapid	10-20 min	2-3 hr	3-4 hr

! meperidine hydrochloride

Meperidine hydrochloride (Demerol) is a synthetic opioid analgesic (Schedule II). Meperidine must be used with caution, if at all, in older adult patients and in patients who require long-term analgesia or who have kidney dysfunction. An active metabolite, normeperidine, can accumulate to toxic levels and lead to seizures. For this reason, meperidine is now used less commonly than before and is not recommended for long-term pain treatment. However, it is still used in emergency department settings for acute migraine headaches and in the immediate postoperative period to reduced shivering. Meperidine is available in oral and injectable forms. For dosage information, see the table on p. 154.

Pharmacokinetics: Meperidine

Route	Onset of Action	Peak Plasma Concentration	Elimination Half-life	Duration of Action
IM	Rapid	30-60 min	3-5 hr	2-4 hr

!methadone hydrochloride

Methadone hydrochloride (Dolophine) is a synthetic opioid analgesic (Schedule II). It is the opioid of choice for the detoxification treatment of opioid addicts in methadone maintenance programs. There has been renewed interest in the use of methadone for chronic (e.g., neuropathic) and cancer-related pain. The drug is readily absorbed through the GI tract with peak plasma concentrations at 4 hours for single dosing. Methadone is unique in that its half-life is longer than its duration of action because it is bound into the tissues of the liver, kidneys, and brain. With repeated doses, the drug accumulates in these tissues and is slowly released, thus allowing for 24-hour dosing. Methadone is eliminated through the liver, which makes it a safer choice than some other opioids for patients with renal impairment. Recent FDA reports have cited the prolonged half-life of the drug as a cause of unintentional overdoses and deaths. There is also concern that methadone may cause cardiac dysrhythmias. Methadone is available in oral and injectable forms. For dosage information, see the table on p. 154.

Pharmacokinetics: Methadone

Route	Onset of Action	Peak Plasma Concentration	Elimination Half-life	Duration of Action
PO	30-60 min	1.5-2 hr	25 hr	22-48 hr

♦!morphine sulfate

Morphine, a naturally occurring alkaloid derived from the opium poppy, is the drug prototype for all opioid drugs. It is classified as a Schedule II controlled substance. Morphine is indicated for severe pain and has a high abuse potential. It is available in oral, injectable, and rectal dosage forms. Extended-release forms include MS Contin and Kadian. Morphine also has a potentially toxic metabolite known as *morphine-6-glucuronide*. Accumulation of this metabolite is more likely to occur in patients with renal impairment. For this reason, other Schedule II opioids such as hydromorphone (Dilaudid), fentanyl, and oxymorphone (Opana) may be safer analgesic choices for patients with renal insufficiency. Morphine is available in oral, rectal, epidural, and injectable dosage forms, including PCA cartridges. Embeda (morphine and naltrexone) is the newest morphine product. For dosage information, see the table on p. 154.

Pharmacokinetics: Morphine Sulfate

Route	Onset of Action	Peak Plasma Concentration	Elimination Half-life	Duration of Action
IV	5-10 min	30 min	2-4 hr	4 hr

!oxycodone hydrochloride

Oxycodone hydrochloride is an analgesic drug that is structurally related to morphine and has comparable analgesic activity (Schedule II). It is also commonly combined in tablets with acetaminophen (Percocet) and with aspirin (Percodan). Oxycodone is also available in immediate-release formulations (Oxy IR) and sustained-released formulations (OxyContin). A somewhat weaker but commonly used opioid is hydrocodone, which is available only in tablet form, most commonly in combination with acetaminophen (Vicodin, Norco). In 2014, hydrocodone was rescheduled as a CII drug. For dosage information, see the table on p. 154.

Pharmacokinetics (Immediate Release): Oxycodone Hydrochloride

Route	Onset of Action	Peak Plasma Concentration	Elimination Half-life	Duration of Action
PO	10-15 min	1 hr	2-3 hr	3-6 hr

OPIOID AGONISTS-ANTAGONISTS

Opioids with mixed actions are often called *agonists-antagonists* (Schedule IV). They bind to the mu receptor and compete with other substances for these sites. They either exert no action (i.e., they are competitive antagonists) or have only limited action (i.e., they are partial agonists). They are similar to the opioid agonists in terms of their therapeutic indications; however, they have a lower risk for misuse and addiction. The antagonistic activity of this group can produce withdrawal symptoms in opioid-dependent patients. Their use is contraindicated in patients who have shown hypersensitivity reactions to the drugs.

These drugs have varying degrees of agonist and antagonist effects on the different opioid receptor subtypes. They are used in situations requiring short-term pain control, such as after obstetric procedures. They are sometimes chosen for patients who have a history of opioid addiction. These medications can both help prevent overmedication and reduce posttreatment addictive cravings in these patients. Combination products of buprenorphine and naloxone offer physicians an in-office treatment of addiction (see Chapter 17). These drugs are normally not strong enough for management of longer-term chronic pain (e.g., cancer pain, chronic lower back pain). They are *not* to be given concurrently with full opioid agonists, because they may both reduce analgesic effects and cause withdrawal symptoms in opioid-tolerant patients. Adverse reactions are similar to opioids but with a lower incidence of respiratory depression. Four opioid agonists-antagonists are currently available: buprenorphine (Buprenex), butorphanol (Stadol), nalbuphine (Nubain), and pentazocine (Talwin). They are available in various oral, injectable, and intranasal dosage forms. A new transdermal form of buprenorphine (Butrans) is also available.

OPIOID ANTAGONISTS

Opioid antagonists produce their antagonistic activity by competing with opioids for CNS receptor sites.

♦naloxone hydrochloride

Naloxone hydrochloride (Narcan) is a pure opioid antagonist. It has no agonistic morphine-like properties and works as a blocking drug for the opioid drugs. Accordingly, the drug does not produce analgesia or respiratory depression. Naloxone is the drug of choice for the complete or partial reversal of opioid-induced respiratory depression. It is also indicated in cases of suspected acute opioid overdose. Failure of the drug to significantly reverse the effects of the presumed opioid overdose indicates that the condition may not be related to opioid overdose. The primary adverse effect is opioid withdrawal syndrome, which can occur with abrupt over-reversal in opioid-tolerant patients. Naloxone is available only in injectable dosage forms. Use of the drug is contraindicated in patients with a history of hypersensitivity to it. For dosage information, see the table on p. 154.

Pharmacokinetics: Naloxone Hydrochloride

Route	Onset of Action	Peak Plasma Concentration	Elimination Half-life	Duration of Action
IV	Less than 2 min	Rapid	64 min	0.5-2 hr

naltrexone hydrochloride

Naltrexone hydrochloride is an opioid antagonist used as an adjunct for the maintenance of an opioid-free state in former opioid addicts. It is also indicated as an adjunct to psychosocial treatments of alcoholism and for reversal of postoperative opioid-induced respiratory depression. Nausea and tachycardia are the most common adverse effects and are related to reversal of the opioid effect. Use of naltrexone hydrochloride is contraindicated in cases of known drug allergy and in patients with hepatitis or other severe liver dysfunction. It is available only for oral use. For dosage information, see the table on p. 154.

Pharmacokinetics: Naltrexone Hydrochloride

Route	Onset of Action	Peak Plasma Concentration	Elimination Half-life	Duration of Action
PO	Rapid	1 hr	4-13 hr	24-72 hr

NONOPIOID AND MISCELLANEOUS ANALGESICS

Acetaminophen (Tylenol) is the most widely used nonopioid analgesic. Acetaminophen is commonly abbreviated APAP in the United States; however, this abbreviation is not recognized in Canada. There is a current movement to stop using APAP as an abbreviation, because of the potential that patients will not realize they are receiving a prescription with acetaminophen and may take additional over-the-counter acetaminophen.

All of the drugs in the NSAID class (which includes aspirin, ibuprofen, naproxen, the cyclooxygenase-2 [COX-2] inhibitor celecoxib [Celebrex], and others) are nonopioid analgesics. These drugs are discussed in greater detail in Chapter 44. They are used for management of pain, especially pain associated with inflammatory conditions such as arthritis, because they have significant antiinflammatory effects in addition to their analgesic effects.

Miscellaneous analgesics include tramadol and transdermal lidocaine and are discussed in depth in their respective drug profiles in this chapter. Capsaicin is a topical product made from several different types of peppers. It works by decreasing or interfering with substance P, a pain signal in the brain. Capsaicin is available over the counter. It can be used for muscle pain, joint pain, and nerve pain. Milnacipran (Savella) is a selective serotonin and norepinephrine dual-uptake inhibitor. It is indicated for the treatment of fibromyalgia. It is thought that patients with fibromyalgia have reduced levels of norepinephrine in their brains, and milnacipran increases norepinephrine levels, which helps reduce pain associated with the disease.

Mechanism of Action and Drug Effects

The mechanism of action of acetaminophen is similar to that of the salicylates. It blocks peripheral pain impulses by inhibition of prostaglandin synthesis. Acetaminophen also lowers febrile body temperatures by acting on the hypothalamus, the structure in the brain that regulates body temperature. Heat is dissipated through vasodilation and increased peripheral blood flow. In contrast to NSAIDs, acetaminophen lacks antiinflammatory effects. Although acetaminophen shares the analgesic and antipyretic effects of the salicylates and other NSAIDs, it does not have many of the unwanted effects of these drugs. For example, acetaminophen products are not usually associated with cardiovascular effects (e.g., edema) or platelet effects (e.g., bleeding), as are aspirin and other NSAIDs. It also does not cause the aspirin-related GI tract irritation or bleeding, nor any of the aspirin-related acid-base changes.

Indications

Acetaminophen is indicated for the treatment of mild to moderate pain and fever. It is an appropriate substitute for aspirin because of its analgesic and antipyretic properties. Acetaminophen is also the antipyretic (antifever) drug of choice in children and adolescents with flu syndromes, because the use of aspirin in these populations is associated with a condition known as *Reye's syndrome*. It is also a valuable alternative for patients who cannot tolerate aspirin.

Contraindications

Contraindications to acetaminophen use include known drug allergy, severe liver disease, and the genetic disease known as *glucose-6-phosphate dehydrogenase (G6PD) deficiency*.

Adverse Effects

Acetaminophen is generally well tolerated and is therefore available over the counter and in many combination prescription drugs. Possible adverse effects include skin disorders, nausea, and vomiting. Much less common but more severe are the adverse effects of blood disorders or dyscrasias (e.g., anemias) and nephrotoxicities, and hepatotoxicity. Hepatotoxicity is the most serious adverse effect of acetaminophen. Hepatotoxicity is associated with excessive doses. Acetaminophen is combined with hydrocodone (Vicodin, Norco) or oxycodone (Percocet, Tylox), and patients may exceed the recommended limit of acetaminophen without knowing these products also contain acetaminophen. In 2011, the FDA announced that combination products are to be limited to 325 mg of acetaminophen.

Currently, the FDA limits total daily doses to 4000 mg; however, the manufacturer of Tylenol suggests a limit of 3000 mg per day. Patients with liver disease or chronic alcohol consumption are advised not to exceed 2000 mg per day.

Toxicity and Management of Overdose

Many people do not realize that acetaminophen, despite its over-the-counter status, is a potentially lethal drug when taken in overdose. Depressed patients (especially adolescents) may intentionally overdose on the drug as an attention-seeking gesture without realizing the grave danger involved.

The ingestion of large amounts of acetaminophen, as in acute overdose, or chronic unintentional misuse can cause hepatic necrosis. Acute ingestion of acetaminophen doses of 150 mg/kg (approximately 7 to 10 grams) or more may result in hepatotoxicity. Acute hepatotoxicity can usually be reversed with acetylcysteine, whereas long-term toxicity is more likely to be permanent.

The long-term ingestion of large doses of acetaminophen is likely to result in severe hepatotoxicity, which may be irreversible. Because the reported quantity of drug ingested is often inaccurate, a serum acetaminophen concentration is determined no sooner than 4 hours after ingestion. If a serum acetaminophen level cannot be determined, it is assumed that the overdose is potentially toxic and treatment with acetylcysteine needs to be started. Acetylcysteine is the recommended antidote for acetaminophen toxicity and works by preventing the hepatotoxic metabolites of acetaminophen from forming. It is most effective when given within 10 hours of an overdose. Historically, the usual dosage regimen is a 140 mg/kg oral loading dose, followed by 70 mg/kg every 4 hours for 17 additional doses. This drug is notoriously bad tasting with an odor of rotten eggs, and vomiting of an oral dose is common. It is recommended that the dose be repeated if vomiting occurs within 1 hour of dosing. An intravenous dosage formulation of acetylcysteine (Acetadote) is also available and much better tolerated by the patient.

Interactions

A few drugs interact with acetaminophen. Alcohol is potentially the most dangerous. Chronic heavy alcohol abusers may be at increased risk of liver toxicity from excessive acetaminophen use. For this reason, a maximum daily dose of 2000 mg is generally recommended for such patients. Health care professionals need to warn patients with regular intake of alcohol not to exceed recommended dosages of acetaminophen because of the risk for liver dysfunction and possible liver failure. Ideally, alcohol consumption is not to exceed three drinks daily. Other hepatotoxic drugs need to be avoided. Other drugs that potentially can interact with acetaminophen include phenytoin, barbiturates, warfarin, isoniazid, rifampin, beta blockers, and anticholinergic drugs, all of which are discussed in greater detail in later chapters.

DRUG PROFILES

◆ acetaminophen

Acetaminophen (Tylenol) is an effective and relatively safe nonopioid analgesic used for mild to moderate pain relief. It is best avoided in patients who are alcoholic or who have hepatic disease. Acetaminophen is available in oral, rectal, and most recently, IV form. Acetaminophen is also a component of several prescription combination drug products, including hydrocodone/acetaminophen (Vicodin) and oxycodone/acetaminophen (Percocet).

Pharmacokinetics: Acetaminophen

Route	Onset of Action	Peak Plasma Concentration	Elimination Half-life	Duration of Action
PO	10-30 min	0.5-2 hr	1-4 hr	3-4 hr

‼ tramadol hydrochloride

Tramadol hydrochloride (Ultram) is categorized as a miscellaneous analgesic due to its unique properties. It is a centrally acting analgesic with a dual mechanism of action. It creates a weak bond to the mu opioid receptors and inhibits the reuptake of both norepinephrine and serotonin. Although it does have weak opioid receptor activity, tramadol is not currently classified as a controlled substance. Tramadol is indicated for the treatment of moderate to moderately severe pain. Tramadol is rapidly absorbed, and its absorption is unaffected by food. It is metabolized in the liver to an active metabolite and eliminated via renal excretion. Adverse effects are similar to those of opioids and include drowsiness, dizziness, headache, nausea, constipation, and respiratory depression. Seizures have been reported in patients taking tramadol and can occur in patients taking both normal and excessive dosages. Patients who may be at greatest risk are those receiving tricyclic antidepressants, selective serotonin reuptake inhibitors (SSRIs), monoamine oxidase inhibitors, neuroleptics, or other drugs that reduce the seizure threshold. There is also an increased risk for developing serotonin syndrome when tramadol is taken concurrently with SSRIs (see Chapter 16). In 2014, tramadol was rescheduled to a class CIV narcotic by the federal government, although certain states consider tramadol a CII or CIII drug. Use of tramadol is contraindicated in cases of known drug allergy, which may include allergy to opioids due to potential cross-reactivity. The drug is only available in oral dosage forms, including a combination with acetaminophen (Ultracet), as well as extended-release formulation (ConZip, Ryzolt, Ultram ER) and as an orally disintegrating tablet called Rybix. A new drug, tapentadol (Nucynta), is structurally related to tramadol with a dual mechanism of action. It is a mu agonist and a norepinephrine reuptake inhibitor. It is a Schedule II narcotic.

Pharmacokinetics: Tramadol

Route	Onset of Action	Peak Plasma Concentration	Elimination Half-life	Duration of Action
PO	30 min	2 hr	5-8 hr	6 hr

lidocaine, transdermal

Transdermal lidocaine is a topical anesthetic (see Chapter 11) that is formulated into a patch (Lidoderm) and is placed onto painful areas of the skin. It is indicated for the treatment of postherpetic neuralgia, a painful skin condition that remains after a skin outbreak of shingles. Lidocaine patches provide local pain relief, and up to three patches may be placed on a large painful area. The patches are not to be worn for longer than 12 hours a day to avoid potential systemic drug toxicity (e.g., cardiac dysrhythmias). Because they act topically, there are minimal systemic adverse effects. However, the skin at the site of treatment may develop redness or edema, and unusual skin sensations may occur. These reactions are usually mild and transient and resolve within a few minutes to hours. Patches are applied only to intact skin with no blisters. They can be used either alone or as part of adjunctive treatment with systemic therapies such as antidepressants (see Chapter 16), opioids, or anticonvulsants (see Chapter 14). Used patches must be disposed of securely because they may be dangerous to children or pets. Specific pharmacokinetic data are not listed due to the continuous nature of dosing. Studies have demonstrated that a patch can provide varying degrees of pain relief for 4 to 12 hours.

NURSING PROCESS

Pain may be acute or chronic and occurs in patients in all settings and across the lifespan, thus leading to much suffering and distress. Patients experiencing pain pose many challenges to the nurse, prescribers, and other members of the health care team involved in their care. The challenge is that pain is a complex and multifaceted problem and demands astute assessment skills with appropriate interventions based on the individual, the specific type of pain, related diseases, and/or health status.

Medical associations, health care organizations, governing bodies, and professional nursing organizations have been involved in defining standards and outcomes of care related to assessment and management of pain. For example, The Joint Commission (www.jointcommission.org) and the Agency for Healthcare Research and Quality (www.ahrq.gov/whatsnew.asp#qt) have developed such standards. In addition, the WHO (www.who.int/en) has developed standards related specifically to cancer pain. Professional nursing organizations, such as the Oncology Nursing Society and the American Nurses Association, have also created standards of care related to pain assessment and management. In 2009, the American Pain Society published guidelines for opioid therapy in chronic noncancer pain. (See *www.americanpainsociety.org* for more guidelines.)

ASSESSMENT

Adequate analgesia requires a holistic, comprehensive, and individualized patient assessment with specific attention to the type, intensity, and characteristics of the pain and the levels of comfort. Comfort, in this situation, is defined as the extent of physical and psychologic ease that an individual experiences. Perform a thorough health history, nursing assessment, and medication history as soon as possible or upon the first encounter with the patient, including questions about the following: (1) allergies to nonopioids, opioids, partial or mixed agonists, and/or opioid antagonists (see previous pharmacologic discussion for examples of specific drugs); (2) potential drug-drug and/or drug-food interactions; (3) presence of diseases or CNS depression; (4) history of the use

of alcohol, street drugs, or any illegal drug or substance and/or history of substance abuse, with information about the substance, dose, and frequency of use; (5) results of laboratory tests ordered, such as levels of serum ALT, ALP, GGT, 5′-nucleotidase, and bilirubin (indicative of liver function), and/or levels of BUN and creatinine (reflective of renal function); abnormal liver or renal function may require that lower doses of analgesic be used to prevent toxicity or overdosage (see the Safety: Laboratory Values related to Drug Therapy box); (6) character and intensity of the pain, including onset, location, and quality (e.g., stabbing/knifelike, throbbing, dull ache, sharp, diffuse, localized, or referred); actual rating of the pain using a pain assessment scale (see later); and any precipitating, aggravating, and/or relieving factors; (7) duration of the pain (acute versus chronic); and (8) types of pharmacologic, nonpharmacologic, and/or adjunctive measures that have been implemented, with further explanation of the treatment's duration of use and overall effectiveness.

To be thorough and effective, include in your assessment the factors or variables that may impact an individual's pain experience, such as physical factors (e.g., age, gender, pain threshold, overall state of health, disease processes, or pathologies) and emotional, spiritual, and cultural variables (e.g., reaction to pain, pain tolerance, fear, anxiety, stressors, sleep patterns, societal influences, family roles, phase of growth and development, and religious, racial, and/or ethnic beliefs or practices). Age-appropriate assessment tools are recommended in assessing pain across the lifespan (see later discussion). For pediatric and older adult patients, nonverbal behavior or cues and information from family members or caregivers may be helpful in identifying pain levels. In an older adult individual, physical and cognitive impairments may affect reporting of pain; however, this does not mean that the older adult patient is not experiencing pain—the patient's reporting may just be altered. Chronic pain and pain associated with cancer are both complex and multifactorial problems requiring a holistic approach with attention to other patient complaints, such as a decrease in activities of daily living, insomnia, depression, social withdrawal, anxiety, personality changes, and quality of life issues.

Perform a system-focused nursing assessment with collection of both subjective and objective data as follows: neurologic status (e.g., level of orientation and alertness, level of sedation, sensory and motor abilities, reflexes); respiratory status (e.g., respiratory rate, rhythm, and depth; breath sounds); GI status (e.g., presence of bowel sounds; bowel patterns; complaints of constipation, diarrhea, nausea, vomiting, or abdominal discomfort); genitourinary status (e.g., urinary output; any burning or discomfort on urination; urinary retention); and cardiac status (e.g., pulse rate and rhythm, blood pressure, any problems with dizziness or syncope). Assess and document vital signs, including blood pressure, pulse rate, respirations, temperature, and level of pain (now considered the fifth vital sign). It is important to pull from one's knowledge base and remember that during the acute pain response, stimulation of the sympathetic nervous system may result in elevated values for vital signs, with an increase in blood pressure (120/80 mm Hg or higher), pulse rate (100 beats/min or higher), and respiratory rate and depth (20 breaths/min or higher and shallow breathing).

Opioid Use

- Assessment of the pediatric patient is challenging, and all types of behavior that may indicate pain, such as muscular rigidity, restlessness, screaming, fear of moving, and withdrawn behavior, must be carefully considered.
- Adequacy of pain management is more difficult to determine in children because of their inability to express themselves. Frequently the reason older pediatric patients do not verbalize their pain is their fear of treatment, such as injections. Compassionate and therapeutic communication skills, as well as the use of alternate routes of administration, as ordered, will help in these situations.
- The "ouch scale" is often used to determine the level of pain in children. This scale is used to obtain the child's rating of the intensity of pain from 0 to 5 by means of simple face diagrams, from a very happy face for level 0 (no pain) to a sad, tearful face for level 5 (severe pain). Pain assessment is very important in pediatric patients because they are often undermedicated. Always thoroughly assess the pediatric patient's verbal and nonverbal behavior, and never underestimate the patient's complaints! Remember that parents and caregivers can play a very important role in this assessment.
- The patient's baseline age, weight, and height are important to document, because drug calculations are often based on these variables. With the pediatric patient, check and double-check *all* mathematical calculations for accuracy to avoid excessive dosages; this is especially true for opioids.
- Analgesics must be given, as ordered, before pain becomes severe, with oral dosage forms used first, if appropriate.
- If suppositories are used, be careful to administer the exact dose and not to split, halve, or divide an adult dose into a child's dose. This may result in the administration of an unknown amount of medication and possible overdose.

- When subcutaneous, intramuscular, and intravenous medications are used, the principle of atraumatic care in the delivery of nursing care must be followed. One technique used to help ensure atraumatic care is the application of a mixture of local anesthetics or other prescribed substances to the injection site before the injection is given. EMLA (lidocaine/prilocaine) is a topical cream that anesthetizes the site of the injection; if ordered, apply 1 to 2½ hours before the injection. Consult policies and procedures for further instructions regarding its use.
- Distraction and creative imagery may be used for older children such as toddlers or preschool-age children.
- Always monitor pediatric patients very closely for any unusual behavior while receiving opioids.
- Report the following signs and symptoms of central nervous system changes to the prescriber immediately if they occur: dizziness, lightheadedness, drowsiness, hallucinations, changes in level of consciousness, and sluggish pupil reaction. Do not administer further medication until the nurse receives further orders from the prescriber.
- Always monitor and document vital signs before, during, and after the administration of opioid analgesics. An opioid medication is usually withheld if a patient's respirations are less than 12 breaths/min or if there are any changes in the level of consciousness. Always follow protocol, and never ignore a patient's status!
- Generally speaking, smaller doses of opioids, with very close and frequent monitoring, are indicated for the pediatric patient. Giving oral medications with meals or snacks may help to decrease GI upset.

A variety of pain assessment tools are available that may be used to gather information about the fifth vital sign. One very basic assessment tool is the Numeric Pain Intensity Scale (0 to 10 pain rating scale); patients are asked to rate their pain intensity by picking the number that most closely represents their level of pain. The Verbal Rating Scale, another pain assessment tool, uses verbal descriptors for pain, including words such as *mild, moderate, severe, aching, agonizing,* or *discomfort*. The FACES Pain Rating Scale is helpful in assessing pain in patients of all ages and educational levels because it relies on a series of faces ranging from happy to sad to sad with tears. The patient is asked to identify the face that best represents the pain he or she is experiencing at that moment. When the patient is in acute pain, when pain intensity is a primary focus for assessment, and/or when the need is to determine the efficacy of pain management intervention, the simple, one-dimensional scales (e.g., the Numeric Pain Intensity Scale) work best. The FLACC pain assessment scale may be used in children who are non-verbal but could also be used in any age of patient who is experiencing trauma or nonverbal. Zero, one, or two points are assigned to the five categories of Face, Legs, Activity, Cry, and Consolability. Further information is available at http://www.nhpco.org/flacc-scores. The older adult, especially those with cognitive impairment, may need more time to respond to the assessment tool and may also require large-print versions of written tools. There are other assessment tools that are multidimensional scales and are more beneficial in assessing patients who experience chronic rather than acute pain. One example is the Brief Pain Inventory

assessment tool, which includes a body map so that the patient can identify on the figure the exact area where pain is felt. This tool also helps in obtaining information about the impact of pain on functioning. Assess pain before, during, and after the pain intervention, as well as the level of pain during activity and at rest. The following sections provide assessment information for specific drug classes.

▮ NONOPIOIDS

For patients receiving *nonopioid analgesics*, focus the assessment not only on general data as described earlier but also on the specific drug being given. For example, in those patients taking acetaminophen, begin the assessment by determining whether the patient has allergies, is pregnant, and/or is breastfeeding. As mentioned in the pharmacology section, *acetaminophen* is contraindicated in those with severe liver disease and in patients with G6PD deficiency. Additionally, cautious use is necessary due to possible adverse effects of blood disorders (anemias) and liver or kidney toxicity. See the pharmacology discussion for more information about acute overdose and chronic unintentional misuse. Also assess for any other medications the patient is taking, because of the risk for excessive doses when taking combination products consisting of acetaminophen. Inadvertent overdosing is a possible consequence of this situation. Other drug interactions and concerns are addressed in the pharmacology discussion.

Once therapy has been initiated, closely monitor for chronic acetaminophen poisoning, looking for symptoms such as rapid, weak pulse, dyspnea, and cold and clammy extremities. Long-term daily use of acetaminophen may lead to increased risk for permanent liver damage, and therefore you must frequently monitor the results of liver function studies. Adults who ingest higher than recommended dosages may be at higher risk for liver dysfunction as well as other adverse effects such as loss of appetite, jaundice, nausea, and vomiting. Children are also at high risk for liver dysfunction if the recommended dosage ranges are exceeded. With the use of *NSAIDs* (e.g., *ibuprofen, aspirin, COX-2 inhibitors*), assess kidney and liver functioning and gather information about GI disorders such as ulcers (see Chapter 44 for more information on antiinflammatory drugs). With *aspirin*, age is important; this drug is not to be given to children and adolescent patients because of the risk of Reye's syndrome. Aspirin may also lead to bleeding and ulcers, so ruling out conditions that represent contraindications and cautions to its use before therapy begins is important to patient safety. With *tramadol hydrochloride*, assessment of age is important because this drug is not recommended for use in individuals 75 years of age or older.

A *miscellaneous nonopioid analgesic, lidocaine transdermal*, is another option for managing different types of pain. For lidocaine transdermal patches, understand that this transdermal drug is indicated in those with postherpetic neuralgia, and thus assess the herpetic lesion(s) and surrounding skin. When these patches are used, they must be kept away from children and are not to be prescribed for very young, small, or debilitated patients because these patients are at higher risk for toxicity. Liver function also needs to be assessed and monitored.

OPIOIDS

When *opioid analgesics,* or any other CNS depressants, are prescribed, focus assessment on vital signs; allergies; respiratory disorders; respiratory function (rate, rhythm, depth, and breath sounds); presence of head injury (which will mask signs and symptoms of increasing intracranial pressure); neurologic status, with attention to level of consciousness or alertness and the level of sedation; sensory and motor functioning; GI tract functioning (bowel sounds and bowel patterns); and genitourinary functioning (intake and output). In addition, all opioids may cause spasms of the sphincter of Oddi. If renal and liver function studies are ordered, monitor results, because the risk for toxicity increases with diminished function of these organs. An additional concern is any past or present history of neurologic disorders such as Alzheimer's disease, dementia, multiple sclerosis, muscular dystrophy, myasthenia gravis, or cerebrovascular accident or stroke, because the use of opioids may alter symptoms of the disease process, possibly masking symptoms or worsening the clinical presentation when no actual pathologic changes have occurred. In these situations, use of another analgesic or pain protocol may be indicated. Attention to age is also important, because both older adult and very young patients are more sensitive to opioids—and holds true for many other medications. In fact, old or young age may be a contraindication to opioid use, depending on the specific drug. See the earlier pharmacology discussion regarding cautions, contraindications, and drug interactions.

OPIOID AGONISTS-ANTAGONISTS

In patients taking *opioid agonists-antagonists,* such as *buprenorphine hydrochloride,* assess vital signs with attention to respiratory rate and breath sounds. The opioid agonists-antagonists still possess opioid agonist effects; therefore, the assessment information related to opioids is applicable to these drugs as well. It is also very important to remember during assessment that these drugs are still effective analgesics and still have CNS depressant effects but are subject to a ceiling effect (see earlier definition). Given the action of these drugs, the assessment may help determine whether the patient is an abuser of opioids. This is important because the simultaneous administration of agonists-antagonists with another opioid will lead to reversal of analgesia and possible opioid withdrawal. Age is another factor to assess, because these drugs are not recommended for use in patients 18 years of age or younger. See the previous discussion for a listing of contraindications, cautions, and drug interactions.

OPIOID ANTAGONISTS

Remember that the *opioid antagonists* are used mainly in reversing respiratory depression secondary to opioid overdosage. *Naloxone* may be used in patients of all ages, including neonates and children. Assess and document vital signs before, during, and after the use of the antagonist so that the therapeutic effects can be further assessed and documented and the need for further doses determined. In addition, remember that the antagonist drug may not work with just one dosing and that repeated doses are generally needed to reverse the effects of the opioid. See the pharmacology section for information about contraindications, cautions, and drug interactions.

NURSING DIAGNOSES

1. Impaired gas exchange related to opioid-induced CNS effects and respiratory depression
2. Acute pain related to specific disease processes or conditions and other pathologies leading to various levels and types of pain
3. Chronic pain related to various disease processes, conditions, or syndromes causing pain
4. Constipation related to the CNS depressant effects on the GI system
5. Deficient knowledge related to lack of familiarity with opioids, their use, and their adverse effects

PLANNING: OUTCOME IDENTIFICATION

1. Patient regains/maintains a respiratory rate between 10 and 20 breaths per minute without respiratory depression while increasing fluid intake and coughing/deep breathing while taking opioids and/or other analgesics for pain.
2. Patient relates increased comfort levels from acute or chronic pain as seen by decreased use of analgesics, increased activity and performance of activities of daily living, decreased complaints of acute pain, as well as decreased levels of pain as rated on a scale of 1 to 10 or alternative pain scales.

Patient uses nonpharmacologic measures such as relaxation therapy, distraction, and music therapy to help improve comfort and enhance any drug therapy regimens for chronic pain.

3. Patient identifies measures to help maintain normal bowel elimination patterns and avoids/minimizes opioid-induced constipation by increasing fluids and fiber in the diet and increasing mobility.

4. Patient reports appropriate use of analgesics with minimal complications/adverse effects and is able to state the drug's rationale, action, and therapeutic effects.

IMPLEMENTATION

Once the cause of pain has been diagnosed or other assessment and data gathering have been completed, begin pain management immediately and aggressively in conformity with the needs of each individual patient and situation. Pain management is varied and multifaceted and needs to incorporate pharmacologic as well as nonpharmacologic approaches (see Box 10-1 and the Safety: Herbal Therapies and Dietary Supplements box). Pain management strategies must also include consideration of the type of pain and pain rating as well as pain quality, duration, and precipitating factors, and interventions that help the pain. Some general principles of pain management are as follows: (1) Individualize a plan of care based on the patient as a holistic and cultural being (see the Patient-Centered Care: Cultural Implications box on p. 144). (2) Manage mild pain with the use of nonopioid drugs such as acetaminophen, tramadol, and NSAIDs (see Chapter 44). (3) Manage moderate to severe pain with a stepped approach using opioids. Other analgesics or types of analgesics may be used in addition to other categories of medication (see pharmacology discussion). (4) Administer analgesics as ordered but before the pain gets out of control. (5) Always consider the use of nonpharmacologic comfort measures (see Box 10-1) such as ice, heat, elevation, rest, homeopathic and folk remedies, exercise, distraction, music or pet therapy, massage, and transcutaneous electrical stimulation. Although not always effective, these measures may prove beneficial for some patients. See Patient-Centered Care: Patient Teaching on p. 168 for more information related to analgesics.

NONOPIOIDS

Give *nonopioid analgesics* as ordered or as indicated for fever or pain. *Acetaminophen* is to be taken as prescribed and within the recommended dosage range over a 24-hour period because of the risk for liver damage and acute toxicity. If a patient is taking other over-the-counter medications with acetaminophen, he or she needs to understand the importance of reading the labels very carefully (of other medications) to identify the total amount of acetaminophen taken and any other drug-drug interactions. In educating the patient, emphasize the signs and symptoms of acetaminophen overdose: bleeding, loss of energy, fever, sore throat, and easy bruising (due to hepatotoxicity). These must be reported immediately by the patient, family member, or caregiver to the nurse and/or prescriber. Any

---

🍃 SAFETY: HERBAL THERAPIES AND DIETARY SUPPLEMENTS   QSEN

Feverfew (Chrysanthemum parthenium)

Overview
A member of the marigold family known for its antiinflammatory properties

Common Uses
Treatment of migraine headaches, menstrual cramps, inflammation, and fever

Adverse Effects
Nausea, vomiting, constipation, diarrhea, altered taste sensations, muscle stiffness, and joint pain

Potential Drug Interactions
Possible increase in bleeding with the use of aspirin and other nonsteroidal antiinflammatory drugs, dipyridamole, and warfarin

Contraindications
Contraindicated in those allergic to ragweed, chrysanthemums, and marigolds, as well as those about to undergo surgery.

---

worsening or changing in the nature and/or characteristic of pain must also be reported. Suppository dosage forms of acetaminophen—like suppository forms of other drugs—may be placed into a medicine cup of ice to prevent melting of the dosage form. Once the suppository is unwrapped, cold water may be run over it to moisten the suppository for easier insertion. The suppository is inserted into the rectum using a gloved finger and water-soluble lubricating gel, if necessary. Acetaminophen tablets may be crushed if needed. Adult patients who take 3000 mg/day or greater of acetaminophen are at increased risk for acute hepatotoxicity. Death may occur after ingestion of more than 15 g. Liver damage from acetaminophen may be minimized by timely dosing with acetylcysteine (see previous discussion). If acetylcysteine is indicated, warn the patient about the drug's foul taste and odor. Many patients report that the drug smells and tastes like rotten eggs. Acetylcysteine is better tolerated if it is disguised by mixing with a drink such as cola or flavored water to increase its palatability. Use of a straw may help minimize contact with the mucous membranes of the mouth and is recommended. This antidote may be given through a nasogastric or orogastric tube or intravenously, if necessary.

If a patient is receiving acetaminophen or taking it at home and has also been prescribed hydrocodone (Vicodin, Norco) or oxycodone (Percocet, Tylox), there is danger of overdosage with the acetaminophen. This overdosage may occur if the patient is not aware of the fact that acetaminophen is in the prescribed medication. Hepatotoxicity would be of concern, so it is critical to patient safety to educate about the ingredients of over-the-counter medications as well as prescribed medications. As discussed in the pharmacology section, the FDA announced that combination products are to be limited to 325 mg of acetaminophen, and they currently limit total daily doses to 4000 mg; however, the manufacturer of Tylenol suggests a limit of 3000 mg per day. Patients with liver disease or alcohol consumption are advised not to exceed 2000 mg per day.

Tramadol may cause drowsiness, dizziness, headache, nausea, constipation, and respiratory depression. If dizziness, blurred vision, or drowsiness occur, be sure to assist the patient with ambulation (as with the use of any analgesic that may lead to dizziness or lightheadedness) to minimize the risk for fall and injury. Educate the patient about injury prevention, including the need to dangle the feet over the edge of the bed before full ambulation, changing positions slowly, and asking for assistance when ambulating. In addition, while the patient is taking tramadol—as well as any other analgesics, and especially opioids—the patient needs to avoid any tasks that require mental clarity and alertness. Increasing fluids and fiber in the diet may help with constipation. Use of flat cola, ginger ale, or dry crackers may help to minimize nausea.

OPIOIDS

When *opioids* (and other analgesics) are prescribed, administer the drug as ordered after checking for the "Nine Rights" of medication administration (see Chapter 1). After the prescriber's order has been double-checked, closely examine the medication profile and documentation to determine the last time the medication was given before another dose is administered. Monitor the patient's vital signs at frequent intervals with special attention to respiratory changes. A respiratory rate of 10 breaths/min (some protocols still adhere to the parameter of 12 breaths/min) may indicate respiratory depression and must be reported to the prescriber. The drug dosage, frequency, and/or route may need to be changed or an antidote (opioid antagonist) given if respiratory depression occurs. Naloxone must always be available, especially with the use of intravenous and/or other parenteral dosage forms of opioids, such as PCA (see Chapter 9 and the discussion to follow), and/or epidural infusions. Naloxone is indicated to reverse CNS depression, specifically respiratory depression, but remember that this antidote also reverses analgesia. Monitor the patient's urinary output as well; it should be at least 600 mL/24 hr. Monitor bowel sounds during therapy; decreased peristalsis may indicate the need for a dietary change,

such as increased fiber, or use of a stool softener or mild laxative (see Box 10-2). Assess the patient's pupillary reaction to light. Pinpoint pupils indicate a possible overdose.

It is crucial to patient safety to re-emphasize the importance of understanding equianalgesia. For example, *hydromorphone (Dilaudid)* is seven times more potent than *morphine*. Deaths have been reported where a nurse gave the patient morphine and did not realize the equialanagesic equivalency (See previous discussion in the pharmacology section).

Opioids or any analgesic must be given before the pain reaches its peak to help maximize the effectiveness of the opioid or other analgesic. Once the drug is administered, return at the appropriate time (taking into consideration the times of onset and peak effect of the drug and the route) to assess the effectiveness of the drug and/or other interventions as well as observe for the presence of adverse effects (see previous discussion of pain assessment tools). With regard to the route of administration, the recommendation is that oral dosage forms be used first, but only if ordered and if there is no nausea or vomiting. Taking the dose with food may help minimize GI upset. Should nausea or vomiting be problematic, an antiemetic may be ordered for administration before or with the dosing of medication. Crucial safety measures include keeping the bed's side rails up, turning on bed alarms (depending on the policies and procedures of the specific health care institution), and making sure the call bell/alarm is within the patient's reach. These measures will help to prevent falls or injury related to opioid use. Opioids and similar drugs lead to CNS depression with possible confusion, altered sensorium or alertness, hypotension, and altered motor functioning. Because of these drug effects, all patients are at risk for falls or injury, and the older adult is at higher risk (see Box 10-2 and the Patient-Centered Care: Lifespan Considerations for the Older Adult Patient box). See Box 10-4 for more specific information concerning the handling of controlled substances and opioid counts.

When managing pain with *morphine* and similar drugs, withhold the dose and contact the prescriber if there is any decline in the patient's condition or if the vital signs are abnormal (see parameters mentioned earlier), especially if the

---

BOX 10-4   Controlled Substance/Opioid Counts—A Must-Do!

Any medication that has the potential for abuse or is a controlled substance—often opioids—is handled differently from other medications. Opioids are delivered to a nursing unit by the pharmacy, and these and other controlled substances (see Chapter 4) are kept in a locked cabinet or in an automated dispensing system (see Chapter 9). At the beginning of each shift, two registered nurses must count all of the opioids and/or other controlled substances located in the locked cabinet and record the count on a controlled substance and/or opioid administration record. When opioids and other controlled substances are dispensed through an automated medication-dispensing system, the drug is counted before the nurse removes the dose from the system. Any discrepancies found in the count of opioids or other controlled substances are investigated by registered nurses. If any opioids are unaccounted for, the nurse manager or supervisor needs to be contacted immediately. The following guidelines must be adhered to when giving opioids and other controlled substances: (1) Check the opioid administration record for the number left in stock. (2) Compare this number with the actual supply available. (3) If the count is accurate, obtain the desired dose of drug. (4) If the count is incorrect, notify the nurse manager or supervisor and follow the health care setting's policies and procedures. (5) Record the count of the remaining supply. Once the dose is removed, the nurse may be required to record the patient's name, prescriber's name, patient's medical record number, dose of medication ordered, and the nurse's signature. (6) Administer the drug according to policy and procedures. If the controlled substance cannot be given to the patient because of patient refusal, medication contamination, changes in vital signs or status, or some other reason, the medication will need to be "wasted." However, wasting of controlled substances requires the signature of another nurse who witnesses the discarding or wasting of the medication and documentation on the appropriate form. Automated systems record this information within the computer system.

Opioid Use

- Record the patient's weight and height before opioid therapy is begun, if appropriate. Monitor the patient carefully for any changes in vital signs, level of consciousness, or respiratory rate, as well as any changes indicative of central nervous system depression, and report and document any such changes.
- Many institutionalized or hospitalized older adult patients are very stoic about pain; older adult patients may also have altered presentations of common illnesses so that the pain experience manifests in a different way or may simply be unable to state how they feel in a clear manner. Each and every patient—regardless of age—has the right to a thorough pain assessment and adequate and appropriate pain management. It is a myth that aging increases one's pain threshold. The problem is that cognitive impairment and dementia are often major barriers to pain assessment. Nevertheless, many older adult patients are still reliable in their reporting of pain, even with moderate to severe cognitive impairment.
- Over time, the older adult patient may lose reliability in recalling and accurately reporting chronic pain. The older adult patient, especially those 75 years of age or older, are at higher risk for too much or too little pain management, so you must remember that drugs have a higher peak and longer duration of action in these patients than in their younger counterparts.
- Smaller dosages of opioids are generally indicated for older adult patients because of their increased sensitivity to the central nervous system depressants and diminished renal and hepatic function. Paradoxical (opposite) reactions and/or unexpected reactions may also be more likely to occur in patients of this age group.

- In older adult male patients, benign prostatic hyperplasia or obstructive urinary diseases must be considered because of the urinary retention associated with the use of opioids. Urinary outflow can become further diminished in these patients and result in adverse reactions or complications. Dosage adjustments may need to be made by the prescriber.
- Polypharmacy is often a problem in older adults; therefore, have a complete list of all medications the patient is currently taking, and assess for drug interactions and treatment (drug) duplication.
- Frequent assessment of older adult patients is needed. Pay attention to level of consciousness, alertness, and cognitive ability while ensuring that the environment is safe by keeping a call bell or light at the bedside. Using bed alarms and/or raising side rails are indicated when appropriate.
- Decreased circulation causes variation in the absorption of intramuscular or intravenous dosage forms and often results in the slower absorption of parenteral forms of opioids.
- As stated by the American Geriatric Society on the Management of Pain, nonsteroidal antiinflammatory drugs must be used with caution because of their potential for renal and gastrointestinal toxicity. Acetaminophen is the drug of choice for relieving mild to moderate pain, but with cautious dosing because of hepatic and renal concerns. The oral route of administration is preferred for analgesia. The regimen needs to be as simple as possible to enhance compliance. Be sure to note, report, and document any unusual reactions to the opioid drugs. Hypotension and respiratory depression may occur more frequently in older adult patients taking opioids; thus very careful vital sign monitoring is needed.

respiratory rate is less than 10 breaths/min. Intramuscular injections are rarely used because of the availability of other effective and convenient dosage forms, such as PCA pumps, transdermal patches, continuous subcutaneous infusions, and epidural infusions.

For transdermal patches (e.g., *transdermal fentanyl*), two systems are used. The oldest type of patch contains a reservoir system consisting of four layers beginning with the adhesive layer and ending with the protective backing. Between these two layers are the permeable rate-controlling membrane and the reservoir layer, which holds the drug in a gel or liquid form. The newer type of patch has a matrix system consisting of two layers: one layer containing the active drug with the releasing and adhesive mechanisms, and the protective impermeable backing layer. The advantages of the matrix system over the reservoir system are that the patch is slimmer and smaller, it is more comfortable, it is worn for up to 7 days (the older reservoir system patch is worn for up to 3 to 4 days), and it appears to result in more constant serum drug levels. In addition, the matrix system is alcohol-free; the alcohol in the reservoir system often irritates the patient's skin. It is important to know what type of delivery system is being used so that proper guidelines are followed to enhance the system's and drug's effectiveness.

Apply transdermal patches to only a clean, nonhairy area. When the patch is changed, place the new patch on a new site, but only after the old patch has been removed and the old site cleansed of any residual medication. Rotation of sites helps to

decrease irritation and enhance drug effects. Transdermal patches require special discarding of old/used patches (see the Safety and Quality Improvement: Preventing Medication Errors box on p. 151). Transdermal systems are beneficial for the delivery of many types of medications, especially analgesics, and have the benefits of allowing multiday therapy with a single application, avoiding first-pass metabolism, improving patient compliance, and minimizing frequent dosing. However, the patient must be watched carefully for the development of any type of contact dermatitis caused by the patch (the prescriber is to be contacted immediately if this occurs) and maintain his or her own pain journal when at home. Journal entries are a valid source of information for the nurse, other health care professionals, the patient, and family members to assess the patient's pain control and to monitor the effectiveness not only of transdermal analgesia but also any medication regimen.

With the intravenous administration of *opioid agonists*, follow manufacturer guidelines and health care institution policy regarding specific dilutional amounts and solutions as well as the time period for infusion. When PCA is used, the amounts and times of dosing must be noted in the appropriate records and tracked by appropriate personnel. The fact that a pump is being used, however, does not mean that it is 100% reliable or safe. Closely monitor and frequently check all equipment. Additionally, frequently monitor pain levels, response to medication, and vital signs with the use of other parenteral opioid administration. Always follow dosage ranges for all

TABLE 10-8 Opioid Administration Guidelines

Opioid	Nursing Administration
buprenorphine and butorphanol	When giving IV, infuse over the recommended time (usually 3-5 min). Always assess respirations before, during, and after use. Give IM as ordered.
codeine	Give PO doses with food to minimize GI tract upset; ceiling effects occur with oral codeine resulting in no increase in analgesia with increased dosage.
fentanyl	Administer parenteral doses over 1-2 minutes as ordered and as per manufacturer guidelines in regard to mg/min to prevent CNS depression and possible cardiac or respiratory arrest. Transdermal patches come in a variety of dosages. Fentanyl lozenges on a stick are also available. Be sure to remove residual amounts of the old patch before application of a new patch. Dispose of patches properly to avoid inadvertent contact with children or pets. Patches are to be folded and flushed down the toilet.
hydromorphone	May be given subcut, rectally, IV, PO, or IM.
meperidine	Given by a variety of routes: IV, IM, or PO; highly protein bound, so watch for interactions and toxicity. Monitor older adult patients for increased sensitivity.
morphine	Available in a variety of forms: subcut, IM, PO, IV, extended- and immediate-release; morphine sulfate (Duramorph) for epidural infusion. Always monitor respiratory rate.
nalbuphine	IV doses of 10 mg given undiluted over 5 min.
naloxone	Antagonist given for opioid overdose; 0.4 mg usually given IV over 15 sec or less. Reverses analgesia as well.
oxycodone	Often mixed with acetaminophen or aspirin; PO and suppository dosage forms. Now available in both immediate and sustained-release tablets.

opioid agonists, and pay special attention to the dosages of morphine and morphine-like drugs. For intravenous infusions, you are responsible for monitoring the intravenous needle site and infusion rates and documenting any adverse effects or complications. Another point to remember when administering opioids—as well as any other analgesic—is that each medication has a different onset of action, peak, and duration of action, with the intravenous route producing the most rapid onset (e.g., within minutes) (Table 10-8).

To reverse an opioid overdose or opioid-induced respiratory depression, an *opioid antagonist,* such as *naloxone,* must be administered. Naloxone is given intravenously in diluted form and administered slowly (such as over 15 seconds, or as ordered; see Table 10-7). However, consider the packaging and manufacturer guidelines. Emergency resuscitative equipment must always be available in the event of respiratory or cardiac arrest.

OPIOID AGONISTS-ANTAGONISTS

Remember when giving *agonists-antagonists* that they react very differently depending on whether they are given by themselves or with other drugs. When administered alone, they are effective analgesics because they bind with opiate receptors and produce an agonist effect (see discussion in the pharmacology section). If given at the same time as other opioids, however, they lead to reversal of analgesia and acute withdrawal because of the blocking of opiate receptors. Be very careful to check dosages and routes as well as to perform the interventions mentioned for opioid agonist drugs, including closely assessing vital signs, especially respiratory rate. Emphasize the importance of reporting any dizziness, unresolved constipation, urinary retention, and sedation. See Table 10-6 for additional adverse effects of opioid agonists as they are similar to the opioid agonist-antagonist drugs. Other points to emphasize with the patient include that the drug also has the ability to reverse analgesia as

well as precipitate withdrawal (if taken with other opioid agonists). A list of other opioid agonists must be shared with the patient, as well.

OPIOID ANTAGONISTS

Opioid antagonists must be given as ordered and be readily available, especially when the patient is receiving PCA with an opioid, is opioid naïve, or is receiving continuous doses of opioids. Several doses of these drugs are often required to ensure adequate opioid agonist reversal (see earlier discussion). Encourage patients to report any nausea or tachycardia.

GENERAL CONSIDERATIONS

You are always responsible and accountable to maintain a current, updated knowledge base on all forms of analgesics as well as protocols for pain management with focus on the specific drug(s) as well as differences in the treatment of mild to moderate pain, severe pain, and pain in special situations (e.g., cancer pain). The WHO's three-step analgesic ladder provides a standard for pain management in cancer patients and must be reviewed and considered, as needed.

Dosing of medications for pain management is very important to the treatment regimen. As noted earlier, once a thorough assessment has been performed, it is best to treat the patient's pain before it becomes severe, which is the rationale for considering pain to be the fifth vital sign. When pain is present for more than 12 hours a day, analgesic doses are individualized and are best administered around the clock rather than on an as-needed basis, while always staying within safe practice guidelines for each drug used. Around-the-clock (or scheduled) dosing maintains steady-state levels of the medication and prevents drug troughs and pain escalation. No given dosage of an analgesic will provide the same level of pain relief for every patient; thus there is a need for a process of titration—upward or even downward—to be carried out based on the individual's needs. Aggressive titration may be necessary in difficult pain control cases and in cancer pain situations. Patients with severe pain, metastatic pain, or bone metastasis pain may need increasingly higher dosages of analgesic. These special pain situations may require an opiate such as morphine that needs to be titrated until the desired response is achieved or until adverse effects occur. A patient-rated pain level of less than 4 on a scale of 1 to 10 is considered to indicate effective pain relief. However, this may vary depending on the health care provider, health care setting, and/or unit.

If pain is not managed adequately by monotherapy, other drugs or adjuvants may need to be added to enhance analgesic efficacy. This includes the use of NSAIDs (for analgesic, antiinflammatory effects), acetaminophen (for analgesic effects), corticosteroids (for mood elevation and antiinflammatory, antiemetic, and appetite stimulation effects), anticonvulsants (for treatment of neuropathic pain), tricyclic antidepressants (for treatment of neuropathic pain and for their innate analgesic properties and opioid-potentiating effects), neuroleptics (for treatment of chronic pain syndromes), local anesthetics (for treatment of neuropathic pain), hydroxyzine (for mild antianxiety properties as well as sedating effects and antihistamine and mild antiemetic actions), or psychostimulants (for reduction of opioid-induced sedation when opioid dosage adjustment is not effective). Table 10-9 provides a listing of drugs that are *not* to be used in patients experiencing cancer pain.

Dosage forms are also important, especially with chronic pain and cancer pain. Oral administration is always preferred but is not always tolerated by the patient and may not even be a viable option for pain control. If oral dosing is not appropriate, less invasive routes of administration include rectal and transdermal routes. Rectal dosage forms are safe, inexpensive, effective, and helpful if the patient is experiencing nausea or vomiting or altered mental status; however, this route is not suitable for those with diarrhea, stomatitis, and/or low white blood cell counts. Transdermal patches may provide up to 7 days of pain control but are not for rapid dose titration and are used only when stable analgesia has been previously achieved. Long-acting forms of morphine and fentanyl may be delivered via transdermal patches when a longer duration of action is needed. Intermittent injections or continuous infusions via the intravenous or subcutaneous route are often used for opioid delivery and may be administered at home in special pain situations, such as in hospice care or management of chronic cancer pain. Subcutaneous infusions are often used when there is no intravenous access. PCA pumps may be used to help deliver opioids intravenously, subcutaneously, or even intraspinally and can be managed in home health care or hospice care for the patient at home. Use of the intrathecal or epidural route requires special skill and expertise, and delivery of pain medications using these routes is available only from certain home health care agencies for at-home care. The main reason for long-term intraspinal opioid administration is intractable pain. Transnasal dosage forms are approved only for *butorphanol*, an *agonist-antagonist drug*, and this dosage form is generally not used or recommended. Regardless of the specific drug or dosage form used, a fast-acting rescue drug needs to be ordered and available for patients with cancer pain and patients presenting other special challenges in pain management.

Regardless of the drug(s) used for the pain management regimen, always remember that individualization of treatment is one of the most important considerations for effective and quality pain control. Also consider implementing the following:
- At the initiation of pain therapy, conduct a review of all relevant histories, laboratory test values, nurse-related charting entries, and diagnostic study results in the patient's medical record. If there are underlying problems, consider these variables while never forgetting to treat the patient with dignity and empathy. Never let compounding variables

TABLE 10-9 Drugs Not Recommended for Treatment of Cancer Pain

Class	Drug	Reason for Not Recommending
Opioids with short durations of action	meperidine	Short (2-3 hr) duration of analgesia; administration may lead to CNS toxicity (tremor, confusion, or seizures)
Miscellaneous	Cannabinoids	Adverse effects of dysphoria, drowsiness, hypotension, and bradycardia: may be indicated for use in treating severe chemotherapy-induced nausea and vomiting
Opioid agonists-antagonists	Pentazocine, butorphanol, nalbuphine	May precipitate withdrawal in opioid-dependent patients; analgesic ceiling effect; possible production of unpleasant psychologic adverse effects, including dysphoria, delusions, and hallucinations
	buprenorphine	Analgesic ceiling effect; can precipitate withdrawal if given with an opioid
Opioid antagonists	Naloxone, naltrexone	Reverses analgesia as well as CNS depressant effects, such as respiratory depression
Combination preparations	Brompton cocktails	No evidence of analgesic benefit over use of a single opioid analgesic
	DPT* (meperidine, promethazine, and chlorpromazine)	Efficacy poor compared with that of other analgesics; associated with a higher incidence of adverse effects
Anxiolytics (as monotherapy) or sedatives-hypnotics (as monotherapy)	Benzodiazepines (e.g., alprazolam)	Analgesic properties not associated with these drugs. Risk for sedation, which may put some patients at higher risk for neurologic complications
	Barbiturates	Analgesic properties not demonstrated; sedation is problematic and limits use

CNS, Central nervous system.
*DPT is the abbreviation for the trade names Demerol, Phenergan, and Thorazine.

CASE STUDY

Safety: What Went Wrong? Opioid Administration

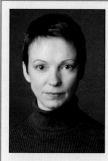

You are the home health nurse assigned to care for a patient who is in the terminal phases of breast cancer. Mrs. D. is 48 years of age and underwent bilateral mastectomy 4 years ago. She had lymph node involvement at the time of surgery, and recently has been diagnosed with metastasis to the bone. She has been taking oxycodone (one 5-mg tablet every 6 hours) at home but is not sleeping through the night and is now complaining of increasing pain to the point that her quality of life has decreased significantly. She wants to stay at home during the terminal phases of her illness but needs to have adequate and safe pain control. Her husband of 18 years is very supportive. They have no children. They are both college graduates and have medical insurance.

1. Mrs. D.'s recent increase in pain has been attributed to bone metastasis in the area of the lumbar spine. At this time, the oxycodone is not beneficial, and you as the home health care nurse need to advocate for Mrs. D. to receive adequate pain relief. When discussing her pain medications with her physician, what type of medication would you expect to be ordered to relieve the bone pain, and what is the rationale for this medication? (Provide references from within this chapter to support the selection of the specific opioid drug.)

   Mrs. D. visits her physician and receives a different opioid medication that is given around-the-clock, plus an additional immediate-release opioid medication to help with any breakthrough pain.
2. After 1 week, Mr. D. finds Mrs. D. awake but lethargic, and speaking with slurred words. What do you think has happened? What should Mr. D. do?
3. Mrs. D. is taken to the emergency department and is treated for oversedation. Her physician is contacted, and the medication doses are adjusted to a lower dose. How can this problem be prevented in the future?

For answers, see *http://evolve.elsevier.com/Lilley.*

and any other problems overshadow the fact that there is a patient who is in pain and deserving of safe, quality care. Always look and listen!

- Develop goals for pain management in conjunction with the patient, family members, significant others, and/or caregiver. These goals include improving the level of comfort with increased levels of activities of daily living and ambulation.
- Collaborate with other members of the health care team to select a regimen that will be easy for the patient to follow while in the hospital and, if necessary, at home (e.g., for cancer patients and other patients with chronic pain).
- Be aware that most regimens for acute pain management include treatment with short-acting opioids plus the addition of other medications such as NSAIDs.
- Be familiar with equianalgesic doses of opioids, because lack of knowledge may lead to inadequate analgesia or overdose.
- Use an analgesic appropriate for the situation (e.g., short-acting opioids for severe pain secondary to a myocardial infarction, surgery, or kidney stones). For cancer pain, the regimen usually begins with short-acting opioids with eventual conversion to sustained-release formulations.

- Use preventative measures to manage adverse effects. In addition, a switch is made to another opioid as soon as possible if the patient finds that the medication is not controlling the pain adequately.
- Consider the option of analgesic adjuvants, especially in cases of chronic pain or cancer pain; these might include other prescribed drugs such as NSAIDs, acetaminophen, corticosteroids, anticonvulsants, tricyclic antidepressants, neuroleptics, local anesthetics, hydroxyzine, and/or psychostimulants. Over-the-counter drugs and herbals may be helpful.
- Be alert to patients with special needs, such as patients with breakthrough pain. Generally, the drug used to manage such pain is a short-acting form of the longer-acting opioid being given (e.g., immediate-release morphine for breakthrough pain while sustained-release morphine is also used).
- Identify community resources that can assist the patient, family members, and/or significant others. These resources may include various websites for patient education such as *www.theacpa.org, www.painconnection.org,* and *www.painaction.com.* Many other pain management sites may be found on the Internet by using the search terms *pain, pain clinic,* or *pain education* and looking for patient-focused materials/sites.
- Conduct frequent online searches to remain current on the topic of pain management, pain education, drug and non-drug therapeutic regimens for pain, and special pain situations. The following professional nurse and/or prescriber-focused websites are listed at *www.painedu.org/resources.asp* as resources for the topic of general pain management: *www.aapainmanage.org, www.painmed.org, www.painfoundation.org, www.ampainsoc.org, www.aspmn.org, www.asam.org, www.paineducators.org, www.asra.com, www.iasp-pain.org, www.painpolicy.wisc.edu, www.painmedicinenews.com, www.pain-topics.org, www.pain.com,* and *www.painandhealth.org.* On the topic of chronic pain, websites are as follows: *www.theacpa.org* and *www.arthritis.org.* On the topic of cancer pain, websites are as follows: *www.cancer.org, www.apos-society.org, www.asco.org, www.cancercare.org, www.cancer.gov,* and *www.ons.org.*
- Because fall prevention is of utmost importance in patient care (after the ABCs [airway, breathing, circulation] of care are addressed), monitor the patient frequently after an analgesic is given. Frequent measurement of vital signs, inclusion of the patient in a frequent watch program, and/or use of bed alarms is encouraged.
- Restraints may cause many injuries; therefore, if restraints are necessary, follow the appropriate policies and procedures. Assess, monitor, evaluate, and document the reason for the restraint; also document the patient's behavior, the type of restraint used, and the assessment of the patient after the placement of restraints. Use of restraints has been largely replaced with a bed watch system and the use of bed and/or wheelchair alarms. Give instructions to the patient, family members, and/or caregivers about the risk for falls and the need for safety measures. Restraints are not used in long-term health care settings.

EVALUATION

Positive therapeutic outcomes of acetaminophen use are decreased symptoms, fever, and pain. Monitor for the adverse reactions of anemias and liver problems due to hepatotoxicity, and report patient complaints of abdominal pain and/or vomiting to the prescriber. During and after the administration of *nonopioid analgesics*, such as tramadol, as well as *opioids* and *mixed opioid agonists*, monitor the patient for both therapeutic effects and adverse effects frequently and as needed. Therapeutic effects of analgesics include increased comfort levels as well as decreased complaints of pain and longer periods of comfort, with improvements in performance of activities of daily living, appetite, and sense of well-being. Monitoring for adverse effects will vary with each drug (see earlier discussions), but effects may consist of nausea, vomiting, constipation, dizziness, headache, blurred vision, decreased urinary output, drowsiness, lethargy, sedation, palpitations, bradycardia, bradypnea, dyspnea, and hypotension. If the patient's vital signs change, the patient's condition declines, or pain continues, contact the prescriber immediately and continue to closely monitor the patient. Respiratory depression may be manifested by a respiratory rate of less than 10 breaths/min, dyspnea, diminished breath sounds, and/or shallow breathing. Include a review of the effectiveness of multimodal and nonpharmacologic approaches to pain management in your evaluation.

PATIENT-CENTERED CARE: PATIENT TEACHING

- Capsaicin is a topical product made from different types of peppers that may help with muscle pain and joint/nerve pain. It may cause local topical reactions, so be sure to share information with the patient about its safe use.
- Opioids are not to be used with alcohol or with other CNS depressants, unless ordered, because of worsening of the depressant effects. Emphasize the importance of patients and caregivers knowing the ingredients of over-the-counter as well as prescribed medications. This is especially important if a patient is taking acetaminophen and also a combination opioid prescribed medication such as hydrocodone (Vicodin, Norco) or oxycodone (Percocet, Tylox) because of danger of overdosage with the acetaminophen (see previous discussions in this chapter).
- A holistic approach to pain management may be appropriate, with the use of complementary modalities including the following: biofeedback, imagery, relaxation, deep breathing, humor, pet therapy, music therapy, massage, use of hot or cold compresses, and use of herbal products.
- Dizziness, difficulty breathing, low blood pressure, excessive sleepiness (sedation), confusion, or loss of memory must be promptly reported to the nurse, prescriber, or other health care providers.
- Opioids may result in constipation, so forcing fluids (up to 3 L/day unless contraindicated), increasing fiber consumption, and exercising as tolerated is recommended. Stool softeners may also be necessary.
- Report any nausea or vomiting. Antiemetic drugs may be prescribed.
- Any activities requiring mental clarity or alertness may need to be avoided if experiencing drowsiness or sedation. Ambulate with caution and/or assistance as needed.

- It is important for the patient to share any history of addiction with health care providers, but when such a patient experiences pain and is in need of opioid analgesia, understand that the patient has a right to comfort. Any further issues with addiction may be managed during and after the use of opioids. Keeping an open mind regarding the use of resources, counseling, and other treatment options is important in dealing with addictive behaviors.
- If pain is problematic and not managed by monotherapy, a combination of a variety of medications may be needed. Other drugs that may be used include antianxiety drugs, sedatives, hypnotics, or anticonvulsants.
- For the cancer patient or patient with special needs, the prescriber will monitor pain control and the need for other options for therapy or for dosing of drugs. For example, the use of transdermal patches, buccal tablets, and continuous infusions while the patient remains mobile or at home is often helpful in pain management. It is also important to understand that if morphine or morphine-like drugs are being used, the potential for addiction exists; however, in specific situations, the concern for quality of life and pain management is more important than the concern for addiction.
- Most hospitals have inpatient and outpatient resources such as pain clinics. Patients need to constantly be informed and aware of all treatment options and remain active participants in their care for as long as possible.
- Tolerance does occur with opioid use, so if the level of pain increases while the patient remains on the prescribed dosage, the prescriber or health care provider must be contacted. Dosages must not be changed, increased, or doubled unless prescribed.

KEY POINTS

- Pain is individual and involves sensations and emotions that are unpleasant. It is influenced by age, culture, race, spirituality, and all other aspects of the individual.

- Pain is associated with actual or potential tissue damage and may be exacerbated or alleviated depending on the treatment and type of pain.

- Types of analgesics include the following:
  - Nonopioids, including acetaminophen, aspirin, and NSAIDs
  - Opioids, which are natural or synthetic drugs that either contain or are derived from morphine (opiates) or have opiate-like effects or activities (opioids), and opioid agonist-antagonist drugs
- Pediatric dosages of morphine must be calculated very cautiously with close attention to the dose and kilograms of body weight. Cautious titration of dosage upward is usually the standard.

- Older adult patients may react differently than expected to analgesics, especially opioids and opioid agonists-antagonists.
- In treating older adults, remember that these patients experience pain the same as the general population does, but they may be reluctant to report pain and may metabolize opiates at a slower rate and thus are at increased risk for adverse effects such as sedation and respiratory depression. The best rule is to start with low dosages, reevaluate often, and go slowly during upward titration.

NCLEX® EXAMINATION REVIEW QUESTIONS

1. For best results when treating severe pain associated with pathologic spinal fractures related to metastatic bone cancer, the nurse should remember that the best type of dosage schedule is to administer the pain medication
   a. as needed.
   b. around the clock.
   c. on schedule during waking hours only.
   d. around the clock, with additional doses as needed for breakthrough pain.
2. A patient is receiving an opioid via a PCA pump as part of his postoperative pain management program. During rounds, the nurse finds him unresponsive, with respirations of 8 breaths/min and blood pressure of 102/58 mm Hg. After stopping the opioid infusion, what should the nurse do next?
   a. Notify the charge nurse
   b. Draw arterial blood gases
   c. Administer an opiate antagonist per standing orders
   d. Perform a thorough assessment, including mental status examination
3. A patient with bone pain caused by metastatic cancer will be receiving transdermal fentanyl patches. The patient asks the nurse what benefits these patches have. The nurse's best response includes which of these features?
   a. More constant drug levels for analgesia
   b. Less constipation and minimal dry mouth
   c. Less drowsiness than with oral opioids
   d. Lower dependency potential and no major adverse effects
4. Intravenous morphine is prescribed for a patient who has had surgery. The nurse informs the patient that which common adverse effects can occur with this medication? *(Select all that apply.)*
   a. Diarrhea
   b. Constipation
   c. Pruritus
   d. Urinary frequency
   e. Nausea

5. Several patients have standard orders for acetaminophen as needed for pain. While reviewing their histories and assessments, the nurse discovers that one of the patients has a contraindication to acetaminophen therapy. Which patient should receive an alternate medication?
   a. A patient with a fever of 103.4° F (39.7° C)
   b. A patient admitted with deep vein thrombosis
   c. A patient admitted with severe hepatitis
   d. A patient who had abdominal surgery 1 week earlier
6. The nurse is administering an intravenous dose of morphine sulfate to a 48-year-old postoperative patient. The dose ordered is 3 mg every 3 hours as needed for pain. The medication is supplied in vials of 4 mg/mL. How much will be drawn into the syringe for this dose?
7. An opioid analgesic is prescribed for a patient. The nurse checks the patient's medical history knowing this medication is contraindicated in which disorder?
   a. Renal insufficiency
   b. Severe asthma
   c. Liver disease
   d. Diabetes mellitus
8. A patient with renal cancer needs an opiate for pain control. Which opioid medication would be the safest choice for this patient?
   a. fentanyl
   b. hydromorphone (Dilaudid)
   c. morphine sulfate
   d. methadone (Dolophine)

1. d, 2. c, 3. a, 4. b, c, e 5. c, 6. 0.75 mL, 7. b, 8. d

CRITICAL THINKING AND PRIORITIZATION QUESTIONS

1. The nurse is about to administer 5 mg of morphine sulfate intravenously to a patient with severe postoperative pain, as ordered. What priority assessment data must be gathered before and after administering this drug? Explain your answer.

2. A young woman is brought by ambulance to the emergency department because she was found unconscious next to an empty bottle of acetaminophen. While the medical team assesses her, the nurse goes to question the family about the situation. What is the most important piece of information to know about this possible overdose?

For answers, see *http://evolve.elsevier.com/Lilley.*

ⓔ EVOLVE WEBSITE

http://evolve.elsevier.com/Lilley
- Animations
- Answer Keys for Textbook Case Studies and Textbook Critical Thinking and Prioritization Questions

- Content Updates
- Key Points
- Review Questions
- Student Case Studies

General and Local Anesthetics

http://evolve.elsevier.com/Lilley

OBJECTIVES

When you reach the end of this chapter, you will be able to do the following:

1. Define anesthesia.
2. Describe the basic differences between general and local anesthesia.
3. List the most commonly used general and local anesthetics and associated risks.
4. Discuss the differences between depolarizing neuromuscular blocking drugs and nondepolarizing blocking drugs and their impact on the patient.
5. Compare the mechanisms of action, indications, adverse effects, routes of administration, cautions, contraindications, and drug interactions for general and local anesthesia as well as drugs used for moderate or conscious sedation.
6. Develop a nursing care plan for patients before anesthesia (preanesthesia), during anesthesia, and after anesthesia (postanesthesia) related to general anesthesia.
7. Develop a nursing care plan for patients undergoing local anesthesia and/or moderate or conscious sedation.

DRUG PROFILES

!dexmedetomidine, p. 174
!ketamine, p. 174
♦lidocaine, p. 178
nitrous oxide, p. 174
♦!propofol, p. 174
♦!rocuronium, p. 181

sevoflurane, p. 175
♦!succinylcholine, p. 180

—————
♦ = *Key drug*
! = *High-alert drug*

KEY TERMS

Adjunct anesthetics Drugs used in combination with anesthetic drugs to control the adverse effects of anesthetics or to help maintain the anesthetic state in the patient. (See *balanced anesthesia*.) (p. 172)

Anesthesia The loss of the ability to feel pain resulting from the administration of an anesthetic drug. (p. 172)

Anesthetics Drugs that depress the central nervous system (CNS) or peripheral nerves to produce decreased or loss of consciousness, or muscle relaxation. (p. 172)

Anesthesia provider A health care professional who is licensed to provide anesthesia. Can be an anesthesiologist (MD), a Certified Registered Nurse Anesthetist (CRNA), or an anesthesia assistant. (p. 172)

Balanced anesthesia The practice of using combinations of different drug classes rather than a single drug to produce anesthesia. (p. 172)

General anesthesia A drug-induced state in which the CNS nerve impulses are altered to reduce pain and other sensations throughout the entire body. It involves complete loss of consciousness and depression of respiratory drive. (p. 172)

Local anesthesia A drug-induced state in which peripheral or spinal nerve impulses are altered to reduce or eliminate pain and other sensations in tissues innervated by these nerves. (p. 172)

Malignant hyperthermia A genetically linked major adverse reaction to general anesthesia characterized by a rapid rise in body temperature, as well as tachycardia, tachypnea, and sweating. (p. 174)

Moderate sedation A milder form of general anesthesia that causes partial or complete loss of consciousness but does not generally reduce normal respiratory drive (also referred to as *conscious sedation*). (p. 175)

Overton-Meyer theory A theory that describes the relationship between the lipid solubility of anesthetic drugs and their potency. (p. 172)

Spinal anesthesia Local anesthesia induced by injection of an anesthetic drug near the spinal cord to anesthetize nerves that are distal to the site of injection (p. 175)

OVERVIEW

Anesthetics are drugs that reduce or eliminate pain by depressing nerve function in the central nervous system (CNS) and/or the peripheral nervous system (PNS). This state of reduced neurologic function is called anesthesia. Anesthesia is further classified as *general* or *local*. General anesthesia involves complete loss of consciousness and loss of body reflexes, including respiratory muscles. This loss of normal respiratory function requires mechanical or manual ventilatory support to avoid brain damage and suffocation (death from respiratory arrest). Local anesthesia does not involve paralysis of respiratory function, only elimination of pain sensation in the tissues innervated by *anesthetized* nerves. Functions of the parasympathetic nervous system, which is a branch of the *autonomic nervous system*, may also be affected.

GENERAL ANESTHETICS

General anesthetics are drugs that are used to produce profound neurosensory depression to allow for surgical procedures. General anesthetics are given only under controlled situations by anesthesia providers (either an anesthesiologist, a nurse anesthetist [CRNA], or anesthesia assistant). General anesthesia is achieved by the use of one or more drugs. Often a synergistic combination of drugs is used, which allows for smaller doses of each drug and better control of the patient's anesthetized state. Inhalational anesthetics are volatile liquids or gases that are vaporized or mixed with oxygen or medical air to induce anesthesia. Box 11-1 offers a historical perspective on general anesthesia.

Parenteral anesthetics (Table 11-1) are given intravenously and are used for induction and/or maintenance of general anesthesia, induction of amnesia, and as adjuncts to inhalation-type anesthetics (Table 11-2). The specific goal varies with the drug. Common intravenous anesthetic drugs include drugs classified solely as general anesthetics, such as etomidate and propofol.

Adjunct anesthetics or simply adjuncts are also used. *Adjunct* is a general term for any drug that enhances clinical therapy when used simultaneously with another drug. Adjunct drugs can be thought of as "helper drugs." They are used simultaneously with general anesthetics for anesthesia initiation (induction), sedation, reduction of anxiety, and amnesia. Adjuncts include neuromuscular blocking drugs (NMBDs; see Neuromuscular Blocking Drugs later in the chapter), sedative-hypnotics or anxiolytics (see Chapter 12) such as propofol (this chapter), benzodiazepines (e.g., diazepam, midazolam), barbiturates (e.g., thiopental; see Chapter 12), opioid analgesics (e.g., fentanyl; see Chapter 10), anticholinergics (e.g., atropine; see Chapter 21), and antiemetics (e.g., ondansetron; see Chapter 52). Note that propofol can be used as a general anesthetic and/or sedative-hypnotic, depending on the dose. The simultaneous use of both general anesthetics and adjuncts is called balanced anesthesia. Common adjunctive anesthetic drugs are listed in Table 11-3.

BOX 11-1 General Anesthesia: A Historical Perspective

Until recently, general anesthesia was described as having several definitive stages. This was especially true with the use of many of the ether-based inhaled anesthetic drugs. Features of these distinctive stages were easily observable to the trained eye. They included specific physical and physiologic changes that progressed gradually and predictably with the depth of the patient's anesthetized state. Gradual changes in pupil size, progression from thoracic to diaphragmatic breathing, vital sign changes, and several other changes all characterized the various stages. Newer inhalational and intravenous general anesthetic drugs, however, often have a much more rapid onset of action and body distribution. As a result, the specific stages of anesthesia once observed with older drugs are no longer sufficiently well-defined to be observable. Thus, the concept of stages of anesthesia is an outdated one in most modern surgical institutions. Registered nurses who pursue advanced training to become anesthesia providers often find this to be a rewarding and interesting area of nursing practice. Some nurses also find that this type of work offers greater flexibility in their work schedule than do other practice areas.

TABLE 11-1 Parenteral General Anesthetics

Generic Name	Trade Name
etomidate	Amidate
ketamine	Ketalar
methohexital	Brevital
propofol	Diprivan
thiopental	Pentothal

TABLE 11-2 Inhalational General Anesthetics

Generic Name	Trade Name
Inhaled Gas	
nitrous oxide (laughing gas)	
Inhaled Volatile Liquid	
desflurane	Suprane
isoflurane	Forane
sevoflurane	Ultane

Mechanism of Action and Drug Effects

Many theories have been proposed to explain the actual mechanism of action of general anesthetics. The drugs vary widely in their chemical structures, and their mechanism of action is not easily explained by a structure-receptor relationship. The concentrations of various anesthetics required to produce a given state of anesthesia also differ greatly. The Overton-Meyer theory has been used to explain some of the properties of anesthetic drugs. It proposes that, for all anesthetics, potency varies directly with lipid solubility. In other words, fat-soluble drugs

TABLE 11-3   **Adjunctive Anesthetic Drugs**

Drug	Pharmacologic Class	Indications/Uses
alfentanil (Alfenta), fentanyl (Sublimaze), sufentanil (Sufenta)	Opioid analgesic	Anesthesia induction
diazepam (Valium), midazolam (Versed)	Benzodiazepine	Amnesia and anxiety reduction
Atropine, glycopyrrolate (Robinul)	Anticholinergic	Drying up of excessive secretions
meperidine (Demerol), morphine	Opioid analgesic	Pain prevention and pain relief
hydroxyzine (Atarax, Vistaril), promethazine (Phenergan)	Antihistamine	Sedation, prevention of nausea and vomiting, anxiety reduction
pentobarbital (Nembutal), secobarbital (Seconal)	Sedative-hypnotic	Amnesia and sedation
dexmedetomidine (Precedex)	Alpha$_2$ agonist	Sedation

TABLE 11-4   **Effects of Inhaled and Intravenous General Anesthetics**

Organ/System	Reaction
Respiratory system	Impaired oxygenation; depressed airway-protective mechanisms; airway irritation and possible laryngospasm
Cardiovascular system	Depressed myocardium; hypotension and tachycardia; bradycardia in response to vagal stimulation
Cerebrovascular system	Increased intracranial pressure
Gastrointestinal system	Reduced hepatic blood flow and thus reduced hepatic clearance
Renal system	Decreased glomerular filtration
Skeletal muscles	Skeletal muscle relaxation
Cutaneous circulation	Vasodilation
Central nervous system (CNS)	CNS depression; blurred vision; nystagmus; progression of CNS depression to decreased alertness, sensorium, and decreased level of consciousness

are stronger anesthetics than water-soluble drugs. Nerve cell membranes have high lipid content, as does the brain, the spinal cord, and the blood-brain barrier (see Chapter 2). Lipid-soluble anesthetic drugs can therefore easily cross the blood-brain barrier to concentrate in nerve cell membranes.

The overall effect of general anesthetics is a progressive reduction of sensory and motor CNS functions. The degree and speed of this process vary with the anesthetics and adjuncts used along with their dosages and routes of administration. General anesthesia initially produces a loss of the senses of sight, touch, taste, smell, and hearing, along with loss of consciousness. Cardiac and pulmonary functions are usually the last to be interrupted, because they are controlled by the *medulla* of the *brainstem*. These are the classical "stages" of anesthesia. Mechanical ventilatory support is absolutely necessary. In more extensive surgical procedures, especially those involving the heart, pharmacologic cardiac support involving adrenergic drugs (see Chapter 18) and inotropic drugs (see Chapter 24) may also be required. The reactions of various body systems to general anesthetics are further described in Table 11-4.

Indications

General anesthetics are used to produce unconsciousness as well as some degree of relaxation of skeletal and visceral smooth muscles for surgical procedures, as well as in electroconvulsive therapy for severe depression (see Chapter 16).

Contraindications

Contraindications to the use of anesthetic drugs include known drug allergy. Depending on the drug type, contraindications may also include pregnancy, narrow-angle glaucoma, acute

porphyria, and known susceptibility to malignant hyperthermia (see Adverse Effects).

PATIENT-CENTERED CARE: LIFESPAN CONSIDERATIONS FOR THE OLDER ADULT PATIENT   [QSEN]

Anesthesia

- The older adult patient is affected more adversely by anesthesia than the young or middle-aged adult. With aging comes organ system deterioration. Declining liver function results in decreased metabolism of drugs, and a decline in renal functioning leads to decreased drug excretion. Either of these can lead to drug toxicity, unsafe levels, and/or overdose. If both of these organs are not functioning properly, the risk for drug toxicity or overdose is even greater. In addition, older adult patients are more sensitive to the effects of drugs affecting the central nervous system.
- Presence of cardiac and respiratory diseases places the older adult patient at higher risk for cardiac dysrhythmias, hypotension, respiratory depression, atelectasis, and/or pneumonia during the postanesthesia and postoperative phases.
- The practice of polypharmacy is yet another concern in the older adult patient with regard to administration of any type of anesthetic. Because of the presence of various age-related diseases, the older adult patient is generally taking more than one medication. The more drugs a patient is taking, the higher the risk for adverse reactions and drug-drug interactions, including interactions with anesthetics.

Adverse Effects

Adverse effects of general anesthetics are dose dependent and vary with the individual drug. The heart, peripheral circulation, liver, kidneys, and respiratory tract are the sites primarily affected. One major complication of general anesthesia is hypotension affecting perfusion of the organs mentioned earlier. With the development of newer drugs, many of the unwanted adverse effects characteristic of the older drugs (such as hepatotoxicity and myocardial depression) are now less frequent. In addition, many of the bothersome adverse effects such as nausea, vomiting, and confusion are less common since balanced anesthesia is widely used. Even with the use of the newer anesthetic agents, the incidence of postoperative nausea and vomiting (PONV) remains one of the most common reasons children and adults have extended/protracted stays in the postanesthesia care units/recovery rooms. There is no exact cause of PONV, and the cause is thought to be multifactorial. Pain is associated with PONV, and the adequate treatment of pain frequently decreases nausea. Substance abuse can predispose a patient to anesthetic-induced complications.

Malignant hyperthermia is an uncommon, but potentially fatal, genetically linked adverse metabolic reaction to general anesthesia. It is classically associated with the use of volatile inhalational anesthetics as well as the depolarizing neuromuscular blocker, NMBD succinylcholine. Signs include rapid rise in body temperature, tachycardia, tachypnea, and muscular rigidity. Patients known to be at greater risk for malignant hyperthermia include children, adolescents, and individuals with muscular and/or skeletal abnormalities. Malignant hyperthermia is treated with cardiorespiratory supportive care as needed to stabilize heart and lung function along with the skeletal muscle relaxant dantrolene (see Chapter 12). In fact, by law, all health care institutions that provide general anesthesia must maintain a certain amount of dantrolene on hand in case of malignant hyperthermia.

Toxicity and Management of Overdose

In large doses, anesthetics are potentially life threatening, with cardiac and respiratory arrest as the ultimate causes of death. However, these drugs are almost exclusively administered in a very controlled environment by personnel trained in advanced cardiac life support. General anesthetics are very quickly metabolized. The newer drugs are much more lipophilic than the older drugs, and this contributes to the "fast on" and "fast off" action of these drugs. These factors combined make an anesthetic overdose rare and easily reversible. Anesthesia is safer today than it is has ever been before due to advances in pharmacology.

Interactions

Some of the drugs that interact with general anesthetics are antihypertensives and beta blockers, which have additive effects when combined with general anesthetics (i.e., increased hypotensive effects from antihypertensives, and increased myocardial depression with beta blockers). No significant laboratory test interactions have been reported.

DRUG PROFILES

The dose of any anesthetic depends on the complexity of the surgical procedure to be performed and the physical characteristics of the patient. All of the general anesthetics have a rapid onset of action and rapid elimination upon discontinuation.

Anesthesia is maintained intraoperatively by continuous administration of the drug.

❗dexmedetomidine

Dexmedetomidine (Precedex) is an alpha-2 adrenergic receptor agonist (see Chapter 18). It produces dose-dependent sedation, decreased anxiety, and analgesia without respiratory depression. It is used for procedural sedation and for surgeries of short duration. It has a short half-life, and the patient awakens quickly upon withdrawal of the drug. Dexmedetomidine is also used in the intensive care setting for sedation of mechanically ventilated patients. Lower doses may be needed with concurrent anesthetics, sedatives, or opioids. Side effects include hypotension, bradycardia, transient hypertension, and nausea. Although the prescribing information states that dexmedetomidine is to be used for only 24 hours, multiple studies have shown it to be safe and effective at longer durations.

❗ketamine

Ketamine is a unique drug with multiple properties. Given intravenously most commonly, it can also be given IM or SubQ and is used for both general anesthesia and moderate sedation. It is commonly used in the emergency department for setting broken bones. It binds to receptors in both central and peripheral nervous systems, including opioid receptors and most importantly, the N-methyl-D-aspartate (NMDA) receptors located in the dorsal horn of the spinal cord. The drug is highly lipid soluble and penetrates the blood-brain barrier rapidly, which results in a rapid onset of action. It has a low incidence of reduction of cardiovascular, respiratory, and bowel function. Ketamine actually has bronchodilating properties, which makes it an excellent choice for the induction of anesthesia in the asthmatic patient. Adverse effects can include disturbing psychomimetic effects, including hallucinations. However, these are less likely to occur when benzodiazepines (see Chapter 12) are coadministered with the drug. Ketamine is contraindicated in cases of known drug allergy.

nitrous oxide

Nitrous oxide, also known as *laughing gas,* is the only inhaled gas currently used as a general anesthetic. It is the weakest of the general anesthetic drugs but has very good analgesic properties and is used primarily for dental procedures or as a supplement to other, more potent anesthetics. Due to its low potency, nitrous oxide is rarely administered as the sole anesthetic for major surgeries and is often administered in addition to one of the other commonly used inhaled agents (sevoflurane and desflurane). High concentrations of nitrous oxide have also been linked to increased incidence of postoperative nausea and vomiting in operations that require more than 1 hour.

♦❗propofol

Propofol (Diprivan) is a parenteral general anesthetic used for the induction and maintenance of general anesthesia and also for sedation for mechanical ventilation in intensive care unit (ICU) settings. In lower doses, it can also be used as a sedative-hypnotic for moderate sedation. Some states allow nurses to administer propofol as part of a moderate sedation protocol. However, many state boards of nursing prohibit administration by nurses. Propofol also is typically well tolerated, producing few undesirable effects. Propofol is a lipid-based emulsion, and if given for prolonged times or if given in conjunction with total parenteral nutrition, serum lipids need to be monitored.

sevoflurane

Sevoflurane (Ultane) and desflurane (Suprane) are inhaled volatile anesthetics that are widely used. Both drugs have rapid onset and elimination, which make them especially useful in all surgical settings. Unlike inhaled anesthetics of the past that left the patient drowsy after awakening from anesthesia, these two commonly used anesthetics are eliminated very quickly from the body. Due to this rapid elimination, there is less incidence of PONV and complications from respiratory difficulty (such as airway obstruction). Unlike sevoflurane, desflurane has been known to cause some airway irritation and coughing.

DRUGS FOR MODERATE SEDATION

Moderate sedation, *conscious sedation*, and *procedural sedation* are synonymous terms for anesthesia that does not cause complete loss of consciousness and does not normally cause respiratory arrest. As more minor surgical procedures move from traditional operating room settings to outpatient surgery centers or office-based practices, the use of moderate sedation will continue to increase. Moderate sedation allows the patient to relax and have markedly reduced or no anxiety, yet still maintain his or her own airway, and respond to verbal commands. Standards must be followed when providing moderate sedation. Health care personnel who administer moderate sedation are required to have advanced cardiac life support training; one professional must have no duties other than to monitor the patient, and someone with the ability to intubate the patient must be present in case the patient slips into a deeper state of sedation and is unable to maintain an open airway. The American Society of Anesthesia has published guidelines on moderate sedation, which can be found at *www.asahq.org*.

The most commonly used drugs for moderate sedation include a short-acting benzodiazepine, usually midazolam (see Chapter 12), with an short-acting opioid, usually fentanyl or morphine. Propofol is also commonly used. Propofol, when used for moderate sedation, is usually given by an anesthesia provider, although there is some debate among physician specialties as to who should be allowed to administer propofol. If midazolam is combined with an opioid such as fentanyl or morphine, the dose should be reduced by 30% to 50%. Mild amnesia is also a common effect, due to the midazolam. This is often desirable for helping patients not to remember painful medical procedures. However, amnesia is not guaranteed. Benzodiazepines (i.e., midazolam) work very similarly to alcohol in the body. If the patient regularly consumes alcohol, this sensitization may require a higher dose to achieve amnesia. **Regardless, the nurse should not assume that the patient will remember things that are said during sedation/anesthesia.** The nurse should always behave and speak as though the patient

was completely awake regardless if the patient is mildly sedated or under a general anesthetic. Moderate sedation is associated with a more rapid recovery time than general anesthesia as well as a better safety profile because of lower cardiopulmonary risks.

The oral route of drug administration is commonly used in pediatric patients. This often involves administering an oral syrup form of midazolam with or without concurrent use of injected medications such as opiates. This is especially helpful for pediatric patients who must undergo uncomfortable procedures such as wound suturing or diagnostic procedures requiring reduced movement such as computed tomography and magnetic resonance imaging. See the Patient-Centered Care: Lifespan Considerations for the Pediatric Patient box for other considerations.

LOCAL ANESTHETICS

Local anesthetics are the second major class of anesthetics. They reduce pain sensations at the level of *peripheral* nerves, although this can involve *neuraxial* or *central* anesthesia (see later). They are also called *regional anesthetics* because they render a specific portion of the body insensitive to pain. They work by interfering with nerve transmission in specific areas of the body, blocking nerve conduction only in the area in which they are applied without causing loss of consciousness. They are most commonly used in clinical settings in which loss of consciousness is undesirable or unnecessary. These include childbirth and other situations in which spinal anesthesia is desired, dental procedures, suturing of skin lacerations, and diagnostic procedures.

Most local anesthetics belong to one of two major groups of organic compounds: esters and amides. They are classified as either *parenteral* (injectable) or *topical* anesthetics. Parenteral anesthetics are most commonly given intravenously but may also be administered by various spinal injection techniques (Box 11-2). Topical anesthetics are applied directly to the skin and mucous membranes. They are available in the form of solutions, ointments, gels, creams, powders, suppositories, and ophthalmic drops. Their dosage strengths are listed in Table 11-5.

The injection of parenteral anesthetic drugs into the area near the spinal cord is known as *spinal* or *neuraxial* anesthesia. This type of anesthesia is generally used to block all peripheral nerves that branch out distal to the injection site. The result is elimination of pain and paralysis of the skeletal and smooth muscles of the corresponding innervated tissues. Some of the medications used for spinal anesthesia include the opioids morphine, hydromorphone, fentanyl, and meperidine (See Chapter 10), and the local anesthetics lidocaine and bupivacaine. Because spinal anesthesia does not depress the CNS at a level that causes loss of consciousness, it can be thought of as a large-scale type of *local* rather than *general* anesthesia. Common types of local anesthesia are described in Box 11-2. The parenteral local anesthetic drugs and their pharmacokinetics are summarized in Table 11-6.

Local anesthesia of specific peripheral nerves is accomplished by *nerve block anesthesia* or *infiltration anesthesia*. Nerve block anesthesia involves relatively deep injections of drugs into

BOX 11-2 Types of Local Anesthesia

Central

- **Spinal or neuraxial or central anesthesia:** Anesthetic drugs are injected into the area near the spinal cord within the vertebral column. Neuraxial or central anesthesia is commonly accomplished by one of two injection techniques: intrathecal and epidural.
  - **Intrathecal anesthesia** involves injection of anesthetic into the subarachnoid space. Intrathecal anesthesia is commonly used for patients undergoing major abdominal or limb surgery for whom the risks of general anesthesia are too high or for patients who prefer this technique instead of complete loss of consciousness during their surgical procedure. More recently, intrathecal injection of anesthetics through implantable drug pumps is even being used on an outpatient basis in patients with severe chronic pain syndromes, such as those resulting from occupational injuries.
  - **Epidural anesthesia** involves injection of anesthetic via a small catheter into the epidural space without puncturing the dura. Epidural anesthesia is commonly used to reduce maternal discomfort during labor and delivery and to manage postoperative acute pain after major abdominal or pelvic surgery. This route is becoming more popular for the administration of opioids for pain management.

Peripheral

- **Infiltration:** Small amounts of anesthetic solution are injected into the tissue that surrounds the operative site. This approach to anesthesia is commonly used for such procedures as wound suturing and dental surgery. Often drugs that cause constriction of local blood vessels (e.g., epinephrine, cocaine) are also administered to limit the site of action to the local area.
- **Nerve block:** Anesthetic solution is injected at the site where a nerve innervates a specific area such as a tissue. This allows large amounts of anesthetic drug to be delivered to a very specific area without affecting the whole body. This method is often reserved for more difficult-to-treat pain syndromes such as cancer pain and chronic orthopedic pain.
- **Topical anesthesia:** The anesthetic drug is applied directly onto the surface of the skin, eye, or any mucous membrane to relieve pain or prevent it from being sensed. It is commonly used for diagnostic eye examinations and skin suturing.

TABLE 11-5 Selected Topical Anesthetics

Drug	Route	Dose Strength
benzocaine (Dermoplast, Lanacane, Solarcaine)	Topical, aerosol, and spray	0.5%-20% ointment or cream
cocaine	Topical	4%-10% solution, jelly
dibucaine (Nupercainal)	Injection and topical	0.5%-1% solution, ointment, or cream
dibucaine	Topical	1% ointment
dyclonine (Dyclone, Sucrets)	Topical	0.5%-1% solution
ethyl chloride (Chloroethane)	Topical	Spray
lidocaine (Lidoderm)	Topical	5% patch
proparacaine (Alcaine, Ophthetic)	Ophthalmic	0.5% solution
prilocaine/lidocaine (EMLA)	Topical	2.5% prilocaine and 2.5% lidocaine cream
tetracaine (Pontocaine)	Injection, topical, and ophthalmic	0.5%-2% solution, ointment, or cream

TABLE 11-6 Selected Parenteral Local Anesthetic Drugs*

Generic Name	Trade Name	Potency	Onset	Duration
lidocaine	Xylocaine	Moderate	Immediate	60-90 min
mepivacaine	Carbocaine	Moderate	Immediate	120-150 min
procaine	Novocain	Lowest	2-5 min	30-60 min
tetracaine	Pontocaine	Highest	5-10 min	90-120 min

*Other common parenteral anesthetic drugs include bupivacaine (Marcaine, Sensorcaine), chloroprocaine (Nesacaine), etidocaine (Duranest), propoxycaine (Ravocaine), and ropivacaine (Naropin).

QSEN ☒ PATIENT-CENTERED CARE: LIFESPAN CONSIDERATIONS FOR THE PEDIATRIC PATIENT

Moderate or Conscious Sedation

- The American Academy of Pediatrics recommends that moderate or conscious sedation be used to reduce anxiety, pain, and fear in the pediatric patient. The use of moderate sedation in the pediatric patient allows a procedure to be performed restraint free in most situations while keeping the patient responsive.
- Pediatric dosing often conforms to the following guidelines:
  - Morphine—pediatric dosing per intravenous (IV) route is to occur over a 2-minute period and is ideal for long procedures or cases in which pain is anticipated after the procedure.
  - Fentanyl—too rapid an IV injection may result in chest rigidity, which may need to be treated with muscle relaxants and possibly mechanical ventilation. Fentanyl is used often for short procedures.
  - Meperidine—pediatric dosing is usually given IV over at least 2 minutes.
- Discharge status of the pediatric patient depends on the type of drugs and drug combinations used. Discharge after conscious or moderate sedation is based mainly on whether the following criteria are met:
  - Patient is alert and oriented compared with the baseline neurologic assessment.

- Protective swallowing and gag reflexes are intact.
- Vital signs are stable and consistent with baseline values for at least 30 minutes after the last dosing. Different health care institutions set different criteria that must be met and documented (blood pressure and pulse rate within normal limits or within 20 points of baseline, temperature lower than 101° F [38.3° C]).
- Oxygen saturation is at least 95% on room air 30 minutes after the last dose.
- Pain rating is at baseline levels or less.
- Ambulation is at baseline level.
- An adult is present to get the patient home and remain with the patient for at least two half-lives of the various drugs used for the anesthesia.
- If a reversal drug was administered, there has been time for the drug to be excreted.

NOTE: Drugs given as anesthesia for moderate sedation procedures are given only under controlled situations by anesthesia providers.

locations adjacent to major nerve trunks or ganglia. It focuses on a relatively large body region but not necessarily as extensive as that affected by spinal anesthesia. In contrast, infiltration anesthesia involves multiple small injections (intradermal, subcutaneous, submucosal, or intramuscular) to produce a more limited or "local" anesthetic field. Another subtype of local anesthesia involves *topical* application of a drug (e.g., lidocaine) onto the surface of the skin, mucous membranes, or eye. A new method of administering local anesthetics is via a peripheral nerve catheter attached to a pump containing the local anesthetic. These pumps are designed to infuse local anesthetic around the nerves that innervate the surgical site for several days postoperatively. The catheter is implanted during surgery and is normally taken out by the patient at home once the anesthetic has been infused. Common trade names include Pain Buster and On-Q pump.

Mechanism of Action and Drug Effects

Local anesthetics work by rendering a specific portion of the body insensitive to pain by interfering with nerve transmission. Nerve conduction is blocked only in the area in which the anesthetic is applied, and there is no loss of consciousness. Local anesthetics block both the generation and conduction of impulses through all types of nerve fibers (autonomic, sensory, and motor) by blocking the movement of certain ions (sodium, potassium, and calcium) important to this process. Some of these drugs are also described as *membrane-stabilizing* because they alter the cell membrane of the nerve so that the free movement of ions is inhibited. The membrane-stabilizing effects occur first in the small fibers, then in the large fibers. In terms of paralysis, usually autonomic activity is affected first, and then pain and other sensory functions are lost. Motor activity is the last to be lost. When the effects of the local anesthetic wear off, recovery occurs in reverse order: motor activity returns first, then sensory functions, and finally autonomic activity.

Possible systemic effects of local anesthetics include effects on circulatory and respiratory function. The systemic adverse effects depend on where and how the drug is administered (e.g., injection at a certain level in the spinal cord or topical application of a drug that gains access to the circulation). Such adverse effects are unlikely unless large quantities of a drug are injected. Local anesthetics also produce *sympathetic blockade*; that is, they block the action of the two *neurotransmitters* of the sympathetic nervous system: *norepinephrine* and *epinephrine* (see Chapter 18).

Indications

Local anesthetics are used for surgical, dental, or diagnostic procedures, as well as for the treatment of various types of chronic pain. Spinal anesthesia is used to control pain during surgical procedures and childbirth. Nerve block anesthesia is used for surgical, dental, and diagnostic procedures and for the therapeutic management of chronic pain. Infiltration anesthesia is used for relatively minor surgical and dental procedures.

Contraindications

Contraindications for local anesthetics include known drug allergy. Only specially formulated dosage forms are intended for ophthalmic use (see Chapter 57).

Adverse Effects

The adverse effects of the local anesthetics are limited and of little clinical importance in most circumstances. The undesirable effects usually occur with high plasma concentrations of the drug, which result from inadvertent intravascular injection, an excessive dose or rate of injection, slow metabolic breakdown, or injection into a highly vascular tissue. One notable complication of spinal anesthesia is *spinal headache.* Spinal headache occurs in up to 70% of patients who either experience inadvertent dural puncture during epidural anesthesia or undergo intrathecal anesthesia. Spinal headache is most often self-limiting and is treated with bed rest and conventional analgesic medications. Oral or intravenous forms of the CNS stimulant caffeine (see Chapter 13) are also sometimes used. Severe cases of spinal headache may be treated by the anesthetist by injection of a small volume (roughly 15 mL) of venous sample of the patient's own blood into the patient's epidural space. The exact mechanism by which this *blood patch* provides relief is unknown, but it is effective in treating spinal headache in over 90% of cases (see Box 11-9 for more information on spinal headaches.)

True allergic reactions to local anesthetics are rare. However, allergic reactions can occur, ranging from skin rash, urticaria, and edema to anaphylactic shock. Such allergic reactions are generally limited to a particular chemical class of anesthetics called the *ester type.* Box 11-3 categorizes the local anesthetic drugs into the ester and amide chemical families. A study tip to differentiate amides versus ester local anesthetics is to remember that amides all have the letter "I" in their name before the suffix "-caine," whereas esters do not.

Different enzymes are responsible for the breakdown of these two groups of anesthetics in the body. Anesthetics belonging to the ester family are metabolized by cholinesterase in the plasma and liver. They are converted into a para-aminobenzoic acid (PABA) compound. This compound is responsible for the allergic reactions. In contrast, the *amide type* of anesthetics is metabolized uneventfully to active and inactive metabolites in the liver by other enzymes. Often when an individual has an adverse reaction to one of the local anesthetics, using a drug from the alternate chemical class avoids this problem.

Toxicity and Management of Overdose

Local anesthetics have little opportunity to cause toxicity under most circumstances. However, systemic reactions are possible if

BOX 11-3 Chemical Groups of Local Anesthetics	
Ester Type	**Amide Type**
benzocaine	bupivacaine
chloroprocaine	dibucaine
cocaine	etidocaine
procaine	lidocaine
proparacaine	mepivacaine
propoxycaine	prilocaine
tetracaine	

sufficiently large quantities are absorbed into the systemic circulation. To prevent this from occurring, a *vasoconstrictor* such as epinephrine is often coadministered with the local anesthetic to maintain localized drug activity (e.g., lidocaine/epinephrine or bupivacaine/epinephrine). This property of epinephrine also serves to reduce local blood loss during minor surgical procedures. If significant amounts of the locally administered anesthetic are absorbed systemically, cardiovascular and respiratory function may be compromised.

Interactions

Few clinically significant drug interactions occur with the local anesthetics. When given with enflurane, halothane, or epinephrine, these drugs can lead to dysrhythmias.

DRUG PROFILES

Local anesthetics include lidocaine, bupivacaine, chloroprocaine, mepivacaine, prilocaine, procaine, propoxycaine, ropivacaine, and tetracaine. There are two major types of local anesthetics as determined by chemical structure: amides and esters (remember that all amides have the "I" located before the "-caine" and esters have no "I" before the "-caine").

◆ lidocaine

Lidocaine belongs to the amide class of local anesthetics. Some patients may report that they have allergic or anaphylactic reactions to the "caines," as they may refer to lidocaine and the other amide drugs. In these situations, it may be wise to try a local anesthetic of the ester type.

Lidocaine (Xylocaine) is one of the most commonly used local anesthetics. It is available in several strengths, both alone and in different concentrations with epinephrine, and is used for both infiltration and nerve block anesthesia. Lidocaine is also available in topical forms, including the unique product EMLA. This is a cream mixture of lidocaine and prilocaine that is applied to skin to ease the pain of needle punctures (e.g., starting an intravenous line). There is also a transdermal lidocaine patch for relief of *postherpetic neuralgia* (see Chapter 10). Parenteral lidocaine is also used to treat certain cardiac dysrhythmias (see Chapter 23). Contraindications include known drug allergy. Lidocaine is classified as a pregnancy category B drug.

NEUROMUSCULAR BLOCKING DRUGS

Neuromuscular blocking drugs (NMBDs) prevent nerve transmission in skeletal and smooth muscles, leading to paralysis. They are often used as adjuncts with general anesthetics for surgical procedures. Neuromuscular blocking drugs also paralyze the skeletal muscles required for breathing: the *intercostal* muscles and the *diaphragm*. The patient is rendered unable to breathe on his or her own, and mechanical ventilation is required to prevent brain damage or death by suffocation. Deaths have been reported when an NMBD is accidentally mistaken for a different drug and given to a patient who is not mechanically ventilated. Most hospitals have taken extra precautions to keep NMBDs separated from other drugs, or marked

with warning stickers. It is essential that the nurse ensure that the patient is ventilated before giving an NMBD and double-check that an NMBD is not inadvertently given. In the event of an error, the patient would experience a horrendous death, because the mind is alert but the patient cannot speak or move (see the Safety and Quality Improvement: Preventing Medication Errors box).

> ⚡ **SAFETY AND QUALITY IMPROVEMENT:**   ▣ QSEN
> **PREVENTING MEDICATION ERRORS**
>
> ### *Neuromuscular Blocking Drugs*
>
> Neuromuscular blocking drugs are considered high-alert drugs, because improper use may lead to severe injury or death. The Institute for Safe Medication Practices has reported several cases of patient death or injury as a result of medication errors involving neuromuscular blocking drugs. Because these drugs paralyze the respiratory muscles, incorrect administration without sufficient ventilator support has resulted in patient deaths. There have been medication errors due to "sound-alike" drug names as well (e.g., vancomycin and vecuronium). Most institutions have followed recommendations to restrict access to these drugs, provide warning labels and reminders, and increase staff awareness of the dangers of these drugs.

For more information, visit *www.ismp.org*.

Historically, snakes and plants have played a role in the discovery of substances that cause paralysis and the related receptor proteins in humans. Curare is considered the grandfather of modern NMBDs. Several curare-like drugs are now used in clinical practice. The first drug to be used medicinally was d-tubocurarine, which was introduced into anesthesia practice in 1940; it has now been replaced by newer drugs.

Mechanism of Action and Drug Effects

NMBDs are classified into two groups based on mechanism of action: depolarizing and nondepolarizing. Depolarizing NMBDs work similarly to the neurotransmitter acetylcholine (ACh). They bind in place of ACh to cholinergic receptors at the motor endplates of muscle nerves or neuromuscular junctions. Thus they are competitive agonists (see Chapter 2). There are two phases of depolarizing block. During phase I (depolarizing phase), the muscles fasciculate (twitch). Eventually, after continued depolarization has occurred, muscles are no longer responsive to the ACh released; thus muscle tone cannot be maintained and the muscle becomes paralyzed. This is phase II, or the desensitizing phase. Succinylcholine is the only depolarizing NMBD. The duration of action of succinylcholine after a single dose is only 5 to 9 minutes because of its rapid breakdown by cholinesterase, the enzyme responsible for metabolizing succinylcholine.

Nondepolarizing NMBDs also bind to ACh receptors at the neuromuscular junction, but instead of mimicking ACh, they block its actions. Therefore, these drugs are *competitive antagonists* (see Chapter 2) of ACh. Consequently, the nerve cell membrane is not depolarized, the muscle fibers are not stimulated, and skeletal muscle contraction does not occur. Nondepolarizing NMBDs include cisatricurium, rocuronium, vecuronium, and pancuronium and are typically classified into three groups based on their duration of action: short-acting, intermediate-acting, and long-acting drugs. Cisatricurium has a unique bio-transformation process. Most drugs are biotransformed in the liver and eliminated by the kidneys. Cisatricurium is broken down by Hoffman elimination, which is a process that is dependent on pH and temperature. This makes it the drug of choice for patients with end-stage renal disease.

The typical time course of NMBD-induced paralysis during a surgical procedure is as follows: The first sensation that is typically felt is muscle weakness. This is usually followed by a total flaccid paralysis. Small, rapidly moving muscles such as those of the fingers and eyes are generally the first to be paralyzed. The next are those of the limbs, neck, and trunk. Finally, the intercostal muscles and the diaphragm are paralyzed, which causes respiratory arrest. The patient can no longer breathe on his or her own. It must be noted that NMBDs, when used alone, do *not* cause sedation or relieve pain or anxiety. Therefore, the patient needs to also receive appropriate medications to manage pain and/or anxiety. Recovery of muscular activity after discontinuation of anesthesia usually occurs in the reverse order of the paralysis, and thus the diaphragm is ordinarily the first to regain function.

Indications

The main therapeutic use of NMBDs is for maintaining skeletal muscle paralysis to facilitate controlled ventilation during surgical procedures. Shorter-acting NMBDs are often used to facilitate intubation with an endotracheal tube. This is commonly done for a variety of diagnostic procedures such as laryngoscopy and bronchoscopy, or when the patient requires mechanical ventilation. When used for this purpose, NMBDs are frequently combined with anxiolytics, analgesics, and anesthetics.

Contraindications

Contraindications to depolarizing NMBDs include known drug allergy and also may include previous history of malignant hyperthermia, penetrating eye injuries, and narrow-angle glaucoma, burns, recent cerebrovascular accident, and crush injuries.

Adverse Effects

The muscle paralysis induced by depolarizing NMBDs (e.g., succinylcholine) is sometimes preceded by muscle spasms, which may damage muscles. These muscle spasms are termed *muscle fasciculations* and are most pronounced in the muscle groups of the hands, feet, and face. Injury to muscle cells may cause postoperative muscle pain and release potassium into the circulation, resulting in hyperkalemia. Hyperkalemia is the primary concern for the anesthesia provider. The nurse should make every effort to be aware of the patient's potassium status. Small doses of nondepolarizing NMBDs are sometimes administered with succinylcholine to minimize these muscle fasciculations. In spite of these disadvantages, succinylcholine is still popular due to its rapid onset of action, its depth of neuromuscular blockade, and its short duration of action. For these

reasons, it is often preferred to nondepolarizing NMBDs for *rapid-sequence induction* of anesthesia (e.g., for emergency intubation).

The effects on the cardiovascular system vary depending on the NMBD used and the individual patient. Some NMBDs cause a release of histamine, which can result in bronchospasm, hypotension, and excessive bronchial and salivary secretion. The gastrointestinal tract is seldom affected by NMBDs. When it is affected, decreased tone and motility typically result, which can lead to constipation or even ileus. Use of succinylcholine has been associated with hyperkalemia; dysrhythmias; fasciculations; muscle pain; myoglobinuria; increased intraocular, intragastric, and intracranial pressure; and malignant hyperthermia.

The key to limiting adverse effects with most NMBDs is to use only enough of the drug to block the neuromuscular receptors. If too much is used, the risk is increased that other ganglionic receptors will be affected. Blockade of these other ganglionic receptors leads to most of the undesirable effects of NMBDs. The effects of ganglionic blockade in various areas of the body are listed in Table 11-7.

Toxicity and Management of Overdose

The primary concern when NMBDs are overdosed is prolonged paralysis requiring prolonged mechanical ventilation (see the Safety and Quality Improvement: Preventing Medication Errors box). Cardiovascular collapse may be seen and is thought to be the result of histamine release. Multiple medical conditions can predispose an individual to toxicity. These conditions increase the sensitivity of the individual to NMBDs and prolong their effects. These predisposing conditions are listed in Box 11-4. Some conditions make it more difficult for NMBDs to work, and therefore higher doses of NMBDs are required in these

TABLE 11-7 Effects of Ganglionic Blockade by Neuromuscular Blocking Drugs

Site	Part of Nervous System Blocked	Physiologic Effect
Arterioles	Sympathetic	Vasodilation and hypotension
Veins	Sympathetic	Dilation
Heart	Parasympathetic	Tachycardia
Gastrointestinal tract	Parasympathetic	Reduced tone and motility; constipation
Urinary bladder	Parasympathetic	Urinary retention
Salivary glands	Parasympathetic	Dry mouth

BOX 11-4 Conditions That Predispose Patients to Toxic Effects from Neuromuscular Blocking Drugs

Acidosis	Myasthenia gravis
Hypocalcemia	Neonatal status
Hypokalemia	Paraplegia
Hypothermia	

BOX 11-5   Conditions That Oppose the Effects of Neuromuscular Blocking Drugs

Cirrhosis with ascites	Hyperkalemia
Clostridial infections	Peripheral nerve transection
Hemiplegia	Peripheral neuropathies
Hypercalcemia	Thermal burns

BOX 11-6   Drugs That Interact with Neuromuscular Blocking Drugs

Additive Effects
Aminoglycosides
Calcium channel blockers
clindamycin
cyclophosphamide
cyclosporine
dantrolene
furosemide
Inhalation anesthetics

Local anesthetics
magnesium
quinidine

Opposing Effects
carbamazepine
corticosteroids
phenytoin

cases. Although these conditions do not necessarily lead to toxicity or overdose, they are listed in Box 11-5.

Anticholinesterase drugs such as neostigmine, pyridostigmine, and edrophonium are antidotes for nondepolarizing NMBDs such as vecuronium, rocuronium, and cistatricurium. Antichoinesterase drugs work by preventing the enzyme cholinesterase from breaking down ACh. This causes ACh to build up at the motor endplate, and it eventually displaces the nondepolarizing NMBD molecule, returning the nerve to its original state. However, succinylcholine is not reversed with acetylcholinesterase inhibitors because of its short duration of action and natural breakdown. Malignant hyperthermia, which is a dysmetabolic syndrome, (see General Anesthetics earlier in the chapter) can also occur with succinylcholine.

BOX 11-7   Classification of Nondepolarizing Neuromuscular Blocking Drugs

Intermediate-Acting Drugs
atracurium (Tracrium)
cisatracurium (Nimbex)
rocuronium (Zemuron)
vecuronium (Norcuron)

Long-Acting Drugs
pancuronium (Pavulon)

DOSAGES

Selected Neuromuscular Blocking Drugs

Drug	Pharmacologic Class	Usual Adult Dosage Range	Indications/ Uses
♦! rocuronium (Zemuron)	Nondepolarizing NMBD (intermediate-acting)	IV: 0.6-1.2 mg/ kg Continuous infusion: 0.8-12 mcg/ kg/minute	Intubation, mechanical ventilation
♦! succinylcholine (Anectine, Quelicin)	Depolarizing NMBD (short-acting)	IV: 0.3-1.1 mg/ kg IM: 3-4 mg/kg	Intubation

NMBD, neuromuscular blocking drug.

Interactions

Many drugs interact with NMBDs, which may lead to either synergistic or opposing effects. Aminoglycoside antibiotics, when given with an NMBD, can have additive effects. The tetracycline antibiotics can also produce neuromuscular blockade, possibly by chelation of calcium, and calcium channel blockers have also been shown to enhance neuromuscular blockade. Other notable drugs that interact with NMBDs are listed in Box 11-6.

Dosages

For dosage information of selected NMBDs, see the table on this page.

DRUG PROFILES

Neuromuscular blocking drugs are one of the most commonly used classes of drugs in the operating room. They are given primarily with general anesthetics to facilitate endotracheal intubation and to relax skeletal muscles during surgery. In addition to their use in the operating room, they are given in the ICU to paralyze mechanically ventilated patients. There are two basic types of NMBDs: depolarizing and nondepolarizing drugs. Nondepolarizing NMBDs are generally classified by their duration of action. Box 11-7 lists examples of currently used nondepolarizing drugs.

DEPOLARIZING NEUROMUSCULAR BLOCKING DRUGS
♦! **succinylcholine**
Succinylcholine is the only currently available drug in the *depolarizing* subclass of NMBDs. Succinylcholine (Anectine, Quelicin) has a structure similar to that of the parasympathetic neurotransmitter ACh. It stimulates the same neurons as ACh and produces the same physiologic responses initially. Compared to ACh, however, succinylcholine is metabolized more slowly. Because of this slower metabolism, succinylcholine subjects the motor endplate to ongoing depolarizing stimulation. Repolarization cannot occur. As long as sufficient succinylcholine concentrations are present, the muscle loses its ability to contract, and flaccid muscle paralysis results. Because of its quick onset of action, succinylcholine is most commonly used to facilitate endotracheal intubation. It is seldom used over long periods because of its tendency to cause muscular fasciculations. It is contraindicated in patients with personal or familial history of malignant hyperthermia, skeletal muscle myopathies,

and known hypersensitivity to the drug. It is available only in injectable form. For dosage information, see the table on the previous page.

Pharmacokinetics: Succinylcholine

Route	Onset of Action	Peak Plasma Concentration	Elimination Half-life	Duration of Action
IV	Rapid, less than 1 min	60 sec	Less than 1 min	4-6 min

NONDEPOLARIZING NEUROMUSCULAR BLOCKING DRUGS

Nondepolarizing NMBDs are commonly used to facilitate endotracheal intubation, reduce muscle contraction, and facilitate a variety of diagnostic procedures. They are often combined with anxiolytics or anesthetics. They may also be used to induce respiratory arrest in patients on mechanical ventilation.

◆!rocuronium

Rocuronium (Zemuron) is a rapid- to intermediate-acting nondepolarizing NMBD. It is used as an adjunct to general anesthesia to facilitate tracheal intubation and to provide skeletal muscle relaxation during surgery or mechanical ventilation. Use of rocuronium is contraindicated in cases of known drug allergy. It is available only in injectable form. For dosage information, see the table on the previous page.

Pharmacokinetics: Rocuronium

Route	Onset of Action	Peak Plasma Concentration	Elimination Half-life	Duration of Action
IV	1-2 min	4 min	50-144 min	30 min

QSEN

TEAMWORK AND COLLABORATION: PHARMACOKINETIC BRIDGE TO NURSING PRACTICE

With moderate (conscious or procedural) sedation or anesthesia, it is always important to understand the pharmacokinetic properties of the drug(s) used. For example, the intravenous form of midazolam has an onset of action of 1 to 5 minutes, a peak plasma effect of 20 to 60 minutes, an elimination half-life of 1 to 4 hours (time it takes for 50% of the drug to be excreted), and a duration of action of 2 to 6 hours. Therefore, if midazolam is used for moderate sedation, you will begin to see the sedating properties within 1 to 5 minutes and peak effects on the patient between 20 to 60 minutes. Since the drug's action only lasts for 2 to 6 hours, midazolam is an attractive option for use in outpatient procedures because of fast onset and short duration of action. Therefore, as noted with this drug's pharmacokinetic properties, you may then be able to predict the drug's onset of action, peak effect, and duration of action.

NURSING PROCESS

ASSESSMENT

It is important to note that *anesthetics* are not drugs that are typically given by the registered nurse unless the nurse is an anesthesia provider. Exceptions to this statement are orders for topical forms, such as oral swish-and-swallow solutions that may be used during chemotherapy and lidocaine patches for pain relief. Associated with each drug used for general and local anesthesia are some very broad as well as specific assessment parameters. First, for any form of anesthesia and during any of the phases of anesthesia, the major parameters to assess are airway, breathing, and circulation (ABCs). Include in your assessment questions regarding allergies and use of prescription as well as over-the-counter drugs, herbals, supplements, and social and/or illegal drugs.

Another important area to assess is the patient's use of alcohol and nicotine. Excessive use of alcohol may alter the patient's response to general anesthesia. If an individual has become tolerant to the effects of alcohol, he or she may typically be more tolerant to anesthetic medication. Also, if the patient has a history of alcohol abuse, withdrawal symptoms generally do not occur in the perioperative period. The critical timeframe for this type of patient will be when he or she has been without alcohol for a couple of days in the postoperative period and is no longer receiving sedation or analgesics. Perform a respiratory assessment (e.g., respiratory rate, rhythm, and depth; breath sounds; oxygen saturation level), especially if the patient has a history of smoking or is currently a smoker. The patient's history of smoking is important because nicotine has a paralyzing effect on the cilia within the respiratory tract. Once they are malfunctioning, these cilia cannot perform their main function of keeping foreign bodies out of the lungs and allowing mucus and secretions to be coughed up with ease. Malfunctioning of the cilia can potentially lead to atelectasis or pneumonia. Other objective data include weight and height, because these parameters are often used in the dosing of anesthesia. Other studies that may be ordered by the anesthesia provider and/or surgeon include an electrocardiogram, chest radiograph, and tests of renal function (e.g., BUN level, creatinine level, urinalysis with specific gravity) and hepatic function (e.g., total protein and albumin levels; bilirubin level; ALP, AST, and ALT levels). Additional laboratory tests may include Hgb, Hct, WBC with differential, and tests that indicate clotting abilities, such as PT-INR, aPTT, and platelet count. Also assess results for serum electrolytes, specifically potassium, sodium, chloride, phosphorus, magnesium, and calcium, because abnormalities may lead to further complications from the anesthesia. You must assess the results of a pregnancy test in females of childbearing age, if ordered, because of the possibility of teratogenic effects (adverse effects on the fetus) related to the anesthetic drug.

Neurologic assessment includes a thorough survey of the patient's mental status. Determine and document level of consciousness, alertness, and orientation to person, place, and time prior to the anesthesia. Additional neurologic assessment includes motor assessments, with left-right and upper-extremity versus lower-extremity comparisons of strength, reflexes, grasp, and ability to move on command. Sensory assessment focuses on the same anatomic areas, with comparisons of the response to various types of stimuli such as sharp, dull, soft, and cold versus warm. Swallowing ability and gag reflexes are also important to assess and document for baseline status and

CASE STUDY

Patient-Centered Care: Moderate (Conscious) Sedation

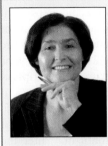 A 53-year-old woman is scheduled to have a colonoscopy this morning, and she is very anxious. The anesthesia provider has explained the moderate (conscious) sedation that is planned, but the patient says after the anesthetist leaves the room, "I'm so afraid of feeling it during the test. Why don't they just put me to sleep?"

1. How does moderate sedation differ from general anesthesia?

2. What is the nurse's best answer to the patient's question?

3. What is important for the nurse to assess before this procedure is performed?

The anesthesia provider prepares to administer morphine and midazolam (Versed) before the procedure.

4. Explain the purpose of these two medications during moderate sedation. How are the dosages adjusted when these are given together?

For answers, see *http://evolve.elsevier.Lilley.*

comparisons. When these motor, sensory, and cognitive parameters are within normal limits, there is proof of an intact neurologic system.

One very significant reaction to assess for in patients receiving *general anesthesia* is that of malignant hyperthermia. This is a rapid progression of hyperthermia that may be fatal if not promptly recognized and aggressively treated. The tendency is inherited, so questions about related signs and symptoms in the family's and patient's medical histories are important to document and report. A familial history of malignant hyperthermia would put the patient at risk. Signs and symptoms of malignant hyperthermia include a rapid rise in body temperature, tachycardia, tachypnea, muscle rigidity, cyanosis, irregular heartbeat, mottling of the skin, diaphoresis (profuse sweating), and an unstable blood pressure. If there is no documented problem with general anesthesia or if the patient is undergoing general anesthesia for the first time, perform an astute and careful examination of all medical and medication histories. With any type of anesthesia, it is often very slight changes in vital signs, other vital parameters, and laboratory test results that may provide nursing and other health care providers with a possible clue to the patient's reaction to anesthesia. Note that malignant hyperthermia occurs during the anesthesia process and in the surgical suite; nevertheless, close observation after anesthesia is still important and much needed. Intravenously administered anesthetic drugs are usually combined with adjuvant drugs (given at the same time) such as sedative-hypnotics, antianxiety drugs, opioid and nonopioid analgesics, antiemetics, and anticholinergics. These drugs are used to decrease some of the undesirable after-effects of inhaled anesthetics. If they are used, perform a complete assessment for each of the drugs, including obtaining a medical history and medication profile. Liver and kidney function studies are important in

these patients as well, so that any risks of toxicity and complications can be anticipated.

For patients about to undergo anesthesia with *neuromuscular blocking drugs (NMBDs)*, perform a complete head-to-toe assessment with a thorough medical and medication history. Which specific drug is being used and whether it is *depolarizing* or *nondepolarizing* will guide your assessment, because of the action of NMBDs on the patient's neuromuscular functioning (see pharmacology discussion). Assess all cautions, contraindications, and drug interactions. Another concern with the use of these drugs is that they are associated with an increase in intraocular pressure and intracranial pressure. Therefore, these anesthetic drugs should not be used or used with extreme caution (close monitoring of these pressures) in patients with glaucoma or closed head injuries.

Complete a thorough respiratory assessment in patients receiving NMBDs because of the effect of these drugs on the respiratory system. In particular, these drugs have a paralyzing effect on the muscles used for breathing and—for this very reason—are used to facilitate intubation for mechanical ventilation. Paralysis of respiratory muscles allows patient relaxation to the point where the patient will not fight against the breaths delivered by the ventilator. Also indicated with the use of NMBDs is careful assessment of serum electrolyte levels, specifically potassium and magnesium levels. Imbalances in these electrolytes may lead to increased action of the NMBD with exacerbation of the drug's actions and toxic effects. Allergic reactions to these drugs are most commonly characterized by rash, fever, respiratory distress, and pruritus. Drug interactions with herbal products are outlined in the following Safety: Herbal Therapies and Dietary Supplements box. For more specific information on the differences between depolarizing and nondepolarizing NMBDs, see the Drug Profiles section of this chapter.

SAFETY: HERBAL THERAPIES AND DIETARY SUPPLEMENTS

QSEN

Possible Effects of Herbal Products When Combined with Anesthetics

Feverfew: Migraine headaches, insomnia, anxiety, joint stiffness, increased risk for bleeding

Garlic: Changes in blood pressure, risk for increased bleeding

Ginger: Sedating effects; risk for bleeding, especially if taken with either aspirin or ginkgo

Ginseng: Irritability and insomnia, risk for cardiac adverse effects

Kava: Sedating effects, potential liver toxicity, risk for additive effects with medications

St. John's Wort: Sedation, blood pressure changes

For more information, visit *www.aana.com*, *www.anesthesiapatient safety.com*, *www.herbalgram.com*, and *http://nccam.NIH.gov.*

With the use of *conscious or moderate sedation,* as with any anesthesia technique, assessment for allergies, cautions, contraindications, and drug interactions is important. Because moderate sedation is commonly used across the lifespan, closely assess organ function and note diseases or conditions that could lead to excessive levels of the drug in the body, such as liver or kidney impairment. See Chapters 10 and 12 for more information about the assessment associated with the use of opioids and sedative-hypnotics/CNS depressants.

Use of *spinal anesthesia* requires thorough assessment with an emphasis on the ABCs, respiratory function, and vital signs, specifically blood pressure. Baseline respirations with attention to rate, rhythm, depth, and breath sounds are important to note, as are oxygen saturation levels obtained via pulse oximetry. Because of possible problems with vasodilatation from the spinal anesthetic, document baseline blood pressure levels and pulse rate. Record history of previous reactions to this form of anesthesia, allergies, and a listing of all medications, and report any abnormal reactions to the anesthesia provider and surgeon. Neurologic assessment with notation of sensory and motor intactness in the lower extremities, as well as documentation of any abnormalities, is important. The use of epidural anesthesia requires special attention to overall hemostasis through monitoring of vital signs and oxygen saturation levels. Assess baseline sensory and motor function in the extremities, and document an intact neurologic system (see Implementation for a more detailed discussion). Spinal headaches may occur with either spinal anesthesia or epidural injections, and thus baseline assessment for the presence of headaches is important.

Local-topical anesthetics, such as *lidocaine,* used for either infiltration or nerve block anesthesia may be administered with or without a vasoconstrictor (e.g., epinephrine). The vasoconstrictors are used to help confine the local anesthetic to the injected area, prevent systemic absorption of the anesthetic, and reduce bleeding. If there is systemic absorption of the vasoconstrictor into the bloodstream, the patient's blood pressure could elevate to life-threatening levels, especially in patients who are at high risk (e.g., those with underlying arterial disease). Therefore, review the patient's medical history to assess for any preexisting illnesses, such as vascular disease, aneurysms, or hypertension, because these may be contraindications to the use of the vasoconstrictor with the anesthetic. In addition, with these local anesthetics, assess for allergies to the drug as well as baseline vital signs. Also assess for possible drug interactions, and note prescription medications, herbal products, supplements, and over-the-counter medications. In summary, it is important with any type of anesthesia to assess the patient's level of homeostasis prior to actual administration of the drug. This assessment may include taking vital signs as well as checking the ABCs. Other parameters of interest may be oxygen saturation levels measured by pulse oximetry, cardiovascular and respiratory function, and neurologic function.

NURSING DIAGNOSES

1. Impaired gas exchange related to the general anesthetic's CNS depressant effect with altered respiratory rate and effort (decreased rate, decreased depth)
2. Decreased cardiac output related to the systemic effects of anesthesia
3. Acute pain related to the adverse effect of spinal headache from epidural anesthesia

4. Deficient knowledge related to lack of information about anesthesia
5. Risk for injury related to the impact of any form of anesthesia on the CNS (e.g., CNS depression, decreased sensorium)

PLANNING: OUTCOME IDENTIFICATION

1. Patient states measures to increase respiratory expansion through coughing, deep breathing, turning, and ambulating (when allowed).
2. Patient remains well hydrated with increase in fluids and remains ambulating to help increase circulation and minimize complications, unless contraindicated.
3. Patient states measures to help minimize and/or prevent acute pain from possible complication of spinal headache with bed rest, hydration, and following postanesthesia/postepidural orders for up to 24 to 48 hours after procedure.
4. Patient experiences maximal effects of anesthesia as noted by following preanesthesia orders, such as remaining NPO, taking medications only as prescribed, as well as experiencing minimal adverse effects from an adequate knowledge about the postanesthesia period and ways to minimize problems (see all measures listed in outcome criteria 1 to 3 and 5).
5. Patient remains free from injury and/or falls by asking for assistance while ambulating or having assistance if at home and recovering alone as well as taking medications only as prescribed, sitting up for brief periods prior to ambulating, forcing fluids, and resuming adequate nutritional intake during the postanesthesia period.

IMPLEMENTATION

Regardless of the type of *anesthesia* used, one of the most important nursing considerations during the preanesthesia, intraanesthesia, and postanesthesia periods is close and frequent observation of all body systems. Begin with a focus on the ABCs of nursing care, vital signs, and oxygen saturation levels as measured by pulse oximetry as well as by the clinical presentation of the patient. Remember that the way a patient looks is very important at any point in time! Document the observations from these interventions, and repeat the interventions as needed, depending on the patient's status and in keeping with the standard of care for the type of anesthesia. Monitor vital signs frequently and as needed, and based on the patient's condition, including assessing the fifth vital sign of pain (see discussion later in this section and in Chapter 10).

For patients undergoing *general anesthesia,* assessing the patient's temperature is especially important because of the risk for malignant hyperthermia, and close monitoring is required if malignant hyperthermia occurred during the anesthesia process. This sudden elevation in the patient's body temperature (e.g., higher than 104° F [40° C]) not only requires critical care during and immediately after anesthesia but also calls for close monitoring even during regular postoperative care (see earlier discussion). When intravenous, inhaled, or other forms of anesthesia are used, resuscitative equipment and medications, including opioid antidotes, are readily available in the surgical and postsurgical areas in case of cardiorespiratory distress or arrest. The anesthesia provider keeps control of the anesthetic drug, and he or she is well prepared for any emergency—as is the entire group of individuals in the surgical suite and postanesthesia recovery area. Continual monitoring of the status of breath sounds is an important intervention, because hypoventilation may be a complication of general and other forms of anesthesia. Oxygen is administered after a patient has received general and/or other forms of anesthesia to compensate for the respiratory depression that may have occurred during the anesthesia and surgical process. Because oxygen is a drug, a doctor's order is needed for its administration. Continuous monitoring of oxygen saturation levels is therefore an important intervention. In addition, hypotension and orthostatic hypotension are possible problems after anesthesia, so postural blood pressure measurements (supine and standing), in addition to regular blood pressure monitoring, may be needed. Additional nursing interventions include monitoring of neurologic parameters such as reflexes, response to commands, level of consciousness or sedation, and pupil reaction to light. Monitor for changes in sensation and movement in the extremities, distal pulses, temperature, and color when nerve blocks and spinal anesthesia are used, because it is important to confirm that areas distal to the anesthetic site have remained intact.

If the patient requires pain management once the anesthesia has been terminated, remember that the anesthetic and any adjuvant drugs used continue to have an effect on the patient until the period of the drugs' action has passed. Therefore, administer sedative-hypnotics, opioids, nonopioids, and other CNS depressants for pain relief cautiously and *only* with close monitoring of vital signs. If the patient has received some of these medications during postanesthesia, document dosages of drugs used, and then pass them on during a report when the patient is transferred to another unit. Additional orders are usually provided by the physician/surgeon or anesthesia provider regarding doses of analgesics to administer once the patient has been transferred or if discharged to home. If such orders have not been provided, however, and the patient is experiencing pain, contact the appropriate prescriber. The concern here is that the patient may receive either too much or not enough analgesic.

Patients who receive *NMBDs* as part of an induction process for mechanical ventilation need to be monitored closely during and after initiation of mechanical ventilation. Patients receiving NMBDs and who are awake may need to receive other medications for sedation and/or pain. These patients are in intensive care or critical care units, and many protocols are provided regarding interventions after the intubation. These include measurement of vital signs and determination of neurologic status, including sensation and hand grasp strength. When mechanical ventilation is used, educate patients and family members about the purpose of the drug-induced paralysis while receiving mechanical ventilation (e.g., to prevent the patient from fighting against the ventilation provided by the machine, resisting the effects of the mechanical ventilatory assistance and possibly leading to hypoventilation). Inform the family and remember in the nursing care of these patients that they can still hear the spoken word. Knowing what to expect is key to helping decrease fear and anxiety—for both the patient and those visiting the patient.

Patients undergoing *moderate sedation* as the method of anesthesia should receive patient education before the procedure. As noted earlier in the chapter, recovery from this type of anesthesia is more rapid, and the safety profile is better than that of general anesthesia with its inherent cardiorespiratory risks. As with general anesthesia, however, monitor the ABCs of care, vital signs, pulse oximetry oxygen saturation levels, and level of consciousness or sedation. Box 11-8 contains more information on moderate sedation.

With *spinal anesthesia,* nursing interventions need to include constant monitoring for a return of sensation and motor activity below the anesthetic insertion site. Because of the risk that the anesthetic drug may move upward in the spinal cord and breathing may be affected, continually monitor respiratory and breathing status. In addition, because positioning is important to the movement of the anesthetic drug, keep the head of the bed elevated. Remember, though, that this complication is usually identified and treated by the anesthesia provider, and patients will not return to their rooms on a nursing unit until all respiratory risks are identified and managed appropriately. Another major area of concern with spinal anesthesia is the risk for a sudden decrease in blood pressure. This drop in blood pressure is secondary to vasodilation caused by the anesthetic block to the sympathetic vasomotor nerves. Vital signs and oxygen saturation levels should return to normal before the patient is transferred out of postanesthesia care; however, continue to monitor these vital signs frequently after transfer.

Another adverse reaction to *neuraxial or central anesthesia* is the occurrence of spinal headaches. These may occur with both intrathecal and epidural injections but are actually more frequent with the latter. Because intrathecal spinal needle designs have been technologically improved, the occurrence of spinal headaches is rare. Larger-bore needles are used to deliver epidural anesthetics, however, and these are more likely to give rise to spinal headache if they are inadvertently passed through the dura mater (the covering of the spinal cord). Keep the patient hydrated and on bed rest as recommended by the anesthesia provider. Box 11-9 offers more information about these headaches and their treatment.

The use of *epidural anesthesia* (also called *regional anesthesia* in some textbooks) does not pose the same risk of respiratory complications as general anesthesia; however, monitoring is still needed to confirm overall homeostasis. You must measure vital signs and pulse oximetry to determine oxygen saturation levels. In addition, patients undergoing this form of anesthesia require monitoring for the return of motor function and tactile sensation. Check the patient frequently for the return of sensation bilaterally along the dermatome (area of the skin innervated by specific segments of the spinal cord); such monitoring is important to ensure patient safety as well as to maximize comfort.

BOX 11-8 Moderate or Conscious Sedation: What to Expect and Questions to Ask

1. What questions do the patient or caregiver need to ask about the technique of moderate or conscious sedation?
   - Who will be providing this type of anesthesia?
   - Who will be monitoring me or my loved one?
   - Will there be constant monitoring of blood pressure, pulse rate, respiratory rate, and temperature?
   - Will there be emergency equipment in the room, in case of need?
   - Are the personnel qualified to administer these drugs? To administer advanced cardiac life support?
   - What do I need to know about care at home? Will I need help? Can I drive after having the procedure?
2. What are the adverse effects of moderate or conscious sedation?
   - Brief periods of amnesia (loss of memory)
   - Headache
   - Hangover feeling
   - Nausea and vomiting
3. What is to be expected immediately following the procedure?
   - Frequent monitoring
   - Written postoperative instructions and care
   - If the patient is of driving age, no driving for at least 24 hours after undergoing moderate sedation
   - A follow-up contact by phone to check on the patient
4. Who administers the conscious sedation?
   - Moderate or conscious sedation is safe when administered by qualified providers. Anesthesia providers, other physicians, dentists, and oral surgeons are qualified to administer conscious sedation.

5. Which procedures generally require moderate sedation?
   - Breast biopsy
   - Vasectomy
   - Minor foot surgery
   - Minor bone fracture repair
   - Plastic or reconstructive surgery
   - Dental prosthetic or reconstructive surgery
   - Endoscopy (such as diagnostic studies and treatment of stomach, colon, and bladder cancer)
6. What are the overall benefits of this type of anesthesia?
   - It is a safe and effective option for patients undergoing minor surgeries or diagnostic procedures.
   - It allows patients to recover quickly and resume normal activities in a relatively short period of time.
7. Are there any concerns about daily medications or herbals if undergoing conscious sedation?
   - As with any form of anesthesia, being open and honest with the anesthesia provider is of significant importance to patient safety.
   - Be sure to follow instructions closely regarding the intake of all medications including herbals, food, or liquids before anesthesia as such substances may react negatively with the drugs being administered.
   - Inquire about any brochures or written pamphlets such as the AANA brochure entitled "Before anesthesia: Your active role makes a difference."

Data from Council for Public Interest in Anesthesia: *Conscious sedation: What patients should expect.* Patient Pamphlet. Available at *www.aana.com.* Accessed March 31, 2015. Publication date unavailable.

BOX 11-9 Spinal Headaches: A Brief Look at a Terrible Pain!

Why do spinal headaches occur? As a result of penetration into and through the dura mater of the spinal cord (the covering of the spinal cord), a leakage of cerebrospinal fluid occurs from the insertion site. If enough of the spinal fluid leaks out, a spinal headache results. These headaches are more likely to be associated with epidural anesthesia than with intrathecal anesthesia because of the larger needles used with epidurals.

What are the symptoms of a spinal headache? Patients say that these headaches are worse than any other type! They are more severe when the patient is in an upright position and improve upon lying down. They may occur up to 5 days after the procedure and may be prevented with bed rest after the epidural procedure.

How are spinal headaches treated? Adequate hydration using intravenous fluids is often tried to help increase cerebral spinal fluid pressure. Other recommendations include the drinking of a beverage high in caffeine and strict bed rest for 24 to 48 hours. If the headaches are intolerable, however, the anesthesia provider may create a "blood patch" to help close up or seal the leak. This requires insertion of a needle into the same space or right next to the area that was injected with the anesthesia. A small amount of blood is then taken from the patient and injected into the epidural space. The blood clots and forms a seal over the hole that caused the leak, and the headache is relieved.

Data from American Association of Nurse Anesthetists: Conscious sedation: what patients should expect, 2005, available at *www.aana.com;* Bezov D, Ashina S, Lipton R: Post-dural puncture headache: part II—prevention, management, and prognosis, *Headache* 50(9):1482-1498, 2010.

Assess touch sensation through hand pressure or a gentle pinch of the skin. You need to know the level at which the epidural anesthesia was given to monitor properly for return of sensation. This monitoring process generally occurs in a postanesthesia care unit, and the patient is not returned to a regular nursing unit until all sensation and/or voluntary movement of the lower extremities is regained.

With regard to the use of *topical or local anesthetics* (e.g., *lidocaine* with or without epinephrine), solutions that are not clear and appear cloudy or discolored are not to be used. Some anesthesia providers mix the solution with sodium bicarbonate to minimize local pain during infiltration, but this also causes a more rapid onset of action and a longer duration of sensory analgesia. If an anesthetic ointment or cream is used, the nurse will thoroughly cleanse and dry the area to be anesthetized before applying the drug. If a topical or local anesthetic is being used in the nose or throat, remember that it may cause paralysis and/or numbness of the structures of the upper respiratory tract, which can lead to aspiration. If the patient receives a solution form of anesthetic, exact amounts of the drug are used and at the exact dosing times or intervals. Local anesthetics are not to be swallowed unless the prescriber has so instructed. Should this occur, closely observe the patient, check for the gag reflex, and expect to withhold food or drink until the patient's sensation and/or gag reflex has returned.

Once the patient has recovered from the anesthesia and procedure and is ready for discharge, complete your patient teaching. Focus the patient education on the patient's needs and how these needs can be met at home. Home health care and/or rehabilitation services may be indicated, and arrangements should be made before the patient is discharged. If additional care or resources are needed at home (e.g., for a patient who lives alone), these arrangements should be completed in a timely fashion. Some examples of procedures for which help might be needed are wound care, dressing changes, surgical site care, drawing of blood for laboratory studies, and administration of various medications through the intravenous, intramuscular, or subcutaneous route. Some patients may also need assistance with taking oral medications at home. Pain management requires thorough and individualized patient teaching and also includes any necessary education for patients who will require home health care. See Chapter 10 for more information on analgesics. Provide simple instructions using age-appropriate teaching strategies (see Chapter 6). Sharing of information about community resources is also important, especially for patients who need transportation, assistance with meals, housekeeping during recovery, and/or the services of additional health care providers (e.g., physical therapists, occupational therapists) in the home setting. Some of these community resources may be agencies that are supported by city or state social service programs. Meals on Wheels, senior citizen support groups, and church-sponsored groups are just a few examples of important resource groups. Many of these resources are free or have income-based fees. Additional suggestions regarding patient education are provided in Patient-Centered Care: Patient Teaching.

EVALUATION

The therapeutic effects of any *general or local anesthesia* include the following: loss of consciousness and reflexes during general anesthesia and loss of sensation to a particular area during local anesthesia (e.g., loss of sensation to the eye during corneal transplantation). Constantly monitor the patient who has undergone general anesthesia for the occurrence of adverse effects of the anesthesia. These may include myocardial depression, convulsions, respiratory depression, allergic rhinitis, and decreased renal or liver function. Constantly monitor patients who have received a local anesthetic for the occurrence of adverse effects, including bradycardia, myocardial depression, hypotension, and dysrhythmias. In addition, as mentioned earlier in this chapter, significant overdoses of local anesthetic drugs or direct injection into a blood vessel may result in cardiovascular collapse or cardiac or respiratory depression. For those receiving spinal anesthesia, therapeutic effects include loss of sensation below the area of administration, and adverse effects include hypotension, hypoventilation, urinary retention, the possibility of a prolonged period of decreased sensation or motor ability, and infection at the site. With *epidural or intrathecal anesthesia,* therapeutic effects are similar and adverse effects include loss of motor function or sensation below the area of administration. Spinal headaches may occur with epidural or spinal anesthesia. *Moderate sedation* provides the therapeutic effect of a decreased sensorium but without the complications of general anesthesia; however, there are CNS depressant effects associated with the drugs used.

QSEN ## PATIENT-CENTERED CARE: PATIENT TEACHING

- Whenever general anesthesia is used, emphasize the prescriber's recommendations/orders about whether any medications should be discontinued or tapered before anesthetic administration.
- Make sure information about the anesthetic, route of administration, adverse effects, and special precautions is included in preprocedure and surgical education.
- Openly discuss with the patient all fears and anxieties about anesthesia and related procedures/surgery.
- Share with the patient and family instructions about the postanesthesia process and the need for close monitoring of vital signs, breath sounds, and neurologic intactness. Patients should expect frequent turning, coughing, and deep breathing to prevent atelectasis or pneumonia.
- Encourage patients to ambulate with assistance as needed and as ordered. Mobility helps increase circulation and improve ventilation to the alveoli of the lungs; consequently, circulation to the legs will be improved (which helps to prevent stasis of blood and possible blood clot formation in the leg veins). Assistance is needed to prevent falls or injury until recovery from the anesthetic.
- Encourage the patient to request pain medication, if needed, before pain becomes moderate to severe. Inform the patient that, even though anesthesia has been administered, there

may still be discomfort or pain from the procedure or surgery. The anesthesia will wear off, and adequate analgesia will be needed. Ask the patient to rate his or her pain on a scale of 0 to 10, with 0 being no pain and 10 being the worst possible pain. See Chapter 10 for more information on pain assessment and its management.
- Explain the rationale for any other treatments or procedures related to the anesthesia (e.g., epidural catheter placement; delivery of oxygen; administration of a gas; use of various tubes, catheters, or intravenous lines). Adequate patient education will help ease fears and anxieties and help in preventing adverse effects or complications.
- For a patient with diminished sensorium, the bed side rails need to be placed in the up position and a call button at the bedside. These actions are critical to patient safety. Note that bed alarms may be used. Everyone involved in the postanesthesia and postsurgical care (e.g., family members) must be educated about these safety measures.
- With local anesthesia, the patient should understand the purpose and action of the local anesthetic as well as adverse effects.
- Inform a patient receiving spinal anesthesia about the need for frequent assessments, measurement of vital signs, and system assessments during and after the procedure.

KEY POINTS

- Anesthesia is the loss of the ability to feel pain resulting from the administration of an anesthetic drug. General anesthesia is a drug-induced state in which the nerve impulses of the CNS are altered to reduce pain and other sensations throughout the entire body and normally involves complete loss of consciousness and respiratory drive depression.
- General anesthetics are drugs that induce general anesthesia, including the administration of specific parenteral anesthetics. Inhalational anesthetic drugs are also general anesthetics and include volatile liquids or gases.
- Local anesthetics are used to induce a state in which peripheral or spinal nerve impulses are altered to reduce or eliminate pain and other sensations. Spinal anesthesia, or regional anesthesia, is a form of local anesthesia.
- Conscious or moderate sedation is a form of general anesthesia resulting in partial or complete loss of consciousness but without reducing normal respiratory drive.

- Adjunct anesthetics are drugs that assist with the induction of general anesthesia and include neuromuscular blocking drugs (NMBDs), sedative-hypnotics, and/or anxiolytics and antiemetics.
- Nondepolarizing NMBDs are used as an adjunct to general anesthesia to provide skeletal muscle relaxation during surgery and/or mechanical ventilation.
- Nursing assessment is very important to patient safety during and after all forms of anesthesia. With general anesthesia, however, one major problem to be concerned with is that of malignant hyperthermia, which may be fatal if not promptly recognized and aggressively treated. Signs and symptoms include rapid rise in body temperature, increased pulse rate (tachycardia)/respiratory rate (tachypnea), muscle rigidity, and unstable blood pressure.

NCLEX® EXAMINATION REVIEW QUESTIONS

1. The physician has requested "lidocaine *with* epinephrine." The nurse recognizes that the most important reason for adding epinephrine is that it
   a. helps to calm the patient before the procedure.
   b. minimizes the risk for an allergic reaction.
   c. enhances the effect of the local lidocaine.
   d. reduces bleeding in the surgical area.

2. The surgical nurse is reviewing operative cases scheduled for the day. Which of these patients is more prone to complications from general anesthesia?
   a. A 79-year-old woman who is about to have hip replacement surgery
   b. A 49-year-old male athlete who quit heavy smoking 12 years ago
   c. A 30-year-old woman who is in perfect health but has never had anesthesia
   d. A 50-year-old woman scheduled for outpatient laser surgery for vision correction

3. Which nursing diagnosis is possible for a patient who is now recovering after having been under general anesthesia for 3 to 4 hours during surgery?
   a. Impaired urinary elimination related to the use of vasopressors as anesthetics
   b. Increased cardiac output related to the effects of general anesthesia
   c. Risk for falls related to decreased sensorium for 2 to 4 days postoperatively
   d. Impaired gas exchange due to the CNS depressant effect of general anesthesia

4. A patient is recovering from general anesthesia. What is the nurse's main concern during the immediate postoperative period?
   a. Airway
   b. Pupillary reflexes
   c. Return of sensations
   d. Level of consciousness

5. A patient is about to undergo cardioversion, and the nurse is reviewing the procedure and explaining moderate sedation with propofol. The patient asks, "I am afraid of feeling it when they shock me." What is the nurse's best response?
   a. "You won't receive enough of a shock to feel anything."
   b. "You will feel the shock but you won't remember any of the pain."
   c. "These medications will help ease any pain during the procedure, and many patients often report having no recollection of the procedure."
   d. "They will give you enough pain medication to prevent you from feeling it."

6. The nurse is administering an NMBD to a patient during a surgical procedure. Number the following phases of muscle paralysis in the order in which the patient will experience them. (Number 1 is the first step.)
   a. Paralysis of intercostals and diaphragm muscles
   b. Muscle weakness
   c. Paralysis of muscles of the limbs, neck, and trunk
   d. Paralysis of small rapidly moving muscles (fingers, eye)

7. During a patient's recovery from a lengthy surgery, the nurse monitors for signs of malignant hyperthermia. In addition to a rapid rise in body temperature, which assessment findings would indicate the possible presence of this condition? *(Select all that apply.)*
   a. Respiratory depression
   b. Tachypnea
   c. Tachycardia
   d. Seizure activity
   e. Muscle rigidity

8. A patient will be receiving diazepam (Valium), 2 mg, IV push as part of preprocedure sedation. The medication is available in an injectable solution of 5 mg/mL. How many milliliters will the nurse give for this dose?

1. d, 2. a, 3. d, 4. a, 5. c, 6. a = 4, b = 1, c = 3, d = 2, 7. b, c, e. 8. 0.4 mL.

CRITICAL THINKING AND PRIORITIZATION QUESTIONS

1. The nurse is assessing a patient who had hip replacement surgery 2 hours earlier and has just arrived to the orthopedic unit from the PACU. The certified nursing assistant reports that the patient's temperature is 104.8° F (40.4° C). The nurse notes that the PACU nurse reported that the patient's temperature was 98.9° F (37.2° C). Another nurse comments that the patient must be developing an infection from the hip replacement. What is the nurse's priority action at this time?

2. The nurse is assessing a patient who is receiving mechanical ventilation because of respiratory problems. The nurse tells the patient's wife that he is receiving medication to keep him relaxed and allow the ventilator to work. The patient's wife asks the nurse, "Is he awake? Can he hear me?" What is the nurse's best answer?

For answers, see *http://evolve.elsevier.com/Lilley.*

ⓔ EVOLVE WEBSITE

http://evolve.elsevier.com/Lilley
- Animations
- Answer Keys for Textbook Case Studies and Textbook Critical Thinking and Prioritization Questions
- Content Updates
- Key Points
- Review Questions
- Student Case Studies

Central Nervous System Depressants and Muscle Relaxants

ⓔ http://evolve.elsevier.com/Lilley

OBJECTIVES

When you reach the end of this chapter, you will be able to do the following:

1. Briefly describe the functions of the central nervous system.
2. Contrast the effects of central nervous system depressant drugs and central nervous system stimulant drugs (see Chapter 13) as relates to their basic actions.
3. Define the terms *hypnotic, rapid eye movement, rapid eye movement sleep interference, rapid eye movement rebound, sedative, sedative-hypnotic, sleep,* and *therapeutic index.*
4. Briefly discuss the problem of sleep disorders.
5. Identify the specific drugs within each of the following categories of central nervous system depressant drugs: benzodiazepines, nonbenzodiazepines, muscle relaxants, and miscellaneous drugs.
6. Contrast the mechanism of action, indications, adverse effects, toxic effects, cautions, contraindications, dosage forms, routes of administration, and drug interactions of the following medications: benzodiazepines, nonbenzodiazepines, muscle relaxants, and miscellaneous drugs.
7. Discuss the nursing process as it relates to the nursing care of a patient receiving any central nervous system depressants and/or muscle relaxant.
8. Develop a thorough nursing care plan related to the use of pharmacologic and nonpharmacologic approaches to the treatment of sleep disorders.

DRUG PROFILES

♦ **baclofen, p. 197**
♦ **cyclobenzaprine, p. 197**
diazepam, p. 193
eszopiclone, p. 193
❗**midazolam, p. 193**

pentobarbital, p. 195
phenobarbital, p. 196
ramelteon, p. 193
temazepam, p. 193

♦ **zaleplon, p. 194**
♦ **zolpidem, p. 194**

_____
♦ = *Key drug*
❗ = *High-alert drug*

KEY TERMS

Barbiturates A class of drugs used to induce sedation; chemical derivatives of barbituric acid. (p. 194)

Benzodiazepines A chemical category of drugs most frequently prescribed as anxiolytic drugs and less frequently as sedative-hypnotic agents. (p. 190)

Gamma-aminobutyric acid (GABA) The primary inhibitory neurotransmitter found in the brain. A key compound affected by sedative, anxiolytic, psychotropic, and muscle-relaxing medications. (p. 191)

Hypnotics Drugs that, when given at low to moderate dosages, calm or soothe the central nervous system (CNS) without inducing sleep but when given at high dosages cause sleep. (p. 190)

Non–rapid eye movement (non-REM) sleep The largest portion of the sleep cycle. It has four stages and precedes REM sleep. (p. 190)

Rapid eye movement (REM) sleep One of the stages of the sleep cycle. Some of the characteristics of REM sleep are rapid movement of the eyes, vivid dreams, and irregular breathing. (p. 190)

REM interference A drug-induced reduction of REM sleep time. (p. 190)

REM rebound Excessive REM sleep following discontinuation of a sleep-altering drug. (p. 190)

Sedatives Drugs that have an inhibitory effect on the CNS to the degree that they reduce nervousness, excitability, and irritability without causing sleep. (p. 190)

Sedative-hypnotics Drugs that can act in the body either as sedatives or as hypnotics. (p. 190)

Sleep A transient, reversible, and periodic state of rest in which there is a decrease in physical activity and consciousness. (p. 190)

Sleep architecture The structure of the various elements involved in the sleep cycle, including normal and abnormal patterns of sleep. (p. 190)

Therapeutic index The ratio between the toxic and therapeutic concentrations of a drug. If the index is low, the difference between the therapeutic and toxic drug concentrations is small, and use of the drug is more hazardous. (p. 194)

OVERVIEW

Sedatives and *hypnotics* are drugs that have a calming effect or that depress the central nervous system (CNS). A drug is classified as either a sedative or a hypnotic drug depending on the degree to which it inhibits the transmission of nerve impulses to the CNS. Sedatives reduce nervousness, excitability, and irritability without causing sleep, but a sedative can become a hypnotic if it is given in large enough doses. Hypnotics cause sleep and have a much more potent effect on the CNS than do sedatives. Many drugs can act as either a sedative or a hypnotic, depending on dose and patient responsiveness, and for this reason are called sedative-hypnotics. Sedative-hypnotics can be classified chemically into three main groups: barbiturates, benzodiazepines, and miscellaneous drugs.

PHYSIOLOGY OF SLEEP

Sleep is defined as a transient, reversible, and periodic state of rest in which there is a decrease in physical activity and consciousness. Normal sleep is cyclic and repetitive, and a person's responses to sensory stimuli are markedly reduced during sleep. During our waking hours, the body is constantly bombarded with stimuli provoking the senses of sight, hearing, touch, smell, and taste. Involuntary and voluntary movements or functions are elicited, but stimuli no longer are part of our awareness during sleep. Sleep research involves study of the patterns of sleep, or what is sometimes referred to as sleep architecture. The architecture of sleep consists of two basic elements that occur cyclically: rapid eye movement (REM) sleep and non–rapid eye movement (non-REM) sleep. The normal cyclic progression of the stages of sleep is summarized in Table 12-1. Various sedative-hypnotic drugs affect different stages of the normal sleep pattern. Prolonged sedative-hypnotic use may reduce the cumulative amount of REM sleep; this is known as REM interference. This can result in daytime fatigue, because REM sleep provides a certain component of the "restfulness" of

sleep. Upon discontinuance of a sedative-hypnotic drug, REM rebound can occur in which the patient has an abnormally large amount of REM sleep, often leading to frequent and vivid dreams. Abuse and misuse of sedative-hypnotic drugs is common and is discussed in Chapter 17.

> ### PATIENT-CENTERED CARE: CULTURAL IMPLICATIONS   QSEN
>
> #### Understanding Your Patient's Sleep Needs
>
> - When questioning your patient about his or her usual sleep patterns and habits, always consider cultural influences on the promotion of sleep.
> - Collect a thorough health, medication, and diet history to identify food, spices and/or supplements or herbal practices used to manage common everyday problems, such as insomnia.
> - Asians, Pacific Islanders, Hispanics, and African Americans have a high incidence of lactose intolerance, so use of warm milk at bedtime to help with sleep may lead to GI distress, abdominal cramping, and bloating. Lactose-free milk may be used.
> - Some Asian Americans believe in the yin and the yang and may practice meditation, herbology, nutritional interventions, and acupuncture for sleep.
> - Chinese patients have been found to require lower doses of the drug class of benzodiazepines including diazepam (Valium) and alprazolam (Xanax).
> - Some Hispanics believe that maintaining a balance in diet and physical activity are methods for preventing evil or poor health. Nondrug therapies and/or home remedies of vegetables and herbs may be used for sleep and other health issues.
> - Jewish Americans may tend to be less accepting of therapeutic touch as compared to some cultures. Nurses must be sensitive to this and find alternatives to massage.

BENZODIAZEPINES AND MISCELLANEOUS HYPNOTIC DRUGS

Historically, benzodiazepines were the most commonly prescribed sedative-hypnotic drugs; however, the nonbenzodiazepine drugs are now more frequently prescribed. Other drugs commonly used for sleep include diphenhydramine (see

TABLE 12-1 **Stages of Sleep**		
Stage	**Characteristics**	**Average Percentage of Sleep Time in Stages (for Young Adult)**
Non-REM Sleep		
1	Dozing or feelings of drifting off to sleep; person can be easily awakened; slow, side-to-side eye movements; insomniacs have longer stage 1 periods than normal.	2%-5%
2	Sleep deepening and a higher arousal threshold being required to awaken the patient.	45%-55%
3	Deep sleep; difficult to wake person; respiratory rates, pulse, and blood pressure may decrease; stages 3 and 4 often combined and referred to as "delta sleep" or "slow-wave sleep"; delta sleep associated with the highest arousal threshold.	3%-8%
4	Very difficult to wake person; person may be very groggy if awakened; dreaming occurs, especially about daily events; sleepwalking or bedwetting may occur.	10%-15%
REM Sleep		
	REMs occur; vivid dreams occur; breathing may be irregular.	25%-33%

NOTE: Four to five cycles are completed during normal sleep for adults. NREM sleep constitutes about the first third of the night and REM sleep is more prominent during the last third of the night.
Modified from Urden LD, Stacy KM, Lough ME: *Priorities in critical care nursing*, ed 6, St Louis, 2012, Mosby.
REM, Rapid eye movement.

TABLE 12-2 Sedative-Hypnotic Benzodiazepines and Miscellaneous Drugs

Generic Name	Trade Name
Long Acting	
clonazepam	Klonopin
diazepam	Valium
flurazepam	Dalmane
Intermediate Acting	
alprazolam	Xanax
lorazepam	Ativan
temazepam	Restoril
Short Acting	
eszopiclone*	Lunesta
midazolam	Versed
ramelteon*	Rozerem
triazolam	Halcion
zaleplon*	Sonata
zolpidem*	Ambien

*These drugs share many characteristics with the benzodiazepines but are classified as miscellaneous hypnotic drugs.

Chapter 36), trazodone, and amitriptyline (see Chapter 16). The benzodiazepines show favorable adverse effect profiles, efficacy, and safety when used appropriately. Benzodiazepines are classified as either sedative-hypnotics or anxiolytics depending on their primary usage. Anxiolytic drugs are used to reduce the intensity of feelings of anxiety. However, any of these drugs can function along a continuum as a sedative and/or hypnotic and/or anxiolytic depending on the dosage and patient sensitivity. See Chapter 16 for a further discussion of the anxiolytic use of benzodiazepines. There are five benzodiazepines commonly used as sedative-hypnotic drugs. In addition, there are several miscellaneous drugs that are used as hypnotics. They function much like benzodiazepines but are chemically distinct from them. All are listed in Table 12-2. Ramelteon is a hypnotic drug not related to any other hypnotics. It has a new mechanism of action and is profiled separately later in the chapter. Two new drugs, suvorexant (Belsomra) and tasimelteon (Hetlioz) became available in 2014. Suvorexant is the first in a new class of drugs called selective oxrexin receptor antagonists. Orexins are neuropeptides involved in the regulation of the sleep-wake cycle. Suvorexant has a half-life of 12 hours, and there are safety concerns regarding daytime somnolence and unconscious nighttime behaviors. Tasimelteon is indicated only for disturbances of sleep-wake cycle in patients who are totally blind.

Mechanism of Action and Drug Effects

The sedative and hypnotic action of benzodiazepines is related to their ability to depress activity in the CNS. The specific areas that are affected include the hypothalamic, thalamic, and limbic systems of the brain. Although the mechanism of action is not certain, research suggests that there are specific receptors in the brain for benzodiazepines. These receptors are thought to be either gamma-aminobutyric acid (GABA) receptors or other adjacent receptors. GABA is the primary inhibitory

neurotransmitter of the brain, and it serves to modulate CNS activity by inhibiting overstimulation. Like GABA itself, benzodiazepine activity appears to be related to their ability to inhibit stimulation of the brain.

Indications

Benzodiazepines have a variety of therapeutic applications. They are commonly used for sedation, relief of agitation or anxiety, treatment of anxiety-related depression, sleep induction, skeletal muscle relaxation, and treatment of acute seizure disorders. Benzodiazepines are often combined with anesthetics, analgesics, and neuromuscular blocking drugs in balanced anesthesia and also moderate sedation (see Chapter 11) for their amnesic properties to reduce memory of painful procedures. Finally, benzodiazepine receptors in the CNS are in the same area as those that play a role in alcohol addiction. Therefore, some benzodiazepines (e.g., diazepam, chlordiazepoxide) are used in the treatment and prevention of the symptoms of alcohol withdrawal (see Chapter 17). When benzodiazepines are used to treat insomnia, it is recommended that they be used short term if clinically feasible to avoid dependency.

Contraindications

Contraindications to the use of benzodiazepines include known drug allergy, narrow-angle glaucoma, and pregnancy.

Adverse Effects

As a class, benzodiazepines have a relatively favorable adverse effect profile; however, they can be harmful if given in excessive doses or when mixed with alcohol. Adverse effects associated with their use usually involve the CNS. Commonly reported undesirable effects are headache, drowsiness, paradoxical excitement or nervousness, dizziness or vertigo, cognitive impairment, and lethargy. Benzodiazepines can create a significant fall hazard in older adults, and the lowest effective dose must be used in this patient population. Although these drugs have comparatively less intense effects on the normal sleep cycle, a "hangover" effect is sometimes reported (e.g., daytime sleepiness). Withdrawal symptoms such as rebound insomnia (i.e., greater insomnia than pretreatment) may occur with abrupt discontinuation.

Toxicity and Management of Overdose

An overdose of benzodiazepines may result in one or all of the following symptoms: somnolence, confusion, diminished reflexes, and coma. Overdose of benzodiazepines alone rarely results in hypotension and respiratory depression. These effects are more commonly seen when benzodiazepines are taken with other CNS depressants such as alcohol or barbiturates. In the absence of the concurrent ingestion of alcohol or other CNS depressants, benzodiazepine overdose rarely results in death.

Treatment of benzodiazepine intoxication is generally symptomatic and supportive. Flumazenil, a benzodiazepine antidote, can be used to acutely reverse the sedative effects of benzodiazepines. It antagonizes the action of benzodiazepines on the CNS by directly competing with the benzodiazepine for binding at the receptors. Flumazenil is used in cases of oral overdose or excessive intravenous sedation. The dosage regimens to be followed for the reversal of conscious sedation or general anesthesia induced by benzodiazepines and the management of suspected overdoses are summarized in Table 12-3.

Interactions

Potential drug interactions with the benzodiazepines are significant because of their intensity, particularly when they involve other CNS depressants (e.g., alcohol, opioids, muscle relaxants). These drugs result in further CNS depressant effects, including reduced blood pressure, reduced respiratory rate, sedation, confusion, and diminished reflexes. This and other major drug interactions are listed in Table 12-4. Herbal supplements that interact with the benzodiazepines include kava and valerian, which may also lead to further CNS depression. Food-drug interactions include interactions with grapefruit and grapefruit juice, which alter drug metabolism via inhibition of the cytochrome P-450 system and can result in prolonged effect, increased effect, and toxicity.

TABLE 12-3 Flumazenil Treatment Regimen

Indication	Recommended Regimen	Duration
Reversal of moderate sedation or general anesthesia	0.2 mg (2 mL) IV over 15 sec, then 0.2 mg if consciousness does not occur; may be repeated at 60-sec intervals prn up to 4 additional times (maximum total dose, 1 mg)	1-4 hr
Management of suspected benzodiazepine overdose	0.2 mg (2 mL) IV over 30 sec; wait 30 sec, then give 0.3 mg (3 mL) over 30 sec if consciousness does not occur; further doses of 0.5 mg (5 mL) can be given over 30 sec at intervals of 1 min up to a cumulative dose of 3 mg	1-4 hr

NOTE: Flumazenil has a relatively short half-life and a duration of effect of 1 to 4 hours; therefore, if flumazenil is used to reverse the effects of a long-acting benzodiazepine, the dose of the reversal drug may wear off and the patient may become sedated again, requiring more flumazenil.

TABLE 12-4 Benzodiazepines: Drug/Food Interactions

Drug	Mechanism	Result
Azole antifungals, verapamil, diltiazem, protease inhibitors, macrolide antibiotics, grapefruit juice	Decreased benzodiazepine metabolism	Prolonged benzodiazepine action
CNS depressants	Additive effects	Increased CNS depression
olanzapine	Unknown	Increased benzodiazepine effects
rifampin	Increased metabolism	Decreased benzodiazepine effects

Dosages

For dosage information, see the table on the next page.

DRUG PROFILES

Benzodiazepines and miscellaneous sedative-hypnotic drugs are prescription-only drugs, and they are designated as Schedule IV controlled substances. Uses for benzodiazepines can vary,

SAFETY: HERBAL THERAPIES AND DIETARY SUPPLEMENTS   QSEN

Kava (Piper Methysticum)

Overview
Kava consists of the dried rhizomes of *Piper methysticum*. The drug contains kava pyrones (kawain). Extended continuous intake can cause a temporary yellow discoloration of the skin, hair, and nails.

Common Uses
Relief of anxiety, stress, restlessness; promotion of sleep

Adverse Effects
Skin discoloration, possible accommodative disturbances and pupillary enlargement, scaly skin (with long-term use)

Potential Drug Interactions
Alcohol, barbiturates, psychoactive drugs

Contraindications
Contraindicated in patients with Parkinson's disease, liver disease, depression, or alcoholism; in those operating heavy machinery; and in pregnant and breastfeeding women

SAFETY: HERBAL THERAPIES AND DIETARY SUPPLEMENTS   QSEN

Valerian (Valeriana Officinalis)

Overview
Valerian root, consisting of fresh underground plant parts, contains essential oil with monoterpenes and sesquiterpenes (valerianic acids).

Common Uses
Relief of anxiety, restlessness, sleep disorders

Adverse Effects
Central nervous system depression, hepatotoxicity, nausea, vomiting, anorexia, headache, restlessness, insomnia

Potential Drug Interactions
Central nervous system depressants, monamine oxidase inhibitors, phenytoin; may have enhanced relative and adverse effects when taken with other drugs (including other herbal products) that have known sedative properties (including alcohol)

Contraindications
Contraindicated in patients with cardiac disease, liver disease, or those operating heavy machinery including treatment of insomnia, moderate sedation (see Chapter 11), muscle relaxation, anticonvulsant therapy (see Chapter 14), and anxiety relief (see Chapter 16). The miscellaneous drugs are normally used only for their hypnotic purposes to treat insomnia. Dosage information appears in the dosages table on this page.

DOSAGES

Selected Benzodiazepine and Other Sedative-Hypnotic Drugs

Drug (Pregnancy Category)	Onset and Duration	Usual Adult Dosage Range	Indications/Uses
diazepam (Valium) (D)	Long acting	PO: 2-10 mg 3-4 times daily IV: 2-10 mg	Muscle relaxation, preprocedure sedation, status epilepticus, acute anxiety/agitation
eszopiclone* (Lunesta) (C)	Short acting	PO: 1-3 mg at bedtime	Sleep induction
ramelteon* (Rozerem) (C)	Short acting	PO: 8 mg at bedtime	Sleep induction
temazepam (Restoril) (D)	Intermediate acting	PO: 7.5-30 mg at bedtime	Sleep induction
♦ zaleplon (Sonata) (C)	Short acting	PO: 5-10 mg at bedtime	Sleep induction
♦ zolpidem* (Ambien) (C)	Short acting	PO: 5 mg at bedtime	Sleep induction

*Nonbenzodiazepine drugs.

BENZODIAZEPINES

diazepam

Diazepam (Valium) was the first clinically available benzodiazepine drug. It has varied uses, including treatment of anxiety, procedural sedation and anesthesia adjunct, anticonvulsant therapy, and skeletal muscle relaxation following orthopedic injury or surgery. It is available in oral, rectal, and injectable forms.

Pharmacokinetics: Diazepam

Route	Onset of Action	Peak Plasma Concentration	Elimination Half-life	Duration of Action
IV	Immediate	8 min	20-50 hr	15-60 min
PO	30 min	1-2 hr	20-60 hr	12-24 hr

!midazolam

Midazolam (Versed) is most commonly used preoperatively and for moderate sedation (see Chapter 11). It is useful for this indication due to its ability to cause amnesia and anxiolysis (reduced anxiety) as well as sedation. The drug is normally given by injection in adults. However, a liquid oral dosage form is also available for children. See Chapter 11 for dosage information.

Pharmacokinetics: Midazolam

Route	Onset of Action	Peak Plasma Concentration	Elimination Half-life	Duration of Action
IV	1-5 minutes	20-60 minutes	1-4 hours	2-6 hours

temazepam

Temazepam (Restoril), an intermediate-acting benzodiazepine, is actually one of the metabolites of diazepam and normally induces sleep within 20 to 40 minutes. Temazepam has a long onset of action, so it is recommended that patients take it about 1 hour prior to going to bed. Although it is still an effective hypnotic, it has been replaced by the newer drugs.

Pharmacokinetics: Temazepam

Route	Onset of Action	Peak Plasma Concentration	Elimination Half-life	Duration of Action
PO	30-60 min	2-3 hr	9.5-12 hr	7-8 hr

NONBENZODIAZEPINES

eszopiclone

Eszopiclone (Lunesta) is the first hypnotic to be FDA-approved for long-term use. It is designed to provide a full 8 hours of sleep. It is considered a short- to intermediate-acting agent. As with other hypnotics, patients should allot 8 hours of sleep time and should avoid taking hypnotics when they must awaken in less than 6 to 8 hours.

Pharmacokinetics: Eszopiclone

Route	Onset of Action	Peak Plasma Concentration	Elimination Half-life	Duration of Action
PO	30-60 min	1 hr	6 hr	8 hr

ramelteon

Ramelteon (Rozerem) is structurally similar to the hormone melatonin, which is believed to regulate circadian rhythms (day-night sleep cycles) in the body. Over-the-counter dietary supplements containing melatonin have been available for several years. Ramelteon works as an agonist at melatonin receptors in the CNS. Technically it is not a CNS depressant, but it is included here because of its use as a hypnotic. It is also not classified as a controlled substance because of its lack of observed dependency risk. It has a shorter duration of action than other hypnotics and is therefore indicated primarily for patients who have difficulty with sleep *onset* rather than sleep maintenance. Its use is contraindicated in cases of severe liver dysfunction. It is best avoided in patients receiving fluconazole or ketoconazole (see Chapter 42), both of which can impede its metabolism. Rifampin (see Chapter 41) can reduce the efficacy of ramelteon by speeding its metabolism via the induction of hepatic enzymes.

Pharmacokinetics: Ramelteon

Route	Onset of Action	Peak Plasma Concentration	Elimination Half-life	Duration of Action
PO	30-60 min	45 min	1-2.5 hr	6-8 hr

♦ zaleplon

Zaleplon (Sonata) is a short-acting nonbenzodiazepine hypnotic. A unique advantage of this drug stems from its very short half-life. Patients whose sleep difficulties include early awakenings can take a dose in the middle of the night as long as it is at least 4 hours before they must arise.

Pharmacokinetics: Zaleplon

Route	Onset of Action	Peak Plasma Concentration	Elimination Half-life	Duration of Action
PO	Rapid	1 hr	1 hr	6-8 hr

♦ zolpidem

Zolpidem (Ambien) is a short-acting nonbenzodiazepine hypnotic. Its relatively short half-life and its lack of active metabolites contribute to a lower incidence of daytime sleepiness compared with benzodiazepine hypnotics; however, the FDA now recommends doses of 5 mg as a maximum dose for women or 5 to 10 mg for men due to risk for next-morning impairment after its use. A unique dosage form, Ambien CR, is a longer-acting form with two separate drug reservoirs. One releases zolpidem faster than the other to induce hypnosis (sleep) more rapidly. The second reservoir also releases zolpidem but does so more slowly throughout the night to help maintain sleep. One special concern with this particular dosage form is the possibility of *somnambulation* or sleepwalking, which has been reported with its use. Nevertheless, Ambien CR is currently one of only two hypnotics to be FDA-approved for long-term use; the other is eszopiclone (Lunesta).

Pharmacokinetics: Zolpidem

Route	Onset of Action	Peak Plasma Concentration	Elimination Half-life	Duration of Action
PO	30 min	1.6 hr	1.4-4.5 hr	6-8 hr

BARBITURATES

Barbiturates were first introduced into clinical use in 1903 and were the standard drugs for treating insomnia and producing sedation. Chemically they are derivatives of barbituric acid. Although 50 different barbiturates are approved for clinical use in the United States, only a few are in clinical use today. This is due to the favorable safety profile and proven efficacy of the benzodiazepines. Barbiturates can produce many unwanted adverse effects. They are physiologically habit forming and have a low **therapeutic index.** Barbiturates can be classified into four groups based on their onset and duration of action. Table 12-5 lists the barbiturates in each category and summarizes their pharmacokinetic characteristics.

TABLE 12-5   Sedative-Hypnotic Barbiturates

Generic Name	Trade Name
Ultrashort Acting	
methohexital	Brevital
thiopental	Pentothal
Short Acting	
pentobarbital	Nembutal
secobarbital	Seconal
Intermediate Acting	
butabarbital	Butisol
Long Acting	
phenobarbital	Generic
mephobarbital	Mebaral

Mechanism of Action and Drug Effects

Barbiturates are CNS depressants that act primarily on the brainstem in an area called the *reticular formation.* Their sedative and hypnotic effects are dose related, and they act by reducing the nerve impulses traveling to the area of the brain called the *cerebral cortex.* Their ability to inhibit nerve impulse transmission is due in part to their ability to potentiate the action of the inhibitory neurotransmitter GABA, which is found in high concentrations in the CNS. Barbiturates also raise the seizure threshold and can be used to treat seizures (see Chapter 14).

Indications

All barbiturates have the same sedative-hypnotic effects but differ in their potency, time to onset of action, and duration of action. It is important to note that the use of barbiturates is no longer recommended for sleep induction. The various categories of barbiturates can be used for the following therapeutic purposes: (1) ultrashort acting: anesthesia for short surgical procedures, anesthesia induction, control of convulsions, and reduction of intracranial pressure in neurosurgical patients; (2) short acting: sedation and control of convulsive conditions; (3) intermediate acting: sedation and control of convulsive conditions; and (4) long acting: epileptic seizure prophylaxis.

Contraindications

Contraindications to barbiturate use include known drug allergy, pregnancy, significant respiratory difficulties, and severe kidney or liver disease. These drugs must be used with caution in older adults due to their sedative properties and increased fall risk.

Adverse Effects

Adverse effects of barbiturates relate to the CNS and include drowsiness, lethargy, dizziness, hangover, and paradoxical restlessness or excitement. Their long-term effects on normal sleep architecture can be detrimental. Barbiturates deprive people of REM sleep, which can result in agitation. When any barbiturate is stopped, a rebound phenomenon may occur. During this

TABLE 12-6	Barbiturates: Adverse Effects
Body System	**Adverse Effects**
Cardiovascular	Vasodilation and hypotension, especially if given too rapidly
Gastrointestinal	Nausea, vomiting, diarrhea, constipation
Hematologic	Agranulocytosis, thrombocytopenia
Nervous	Drowsiness, lethargy, vertigo
Respiratory	Respiratory depression, cough
Other	Hypersensitivity reactions: urticaria, angioedema, rash, fever, Stevens-Johnson syndrome

TABLE 12-7	Barbiturates: Controlled Substance Schedule
Schedule	**Barbiturates**
C-II	pentobarbital, secobarbital
C-III	butabarbital, thiopental
C-IV	mephobarbital, methohexital, phenobarbital

rebound, the proportion of REM sleep is increased, and nightmares often ensue. Common adverse effects of barbiturates are listed in Table 12-6. As is the case with most sedative drugs, barbiturates are associated with an increased incidence of falls when used in older adults. If they are recommended for older adults at all, the usual dose is reduced by half whenever possible.

Toxicity and Management of Overdose

Treatment of an overdose is mainly symptomatic and supportive. The mainstays of therapy are maintenance of an adequate airway, assisted ventilation, and oxygen administration if needed, along with fluid and pressor support as indicated. Activated charcoal may be given; however, recent clinical data does not support its use because no improvement in clinical outcome has been shown. Phenoobarbital and mephobarbital are relatively acidic and can be eliminated more quickly by the kidneys when the urine is alkalized (pH is raised). This keeps the drug in the urine and prevents it from being resorbed back into the circulation. Alkalization, along with forced diuresis using diuretics (e.g., furosemide [see Chapter 28]), can hasten elimination of the barbiturate.

Interactions

Barbiturates as a class are notorious enzyme inducers. They stimulate the action of enzymes in the liver that are responsible for the metabolism or breakdown of many drugs. By stimulating the action of these enzymes, they cause many drugs to be metabolized more quickly, which usually shortens their duration of action. Barbiturates increase the activity of hepatic microsomal or cytochrome P-450 enzymes (see Chapter 2). This process is called *enzyme induction*. Induction of this enzyme system results in increased drug metabolism and breakdown. However, if two drugs are competing for the same enzyme system, the result can be inhibited drug metabolism and possibly increased toxicity for the wide variety of drugs that are metabolized by these enzymes. Other drugs that are enzyme inducers are rifampin and phenytoin.

Additive CNS depression occurs with the coadministration of barbiturates with alcohol, antihistamines, benzodiazepines, opioids, and tranquilizers. Drugs most likely to have marked interactions with the barbiturates include monoamine oxidase inhibitors (MAOIs), tricyclic antidepressants (see Chapter 16), anticoagulants (see Chapter 26), glucocorticoids (see Chapter 30), and oral contraceptives (see Chapter 34) with barbiturates. Coadministration of MAOIs and barbiturates can result in prolonged barbiturate effects. Coadministration of anticoagulants with barbiturates can result in decreased anticoagulation response and possible clot formation. Coadministration of barbiturates with oral contraceptives can result in accelerated metabolism of the contraceptive drug and possible unintended pregnancy. Women taking both types of medication concurrently need to be advised to consider an additional method of contraception as a backup.

Dosages

Barbiturates can act as either sedatives or hypnotics depending on the dosage. For information on selected barbiturates and their recommended sedative and hypnotic dosages, see the table on this page.

DOSAGES

Selected Barbiturates

Drug	Onset and Duration	Usual Dosage Adult Range	Indications/Uses
pentobarbital (Nembutal)	Short acting	IM: 150-200 mg IV: 100 mg	Preoperative sedative
phenobarbital	Long acting	PO: 30-120 mg/day divided IM/IV: 100-200 mg 60-90 min before surgery	Sedative Preoperative sedative

DRUG PROFILES

Like benzodiazepines, barbiturates can also have varied uses, including preoperative sedation, anesthesia adjunct, and anticonvulsant therapy. All barbiturates are controlled substances, but not all are on the same schedule, as illustrated in Table 12-7. Dosage information appears in the dosages table for barbiturates.

pentobarbital

Pentobarbital (Nembutal) is a short-acting barbiturate. Formerly prescribed as a sedative-hypnotic for insomnia, pentobarbital is now principally used preoperatively to relieve anxiety and provide sedation. In addition, it is used occasionally to control status epilepticus. Pentobarbital may also be used to treat withdrawal symptoms in patients who are physically dependent on barbiturates or nonbarbiturate hypnotics. It is available in oral, injectable, and rectal dosage forms.

Pharmacokinetics: Pentobarbital

Route	Onset of Action	Peak Plasma Concentration	Elimination Half-life	Duration of Action
PO	30-60 min	1-2 hr	20-45 min	3-4 hr

phenobarbital

Phenobarbital is considered the prototypical barbiturate and is classified as a long-acting drug. Phenobarbital is used for the prevention of generalized tonic-clonic seizures and fever-induced convulsions. In addition, it has been useful in the treatment of hyperbilirubinemia in neonates. It is only rarely used today as a sedative and is no longer recommended to be used as a hypnotic drug. It is available in oral and injectable forms.

Pharmacokinetics: Phenobarbital

Route	Onset of Action	Peak Plasma Concentration	Elimination Half-life	Duration of Action
IV	5 min	30 min	50-120 hr	6-12 hr
PO	30 min	1-6 hr	50-120 hr	6-12 hr

OVER-THE-COUNTER HYPNOTICS

Nonprescription sleeping aids often contain antihistamines (see Chapter 36). These drugs have a CNS depressant effect. The most common antihistamines contained in over-the-counter sleeping aids are doxylamine (Unisom) and diphenhydramine (Sominex). Analgesics (e.g., acetaminophen [see Chapter 10]) are sometimes added to offer some pain relief if pain is a component of the sleep disturbance (e.g., acetaminophen/ diphenhydramine [Extra Strength Tylenol PM]). As with other CNS depressants, concurrent use of alcohol can cause additive CNS depression.

MUSCLE RELAXANTS

A variety of conditions such as trauma, inflammation, anxiety, and pain can be associated with acute muscle spasms. The muscle relaxants are a group of compounds that act predominantly within the CNS to relieve pain associated with skeletal muscle spasms. Most muscle relaxants are known as *centrally acting* skeletal muscle relaxants because their site of action is the CNS. Centrally acting skeletal muscle relaxants are similar in structure and action to other CNS depressants such as diazepam. It is believed that the muscle relaxant effects are related to this CNS depressant activity. Only one of these compounds, dantrolene, acts directly on skeletal muscle. It belongs to a group of relaxants known as direct-acting skeletal muscle relaxants. It closely resembles GABA.

Mechanism of Action and Drug Effects

The majority of the muscle relaxants work within the CNS. Their beneficial effects are believed to come from their sedative effects rather than from direct muscle relaxation. Dantrolene acts directly on the excitation-contraction coupling of muscle fibers and not at the level of the CNS. It directly affects skeletal muscles by decreasing the response of the muscle to stimuli. It appears to exert its action by decreasing the amount of calcium released from storage sites in the sarcoplasmic reticula of muscle fibers. All other muscle relaxants have no direct effects on muscles, nerve conduction, or muscle-nerve junctions and have a depressant effect on the CNS. Their effects are the result of CNS depression in the brain primarily at the level of the brainstem, thalamus, and basal ganglia and also at the spinal cord. The effects of muscle relaxants are relaxation of striated muscles, mild weakness of skeletal muscles, decreased force of muscle contraction, and muscle stiffness. Other effects include generalized CNS depression manifested as sedation, somnolence, ataxia, and respiratory and cardiovascular depression.

Indications

Muscle relaxants are primarily used for the relief of painful musculoskeletal conditions such as muscle spasms, often following injuries such as low back strain. They are most effective when used in conjunction with physical therapy. They may also be used in the management of spasticity associated with severe chronic disorders such as multiple sclerosis and other types of cerebral lesions. Intravenous dantrolene is used for the management of skeletal muscle spasms that accompany the crisis condition known as *malignant hyperthermia* (see Chapter 11). Baclofen has been shown to be effective in relieving hiccups.

Contraindications

The only usual contraindication to the use of muscle relaxants is known drug allergy, but contraindications for some drugs may include severe renal impairment.

Adverse Effects

The primary adverse effects of muscle relaxants are an extension of their effects on the CNS and skeletal muscles. Euphoria, lightheadedness, dizziness, drowsiness, fatigue, confusion, and muscle weakness are often experienced early in treatment. These adverse effects are generally short-lived, as patients grow tolerant to them over time. Less common adverse effects seen with muscle relaxants include diarrhea, GI upset, headache, slurred speech, muscle stiffness, constipation, sexual difficulties in males, hypotension, tachycardia, and weight gain.

Toxicity and Management of Overdose

The toxicities and consequences of an overdose of muscle relaxants primarily involve the CNS. There is no specific antidote (or reversal drug) for muscle relaxant overdoses. They are best treated with conservative supportive measures. More aggressive therapies are generally needed when muscle relaxants are taken along with other CNS depressant drugs in an overdose. An adequate airway must be maintained, and means of artificial respiration must be readily available. Electrocardiographic monitoring needs to be instituted, and large quantities of intravenous fluids are administered to avoid crystalluria.

Interactions

When muscle relaxants are administered along with other depressant drugs such as alcohol and benzodiazepines, caution needs to be used to avoid overdosage. Mental confusion, anxiety, tremors, and additive hypoglycemic activity have been reported with this combination as well. A dosage reduction and/or discontinuance of one or both drugs is recommended.

Dosages

For dosage information about commonly used muscle relaxants, see the table below.

DOSAGES

Selected Muscle Relaxants

Drug (Pregnancy Category)	Pharmacologic Class	Usual Adult Dosage Range	Indications/ Uses
◆ baclofen (Lioresal) (C)	Centrally acting	PO: 5-20 mg three times daily (max: 20 mg po qid)	Spasticity
◆ cyclobenzaprine (Flexeril) (B)	Centrally acting	PO: 5-10 mg	Spasticity

DRUG PROFILES

With the exception of dantrolene (Dantrium), which acts directly on skeletal muscle tissues, muscle relaxants are classified as centrally acting drugs because of their site of action in the CNS. These include baclofen (Lioresal), carisoprodol (Soma), chlorzoxazone (Paraflex), cyclobenzaprine (Flexeril), metaxalone (Skelaxin), methocarbamol (Robaxin), and tizanidine (Zanaflex). Carisoprodol has become a popular drug of abuse. When combined with an opioid and a benzodiazepine, it is known as "The Holy Trinity." This combination produces a herion-like effect. Despite the abuse potential, it and other muscle relaxants are not controlled substances. Use of all muscle relaxants is contraindicated in patients who have shown a hypersensitivity reaction to them or have compromised pulmonary function, active hepatic disease, or impaired myocardial function. Dosage information appears in the dosages table for muscle relaxants.

◆ baclofen

Baclofen (Lioresal) is available in both oral and injectable dosage forms. The injectable form is for use with an implantable baclofen pump device. This method is sometimes used to treat chronic spastic muscular conditions. With this route, a test dose needs to be administered initially to test for a positive response. The injection is diluted before infusion. Both oral and injectable doses are titrated to a desired response.

Pharmacokinetics: Baclofen

Route	Onset of Action	Peak Plasma Concentration	Elimination Half-life	Duration of Action
PO	0.5-1 hr	2-3 hr	2.5-4 hr	8 hr or longer

◆ cyclobenzaprine

Cyclobenzaprine (Flexeril) is available in a 5-mg and 10-mg dose and an extended-release formulation (Amrix). Cyclobenzaprine is a centrally acting muscle relaxant that is structurally and pharmacologically related to the tricyclic antidepressants. It is the most commonly used drug in this class to reduce spasms following musculoskeletal injuries. It is very common for patients to exhibit marked sedation from its use.

Pharmacokinetics: Cyclobenzaprine

Route	Onset of Action	Peak Plasma Concentration	Elimination Half-life	Duration of Action
PO	1 hr	3-8 hr	8-37 hr	12-24 hr

NURSING PROCESS

ASSESSMENT

Before administering any *CNS depressant drug*, such as a *benzodiazepine, nonbenzodiazepine, miscellaneous drug, muscle relaxant*, or *barbiturate*, perform an assessment focusing on some of the more common parameters and data, including the following: (1) complaints of any insomnia with attention to onset, duration, frequency, and pharmacologic as well as non-pharmacologic measures used; (2) any concerns voiced by the patient or family of sleep disorders, sleep patterns, difficulty in sleeping, or frequent awakenings; (3) the time it takes to fall asleep and the energy level upon awakening; (4) vital signs with attention to blood pressure (both supine and standing measurements); pulse rate and rhythm; respiratory rate, rhythm, and depth; body temperature; and presence of pain; (5) thorough physical assessment/examination for baseline comparisons; (6) neurologic findings with a focus on any changes in mental status, memory, cognitive abilities, alertness, level of orientation (to person, place, and time) or level of sedation, mood changes, depression or other mental disorder, changes in sensations, anxiety, and panic attacks; and (7) miscellaneous information about medical history; allergies; use of alcohol; smoking history; caffeine intake (especially 6 hours prior to bedtime); past and current medication profile, with notation of use of any prescription drugs, over-the-counter drugs, and herbals; alternative or folk practices; and any changes in health status, weight, nutrition, exercise, life stressors (including loss and grief), or lifestyle.

For patients taking *benzodiazepines* or *benzodiazepine-like drugs*, assessment needs to also focus on the identification of disorders or conditions that represent cautions or contraindications to use of these drugs as well as drugs the patient is taking that might interact with benzodiazepines or benzodiazepine-like drugs (see pharmacology discussion). Closely monitor those who are anemic, suicidal, or have a history of abusing drugs, alcohol, or other substances. Other significant cautions pertain to use of these drugs in the very young or in older adults because of their increased sensitivity to these drugs. Cautions are also extended to the pregnant or lactating patient. The very young and older adult patient may require lower dosages due to potential ataxia and excessive sedation. In addition, before initiating drug therapy with the benzodiazepines and other *sedative-hypnotic drugs*, including *barbiturates*, the prescriber may order blood studies such as CBC. Renal function studies (BUN or creatinine levels) and/or hepatic function studies (ALP level) may be ordered to rule out organ impairment and prevent potential toxicity or complications resulting from decreased excretion and/or metabolism. Potential drug interactions for benzodiazepines are presented in Table 12-4. Pay particular attention to the concurrent use of other CNS depressants (e.g., opioids), because this may lead to severe decreases in blood pressure, respiratory rate, reflexes, and level of consciousness.

With the *nonbenzodiazepines* such as *zaleplon* and *zolpidem tartrate*, include a head-to-toe physical assessment and a thorough medication history with measurement of vital signs and other parameters previously mentioned. Assess and document for allergies to these drugs and to aspirin. If the patient is allergic to aspirin, there is an associated risk for allergies to nonbenzodiazepines. Other considerations include the need for assessment of any confusion and lightheadedness, especially in older adults because of their increased sensitivity. Do not use zaleplon and *eszopiclone* in those younger than 18 years of age, and use extreme caution if there is a history of compromised respiratory status or drug, alcohol, or other substance abuse. Drug interactions include other CNS depressants. Gender of the patient is also important to consider in assessment because of the reduced dosage recommended by the FDA for female patients (see pharmacology discussion).

For *muscle relaxants,* always note drug allergies before use, and perform a complete head-to-toe assessment with a focus on the neurologic system. In the older adult, there is increased risk for CNS toxicity with possible hallucinations, confusion, and excessive sedation. Assessment includes taking a thorough health/medication history and examining the complete patient profile with results of associated laboratory studies. See the pharmacology discussion about cautions, contraindications, and drug interactions.

The *miscellaneous* drug *ramelteon* is a newer medication that is used for insomnia but is not associated with CNS depression, does not carry the potential for abuse or dependence, and does not lead to withdrawal symptoms when treatment stops. Therefore, this drug can be used for patients who are likely to be abusers of CNS depressants. Include inquiry into sleep patterns and habits in your assessment. Because this drug is not to be used in patients with liver impairment, liver function studies are needed prior to beginning the medication. Perform respiratory assessment and assessment of other vital signs as well. If the patient has a history of respiratory disorders such as chronic obstructive pulmonary disease or sleep apnea, or if the patient is a child, this medication would not be indicated.

Barbiturates are discussed further in Chapter 14 along with other antiepileptic drugs. However, a brief description is needed to emphasize the importance of conducting a thorough patient assessment as well as evaluating for cautions, contraindications, and drug interactions. Barbiturates are not to be used by pregnant or lactating women. These drugs cross the placenta and breast-blood barriers, posing a risk for respiratory depression in the fetus and neonate. Withdrawal symptoms may appear in neonates born to women who have taken barbiturates during their last trimester of pregnancy. Barbiturates may also produce paradoxical excitement in children and confusion and mental depression in the older adult, so baseline neurologic assessment is needed. Assessment of renal and liver function is also important in those with compromised organ function and in the older adult to help avoid toxicity.

NURSING DIAGNOSES

1. Impaired gas exchange related to respiratory depression associated with CNS depressants
2. Deficient knowledge related to inadequate information about the various CNS drugs and their first-time use
3. Disturbed sleep pattern related to the drug's interference with REM sleep
4. Risk for injury related to the adverse effect of decreased sensorium
5. Risk for injury related to possible drug overdose or adverse reactions related to drug-drug interactions (e.g., combined use of the drug with alcohol, tranquilizers, and/or analgesics) and decreased level of alertness and an unsteady gait
6. Risk for injury related to physical or psychologic dependence on CNS drugs

PLANNING: OUTCOME IDENTIFICATION

1. Patient maintains normal gas exchange and is free from respiratory depression through coughing, deep breathing, and taking medication as prescribed.
2. Patient demonstrates adequate knowledge about the drugs including sedating/hypnotic properties, CNS depressant effects and side effects of decreased respirations, altered cough, confusion, drowsiness, and drug interactions.
3. Patient remains free from further disturbed sleep patterns and implements nonpharmacologic measures for improving sleep such as massage, relaxation therapy, meditation, and music.
4. Patient remains free from self-injury and falls and demonstrates understanding of safety measures such as removing all throw rugs from walking areas (especially at night), changing positions slowly, ambulating with caution, and well-lit rooms at night.
5. Patient remains free from injury due to adequate information about drug interactions that lead to further CNS depression, such as other CNS depressants, herbals, opioids, alcohol, and other sedating over-the-counter products such as diphenhydramine.
6. Patient remains free from injury to self with no drug dependence and reports any problems with drug resistance, excessive sedation, or the need for more medication

IMPLEMENTATION

Patients taking *benzodiazepines* and other CNS depressants experience sedation and possible ataxia, thus there is a need for patient safety measures. Policies at hospitals or health care settings mandate the type of safety precautions to be taken, such as the use of side rails or bed alarms. Ambulation needs to occur safely and with assistance when patients are sedated or are experiencing the adverse effects of these drugs. In addition, dependence may be a problem with the benzodiazepines, but not to the same degree as with the barbiturates. While taking these drugs, patients need to avoid driving or participating in any activities that require mental alertness. It is recommended that these drugs be taken on an empty stomach for faster onset of action; however, this often results in GI upset, so, practically speaking, they may need to be taken with food, a light snack, or meals. Orally administered benzodiazepines have an onset of action of 30 minutes to 6 hours depending on the drug (see the pharmacokinetics tables in the Drug Profiles section), and the appropriate timing and intervals of dosing will be determined by these characteristics. For example, if a patient takes a benzodiazepine or other CNS depresssant drug to induce sleep and the drug's onset of action is 30 to 60 minutes, then the drug needs to be dosed 60 minutes prior to bedtime. In addition, it is crucial to patient compliance and safety that there is understanding about drug tolerance developing to many of these drugs. Because of this tolerance, the patient may require larger dosages to produce the same therapeutic effect, at some point. Interrupting therapy helps to decrease drug tolerance. When administering IV diazepam, do not mix or dilute with other solutions/drugs in syringe or infusion container. If it is not feasible to give diazepam directly IV, it may be injected slowly, at least one minute for each 5 mg given, through the infusion tubing as close as possible to the vein insertion site. Do not use small veins, and be very cautious to avoid intraarterial administration or extravasation.

Among the benzodiazepines, REM interference is less problematic with flurazepam, quazepam, and estazolam, primarily because they produce fewer active metabolites. Educate patients about the REM interference and rebound insomnia that may occur with just a 3- to 4-week regimen of drug therapy. To minimize REM interference, benzodiazepines and other drugs are only used when nonpharmacologic methods fail and must be used with caution in all patients with sleep disorders and for short periods of time. *Zolpidem* is also available in a sustained-release product used for long-term management of sleep disorders. Gradual weaning-off periods are recommended for benzodiazepines and all CNS depressants. Hangover effects are also associated with many of the CNS depressants but occur less frequently with benzodiazepines and nonbenzodiazepines than with barbiturates.

It is recommended that *nonbenzodiazepines* (e.g., *zaleplon*) be taken for the prescribed time. Take zaleplon as directed and immediately before bedtime due to its quick onset of action. Avoid consumption of very heavy and/or high-fat meals within 2 hours of taking this drug because of interference with the drug's action. Zolpidem has optimal absorption if taken at bedtime on an empty stomach with no crushing, chewing, or breaking of the oral dosage form. It is also important to administer these drugs not too late in the night. Generally speaking, dosing before midnight may help prevent daytime drowsiness or difficulty waking. This drug may infrequently lead to temporary memory loss (see the pharmacology discussion about FDA dosage recommendations for women). To help avoid this adverse effect, it is important to encourage the patient to not take a dose of the drug without a full night's sleep (e.g., at least 7 to 8 hours) the previous night. As with any CNS depressant drug, avoid tasks requiring mental alertness until response to the drug is known. Tolerance and dependence are possible with prolonged use, and this drug is to be gradually weaned before discontinuation.

Muscle relaxants have different indications than the barbiturates and benzodiazepines and are not used to treat insomnia. They are generally indicated for some forms of spasticity (see the pharmacology discussion). However, when used they may lead to adverse effects and toxicities, so frequently monitor airway, breathing, and circulation. Early identification of toxicity is critical to provide prompt treatment and to prevent respiratory and other CNS depressant effects. Closely monitor all vital parameters, level of consciousness, and presence of sedation when these muscle relaxants are used. Encourage cautious ambulation. Recommend that the patient change positions purposefully and slowly to prevent syncope or dizziness. The greatest risk for hypotension associated with these drugs is usually within 1 hour of dosing, so the patient must be more cautious about activity during this time.

The *miscellaneous* drug *ramelteon* must be used with caution, with emphasis on the fact that the drug is not to be mixed with alcohol. In the patient education, include that the drug is to be taken 30 minutes before bedtime and is *not* to be taken along with or immediately following a high-fat meal.

Barbiturates are to be used with very close monitoring and extreme caution. Observe and document the patient's level of consciousness or sedation; orientation to person, place, and time; respiratory rate; oxygen saturation; and other vital signs. Advise the patient to take oral doses with food or a light snack, and not to alter dosage forms. Use a bed alarm system or side rails, and provide assistance with ambulation, as needed or indicated, to help prevent injury. Barbiturates also produce a hangover effect, and this residual drowsiness occurs upon awakening and results in impaired reaction times. The intermediate- and long-acting hypnotics are often the culprits for this adverse effect. Abrupt withdrawal of barbiturates after prolonged therapy may produce adverse effects ranging from nightmares, hallucinations, and delirium to seizures. In addition, while the patient is taking barbiturates, monitor the patient's red blood cell count and hemoglobin and hematocrit levels because of the possible adverse effect of anemia. Long-term use of barbiturates also requires monitoring of therapeutic blood levels of the drug. For example, the therapeutic level of *phenobarbital* must range between 10 and 40 mcg/mL. Patients with serum levels above 40 mcg/mL may experience toxicity manifested by cold and clammy skin, respiratory rate of less than 10 breaths/min, and other signs of severe CNS depression.

Intravenous use of *barbiturates* requires dilution of the drug with normal saline or other recommended solutions. Recommendations regarding diluents and rates of intravenous administration must be strictly followed for safe use. Most of the drugs are not to be given any faster than 1 mg/kg per minute, and a maximum amount per minute may be specified. Consult authoritative drug sources (e.g., a current drug handbook/reference or the manufacturer's insert) for the recommended rate of infusion before giving any of these drugs. Too rapid an infusion of a barbiturate may produce profound hypotension and marked respiratory depression. If intravenous infiltration is present, the site may become swollen, erythematous, and tender. Tissue necrosis may occur with infiltration, depending on the irritating qualities of the particular drug. There are antidote protocols for some of the intravenous barbiturates. For example, with *phenobarbital* intravenous infiltration, the solution must be discontinued, a 0.5% procaine solution injected into the affected area, and moist heat applied, as per policy or procedure manuals. Always check protocol for management of infiltration of an intravenous drug before intervening because, in certain situations, the intravenous catheter may be left in place until antidotes are administered. Another area of concern with intravenous drugs is incompatibilities with other intravenously administered medications, and barbiturates have several. Some intravenous drugs that are incompatible with barbiturates include amphotericin B, hydrocortisone, and hydromorphone. Only give these particular drugs after the intravenous line has been adequately flushed with normal saline. With intramuscular injection, give the solution deep into a large muscle mass to prevent tissue sloughing; however, avoid this route and use only when absolutely necessary.

In summary, before giving any *CNS depressant*, it is always important to try nonpharmacologic measures to induce sleep. However, if medication therapy is indicated, preventing respiratory depression and other problems associated with CNS depression is of prime importance, as is maintaining patient safety and preventing injury. Documentation must be timely, clear, and concise and reflect follow-up of the patient's response to the drug. It is also important to document the dose, route, time of administration, and safety measures taken after each dose is given.

CASE STUDY

Patient-Centered Care: Drugs for Sleep

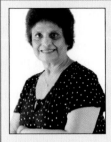

P.S., a 68-year-old retired secretary, comes to the office complaining of feeling "so tired" during the day. She has had trouble sleeping off and on for years, and a few weeks ago received a prescription for the benzodiazepine alprazolam (Xanax) to take "as needed for nerves." Upon closer questioning, the nurse discovers that P.S. has been using alprazolam almost every night for 3 weeks to help her get to sleep. She says, "I just could not fall asleep before! I am sleeping very well, but I'm so tired during the day. I don't understand how I can get such good sleep and still feel tired!"

1. Can you explain the reason for her tiredness?
2. P.S.'s nurse practitioner prescribes a period of decreasing doses of the alprazolam each evening, then every other evening, until the medication is stopped. Explain the rationale behind the tapering dosage schedule.
3. P.S. receives a prescription for ramelteon (Rozerem). How is this drug different from alprazolam?
4. What nonpharmacologic measures can P.S. try to improve her sleep?

For answers, see http://evolve.elsevier.com/Lilley.

EVALUATION

Some of the criteria by which to confirm a patient's therapeutic response to a *CNS depressant* include the following: an increased ability to sleep at night, fewer awakenings, shorter sleep induction time, few adverse effects such as hangover effects, and an improved sense of well-being because of improved sleep. Therapeutic effects related to *muscle relaxants* include decreased spasticity, reduction of choreiform movements in Huntington's chorea, decreased rigidity in parkinsonian syndrome, and relief of pain from trigeminal neuralgia. Constantly watch for and document the occurrence of any of the adverse effects of benzodiazepines, barbiturates, and muscle relaxants. See the previous discussions of adverse effects for each type of drug. Evaluation for CNS depressant toxic effects includes monitoring for severe CNS depression of all body systems, especially respiratory and circulatory collapse, with decrease in respiratory rate/depth and decrease in blood pressure.

PATIENT-CENTERED CARE: PATIENT TEACHING

- Encourage patients to keep a journal recording sleep habits, sleep patterns, and response to both drug and nondrug therapy (Box 12-1).
- Implement nonpharmacologic measures first to enhance sleep. This is important because the use of CNS depressants for treatment of sleep deficit or insomnia often leads to interference with the REM stage of sleep, hangover effects, and/or tolerance, as well as other adverse effects.
- Caffeine takes about 5 to 7 hours for approximately 50% elimination and 8 to 10 hours for 75% of elimination from

the body. Caffeine consumption in the morning won't interfere with sleep at night, however, consuming caffeine later in the day may interfere with sleep. For most individuals, sleep will most likely *not* be affected if caffeine is avoided at least 6 hours before bedtime.
- Always check with the prescriber or pharmacist before taking any over-the-counter medications because of the many drug interactions with CNS depressants.
- Keep these drugs and all medications out of the reach of children.

BOX 12-1   Sleep Diaries and Nonpharmacologic Treatment of Sleep Disorders

Information for a Sleep Diary

- What time do you usually go to bed and wake up?
- How long and how well do you sleep?
- When were you awake during the night, and for how long?
- How easy was it to go to sleep?
- How easy was it to wake up in the morning?
- How much caffeine or alcohol do you consume?
- What time did you last eat or drink (if after dinner)?
- Did you have any bedtime snacks?
- What emotions or stressors are present?
- What medications do you take daily?
- Do you smoke? If so, how much and for how long?
- Do you consume alcohol? If so, how much and for how long?
- Do you take any over-the-counter drugs? If so, what drug and for what reason? How much and for how long?
- Do you take any herbals? If so, which ones? For what and for how long?

Nonpharmacologic Sleep Interventions

- Establish a set sleep pattern with a time to go to bed at night and a regular time to get up in the morning, and stick to it. This will help to reset your internal clock.
- Sleep only as much as you need to feel refreshed and renewed. Too much sleep may lead to fragmented sleep patterns and shallow sleep.
- Keep bedroom temperatures moderate, if possible.
- Avoid caffeine-containing beverages and food within 6 hours of bedtime.
- Decrease exposure to loud noises.
- Avoid daytime napping.
- Avoid exercise late in the evening (i.e., not past 7 PM).
- Avoid alcohol in the evening. Rather than putting you to sleep, it actually results in fragmented sleep.
- Refrain from intake of caffeine beverages and/or caffeine-containing foods at least 6 hours prior to bedtime. Caffeine content may range from 160 mg in some energy drinks to about 4 mg in a 1-ounce serving of a chocolate-flavored beverage. Caffeine is present in some over-the-counter pain/headache relievers, cold medications, and diet pills ranging from as little as 16 mg to 200 mg. Decaffeinated coffee also contains some caffeine.
- Avoid tobacco at bedtime because it disturbs sleep.
- Try to relax before bedtime with soft music, yoga, relaxation therapy, deep breathing, or light reading on a topic that is not intense or anxiety provoking.
  - Drink a warm decaffeinated beverage, such as warm milk or chamomile tea, 30 minutes to 1 hour before bedtime.
  - If you are still awake 20 minutes after going to bed, get up and engage in a relaxing activity (as noted previously) and go back to bed once you feel drowsy. Repeat as necessary.

- Emphasize that medications are to be taken only as prescribed. The patient is usually told that if one dose does not work, not to double up on the dosage unless otherwise prescribed or directed.
- Educate the patient about any time constraints related to driving, operation of heavy machinery or equipment, and participation in activities requiring mental alertness while taking these medications.
- Encourage assistance with ambulation when getting out of bed to help prevent falls.
- Medications taken for sleep are to be given before midnight to prevent difficulty waking in the morning.
- Educate the patient about drug interactions (e.g., pain medications or other CNS depressants) to prevent oversedation.
- Do not abruptly discontinue or withdraw these medications, if possible, to avoid rebound insomnia.

- Sedative-hypnotic drugs (for sleep promotion) are not intended for long-term use because of their adverse effects, interference with REM sleep, and addictive properties.
- Advise the patient that hangover effects may occur with most of these drugs and that this is more problematic in older adults or in patients with altered renal and hepatic function.
- Provide the patient with thorough instructions about safety with these drugs, such as avoiding smoking in bed or when lounging.
- Teach the patient about significant drug/drug and drug/food interactions with all these medications.
- Educate the patient about the effect of grapefruit and grapefruit juice on benzodiazepines. The grapefruit results in decreased drug metabolism via inhibition of the cytochrome P-450 system and may lead to a prolonged effect and possible toxicity (of the benzodiazepine).

KEY POINTS

- Nonpharmacologic measures to improve sleep need to be tried before resorting to treatment with medications.
- Recognize and understand the classification and pharmacokinetic properties of barbiturates. Short-acting barbiturates include pentobarbital and secobarbital. Intermediate-acting barbiturates include butabarbital. Long-acting barbiturates include phenobarbital and mephobarbital.
- The pharmacokinetics of each group of barbiturates lends specific characteristics to the drugs in that group. You need to understand how these drugs are absorbed orally and used parenterally, as well as their onset time, time until peak effect, and duration of action. You must understand the life-threatening potential of these drugs because

too rapid an infusion may precipitate respiratory and/or cardiac arrest.
- Benzodiazepines are commonly used for sedation, relief of anxiety, skeletal muscle relaxation, and treatment of acute seizure disorders.
- Most sedative-hypnotic drugs suppress REM sleep and should be used only for the recommended period of time. This time frame varies, depending on the specific drug used.
- Long-acting benzodiazepines include clonazepam, diazepam, and flurazepam. Intermediate-acting benzodiazepines include alprazolam, lorazepam, and temazepam. Short-acting benzodiazepines include eszopiclone, midazolam, ramelteon, triazolam, zaleplon, and zolpidem.

NCLEX® EXAMINATION REVIEW QUESTIONS

1. A patient has been admitted to the emergency department because of an overdose of an oral benzodiazepine. He is very drowsy but still responsive. The nurse will prepare for which immediate intervention?
   a. Hemodialysis to remove the medication
   b. Administration of flumazenil
   c. Administration of naloxone
   d. Intubation and mechanical ventilation

2. An older adult has been given a benzodiazepine for sleep induction, but the night nurse noted that the patient was awake most of the night, watching television and reading in bed. The nurse documents that the patient has had which type of reaction to the medication?
   a. Allergic
   b. Teratogenic
   c. Paradoxical
   d. Idiopathic

3. The nurse is preparing to administer a medication for sleep. Which intervention applies to the administration of a non-benzodiazepine, such as zaleplon (Sonata)?
   a. These drugs need to be taken about 1 hour before bedtime.
   b. Because of their rapid onset, these drugs need to be taken just before bedtime.
   c. The patient needs to be cautioned about the high incidence of morning drowsiness that may occur after taking these drugs.
   d. These drugs are less likely to interact with alcohol.

4. The nurse will monitor the patient who is taking a muscle relaxant for which adverse effect?
   a. CNS depression
   b. Hypertension
   c. Peripheral edema
   d. Blurred vision

5. A hospitalized patient is complaining of having difficulty sleeping. Which action will the nurse take first to address this problem?

   a. Administer a sedative-hypnotic drug if ordered.
   b. Offer tea made with the herbal preparation valerian.
   c. Encourage the patient to exercise by walking up and down the halls a few times if tolerated.
   d. Provide an environment that is restful, and reduce loud noises.

6. Which considerations are important for the nurse to remember when administering a benzodiazepine as a sedative-hypnotic drug? *(Select all that apply.)*
   a. These drugs are intended for long-term management of insomnia.
   b. The drugs can be administered safely with other CNS depressants for insomnia.
   c. The dose needs to be given about 1 hour before the patient's bedtime.
   d. The drug is used as a first choice for treatment of sleeplessness.
   e. The patient needs to be evaluated for the drowsiness that may occur the morning after a benzodiazepine is taken.

7. A child is to receive phenobarbital 2 mg/kg IV on call as a preoperative sedative. The child weighs 64 pounds. How many milligrams will the child receive for this dose? *(Record your answer using one decimal place.)*

8. The nurse is reviewing the prescriptions for a patient who will be discharged to home after being hospitalized for a hysterectomy. The patient asked for a sleeping pill, and the surgeon wrote a prescription for Ambien, 10 mg at bedtime as needed for sleep. What is the nurse's priority action at this time?
   a. Review the potential adverse effects with the patient.
   b. Suggest that the patient try drinking a glass of wine at bedtime.
   c. Contact the prescriber to question the dose of the Ambien.
   d. Assist the patient to find a pharmacy to fill the prescription on her way home.

1. b, 2. c, 3. b, 4. a, 5. d, 6. c, e, 7. 58.2 mg, 8. c

CRITICAL THINKING AND PRIORITIZATION QUESTIONS

1. During rounds on the night shift, the nurse finds a patient lying in bed wide awake at 4 AM. The patient complains, "I can't sleep. I need my sleeping pill. Can I have it now?" The patient's medication administration sheet has a prn (as needed) order for temazepam (Restoril). What is the nurse's priority action at this time?

2. The nurse is talking to a patient about what adverse effects to expect when taking a muscle relaxant for injuries the

patient received in an automobile accident. What is the priority adverse effect the nurse needs to discuss with the patient? Explain your answer.

For answers, see *http://evolve.elsevier.com/Lilley*.

EVOLVE WEBSITE

http://evolve.elsevier.com/Lilley
- Animations
- Answer Keys for Textbook Case Studies and Textbook Critical Thinking and Prioritization Questions
- Content Updates
- Key Points
- Review Questions
- Student Case Studies

Central Nervous System Stimulants and Related Drugs

http://evolve.elsevier.com/Lilley

OBJECTIVES

When you reach the end of this chapter, you will be able to do the following:

1. Briefly review the anatomy, physiology, and functions of the central nervous system with attention to the stimulant effects on its function.
2. Review the key terms as they relate to the central nervous system and stimulant drugs.
3. Identify the various central nervous system stimulant drugs.
4. Discuss the mechanisms of action, indications, dosages, routes of administration, contraindications, cautions, drug interactions, adverse effects, and any related toxicity for the various central nervous system stimulants and related drugs.
5. Develop a nursing care plan based on the nursing process for patients using central nervous system stimulants and related drugs.

DRUG PROFILES

♦ **amphetamines, p. 206**
atomoxetine, p. 206
caffeine, p. 212
doxapram, p. 212
♦ **methylphenidate, p. 207**
modafinil, p. 207

orlistat, p. 208
♦ **phentermine, p. 208**
♦ **sumatriptan, p. 209**

_____

♦ = *Key drug*
! = *High-alert drug*

KEY TERMS

Amphetamines A class of stimulant drugs that includes amphetamine sulfate and all of its drug derivatives. (p. 205)

Analeptics Central nervous system stimulants that have effects on the brainstem and spinal cord, which produce an increase in responsiveness to external stimuli and stimulate respiration. (p. 211)

Anorexiants Drugs used to control or suppress appetite. (p. 207)

Attention deficit hyperactivity disorder (ADHD) A syndrome characterized by difficulty in maintaining concentration on a given task and/or hyperactive behavior; may affect children, adolescents, and adults. The term *attention deficit disorder (ADD)* has been absorbed under this broader term. (p. 204)

Cataplexy A condition characterized by abrupt attacks of muscular weakness and hypotonia triggered by an emotional stimulus such as joy, laughter, anger, fear, or surprise. (p. 204)

Central nervous system (CNS) stimulants Drugs that stimulate specific areas of the brain or spinal cord. (p. 204)

Ergot alkaloids Drugs that constrict blood vessels in the brain and provide relief of pain for certain migraine headaches. (p. 209)

Migraine A common type of recurring painful headache characterized by a pulsatile or throbbing quality, incapacitating pain, and photophobia. (p. 205)

Narcolepsy A syndrome characterized by sudden sleep attacks, *cataplexy,* sleep paralysis, and visual or auditory hallucinations at the onset of sleep. (p. 204)

Serotonin receptor agonists A class of CNS stimulants used to treat migraine headaches; they are often referred to as *selective serotonin receptor agonists* or *triptans.* (p. 209)

Sympathomimetic drugs CNS stimulants such as noradrenergic drugs whose actions resemble or mimic those of the sympathetic nervous system. (p. 204)

OVERVIEW

The central nervous system (CNS) is a very complex system in the human body. Many drugs either work in the CNS or cause adverse effects in the CNS. Activity of the CNS is regulated by a checks-and-balances system that consists of excitatory and inhibitory neurotransmitters and their corresponding receptors in the brain and spinal cord tissues. CNS stimulation results from either excessive stimulation of excitatory neurons or blockade of inhibitory neurons. Central nervous system (CNS) stimulants are a broad class of drugs that stimulate specific areas of the brain or spinal cord. Most CNS stimulant drugs act by stimulating the excitatory neurons in the brain. These neurons contain receptors for excitatory neurotransmitters, including dopamine (dopaminergic drugs), norepinephrine (adrenergic drugs), and serotonin (serotonergic drugs). Dopamine is a metabolic precursor of norepinephrine, which is also a neurotransmitter in the sympathetic nervous system. Actions of adrenergic drugs often resemble or mimic the actions of the sympathetic nervous system. For this reason, adrenergic drugs (and, to a lesser degree, dopaminergic drugs as well) are also called sympathomimetic drugs. Other sympathomimetic drugs are discussed further in Chapter 18.

CNS stimulant drugs are classified in three ways. The first is based on chemical structural similarities. Major chemical classes of CNS stimulants include amphetamines, serotonin agonists, sympathomimetics, and xanthines (Table 13-1). Second, they can be classified according to their site of action in the CNS (Table 13-2). Finally, they can be categorized according to their therapeutic usage (Table 13-3). These include anti–attention deficit, antinarcoleptic, anorexiant, antimigraine, and analeptic drugs. Anorexiants are drugs used to control obesity by suppression of appetite. Analeptics are drugs used for specific CNS stimulation in certain clinical situations. Some therapeutic overlap exists among these drug categories.

ATTENTION DEFICIT HYPERACTIVITY DISORDER

Attention deficit hyperactivity disorder (ADHD), formerly known as *attention deficit disorder (ADD)*, is the most common psychiatric disorder in children, affecting 4% to 10% of school-age children. Boys are affected two to nine times more often than girls, although the disorder may be underdiagnosed in girls. Primary symptoms of ADHD are inappropriate ability to maintain attention span and/or the presence of hyperactivity and impulsivity. The disorder may involve predominantly attention deficit, predominantly hyperactivity or impulsivity, or a combination of both. It usually begins before 7 years of age, sometimes earlier than 4 years of age. It can officially be diagnosed when symptoms last at least 6 months and occur in at least two different settings (e.g., home and school), according to the *Diagnostic and Statistical Manual of Mental Disorders (DSM-5)*. Many children outgrow ADHD, but adult ADHD is also common. Drug therapy for both childhood and adult ADHD is the same. There is some social controversy regarding possible overdiagnosis of, and overmedication for, this disorder.

NARCOLEPSY

Narcolepsy is an incurable neurologic condition in which patients unexpectedly fall asleep in the middle of normal daily activities. These "sleep attacks" are reported to cause car accidents or near-misses in 70% or more of patients. Cataplexy is an associated symptom in at least 70% of narcolepsy cases. It involves sudden acute skeletal muscle weakness. The condition

TABLE 13-1 Structurally Related CNS Stimulants

Chemical Category	CNS Stimulants and Related Drugs
Amphetamines and related stimulants	dextroamphetamine, methamphetamine, benzphetamine, methylphenidate, dexmethylphenidate
Serotonin agonists	almotriptan, eletriptan, frovatriptan, naratriptan, rizatriptan, sumatriptan, zolmitriptan
Sympathomimetics	phentermine
Xanthines	caffeine, theophylline, aminophylline
Miscellaneous	modafinil, armodafinil, orlistat (lipase inhibitor), doxapram (analeptic)

TABLE 13-2 CNS Stimulants: Site of Action

Primary Site of Action	CNS Stimulants
Cerebrovascular system, 5-HT$_{1D/1B}$ receptors	Serotonin agonists
Cerebral cortex	Amphetamines, phenidates, modafinil, armodafinil
Hypothalamic and limbic regions	Anorexiants
Medulla and brainstem	Analeptics

TABLE 13-3 CNS Stimulants and Related Drugs: Therapeutic Categories

Category	Drugs
Anti-ADHD	dextroamphetamine, lisdexamfetamine, methamphetamine, methylphenidate, atomoxetine (norepinephrine reuptake inhibitor)
Antinarcoleptic	dextroamphetamine, methamphetamine, methylphenidate, modafinil, armodafinil
Anorexiant	methamphetamine, phentermine, phendimetrazine, diethylpropion, benzphetamine, orlistat (lipase inhibitor), loracaserin
Antimigraine	almotriptan, eletriptan, frovatriptan, naratriptan, rizatriptan, sumatriptan, zolmitriptan (serotonin agonists); dihydroergotamine mesylate, ergotamine tartrate with caffeine (ergot alkaloids)
Analeptic	caffeine, doxapram, aminophylline, theophylline, modafinil, armodanafil (antinarcoleptic)

is often associated with strong emotions (e.g., joy, anger), and commonly the knees buckle and the individual falls to the floor while still awake. Men and women are equally affected, with approximately 100,000 cases in the United States. Roughly half of patients with narcolepsy experience migraine headaches as well.

OBESITY

According to the National Institutes of Health and the Centers for Disease Control and Prevention, approximately 30% of Americans are obese and nearly two thirds (64.5%) are overweight. This translates into more than 72 million obese adults, with a higher incidence of obesity among women and minorities. Obesity was formerly defined as being 20% or more above one's ideal body weight based on population statistics for height, body frame, and gender. More recent data are based on a measurement known as the body mass index (BMI), defined as weight in kilograms divided by height in meters squared (i.e., $BMI = weight\ [kg] \div [height\ (m)]^2$). *Overweight* is now defined as a BMI of 25 to 29.9, whereas *obesity* is now defined as a BMI of 30 or higher. Moreover, the incidence of obesity in young people 6 to 19 years of age has more than tripled since 1980. The pathophysiology of obesity is not fully understood, but calorie excess, disordered metabolism, and other factors are hypothesized. Obesity increases the risk for hypertension, dyslipidemia, coronary artery disease, stroke, type 2 diabetes mellitus, gallbladder disease, gout, osteoarthritis, sleep apnea, and certain types of cancer, including breast and colon cancer. An estimated 80% of diabetes risk in the United States can be attributed to excess weight. Some 112,000 deaths each year are linked to obesity. The related health care costs alone are currently estimated at more than $140 billion. Yet many people who attempt weight loss do so for cosmetic reasons rather than health reasons. Obese people are often stigmatized, at times even by the health care professionals treating them.

MIGRAINE

A migraine is a common type of recurring headache, usually lasting from 4 to 72 hours. Typical features include a pulsatile quality with pain that worsens with each pulse. The pain is most commonly unilateral but may occur on both sides of the head. Associated symptoms include nausea, vomiting, *photophobia* (avoidance of light), and *phonophobia* (avoidance of sounds). In addition, some migraines are accompanied by an *aura,* which is a predictive set of altered visual or other senses. However, the majority of migraines are without an aura. Migraines affect about 30 million people in the United States, with a reported incidence in females roughly three times that in males. Migraine headaches have been classified by the World Health Organization as one of the 19 most disabling diseases worldwide, with approximately 64 to 150 million workdays lost annually. Migraines commonly begin after 10 years of age and peak between the mid-twenties and early forties. They often fade after 50 years of age. Familial inheritance of migraine is well recognized. Precipitating factors include stress, hypoglycemia,

menses, endogenous estrogen (including oral contraceptives), exercise, and intake of alcohol, caffeine, cocaine, nitroglycerin, aspartame, and the food additive monosodium glutamate (MSG). Historically, there have been several theories regarding the cause of migraines, including the "vascular hypothesis" and the "neurovascular hypothesis." Most recent evidence points to decreased serotonin levels. Thus, the majority of current investigations involve drugs that can increase serotonin levels.

ANALEPTIC-RESPONSIVE RESPIRATORY DEPRESSION SYNDROMES

Neonatal apnea, or periodic cessation of breathing in newborn babies, is a common condition seen in about 25% of premature infants whose pulmonary and CNS structures, including the medullary centers that control breathing, have not completed their gestational development because of preterm birth. Infants undergoing prolonged mechanical ventilation, especially at high pressures, often develop a chronic lung disease known as *bronchopulmonary dysplasia,* for which caffeine can be helpful. *Postanesthetic respiratory depression* occurs when a patient's spontaneous respiratory drive does not resume adequately and in a timely manner after general anesthesia. Respiratory depression may also be secondary to abuse of some drugs. Hypercapnia, or elevated blood levels of carbon dioxide, is often associated with later stages of chronic obstructive pulmonary disease (COPD). Analeptic drugs such as theophylline, aminophylline, caffeine, and doxapram may be used to treat one or more of these conditions.

DRUGS FOR ATTENTION DEFICIT HYPERACTIVITY DISORDER AND NARCOLEPSY

CNS stimulants are the first-line drugs of choice for both ADHD and narcolepsy. They are potent drugs with a strong potential for tolerance and psychologic dependence (addiction; see Chapter 17), and as such they are classified as Schedule II drugs. Although there has been some public controversy regarding their use in ADHD, these drugs have led to a 65% to 75% improvement in symptoms in treated patients compared with a placebo. In general, CNS stimulants elevate mood, produce a sense of increased energy and alertness, decrease appetite, and enhance task performance impaired by fatigue or boredom. Two of the oldest known stimulants are cocaine and amphetamine, which are prototypical drugs for this class. Caffeine, contained in coffee and tea, is another plant-derived CNS stimulant.

Amphetamine sulfate was first synthesized in the late 1800s. Later derivatives of this drug, which are still used clinically, include its d-isomer dextroamphetamine sulfate, methamphetamine hydrochloride, and mixed amphetamine salts—salts of both amphetamine and dextroamphetamine. They are often collectively referred to simply as amphetamines. Methylphenidate, a synthetic amphetamine derivative, was first introduced for the treatment of hyperactivity in children in 1958 and is also a Schedule II drug. All of the amphetamine-related drugs are used to treat ADHD and/or narcolepsy. Nonamphetamine stimulants include pemoline and modafinil. Atomoxetine is a nonstimulant drug that is also used to treat ADHD. Atomoxetine is a norepinephrine reuptake inhibitor. Because it is not an amphetamine, it is associated with a low incidence of insomnia and has low abuse potential. Another advantage is that phone-in refills are allowed for this drug (as opposed to Schedule C-II drugs, which require a written prescription). One of the newest drugs in the ADHD arsenal is lisdexamfetamine (Vyvanse). It is a prodrug for dextroamphetamine, meaning it is converted in the body to dextroamphetamine. Lisdexamfetamine has the unique FDA-approved indication for the treatment of binge eating disorder.

Mechanism of Action and Drug Effects

Amphetamines stimulate areas of the brain associated with mental alertness, specifically the cerebral cortex and the thalamus. Pharmacologic actions of CNS stimulants are similar to the actions of the sympathetic nervous system, with the CNS and respiratory systems primarily affected. CNS effects include mood elevation or euphoria, increased mental alertness and capacity for work, decreased fatigue and drowsiness, and prolonged wakefulness. The respiratory effects most commonly seen are relaxation of bronchial smooth muscle, increased respiration, and dilation of pulmonary arteries.

The amphetamines and phenidates increase the effects of norepinephrine and dopamine in CNS synapses by increasing their release and blocking their reuptake. As a result, both neurotransmitters are in contact with their receptors longer, which lengthens their duration of action. Modafinil and armodafinil are also classified as an analeptic. It promotes wakefulness like the amphetamines and phenidates but lacks sympathomimetic properties and appears to work primarily by reducing gamma-aminobutyric acid (GABA)–mediated neurotransmission in the brain. GABA is the principal inhibitory neurotransmitter in the brain. The nonstimulant drug atomoxetine works in the CNS by selective inhibition of norepinephrine reuptake.

Indications

Various amphetamine derivatives, including methylphenidate, are currently used to treat both ADHD and narcolepsy. Dexmethylphenidate is currently indicated for ADHD alone. Amphetamine sulfate was used to treat obesity in the early to mid-twentieth century. However, the only amphetamines currently approved for this indication are benzphetamine and methamphetamine (see Anorexiants). The nonamphetamine stimulants modafinil and armodafinil are indicated for narcolepsy.

Specialists sometimes recommend periodic "drug holidays" (e.g., 1 day per week) without medication to diminish the addictive tendencies of the stimulant drugs. School-age children often do not take these drugs on weekends and school vacations.

Contraindications

Contraindications to the use of amphetamine and nonamphetamine stimulants include known drug allergy or cardiac structural abnormalities. These drugs can also exacerbate the following conditions: marked anxiety or agitation, Tourette's syndrome, hypertension, and glaucoma. The drugs must not be used in patients who have received therapy with any monoamine oxidase inhibitor (MAOI) in the preceding 14 days (see Chapter 16). Contraindications specific to atomoxetine include drug allergy, glaucoma, and recent MAOI use.

Adverse Effects

Both amphetamine and nonamphetamine stimulants have a wide range of adverse effects. These drugs tend to "speed up" body systems. For example, effects on the cardiovascular system include increased heart rate and blood pressure. Other adverse effects include angina, anxiety, insomnia, headache, tremor, blurred vision, increased metabolic rate (beneficial in treatment of obesity), gastrointestinal (GI) distress, dry mouth, and worsening of or new onset of psychiatric disorders, including mania, psychoses, or aggression. Common adverse effects associated with atomoxetine include headache, abdominal pain, vomiting, anorexia, and cough.

Interactions

Drug interactions associated with these drugs vary greatly from class to class. Table 13-4 summarizes some of the more common interactions for all drug classes in this chapter.

Dosages

For dosage information, see the table on p. 210.

DRUG PROFILES

AMPHETAMINES AND RELATED STIMULANTS

The principal drugs used to treat ADHD and narcolepsy are amphetamines and nonamphetamine stimulants. Atomoxetine, a nonstimulant drug, is also used for ADHD.

◆ amphetamines

Amphetamine is available in prescription form only for oral use, both as single-component dextroamphetamine sulfate (Dexedrine) and as a mixture of dextroamphetamine sulfate, dextroamphetamine saccharate, amphetamine sulfate, and amphetamine aspartate (Adderall, Adderall XR) and are used to treat ADHD and narcolepsy.

Pharmacokinetics: Dextroamphetamine

Route	Onset of Action	Peak Plasma Concentration	Elimination Half-life	Duration of Action
PO	30-60 min	90-120 min	7-14 hr	10 hr

atomoxetine

Atomoxetine (Strattera) is approved for treating ADHD in children older than 6 years of age and in adults. This medication is not a controlled substance because it lacks addictive properties, unlike amphetamines and phenidates. In September 2005, the FDA issued a warning describing cases of suicidal thinking and behavior in small numbers of adolescent patients receiving this medication.

TABLE 13-4 CNS Stimulants: Common Drug Interactions

Drug	Interacting Drugs	Mechanism	Result
Amphetamine and Nonamphetamine Stimulants			
Amphetamines (various salts) methylphenidate	CNS stimulants	Additive toxicities	Cardiovascular adverse effects, nervousness, insomnia
	MAOIs	Increased release of catecholamines	Headaches, dysrhythmias, severe hypertension
Atomoxetine	Sympathomimetic drugs	Enhanced SNS effects	Cardiovascular adverse effects
	CYP2D6 inhibitors (MAOIs, paroxetine)	Reduced metabolism of atomoxetine	Enhanced atomoxetine toxicity
Anorexiants and Analeptics			
phentermine	CNS stimulants	Additive toxicities	Nervousness, insomnia, dysrhythmias, seizures
	MAOIs	Increased release of catecholamines	Headaches, dysrhythmias, severe hypertension
	Serotonergic drugs	Additive toxicity	Cardiovascular adverse effects, nervousness, insomnia, convulsions
Serotonin Agonists			
sumatriptan and others	Ergot alkaloids, SSRIs, MAOIs	Additive toxicity	Cardiovascular adverse effects, nervousness, insomnia, convulsions
Ergot Alkaloids			
D.H.E.45, Caffergot	Protease inhibitors, azole antifungals, macrolide antibiotics	Increased ergot levels	Acute ergot toxicity; nausea, vomiting, hypotension or hypertension, seizures, coma, death; use with ergot alkaloids is contraindicated

CYP2D6, Cytochrome P-450 enzyme 2D6; *MAOIs,* monoamine oxidase inhibitors.

Pharmacokinetics: Atomoxetine

Route	Onset of Action	Peak Plasma Concentration	Elimination Half-life	Duration of Action
PO	60 min	1-2 hr	5-24 hr	24-120 hr

◆ methylphenidate

Methylphenidate (Ritalin) was the first prescription drug indicated for ADHD and is also used for narcolepsy. Extended-release dosage forms include Ritalin SR, Concerta, and Metadate CD.

Pharmacokinetics (Immediate Release): Methylphenidate

Route	Onset of Action	Peak Plasma Concentration	Elimination Half-life	Duration of Action
PO	30-60 min	6-8 hr	1-3 hr	4-6 hr

modafinil

Modafinil (Provigil) is indicated for improvement of wakefulness in patients with excessive daytime sleepiness associated with narcolepsy and also with *shift work sleep disorder*. It has less abuse potential than amphetamines and methylphenidate and is a Schedule IV drug. A related drug is armodafinil (Nuvigil), which is similar to modafinil.

Pharmacokinetics: Modafinil

Route	Onset of Action	Peak Plasma Concentration	Elimination Half-life	Duration of Action
PO	1-2 months*	2-4 hr	8-15 hr	Unknown

*Therapeutic effects.

ANOREXIANTS

By definition, an *anorexiant* is any substance that suppresses appetite. Anorexiants are CNS stimulant drugs used to promote weight loss in obesity; however, their effectiveness has not been proven. These drugs include phentermine (Ionamin), benzphetamine (Didrex), methamphetamine (Desoxyn), and diethylpropion (Tenuate). In 2010, sibutramine (Meridia) was withdrawn from the market due to safety concerns. Benzphetamine and methamphetamine are the only amphetamines currently approved for treating obesity.

Orlistat (Xenical) is a related nonstimulant drug used to treat obesity. It works locally in the small and large intestines, where it inhibits absorption of caloric intake from fatty foods. Several new drugs have been approved for the treatment of obesity including lorcaserin (Belviq), Qsymia (phentermine and topiramate), and Contrave ER (naltrexone and bupropion). In 2015, the FDA approved liraglutide (Saxenda). Liraglutide is also marketed under the name Victoza and is used for the treatment of diabetes.

Mechanism of Action and Drug Effects

Anorexiants are CNS stimulants that are believed to work by suppressing appetite control centers in the brain. Some evidence suggests that they also increase the body's basal metabolic rate, including mobilization of adipose tissue stores and enhanced cellular glucose uptake, as well as reduce dietary fat absorption.

There are some minor differences between these drugs in terms of their individual actions. Phentermine, diethylpropion, methamphetamine, and benzphetamine resemble amphetamine

CASE STUDY

Patient-Centered Care: Methylphenidate for Attention Deficit Hyperactivity Disorder

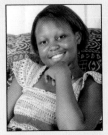

N., a 13-year-old girl, has been diagnosed with attention deficit hyperactivity disorder. She is in the seventh grade at a local middle school and plays the clarinet in the school's after-school band. Her parents have noticed that she has had trouble focusing on assignments and music practice for the last year and have discussed her problems with N.'s pediatrician. The physician has prescribed methylphenidate (Ritalin) 5 mg twice a day for 2 weeks, and then increasing the dose to 10 mg twice a day if no improvement is noted.

1. What are the therapeutic effects of methylphenidate?
2. After 3 weeks, N.'s mother calls the physician's office to say that N. has been doing better at school, as reported by her morning teacher, but the band teacher has reported that N. gets restless during after-school rehearsals. N.'s mother also reports that N. seems unable to get to sleep at night and has been staying up too late. What should the nurse suggest?
3. At the 2-month checkup, the physician suggests that N.'s mother hold the medication on weekends, giving the drug only during the weekdays while N. is at school. In addition, careful height and weight measurements are taken. What is the reason for this "drug holiday," as described by the physician? What is the purpose of the height and weight measurements?
4. When it is time for a refill, N.'s mother calls the pharmacy. However, the pharmacist tells her, "I can't refill this medication by phone. You will need to bring in a new prescription." What is the reason for this?

For answers, see http://evolve.elsevier.com/Lilley.

sulfate in their chemical structures and CNS effects. These drugs are classified as both anorexiants and adrenergic (sympathomimetic) drugs. However, all appear to suppress appetite centers in the CNS through dopamine- and norepinephrine-mediated pathways.

Orlistat differs from other antiobesity drugs in that it is not a CNS stimulant. It works by inhibiting the enzyme lipase. This results in reduced absorption of dietary fat from the intestinal tract and increased fat elimination in the feces. Lorcaserin (Belviq) is a serotonin 2C receptor agonist. Its exact mechanism of action is unknown.

Indications

Anorexiants are used for the treatment of obesity. However, their effects are often minimal without accompanying behavioral modifications involving diet and exercise. Current evidence-based guidelines for the treatment of obesity do not support the use of anorexiants as monotherapy. They are most commonly used in higher-risk patients. These include obese patients with a BMI of 30 or higher, or patients with a BMI of 27 who are also hypertensive or have high cholesterol or diabetes.

Contraindications

Contraindications to anorexiants include drug allergy, severe cardiovascular disease, uncontrolled hypertension, hyperthyroidism, glaucoma, mental agitation, history of drug abuse, eating disorders (e.g., anorexia, bulimia), and use of MAOIs (see Chapter 16) within the previous 14 days. Orlistat is contraindicated in cases of chronic malabsorption syndrome (e.g. Crohn's disease, colitis, short bowel syndrome) or cholestasis.

Adverse Effects

With the exception of diethylpropion, anorexiants may raise blood pressure and cause heart palpitations and even dysrhythmias at higher dosages. Ironically, at therapeutic dosages, they may actually reflexively slow the heart rate. Diethylpropion, however, has little cardiovascular activity. These drugs may also cause anxiety, agitation, dizziness, and headache. The most common adverse effects of orlistat include headache, upper respiratory tract infection (mechanism uncertain), and GI distress, including fecal incontinence and oily stools.

Interactions

See Table 13-4.

Dosages

For dosage information, see the table on p. 210.

DRUG PROFILES

Amphetamine salts are no longer used for treatment of obesity because of their high abuse potential. The nonstimulant drug orlistat, a lipase inhibitor, is available over the counter.

◆ phentermine

Phentermine (Ionamin) is a sympathomimetic anorexiant that is structurally related to amphetamines but with much lower abuse potential. It is classified as a Schedule IV drug. This drug is not to be confused with several other drugs that were recalled by the FDA in the late 1990s (fenfluramine/dexfenfluramine [Phen-Fen]) and in 2000 (phenylpropanolamine) because of case reports of various adverse cardiovascular and/or pulmonary effects.

orlistat

Orlistat (Xenical) is unrelated to other drugs in its category. Allī is an over-the-counter (OTC) version released in 2007. It works by binding to gastric and pancreatic enzymes called *lipases*. Blocking these enzymes reduces fat absorption by roughly 30%. Restricting dietary intake of fat to less than 30% of total calories can help reduce some of the GI adverse effects, which include oily spotting, flatulence, and fecal incontinence in 20% to 40% of patients. Decreases in serum concentrations of vitamins A, D, and E and beta carotene are seen as a result of the blocking of fat absorption. Supplementation with fat-soluble vitamins corrects this deficiency.

Pharmacokinetics: Orlistat

Route	Onset of Action	Peak Plasma Concentration	Elimination Half-life	Duration of Action
PO	3 mo*	6-8 hr	1-2 hr	Unknown

*Therapeutic effects.

ANTIMIGRAINE DRUGS

Serotonin receptor agonists, first introduced in the 1990s, have revolutionized the treatment of migraine headache. They work by stimulating serotonin receptors in the brain. They include sumatriptan (Imitrex), almotriptan (Axert), eletriptan (Relpax), naratriptan (Amerge), rizatriptan (Maxalt), zolmitriptan (Zomig), and frovatriptan (Frova). Collectively, these drugs are referred to as *triptans*. They are to be used cautiously in patients with severe cardiovascular disease. Historically, **ergot alkaloids** were the mainstay of treatment of migraine headaches but have been replaced by the triptans for first-line therapy.

Mechanism of Action and Drug Effects

The chemical name for serotonin is 5-hydroxytryptamine, or 5-HT. Physiologists have further identified two 5-HT receptor subtypes on which these drugs have their greatest effect: 5-HT_{1B} and 5-HT_{1D}. Triptans stimulate these receptors in cerebral arteries, causing vasoconstriction and reducing or eliminating headache symptoms. They also reduce the production of inflammatory neuropeptides. This is known as *abortive* drug therapy because it treats a headache that has already started. Ergot alkaloids constrict blood vessels in the brain. Although the cause of migraines is not fully understood, it is thought to be related to abnormal dilation of the blood vessels within the brain.

Indications

The triptan antimigraine drugs, also referred to as *selective serotonin receptor agonists (SSRAs)*, are indicated for abortive therapy of an acute migraine headache. Although they may be taken during aura symptoms in patients who have auras with their headaches, these drugs are not indicated for *preventive* migraine therapy. Preventive therapy is indicated if migraine attacks occur one or more days per week. A variety of drugs are used for preventive therapy and are discussed in more detail in other chapters. First-line drugs for preventive therapy include propranolol (see Chapter 19), amitriptyline (see Chapter 16), valproic acid, and topiramate (see Chapter 15). Second-line therapies include the ergot alkaloid dihydroergotamine mesylate (D.H.E. 45); nonsteroidal antiinflammatory drugs, including naproxen (see Chapter 44); calcium channel blockers; and angiotensin receptor blockers (see Chapter 22). In many cases, preventive drug therapy is sufficient to prevent a full-blown migraine. However, when prevention fails, treatment is needed and the triptans are the most commonly prescribed drug class. Another frequently used product as abortive therapy is a combination of acetaminophen or aspirin plus the barbiturate butalbital plus the analeptic caffeine, with or without codeine (Fioricet). In addition to potentiating the effects of the analgesics, caffeine can also enhance intestinal absorption of the ergot alkaloids and has a vasoconstricting effect, which can reduce cerebral blood flow to ease headache pain. Caffeine also has a diuretic effect, which may ultimately also reduce cerebral blood flow owing to reduced vascular volume secondary to enhanced urinary output.

Contraindications

Contraindications to triptans include drug allergy and the presence of serious cardiovascular disease, due to their vasoconstrictive potential. Contraindications to the use of ergot alkaloids include uncontrolled hypertension; cerebral, cardiac, or peripheral vascular disease; dysrhythmias; glaucoma; and coronary or ischemic heart disease.

Adverse Effects

Triptans have potential vasoconstrictor effects, including effects on the coronary circulation. Injectable dosage forms may cause local irritation at the site of injection. Other adverse effects include feelings of tingling, flushing (skin warmth and redness), and a congested feeling in the head or chest. Ergot alkaloids are associated with the adverse effects of nausea, vomiting, cold or clammy hands and feet, muscle pain, dizziness, numbness, a vague feeling of anxiety, a bitter or foul taste in the mouth or throat, and irritation of the nose (with the nasal spray dosage form). Overuse of abortive therapy may result in rebound headaches.

Interactions

See Table 13-4.

Dosages

For dosage information, see the table on the next page.

DRUG PROFILES

SEROTONIN RECEPTOR AGONISTS

Serotonin receptor agonists are used to treat migraine headache. They can produce relief from moderate to severe migraines within 2 hours in 70% to 80% of patients. They work by stimulating 5-HT_1 receptors in the brain and are sometimes referred to as *SSRAs* or *triptans*. They are available in a variety of formulations, including oral tablets, sublingual tablets, subcutaneous self-injections, and nasal sprays. Orally administered medications are not tolerated by some patients because of nausea and vomiting associated with migraines. Nonoral (including sublingual) forms are advantageous for this reason. They also often have a more rapid onset of action, producing relief in some patients in 10 to 15 minutes, compared with 1 to 2 hours for tablets taken orally. For dosage information, see the table on the next page.

◆ sumatriptan

Sumatriptan (Imitrex) was the original prototype drug for this class. As noted earlier, there are now seven triptans. Slight pharmacokinetic differences exist among some of these products, but their effects are comparable overall.

Pharmacokinetics: Sumatriptan

Route	Onset of Action	Peak Plasma Concentration	Elimination Half-life	Duration of Action
PO	0.5-1 hr	2.5 hr	2.5 hr	4 hr

ERGOT ALKALOIDS

Ergot alkaloids, such as ergotamine, are still used in the treatment and prevention of migraines, but not frequently.

EVIDENCE-BASED PRACTICE

First TENS Device for Migraine Prevention Approved

Review

More than 30 million people in the U.S. have 1 or more migraine headaches per year. Migraine headaches account for 64% of severe headaches in females and 43% in males. Currently, 1 in 6 women suffer from migraine headaches. The economic impact resulting from migraine-related loss of productive time in the U.S. workforce is more than $13 billion per year. The prevalence of migraine seems to be lower among African Americans and Asian Americans as compared to whites. The World Health Organization (WHO) estimates that migraine is 19th among all causes of years lived with disability. So with migraine headache being a common, disabling condition on the individual, health care services, and society, an effective nonpharmacologic approach to treating this health issue would be significant. The device is the first of its kind developed specifically for patient use prior to the onset of migraine pain. The device is a small, portable, battery-powered prescription device worn across the forehead with a self-adhesive electrode. An electric current is transmitted from the device to the skin and subsequently to underlying tissues stimulating the trigeminal nerve branches that are often associated with migraine headaches.

Type of Evidence

The FDA marketing approval of the first transcutaneous electrical nerve stimulation (TENS) device was based on a clinical study out of Belgian. The clinical study included 67 participants and a patient satisfaction study of 2313 Cefaly Technology device users in Belgium and France. The review conducted by the FDA was via the *de novo* or what is a premarket approval pathway for generally low- to moderate-risk medical devices that are not "substantially equivalent" to an already marketed device. The FDA also reviewed a study out of Belgium consisting of 67 people who were having at least two migraines per month and had ceased taking migraine medication up to 3 months prior to the trial. Results showed that, when compared to participants using a "dummy" device, those using the Cefaly unit reported significantly fewer days/month with migraines and using less migraine medication. As stated earlier, the Cefaly unit did not completely prevent migraines or reduce their intensity when they did occur. The patient satisfaction associated with the 2313 Cefaly users in France and Belgium was found to be at 53% with the treatment. No serious adverse effects were reported.

Link of Evidence to Nursing Practice

With the millions of people impacted by migraine headaches that may last for up to 72 hours and the accompanying symptoms of intense pain, nausea, vomiting, and sensitivity to light and sound, it is significant that a nonpharmacologic therapy has been made available to those who suffer (with these attacks). It is a significant step in the treatment of migraines and may be of help to patients who cannot tolerate current migraine prevention and/or treatment regimens. In fact, this is the first TENS device approved specifically for use prior to the onset of pain. Nurses may be involved in the teaching and application of these devices as well as conducting future research on the device's effectiveness and its impact on patients' quality of life.

Paddock, C. First device to prevent migraine headaches wins FDA approval. Medical News Today. MediLexicon, Intl. March 12, 2014. Available at http://www.medicalnewstoday.com/articles/273894.

DOSAGES

Selected CNS Stimulants and Related Drugs

Drug (Pregnancy Category)	Pharmacologic Class	Usual Dosage Range
◆amphetamine/dextroamphetamine (Adderall) (C)	CNS stimulant	**Pediatric 3-5 yr** PO: 2.5 mg/day, increased weekly until desired effect **Pediatric 6 yr and older and adult** PO: 5 mg once or twice daily, increased weekly until desired effect to a daily max of 40 mg
atomoxetine (Strattera) (C)	Selective norepinephrine reuptake inhibitor	**Pediatric (less than 70 kg)** PO: 0.5-1.2 mg/kg/day divided once or twice daily **Adult (70 kg or more)** PO: 40-100 mg/day divided once or twice daily
caffeine (B)	Xanthine cerebral stimulant	**Adult** PO: 300-400 mg IV: 500 mg **Premature infant** IV (caffeine citrate only): 20 mg/kg load followed by 5 mg/kg once daily
doxapram (Dopram) (B)	Respiratory stimulant (analeptic)	**Adult and pediatric older than 12 yr** IV: 0.5-1 mg/kg, may repeat up to 2 mg/kg Infusion of 1-2 mg/min for up to 2 hr
◆methylphenidate, extended release (Concerta) (C)	CNS stimulant	**Pediatric and adult** 18-72 mg/day in a single dose
◆methylphenidate (Ritalin) (C)	CNS stimulant	**Pediatric 6 yr and older** PO: 5 mg bid before breakfast and lunch and increased weekly until desired effect to max of 60 mg/day **Adult** PO: 20-60 mg/day divided bid-tid
◆methylphenidate, extended release (Ritalin-SR) (C)	CNS stimulant	**Pediatric and adult** 20-60 mg/day in a single dose

DOSAGES

Selected CNS Stimulants and Related Drugs—cont'd

Drug (Pregnancy Category)	Pharmacologic Class	Usual Dosage Range
modafinil (Provigil) (C)	CNS stimulant	**Adult** PO: 200 mg q AM; if second dose needed, give at noon
orlistat (Xenical, Alli) (B)	Lipase inhibitor	**Adult** PO: 120 mg tid with each meal containing fat
◆ sumatriptan (Imitrex) (C)	Serotonin receptor agonist	**Adult** PO: 25, 50, or 100 mg; can repeat after 2 hr (max 200 mg/day) Subcut: 4-6 mg; can repeat in 1 hr (max 2 injections/day) Nasal spray: 5, 10, or 20 mg; can repeat after 2 hr (max 40 mg/day)

Dihydroergotamine mesylate (D.H.E. 45) is available in injectable form and as a nasal spray (Migranal). Ergotamine tartrate with caffeine (Cafergot) is available in tablet form.

DRUGS FOR SPECIFIC RESPIRATORY DEPRESSION SYNDROMES: ANALEPTICS

Analeptics include doxapram (Dopram) and the methylxanthines aminophylline, theophylline, and caffeine. These drugs are sometimes used to treat neonatal and postoperative respiratory depression. Neonatal uses are more common.

Mechanism of Action and Drug Effects

Analeptics work by stimulating areas of the CNS that control respiration, mainly the medulla and spinal cord. Methylxanthine analeptics (caffeine, aminophylline, and theophylline) also inhibit the enzyme *phosphodiesterase.* This enzyme breaks down a substance called *cyclic adenosine monophosphate (cAMP).* When analeptics block this enzyme, cAMP accumulates. This results in relaxation of smooth muscle in the respiratory tract, dilation of pulmonary arterioles, and stimulation of the CNS in general. Aminophylline is a *prodrug,* and it is *hydrolyzed* to theophylline in the body. Theophylline, in turn, is metabolized to caffeine. Caffeine is inherently a stronger CNS stimulant, hence its popularity in coffee, tea, and soft drinks. It also helps to potentiate the effects of analgesics used for migraine therapy and has a diuretic effect. The stimulant effects of caffeine are attributed to its antagonism (blocking) of adenosine receptors in the brain, which is associated with sleep promotion. The mechanism of action of doxapram is similar to that of the methylxanthines, but it has a greater stimulant effect in the area of the brain that senses carbon dioxide content. When the carbon dioxide content of the blood is high, the respiratory center in the brain is stimulated to induce deeper and faster breathing in an attempt to exchange more carbon dioxide for inhaled oxygen.

Indications

Currently listed indications for analeptics include neonatal apnea, bronchopulmonary dysplasia, hypercapnia associated with COPD, postanesthetic respiratory depression, and respiratory depression secondary to drugs of abuse (e.g., opioids, alcohol, or barbiturates). In newborns, administration of caffeine is associated with less tachycardia, CNS stimulation, and feeding intolerance than administration of theophylline or aminophylline. The latter are also used to treat neonatal bradycardia and are infrequently used to treat asthma in older children and adults.

Contraindications

Contraindications to the use of analeptics include drug allergy, peptic ulcer disease (especially for caffeine), and serious cardiovascular conditions. Concurrent use of other phosphodiesterase-inhibiting drugs such as sildenafil (see Chapter 35) and similar drugs is also not recommended.

Doxapram use is contraindicated in newborns because of the benzyl alcohol contained in the injectable formulation of the drug. Benzyl alcohol is associated with *gasping syndrome* in infants and may also displace bilirubin into the blood from albumin binding sites in the circulation. This, in turn, could cause or worsen hyperbilirubinemia, a common condition in high-risk infants. Its use is also contraindicated in patients with epilepsy, allergy, head injury, cardiovascular impairment or severe hypertension, and stroke.

Adverse Effects

At higher dosages, analeptics stimulate the vagal, vasomotor, and respiratory centers of the medulla in the brainstem, as well as increasing blood flow to skeletal muscles. Vagal effects include stimulation of gastric secretions, diarrhea, and reflex tachycardia. Vasomotor effects include flushing (warmth, redness) and sweating of the skin. Respiratory effects include elevated respiratory rate (which is normally desired). Skeletal muscle effects include muscular tension and tremors. Neurologic effects include reduced deep tendon reflexes.

Interactions

See Table 13-4.

Dosages

For dosage information, see the table on p. 210.

DRUG PROFILES

Analeptic drugs include doxapram (Dopram), aminophylline, theophylline, and caffeine. The profiles for aminophylline and theophylline can be found in Chapter 37. The antinarcoleptic analeptic drugs modafinil and armodafinil were discussed earlier in the narcolepsy section of this chapter. For dosage information, see the table on p. 210.

TABLE 13-5 Caffeine-Containing Beverages and Drugs

Medication or Beverage	Amount of Caffeine
Nonprescription Medications	
Analgesics	
Anacin	32 mg/tab
Excedrin, Excedrin Aspirin-Free, Excedrin Migraine	65 mg/tab
Stimulants	
NoDoz Maximum Strength	100 mg/tab
Vivarin	200 mg/tab
Zantrex-3 (marketed as anorexiant)	200 mg/tab
Prescription Medications (for Migraines)	
Fioricet, Fiorinal	40 mg/tab
Esgic	40 mg/tab
Cafergot	10 mg/suppository
Beverages	
Coffee (brewed, instant)	80-150 mg/5-oz cup
Coffee (decaffeinated)	2-20 mg/5-oz cup
Tea (brewed)	30-75 mg/5-oz cup
Soft drinks	35-60 mg/12-oz cup
Cocoa	5-40 mg/5-oz cup
Supplemented water (Red Bull, Propel, Vitamin Water)	~50 mg/12-oz cup
Coffee-flavored or chocolate ice cream	30-45 mg/0.5-oz cup

caffeine

Caffeine is a CNS stimulant that can be found in OTC drugs (e.g., NoDoz) and combination prescription drugs (e.g., Fioricet, Fiorinal). It is also contained in many beverages and foods. A few of the many foods and drugs that contain caffeine are listed in Table 13-5. Caffeine is contraindicated in patients with a known hypersensitivity to it and is used with caution in patients who have a history of peptic ulcers or cardiac dysrhythmias or who have recently experienced a myocardial infarction. Caffeine is available in oral and injectable dosage forms.

Pharmacokinetics: Caffeine

Route	Onset of Action	Peak Plasma Concentration	Elimination Half-life	Duration of Action
PO	15-45 min	1 hr	3-4 hr	6 hr

There are two forms of intravenous caffeine: caffeine citrate and caffeine sodium benzoate. Caffeine citrate is recommended for neonatal apnea. Caffeine sodium benzoate is used for respiratory depression in adults only, because it contains the preservative benzyl alcohol.

doxapram

Doxapram (Dopram) is an analeptic that can be used in conjunction with supportive measures in cases of respiratory depression that involve anesthetics or drugs of abuse and in COPD-associated hypercapnia. Deep tendon reflexes, in addition to vital signs and heart rhythm, are monitored to prevent overdosage of this drug.

Pharmacokinetics: Doxapram

Route	Onset of Action	Peak Plasma Concentration	Elimination Half-life	Duration of Action
IV	Less than 30 sec	Less than 2 min	2-4 hr	5-12 min

NURSING PROCESS

ASSESSMENT

CNS stimulants are used for a variety of conditions and disorders. They have addictive potential, and so the following assessment data need to be collected before their use, regardless of indication: (1) a thorough medical history with attention to preexisting diseases or conditions, especially those of the cardiovascular, cerebrovascular, neurologic, renal, and liver systems; (2) past and current history of addictive or substance abuse behaviors; (3) complete medication profile with a listing of prescription, OTC, and herbal drugs and any use of alcohol, nicotine, and/or social or illegal drugs; and (4) a complete nutritional and dietary history. Assess all of these areas because of the mechanism of action of CNS stimulants, which increases pulse rate and blood pressure, and can lead to seizures, intracerebral bleeding, and toxicity (due to decreased drug metabolism and excretion). Stimulation of the respiratory system is actually desirable, and this action is beneficial in those patients suffering from CNS depression, such as postoperatively. Improvement of attention span is beneficial for those in need of the medication, but the possibility of adverse effects requires a thorough assessment to obtain baseline information. The anorexiant action may cause complications if the drugs are used or ordered inappropriately. When these drugs are taken for appetite suppression, assess and document baseline height, weight, and dietary intake. Measure vital signs with specific attention to blood pressure and pulse rate whenever these drugs are used.

To add to the thoroughness of the assessment, include in your nursing history the following information: inquiry about lifestyle, exercise, nutritional habits and patterns (e.g., a reduction in fat-soluble vitamins, history of any type of eating disorder), educational level, previous teaching and learning successes and failures, available support structures (e.g., family and friends), self-esteem, stress levels, mental status and mental health problems (drugs may exacerbate psychosis), presence of diabetes (diabetic patients need closer monitoring and tighter glucose control when taking stimulant medications due to increased glucogenolysis), and information related to contraindications, cautions, and drug interactions (see Table 13-4).

With *drugs used for the management of attention deficit hyperactivity disorder*, continuous and very cautious patient assessment is needed. For the pediatric patient, gather the following information during assessment: baseline weight, height, growth and development patterns, vital signs, complete blood cell counts (if ordered), cardiac assessment, baseline emotional/mental status, and sleep habits/patterns. Atypical behavior, loss of attention span, and history of social problems or problems in school are also important to assess and document before and during therapy for baseline comparison. For children with ADHD, parental support is important to the success of treatment, so a home assessment may be needed. Attention to and documentation of daily dietary intake before drug therapy is important because of the risk for drug-related weight loss. It is also important that the pediatric patient not experience too rapid or too much weight loss; a thorough nutritional and dietary assessment is needed.

Adult patients requiring these medications also need thorough assessment of baseline weight, height, and vital signs. Assess and document usual sleep habits and patterns so that sleep disturbances may be anticipated and managed appropriately. Cardiac assessment and determining any preexisting cardiac symptoms/disease is important because of the CNS stimulation. Blood pressure, pulse rate, heart sounds, and any history of chest pain or palpitations must be noted. Other data to gather during assessment include possible contraindications, cautions, and drug interactions (see previous discussion). Document findings, and note the patient's use of any prescription drugs, OTC drugs (e.g., nasal decongestants, which are also stimulants), and herbal preparations, specifically ginseng and caffeine (see the Safety: Herbal Therapies and Dietary Supplements box).

QSEN ✍ SAFETY: HERBAL THERAPIES AND DIETARY SUPPLEMENTS

Selected Herbal Compounds Used for Nervous System Stimulation

Common Name(s)	Uses	Possible Drug Interactions (Avoid Concurrent Use)
Ginkgo biloba, ginkgo	To enhance mental alertness; to improve memory or dementia	Warfarin, aspirin
Ginseng	To enhance impaired mental function and concentration	Drugs for diabetes that lower blood sugar (e.g., insulin, oral hypoglycemic drugs), monoamine oxidase inhibitors

The *serotonin agonists* commonly used in the treatment of migraines are not without adverse reactions, contraindications, cautions, and drug interactions (see earlier discussion). Include in your assessment a thorough cardiac history as well as measurement of blood pressure and pulse rate and rhythm. If a patient has a history of hypertension, there is risk for further increases in blood pressure to dangerous levels with use of these drugs, thus the need for careful assessment and documentation. In fact, generally these drugs are not prescribed for patients with migraines who also have coronary artery disease unless a thorough cardiac evaluation has been performed. Conduct a careful assessment to identify other drugs the patient is taking that might lead to significant drug interactions, such as ergot alkaloids, selective serotonin receptor inhibitors, and MAOIs. If serotonin agonists are taken within 2 weeks of the use of these drugs, there is high risk for additive toxicity. Such toxicity would

be manifested by nervousness, insomnia, cardiovascular complications, and convulsions (serotonin syndrome).

Ergot alkaloids also have cautions, contraindications, and drug interactions (see earlier discussion), which need to be assessed and documented. Obtain a history of the migraines and their pattern, exacerbating factors, measures that provide relief, and previous treatments with associated successes and failures. Success and failure with antimigraine drug therapy (i.e., serotonin agonists and ergot alkaloids) need to be assessed and documented.

An *analeptic*, such as *doxapram*, is used as a central respiratory stimulant; therefore, it is most likely to be used in a hospital setting, specifically in intensive care units or postanesthesia units. The same concerns regarding contraindications, cautions, and drug interactions exist for this drug as for all CNS stimulants, and even closer attention must be paid to vital signs, especially heart rate and rhythm, and blood pressure. Any elevations in blood pressure and pulse rate may put the patient at a higher risk for complications. Perform a thorough neurologic assessment with specific attention to any possibility of seizures. Assess baseline deep tendon reflexes, and document for comparative purposes.

▌NURSING DIAGNOSES

1. Decreased cardiac output related to adverse effects of CNS stimulants (e.g., palpitations and tachycardia)
2. Imbalanced nutrition, less than body requirements, related to adverse effects of CNS stimulants (e.g., amphetamines and anorexiants)
3. Chronic pain related to the experience of or a history of migraine headaches
4. Disturbed sleep pattern related to the action and adverse effects of CNS stimulants

▌PLANNING: OUTCOME IDENTIFICATION

1. Patient maintains normal ranges of blood pressure (120/80) and pulse rate (60 to 100) while remaining free from cardiac symptoms and adverse effects, such as palpitations and chest pain, which need to be reported to the prescriber immediately.
2. Patient's nutritional status remains intact with near-normal body weight and BMI during therapy.
3. Patient regains adequate comfort level with adequate and efficient management of migraines and a reported decrease in headaches, with improved quality of life and well-being and minimal adverse effects while taking medications as prescribed.
4. Patient experiences minimal disturbed sleep patterns and more restful sleep during drug therapy with use of nonpharmacologic measures such as massage, biofeedback, music therapy, and relaxation techniques

▌IMPLEMENTATION

With *drugs used for the treatment of attention deficit hyperactivity disorder,* some pediatric patients may respond better to certain dosage forms such as immediate release. However, dosing needs to be individualized and based on the patient's needs at different times during the school day (e.g., a noon dose to help with music lessons later in the afternoon). Well-planned scheduling of these medications and close communication among the school, teachers, school nurse, and the family and patient is very important to successful treatment. It is also important to time the dosing of medications—but as ordered—for periods in which symptom control is most needed but without causing alterations in sleep patterns. Generally speaking, once-a-day dosing is used with extended-release or long-acting preparations. Adequate and proper dosing will be manifested by good control of inattentive/impulsive behavior during school time. If extended-release dosage forms lead to acceptable outcomes for the pediatric patient, taking medications at school may not be necessary. Many times a stigma is associated with taking medications at school. This may be preventable with use of long-acting preparations or other scheduling. To help decrease the occurrence of insomnia, it is recommended that the last daily dose be taken 4 to 6 hours before bedtime, as ordered. During therapy, monitor the patient for continued physical growth, with specific attention to weight and height. The prescriber may order medication-free times on weekends, holidays, and/or vacations; that is, the drug may be discontinued periodically so that the need for the medication can be reassessed and sensitivity increased.

Because *anorexiants* are generally used for a short period of time, emphasize to the patient and all members of the patient's support system that a suitable diet, appropriate independent and/or supervised exercise program, and behavioral modifications are necessary to support a favorable result and to help the patient cease overeating and experience healthy weight loss. With a drug regimen, medications are usually taken first thing in the morning, as ordered, to minimize interference with sleep. Therefore, it is recommended that these drugs not be taken within 4 to 6 hours of sleep. If the patient has been taking these drugs for a prolonged period, an interval period of weaning before discontinuation is needed to avoid withdrawal symptoms and to avoid any chance of a rebound increase in appetite. Weights must be assessed weekly or as ordered. Encourage journal keeping so that patients can record food intake as well as responses to the drug regimen, any adverse effects, socialization, exercise, and notes about how they are feeling day to day. Dry mouth may be managed with frequent mouth care, use of sugar-free gum or hard candy, and use of oral care products indicated for dry mouth (available in mouth rinses, gel, spray, and lozenges). Sucking ice chips, as well as keeping a bottle of fresh water on hand at all times, may also be helpful. If headaches occur, acetaminophen will most likely be suggested. Caffeine in any form needs to be avoided including coffee, tea, sodas, and chocolate. Other products that may contain caffeine include some OTC analgesics; OTC compounds to treat menstrual symptoms; OTC products for cough, cold, flu, or congestion; and prescription drugs such as analgesics with ergotamine and caffeine, and butalbital with aspirin and caffeine. Supplementation with fat-soluble vitamins may be indicated with use of these drugs. It is also important to watch for tolerance to the anorexiant during the course of treatment. Other nursing considerations include emphasis on a holistic approach to treatment of obesity, including the possible use of hypnosis, biofeedback, and guided imagery, as ordered. Encourage patients to keep follow-up visits with their prescribers and others involved in their care.

SSRAs come in a variety of dosage forms. *Rizatriptan* is available in oral tablets as well as in a disintegrating tablet or wafer that dissolves on the tongue. The latter dosage form leads to a more rapid absorption. Use of the nasal spray or self-injectable forms of the serotonin agonists is especially desirable in patients experiencing the nausea and vomiting that may occur with migraine headaches. Self-injectable forms and nasal sprays also have the benefit of an onset of action of 10 to 15 minutes compared with 1 to 2 hours for tablet forms. Administration of a test dose of the injectable and all other dosage forms is usually recommended. If the injectable form is prescribed, provide instructions and demonstrations of the technique. See the Patient-Centered Care: Patient Teaching section later in the chapter for more information.

Ergot alkaloids are taken exactly as prescribed; for example, tablets need to be taken with 6 to 8 ounces of water or other fluid and work best when taken at the first sign of a migraine. This allows more successful treatment. With *ergotamine tartrate* and related drugs, the maximum dose is usually 6 tablets for a single headache and 10 tablets in any 7-day period. Dependence may occur with the ergots, and if they are withdrawn suddenly, rebound headaches may occur. Encourage the patient to report to the prescriber any headaches that are uncharacteristic or unusual, as well as any persistent headache, worsening of headaches, severe nausea, vomiting, dizziness, or restlessness. Any of the following also need to be reported immediately to the prescriber: slow, fast, or irregular heartbeat; tingling, pain, or coldness in the fingers or toes; loss of feeling in the fingers or toes; muscle pain or weakness; chest pain; severe stomach or abdominal pain; lower back pain; little or no urine. Emphasize that the patient must seek immediate medical attention if there is any chest pain, vision changes, confusion, or slurred speech. As mentioned earlier, these medications are not to be taken with triptans. Should medication therapy not prove helpful for migraines, the patient may be a candidate for use of the Cefaly unit which is the first TENS device for migraine prevention (see the Evidence-Based practice box). It is worn across the forehead and has a self-adhesive electrode.

The *analeptic doxapram* may be administered intravenously, but at different dosages depending on the purpose. (For dosage information, see the table on p. 210.) Give doxapram infusions using an intravenous pump, and closely monitor the patient. Because the patient's sensorium is generally diminished in this situation, place the patient in the Sims' or semi-Fowler's position to prevent aspiration. The patient's airway, breathing, and circulation (ABCs of care) are of highest priority. If adverse effects occur (see the pharmacology discussion), notify the prescriber.

Evaluation

Therapeutic responses to *drugs for attention deficit hyperactivity disorder* include decreased hyperactivity, increased attention span and concentration, improved behavior, and, for adults, increased effectiveness at work. Adverse effects range from loss of appetite to increased irritability, insomnia, palpitations, nausea, and headaches. Therapeutic effects of *anorexiants* include appetite control and weight loss for the treatment of obesity. Adverse effects of these drugs include dry mouth, headache, insomnia, constipation, tachycardia, cardiac irregularities, hypertension, changes in mental status or sensorium, changes in mood or affect, alteration of sleep patterns, and seizures (all due to excess CNS stimulation).

Evaluating for any increased irritability and withdrawal symptoms (e.g., headache, nausea vomiting) is also important. If the anorexiant affects fat metabolism, then there may be adverse effects such as flatulence with an oily discharge, spotting, and fecal urgency. The patient also needs to be closely evaluated for decreased levels of fat-soluble vitamins (A, D, E, and K), because their levels may be affected by the decreased absorption of fats. For *drugs used to treat narcolepsy*, therapeutic responses include a decrease in daytime sleepiness. Adverse effects for which to monitor include headache, nausea, nervousness, insomnia, and anxiety. Therapeutic responses to the *serotonin agonists* include aborting of migraine headache with improved daily functioning and performance because of the reduction in headaches. Adverse effects for which to monitor include pain at the injection site (if a self-injectable form is used; such pain is temporary), flushing, chest tightness or pressure, weakness, sedation, dizziness, sweating, increase in blood pressure and pulse rate, and bad taste with the nasal spray formulation, which may precipitate nausea.

QSEN ➤ **TEAMWORK AND COLLABORATION: LEGAL AND ETHICAL PRINCIPLES**

Handling of Prescription Drugs

It is important for the nurse to understand the following amendments to the federal laws that apply to the handling of all prescription drugs by the registered nurse. (NOTE: This is a summary and does not reflect the laws in their entirety.) The registered nurse is prohibited from doing the following:

• Compounding or dispensing the designated drugs for legal distribution and administration.
• Distributing the drugs to any individuals who are not licensed or authorized by federal or state law to receive the drugs (e.g., those outside the health care provider–patient relationship); the penalties for such actions are generally severe.
• Making, selling, keeping, or concealing any counterfeit drug equipment.
• Possessing any type of stimulant or depressant drug unless authorized to do so by a legal prescription (as a patient); any unauthorized possession is illegal.

It is important to adhere to these legal guidelines in the practice of drug administration to avoid legal penalties, including possible loss of license or other severe penalties.

PATIENT-CENTERED CARE: PATIENT TEACHING

General Information

• With any of the CNS stimulant medications, keep out of the reach of small children for safety concerns and with teenagers who may abuse or sell them.
• Serotonin agonists are to be taken as prescribed on a prn (as needed) basis at the onset of the migraine but within the frequency and dosage amount prescribed.
• Medications need to be taken exactly as prescribed without skipping, omitting, or adding doses.
• Alcohol, OTC cold products, cough syrups that contain alcohol, nicotine, and caffeine-containing food items and/or beverages must be avoided.
• Keeping a journal of daily activities and response to drug therapy and any adverse effects is encouraged. Medications or foods/beverages identified as triggers to a migraine may vary from person to person. Encourage the patient to track food/beverage intake as well as sleep habits and other practices/factors that may be identified as precipitators of migraines.
• Avoid any abrupt or sudden withdrawal of medications.

Drugs Used to Treat Attention Deficit Hyperactivity Disorder

• For maximal drug effects, medications are to be taken on an empty stomach 30 to 45 minutes before eating.

• Keeping all follow-up appointments is important to monitoring drug therapy.
• If the prescriber decides to discontinue the medication, a weaning process with careful supervision is recommended.
• Extended-release or long-acting preparations are to be taken in their original dosage form and only as directed. They are not to be crushed, chewed, broken, or altered in any way.
• Dosage amounts are not to be increased or decreased by the patient or family, because this may lead to drug-related complications. If there is any concern about the drug and its dosage amount or adverse effects, encourage parents or caregivers to contact the prescriber.

Anorexiants

• The patient must follow all prescriber instructions regarding medications, diet, and exercise.
• Some of these medications may impair alertness and the ability to think, so patients need to remain very cautious if engaging in activities that may be adversely affected until these impairments are resolved.
• An unpleasant taste of the medicine and/or dry mouth may be minimized by the use of mouth rinses, ice chips, sugarless chewing gum, and/or hard candies.

Antimigraine Drugs

- Encourage patients who experience migraines to avoid foods/beverages that are known triggers to severe or other forms of migraine headache.
- Other triggers for some individuals may include food additives, preservatives (including MSG, nitrates, and nitrites), artificial sweeteners (especially aspartame when used for extended periods of time), and chocolate.
- Before using a nasal spray dosage form of an antimigraine drug, instruct the patient to first gently blow the nose to clear the nasal passages. With the head upright, the patient then closes one nostril and inserts the nozzle into the open nostril. While a breath is taken through the nose, the spray is released. The nozzle is removed, and then the patient gently breathes in through the nose and out through the mouth for 10 to 20 seconds. Some bad taste may be experienced.
- Until migraine is resolved, the patient may find comfort by avoiding doing things that require alertness and rapid skilled movements. It may be helpful to keep the room darkened and noise to a minimum. If the headache is not resolved and/or vomiting occurs, the patient may need further medical attention to help avoid additional problems, such as dehydration.
- Encourage keeping a journal about the experience of all headaches, precipitators/relievers, and the rating of each headache on a scale of 0 to 10 (where 0 is no pain and 10 is the worst pain ever). Recording of other symptoms (e.g., photophobia, nausea, and vomiting) as well as their frequency and duration is recommended.

- When taking SSRAs, the patient must understand the importance of contacting the prescriber immediately if there are any problems with palpitations, chest pain, and/or pain or weakness in the extremities.
- Injectable forms of sumatriptan are to be given subcutaneously and as ordered. Have the patient practice administering injections (without the medication) with you at the prescriber's office so that proper technique is used and a moderate comfort level is achieved.
- Autoinjectors with prefilled syringes may be used. The syringe needs to be discarded in an appropriate container or receptacle after use and kept out of the reach of children.
- Administer no more than two injections of sumatriptan during a 24-hour period, and allow at least 1 hour between injections.
- When using injectable sumatriptan, contact the prescriber or emergency services immediately if there is swelling around the eyes, pain or tightness in the chest or throat, wheezing, and/or heart throbbing.
- Treatment for migraine headaches may relieve the pain and symptoms of a migraine attack as well as prevent further migraine attacks. Some abortive therapies, such as sumatriptan, may offer rapid relief if drugs are given as ordered and before the headache worsens. Drugs may be given orally, sublingually, or by subcutaneous injection in the thigh. When a triptan does not work, an ergot alkaloid (e.g., dihydroergotamine or ergotamine tartrate) may be ordered but is not to be used concurrently. Other drugs that may also be used to try to prevent migraine headache include antidepressants, antiseizure medications, and beta blockers.

KEY POINTS

- CNS stimulants are drugs that stimulate the brain or spinal cord.
- The actions of these stimulants mimic those of the neurotransmitters of the sympathetic nervous system (e.g., norepinephrine, dopamine, and serotonin).
- Included in the family of CNS stimulants are amphetamines, analeptics, and anorexiants with therapeutic uses for attention deficit hyperactivity disorder, narcolepsy, and appetite control. Adverse effects associated with CNS stimulants include changes in mental status or sensorium, changes in mood or affect, tachycardia, loss of appetite, nausea, altered sleep patterns (e.g., insomnia), physical dependency, irritability, and seizures.
- Serotonin agonists may be administered as a subcutaneous injection, as a nasal spray, and as oral tablets. Any chest pain or tightness, tremors, vomiting, or worsening symptoms needs to be reported to the prescriber immediately.

- Anorexiants control or suppress appetite. They are used to stimulate the CNS and result in suppression of appetite control centers in the brain.
- Contraindications to the use of anorexiants, as well as other CNS stimulants, include hypersensitivity, seizure activity, convulsive disorders, and liver dysfunction.
- The SSRAs are a newer class of CNS stimulants and are used to treat migraine headaches. They are not to be given to patients with coronary heart disease.
- Amphetamines elevate mood or produce euphoria, increase mental alertness and capacity for work, decrease fatigue and drowsiness, and prolong wakefulness.
- Journaling is helpful in evaluating the effects of all drugs used to treat attention deficit hyperactivity disorder, obesity, migraines, and narcolepsy.

NCLEX® EXAMINATION REVIEW QUESTIONS

1. A patient with narcolepsy will begin treatment with a CNS stimulant. The nurse expects to see which adverse effect?
   a. Bradycardia
   b. Nervousness
   c. Mental clouding
   d. Drowsiness at night

2. A patient at a weight management clinic who was given a prescription for orlistat (Xenical) calls the clinic hotline complaining of a "terrible side effect." The nurse suspects that the patient is referring to which problem?
   a. Nausea
   b. Sexual dysfunction
   c. Urinary incontinence
   d. Fecal incontinence

3. The nurse is developing a plan of care for a patient receiving an anorexiant. Which nursing diagnosis is most appropriate?
   a. Deficient fluid volume
   b. Sleep deprivation
   c. Impaired memory
   d. Imbalanced nutrition, less than body requirements

4. A patient has a new prescription for sumatriptan (Imitrex). The nurse providing patient teaching on self-administration will include which information?
   a. Correct technique for intramuscular injections
   b. Take the medication before the headache worsens.
   c. Allow at least 30 minutes between injections.
   d. Take no more than 4 doses in a 24-hour period.

5. The nurse is reviewing the history of a patient who will be starting the triptan sumatriptan (Imitrex) as part of treatment for migraine headaches. Which condition, if present, may be a contraindication to triptan therapy?

   a. Cardiovascular disease
   b. Chronic bronchitis
   c. History of renal calculi
   d. Diabetes mellitus type 2

6. The nurse is reviewing medication therapy with the parents of an adolescent with ADHD. Which statement is correct? *(Select all that apply.)*
   a. "Be sure to have your child blow his nose before administering the nasal spray."
   b. "This medication is used only when symptoms of ADHD are severe."
   c. "The last dose should be taken 4 to 6 hours before bedtime to avoid interference with sleep."
   d. "Be sure to contact the physician right away if you notice expression of suicidal thoughts."
   e. "We will need to check your child's height and weight periodically to monitor physical growth."
   f. "If adverse effects become severe, stop the medication for 3 to 4 days."

7. The medication order reads: "Atomoxetine (Strattera) 1.2 mg/kg/day in 2 divided doses." The child weighs 66 lbs. How much will be given with each dose?

8. A patient with narcolepsy is having problems with excessive daytime sleepiness. The nurse expects which drug to be prescribed to improve the patient's wakefulness?
   a. phentermine (Ionamin)
   b. almotriptan (Axert)
   c. modafinil (Provigil)
   d. methylphenidate (Ritalin)

1. b, 2. d, 3. d, 4. b, 5. a, 6. c, d, e, 7. 18 mg per dose, 8. c

CRITICAL THINKING AND PRIORITIZATION QUESTIONS

1. The parents of a 10-year-old boy are concerned about the effects of the medication their son is taking for ADHD. They ask, "What should we be looking for when he starts this medicine?" What is the nurse's best response?

2. A patient calls the headache clinic because she is unhappy about her medication. She says, "I've been taking zolmitriptan

(Zomig) to prevent headaches, but I am still having them." What is the nurse's priority action at this time?

For answers, see *http://evolve.elsevier.com/Lilley*.

ⓔ EVOLVE WEBSITE

http://evolve.elsevier.com/Lilley
- Animations
- Answer Keys for Textbook Case Studies and Textbook Critical Thinking and Prioritization Questions

- Content Updates
- Key Points
- Review Questions
- Student Case Studies

Antiepileptic Drugs

http://evolve.elsevier.com/Lilley

OBJECTIVES

When you reach the end of this chapter, you will be able to do the following:

1. Briefly describe the pathophysiology of epilepsy.
2. Discuss the rationale for the use of the various classes of antiepileptic drugs (AEDs) in the management of the different forms of epilepsy.
3. Identify the various drugs in each of the following drug classes: iminostilbenes, benzodiazepines, barbiturates, hydantoins, and miscellaneous drugs.
4. Identify the mechanisms of action, indications, cautions, contraindications, dosages, routes of administration, adverse effects, toxic effects, therapeutic blood levels, and drug interactions for each antiepileptic drug.
5. Develop a nursing care plan, including patient education, based on the nursing process for patients receiving AEDs.

DRUG PROFILES

♦ carbamazepine, p. 226
ethosuximide, p. 226
♦ gabapentin, p. 227
lamotrigine, p. 227
levetiracetam, p. 227
oxcarbazepine, p. 226
♦ phenobarbital and ♦ primidone, p. 224
♦ ! phenytoin and ♦ fosphenytoin, p. 225

pregabalin, p. 227
tiagabine, p. 227
topiramate, p. 228
♦ valproic acid, p. 228

___

♦ = *Key drug*
! = *High-alert drug*

KEY TERMS

Anticonvulsants Substances that prevent or reduce the severity of *epileptic* or other *convulsive* seizures. (p. 220)

Antiepileptic drugs Prescription drugs that prevent or reduce the severity of epilepsy and different types of epileptic seizures, not just convulsive seizures. (p. 220)

Autoinduction A metabolic process in which a drug stimulates the production of enzymes that enhance its own metabolism, which leads to a reduction in drug concentrations. (p. 226)

Convulsion A type of seizure involving excessive stimulation of neurons in the brain and characterized by the spasmodic contraction of voluntary muscles. (See also *seizure.*) (p. 219)

Electroencephalogram (EEG) A recording of the electrical activity that arises from spontaneous currents in nerve cells in the brain. (p. 219)

Epilepsy A general term for any of a group of neurologic disorders characterized by *recurrent* episodes of *convulsive seizures*, sensory disturbances, abnormal behavior, loss of consciousness, or any combination of these. (p. 219)

Generalized onset seizures Seizures originating simultaneously in both cerebral hemispheres. (p. 219)

Gingival hyperplasia Overgrowth of gum tissue and often a side effect of phenytoin. (p. 225)

Partial onset seizures Seizures originating in a more localized region of the brain (also called *focal* seizures). (p. 219)

Primary epilepsy Epilepsy in which there is no identifiable cause. Also known as *idiopathic*. (p. 219)

Seizure Excessive stimulation of neurons in the brain leading to a sudden burst of abnormal neuron activity that results in temporary changes in brain function, primarily affecting sensory and motor activity. (p. 219)

Status epilepticus A seizure disorder characterized by generalized tonic-clonic convulsions that occur repeatedly; considered a true medical emergency. (p. 220)

Tonic-clonic seizures Seizures involving initial muscular contraction throughout the body (tonic phase), progressing to alternating contraction and relaxation (clonic phase). (p. 219)

EPILEPSY

Epilepsy is a syndrome of central nervous system (CNS) dysfunction that can cause symptoms ranging from momentary sensory disturbances to convulsive seizures. It is the most common chronic neurologic illness, affecting 3 million people in the United States and 50 million people worldwide. It results from excessive electrical activity of neurons (nerve cells) located in the superficial area of the brain known as the *cerebral cortex* or *gray matter*. The terms *seizure, convulsion,* and *epilepsy* are often used interchangeably, but they do not have the same meaning. A seizure is a brief episode of abnormal electrical activity in the nerve cells of the brain, which may or may not lead to a convulsion. A convulsion is a more severe seizure characterized by involuntary spasmodic contractions of any or all voluntary muscles throughout the body. Commonly reported symptoms include abnormal motor function, loss of consciousness, altered sensory awareness, and psychic changes. In contrast, epilepsy is a chronic, recurrent pattern of seizures. Excessive electrical discharges can often be detected by an electroencephalogram (EEG), which is obtained to help diagnose epilepsy. Up to 50% of patients with epilepsy have normal EEGs; therefore a careful history is very important for accurate diagnosis. Other applicable diagnostic tests include skull radiography, *computed tomography,* and *magnetic resonance imaging.* These procedures help to rule out structural causes of epilepsy, such as brain tumors.

Epilepsy occurs most commonly in children and older adults. Epilepsy without an identifiable cause is known as primary epilepsy or *idiopathic* epilepsy. Primary epilepsy accounts for roughly 50% of cases. Evidence indicates genetic predispositions. Studies in the field of *pharmacogenomics* (see Chapter 8) are beginning to clarify genetic factors that can help optimize antiepileptic drug therapy.

Secondary or *symptomatic* epilepsy has a distinct cause, such as trauma, infection, cerebrovascular disorder, or other illness. In children and infants, the chief causes of secondary epilepsy are developmental defects, metabolic disease, and injury at birth. *Febrile seizures* occur in children 6 months to 5 years of age, and by definition are caused by fever. Children usually outgrow these seizures and thus febrile seizures do not constitute a chronic illness. Antipyretic drugs (e.g., acetaminophen) are normally adequate for acute treatment. In adults, acquired brain disorder is the major cause of secondary epilepsy. Examples include head injury, disease or infection of the brain and spinal cord, stroke, metabolic disorders, adverse drug reactions (e.g., meperidine [see Chapter 10], theophylline [see Chapter 37]), brain tumor, or other nonspecific neurologic diseases. Older adults have the highest incidence of new-onset epilepsy, and seizures are often well controlled with drug therapy.

Seizures are classified into different categories based on their presenting features. There are three major categories: *partial onset, generalized onset,* and *unclassified* seizures (Box 14-1). Generalized onset seizures, formerly called *grand mal* seizures, are characterized by neuronal activity that originates simultaneously in the gray matter of both hemispheres. There are several

---

BOX 14-1   Classification of Seizures

Partial Seizures

Short alterations in consciousness, repetitive unusual movements (chewing or swallowing movements), psychologic changes, and confusion

Simple Seizures
- No impaired consciousness
- Motor symptoms (most commonly related to the face, arm, or leg)
- Hallucinations of sight, hearing, or taste along with somatosensory changes (tingling)
- Autonomic nervous system responses
- Personality changes

Complex Seizures
- Impaired consciousness
- Memory impairment
- Behavioral effects
- Purposeless behaviors
- Aura, chewing and swallowing movements, unreal feelings, and bizarre behavior
- Tonic, clonic, or tonic-clonic seizures

Generalized Seizures

Most often seen in children and commonly characterized by temporary lapses in consciousness lasting a few seconds. Staring off into space, daydreaming, and inattentive look are common symptoms. Patients may exhibit rhythmic movements of their eyes, head, or hands but do not experience convulsions. Patients may have several attacks per day.
- Both cerebral hemispheres involved
- Tonic, clonic, myoclonic, atonic, or tonic-clonic seizures and infantile spasms possible
- Brief loss of consciousness for a few seconds with no confusion
- Head drop or falling-down symptoms

Unclassified Seizures

Seizures that are not officially classified due to inadequate data, as well as seizures that do not fit into the above categories. These include neonatal seizures such as those manifested by rhythmic eye movements, chewing, and swimming movements.

---

subtypes of generalized seizures. Tonic-clonic seizures begin with muscular contraction throughout the body (tonic phase) and progress to alternating contraction and relaxation (clonic phase). *Tonic* seizures involve spasms of the upper trunk with flexion of the arms. *Clonic* seizures are the same as tonic-clonic seizures but without the tonic phase. *Atonic* seizures, also known as *drop attacks,* involve sudden global muscle weakness and syncope. *Myoclonic* seizures are characterized by brief muscular jerks, but not as extreme as in other subtypes. Finally, *absence* seizures involve a brief loss of awareness that commonly occurs with repetitive spasmodic eye blinking for up to 30 seconds. This type occurs primarily in childhood and rarely after 14 years of age.

Partial onset seizures originate in a localized or *focal* region (e.g., one lobe) of the brain. There are three types of partial onset seizures. *Simple partial onset seizure,* formerly called *petit mal* seizure, is characterized by brief loss of awareness (e.g., blank stare) but without loss of consciousness or spasmodic eye blinking. In *complex partial onset seizure,* the level of consciousness is reduced but is not completely lost. Partial onset seizures can progress to generalized tonic-clonic seizures in up to 40% of patients. This third type is known as a *secondary generalized tonic-clonic seizure.* The latter two types are also associated with *postictal confusion,* a term for the confused mental state that follows seizure activity. *Unclassified seizures* are those that do not clearly fit into any of the other categories.

Seizure episodes can start off as partial and then become generalized. If the partial component is not noticed, the patient may be misdiagnosed and receive suboptimal drug therapy. Another important seizure condition is status epilepticus. In status epilepticus, multiple seizures occur with no recovery between them. If appropriate therapy is not started promptly, hypotension, hypoxia, brain damage, and death can quickly ensue. Thus, status epilepticus is considered a true medical emergency (see Table 14-3 for drugs used to treat status epilepticus).

ANTIEPILEPTIC DRUGS

Antiepileptic drugs are also called *anticonvulsants.* Antiepileptic drugs is a more appropriate term, because many of these medications are indicated for the management of all types of epilepsy, and not necessarily just convulsions. Anticonvulsants, on the other hand, are medications that are used to prevent the *convulsive* seizures typically associated with epilepsy.

The goal of antiepileptic drug therapy is to control or prevent seizures while maintaining a reasonable quality of life. Approximately 70% of patients can expect to become seizure free while taking only one drug. The remaining 30% of cases are more complicated, and often require multiple medications. Antiepileptic drugs have many adverse effects, and it is often difficult to achieve seizure control while avoiding adverse effects. In most cases, the therapeutic goal is not to eliminate seizure activity but rather to maximally reduce the incidence of seizures while minimizing drug-induced toxicity. Many patients must take these drugs for their entire lives; however, the majority of pediatric and adult epilepsy patients who have been seizure free for 1 to 2 years while taking antiepileptic drugs can eventually stop taking them with medical supervision. Abrupt discontinuation of these drugs can result in withdrawal seizures.

In both children and adults, there is only a 40% chance of recurrence after the first partial or generalized seizure. Therefore, antiepileptic drug therapy is *not* recommended after a single isolated seizure event. There are numerous antiepileptic drugs available. To optimize drug selection, neurologists must consider the known efficacy of a drug for a certain type of seizure, the adverse effects and drug interaction profile, the cost, ease of use, and the availability of pediatric dosage forms. Many antiepileptic drugs are also used to treat other types of illnesses, including psychiatric disorders (see Chapter 16), migraine headaches (see Chapter 13), and neuropathic pain syndromes (see Chapter 10).

Single-drug therapy must fail before multidrug therapy is attempted. Patients are normally started on a single antiepileptic drug, and the dosage is slowly increased until the seizures are controlled or until clinical toxicity occurs. If the first antiepileptic drug is not effective, the drug is tapered slowly while a second drug is introduced. Antiepileptic drugs are never to be stopped abruptly unless a severe adverse effect occurs.

Therapeutic drug monitoring (see Chapter 2) of serum drug concentrations provides a useful guideline in assessing the effectiveness of and adherence to therapy. For example, if a patient has a very low serum level, it may mean the patient is not taking the medication as prescribed. This gives the nurse an opportunity to ask about why the patient may not be taking the medication. If the level is above normal, the nurse needs to contact the prescriber before giving the next dose. Maintaining serum drug levels within therapeutic ranges helps not only to control seizures but also to reduce adverse effects. There are established normal therapeutic ranges for many antiepileptic drugs, but these are only guidelines (see Table 14-6). The serum concentrations of phenytoin, phenobarbital, carbamazepine, and primidone correlate better with seizure control and toxicity than do those of valproic acid, ethosuximide, and clonazepam. Each patient must be monitored and dosed based on the individual case. In many patients, maintenance is successful at levels below or above the usual therapeutic range. The goal is to slowly titrate to the lowest effective serum drug level that controls the seizure disorder. This reduces the risk for adverse drug effects and drug interactions. Successful control of a seizure disorder hinges on selection of the appropriate drug class and drug dosage, avoidance of drug toxicity, and patient compliance with the treatment regimen.

Antiepileptic drugs traditionally used to manage seizure disorders include barbiturates, hydantoins, and iminostilbenes, plus valproic acid. Second- and third-generation antiepileptics are also available (Table 14-1) and tend to have fewer adverse effects and drug interactions than the original drugs. This may benefit older adults, who are more likely to be taking multiple medications and, therefore, are more prone to drug interactions. However, there is currently debate in the literature as to whether patients actually benefit more from newer drugs.

Many of the antiepileptic drugs are available in generic forms. All generic drug manufacturers are required to provide research data that demonstrate *bioequivalency* of their generic drugs to the corresponding original brand-name drugs (see Chapter 2). Despite these requirements, the American Academy of Neurology and the American Epilepsy Society are concerned that generic drug products may be less clinically efficacious than brand-name drug products. Of particular concern is the common requirement of health insurance companies that patients receive generic drugs when available. Increased monitoring of patients is necessary when switching from brand-name products to generics.

Mechanism of Action and Drug Effects

As with many classes of drugs, the exact mechanism of action of the antiepileptic drugs is not known with certainty. However, evidence indicates that they alter the movement of sodium, potassium, calcium, and magnesium ions. The changes in the movement of these ions result in more stabilized and less excitable cell membranes.

TABLE 14-1 Currently Available Antiepileptic Drugs

Generic Name	Trade Name	Route
Traditional Antiepileptic Drugs		
Barbiturates		
phenobarbital	Generic	PO, IV
primidone	Mysoline	PO
Hydantoins		
phenytoin	Dilantin	PO, IV
fosphenytoin	Cerebyx	IV, IM
Iminostilbenes		
carbamazepine	Tegretol, Carbatrol	PO
oxcarbazepine	Trileptal	PO
Miscellaneous Antiepileptic Drugs		
ezogabine	Potiga	PO
eslicarbazepine	Aptiom	PO
gabapentin	Neurontin	PO
lacosamide	Vimpat	PO, IV
lamotrigine	Lamictal	PO
levetiracetam	Keppra	PO
pregabalin	Lyrica	PO
permapanel	Fycompa	PO
tiagabine	Gabitril	PO
topiramate	Topamax	PO
valproic acid	Depakene, Depakote	PO
	Depacon	IV
zonisamide	Zonegran	PO
vigabatrin	Sabril	PO

PATIENT-CENTERED CARE: LIFESPAN CONSIDERATIONS FOR THE PEDIATRIC PATIENT   [QSEN]

Antiepileptic Drugs

- If a skin rash develops in a child or infant taking phenytoin, discontinue the drug immediately and notify the prescriber.
- Chewable dosage forms of antiepileptic drugs are not recommended for once-a-day administration. Intramuscular injections of barbiturates or phenytoin must never be used.
- Encourage family members, parents, significant others, or caregivers to keep a journal with a record of the signs and symptoms before, during, and after a seizure and before, during, and after treatment with an antiepileptic drug.
- Encourage the wearing of a medical alert bracelet or necklace at all times with information about the diagnosis, drug therapy, and any drug allergies.
- Shake suspension dosage forms thoroughly before use. A graduated device or oral syringe may be used for more accurate dosing of this liquid.
- Pediatric patients are more sensitive to barbiturates and may respond to lower than expected dosages. They may also experience more profound central nervous system depressive effects related to the antiepileptic drug or show depression, confusion, or excitement (a paradoxical reaction).
- Any excessive sedation, confusion, lethargy, hypotension, bradypnea, tachycardia, and/or decreased movement in pediatric patients taking any antiepileptic drug must be reported to the prescriber immediately.
- Carbamazepine may be given with meals to reduce the risk for gastrointestinal distress. All suspension forms are to be shaken and mixed thoroughly before use.
- Oral forms of valproic acid are not to be given with milk, because this may cause the drug to dissolve early and irritate the mucosa. Carbonated beverages must also be avoided.

The major pharmacologic effects of antiepileptics are three-fold. First, they *increase the threshold* of activity in the *motor cortex.* In other words, they make it more difficult for a nerve to be excited, or they reduce the nerve's response to incoming electrical or chemical stimulation. Second, they act to *limit the spread* of a seizure discharge from its origin, by suppressing the transmission of impulses from one nerve to the next. Third, they can *decrease the speed* of nerve impulse conduction within a given neuron. Some drugs work by enhancing the effects of the inhibitory neurotransmitter gamma-aminobutyric acid (GABA), which plays a role in regulating neuron excitability in the brain.

Low levels of GABA are associated with seizures. Many antiepileptic drugs increase GABA levels to the normal range, and thus reduce the potential for seizures. Regardless of the mechanism, the overall effect is that antiepileptics stabilize neurons and keep them from becoming hyperexcited and generating excessive nerve impulses to adjacent neurons.

Indications

Antiepileptic drugs are used to prevent or control seizure activity. As evidenced by the wide range of seizure disorders listed in Box 14-1, epilepsy is a very diverse disorder. As a result, specific indications vary among drugs. The most recent indications are noted in Table 14-2, in the dosages table on p. 225, and in specific drug profiles. It is important to have an accurate diagnosis of the seizure type, because some drugs may not be ideal for specific seizures. For example, it is known that carbamazepine may worsen myoclonic or absence seizures. Specific antiepileptic drugs and the seizure disorders they are used to treat are listed in Table 14-2.

Antiepileptics are used for the long-term maintenance treatment of epilepsy. However, they are also useful for the acute treatment of status epilepticus. In this case, diazepam or lorazepam are considered to be the drugs of choice. Other commonly used drugs in status epilepticus are listed in Table 14-3. Once status epilepticus is controlled, long-term drug therapy is begun with other drugs for the prevention of future seizures. Patients who undergo brain surgery or who have experienced severe head injuries may receive prophylactic antiepileptic therapy.

Contraindications

The only usual contraindication to antiepileptics is known drug allergy. Pregnancy is also a contraindication; however, the prescriber must consider the risks to mother and infant of untreated maternal epilepsy. Many women take antiepileptics throughout their pregnancy. The newer-generation antiepileptic drugs appear to be safer in pregnancy than the traditional drugs.

TABLE 14-2 Common Seizure Indications for Antiepileptic Drugs

Partial	Secondary General	Generalized Tonic-Clonic	Absence	Myoclonic
carbamazepine	carbamazepine	carbamazepine	ethosuximide	clonazepam
clonazepam	clonazepam	clonazepam	lamotrigine	lamotrigine
clorazepate	fosphenytoin	fosphenytoin	valproic acid	valproic acid
fosphenytoin	gabapentin	lamotrigine	zonisamide	zonisamide
gabapentin	lamotrigine	phenobarbital		
lamotrigine	levetiracetam	phenytoin		
levetiracetam	oxcarbazepine	primidone		
oxcarbazepine	phenobarbital	topiramate		
phenobarbital	phenytoin	valproic acid		
phenytoin	primidone	zonisamide		
pregabalin	tiagabine			
primidone	topiramate			
tiagabine	zonisamide			
topiramate				
zonisamide				

TABLE 14-3 Antiepileptic Drugs Used to Treat Status Epilepticus

Drug	IV Dose	Onset	Duration	Half-Life	Adverse Effects
diazepam	5-30 mg	Immediate	15-60 min	20-50 hr	Apnea, hypotension, somnolence
fosphenytoin	15-20 phenytoin equivalents/kg	15-30 min	12-24 hr	10-60 hr	Comparable to those for phenytoin (see below)
lorazepam*	4 mg	5 min	Hours	15 hr	Apnea, hypotension, somnolence
phenobarbital	15-20 mg/kg	5 min	6-12 hr	50-120 hr	Apnea, hypotension, somnolence
phenytoin	15-20 mg/kg	1-2 hr	12-24 hr	7-42 hr	Cardiac dysrhythmias, hypotension

*Off-label use (not a Food and Drug Administration–approved indication), but still used for this purpose.

Adverse Effects

Antiepileptic drugs are plagued by many adverse effects, which often limit their usefulness. Many patients cannot tolerate the adverse effects, and therapy must be withdrawn. Birth defects in infants of epileptic mothers are higher than normal, regardless of whether the mother was receiving drug therapy. Epileptic women need to be monitored closely during pregnancy by both an obstetrician and a neurologist. Each antiepileptic drug is associated with its own diverse set of adverse effects. The various antiepileptic drugs and their most common adverse effects are listed in Table 14-4. Gastrointestinal side effects, such as nausea, vomiting, or diarrhea are common side effects of most antiepileptic drugs.

In December 2008, the U.S. Food and Drug Administration (FDA) required black box warnings on all antiepileptic drugs regarding the risk for suicidal thoughts and behavior. Patients being treated with antiepileptic drugs for any indication need to be monitored for the emergence or worsening of depression, suicidal thoughts or behavior, or any unusual changes in mood or behavior.

Interactions

Drug interactions that can occur with antiepileptic drugs are numerous and are summarized in Table 14-5. Many of the antiepileptic drugs can interact with each other, requiring close monitoring of the patient. Since many of these drugs induce hepatic metabolism, the effects of other drugs may be reduced, including oral contraceptives. There is a prime opportunity to counsel the patient about the need for alternative birth control methods due to reduced efficacy. Carbamazepine is not to be given with grapefruit because this leads to increased toxicity of the antiepileptic drug.

Dosages

Certain antiepileptic drugs have a narrow therapeutic index. Table 14-6 lists the various drugs for which monitoring of therapeutic plasma levels is required and their corresponding therapeutic values. For dosage information see the table on p. 225.

DRUG PROFILES

After valproic acid was introduced in 1978, no major new drugs for the treatment of epilepsy were introduced in the United States until the 1990s, at which time Gabapentin (Neurontin), lamotrigine (Lamictal), and felbamate (Felbatol) all were approved. Antiepileptic drugs approved in the 2000s include levetiracetam (Keppra), topiramate (Topamax), zonisamide (Zonegran), tiagabine (Gabitril), and pregabalin (Lyrica). Several new drugs were approved in 2014 including permapanel (Fycompa,) ezogabine (Potiga), vigabatrin (Sabril), and eslicarbazepine (Aptiom). These drugs fall into the miscellaneous

TABLE 14-4 Adverse Effects of Selected Antiepileptic Drugs

Drug or Drug Class	Adverse Effects
Barbiturates: phenobarbital, primidone	Dizziness, drowsiness, lethargy, paradoxical restlessness, GI upset
Hydantoins: phenytoin, fosphenytoin	Nystagmus, ataxia, drowsiness, rash, gingival hyperplasia, thrombocytopenia, agranulocytosis, hepatitis, GI upset
Iminostilbenes: carbamazepine, oxcarbazepine	Nausea, headache, dizziness, unusual eye movements, visual change, behavioral changes, rash, abdominal pain, abnormal gait, GI upset
valproic acid and derivatives, including valproate sodium and divalproex sodium	Dizziness, drowsiness, GI upset, weight gain, hepatotoxicity, pancreatitis
ethosuximide	Nausea, abdominal pain, dizziness, drowsiness
gabapentin	Dizziness, drowsiness, nausea, visual and speech changes, edema
pregabalin	Dizziness, drowsiness, peripheral edema, blurred vision
lamotrigine	Drowsiness, ataxia, headache, nausea, blurred or double vision
levetiracetam	Dizziness, drowsiness, hyperactivity, behavior changes such as anxiety, hostility, agitation, or suicidal ideation
tiagabine	Dizziness, drowsiness, agitation, asthenia, GI upset, abdominal pain, rash, tremor
topiramate	Dizziness, drowsiness, GI upset, ataxia
zonisamide	Drowsiness, anorexia, ataxia, confusion, agitation, cognitive impairment

TABLE 14-5 Significant Drug Interactions of Antiepileptic Drugs

AED Drug or Drug Class	Interacting Drug	Mechanism	Results
Barbiturates			
	Beta blockers, corticosteroids, oral contraceptives, calcium channel blockers, metronidazole, theophylline	Altered CYP450 enzyme metabolism	Reduced effects of listed drugs
	ethanol (alcohol)	Enhanced CNS depression	Can be fatal
Hydantoins			
phenytoin	amiodarone, benzodiazepines, azole antifungals, isoniazid, proton pump inhibitors, sulfonamide antibiotics	Altered CYP450 enzyme metabolism	Reduced phenytoin clearance and increased effects
	carbamazepine	Altered CYP450 enzyme metabolism	Increased phenytoin clearance and reduced effects
	cyclosporine, meperidine, rifampin, quetiapine, theophylline	Increased metabolism	Reduced effects of listed drugs
	warfarin	Displacement of warfarin from plasma protein binding sites	Increased free warfarin levels and bleeding risk
Iminostilbenes			
carbamazepine	Azole antifungals, diltiazem, isoniazid, macrolides, protease inhibitor antiretrovirals, SSRIs, valproic acid, verapamil	Altered CYP450 enzyme metabolism	Increased carbamazepine levels and toxicity risk
	Barbiturates, hydantoins, rifampin, succinimides, theophylline	Altered CYP450 enzyme metabolism	Reduced carbamazepine levels and efficacy
	acetaminophen	Altered CYP450 enzyme metabolism	Increased hepatic metabolism of acetaminophen and toxicity risk, and reduced efficacy
	Antipsychotics, antidepressants, benzodiazepines, cyclosporine, oral contraceptives	Altered CYP450 enzyme metabolism	Reduced efficacy; patient response must be monitored
	Monoamine oxidase inhibitors (MAOIs)	Altered CYP450 enzyme metabolism	Increased MAOI toxicity risk
oxcarbazepine	Barbiturates, hydantoins	Altered CYP450 enzyme metabolism	Increased barbiturate and hydantoin levels and reduced oxcarbazepine levels
	valproic acid, verapamil	Altered CYP450 enzyme metabolism	Reduced oxcarbazepine levels
	lamotrigine	Altered CYP450 enzyme metabolism	Reduced lamotrigine levels
	Oral contraceptives	Altered CYP450 enzyme metabolism	Reduced oral contraceptive levels and increased likelihood of pregnancy

Continued

TABLE 14-5 Significant Drug Interactions of Antiepileptic Drugs—cont'd

AED Drug or Drug Class	Interacting Drug	Mechanism	Results
Valproic Acid and Derivatives			
valproic acid, valproate sodium, and divalproex sodium	aspirin	Displacement of valproic acid from plasma protein binding sites	Increased free valproic acid levels and toxicity risk
	carbamazepine, oxcarbazepine, lamotrigine	Altered CYP450 enzyme metabolism	Reduced valproic acid efficacy; increased lamotrigine levels; increased or decreased carbamazepine levels
	lorazepam	Altered hepatic metabolism	Increased lorazepam toxicity risk
	rifampin	Altered CYP450 enzyme metabolism	Reduced valproic acid efficacy
	Tricyclic antidepressants	Altered CYP450 enzyme metabolism	Increased tricyclic antidepressant toxicity risk
Succinimides			
ethosuximide	Hydantoins, barbiturates, valproic acid	Altered CYP450 enzyme metabolism	Increased or reduced involved drug clearance
Miscellaneous AEDs			
gabapentin	Alcohol	Additive CNS depression	Increased CNS depression
pregabalin	None listed		
lamotrigine	Hydantoins, oral contraceptives, oxcarbazepine, rifampin	Altered CYP450 enzyme metabolism	Reduced lamotrigine levels and efficacy; may need dosage increase
	CNS depressants	Additive effects	Increased CNS depression
	valproic acid	Altered CYP450 enzyme metabolism	Increased lamotrigine levels and toxicity risk; may need dosage reduction
levetiracetam	None listed		
tiagabine	CNS depressants	Additive effects	Increased CNS depression
topiramate	carbamazepine, hydantoins, valproic acid, oral contraceptives	Altered CYP450 enzyme metabolism	Reduced object drug activity
zonisamide	CYP450 enzyme inducers or inhibitors	Altered CYP450 enzyme metabolism	Increased or reduced clearance and effects

AED, Antiepileptic drug; *CYP450,* cytochrome P-450; *SSRIs,* selective serotonin reuptake inhibitors.

TABLE 14-6 Therapeutic Plasma Levels of Antiepileptic Drugs with a Narrow Therapeutic Range

Antiepileptic Drug	Therapeutic Plasma Level (mcg/mL)
carbamazepine	4-12
phenobarbital	15-40
phenytoin	10-20
primidone	5-12
valproic acid	50-125

category of antiepileptics and have greatly expanded the options currently available to treat patients with seizure disorders. Common adverse effects and drug interactions are listed in the individual drug profiles and/or in Tables 14-3 and 14-4 and dosage information.

BARBITURATES

◆phenobarbital and ◆primidone

Historically, two of the most commonly used antiepileptic drugs were the barbiturates phenobarbital and primidone (Mysoline). Primidone is metabolized in the liver to phenobarbital. Use of primidone can provide anticonvulsant activity with a lower serum level of phenobarbital than that attained with phenobarbital itself. This can reduce the likelihood of sedation and fatigue associated with phenobarbital. In third-world countries, oral phenobarbital is often the drug of choice for routine seizure prophylaxis because of its low cost. The most common adverse effect of phenobarbital is sedation, although tolerance to this effect usually develops with continued therapy. Therapeutic effects are generally seen at serum drug levels of 10 to 40 mcg/mL. A major advantage of this drug is its long half-life, which allows once-a-day dosing. This can be a substantial advantage for patients who have a difficult time remembering to take their medication or for those who have erratic schedules. Even if a patient takes his or her dose 12 or even 24 hours late, therapeutic blood levels may still be maintained. Contraindications include known drug allergy, porphyria (a disorder of the synthesis of *heme,* a component of hemoglobin), liver or kidney impairment, and respiratory illness. Adverse effects include cardiovascular, CNS, gastrointestinal (GI), and dermatologic reactions (see Table 14-4). Phenobarbital interacts with many drugs because it is a major inducer of hepatic microsomal enzymes, including the cytochrome P-450 system enzymes (see Chapter 2), which causes more rapid clearance of some

DOSAGES

Selected Antiepileptic Drugs*

Drug (Pregnancy Category)	Pharmacologic Class	Usual Adult Dosage Range
◆carbamazepine (Tegretol, Tegretol XR) (D)	Iminostilbene	PO: 400-1200 mg/day
ethosuximide (Zarontin) (C)	Succinimide	PO: 500 mg/day, then adjust
◆fosphenytoin (Cerebyx) (D)	Hydantoin	IV: 10-20 PE†/kg loading dose; maintenance dose 4-6 PE/kg/day
◆gabapentin (Neurontin) (C)	Miscellaneous	PO: 900-3600 mg/day
lamotrigine (Lamictal) (C)	Miscellaneous	PO: 50-600 mg/day
levetiracetam (Keppra) (C)	Miscellaneous	PO: 500 mg bid to 3000 mg/day
oxcarbazepine (Trileptal) (C)	Iminostilbene	600-2400 mg/day
◆phenobarbital (oral, injectable) (D)	Barbiturate	PO/IV: 1-3 mg/kg/day
◆!phenytoin (Dilantin) (D)	Hydantoin	PO: 300-400 mg/day
pregabalin (Lyrica) (C)	Miscellaneous	PO: 150-600 mg/day divided into 2 or 3 doses
◆primidone (Mysoline) (D)	Barbiturate	PO: 750-1500 mg/day
topiramate (Topamax) (C)	Miscellaneous	PO: 25-400 mg/day
◆valproic acid derivatives (Depacon, IV Depakote, Depakene oral) (D)	Miscellaneous	PO/IV: 30-60 mg/kg/day
zonisamide (Zonegran) (C)	Miscellaneous	100-400 mg/day

AED, Antiepileptic drug; *PE*, phenytoin equivalent.
*See Table 14-3 for doses of drugs used for status epilepticus.
†One PE = 1.5 mg fosphenytoin = 1 mg phenytoin. Therefore, 1.5 mg fosphenytoin is given for each milligram of phenytoin desired.

drugs (see Table 14-5). Phenobarbital is available in oral and injectable forms, whereas primidone is available only for oral use.

Pharmacokinetics: Phenobarbital

Route	Onset of Action	Peak Plasma Concentration	Elimination Half-life	Duration of Action
PO	20-60 min	8-12 hr	50-120 hr	6-12 hr
IV	5 min	30 min	50-120 hr	6-12 hr

Pharmacokinetics: Primidone

Route	Onset of Action	Peak Plasma Concentration	Elimination Half-life	Duration of Action
PO	Unknown	3-4 hr	10-12 hr*	Unknown

*Longer for active metabolites, including phenobarbital

HYDANTOINS
◆!phenytoin and ◆fosphenytoin

Phenytoin (Dilantin) has been used as a first-line drug for many years and is the prototypical drug. It is indicated for the management of tonic-clonic and partial seizures. Contraindications include known drug allergy and heart conditions that involve bradycardia. Adverse effects and drug interactions both are numerous and are listed in Tables 14-4 and 14-5, respectively. The most common adverse effects are lethargy, abnormal movements, mental confusion, and cognitive changes. Gingival hyperplasia is a well-known adverse effect of long-term oral phenytoin therapy. Scrupulous dental care can help prevent this. Other adverse effects associated with long-term phenytoin therapy can cause acne, hirsutism, and hypertrophy of subcutaneous facial tissue resulting in an appearance known as *Dilantin facies* and osteoporosis. Therapeutic drug levels are usually 10 to 20 mcg/mL. At toxic levels, phenytoin can cause nystagmus, ataxia, dysarthria, and encephalopathy. Phenytoin can interact with other medications for two main reasons. First, it is highly bound to plasma proteins and competes with other highly protein-bound medications for binding sites. Second, it induces hepatic microsomal enzymes, mainly cytochrome P-450 enzymes (see Chapter 2). This increases the metabolism of other drugs that are metabolized by these enzymes and reduces their blood levels.

Because phenytoin is highly protein bound, exaggerated phenytoin levels can be seen in patients with very low serum albumin concentrations. With lower levels of albumin, more of the free, unbound, pharmacologically active phenytoin molecules will be present in the blood. This most commonly occurs in patients who are malnourished or have chronic renal failure. It is generally necessary to maintain phenytoin levels well below 20 mcg/mL in such patients. Phenytoin has many advantages for long-term therapy. It is usually well tolerated, highly effective, and relatively inexpensive. It can also be given intravenously if needed. Most often, however, phenytoin is taken orally. The long half-life of the drug allows for twice- or even once-daily dosing. This encourages patient adherence to drug therapy.

Parenteral phenytoin is adjusted chemically to a pH of 12 with propylene glycol (antifreeze) for drug stability. It is very irritating to veins when injected and must be given by slow intravenous (IV) push (not exceeding 50 mg/min in adults) directly into a large vein through a large-gauge (20-gauge or larger) venous catheter. Phenytoin is only to be diluted in normal saline (NS) for IV infusion, and a filter must be used. Follow each dose by an injection of a saline flush to avoid local venous irritation. Soft-tissue irritation and inflammation can occur at the site of injection with or without extravasation. This can vary from slight tenderness to extensive necrosis and sloughing, and in rare instances can require amputation. Avoid improper administration, including subcutaneous or perivascular injection, to prevent the possibility of such occurrences.

Fosphenytoin (Cerebyx) is an injectable prodrug of phenytoin that was developed in an attempt to overcome some of the chemical disadvantages of phenytoin injection. Fosphenytoin is a water-soluble phenytoin derivative that can be given intramuscularly or intravenously—by IV push or continuous infusion—without causing burning on injection associated with phenytoin. Fosphenytoin is dosed in *phenytoin equivalents (PE)* as indicated in Table 14-7. Fosphenytoin is given at a rate of 150 mg PE/min or less to avoid hypotension or cardiorespiratory depression. Implement fall-prevention measures after infusion of either phenytoin or fosphenytoin because of possible ataxia and dizziness. Check available references, and/or consult with a pharmacist before administering because there are numerous IV incompatibilities with both drugs.

IMINOSTILBENES
◆ carbamazepine

Carbamazepine (Tegretol) is the second most commonly prescribed antiepileptic drug in the United States, after phenytoin. It was originally marketed in the late 1960s for the treatment of *trigeminal neuralgia* (a painful facial nerve condition). It is chemically related to the *tricyclic* antidepressants (see Chapter 16) and is considered a first-line treatment for partial seizures and generalized tonic-clonic seizures. It may actually worsen myoclonic or absence seizures. Therefore its use is contraindicated in both of these conditions as well as in cases of known drug allergy and bone marrow depression. Carbamazepine is associated with autoinduction of hepatic enzymes. Autoinduction is a process in which, over time, a drug stimulates the production of enzymes that enhance its own metabolism, and leads to lower than expected drug concentrations. With carbamazepine, this process usually occurs within the first 2 months after starting the drug. Carbamazepine has numerous adverse reactions and drug interactions; examples are given in Tables 14-4 and 14-5. It is available for oral use only.

Pharmacokinetics: Carbamazepine

Route	Onset of Action	Peak Plasma Concentration	Elimination Half-life	Duration of Action
PO	Slow	4-8 hr	25-65 hr	12-24 hr

oxcarbazepine

Oxcarbazepine (Trileptal) is a chemical analogue of carbamazepine. Its precise mechanism of action has not been identified, although it is known to block voltage-sensitive sodium channels, which aids in stabilizing excited neuronal membranes. It is indicated for partial seizures and secondarily generalized seizures. Contraindications include known drug allergy. Common adverse reactions include headache, dizziness, and nausea (see also Table 14-4). Unlike carbamazepine, this drug is not a hepatic enzyme inducer. As a result, it is associated with far fewer common drug interactions than is carbamazepine (see Table 14-5). Oxcarbazepine is available for oral use only.

Pharmacokinetics: Oxcarbazepine

Route	Onset of Action	Peak Plasma Concentration	Elimination Half-life	Duration of Action
PO	2-4 hr	2-3 days	2-9 hr	Unknown

SUCCINIMIDE
ethosuximide

Ethosuximide (Zarontin) is used in the treatment of uncomplicated absence seizures. It is not effective for secondary generalized tonic-clonic seizures. The only listed contraindication for either use is known drug allergy. Adverse effects include GI and CNS effects (see Table 14-4). Drug interactions most commonly involve hepatic enzyme–inducing drugs (see Table 14-5).

Pharmacokinetics: Phenytoin

Route	Onset of Action	Peak Plasma Concentration	Elimination Half-life	Duration of Action
PO	Unknown	12 hr	7-42 hr	12-36 hr
IV	1-2 hr	2-3 hr	7-42 hr	12-24 hr

TABLE 14-7 Comparison of Phenytoin Sodium and Fosphenytoin Sodium

	Phenytoin Sodium (Dilantin IV)	Fosphenytoin Sodium (Cerebyx IM/IV)
pH	12	8.6-9
Maximum infusion rate	50 mg/min	150 mg PE*/min
Admixtures	0.9% saline	0.9% saline or 5% dextrose

PE, Phenytoin sodium equivalents.

*150 mg fosphenytoin sodium = 100 mg phenytoin sodium.

Pharmacokinetics: Ethosuximide

Route	Onset of Action	Peak Plasma Concentration	Elimination Half-life	Duration of Action
PO	Unknown	4 hr	60 hr	Unknown

MISCELLANEOUS DRUGS

Four new miscellaneous drugs were recently approved. Ezogabine (Potiga) is indicated for adjunctive therapy for partial-onset seizures and can cause potential vision loss and skin discoloration, both which may be permanent. The FDA recommends it be used only in patients who have not responded to other drugs. Perampanel (Fycompa) is also indicated as adjunctive therapy for partial-onset seizures. It is associated with a high incidence of dizziness. Vigabatrin (Sabril) is indicated for refractory complex partial seizures. It carries the risk for visual impairment and as such is only available through a restricted distribution program. Eslicarbazepine (Aptiom) was recently approved and is indicated as adjunctive therapy for partial-onset seizures.

♦ gabapentin

Gabapentin (Neurontin) is a chemical analogue of *GABA,* a neurotransmitter that inhibits brain activity. The exact mechanism of action is unknown, but is believed to work by increasing the synthesis and synaptic accumulation of GABA between neurons. It is indicated as an adjunct drug for the treatment of partial seizures and for prophylaxis of partial seizures. Evidence also shows gabapentin to be effective as single-drug therapy for new-onset epilepsy. It is most commonly used to treat neuropathic pain (see Chapter 10). Contraindications include known drug allergy. Adverse effects include CNS and GI symptoms (see Table 14-4). Drug interactions are listed in Table 14-5. Gabapentin is available for oral use only.

Pharmacokinetics: Gabapentin

Route	Onset of Action	Peak Plasma Concentration	Elimination Half-life	Duration of Action
PO	Unknown	Unknown	5-7 hr	Unknown

lamotrigine

Lamotrigine (Lamictal) is indicated for simple or complex partial seizures, for generalized seizures related to *Lennox-Gastaut syndrome* (an atypical form of absence epilepsy that may persist into adulthood), and, most recently, for primary generalized tonic-clonic seizures. It is also used for the treatment of bipolar disorder. The only contraindication is known drug allergy. Common adverse effects include relatively minor CNS and GI symptoms (see Table 14-4). One potentially serious adverse effect is a rash that can progress to the major dermatologic reaction known as *Stevens-Johnson syndrome.*

This condition involves inflammation and sloughing of skin, potentially over the entire body, in a manner that resembles a third-degree burn. It is often reversible but can also be fatal. To avoid this condition, doses are very slowly titrated over several weeks. Drug interactions chiefly involve other antiepileptic drugs as well as other CNS depressants and oral contraceptives (see Table 14-5). Lamotrigine is available for oral use only.

Pharmacokinetics: Lamotrigine

Route	Onset of Action	Peak Plasma Concentration	Elimination Half-life	Duration of Action
PO	Unknown	1.4-2.3 hr	24 hr	Unknown

levetiracetam

Levetiracetam (Keppra) is indicated as adjunct therapy for partial seizures with and without secondary generalization. It is contraindicated in cases of known drug allergy. Its mechanism of action is unknown. It is generally well tolerated, with the most common adverse effects being CNS related (see Table 14-4). No drug interactions are currently listed; however, like all antiepileptic drugs, the potential for excessive CNS depression exists when it is used in combination with other sedating drugs. Levetiracetam is available in both oral and injectable forms.

Pharmacokinetics: Levetiracetam

Route	Onset of Action	Peak Plasma Concentration	Elimination Half-life	Duration of Action
PO	Rapid	1 hr	6-8 hr	Unknown

pregabalin

Pregabalin (Lyrica), like gabapentin, is structurally related to GABA. However, it does not bind to GABA receptors but rather to the alpha$_2$-delta receptor sites, which affect calcium channels in CNS tissues. Its mechanism of action is still not fully understood. Pregabalin is a Schedule V controlled substance. The drug is indicated as adjunct therapy for partial seizures, although it is most commonly used for *neuropathic pain* (see Chapter 10), and *postherpetic neuralgia* (see Chapter 40) and fibromyalgia. Contraindications include known drug allergy. Adverse drug reactions are primarily CNS related (see Table 14-4). No clinically significant drug interactions are listed to date; however, as with all antiepileptic drugs, the potential for additive CNS depression exists when other sedating drugs are used. Pregabalin is available for oral use only.

Pharmacokinetics: Pregabalin

Route	Onset of Action	Peak Plasma Concentration	Elimination Half-life	Duration of Action
PO	Unknown	1.5 hr	6 hr	Unknown

tiagabine

Tiagabine (Gabitril) is indicated as adjunct therapy for partial seizures. Contraindications include known drug allergy. Its exact mechanism of action has not been identified, but is known to have beneficial effects by inhibiting the reuptake of GABA from the neuronal synapses (spaces between neurons) in the brain. Although tiagabine is effective in controlling epileptic seizures, there have been several case reports of *paradoxical* seizures (opposite of what would intuitively be expected) in nonepileptic patients who are treated with the drug for other indications. Most of these cases involved patients being treated for bipolar disorder. Of even greater concern is that in some of these cases the seizure episodes progressed to status epilepticus. For these reasons, prescribers are currently advised to avoid off-label use of tiagabine. Common adverse effects are CNS and GI symptoms (see Table 14-4). Drug interactions chiefly involve other CNS depressant drugs (see Table 14-5). Tiagabine is available for oral use only.

Pharmacokinetics: Tiagabine

Route	Onset of Action	Peak Plasma Concentration	Elimination Half-life	Duration of Action
PO	Rapid	45 min	7-9 hr	Unknown

topiramate

Topiramate (Topamax) is a structurally unique drug chemically related to fructose. It is indicated as adjunct therapy for partial and secondarily generalized seizures, for generalized tonic-clonic seizures, and for drop attacks in Lennox-Gastaut syndrome. Contraindications include known drug allergy. Its exact mechanism of action is unknown. Common adverse effects are primarily CNS related (see Table 14-4). Angle-closure glaucoma can also occur, and the patient must immediately report any visual changes. Common drug interactions involve chiefly other antiepileptic drugs and oral contraceptives (see Table 14-5). Topiramate is available for oral use only. In 2011, the FDA notified health care professionals about an increased risk for cleft palate in children born to mothers who were taking topiramate during pregnancy.

Pharmacokinetics: Topiramate

Route	Onset of Action	Peak Plasma Concentration	Elimination Half-life	Duration of Action
PO	Unknown	2-4 hr	21 hr	Unknown

♦valproic acid

Valproic acid is used primarily in the treatment of generalized seizures (absence, myoclonic, and tonic-clonic). It is also used for bipolar disorder (see Chapter 16) and has been shown to be effective in controlling partial seizures. Contraindications include known drug allergy, liver impairment, and *urea cycle disorders* (genetic disorders of urea metabolism). Common adverse effects include drowsiness; nausea, vomiting, and other GI disturbances; tremor; weight gain; and transient hair loss (see Table 14-4). The most serious adverse effects are hepatotoxicity and pancreatitis. Valproic acid can interact with many medications (see Table 14-5). Valproic acid is highly protein bound and competes with other highly protein-bound

medications for binding sites. It also is metabolized by hepatic microsomal enzymes and competes for metabolism with other drugs. In contrast to phenobarbital and phenytoin, it is not a hepatic enzyme inducer. It is available in both oral and injectable forms. Valproic acid itself is chemically the simplest dosage form and is available as an oral liquid. Long-acting oral dosage forms are also available as divalproex sodium (Depakote), which comes in delayed- and extended-release tablets as well as capsules with long-acting granules (Depakote Sprinkles) that can be opened and sprinkled onto food. The injectable form is the salt valproate sodium (Depacon).

Pharmacokinetics: Valproic Acid

Route	Onset of Action	Peak Plasma Concentration	Elimination Half-life	Duration of Action
PO, IV	15-30 min	1-4 hr	6-16 hr	4-6 hr

zonisamide

Zonisamide (Zonegran) is a sulfonamide derivative (see Chapter 38) indicated for a variety of seizure types, including partial and secondary generalized, primary generalized, absence, and myoclonic. It is contraindicated in patients with known drug allergy to the drug itself or to sulfa drugs (see Chapter 38). Common adverse effects include CNS and GI symptoms (see Table 14-4). Zonisamide interacts with a number of drugs metabolized by cytochrome P-450 enzymes, which increase or decrease clearance of zonisamide (see Table 14-5). Zonisamide is available for oral use only.

Pharmacokinetics: Zonisamide

Route	Onset of Action	Peak Plasma Concentration	Elimination Half-life	Duration of Action
PO	Rapid	2-6 hr	63 hr	Unknown

⚡ SAFETY AND QUALITY IMPROVEMENT: PREVENTING MEDICATION ERRORS · QSEN

Look-Alike/Sound-Alike Drugs: Cerebyx and Celebrex

Be careful with drug names! When using their trade names, Cerebyx and Celebrex sound and look very much alike. However, they are quite different. Cerebyx is a trade name for fosphenytoin, a hydantoin class antiepileptic drug. It is used to treat a variety of seizure disorders. Celebrex is the trade name for celecoxib, a COX-2 inhibitor antiinflammatory drug used for pain and various disorders such as osteoarthritis and rheumatoid arthritis (see Chapter 44). Think about what would happen if a patient with a seizure disorder received an anti-inflammatory drug instead of an antiepileptic drug. Although the trade names are very similar, the indications are very different! These two drugs illustrate the importance of using both the trade name and generic name when ordering medications.

NURSING PROCESS

ASSESSMENT

With use of any of the *antiepileptic drugs,* a thorough physical assessment needs to be obtained as well as a comprehensive health and medication history. Any possible allergies, drug interactions, adverse reactions, cautions, and contraindications can be identified at this time. Thoroughly review the patient's medical history, and be astute to the occurrence of any type of seizure disorder/activity. If there has been evidence of any type of seizure activity, be sure to assess for the occurrence of an aura, precipitating events, location of symptoms, duration, frequency, and intensity. Some patients experience an aura or a distinctive feeling or some other warning sign when a seizure is about to occur. Some auras are reported to be unpleasant but may be very helpful because they can give patients time to prepare for a seizure and keep themselves from being injured. Auras vary greatly between people and may occur right before the seizure or several minutes to hours earlier. Patients experiencing an aura, or common warning sign before a seizure, report changes in bodily sensations and in their ability to interact with the outside world. Other warning signs may include depression, irritability, sleep disruption, nausea, and headache (visit *www.epilepsy.com/epilepsy* for more information).

Other information to assess for includes the occurrence of any other problems or signs and symptoms occurring before, during, or after the seizure. Question the patient about the occurrence of panic attacks because of the possible association between high levels of anxiety or stress and the precipitation of seizures in those at risk. Assess the patient for signs and symptoms of autonomic nervous system responses associated with anxiety or stress such as cold, clammy hands, excessive sweating (diaphoresis), agitation, and trembling of the extremities. Additional assessment about other problems or symptoms is important because some antiepileptic medications may be indicated for other medical diagnoses, such as prevention of migraines or treatment of postherpetic neuralgia and neuropathic pain. A complete neurologic assessment with documentation of baseline CNS functioning is also important before administering antiepileptic drugs. This may include testing and grading the response of deep tendon reflexes, bilateral and upper- and lower-extremity sensory and motor testing, and questioning about the presence of any headaches, photosensitivity, occurrence of auras, or visual changes.

Before giving these drugs, review laboratory test results, which may include red blood cell and white blood cell counts, clotting studies, and renal and/or liver function studies. Knowing baseline levels of these laboratory values is important to help identify any initial abnormalities as well as to provide a comparison value when assessing for possible adverse effects, cautions, contraindications, and interactions. Assess urinary output for at least 30 mL/hr and urine specific gravity. Another measurement of urinary output may be the parameter of 0.5 mL/kg/hr to take in account the age and size of the patient. Conditions other than epilepsy or seizure disorders may also cause loss of or alterations in consciousness and are worthy of consideration during assessment. These conditions include syncope, breath-holding practices, transient ischemic attacks, drug use, metabolic disorders, infections, head trauma, tumors, and psychogenic problems. Therefore, an attempt will most likely be made to rule out or eliminate many of these disorders or conditions during the diagnosing of epilepsy, and therein lies the importance of analyzing all available points of data. An EEG may also be ordered to provide more information related to the diagnosis of epilepsy. Another diagnostic procedure, magnetic resonance imaging (MRI), may be performed for neuroimaging and further data gathering.

If *barbiturates* have been ordered, carefully assess not only the neurologic system but also vital signs because of the CNS depression associated with this class of drugs. Obtain and document all of the aforementioned general assessment data when barbiturates are prescribed. In addition, identify patients at high risk for excessive sedation for safety purposes. If the patient is in an acute care institution, assess the room and environment to ensure that safety measures are in place (e.g., side rails up or a bed alarm system in use depending on health care institution policy), noise level is controlled, and seizure precautions are available (oxygen, suctioning equipment, and airway devices nearby; padded side rails being used; and IV access obtained per health care instituion policy). Note the patient's age, because the very young and the older adult react with more sensitivity to these drugs with paradoxical reactions, irritability, and hyperactivity (as compared to CNS depressant effects). Cautions, contraindications, and drug interactions are discussed earlier in the chapter.

With *hydantoins* like *phenytoin*, the previously mentioned assessment data are also appropriate. Perform a skin assessment, and document intactness and the presence or absence of any rashes, because of the possibility of a measles-like rash. In addition, baseline dental hygiene habits and an oral assessment, such as the status of the patient's gums and teeth, are important because of the adverse effects of gingival hyperplasia. Assessment of baseline neurologic functioning is crucial with the use of these CNS-altering medications and needs to include the following: (1) a focus on vision with attention to any abnormalities, especially those related to eye movement; (2) baseline neuromuscular stability with attention to coordinated movements, gait, and reflexes; and (3) assessment of speech for clarity and ability to form and express words appropriately. In addition, when the phenytoins are administered, baseline liver function studies and complete blood counts are needed. Attention must also be given to specific drug-related cautions, contraindications, and drug interactions.

Before administering the *iminostilbene carbamazepine,* a CBC is often ordered. Document these laboratory findings for baseline comparisons because of the possible adverse effect of drug-related anemias (e.g., aplastic anemia). Measure baseline vision and any abnormalities because of the potential visual changes. Significant contraindications include conditions or drugs involving and/or precipitating bone marrow suppression because of carbamazepine's adverse effect (though rare) of the same.

The use of a *succinimide,* such as *ethosuximide,* requires assessment for the specific indication for this medication, that is, generalized absence seizures. In addition to performing a baseline neurologic assessment, other questions to pose to the patient include inquiring about any problems with nausea, abdominal pain, or dizziness. Always assess for any allergies to this drug.

Miscellaneous drugs such as tiagabine, topiramate, and zonisamide are some of the more recently available antiepileptic drugs and have significant contraindications, cautions, and drug interactions, which are discussed earlier in this chapter and are summarized in Tables 14-4 and 14-5. Assess vital signs and mental status with attention to the patient's sensorium, level of alertness or consciousness, and any mental depression before, during, and after drug therapy and/or seizure activity. Document any of the following baseline problems if administering tiagabine or topiramate: dizziness, drowsiness, GI upset, ataxia, and/or agitation.

There are several *miscellaneous antiepileptic drugs* also associated with cautious assessments. *Gabapentin* requires a thorough neurologic assessment with attention to baseline energy levels, visual intactness, sensory and motor functioning, and any changes in speech. It is also important to understand the rationale for gabapentin's use so that appropriate education and instructions can be shared with the patient and family. For example, gabapentin may be used for seizure therapy, but it is also used to treat postherpetic neuralgia and neuropathic pain and to prevent migraines. Thus, an individualized plan of care with proper education needs to be developed from the appropriate assessment data. *Pregabalin* is similar to gabapentin and requires the same assessment.

Lamotrigine use requires a thorough neurologic assessment and documentation of baseline energy levels, vision acuity, and history of headaches for comparative purposes due to common adverse effects of headaches, vision changes, and drowsiness. Several other *miscellaneous antiepileptic drugs* are available, such as *levetiracetam, topiramate, zonisamide, tiagabine,* and *pregabalin.* These drugs require the same thorough, general assessment as with other antiepileptic drugs. A few additional points must be kept in mind. For example, in patients taking levetiracetam, you must document the presence of any neuropsychiatric symptoms because of the potential for drug-related agitation, depression, anxiety, and other mood or behavioral changes. Although these adverse effects are rare, the assessment data must still be thorough. One interesting fact, as noted in the pharmacology section, is the lack of drug interactions with levetiracetam; however, it does depress the CNS, as with all antiepileptic drugs, and so assessment of the use of other CNS depressant drugs is important to note. Liver and renal functioning also need monitoring before therapy is initiated. Topiramate is used for management of seizures as well as for cluster migraine headaches and neuropathic pain. Therefore, include a thorough review of the patient's medical and medication history to better understand the reason for the drug's use. Document energy levels with this and all antiepileptic drugs.

Valproic acid requires a careful assessment, as well. Gather and document information about the patient's medical history, medication profile, and neurologic system with information about seizure activity (see previous discussion). Assessment for drug allergies, cautions, contraindications, and drug interactions has been previously discussed. Other assessment areas include baseline weight, liver function studies, and notation of a history of pancreatitis.

CASE STUDY

Safety: What Went Wrong? Monitoring Antiepileptic Drug Therapy

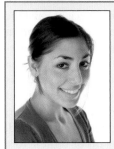

D., a 21-year-old college student, has been brought to the emergency department in status epilepticus. Measures are taken to ensure her safety and prevent injury, and an intravenous (IV) line is started. The emergency department physician has ordered diazepam (Valium) 8 mg IV push, STAT.

1. The diazepam is supplied in a vial of 5 mg/mL. How much medication will the nurse draw up into the syringe?

    The IV diazepam is given at a rate of 2 mg/min. Soon after the IV diazepam is given, D.'s seizures stop, and she regains consciousness. She is admitted to a medical-surgical unit, and her mother goes to the room with her. The admitting orders call for an initial IV dose of phenytoin, followed by oral doses twice a day.

2. Why was the loading dose given intravenously?

    After 2 days of observation, D. is ready for discharge to her mother's home. Her phenytoin level is 16 mcg/mL. She is very concerned about how the phenytoin will affect her.

3. Evaluate the phenytoin level of 16 mcg/mL. Would there be a safety concern if the level were 8 mcg/mL?

4. What teaching should the patient receive regarding self-care and the adverse effects of phenytoin?

5. After 4 months, the patient's mother calls to report that D. has seemed "very sad lately" and has not wanted to join her friends or family for evenings out. "She just goes to school, then comes home and stays in her room." What is the safety priority in this situation?

For answers, see *http://evolve.elsevier.com/Lilley.*

NURSING DIAGNOSES

1. Deficient knowledge related to lack of familiarity and minimal experience with and lack of information concerning the use of antiepileptic drugs
2. Noncompliance with the therapeutic regimen related to the patient's misuse of drugs or lack of understanding about the seizure disorder and its treatment
3. Chronic low self-esteem related to diagnosis of a lifelong disease and the adverse effects associated with antiepileptic drugs
4. Risk for injury related to decreased sensorium and CNS depression associated with the actions and adverse effects of antiepileptic drugs

PLANNING: OUTCOME IDENTIFICATION

1. Patient demonstrates adequate knowledge about diagnosis and associated drug therapy through stating the therapeutic, adverse, and toxic effects of the drug as well as safety measures to initiate.
2. Patient remains compliant with the therapy regimen, minimizes adverse effects as much as possible, and maximizes therapeutic effectiveness.
    - Patient states the dangers, such as rebound seizure activity, associated with sudden withdrawal of antiepileptic drugs.

3. Patient maintains positive self-esteem and body image through open and frequent communication about diagnosis and related treatment.
4. Patient remains free from injury related to drug therapy through implementation of safety measures while at home/work and reports symptoms of excessive sedation, confusion, lethargy, and dizziness to prescriber.

IMPLEMENTATION

For patients taking *antiepileptic* drugs, interventions focus on monitoring the patient while providing safety measures (see previous discussion) and securing the airway, breathing, and circulation. Airway maintenance is of critical importance for epileptic patients because the tongue relaxes during seizure activity, falling backward and subsequently blocking the airway. Maintain the patient's airway in the same way as during cardiopulmonary resuscitation, using the chin lift or jaw thrust method. Provide rescue breathing, if the patient is not breathing on his or her own, at a rate of 1 breath every 5 seconds. If the patient is breathing, keep the airway open through proper positioning (as just described). In addition to performing these critical components of care, maintain seizure precautions according to health care institution policy. This may include making sure the patient is gently kept in bed or kept from falling, putting the side rails up, and placing the patient in a side-lying position if needed. Avoid use of a tongue blade or other instrument to pry open the patient's mouth or clenched teeth, and ensure quick access to oxygen and suctioning equipment at all times.

With antiepileptic drug administration, adhere closely to the drug dose and frequency of dosing, as ordered. Close monitoring of dosing is important to attain therapeutic blood levels. For example, if an antiepileptic drug is ordered to be administered every 6 hours, it is crucial to dose the drug so that it is given around the clock to maintain blood levels. Administering the antiepileptic drug at the same time every day is also important to maintain blood levels. Educate patients on the importance of adhering to the medication regimen due to the impact one dose may have on maintaining steady states and therapeutic blood levels (see Chapter 2). If one or more doses of the antiepileptic drug is missed, the prescriber must be contacted immediately due to the increased risk for seizure activity. See Patient-Centered Care: Patient Teaching for more information.

With oral dosing, it is recommended that these drugs be taken with at least 6 to 8 ounces of fluid, preferably water, and with food, meals, or a snack to help decrease the risk for gastrointestinal upset, a frequently encountered adverse effect. Some beverages need to be avoided with some of the anticonvulsants to avoid an interaction. Grapefruit or related citrus fruits or pomegranate juice needs to be avoided with *carbamazepine (Tegretol)*. Always check for drug-drug and drug-food/beverage interactions. Oral suspensions are to be shaken and the solution mixed thoroughly. Capsules are *not* to be crushed, opened, or chewed—especially if they are extended- or long-release forms; *Depakote Sprinkles* are the exception. Chewing or altering these long-release type formulations would allow for the entire dosage to be released at once versus over a period of time. Extended-release dosage forms are usually ordered once a day, and so checking and double-checking the dosage and frequency is critical to patient safety. These actions will help to prevent the patient from experiencing either too high or too low drug serum levels. An exception to this is with *divalproex sodium sprinkles (Depakote Sprinkles)*. This dosage form may be opened and the medication sprinkled into a spoonful of applesauce or pudding to facilitate swallowing. It is recommended to swallow this mixture immediately.

If there are any questions regarding the type of capsule, pill, or tablet or questions about other dosage forms and recommended administration guidelines, use appropriate authoritative sources. These sources would include a licensed pharmacist, the manufacturer-package insert, and/or a current (within last 3 years) nursing drug handbook or pharmacology book. If there are any questions about the medication order or the medication prescribed, contact the prescriber immediately for clarification. *Topiramate* and *valproic acid* tablets and delayed- or extended-release dosage forms are not to be altered in any way and must be given as prescribed.

The following interventions are specific to drugs and/or drug classes:

- *Barbiturates* (e.g., *phenobarbital*): Abrupt withdrawal of these drugs, as well as any antiepileptic drugs, must be avoided due to possible rebound seizure activity. Most of the oral dosage forms of this class of drugs are to be taken with water. Elixir dosage forms may be safely mixed with fruit juice, milk, or water. If IV infusions are indicated, calculate the dose carefully and use an IV infusion pump to administer the drug. Too rapid an infusion of IV dosage forms may lead to cardiovascular collapse and respiratory depression. In addition, frequently monitor vital signs and IV infusion rates, and document in the patient's chart. If any signs or symptoms of cardiovascular or respiratory depression are noted, withhold the drug and contact the prescriber immediately while providing supportive care through maintenance of the airway, breathing, and circulation.

- *Hydantoins:* As a point of reference, 150 mg of *fosphenytoin* is the equivalent of 100 mg of *phenytoin*, and the dose, concentration, solution, and infusion rate of fosphenytoin is expressed as a *phenytoin equivalent (PE)*. With parenteral forms, the only dilutional fluid to use with these drugs is normal saline (NS). A filter must also be used. Rates of infusion must follow manufacturer's guidelines and are usually 150 mg PE/min or less to avoid hypotension and cardiorespiratory depression. If dysrhythmias or hypotension occur, discontinue the infusion immediately, monitor patient vital signs, and contact the prescriber immediately. Implement safety measures, such as assisting the patient with ambulation and having the patient move slowly and purposefully, when this drug (or any other antiepileptic drug) is given because of the adverse effects of ataxia and dizziness. IV dose administration requires even more cautious use because of the rapid onset of action. CNS depression is always a concern; thus, there is a need to frequently monitor the patient's vital signs. If existing IV lines contain D_5W or other solutions, the line must be flushed with normal saline before and after dosing to avoid precipitate formation. If infiltration of the IV site leads to subcutaneous tissue access, ischemia and sloughing may occur because of the high alkalinity of the drug. Review health care institution policy as well as manufacturer's guidelines regarding the use of possible antidotes. If infiltration occurs, discontinue infusion of the solution immediately, but leave the IV catheter/needle in place until all orders from the prescriber have been received. This practice allows any antidote medication to be administered through the IV catheter, if ordered. Sustained- or extended-release oral dosage forms are never to be opened, punctured, chewed, or broken in pieces. Other regular forms of the drug may be crushed, as needed. Gingival hyperplasia is an adverse effect and requires that the patient receive daily oral care as well as frequent dental visits. Complete blood counts are often monitored very closely within the first year of therapy (e.g., measured monthly for 1 year, then every 3 months).

- *Carbamazepine* (an *iminostilbene*): This drug is *not* to be given with grapefruit/grapefruit juice because this leads to increased toxicity of the antiepileptic drug. If the drug is to be replaced with another antiepileptic drug, a plan needs to be in place to decrease the dosages of the older drug before beginning low doses (at first) of the newer drug. Serum therapeutic levels are given in Table 14-6.
- *Gabapentin:* This is one of the antiepileptic drugs that can be taken without regard to meals. If discontinuation of the drug is indicated, taper the dosage, as ordered, over at least 1 week to avoid rebound seizures.
- *Lamotrigine:* The dosing regimen must be followed, as ordered. Checking for possible drug interactions is important to patient safety. If the patient shares any suicidal thoughts or actions, contact the prescriber immediately.
- *Levetiracetam:* The most common adverse effect is sleepiness. Contact the prescriber if any extreme adverse effects or any problems with moving, walking, or changes in mood/behavior occur. Any suicidal thoughts or psychotic symptoms must also be reported immediately. With the beginning of antiepileptic therapy, encourage the patient not to drive, operate heavy machinery, or make major decisions due to the sedation and CNS depression.
- *Oxcarbazepine:* This drug is to be taken as prescribed and is usually given in two divided doses. Always check for any potential drug interactions before administering (see previous discussion). The drug must be taken with food or snacks. Rash, abnormal walking or moving, or abdominal pain must also be reported, if present.
- *Pregabalin:* The daily dosage is usually given in two or three divided doses. Sudden or abrupt withdrawal is to be avoided. Monitor the patient for any excessive dizziness, ocular or visual changes, or edema. If these are present, report immediately.
- *Tiagabine:* This drug is to be taken with food. Report any problems with tremors, rash, or abdominal pain.
- *Valproic acid:* Oral dosage forms are not to be taken with carbonated beverages. It is recommended that this drug be taken with at least 4 to 6 oz of water, food, or a snack to minimize GI upset.
- *Miscellaneous new drugs:* With *ezogabine (Potiga)*, patient education is critical about the occurrence of any statements about suicide. Skin discoloration may occur and is permanent, and its use is recommended only if patient has not responded to other drugs. *Perampanel (Fycompa)* has concerns of suicidal thoughts/behaviors and a Black Box Warning of bipolar disorder, psychosis, and schizophrenia. With *vigabatrin (Sabril)*, any onset of visual changes or disturbances must be reported to the prescriber immediately.

Evaluation

A therapeutic response to *antiepileptic drug therapy* does not mean that the patient has been cured of the seizures but only that seizure activity is decreased or absent. Thoroughly document any response to the medication in the nurse's notes. These classes of medications have other indications, such as management of chronic pain and migraines, so the existing problem or disorder would show improvement with minimal adverse effects. In addition, when monitoring and evaluating the effects of antiepileptic drugs, constantly assess the patient for changes in mental status/level of consciousness, affect, eye problems, or visual disorders. Monitoring CBC is also important because of the occurrence of blood dyscrasias. Measurements of serum levels of the specific antiepileptic drug are ordered at baseline or at the start of therapy and frequently thereafter to determine if subsequent serum levels are subtherapeutic, therapeutic, or toxic. Subtherapeutic levels indicate that the dosage may need to be increased (by the prescriber), and toxic levels require withholding or decreasing the dose—but only if prescribed! Serum therapeutic levels are found in Table 14-6.

PATIENT-CENTERED CARE: PATIENT TEACHING

- Educate the patient about the sedating effects of drug therapy so that appropriate steps may be taken to ensure patient safety until a steady state is achieved (usually after four or five drug half-lives). The patient is not to drive, operate heavy machinery, or make major decisions until steady state is achieved or as instructed by the prescriber.
- With any of the antiepileptic drugs, the patient needs to understand the importance of reporting any suicidal thoughts or ideas immediately.
- The intake of alcohol and caffeine are to be avoided, as is smoking.
- Antiepileptic drugs must never be abruptly discontinued as this may precipitate rebound seizure activity.

- The adverse effects most commonly associated with these drugs are drowsiness, GI upset, and CNS-depressing effects. Remind the patient that these adverse effects often decrease after the drug has been taken for several weeks. Taking the antiepileptic drug with food and/or 6 to 8 ounces of fluids will help to minimize GI upset, unless otherwise noted.
- Advise the female patient contemplating pregnancy to seek education and medical advice from the prescriber due to the teratogenic effects of some of the medications.
- Educate the patient about drug interactions between antiepileptic drugs and beta blockers, corticosteroids, calcium channel blockers, ethanol (alcohol), and other CNS depressants.
- Inform the patient that a recurrence of seizure activity is usually due to a lack of compliance with the drug regimen. If a dose or doses of medication are missed, the prescriber needs to be contacted for further instructions. Adherence to medication regimen is critical to the prevention of seizure activity.
- Emphasize to the patient that treatment of epilepsy is life-long and that compliance with the treatment regimen is important for effective therapy. Share information with the patient and family about community and other appropriate resources (e.g., national and local support groups).
- Discuss with the patient important ways to improve *safety* in day-to-day activities while taking antiepileptic drugs: *In the kitchen:* Use an electric stove with no open flame, wear oven mitts, and cook only on rear burners. Cook in the microwave—it is the safest option. Have a plumber install a heat-control device on faucets to avoid burns. Carpet floors to help cushion falls, and use plastic dishes and containers instead of glass when possible. *In the bathroom:* Use heat-control devices on faucets. Carpet floors instead of using tile. Do not put a lock on the bathroom door so that help can be obtained if needed. Bathe with only a few inches of water in the tub, and if seizure activity has not been fully controlled, bathe while someone else is present in the home. *During activities:* Always have someone along when engaging in sports, and make sure the person is knowledgeable about the management of airway and seizures. Bike riding with a helmet, swimming, and water sports are okay if an accompanying adult is present who knows how to manage seizure activity and its consequences.
- Each state has different driving regulations for individuals with epilepsy, and the Waiting Period for Drivers License Following Seizures provides specific requirements/guidelines. Contact each state's Division of Motor Vehicles for current and relevant information.
- Many people with epilepsy work at steady jobs and have successful careers. Some are unable to work, but epilepsy should not prevent the individual from getting a job; such discrimination has been outlawed by the Americans with Disabilities Act of 1990 (Public Law 101-336).
- Encourage the patient to wear a medical alert bracelet or necklace and to keep a medical alert card on his or her person at all times.
- Keeping a daily diary or journal is important and is a helpful tool for the patient, prescriber, and/or caregivers. Entries need to include the date and time of any seizure as well as any details such as omitted drug doses, illnesses, and so on. The location, type, and duration of any type of seizure activity needs to be documented as well as the occurrence of any aura.

▌ K E Y   P O I N T S

- *Epilepsy* is a disorder of the brain manifested as a chronic, recurrent pattern of seizures. A *seizure* is abnormal electrical activity in the brain.
- Seizures are classified as follows: partial-onset seizures or those originating in a more localized region of the brain; status epilepticus, characterized by generalized tonic-clonic convulsions that occur repeatedly in succession; and tonic-clonic seizures involving initial muscular contraction throughout the body (tonic) and progressing to alternating contraction and relaxation (clonic phase).
- You must be able to distinguish between the different types of seizure, and assess/document all symptoms, events, and problems that occur before, during, and after any seizure activity. This information may aid in the diagnosis of the type of seizure the patient is experiencing.
- Noncompliance with the drug regimen is the most important factor leading to treatment failure.
- Monitor therapeutic blood levels at all times. Avoid abrupt withdrawal of the antiepileptic drug to prevent rebound seizure activity.
- IV infusions of antiepileptic drugs are very dangerous and must be managed cautiously, with adherence to health care institution policy and manufacturer's guidelines. Avoid rapid infusions because of the risk for cardiac and/or respiratory arrest.
- Older adult patients may experience paradoxical reactions to antiepileptic drugs, resulting in hyperactivity and irritability versus sedation.

NCLEX® EXAMINATION REVIEW QUESTIONS

1. The nurse is preparing to give medications. Which is the most appropriate nursing action for intravenous (IV) phenytoin (Dilantin)?
   a. Give IV doses via rapid IV push.
   b. Administer in normal saline solutions.
   c. Administer in dextrose solutions.
   d. Ensure continuous infusion of the drug.

2. The nurse is reviewing the drugs currently taken by a patient who will be starting drug therapy with carbamazepine (Tegretol). Which drug may raise a concern for interactions?
   a. digoxin (Lanoxin)
   b. acetaminophen (Tylenol)
   c. diazepam (Valium)
   d. warfarin (Coumadin)

3. Which response would the nurse expect to find in a patient with a phenytoin (Dilantin) level of 25 mcg/mL?
   a. Ataxia
   b. Hypertension
   c. Seizures
   d. No unusual response; this level is therapeutic.

4. A patient is taking pregabalin (Lyrica) but does not have a history of seizures. The nurse recognizes that this drug is also indicated for
   a. postherpetic neuralgia.
   b. viral infections.
   c. Parkinson's disease.
   d. depression.

5. The nurse is assessing a newly admitted patient who has a history of seizures. During the assessment, the patient has a generalized seizure that does not stop for several minutes. The nurse expects that which drug will be ordered for this condition?
   a. valproic acid (Depakote)
   b. neurontin (Gabapentin)
   c. carbamazepine (Tegretol)
   d. diazepam (Valium)

6. The nurse is administering an antiepileptic drug and will follow which guidelines? *(Select all that apply.)*
   a. Monitor the patient for drowsiness.
   b. Medications may be stopped if seizure activity disappears.
   c. Give the medication at the same time every day.
   d. Give the medication on an empty stomach.
   e. Notify the prescriber if the patient is unable to take the medication.

7. The nurse is preparing to administer valproic acid to a child. The order reads: "Give valproic acid, 15 mg/kg/day PO in three divided doses." The child weighs 33 pounds. How many milligrams will the child receive with each dose?

8. The nurse is providing education for a patient who will be taking an antiepileptic drug for the first time. Which statement by the patient indicates that further teaching is indicated?
   a. "I will take the medicine at the same time every day."
   b. "I will check with my doctor before taking any over-the-counter drugs."
   c. "I will keep the appointments to check my bloodwork."
   d. "I can drive to work again once my drug levels are normal."

1. b, 2. b, 3. a, 4. a, 5. d, 6. a, c, e, 7. 75 mg per dose, 8. d

CRITICAL THINKING AND PRIORITIZATION QUESTIONS

1. The nurse is about to administer the morning dose of phenobarbital to a patient with a history of seizures. Before the dose is given, the laboratory calls to report that the patient's phenobarbital blood level is 8 mcg/mL. What is the nurse's priority action at this time?

2. The laboratory results indicate that the patient's valproic acid level is at toxic levels, but the patient insists that he has not taken extra doses of medication. "I take it the same way at the same time every morning," he states emphatically. Upon further questioning, the patient mentions that he also takes aspirin three or four times a day for muscle aches. "Could that have any effect on my drug level?" he asks. What is the nurse's best response?

For answers, see *http://evolve.elsevier.com/Lilley.*

Ⓔ EVOLVE WEBSITE

http://evolve.elsevier.com/Lilley
- Animations
- Answer Keys for Textbook Case Studies and Textbook Critical Thinking and Prioritization Questions
- Content Updates
- Key Points
- Review Questions
- Student Case Studies

Antiparkinson Drugs

http://evolve.elsevier.com/Lilley

OBJECTIVES

When you reach the end of this chapter, you will be able to do the following:

1. Briefly discuss the impact of acetylcholine and dopamine on the brain.
2. Describe the pathophysiology of Parkinson's disease.
3. Identify the different classes of medications used to manage Parkinson's disease, and list the drugs in each class.
4. Discuss the mechanisms of action, dosages, indications, routes of administration, contraindications, cautions, drug interactions, adverse effects, and toxic effects of antiparkinson drugs.
5. Develop a nursing care plan that includes all phases of the nursing process for patients taking antiparkinson drugs.

DRUG PROFILES

amantadine, p. 240
♦ benztropine mesylate, p. 243
bromocriptine, p. 242
♦ carbidopa-levodopa, p. 243
entacapone, p. 241

♦ ropinirole, p. 242
rasagiline and selegiline, p. 238

_____
♦ = *Key drug*
! = *High-alert drug*

KEY TERMS

Adjunctive drugs Drugs that are added as a second drug for combined therapy with a primary drug and may have additive or independent properties. (p. 238)

Akinesia Classically defined as "without movement." Absence or poverty of movement that results in a masklike facial expression and impaired postural reflexes. (p. 237)

Bradykinesia Slowness of movement; a classic symptom of Parkinson's disease. (p. 237)

Chorea A condition characterized by involuntary, purposeless, rapid motions such as flexing and extending the fingers, raising and lowering the shoulders, or grimacing. (p. 237)

Dyskinesia Abnormal involuntary movements; inability to control movements. (p. 237)

Dystonia Impaired or distorted voluntary movement, involving the head, neck, or feet. (p. 237)

Exogenous A term describing any substance produced outside of the body that may be taken into the body (e.g., a medication, food, or environmental toxin). (p. 242)

On-off phenomenon A common experience of patients taking medication for Parkinson's disease in which they experience periods of greater symptomatic control ("on" time) alternating with periods of lesser symptomatic control ("off" time). (p. 237)

Parkinson's disease A slowly progressive, degenerative neurologic disorder characterized by resting tremor, pill-rolling of the fingers, masklike facies, shuffling gait, forward flexion of the trunk, loss of postural reflexes, and muscle rigidity and weakness. (p. 236)

Postural instability A decrease or change in motor and muscle movements that leads to unsteadiness and hesitation in movement and gait when the individual starts or stops walking, or causes leaning to the left or right when sitting; occurs in Parkinson's disease. (p. 237)

Presynaptic Drugs that exert their antiparkinson effects before the nerve synapse. (p. 240)

Rigidity Resistance of the muscles to passive movement; leads to the "cogwheel" rigidity seen in Parkinson's disease. (p. 237)

TRAP (*T*remor, *R*igidity, *A*kinesia, *P*ostural instability); an acronym for symptoms of Parkinson's disease. (p. 237)

Tremor In Parkinson's disease, shakiness of the extremities seen mostly at rest. (p. 237)

Wearing-off phenomenon A gradual worsening of parkinsonian symptoms as a patient's medications begin to lose their effectiveness, despite maximal dosing with a variety of medications. (p. 237)

PATHOPHYSIOLOGY OF PARKINSON'S DISEASE

Parkinson's disease is a chronic, progressive, neurodegenerative disorder affecting the dopamine-producing neurons in the brain. Parkinson's disease was initially recognized in 1817, at which time it was called *shaking palsy.* James Parkinson later described in more detail the symptoms of both the early and advanced stages of the disease. The underlying pathologic defect was not discovered until the 1960s. It was then recognized that Parkinson's disease involves a dopamine deficit in the area of the cerebral cortex called the *substantia nigra,* which is contained within another brain structure known as the *basal ganglia.* Also relevant is the adjacent structure called the *globus pallidus.* All three structures are parts of the brain that make up the *extrapyramidal system,* which is involved in motor function, including posture, muscle tone, and smooth muscle activity. In addition, the *thalamus* serves as a relay station for brain impulses, whereas the *cerebellum* regulates muscle coordination (Figure 15-1).

Dopamine is an inhibitory neurotransmitter, and *acetylcholine* is an excitatory neurotransmitter in this area of the brain. A correct balance between these two neurotransmitters is needed for the proper regulation of posture, muscle tone, and voluntary movement. Parkinson's disease results from an imbalance in these two neurotransmitters in the basal ganglia. This imbalance is caused by failure of the nerve terminals in the substantia nigra to produce dopamine. Dopamine acts in the basal ganglia to control movements. Destruction of the substantia nigra by Parkinson's disease leads to dopamine depletion. This often results in excessive, unopposed acetylcholine (cholinergic) activity. Figure 15-2 illustrates the difference in neurotransmitter concentrations in persons with normal balance and in patients with Parkinson's disease.

Some theorize that Parkinson's disease is the result of an earlier head injury or of excess iron in the substantia nigra, which undergoes oxidation and causes the generation of toxic free radicals. Another theory postulates that Parkinson's disease represents a premature aging of the *nigrostriatal cells* of the substantia nigra resulting from environmental or intrinsic biochemical factors, or both.

Parkinson's disease affects at least 1 million Americans and 4 million people worldwide. It is the second most common neurodegenerative disease after Alzheimer's disease. Some patients may have symptoms of both conditions. In most patients, the disease becomes apparent between 45 and 65 years of age, with a mean age of onset of 56 years. The number of patients with Parkinson's disease is expected to continue to increase as our older adult population grows. The disease occasionally occurs in younger people, especially after acute encephalitis, or carbon monoxide or metallic poisoning. However, it is usually idiopathic (of no known cause). Overall, there is a 2% chance of developing the disease in one's lifetime. Men are affected more often than women in a ratio of up to 3:2. Evidence now suggests a possible genetic link, with up to 20% of patients having a family history of the disease.

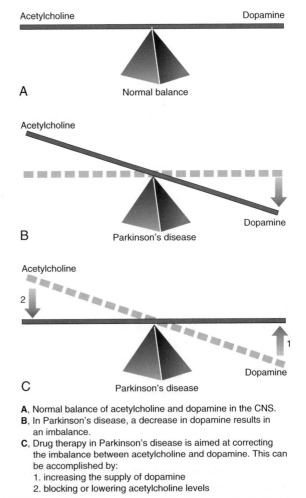

A, Normal balance of acetylcholine and dopamine in the CNS.
B, In Parkinson's disease, a decrease in dopamine results in an imbalance.
C, Drug therapy in Parkinson's disease is aimed at correcting the imbalance between acetylcholine and dopamine. This can be accomplished by:
1. increasing the supply of dopamine
2. blocking or lowering acetylcholine levels

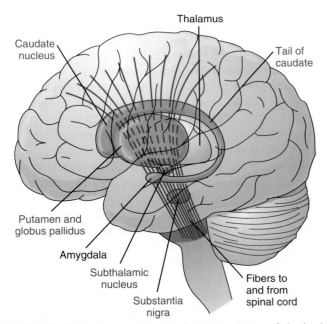

FIGURE 15-1 Basal ganglia and related structures of the brain. (From Copstead-Kirkhorn LC, Banasik JL: *Pathophysiology,* ed 4, St Louis, 2010, Saunders.)

FIGURE 15-2 The neurotransmitter abnormality in Parkinson's disease.

TABLE 15-1 Classic Parkinsonian Symptoms

Symptom	Description
Akinesia	Absence of psychomotor activity resulting in masklike facial expression
Bradykinesia	Slowness of movement
Rigidity	"Cogwheel" rigidity, resistance to passive movement
Tremor	Pill rolling: tremor of the thumb against the forefinger, seen mostly at rest and less severe during voluntary activity; usually starts on one side then progresses to the other; is the presenting sign in 70% of cases; also seen as tremor of the hand and extremities.
Postural instability	Unsteadiness (associated with bradykinesia and rigidity) that leads to danger of falling; leaning to one side, even when sitting

There are no readily available laboratory tests that can detect or confirm Parkinson's disease. The diagnosis is usually made on the basis of the classic symptoms and physical findings. The classic symptoms of Parkinson's disease include bradykinesia, postural instability, rigidity, and tremors (TRAP [Tremor, Rigidity, Akinesia, Postural instability] with akinesia really manifesting as bradykinesia) (Table 15-1). Unfortunately, Parkinson's disease is a progressive condition, and over time there is substantial reduction in the number of surviving dopaminergic terminals that can take up pharmacologically administered levodopa and convert it into dopamine. Rapid swings in the response to levodopa, called the on-off phenomenon, also occur. The result is worsening of the disease when too little dopamine is present, or dyskinesias when too much is present. In contrast, the wearing-off phenomenon occurs when anti–Parkinson's disease medications begin to lose their effectiveness, despite maximal dosing, as the disease progresses. Dyskinesia is the difficulty in performing voluntary movements and is commonly seen in the disease. The two dyskinesias most frequently associated with antiparkinson therapy are chorea (irregular, spasmodic, involuntary movements of the limbs or facial muscles) and dystonia (abnormal muscle tone leading to impaired or abnormal movements). Dystonia commonly involves the head, neck, or feet and is a symptom common to patients with Parkinson's disease. These motor complications make Parkinson's disease a prominent cause of disability. Dementia may also be a result of the disease and is referred to as *Parkinson's disease–associated dementia.*

Symptoms of Parkinson's disease do not appear until approximately 80% of the dopamine store in the substantia nigra has been depleted. This means that by the time the disease is diagnosed, only approximately 20% of the patient's original dopaminergic terminals are functioning normally.

TREATMENT OF PARKINSON'S DISEASE

The first step in the treatment of Parkinson's disease is to provide a full explanation of the disease to the patient. Physical therapy, speech therapy, and occupational therapy are almost always needed when the patient is in the later stages of the disease. Treatment of the disease centers on drug therapy. However, physical activity is a must for these patients. Many experts believe that physical activity is as important as any drug therapy, and together they greatly improve mobility. For severe cases, the surgical technique of *deep brain stimulation* may be used.

PHARMACOLOGY OVERVIEW

Because Parkinson's disease is thought to be due to an imbalance of dopamine and acetylcholine with a deficiency of dopamine in certain areas of the brain, it seems logical that drug therapies are aimed at increasing the levels of dopamine and/or antagonizing the effects of acetylcholine. Unfortunately, current drug therapy does not slow the progression of the disease, but rather is used to slow the progression of symptoms. The drugs available for the treatment of Parkinson's disease are listed in Table 15-2. In patients with advanced disease, there is some concern when switching from brand name to generic drugs. Patients must be observed closely for adverse effects and changes in drug efficacy.

INDIRECT-ACTING DOPAMINERGIC DRUGS

MONOAMINE OXIDASE INHIBITORS

The enzyme *monoamine oxidase (MAO)* causes the breakdown of *catecholamines* in the body. Catecholamines include dopamine, norepinephrine, and epinephrine. There are two subclasses of MAO in the body: MAO-A and MAO-B. As early as 1965, nonselective monoamine oxidase inhibitors (MAOIs), which inhibit both MAO-A and MAO-B, were being used to improve the therapeutic effect of levodopa by preventing its metabolic breakdown. A major adverse effect of the nonselective MAOIs is that they interact with tyramine-containing foods (cheese, red wine, beer, and yogurt) because of their inhibitory activity against MAO-A. This has been called the *cheese effect,* and can result in severe hypertension. Rasagiline and selegiline are selective MAO-B inhibitors and are much less likely to elicit the classic cheese effect. Drug interactions and adverse effects are similar for both drugs.

Mechanism of Action and Drug Effects

The MAO enzymes are widely distributed throughout the body, with the highest concentrations found in the liver, kidney, stomach, intestinal wall, and brain. The primary role of MAO enzymes is the breakdown of catecholamines, such as dopamine, norepinephrine, and epinephrine, as well as serotonin. Giving an MAO-B inhibitor such as rasagiline or selegiline causes an increase in the levels of dopaminergic stimulation in the CNS. This helps to counter the dopaminergic deficiency seen in Parkinson's disease. Administration of rasagiline or selegiline can also allow the dose of levodopa (discussed later in this chapter) to be reduced. Improvement in functional ability and decreased severity of symptoms can occur; however, only approximately 50% to 60% of patients show a positive response.

TABLE 15-2   Review of Pharmacologic Therapy for Parkinson's Disease

Generic Name	Trade Name	Route	Indications
Indirect-Acting Dopamine Receptor Agonists (MAO-B Inhibitors)			
Rasagiline	Azilect	PO	Used alone or in conjunction with carbidopa-levodopa in early stages of disease;
selegiline	Eldepryl, Zelapar*	PO	helpful with symptom fluctuations
Dopamine Modulator			
amantadine	Symmetrel	PO	Used in early stages; can be effective in moderate or advanced stages; reduces tremor or muscle rigidity
COMT Inhibitors			
Entacapone	Comtan	PO	Usually added to carbidopa-levodopa to treat symptom fluctuations; delays "off" periods; has levodopa dose-sparing effect
tolcapone	Tamsar	PO	
Direct-Acting Dopamine Receptor Agonists			
Ergot			
bromocriptine	Parlodel	PO	Usually used as drug of choice for young patients; first- or second-line therapy of choice for older adults; can be used as adjunct to levodopa for "off" periods; can be used to reduce dyskinesia associated with later stages
Nonergot			
pramipexole	Mirapex	PO	
ropinirole	Requip	PO	
rotigotine	Neupro	Transdermal	
Dopamine Replacement Drugs			
carbidopa-levodopa	Sinemet, Rytary	PO	Usually started as soon as patient becomes functionally impaired; drug of choice for most older adults
Anticholinergic Drugs†			
benztropine	Cogentin	PO, IV	Used as secondary drug for tremor/muscle rigidity
trihexyphenidyl	Generic only	PO	
Antihistamines‡			
diphenhydramine	Benadryl	PO, IV	Used as secondary drug for tremor/muscle rigidity

COMT, Catechol ortho-methyltransferase; *MAO-B,* monoamine oxidase type B.
*Orally disintegrating tablet (see Chapter 2).
†See Chapter 21.
‡See Chapter 36.

Indications

Rasagiline and selegiline are used as monotherapy or in conjunction with levodopa therapy (as adjunctive drugs) in the treatment of Parkinson's disease. Rasagiline is given once a day, whereas selegiline is given twice a day with breakfast and lunch. Studies have shown that selegiline-treated patients required levodopa therapy approximately 1.8 times later than control patients.

Contraindications

Rasagiline and selegiline are contraindicated in cases of known drug allergy. Concurrent use with the opioid analgesic meperidine (see Chapter 10) is also contraindicated due to a drug interaction between MAOIs and meperidine.

Adverse Effects

The most common adverse effects associated with rasagiline and selegiline use are mild and are listed in Table 15-3. At recommended dosages, both drugs maintain their selective MAO-B inhibition. However, at higher doses they become nonselective MAOIs.

Interactions

Rasagiline and selegiline interact with meperidine and have been associated with delirium, muscle rigidity, and hyperpyrexia. Other reported reactions are listed in Table 15-4. Both drugs may be safely taken concurrently with catechol ortho-methyltransferase (COMT) inhibitors (see later drug section). Patients taking higher doses of either drug need to avoid tyramine-containing foods such as aged cheese, sausages, and draft beer.

Dosages

For dosage information, see the table on the next page. Also see the Safety and Quality Improvement: Preventing Medication Errors box on p. 240.

DRUG PROFILES

rasagiline and selegiline

Rasagiline (Azilect) and selegiline (Eldepryl) are selective MAO-B inhibitors, which are indicated for Parkinson's disease. Adverse effects increase with higher than recommended doses as they lose their selectivity for MAO-B, and are listed in Table 15-3. Drug interactions are listed in Table 15-4. Selegiline is

TABLE 15-3   Adverse Effects of Selected Antiparkinson Drugs

Drug or Drug Class	Adverse Effects
MAO-B inhibitor: selegiline	Headache, insomnia, dizziness, nausea, hypotension, confusion, rash, weight loss, diarrhea, stomatitis, dyskinesia, back pain, somnolence, impulse control disorders
Dopamine modulator: amantadine	Orthostatic hypotension, peripheral edema, dizziness, insomnia, agitation, anxiety, headache, hallucinations, nausea, dry mouth
COMT inhibitor: entacapone	GI upset, dyskinesia, orthostatic hypotension, syncope, dizziness, fatigue, hallucinations, anxiety, somnolence, rash, dyspnea, worsening of dyskinesia, urine discoloration
Anticholinergic agent: benztropine	Tachycardia, confusion, memory impairment, rash, hyperthermia, constipation; dry throat, nausea, vomiting, urinary retention, blurred vision, fever
Ergot derivative: bromocriptine	Ataxia, dizziness, headache, depression, drowsiness, GI upset, visual changes
Nonergot derivatives: pramipexole, ropinirole	Edema, fatigue, syncope, dizziness, drowsiness, GI upset
Dopamine replacement drugs: levodopa, carbidopa-levodopa combination	Palpitations, hypotension, urinary retention, depression, dyskinesia

TABLE 15-4   Selected Drug Interactions of Antiparkinson Drugs

Drug or Drug Class	Interacting Drug	Mechanism	Result
MAO-B inhibitor: selegiline	meperidine and other opioids, tramadol, cyclobenzaprine, dextromethorphan, other MAOIs, serotonergic antidepressants, oxcarbazepine	Additive CNS stimulation	Serotonin syndrome
	carbamazepine, oral contraceptives	Reduced selegiline clearance	Potential selegiline toxicity
	buspirone	Uncertain	Hypertension
Dopamine modulator: amantadine	Anticholinergics	Additive effects	Increased anticholinergic adverse effects
COMT inhibitor: entacapone	MAOIs, catecholamines	Reduced catecholamine metabolism	Tachycardia, cardiac dysrhythmias, hypertension
Ergot derivative: bromocriptine	erythromycin	Cytochrome P-450 interactions	Increased bromocriptine effects with risk for toxicity
	Sympathomimetics	Additive effects	Hypertension, cardiac dysrhythmias
	Antihypertensives	Additive effects	Hypotension
Nonergot derivative: ropinirole	warfarin, ciprofloxacin	Cytochrome P-450 interactions	Reduced ropinirole clearance with risk for toxicity
	Antipsychotics	Antidopaminergic activity	Reduced efficacy of ropinirole
Dopamine replacement: levodopa, carbidopa	Nonselective MAOIs	Additive toxicity	Hypertensive reactions
	Benzodiazepines, antipsychotics	Reduced levodopa effects	Reduced therapeutic effects

COMT, Catechol ortho-methyltransferase; *MAO-B,* monoamine oxidase type B; *MAOI,* monoamine oxidase inhibitor.

DOSAGES

Selected Antiparkinson Drugs

Drug (Pregnancy Category)	Pharmacologic Class	Usual Adult Dosage Range	Indications
amantadine (Symmetrel) (C)	Dopamine modulator	PO: 100-400 mg/day divided every 12 hr	
◆benztropine (Cogentin) (C)	Anticholinergic	PO: 0.5-6 mg/day	
bromocriptine (Parlodel) (D)	Direct-acting dopamine agonist; ergot derivative	PO: 2.5-100 mg/day	
◆carbidopa-levodopa (Sinemet, Sinemet CR) (C)	Antiparkinson agent	PO: 10/100, 1 tab 3-8 times/day; 25/100, 1 tab 3-6 times/day; 25/250, 1 tab tid-qid CR: 50/200 mg; initial dose of 1 tab bid at 4-8 hr intervals during waking hours	Parkinson's disease
entacapone (Comtan) (C)	COMT inhibitor	PO: 200 mg with each dosage of levodopa, up to max dose of 1600 mg/day	
◆ropinirole (Requip) (C)	Direct-acting dopamine agonist; nonergot derivative	PO: 0.25 mg tid, slowly titrating to max dose of 24 mg/day	
selegiline (Eldepryl, Zelapar) (C)	Selective MAO-B inhibitor	PO: 5 mg bid with breakfast and lunch; PO (orally disintegrating tablet [Zelapar]): 1.25-2.5 mg once daily before breakfast	

CR, Controlled release.

available as an oral tablet and an orally disintegrating tablet for buccal use known as Zelapar, which can provide improved drug absorption. In addition, a transdermal form of the drug known as Emsam is available, which is indicated only for major depressive disorder (see Chapter 16). Rasagiline (Azilect) is available as an oral tablet. Rasagiline is FDA approved for monotherapy, but selegiline is also being used in such a manner. Both are approved as adjunctive therapy with levodopa.

Pharmacokinetics: Selegiline

Route	Onset of Action	Peak Plasma Concentration	Elimination Half-life	Duration of Action
PO	1 hr	0.5-2 hr	2 hr	1-3 days

QSEN ⚡ SAFETY AND QUALITY IMPROVEMENT: PREVENTING MEDICATION ERRORS

Look-Alike/Sound-Alike Drugs: Selegiline and Salagen

Be careful with look-alike/sound-alike drugs! Medication errors often occur when drug names are similar.

Selegiline is a monoamine oxidase inhibitor that is used to treat Parkinson's disease. Salagen, an oral form of pilocarpine hydrochloride, is prescribed for relief of dry mouth symptoms, also known as *xerostomia*, in patients who have Sjögren's syndrome or who have received radiation therapy. To make it more confusing, both drugs are available in 5-mg dosage forms. Be sure to double-check the name and use of these drugs when receiving orders, and instruct patients to check the drug names when getting these drugs filled at pharmacies. They should also immediately report any difference in the appearance of their medications.

For more information, visit *www.ismp.org*.

DOPAMINE MODULATOR

Only one drug is currently known to function as a dopamine modulator. Amantadine (Symmetrel) was first recognized as an antiviral drug and was used for treating influenza virus infections. It is still used for this purpose (see Chapter 40) as well as for management of Parkinson's disease.

Mechanism of Action and Drug Effects

Amantadine appears to work by causing the release of dopamine and other catecholamines from their storage sites in the presynaptic fibers of nerve cells within the basal ganglia that have not yet been destroyed by the disease process. Amantadine also blocks the reuptake of dopamine into the nerve fibers. This results in higher levels of dopamine in the synapses between nerves and improved dopamine neurotransmission between neurons. Because amantadine does not directly stimulate dopaminergic receptors, it is considered to be indirect acting. Amantadine also has some anticholinergic properties (see Chapter 21). This may further help by controlling symptoms of dyskinesia.

Indications

Amantadine is generally indicated in the early stages of Parkinson's disease while there are still some intact neurons in the basal ganglia. It is usually effective for only 6 to 12 months, after which it often fails to relieve hypokinesia and rigidity. It is often used to treat dyskinesia associated with carbidopa-levodopa. It is also indicated for influenza virus infection (see Chapter 40).

Contraindications

Amantadine is contraindicated in cases of known drug allergy.

Adverse Drug Effects

Common adverse effects associated with amantadine are relatively mild and include dizziness, insomnia, and nausea.

Drug Interactions

Amantadine causes increased anticholinergic adverse effects when given with anticholinergic drugs.

Dosage

For dosage information, see the table on the previous page.

DRUG PROFILE

amantadine

Amantadine (Symmetrel) is an antiviral drug most often for influenza virus infection (see Chapter 40). It is also indicated for treatment of mild to moderate Parkinson's disease. It helps to control symptoms of tremor, including motor rigidity, by virtue of both its dopaminergic and anticholinergic effects. Common adverse reactions include dizziness, insomnia, and nausea. Interacting drugs include anticholinergics (additive effects) (see Table 15-4). Amantadine is available only for oral use.

Pharmacokinetics: Amantadine

Route	Onset of Action	Peak Plasma Concentration	Elimination Half-life	Duration of Action
PO	48 hr	2-4 hr	11-15 hr	6-12 wk

CATECHOL ORTHO-METHYLTRANSFERASE INHIBITORS

The third category of indirect-acting dopaminergic drugs is the *catechol ortho-methyltransferase (COMT)* inhibitors. There are currently two drugs in this category: entacapone (Comtan) and tolcapone (Tasmar).

Mechanism of Action and Drug Effects

Entacapone and tolcapone, like amantadine, work presynaptically. Both drugs block COMT. COMT is the enzyme that catalyzes the breakdown of the body's catecholamines. Tolcapone acts both centrally and peripherally, whereas entacapone cannot cross the blood-brain barrier and therefore can act only peripherally. The positive effect of these drugs is that they prolong the duration of action of levodopa. This is especially true when levodopa is given with carbidopa (see section on dopamine replacement drugs later in the chapter). This results in reduction of the wearing-off phenomenon.

Indications

COMT inhibitors are indicated for the treatment of Parkinson's disease.

Contraindications

Both COMT inhibitors (entacapone and tolcapone) are contraindicated in cases of known drug allergy. Tolcapone is also contraindicated in cases of liver failure.

Adverse Effects

Commonly reported adverse effects with both COMT inhibitors include gastrointestinal (GI) upset and urine discoloration. In addition, they also can worsen dyskinesia that may already be present (see Table 15-3). Tolcapone has been associated with cases of severe liver failure, and the FDA announced in 1998 that it is to be considered only in patients who do not respond to other Parkinson's disease drug therapy.

Interactions

Neither entacapone nor tolcapone are to be taken with nonselective MAOIs because of cardiovascular risk due to reduced catecholamine metabolism. However, the selective MAO-B inhibitors rasagiline and selegiline may be safely taken concurrently with COMT inhibitors.

Dosages

For dosage information, see the table on p. 239.

DRUG PROFILE

Inhibition of the enzyme in the body known as COMT is a strategy for prolonging the duration of action of levodopa. Entacapone (Comtan) and tolcapone (Tasmar) are reversible inhibitors of COMT. Tolcapone has been associated with severe liver failure and is rarely used.

entacapone

Entacapone (Comtan) is a COMT inhibitor indicated for the adjunctive treatment of Parkinson's disease. Entacapone is taken with levodopa and is effective from the first dose, and benefits are seen within a few days. Entacapone helps minimize the wearing-off effect, and when used with levodopa, it can also reduce on-off effects. The levodopa dosage can often be reduced when taken with entacapone. Adverse reactions include GI upset, dyskinesias, and urine discoloration (see Table 15-3). Entacapone is contraindicated in patients with known drug allergy and used with caution in patients with preexisting liver disease. Entacapone is available only for oral use. It is also available in combination tablets that contain various doses of entacapone, carbidopa, and levodopa (Stalevo).

Pharmacokinetics: Entacapone

Route	Onset of Action	Peak Plasma Concentration	Elimination Half-life	Duration of Action
PO	1 hr	0.5-1.5 hr	1-5.3.5 hr	6 hr

DIRECT-ACTING DOPAMINE RECEPTOR AGONISTS

Direct-acting dopamine receptor agonists are drugs used to treat Parkinson's disease, often as first-line agents used upon diagnosis. These drugs include two subclasses: *nondopamine dopamine receptor agonists (NDDRAs)* and *dopamine replacement drugs*. NDDRAs are further subdivided into the ergot derivatives bromocriptine (Parlodel) and the nonergot drugs pramipexole (Mirapex), ropinirole (Requip), and rotigotine (Neupro).

NONDOPAMINE DOPAMINE RECEPTOR AGONISTS

Mechanism of Action and Drug Effects

All of the NDDRAs work by direct stimulation of presynaptic and/or postsynaptic dopamine receptors in the brain. They may be used in early or late stages of the disease.

Chemically, bromocriptine is an ergot alkaloid similar to ergotamine (see Chapter 13). Bromocriptine works by activating presynaptic dopamine receptors to stimulate the production of more dopamine. Its chief site of activity is the D_2 subclass of dopamine receptors. Pramipexole, ropinirole, and rotigotine are *nonergot* NDDRAs. Both are effective in early and late stages of Parkinson's disease.

Indications

Both ergot and nonergot NDDRAs are used to treat various stages of Parkinson's disease, either alone or in combination with other drugs. Bromocriptine also inhibits the production of the hormone *prolactin*, which stimulates normal lactation and can be used to treat women with excessive or undesired breast milk production (*galactorrhea*) and for treatment of prolactin-secreting tumors. Ropinirole and rotigotine are also used to treat a disorder known as *restless legs syndrome*, a nocturnal movement of the legs that disrupts sleep.

Contraindications

Known allergy is a contraindication to dopaminergic drug therapy. These drugs are not to be used concurrently with adrenergic drugs (see Chapter 18) due to the cardiovascular risk for excessive catecholamine activity.

Adverse Effects

Many potential adverse effects are associated with the dopaminergic drugs. They are listed in Table 15-3.

Interactions

Interactions vary among drugs and are listed in Table 15-4.

Dosages

For dosage information, see the table on p. 239.

DRUG PROFILES

The traditional role of the NDDRAs bromocriptine, pramipexole, ropinirole, and rotigotine has been as adjuncts to levodopa for management of motor fluctuations; however, they are now often used as first-line therapy. These drugs differ from levodopa in that they do not replace dopamine itself but act by stimulation of dopaminergic receptors in the brain. They have been used as initial monotherapy and as combination therapy with low-dose levodopa in an attempt to either delay levodopa therapy or reduce the dosage of levodopa and its associated motor complications (see drug profile for levodopa).

bromocriptine

Bromocriptine stimulates only the D_2 receptors and antagonizes the D_1 receptors. The use of amantadine or a nondopamine agonist until it fails may postpone the need for levodopa therapy. Bromocriptine may also be given with carbidopa-levodopa so that lower dosages of the levodopa are needed. This often results in prolonging the "on" periods and minimizing the "off" periods of the disease. Bromocriptine is indicated for Parkinson's disease as well as hyperprolactinemia. It is contraindicated in known drug allergy to any ergot alkaloids and in patients with severe ischemic disease of any kind (e.g., peripheral vascular disease). Bromocriptine can stimulate dopamine receptors in the peripheral tissues outside of the brain, which can result in vasoconstriction, which, in turn, can worsen peripheral vascular disease. Adverse reactions include GI upset, dyskinesias, sleep disturbances, and others as listed in Table 15-3. Drug interactions occur with erythromycin (see Chapter 38) and adrenergic drugs (see Chapter 18). Drug interactions are listed in Table 15-4. Bromocriptine is available only for oral use.

Pharmacokinetics Bromocriptine

Route	Onset of Action	Peak Plasma Concentration	Elimination Half-life	Duration of Action
PO	0.5-1.5 hr	1-3 hr	3-5 hr	4-8 hr

◆ropinirole

Ropinirole (Requip) is a nonergot NDDRA. Similar drugs include pramipexole (Mirapex) and rotigotine (Neupro). These nonergot drugs have a better adverse effects profile (e.g., fewer dyskinesias) than bromocriptine. Ropinirole, pramipexole, and rotigotine are more specific than bromocriptine for the D_2 subfamily of dopamine receptors (D_2, D_3, and D_4). This, in turn, results in more specific antiparkinson effects with fewer of the adverse effects. These drugs (ropinirole, pramipexole, and rotigotine) can be effective in both early- and late-stage Parkinson's disease and appear to delay the need for levodopa therapy. They can be used as monotherapy and adjunctive therapy with levodopa. Ropinirole and rotigotine are also indicated for treatment of moderate to severe primary restless legs syndrome. All drugs are contraindicated in patients with known drug allergy. Adverse effects include dizziness, GI upset, and somnolence (see Table 15-3). Drug interactions occur with any drug metabolized by cytochrome P-450 enzyme 1A2 (e.g., warfarin, ciprofloxacin) (see Table 15-4). Ropinirole and pramipexole are available only for oral use, while rotigotine is available as a transdermal patch, providing 24-hour continuous therapy.

Pharmacokinetics: Ropinirole

Route	Onset of Action	Peak Plasma Concentration	Elimination Half-life	Duration of Action
PO	30 min	1-2 hr	3-5 hr	6-10 hr

DOPAMINE REPLACEMENT DRUGS

The traditional cornerstone of therapy for Parkinson's disease has been with the drug levodopa. It is a biologic precursor of dopamine required by the brain for dopamine synthesis. However, levodopa is significantly metabolized before it reaches the brain, so it is combined with another substance, carbidopa. Carbidopa it is a levodopa enhancer and allows for much lower doses of levodopa to be used and reduces the side effects associated with high-dose levodopa. Using the analogy that carbidopa is the car that drops off levodopa in the brain may be helpful. The combination product carbidopa-levodopa provides exogenous sources of dopamine that directly replace dopamine in the substantia nigra. These drugs are classified as *dopamine replacement* drugs and are drugs of choice in the later stages of Parkinson's disease. As Parkinson's disease progresses, it becomes more difficult to manage it with levodopa. Ultimately, levodopa no longer controls the disease, and the patient is seriously debilitated. This generally occurs between 5 and 10 years after the start of levodopa therapy.

Mechanism of Action and Drug Effects

Dopamine replacement drugs stimulate presynaptic dopamine receptors to increase brain levels of dopamine. Dopamine must be administered orally as levodopa, because exogenously administered dopamine cannot pass through the blood-brain barrier. Levodopa is the biologic precursor of dopamine and can penetrate into the CNS. Levodopa is broken down outside the CNS by the enzyme dopa decarboxylase, and very large oral doses of levodopa are required to obtain adequate levels. The large doses needed result in high peripheral levels of dopamine and lead to many unwanted adverse effects (see Table 15-3). These adverse effects include confusion, involuntary movements, GI distress, hypotension, and cardiac dysrhythmias. Therefore, levodopa is given with carbidopa. Carbidopa is a peripheral decarboxylase inhibitor with little or no pharmacologic activity when given alone. When given in combination with levodopa, carbidopa inhibits the breakdown of levodopa in the periphery and thus allows smaller doses of levodopa to be used. Lesser amounts of levodopa result in fewer unwanted adverse effects.

Indications

Dopamine replacement drugs are used to directly restore dopaminergic activity in Parkinson's disease. Dopamine itself is also given by injection in critical care settings (see Chapter 18).

Contraindications

Levodopa and carbidopa are both contraindicated in cases of angle-closure glaucoma; however, they may be used cautiously in patients with open-angle glaucoma (see Chapter 57). Neither drug is to be used in patients with any undiagnosed skin condition, because both drugs can activate malignant melanoma.

Adverse Effects

Adverse effects of dopamine replacement drugs include cardiac dysrhythmias, hypotension, chorea, muscle cramps, and GI distress (see Table 15-3).

Interactions

A possible drug interaction can occur with pyridoxine (vitamin B_6). Pyridoxine reduces the effectiveness of carbidopa-levodopa; however, the dose can usually be adjusted to overcome this interaction. See the nursing implementation section for discussion of the possible interaction of carbidopa-levodopa with dietary protein. Other interactions are listed in Table 15-4.

DRUG PROFILE

♦ carbidopa-levodopa

Carbidopa-levodopa (Sinemet), available orally, is one of the most commonly used drugs for Parkinson's disease. Carbidopa (Lodosyn) alone is not used as therapy, rather as an adjunct to treat nausea associated with Sinemet. A variety of studies have shown that the controlled-release product Sinemet CR (or generic) increases "on" time and decreases "off" time. As with all sustained-release products, Sinemet CR must not be crushed; however, it can be split one time, unlike most other CR or XR drugs on the market. Drug interactions occur with tricyclic antidepressants and other drugs (see Table 15-4). Carbidopa-levodopa is best taken on an empty stomach; however, to minimize GI side effects, it can be taken with food. A new extended release formulation of carbidopa-levodopa (Rytary) was recently released.

Pharmacokinetics: Carbidopa-Levodopa

Route	Onset of Action	Peak Plasma Concentration	Elimination Half-life	Duration of Action
PO	2-3 wk*	0.5-2 hr	1.5 hr	5 hr

*Therapeutic effect.

ANTICHOLINERGIC DRUGS

Anticholinergic drugs block the effects of the neurotransmitter acetylcholine at cholinergic receptors in the brain as well as in the rest of the body. They are discussed in greater detail in Chapter 21. Anticholinergics are used as adjunct drug therapy in Parkinson's disease due to their antitremor properties. The purpose of their use is to reduce excessive cholinergic activity in the brain. Accumulation of acetylcholine in Parkinson's disease causes an overstimulation of the cholinergic excitatory pathways, which results in tremors and muscle rigidity. Cogwheel rigidity is an example and is defined as resistance to passive movement. It can be observed when an arm that is flexed toward the body is then extended at the elbow. Muscle tremors are usually worse when the patient is at rest and consist of a pill-rolling movement and bobbing of the head. Anticholinergic drugs help to alleviate these bothersome and often disabling symptoms. Anticholinergics do little to relieve the *bradykinesia* (extremely slow movements).

Acetylcholine is responsible for causing increased *s*alivation, *l*acrimation (tearing of the eyes), *u*rination, *d*iarrhea, increased *G*I motility, and possibly *e*mesis (vomiting). The acronym *SLUDGE* is often used to describe these cholinergic effects. Anticholinergics have the opposite effects. They cause dry mouth or decreased salivation, urinary retention, decreased GI motility (constipation), dilated pupils (mydriasis), and smooth muscle relaxation. Anticholinergic drugs readily cross the blood-brain barrier and therefore can get to the site of Parkinson's disease pathology in the brain, the substantia nigra.

Historically, the anticholinergic drugs atropine and scopolamine were used. However, the anticholinergic adverse effects of dry mouth, urinary retention, and blurred vision associated with these original anticholinergics can be excessive. Therefore, synthetic anticholinergics were developed that have better adverse effect profiles. The anticholinergics most commonly used include benztropine (Cogentin) and trihexyphenidyl. Antihistamines (see Chapter 36) also have significant anticholinergic properties; they can also be used to manage cholinergic symptoms in Parkinson's disease. Anticholinergics must be used cautiously in older adults because of significant potential adverse effects such as confusion, urinary retention, visual blurring, palpitations, and increased intraocular pressure.

DRUG PROFILE

♦ benztropine mesylate

Benztropine (Cogentin) is an anticholinergic drug used for Parkinson's disease and also for extrapyramidal symptoms from antipsychotic drugs (see Chapter 16). Benztropine is to be used with caution in hot weather or during exercise because it may cause hyperthermia. Other adverse effects include tachycardia, confusion, disorientation, toxic psychosis, urinary retention, dry mouth, constipation, nausea, and vomiting. Anticholinergic syndrome can occur when it is given with other drugs that are associated with a high incidence of anticholinergic effects. Alcohol is to be avoided. Benztropine is available as tablets and in injectable form.

Pharmacokinetics: Benztropine

Route	Onset of Action	Peak Plasma Concentration	Elimination Half-life	Duration of Action
PO	1 hr	2-4 hr	4-8 hr	6-10 hr

NURSING PROCESS

ASSESSMENT

After patients are confronted with the diagnosis of Parkinson's disease, they soon experience the impact of the disease with every movement and activity of daily living. Not only will their lives never be the same, they will soon learn that their quality of life depends on drug therapy and nondrug measures. Before medications for Parkinson's disease are given, assess and document vital signs (e.g., blood pressure, pulse, respirations, temperature, pain) and ABCs (airway, breathing, and circulation). In addition, obtain a complete nursing history with a thorough physical assessment, including compiling a comprehensive medication profile. Because it may take several weeks to see a therapeutic response to medication regimens, a keen assessment and careful patient monitoring are even more critical to quality nursing care. A thorough assessment includes a health history, review of systems, and determination of sensory and motor abilities. Also gather the following information: complaint(s) upon admission or the symptom(s)/event that led the patient to obtain medical treatment; past and current medical history with a focus on the presence or absence of head injury, seizures, diabetes, hypertension, heart disease, and/or cancer; family history of any neuromuscular or neurologic disorders, heart disease, diabetes, cancer, seizures, cerebrovascular accident (stroke), and/or Parkinson's disease. Additionally, complete a thorough systems assessment with gathering of subjective and objective data in the following areas as related to the possible impact of Parkinson's disease:

- *Central nervous system*—Inquire about any headaches, fatigue, weakness, paralysis, dizziness, and/or syncope. Note any changes in walking or mobility, increase in rigidity or muscle movements, and/or changes in the ability to carry out activities of daily living. Also important are any changes in sensation in the extremities, changes in vision or hearing, loss of or changes in coordination, changes in gait and balance, and/or any changes in energy level. Include questions about any changes in baseline levels of alertness; changes in memory (short-term or long-term); blackouts or seizures; numbness, tingling, or abnormal sensations in the extremities; changes in mood; changes in muscle movement or strength (e.g., paralysis) or voluntary versus involuntary motor control; and any muscle rigidity or tremors. Assess response to stimuli, and assess pupils with attention to size, shape, response to light, and symmetry (in reactions). Assess deep tendon reflexes with attention to strength bilaterally. Observe and document the patient's ability to walk, his or her gait, and upper/lower, left/right extremity strength. Also assess and document ability to feed self and carry out activities of daily living.
- *Genitourinary and gastrointestinal systems*—Perform a general survey of the abdominal area with inspection, auscultation of bowel sounds, and palpation for any distention or tenderness. Determine daily baseline urinary and bowel patterns with attention to any changes in or loss of control of bladder or bowel functioning as well as the patient's ability to engage in toileting activities. Inquire about the need for assistance with these daily functions. Ask the patient about any difficulty in swallowing (dysphagia) and any problems in feeding self or preparing meals. If such difficulties are identified, assess further for any subsequent nutritional excesses or deficits.
- *Skin and oral mucus membranes*—Assess the skin's color, texture, turgor, and fragility, and note any breaks in the skin, bruises, lesions, masses, and/or swelling. Assess the mouth and mucus membranes for intactness, color, and hydration status.

- *Respiratory system*—Focus assessment on respiratory rate, rhythm, depth, effort, and breath sounds and the presence/absence of adventitious (abnormal) breath sounds. Inquire about any respiratory difficulties.
- *Psychological and emotional status*—Assess the patient for any recent or past changes in mood, affect, or personality. Be astute to any disease-related concerns such as depression, emotional ups and downs, increase in irritability, social withdrawal, or changes in sexual functioning or intimacy.
- *Functional abilities*—Inquire about any changes in everyday function in the patient's personal and/or professional life. Assess and note any changes in daily task performance at the place of employment or need to take sick leave or sick days, as well as the patient's ability to exercise, drive, and/or shop for groceries and other necessities.

With *indirect-acting dopamine receptor agonists,* such as *amantadine,* and *direct-acting dopamine receptor agonists,* such as *carbidopa-levodopa* and *ropinirole,* assess vital signs with supine and standing blood pressures (because of drug-related postural hypotension), height, weight, medication and medical history, and nursing history. Include family, significant others, and/or caregiver in the assessment and data collection process. Note contraindications, cautions, and drug interactions prior to administering these drugs (see previous pharmacology discussion). Assess motor skills, including abilities and deficiencies, and for the presence of akinesia, bradykinesia, postural instability, rigidity, tremors, staggering gait, or drooling (see Table 15-1 for a review of classic symptoms of Parkinson's disease). Assessment for changes in urinary patterns is also important because of the possibility of drug-induced urinary retention. If BUN and creatinine measurements are ordered, the results need to be routinely examined because these values are indicators of renal function. Alkaline phosphatase levels are indicators of liver function and need to be assessed, if ordered. These laboratory values are important to determine in patients with decreased renal or liver function because the dosage amounts of antiparkinson drugs may be altered by the prescriber.

As related to lifespan considerations, it is important to understand the gynecologic history of the patient and to know if the patient is pregnant and/or lactating. Some of the *dopamine replacement drugs* cross into the placenta and into breast milk and have unknown actions in the pediatric patient. See Table 15-2 for a review of drugs used in Parkinson's disease. Drug interactions are listed in Table 15-4.

When *anticholinergic drugs* are prescribed, assess the patient carefully to determine gross level of organ functioning—especially in those systems most affected by Parkinson's disease. These include the gastrointestinal, genitourinary, eye/visual, cardiac, and neurologic systems. Be astute to any present or past changes in mental status such as the presence of confusion, disorientation, or psychotic-like behavior. This is especially important to consider in older adult patients because of decline in liver function and subsequent higher risk for adverse effects and possible toxicity (with *antiparkinson drugs* and drugs in general) as well as an overall increased sensitivity to the effects of drugs (see Chapter 3 and Patient-Centered Care box below). Cautions, contraindications, and drug interactions have been previously discussed.

For the *indirect-acting dopamine receptor agonist drugs* (a subclass of *presynaptic dopamine release enhancers*) that are also antiviral (e.g., *amantadine*), the previously discussed baseline and general assessment information is also applicable. Assess the patient's knowledge of the drug's use for Parkinson's disease (versus its use as an antiviral) and awareness of its delayed onset of several days or longer. Continual assessment of the patient's status and improvement of disease-related symptoms is important because a decline in this drug's effectiveness (specifically a failure in the ability to control hypokinesia and rigidity of Parkinson's) may occur within 6 to 12 months after initiation of therapy.

PATIENT-CENTERED CARE: LIFESPAN CONSIDERATIONS FOR THE OLDER ADULT PATIENT

Antiparkinson Drugs

- Carbidopa-levodopa must be used cautiously and with close monitoring in older adult patients, especially those with a history of cardiac, renal, hepatic, endocrine, pulmonary, ulcer, or psychiatric disease.
- Older adult patients taking carbidopa-levodopa are at an increased risk for experiencing adverse effects, especially confusion, loss of appetite, and orthostatic hypotension.
- Carbidopa-levodopa is often started at a low dose because of the increased sensitivity of older adult patients to these medications and the need to save higher dosages for a later time during treatment.
- Overheating is a problem in patients taking anticholinergics. Older adult patients or anyone with heat sensitivity and taking anticholinergics must avoid excessive exercise during warm weather and excessive heat exposure.
- One of the main problems with the long-term use of carbidopa-levodopa is that its duration of effectiveness decreases over time; this is even more problematic in the older adult patient. Catechol ortho-methyltransferase (COMT) inhibitors hold much promise for the older adult patient experiencing the wearing-off phenomenon; they help turn the "off" times into "on" times so that the drug begins to work throughout the day.

If *amantadine* (also a prolactin inhibitor) is prescribed, you must understand that this drug is also used for suppression of lactation and must assess for the appropriateness of its use. Patients taking these drugs also require additional CNS assessment because of the possible adverse effects of dizziness, headache, insomnia, and anxiety. Also, if the patient is taking this medication long term, assessment for orthostatic hypotension and dizziness is crucial to patient safety.

The antiparkinson drugs classified as *indirect-acting dopamine receptor agonists* (a subclass of *MAO-B inhibitors*), such as *selegiline*, require assessment of many of the same parameters discussed earlier. In addition, however, cardiac status is important to assess and document because of the possible adverse effects of hypotension. Assessment of dosing is also important because, as with other antiparkinson drugs, a low dose is used initially with gradual increases over approximately a 3- to

4-week period. The lowest possible dose is recommended for initiation of therapy so that plenty of room exists for further increases in dosing as the disease progresses. These drugs also require careful neurologic assessment due to drug-adverse effects of headache, insomnia, and confusion (see Table 15-3).

For the *indirect-acting dopamine receptor agonist-COMT inhibitors* (e.g., *entacapone, tolcapone*), assess baseline vital signs with additional standing and supine blood pressure readings. Vital signs and postural blood pressure readings are important because of the adverse effects of orthostatic hypotension and syncope. These postural changes in blood pressure occur more frequently with the COMT inhibitors than with the other antiparkinson drugs, and so increased caution and concern is needed. Assessment of dosing time is also important because if these drugs are not given 1 hour before or 2 hours after meals, the bioavailability of the drug may be adversely affected. Assess serum transaminase levels before and during drug therapy with tolcapone because of the adverse effect of liver failure. If the patient's ALT level is elevated to the upper range of normal or higher, the prescriber will most likely discontinue the drug because of the increased risk for hepatic failure.

NURSING DIAGNOSES

1. Urinary retention related to the pathophysiologic effects of the disease process on the bladder with incomplete emptying
2. Constipation related to decreased GI peristalsis associated with the disease process
3. Imbalanced nutrition, less than body requirements, related to the disease process as well as adverse effects of drug therapy
4. Impaired physical mobility related to the disease process and adverse effects of the various antiparkinson medications
5. Disturbed body image related to changes in appearance and mobility due to the disease process
6. Deficient knowledge related to lack of exposure to and experience with a complex and long-term treatment regimen

PLANNING: OUTCOME IDENTIFICATION

1. Patient discusses ways to maximize normal bladder elimination patterns and minimize problems associated with drug-induced alterations in bladder elimination patterns (retention) such as forcing fluids, taking medications as prescribed, attempting to empty the bladder at regular intervals, and reporting any unresolved urinary problems.
2. Patient implements various measures to maintain normal bowel elimination patterns such as increasing bulk and fiber in the diet with fruits and vegetables, forcing fluids, and remaining as active as possible.
3. Patient maintains balanced nutritional status with implementing daily menus for increased dietary protein; increased intake from the major food groups divided in six small, frequent meals; and use of nutritional supplements and vitamins.

4. Patient participates in activities of daily living with proper use of assistive devices, removal of any barriers to safe mobility in the home environment, use of active/passive range-of-motion exercises, and/or use of physical and/or occupational therapy resources at home.

5. Patient maintains positive self-image and verbalizes fears, anxieties, and bodily changes with members of the health care team, supportive staff, family, and support groups.

6. Patient (and family, significant others, and/or caregiver) openly discusses impact of the disease process on relationships, daily activities, future activities; the lifelong need for daily medication; and monitoring for adverse and toxic effects (e.g., dizziness, nausea, vomiting, GI upset, palpitations).

CASE STUDY

Patient-Centered Care: Drugs for Parkinson's Disease

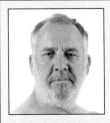 B., a 62-year-old retired contractor, is undergoing surgery to repair an umbilical hernia. He has had Parkinson's disease for 5 years and is currently taking carbidopa-levodopa (Sinemet CR) and selegiline (Eldepryl). Other than the Parkinson's disease, he has no health problems. He has enjoyed fairly good control up until this week but is now experiencing more "bad times," as he calls them.

1. Patients who are taking long-term levodopa treatment often experience an "on-off" phenomenon in symptoms. Explain the physiology behind this phenomenon.
2. Explain the reason for giving selegiline along with the carbidopa-levodopa. Ben undergoes the surgery without any difficulties, and the following medication orders are noted on the medical record:

      Continue previous orders for carbidopa-levodopa (Sinemet CR) 1 tablet bid and selegiline (Eldepryl) 5 mg bid (taken with the Sinemet CR)
      Meperidine (Demerol) 10 mg IV every 4 hours as needed for pain
      Ondansetron (Zofran) 4 mg IV one time if needed for nausea
      Begin entacapone (Comtan) 200 mg bid with each dose of Sinemet
3. Are there any concerns regarding drug interactions? Explain your answer.
4. What is the purpose of the entacapone?
5. Before administering the entacapone, the nurse reviews B.'s history for any potential contraindications. What condition(s) would be a potential contraindication to entacapone?

For answers, see *http://evolve.elsevier.com/Lilley.*

IMPLEMENTATION

Nursing interventions associated with the various *antiparkinson drugs* will vary somewhat depending on the drug class, but close monitoring and comprehensive patient education are required for the safe and effective use of these medications. With the onset of drug therapy, encourage patients, family, or caregivers to begin keeping a daily drug calendar or journal with entries including the drugs prescribed, dosage, frequency/timing, therapeutic changes, and adverse effects. During the start of *dopaminergic replacement drug* therapy, the patient may need assistance when walking because of the dizziness and possible syncope caused by these drugs. Doses are given several hours before bedtime to decrease the incidence of insomnia, a known adverse effect of these drugs. Oral doses are given with food to help minimize GI upset. Interaction of vitamin B_6 (pyridoxine) with levodopa was once a major concern because this vitamin was found to block the uptake of plain *levodopa*. However, a majority of patients taking a *carbidopa-levodopa* combination drug were found to have no problems with vitamin B_6. The National Parkinson's Disease Foundation (available at *www.pdf.org*) reports that only patients who are very sensitive to the effects of any of these drugs will have problems with vitamin B_6. If it is a problem, the prescriber needs to be consulted for further instructions. In addition, a high-protein diet can slow or prevent absorption of this medication. So it is important to make sure that the patient, family and/or caregivers understand that the while taking carbidopa-levodopa, the patient may continue to eat high-protein foods (e.g., meat, fish, poultry, and dairy products) but with the following special instructions: use portion control (meat portion about the size of a deck of cards) and take the drug dose one-half hour before eating a protein-containing meal or 1 hour after. Emphasize to the patient that he or she may want to eat higher-protein foods later in the day or in small amounts over the course of the day. Timing is the issue! A nutritional consult may be beneficial to assist the patient in menu planning. A nutritionist may also be helpful in teaching the patient about how to divide the total quantity of protein among small frequent meals so that minimal amounts of protein are ingested throughout the day and are consumed at the proper time. Consumption of well-balanced meals is important, as is increasing fluids. Patients need to aim at drinking at least 3000 mL/day unless contraindicated. Drinking water is important, even if the patient is not thirsty or in need of hydration, to prevent and manage the adverse effect of constipation. Encourage the intake of foods that have plenty of grain products, vegetables, and fruits that provide the vitamins, minerals, fiber, and complex carbohydrates. If the adverse effect of dry mouth is problematic, taking fluids and sucking on hard candy or lozenges may be helpful. If nausea or vomiting occurs or problems with edema are persistent (the patient gains 2 pounds or more in 24 hours or 5 pounds or more in 1 week), the prescriber must be contacted immediately.

With *anticholinergic drugs,* patients need to take the medication as prescribed, after meals or at bedtime and not at the same time as with other medications. Patients also need to know that it may take a few days to several weeks for the drugs to show their therapeutic effectiveness (e.g., improvement in tremors). Because of the risk for stomach upset (i.e., nausea, vomiting), it is recommended that these drugs be taken with a snack, such as ginger ale, graham crackers, or soda crackers. Ginger tea is sometimes a good choice to help with the GI upset. These medications are generally taken at night because of their sedating properties. Measures to help prevent and treat dry mouth are encouraged, such as increasing fluids and sucking on sugar-free hard candies. See Chapter 21 for further information about the use of these drugs, interventions, and adverse effects to report. *Bromocriptine* is to be taken as prescribed and not abruptly stopped. Because this drug may cause GI upset, it is best taken with a snack. Any severe dizziness, GI upset, ataxia, excess drowsiness, or visual changes must be reported immediately.

MAO-B inhibitors, such as *selegiline,* are to be given exactly as ordered. Selegiline is often given in upwardly titrated dosages while carbidopa-levodopa dose amounts are decreased. Place oral disintegrating dosage forms on the tongue, and do not swallow the dosage form until it is completely melted. This dosage form is to be taken without liquids and given in the morning before breakfast. Foods and fluids are not to be consumed for 5 minutes before or after the drug is taken. Postural hypotension may be a transient problem, and so the patient needs to move and change positions slowly and purposely. If dizziness is severe or if the patient experiences hallucinations, the prescriber must be contacted for further instructions.

The newer *COMT inhibitors* have been shown to have greater efficacy in patients with advanced forms of Parkinson's disease. After treatment using the various dosage forms of levodopa or carbidopa-levodopa, a COMT inhibitor may then be added to the therapeutic regimen. Onset of therapeutic effects is rapid. These drugs are to be administered as prescribed and may be taken without regard to meals or food. These and other antiparkinson drugs are never to be discontinued abruptly and require a gradual weaning period to avoid worsening of Parkinson's disease or other dangerous effects. Emphasize to patients and caregivers that all appointments with the prescriber must be kept and all laboratory testing performed, as ordered. Patients need to also understand the importance of changing positions slowly and with purpose to avoid syncope due to drug-related orthostatic hypotension. Inform patients that *entacapone* may turn their urine brownish-orange but that this is not harmful. As with all medications, patients must keep on their person a written list of prescription drugs, over-the-counter drugs, vitamins, minerals, and herbal therapies they are taking at all times. This list of medications needs updating frequently and should be taken each time the prescriber is visited and/or the patient is hospitalized. This allows continuity of information with health care providers and helps to prevent errors or omission of medications. Encourage patients to report to the prescriber any back and/or abdominal pain (especially in the right upper quadrant), bruising, or jaundice as these may be indicative of liver dysfunction associated with *tolcapone* (see Table 15-3).

It is most important in the care of patients with Parkinson's disease to be aware of all other forms of therapies that may be beneficial, such as support groups, water aerobics, and occupational and physical therapy. Some community resources that are available are community-wide recreation facilities, transportation services, and Meals on Wheels. Educational materials and emotional support resources need to be made available and shared with family members, caregivers, and significant others because of the long-term and progressive nature of the disease. Contacting research institutes about new treatment protocols may be a viable option for patients and family members during the course of the disease. See Patient-Centered Care: Patient Teaching for more information.

EVALUATION

Monitoring the patient's response to any of the *antiparkinson drugs* is crucial to documenting treatment success or failure. Therapeutic responses to the antiparkinson drugs include an improved sense of well-being, improved mental status, increased appetite, ability to perform activities of daily living, improved concentration and ability to think more clearly, and a decrease in the intensity of parkinsonian symptoms (e.g., less tremor, shuffling of gait, and muscle rigidity, and fewer involuntary movements). In addition to monitoring for therapeutic responses, also monitor for adverse effects such as dizziness, hallucinations, nausea, insomnia (associated with *indirect-acting dopamine receptor agonists* such as *selegiline, amantadine, entacapone,* and *tolcapone*), ataxia, depression (associated with *direct-acting dopamine receptor agonists* such as *bromocriptine* and *dopamine replacement drugs* such as *levodopa* and *carbidopa*), palpitations, hypotension, and urinary retention. Patients need to understand the importance of immediately reporting to their prescriber any of the following signs and symptoms indicating possible overdose: excessive twitching, drooling, or eye spasms. Therapeutic effects of *COMT inhibitors* (e.g., *entacapone*) may be noticed within a few days, whereas therapeutic effects of other antiparkinson drugs may take weeks to manifest. Adverse effects for which to monitor with COMT inhibitors include those mentioned previously, but fewer dyskinesias are seen than with dopamine agonists.

PATIENT-CENTERED CARE: PATIENT TEACHING

- All medications must be taken exactly as ordered. Around-the-clock dosing is usually prescribed to achieve steady blood levels, especially with dopamine agonists.
- Some patients will be allowed a certain amount of freedom in the dosing of their medications depending on their individual needs. An example is when a patient is traveling or attending a function where an extra dose of medication may be indicated/needed to help with movement disorder.
- Alcohol, over-the-counter drugs, and herbals are to be avoided unless approved by the prescriber.
- Emphasize the importance of taking the medication as prescribed and not quitting the medication. It is important for

the patient/family/caregiver to understand that medication(s) must be taken at the dosage and time prescribed. Inability to adhere to or remain compliant may lead to exacerbation of symptoms and development of complications. Missing a dose by even 30 minutes may lead to an "off" period and last hours.

- If the patient misses a dose of medication, the prescriber must be notified for further instructions. Some prescribers tell patients initially that if they miss a dose to take it as soon as they remember, and if it is close to the next dose time, then to skip the missed dose and take the next dose.

- If experiencing postural hypotension, the patient needs to understand the rationale for changing positions slowly and the need to increase fluids and wear compression stockings, unless contraindicated. If the patient has a history of congestive heart failure, fluid intake must be done very cautiously.
- Sustained-released drug forms are not to be crushed, chewed, or altered in any way. The drug is to be taken in its whole form. The exception to this standard of care is with Sinemet CR, which may be split only once and is available in scored dosage form for this reason (see pharmacology discussion).
- With anticholinergics, warn the patient about the adverse effect of dry mouth. Use of artificial saliva drops/gum, frequent mouth care, fluids, and sucking on sugarless gum or hard candy may be helpful.
- Inform the patient that urine color may darken if taking entacapone and that this adverse effect is harmless.
- Encourage the patient to report any change in vision (e.g., blurring), decline in mental alertness, confusion, or lethargy experienced while taking any of the antiparkinson drugs. Any difficulty with urination, irregular pulse rate, or severe, uncontrolled movements of the arms or legs must also be reported.
- The patient and family must understand that some antiparkinson drugs are often titrated to the patient's response and that it may take 3 to 4 weeks for a therapeutic response to become evident.
- The nonergot drug ropinirole may result in drowsiness, fatigue, and syncope. Emphasis on safety and how to handle these adverse effects is important.
- Fluids and dietary fiber, such as fruits and vegetables, need to be increased to help prevent constipation associated with the disease process as well as with drug therapy.
- Inform the patient that the COMT inhibitors entacapone and tolcapone need to be taken with food, meals, or a snack to minimize GI upset. Other instructions with the use of entacapone include reporting any signs and symptoms of possible liver dysfunction such as jaundice and back or abdominal pain.

- Any abnormal contractions of the head, neck, or trunk, as well as any syncope, falls, itching, and/or jaundice must be reported immediately to the prescriber.
- Educate the patient about the goal of therapy, especially if entacapone is being used to help manage the wearing-off phenomenon. The wearing-off phenomenon is a waning of the effects of a dose of levodopa before the scheduled time of the next dose, resulting in diminished motor ability and the experience of more disease symptoms. If a COMT inhibitor is added to carbidopa-levodopa, the wearing-off phenomenon is minimized, and the therapeutic effects of the regimen are maximized. The patient can then expect that the "off" time will be minimized and that the drugs will work throughout the day, which is the goal in the treatment of Parkinson's disease.
- There are generic formulations of carbidopa/levodopa, dopamine agonists, monoamine oxidase inhibitors (MAOI), and anticholinergics. Patients must understand that if they have Parkinson's disease and are taking a brand name medication and then are offered a generic substitution (for one of their Parkinson's medications), the FDA requires that generic drugs must show an "essential similarity" to the branded drug prior to market approval. In some cases, this standard is not enough. A review supported by the National Parkinson's Foundation chronicles "compelling evidence that if a patient is in more advanced stages of the disease, switching from branded drugs to generic, or from one generic to another, may have adverse effects." (See *www.parkinson.org/professionals.aspx* for more information or contact 1-800-4PD-INFO or 1-800-473-4636.)
- For patients taking a carbidopa-levodopa combination drug, it is important that they understand the interaction with protein intake and interaction with the medication. The patient may continue to eat high-protein foods (e.g., meat, fish, poultry, and dairy products) with use of portion control and to take the drug dose one-half hour before eating a protein-containing meal or one hour after. Encourage patients to eat higher protein–containing foods later in the day or in small amounts over the course of the day.

KEY POINTS

- The neurotransmission-related abnormalities in Parkinson's disease include the chronic, progressive degeneration of dopamine-producing neurons in the brain. Patients with this disease also have elevated acetylcholine levels and lowered dopamine levels.
- Signs and symptoms of this disease process include bradykinesia (slow movements), muscle rigidity (cogwheel rigidity), tremor (pill rolling), postural instability, and dystonias (abnormal muscle tone in any tissue).
- Dyskinesias occur as adverse effects of some of the antiparkinson drugs. Dyskinesias include motor difficulties while performing voluntary movements.
- Drugs used in the treatment of Parkinson's disease include amantadine, benztropine, bromocriptine, carbidopa-levodopa, entacapone, ropinirole, and selegiline. They have a variety

of mechanisms of action and many adverse effects, drug interactions, and dosing concerns. Nutritional concerns include making sure the patient is taking adequate fiber, vegetables, and fruit as well as increasing fluid intake, if not contraindicated. Additional concerns include distribution of protein intake over the course of the day if taking levodopa/carbidopa. The drug is to be taken one-half hour before eating a protein-containing meal or 1 hour after.
- Patient considerations include providing individual and family support along with options for care of the family member with Parkinson's disease. The disease is long-term and lifelong, as well as debilitating. A holistic approach in which all aspects of the patient and family are considered and respected is the key to quality nursing care.

NCLEX® EXAMINATION REVIEW QUESTIONS

1. Which condition will alert the nurse to a potential caution or contraindication regarding the use of a dopaminergic drug for treatment of mild Parkinson's disease?
   a. Diarrhea
   b. Tremors
   c. Angle-closure glaucoma
   d. Unstable gait
2. A patient is taking entacapone (Comtan) as part of the therapy for Parkinson's disease. Which intervention by the nurse is appropriate at this time?
   a. Notify the patient that this drug causes discoloration of the urine.
   b. Limit the patient's intake of tyramine-containing foods.
   c. Monitor the results of renal studies because this drug can seriously affect renal function.
   d. Force fluids to prevent dehydration.
3. During a patient teaching session about antiparkinson drugs, the nurse will include which statement?
   a. "The drug will be stopped when tremors and weakness are relieved."
   b. "If a dose is missed, take two doses to avoid significant decreases in blood levels."
   c. "Be sure to notify your physician if your urine turns brownish-orange in color."
   d. "Take care to change positions slowly to prevent falling due to a drop in blood pressure."
4. A patient will be taking selegiline (Eldepryl), 10 mg daily, in addition to dopamine replacement therapy for Parkinson's disease. The nurse will implement which precautions regarding selegiline?
   a. Teach the patient to avoid foods containing tyramine.
   b. Monitor for dizziness.
   c. Inform the patient that this drug may cause urine discoloration.
   d. Monitor for weight gain.

5. A patient with Parkinson's disease will start taking entacapone (Comtan) along with the carbidopa-levodopa (Sinemet) he has been taking for a few years. The nurse recognizes that the advantage of taking entacapone is that
   a. the entacapone can reduce on-off effects.
   b. the levodopa may be stopped in a few days.
   c. there is less GI upset with entacapone.
   d. it does not cause the cheese effect.
6. The nurse is assessing a patient who has begun therapy with amantadine (Symmetrel) for Parkinson's disease. The nurse will look for which possible adverse effects? *(Select all that apply.)*
   a. Nausea
   b. Palpitations
   c. Dizziness
   d. Insomnia
   e. Fatigue
7. The order reads: bromocriptine (Parlodel) 10 mg per day PO. The medication is available in 2.5-mg tablets. How many tablets will the nurse give per dose?
8. A patient who has been taking carbidopa-levodopa for Parkinson's disease for over 1 year wants to start a low-carbohydrate/high-protein weight-loss diet. The nurse tells the patient that this type of diet may have what effect on his drug therapy?
   a. There will be no problems with this diet while on this medication.
   b. The high-protein diet can slow or prevent absorption of this medication.
   c. The high-protein diet may cause increased blood levels of this medication.
   d. The high-protein diet will cause no problems as long as the patient also takes pyridoxine (vitamin B$_6$).

1. c, 2. a, 3. d, 4. b, 5. a, 6. a, c, d, 7. 4 tablets, 8. b

CRITICAL THINKING AND PRIORITIZATION QUESTIONS

1. A patient with Parkinson's disease will be starting therapy with amantadine (Symmetrel). He asks the nurse, "How long will I have to take this medicine?" What would be the nurse's best response?
2. The nurse is assessing a patient who is visiting the clinic for a 2-month follow-up appointment after starting selegiline (Eldepryl), 10 mg daily. The patient is pleased with the

improvement in his Parkinson's disease symptoms but states, "My wife looked up this drug and told me that I can't eat cheese or drink wine anymore. I hate that, and I really don't want to take this medicine." What is the nurse's priority action at this time?

For answers, see *http://evolve.elsevier.com/Lilley*.

ⓔ EVOLVE WEBSITE

http://evolve.elsevier.com/Lilley
- Animations
- Answer Keys for Textbook Case Studies and Textbook Critical Thinking and Prioritization Questions
- Content Updates
- Key Points
- Review Questions
- Student Case Studies

Psychotherapeutic Drugs

http://evolve.elsevier.com/Lilley

OBJECTIVES

When you reach the end of this chapter, you will be able to do the following:

1. Briefly discuss the various mental illnesses.
2. Identify the various psychotherapeutic drug classes, such as anxiolytic drugs, antidepressants, mood-stabilizing drugs, and antipsychotics.
3. Discuss the mechanisms of action, indications, therapeutic effects, adverse effects, toxic effects, drug interactions, contraindications, and cautions associated with the various psychotherapeutic drugs.
4. Develop a nursing care plan that includes all phases of the nursing process for patients taking psychotherapeutic drugs.
5. Develop patient education guidelines for patients taking psychotherapeutic drugs.

DRUG PROFILES

♦ alprazolam, p. 253
♦ amitriptyline, p. 258
♦ aripiprazole, p. 266
♦ bupropion, p. 261
buspirone, p. 254
♦ citalopram, p. 262
clozapine, p. 266
♦ diazepam, p. 254
duloxetine, p. 262
♦ fluoxetine, p. 262

haloperidol, p. 265
♦ lithium, p. 255
♦ lorazepam, p. 254
♦ mirtazapine, p. 262
♦ risperidone, p. 267
selegiline transdermal patch, p. 260
trazodone, p. 262

♦ = *Key drug*
! = *High-alert drug*

KEY TERMS

Affective disorders Emotional disorders that are characterized by changes in mood. (p. 252)

Agoraphobia An anxiety disorder that involves an intense fear of being in unfamiliar situations or places. (p. 252)

Akathisia A movement disorder in which there is an inability to sit still; motor restlessness. It can occur as an adverse effect of psychotropic medications. (p. 264)

Anxiety The unpleasant state of mind in which real or imagined dangers are anticipated and/or exaggerated. (p. 252)

Biogenic amine hypothesis A theory suggesting that depression and mania are caused by alterations in the concentrations of dopamine and norepinephrine, and of serotonin and histamine in the brain. (p. 256)

Bipolar disorder A psychological disorder characterized by episodes of *mania* or *hypomania,* cycling with depression; formerly called *manic-depressive illness.* (p. 252)

Depression An abnormal emotional state characterized by exaggerated feelings of sadness, melancholy, dejection, worthlessness, emptiness, and hopelessness. Signs include withdrawal from social contact, loss of appetite, and insomnia. (p. 252)

Dopamine hypothesis A theory suggesting that dopamine dysregulation in certain parts of the brain is one of the primary contributing factors to the development of psychotic disorders (psychoses). (p. 252)

Dyskinesia Term for abnormal and distressing involuntary movements; inability to control movements. (p. 264)

Dysregulation hypothesis A theory that views depression and affective disorders by failure of the brain to *regulate* the levels of neurotransmitters. (p. 256)

Dystonia A syndrome of abnormal muscle contraction that produces repetitive involuntary twisting movements and abnormal posturing of the neck, face, trunk, and extremities; often caused as an adverse reaction to psychotropic medications. (p. 264)

Extrapyramidal symptoms The term for signs and symptoms that resemble pathologic changes to the *pyramidal* portions of the brain. Such symptoms include various motion disorders similar to those seen in

Parkinson's disease, and are an adverse effect associated with use of various antipsychotic drugs. (p. 264)

Gamma-aminobutyric acid An amino acid in the brain that functions to inhibit nerve transmission in the central nervous system. (p. 251)

Hypertensive crisis A term referring to severely elevated blood pressure; can present as hypertensive urgency or hypertensive emergency. (p. 258)

Hypomania A less severe and less potentially hazardous form of mania. (p. 252)

Mania An acute illness characterized by an expansive emotional state, including extreme excitement, elation, hyperactivity, agitation, talkativeness, flight of ideas, reduced attention span, increased psychomotor activity, impulsivity, insomnia, anorexia, and sometimes violent, destructive, and self-destructive behavior. (p. 252)

Metabolic syndrome A cluster of conditions (increased glucose level, increased blood pressure, abnormal cholesterol levels, excess body fat around the waist) occurring together that increases the risk for heart disease, stroke, and diabetes. (p. 264)

Neuroleptic malignant syndrome An uncommon but serious adverse effect associated with the use of antipsychotic drugs and characterized by symptoms such as fever, cardiovascular instability, and myoglobinemia (presence in the blood of muscle breakdown proteins). (p. 264)

Neurotransmitters Endogenous chemicals in the body that serve to conduct nerve impulses between nerve cells (neurons). (p. 251)

Permissive hypothesis A theory postulating that reduced concentrations of serotonin (5-hydroxytriptamine) is the predisposing factor in individuals with affective disorders. (p. 256)

Psychosis (Plural: *psychoses*) A type of serious mental illness that is associated with being out of touch with reality; that is, the individual is unable to distinguish imaginary from real circumstances and events. (p. 252)

Psychotherapeutics The treatment of emotional and mental disorders. (p. 252)

Psychotropic Capable of affecting mental processes; usually said of a medication. (p. 252)

Serotonin syndrome A collection of symptoms resulting from elevated levels of the neurotransmitter *serotonin;* may occur with the use of any psychotropic drug (e.g., antidepressants, buspirone, tramadol) that enhances brain serotonin activity (see Box 16-1). (p. 261)

Tardive dyskinesia A serious drug adverse effect characterized by abnormal and distressing involuntary body movements and muscle tension that is associated with the use of antipsychotic medications. (p. 264)

OVERVIEW

Most people experience the normal emotions of anxiety, depression, excitement, and grief as part of life or due to certain situations. Treatment, if any, is often limited to psychotherapy, and possibly short-term drug therapy. However, longer-term pharmacotherapy in conjunction with psychotherapy is usually recommended when a person's emotions or behaviors compromise his or her quality of life, ability to carry out normal activities of daily living, social functioning, or occupational functioning over a prolonged period (at least several months).

The exact causes of mental disorders are not fully understood. There are many theories that attempt to explain the etiology and pathophysiology of mental dysfunction. In the biochemical imbalance theory, mental disorders are thought to arise as the result of abnormal levels of endogenous chemicals in the brain known as neurotransmitters. The proposed mechanisms of both the pathology of and drug therapy for mental illness center around neurotransmission within the brain. There is evidence indicating that the brain levels of catecholamines (especially dopamine and norepinephrine; see Chapter 18) and indolamines (serotonin and histamine) play an important role in maintaining mental health. Other biochemical substances necessary for the maintenance of normal mental function are the inhibitory neurotransmitter gamma-aminobutyric acid, the cholinergic neurotransmitter acetylcholine (see Chapter

20), and some inorganic ions such as sodium, potassium, and magnesium. Drugs used to treat mental illnesses, including anxiety, affective disorders, and psychoses, work by blocking or stimulating the release of various endogenous neurotransmitters.

The symptoms of the different psychiatric disorders often overlap, which can make them difficult to accurately diagnose. Complicating this issue further is the subjectivity of patients' experience of their symptoms. The *Diagnostic and Statistical Manual of Mental Disorders*, 5th edition, *(DSM-V)* is a widely used reference published by the American Psychiatric Association. It presents demographic information and diagnostic criteria for recognized psychiatric disorders. Research shows that more than half of chronically depressed adults also have a comorbid personality disorder, and one third have a comorbid anxiety disorder and/or a substance abuse disorder. Patients with mental illness may be more susceptible to various physical health problems than the general population. Obesity and tobacco use is significantly more common in patients with certain mental disorders. Economic, educational, and psychosocial issues may preclude a mentally ill person from seeking psychiatric health care. Thus, many patients self-medicate with substances of abuse, including alcohol, tobacco, and illegal or unauthorized prescription drugs. This compounds the problem of their baseline psychiatric illness.

The treatment of mental disorders is called **psychotherapeutics.** Ideal mental health care involves many components, including a carefully detailed patient interview (to help ensure accurate and complete diagnosis) and carefully chosen and regularly monitored drug therapy. Nonpharmacologic treatments include psychotherapy, support groups, social and family support systems, and often spiritual support systems. Other practices that promote mental health include physical exercise, good nutrition, and mental exercises such as meditation and visualization.

This chapter focuses on three common types of mental illness: anxiety, affective, and psychotic disorders. The drugs used to treat anxiety are anxiolytics. Mood stabilizers and antidepressants are used to treat affective disorders, while antipsychotics are used to treat psychotic disorders.

Anxiety is the unpleasant state of mind characterized by a sense of dread and fear. It may be based on anticipated or past experiences. Persistent anxiety is divided clinically into several distinct disorders, including the following:
- Obsessive-compulsive disorder
- Posttraumatic stress disorder
- Generalized anxiety disorder (GAD)
- Panic disorder with or without agoraphobia
- Social phobia (also called social anxiety disorder)
- Simple phobia

Anxiety is a normal reaction to stress; however, results of epidemiologic studies show that 5% to 8% of adults suffer from generalized anxiety disorder, 2.7% from panic disorder, 6.8% to 12% from posttraumatic stress disorder, and 3.8% from **agoraphobia.** Obsessive-compulsive disorder is twice as common as schizophrenia or panic disorder in the general population. Anxiety may occur as a result of medical illnesses (e.g., cardiovascular or pulmonary disease, hypothyroidism, hyperthyroidism, and hypoglycemia).

Affective disorders, also called *mood disorders,* are characterized by changes in mood and range from **mania** (exaggerated emotions) to **depression** (fewer emotions or emotional range). Some patients may exhibit both mania and depression, and this is referred to as **bipolar disorder.** **Hypomania** is a form of mania that is less severe.

Bipolar disorder occurs in an estimated 2% of the population. Depression is currently reported to have prevalence rates ranging from 8% to 12%. Major depressive disorders are expected to become the second leading cause of disability by 2020. Common depressive symptoms include feelings of worthlessness, loss of interest in normally pleasurable activities, reduced energy level, reduced motivation, drastic increase or decrease in appetite, insomnia or hypersomnia, and recurrent thoughts of death or suicide. In addition to being associated with reductions in quality of life and occupational and social functioning, depression is also accompanied by the occurrence of major sleep disturbances in up to 80% of patients. Despite recent advances in pharmacotherapy for depression, it remains undertreated in many cases.

Psychosis is a severe mental disorder that often impairs mental function to the point of causing significant disability in performing the activities of daily living. A hallmark of psychosis is a loss of contact with reality. The primary psychotic disorders are schizophrenia and depressive and drug-induced psychoses. Schizophrenia may trigger hallucinations, paranoia, and delusions (false beliefs), and it is estimated to affect 1% of the population. The **dopamine hypothesis** of psychotic illness suggests that psychotic patients often have excessive dopaminergic activity in the brain. Drug therapy is therefore aimed at reducing this activity. Note that this is in direct contrast to the treatment of Parkinson's disease (see Chapter 15).

PHARMACOLOGY OVERVIEW

Psychotropic drugs are widely prescribed in the United States. Because of the inherent variability in symptoms and diagnoses of mental disorders, the effects of these drugs are less easily quantified than other types of medications. The effectiveness of psychotropic drug therapy is often measured by verbal reports from patients regarding the level of improvement (if any) in their social and occupational functioning. Drug selection is often a trial-and-error process, which can be long and frustrating for both prescribers and patients.

It is hoped that the emerging field of pharmacogenomics (see Chapter 8) will eventually allow more proactive and improved customization of psychotropic drug therapy. As more information is learned about a drug after initial marketing, it is common for the approved indications for a given drug to expand. For example, a drug initially approved to treat depression may later be approved to treat social anxiety disorder or additional conditions.

A common problem with psychotropic drug therapy, as with other types of drug therapy, is nonadherence to the prescribed regimen. Patients may have legitimate fears about adverse effects, as well as fear of the unknown regarding their illness. For example, the weight gain that is associated with antipsychotics can be a reason for patient noncompliance.

ANXIETY DISORDERS

ANXIOLYTIC DRUGS

Primary anxiolytic drugs include the benzodiazepine drug class and the miscellaneous drug buspirone (Table 16-1). The benzodiazepines, including alprazolam, diazepam, and lorazepam, are commonly used as first-line drug therapy for both acute and chronic anxiety disorders.

Mechanism of Action and Drug Effects

Anxiolytic drugs decrease anxiety by reducing overactivity in the CNS. Benzodiazepines increase the action of gamma-aminobutyric acid (GABA), which is an inhibitory neurotransmitter in the brain that blocks nerve transmission in the CNS. Benzodiazepines work by depressing activity in the areas of the brain called the *brainstem* and the *limbic system.* The drug buspirone is a miscellaneous anxiolytic in its own class and is described in further detail in its drug profile.

TABLE 16-1 Currently Available Anxiolytic Drugs

Generic Name	Trade Name	Route
Benzodiazepines		
alprazolam	Xanax	PO
clorazepate	Tranxene T-Tab	PO
chlordiazepoxide	Librium	PO, IM, IV
clonazepam	Klonopin	PO
diazepam	Valium	PO, PR, IM, IV
lorazepam	Ativan	PO, IM, IV
oxazepam	Serax	PO
Miscellaneous		
buspirone	BuSpar	PO
meprobamate	Miltown	PO
hydroxyzine	Vistaril	PO, IM

TABLE 16-2 Adverse Effects of Selected Anxiolytic Drugs

Drug or Drug Class	Adverse Effects
Benzodiazepines	Amnesia, anorexia, sedation, lethargy, fatigue, confusion, drowsiness, dizziness, ataxia, headache, visual changes, hypotension, weight gain or loss, nausea, weakness
Miscellaneous	
buspirone	Paradoxical anxiety, dizziness, blurred vision, headache, nausea

Indications

Benzodiazepines are the largest and most commonly prescribed anxiolytic drug class. They are also used to treat ethanol withdrawal (see Chapter 17), insomnia and muscle spasms (see Chapter 12), seizure disorders (see Chapter 14), and as adjuncts in anesthesia (see Chapter 11). They are commonly used as adjunct therapy for depression because depressive and anxious symptoms often occur together.

Contraindications

Contraindications to benzodiazepines include known drug allergy; narrow-angle glaucoma, and pregnancy, due to their sedative properties and risk for teratogenic effects.

Adverse Effects

The most common adverse effects are due to an overexpression of their therapeutic effects, in particular CNS depression. Benzodiazepines can also cause hypotension. Paradoxical reactions (opposite of those that would normally be expected) rarely occur with the benzodiazepines and include hyperactivity and aggressive behavior. They are more likely to occur in children, adolescents, and in the older adult with dementia. Rebound disinhibition can occur in older adults upon tapering of doses or discontinuation of the benzodiazepines. In rebound disinhibition, the patient experiences marked sedation for 1 to 2 hours, followed by marked agitation and confusion for several hours afterward. All benzodiazepines are potentially habit-forming and addictive (Schedule IV). Although they can provide significant symptom relief, they must be used judiciously and at the lowest effective doses needed for symptom control. Table 16-2 contains more information on adverse effects. Older adults tend to be more sensitive to the sedating effects of benzodiazepines, which can increase their risk for falls; thus lower doses are usually needed.

Toxicity and Management of Overdose

When benzodiazepines are taken alone, an overdose is generally not life threatening. When they are combined with alcohol or other CNS depressants, the outcome is much more severe. An overdose of benzodiazepines may result in any of the following symptoms: somnolence, confusion, coma, and respiratory depression. The treatment of benzodiazepine intoxication is generally symptomatic and supportive. Flumazenil (Romazicon) is a benzodiazepine receptor blocker (antagonist) that is used to reverse the effects of benzodiazepines. The treatment regimen for the acute reversal of benzodiazepine effects is summarized in Chapter 12. Flumazenil may cause acute withdrawal syndrome, including seizures in patients taking long-term benzodiazepine therapy.

Interactions

Several notable drug interactions occur with the use of benzodiazepines. Alcohol and CNS depressants can result in additive CNS depression and even death. This serious consequence is more likely to occur in patients with renal and/or hepatic compromise. Other drug interactions are listed in Table 16-3.

Dosages

Recommended dosages of selected anxiolytic drugs are given in the table on the next page.

DRUG PROFILES

BENZODIAZEPINES

Benzodiazepines are widely used anxiolytic drugs. Benzodiazepines are all classified as Schedule IV controlled substances. For dosage and indication information, see the table on the next page.

◆ alprazolam

Alprazolam (Xanax) is most commonly used as an anxiolytic. It is indicated for generalized anxiety disorder (GAD), short-term relief of anxiety symptoms, panic disorder, and anxiety associated with depression. Adverse effects include confusion, ataxia, headache, and others listed in Table 16-2. Interacting drugs include alcohol, oral contraceptives, and others listed in Table 16-3. Alprazolam is available only for oral use, in both tablet and orally dissolving tablet forms.

Pharmacokinetics: Alprazolam

Route	Onset of Action	Peak Plasma Concentration	Elimination Half-life	Duration of Action
PO	30-60 min	1-2 hr	10-15 hr	6 hr

TABLE 16-3	Drug Interactions of Selected Anxiolytic Drugs		
Drug Class	**Interacting Drug(s)**	**Mechanism**	**Result**
Benzodiazepines	CNS depressants (e.g., alcohol, opioids)	Additive effects	Enhanced CNS depression (e.g., sedation, confusion, ataxia)
	Oral contraceptives, azole antifungals, SSRIs, verapamil, diltiazem, opioids, valproic acid	Impaired hepatic elimination of benzodiazepine	Enhanced benzodiazepine effects (e.g., CNS depression)
	rifampin	Enhanced benzodiazepine clearance	Reduced therapeutic effects
	theophylline	Antagonistic effects	Reduced sedative effects
	phenytoin	Reduced clearance	Potential for benzodiazepine toxicity
Miscellaneous buspirone	CYP3A4 inhibitors, azole antifungals, verapamil, diltiazem	Impaired hepatic metabolism of buspirone	Enhanced buspirone effects
	rifampin	Enhanced buspirone clearance	Reduced therapeutic effects
	MAOIs	Unknown	Increased blood pressure

CNS, Central nervous system; *CYP3A4,* cytochrome P-450 enzyme 3A4; *MAOIs,* monoamine oxidase inhibitors; *NSAIDs,* nonsteroidal antiinflammatory drugs; *SSRIs,* selective serotonin reuptake inhibitors.

DOSAGES

Selected Anxiolytic Drugs

Drug (Pregnancy Category)	Pharmacologic Class	Usual Adult Dosage Range	Current FDA-Approved Indications/Uses
◆ alprazolam (Xanax) (D)	Benzodiazepine	PO: 0.25-0.5 mg tid; do not exceed 4 mg/day	Anxiety
◆ diazepam (Valium) (D)	Benzodiazepine	PO: 2-10 mg 2-4 times/day	Anxiety
◆ lorazepam (Ativan) (D)	Benzodiazepine	PO: 2-6 mg/day in 2-3 divided doses	Anxiety, alcohol withdrawal, agitation

◆diazepam

Diazepam (Valium) used to be the most commonly prescribed benzodiazepine; however, for treatment of anxiety, it has been replaced by the shorter-acting benzodiazepines alprazolam and lorazepam. Diazepam is indicated for the relief of anxiety, management of alcohol withdrawal, reversal of status epilepticus, preoperative sedation, and as an adjunct for the relief of skeletal muscle spasms. Diazepam has active metabolites that can accumulate in patients with hepatic dysfunction, because it is metabolized primarily in the liver. This can result in additive effects and is best avoided in patients with major hepatic compromise. Adverse drug effects include headache, confusion, slurred speech, and others listed in Table 16-2. Diazepam interacts with alcohol, oral contraceptives, and others as shown in Table 16-3. Diazepam is available in oral, rectal, and injectable dosage forms.

Pharmacokinetics: Diazepam

Route	Onset of Action	Peak Plasma Concentration	Elimination Half-life	Duration of Action
PO	30-60 min	1-2 hr	20-80 hr	12-24 hr

◆lorazepam

Lorazepam (Ativan) is an intermediate-acting benzodiazepine, whereas alprazolam is the shortest acting, and diazepam is the longest acting. Lorazepam is available in oral and injectable forms. It may be given intravenously or intramuscularly. It has excellent absorption and bioavailability when given intramuscularly, but it is irritating to the muscle and must be diluted. The conversion between injectable and oral dosage forms is 1:1. Lorazepam can be given by intravenous push, which is useful in the treatment of an acutely agitated patient. It is often administered as a continuous infusion to agitated patients who are undergoing mechanical ventilation. It is also used to treat or prevent alcohol withdrawal (see Chapter 17). Indications, contraindications, and adverse effects are similar to those of alprazolam.

Pharmacokinetics: Lorazepam

Route	Onset of Action	Peak Plasma Concentration	Elimination Half-life	Duration of Action
PO	30-60 min	2 hr	11-16 hr	8 hr

MISCELLANEOUS DRUG

buspirone

Buspirone (BuSpar) is an anxiolytic drug that is different both chemically and pharmacologically from the benzodiazepines. Its precise mechanism of action is unknown, but it appears to have agonist activity at both serotonin and dopamine receptors. It is indicated for the treatment of anxiety. It needs to be administered on a scheduled (not "as-needed") basis, as opposed to the benzodiazepines, which may be administered as needed or on a schedule. The only reported contraindication is known drug allergy. Buspirone lacks the sedative properties and dependency potential of the benzodiazepines. Adverse effects include paradoxical anxiety, dizziness, blurred vision, headache, and nausea. Potential drug interactions include a risk for serotonin syndrome (see section on antidepressants). A waiting period of at least 14 days after discontinuation of MAOI therapy must be allowed before buspirone is started. Other drugs that interact with buspirone include *inhibitors* of the cytochrome P-450 enzyme system (see Chapter 2)—specifically with CYP3A4 (e.g., ketoconazole [see Chapter 42], clarithromycin [see Chapter 38])—which can reduce buspirone clearance; and *inducers* of these same enzymes, which can enhance buspirone clearance and decrease its therapeutic effect. In either case, the buspirone dosage may need to be adjusted. Other interactions are listed in Table 16-3. Buspirone is available only for oral use.

Pharmacokinetics: Buspirone

Route	Onset of Action	Peak Plasma Concentration	Elimination Half-life	Duration of Action
PO	2-3 wk	40-60 min	2-3 hr	unknown

AFFECTIVE DISORDERS

Several classes of drugs are used in the treatment of the affective (emotional) disorders. The two main drug categories are mood-stabilizing drugs and antidepressant drugs.

MOOD-STABILIZING DRUGS

Mood stabilizers are drugs used to treat bipolar illness (cycles of mania, hypomania, and depression). Clinical evidence indicates that the catecholamines (dopamine and norepinephrine) play an important pathophysiologic role in the development of mania. Serotonin also appears to be involved. The antiepileptic drugs valproic acid, lamotrigine, oxcarbazepine, and topiramate (see Chapter 14) are often the drugs of choice for bipolar illness. The aforementioned drugs are effective in treating mania, hypomania, and, to a lesser degree, depressive symptoms. Current evidence has shown that the atypical antipsychotic drugs aripiprazole,asenapine, lurasidone, risperidone, olanzapine, quetiapine, and ziprasidone (see later) can also be effective in treating mania and hypomania. Lithium has been in use for many years to alleviate the symptoms of acute mania and for maintenance treatment of bipolar disorder. Lithium is available in two salt forms: lithium carbonate and lithium citrate. Lithium is thought to potentiate serotonergic neurotransmission. Lithium has a narrow therapeutic range and requires blood level monitoring. Available mood-stabilizing drugs are listed in Table 16-4.

DRUG PROFILE

♦ lithium

The antimanic effect of lithium is not fully understood. Research indicates that lithium ions alter sodium ion transport in nerve cells, which results in a shift in catecholamine metabolism. Both

TABLE 16-4 Currently Available Mood Stabilizers and Antidepressants

Generic Name	Trade Name	Route
Mood Stabilizers		
lithium carbonate, lithium citrate	Lithobid, generic	PO
Antiepileptics (valproic acid, lamotrigine, topiramate, oxcarbazepine)	Depakote, Depakene, Lamictal, Topamax, Trileptal	PO
Atypical antipsychotics (aripiprazole, lurasidone, others)	Abilify, Latuda	PO
Antidepressants		
First Generation		
Tricyclics		
amitriptyline	Elavil	PO
amoxapine	Generic	PO
clomipramine	Anafranil	PO
desipramine	Norpramin	PO
doxepin	Sinequan	PO
imipramine	Tofranil	PO
nortriptyline	Pamelor	PO
protriptyline	Vivactil	PO
trimipramine	Surmontil	PO
Tetracyclics		
maprotiline (first generation)	Generic	PO
mirtazapine (second generation)	Remeron	PO
MAOIs		
isocarboxazid	Marplan	PO
phenelzine	Nardil	PO
tranylcypromine	Parnate	PO
Second Generation		
SSRIs		
citalopram	Celexa	PO
escitalopram	Lexapro	PO
fluoxetine	Prozac	PO
fluvoxamine	Generic	PO
paroxetine	Paxil	PO
sertraline	Zoloft	PO
Vortioxetine	Brintellix	PO
SNRIs		
duloxetine	Cymbalta	PO
Levomilnacipran	Fetzima	PO
venlafaxine	Effexor	PO
desvenlafaxine	Pristiq, Aptryxol	PO
Miscellaneous		
bupropion	Wellbutrin	PO
nefazodone	Generic	PO
trazodone	Generic, Oleptro	PO
vilazodone	Viibryd	PO

sodium and lithium are monovalent positive ions, and one can affect the other. Therefore, the patient's serum sodium levels need to be kept in the normal range which helps to maintain therapeutic lithium levels. Patients should be advised not to drastically change their sodium intake while taking lithium and to avoid overhydration as well as dehydration.

The levels of lithium required to produce a therapeutic effect are close to the toxic levels. Lithium is indicated for the treatment of manic episodes in bipolar disorder as well as for maintenance therapy to prevent such episodes. Contraindications to lithium therapy are relative and include dehydration, known sodium imbalance, and major renal or cardiovascular disease. Renal dysfunction of any degree can increase lithium levels. Adverse effects tend to correlate with serum levels and include gastrointestinal discomfort, tremor, confusion, somnolence, seizures, and possibly death. The most serious adverse effect is cardiac dysrhythmia. Other adverse effects include drowsiness, slurred speech, epilepsy-type seizures, choreoathetotic movements (involuntary wavelike movements of the extremities), ataxia (generalized disturbance of muscular coordination), and hypotension. Potentially interacting drugs include the thiazide diuretics (see Chapter 28), angiotensin-converting enzyme inhibitors (see Chapter 22), and nonsteroidal antiinflammatory drugs (see Chapter 44), all of which can increase lithium toxicity. Lithium carbonate is available only for oral use. As mentioned above, the use of lithium has been replaced with antiepileptic drugs such as lamotrigine.

Pharmacokinetics (Immediate Release): Lithium Carbonate

Route	Onset of Action	Peak Plasma Concentration	Elimination Half-life	Duration of Action
PO	7-14 days*	0.5-2 hr	7-20 hr	2-24 hr

*Therapeutic benefit for maintenance control of mania.

ANTIDEPRESSANT DRUGS

Antidepressants are the pharmacologic treatment of choice for major depressive disorders. They are very effective in treating depression, and they are also useful in treating other disorders, such as dysthymia (chronic low-grade depression), schizophrenia (as an adjunctive drug), eating disorders, and personality disorders. Some antidepressants are also used in the treatment of various medical conditions, including migraine headaches, chronic pain syndromes, sleep disorders, premenstrual syndrome, and hot flashes associated with menopause. Available antidepressants are listed in Table 16-4.

Antidepressants increase the levels of neurotransmitter concentrations in the CNS; these neurotransmitters include serotonin (also known as 5-hydroxytryptamine, or 5-HT), dopamine, and norepinephrine. Treatment is based on the belief that alterations in the levels of these neurotransmitters are responsible for causing depression. A widely held hypothesis advanced to explain depression in these terms is the biogenic amine hypothesis. It postulates that depression results from a deficiency of neuronal and synaptic catecholamines (primarily norepinephrine) and mania from an excess of amines at the adrenergic receptor sites in the brain. This hypothesis is illustrated in Figure 16-1.

Another hypothesis regarding the cause of depression is the permissive hypothesis, which led to the creation of the selective serotonin reuptake inhibitor (SSRI) drug class. The permissive theory postulates that reduced concentrations of serotonin

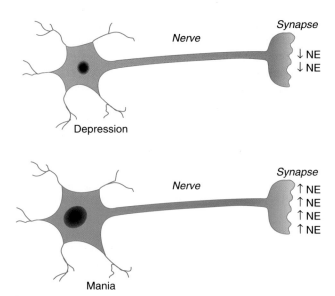

FIGURE 16-1 Biogenic amine hypothesis. *NE*, Norepinephrine.

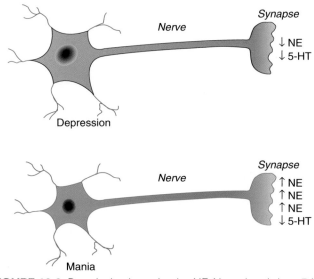

FIGURE 16-2 Permissive hypothesis. *NE*, Norepinephrine; *5-HT*, serotonin.

are the predisposing factor in patients with affective disorders. Depression results from decreases in both the serotonin and catecholamine levels, whereas mania results from increased dopamine and norepinephrine levels but decreased serotonin levels. The permissive hypothesis is illustrated in Figure 16-2. The dysregulation hypothesis is essentially a reformulation of the biogenic amine hypothesis. This theory views depression and other affective disorders not simply in terms of decreased or increased catecholamine activity but as a failure of the regulation of these systems.

Research indicates that early and aggressive antidepressant treatment increases the chances for full remission. The first 6 to 8 weeks of therapy constitute the acute phase. The primary goals during this time are to obtain a response to drug therapy and to improve the patient's symptoms. It is currently recommended that antidepressant drug therapy be maintained at the effective dose for an additional 8 to 14 months after remission of depressive symptoms. In choosing an antidepressant, the patient's previous psychotropic drug response history (if any) needs to be considered as well as family history. Therapeutic response is measured primarily by subjective patient feedback. In addition, a few measurement tools are available that attempt to quantify the patient's response to drug therapy, such as the Hamilton Rating Scale for Depression and the Symptom Checklist-90 anxiety factor scale.

Anxiety and depression commonly occur together and reinforce each other. Similarly, there is much crossover in terms of symptom control between antidepressant and anxiolytic drugs. A nonresponse to antidepressant drug therapy is defined as failure to respond to at least 6 weeks of therapy with adequate drug dosages. Twenty percent to 30% of patients who do not respond to the usual dosage of an antidepressant will respond to higher dosages. Therefore, dosage optimization, which involves careful upward titration of dose for several weeks, is recommended before concluding that a given drug is ineffective. Oftentimes a switch to a different pharmacologic class of antidepressant is necessary. Forty percent to 60% of patients will respond to the second drug class tried. Anxiolytic and antipsychotic drugs may also be used, either alone or as adjunct therapy. Evidence suggests that psychotherapy given with antidepressant medication is more effective than medication alone.

The most severe cases of depression that do not respond to drug therapy may warrant an attempt at treatment with electroconvulsive therapy. Electroconvulsive therapy treatment is generally carried out in a postanesthesia care unit setting under brief general anesthesia. Seizure activity is induced in the anesthetized patient via externally applied electric shocks to the brain.

Treatment failure in cases of depression may be due to a misdiagnosis or failure to treat comorbid mental illness (e.g., anxiety disorder, substance abuse) and/or comorbid nonpsychiatric illness (e.g., hypothyroidism). It may also be due to nonadherence to drug therapy. Careful choice of drug therapy to minimize adverse effects may improve patient adherence. Another reason for treatment failure may be the discouragement associated with depression itself. This alone may cause patients to give up prematurely on their drug therapy, especially because antidepressants often take several weeks to reach their full effect. Effective psychotherapy and support groups can help encourage patients to be consistent with prescribed psychotropic drug therapy.

In 2005, the U.S. Food and Drug Administration (FDA) issued black box warnings regarding the use of all classes of antidepressants in both adult and pediatric patient populations. Data from the FDA indicated a higher risk for suicide in patients receiving these medications. As a result, current recommendations for all patients receiving antidepressants include regular monitoring for signs of worsening depressive symptoms, especially when the medication is started or the dosage is changed.

TRICYCLIC ANTIDEPRESSANTS

Tricyclic antidepressants (TCAs) were the original first-generation antidepressants. The TCAs are so named because of their characteristic three-ring chemical structure. Their use has largely been replaced with the selective serotonin reuptake inhibitors (SSRIs) and serotonin-norepinephrine reuptake inhibitors (SNRIs).

Mechanism of Action and Drug Effects

TCAs work by correcting imbalance in the neurotransmitter concentrations of serotonin and norepinephrine at the nerve endings in the CNS (the biogenic amine hypothesis). This is accomplished by blocking the presynaptic reuptake of the neurotransmitters, which makes them available to transmit nerve impulses to adjacent neurons in the brain. Some also believe that these drugs may help regulate malfunctioning neurons (the dysregulation hypothesis).

Indications

Originally used to treat depression, currently TCAs are most commonly used to treat neuropathic pain syndromes and insomnia. Some of the TCAs have additional specific indications. For example, imipramine is used as an adjunct in the treatment of childhood enuresis (bedwetting), and clomipramine is useful in the treatment of obsessive-compulsive disorder. Because TCAs tend to increase appetite leading to weight gain, they are sometimes used to treat anorexia nervosa.

Contraindications

Contraindications for TCAs include known drug allergy, use of MAOIs within the previous 14 days, and pregnancy. TCAs are not recommended in patients with any acute or chronic cardiac problems or history of seizures, because both conditions are associated with a greater likelihood of death upon TCA overdose.

Adverse Effects

Undesirable effects of TCAs are a result of their effects on various receptors. Blockade of cholinergic receptors results in undesirable anticholinergic adverse effects, the most common being constipation and urinary retention. Nortriptyline and desipramine have less anticholinergic activity, and they are preferred for use in older adults. Adrenergic and dopaminergic receptor blockade can lead to disturbances in cardiac conduction and hypotension. Histaminergic blockade can cause sedation, and serotonergic blockade can alter the seizure threshold and cause sexual dysfunction (Table 16-5).

Toxicity and Management of Overdose

Tricyclic antidepressant overdoses are notoriously lethal. It is estimated that 70% to 80% of patients who die of TCA overdose do so before reaching the hospital, especially if the drugs are taken with alcohol. The primary organ systems affected are the CNS and cardiovascular system. Death usually results from either seizures or dysrhythmias.

There is no specific antidote for TCA poisoning. Management efforts are aimed at reducing drug absorption by administering multiple doses of activated charcoal. Sodium bicarbonate may be given as it speeds up elimination of the TCA by alkalinizing the urine. CNS damage may be minimized by the

TABLE 16-5   Adverse Effects of Selected Mood Stabilizers and Antidepressants

Drug or Drug Class	Adverse Effects
Mood Stabilizers	
lithium salts	GI discomfort, tremor, confusion, sedation, seizures, cardiac dysrhythmia, drowsiness, slurred speech, slowed motor abilities, weight gain, ataxia, hypotension
Antiepileptic drugs	Dizziness, drowsiness, GI upset, weight gain, hepatotoxicity, pancreatitis, unusual eye movements, visual changes, behavioral changes, ataxia
Antidepressants	
First Generation	
Tricyclics	Anorexia, dry mouth, blurred vision, constipation, gynecomastia, sexual dysfunction, altered blood glucose level, urinary retention, agitation, anxiety, ataxia, cognitive impairment, sedation, headache, insomnia, skin rash, photosensitivity, weight changes, orthostatic hypotension, blood dyscrasias
MAOIs	Dizziness, dyskinesias, nausea, syncope, hypotension
Second Generation	
Tetracyclics	
mirtazapine, maprotiline	Drowsiness, abnormal dreams, dry mouth, constipation, increased appetite, asthenia (muscle weakness)
SSRIs	Anxiety, dizziness, drowsiness, headache, mild GI disturbance, sexual dysfunction, asthenia, tremor
SNRIs	Dizziness, drowsiness, headache, GI upset, anorexia, hepatotoxicity
Miscellaneous	
trazodone, bupropion	Dizziness, headache, sedation, nausea, blurred vision, tachycardia

administration of diazepam, and cardiovascular events may be minimized by giving antidysrhythmics. Other care includes basic life support in an intensive care setting to maintain vital organ functions. These interventions must continue until enough of the TCA is eliminated to permit restoration of normal organ function.

Interactions

Increased anticholinergic effects are seen when TCAs are taken with anticholinergics and phenothiazines. When MAOIs are taken with TCAs, the result may be increased therapeutic and toxic effects, including hyperpyretic crisis (excessive fever). Other drug interactions are listed in Table 16-6.

Dosages

Recommended dosages of selected TCA drugs are given in the table on the next page.

DRUG PROFILE

TCAs are effective drugs in the treatment of various affective disorders, but they are associated with serious adverse effects. Some herbal products used to treat depression, such as St. John's wort (see the Safety: Herbal Therapies and Dietary Supplements box on p. 260), are available over the counter but should not be taken with prescription antidepressants. Most TCAs are rated as pregnancy category D drugs, which makes their use by pregnant women relatively more hazardous than that of most of the newer drugs.

♦ amitriptyline

Amitriptyline (Elavil) is the oldest and most widely used of all the TCAs. Its original indication was depression, but it is now more commonly used to treat insomnia and neuropathic pain. Contraindications include known drug allergy, pregnancy, and recent myocardial infarction. It has very potent anticholinergic properties, which can lead to many adverse effects such as dry mouth, constipation, blurred vision, urinary retention, and dysrhythmias (see Table 16-5). Drug interactions are listed in Table 16-6. Amitriptyline is available only for oral use.

Pharmacokinetics: Amitriptyline

Route	Onset of Action	Peak Plasma Concentration	Elimination Half-life	Duration of Action
PO	7-21 days	2-12 hr	10-50 hr	6-12 hr

MONOAMINE OXIDASE INHIBITORS

Monoamine oxidase inhibitors (MAOIs), along with TCAs, represent the first generation of antidepressant drug therapy. They are rarely used as antidepressants, but are used to treat Parkinson's disease. A serious disadvantage to MAOI use is their potential to cause a hypertensive crisis when taken with stimulant medications or with substances containing tyramine, which is found in many common foods and beverages (Table 16-7). Hypertensive crisis can present as either hypertensive urgency (BP greater than 180/110) or hypertensive emergency (BP greater than 180/120). Patients must seek emergency medical treatment.

Currently four MAOI antidepressants are available. Isocarboxazid, phenelzine, and tranylcypromine are nonselective inhibitors of both MAO type A and MAO type B. Selegiline is a selective MAO-B inhibitor that comes in a transdermal dosage form. An oral form selegiline is used to treat Parkinson's disease (see Chapter 15). These drugs inhibit the MAO enzyme system

TABLE 16-6   Drug Interactions of Selected Mood-Stabilizing and Antidepressant Drugs

Drug Class	Interacting Drug(s)	Mechanism	Result
Mood Stabilizers			
lithium salts	Thiazide diuretics, angiotensin converting enzyme inhibitors, verapamil, diltiazem, NSAIDs	Decreased lithium excretion	Increased lithium toxicity
Antiepileptic drugs	See Table 14-5.		
Antidepressants			
First Generation			
Tricyclics	carbamazepine, rifamycins	Enhanced TCA clearance	Reduced therapeutic effects
	carbamazepine	Reduced carbamazepine clearance	Potential for carbamazepine toxicity
	MAOIs	Enhance serotonergic effects	Potential for serotonin syndrome
	valproic acid	Reduced TCA clearance	Potential for TCA toxicity
	Anticholinergics	Additive anticholinergic effects	Potential for paralytic ileus
	Sympathomimetics	Enhanced sympathomimetic effects	Potential for cardiac dysrhythmias
Second Generation			
Tetracyclics			
mirtazapine, maprotiline	Alcohol, CYP inhibitors	Additive effects	Increased toxicity
SSRIs	MAOIs, linezolid, lithium, metoclopramide, buspirone, sympathomimetics, tramadol	Additive effects	Potential for serotonin syndrome
	Benzodiazepines	Reduced metabolism	Potential benzodiazepine toxicity
	warfarin, phenytoin	Protein-binding displacement	Potential for warfarin or phenytoin toxicity
	propafenone	Increased propafenone levels	Potential for propafenone toxicity
SNRIs			
duloxetine	SSRIs, triptans	Additive effects	Risk for serotonin syndrome
	NSAIDs, warfarin	Additive effects	Risk for bleeding
	Alcohol	Additive liver toxicity	Increased risk for hepatotoxicity
Miscellaneous			
trazodone, bupropion	Azole antifungals, phenothiazines, protease inhibitors	Impaired hepatic metabolism	Increased effects
	Carbamazepine	Increased metabolism	Decreased therapeutic effects
	Alcohol, CNS depressants	Additive effects	Increased CNS depression

CYP, Cytochrome P-450; *MAOIs*, monoamine oxidase inhibitors; *NSAIDs*, nonsteroidal antiinflammatory drugs; *SNRIs*, serotonin-norepinephrine reuptake inhibitors; *SSRIs*, selective serotonin reuptake inhibitors.

DOSAGES

Selected Mood-Stabilizing and Antidepressant Drugs

Drug (Pregnancy Category)	Pharmacologic Class	Usual Dosage Range	Current FDA-Approved Indications/Uses
Mood Stabilizers			
◆ lithium carbonate (D)	Inorganic salt	600-1800 mg/day divided bid-tid	Acute mania, prevention of mania
Antidepressants			
First Generation			
◆ amitriptyline (generic only; formerly Elavil) (C)	Tricyclic	PO: 10-300 mg/day	Depression (more commonly used for insomnia and neuropathic pain)
Second Generation			
◆ bupropion (Wellbutrin) (C)	Miscellaneous	PO: 200-450 mg/day, divided bid PO/SR: 200-400 mg/day	Depression (Wellbutrin) Smoking cessation (Zyban)
duloxetine (Cymbalta) (C)	SNRI	PO: 20-40 mg/day or 60 mg/day divided bid	Depression, GAD, diabetic peripheral neuropathy
◆ fluoxetine (Prozac) (C)	SSRI	PO: 10-20 mg/day; higher doses up to 80 mg/day divided bid	Depression, OCD, bulimia nervosa, panic disorder, premenstrual dysphoric disorder
◆ mirtazapine (Remeron) (C)	Tetracyclic	PO: 15-45 mg at bedtime	Depression, bipolar disorder
trazodone (Desyrel) (C)	Triazolopyridine	PO: 25-600 mg/day, with larger doses divided	Depression (more commonly used for insomnia)

TABLE 16-7   Food and Drink to Avoid When Taking Monoamine Oxidase Inhibitors

Food/Drink	Examples
High Tyramine Content (Not Permitted)	
Aged mature cheeses	Cheddar, blue, Swiss
Smoked or pickled meats	Herring, sausage, corned beef, smoked fish or poultry, salami, pepperoni
Aged or fermented meats	Chicken or beef liver pâté, game fish or poultry
Yeast extracts	Brewer's yeast
Red wines	Chianti, burgundy, sherry, vermouth
Italian broad beans	Fava beans
Moderate Tyramine Content (Limited Amounts Allowed)	
Meat extracts	Bouillon, consommé
Pasteurized light and pale beer	
Ripe avocado	
Low Tyramine Content (Permissible)	
Distilled spirits	Vodka, gin, rye, scotch (in moderation)
Non-aged cheeses	American cheese, mozzarella, cottage cheese, cream cheese
Chocolate and caffeinated beverages	
Fruit	Figs, bananas, raisins, grapes, pineapple, oranges
Soy sauce	
Yogurt, sour cream	

QSEN | **SAFETY: HERBAL THERAPIES AND DIETARY SUPPLEMENTS**

St. John's Wort (Hypericum perforatum)

Overview
St. John's wort herbal preparations consist of the dried above-ground parts of the plant species *Hypericum perforatum*. The herb is available over the counter in numerous oral dosage forms. St. John's wort is sometimes referred to as the *herbal Prozac.*

Common Uses
Depression, anxiety, sleep disorders, nervousness

Adverse Effects
Gastrointestinal upset, allergic reactions, fatigue, dizziness, confusion, dry mouth, possible photosensitivity (especially in fair-skinned individuals)

Potential Drug Interactions
Monoamine oxidase inhibitors, selective serotonin reuptake inhibitors, tricyclic antidepressants, benzodiazepines, phenytoin, valproic acid, phenobarbital, zolpidem and other hypnotic drugs, cyclosporine and other immunosuppressants, sympathomimetic amines, tyramine-containing foods, opioids, digoxin, estrogens, theophylline, warfarin, triptans, dextromethorphan, loratadine, cetirizine, fexofenadine, HIV drugs, and oral contraceptives

Contraindications
Contraindicated in patients with bipolar depression, schizophrenia, Alzheimer's disease, and dementia

in the CNS, therefore, dopamine, serotonin, and norepinephrine are not broken down, and therefore higher levels of these substances occur. This, in turn, alleviates the symptoms of depression.

Most adverse effects of MAOIs stem from their interactions with food and other medications. A variety of over-the-counter drugs (especially for cough and cold) also can interact with MAOIs to cause adverse cardiovascular effects. Patients taking MAOIs need to read labels and/or consult the pharmacist when using any such products. Dosage information for selected MAOIs is given in the table on the previous page.

Sympathomimetic drugs can also interact with MAOIs, and together these drugs can cause a hypertensive crisis. MAOIs can markedly potentiate the effects of meperidine, and therefore their concurrent use is contraindicated. In addition, concurrent use of MAOIs with SSRIs carries the risk for serotonin syndrome. A "washout" period of 2 to 5 weeks between drugs is recommended.

DRUG PROFILE

selegiline transdermal patch
The selegiline transdermal patch (Emsam) is a selective MAO-B inhibitor. It is currently indicated for major depression. The lowest strength of the selegiline transdermal patch (6 mg/24 hr) can be used without dietary restrictions. However, to date there are insufficient data to permit the same dietary freedom with the 9- and 12-mg patch strengths. Contraindications include known drug allergy. Adverse drug effects and drug interactions are the same as for the oral dosage form and can be found earlier in the discussion of MAOIs in general and in Chapter 15 for selegiline in particular. Patients need to avoid exposing the patch to external sources of heat or prolonged direct sunlight, as heat speeds absorption. Standard pharmacokinetic parameters for the transdermal dosage form are not known at this time.

SECOND-GENERATION ANTIDEPRESSANTS

Second generation antidepressants were introduced in the 1980s and continue to be introduced today. Currently available second-generation drugs are listed in Table 16-4. The second-generation antidepressants are generally considered superior to TCAs and MAOIs in terms of their adverse-effect profiles. They are associated with significantly fewer adverse effects, especially anticholinergic and cardiovascular adverse effects. It takes the same amount of time to reach maximum clinical effectiveness with the second-generation antidepressants as it does with the TCAs and MAOIs, typically 4 to 6 weeks.

Mechanism of Action and Drug Effects
The inhibition of serotonin reuptake is the primary mechanism of action of the SSRIs, although SSRIs may also have weak effects on norepinephrine and dopamine reuptake. SNRIs inhibit the reuptake of both serotonin and norepinephrine.

Indications
Although depression is their primary indication, they have shown benefit in treating a variety of other mental and physical

disorders. Examples include bipolar disorder, obesity, eating disorders, obsessive-compulsive disorder, panic attacks or disorders, social anxiety disorder, posttraumatic stress disorder, premenstrual dysphoric disorder, the neurologic disorder myoclonus, and various substance abuse problems such as alcoholism. This list is expanding with continued research on these drugs. In treatment-resistant depression, addition of an atypical antipsychotic (see later) has been shown to be beneficial.

Contraindications

Contraindications include known drug allergy, use of MAOIs in the previous 14 days, and therapy with certain antipsychotic drugs such as thioridazine or mesoridazine. Bupropion is contraindicated in cases of seizure disorders because it can lower the seizure threshold.

Adverse Effects

The second-generation antidepressants offer advantages over TCAs and MAOIs due to their improved adverse-effect profiles. However, up to two thirds of all depressed patients may still discontinue therapy due to drug adverse effects. Some of the most common adverse effects are insomnia (partly due to reduced rapid eye movement sleep), weight gain, and sexual dysfunction. Sexual dysfunction caused by the SSRIs is primarily related to inability to achieve orgasm. One potentially hazardous adverse effect of any drug or combination of drugs that have serotoninergic activity is known as serotonin syndrome. The symptoms of this condition are listed in Box 16-1. Fortunately, it is usually self-limiting on discontinuation of the causative drugs. (See also Table 16-5.) SSRIs are associated with a discontinuation syndrome or withdrawal syndrome, and the drugs must be very slowly tapered. SSRIs with the shortest half-lives (citalopram, escitalopram, sertraline, paroxetine) are most commonly associated with the discontinuation syndrome. Symptoms include flulike feeling, difficulty concentrating, faintness, and GI symptoms. Often, even with slow reduction

in dose, patients decide to go back on the SSRI due to the withdrawal symptoms. Once the drug is restarted, the symptoms abate. While the syndrome is most commonly associated with the SSRIs, it can occur with the SNRIs (venlafaxine, desvenlafaxine, duloxetine).

Interactions

The second-generation antidepressants are highly bound to albumin. When given with other drugs that are also highly protein bound (e.g., warfarin and phenytoin), they compete for binding sites on the surface of albumin. This results in more free, unbound drug and therefore a more pronounced drug effect. To prevent the potentially fatal pharmacodynamic interactions that can occur between these drugs and the MAOIs, a 2- to 5-week "washout" period is recommended between uses of these two classes of medications. The antibiotic linezolid (Zyvox) is structurally related to MAOIs, as such it is best to avoid concurrent use of linezolid and SSRIs. The herbal product, St. John's wort can interact with antidepressants and is best avoided. Other drug interactions are listed in Table 16-6.

Dosages

Recommended dosages of selected newer-generation antidepressants are given in the table on p. 259.

DRUG PROFILES

The second-generation drugs are effective antidepressants with better adverse-effect profiles than first-generation antidepressants. They are considered first-line drugs in the treatment of patients with depression, including patients with concurrent symptoms of anxiety and patients with depression with suicidal ideation.

◆ bupropion

Bupropion is a unique antidepressant in terms of both its structure and mechanism of action. It has weak effects on brain serotonin activity, and little to no effect on monoamine oxidase. Its strongest therapeutic activity appears to be primarily dopaminergic and noradrenergic.

Bupropion was originally indicated for treatment of depression but is now also indicated as an aid in smoking cessation. It is sometimes added as an adjunct antidepressant for patients experiencing sexual adverse effects secondary to SSRI therapy. A sustained-release form of bupropion, Zyban, is approved for smoking cessation treatment. Its exact mechanism of action in treating nicotine dependence is unknown, but it is believed to be related to the drug's ability to modulate dopamine and norepinephrine levels in the brain. Both of these neurotransmitters are believed to play an important role in maintaining nicotine addiction. The newer smoking cessation drug varenicline (Chantix; see Chapter 17) is becoming popular for this purpose.

Bupropion is contraindicated in patients who have a known drug allergy, those with a seizure disorder (bupropion can lower the seizure threshold), and those currently taking an MAOI. Common adverse effects include dizziness, confusion, tachycardia, agitation, tremor, and dry mouth. Drugs that interact with bupropion include the azole antifungals (see Chapter 42) as well

---

BOX 16-1 Common Symptoms of Serotonin Syndrome

Common symptoms include:
- Delirium
- Agitation
- Tachycardia
- Sweating
- Myoclonus (muscle spasms)
- Hyperreflexia
- Shivering
- Coarse tremors
- Extensor plantar muscle (sole of foot) responses

In more severe cases, the following may occur:
- Hyperthermia
- Seizures
- Rhabdomyolysis
- Renal failure
- Cardiac dysrhythmias
- Disseminated intravascular coagulation

as other drugs metabolized by the cytochrome P-450 enzyme system (see Chapter 2) and CNS depressants. Other drug interactions are listed in Table 16-6. Bupropion is available only for oral use.

Pharmacokinetics: Bupropion

Route	Onset of Action	Peak Plasma Concentration	Elimination Half-life	Duration of Action
PO	Up to 4 wk	3 hr	10-14 hr	Weeks to months

◆ citalopram

Citalopram (Celexa) is one of the most commonly used SSRIs. It is FDA approved for the treatment of depression, but is also used for obsessive-compulsive disorder. It has a short half-life (24 to 48 hours), similar to escitalopram, sertraline, and paroxetine. Because of the short half-life, it is commonly associated with the discontinuation syndrome. Adverse effects include anxiety, dizziness, drowsiness, insomnia, and others listed in Table 16-5. Drug interactions are similar for all SSRIs and are listed in Table 16-6.

Pharmacokinetics: Citalopram

Route	Onset of Action	Peak Plasma Concentration	Elimination Half-life	Duration of Action
PO	1-4 wk	1-6 hr	24-48 hours	unknown

duloxetine

Duloxetine (Cymbalta), like venlafaxine, is a serotonin-norepinephrine reuptake inhibitor (SSNRI). It is indicated for depression and generalized anxiety disorder. It is also indicated for pain resulting from diabetic peripheral neuropathy or fibromyalgia. It is contraindicated in cases of known drug allergy and concurrent MAOI use, and it can worsen uncontrolled angle-closure glaucoma. Adverse effects include dizziness, drowsiness, headache, gastrointestinal upset, anorexia, and hepatotoxicity. Drug interactions include SSRIs and triptans (increased risk for serotonin syndrome) and alcohol (increased risk for liver injury). Duloxetine is available only for oral use. Levomilnacipran (Fetzima) is the newest SSNRI approved. Notable side effects include hyperhidrosis, tachycardia and urinary retention.

Pharmacokinetics: Duloxetine

Route	Onset of Action	Peak Plasma Concentration	Elimination Half-life	Duration of Action
PO	2-6 weeks	6 hr	12 hr	unknown

◆ fluoxetine

Fluoxetine (Prozac) was the first SSRI marketed for the treatment of depression and is considered the prototypical SSRI. Although it was initially indicated for the treatment of depression, the indications for fluoxetine have expanded to include bulimia, obsessive-compulsive disorder, panic disorder, and premenstrual dysphoric disorder. Contraindications include

known drug allergy and concurrent MAOI therapy. Adverse effects include anxiety, dizziness, drowsiness, insomnia, and others listed in Table 16-5. Drug interactions are listed in Table 16-6. Fluoxetine is available only for oral use.

Pharmacokinetics: Fluoxetine

Route	Onset of Action	Peak Plasma Concentration	Elimination Half-life	Duration of Action
PO	1-4 wk	6-8 hr	1-3 days*	2-4 weeks

*Active metabolite has a half-life of 7 to 10 days.

◆ mirtazapine

Mirtazapine (Remeron) is unique in that it promotes the presynaptic release of serotonin and norepinephrine in the brain. This is due to its antagonist activity in the presynaptic alpha$_2$-adrenergic receptors. It does not inhibit the reuptake of either of these neurotransmitters. It is strongly associated with sedation in more than 50% of patients due to its histamine 1 (H$_1$) receptor activity and therefore is usually dosed once daily at bedtime. Mirtazapine is indicated for treatment of depression, including that associated with bipolar disorder. It is also helpful (mechanism unknown) in reducing the sexual adverse effects in male patients receiving SSRI therapy. Mirtazapine is known to be an appetite stimulant and thus can be helpful in underweight depressed patients or harmful in those who are already overweight. Mirtazapine is contraindicated in cases of known drug allergy and concurrent use of MAOIs. Adverse effects include drowsiness, abnormal dreams, dry mouth, constipation, increased appetite, and asthenia. Drug interactions include additive CNS depressant effects with alcohol and CYP inhibitors (see Chapter 2). Mirtazapine is available only for oral use.

Pharmacokinetics: Mirtazapine

Route	Onset of Action	Peak Plasma Concentration	Elimination Half-life	Duration of Action
PO	1-3 wk	2 hr	20-40 hr	Unknown

trazodone

Trazodone (Desyrel, Oleptro) is in the triazolopyridine drug class. It was the first of the second-generation antidepressants that could selectively inhibit serotonin reuptake but minimally affect norepinephrine reuptake. Trazodone has minimal adverse effects on the cardiovascular system. It is indicated for the treatment of depression, and it is also commonly used for insomnia. Contraindications include known drug allergy. Adverse effects include strongly sedative qualities. These can be severe and can impair cognitive function in older adults. However, the sedating effect of trazodone is often advantageous in helping depressed patients, who commonly have comorbid anxiety and/or insomnia, obtain effective sleep. Trazodone also has been associated in rare cases with transient nonsexual *priapism*. This is a dangerously sustained penile erection that is the result of alpha-adrenergic blockade. Drug interactions are listed in Table 16-6. Trazodone is available only for oral use. Vilazodone (Viibryd) is similar to trazodone, although it has a dual mechanism of action; it is a SSRI and a 5-HT$_{1A}$ receptor agonist.

Pharmacokinetics: Trazodone

Route	Onset of Action	Peak Plasma Concentration	Elimination Half-life	Duration of Action
PO	1-2 wk	2-4 wk	6-9 hr	Several weeks

PSYCHOTIC DISORDERS

ANTIPSYCHOTIC DRUGS

Antipsychotic drugs are used to treat serious mental illnesses such as drug-induced psychoses, schizophrenia, and autism. Antipsychotics are also used to treat extreme mania (as an adjunct to lithium), bipolar disorder, depression that is resistant to other therapy, certain movement disorders (e.g., Tourette's syndrome), and certain other medical conditions (e.g., nausea, intractable hiccups). Antipsychotics have also been referred to as *tranquilizers* or *neuroleptics* because they produce a state of tranquility and act on abnormally functioning nerves. However, these are both older terms that are now less commonly used.

Antipsychotic drugs represent a significant advance in the treatment of mental illnesses, as evidenced by the fact that the early treatment of mental illnesses (before the 1950s) consisted of such extreme measures as isolation, physical restraint, shock therapy, and even lobotomy.

The phenothiazines are the largest chemical class of antipsychotic drugs, constituting about two thirds of all antipsychotics. They were also the original drugs in this category. The currently available antipsychotics are listed in Table 16-8.

Overall, there are few differences between conventional, or first-generation, antipsychotics in terms of mechanism of action. Therefore, selection of an antipsychotic is based primarily on the patient's tolerance and the need to minimize adverse effects. Antipsychotic drug therapy does not normally provide a cure for psychoses but is a way of chemically controlling the symptoms of the illness.

More recently, a new generation of antipsychotic medications has evolved. These are referred to as *atypical antipsychotics*. Atypical antipsychotics differ from conventional drugs in that they tend to have better adverse-effect profiles. They still have adverse effects, but they are usually not as severe as seen with the conventional antipsychotic drugs.

Mechanism of Action and Drug Effects

All antipsychotics block dopamine receptors in the brain, which decreases the dopamine concentration in the CNS. Specifically, the conventional phenothiazines block the dopamine receptors postsynaptically in certain areas of the CNS, such as the limbic system and the basal ganglia. These are the areas associated with emotions, cognitive function, and motor function. This receptor blocking produces a tranquilizing effect in psychotic patients. Both the therapeutic and toxic effects of these drugs are the direct result of the dopamine blockade in these areas. The atypical antipsychotic drugs block specific dopamine receptors called

TABLE 16-8   Currently Available Antipsychotic Drugs

Generic Name	Trade Name	Route
Conventional		
Phenothiazines		
chlorpromazine	Thorazine	PO, PR, IM, IV
fluphenazine	Generic	PO, IM
perphenazine	Generic	PO
prochlorperazine	Compazine	PO, PR, IM, IV
trifluoperazine	Generic	PO
thioridazine	Generic	PO
Thioxanthene		
thiothixene	Navane	PO
Phenylbutylpiperidines		
haloperidol	Haldol	PO, IM
pimozide	Orap	PO
Dihydroindolone		
molindone	Moban	PO
Atypical		
Dibenzodiazepines		
clozapine	Clozaril	PO
loxapine	Loxitane	PO
olanzapine	Zyprexa	PO, IM
quetiapine	Seroquel	PO
asenapine	Saphris	sublingual
Benzisoxazoles		
lurasidone	Latuda	PO
paliperidone	Invega	PO
risperidone	Risperdal	PO, IM
ziprasidone	Geodon	PO, IM
iloperidone	Fanapt	PO
Quinolinone		
aripiprazole	Abilify	PO, IM

MAOIs, Monoamine oxidase inhibitors; *SNRIs,* serotonin-norepinephrine reuptake inhibitors; *SSRIs,* selective serotonin reuptake inhibitors.

dopamine 2 (D$_2$) receptors, as well as specific serotonin receptors in the brain known as serotonin 2 (5-HT$_2$) receptors. These more refined mechanisms of action of the atypicals are responsible for their improved efficacy and safety profiles, compared with the conventional drugs (see Adverse Effects).

All antipsychotics show efficacy in improving the positive symptoms of schizophrenia. So-called *positive symptoms* include hallucinations, delusions, and conceptual disorganization. Unfortunately, conventional drugs are less effective in managing negative symptoms. Negative symptoms are apathy, social withdrawal, blunted affect, monotone speech, and catatonia. It is these negative symptoms that account for most of the social and vocational disability caused by schizophrenia. Fortunately, atypical antipsychotics have improved efficacy in treating both positive and negative symptoms.

Indications

Antipsychotic drugs are indicated for psychotic illness, most commonly schizophrenia. Several of the atypical antipsychotic drugs are also used as adjunctive therapy for depression. Certain antipsychotics (e.g., prochlorperazine) are used as antiemetics (see Chapter 52). They block serotonin receptors and dopamine receptors in the chemoreceptor trigger zone in the brain and inhibit neurotransmission in the vagus nerve in the gastrointestinal tract. Additional blocking of dopamine receptors in the brainstem reticular system also allows atypical drugs to have anxiolytic or antianxiety effects.

Contraindications

Contraindications to the use of antipsychotic drugs include known drug allergy, significant CNS depression, brain damage, liver or kidney disease, blood dyscrasias, or uncontrolled epilepsy.

Adverse Effects

Adverse effects are caused by blockade of the alpha-adrenergic, dopamine, endocrine, histamine, and muscarinic (cholinergic) receptors and are listed in Table 16-9. Possible severe hematologic effects include agranulocytosis (lack of granulocytes in the blood) and hemolytic anemia. CNS effects include drowsiness, neuroleptic malignant syndrome, extrapyramidal symptoms, and tardive dyskinesia. Neuroleptic malignant syndrome is a potentially life-threatening adverse effect that may include high fever, unstable blood pressure, and myoglobinemia. Extrapyramidal symptoms are involuntary motor symptoms similar to those associated with Parkinson's disease (see Chapter 15). This drug-induced state is known as *pseudoparkinsonism* and is characterized by symptoms such as akathisia (distressing motor restlessness) and acute dystonia (painful muscle spasms). Two anticholinergic medications, benztropine (Cogentin) and trihexyphenidyl (Artane), are commonly used to treat these symptoms (see Chapter 15). *Tardive* is a word that means "late appearing." Tardive dyskinesia is characterized by involuntary contractions of oral and facial muscles (e.g., involuntary tongue thrusting) and choreoathetosis (wavelike movements of the extremities) and usually appears after continuous long-term antipsychotic therapy. Theoretically these effects are possible

with atypical antipsychotics as well; however, evidence suggests that the incidence is lower.

Adverse effects on the endocrine system associated with antipsychotics include insulin resistance, weight gain, and changes in serum lipid levels. Antipsychotics are associated with development of metabolic syndrome, which can cause serious long-term health problems.

All antipsychotics carry a black box warning regarding the use in older adults with dementia where an increased risk for death is seen. They also have a black box warning of increased risk for suicidal thinking in children through young adults. In addition, in 2011, the FDA required manufacturers to include stronger wording regarding the use of antipsychotics in pregnant women. The new labeling includes more consistent information about the potential risk for abnormal muscle movements (extrapyramidal symptoms) and withdrawal symptoms in newborns whose mothers were treated with these drugs during the third trimester of pregnancy. Other adverse effects are listed in Table 16-10.

Interactions

Major drug interactions are listed in Table 16-11. Antihypertensives may have additive hypotensive effects, and CNS depressants may have additive CNS depressant effects when taken with antipsychotics. Grapefruit juice can enhance the effects of clozapine (by reducing its metabolism via the cytochrome P-450 enzyme system). Because grapefruit juice affects many enzymes in the P-450 system, it is wise to avoid this food for patients taking multiple medications.

Dosages

Recommended dosages of selected antipsychotic drugs are given in the table on this page.

DRUG PROFILES

The conventional antipsychotic drugs are currently still available on the U.S. market (see Table 16-8). However, much of

---

TABLE 16-9 Antipsychotics: Receptor-Related Adverse Effects

Receptor	Adverse Effects
Alpha-adrenergic	Postural hypotension, lightheadedness, reflex tachycardia
Dopamine	Extrapyramidal movement disorders, dystonia, parkinsonism, akathisia, tardive dyskinesia
Endocrine	Prolactin secretion (galactorrhea, gynecomastia), menstrual changes, sexual dysfunction
Histamine	Sedation, drowsiness, hypotension, weight gain
Muscarinic (cholinergic)	Blurred vision, worsening of angle-closure glaucoma, dry mouth, tachycardia, constipation, urinary retention, decreased sweating

---

TABLE 16-10 Adverse Effects of Selected Psychotropic Drugs

Drug or Drug Class	Adverse Effects
Conventional (e.g., haloperidol)	Akathisia, extrapyramidal symptoms, hypotension, neuroleptic malignant syndrome, confusion, headache, mild GI disturbance, dry mouth, amenorrhea, gynecomastia, visual disturbances, hyperpyrexia, edema, tardive dyskinesia, skin rash, photosensitivity, weight gain, urinary retention, tardive dyskinesia
Atypical (e.g., clozapine, risperidone)	Sedation, somnolence, tachycardia, akathisia, agitation, asthenia, ataxia, seizures, dyskinesia, dizziness, drowsiness, headache, insomnia, dry mouth, dyspepsia, anxiety, increased appetite, weight gain, extrapyramidal symptoms and tardive dyskinesia (lower risk than conventional agents)

TABLE 16-11   Drug Interactions of Selected Antipsychotics

Drug Class	Interacting Drug(s)	Mechanism	Result
Conventional and Atypical	Alcohol, other CNS depressants	Additive drug effects	Enhanced CNS depression; dystonia with alcohol
	Antihypertensives	Enhanced antihypertensive effects	Potential for hypotension
Conventional: Phenothiazines	Anticholinergics	Additive and antagonistic drug effects	Reduced phenothiazine efficacy; enhanced anticholinergic effects
	Beta blockers	Additive drug effects	Potential toxicity of either drug
	Opioids	Additive drug effects	Excessive sedation, hypotension
	levodopa/carbidopa	Uncertain	Diminished antiparkinson effects
	phenytoin	Uncertain	Can increase or reduce phenytoin levels
	Thiazide diuretics	Reduced diuretic clearance	Potential for hypotension
Atypicals	CYP3A4 inhibitors (e.g., ketoconazole)	Reduced antipsychotic clearance	Potential for antipsychotic toxicity
	carbamazepine	Enhanced antipsychotic clearance	Reduced therapeutic effects

CYP3A4, Cytochrome P-450 enzyme 3A4.

their use in clinical practice has been replaced by the atypical antipsychotic drugs. No single drug stands out as being either more or less effective in the treatment of the symptoms of psychosis. Some of the factors to be considered before selecting an antipsychotic are the patient's history of response to a drug and the possible adverse-effect profile. Starting at a low dose with titration to the lowest effective dose helps achieve a balance between symptom relief and adverse effects. For dosage information on profiled drugs, see the table on this page.

BUTYROPHENONE
haloperidol

Haloperidol (Haldol) is structurally different from the thioxanthenes and the phenothiazines but has similar antipsychotic properties.

It is indicated primarily for the long-term treatment of psychosis. Low doses can also be used for nausea. However, it has been largely replaced by the atypical antipsychotics because of its adverse effects (see later). Haloperidol is contraindicated with known hypersensitivity, Parkinson's disease (due to its antidopaminergic effects), and in those patients taking large amounts of CNS depressants. Haloperidol is a high-potency neuroleptic drug that has a favorable cardiovascular, anticholinergic, and sedative adverse-effect profile, but it can cause extrapyramidal symptoms as well as tardive dyskinesia. Haloperidol is available in three salt forms: base (for oral use), decanoate injection (for IM only), and lactate injection (IM or IV). Haloperidol decanoate has an extremely long duration of action, which makes it useful in treating patients with schizophrenia who were nonadherent with their drug regimen. The lactate formulation is commonly given intravenously in acute situations. It is important to note that, although the manufacturer states that it is not to be given intravenously, clinical experience and case reports have shown the intravenous route to be safe and effective. Other adverse effects are listed in Table 16-10. Drugs with which haloperidol interacts are listed in Table 16-11.

DOSAGES

Selected Antipsychotic Drugs

Drug (Pregnancy Category)	Pharmacologic Class	Usual Dosage Range	Current FDA-Approved Indications/Uses
First Generation (Conventional)			
haloperidol (Haldol) (C)	Butyrophenone, phenylbutylpiperidine	PO, IM/IV: 0.5-5 mg bid-tid	Schizophrenia, Tourette's syndrome, severe refractory behavioral problems or hyperactivity
Second Generation (Atypical)			
◆ aripiprazole (Abilify) (C)	Quinolinone	PO: 10-15 mg/day IM: 400 mg monthly	Schizophrenia, bipolar disorder, major depressive disorder, irritability associated with autistic disorder
clozapine (Clozaril) (B)	Dibenzodiazepine	PO: 12.5 mg bid, titrate up to maximum of 900 mg/day. Larger doses divided tid	Schizophrenia, recurrent suicidal behavior in patients with schizophrenia or schizoaffective disorder
◆ risperidone (Risperdal) (C)	Benzisoxazole	PO: 2-8 mg/day in either one or two doses IM depot form (Risperdal Consta): 25-50 mg every 2 wk	Schizophrenia, mania, irritability associated with autism

Pharmacokinetics: Haloperidol

Route	Onset of Action	Peak Plasma Concentration	Elimination Half-life	Duration of Action
PO	2 hr	2-6 hr	13-35 hr	8-12 hr
IM	Lactate: 20-30 min	Lactate: 30-45 min	13-35 hr	Lactate: 4-8 hr
	Decanoate: 3-9 days	Decanoate: unknown		Decanoate: 1 mo

ATYPICAL ANTIPSYCHOTICS

Between 1975 and 1990, not a single new antipsychotic drug was approved in the United States. In 1990, clozapine (Clozaril), the first of the atypical antipsychotics, was approved. Clozapine was followed by risperidone (Risperdal), olanzapine (Zyprexa), quetiapine (Seroquel), ziprasidone (Geodon), aripiprazole (Abilify), paliperidone (Invega), iloperidone (Fanapt), asenapine (Saphris), and lurasidone (Latuda).

The term *atypical antipsychotics* refers to advantageous properties of these drugs over conventional drugs: reduced effect on prolactin levels; improvement in the negative symptoms associated with schizophrenia; and lower risk for neuromuscular malignant syndrome, extrapyramidal adverse effects, and tardive dyskinesia. The atypical antipsychotic drugs block specific dopamine receptors called dopamine 2 (D_2) receptors, as well as specific serotonin receptors in the brain known as serotonin 2 ($5-HT_2$) receptors. D_2 receptor antagonism is believed to be the mechanism of their antimanic activity. Serotonergic (serotonin agonist) activity at 5-HT receptor subtypes and alpha$_2$-adrenergic (agonist) activity are associated with antidepressant activity. Alpha$_1$-adrenergic receptor antagonist activity is associated with orthostatic hypotension, and histamine (H_1) receptor antagonist activity is associated with both sedative and appetite-stimulating effects.

Weight gain is a common adverse effect of antipsychotics and varies among drugs. Clozapine and olanzapine are associated with the most weight gain, lurasidone, risperidone and quetiapine with less, and ziprasidone is considered weight-neutral. Other atypical antipsychotics fall between the aforementioned drugs. All antipsychotics, both conventional and atypical, have been associated with development of metabolic syndrome. Sedative effects may diminish over time and can actually be helpful for patients with insomnia. Although these drugs all have similar pharmacologic properties, they vary in the degree of affinity for the various types of receptors. These subtle pharmacologic differences explain why some patients respond better (or do not respond) to one medication versus another. Atypical antipsychotics can also be used in bipolar disorder or depression. Aripiprazole (Abilify) and lurasidone (Latuda) are the two most aggressively marketed for these additional indications.

In April 2005, the FDA issued a special public health advisory concerning the use of atypical antipsychotic drugs in older adults for off-label (non–FDA-approved) uses. These medications are currently approved for the treatment of schizophrenia and mania. In practice, however, they are commonly used to control behavioral symptoms of agitation in older adults with dementia, including dementia related to Alzheimer's disease. The FDA data found that older adult patients given atypical antipsychotics for this reason were up to 1.7 times more likely to die during treatment.

Dosage information for atypical antipsychotics is given in the table on the previous page.

◆ aripiprazole

Aripiprazole (Abilify) is the only quinolinone atypical antipsychotic. It is indicated for schizophrenia, bipolar disorder, major depressive disorder, and for agitation associated with autistic disorder. It is similar to the other atypical antipsychotics and shares the same black box warnings (increased risk for suicide in children, adolescents, and young adults; increased risk for death in older adults with dementia). It is classified as a pregnancy category C drug. Side effects are similar to those seen with other atypical antipsychotics. It is available orally and as an extended release IM injection (Abilify Maintena) which is given once a month.

Pharmacokinetics: Aripiprazole

Route	Onset of Action	Peak Plasma Concentration	Elimination Half-life	Duration of Action
PO	1-3 weeks	3-5 hours	75-94 hours	N/A

clozapine

Clozapine (Clozaril) was the first of the *atypical* antipsychotics. Atypical antipsychotics selectively block the dopaminergic receptors in the *mesolimbic* region of the brain. Conventional antipsychotic drugs block dopamine receptors in an area of the brain called the *neostriatum*, which is associated with extrapyramidal adverse effects. Because clozapine and other atypical antipsychotics have weak dopamine-blocking abilities in this area of the brain, they are associated with minor or no extrapyramidal symptoms. This often makes atypical antipsychotics the drug of choice in patients who also have Parkinson's disease, because they do not worsen motor symptoms.

Adverse effects of clozapine include the potential for agranulocytosis, a dangerous disorder of white blood cell (WBC) underproduction that is drug induced. For this reason, patients beginning clozapine therapy require weekly monitoring of WBC counts for the first 6 months of therapy. Clozaril is available only through the Clozapine National Registry, with which the patient and prescriber must be registered. Other adverse effects are listed in Table 16-10. Clozapine is contraindicated in patients with known drug allergy and in those with myeloproliferative disorders, severe granulocytopenia, CNS depression, or angle-closure glaucoma. Drug interactions are listed in Table 16-11. Clozapine is available only for oral use.

Other atypical antipsychotics (see Table 16-8) have features comparable to those of clozapine but do not require extensive WBC monitoring. Risperidone is described in the following profile as an example of these drugs. Orally disintegrating tablets are available for many of the atypical antipsychotics which may improve compliance. The dosage is the same as that for regular tablets (see the Dosages table on the previous page).

Pharmacokinetics: Clozapine

Route	Onset of Action	Peak Plasma Concentration	Elimination Half-life	Duration of Action
PO	1-6 hr	Weeks	6 hr	4-12 hr

◆ risperidone

Risperidone (Risperdal) is an atypical antipsychotic that was introduced a few years after clozapine. It is even more active than clozapine at the serotonin (5-HT$_{2A}$ and 5-HT$_{2C}$) receptors. It also has a high affinity for alpha$_1$- and alpha$_2$-adrenergic receptors and histamine H$_1$ receptors. This drug is indicated for schizophrenia, including negative symptoms, and causes minimal extrapyramidal adverse effects at therapeutic dosages of 1 to 6 mg/day.

Risperidone is contraindicated in cases of known drug allergy. Adverse effects are listed in Table 16-10. Drugs interacting with risperidone include CNS depressants and others listed in Table 16-11. Risperidone is available for oral and injectable use. The long-acting injectable form is called Risperdal Consta, and one intramuscular injection lasts approximately 2 weeks. This is one option for helping patients maintain adherence with the prescribed drug regimen. Patients must continue to take oral risperidone for 3 weeks after the first injection of the Consta dosage form to ensure adequate blood levels from the injection. Paliperidone also comes as a long-acting injection (Invega Sustenna), which lasts 1 month.

Pharmacokinetics: Risperidone

Route	Onset of Action	Peak Plasma Concentration	Elimination Half-life	Duration of Action
PO	1-2 wk	1-2 hr	20-30 hr	7 days
IM	3 wk	Unknown	20-30 hr	2 wk

NURSING PROCESS

ASSESSMENT

Before administering any of the *psychotherapeutic drugs*, perform a complete head-to-toe physical assessment and mental status examination. Document your findings. This data will serve as a comparative baseline for the patient during and after initiation of therapy.

Thoroughly assess the patient's neurologic functioning, including level of consciousness, mental alertness, and level of motor and cognitive functioning. The Mini-Mental State Examination (MMSE) is one tool that you may use to assess cognitive status and help identify impairments often found in mental illnesses. The MMSE is simple to use, cost-effective, and may be completed in about 20 minutes. The MMSE is available in most nursing assessments, nursing fundamentals, and/or psychiatric or mental health nursing textbooks. Points are scored in the areas of level of orientation, attention and calculation ability, recall, and language skills. Other mental health assessment tools include the six-item Blessed Orientation-Memory-Concentration Test, clock-drawing tasks, and Functional Activities Questionnaire (for those with dementia), Alzheimer's Disease Assessment Scale, Mattis Dementia Rating Scale, Severe Impairment Battery, and the Hamilton Rating Scale for Depression. In addition to performing examinations such as these, note baseline levels of motor responses and reflexes as well as the presence of any tremors and/or personality changes. Assess for the presence of cold clammy hands, sweating, and/or pallor. These particular findings may be indicative of an altered autonomic nervous system response.

Constantly assess the patient for any suicidal ideation or tendencies, with attention not only to overt cues and behaviors but also to covert thoughts and ideation. This is important because of the potential for suicide with the use of psychotherapeutic drugs, with or without the concurrent use of other medications or alcohol. Suicide assessment tools are available and may help you identify an individual's risk for suicidal behaviors. One such tool, the Suicide Assessment Scale, has been found to be valid, reliable, and easy to use. The following are some questions that may be helpful: "What brings you to the doctor's office today?" "How has life been treating you?" "What are some of your worries or concerns?" "How would you describe your mood?" "Tell me about your thoughts." If an assessment reveals any concerns and/or the patient acknowledges suicidal thoughts, make an appropriate referral for immediate assessment and/or treatment.

Remember that many of the patients who require psychotherapeutic drugs are depressed and, as such, suffer from insomnia and possibly from self-neglect. Deterioration in health status and weight loss or gain may also occur. Therefore, it is important to assess sleep habits and nutritional intake and to perform a head-to-toe physical examination for baseline and comparative purposes. Note any drug allergies as well as any contraindications, cautions, and potential drug interactions (see pharmacology discussion and Tables 16-3, 16-6, and 16-11). Assess and document blood pressure and pulse rate before, during, and after drug therapy. Postural blood pressures (i.e., blood pressure taken supine then standing) are particularly important to note because of the possible drug-related adverse effects of postural hypotension and dizziness. The more potent older drugs (e.g., *MAOIs* or *TCAs*) may lead to a significant drop in blood pressure and possible syncope, warranting even more skillful assessment and close monitoring (of blood pressure readings).

Review the results of any laboratory studies performed before and during the drug therapy. This is especially important for patients who are receiving long-term drug therapy to prevent or identify any early complications or other possible adverse effects or toxicity. Laboratory studies may include, but are not limited to, tests to confirm therapeutic serum levels of the specific drug and, if appropriate, a complete blood count, erythrocyte sedimentation rate, serum electrolyte and glucose levels, BUN, liver function studies, serum level of vitamin B$_{12}$, and thyroid studies. If the patient is experiencing forms of dementia, other types of testing may be needed, such as genetic studies, computed tomography, or magnetic resonance imaging.

With psychotherapeutic drug therapy, assess the patient's mouth and oral cavity to make sure the patient has swallowed the entire oral dosage. This helps to prevent hoarding or "cheeking" of medications, a form of noncompliance that may lead to drug toxicity or overdose. If the assessment shows that this is a potential risk, using liquid dosage forms, when available, may minimize such problems. Other areas to assess include the patient's appetite, sleeping patterns, addictive behaviors, elimination difficulties, and allergic reactions. Note any new symptoms or problems.

ANXIOLYTIC DRUGS

Anxiety disorders are treated with the anxiolytic drugs. *Anxiolytic drugs*, specifically the benzodiazepines, are associated with many contraindications, cautions, and drug interactions (see pharmacology discussion). When these drugs are used, the prescriber may order laboratory studies, such as complete blood counts, serum electrolyte levels, and hepatic/renal function studies (see earlier discussion).

QSEN

PATIENT-CENTERED CARE: LIFESPAN CONSIDERATIONS FOR THE OLDER ADULT PATIENT

Psychotherapeutic Drugs

- Older adult patients show higher serum levels of psychotherapeutic drugs because they have age-related changes in drug distribution and metabolism, less serum albumin, decreased lean body mass, less water in tissues, and increased body fat. They also have decreased renal function. Because of these changes, older adult patients generally require lower dosages of antipsychotic and antidepressant drugs and are at greater risk for toxicity.
- Orthostatic hypotension, anticholinergic adverse effects, sedation, and extrapyramidal symptoms are more common in older adult patients taking psychotherapeutic drugs.
- Careful evaluation and documentation of baseline parameters, including neurologic findings, are important to the safe use of these drugs.
- Increased anxiety is often associated with the use of tricyclic antidepressants.
- Patients with a history of cardiac disease may be at a greater risk for experiencing dysrhythmias, tachycardia, stroke, myocardial infarction, or heart failure.
- Lithium toxicity is more common in older adult patients, and lower dosages are often necessary to achieve therapeutic levels. Close monitoring is important to its safe use in this age group. Central nervous system toxicity, lithium-induced goiter, and hypothyroidism are also more common in older adult patients.

Blood pressure readings are also very important to assess because of drug-related postural hypotension. The baseline neurologic examination needs to include assessment of alertness, orientation, and sensory/motor functioning as well as any complaints of ataxia, headache, or other neurologic abnormalities. To complete a thorough medication profile, create a list of all medications taken along with any other psychotherapeutic drugs, all prescription drugs, over-the-counter drugs, vitamins, minerals, and herbal products. *Diazepam*, although one of the more commonly prescribed *benzodiazepines*, is generally used for seizure disorders and preoperative sedation and requires

---

QSEN

PATIENT-CENTERED CARE: LIFESPAN CONSIDERATIONS FOR THE PEDIATRIC PATIENT

Psychotherapeutic Drugs

- Pediatric patients are more likely to experience adverse effects from psychotropic drugs, especially extrapyramidal effects.
- The incidence of Reye's syndrome and other adverse reactions is greater in pediatric patients who have had chickenpox, central nervous system infections, measles, acute illnesses, or dehydration and are taking psychotropic drugs.
- Lithium may lead to decreased bone density or bone formation in children; therefore, children receiving it need to be closely monitored for signs and symptoms of lithium toxicity and bone disorders. The safety and efficacy of lithium dosing for those younger than 6 years of age is not established.
- Tricyclic antidepressants generally are not prescribed for patients younger than 12 years of age. However, some antidepressants are used in children with enuresis, attention deficit disorders, and major depressive disorders, and may be associated with adverse reactions such as electrocardiographic changes, nervousness, sleep disorder, fatigue, elevated blood pressure, and gastrointestinal upset.
- Pediatric patients are generally more sensitive to the effects of most drugs, and psychotherapeutic drugs are no exception. Be aware of the risk for toxicity, which can be fatal. If confusion, lethargy, visual disturbances, insomnia, tremors, palpitations, constipation, or eye pain occur, contact the prescriber immediately.

---

assessment related to these uses (see Chapters 11 and 14). Specific concerns for pediatric and older adult patients are presented in the boxes on this page. Closely observe and assess older adult patients for oversedation and/or profound CNS depression during drug therapy. Patients of this age are often more sensitive to drugs and therefore more likely to experience adverse effects. The patient's safety needs to be a constant concern.

Since eye problems may occur with use of *benzodiazepines*, baseline visual testing using a Snellen chart or an eye examination conducted by the appropriate health care provider (e.g., an ophthalmologist or optometrist) is recommended. Allergic reactions to some of these medications (e.g., *clonazepam*) are characterized by a red raised rash. In addition, obese patients may experience toxicity in a shorter period of time than those who are not obese. This occurs because several anxiolytic drugs are lipid soluble and have greater affinity for fatty tissues; therefore, their half-life is increased in patients who are obese. Give *lorazepam* cautiously (under very close supervision) if the patient is suicidal, because its use may be associated with suicide attempts. Administer *alprazolam* only after very careful assessment of mental status, mood, sensorium, and sleep patterns.

Some benzodiazepines are also associated with medication errors because of the existence of sound-alike or look-alike drugs. Assessing the drug order for the right drug is important because of the possibility of such an error and the negative consequences to the patient. Benzodiazepine drugs and the sound-alike medications with which they could be confused include the following: *Klonopin* (*clonazepam*) and *clonidine*;

diazepam and *Ditropan (oxybutynin); lorazepam* and *alprazolam*; and *Versed (midazolam), VePesid (etoposide)*, and *Vistaril (hydroxyzine)*.

Buspirone is another anxiolytic drug that is not a benzodiazepine. It is used because it has fewer adverse effects, such as decreased sedation and lack of dependency potential. However, it is associated with many drug interactions, cautions, and contraindications (see pharmacology discussion). General assessment of the neurologic system and a mental health assessment are also important to complete.

OSEN ⚡ SAFETY AND QUALITY IMPROVEMENT: PREVENTING MEDICATION ERRORS

Sound-Alike Drugs: Bupropion and Buspirone

Is it bupropion or buspirone? Be careful—these two central nervous system drugs have sound-alike names but very different uses.

Bupropion (Wellbutrin) is an antidepressant that is used to relieve depression. The Zyban formulation of bupropion is given to treat nicotine withdrawal symptoms. Bupropion is available in various formulations ranging from 75- to 100-mg tablets to extended- or sustained-release formulations of 100-mg, 150-mg, 200-mg, and 300-mg tablets.

Buspirone hydrochloride (BuSpar) is an anxiolytic drug that is used for short-term treatment of anxiety symptoms or long-term management of anxiety disorders. It is available in tablets ranging from 5 mg to 30 mg.

▌MOOD-STABILIZING DRUGS

As previously discussed in the pharmacology section, affective disorders are treated with *mood-stabilizing drugs* and antidepressant drugs. Before *antimanic drugs*, such as *lithium*, are administered, perform a thorough neurologic examination. Also assess vital signs, especially blood pressure, hydration status, dietary intake, skin tone, and presence of edema. Baseline levels of consciousness and alertness, gait and mobility levels, and overall motor functioning are also important to assess. These are particularly important to assess because poor coordination, tremors, and weakness may be symptoms of toxic blood levels of antimanic drugs. Laboratory studies often ordered before and during drug therapy include serum sodium, albumin, and uric acid levels. Serum levels of sodium are important to know because lithium toxicity is potentiated by the presence of hyponatremia and hypovolemia. During the initial phase of therapy, serum lithium levels must be assessed every 3 to 4 days (therapeutic levels are 0.6 mEq/L to 1.2 mEq/L; toxic levels are above 1.5 mEq/L). A urinalysis with specific gravity may also be ordered to assess volume status.

▌ANTIDEPRESSANTS

You must assess for many cautions, contraindications, and drug interactions before giving *antidepressants* (see pharmacology discussion). Continuous assessment for any suicidal ideation or tendencies is important because indicators of suicide risk may be covert as well as overt. Suicide must always be considered a potential risk when any psychotherapeutic medication, whether an antidepressant or other CNS-altering drug, is taken alone or in combination with other drugs or alcohol.

TCAs, as an older class of antidepressants, are effective drugs but are associated with serious adverse effects. However, some patients do tolerate the TCAs. When patients are taking TCAs, monitor closely for potential adverse effects. Use with the herbal product, St. John's wort, is not recommended. Amitriptyline is not to be used in patients with recent myocardial infarction and is associated with potent anticholinergic properties leading to dry mouth, constipation, blurred vision, urinary retention, and alterations in cardiac rhythm.

Closely monitor patients receiving *MAOIs* who have a history of suicide attempts or suicidal ideation. Suicidal thoughts and suicide attempts are important to consider, because these drugs may be hoarded by the patient and then used to carry out suicide. These patients must be under the care of a health care professional (e.g., psychiatrist, physician, or nurse practitioner) so that they may be closely monitored for destructive behaviors. MAOIs are also known for their significant drug interactions (see Table 15-4) such as with meperidine, other opioids, other MAOIs, SSRIs, oral contraceptives, and buspirone. MAOIs, if taken with foods high in tyramine (see Table 16-7), are associated with a hypertensive crisis; therefore, closely monitor blood pressure readings, including postural blood pressure measurements. Postural hypotension, an adverse effect of MAOIs, may lead to a high risk for dizziness, fainting, and possible falls or injury. If the patient is hospitalized, monitor supine/standing or sitting blood pressures at least every 8 hours or more frequently, if needed. A period of 1 to 2 minutes needs to elapse after taking the supine blood pressure before measuring standing or sitting pressures and pulse rate. Laboratory tests that are often ordered for patients taking these drugs include complete blood counts and renal and liver function studies. In addition, it is crucial to understand that the older adult patient must be given these medications only if it is deemed absolutely necessary by the prescriber and only with careful monitoring.

🍃 SAFETY: HERBAL THERAPIES AND DIETARY SUPPLEMENTS OSEN

Ginseng

Overview
Comes from the *Panax quinquefolius* plant in North America (American ginseng), the *Panax ginseng* plant in Asia (Panax ginseng), and the *Acanthopanax senticosus* plant in Russia (Siberian ginseng).

Common Uses
Improvement of physical endurance and concentration, stress reduction (NOTE: This is a very abbreviated list of uses for these products.)

Adverse Effects
Elevated blood pressure, chest pain or palpitations, anxiety, insomnia, headache, nausea, vomiting, diarrhea

Potential Drug Interactions
May reduce the effectiveness of anticoagulants and immunosuppressants, but enhance the effectiveness of anticonvulsants and antidiabetic drugs

Contraindications
Contraindicated in children and pregnant women

The *second-generation antidepressants* are associated with fewer and less severe adverse effects as compared to the older TCA and MAOI antidepressants. These second-generation drugs include *SSRIs (fluoxetine [Prozac])* and *SNRIs (duloxetine [Cymbalta])*. However, with SSRIs it is still important to assess and document neuromuscular and gastrointestinal systems. Cautious use in the older adult patient is recommended due to their increased risk for toxicity. Additionally, there is concern for the occurrence of serotonin syndrome. Serotonin syndrome (see Box 16-1) includes symptoms such as agitation, tachycardia, sweating, and muscle tremors. Contraindications include the use of these drugs within 14 days of use of MAOIs and with some antipsychotic drugs. Assess for significant drug interactions, such as warfarin and phenytoin, due to their increased protein binding. Do not give *SNRIs*, such as *duloxetine (Cymbalta)*, to patients with closed-angle glaucoma or those taking MAOIs. Liver function studies may be ordered prior to use of this drug because of the risk for liver toxicity. The *miscellaneous antidepressant bupropion* may be preferred over some of the other antidepressants because of fewer anticholinergic, antiadrenergic, and cardiotoxic effects (see pharmacology discussion). Assess the patient's baseline neurologic, mental, and cardiac status before the drug is used. Because of delayed therapeutic effects, closely assess the patient for any suicidal tendencies or ideation. Assess the availability of family support systems as well as the need for any supportive resources.

ANTIPSYCHOTICS

The use of *antipsychotics* requires careful assessment of all body systems. Assessment of cardiovascular, cerebrovascular, neurologic, gastrointestinal, genitourinary, renal, hepatic, and hematologic functioning is important to safe and efficacious drug therapy. The presence of significant disease in one or several organ systems may lead to a more adverse response to a drug and may even be dose limiting; therefore, perform a careful and skillful assessment of the patient before and during drug therapy. Weight gain may occur, and if the patient is experiencing deleterious health effects because of this, another drug may be ordered. Suicidal ideation, orthostatic changes in blood pressure, extrapyramidal symptoms, confusion, headache, gastrointestinal upset, abnormal muscle movements, rashes, and dry mouth may be associated with many of these drugs; therefore, perform and document a thorough nursing history and mental status examination prior to the initiation of drug therapy. Identify possible drug interactions with any prescription drugs, over-the-counter medications, and/or herbals the patient is taking, as well as any conditions that represent cautions or contraindications to use of the antipsychotic drug (see pharmacology discussion). The *phenothiazine antipsychotics* may still be prescribed in some situations but are mentioned here mainly for historical purposes. These antipsychotics are associated with significant extrapyramidal adverse effects (see earlier discussion) as well as anticholinergic adverse effects such as dry mouth, urinary hesitancy, and constipation.

Haloperidol is similar to other high-potency antipsychotics because its sedating effects are low but the incidence of extrapyramidal symptoms is high. Assessment of baseline motor, sensory, and neurologic functioning is therefore very important to patient safety. With some of the antipsychotic drugs, patients may experience adverse effects of tremors and muscle twitching from the drug's blockade of dopamine receptors (dopamine generally has an inhibitory effect on specific motor activity in the musculoskeletal system). These extrapyramidal movements are like those in parkinsonism (see Chapter 15) and may be very bothersome and uncomfortable.

Atypical antipsychotics, such as *aripiprazole (Abilify)*, *clozapine (Clozaril)*, *lurasidone (Latuda)*, and *risperidone (Risperdal)*, have many contraindications, cautions, and drug interactions (see pharmacology discussion). Perform a thorough mental status examination, and document the findings prior to initiation of treatment with these and other antipsychotic drugs. An assessment of musculoskeletal functioning and monitoring for any extrapyramidal reaction is also important to patient safety. Monitor liver and renal function studies, complete blood count, and urinalysis before and during therapy. Make sure to document blood pressure readings with close attention to postural readings because of the potential for the adverse effect of postural hypotension. A drop of 20 mm Hg or more in the systolic blood pressure requires immediate attention and implementation of safety precautions. In addition, for the older adult patient, the prescriber may order reduced dosages to help prevent toxicity. These drugs are also associated with a high degree of sedation and must be used only when absolutely necessary and with extreme caution (close monitoring) in the older adult patient and other patients who are at risk for falls or have limited motor and sensory capabilities. Carefully monitor heart sounds, and observe for any abnormal heart rhythms in patients taking these drugs.

NURSING DIAGNOSES

1. Imbalanced nutrition, less than body requirements, related to the consequences of the mental health disorder and/or the use of psychotherapeutic drugs
2. Urinary retention related to the adverse effects of psychotherapeutic drugs
3. Constipation related to the adverse effects of psychotherapeutic drugs
4. Sexual dysfunction related to the adverse effects associated with psychotherapeutic drugs
5. Sleep deprivation related to the mental health disorder and/or related drug therapy
6. Deficient knowledge related to lack of information about the specific psychotherapeutic drugs and their adverse effects
7. Impaired social interaction related to various inadequacies felt by the patient due to illness or isolation from others
8. Situational low self-esteem related to the mental health disorder and from the adverse effects of psychotherapeutic drugs, including sexual dysfunction
9. Risk for injury to self related to the mental health disorder and/or possible adverse effects of psychotherapeutic drugs

PLANNING: OUTCOME IDENTIFICATION

1. Patient shows improved nutritional status/healthy nutritional habits with appropriate weight gain and a diet that includes foods from the U.S. Department of Agriculture MyPlate (*www.choosemyplate.gov*).
2. Patient minimizes alterations in urinary elimination with adequate fluid intake and reporting of any problems with urinary hesitancy, urgency, retention, or discomfort over the lower abdominal area.
3. Patient states measures to maintain healthy bowel elimination patterns with an increase in fluids and dietary bulk/fiber with fruits and vegetables.
4. Patient openly identifies/discusses with the prescriber options for improving sexual functioning to assist with any altered patterns of sexual behavior.
5. Patient reports measures to maintain healthy sleeping patterns/sleeping habits through use of nondrug sleep-enhancement measures such as going to bed at a regular time nightly, decreasing room noise/light, listening to calming music, using aromatherapy, and avoiding caffeine in the late afternoon/evening (see Chapter 12 for more interventions related to sleep).
6. Patient states importance for compliance to medication regimen, as well as the need to take the medication exactly as prescribed, and related drug safety measures.
7. Patient demonstrates improved or no further deterioration in social integration with healthier patterns of communication and participation in activities with family, friends, significant others, and members of the health care team without suspicion or paranoia.
8. Patient maintains healthy and positive self-concept/self-esteem in daily interactions with family/friends/significant others while experiencing fewer episodes of self-destructive and negative behaviors.
9. Patient remains free from injury and demonstrates safety with activities of daily living and self-care measures by moving slowly, changing positions slowly, and reporting excess dizziness as well as fainting episodes.

IMPLEMENTATION

Regardless of the *psychotherapeutic drug* prescribed, several general nursing actions are important for safe administration. First and foremost, demonstrate a firm, calm, and empathic attitude with use of therapeutic communication skills while establishing a therapeutic relationship. Once the patient's reading level and effective means of teaching and learning are identified, provide the patient with simple explanations about the drug, its action, and the length of time before therapeutic effects can be expected. Always use a thorough psychosocial and holistic approach when caring for any patient with any illness. Monitor vital signs and document findings, especially during the initiation of drug therapy. Of great concern is administration of these medications to the older adult patient and to patients with a history of hypertension and cardiac disease. All of the psychotherapeutic drugs are to be taken exactly as prescribed and at the same time every day without failure. If omission occurs, the patient should have previous instructions in how to handle this or to contact the prescriber immediately. Abrupt withdrawal may have negative effects on the patient's physical and mental status. Solicit help from family members or others providing support in the care of the patient so that there are options for assistance with drug administration. Adherence to the medication regimen is crucial to effective management; identify and utilize all support systems and resources to accomplish this.

ANXIOLYTIC DRUGS

Specific nursing interventions related to the use of *anxiolytic drugs* include frequent monitoring of vital signs with special attention to blood pressure and postural blood pressures readings. Encourage the use of elastic compression stockings and changing positions slowly to minimize dizziness and falls from orthostatic hypotension. Create a therapeutic environment for open communication—especially for the patient's verbalizing of all disturbing thoughts, including those of suicide. Check the patient's oral cavities for hoarding or cheeking of drugs. Use intravenous routes of administration only as prescribed, and give the drug over the recommended time with the proper diluent and at a rate indicated by the manufacturer and prescriber. Always administer intramuscular dosage forms in a large muscle mass and only as ordered or indicated (see Chapter 9 for more information on parenteral administration). See Patient Centered Care: Patient Teaching for more information.

MOOD-STABILIZING DRUGS

Safe use of the *mood-stabilizing drug lithium* depends on adequate hydration and electrolyte status, because lithium levels may become toxic with dehydration and hyponatremia. See Patient Centered Care: Patient Teaching for more information.

ANTIDEPRESSANTS

Administer all antidepressants carefully and exactly as ordered. It is important to remember that it may take 4 to 6 weeks before therapeutic effects are evident with *TCAs*, *MAOIs*, and *second-generation antidepressants*. Make sure the patient understands this and continues to take the medication as prescribed—even if the patient feels his or her condition is not improving. Carefully monitor the patient, be readily available, and provide supportive care during this time. The period before therapeutic effects are seen may be the time the patient is at highest risk for self-harm and/or suicide. Advise the patient to take the drug(s) with food and at least 4 to 6 ounces of fluid. Assist with ambulation and other activities if the patient is weak, an older adult, or dizzy (from postural hypotension). Counsel the patient about potential sexual dysfunction (if appropriate). If sexual dysfunction occurs, encourage the patient to talk to his or her prescriber to discuss possible options. Abrupt withdrawal of the drug or discontinuing it without first contacting the prescriber is to be avoided. *Citalopram (Celexa)*, one of the most commonly prescribed *SSRIs*, has a short-half life and is therefore associated more frequently with discontinuation syndrome. See previous pharmacology discussion and Patient-Centered Care:

Patient Teaching for more specific information regarding *SSRIs* and *SNRIs*.

With the use of *TCAs* and *MAOIs*, educate patients on adverse effects and drug/food interactions. Emphasize the importance of keeping a list of all medications on their person at all times. Advise to change positions purposely and slowly. All health care providers need to be informed that the patient is taking these drugs and that weaning must occur when these drugs are to be discontinued. With TCAs, advise the patient to report any of the following to the prescriber if they occur: blurred vision, excessive drowsiness, sleepiness, urinary retention, constipation, and cognitive impairment. It is also important to inform patients that tolerance to sedation will occur with some *second-generation antidepressants.*

🌐 PATIENT-CENTERED CARE: CULTURAL IMPLICATIONS

Psychotherapeutic Drugs

Many racial and ethnic groups respond to drugs differently. For example, Asians have lower drug metabolism activity than whites related to lower levels of various enzymes. Asians often require lower dosages of benzodiazepines and tricyclic antidepressants because they have lower levels of the enzymes metabolizing these drugs (e.g., CYO2D6) and are therefore more sensitive to the drugs.

Diazepam follows a different metabolic pathway in the Chinese and Japanese populations. These two groups are found to be poor metabolizers of this drug and its metabolite. Approximately 20% of Chinese and Japanese individuals metabolize diazepam poorly, which results in rapid drug accumulation. To prevent possible toxicity, lower dosages are generally required. Nurses need to be aware of this cultural variable and assess these patients for sedation, overdosage, and other adverse reactions.

Researchers have also identified genetic factors that help predict a response to antidepressants. A study of some 80 Mexican Americans with depression found that depressed and highly anxious patients with certain variant genes had a 70% higher reduction in anxiety and a 30% higher reduction in depression in response to treatment with fluoxetine than did other racial and ethnic groups without the specific gene variation.

From ISMP Medication Safety Alert: *Cultural diversity and medication safety,* September 4, 2003. Available at *www.ismp.org/newsletters/acutecare/articles/20030904.asp.* Accessed April 4, 2014.

ANTIPSYCHOTICS

Patients need to be aware that *antipsychotic drugs* are to be taken exactly as prescribed to be effective. Different levels of paranoia or delusions may lead the patient to mistrust you and other members of the health care team, so maintain a sufficient level of trust through consistency, empathy, and the establishment of therapeutic communication to help ensure compliance. Adherence/compliance is always a critical issue for patients with psychotic illnesses, because these patients are at higher risk for not taking medications, not keeping follow-up appointments, and lacking trust needed for establishing therapeutic and social relationships. Nonadherence to the medical and treatment regimen is of major concern because the serum levels of drugs such as *haloperidol* must be within a specified therapeutic range for the patient to feel better and be functional. If serum levels of haloperidol are less than 4 ng/mL, the patient may show symptoms of the mental disorder, whereas levels higher than

22 ng/mL may result in toxicity. Therefore, selection of an antipsychotic drug and its dosage, route of administration, risk for toxicity, and/or suicidal potential, as well as therapeutic communication and patient education, are all important factors for successful therapy. Because most antipsychotic drugs are quite potent, be sure that oral dosage forms have actually been swallowed and have not been intentionally hidden in the side of the mouth (see previous discussion on cheeking of medications). Oral forms of the antipsychotics are generally well absorbed and will cause less gastrointestinal upset if taken with food or a full glass of water. Sucking on sugar-free hard candy or gum and/or use of artificial saliva drops/gum may help to relieve dry mouth. With any of the dosage forms, perspiration may be increased; therefore, encourage the patient to avoid engaging in excessive activity or being exposed to heat or humidity. Excessive sweating can lead to dehydration and subsequent drug toxicity.

Haloperidol may not necessarily be the best drug to use because of the risk for undermedication or overmedication and troubling adverse effects (see Table 16-10). Therefore, other antipsychotics (e.g., *clozapine, risperidone*) may be preferred, as previously discussed. Clozapine and risperidone are therapeutically effective and carry a minimal risk for tardive dyskinesia and extrapyramidal symptoms. In addition, they usually lead to improvement in cognitive behavior. Clozapine is to be taken as ordered and usually given in divided doses; proper dosing is very important to therapeutic effectiveness. If any changes in blood counts (e.g., leukopenia) are noted or if abnormal cardiac functioning (e.g., tachycardia) is identified, contact the prescriber immediately. In such a case, the medication may need to be discontinued, but only as ordered, and the patient monitored closely. Titration of doses of clozapine, either upward or downward, needs to be done very carefully with close monitoring of the patient for any exacerbation of the mental illness or suicidal tendencies.

Risperidone is to be given as ordered and administered by injection into a deep muscle mass. Always check health care institution and/or drug insert guidelines regarding the administration of this drug. Intramuscular injection dosage forms may be ordered along with oral doses of risperidone or possibly of another antipsychotic drug for several weeks, with maintenance doses of an intramuscular injection given every 2 to 4 weeks, as ordered. Always alternate intramuscular injection sites to maintain tissue integrity and muscle mass, and be sure that the site is not red, swollen, or irritated. Document and report any changes. Oral solution, tablets, and orally disintegrating tabs are other available dosage forms. Do not give oral solutions with cola or tea. Disintegrating tabs need to be dissolved under the tongue before swallowing with or without liquid. Always follow the prescriber's orders for administering this and all other drugs. The daily amount is usually given in two divided doses, with dosage decreased in the older adult patient and in those with impaired renal or hepatic function. Make sure you report any excess sedation, anxiety, extrapyramidal symptoms, tardive dyskinesia, seizures, or strokelike symptoms immediately. Measuring vital signs and monitoring for any postural hypotension is also important during treatment.

Once therapy with any of the *antipsychotic drugs* has been initiated, it is important for you and other health care providers involved in the patient's care to monitor drug therapy closely, including measuring serum drug levels during follow-up visits. If the patient is suspected of being nonadherent and serum drug levels are subtherapeutic, the patient needs to be reevaluated by the prescriber for a possible change of drug or dosage form. The parenteral dosage forms usually come in a depot (longer-releasing) dosage formulation that releases the drug over 2 to 4 weeks, leading to increased compliance and often a better therapeutic outcome.

Patient education (see Patient Centered Care: Patient Teaching) and patient adherence with the drug regimen are keys to successful treatment, regardless of the mental illness. Often it is the mental disorder itself that causes patient nonadherence. Keeping communication open with the patient, family, and/or caregiver is important to develop trust and a sense of empathy. Although patient education may have been thorough, emphasize that the patient may call the prescriber, clinic, or hotline 24 hours a day. Keep phone numbers continually updated. Make constant and ongoing professional counseling available with a mental health care provider (psychiatrist, nurse practitioner, or other licensed mental health professional) so that the patient's progress is consistently monitored. Group therapy and support groups are also available for the patient and significant others.

EVALUATION

Monitor the therapeutic effects of *psychotherapeutic medications* and the patient's progress before and during drug therapy. Mental alertness, cognition, affect, mood, ability to carry out activities of daily living, appetite, and sleep patterns are all areas that need to be closely monitored and documented. The patient must continue with other forms of therapy, in addition to drug therapy, with the goal of acquiring more effective coping skills. Other forms of treatment may include intense psychotherapy, relaxation therapy, stress reduction, and lifestyle changes. It is important to mention that blood levels of these drugs will be measured during follow-up visits to ensure that therapeutic levels are maintained. Such monitoring of serum drug levels helps identify both subtherapeutic and toxic levels.

The therapeutic effects of *anxiolytic drugs* are evidenced by improved mental alertness, cognition, and mood; fewer anxiety and panic attacks; improved sleep patterns and appetite; more interest in self and others; less tension and irritability; and fewer feelings of fear, impending doom, and stress. Watch for the adverse effects of hypotension, lethargy, fatigue, drowsiness, and confusion in patients taking anxiolytic drugs.

Therapeutic effects of the *mood stabilizer lithium* are decreased mania and stabilization of the patient's mood.

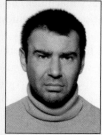
Lithium is usually better tolerated by the patient during the manic phase. Adverse reactions to lithium include dysrhythmias, hypotension, sedation, slurred speech, slowed motor abilities, and weight gain. Gastrointestinal adverse effects include GI discomfort.

In general, adverse reactions to *antidepressants* consist of drowsiness, dry mouth, constipation, dizziness, postural hypotension, sedation, blood dyscrasias, sexual dysfunction, and dyskinesias. Overdose is evidenced by seizures or dysrhythmias.

When used as antidepressants, *SSRIs* and *SNRIs* may take 4 to 6 weeks to reach full therapeutic effect. A therapeutic response to these drugs includes improved depression or mental status, improved ability to carry out activities of daily living, less insomnia, and improved mood disorder with minimal adverse effects of weight gain, headache, gastrointestinal upset, insomnia, dizziness, drowsiness, and sexual dysfunction. Monitor the patient for symptoms of serotonin syndrome such as agitation, tachycardia, hyperreflexia, and tremors (see Box 16-1).

The therapeutic effects of the *antipsychotic drugs* include improvement in mood and affect, and alleviation or decrease in psychotic symptoms (decrease in hallucinations, paranoia, delusions, garbled speech) once the patient has been taking the medication for several weeks. Careful monitoring of the patient's potential to injure self or others during the delay between the start of therapy and symptomatic improvement is critical. Evaluation for adverse effects includes monitoring blood counts (*clozapine*) as well as ticlike trembling movements of the hands, face, neck, and head; hypotension; and dry mouth (*haloperidol*).

PATIENT-CENTERED CARE: PATIENT TEACHING

Anxiolytic Drugs

- Encourage patients to avoid operating heavy machinery and driving until the adverse effects of sedation or drowsiness have resolved.
- Educate about the development of tolerance to the sedating properties of benzodiazepines with chronic use (see Chapter 12).
- Instruct patients not to take over-the-counter drugs or herbals without seeking advice from the prescriber.
- Keep these and all psychotherapeutic drugs out of the reach of children.
- Concurrent use of alcohol with psychotherapeutic drugs and other CNS depressants must be avoided.
- Advise patients to carry a medical alert or other identification bracelet/necklace with their diagnoses and a list of their drugs and allergies at all times. The drug list needs to be updated at least every 3 months.
- Medications must always be taken exactly as ordered. Avoid sudden withdrawal. If withdrawal of a drug is necessary, tapering/weaning of doses is needed and under supervision/advice of prescriber.

Mood-Stabilizing Drugs

- Instruct the patient that lithium must be taken at the same time each day, and give specific instructions on how to handle missed doses. Make sure the patient understands the importance of adequate hydration.
- Inform the patient that the adverse effects of lithium are usually transient; however, excessive tremors, seizures, confusion, ataxia, and excessive sedation must be reported to the prescriber immediately.

Monoamine Oxidase Inhibitors and Tricyclic Antidepressants

- Advise the patient taking MAOIs to contact the prescriber immediately if any of the following signs and symptoms of overdosage or toxicity occur: tachycardia, hyperthermia, or seizures.
- If the patient is taking an MAOI, caution him or her about avoiding over-the-counter cold and flu products. Foods or beverages high in tyramine are to be avoided (see Table 16-7).
- When the patient is taking a TCA, any blurred vision, agitation, urinary retention, or ataxia needs to be reported to the prescriber immediately.
- Encourage wearing of a medical alert necklace or bracelet showing the diagnosis and a list of current drugs.

Selective Serotonin Reuptake Inhibitors and Serotonin-Norepinephrine Reuptake Inhibitors (Antidepressants)

- Consumption of fiber supplements must occur at least 2 hours before or after the dosing of medication to avoid interference with drug absorption; however, dietary fiber intake is appropriate.
- Encourage the patient to openly discuss any concerns about the medication and adverse effects such as gastrointestinal upset, sexual dysfunction, or tremors.
- Provide a listing of drug-drug interactions, such as the strong interaction between SSRIs and MAOIs, St. John's wort (an herbal product), and tryptophan (a serotonin precursor found in foods). Such interactions may pose a risk for serotonin syndrome (see earlier discussion). Cold products and over-the-counter medications must be approved by the prescriber.
- SSRIs must be taken carefully and as prescribed. Any increase in suicidal thoughts or extreme changes in mood must be reported immediately to the prescriber.
- Emphasize that all follow-up visits must be kept and prescriber contacted if there are any concerns. Educate that discontinuation of SSRIs and SNRIs requires a tapering period of up to 1 to 2 months, as ordered. Discontinuation syndrome may occur with or without a tapering period; this syndrome is exhibited by flulike symptoms, difficulty concentrating, feeling dizzy, fainting, and GI symptoms such as diarrhea. The prescriber needs to be contacted immediately if these symptoms occur.
- Citalopram (Celexa), one of the most commonly used SSRIs, is commonly associated with this discontinuation syndrome.
- If there is ever doubt that too much of an antidepressant has been taken, contact the prescriber and/or seek emergency medical treatment immediately. For a poison emergency, always have this number available: In the United States, call 1-800-222-1222. If transdermal patches are the dosage form used, emphasize the importance of rotating the patch site with each application and placing the patch on a nonhairy, healthy, intact area. Any residue from the previous patch is to be gently cleansed off prior to application of a new patch.
- Advise patients to avoid hot baths, saunas, and hot climates with antipsychotics because of the risk for further drop in blood pressure, especially upon standing (postural hypotension). Injury to self may occur due to dizziness or fainting.
- Haloperidol and other antipsychotics must never be stopped abruptly because of the high risk for inducing a withdrawal psychosis.
- Drug interactions with clozapine include alcohol, CNS depressants, levodopa, and antihypertensives.
- Any sore throat, malaise, fever, or bleeding must be reported to the prescriber immediately because of the drop in WBC counts with clozapine.

KEY POINTS

- Psychosis is a major emotional disorder that impairs mental function. A person experiencing psychosis cannot participate in everyday life and shows the hallmark sign of loss of contact with reality.
- Affective disorders are emotional disorders characterized by changes in mood. They range from mania (abnormally elevated emotions) to depression (abnormally reduced emotions) and include anxiety, a normal emotion that may be a healthy reaction but becomes pathologic when it is life-altering.
- Situational anxiety arises in response to specific life events, and nursing assessment is key to identifying patients at risk.
- SSRIs and SNRIs are often prescribed because of their superiority to older antidepressants.
- Atypical antipsychotics can be used in bipolar disorder or depression including drugs such as aripiprazole (Abilify) and lurasidone (Latuda).
- Nursing considerations related to psychotherapeutic drugs include the need for skillful patient assessment with an emphasis on past and present medical history, physical examination, and a thorough medication history and profile.

NCLEX® EXAMINATION REVIEW QUESTIONS

1. In caring for a patient experiencing ethanol withdrawal, the nurse expects to administer which medication or medication class as treatment for this condition?
   a. lithium (Eskalith)
   b. Benzodiazepines
   c. buspirone (BuSpar)
   d. Antidepressants

2. Patient teaching for a patient receiving an MAOI would include instructions to avoid which food product?
   a. Orange juice
   b. Milk
   c. Shrimp
   d. Swiss cheese

3. After a patient has been treated for depression for 4 weeks, the nurse calls the patient to schedule a follow-up visit. What concern will the nurse assess for during the conversation with the patient?
   a. Weakness
   b. Hallucinations
   c. Suicidal ideation
   d. Difficulty with urination

4. The nurse is caring for a patient who has been taking clozapine (Clozaril) for 2 months. Which laboratory test(s) should be performed regularly while the patient is taking this medication?
   a. Platelet count
   b. WBC count
   c. Liver function studies
   d. Renal function studies

5. The nurse is giving medications to a patient. Which drug or drug class, when administered with lithium, increases the risk for lithium toxicity?

   a. Thiazides
   b. levofloxacin
   c. calcium citrate
   d. Beta blockers

6. The nurse is teaching a patient about treatment with an SSRI antidepressant. Which teaching considerations are appropriate? (Select all that apply.)
   a. The patient should be told which foods contain tyramine and instructed to avoid these foods.
   b. The patient should be instructed to use caution when standing up from a sitting position.
   c. The patient should not take any products that contain the herbal product St. John's wort.
   d. This medication should not be stopped abruptly.
   e. Drug levels may become toxic if dehydration occurs.
   f. The patient should be told to check with the prescriber before taking any over-the-counter medications.

7. A patient with a feeding tube will be receiving risperidone (Risperdal) 8 mg in 2 divided doses via the feeding tube. The medication is available in a 1 mg/mL solution. How many milliliters will the nurse administer for each dose?

8. A patient who has been taking lithium for 6 months has had severe vomiting and diarrhea from a gastrointestinal flu. The nurse will assess for which potential problem at this time?
   a. Anxiety
   b. Chest pain
   c. Agitation
   d. Dehydration

1. b, 2. d, 3. c, 4. b, 5. a, 6. b, c, d, f, 7. 4 mL per dose, 8. d

CRITICAL THINKING AND PRIORITIZATION QUESTIONS

1. A 68-year-old patient has been taking an SSRI antidepressant for 3 weeks. His wife calls and expresses concern because he has started to give away some of his keepsakes. What is the nurse's priority action at this time?

2. A patient has been admitted to the hospital because of a suspected overdose of a tricyclic antidepressant. What two problems are the nurse's priorities at this time?

For answers, see *http://evolve.elsevier.com/Lilley.*

ⓔ EVOLVE WEBSITE

http://evolve.elsevier.com/Lilley

- Animations
- Answer Keys for Textbook Case Studies and Textbook Critical Thinking and Prioritization Questions

- Content Updates
- Key Points
- Review Questions
- Student Case Studies

Substance Abuse

e http://evolve.elsevier.com/Lilley

OBJECTIVES

When you reach the end of this chapter, you will be able to do the following:

1. Discuss substance abuse and the significance of the problem in the United States.
2. Identify the drugs or chemicals that are most frequently abused.
3. Contrast the signs and symptoms of the most commonly abused drugs/chemicals.
4. Compare the treatments for drug withdrawal for the most commonly abused opioids (narcotics), central nervous system (CNS) depressants, amphetamines and other CNS stimulants, nicotine, and alcohol.
5. Describe alcohol abuse syndrome with a focus on signs and symptoms, mild to severe alcohol withdrawal symptoms, and associated treatment.
6. Describe other drug abuse syndromes, signs and symptoms, withdrawal symptoms, and treatment regimens.
7. Identify various assessment tools used in the nursing assessment of substance abuse.
8. Develop a nursing care plan encompassing all phases of the nursing process for a patient undergoing treatment for substance abuse and dependency.

KEY TERMS

Addiction Psychologic or physical dependence on a drug or psychoactive substance. (p. 278)

Amphetamine A drug that stimulates the central nervous system. (p. 280)

Detoxification A process of eliminating a toxic substance from the body; a medically supervised program for alcohol, benzodiazepine, methamphetamine, or opioid addiction. (p. 279)

Enuresis Urinary incontinence. (p. 280)

Habituation Development of tolerance to a substance following prolonged medical use but without psychologic or physical dependence (addiction). (p. 278)

Illicit drug use The use of a drug or substance in a way that it is not intended to be used or the use of a drug that is not legally approved for human administration. (p. 279)

Intoxication Stimulation, excitement, or stupefaction produced by a chemical substance. (p. 278)

Korsakoff's psychosis A syndrome of amnesia with confabulation (making up of stories) associated with chronic alcohol abuse; it often occurs together with *Wernicke's encephalopathy.* (p. 283)

Micturition Urination, the desire to urinate, or the frequency of urination. (p. 280)

Narcolepsy A sleep disorder characterized by sleeping during the day, disrupted nighttime sleep, cataplexy, sleep paralysis, and hallucinations. (p. 281)

Physical dependence A condition characterized by physiologic reliance on a substance, usually indicated by tolerance to the effects of the substance and development of withdrawal symptoms when use of the substance is terminated. (p. 278)

Psychoactive properties Drug properties that affect mood, behavior, cognitive processes, and mental status. (p. 280)

Psychologic dependence A condition characterized by strong desires to obtain and use a substance. (p. 278)

Raves Increasingly popular all-night parties that typically involve dancing, drinking, and the use of various illicit drugs. (p. 280)

Roofies Pills that are classified as benzodiazepines. They have recently gained popularity as a recreational drug; chemically known as *flunitrazepam.* (p. 281)

Substance abuse The use of a mood- or behavior-altering substance in a maladaptive manner that often compromises health, safety, and social and occupational functioning, and causes legal problems. (p. 278)

Wernicke's encephalopathy A neurologic disorder characterized by apathy, drowsiness, ataxia, nystagmus, and ophthalmoplegia; it is caused by thiamine (vitamin B_1) deficiency secondary to chronic alcohol abuse. (p. 283)

Withdrawal A substance-specific mental disorder characterized by physical symptoms, following the cessation or reduction in use of a psychoactive substance that has been taken regularly to induce a state of intoxication. (p. 278)

OVERVIEW

Substance abuse affects people of all ages, sexes, and ethnic and socioeconomic groups. Physical dependence and psychologic dependence on a substance are chronic disorders with remissions and relapses common. Relapses are not to be seen as failures but as indications to intensify treatment. Recognizing physical or psychologic dependence and understanding the various treatment guidelines are important skills for those caring for these patients. Habituation refers to situations in which a patient becomes accustomed to a certain drug (develops tolerance) and may have mild psychologic dependence on it but does not show compulsive dose escalation, drug-seeking behavior, or major withdrawal symptoms on drug discontinuation. This might occur, for example, in a postsurgical patient who receives opioid pain therapy regularly for only a few weeks.

According to the most recently updated statistics from The Substance Abuse and Mental Health Services Administration in 2013, 23.1 million Americans 12 years of age or older were current illicit drug users. Heroin and prescription drugs showed the biggest increase in use, while marijuana was identified as the most commonly used illicit drug. Tobacco use has shown a consistent decline, falling from 15.2% in 2002 to 8.6% in 2012. Illicit prescription drug use includes psychotherapeutic drugs (primarily stimulants), pain relievers, tranquilizers, and sedatives.

Nearly 50% of the adult patients seen in many family practice clinics have an alcohol or drug disorder. Some 25% to 40% of hospital admissions are related to substance abuse and its sequelae. Substance abuse is strongly associated with many types of mental illness. Treatment of both disorders is often very difficult, in part because of the high risk for drug interactions with the abused substances. Assessment, intervention, use of certain medications, specific addiction treatment strategies, and monitoring of recovery are essential to the care of this patient population.

This chapter focuses on commonly abused substances. A description of the category or the individual drug, possible effects, signs and symptoms of intoxication and withdrawal, peak period and duration of withdrawal symptoms, and drugs used to treat withdrawal are discussed. The list of substances of abuse in Box 17-1 is not all-inclusive, but it contains some of the substances most commonly abused at this time. Not all of these substances are discussed in this chapter. Refer to The National Institute on Drug Abuse, available at *www.nida.nih.gov/nidahome.html* for further information.

Pharmacologic therapies are indicated for patients with addictive disorders to prevent life-threatening withdrawal complications, such as seizures and delirium tremens, and to increase compliance with psychosocial forms of addiction treatment.

OPIOIDS

Opioid analgesics are synthetic versions of pain-relieving substances that were originally derived from the opium poppy plant (see Chapter 10). Diacetylmorphine (better known as *heroin*) and opium are classified as Schedule I drugs and are not

---

BOX 17-1   Commonly Abused Substances

Major Categories
Opioids
Stimulants
Depressants

Individual Drugs
Alcohol
Anabolic steroids (see Chapter 35)
Dextromethorphan
Lysergic acid diethylamide (LSD)
Marijuana
Methamphetamine
Methylenedioxymethamphetamine (MDMA, ecstasy, Molly)
Nicotine
Phencyclidine (PCP)

---

available in the United States for therapeutic use. Heroin was banned in the United States in 1924 because of its high potential for abuse and the increasing number of heroin addicts. In Europe, heroin is available for medical treatment of pain, and governmental programs also exist to provide heroin to addicts with the goal of reducing crime.

Heroin is one of the most commonly abused opioids. Other commonly abused opioids are codeine, hydrocodone, hydromorphone, meperidine, morphine, and oxycodone. Currently, heroin remains one of the top 10 most abused drugs in the United States and often is used in combination with the stimulant drug cocaine (discussed later in the Stimulants section). When heroin is injected (called *mainlining* or *skin popping*), sniffed (known as *snorting*), or smoked, it binds with opiate receptors found in many regions of the brain. The result is intense euphoria, often referred to as a *rush*. This rush lasts only briefly and is followed by a relaxed, contented state that persists for a couple of hours. In large doses, heroin, like other opioids, can reduce or stop respiration. Krokodil is a toxic homemade heroin substitute made by combining codeine tablets with various toxic chemicals including lighter fluid. At the time of this writing, the DEA has not yet confirmed krokodil in the United States, despite reports to the contrary. The combination of an opioid, a benzodiazepine, and the muscle relaxant carisprodol (Soma) is commonly abused and is known as the "Holy Trinity." This combination produces herion-like effects.

Mechanism of Action and Drug Effects

Opioids bind to specific opioid pain receptors in the brain and cause an analgesic response—the reduction of pain sensation. There are three main receptor types to which opioids bind and are discussed in detail in Chapter 10. One of the reasons that opioids are abused is their ability to produce euphoria.

The drug effects of opioids are primarily centered in the CNS. However, these drugs also act outside the CNS, and many of their unwanted effects stem from these actions. In addition to analgesia, opioids produce drowsiness, euphoria, tranquility, and other alterations in mood. The effects of opioids can be collectively referred to as *narcosis* or *stupor*, which involves reduced sensory response, especially to painful stimuli. For this reason, opioid analgesics are also referred to as *narcotics* (see Chapter 4), especially by law enforcement authorities.

Indications

The intended drug effects of opioids are to relieve pain, reduce cough, relieve diarrhea, and induce anesthesia. Many have a high potential for abuse and are therefore classified as Schedule II controlled substances. Relaxation and euphoria are the most common drug effects that lead to abuse and psychologic dependence. Sustained-release oxycodone (e.g., OxyContin) is an example of an opioid that is controversial because it is often overprescribed, misused, and grossly abused. Numerous deaths have been reported when sustained-release oxycodone was crushed and the entire 12-hour supply was released at one time. Several new abuse deterrent formulations of opioids have recently been approved by the FDA. Abuse deterrents are divided into the following techniques: chemical/physical barriers, agonist/antagonist combinations, aversion, delivery system, and prodrug. Each of these techniques targets known or expected routes of abuse.

Certain opioid drugs are themselves used to treat opioid dependence. Methadone has been used most commonly for this purpose. Its long half-life of up to 12 to 24 hours allows patients to be dosed once daily at federally approved methadone maintenance clinics. In theory, the goal of such programs is to reduce the patient's dosage gradually so that eventually the patient can live permanently drug free. Unfortunately, relapse rates are often high in these programs.

Contraindications

Contraindications to the therapeutic use of opioid medications include known drug allergy, pregnancy (high dosage or prolonged use is contraindicated), respiratory depression or severe asthma when resuscitative equipment is not available, and *paralytic ileus* (bowel paralysis).

Adverse Effects

Adverse effects of opioids can be broken down into two groups: CNS and non-CNS. The primary adverse effects of opioids are related to their actions in the CNS. The major CNS-related adverse effects include diuresis, miosis, convulsions, nausea, vomiting, and respiratory depression. Many of the non-CNS adverse effects are secondary to the release of histamine. Histamine release can cause vasodilation leading to hypotension, spasms of the colon leading to constipation, increased spasms of the ureter resulting in urinary retention, and dilation of cutaneous blood vessels leading to flushing of the skin of the face, neck, and upper thorax. The release of histamine is also thought to cause sweating, urticaria, and pruritus.

Management of Withdrawal, Toxicity, and Overdose

Box 17-2 lists the signs and symptoms of opioid withdrawal. Many patients require a formal detoxification program while withdrawal symptoms are occurring. See Chapter 10 for a detailed discussion of physical dependence and the management of acute intoxication, toxicity, and overdose. Withdrawal symptoms include nausea, dysphoria, muscle aches, lacrimation, rhinorrhea, pupillary dilation, piloerection (hair standing

---

BOX 17-2   Signs and Symptoms of Opioid Withdrawal

Peak Period
1 to 3 days

Duration
5 to 7 days

Signs
Drug seeking, mydriasis, piloerection, diaphoresis, rhinorrhea, lacrimation, vomiting, diarrhea, insomnia, elevated blood pressure and pulse rate

Symptoms
Intense desire for drugs, muscle cramps, arthralgia, anxiety, nausea, malaise

---

BOX 17-3   Medications for Treatment of Opioid Withdrawal

Clonidine (Catapres) Substitution
Clonidine, 0.1 or 0.2 mg orally, is given every 4 to 6 hours as needed for signs and symptoms of withdrawal for 5 to 7 days. Days 2 to 4 are typically the most difficult days for the patient in detoxification. Check blood pressure before each dose, and do not give medication if patient is hypotensive.

Methadone Substitution
A single dose of 20 to 30 mg of methadone is usually sufficient to suppress symptoms. If needed, 5 to 10 mg every 2 to 4 hours as needed may be given. Range for total daily dose is 15 to 30 mg. Repeat total first-day dose in two divided doses (stabilization dose) for 2 to 3 days, then reduce dosage by 5 to 10 mg/day until medication is completely withdrawn.

---

on end) or sweating, diarrhea, yawning, fever, and insomnia. Medications listed in Box 17-3 are intended to help decrease the desire for the abused opioid and reduce the severity of these withdrawal symptoms. The most serious adverse effect and the most common cause of death with opioids is respiratory depression.

Certain medications are used to prevent relapse use once an initial remission is achieved. They are useful only when concurrent counseling is provided and offer additional insurance against return to illicit drug use. For opioid abuse or dependence, naltrexone, an opioid antagonist, is administered. Naltrexone, which is also available as an injection called Vivitrol, works by blocking the opioid receptors so that use of opioid drugs does not produce euphoria. When euphoria is eliminated, the reinforcing effect of the drug is lost. The patient needs to be free from opioids for at least 1 week before beginning this medication, because naltrexone can produce withdrawal symptoms if given too soon. Naltrexone is also approved for use by alcohol-dependent patients to reduce cravings for alcohol and the likelihood of a full relapse if a slip occurs. Another opioid antagonist, naloxone, is used for opioid dependence. It is combined with buprenorphine (Subutrex) or used alone (Suboxone) (see Chapter 10). Although dextromethorphan failed as an opioid, it is widely used as an over-the-counter cough suppressant. It is becoming an increasingly popular drug of abuse. It can produce a "high" associated with very large doses. It also produces hallucinations, which is documented to be similar to phencyclidine (PCP).

STIMULANTS

The abuse of stimulants is related to their ability to cause elevation of mood, reduction of fatigue, a sense of increased alertness, and invigorating aggressiveness. Amphetamine is a stimulant drug that is commonly abused. Chemically, three classes of amphetamine exist: salts of racemic amphetamine, dextroamphetamine, and methamphetamine. These classes vary with respect to their potency and peripheral effects. Another stimulant drug of abuse is cocaine, which also produces strong CNS stimulation. Cocaine was originally classified as a narcotic. It is considered a narcotic by the penal system and is treated as a narcotic in terms of secured storage in health care facilities. However, unlike the opioid analgesics, cocaine does not induce a state of narcosis or stupor and is therefore more correctly categorized as a stimulant drug. Other commonly abused substances in this category include methylphenidate, dextroamphetamine, phenmetrazine, and methamphetamine. Multiple slight chemical variants of amphetamine exist. They are commonly referred to as "designer drugs," which have psychoactive properties along with their stimulant properties, which further enhances their abuse potential. Table 17-1 lists commonly abused forms of amphetamine and cocaine with their street names.

Methamphetamine is a chemical class of amphetamine, but it has a much stronger effect on the CNS than the other two classes of amphetamine. Methamphetamine is generally used in pill form orally or in powder form by snorting or injecting. It has 15 to 20 times the potency of amphetamine sulfate, the original drug in this class. Crystallized methamphetamine, known as *ice, crystal,* or *crystal meth,* is a smokable and more powerful form of the drug. Methamphetamine users who inject the drug and share needles are at risk for acquiring human immunodeficiency virus (HIV) infection and acquired immunodeficiency syndrome (AIDS), as well as hepatitis B and C. Marijuana and alcohol are commonly listed as additional drugs of abuse in those admitted for treatment of methamphetamine

abuse. Most of the recorded methamphetamine-related deaths involved the use of methamphetamine in combination with at least one other drug, such as alcohol, heroin, or cocaine. The over-the-counter (OTC) decongestant pseudoephedrine is commonly used to synthesize methamphetamine in illegal drug laboratories, often in private homes. The Combat Methamphetamine Epidemic Act of 2005 required restricted retail sales of all nonprescription drug products containing pseudoephedrine. Specific restrictions include allowing sales only from *behind* the pharmacy counter, requiring photo identification and electronic or paper record keeping of purchasers (which must remain on file for 2 years), and setting maximum allowable amount (in grams) of pseudoephedrine that can be sold per consumer per month.

Another synthetic amphetamine derivative is methylenedioxymethamphetamine (MDMA, "ecstasy," or "E"), which is also usually prepared in illegal home laboratories. This drug tends to have more calming effects than other amphetamine drugs. It is usually taken in pill form but can also be snorted or injected. Users often feel a strong sense of social bonding with and acceptance of other people, hence the nickname "love drug." The drug can also be very energizing, which makes it popular at raves (all-night dance parties). Molly is an increasingly popular drug of abuse and it is the pure crystalline powder of MDMA. As a central nervous system stimulant, Molly produces euphoric highs. It may also lead to rapid heartbeat, high blood pressure, blood vessel constriction, and sweating, and dangerously affect body temperature. Confusion, depression, and sleep problems may also occur.

In addition to the aforementioned substances, cocaine has demonstrated its danger in illicit use. Cocaine is a white powder that is derived from the leaves of the South American coca plant. Cocaine is either snorted or injected intravenously. Cocaine tends to give a temporary illusion of limitless power and energy but afterward leaves the user feeling depressed, edgy, and craving more. Crack is a smokable form of cocaine that has been chemically altered. Cocaine and crack are highly addictive. The psychologic and physical dependence can erode physical and mental health and can become so strong that these drugs dominate all aspects of the addict's life.

Mechanism of Action and Drug Effects

Stimulants work by releasing the *biogenic amine,* norepinephrine from its storage sites in the nerve terminals. This results in CNS stimulation, as well as cardiovascular stimulation, which results in increased blood pressure and heart rate and possibly cardiac dysrhythmias. The effect on smooth muscle is seen primarily in the urinary bladder and results in contraction of the sphincter. This is helpful in treating enuresis (urinary incontinence) but results in painful and difficult micturition (voiding or urination) otherwise.

Stimulants, particularly amphetamines, are very potent CNS stimulants. This CNS stimulation commonly results in wakefulness, alertness, and a decreased sense of fatigue; elevation of mood, with increased initiative, self-confidence, and ability to concentrate; often elation and euphoria; and an increase in motor and speech activity.

TABLE 17-1 **Various Forms of Amphetamine and Cocaine with Street Names**	
Chemical Name	**Street Names**
dimethoxymethylamphetamine	DOM, STP
methamphetamine (crystallized form)	Ice, crystal, glass
methamphetamine (powdered form)	Speed, meth, crank
methylenedioxyamphetamine	MDA, love drug
methylenedioxymethamphetamine	MDMA, ecstasy, Molly
cocaine (powdered form)	Coke, dust, snow, flake, blow, girl
cocaine (crystallized form)	Crack, crack cocaine, freebase rocks, rock

Indications

Many therapeutic uses for stimulants exist. Currently their most common use is in the treatment of attention deficit hyperactivity disorder (see Chapter 13). Stimulants may be used to prevent or reverse fatigue and sleep, such as when they are used to treat narcolepsy (episodes of acute sleepiness). Stimulants are also used to reduce food intake and treat obesity; however, this therapeutic effect is limited because of rapid development of tolerance.

Contraindications

Contraindications to the therapeutic use of stimulant medications include drug allergy, diabetes, cardiovascular disorders, states of agitation, hypertension, known history of drug abuse, and Tourette's syndrome.

Adverse Effects

Adverse effects of stimulants are commonly an extension of their therapeutic effects. The CNS-related adverse effects are restlessness, syncope (fainting), dizziness, tremor, hyperactive reflexes, talkativeness, tenseness, irritability, weakness, insomnia, fever, and sometimes euphoria. Confusion, aggression, increased libido, anxiety, delirium, paranoid hallucinations, panic states, and suicidal or homicidal tendencies occur, especially in mentally ill patients. Fatigue and depression usually follow the CNS stimulation. Cardiovascular effects are common and include headache, pallor or flushing, palpitations, tachycardia, cardiac dysrhythmias, hypertension or hypotension, and circulatory collapse. Excessive sweating can also occur. Gastrointestinal (GI) effects include dry mouth, anorexia, nausea, vomiting, diarrhea, and abdominal cramps. A sometimes fatal hyperthermia can also occur, driven partly by excessive drug-induced muscular contractions.

Management of Withdrawal, Toxicity, and Overdose

Box 17-4 lists the signs and symptoms of withdrawal from stimulants. Death due to poisoning or toxic levels is usually a result of convulsions, coma, or cerebral hemorrhage and may occur during periods of intoxication or withdrawal. Treatment

---

BOX 17-4 Signs and Symptoms of Stimulant Withdrawal

Peak Period
1 to 3 days

Duration
5 to 7 days

Signs
Social withdrawal, psychomotor retardation, hypersomnia, hyperphagia

Symptoms
Depression, suicidal thoughts and behavior, paranoid delusions

Treatment
No specific pharmacologic treatments to reduce cravings or reverse acute toxicity and no known antidotes

---

of overdose is supportive and generally requires sedation of the patient.

DEPRESSANTS

Depressants are drugs that relieve anxiety, irritability, and tension when used as intended. They are also used to treat seizure disorders and induce anesthesia. The two main pharmacologic classes of depressant are benzodiazepines and barbiturates. Both of these drug classes are discussed further in Chapter 12.

Benzodiazepines are relatively safe. However, they are often intentionally and unintentionally misused. Ingestion of benzodiazepines together with alcohol can be lethal. Another depressant that is neither a benzodiazepine nor a barbiturate is marijuana. Derived from the cannabis plant, marijuana ("pot," "grass," "weed") is the most commonly abused drug worldwide. Marijuana is generally smoked as a cigarette ("joint") or in a pipe ("bong") but can be mixed in food or tea.

A benzodiazepine that has gained popularity as a recreational drug is flunitrazepam. Flunitrazepam is not legally available for prescription in the United States, but it is legally sold in over 60 countries for treatment of insomnia. The drug, known as roofies among young people, creates a sleepy, relaxed, drunken feeling that lasts 2 to 8 hours. Roofies are commonly used in combination with alcohol and other drugs. They are sometimes taken to enhance a heroin high or to mellow or ease the experience of coming down from a cocaine or crack high. Used with alcohol, roofies produce disinhibition and amnesia.

Roofies have recently gained a reputation as a "date rape" drug. Victims, both men and women, around the country have reported being raped after being involuntarily sedated with roofies, which were often slipped into their drinks by their attackers. The drug has no taste or odor, so the victims do not realize what is happening. About 10 minutes after ingesting the drug, the victim may feel dizzy and disoriented, simultaneously too hot and too cold, nauseous, have difficulty speaking and moving, and then pass out. Such a victim will have no memories of what happened while under the influence of the drug. Another popular date rape drug used in similar fashion is gamma-hydroxybutyric acid (GHB). GHB works by mimicking the natural inhibitory brain neurotransmitter gamma-aminobutyric acid (GABA). It is also known as "liquid ecstasy." These drugs are also used simply for their depressant and hallucinogenic effects.

Mechanism of Action and Drug Effects

Benzodiazepines and barbiturates work by increasing the action of GABA. GABA is an amino acid in the brain that inhibits nerve transmission in the CNS. This results in relief of anxiety, sedation, and muscle relaxation. The effects of depressants are primarily limited to the CNS, where they can cause amnesia and unconsciousness. They have moderate effects outside the CNS, causing slight blood pressure decreases.

The active ingredients of the marijuana plant are known as cannabinoids, the most active of which is delta-9-trans-tetrahydrocannabinol, abbreviated *THC*. THC exerts its effects on the body by chemically binding to and stimulating two cannabinoid receptors in the CNS. Smoking it leads to acute sensorial changes that start within 3 minutes, peak in 20 to 30 minutes, and last for 2 to 3 hours. Effects are longer when the drug is taken via the oral route. Specific effects include mild euphoria, memory lapses, dry mouth, enhanced appetite, motor awkwardness, and distorted sense of time and space. THC also stimulates sympathetic receptors and inhibits parasympathetic receptors in cardiac tissue, which leads to tachycardia. Other effects include hallucinations, anxiety, paranoia, and unsteady gait.

Indications

Benzodiazepines are used primarily to relieve anxiety, to induce sleep, to sedate, and to prevent seizures. Barbiturates are used as sedatives and anticonvulsants and to induce anesthesia. Controversial medical uses for marijuana include treatment of chronic pain, reduction of nausea and vomiting associated with cancer treatment, and appetite stimulation in those with wasting syndromes, such as patients with cancer or AIDS. In 1996 California became the first state to legalize the medical use of marijuana. Since that time, 23 other states have legalized the use of marijuana for medical purposes, and others have legislation pending. Dronabinol is a synthetic THC prescription capsule approved by the Food and Drug Administration (FDA) for the previously mentioned indications (see Chapter 52 for further discussion of this drug).

Contraindications

Contraindications to the therapeutic use of depressant medications include known drug allergy, dyspnea or airway obstruction, narrow-angle glaucoma, and porphyria (a metabolic disorder).

Adverse Effects

The most common undesirable effect of benzodiazepines and barbiturates is an overexpression of their therapeutic effects. The CNS is the primary area of the body adversely affected by these drugs. Drowsiness, sedation, loss of coordination, dizziness, blurred vision, headaches, and paradoxical reactions (insomnia, increased excitability, hallucinations) are the primary CNS adverse effects. Occasional GI effects include nausea, vomiting, constipation, dry mouth, and abdominal cramping. Long-term use of marijuana may result in chronic respiratory symptoms (similar to those of tobacco abuse) and memory and attention deficit problems. A chronic depressive "amotivational" syndrome has also been observed, especially among younger users.

Management of Withdrawal, Toxicity, and Overdose

Box 17-5 lists the signs, symptoms, and treatment of withdrawal from depressants. Fatal poisoning is unusual with benzodiazepines when they are taken alone. When benzodiazepines are ingested with alcohol or barbiturates, however, the combination can be lethal. Death is typically due to respiratory arrest. Abrupt withdrawal of benzodiazepines after prolonged use has resulted in autonomic withdrawal symptoms, seizures,

---

> ### BOX 17-5 Signs, Symptoms, and Treatment of Depressant Withdrawal
>
> **Peak Period**
> 2 to 4 days for short-acting drugs
> 4 to 7 days for long-acting drugs
>
> **Duration**
> 4 to 7 days for short-acting drugs
> 7 to 12 days for long-acting drugs
>
> **Signs**
> Increased psychomotor activity; agitation; muscular weakness; hyperthermia; diaphoresis; delirium; convulsions; elevated blood pressure, pulse rate, and temperature; tremors of eyelids, tongue, and hands
>
> **Symptoms**
> Anxiety; depression; euphoria; incoherent thoughts; hostility; grandiosity; disorientation; tactile, auditory, and visual hallucinations; suicidal thoughts
>
> **Treatment of Benzodiazepine Withdrawal**
> A 7- to 10-day taper (10- to 14-day taper with long-acting benzodiazepines). Treat with diazepam (Valium) 10 to 20 mg orally qid on day 1, then taper until the dosage is 5 to 10 mg orally on the last day. Avoid giving the drug "as needed." Adjustments in dosage according to the patient's clinical state may be indicated.
>
> **Treatment of Barbiturate Withdrawal**
> A 7- to 10-day taper or a 10- to 14-day taper. Calculate barbiturate equivalence, and give 50% of the original dosage (if actual dosage is known before detoxification); taper. Avoid giving the drug "as needed."

---

delirium, rebound anxiety, myoclonus (involuntary muscle contractions), myalgia, and sleep disturbances.

Flumazenil is a benzodiazepine reversal agent. Flumazenil antagonizes the action of benzodiazepines on the CNS by directly competing with them for binding at the benzodiazepine receptor in the CNS and thus reversing sedation. The dosage regimens are summarized in Chapter 12 (Table 12-3).

Barbiturates and benzodiazepines are commonly implicated in suicides, especially in combination with alcohol. Generally speaking, depressants are not prescribed for long periods. Combinations of sedative-hypnotic drugs or in combination with alcohol need to be avoided. Long-term use of hypnotic drugs leads to ineffective control of insomnia, decrease in rapid eye movement sleep, dependence, and drug withdrawal symptoms.

Effects of marijuana use are usually self-limiting and resolve within a few hours.

ALCOHOL

Alcoholic beverages have been used since the beginning of human civilization. Long-term ingestion of excessive amounts presents major social and medical problems.

Mechanism of Action and Drug Effects

Alcohol, which is more accurately known as *ethanol* and abbreviated as *ETOH*, is a CNS depressant. It results in CNS depression by dissolving in the lipid membranes within the CNS. Some also believe that ethanol may augment GABA-mediated synaptic inhibition and fluxes of chloride, which causes CNS depression. The CNS is continuously depressed in the presence of ethanol. Moderate amounts of ethanol may stimulate or depress respirations. Effects of ethanol on the circulation are relatively minor. In moderate doses, ethanol causes vasodilation, especially of the cutaneous vessels, and produces warm, flushed skin. Ingestion of ethanol causes a feeling of warmth because it enhances cutaneous and gastric blood flow. Increased sweating may also occur. Heat is therefore lost more rapidly, and the internal body temperature consequently falls. The short-term (versus long-term) ingestion of ethanol, even in intoxicating doses, produces little lasting change in hepatic function. However, long-term ingestion of ethanol is one of the primary causes of liver failure. Ethanol exerts a diuretic effect by virtue of its inhibition of antidiuretic hormone secretion and the resultant decrease in renal tubular reabsorption of water.

Indications

Few legitimate uses of ethanol and alcoholic beverages exist. Ethanol is an excellent solvent for many drugs and is commonly employed as a vehicle for medicinal mixtures. When applied topically to the skin, ethanol acts as a coolant. It may be used in liniments (oily medications used on the skin). Applied topically, ethanol is the most popular skin disinfectant. More commonly, however, the type of alcohol used on the skin is isopropyl alcohol, which is similar in structure to ethanol but is more toxic and is not drinkable.

Systemic uses of ethanol are limited to the treatment of methyl alcohol and ethylene glycol intoxication (e.g., from drinking automotive antifreeze solution). However, small amounts of ethanol preparations (such as red wine) have been shown to have cardiovascular benefits.

Adverse Effects

Long-term excessive ingestion of ethanol is directly associated with serious neurologic and mental disorders. These neurologic disorders can result in seizures. Nutritional and vitamin deficiencies, especially of the B vitamins, can occur and can lead to Wernicke's encephalopathy, Korsakoff's psychosis, polyneuritis, and nicotinic acid deficiency encephalopathy.

Moderate amounts of ethanol may stimulate or depress respirations. Large amounts produce dangerous or lethal depression of respiration. Although circulatory effects of ethanol are relatively minor, acute severe alcoholic intoxication may cause cardiovascular depression. Long-term excessive use of ethanol has largely irreversible effects on the heart, such as cardiomyopathy.

When consumed on a regular basis in large quantities, ethanol produces a constellation of dose-related negative effects such as alcoholic hepatitis or its progression to cirrhosis. Teratogenic effects can be devastating and are caused by the direct action of ethanol, which inhibits embryonic cellular proliferation early in gestation. This often results in a condition known as *fetal alcohol syndrome,* which is characterized by craniofacial abnormalities, CNS dysfunction, and both prenatal and postnatal growth retardation in the infant. Pregnant women need to be strongly advised not to consume alcohol during pregnancy, and appropriate treatment and counseling need to be arranged for pregnant women addicted to alcohol or any other drug of abuse.

Interactions

Alcohol can intensify the sedative effects of any medications that work in the CNS (e.g., sedative-hypnotics, benzodiazepines, antidepressants, antipsychotics, opioids). It can interact with the antibiotic metronidazole, causing a disulfiram reaction. Alcohol can also cause severe hepatotoxicity when taken with acetaminophen. Acute ingestion of alcohol can increase the bioavailability of the blood thinner warfarin, which increases the chances of bleeding. Chronic ingestion can cause warfarin to be less effective, leading to increased risk for clots.

Management of Withdrawal, Toxicity, and Overdose

Box 17-6 lists the common signs and symptoms of ethanol (alcohol) withdrawal. Signs and symptoms may vary depending on the individual's usage pattern, the preferred type of ethanol, and the presence of comorbidities. Treatment of ethanol toxicity is supportive and strives to stabilize the patient and maintain the airway. Ethanol withdrawal can be life threatening.

BOX 17-6 Signs, Symptoms, and Treatment of Ethanol Withdrawal

Signs and Symptoms
Mild Withdrawal
Systolic blood pressure higher than 150 mm Hg, diastolic blood pressure higher than 90 mm Hg, pulse rate higher than 110 beats/min, temperature above 100° F (37.7° C), tremors, insomnia, agitation

Moderate Withdrawal
Systolic blood pressure 150 to 200 mm Hg, diastolic blood pressure 90 to 140 mm Hg, pulse rate 110 to 140 beats/min, temperature 100° to 101° F (37.7° to 38.3° C), tremors, insomnia, agitation

Severe Withdrawal (Delirium Tremens)
Systolic blood pressure higher than 200 mm Hg, diastolic blood pressure higher than 140 mm Hg, pulse rate higher than 140 beats/min, temperature above 101° F (38.3° C), tremors, insomnia, agitation

Treatment
Benzodiazepines are the treatment of choice for ethanol withdrawal. Lower dosages are used for mild symptoms, and higher dosages are needed for severe withdrawal. The oral route is preferred; however, it is often necessary to use the intravenous route for patients experiencing severe withdrawal. Patients who are experiencing severe withdrawal often require monitoring in an intensive care unit for cardiac and respiratory function, fluid and nutrition replacement, vital signs, and mental status. Restraints are indicated for a patient who is confused or agitated to protect the patient from self and to protect others (delirium tremens can be a terrifying and life-threatening state). Thiamine administration, hydration, and magnesium replacement may be indicated depending on the severity of the withdrawal state.

TABLE 17-2   Disulfiram Adverse Effects: Acetaldehyde Syndrome

Body System Affected	Result
Cardiovascular	Vasodilation over the entire body, hypotension, orthostatic syncope, chest pain
Central nervous	Intense throbbing of the head and neck leading to a pulsating headache, sweating, uneasiness, weakness, vertigo, blurred vision, confusion
Gastrointestinal	Nausea, copious vomiting, thirst
Respiratory	Difficulty breathing

One pharmacologic option for the treatment of alcoholism is disulfiram (Antabuse). Disulfiram works by altering the metabolism of alcohol. It is not a cure for alcoholism, but it helps patients who have a sincere desire to stop drinking. The rationale for its use is that patients know that if they are to avoid the devastating experience of *acetaldehyde syndrome,* they cannot drink for at least 3 or 4 days after taking disulfiram. Table 17-2 outlines acetaldehyde syndrome. These adverse effects are obviously very uncomfortable and potentially dangerous for someone with any other major illnesses. For this reason, disulfiram is usually reserved as the treatment of last resort for alcoholic patients for whom other treatment options (e.g., Alcoholics Anonymous, psychotherapy) have failed but who still hope to avoid continued alcohol abuse. When ethanol is ingested by an individual previously treated with disulfiram, the blood acetaldehyde concentration rises 5 to 10 times higher than in an untreated individual. Within about 5 to 10 minutes of alcohol ingestion, the individual's face feels hot, and soon afterward it is flushed and scarlet. After this, throbbing in the head and neck, nausea, copious vomiting, diaphoresis, dyspnea, hyperventilation, vertigo, blurred vision, and confusion occur. As little as 7 mL of alcohol will cause mild symptoms in a sensitive person. The effects last from 30 minutes to several hours. After the symptoms wear off, the patient is exhausted and may sleep for several hours. Most of the signs and symptoms observed after the ingestion of disulfiram plus alcohol are attributable to the resulting increase in the concentration of acetaldehyde in the body.

A less noxious drug therapy option is the use of naltrexone, as mentioned in the Opioids section earlier in this chapter. The newest drug treatment indicated for alcoholism is acamprosate. It is used to maintain abstinence from alcohol in patients who are abstinent when starting the drug and who have additional psychosocial support. Its mechanism of action is not completely understood, but it may interact with *glutamate* and *GABA* receptors in the brain

NICOTINE

Nicotine was first isolated from the leaves of tobacco in 1828. The medical significance of nicotine grows out of its toxicity, presence in tobacco, and propensity for eliciting dependence in its users. The long-term effects of nicotine and the untoward effects of the long-term use of tobacco are considerable. Although many people smoke because they believe cigarettes calm their nerves, smoking releases epinephrine, a hormone that creates physiologic stress in the smoker rather than relaxation. The apparent calming effects may be related to the increased deep breathing associated with smoking. The use of tobacco is addictive. Most users develop tolerance for nicotine and need greater amounts to produce the desired effect. Smokers become physically and psychologically dependent and will suffer withdrawal symptoms in its absence. Smoking is particularly dangerous in adolescents because their bodies are still developing and changing. The chemicals, including 200 known poisons, present in cigarette smoke can adversely affect this maturation. More than 60% of people who start smoking in high school are still smoking 7 to 9 years later.

Mechanism of Action and Drug Effects

Nicotine works by directly stimulating the autonomic ganglia of the nicotinic receptors (see Chapter 20). Its site of action is the ganglion itself rather than the preganglionic or postganglionic nerve fiber. The organs throughout the body that are innervated by nerves stimulated by nicotine actually contain nicotinic receptors. Nicotine can have multiple unpredictable and dramatic effects on the body because nicotinic receptors are found in several systems, including the adrenal glands, skeletal muscles, and CNS.

The major action of nicotine is transient stimulation, followed by more persistent depression of all autonomic ganglia. Nicotine markedly stimulates the CNS, including respiratory stimulation. This stimulation of the CNS is followed by depression. Nicotine can have dramatic effects on the cardiovascular system as well, resulting in increases in heart rate and blood pressure. The GI system is stimulated by nicotine, which produces increased tone and activity in the bowel. This often leads to nausea and vomiting and occasionally to diarrhea.

Indications

The nicotine found in nature (i.e., tobacco plants) has no known therapeutic uses. It is medically significant because of its addictive and toxic properties. However, nicotine that is formulated into various drug products to reduce cravings and promote smoking cessation can be considered a therapeutic drug. It is available for this purpose as chewing gum, transdermal patches, vaporizer, and nasal spray.

Adverse Effects

Nicotine primarily affects the CNS. Large doses can produce tremors and even convulsions. Respiratory stimulation also commonly occurs. The initial CNS stimulation is quickly followed by depression. Death can result from respiratory failure, which is thought to be due to both central paralysis and peripheral blockade of respiratory muscles. The cardiovascular effects of nicotine are an increase in heart rate and blood pressure. The effects of nicotine on the GI system are largely due to parasympathetic stimulation, which results in increased tone and motor activity of the bowel. Nicotine induces vomiting by both central and peripheral actions. Centrally, nicotine's emetic effects are due to stimulation of the *chemoreceptor trigger zone* in the brain.

Management of Withdrawal, Toxicity, and Overdose

Acute nicotine toxicity generally occurs in children who accidentally ingest cigarettes. Treatment is supportive and may include treatment with activated charcoal. Smoking cessation is the primary cause of nicotine withdrawal, although discontinuation of any tobacco product can lead to this syndrome. An important and often overlooked problem in hospitalized patients is nicotine withdrawal, which manifests largely as cigarette craving. Irritability, restlessness, and a decrease in heart rate and blood pressure occur. Cardiac symptoms resolve over 3 to 4 weeks, but cigarette craving may persist for months or even years.

The nicotine transdermal system (patch), nicotine polacrilex (gum), and inhalers or nasal spray can be used to provide nicotine without the carcinogens in tobacco and are now available OTC. The patch system uses a stepwise reduction in subcutaneous delivery to gradually decrease the nicotine dose, and patient treatment compliance seems higher than with the gum. Acute relief from withdrawal symptoms is most easily achieved with the use of the gum, because rapid chewing releases an immediate dose of nicotine. The dose is approximately half the dose the average smoker receives in one cigarette, however, and the onset of action is 30 minutes versus 10 minutes or less from smoking. These pharmacologic changes in delivery minimize the immediate reinforcement and self-reward effects that are prominent with the rapid nicotine delivery of cigarette smoking.

A sustained-release form of the antidepressant bupropion (see Chapter 16) called *Zyban* has been approved as first-line therapy to aid in smoking cessation treatment. Sustained-release bupropion was the first nicotine-free prescription medicine to treat nicotine dependence. Table 17-3 lists the currently available drugs for nicotine withdrawal therapy.

Varenicline (Chantix) is indicated for smoking cessation. It both activates and antagonizes the *alpha-4-beta-2* nicotinic receptors in the brain. This effect provides some stimulation to nicotine receptors, while also reducing the pleasurable effects of nicotine from smoking. This drug has demonstrated greater efficacy than bupropion. An optional second 12-week regimen may be prescribed to help the patient maintain tobacco abstinence. The most common adverse effects are nausea, vomiting, headache, flatulence, insomnia, and taste disturbances. Drowsiness has also been reported, which prompted the FDA to recommend caution in driving and engaging in other potentially hazardous activities. Many highly addicted smokers have reported significant success with varenicline. In 2008, the FDA issued warnings regarding its use. Specifically, case reports of psychiatric symptoms including agitation, depression, and suicidality, as well as worsening of preexisting psychiatric illness while using the drug have emerged. Recent studies do not show a difference in the psychiatric symptoms when compared to placebo. Varenicline is classified as a pregnancy category C drug.

TABLE 17-3 Nicotine Withdrawal Therapies		
Drug	**Dosage**	**Recommended Duration of Use**
Transdermal Nicotine Systems		
Habitrol,	7 mg/24 hr	2-4 wk
Nicoderm	14 mg/24 hr	2-4 wk
	21 mg/24 hr	4-8 wk
Nicotrol	5 mg/16 hr	2-4 wk
	10 mg/16 hr	2-4 wk
	15 mg/16 hr	4-12 wk
Nicotrol inhaler	6-16 cartridges inhaled/ day, then taper	6-12 wk
Nicotrol NS nasal spray	1 spray each nostril 1-2 times/hr to max of 5 times/hr or 40 times/day	
nicotine gum	1 stick of gum when having strong urge to smoke; max 24 pieces/day	
nicotine lozenge	1 lozenge when having strong urge to smoke; max 20 lozenges/day	
Antidepressant		
bupropion (Zyban)	150-mg sustained-release tabs	150 mg on days 1-3, then 150 mg bid for 7-12 wk
Partial Nicotine Agonist		
varenicline (Chantix)	0.5 or 1 mg tabs	12-wk regimen, beginning with 0.5 mg orally bid, titrated to 1 mg bid by day 8

NURSING PROCESS

ASSESSMENT

The purpose of a substance abuse assessment is to determine whether substance abuse exists (or existed), to evaluate the relationship between the abuse and other health concerns, and to begin the implementation of an effective health promotion and health restoration plan. Because of the prevalence of substance abuse and the role played by the professional nurse in a variety of settings, the nurse may be the first one to identify the risky behavior in a patient. Indications of abuse problems in patients may also present themselves during an abuser's hospitalization for an injury, illness, or surgery. However, even when substance abuse is not suspected, it is important to include questions about use of alcohol, nicotine, opioids, and substances during a general nursing assessment and medication history (see the pharmacology discussion). Question all patients about the use and misuse of substances, because addiction is found across the lifespan, in all cultures and in all types of individuals, and may therefore be encountered in all clinical specialties. Additionally, abuse/misuse of substances/prescription medications may need to be assessed in family members because adolescents and other individuals in the home may be stealing their parents' prescription drugs.

The nurse's responsibilities relative to drug abuse and the nursing process must begin with the cultivation of excellent interpersonal communication skills. It is important for you to acknowledge and address your own individual beliefs about drug and alcohol use and/or abuse as well as any personal history of coping with addiction or dealing with addicted family members. This process will allow you to anticipate potential responses and behaviors toward this patient population and seek out resolution about these feelings. Acknowledging feelings and beliefs about this group of patients within a proper perspective and ethical framework will allow you to resolve any personal animosity, judgmental attitudes, rejection, and/or enabling behaviors. Once detrimental behaviors and possible barriers to responsible and nonjudgmental care have been dealt with, focus on the patient and avoid being drawn into the manipulative and other negative behaviors of the abuser.

A thorough patient assessment and history must include specific questions about the substance(s) being used, the duration of abuse, related physical and mental health concerns, and withdrawal potential. In patients with suspected or confirmed substance abuse, honesty—on the part of the patient as well as the family or significant other—may be problematic when it comes to answering questions about the abused substance. Therefore, establishing a more communicative, nonjudgmental environment is needed and may be possible through the use of open-ended questions during assessment. A medication history needs to include information about all drugs being used, including prescription drugs, OTC drugs, herbals, dietary supplements, and illegal or street drugs. Include the names of these drugs, doses, frequency, and duration of use. Be attentive to any clues the patient, family, or significant other may reveal, including behavioral and mood changes. A patient's reported use of multiple prescribed drugs as well as contact with multiple prescribers raises a red flag as a possible sign of drug abuse. In addition, laboratory findings are important to assess, including results of renal and liver function studies and any drug screening studies. Assess and monitor results of HIV and hepatitis laboratory tests, once ordered. Measure and document baseline vital signs.

A number of assessment tools with established validity and reliability are available to nurses and health care professionals for use with patients suspected of drug or substance abuse. The goal of adequate screening for alcohol and other drug abuse or addiction is to identify patients who have or are at risk for developing alcohol or drug-related problems and to further engage them in discussion. This may help in further diagnosing and more accurately treating the patient's abuse problem. Laboratory tests are available to detect alcohol and other drugs in the blood and/or urine. These are used to identify more recent drug abuse rather than long-term use or dependence. However, there are other tests that are best used when assessing someone for confirmation of a diagnosis rather than screening (Box 17-7). The CAGE Questionnaire is available as a screening tool for alcohol use in adults and is used by many health care professionals in the field of alcohol addiction. Even though it is simple and brief (consisting of only four questions), it has a noted 93% accuracy rate. The CAGE Questionnaire has also been adapted to include drug use in adults (CAGE-AID). Other available screening tools include the Substance Abuse Subtle Screening Inventory (SASSI), the Michigan Alcoholism Screening Test (MAST-G)

BOX 17-7　Diagnosis of Dependence

In the most current edition of the *Diagnostic and Statistical Manual of Mental Disorders (DSM-5)*, there are substantive changes to the chapter "Substance-Related and Addictive Disorders." Substance use disorder in the *DSM-5* combines the categories of substance abuse and substance dependence categories found in the *DSM-IV* into a single disorder measured from mild to severe. Each specific substance is now addressed as a separate "use disorder (e.g., alcohol use disorder, stimulant use disorder...) with nearly all the substances based upon the same overarching criteria. With this overarching disorder, criteria have been combined and strengthened. Where previously a diagnosis of substance abuse required one symptom, in the *DSM-5*, a mild substance use disorder requires two to three symptoms from a list of 11. It is thought that there will be a better match of symptoms to what a patient is actually experiencing with use of the *DSM-5* criteria. For more information, please visit *www.DSM5.org*, *www.psychiatry.org*, and/or *www.healthyminds.org*.

Source: American Psychiatric Association: Substance-related and addictive disorders, 2013. Available at *www.dsm5.org/Documents/ Substance%20Use%20Disorder%20Fact%20Sheet.pdf*. Accessed November 9, 2014.

---

for use in geriatric patients, and the Problem Oriented Screening Instrument for Teenagers (POSIT). If the findings of an assessment questionnaire are positive, the next step would be to explore the history of the patient's alcohol or drug use and problems. Substance use disorder and addictive disorders are identified thoroughly and with updated diagnostic criteria in the *DSM-5* (see Box 17-7). Further observation is needed to identify any physical, psychologic, and social signs of dependence and dysfunction. Maintaining communication with family members may also provide useful information. If abuse is identified by a history-taking process, physical assessment, drug history profile, screening tests, or patient's confession of abuse, then confidentiality, privacy, and nonjudgmental behavior are keys to ethical nursing practice. Although the substance abuse must be reported to the necessary health care professionals, adhere to the American Nurses Association *Code of Ethics for Nurses* in making this report (see Chapter 4).

Assessment of *opioid* abuse includes, in addition to the previously discussed assessment information, determination of the route being used for drug delivery (e.g., oral versus intravenous use). The use of intravenous drugs raises major health risks/ concerns such as HIV/AIDS or hepatitis. Respiratory assessment with attention to rate and rhythm are important because of the risk for respiratory depression with opioid overdose or overuse. Other more specific signs and symptoms are described earlier in the chapter. Any baseline laboratory values need to also be assessed, if ordered.

Assessment of *CNS stimulant* abuse requires careful questioning about and observation for adverse effects, toxicity, and withdrawal signs and symptoms. Some of the more commonly abused CNS stimulants are *dextroamphetamine, methamphetamine* (crystallized and powdered forms), and *cocaine* (see Table 17-1). Based on the signs and symptoms of stimulant abuse (see the pharmacology discussion), the following need to be assessed and documented: (1) frequent vital signs; (2) thorough head-to-toe physical examination; (3) assessment of neurologic functioning with attention to mydriasis (pupil dilation), hyperactive reflexes, headache, increased motor/speech activity, agitation, syncope, tremors, altered level of consciousness, and seizure activity; and (4) cardiac assessment with attention to increased heart rate (tachycardia), irregular heart rhythm (dysrhythmia), and hypertension or hypotension. Document and immediately report any abnormal assessment findings and/or the presence of an elevated temperature (hyperthermia, which may be fatal), complaints of vomiting, headache, flushing of the face, and/or elevated temperature.

The most dangerous substances in terms of withdrawal are the *CNS depressants*, including *barbiturates*, *benzodiazepines*, and *cannabinoids*. Abuse of CNS depressants is manifested by a decrease in vital signs and mental functioning (see previous discussion); therefore, frequent monitoring of vital signs and neurologic status is needed for safe and prudent care. As with any drug, obtain a comprehensive, thorough nursing history and medication profile. Additional signs and symptoms of abuse are tremors and agitation with possible progression to hallucinations and sometimes death with continued abuse. Early withdrawal may be manifested by increased blood pressure and pulse rate and altered mental status. Because of the risk for respiratory and circulatory depression, always perform an assessment of the patient's ABCs (*airway, breathing, and circulation*). See the pharmacology discussion for more specific information. *Marijuana*, as a depressant, may cause dizziness, disorientation, euphoria, and difficulty with speech and motor activities. Long-term use of marijuana may lead to a chronic, depressive, amotivational behavior. Be sure to always assess for any different or unusual behavioral changes. Assessment of marijuana use includes appraisal of cognitive and motor function and assessment for the inability to carry out minor tasks.

The signs and symptoms of *ethanol* withdrawal and toxicity are presented in Box 17-6. Include gathering data about possible drug interactions, especially the use of other CNS depressants such as opioids, sedatives, and hypnotics in the assessment. Blood alcohol levels are important to monitor, because the health issues and signs and symptoms that appear are directly related to the blood alcohol level.

Abuse of *nicotine* (a *CNS stimulant*) is associated with adverse effects such as increase in heart rate and blood pressure. It can also result in vomiting and increased bowel tone and motor activity. If the patient has a history of malnutrition, chronic lung disease, stroke, cancer, cardiac disease, or renal or liver dysfunction, relevant laboratory tests are generally ordered, and their results need to be examined by the nurse and those involved in the patient's care. Assessment needs to include vital signs, breath sounds, oxygen saturation levels, and monitoring for changes in neurologic functioning (e.g., level of consciousness, sensory/motor problems). Remember that smoking cessation and signs and symptoms of nicotine withdrawal may happen abruptly in hospitalized patients. Signs and symptoms of a craving for nicotine include irritability, restlessness, and decrease in pulse rate and blood pressure, which will help in early identification of more serious problems.

CASE STUDY

Patient-Centered Care: Substance Abuse and Adolescents

 You are having a discussion with a neighbor who has a 14-year-old son. The neighbor expresses concern about his son and substance abuse problems he has heard about.

1. The neighbor describes his son's friend, who was a bright and motivated student but has become sullen and withdrawn, and lacks the motivation he once had. In addition, he has a chronic cough but denies that he smokes cigarettes. This behavior change may indicate abuse of what substance? Are there any long-term effects?

2. The neighbor mentions that his son has told him that his friends have been playing drinking games at parties. Your neighbor asks, "I had not thought about kids his age drinking. Is that really a concern? It's not the same as taking cocaine, right?" What do you tell him?

    A few weeks later, the neighbor calls you because his son is extremely drowsy and unable to speak. The neighbor notes that his bottle of alprazolam (Xanax) is almost empty and worries that his son has taken an overdose.

3. What will you do first? What treatment would you expect his son to receive?

For answers, see http://evolve.elsevier.com/Lilley.

NURSING DIAGNOSES

1. Ineffective health management of self related to perceived barriers of care due to substance abuse
2. Deficient knowledge related to lack of information about addictive behaviors and drugs being abused
3. Chronic low self-esteem related to the influence of substance abuse
4. Risk for injury and falls related to substance abuse and/or abrupt withdrawal

PLANNING: OUTCOME IDENTIFICATION

1. Patient demonstrates patterns of more effective health maintenance with healthy participation and cooperation with therapeutic regimen for addictive/abusive behaviors.
2. Patient openly discusses his or her substance abuse and the benefits of a treatment regimen with expectations of recovery and short-/long-term effects (of treatment).
3. Patient gains improved self-esteem during and after treatment for substance abuse.
4. Patient remains free from injury during and after treatment for substance abuse and addictive disorder.

IMPLEMENTATION

The nurse plays a vital role in the care of patients manifesting abuse behaviors, intoxication, and withdrawal. It is also the nurse who, through the nursing process, helps to meet the patient's basic needs after developing a therapeutic relationship and teaches the patient, family, and/or significant others about addiction and its effect on the entire family. Nursing strategies for meeting actual or potential health problems are implemented for nursing diagnoses generated from assessment data. Nurses working with substance abuse patients need their own sound knowledge base as well as special understanding and empathy. Participation in training, seminars, and education about the process of substance abuse and related lifestyles is encouraged to assist in understanding the patient and developing a comprehensive plan of care. In general, nursing interventions involve maximizing all of the therapeutic plans and minimizing those factors contributing to the abusive behaviors. Once a therapeutic rapport has been established and a patient–nurse–health care provider contract has been agreed upon, maximizing recovery is the plan. Interventions are based on the patient's specific physical and emotional problems and are carried out accordingly and in order of priority of basic needs. For example, if a patient is experiencing hallucinations (from either use of a substance or from its withdrawal), manage the ABCs of care and monitor vital signs and neurologic and mental status while providing a calm, quiet, nonjudgmental, and non-threatening environment. Seizures may occur, so safety precautions are needed, including the use of protective measures such as attention to the airway, padding of side rails, and implementation of other seizure precautions. (Consult health care institution policies and procedures.) For more information related to lifespan considerations for adolescent and older adult patients, see the boxes below.

QSEN   PATIENT-CENTERED CARE: LIFESPAN CONSIDERATIONS FOR THE OLDER ADULT PATIENT

Alcohol and Substance Abuse

Alcohol and substance abuse among older adult patients is a hidden national epidemic. A substantial number of older adults are drinking at higher than recommended levels; thus, alcohol abuse is becoming a growing problem in this population and is one that is often ignored and/or missed by many health care providers.

Alcohol abuse and alcoholism cut across gender, race, and nationality. The National Survey on Drug Use and Health (2010) found that nearly 40% of adults 65 years of age and older drink alcohol. A study conducted in 2011 by the Substance Abuse and Mental Health Services Administration found that adults 50 to 59 years of age had a rate increase of current illicit drug use of 6.3% in 2011 from 2.7% in 2002. The most commonly abused drugs were alcohol, opiates, cocaine, and marijuana. To appreciate the sense of magnitude of this mental health crisis, in 2010 the best estimates were 6 to 8 million older Americans—or about 14 to 20 percent of the overall older adult population—had one or more substance abuse or mental disorders. The number of older adults 65 years of age and older is projected to increase from 40 million to 73 million between 2010 and 2030, with a tremendous impact on the country's mental health system with the increased numbers needing treatment. Obviously, alcohol abuse is of major concern for the older population and renders the necessity of thorough assessment for drug/chemical abuse in this group of patients.

Abuse of other substances by older adults is also an overlooked and often ignored problem. Older drug abusers are often poor, frail, and hidden from health professionals and service providers. The stigma associated with these problems keeps them, as well as family members, from coming forward to report problems. Although the overall rate of substance abuse is lower in older adults than in younger people, substance abuse in the older adult is a significant and growing problem. Alcohol abuse in the older adult is complicated by the fact that many abusers in this age group also use prescription and OTC medications. OTC drugs may cause adverse effects even when taken alone, with serious consequences resulting when taken with alcohol. The main problems are seen when the combining of alcohol with a drug results in intensification of the drug's action (e.g., heightened hypotensive effects when an antihypertensive drug is taken with alcohol); this can lead to increased adverse effects with significant negative consequences (such as dizziness and possible syncope due to the greater drop in blood pressure, which can result in falls and injury). Some of the signals indicating an alcohol- or alcohol and medication–related problem in the older adult patient include trouble with memory after having a drink or taking a medication; loss of coordination, unsteadiness in walking, or frequent falls; changes in sleeping habits; unexplained bruises; and irritability, sadness, depression, and being unsure of oneself.

QSEN   PATIENT-CENTERED CARE: LIFESPAN CONSIDERATIONS FOR THE PEDIATRIC PATIENT

Substance Abuse

The CBHSQ Report: A Day in the Life of American Adolescents: Substance Use Facts Update. This Report presents facts about adolescent substance use including information on the initiation of the substance use, past year use, emergency department visits, and related treatment. In 2011, there were an estimated 25.1 million adolescents 12 to 17 years of age in the United States. In the past year, more than one quarter of adolescents drank alcohol, an estimated one fifth used an illicit drug, and almost one eighth smoked cigarettes. There has been a decline in adolescent use of alcohol, cigarettes, and illicit drugs between 2008 and 2011; however, the percentage of adolescents 12 to 17 years of age receiving abuse treatment has remained fairly stable. Additionally, the number of adolescents seen in an emergency department (ED) for the use of illicit drugs and the misuse/abuse of pharmaceuticals remained stable from 2004 to 2011. According to combined 2010 and 2011 National Surveys on Drug Use and Health (NSDUH) data, in the past year, approximately 7 million adolescents 12 to 17 years of age drank alcohol, nearly 5 million used an illicit drug, and 3 million smoked cigarettes. In addition, on an average day during this same time frame, adolescents 12 to 17 years of age used the following substances: 881,684 smoked cigarettes; 646,702 used marijuana; 57,672 drank alcohol; 38,540 used inhalants; 1775 used hallucinogens; 6747 used cocaine; and 5602 used heroin. It is obviously a major health concern for the United States, and education is a key factor to tackling this concern. Education needs to begin early on in elementary school so that children learn of the problem and the related damaging effects to the brain before actual exposure to the practice. Education and awareness are important to prevent abuse and abuse behaviors, and a child is never too young to learn about these types of dysfunctional and life-threatening behaviors. Parents, other family members and relatives, and caregivers need to be actively involved in any educational sessions about this specific practice, as well as about other drugs that are abused, and related signs and symptoms.

From SAMSHA, Center for Behavioral Health Statistics and Quality: The CBHSQ report: A day in the life of American adolescents: substance use facts update, August 29, 2013. Available at *www.SAMSHA.org*. Accessed March 28, 2014.

Substance withdrawal is treated with a multimodal approach that includes pharmacologic and nonpharmacologic interventions. You have the responsibility to remain nonjudgmental while assisting in the patient's recovery and rehabilitation. You need to remain current in your knowledge about the different substances being abused as well as the various treatment and rehabilitation protocols. Of all interventions, ensuring patient safety is of utmost importance. The patient's movement through the plan of care for withdrawal, recovery, and rehabilitation must be individualized and in a safe, secure, and nonthreatening environment. Patient education remains an essential part of patient care to help the patient, family, and/or significant others understand the need for long-term lifestyle changes. Whether it is disulfiram treatment for alcohol abuse or bupropion therapy for nicotine withdrawal, patients need careful instructions and information about their treatment regimen.

Substance abuse has a major impact on family members and significant others. The family will also be in need of treatment and therapeutic support. But it is the caring, empathic, supportive, and educative responses by the nurse that will convey acceptance to the patient and family and help in the overall process of recovery and rehabilitation. A nonjudgmental attitude, caring, empathy, and quality care must always be the center of Patient Rights as well as the American Nurses Association *Code of Ethics for Nurses* (see Chapter 4), regardless of the admitting diagnosis and/or the type of substance being abused. Lifelong treatment is often indicated; the need for support during the long-term process of recovery must be emphasized and support recommended from within the family unit and extending outward to the community. (Box 17-8 provides a listing of various organizations and resources.) Methods to encourage recovery and minimize relapse need to be individualized for each patient and draw on all available resources, whether private or public. Communication techniques must be reinforcing and firm, yet sensitive to the patient's values and beliefs. Family members must be an integral part of all treatment and must participate in all educational sessions.

BOX 17-8   Organizations and Agencies Concerned with Substance Abuse

Alcoholics Anonymous
American Council for Drug Education
American Society of Addiction Medicine
International Nurses Society on Addictions
National Center on Addiction and Substance Abuse at Columbia University
National Clearinghouse for Alcohol and Drug Information
National Council on Alcoholism and Drug Dependence
National Inhalant Prevention Coalition
National Institute on Alcohol Abuse and Alcoholism
National Institute on Drug Abuse
Partnership for a Drug-Free America
Substance Abuse and Mental Health Services Administration
U.S. Drug Enforcement Administration

EVALUATION

Patient safety is of utmost importance at all times during patient care but especially when the patient is experiencing the signs and symptoms of withdrawal. Patients may go from mild withdrawal to severe withdrawal and enter into life-threatening situations within a period of a day or two, and therefore complete evaluation of the patient and environment must be ongoing. Evaluation of the recovery and rehabilitation process is important as well, with monitoring of the therapeutic effects of the treatment regimen and monitoring for any ill effects from the physiologic and/or psychologic withdrawal of the substance. Part of this evaluation process also is appraisal of the support provided by others such as family members, as well as review of the availability of needed resources during and after hospitalization. In addition, report any abnormality in vital signs, laboratory test results, mental status, or other parameters immediately. An ongoing evaluation needs to also examine the availability of emotional, social, cultural, spiritual, and financial support, and revise the nursing care plan as needed.

PATIENT-CENTERED CARE: PATIENT TEACHING TIPS

- Ensure that relevant, nondiscriminatory, current, and accurate information—at various reading levels—is available to the patient, family, or significant others regarding the specific abuse disorder, signs and symptoms, withdrawal, and treatment regimens. Making an informed decision is best for everyone involved in the process of recovery and rehabilitation.
- Educate the patient, family, and/or significant other about available support groups and community resources. Make information available in various formats such as written materials, videos, and community resources.
- Be sure that the patient understands the importance of having—on his or her person at all times—a current list of all medications, including treatment regimens for the abuse disorder. Include information about the drug, its action, why it is used and how, adverse effects, cautions, drug-drug and drug-food interactions, cautions, contraindications, dosing, and consequences of any missed doses.
- Patients must be educated about their rights to ethical and empathic treatment, regardless of the reason for treatment. One online resource is available at *www.healthline.com/galecontent/center-for-substance-abuse-prevention.* This site provides written information, resources, and video clips about drug/chemical abuse.

KEY POINTS

- Physical dependence is a condition characterized by physiologic reliance on a substance, usually indicated by tolerance to the effects of the substance and development of withdrawal symptoms when use of the substance is terminated.
- Psychologic dependence is a condition characterized by strong desires to obtain and use a substance.
- Habituation refers to situations in which a patient becomes accustomed to a certain drug (develops tolerance) and may have mild psychologic dependence on it but does not show compulsive dose escalation, drug-seeking behavior, or major withdrawal symptoms upon drug discontinuation.
- Acamprosate is used to maintain abstinence from alcohol in patients who are abstinent when starting the drug and who have additional psychosocial support. Its mechanism of action is not completely understood.
- A new medication for smoking cessation is varenicline, which has shown better efficacy than bupropion.
- Drug withdrawal symptoms vary with the class of drug and may even be the opposite of the drug's action. Signs and symptoms of *opioid withdrawal* include seeking the drug from more than one prescriber, mydriasis (pupil dilatation), rhinorrhea, diaphoresis, piloerection (goose bumps), lacrimation, diarrhea, insomnia, and elevated blood pressure and pulse rate. Signs and symptoms of *CNS stimulant withdrawal* include social isolation or withdrawal, psychomotor retardation, and hypersomnia. Signs and symptoms of *CNS depressant withdrawal* include increased psychomotor activity; agitation; muscular weakness; hyperthermia; diaphoresis; delirium; convulsions; elevated blood pressure, pulse rate, and temperature; and eyelid tremors. *Ethanol withdrawal* produces varying degrees of signs and symptoms depending on the specific blood alcohol level. Delirium tremens are characterized by hypertensive crisis, tachycardia, and hyperthermia and may be life threatening.
- Evaluation of the recovery and rehabilitation process is important, including monitoring of the therapeutic effects of the treatment regimen and monitoring for any physiologic and/or psychologic ill effects from the withdrawal of the abused substance.

NCLEX® EXAMINATION REVIEW QUESTIONS

1. A patient is experiencing withdrawal from opioids. The nurse expects to see which assessment finding most commonly associated with acute opioid withdrawal?
   a. Elevated blood pressure
   b. Decreased pulse
   c. Lethargy
   d. Constipation

2. During treatment for withdrawal from opioids, the nurse expects which medication to be ordered?
   a. amphetamine (Dexedrine)
   b. clonidine (Catapres)
   c. diazepam (Valium)
   d. disulfiram (Antabuse)

3. The nurse is presenting a seminar on substance abuse. Which drug is the most commonly used illicit drug in the United States?
   a. Crack cocaine
   b. Heroin
   c. Marijuana
   d. Methamphetamine

4. A patient who is taking disulfiram as part of an alcohol treatment program accidentally takes a dose of cough syrup that contains a small percentage of alcohol. The nurse expects to see which symptom as a result of acetaldehyde syndrome?
   a. Lethargy
   b. Copious vomiting
   c. Hypertension
   d. No ill effect because of the small amount of alcohol in the cough syrup

5. The nurse is assessing a patient for possible substance abuse. Which assessment finding indicates possible use of amphetamines?
   a. Lethargy and fatigue
   b. Cardiovascular depression
   c. Talkativeness and euphoria
   d. Difficulty swallowing and constipation

6. A patient experiencing ethanol withdrawal is beginning to show severe manifestations of delirium tremens. The nurse will plan to implement which interventions for this patient? *(Select all that apply.)*
   a. Doses of an oral benzodiazepine
   b. Doses of an intravenous benzodiazepine
   c. Restraints if the patient becomes confused, agitated, or a threat to himself or others
   d. Thiamine supplementation
   e. Oral disulfiram (Antabuse) treatment
   f. Monitoring in the intensive care unit

7. A patient has been admitted to the emergency department after a suspected overdose of benzodiazepines mixed with alcohol. The patient is lethargic and cannot speak. The nurse expects which immediate measures to be implemented? *(Select all that apply.)*
   a. Prepare to administer naloxone (Narcan).
   b. Prepare to administer flumazenil.
   c. Monitor the patient for convulsions.
   d. Prepare for potential respiratory arrest.
   e. Apply restraints.

8. The nurse is teaching a class about the effects of alcohol. Long-term excessive use of alcohol is associated with which of these problems? *(Select all that apply.)*
   a. Coronary artery disease
   b. Wernicke's encephalopathy
   c. Polyneuritis
   d. Seizures
   e. Cirrhosis of the liver
   f. Korsakoff's psychosis

1. a, 2. b, 3. c, 4. b, 5. c, 6. b, c, 7. b, d, f, 8. b, c, d, e, f

CRITICAL THINKING AND PRIORITIZATION QUESTIONS

1. A friend has revealed to the nurse that she has used crack cocaine often in the past few months and states that even though she enjoys the sensations she can "stop at any time." What is the nurse's priority action in this situation?
2. A patient is admitted to the hospital for major abdominal surgery, and the physician has ordered that a transdermal nicotine patch be used while the patient is hospitalized because the patient was a heavy smoker. While the patch is applied, the patient asks, "Why in the world would you want to give me nicotine when I'm trying to stop smoking?" What is the nurse's priority when answering the patient's question?

For answers, see *http://evolve.elsevier.com/Lilley*.

EVOLVE WEBSITE

http://evolve.elsevier.com/Lilley
- Animations
- Answer Keys for Textbook Case Studies and Textbook Critical Thinking and Prioritization Questions
- Content Updates
- Key Points
- Review Questions
- Student Case Studies

PART 3

Drugs Affecting the Autonomic Nervous System

Learning Strategies

VOCABULARY

Learning pharmacology in nursing means that there is an abundance of new terminology that you, the student, will encounter in your readings. It is important that you study the vocabulary so that you will have a deeper understanding of the content being taught. You may already be familiar with some of the vocabulary from other courses. Each chapter opens with a list of **Key Terms** or significant vocabulary that will be introduced in that chapter. Oftentimes these words will appear in future chapters, so it is imperative that time is spent not just memorizing the terms but putting the terms into use and applying their meaning. Remember application is important in nursing. The vocabulary words will appear in the text in colored boldface font and alert you to the fact that it is a Key Term. Each vocabulary word is defined in the Key Terms section at the beginning of the chapter. When you see the word again in the content of the chapter, it is further defined either by explanation or application. For example in Chapter 19, the term **First-dose phenomena** is defined *as a severe and sudden drop in blood pressure after the administration of the first dose of an alpha-adrenergic blocker.* The page notation after the term alerts you that this term is used on page 311. If you look on that page, the word is used under the heading "adverse effects," so it is helpful for you to realize that the first-dose phenomena is not something good. It is further explained in the text that this adverse effect may cause patients to fall or pass out. This example demonstrates that when you are learning a key term, it is helpful to fully comprehend the implications and application for nursing practice. Taking your learning further, you can now associate this term with patient safety and a nursing diagnosis of Risk for Falls. All of a sudden, a simple key term means so much more to you as a student. You can now see the application to the nursing process and the bigger picture.

Other key terms are straightforward vocabulary words that you can learn and understand by looking at the prefix or suffix. For example, *osteoarthritis* and *osteoporosis* both begin with the prefix *osteo*, which means "bone." Learning the meaning of prefixes like *osteo* will help you decipher other words too. The words *agonist* and *antagonist* are similar; both have the word *agonist* in them. You will want to question how these words are related as well as what difference exists between the two words.

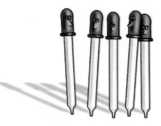

Many students find that writing out flash cards helps them to study and learn the Key Terms. If you choose this method, remember to also include some type of application of the word or phrase. That way you are not just memorizing, but rather making connections to previous learning and relating it to the nursing process. Memorizing is lower-level learning, whereas application is higher-level learning.

Some ebooks have built-in flash cards of all the vocabulary words, which make quizzing yourself easy. Just remember they may not be as in-depth as the flash cards you can make yourself. There are also applications that you can download on your computer, smart phone, or tablet that will allow you to type your flash cards and bring them up on your device anywhere to study instantly. That way you can learn any time you want.

TEXT NOTATION

Text notation is a way for students to pick out the important content as they are reading the chapters. Many students accomplish this by underlining or highlighting the text as they read. A major mistake is to begin underlining or highlighting the text the first time through. What happens on the first read through, is that everything seems important and before you know it you have marked whole paragraphs as important. The best way to prevent this from occurring is to first read through the material once without underlining or highlighting. You need to see where the author is leading you and what content is being presented in the chapter. Then you need to be aware of the author's language. You can usually tell when a concept is important. Many times those key terms are part of the content you will need to underline or highlight. While reading the text a second time, you will be able to be more selective in what you underline or highlight. The following are three paragraphs from Chapter 10 that have been underlined. The underlining should be viewed as an example of what can be done. Each reader will mark the text somewhat differently based on his or her background and experience. As you study this example, think not only about what has been underlined but also about why that material was chosen.

> ***Pain*** *is* <u>*most commonly defined*</u> *as an* <u>*unpleasant sensory*</u> <u>*and emotional experience*</u> *associated with either actual or potential tissue damage. It is a very personal and individual experience. Pain can be defined as whatever the patient says it is, and it exists whenever the patient says it does. Although the mechanisms of pain are becoming better understood, a* <u>*patient's perception of pain is a complex process. Pain*</u> <u>*involves physical, psychologic, and even cultural factors.…*</u> *Because pain intensity cannot be precisely quantified, health care providers must cultivate relationships of mutual trust with their patients to provide optimal care.*
>
> *There is* <u>*no single approach to effective pain management*</u>*. Instead, pain management is tailored to each patient's needs. The cause of the pain, the existence of concurrent medical conditions; the characteristics of the pain; and the psychologic and cultural characteristics of the patient need to be considered. It also requires ongoing reassessment of the pain and the effectiveness of treatment. The patient's* <u>*emotional response to pain depends*</u> *on his or her* <u>*psychological*</u> <u>*experiences of pain*</u>*.* <u>*Pain results from the stimulation of*</u> <u>*sensory nerve fibers*</u> *known as* ***nociceptors****. These receptors* <u>*transmit pain signals*</u> *from various body regions to the* <u>*spinal*</u> <u>*cord and brain, which leads to the sensation of pain, or*</u>

<u>*nociception.…*</u> *The* <u>*physical impulses*</u> *that signal pain* <u>*activate various nerve pathways*</u> *from the* <u>*periphery to the*</u> <u>*spinal cord and to the brain*</u>*. The level of stimulus needed to produce a* <u>*painful sensation is referred to as the*</u> ***pain*** ***threshold***. *Because this is a* <u>*measure of the physiologic*</u> <u>*response*</u> *of the nervous system, it is* <u>*similar for most persons*</u>*. However,* <u>*variations in pain sensitivity*</u> *may result from* <u>*genetic factors*</u>*.*

When students highlight in an effective manner, it makes the learning easier, because they can just review chunks of content versus studying entire sections. Highlighting is a feature that is included in most online formats of textbooks. So if you read your textbook in online format, highlighting is very easy. In some e-books you can choose different highlight colors to mean different things. For example, yellow is important, red is needs clarification, blue is a definition. Some e-books also automatically take your highlighted text and place it into your notes, turning your note taking into study guides.

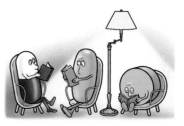

When using e-books, students have the capability of adding notes as they read along. This will enhance learning and make studying for tests easier. Students can add information that they obtain in the classroom right into the notes in their e-book. Also, you can add a note with a question about the content if there is something you read that is not clear. Later in class, you can use your note to ask the instructor for clarification.

ENHANCED TYPEFACE

Throughout your textbook, the authors have used several types of enhanced typeface and color to bring to your attention or to focus in on something that they feel is important for you to understand. When key terms first appear in text, they are set in a colored boldface font. This will help you make connections to the definitions you read in the beginning with the application of the terms used in the text. In the text, there are also words or phrases in italics. These are words or phrases that are not included in key terms but are important in their own right. They signal a term or phrase that the student needs to learn to comprehend the content. For example, in Chapter 10 students will see the phrase *PCA by Proxy* italicized. This phrase is an important concept for maintaining patient safety. Further in that chapter, the term *allodynia* is also italicized and defined. Again this word is not in the Key terms, but a student should understand the meaning of the word, which is given in the text.

The chapter headings are like signs that tell you what is going to be discussed. The authors begin each section with a boldface heading, and these will appear in the same order in every chapter. In this way, students can recognize the general flow of the content. This helps them to organize the drug information in a consistent fashion. You will notice that there are subheadings that also occur in an orderly fashion. In Chapter 10, there is a section entitled Treatment of Pain in Special Situations. This section is different in that it doesn't follow the usual chapter format. This informs the reader that there is additional information to be conveyed that did not neatly fit into the previous section.

As you read your textbook, use these strategies and the authors' chapter headings to guide your learning.

Adrenergic Drugs

OBJECTIVES

When you reach the end of this chapter, you will be able to do the following:

1. Briefly describe the functions of the sympathetic nervous system and the specific effects of adrenergic stimulation.
2. List the various drugs classified as adrenergic agonists or sympathomimetics.
3. Discuss the mechanisms of action, therapeutic effects, indications, adverse and toxic effects, cautions, contraindications, drug interactions, and available antidotes to overdosage for the various adrenergic agonists or sympathomimetic drugs.
4. Develop a nursing care plan that includes all phases of the nursing process for patients taking adrenergic agonists.

DRUG PROFILES

♦ **dobutamine**, p. 301
♦! **dopamine**, p. 301
♦! **epinephrine**, p. 302
♦ **fenoldopam**, p. 302
♦ **midodrine**, p. 302
♦ **mirabegron**, p. 302

♦! **norepinephrine**, p. 302
♦! **phenylephrine**, p. 303

_____

♦ = *Key drug*
! = *High-alert drug*

KEY TERMS

Adrenergic agonists Drugs that stimulate and mimic the actions of the sympathetic nervous system. Also called *sympathomimetics.* (p. 296)

Adrenergic receptors Receptor sites for the sympathetic neurotransmitters norepinephrine and epinephrine. (p. 296)

Alpha-adrenergic receptors A class of adrenergic receptors that are further subdivided into alpha$_1$- and alpha$_2$-adrenergic receptors. (p. 296)

Autonomic functions Bodily functions that are involuntary and result from the physiologic activity of the autonomic nervous system. The functions often occur in pairs of opposing actions between the sympathetic and parasympathetic divisions of the autonomic nervous system. (p. 296)

Autonomic nervous system A branch of the peripheral nervous system that controls autonomic bodily functions. It consists of the sympathetic nervous system and the parasympathetic nervous system. (p. 296)

Beta-adrenergic receptors Receptors located on postsynaptic cells that are stimulated by specific autonomic nerve fibers. Beta$_1$-adrenergic receptors are located primarily in the heart, whereas beta$_2$-adrenergic receptors are located in the smooth muscle fibers of the bronchioles, arterioles, and visceral organs. (p. 296)

Catecholamines Substances that can produce a sympathomimetic response. They are either endogenous catecholamines (such as epinephrine, norepinephrine, and dopamine) or synthetic catecholamine drugs (such as dobutamine). (p. 296)

Dopaminergic receptor A third type of adrenergic receptor (in addition to alpha-adrenergic and beta-adrenergic receptors) located in various tissues and organs and activated by the binding of the neurotransmitter dopamine, which can be either endogenous or a synthetic drug form. (p. 296)

Mydriasis Pupillary dilation, whether natural (physiologic) or drug induced. (p. 299)

Ophthalmics Drugs that are used in the eye. (p. 299)

Positive chronotropic effect An increase in heart rate. (p. 299)

Positive dromotropic effect An increase in the conduction of cardiac electrical impulses through the atrioventricular node, which results in the transfer of nerve action potentials from the atria to the ventricles. This ultimately leads to a systolic heartbeat (ventricular contractions). (p. 299)

Positive inotropic effect An increase in the force of contraction of the heart muscle (myocardium). (p. 299)

OVERVIEW

The body's nervous system is divided into two major branches: the central nervous system and the peripheral nervous system (Figure 18-1). The central nervous system contains the brain and the spinal cord. The peripheral nervous system is further subdivided into somatic and autonomic. The autonomic nervous system is yet further subdivided into the parasympathetic (cholinergic) and the sympathetic (adrenergic). Understanding the autonomic nervous system and its subclasses is critical in the study of pharmacology, as numerous drugs act in these systems. This chapter will focus on the adrenergic nervous system and related compounds.

Adrenergic compounds include several exogenous (synthetic) and endogenous (produced in the body naturally) substances. They have a wide variety of therapeutic uses depending on their site of action and their effect on different types of adrenergic receptors. Adrenergics stimulate the sympathetic nervous system (SNS) and are also called adrenergic agonists. They are also known as sympathomimetics, because they mimic the effects of the SNS neurotransmitters norepinephrine, epinephrine, and dopamine. These three neurotransmitters are chemically classified as catecholamines. In considering the adrenergic class of medications, it is helpful to understand how the SNS operates in relation to the rest of the nervous system.

SYMPATHETIC NERVOUS SYSTEM

Figure 18-1 depicts the divisions of the nervous system and shows the relationship of the SNS to the entire nervous system. The SNS is the counterpart of the parasympathetic nervous system; together they make up the autonomic nervous system. They provide a checks-and-balances system for maintaining the normal homeostasis of the autonomic functions of the human body.

There are receptor sites for the catecholamines norepinephrine and epinephrine throughout the body. These are referred to as adrenergic receptors. It is at these receptor sites that adrenergic drugs bind and produce their effects. Many physiologic responses are produced when they are stimulated or blocked. Adrenergic receptors are further divided into alpha-adrenergic receptors and beta-adrenergic receptors, depending on the specific physiologic responses caused by their stimulation. Both types of adrenergic receptors have subtypes (designated 1 and 2), which provide a further means of checks and balances that control stimulation and blockade, vasoconstriction and vasodilation of blood vessels, and the increased and decreased production of various substances. The alpha$_1$- and alpha$_2$-adrenergic receptors are differentiated by their location relative to nerves. The alpha$_1$-adrenergic receptors are located on postsynaptic effector cells (the tissue, muscle, or organ that the nerve stimulates). The alpha$_2$-adrenergic receptors are located on the presynaptic nerve terminals. They control the release of neurotransmitters. The predominant alpha-adrenergic agonist response is vasoconstriction and central nervous system (CNS) stimulation.

The beta-adrenergic receptors are all located on postsynaptic effector cells. The beta$_1$-adrenergic receptors are primarily located in the heart, whereas the beta$_2$-adrenergic receptors are located in the smooth muscle fibers of the bronchioles, arterioles, and visceral organs. A beta-adrenergic agonist response results in bronchial, gastrointestinal (GI), and uterine smooth muscle relaxation; glycogenolysis; and cardiac stimulation. Table 18-1 provides a more detailed listing of the adrenergic receptors and the responses elicited when they are stimulated by a neurotransmitter or a drug that acts like a neurotransmitter (Figure 18-2). Recently identified, beta$_3$ receptors are located in the human urothelium muscle and detrusor muscle.

Another type of adrenergic receptor is the dopaminergic receptor. When stimulated by dopamine, these receptors cause the vessels of the renal, mesenteric, coronary, and cerebral arteries to dilate, which increases blood flow to these tissues. Dopamine is the only substance that can stimulate these receptors.

Catecholamine neurotransmitters are produced by the SNS and are stored in vesicles or granules located in the ends of

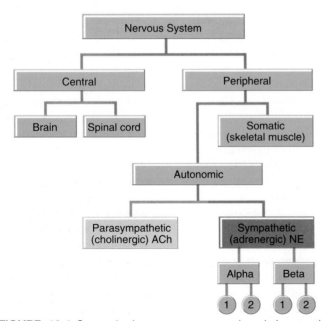

FIGURE 18-1 Sympathetic nervous system in relation to the entire nervous system. *ACh,* Acetylcholine; *NE,* norepinephrine.

TABLE 18-1   Adrenergic Receptor Responses to Stimulation

Location	Receptor	Response
Cardiovascular		
Blood vessels	Alpha$_1$	Vasoconstriction
	Beta$_2$	Vasodilation
Cardiac muscle	Beta$_1$	Increased contractility
Atrioventricular node	Beta$_1$	Increased heart rate
Sinoatrial node	Beta$_1$	Increased heart rate
Endocrine		
Liver	Alpha$_1$, beta$_2$	Glycogenolysis
Kidney	Beta$_1$	Increased renin secretion
Gastrointestinal		
Muscle	Alpha$_1$, beta$_2$	Decreased motility (relaxation of gastrointestinal smooth muscle)
Genitourinary		
Bladder sphincter	Alpha$_1$	Constriction
Penis	Alpha$_1$	Ejaculation
Uterus	Alpha$_1$	Contraction
	Beta$_2$	Relaxation
Respiratory		
Bronchial muscles	Beta$_2$	Dilation (relaxation of bronchial smooth muscles)
Ocular		
Pupillary muscles of the iris	Alpha$_1$	Mydriasis (dilated pupils)

nerves. Here the transmitter waits until the nerve is stimulated, then the vesicles move to the walls of nerve endings and release their contents into the space between the nerve ending and the effector organ, known as the synaptic cleft or *synapse*. The released contents of the vesicles (catecholamines) then have the opportunity to bind to the receptor sites located all along the effector organ (see Figure 18-2). Once the neurotransmitter binds to the receptors, the effector organ responds. Depending on the function of the particular organ, this response may involve smooth muscle contraction (e.g., skeletal muscles) or relaxation (e.g., GI and airway smooth muscles), an increased heart rate, the increased production of one or more substances (e.g., stress hormones), or constriction of a blood vessel.

This process is halted by the action of specific enzymes and by reuptake of the neurotransmitter molecules back into the nerve cell (neuron). Catecholamines are metabolized by two enzymes, monoamine oxidase (MAO) and catechol ortho-methyltransferase (COMT). Each enzyme breaks down catecholamines but is responsible for doing it in different areas. MAO breaks down the catecholamines that are in the nerve ending, whereas COMT breaks down the catecholamines that are outside the nerve ending at the synaptic cleft (see Figure 18-2). Neurotransmitter molecules may also be taken back up into the presynaptic nerve fiber by various protein pumps within the cell membrane. This phenomenon is known as *active*

transport. This restores the catecholamine to the vesicle and provides another means of maintaining an adequate supply of the substance for future sympathetic nerve impulses. This process is illustrated in Figure 18-2. The sympathetic branch of the autonomic nervous system is often described as having a "fight-or-flight" function, because it allows the body to respond in a self-protective manner to dangerous situations.

ADRENERGIC DRUGS

Adrenergics are drugs with effects that are similar to or mimic the effects of the SNS neurotransmitters norepinephrine, epinephrine, and dopamine. These neurotransmitters are known as *catecholamines.* Catecholamines produce a sympathomimetic response. They are either endogenous substances such as epinephrine, norepinephrine, and dopamine or synthetic substances such as dobutamine and phenylephrine. The three endogenous catecholamines, (epinephrine, norepinephrine, and dopamine) are also available in synthetic drug form.

Catecholamine drugs that are used therapeutically produce the same result as endogenous catecholamines. When any of the adrenergic drugs is given, it bathes the area between the nerve and the effector cell (i.e., the synaptic cleft). Once there, the drug has the opportunity to induce a response. This can be accomplished in one of three ways: by direct stimulation, by indirect stimulation, or by a combination of the two (mixed-acting).

A direct-acting sympathomimetic binds directly to the receptor and causes a physiologic response (Figure 18-3). Epinephrine is an example of such a drug. An indirect-acting sympathomimetic causes the release of the catecholamine from the storage sites (vesicles) in the nerve endings; it then binds to the receptors and causes a physiologic response (Figure 18-4). Amphetamine and other related anorexiants (see Chapter 13) are examples of such drugs. A mixed-acting sympathomimetic both directly stimulates the receptor by binding to it and indirectly stimulates the receptor by causing the release of the neurotransmitter stored in vesicles at the nerve endings (Figure 18-5). Ephedrine is an example of a mixed-acting adrenergic drug.

There are also noncatecholamine adrenergic drugs such as phenylephrine, metaproterenol, and albuterol. These are structurally dissimilar to the endogenous catecholamines and have a longer duration of action than either the endogenous or synthetic catecholamines. The noncatecholamine drugs show similar patterns of activity.

Adrenergic agents can also be classified as either selective or nonselective in their actions. For example, phenylephrine and clonidine are considered selective agonists, meaning they only affect one receptor subtype. Epinephrine and norepinephrine are considered nonselective agonists, because they have action at both alpha and beta receptors. Adrenergic drugs can also act at different types of adrenergic receptors depending on the amount of drug administered. For example, dopamine may produce dopaminergic, beta$_1$, or alpha$_1$ effects, depending on the dose given. Other examples of catecholamines and the dose-specific selectivity can be found in Table 18-2.

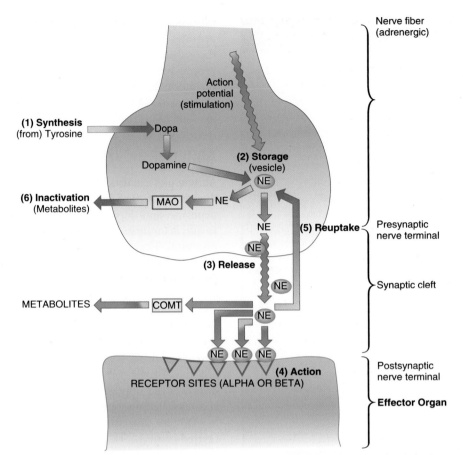

FIGURE 18-2 Mechanism by which stimulation of a nerve fiber results in a physiologic process; adrenergic drugs mimic this same process. *COMT*, Catechol ortho-methyltransferase; *MAO*, monoamine oxidase; *NE*, norepinephrine.

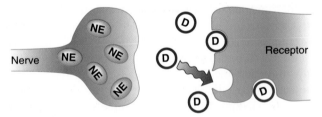

FIGURE 18-3 Mechanism of physiologic response to direct-acting sympathomimetics. *D*, Drug; *NE*, norepinephrine.

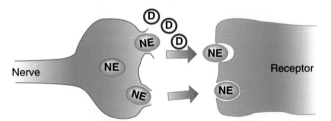

FIGURE 18-4 Mechanism of physiologic response to indirect-acting sympathomimetics. *D*, Drug; *NE*, norepinephrine.

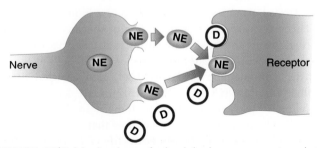

FIGURE 18-5 Mechanism of physiologic response to mixed-acting sympathomimetics. *D*, Drug; *NE*, norepinephrine.

TABLE 18-2	Catecholamines and Their Dose-Response Relationship	
Drug	**Dosage**	**Receptor**
dobutamine (Dobutrex)	Maintenance: 2-20 mcg/kg/min	Beta$_1$ more than beta$_2$
dopamine (Intropin)	Low: 0.5-2 mcg/kg/min	Dopaminergic
	Moderate: 2-4 or less than 10 mcg/kg/min	Beta$_1$
	High: 20-30 mcg/kg/min	Alpha$_1$
epinephrine (Adrenalin)	Low: 1-4 mcg/min	Beta$_1$ more than beta$_2$ more than alpha$_1$
	High: 4-40 mcg/min	Alpha$_1$ more than/equal to beta$_1$

Although adrenergics work primarily at postganglionic receptors (the receptors that immediately innervate the effector organ, gland, or muscle) peripherally, they may also work more centrally in the nervous system at the preganglionic sympathetic nerve trunks. The ability to do so depends on the potency of the specific drug and the dose used.

Adrenergic drugs are classified most technically by their specific receptor activities. They may also be categorized in terms of their clinical effects. For example, phenylephrine is both an alpha$_1$ agonist and a vasopressive drug (pressor), whereas albuterol is both a beta$_2$ agonist and a bronchodilator. Both classifications are suitable for most clinical purposes. Clinically, it may be necessary to carefully choose an adrenergic drug with greater selectivity for a particular receptor type to avoid undesired clinical effects. In such a situation, detailed knowledge of the type and degree of receptor selectivity of different drugs becomes important.

Mechanism of Action and Drug Effects

To fully understand the mechanism of action of adrenergics, one must have a working knowledge of normal adrenergic transmission. This transmission takes place at the junction between the nerve (postganglionic sympathetic neuron) and the receptor site of the innervated organ or tissue (effector). The process of SNS stimulation is illustrated in Figure 18-2 and is discussed earlier in this chapter. When adrenergic drugs stimulate alpha$_1$-adrenergic receptor sites located on smooth muscles, vasoconstriction usually occurs. Binding to these alpha$_1$ receptors can also cause the relaxation of GI smooth muscle, contraction of the uterus and bladder, male ejaculation, and contraction of the pupillary muscles of the eye, which causes the pupils to dilate (see Table 18-1). Stimulation of alpha$_2$-adrenergic receptors, on the other hand, actually tends to reverse sympathetic activity but is not of great significance either physiologically or pharmacologically.

There are beta$_1$-adrenergic receptors on the myocardium and in the conduction system of the heart, including the sinoatrial node and the atrioventricular node. When these beta$_1$-adrenergic receptors are stimulated by an adrenergic drug, three things result: (1) an increase in the force of contraction (*positive inotropic effect*), (2) an increase in heart rate (*positive chronotropic effect*), and (3) an increase in the conduction of cardiac electrical nerve impulses through the atrioventricular node (*positive dromotropic effect*). In addition, stimulation of beta$_1$ receptors in the kidney causes an increase in renin secretion. Activation of beta$_2$-adrenergic receptors produces relaxation of the bronchi (bronchodilation) and uterus, and also causes increased glycogenolysis (glucose release) from the liver (see Table 18-1). Stimulation of beta$_3$ receptors decreases the frequency of bladder contractions during the filling phase, which leads to increased bladder capacity.

Indications

Adrenergics, or sympathomimetics, are used in the treatment of a wide variety of illnesses and conditions. Their selectivity for either alpha- or beta-adrenergic receptors and their affinity for certain tissues or organs determine the settings in which they are most commonly used. Some adrenergics are used as adjuncts to dietary changes in the short-term treatment of obesity. These drugs are discussed in more detail in Chapter 13.

Respiratory Indications

Bronchodilators are adrenergic drugs that have an affinity for the adrenergic receptors located in the respiratory system. They tend to preferentially stimulate the beta$_2$-adrenergic receptors and cause bronchodilation. Of the two subtypes of beta-adrenergic receptors, these drugs are attracted more to the beta$_2$-adrenergic receptors located on the bronchial, uterine, and vascular smooth muscles as opposed to the beta$_1$-adrenergic receptors located on the heart. The beta$_2$ agonists are helpful in treating conditions such as asthma and bronchitis. Common bronchodilators that are classified as predominantly beta$_2$-selective adrenergic drugs include albuterol, ephedrine, formoterol, levalbuterol, metaproterenol, pirbuterol, salmeterol, and terbutaline. These drugs are discussed in more detail in Chapter 37.

Indications for Topical Nasal Decongestants

The intranasal application of certain adrenergics can cause the constriction of dilated arterioles and a reduction in nasal blood flow, which thus decreases congestion. These adrenergic drugs work by stimulating alpha$_1$-adrenergic receptors and have little or no effect on beta-adrenergic receptors. The nasal decongestants include ephedrine, naphazoline, oxymetazoline, phenylephrine, and tetrahydrozoline. They are discussed in more detail in Chapter 36.

Ophthalmic Indications

Some adrenergics are applied to the surface of the eye. These drugs are called ophthalmics. They work in much the same way as nasal decongestants except that they affect the vasculature of the eye. They stimulate alpha-adrenergic receptors located on small arterioles in the eye and temporarily relieve conjunctival congestion by causing arteriolar vasoconstriction. The ophthalmic adrenergics include epinephrine, naphazoline, phenylephrine, and tetrahydrozoline.

Adrenergics can also be used to reduce intraocular pressure, which makes them useful in the treatment of open-angle glaucoma. They can also dilate the pupils (mydriasis), which makes them useful for diagnostic eye examinations. They produce these effects by stimulating alpha- or beta$_2$-adrenergic receptors, or both. The two adrenergics used for this purpose are epinephrine and dipivefrin. Ocular adrenergic drugs are discussed in more detail in Chapter 57.

Overactive Bladder Indications

The beta$_3$ agonist, mirabegron (Myrbetriq), relaxes the detrusor muscle during the storage phase of the bladder fill cycle, which leads to an increase in bladder storage capacity. This new mechanism of action is an improvement over other drugs for overactive bladder, which are discussed in Chapter 21.

Cardiovascular Indications

The final group of adrenergic agents is used to support the cardiovascular system during cardiac failure or shock. These drugs are referred to as *vasoactive sympathomimetics, vasoconstrictive drugs* (also known as *vasopressive drugs,* or *pressors),* *inotropes,* or *cardioselective sympathomimetics.* They have a variety of effects on the various alpha- and beta-adrenergic receptors, and the effects can be related to the specific dose of the adrenergic drug. Common vasoactive adrenergic drugs include dobutamine, dopamine, ephedrine, epinephrine, fenoldopam, midodrine, norepinephrine, and phenylephrine.

It is important to note that a common medication error is confusion between norepinephrine and the brand name for phenylephrine, which is Neo-Synephrine. These drugs are often both ordered for a patient at the same time, and, because the names sound alike, the wrong drug may be given. To avoid this confusion, many pharmacies list these drugs by their trade names as well: norepinephrine is called *Levophed,* and phenylephrine is called *Neo-Synephrine.*

Contraindications

The only usual contraindications to the use of adrenergic drugs are known drug allergy and severe hypertension.

Adverse Effects

Unwanted CNS effects of the alpha-adrenergic drugs include headache, restlessness, excitement, insomnia, and euphoria. Possible cardiovascular adverse effects of the alpha-adrenergic drugs include chest pain, vasoconstriction, hypertension, reflexive bradycardia, and palpitations or dysrhythmias. Effects on other body systems include anorexia (loss of appetite), dry mouth, nausea, vomiting, and, rarely, taste changes.

The beta-adrenergic drugs can adversely stimulate the CNS, causing mild tremors, headache, nervousness, and dizziness. These drugs can also have unwanted effects on the cardiovascular system, including increased heart rate (positive chronotropy), palpitations (dysrhythmias), and fluctuations in blood pressure. Other significant effects include sweating, nausea, vomiting, and muscle cramps. See the Patient-Centered Care: Lifespan Considerations for the Older Adult Patient box on this page for additional information.

Toxicity and Management of Overdose

The toxic effects of adrenergic drugs are an extension of their common adverse effects (e.g., seizures from excessive CNS stimulation, hypotension or hypertension, dysrhythmias, palpitations, nervousness, dizziness, fatigue, malaise, insomnia, headache, tremor, dry mouth, and nausea). The two most life-threatening effects involve the CNS and cardiovascular system. In the acute setting, seizures can be effectively managed with diazepam. Intracranial bleeding can also occur, often as the result of an extreme elevation in blood pressure. Such elevated blood pressure poses the risk for hemorrhage not only in the brain but elsewhere in the body as well. The best and most effective treatment in this situation is to lower the blood pressure using a rapid-acting sympatholytic drug (e.g., esmolol; see Chapter 19). This can directly reverse the adrenergic-induced state.

The majority of the adrenergic compounds have very short half-lives, and thus their effects are short-lived. Therefore, when these drugs are taken in overdose or toxicity develops, stopping the drug causes the toxic symptoms to subside in a relatively short period of time. The recommended treatment for overdose is often to manage the symptoms and support the patient. If death occurs, it is usually the result of either respiratory failure or cardiac arrest. The treatment of overdose is therefore aimed at supporting the respiratory and cardiac systems.

Interactions

Numerous drug interactions can occur with adrenergic drugs. Although many of the interactions result only in a diminished effect because of direct antagonism at and competition for receptor sites, some reactions can be life-threatening. The following are some of the more serious drug-drug interactions involving adrenergic drugs: When alpha- and beta-adrenergic drugs are given with adrenergic antagonists (e.g., some classes of antihypertensive drugs), the drugs directly antagonize each other, which results in reduced therapeutic effects. Administration of adrenergics with anesthetic drugs (see Chapter 11)

QSEN ⬛ **PATIENT-CENTERED CARE: LIFESPAN CONSIDERATIONS FOR THE OLDER ADULT PATIENT**

Use of Beta-Adrenergic Agonists

- Several physiologic changes occur in the cardiovascular system of the older adult, including a decline in the efficiency and contractile ability of the heart muscle, decrease in cardiac output, and diminished stroke volume. In most cases, the older adult adjusts to these changes without too much difficulty, but if unusual demands are placed on the aging heart, problems and complications may arise. Examples of unusual demands include strenuous activities, excess stress, heat, and use of types of medications. For example, stress, heat, and use of beta-adrenergic agonists may lead to significant increases in blood pressure and pulse rate. The older adult may react negatively with a diminished ability to compensate and/or respond appropriately and adequately for these changes.
- Baroreceptor activity does not work as effectively in the older adult patient. Reduced baroreceptor activity may lead to orthostatic hypotension, even without the impact of certain medications and their adverse effects. Medications that lead to drops in blood pressure or pulse rate may then have negative consequences.
- Because of the possible presence of concurrent medical conditions in the older adult (e.g., hypertension, diabetes, chronic lung disease, peripheral

- vascular disease, cardiovascular disease, and/or cerebrovascular disease), monitor them carefully before, during, and after administration of adrenergic drugs.
- Advise patients that the occurrence of chest pain, palpitations, headache, or seizures must be reported immediately to the prescriber and/or emergency care accessed.
- Caution the patient about the use of over-the-counter drugs, herbals, supplements, and other medications. This caution is due to possible drug-drug interactions as well as the older adult's increased sensitivity to many drugs and other chemicals.
- Frequently monitor vital signs, especially blood pressure and pulse rate, when the patient is taking any of the adrenergic drugs because of their cardiovascular and cerebrovascular effects.
- The older adult patient may have decreased motor and cognitive functioning. Therefore, recommend use of appropriate aids or equipment for facilitation of activities of daily living. Provide written and verbal instructions to help ensure proper dosing of medications.

DOSAGES

Selected Vasoactive Adrenergics

Drug	Pharmacologic Class	Usual Adult Dosage Range	Indications
◆ dobutamine (Dobutrex) (D)	Beta$_1$-adrenergic	IV infusion: 2.5-40 mcg/kg/min	Cardiac decompensation
◆! dopamine (Intropin) (C)	Beta$_1$-adrenergic	IV infusion: 1-50 mcg/kg/min	Shock syndrome, cardiopulmonary arrest
◆! epinephrine (Adrenalin) (C)	Alpha- and beta-adrenergic	Subcut: 0.3-0.5 mg repeated every 10-15 min if required	Anaphylaxis
		IV: 1 mg every 3-5 min if required	Cardiopulmonary arrest
◆ fenoldopam (Corlopam) (C)	Dopamine 1 agonist	IV: 0.1-1.6 mcg/kg/min for up to 48 hr	Hypertensive emergency in hospital setting
◆ midodrine (ProAmatine) (C)	Alpha$_1$-adrenergic	PO: 10 mg tid; max 40 mg/day	Orthostatic hypotension
◆ mirabegron (Myrbetriq) (C)	Beta$_3$-adrenergic	PO: 25-50 mg/day	Overactive bladder
◆! norepinephrine (Levophed) (C)	Alpha- and beta-adrenergic	IV infusion: 2-30 mcg/min	Hypotensive states
◆! phenylephrine (Neo-Synephrine) (C)	Alpha-adrenergic	IV infusion: Start at 100-180 mcg/min, and titrate down to 40-60 mcg/min IM/subcut: 2-5 mg per dose IV: 0.1-0.5 mg every 10-15 min	Hypotension or shock

can increase the risk for cardiac dysrhythmias. Administration of adrenergic drugs with monoamine oxidase inhibitors (MAOIs) may cause a possibly life-threatening hypertensive crisis (see Chapter 16). Antihistamines (see Chapter 36) and thyroid preparations (see Chapter 31) can also increase the effects of adrenergic drugs.

Laboratory Test Interactions

Alpha-adrenergic drugs can cause an increase in serum levels of endogenous corticotropin (i.e., adrenocorticotropic hormone), corticosteroids, and glucose.

Dosages

For dosage information on various adrenergic drugs, see the table on this page.

DRUG PROFILES

The four frequently used classes of adrenergic drugs are bronchodilators (see Chapter 37), ophthalmic drugs (see Chapter 57), nasal decongestants (see Chapter 36), and vasoactive drugs, which are emphasized in this chapter (see Drug Profiles) and in Chapter 24. The receptor selectivity for the alpha$_1$, beta$_1$, and beta$_2$ receptor subtypes is *relative* (as opposed to *absolute*). Thus, there may be some overlap of drug effects between the different adrenergic classes of drugs, especially at higher dosages. In contrast, dopamine receptors are more specific for dopamine itself and/or specific dopaminergic drugs.

VASOACTIVE ADRENERGICS

Adrenergics that have primarily cardioselective effects are referred to as *vasoactive adrenergics*. They are used to support a failing heart or to treat shock. They may also be used to treat orthostatic hypotension. These drugs have a wide range of effects on alpha- and beta-adrenergic receptors, depending on the dosage. The vasoactive adrenergics are very potent, quick-acting, injectable drugs. Although dosage recommendations are given in the table above, all of these drugs are titrated to the desired physiologic response. All of the vasoactive adrenergics (with the exception of midodrine) are rapid in onset, and their effects very quickly cease when administration is stopped. Therefore, careful titration and monitoring of vital signs and electrocardiogram (ECG) are required.

◆dobutamine

Dobutamine (Dobutrex) is a beta$_1$-selective vasoactive adrenergic drug that is structurally similar to the naturally occurring catecholamine dopamine. Through stimulation of the beta$_1$ receptors on heart muscle (myocardium), it increases cardiac output by increasing contractility (positive inotropy), which increases the stroke volume, especially in patients with heart failure. Dobutamine is available only as an intravenous drug and is given by continuous infusion. (See the dosages table above.)

Pharmacokinetics: Dobutamine

Route	Onset of Action	Peak Plasma Concentration	Elimination Half-life	Duration of Action
IV	Less than 2 min	Less than 10 min	2-5 min	Less than 10 min

◆!dopamine

Dopamine (Intropin) is a naturally occurring catecholamine neurotransmitter. It has potent dopaminergic as well as beta$_1$- and alpha$_1$-adrenergic receptor activity, depending on the dosage. Dopamine, when used at low dosages, can dilate blood vessels in the brain, heart, kidneys, and mesentery, which increases blood flow to these areas (dopaminergic receptor activity). At higher infusion rates, dopamine can improve cardiac contractility and output (beta$_1$-adrenergic receptor activity). At highest doses, dopamine causes vasoconstriction (alpha$_1$-adrenergic receptor activity). Use of dopamine is contraindicated in patients who have a catecholamine-secreting tumor of the adrenal gland known as a *pheochromocytoma*. The drug is available only as an intravenous injectable drug and is given by continuous infusion. (See the Dosages table on the previous page.)

Pharmacokinetics: Dopamine

Route	Onset of Action	Peak Plasma Concentration	Elimination Half-life	Duration of Action
IV	2-5 min	Rapid	Less than 2 min	10 min

♦! epinephrine

Epinephrine (Adrenalin) is an endogenous vasoactive catecholamine. It acts directly on both the alpha- and beta-adrenergic receptors of tissues innervated by the SNS. It is considered the prototypical nonselective adrenergic agonist. Epinephrine is administered in emergency situations and is one of the primary vasoactive drugs used in many advanced cardiac life support protocols. The physiologic response is dose related. At low dosages, it stimulates mostly beta$_1$-adrenergic receptors, increasing the force of contraction and heart rate. It is also used to treat acute asthma (see Chapter 37) and anaphylactic shock at these dosages because it has significant bronchodilatory effects via the beta$_2$-adrenergic receptors in the lungs. At high dosages (e.g., intravenous drip), it stimulates mostly alpha-adrenergic receptors, causing vasoconstriction, which elevates the blood pressure. (See the Dosages table on the previous page.) Epinephrine is available in two strengths for IV use, which has led to many medication errors. It is available as 1:1000 (1 mg/mL) and also as 1:10,000 (0.1 mg/mL). Be aware of these differences in strength and associated indications. Reading the label carefully before administering the drug is critical to patient safety.

Pharmacokinetics: Epinephrine

Route	Onset of Action	Peak Plasma Concentration	Elimination Half-life	Duration of Action
Subcut	5-10 min	20 min	Variable	Unknown
IV	Less than 2 min	Rapid	Less than 5 min	5-30 min

♦ fenoldopam

Fenoldopam (Corlopam) is a peripheral dopamine 1 (D$_1$) agonist indicated for parenteral use in lowering blood pressure. Fenoldopam produces its blood pressure–lowering effects by inducing arteriolar vasodilation mainly through stimulation of D$_1$ receptors. It appears to be as effective as sodium nitroprusside for short-term treatment of severe hypertension and may have beneficial effects on renal function because it increases renal blood flow. It is available as a 10-mg/mL injection. (See the Dosages table on the previous page.)

Pharmacokinetics: Fenoldopam

Route	Onset of Action	Peak Plasma Concentration	Elimination Half-life	Duration of Action
IV	5 min	20 min	More than 5 min	10 min

♦ midodrine

Midodrine (ProAmatine) is a prodrug that is converted in the liver to its active form, desglymidodrine. This active metabolite is responsible for the primary pharmacologic action of midodrine, which is alpha$_1$-adrenergic receptor stimulation. This alpha$_1$ stimulation causes constriction of both arterioles and veins, resulting in peripheral vasoconstriction. Midodrine is primarily indicated for the treatment of symptomatic orthostatic hypotension. Midodrine is available as 2.5- and 5-mg tablets (see the Dosages table on the previous page.) Midodrine is usually given two to three times per day. Due to the possibility of supine hypertension, the last dose of the day should not be given after 6 PM, or at least four hours before bedtime.

Pharmacokinetics: Midodrine

Route	Onset of Action	Peak Plasma Concentration	Elimination Half-life	Duration of Action
PO	45-90 min	1 hr	More than 3-4 hr	6-8 hr

♦ mirabegron

Mirabegron (Myrbetriq) is a beta$_3$ agonist. It represents a new mechanism of action. It targets the beta$_3$ receptors that are found in the urothelium and detrusor muscles. By stimulating the beta$_3$ receptor, it relaxes the detrusor muscle during the storage phase of the bladder fill cycle, which increases the bladder capacity. It is indicated for relief of overactive bladder. Other drugs used for this condition are discussed in Chapter 21. Mirabegron is available as a sustained-release tablet and cannot be chewed or crushed. There are no reported contraindications for this drug. Mirabegron does not have same side effects as other drugs to treat overactive bladder since it is a beta$_3$ agonist as compared to being a muscarinic blocker (see Chapter 21). The most common adverse effects are hypertension, urinary tract infection, headache, nasopharyngitis, nausea, and dizziness. It is an inhibitor of CYP2D6 and can interact with metoprolol and desipramine; it can also interact with digoxin. Mirabegron is classified as a pregnancy category C drug.

Pharmacokinetics: Mirabegron

Route	Onset of Action	Peak Plasma Concentration	Elimination Half-life	Duration of Action
PO	NA	3.5 hours	50 hours	NA

♦! norepinephrine

Norepinephrine (Levophed) acts predominantly by directly stimulating alpha-adrenergic receptors, which leads to vasoconstriction. It also has some direct-stimulating beta-adrenergic effects on the heart (beta$_1$-adrenergic receptors) but none on the lung (beta$_2$-adrenergic receptors). Norepinephrine is directly metabolized to dopamine and is used primarily in the treatment of hypotension and shock. It is given only by continuous infusion. (See the Dosages table on p. 301.) In 2014, a new oral drug called Droxidpa (Northera) was approved for the treatment of neurogenic orthostatic hypotension. Droxidopa is converted to norepinephrine in the body. The most common adverse events are headache, dizziness, nausea, hypertension, and fatigue. Droxidopa has a black box warning about the risk for supine hypertension. Patients must sleep with the head and upper body elevated, and the last dose of the day should be taken at least 3 hours prior to bedtime. Droxidopa has been associated with neuroleptic malignant syndrome.

Pharmacokinetics: Norepinephrine

Route	Onset of Action	Peak Plasma Concentration	Elimination Half-life	Duration of Action
IV	Rapid	1-2 min	Less than 5 min	1-2 min

♦!phenylephrine

Phenylephrine (Neo-Synephrine) works almost exclusively on the alpha-adrenergic receptors. It is used primarily for short-term treatment to raise blood pressure in patients in shock, to control some dysrhythmias (supraventricular tachycardias), and to produce vasoconstriction in regional anesthesia. It is also administered topically as an ophthalmic drug (see Chapter 57) and as a nasal decongestant (see Chapter 36). (See the Dosages table on p. 301.)

Pharmacokinetics: Phenylephrine

Route	Onset of Action	Peak Plasma Concentration	Elimination Half-life	Duration of Action
IV	Rapid	Rapid	Less than 5 min	15-20 min

▌NURSING PROCESS

▌ASSESSMENT

Adrenergic agonist drugs have a variety of effects depending on the receptors they stimulate. Stimulation of the alpha-adrenergic receptors results in vasoconstriction of blood vessels. Stimulation of beta$_1$-adrenergic receptors produces cardiac stimulation, and beta$_2$-adrenergic receptor stimulation results in bronchodilation. Because of these sympathomimetic properties, use of adrenergic agonists requires careful patient assessment and monitoring to maximize therapeutic effects and minimize possible adverse effects. Focus assessment on a comprehensive health history with past and present medical history.

Obtain a past and present medication history. Also include specific system-based questions, and identify cautions, contraindications, and drug interactions. Include the following health history questions in your assessment: (1) Medication history and allergies: What prescription medications are taken regularly? What about the self-administration of over-the-counter medications and herbal products? Are there allergies to any

Ratio Solutions: Which Strength Is Stronger?

- When giving epinephrine, it is important to choose the correct dosage form. Ratio solutions indicate the number of grams of the medication per total milliliters of solution. Be sure you know what the numbers mean!
- A medication that is designated 1:1000 has 1 gram of medication per 1000 mL of solution.
- A medication that is designated 1:10,000 has 1 gram of medication per 10,000 mL of solution.
- Which is the more potent dose? 1:1000 or 1:10,000? 1:10,000 strength contains 0.1 mg/mL of medication; 1:1000 strength contains 1 mg/mL of medication, which is ten times stronger than the 1:10,000 strength. Therefore, the solution with the smaller number of milliliters is actually the more potent dose!
- Epinephrine solution for injection comes in vials and ampules that are labeled 1:1000 or 1:10,000. Be certain that you have the correct strength when giving this medication!

medications, over-the-counter drugs, herbal products, foods, topical products, and/or environmental pollutants/products? Are you aware of specific concerns, cautions, and contraindications related to the medication(s)? (2) Respiratory: Is there a history of asthma, and, if present, how frequent and severe are the acute episodes? What factors exacerbate or help to alleviate asthma? Are there any other asthma-related symptoms such as dyspnea or chest pain? What treatments have been used for asthma, and what are their associated successes or failures? (3) Cardiovascular: Is there a history of transient ischemic attacks or cerebrovascular accident or stroke? Is there a history of hypertension, hypotension, postural hypotension, or orthostatic hypotension (Inquire if the patient gets dizzy when standing up too quickly), cardiac irregularities, or other cardiovascular disease? (4) Renal/liver: Is there a history of kidney problems? Has anyone ever reported that kidney/liver function studies are abnormal? Is there a history of chronic kidney infections? History of liver disorders? Any jaundice? It is important to remember that with altered renal/liver function, there is the risk for altered excretion/metabolism of drugs thus leading to possible toxicity.

Performing a thorough head-to-toe physical assessment is also a very important part of data collection with these drugs. Thorough assessment of the cardiac system is important because adrenergic agonist drugs may exacerbate preexisting cardiac disorders. Other parameters that need to be thoroughly assessed include baseline vital signs. Assess and document breath sounds, heart sounds, peripheral pulses, skin color, and capillary refill. With the use of *mitodrine*, assess postural blood pressures and pulse rates in supine, sitting, and standing positions before, during, and after drug administration. Additionally, make sure to inquire about other significant symptoms such as dizziness, lightheadedness, and syncope. Your thorough assessment of the patient's symptoms as well as their perception of either disease progression or a decrease in symptoms is very important for effective and successful treatment.

With other *adrenergic drugs*, such as those used for bronchodilating effects, perform a thorough respiratory assessment. This includes assessing the patient's respiratory rate, rhythm, and depth as well as the presence of normal and/or adventitious (abnormal) breath sounds. Inquire about any complaints of difficulty in breathing, shortness of breath, and level of tolerance for activity/exercise. Assess and document pulse oximetry readings for oxygen saturation levels. Include in the assessment measurement of respiratory peak flow using a flow meter as well as measurement of the anterior-posterior diameter of the chest wall. A decrease in peak flow readings may indicate bronchospasms, whereas an increased anterior-posterior chest wall diameter is seen in chronic lung disorders such as emphysema. Prescribers may also order additional respiratory function studies such as measurement of arterial blood gas levels.

Older adult and pediatric patients may react with increased sensitivity to these drugs. In addition, some of these drugs are used only for acute episodes of asthma, whereas other drugs are used year-round as preventive drugs. For example, the drugs *salmeterol* (see Chapter 37) and *formoterol* (longer acting) are *not* used to treat acute asthmatic episodes, whereas *albuterol* (short acting) is indicated for treatment of acute episodes.

Epinephrine and similar drugs are used for their cardiac, bronchial, anti-allergic, ophthalmic, and vasopressor effects. Focus assessment on vital signs and breath sounds and, if ordered, arterial blood gas levels and ECG findings. Assess and document liver and renal function test results. In addition, assess each system related to the specific action of the drug. *Mirabegron (Myrbetriq)*, a newer adrenergic drug, works by stimulating the beta$_3$ receptors (see pharmacology discussion). Assess urinary patterns and pretherapy occurrence of urinary distention, frequency, urgency, and incontinence. Blood pressure readings are important to assess and document due to the side effect of hypertension. Assess for potential drug interactions with metoprolol, desipramine, and digoxin.

Overall, adrenergic drugs work in similar ways, but individual drugs may have some differences with regard to action, indications, and overall considerations. If the general class of drugs and the way in which they work is known, then the relevant assessment parameters, cautions, contraindications, drug interactions, and lifespan considerations are easy to determine. If the drug is a *pure adrenergic agonist*, the net effect is stimulation of alpha-adrenergic receptors with vasoconstriction of blood vessels and subsequent elevation of blood pressure and heart rate. You would then know to expect specific actions from the drug as well as to anticipate certain adverse effects. The drug may be used for the therapeutic effect of increased blood pressure, but an unwanted adverse effect could then be a hypertensive crisis. If the drug is a *beta-adrenergic agonist*, it will stimulate both beta$_1$ and beta$_2$ receptors, which will lead to cardiac stimulation and bronchodilation. This beta$_1$ action can also result in too much stimulation with severe tachycardia and possibly chest pain, especially if coronary artery disease is present. Thus, by knowing the actions of a given drug, you may draw conclusions about, anticipate, and be very alert to the drug's therapeutic action, adverse effects, cautions, contraindications, drug interactions, and toxicity.

NURSING DIAGNOSES

1. Impaired gas exchange related to asthma-induced bronchospasms
2. Decreased cardiac output related to cardiovascular adverse effects of adrenergic agonist drugs
3. Ineffective peripheral tissue perfusion related to intense vasoconstrictive actions of medications
4. Acute pain related to adverse effects of tachycardia and palpitations
5. Disturbed sleep patterns related to CNS stimulation caused by adrenergic drugs
6. Deficient knowledge of the therapeutic regimen, adverse effects, drug interactions, and precautions related to the use of adrenergic drugs
7. Noncompliance with drug therapy related to lack of information about the importance of taking the medication as ordered
8. Risk for injury related to possible adverse effects (nervousness, vertigo, hypertension, or tremors) or to potential drug interactions

PLANNING: OUTCOME IDENTIFICATION

1. Patient shows improvement in gas exchange and respiratory status with a return to normal respiratory rate (12 to 20 breaths/minute), regular rhythm and depth, clearing breath sounds, and pulse oximetry reading above 90%.
2. Patient maintains normal cardiac output status with blood pressure and pulse rate readings within normal limits (BP 120/80; pulse 60 to 100 beats/min) and capillary refill less than 5 seconds in fingers and toes.
3. Patient's circulation/tissue perfusion remains intact in extremities with strong pedal pulses and are pink in color and warm.
4. Patient experiences relief of pain and remains comfortable during drug therapy.
5. Patient experiences improved sleep patterns with use of relaxation therapy and massage while taking medication as prescribed.
6. Patient demonstrates adequate knowledge about drug regimen by stating therapeutic and adverse effects of medications as well as the importance of timing/dosing and scheduling (of drug therapy).
7. Patient remains adherent to drug therapy with minimal to no adverse effects and no toxicity.
8. Patient remains free from injury to self due to safe and as-prescribed self-administration of drug therapy.

IMPLEMENTATION

There are several nursing interventions that may maximize the therapeutic effects of *adrenergic drugs* and minimize their adverse effects. These interventions include checking package

CASE STUDY

Safety: What Went Wrong? Dopamine Infusion

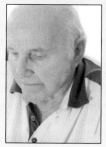

Mr. P., 82 years of age, is receiving dopamine at a dose of 5 mcg/kg/min for heart failure. He has a history of hypothyroidism and takes a daily dose of thyroid replacement hormone. Yesterday, Mr. P's vital signs were as follows:

Blood pressure: 150/88 mm Hg

Pulse rate: 92 beats/min

Respiration rate: 16 breaths/min

His heart rhythm showed sinus rhythm with rare ectopic beats. While at rest, he had no shortness of breath but did experience some dyspnea when getting up to the bedside commode. He has edema in his lower legs rated as 2+ edema.

1. Explain how this dose of dopamine works to help treat Mr. P's heart failure.

    This morning, you make rounds and find that Mr. P's vital signs are as follows:

    Blood pressure: 170/94 mm Hg

    Pulse rate: 120 beats/min

    Respiration rate: 22 breaths/min

    The heart monitor shows sinus tachycardia with two to three ectopic beats per minute. Mr. P. is complaining of palpitations and some shortness of breath at rest but says, "I've felt this before when I've had bad spells with my heart. I'm sure it will pass."

2. Do you think there is a concern at this time? Explain your reasoning and what should be done.

    The physician decides to titrate the dopamine infusion to 3 mcg/kg/min, which you do immediately.

3. How quickly should you see a response from the patient to this decrease in dosage?

    Later in the day, while making rounds, you check the insertion site of Mr. P.'s dopamine infusion and find the area swollen and cool to the touch.

4. What went wrong? What is your priority action, and what treatment will you expect to be given?

For answers, see *http://evolve.elsevier.com/Lilley.*

inserts for the types and amounts of dilutional solutions to use with parenteral dosage forms (and for all dosage forms). For example, subcutaneous administration of the adrenergic agonist epinephrine to patients with asthma requires safe calculations and accurate dosing. A tuberculin syringe may be used for subcutaneous administration of epinephrine to help in accurate dosing for both adult and pediatric patients.

Use of *epinephrine* and some of the other pure *alpha-adrenergics* may not be indicated for shock-related symptoms because these drugs lead to vasoconstriction of the renal vessels and subsequent renal damage or shutdown. Therefore, when a patient is in shock and requires medications, *dopamine* is generally the drug of choice (rather than epinephrine). Dopamine is used because, in specific dosage ranges, it helps treat a shock-related syndrome through its ability to produce vasoconstriction of peripheral blood vessels and increase blood pressure, but without vasoconstriction of the renal vasculature. This lack of renal vasculature vasoconstriction helps improve perfusion through the kidneys and thus salvages the kidneys (while increasing blood pressure). With administration of dopamine

and similar drugs, check the intravenous site frequently for infiltration (e.g., every hour, as needed) to be sure that the site remains intact and that the drug is being infused at the proper rate. Infiltration of an intravenous solution containing an adrenergic drug may lead to tissue necrosis from excessive vasoconstriction around the intravenous site. *Phentolamine* is often used for the treatment of infiltration (see Chapter 19). Also, with intravenous infusions, use only clear solutions and a proper dilutional fluid, always administer the drug with an intravenous infusion pump, and closely monitor the cardiac system (e.g., vital signs, heart sounds, and/or ECG monitoring). Give all of these drugs per the manufacturer's instructions and suggested infusion rates to avoid precipitating dangerously high blood pressure and pulse rate and subsequent complications.

When these drugs are given via an inhaler or nebulizer, provide the patient with complete, thorough, and age-appropriate instructions about correct use, storage, and care of equipment. Instruct the patient on how to use a spacer correctly, because use of this device with the inhaler is often ordered. A spacer provides more effective delivery of inhaled doses of drug (see Patient-Centered Care: Patient Teaching, as well as Chapter 9). When the *adrenergics* are dosed for bronchodilating effects, often two adrenergics are prescribed. This is because different medications are associated with different pharmacokinetics and actions. One inhaler may be for use in *acute* situations, and the other may be for *long-term* and/or *preventative* use. With this type of treatment regimen, the patient needs to receive thorough, simple, and complete instructions and explanations about the method of delivery as well as the drugs used. This will help to minimize overdosage and reduce the risk for severe adverse effects such as hypertension, severe tachycardia, tremors, and CNS overstimulation.

Emphasize in patient teaching that these medications are to be used only as prescribed with regard to amount, timing, and spacing of doses. Because of their synergistic effects, when these medications (especially asthmatics) are used in combination with other types of bronchodilators, the patient must be very clear about what to do before, during, and after the dose is delivered. If the patient is taking an inhaled dosage form, he or she may also be taking an oral or parenteral form of the same or a similar drug. The reason for the use of more than one drug of the same drug class and the use of more than one route of administration is to achieve combined therapeutic effects. In educating the patient, pay extremely close attention to these regimens because of the need to prevent exacerbation of adverse effects, minimize drug interactions, and prevent severe vascular and cardiovascular adverse effects. Advise the patient to immediately report any complaints of chest pain, palpitations, headache, or seizures.

Patients with chronic lung disease who are receiving *adrenergic drugs* also need to avoid anything that may exacerbate their respiratory condition (e.g., food or other allergens, cigarette smoking) and implement measures that may help diminish the risk for respiratory infection. These measures may include avoiding those who are ill with colds or flu, avoiding crowded areas, remaining well-nourished and rested, and maintaining fluid intake of up to 3000 mL/day to ensure adequate hydration (unless contraindicated). Keeping a journal of symptoms and noting any improvement or worsening in the treated condition while taking the medications may also be very helpful.

Salmeterol is not to be used for relief of acute symptoms, and education about its dosing is important. The dosage of salmeterol is usually 1 puff twice daily, 12 hours apart. Always recheck these orders and directions. If another type of inhalant is used, such as a corticosteroid, instruct the patient to use the bronchodilator first, with a 5-minute waiting period prior to taking the second drug. All equipment must be rinsed after use. Provide patients with instructions about the importance of rinsing their mouth thoroughly after the use of any inhalant form of medication. Oral rinsing and mouth care after use of the inhaled drug is needed to prevent irritation and infection. See Chapter 37 for further discussion of salmeterol.

If ophthalmic forms of these drugs are used, make sure that the medication has not expired and is a clear solution. Do not allow the eyedropper to touch the eye when the drug is applied to help prevent contamination of the remaining solution. With ophthalmic administration, apply drops and ointments into the conjunctival sac—not directly onto the eye (cornea) itself.

Oral *midodrine* is to be taken exactly as prescribed. This medication is usually ordered to be given with increase in fluids before the patient gets out of bed in the morning. Doses of the drug are often front-loaded in their dosing schedule so that most of the doses occur in the morning when patients with orthostatic intolerance are usually more symptomatic. Patients need to avoid taking this medication after 6 PM *if at all possible* to prevent insomnia and possible supine hypertension.

With *mirabegron (Myrbetriq)*, make sure the patient knows to take the tablet in its whole dosage form and is not broken, chewed, or crushed. It is a timed-release product, and altering its dosage form can lead to potential toxic effects. Mirabegron may be taken with or without food/meals.

EVALUATION

Therapeutic effects of *adrenergic drugs* include the following: For vasoactive drugs, therapeutic effects include improved cardiac output (with increased urinary output), return to normal vital signs (e.g., blood pressure of 120/80 mm Hg or higher or gradual increases in blood pressure as indicated, pulse rate greater than 60 but less than 100 beats/min), improved skin color (pallor to pink) and temperature (cool to warm) in the extremities, improved peripheral pulses, and increased level of consciousness. Therapeutic effects of drugs given for bronchial indications include a return to normal respiratory rate (more than 12 but fewer than 20 breaths/min), improved breath

---

QSEN ➤ **TEAMWORK AND COLLABORATION: LEGAL AND ETHICAL PRINCIPLES**

Infiltrating Intravenous Infusions

Nurses often encounter infiltrating intravenous (IV) infusions in the routine care of many of their patients. Every action taken is very important in meeting the standard of care for the patient and in ensuring that the nurse has acted as any prudent nurse would. The assessment and action of the nurse can be important for the patient, as in the case of *Macon-Bibb County Hospital Authority v. Ross* (335 SE2d 633-GA).

Situation and Outcome

At approximately 2:52 PM, Ms. Ross arrived at the emergency department with dyspnea, bradycardia, and a blood pressure (BP) of 250/150 mm Hg. She became unresponsive, and at 2:55 PM went into respiratory arrest. She was intubated by a respiratory therapist. At approximately 2:58 PM, she received intravenous (IV) Nipride in an IV site in her right wrist. Nipride was used to decrease the severely elevated blood pressure. By 3:13 PM, the patient's blood pressure was 120/90 and the Nipride was discontinued as prescribed by the physician. Actual events are documented as follows: At 3:28 PM, the patient had no blood pressure at all and the physician had prescribed IV administration of dopamine to elevate her blood pressure; dopamine was actually administered at 3:31 PM to increase the then nonexistent blood pressure. She was then transferred to the cardiac care unit at approximately 4:30 PM after her blood pressure had stabilized. At midnight, a nurse noted that the IV catheter site had a "bruise bluish in color." The next notation was at 11:00 AM that morning. The patient's right arm was noted to be swollen, sore, and with a large blistered area located around the IV catheter site. The same description was noted again at 4:00 PM. There was no evidence that a physician was consulted or informed until 6:50 PM. At this time, the blistered area was shown to a physician but it wasn't until later in the evening that another physician cleansed the blistered area and treated it as a burn. The patient's lower right arm was permanently scarred and, it was undisputed, that the injury was a result of the infiltration of the dopamine. A nurse expert testified that she believed that the hospital personnel had been negligent in inserting the IV in the smaller vein at the patient's wrist or at least in the failure to document why it was not placed in the recommended vein initially or subsequently. However, most significant was the fact that there was a failure to notify the physician of the swollen and blistered arm. On a jury verdict, the court entered judgment for the patient. The hospital appealed.

The court of appeals affirmed the judgment of the lower court. It was noted that, although an infiltration may result from an improper technique, it may also be due to the size of the needle, the status of the patient's veins, or specific intolerance to an IV catheter. However, according to the expert nurse's testimony, supported by suitable references, dopamine must be infused into a large vein such as a vein in the antecubital fossa, to minimize the risk for extravasation. In addition, a dopamine infusion needs to be monitored continuously and the infusion very closely regulated. The antidote to counter the effects of dopamine extravasation is phentolamine (Regitine), and damage may be decreased or reversed if given within a specified time period. The nurses were criticized for not being sufficiently knowledgeable regarding dopamine, which resulted in their failure to notify a physician of the patient's impaired tissue integrity.

Data from *Macon-Bibb County Hospital Authority v Ross*, 70785 (176 Ga. App. 221) (335 SE2d 633), 1985. Available at *www.lawskills.com/case/ga/id/427/29/index.html.* Accessed November 2, 2011.

sounds throughout the lung field with fewer adventitious (abnormal) sounds, increased air exchange in all areas of the lungs, decreased to no coughing, less dyspnea, improved partial pressure of oxygen and pulse oximeter readings, and tolerance of slowly increasing levels of activity. Therapeutic effects of *midodrine* include improved level of functioning and improved performance of the activities of daily living, fewer episodes of postural intolerance (dizziness, lightheadedness, and syncopal episodes), and more energy.

To evaluate for the occurrence of adverse effects with *adrenergic drugs*, monitor for stimulation of the systems that are affected, such as the cardiac system and the CNS. Adverse effects such as cardiac irregularities, hypertension, and tachycardia may occur. Be sure to monitor for chest pain.

PATIENT-CENTERED CARE: PATIENT TEACHING

- Medications are to be taken as prescribed. Excessive dosing may cause CNS and cardiovascular stimulation with tremors, nervousness, tachycardia, and palpitations.
- Instructions must be clear and concise for use of inhaled forms of medication, including nebulizers, inhalers, and metered-dose inhalers (see Chapter 9).
- Instruct the patient to report any worsening of respiratory symptoms, dyspnea, distress, chest pain, and/or cardiac palpitations to the prescriber immediately and/or seek immediate emergency medical assistance. Other symptoms to report include headache and/or blurred vision.

- Over-the-counter medications and herbal supplements are to be avoided unless the prescriber's approval is obtained.
- Myrbetriq, a newer drug for overactive bladder, is associated with dizziness, and so encourage the patient to avoid hazardous activities if this occurs. As with any patient with overactive bladder (see Chapter 21), avoid liquids before bedtime.
- Midodrine requires careful dosing, as ordered. Encourage the patient to keep a journal to record adverse effects, improvements in symptoms, and any worsening of symptoms.

KEY POINTS

- Catecholamines are substances that produce a sympathomimetic response (stimulate the SNS). The naturally occurring or endogenous catecholamines include epinephrine, norepinephrine, and dopamine. An example of an exogenous catecholamine is dobutamine.
- If the patient has a chronic respiratory disease, such as emphysema or chronic asthma or bronchitis, it is important for the patient to avoid contact with individuals who may have infections to help minimize situations that would exacerbate the original problem. Respiratory irritants must be avoided.

- Midodrine use requires careful blood pressure monitoring, so patient education about supine blood pressure measurement and journaling of measured blood pressure values is very important to the effective use of the drug.
- Inhaled forms of beta$_2$ agonists are used for their bronchodilating action and must be taken only as prescribed, with caution to avoid any overuse of the drug. Overdosage of these drugs may lead to severe cardiovascular, CNS, and cerebrovascular adverse effects and stimulation.
- Mirabegron is a newer drug that is a beta$_3$ agonist and used for overactive bladder.

NCLEX® EXAMINATION REVIEW QUESTIONS

1. The nurse caring for a patient who is receiving beta$_1$ agonist drug therapy needs to be aware that these drugs cause which effect?
   a. Increased cardiac contractility
   b. Decreased heart rate
   c. Bronchoconstriction
   d. Increased GI tract motility
2. During a teaching session for a patient who is receiving inhaled salmeterol, the nurse emphasizes that the drug is indicated for which condition?
   a. Rescue treatment of acute bronchospasms
   b. Prevention of bronchospasms
   c. Reduction of airway inflammation
   d. Long-term treatment of sinus congestion
3. For a patient receiving a vasoactive drug such as intravenous dopamine, which action by the nurse is most appropriate?
   a. Monitor the gravity drip infusion closely, and adjust as needed.

   b. Assess the patient's cardiac function by checking the radial pulse.
   c. Assess the intravenous site hourly for possible infiltration.
   d. Administer the drug by intravenous boluses according to the patient's blood pressure.
4. A patient is receiving dobutamine for shock and is complaining of feeling more "skipping beats" than yesterday. What will the nurse do next?
   a. Monitor for other signs of a therapeutic response to the drug.
   b. Titrate the drug to a higher dose to reduce the palpitations.
   c. Discontinue the dobutamine immediately.
   d. Assess the patient's vital signs and cardiac rhythm.
5. When a drug is characterized as having a negative chronotropic effect, the nurse knows to expect which effect?
   a. Reduced blood pressure
   b. Decreased heart rate
   c. Decreased ectopic beats
   d. Increased force of cardiac contractions

6. The nurse is monitoring a patient who is receiving an infusion of a beta-adrenergic agonist. Which adverse effects may occur with this infusion? *(Select all that apply.)*
   a. Mild tremors
   b. Bradycardia
   c. Tachycardia
   d. Palpitations
   e. Drowsiness
   f. Nervousness

7. The order reads: "Dopamine 3 mcg/kg/min IV." The solution available is 400 mg in 250 mL D$_5$W, and the patient weighs 176 pounds. The nurse will set the IV infusion pump to run at how many mL/hour?

8. The nurse is reviewing the home medications for a newly admitted patient, and notes that the patient takes Mirabegron (Myrbetriq). The nurse will conclude that the patient has which condition?
   a. Asthma
   b. Overactive bladder
   c. Urinary retention
   d. Orthostatic hypotension

1. a, 2. b, 3. c, 4. d, 5. b, 6. a, c, d, f, 7. 9 mL/hr, 8. b.

CRITICAL THINKING AND PRIORITIZATION QUESTIONS

1. A patient is experiencing a severe anaphylactic reaction after a dose of an antibiotic, and the emergency team is present. The nurse is expecting to give what drug first? Explain your answer.

2. The nurse is assessing a 63-year-old patient who is taking mirabegron (Myrbetriq). What safety issues are most important to monitor while the patient is taking this medication? Explain your answer.

For answers, see *http://evolve.elsevier.com/Lilley*.

ⓔ EVOLVE WEBSITE

http://evolve.elsevier.com/Lilley
- Animations
- Answer Keys for Textbook Case Studies and Textbook Critical Thinking and Prioritization Questions
- Content Updates
- Key Points
- Review Questions
- Student Case Studies

Adrenergic-Blocking Drugs

http://evolve.elsevier.com/Lilley

OBJECTIVES

When you reach the end of this chapter, you will be able to do the following:

1. Briefly review the functions of the sympathetic nervous system and the specific effects of adrenergic-blocking drugs.
2. List the various drugs classified as adrenergic antagonists (blockers) or sympatholytics.
3. Discuss the mechanisms of action, therapeutic effects, indications, adverse and toxic effects, cautions, contraindications, drug interactions, dosages, routes of administration, and any antidotal management for the various alpha antagonists (blockers), beta nonselective blockers, and the beta$_1$ and beta$_2$ blockers.
4. Develop a nursing care plan that includes all phases of the nursing process for patients taking adrenergic antagonists.

DRUG PROFILES

⬥atenolol, p. 314
carvedilol, p. 315
⬥esmolol, p. 315
labetalol, p. 315
⬥metoprolol, p. 315
⬥phentolamine, p. 312

⬥propranolol, p. 315
sotalol, p. 316
tamsulosin, p. 313

_____
⬥ = *Key drug*
❗ = *High-alert drug*

KEY TERMS

Acrocyanosis Decreased amount of oxygen delivered to the extremities, causing the feet or hands to turn blue. (p. 311)

Adrenergic receptors Specific receptor sites located throughout the body for the endogenous sympathetic neurotransmitters norepinephrine and epinephrine. (p. 310)

Agonists Drugs with a specific receptor affinity that mimic the body's natural chemicals (e.g., hormones, neurotransmitters). (p. 310)

Angina Paroxysmal (sudden) chest pain caused by myocardial ischemia. (p. 313)

Antagonists Drugs that bind to specific receptors and inhibit or block the response of the receptors. (p. 310)

Dysrhythmias Irregular heart rhythms; generally called *arrhythmias* in clinical practice. (p. 313)

Extravasation The leaking of fluid from a blood vessel into the surrounding tissues, as in the case of an infiltrated intravenous infusion. (p. 311)

First-dose phenomenon Severe and sudden drop in blood pressure after the administration of the first dose of an alpha-adrenergic blocker. (p. 311)

Intrinsic sympathomimetic activity The paradoxical action of some beta-blocking drugs (e.g., acebutolol) that mimics the action of the sympathetic nervous system. (p. 313)

Lipophilicity The chemical attraction of a substance (e.g., drug molecule) to lipid or fat molecules. (p. 314)

Orthostatic hypotension A sudden drop in blood pressure when a person stands up. Also referred to as *postural hypotension* or *orthostasis.* (p. 311)

Pheochromocytoma A vascular adrenal gland tumor that is usually benign but secretes epinephrine and norepinephrine and thus often causes central nervous system stimulation and substantial blood pressure elevation. (p. 311)

Raynaud's disease A narrowing of small arteries that limits the amount of blood circulation to the extremities, causing numbness of the nose, fingers, toes, and ears in response to cold temperatures or stress. (p. 311)

Sympatholytics Drugs that inhibit the postganglionic functioning of the sympathetic nervous system. (p. 310)

OVERVIEW

The autonomic nervous system consists of the parasympathetic and sympathetic nervous systems. The class of drugs discussed in this chapter works primarily on the sympathetic nervous system (SNS). As discussed in Chapter 18, the adrenergic agonist drugs stimulate the SNS. Those drugs are called **agonists** because they bind to receptors and cause a response. Adrenergic blockers have the opposite effect and are therefore referred to as **antagonists**. They bind to adrenergic receptors, but in doing so inhibit or block stimulation by the SNS. They are also referred to as **sympatholytics** because they "lyse," or inhibit, SNS stimulation.

Throughout the body, there are receptor sites for the endogenous sympathetic neurotransmitters norepinephrine and epinephrine. Such receptors are known as **adrenergic receptors**, and two basic types are found: alpha and beta. There are subtypes of the alpha- and beta-adrenergic receptors, designated 1 and 2. The alpha$_1$- and alpha$_2$-adrenergic receptors are differentiated by their location on nerves. The alpha$_1$-adrenergic receptors are located on the tissue, muscle, or organ that the nerve is stimulating (postsynaptic effector cells). The alpha$_2$-adrenergic receptors are located on the actual nerves that stimulate the presynaptic effector cells. The alpha$_2$ receptors are inhibitory in nature. Thus, it is actually the stimulation of alpha$_2$ receptors that causes the inhibitory effects of the SNS. Alpha$_2$-active drugs (e.g., clonidine) are discussed in Chapter 22. The beta$_1$-adrenergic receptors are located primarily in the heart. The beta$_2$-adrenergic receptors are located primarily on the smooth muscles of the bronchioles and blood vessels. It is at these various receptors that adrenergic blockers act. They are classified by the type of adrenergic receptor they block—alpha or beta or, in a few cases, both. Hence, they are called alpha blockers, beta blockers, or alpha/beta blockers.

ALPHA BLOCKERS

Mechanism of Action and Drug Effects

The alpha-adrenergic–blocking drugs, or alpha blockers, interrupt stimulation of the SNS at the alpha$_1$-adrenergic receptors. More specifically, alpha blockers work either by direct competition with norepinephrine or by a noncompetitive process. Figure 19-1 illustrates these two mechanisms. Alpha blockers have a greater affinity for the alpha-adrenergic receptor than norepinephrine does and therefore can chemically displace norepinephrine molecules from the receptor. Adrenergic blockade at these receptors leads to effects such as vasodilation, reduced blood pressure, miosis (pupillary constriction), and reduced smooth muscle tone in organs such as the bladder and prostate. Currently available alpha blockers are listed in Table 19-1.

Indications

The alpha blockers such as doxazosin, prazosin, and terazosin cause both arterial and venous dilation, which reduces peripheral vascular resistance and blood pressure. These drugs are used to treat hypertension (see Chapter 22). There are also

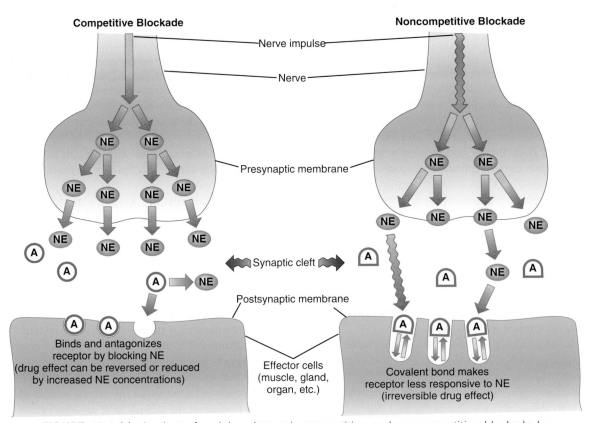

FIGURE 19-1 Mechanisms for alpha-adrenergic competitive and noncompetitive blockade by alpha blocker drugs. *A,* Alpha blocker; *NE,* norepinephrine.

TABLE 19-1 Currently Available Adrenergic-Blocking Drugs

Generic Name	Trade Name	Route
Alpha₁ Blockers		
alfuzosin	Uroxatral	PO
doxazosin	Cardura	PO
phenoxybenzamine	Dibenzyline	PO
phentolamine	Generic	IV, IM, IM/subcut/intradermal (for extravasation wounds)
prazosin	Minipress	PO
terazosin	Hytrin	PO
tamsulosin	Flomax	PO
Beta Blockers		
Nonselective		
carvedilol*	Coreg, Coreg CR	PO
labetalol*	Normodyne, Trandate	PO, IV
nadolol	Corgard	PO
penbutolol	Levatol	PO
pindolol	Visken	PO
propranolol*	Inderal, Inderal LA	PO, IV
sotalol	Betapace	PO
timolol	Blocadren, Timoptic	PO, IV, ophthalmic
Cardioselective		
acebutolol	Sectral	PO
atenolol	Tenormin	PO
betaxolol	Kerlone	PO
bisoprolol	Zebeta	PO
esmolol	Brevibloc	IV
nebivolol	Bystolic	PO
metoprolol	Lopressor, Toprol-XL	PO, IV

*Has antagonist activity at alpha₁, beta₁, and beta₂ receptors.

TABLE 19-2 Alpha Blockers: Adverse Effects

Body System	Adverse Effects
Cardiovascular	Palpitations, orthostatic hypotension, tachycardia, edema, chest pain
Central nervous	Dizziness, headache, anxiety, depression, weakness, numbness, fatigue
Gastrointestinal	Nausea, vomiting, diarrhea, constipation, abdominal pain
Other	Incontinence, dry mouth, pharyngitis

is an alpha blocker that is beneficial in the treatment of these syndromes, although its use is uncommon.

Still other alpha blockers (e.g., phentolamine) are effective at counteracting the effects of injected epinephrine and norepinephrine. They do this by causing peripheral vasodilation and reducing peripheral resistance by blocking catecholamine-stimulated vasoconstriction. Because of their potent vasodilating properties and their fast onset of action, they are used to prevent skin necrosis and sloughing after the extravasation of vasopressors such as norepinephrine or epinephrine. When these drugs extravasate (leak out of the blood vessel into the surrounding tissue), they cause vasoconstriction and ultimately tissue death, or necrosis. If the vasoconstriction is not reversed quickly, the entire limb can be lost. Phentolamine, in particular, can reverse this potent vasoconstriction and restore blood flow to the ischemic tissue.

Contraindications

Contraindications to the use of alpha-blocking drugs include known drug allergy and peripheral vascular disease and may include hepatic and renal disease, coronary artery disease, peptic ulcer, and sepsis.

Adverse Effects

The primary adverse effects of alpha blockers are those related to their effects on the vasculature. First-dose phenomenon, which is a severe and sudden drop in blood pressure after the administration of the first dose of an alpha-adrenergic blocker, can cause patients to fall or pass out. All patients must be warned about this adverse effect before they take their first dose of an alpha blocker. Orthostatic hypotension can occur with any dose of an alpha blocker, and patients must be warned to get up slowly from a supine position. Common adverse effects include dizziness, headache, and constipation. Other adverse effects of the alpha blockers are listed by body system in Table 19-2.

Toxicity and Management of Overdosec

With overdoses of both oral and injectable forms, symptomatic and supportive measures are to be instituted as needed. Blood pressure is supported with the administration of fluids, volume expanders, and vasopressor drugs, and anticonvulsants such as diazepam are administered for the control of seizures.

alpha-adrenergic receptors in the prostate and bladder. By blocking stimulation of alpha₁ receptors, these drugs reduce smooth muscle contraction of the bladder neck and the prostatic portion of the urethra. For this reason, alpha blockers are given to patients with benign prostatic hyperplasia (BPH) to decrease resistance to urinary outflow. This reduces urinary obstruction and relieves some of the effects of BPH. Tamsulosin and alfuzosin are used exclusively for treating BPH, whereas terazosin and doxazosin can be used for both hypertension and BPH.

Other alpha blockers can inhibit responses to adrenergic stimulation. These drugs noncompetitively block alpha-adrenergic receptors on smooth muscle and various exocrine glands. Because of this action, they are very useful in controlling or preventing hypertension in patients who have a pheochromocytoma, a tumor that forms on the adrenal gland on top of the kidney and secretes norepinephrine, thus causing SNS stimulation. The alpha blockers are also useful in the treatment of patients who have increased endogenous alpha-adrenergic agonist activity, which results in vasoconstriction. Three conditions in which this occurs are Raynaud's disease, acrocyanosis, and frostbite. Phenoxybenzamine, in particular,

TABLE 19-3 Alpha Blockers: Common Drug Interactions

Drug	Interacting Drug	Mechanism	Result
phentolamine	Beta blockers, alcohol, erectile dysfunction drugs	} Additive effects	} Profound hypotension
	Epinephrine	Antagonism	Reduced phentolamine effects
tamsulosin	Warfarin	Competition for plasma protein-binding sites	Risk for bleeding
	Antihypertensives, erectile dysfunction drugs, alcohol	} Additive effects	} Risk for hypotension

DOSAGES

Selected Alpha-Adrenergic–Blocking Drugs

Drug (Pregnancy Category)	Pharmacologic Class	Usual Adult Dosage Range	Indications
◆ phentolamine (Regitine) (C)	Alpha blocker	IM/IV: 5 mg; repeat if necessary	Hypertensive episodes with pheochromocytoma
		5-10 mg diluted in 10 mL NS injected into extravasation site	Alpha-adrenergic drug extravasation
tamsulosin (Flomax) (B)*	Alpha₁ blocker	PO: 0.4 mg once daily; max dose 0.8 mg	Benign prostatic hyperplasia

*Not indicated for use in women; however, it is sometimes used for kidney stones.

Interactions

The most severe drug interactions with alpha blockers are those that potentiate the effects of the alpha blockers. The alpha blockers are very highly protein bound and compete for binding sites with other drugs that are highly protein bound (see Chapter 2). Because of the limited sites for binding on proteins and the increased competition for these sites, more free alpha blocker molecules circulate in the bloodstream. More active drug results in a more pronounced drug effect. Some of the common drugs that interact with alpha blockers and the results of these interactions are listed in Table 19-3.

Dosages

For dosage information on alpha blockers, see the Dosages table above.

DRUG PROFILES

The alpha blockers are commonly used to treat hypertension and/or benign prostatic hyperplasia. They include phentolamine, phenoxybenzamine, terazosin, alfuzosin, tamsulosin, silodosin, and prazosin. Prazosin is discussed in Chapter 22.

◆ phentolamine

Phentolamine (Regitine) is an alpha blocker that reduces peripheral vascular resistance and is also used to treat hypertension. Like phenoxybenzamine, it is used to treat the high blood pressure caused by pheochromocytoma, but phentolamine can also be used in the diagnosis of this catecholamine-secreting tumor. To help establish a diagnosis of pheochromocytoma, a single intravenous dose of phentolamine is given to the hypertensive patient. If the blood pressure declines rapidly, it is highly likely that the patient has a pheochromocytoma. Phentolamine is available only as an injectable preparation. It is most commonly used to treat the extravasation of vasoconstricting drugs such as norepinephrine, epinephrine, and dopamine, which when given intravenously can leak out of the vein, especially if the intravenous tube is not correctly positioned. If such a drug is allowed to extravasate into the surrounding tissue, the result is intense vasoconstriction, decreased blood flow, necrosis, and potential loss of the limb. When phentolamine is injected subcutaneously in a circular fashion around the extravasation site, it causes alpha-adrenergic receptor blockade and vasodilation, which in turn increases blood flow to the ischemic tissue and thus prevents permanent damage. Its use is contraindicated in known hypersensitivity, myocardial infarction (MI), and coronary artery disease. Adverse effects include tachycardia, dizziness, gastrointestinal upset, and others listed in Table 19-2. Drugs with which phentolamine interacts include alcohol (a disulfiram-like reaction; see Chapter 17) and erectile dysfunction medications such as sildenafil (additive hypotensive effects; see Chapter 35). Epinephrine and ephedrine can counteract the desired effects of phentolamine. The recommended dosages are given in the table above.

Pharmacokinetics: Phentolamine

Route	Onset of Action	Peak Plasma Concentration	Elimination Half-life	Duration of Action
IV	1 hr	4-6 hr	24 hr	3-4 days

tamsulosin

Tamsulosin (Flomax) is an alpha blocker used primarily to treat BPH and is exclusively indicated for male patients. Similar drugs with the same indication are alfuzosin and silodosin. These drugs block alpha-adrenergic receptors on smooth muscle within the prostate and bladder. This results in relaxation of these smooth muscle fibers and improved urinary flow. Other similar drugs include terazosin and doxazosin, which can be used to treat both BPH and hypertension. Contraindications to tamsulosin include known drug allergy and concurrent use of erectile dysfunction drugs such as sildenafil. Adverse effects include headache, abnormal ejaculation, rhinitis, and others listed in Table 19-2. Interacting drugs include other alpha blockers, calcium channel blockers, and erectile dysfunction drugs (additive hypotensive effects); drugs that induce or inhibit hepatic enzymes may reduce or enhance the effects of tamsulosin. It is available only for oral use.

Pharmacokinetics: Tamsulosin

Route	Onset of Action	Peak Plasma Concentration	Elimination Half-life	Duration of Action
PO	Unknown	4-7 hr	15 hr	Unknown

BETA BLOCKERS

Mechanism of Action and Drug Effects

The beta-adrenergic–blocking drugs (beta blockers) block SNS stimulation of the beta-adrenergic receptors by competing with norepinephrine and epinephrine. The beta blockers can be either selective or nonselective, depending on the type of beta-adrenergic receptors they antagonize. $Beta_1$-adrenergic receptors are located primarily in the heart. Beta blockers that are selective for these receptors are called *cardioselective beta blockers* or *beta₁-blocking drugs*. Other beta blockers block both beta₁- and beta₂-adrenergic receptors and are referred to as *nonselective beta blockers*. $Beta_2$ receptors are located primarily on the smooth muscles of the bronchioles and blood vessels. In addition, beta blockers can be further categorized according to whether or not they have **intrinsic sympathomimetic activity**. Drugs with intrinsic sympathomimetic activity (acebutolol, penbutolol, pindolol) not only block beta-adrenergic receptors but also partially stimulate them. This was initially believed to be an advantageous characteristic, but clinical experience has not shown this to be useful. Two beta blockers, carvedilol and labetalol, also have alpha-receptor–blocking activity, especially at higher dosages. Table 19-1 lists the currently available beta blockers.

Cardioselective $beta_1$ blockers block the $beta_1$ receptors on the surface of the heart. This reduces myocardial stimulation, which in turn reduces heart rate, slows conduction through the atrioventricular (AV) node, prolongs sinoatrial (SA) node recovery, and decreases myocardial oxygen demand by decreasing myocardial contractile force (contractility). Nonselective beta blockers not only have these cardiac effects, but they block $beta_2$ receptors on the smooth muscle of the bronchioles and blood vessels as well.

Smooth muscle that surrounds the airways in the lungs is called the *bronchioles*. When the $beta_2$ receptors in the bronchioles are blocked, the end result is bronchial smooth muscle contraction and narrowing of the airways. This may lead to shortness of breath. The smooth muscle that surrounds blood vessels can cause dilation or constriction, depending on whether the $beta_1$ or $beta_2$ receptors are stimulated. When this $beta_2$ stimulation is blocked, the muscles are then stimulated by unopposed sympathetic activity at the $beta_1$ receptors, which causes them to contract. This causes increased peripheral vascular resistance. $Beta_2$ receptors promote *glycogenolysis* (the production of glucose from glycogen) and mobilize glucose in response to hypoglycemia. Nonselective beta blockers block glycogenolysis and can delay recovery from hypoglycemia and mask or blunt the perception of symptoms associated with hypoglycemia such as tachycardia, tremor, or nervousness. In addition, they also can impede the secretion of insulin from the pancreas, which results in elevation of blood glucose levels. Therefore, nonselective beta blockers can cause either hypoglycemia or hyperglycemia.

Finally, beta blockers can cause the release of free fatty acids from adipose tissue. This may result in moderately elevated blood levels of triglycerides and reduced levels of the "good cholesterol" known as *high-density lipoprotein (HDL)*.

Indications

Indications for beta blockers include angina, MI, cardiac dysrhythmias, hypertension, and heart failure.

Beta blockers are commonly used in the treatment of **angina**, or chest pain (see Chapter 23). These drugs work by decreasing the demand for myocardial energy and oxygen consumption, which helps shift the supply/demand ratio to the supply side and allows more oxygen to get to the heart muscle. This in turn helps to relieve the pain in the heart muscle caused by the lack of oxygen.

Beta blockers are also considered to be *cardioprotective* because they inhibit stimulation of the myocardium by circulating catecholamines. Myocardial infarction causes catecholamines to be released. Unopposed stimulation by catecholamines would further increase the heart rate and the contractile force and thereby increase myocardial oxygen demand. When a beta blocker occupies myocardial $beta_1$ receptors, circulating catecholamine molecules are prevented from binding to the receptors. Thus, the beta blockers protect the heart from being stimulated by these catecholamines. Because of this characteristic, beta blockers are commonly given to patients after they have experienced an MI to protect the heart.

Beta blockers have a profound effect on the conduction system of the heart. The AV node normally receives impulse stimulation from the SA node and slows it down so that the ventricles have time to fill before they are stimulated to contract. Conduction in the SA node is slowed by beta blockers, which results in a decreased heart rate. These drugs also slow conduction through the AV node. These effects of the beta blockers on the conduction system of the heart make them useful in the treatment of various types of irregular heart rhythms called **dysrhythmias** (see Chapter 25).

Beta blockers are useful in treating hypertension because of their ability to reduce SNS stimulation of the heart, including reducing heart rate and the force of myocardial contraction (systole). Certain beta blockers such as carvedilol and metoprolol have been shown to be useful in heart failure.

Because of their lipophilicity (attraction to lipid or fat), some beta blockers (e.g., propranolol) can easily gain entry into the central nervous system and are used to treat migraine headaches. In addition, the topical application of timolol to the eye has been very effective in treating ocular disorders such as glaucoma (see Chapter 57).

Contraindications

Contraindications to the use of beta blockers include known drug allergies and may include uncompensated heart failure, cardiogenic shock, heart block or bradycardia, pregnancy, severe pulmonary disease, and Raynaud's disease. All beta blockers share a black box warning stating that therapy should not be withdrawn abruptly, but should be tapered over 1 to 2 weeks.

Adverse Effects

The adverse effects of beta blockers are primarily extensions of their pharmacologic activity. Most such effects are mild and diminish with time. The most common adverse effects of beta blockers include bradycardia, depression, impotence, constipation and fatigue. Some of the most serious undesirable effects can be caused by acute withdrawal of the drug. For example, such sudden withdrawal may exacerbate underlying angina, precipitate an MI, or cause rebound hypertension. Beta blockers also delay the recovery from hypoglycemia in patients with type 1 diabetes (rarely in those with type 2). Adverse effects induced by beta blockers are listed by body system in Table 19-4.

Toxicity and Management of Overdose

For overdoses of both oral and injectable dosage forms, treatment consists primarily of symptomatic and supportive care. Atropine may be given intravenously for the management of bradycardia. If the bradycardia still persists, placement of a transvenous cardiac pacemaker may be considered. For the treatment of severe hypotension, vasopressors are titrated until the desired blood pressure and heart rate are achieved. Most beta blockers are dialyzable; therefore, hemodialysis may be useful in enhancing elimination in the event of severe overdose.

Interactions

Most of the drug interactions with beta blockers result from either the additive effects of coadministered medications with similar mechanisms of action or the antagonistic effects of various drugs. Nonselective beta blockers may mask the tachycardia from hypoglycemia caused by insulin and sulfonylureas, and the hypoglycemic effect of insulin and sulfonylureas may be enhanced (see Chapter 32). Some of the common drugs that interact with beta blockers and the resulting effects are given in Table 19-5.

Dosages

For dosage information on selected beta blockers, see the table on this page.

DRUG PROFILES

Numerous beta blockers currently available are listed in Table 19-1. Several beta blockers are profiled in the following sections. Contraindications, adverse reactions, and drug interactions are comparable for these drugs and are listed in the previous text, Table 19-4, and Table 19-5, respectively.

♦ atenolol

Atenolol (Tenormin) is a cardioselective beta blocker that is commonly used to prevent future heart attacks in patients who have had one. It is also used in the treatment of hypertension and angina and in the management of thyrotoxicosis to help block the symptoms of excessive thyroid activity. Atenolol is available for oral use. Recommended dosages are given in the table on the next page.

Pharmacokinetics: Atenolol

Route	Onset of Action	Peak Plasma Concentration	Elimination Half-life	Duration of Action
PO	1 hr	2-4 hr	6-7 hr	24 hr

TABLE 19-4 Beta Blockers: Common Adverse Effects

Body System	Adverse Effects
Cardiovascular	Atrioventricular block, bradycardia, heart failure
Central nervous	Dizziness, fatigue, depression, drowsiness, unusual dreams
Gastrointestinal	Nausea, vomiting, constipation, diarrhea
Hematologic	Agranulocytosis, thrombocytopenia
Metabolic	Delayed hypoglycemia recovery, masked symptoms of hypoglycemia, hyperlipidemia
Other	Impotence, alopecia, bronchospasm, wheezing, dry mouth

TABLE 19-5 Beta Blockers: Drug Interactions

Interacting Drug	Mechanism	Result
Antacids (aluminum hydroxide type)	Decrease absorption	Decreased beta blocker activity
Antimuscarinics, anticholinergics	Antagonism	Reduced beta blocker effects
digoxin	Additive effect	Enhanced bradycardic effects of digoxin
Diuretics, cardiovascular drugs, alcohol	Additive effect	Additive hypotensive effects
Neuromuscular blocking drugs	Additive effect	Prolonged neuromuscular blockade
Oral hypoglycemic drugs, insulin	Mask signs of hypoglycemia	Delayed recovery from hypoglycemia

DOSAGES

Selected Beta-Adrenergic–Blocking Drugs

Drug (Pregnancy Category)	Pharmacologic Class	Usual Adult Dosage Range	Indications
◆ atenolol (Tenormin) (C)	Beta$_1$ blocker	PO: 50-200 mg/day daily or divided bid; max 200 mg/day	Hypertension, angina
carvedilol (Coreg) (C)	Alpha and beta blocker	PO: 6.25-100 mg/day depending on indication PO: CR: 10-80 mg/day	Heart failure, angina, hypertension
labetalol (Normodyne, Trandate) (C)	Alpha$_1$ and beta blocker	PO: 100-400 mg bid; max 2400 mg/day IV: 20 mg with additional doses of 40-80 mg at 10-min intervals until desired effect or a total dose of 300 mg is injected; maintenance infusion of 2 mg/min initially and titrated to response	Hypertension Severe hypertension
◆ metoprolol (Lopressor, Toprol XL) (C)	Beta$_1$ blocker	PO: 50-400 mg/day depending on form used IV/PO: 3 bolus injections of 5 mg at 2-min intervals followed in 15 min by 50 mg PO every 6 hr for 48 hr; thereafter 50-100 mg PO bid	Hypertension, Late MI Early MI
◆ propranolol (Inderal, Inderal LA) (C)	Beta blocker	PO: 80-320 mg/day divided bid-qid 120-640 mg/day divided bid-tid 30-120 mg/day divided tid-qid 180-240 mg/day divided tid-qid 160-240 mg/day divided	Angina Hypertension Dysrhythmias Post-MI Migraine

carvedilol

Carvedilol (Coreg) has many effects, including acting as a non-selective beta blocker, an alpha$_1$ blocker, a calcium channel blocker, and possibly an antioxidant. It is used primarily in the treatment of heart failure but is also beneficial for hypertension and angina. It has been shown to slow the progression of heart failure and to decrease the frequency of hospitalization in patients with mild to moderate (class II or III) heart failure. Carvedilol is most commonly added to digoxin, furosemide, and angiotensin-converting enzyme inhibitors when used to treat heart failure. Carvedilol is available as immediate release and controlled-release formulations. Recommended dosages are given in the table above.

Pharmacokinetics: Carvedilol

Route	Onset of Action	Peak Plasma Concentration	Elimination Half-life	Duration of Action
PO	20-120 min	1-4 hr	6-8 hr	8-24 hr

◆ esmolol

Esmolol (Brevibloc) is a very strong short-acting beta$_1$ blocker. It is primarily used in acute situations to provide rapid temporary control of the ventricular rate in patients with supraventricular tachydysrhythmias. Because of its very short half-life, it is given only as an intravenous infusion and is titrated to achieve the serum levels that control the patient's symptoms.

Pharmacokinetics: Esmolol

Route	Onset of Action	Peak Plasma Concentration	Elimination Half-life	Duration of Action
IV	Immediate	6 min	9 min	15-20 min

labetalol

Labetalol (Normodyne) is unusual in that it can block both alpha- and beta-adrenergic receptors. It is used in the treatment of severe hypertension and hypertensive emergencies to quickly lower the blood pressure before permanent damage is done. Labetalol is available for oral and injectable use. Recommended dosages are given in the table above.

Pharmacokinetics: Labetalol

Route	Onset of Action	Peak Plasma Concentration	Elimination Half-life	Duration of Action
IV	2-5 min	5-15 min	2.5-8 hr	2-4 hr
PO	20-120 min	1-4 hr	2.5-8 hr	8-24 hr

◆ metoprolol

Metoprolol (Lopressor) is the most commonly used beta$_1$ blocker. Recent studies of metoprolol have shown increased survival in patients given the drug after they have experienced an MI. Metoprolol is available for oral and injectable use. When metoprolol is given IV, it is considered a high-alert drug and the patient should be monitored. Recommended dosages are given in the table above.

Pharmacokinetics: Metoprolol

Route	Onset of Action	Peak Plasma Concentration	Elimination Half-life	Duration of Action
IV	1 min	20 min	3-8 hr	5-8 hr
PO	1 hr	2-4 hr	3-8 hr	10-20 hr

◆ propranolol

Propranolol (Inderal) is the prototypical nonselective beta$_1$- and beta$_2$-blocking drug. It was one of the very first beta blockers. Lengthy experience has revealed many uses for it. In addition to the indications mentioned for metoprolol, propranolol has been used for the treatment of tachydysrhythmias associated with cardiac glycoside intoxication and for the treatment of hypertrophic subaortic stenosis, pheochromocytoma, thyrotoxicosis, migraine headache, essential tremor, and many other conditions. The same contraindications that apply to the cardioselective beta blockers discussed earlier hold for propranolol as well. In addition, its use is contraindicated in patients with bronchial asthma. Propranolol is available for oral and injectable use. Recommended dosages are given in the table on the previous page.

Pharmacokinetics: Propranolol

Route	Onset of Action	Peak Plasma Concentration	Elimination Half-life	Duration of Action
IV	2 min	1-4 hr	3-5 hr	3-6 hr
PO	1-2 hr	1-4 hr	3-5 hr	6-12 hr

sotalol

Sotalol (Betapace) is a nonselective beta blocker that has very potent antidysrhythmic properties. It is commonly used for the management of difficult-to-treat dysrhythmias. Often these dysrhythmias are life-threatening ventricular dysrhythmias such as sustained ventricular tachycardia. It has properties characteristic of both a class II and class III antidysrhythmic drug (see Chapter 25). Because it is a nonselective beta blocker, it causes some of the unwanted adverse effects typical of these drugs (e.g., hypotension). Sotalol is available only for oral use.

Pharmacokinetics: Sotalol

Route	Onset of Action	Peak Plasma Concentration	Elimination Half-life	Duration of Action
PO	1-2 hr	2.5-4 hr	12 hr	8-16 hr

NURSING PROCESS

ASSESSMENT

Adrenergic-blocking drugs, or *sympatholytics,* produce a variety of effects on the patient, depending on the type of receptor(s) blocked. Because of the impact of these drugs, primarily on the cardiac and respiratory systems, their use requires careful assessment to help minimize the adverse effects and maximize the therapeutic effects. Understanding the basic anatomy and physiology of adrenergic receptors and their subsequent actions if stimulated or blocked is also critical in carrying out assessment and other aspects of the nursing process and drug therapy.

If an *adrenergic-blocking drug* is *nonselective,* it blocks both alpha and beta (beta$_1$ and beta$_2$) receptors. Alpha receptor blocking affects blood vessels, whereas beta$_1$ receptor blocking

affects heart rate and beta$_2$ blocking affects bronchial smooth muscle. Therefore, a nonselective adrenergic blocker will have the following actions: (1) alpha blocking leading to blockade of the sympathetic stimulation of blood vessels (i.e., vasoconstriction) and resulting in vasodilation and a subsequent decrease in blood pressure; (2) beta$_1$ blocking leading to blockade of the sympathetic effects on heart rate, contractility, and conduction with resulting bradycardia, negative inotropic effects (i.e., decrease in contractility), and a decrease in conduction; and (3) beta$_2$ blocking leading to blockade of the sympathetic effects on bronchial smooth muscle with the net effect of bronchoconstriction. However, if the drug is only an *alpha, beta$_1$,* or *beta$_2$ blocker,* the resulting effect will be related to the specific receptor being blocked (or combination of receptors, depending on the drug). An understanding of these basic physiologic concepts is necessary to critical thinking and decision making in the administration of these drugs.

Begin a thorough assessment by gathering information about the patient's allergies and past and present medical conditions. Conducting a system overview and taking a thorough medication history is also a part of this process. Pose the following questions, and document the findings: Are there any allergies to medications and/or foods? Is there a history of chronic obstructive pulmonary disease (e.g., emphysema, asthma, chronic bronchitis), other respiratory diseases, hypertension or hypotension, cardiac disease, bradycardia, heart failure, and/or cardiac dysrhythmias? This information is crucial because the action and adverse effects of alpha and beta blockers may pose additional health risks to individuals with these problems. For example, *alpha blockers* may precipitate hypotension, thus patients with baseline low blood pressure readings need more frequent blood pressure monitoring, or they may not tolerate the drug at all. *Beta-blocking drugs* may precipitate bradycardia, hypotension, heart block, heart failure, bronchoconstriction, and/or increased airway resistance. Therefore, any preexisting condition that might be worsened by the concurrent use of any of these medications may then represent a contraindication or caution. More specifically, with *beta₁-blocking drugs*, patients with preexisting bradycardia, decreased cardiac contractility, heart failure, and/or decreased conduction with heart block cannot take these drugs without further worsening of these conditions. Trends in vital signs, specifically blood pressure and heart rate, as well as current findings of these parameters are important to assess prior to giving these medications. As another example, patients with a history of asthma, emphysema, bronchitis, or any condition with increased airway resistance or bronchoconstriction cannot take *beta₂-blocking drugs* without experiencing further bronchoconstriction and negative effects on their underlying disease condition. Given the actions and adverse effects of the drug, it is also important to assess intake and output, daily weights, breath sounds, and blood glucose levels, especially if the patient has diabetes. For a complete listing of drug interactions, see Tables 19-3 and 19-5.

NURSING DIAGNOSES

1. Ineffective airway clearance related to the adverse effect of bronchoconstriction caused by beta-adrenergic drugs as well as any underlying restrictive airway conditions
2. Ineffective peripheral tissue perfusion related to the adverse effects of the disease of hypertension and the adverse effects of the adrenergic-blocking drugs (hypotension)
3. Imbalanced nutrition, less than body requirements, due to nausea and vomiting related to the adverse effects of the adrenergic blockers
4. Deficient knowledge related to lack of information about the therapeutic regimen, drug adverse effects, drug interactions, and precautions to be taken during drug treatment
5. Risk for injury related to possible adverse effects of the adrenergic-blocking drugs (e.g., postural hypotension, dizziness, syncope, numbness and tingling of the fingers and toes)

PLANNING: OUTCOME IDENTIFICATION

1. Patient maintains/regains effective airway clearance and airway exchange evidenced with ease of respirations and without any bronchospasm, wheezing, or difficulty.
2. Patient maintains adequate peripheral tissue perfusion as noted by blood pressure readings within normal ranges and minimal adverse effects of hypotension.
3. Patient maintains adequate nutritional status with adequate dietary intake of the following: grains, vegetables, fruits, dairy, and protein foods (see *www.choosemyplate.gov*).
4. Patient states the rationale for both pharmacologic and nonpharmacologic treatment of hypertension, importance of taking medication as prescribed, and reporting adverse effects.
5. Patient remains free from injury by adhering to prescribed medication regimen and reporting adverse reactions.

IMPLEMENTATION

Several nursing interventions may help maximize therapeutic effects of *adrenergic-blocking drugs* and minimize their adverse

effects. To help minimize dry mouth, encourage intake of water within any restrictions and frequent rinsing/spraying of mouth with over-the-counter dental products indicated for dry mouth. Sugarless gum/candy may also be helpful with dry mouth. If any of the medications are given intravenously, an ECG monitor/cardiac monitoring is usually recommended. Encourage patients taking alpha blockers to change positions slowly and with purpose to prevent or minimize postural hypotension with subsequent dizziness and/or syncope. *Alpha adrenergic blockers* and their indications in treatment of hypertensive disease and/or hypertensive crises are discussed further in Chapter 22. Use of the newer alpha blocker, *tamsulosin*, in patients with BPH is quite common, and patients taking this drug need to inform all health care providers—including dentists—that this is part of their medical regimen, especially before any type of surgery. In addition, anything leading to vasodilation needs to be avoided to prevent postural hypotension with resultant dizziness, lightheadedness, and syncope. This includes alcohol intake, excessive exercise, exposure to hot climates, and use of saunas, hot tubs, and heated showers or baths. See Patient Centered Care: Patient Teaching for more information.

When either an *alpha blocker* or *beta blocker* is used, count the apical pulse for 1 full minute. Measure and document both supine and standing blood pressures. Contact the prescriber

CASE STUDY

Safety: What Went Wrong? Beta Blockers

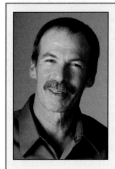 F., a 58-year-old high school orchestra teacher, has been hospitalized after experiencing a myocardial infarction. He is married with two teenage children. His physician told him that his myocardial infarction was "mild" but that F. must make some lifestyle changes, including exercise and dietary changes. F. has a history of asthma; he had stopped smoking 5 years earlier and has had no recent problems. His history also includes gallbladder removal at 50 years of age. F.'s pulse rate has ranged from 78 to 112 beats/min; his blood pressure has been within normal range, 118/74 to 122/80 mm Hg. He is preparing for discharge and has the following prescriptions:

Aspirin, enteric-coated, 81 mg once a day, PO
Propranolol (Inderal) 40 mg three times a day, PO

1. Explain the purpose of the propranolol order for F.

After F. has been home for a week, the home health nurse calls F. to check on how he is doing. F. tells the nurse that he was "about to call the doctor" because he has been feeling more and more short of breath, even though he has been resting at home.

2. What could be causing this problem? What do you expect will happen as a result?

Two months later, F. is in the office for a follow-up visit. He seems upset, even though his blood pressure is within normal range, his cardiac function is stable, and he has had no further breathing problems. He tells the nurse, "I don't care what the doctor tells me, I'm going to stop that new pill. I'm having a terrible problem and I know it's because of that medicine."

3. What went wrong to cause F. to be so upset, and what will be done about it? Will the beta blocker be discontinued today? Explain your answer.

For answers, see *http://evolve.elsevier.com/Lilley*.

immediately if the patient has any problems with dizziness, fainting, or lightheadedness, or if the systolic blood pressure is lower than 100 mm Hg or the pulse rate is lower than 60 beats/min.

Recording daily weights is important to monitor the progress of therapy and check for the adverse effect of edema. A standard of care to acknowledge is that the prescriber needs to be contacted if the patient shows an increase of 2 pounds or more over a 24-hour period or 5 pounds or more within 1 week. Keeping a daily journal documenting daily weights, blood pressure readings, pulse rates, adverse effects, and overall feelings of wellness or lack thereof will be important to the monitoring of the therapeutic regimen. Other symptoms to report to the prescriber include muscle weakness, shortness of breath, and collection of fluid in the lower extremities as manifested by difficulty in putting on shoes or socks and weight gain. Patients taking any of these medications must be weaned off the drug slowly because an abrupt discontinuation could lead to rebound hypertension or chest pain. The prescriber will designate a period of time for weaning; however, it is generally over a period of 1 to 2 weeks. Understanding basic anatomy and physiology and how receptors work will help guide nursing actions related to these drugs. See Patient Centered Care: Patient Teaching for more specific information.

EVALUATION

Therapeutic effects associated with the *adrenergic-blocking drugs* include, but are not limited to, a decrease in blood pressure, pulse rate, and palpitations (in patients with these specific problems before drug therapy); alleviation of the symptoms of the disorder for which the drug was indicated; a return to normal blood pressure and pulse with lowering of the blood pressure toward 120/80 mm Hg and the pulse toward 60 beats/min in patients with diagnosed hypertension; and a decrease in chest pain in patients with angina. Also monitor patients for adverse effects associated with these medications, including bradycardia, depression, fatigue, and hypotension. See Tables 19-2 and 19-4 for other potential adverse effects.

PATIENT-CENTERED CARE: PATIENT TEACHING

- Give patients written and verbal information about drug indications, actions, adverse effects, cautions, contraindications, and drug interactions. This information needs to be age-specific and tailored to the specific learning needs of the patient.
- Emphasize the need to wear a medical alert bracelet or necklace identifying the specific medical diagnoses, and provide a list of all medications. The patient needs to understand the importance of carrying this information in written form on his or her person at all times and updating the information at least every few months or whenever there are major changes in the diagnosis and treatment regimen. Recommend to the patient that he or she also keep a card in his or her wallet or purse to record blood pressure readings by date and time. This information may then be shared with other health care professionals. A few examples of patient drug cards can be found at *www.ahrq.gov/patients-consumers/diagnosis-treatment/treatments/pillcard/pillcard.pdf* and *http://macoalition.org/Initiatives/RMToolkit.shtml.*
- Caution the patient to take medications exactly as prescribed and to never abruptly discontinue them due to the risk for rebound hypertension. If there is concern about omitted or skipped doses, the patient needs to contact the prescriber immediately.
- Caffeine and other central nervous system stimulants must be avoided while taking adrenergic-blocking drugs to prevent further irritability of the cardiac and central nervous systems and subsequent negative effects on health status.
- Alcohol ingestion is to be avoided because it causes vasodilation, which increases the risk for hypotension and postural blood pressure changes.
- Encourage the patient to contact the prescriber if he or she experiences palpitations, chest pain, confusion, weight gain (2 pounds or more in 24 hours or 5 pounds or more in 1 week), dyspnea, nausea, or vomiting. Other problems to report include swelling in the feet and ankles, shortness of breath, excessive fatigue, dizziness, and syncope.
- The alpha blocker tamsulosin must be taken as directed and with caution in patients with blood pressure problems (e.g., hypotension). The drug must also be used with caution by the older adult patient and while driving or engaging in other activities requiring alertness, because the adverse effects of this drug include blurred vision, dizziness, and drowsiness.
- Caution patients to change positions slowly to avoid dizziness and/or syncope. Excessive exercise, exposure to hot climates, use of a sauna or tanning bed, and alcohol consumption exacerbate vasodilation from the adrenergic-blocking drugs and lead to a greater drop in blood pressure with even more risk for dizziness and syncope.
- Constipation may develop as an adverse effect with alpha and beta blockers. Increasing fluids as well as fiber may help to prevent constipation.

KEY POINTS

- Adrenergic-blocking drugs block the stimulation of the alpha-, beta$_1$-, and/or beta$_2$-adrenergic receptors, with the net result of blocking the effects of either norepinephrine or epinephrine on the receptors. This blocking action leads to a variety of physiologic responses depending on which receptors are blocked. Knowing how these receptors work allows the nurse to understand and predict the expected therapeutic effects of the drugs as well as the expected adverse effects.
- With alpha blockers, the predominant response is vasodilation. This is due to blocking of the alpha-adrenergic

effect of vasoconstriction, which results in blood vessel relaxation.

- Vasodilation of blood vessels with the alpha blockers results in a drop in blood pressure and a reduction in urinary obstruction, which may lead to increased urinary flow rates. Monitor for these effects in patients taking alpha blockers.
- Beta blockers inhibit the stimulation of beta-adrenergic receptors by blocking the effects of the SNS neurotransmitters norepinephrine, epinephrine, and dopamine. Stimulation of beta$_1$ receptors leads to an increase in heart rate, conduction, and contractility. Stimulation of beta$_2$ receptors results in bronchial smooth muscle relaxation or bronchodilation. Blocking of beta$_1$ receptors results in a *decrease* in heart rate, conduction, and contractility. Blocking of beta$_2$ receptors leads to a *decrease* in bronchial smooth muscle relaxation, or bronchoconstriction.
- Beta blockers are classified as either selective or nonselective. Selective beta blockers are also called *cardioselective beta blockers* and block only the beta-adrenergic receptors in the heart that are located on the postsynaptic effector cells (i.e., the cells that nerves stimulate). The beneficial effects of the cardioselective beta blockers include decreased heart rate, reduced cardiac conduction, and decreased myocardial contractility with no bronchoconstriction. These drugs are a good choice for patients with hypertension who also have bronchospastic airway disease or other pulmonary disease.
- Nonselective beta blockers block both beta$_1$- and beta$_2$-adrenergic receptors and affect the heart and bronchial smooth muscle. These drugs are used to treat patients with hypertension who do not have a problem with bronchospasm or pulmonary airway disease.
- Nursing considerations for patients taking alpha and beta blockers include teaching patients that they must weigh themselves daily, avoid sudden changes in position, and increase intake of fluids and fiber. Weight gain, dizziness, fainting, and/or a decrease in heart rate below 60 beats/min or a blood pressure of less than 100 mm Hg systolic or less than 80 mm Hg diastolic need to be reported immediately.

NCLEX® EXAMINATION REVIEW QUESTIONS

1. When a patient has experienced extravasation of a peripheral infusion of dopamine, the nurse will inject the alpha blocker phentolamine (Regitine) into the area of extravasation and expect which effect?
   a. Vasoconstriction
   b. Vasodilation
   c. Analgesia
   d. Hypotension
2. When administering beta blockers, the nurse will follow which guideline for administration and monitoring?
   a. The drug may be discontinued at any time.
   b. Postural hypotension rarely occurs with this drug.
   c. Tapering off the medication is necessary to prevent rebound hypertension.
   d. The patient needs to stop taking the medication at once if he or she gains 3 to 4 pounds in a week.
3. The nurse providing teaching for a patient who has a new prescription for beta$_1$ blockers will keep in mind that these drugs may result in which effect?
   a. Tachycardia
   b. Tachypnea
   c. Bradycardia
   d. Bradypnea
4. A patient who has recently had a myocardial infarction (MI) has started therapy with a beta blocker. The nurse explains that the main purpose of the beta blocker for this patient is to
   a. cause vasodilation of the coronary arteries.
   b. prevent hypertension.
   c. increase conduction through the SA node.
   d. protect the heart from circulating catecholamines. ✳

5. Before initiating therapy with a nonselective beta blocker, the nurse will assess the patient for a history of which condition?
   a. Hypertension
   b. Liver disease
   c. Pancreatitis
   d. Asthma
6. A patient is taking an alpha blocker as treatment for benign prostatic hyperplasia. The nurse will monitor for which potential drug effects? *(Select all that apply.)*
   a. Orthostatic hypotension
   b. Increased blood pressure
   c. Increased urine flow
   d. Headaches
   e. Bradycardia
7. A child in the pediatric ICU has been receiving a dopamine infusion. This morning while on rounds, the nurse noted that the IV has infiltrated. After stopping the infusion, the nurse prepares to administer phentolamine (Regitine). The ordered dose is 0.2 mg/kg, to be injected into the area of extravasation. The child weighs 39 lb. How many milligrams will the nurse administer? *(Record your answer using one decimal place.)*
8. The nurse is reviewing the mechanism of action of alpha adrenergic drugs. Adrenergic blockade at the alpha receptors leads to which effects? *(Select all that apply).*
   a. Miosis
   b. Vasodilation
   c. Vasoconstriction
   d. Bradycardia
   e. Reduced blood pressure

1. b, 2. c, 3. c, 4. d, 5. d, 6. a, c, d, 7. 3.5 mg, 8. a, b, e.

CRITICAL THINKING AND PRIORITIZATION QUESTIONS

1. A 46-year-old woman is now taking propranolol (Inderal) for the control of tachycardia and hypertension. What is the nurse's priority in answering if the patient states, "Well, if it doesn't work after a month or two, I'll just quit taking it!"

2. A 73-year-old man is given a new prescription for tamsulosin (Flomax) for treatment of BPH. He lives at home with his wife and uses a cane to help him walk because of the effects of a stroke he had 5 years ago. During the patient education session, the nurse should emphasize which issue of highest priority?

For answers, see *http://evolve.elsevier.com/Lilley.*

ⓔ EVOLVE WEBSITE

http://evolve.elsevier.com/Lilley
- Animations
- Answer Keys for Textbook Case Studies and Textbook Critical Thinking and Prioritization Questions

- Content Updates
- Key Points
- Review Questions
- Student Case Studies

Cholinergic Drugs

OBJECTIVES

When you reach the end of this chapter, you will be able to do the following:

1. Briefly review the functions of the autonomic nervous system and the impact of the parasympathetic division.
2. List the various drugs classified as cholinergic agonists (also called *parasympathomimetics*).
3. Discuss the mechanisms of action, therapeutic effects, indications, adverse and toxic effects, drug interactions, cautions, contraindications, dosages, routes of administration, and any antidotal management for the various cholinergic agonists (or parasympathomimetics).
4. Develop a nursing care plan that includes all phases of the nursing process for patients taking cholinergic agonists.

DRUG PROFILES

♦ **bethanechol, p. 324**
♦ **donepezil, p. 325**
♦ **memantine, p. 325**
♦ **pyridostigmine, p. 325**

♦ = *Key drug*
❗ = *High-alert drug*

KEY TERMS

Acetylcholine The neurotransmitter responsible for transmission of nerve impulses to effector cells in the parasympathetic nervous system. (p. 321)

Acetylcholinesterase The enzyme responsible for the breakdown of acetylcholine. (p. 322)

Alzheimer's disease A disease of the brain that is characterized by progressive mental deterioration manifested by confusion, disorientation, and loss of memory, ability to calculate, and visual-spatial orientation. (p. 323)

Atony A lack of normal muscle tone. (p. 323)

Cholinergic crisis Severe muscle weakness and respiratory paralysis due to excessive acetylcholine; often seen in patients with myasthenia gravis as an adverse effect of drugs used to treat the disorder. (p. 324)

Cholinergic receptor A nerve receptor that is stimulated by acetylcholine. (p. 321)

Miosis The contraction of the pupil. (p. 323)

Muscarinic receptors Cholinergic receptors that are located postsynaptically in the *effector organs* such as smooth muscle, cardiac muscle, and glands supplied by parasympathetic fibers. (p. 321)

Nicotinic receptors Cholinergic receptors located in the *ganglia* (where presynaptic and postsynaptic nerve fibers meet) of both the parasympathetic nervous system and the sympathetic nervous system; so named because they can be stimulated by the alkaloid nicotine. (p. 321)

Parasympathomimetics Drugs that mimic the parasympathetic nervous system; also referred to as *cholinergic agonist drugs*. (p. 322)

OVERVIEW

Cholinergic drugs, cholinergic agonists, and *parasympathomimetics* are all terms that refer to the class of drugs that stimulate the parasympathetic nervous system.

PARASYMPATHETIC NERVOUS SYSTEM

The parasympathetic nervous system (PNS) is the branch of the autonomic nervous system with functions opposite those of the sympathetic nervous system (Figure 20-1). Acetylcholine is the neurotransmitter responsible for the transmission of nerve impulses to effector cells in the parasympathetic nervous system. A cholinergic receptor is a receptor that binds acetylcholine and mediates its actions. There are two types of cholinergic receptors, as determined by their location and their action. Nicotinic receptors are located in the ganglia of both the parasympathetic nervous system and sympathetic nervous system. They are called *nicotinic* because they can also be stimulated by nicotine. The other type of cholinergic receptor is the muscarinic receptor. Muscarinic receptors are located postsynaptically in the effector organs (i.e., smooth muscle,

321

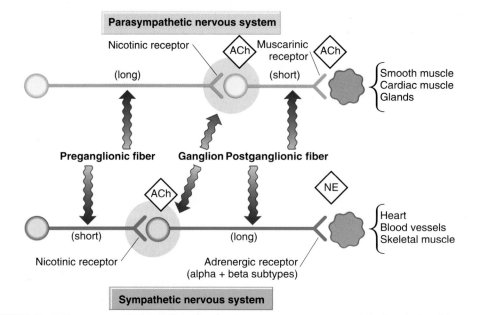

FIGURE 20-1 Parasympathetic and sympathetic nervous systems and their relationship to one another. *ACh*, Acetylcholine; *NE*, norepinephrine.

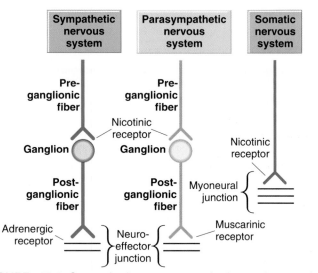

FIGURE 20-2 Sympathetic, parasympathetic, and somatic nervous systems. Note the location of the nicotinic and muscarinic receptors in the parasympathetic nervous system.

BOX 20-1   Cholinergic Drugs

Direct-Acting Drugs
bethanechol (Urecholine)
carbachol (Carboptic, others)
cevimeline (Evoxac)
pilocarpine (Salagen, Pilocar [see Chapter 57], others)
succinylcholine (Anectine, Quelicin; see Chapter 11)

Indirect-Acting Drugs
donepezil (Aricept)
echothiophate (Phospholine Iodide; see Chapter 57)
edrophonium (Tensilon, others)
galantamine (Razadyne)
neostigmine (Prostigmin)
physostigmine (Antilirium)
pyridostigmine (Mestinon)
rivastigmine (Exelon)

---

cardiac muscle, and glands) supplied by the parasympathetic fibers. They are called *muscarinic* because they are stimulated by the alkaloid muscarine, a substance isolated from mushrooms. Figure 20-2 shows how the nicotinic and muscarinic receptors are arranged in the parasympathetic nervous system.

CHOLINERGIC DRUGS

Cholinergic drugs, also known as cholinergic *agonists* or para-sympathomimetics, mimic the effects of acetylcholine. These drugs can stimulate cholinergic receptors either directly or indirectly. *Direct-acting* cholinergic agonists bind directly to

cholinergic receptors and activate them. *Indirect-acting* cholinergic agonists stimulate the postsynaptic release of acetylcholine at the receptor site. This then allows acetylcholine to bind to and stimulate the receptor. Indirect-acting cholinergic drugs (also known as *cholinesterase inhibitors*) work by inhibiting the action of acetylcholinesterase. Acetylcholinesterase is the enzyme responsible for breaking down acetylcholine and is also referred to as *cholinesterase*. There are two categories of cholinesterase inhibitors: reversible inhibitors and irreversible inhibitors. *Reversible* cholinesterase inhibitors bind to cholinesterase for a short period, whereas *irreversible* cholinesterase inhibitors have a long duration of activity, and the body must generate new cholinesterase enzymes to override the effects of the irreversible drugs. Box 20-1 lists the direct- and indirect-acting cholinergics.

Mechanism of Action and Drug Effects

When acetylcholine directly binds to its receptor, stimulation occurs. Once binding takes place on the membranes of an effector cell (cell of the target tissue or organ), the permeability of the cell changes, and calcium and sodium are permitted to flow into the cell. This then depolarizes the cell membrane and stimulates the effector organ.

The effects of direct- and indirect-acting cholinergic drugs are seen when the parasympathetic nervous system is stimulated. There are many mnemonics to aid in remembering these effects. One is to think of the parasympathetic nervous system as the "rest and digest" system, in contrast to the "flight or fight" sympathetic nervous system.

Cholinergic drugs are used primarily for their target effects on the gastrointestinal (GI) tract, bladder, and eye. These drugs stimulate the intestine and bladder, which results in increased gastric secretions, GI motility, and urinary frequency. They also stimulate constriction of the pupil, termed miosis. This helps decrease intraocular pressure. In addition, cholinergic drugs cause increased salivation and sweating. Cardiovascular effects include reduced heart rate and vasodilation. Pulmonary effects include causing the bronchi of the lungs to constrict and the airways to narrow.

At recommended dosages, cholinergic drugs primarily affect the muscarinic receptors, but at high dosages, the nicotinic receptors can also be stimulated. The desired effects come from muscarinic receptor stimulation; many of the undesirable adverse effects are due to nicotinic receptor stimulation. The various effects of the cholinergic drugs are listed in Table 20-1 according to the receptors stimulated.

Indications

Direct-Acting Drugs

Direct-acting drugs, such as carbachol, pilocarpine, and echothiophate, are used topically to reduce intraocular pressure in patients with glaucoma or in those undergoing ocular surgery (see Chapter 57). They are poorly absorbed orally, which limits their use mostly to topical application. One exception is the direct-acting cholinergic drug bethanechol, which is administered orally. Bethanechol affects the detrusor muscle of the urinary bladder and also the smooth muscle of the GI tract. It causes increased bladder and GI tract tone and motility, which increases the movement of contents through these areas. It also causes the sphincters in the bladder and the GI tract to relax, allowing them to empty. Bethanechol is also used postoperatively to treat atony of the bladder and GI tract. The direct-acting drug, cevimeline, is used to treat excessively dry mouth (xerostomia) resulting from a disorder known as *Sjögren's syndrome*. Oral pilocarpine can also be used for this purpose. Another direct-acting cholinergic is succinylcholine, which is used as a neuromuscular blocker in general anesthesia (see Chapter 11).

Indirect-Acting Drugs

Indirect-acting drugs work by increasing acetylcholine concentrations at the receptor sites, which leads to stimulation of the effector cells. Indirect-acting drugs cause skeletal muscle contraction and are used for the diagnosis and treatment of myasthenia gravis.

TABLE 20-1	Cholinergic Agonists: Drug Effects	
	RESPONSE TO STIMULATION	
Body Tissue/Organ	**Muscarinic**	**Nicotinic**
Bronchi (lung)	Increased secretions, constriction	None
Cardiovascular		
Blood vessels	Dilation	Constriction
Heart rate	Slowed	Increased
Blood pressure	Decreased	Increased
Eye	Miosis (pupil constriction), decreased accommodation	Miosis (pupil constriction), decreased accommodation
Gastrointestinal		
Tone	Increased	Increased
Motility	Increased	Increased
Sphincter	Relaxed	None
Genitourinary		
Tone	Increased	Increased
Motility	Increased	Increased
Sphincter	Relaxed	Relaxed
Glandular secretions	Increased intestinal, lacrimal, salivary, and sweat gland secretion	—
Skeletal muscle	—	Increased contraction

Their ability to inhibit acetylcholinesterase makes them useful for the reversal of neuromuscular blockade produced either by neuromuscular blocking drugs or by anticholinergic poisoning. The indirect-acting drug physostigmine is considered the antidote for anticholinergic poisoning as well as poisoning by irreversible cholinesterase inhibitors such as the organophosphates and carbamates, which are common classes of insecticides.

Indirect-acting drugs are also used to treat Alzheimer's disease, which is a neurologic disorder in which patients have decreased levels of acetylcholine. In the treatment of Alzheimer's disease, cholinergic drugs increase concentrations of acetylcholine in the brain by inhibiting cholinesterase. This increase in acetylcholine levels helps to enhance and maintain memory and learning capabilities. There are three cholinesterase inhibitors used to treat Alzheimer's disease, including donepezil (Aricept), galantamine (Razadyne), and rivastigmine (Exelon); all are indirect-acting cholinergic drugs. Although their therapeutic efficacy is often limited (it has been reported that only 15% to 30% of patients treated see benefits), these drugs may enhance a patient's mental status enough to cause a noticeable, if temporary, improvement in the quality of life for patients as well as caregivers and family members. Patient response to these drugs is highly variable. Failure to respond to maximally titrated dosages of one of these drugs does not necessarily rule out an attempt at therapy with another drug in this same class. Memantine (Namenda) is also used to treat Alzheimer's disease, but it is not a cholinesterase inhibitor. For dosage information on these drugs, see the table on the next page.

Contraindications

Contraindications to the use of cholinergic drugs include known drug allergy, GI or genitourinary (GU) tract obstruction, bradycardia, defects in cardiac impulse conduction, hyperthyroidism, epilepsy, hypotension, or chronic obstructive pulmonary disease. Parkinson's disease (see Chapter 15) is listed as a precaution to these drugs; however, rivastigmine (Exelon) is used in patients with Parkinson's disease who also have dementia.

Adverse Effects

The primary adverse effects of cholinergic drugs are the consequence of overstimulation of the parasympathetic nervous system. The major effects are listed by body system in Table 20-2. The effects on the cardiovascular system are complex and may include syncope, hypotension with reflex tachycardia, hypertension, or bradycardia, depending on if the muscarinic or nicotinic receptors are stimulated.

Toxicity and Management of Overdose

The most severe consequence of an overdose of an orally administered cholinergic drug is a cholinergic crisis. Symptoms include circulatory collapse, hypotension, bloody diarrhea,

shock, and cardiac arrest. Early signs include abdominal cramps, salivation, flushing of the skin, nausea, and vomiting. Transient syncope, transient complete heart block, dyspnea, and orthostatic hypotension may also occur. These can be reversed promptly by the administration of atropine, a cholinergic antagonist. Severe cardiovascular reactions or bronchoconstriction may be alleviated by epinephrine, an adrenergic agonist. One way of remembering the effects of cholinergic poisoning is to use the acronym *SLUDGE*, which stands for *s*alivation, *l*acrimation, *u*rinary incontinence, *d*iarrhea, GI cramps, and *e*mesis.

Interactions

Anticholinergics (such as atropine), antihistamines, and sympathomimetics may antagonize cholinergic drugs and lead to a reduced response to them. Other cholinergic drugs may have additive effects.

Dosages

For the recommended dosages of the cholinergic drugs, see the dosages table below.

DRUG PROFILES

◆bethanechol

Bethanechol (Urecholine) is a direct-acting cholinergic agonist. It is used in the treatment of acute postoperative and postpartum nonobstructive urinary retention and for the management of urinary retention associated with neurogenic atony of the bladder. Bethanechol is available orally. Contraindications include known drug allergy, hyperthyroidism, peptic ulcer, active bronchial asthma, cardiac disease or coronary artery disease, epilepsy, and parkinsonism. It is to be avoided in patients in whom the strength or integrity of the GI tract or bladder wall is questionable.

TABLE 20-2	Cholinergic Agonists: Adverse Effects	
Body System	**Adverse Effects**
Cardiovascular	Bradycardia or tachycardia, hypotension or hypertension, syncope, conduction abnormalities
Central nervous	Headache, dizziness, convulsions, ataxia
Gastrointestinal	Abdominal cramps, increased secretions, nausea, vomiting, diarrhea
Respiratory	Increased bronchial secretions, bronchospasm
Other	Lacrimation, sweating, salivation, miosis

DOSAGES

Selected Cholinergic Agonist Drugs

Drug (Pregnancy Category)	Pharmacologic Class	Usual Adult Dosage Range	Indications/Uses
◆bethanechol (Urecholine) (C)	Muscarinic (direct-acting)	PO: 10-50 mg tid-qid (usually start with 5-10 mg, repeating hourly until urination, max 50 mg/cycle)	Postoperative and postpartum functional urinary retention
◆donepezil (Aricept) (C)	Anticholinesterase (indirect-acting)	PO: 5-23 mg/day as a single dose	Alzheimer's dementia
◆memantine (Namenda, Namenda XR) (B)	NMDA-receptor antagonist	PO: Initial dose is 5 mg/day; titrate by 5 mg/wk up to a target dose of 10 mg/bid (20 mg/day) Namenda XR: 7-28 mg/day	Alzheimer's dementia
physostigmine (Antilirium) (C)	Anticholinesterase (indirect-acting)	IM/IV; 0.5-2 mg repeated every 10-30 min if needed	Reversal of anticholinergic drug effects and tricyclic antidepressant overdose
◆pyridostigmine (Mestinon) (C)	Anticholinesterase (indirect-acting)	PO: 600 mg/day in divided doses IV: 0.1-0.25 mg/kg/dose	Myasthenia gravis Antidote for neuromuscular blocker toxicity

NMDA, N-methyl-d-aspartate.

Adverse effects include syncope, hypotension with reflex tachycardia, headache, seizure, GI upset, and asthmatic attacks. Drugs that interact with bethanechol include acetylcholinesterase inhibitors (i.e., indirect-acting cholinergics), which can enhance the adverse effects of bethanechol. Recommended dosages are given in the table on the previous page.

Pharmacokinetics: Bethanechol

Route	Onset of Action	Peak Plasma Concentration	Elimination Half-life	Duration of Action
PO	30-90 min	Less than 30 min	Unknown	1-6 hr

◆ donepezil

Donepezil (Aricept) is a cholinesterase inhibitor that works centrally in the brain to increase levels of acetylcholine by inhibiting acetylcholinesterase. It is used in the treatment of mild to moderate Alzheimer's disease. Similar cholinesterase inhibitors include galantamine and rivastigmine. Rivastigmine is also approved for treating dementia associated with Parkinson's disease. Contraindications for donepezil include known drug allergy. Adverse effects are normally mild and resolve on their own and can often be avoided by careful dose titration. They include GI upset (including ulcer risk due to increased gastric secretions), drowsiness, dizziness, insomnia, and muscle cramps. The effects on the cardiovascular system are complex and may include bradycardia, syncope, hypotension with reflex tachycardia, or hypertension. Interacting drugs include anticholinergics (counteract donepezil effects) and nonsteroidal antiinflammatory drugs (see Chapter 44). Donepezil is available only for oral use as both a tablet and a rapid-acting, orally disintegrating tablet. Recommended dosages are given in the table on the previous page.

Pharmacokinetics: Donepezil

Route	Onset of Action	Peak Plasma Concentration	Elimination Half-life	Duration of Action
PO	3 wk	3-4 hr	70 hr	2 wk

◆ memantine

Memantine (Namenda) is not a cholinergic drug, but it is being included here in the discussion of drugs for Alzheimer's dementia. It is classified as an N-methyl-D-aspartate (NMDA) receptor antagonist owing to its inhibitory activity at the NMDA receptors in the central nervous system. Stimulation of these receptors is believed to be part of the Alzheimer's disease process. Memantine blocks this stimulation and thereby helps to reduce or arrest the patient's degenerative cognitive symptoms. As with all other currently available medications for this debilitating illness, the effects of this drug are likely to be temporary but may still afford some improvement in quality of life and general functioning for some patients. Its only current contraindication is known drug allergy. Reported adverse effects are relatively uncommon but include hypotension, headache, GI upset, musculoskeletal pain, dyspnea, ataxia, and fatigue. No clearly defined drug interactions are listed.

Memantine is available only for oral use. The recommended dosage is given in the table on the previous page.

Pharmacokinetics: Memantine

Route	Onset of Action	Peak Plasma Concentration	Elimination Half-life	Duration of Action
PO	Unknown	5 hr	70 hr	Unknown

◆ pyridostigmine

Pyridostigmine (Mestinon) is a synthetic quaternary ammonium compound that is similar in structure to other drugs in this class, including edrophonium, physostigmine, and neostigmine. All are indirect-acting cholinergic drugs that work to increase acetylcholine by inhibiting acetylcholinesterase. Pyridostigmine has been shown to improve muscle strength and is used to relieve the symptoms of myasthenia gravis, and it is the most commonly used drug for symptomatic treatment of myasthenia gravis. Edrophonium (Tensilon) is an indirect-acting cholinergic drug that is used to diagnose myasthenia gravis. It can also be used to differentiate between myasthenia gravis and cholinergic crisis. Neostigmine, pyridostigmine, and physostigmine are also useful for reversing the effects of nondepolarizing neuromuscular blocking drugs (see Chapter 11) after surgery. They are also used in the treatment of severe overdoses of tricyclic antidepressants because of the significant anticholinergic effects associated with the tricyclic antidepressants. Physostigmine, neostigmine, and pyridostigmine are also used as an antidote after toxic exposure to nondrug anticholinergic agents, including those used in chemical warfare. Contraindications to these drugs include known drug allergy, prior severe cholinergic reactions, asthma, gangrene, hyperthyroidism, cardiovascular disease, and mechanical obstruction of the GI or GU tracts. Adverse effects include GI upset and excessive salivation. Interacting drugs include the anticholinergic drugs, which counteract the therapeutic effects of indirect-acting cholinergic drugs. Pyridostigmine is available in oral and injectable forms. Recommended dosages are given in the table on the previous page.

Pharmacokinetics: Pyridostigmine

Route	Onset of Action	Peak Plasma Concentration	Elimination Half-life	Duration of Action
Oral/IM	15-45 min	1-2 hours	3-4 hr	Up to 6 hr
IV	2-5 min	Immediate	1-2 hr	2-3 hr

NURSING PROCESS

ASSESSMENT

Cholinergic drugs, or *parasympathomimetics,* produce a variety of effects stemming from their ability to stimulate the parasympathetic nervous system and mimic the action of acetylcholine. These effects include a decrease in heart rate, increase in gastrointestinal (GI) and genitourinary (GU) tone through increased contractility of the smooth muscle of the bowel and bladder, increase in the contractility and tone of bronchial smooth muscle, increased respiratory secretions, and miosis or pupillary constriction. Therefore, if the patient has any preexisting conditions, such as heart block, or if the patient is taking other drugs that mimic the actions of the parasympathetic nervous system, adverse effects or toxicity may be increased. Before *cholinergic drugs* are given, perform a thorough head-to-toe physical examination, and obtain a nursing history and medication history (including prescription drugs, over-the-counter drugs, and herbals; see Chapter 7). Document drug allergies and past and present medical conditions. Identify cautions, contraindications, and drug interactions. Assess vital signs, and document with special attention to baseline blood pressure readings because of the potential for orthostatic hypotension.

Before a drug for Alzheimer's disease, such as *donepezil* or *memantine*, is used, assess the patient for allergies, cautions, contraindications, and drug interactions. Perform a close assessment and documentation of the patient's neurologic status with attention to short- and long-term memory; level of alertness; motor, cognitive, and sensory functioning; any suicidal tendencies or thoughts; musculoskeletal intactness; and GI, GU, and cardiovascular functioning. Assess urinary patterns so that any problems with urinary retention may be identified. Report any abnormalities and/or complaints to the prescriber immediately. It is important to note the presence or absence of family support systems because of the chronic nature of this illness. Once the patient has begun taking medication, it is critical for you to continue to assess the patient's response to the drug. Especially note any changes in symptoms within the first 6 weeks of therapy. Journaling may be helpful to the prescriber to assess any positive changes and any adverse effects and/or lack of improvement. Ginkgo may be used by some health care providers for organic brain syndrome (see the Safety: Herbal Therapies and Dietary Supplements box).

NURSING DIAGNOSES

1. Decreased cardiac output related to adverse cardiovascular effects of hypotension and bradycardia
2. Deficient knowledge of the therapeutic regimen, adverse effects, drug interactions, and precautions for cholinergic drugs related to lack of experience with drug therapies
3. Risk for injury related to the possible adverse effects of cholinergic drugs, such as bradycardia and hypotension, with subsequent risk for falls or syncope

PLANNING: OUTCOME IDENTIFICATION

1. Patient maintains normal cardiac output/status through safe, self-administration of medication, monitoring blood pressure and pulse rate daily, and reporting adverse effects of dizziness, syncope, excess fatigue, and lightheadedness.
2. Patient, caregiver, or family member demonstrates adequate knowledge about use of prescribed medication with onset of action (for Alzheimer's disease) of several weeks and its use for symptomatic control not curative action.
3. Patient, caregiver, or family member demonstrates an understanding about the need to implement safety measures to

CASE STUDY

Patient-Centered Care: Donepezil (Aricept) for Alzheimer's Disease

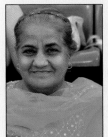

E. is a 72-year-old woman married to G., who is 73 years of age. G. has noticed that E. is becoming more forgetful but did not worry about it until she got lost while driving home from the grocery store. G. makes an appointment for E. to see their primary care physician, Dr. S. After the examination, Dr. S. tells G., in private, that she thinks that E. is in the early stages of Alzheimer's disease but will order some tests to rule out other problems. G. then accompanies Dr. S. while she tells E. of the tentative diagnosis. Understandably, E. is upset to hear this news.

1. In her discussion with E. and her husband, Dr. S. mentioned a drug called donepezil (Aricept) that can be used in the early stages of Alzheimer's disease. It may be started after a few diagnostic tests are performed. After Dr. S. leaves the room, E. asks the nurse, "What will this drug do for me? Will it stop the Alzheimer's disease?" How will the nurse reply?

   Several diagnostic tests are performed, including a complete blood count, serum electrolyte levels, vitamin B_{12} levels, liver and thyroid function tests, and a magnetic resonance imaging scan to rule out other neurologic diseases. Results of all tests are within normal limits. Dr. S. decides to prescribe donepezil, 5 mg, daily, for E. with an oral dissolving tablet.

2. G. is not sure about the oral dissolving tablet. "Can't she just swallow it?" What will the nurse teach them about taking this form of the drug?

3. After 6 weeks, G. brings E. back to the doctor's office for a follow-up appointment. G. privately tells Dr. S. that he is "upset" because he has noticed very little improvement. E. tells Dr. S. that she feels "fine" and has not noticed any problems. What do you think will be Dr. S.'s next order at this time? Is E.'s response to the donepezil typical? Explain your answer.

For answers, see *http://evolve.elsevier.com/Lilley.*

SAFETY: HERBAL THERAPIES AND DIETARY SUPPLEMENTS

Ginkgo (Ginkgo biloba)

Overview
The dried leaf of the ginkgo plant contains flavonoids, terpenoids, and organic acids that help ginkgo preparations exert their positive effects as an antioxidant and inhibitor of platelet aggregation.

Common Uses
To prevent memory loss, peripheral arterial occlusive disease, vertigo, tinnitus

Adverse Effects
Stomach or intestinal upset, headache, bleeding, allergic skin reaction

Potential Drug Interactions
Aspirin, nonsteroidal antiinflammatory drugs, warfarin, heparin, anticonvulsants, ticlopidine, clopidogrel, dipyridamole, antidepressants, antihypertensives, insulin, thiazide diuretics

Contraindications
None

avoid falls such as taking time to move slowly from lying/sitting to standing, taking purposeful movements, and using compression stockings.

IMPLEMENTATION

Several nursing interventions may help to maximize the therapeutic effects and minimize the adverse effects of *cholinergic drugs*. If the indication for use of the cholinergic drug is for postoperative-related decreased GI peristalsis, make sure to encourage ambulation and increased intake of fluids and fiber, unless contraindicated. Early postoperative ambulation helps to increase GI peristalsis and may even possibly prevent the need for these cholinergic drugs (i.e., *bethanechol*). However, do not administer these drugs if there is suspicion that there may be a mechanical obstruction. This diagnosis would be confirmed by a variety of diagnostic testing and clinical signs and symptoms. Some of these symptoms would include abdominal distention, hypoactive to no bowel sounds, inability to pass flatus or bowel movements, nausea, vomiting, and abdominal pain. Use of cholinergic drugs, in a mechanical obstruction, may result in bowel perforation and peritonitis. It is always preferable to use nonpharmacologic measures rather than pharmacologic regimens to treat the anticipated postoperative problems of decreased peristalsis and/or urinary retention. For drugs used to treat myasthenia gravis, give the oral medication about 30 minutes before meals to allow for onset of action and therapeutic effects (e.g., decreased dysphagia or decreased difficulty swallowing). Atropine is the antidote to a cholinergic overdose; therefore, this medication needs to be readily available and given per the prescriber's order.

Drugs used in the treatment of Alzheimer's disease are not for curative purposes. It is important to compassionately and empathically discuss with patients, family, and caregivers that there is no cure for the disease but some improvement of function and cognition may occur with drug therapy. The diagnosis of Alzheimer's disease and/or dementia is shocking, at best. Those involved in the care of the patient need to be honest in sharing information with the patient, family, significant others, and caregivers. Always follow ethical standards of practice when working with patients, and adhere to the American Nurses Association *Code of Ethics for Nurses*. This code outlines behaviors required to maintain a high level of professionalism and specific actions that demonstrate respect for patient rights in any patient care situation. However, any sharing of information with the patient, family, significant others, and caregivers must be done with the approval of the prescriber, with good intent, in compliance with any research protocol, and/or with the goal of being a patient advocate.

With the starting of drug therapy for Alzheimer's disease, the patient will most likely need continued assistance and help with activities of daily living (ADLs) and ambulation. At the initiation of drug therapy, the patient will continue to need assistance because of drug-related dizziness and subsequent gait imbalances. The patient, family members, and caregivers also need to understand the importance of taking the medication exactly as ordered. Dosages and exact scheduling of medications is critical for the patient and family/caregiver to understand in order to

achieve the drug's maximum therapeutic effects. In addition, instruct the patient and anyone involved in the patient's daily care about how to take the medication (e.g., taking the drug with food to decrease GI upset). Encourage the patient and family/caregiver to educate themselves about the use of the drug, its adverse effects, possible interactions, and potential for harm, and emphasize the importance of *not* withdrawing the medication abruptly. If discontinuing of the drug is ordered, the patient must be weaned off over a period as designated by the prescriber. If weaning does not occur, there is the potential for a rapid decline in cognitive functioning and the patient's condition. Dissolving forms of the medication *donepezil* are to be placed on the tongue and allowed to dissolve before the patient drinks fluids or swallows.

Most of the *cholinergic agonists* have dose-limiting adverse effects that include severe GI disturbances such as nausea and vomiting. Blood pressure readings and pulse rates need to be taken and recorded before, during, and after initiation of drug therapy. Dizziness may occur with therapy, resulting in the need for assistance with ambulation and other ADLs. Maintenance of a daily journal by the patient, family, or caregiver is helpful in recording daily doses of drugs, ability of the patient to participate in ADLs, motor ability, gait, mental status, cognition, and any adverse effects. This would provide valuable information to any health care provider or caregiver involved in the patient's day-to-day care.

Dosages of these medications may be changed by the prescriber after about 6 weeks if no therapeutic response occurs. For patient safety, blood pressure, pulse rate, and electrocardiogram need to be carefully monitored throughout therapy. Instruct the patient, family, or caregiver to report any cardiac problems such as decrease in pulse rate (less than 60 beats/min) and/or drop in blood pressure. An overdose of cholinergic drugs may result in a cholinergic crisis. Early signs include abdominal cramping, flushing of the skin, nausea and vomiting, and salivation progressing to circulatory collapse, hypotension, and cardiac arrest. Transient syncope, orthostatic hypotension, and dyspnea may also occur. *SLUDGE* is an acronym used to remember the effects of cholinergic crisis (see pharmacology discussion).

In summary, because most of the cholinergic drugs are used to treat patients diagnosed with Alzheimer's disease, closely monitor the patient's family, significant others, and caregivers. Be sure that there is ample opportunity for time to answer questions, address short- and long-term concerns, and assess their needs. *Preplanned* educational sessions that address these concerns is an important part of a holistic approach to patient care and to the meeting of patient needs. Often the best place to begin in terms of education is to prepare answers to the following questions that are often posed: What should we expect for our loved one? What will happen to the person emotionally and physically? What treatments are available, and what drugs are deemed safe? What are the common adverse effects of drug therapy, and how can they be minimized? What about diet, fluids, and exercise for our loved one? Are there herbals or any supplements or over-the-counter drugs that would help with the disease, or should they be avoided? What will we need to do for long-term care or other living situations for our loved one?

What are the expected costs of our loved one's care now and in the future? What are the costs of drug therapy? Other costs? What kind of help can we all receive emotionally? What about emotional support for our loved one? How can this disease affect intimate relationships? What type of attorney should we seek out? What about durable power of attorney and living wills? Other types of wills? Are these needed right away if we don't have these legal documents already? How do we all go on with our lives when our loved one is changing so drastically? Will life ever be normal again? What about research and clinical trials for treatment regimens? Should we pursue other treatments or do nothing new? What about drugs that are not yet FDA-approved? How long will this process take? Just what can we expect over time?

EVALUATION

Monitor patients for the following therapeutic effects: (1) in patients with myasthenia gravis, a decrease in the signs and symptoms of the disease; (2) in patients experiencing a decrease in GI peristalsis postoperatively, an increase in bowel sounds, the passage of flatus, and the occurrence of bowel movements (all indicating an increase in peristalsis); and (3) in patients who have a hypotonic bladder with urinary retention, micturition (voiding) within about 60 minutes of the administration of *bethanechol*. Also monitor for adverse effects of these medications, including increased respiratory secretions, bronchospasm, nausea, vomiting, diarrhea, hypotension, bradycardia, and conduction abnormalities. For other adverse effects, see Table 20-2.

Therapeutic effects of the drugs used to manage Alzheimer's disease–related dementia or cognitive impairment include an improvement in the symptoms of the disease. In most cases, it may take up to 6 weeks for these effects to become apparent. Varying degrees of improvement in mood and a decrease in confusion usually occur. Adverse effects include nausea, vomiting, dizziness, and others (see individual drug profiles for specific information).

QSEN ▎**EVIDENCE-BASED PRACTICE**

Walking Stabilizes Cognitive Functioning in Alzheimer's Disease (AD) Across One Year

Review

Alzheimer's disease (AD) seriously impacts cognition, mood, and daily activities. AD is a public health issue affecting 1 out of every 8 Americans 65 years of age and older as well as almost one-half of all Americans 85 years of age and older. In 2010, California alone reported some 480,000 individuals affected by AD with a 50% increase expected in 15 years. The consequences of AD are devastating for the individual and the family with impairment of cognitive-behavioral functioning and disruption of activities of daily living. It is because of these consequences that the identification of promising treatment strategies is needed.

Exercise is one such promising strategy, and several studies involving older adults have suggested that physical activity may slow the progression in the decline of cognitive function, improve performance on cognition and mood tests, and enhance the quality of sleep. Along with these epidemiologic studies are a limited number of clinical studies linked to increased physical activity in healthy older adults to improved cognition. The epidemiologic, clinical, and neuroimaging studies are supported by animal research showing enhanced cerebral function through upregulation of neurotropic factors, increased blood flow, reduced oxidative stress, as well as reduced beta-amyloid in response to exercise. Additionally, the benefits of exercise on cognition are supported in controlled trials in normal aging adults.

Type of Evidence

This study was designed to look at the relationship between exercise and mood in early stage patients with AD from California over a 1-year period. Within California, nine of ten Alzheimer's Research Centers of California (ARCCs) were involved in recruiting cognitively impaired participants for this study. Written consents were obtained from the participants or their designated surrogate. The study used a mixed Analysis of Covariance (ANCOVA) for all of the primary outcome analytical measures. In the repeated measures design, the change in (MMSE) over a 1-year interval was the dependent variable, and age, years of education, and gender were the covariates (see article for a further description). Changes to mood/affect (GDS, POMS), behavior/psychiatric symptoms (NPI), functional abilities (BRDRS and FAQ), and physical activities (YALE) were evaluated only with respect to their effects on change in the MMSE. Separate ANCOVAs were done using each of the previously mentioned tests as the independent variables, while the MMSE was used as the dependent variable. The total YALE score was not used in this study. All significant covariates, main effects, and interactions were reported along with their supporting statistical values.

Results of the Study

The final sample size was 104, with approximately half of the participants being female; 69.8% were Caucasian, and 20.1% were Latino/Hispanic Americans. The participants ranged from 63 to 98 years of age, with a mean age of 81 years of age. The average years in education was 16.67. The physical activities versus cognition level at baseline included the primary activity of walking. According the AD patient informants at baseline, the primary physical activity the AD patients engaged in was walking, with 68% walking one of more hours per week and 32% being sedentary. MMSE scores were significantly higher among the active patients as compared to the sedentary AD patients. The researchers examined the relationship between amount of time spent walking and MMSE scores at baseline and 1 year to try and determine the relationship between physical activity and global cognition. AD patients who were sedentary declined significantly, which was consistent with the literature review. Those participants who walked for 1 hour or more weekly during the year experienced a stabilization in cognitive functioning, and those walking for 2 hours or more showed a significant improvement in MMSE. For further information about all the specific statistical results, please refer to the article. The results from this study support the premise that some level of physical activity is beneficial to the cognitive functioning of those with mild-to-moderate Alzheimer's disease. Limitations of the study included a relatively small sample size and a study conducted in one geographical area.

Link of Evidence to Nursing Practice

The findings from this study conclude that a sedentary lifestyle may correlate to a decline in cognitive functioning; a loss of vigor; and an increase in feelings of

EVIDENCE-BASED PRACTICE

Walking Stabilizes Cognitive Functioning in Alzheimer's Disease (AD) Across One Year—cont'd

anger, confusion, depression, and fatigue. For patients with Alzheimer's disease, this study supported the premise that exercise, such as walking activities, may be one type of intervening strategy that could be helpful in cognitive functioning. A very important achievement of this study is its demonstration of the potential benefit of the simple nonpharmacologic intervention of exercise, which is almost universally available, in the prevention of cognitive decline. For these participants as well as many other patients with physical and/or mental disease, the benefits of exercise go beyond improvement in cognition and include a positive impact on depression, quality of life, and cardiovascular function, as well as a decrease in falls and disability. Although advances are being made in health and

technology and people are living longer, there is a need to find alternative therapies as well as therapies that are nonpharmacologic and simple to implement to prevent and treat diseases such as Alzheimer's dementia and other catastrophic brain disorders. Nurses can educate patients and family members on the importance of habitual exercise as well as encourage the provision of consistent medical care, a suitable environment, adequate nutritional intake, and social interaction to help prevent mental and physical deterioration associated with certain disease states. These simple measures are easy to implement and may contribute significantly to the improvement of the individual's well-being in later life.

Winchester J, Dick MB, Gillen D, et al: Walking stabilizes cognitive functioning in Alzheimer's disease (AD) across one year. *Arch Gerontol Geriatr* 56(1):96-103, 2013.

PATIENT-CENTERED CARE: PATIENT TEACHING

- Medications must be taken exactly as ordered and with meals to minimize GI upset. The dosage of a medication is never to be increased except on the advice of the prescriber. Give specific instructions on what to do if a medication dose has been omitted.
- Intervals between doses of medication need to be timed consistently to optimize therapeutic effects and minimize adverse effects and toxicity.
- Encourage patients, family, significant others, and/or caregivers to call the prescriber or other health care provider if there is any increased muscle weakness, abdominal cramps, diarrhea, dizziness, ataxia, and/or difficulty breathing.
- Share information about community resources with patients, caregiver(s), family, and significant others. Such resources may include, but are not be limited to, Meals on Wheels; local, state, and national chapters of the Alzheimer's Association; adult day care and/or alternate care resources; special prescription services (e.g., Nationwide Prescription Assistance at the toll-free number 888-812-5152 or online at

www.freemedicinefoundation.com); and respite care and/or home health care services.
- Signs and symptoms of improvement of myasthenia gravis include a decrease in or absence of ptosis (eyelid drooping) and diplopia (double vision), less difficulty swallowing and chewing, and an improvement in muscle weakness. If the medication is being taken for myasthenia gravis, the patient needs to take it 30 minutes before meals so that the drug begins to work before the patient chews and swallows. This will help strengthen the muscles for chewing and eating.
- Sustained-released or extended-release dosage forms must be taken in their entirety and should not be crushed, chewed, or broken in any way.
- Encourage the wearing of a medical alert bracelet or necklace and to carry a medical alert card on his or her person at all times. Medical alert jewelry has enough space for a diagnosis, allergies and other critically, pertinent information. A list of medications, other disease related information, additional diseases, and emergency contact phone numbers may be listed on a paper/written/typed form.

KEY POINTS

- *Cholinergics, cholinergic agonists,* and *parasympathomimetics* are all appropriate terms for the class of drugs that stimulate the parasympathetic nervous system, which is the branch of the autonomic nervous system that opposes the sympathetic nervous system.
- The primary neurotransmitter of the parasympathetic nervous system is acetylcholine, and there are two types of cholinergic receptors: nicotinic and muscarinic.
- Nursing considerations for the administration of cholinergic drugs include giving the drug as directed and monitoring the

patient carefully for the occurrence of bradycardia, hypotension, headache, dizziness, respiratory depression, and bronchospasms. If these occur in a patient taking cholinergics, the prescriber must be contacted immediately.
- It may take up to 6 weeks for a therapeutic response to occur with some of the medications used for Alzheimer's disease.
- Patients taking cholinergics need to change positions slowly to avoid dizziness and fainting that may result from the adverse effect of postural hypotension.

NCLEX® EXAMINATION REVIEW QUESTIONS

1. The nurse is reviewing the use of bethanechol (Urecholine) in a patient who is experiencing postoperative urinary retention. Which statement best describes the mechanism of action of bethanechol?
   a. It causes decreased bladder tone and motility.
   b. It causes increased bladder tone and motility.
   c. It increases the sensation of a full bladder.
   d. It causes the sphincters in the bladder to become tighter.

2. The family of a patient who has recently been diagnosed with Alzheimer's disease is asking about the new drug prescribed to treat this disease. The patient's wife says, "I'm so excited that there are drugs that can cure this disease! I can't wait for him to start treatment." Which reply from the nurse is appropriate?
   a. "The sooner he starts the medicine, the sooner it can have this effect."
   b. "These effects won't be seen for a few months."
   c. "These drugs do not cure Alzheimer's disease. Let's talk about what the physician said to expect with this drug therapy."
   d. "His response to this drug therapy will depend on how far along he is in the disease process."

3. The nurse is giving a dose of bethanechol (Urecholine) to a postoperative patient. The nurse is aware that contraindications to bethanechol include:
   a. bladder atony.
   b. peptic ulcer.
   c. urinary retention.
   d. hypothyroidism.

4. A patient took an accidental overdose of a cholinergic drug while at home. He comes to the emergency department with severe abdominal cramping and bloody diarrhea. The nurse expects that which drug will be used to treat this patient?
   a. atropine (generic)
   b. pilocarpine (Salagen)
   c. bethanechol (Urecholine)
   d. phentolamine (Regitine)

5. The nurse is reviewing the orders for a newly admitted patient and sees an order for edrophonium (Tensilon). The nurse expects that this drug is ordered for which reason?
   a. To reduce symptoms and delay the onset of Alzheimer's disease
   b. To treat the symptoms of myasthenia gravis
   c. To aid in the diagnosis of myasthenia gravis
   d. To reverse the effects of nondepolarizing neuromuscular blocking drugs after surgery

6. When giving intravenous cholinergic drugs, the nurse must watch for symptoms of a cholinergic crisis, such as: *(Select all that apply.)*
   a. peripheral tingling.
   b. hypotension.
   c. dry mouth.
   d. syncope.
   e. dyspnea.
   f. tinnitus.

7. A patient who has had an accidental overdose of tricyclic antidepressants is to receive physostigmine (Antilirium), 1.5 mg IM stat. The medication is available in a vial that contains 2 mL, with a concentration of 1 mg/mL. How much medication will the nurse draw up into the syringe for this dose?

8. The nurse is teaching a patient about the possible adverse effects of donepezil (Aricept) for Alzheimer's disease. Which of these are possible adverse effects? *(Select all that apply.)*
   a. Constipation
   b. GI upset
   c. Drowsiness
   d. Dizziness
   e. Blurred vision

1. b, 2. c, 3. b, 4. a, 5. c, 6. b, d, e, 7. 1.5 mL, 8. b, c, d.

CRITICAL THINKING AND PRIORITIZATION QUESTIONS

1. An older adult neighbor wants to take Ginkgo (*Ginkgo biloba*) because he is worried about "losing his mind." He asks you if this drug would help him. He has lived alone since being widowed last year and does not have any family members in the area. What is your best answer for this neighbor? Review the Safety: Herbal Therapies and Dietary Supplements box in this chapter and other sources, if desired.

2. A patient who has been newly diagnosed with myasthenia gravis has received a dose of pyridostigmine (Mestinon) in the morning, just before breakfast. She says, "Oh, I know this won't cure me, but I'm so glad that this drug makes me feel better. Will it last all day?" What is the priority when the nurse is teaching this patient about pyridostigmine?

For answers, see *http://evolve.elsevier.com/Lilley*.

Ⓔ EVOLVE WEBSITE

- Animations
- Answer Keys for Textbook Case Studies and Textbook Critical Thinking and Prioritization Questions
- Content Updates
- Key Points
- Review Questions
- Student Case Studies

Cholinergic-Blocking Drugs

OBJECTIVES

When you reach the end of this chapter, you will be able to do the following:

1. Briefly review the functions of the sympathetic nervous system and the specific effects of blocking cholinergic receptors (parasympatholytic effects).
2. List the various drugs classified as cholinergic antagonists (blocking) or sympatholytics.
3. Discuss the mechanisms of action, therapeutic effects, indications, adverse and toxic effects, drug interactions, cautions, contraindications, dosages, routes of administration, and any antidotal management for the various cholinergic antagonists (blockers).
4. Develop a nursing care plan that includes all phases of the nursing process for patients taking cholinergic antagonists.

DRUG PROFILES

♦ atropine, p. 334
♦ dicyclomine, p. 334
glycopyrrolate, p. 334
oxybutynin, p. 334
scopolamine, p. 335

♦ tolterodine, p. 335

_____
♦ = *Key drug*
! = *High-alert drug*

KEY TERMS

Cholinergic-blocking drugs Drugs that block the action of acetylcholine and substances similar to acetylcholine at receptor sites in the synapse. (p. 331)

Mydriasis Dilation of the pupil of the eye caused by contraction of the dilator muscle of the iris. (p. 332)

Parasympatholytics Drugs that reduce the activity of the parasympathetic nervous system; also called *anticholinergics*. (p. 331)

PARASYMPATHETIC NERVOUS SYSTEM

The parasympathetic nervous system is the branch of the autonomic nervous system with nerve functions opposite those of the sympathetic nervous system (see Chapters 18 and 19 for a discussion of the sympathetic nervous system). Acetylcholine is the neurotransmitter responsible for the transmission of nerve impulses to effector cells in the parasympathetic nervous system. A cholinergic receptor is one that binds acetylcholine and mediates its actions. This chapter focuses on cholinergic-blocking drugs, which inhibit the effects of the parasympathetic nervous system.

CHOLINERGIC-BLOCKING DRUGS

Cholinergic blockers, anticholinergics, parasympatholytics, and *antimuscarinic drugs* are all terms that refer to the class of drugs that block or inhibit the actions of acetylcholine in the parasympathetic nervous system. They are most commonly referred to as anticholinergics in clinical practice. These drugs were first discussed in Chapter 15 in relation to treatment of Parkinson's disease.

Cholinergic blockers have many therapeutic uses and are one of the oldest groups of therapeutic drugs. Originally they were derived from various plant sources. Box 21-1 lists the currently available cholinergic blockers.

Mechanism of Action and Drug Effects

Cholinergic-blocking drugs block the action of the neurotransmitter acetylcholine at the muscarinic receptors in the parasympathetic nervous system (PNS). Acetylcholine that is released from a stimulated nerve fiber is then unable to bind to the receptor site and fails to produce a cholinergic effect. This is why the cholinergic blockers are also referred to as

331

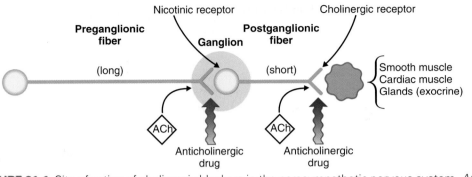

FIGURE 21-1 Site of action of cholinergic blockers in the parasympathetic nervous system. *ACh,* Acetylcholine.

BOX 21-1   Cholinergic Blockers Grouped According to Chemical Class

Natural Plant Alkaloids

atropine (generic)

belladonna (Belladonna tincture)

hyoscyamine (Levsin)

scopolamine (Transderm-Scōp)

Synthetic and Semisynthetic Drugs

benztropine (Cogentin; see Chapter 16)

biperiden (Akineton)

darifenacin (Enablex)

dicyclomine (Bentyl)

fesoterodine (Toviaz)

glycopyrrolate (Robinul)

homatropine (Isopto Homatropine; see Chapter 57)

ipratropium (Atrovent; see Chapter 37)

mepenzolate (Cantil)

methscopolamine (Pamine)

oxybutynin (Ditropan)

procyclidine (Kemadrin)

propantheline (Pro-Banthine)

solifenacin (Vesicare)

tolterodine (Detrol)

trihexyphenidyl (generic; see Chapter 15)

trospium (Sanctura)

TABLE 21-1   Cholinergic Blockers: Drug Effects

Body System	Cholinergic-Blocking Effects
Cardiovascular	Small doses: decrease heart rate
	Large doses: increase heart rate
Central nervous	Small doses: decrease muscle rigidity and tremors
	Large doses: cause drowsiness, disorientation, hallucinations
Eye	Dilate pupils (mydriasis), decrease accommodation by paralyzing ciliary muscles (cycloplegia)
Gastrointestinal	Relax smooth muscle tone of gastrointestinal tract, decrease intestinal and gastric secretions, decrease motility and peristalsis
Genitourinary	Relax detrusor muscle of bladder, increase constriction of internal sphincter; these two effects may result in urinary retention
Glandular	Decrease bronchial secretions, salivation, and sweating
Respiratory	Decrease bronchial secretions, dilate bronchial airways

anticholinergics. Blocking the parasympathetic nerves allows the sympathetic (adrenergic) nervous system to dominate. Because of this, anticholinergics have many of the same effects as the adrenergics (see Chapter 18). Figure 21-1 illustrates the site of action of the cholinergic blockers in the parasympathetic nervous system.

Cholinergic blockers are *competitive antagonists.* They compete with acetylcholine for binding at the muscarinic receptors of the parasympathetic nervous system. Once they have bound to the receptor, they inhibit cholinergic nerve transmission. This occurs at the neuroeffector junction, or the point where the nerve ending reaches the effector organs such as smooth muscle, cardiac muscle, and glands. Cholinergic blockers have little effect at the nicotinic receptors, although at high doses they can have partial blocking effects.

The major sites of action of the anticholinergics are the heart, respiratory tract, gastrointestinal (GI) tract, urinary bladder, eye, and exocrine glands (sweat gland, salivary gland). Anticholinergics have the opposite effects of the cholinergics (see Chapter 20). Anticholinergic effects on the cardiovascular system are seen as an increase in heart rate. Respiratory system effects are dry mucous membranes and bronchial dilation. In the GI tract, cholinergic blockers cause a decrease in GI motility, GI secretions, and salivation. In the genitourinary (GU) system, they lead to decreased bladder contraction, which can result in urinary retention. In the skin they reduce sweating, and, finally, anticholinergics cause the pupils to dilate and increase intraocular pressure. This occurs because the ciliary muscles and the sphincter muscle of the iris are innervated by cholinergic nerve fibers. Cholinergic blockers keep the sphincter muscle of the iris from contracting, which results in dilation of the pupil (**mydriasis**) and paralysis of the ocular lens (cycloplegia). These and other effects are listed by body system in Table 21-1. Many of the cholinergic-blocking drugs are available in a variety of forms, including intravenous, intramuscular, oral, and subcutaneous preparations.

Indications

Anticholinergics are indicated for Parkinson's disease (Chapter 15) and for drug-induced extrapyramidal reactions such as those associated with antipsychotic drugs (see Chapter 16). These conditions involve dysfunction of the extrapyramidal parts of the brain and include motor dysfunctions such as chorea, dystonia, and dyskinesia. Anticholinergics decrease muscle rigidity and diminish tremors.

Cardiovascular effects of anticholinergics are seen on the heart's conduction system. At low dosages, anticholinergics may slow the heart. At high dosages, they block the inhibitory vagal (i.e., parasympathetic or cholinergic) effects on the pacemaker cells, which leads to increased heart rate. Atropine is used primarily in the management of cardiovascular disorders including treatment of symptomatic second-degree atrioventricular block, and provision of advanced life support in the treatment of sinus bradycardia. It also has ophthalmic uses (see Chapter 57).

In the respiratory tract, anticholinergics decrease secretions from the nose, mouth, pharynx, and bronchi. They also cause relaxation of the smooth muscles in the bronchi and bronchioles, which results in decreased airway resistance and bronchodilation. Because of this, the cholinergic blockers are used in treating exercise-induced bronchospasm, chronic bronchitis, asthma, and chronic obstructive pulmonary disease. They are also used preoperatively to reduce salivary secretions, which aids in intubation and other procedures (e.g., endoscopy) involving the oral cavity.

Cholinergic blockers cause reduced GI secretions, relaxation of smooth muscle, and reduced GI motility and peristalsis. For these reasons, cholinergic blockers are commonly used in the treatment of irritable bowel disease and GI hypersecretory states.

Anticholinergics are useful in the treatment of GU tract disorders as reflex neurogenic bladder and incontinence. They relax the detrusor muscles of the bladder and increase constriction of the internal sphincter.

Contraindications

Contraindications to the use of anticholinergic drugs include known drug allergy, angle-closure glaucoma, acute asthma or other respiratory distress, myasthenia gravis, acute cardiovascular instability (some exceptions were listed previously), and GI or GU tract obstruction (e.g., benign prostatic hyperplasia).

Adverse Effects

Anticholinergic drugs cause widely varied adverse effects, with many body systems affected. The various adverse effects of cholinergic blockers are listed by body system in Table 21-2. Certain patient populations are more susceptible to the effects of the anticholinergics. These include infants, children with Down syndrome, those with spastic paralysis or brain damage, and older adults. The older adult patient is extremely sensitive to the

TABLE 21-2 **Cholinergic Blockers: Adverse Effects**	
Body System	**Adverse Effects**
Cardiovascular	Increased heart rate, dysrhythmias (tachycardia, palpitations)
Central nervous	Excitation, restlessness, irritability, disorientation, hallucinations, delirium, ataxia, drowsiness, sedation, confusion
Eye	Dilated pupils (causing blurred vision), increased intraocular pressure
Gastrointestinal	Decreased salivation, gastric secretions, and motility (causing constipation)
Genitourinary	Urinary retention
Glandular	Decreased sweating
Respiratory	Decreased bronchial secretions

CNS effects of anticholinergics, and it is not uncommon for delirium to develop due to anticholinergic effects.

Toxicity and Management of Overdose

The treatment of cholinergic blocker overdose consists of symptomatic and supportive therapy. The patient should be hospitalized, with continuous electrocardiographic monitoring. Activated charcoal is effective in removing from the GI tract any drug that has not yet been absorbed.

Fluid therapy and other standard measures used for the treatment of shock are instituted as needed. Delirium, hallucinations, coma, and cardiac dysrhythmias respond favorably to treatment with the cholinergic drug physostigmine. However, its routine use as an antidote for cholinergic blocker overdose is controversial because it has the potential to produce severe adverse effects (e.g., seizures and cardiac asystole) and is usually reserved for the treatment of patients who show extreme delirium or agitation.

Interactions

Drug interactions most commonly reported are additive anticholinergic effects when taken with other drugs that possess anticholinergic side effects such as amantadine (see Chapter 15), antihistamines (see Chapter 36), and tricyclic antidepressants (see Chapter 16). Increased effects of digoxin (see Chapter 24) are seen when combined with anticholinergics.

Dosages

For dosage information on selected cholinergic blockers, see the table on the next page.

DRUG PROFILES

Among the oldest and best known naturally occurring cholinergic blockers are the belladonna alkaloids. Of these, atropine is the prototypical drug. It has been in use for hundreds of years and continues to be widely administered because of its effectiveness. Besides atropine, scopolamine and hyoscyamine are the other naturally occurring drugs.

Cholinergic blockers are used in the treatment of a variety of illnesses and conditions ranging from irritable bowel syndrome to the symptoms of the common cold and are also administered preoperatively to dry up secretions. They are the synthetic counterparts of the plant-derived belladonna alkaloids and are more specific in binding predominantly with muscarinic receptors. Adverse effects and drug interactions are comparable for the different anticholinergic drugs and are detailed in Table 21-2 and previous text, respectively, unless otherwise noted.

◆ atropine

Atropine is a naturally occurring antimuscarinic. It is more potent than scopolamine in its cholinergic-blocking effects on the heart and in its effects on the smooth muscles of the bronchi and intestines. Because atropine causes increased heart rate, it is used to treat bradycardia and ventricular asystole. Atropine is also used as an antidote for anticholinesterase inhibitor toxicity or poisoning. It is also used preoperatively to reduce salivation and GI secretions, as is glycopyrrolate. Atropine is contraindicated in patients with angle-closure glaucoma, advanced hepatic and renal dysfunction, hiatal hernia associated with reflux esophagitis, intestinal atony, obstructive GI or GU conditions, and severe ulcerative colitis. It is available in injectable, oral, and ophthalmic forms (see Chapter 57). It is also combined with the opiate diphenoxylate to make Lomotil tablets, a common antidiarrheal preparation. Recommended dosages are given in the table on this page.

Pharmacokinetics: Atropine

Route	Onset of Action	Peak Plasma Concentration	Elimination Half-life	Duration of Action
IV	Immediate	2-4 min	2.5 hr	4-6 hr

◆ dicyclomine

Dicyclomine (Bentyl) is a synthetic antispasmodic cholinergic blocker used primarily in the treatment of functional disturbances of GI motility such as irritable bowel syndrome.

It is contraindicated in patients who have a known hypersensitivity to anticholinergics and in those with angle-closure glaucoma, GI tract obstruction, myasthenia gravis, paralytic ileus, GI atony, or toxic megacolon. It is available in injectable and oral form. Recommended dosages are given in the table on this page.

Pharmacokinetics: Dicyclomine

Route	Onset of Action	Peak Plasma Concentration	Elimination Half-life	Duration of Action
PO	1-2 hr	60-90 min	9-10 hr	3-4 hr

glycopyrrolate

Glycopyrrolate (Robinul) is a synthetic antimuscarinic drug that blocks receptor sites in the autonomic nervous system that control the production of secretions. It is used preoperatively to reduce salivation and excessive secretions in the respiratory and GI tracts. It is contraindicated in patients who are hypersensitive to it and in those with angle-closure glaucoma, myasthenia gravis, GI or GU tract obstruction, tachycardia, myocardial ischemia, hepatic disease, ulcerative colitis, or toxic megacolon. Glycopyrrolate is available in injectable and oral form. Recommended dosages are given in the table on this page.

Pharmacokinetics: Glycopyrrolate

Route	Onset of Action	Peak Plasma Concentration	Elimination Half-life	Duration of Action
IV	1 min	10-15 min	Variable	4 hr
PO	Up to 45 min	1 hr	Variable	6 hr

oxybutynin

Oxybutynin (Ditropan) is a synthetic antimuscarinic drug used for the treatment of overactive bladder (OAB). It is also used as an antispasmodic for neurogenic bladder associated with spinal cord injuries and congenital conditions such as spina bifida. Contraindications include drug allergy, urinary or gastric retention, and uncontrolled angle-closure glaucoma. Oxybutynin is

DOSAGES

Selected Cholinergic Antagonist (Anticholinergic) Drugs

Drug (Pregnancy Category)	Usual Adult Dosage Range	Indications/Uses
◆ atropine	IV: 0.5-1 mg given every 3-5 min (max 3 mg)	Treatment of bradycardia, cardiopulmonary resuscitation
◆ dicyclomine (Bentyl) (B)	PO: 80-160 mg/day divided qid	Treatment of irritable bowel syndrome
oxybutynin (Ditropan, Ditropan XL, Oxytrol [transdermal patch])	PO: 5 mg bid-qid; ER tab: 5-30 mg/day in single or divided doses Transdermal patch: 1 patch (3.9 mg/day) applied twice weekly (every 3-4 days) (for overactive bladder)	Antispasmodic for neurogenic bladder (e.g., following spinal cord injury), overactive bladder
scopolamine	IM/IV/subcut: 0.3-0.65 mg Transdermal patch: 1.5 mg patch behind ear every 3 days; apply at least 4 hr before transportation	Preoperative control of secretions Motion sickness prevention
◆ tolterodine (Detrol, Detrol XL) (C)	PO: 1-2 mg bid; ER cap: 2-4 mg daily	Treatment of overactive bladder

ER, Extended release.

available for oral use. A transdermal patch (Oxytrol) is available over-the-counter and is approved for treatment of overactive bladder. Recommended dosages are given in the table on the previous page.

Pharmacokinetics: Oxybutynin

Route	Onset of Action	Peak Plasma Concentration	Elimination Half-life	Duration of Action
PO	Unknown	1 hr	2-3 hr	Unknown

scopolamine

Scopolamine is a naturally occurring cholinergic blocker and one of the principal belladonna alkaloids. It is the most potent antimuscarinic for the prevention of motion sickness. It works by correcting the imbalance between acetylcholine and norepinephrine in the higher centers in the brain, particularly in the vomiting center. Scopolamine is available in several different delivery systems. For the prevention of motion sickness, it is available in a transdermal delivery system (Transderm-Scōp), a patch that can be applied just behind the ear 4 to 5 before travel (see Chapter 52). Transdermal scopolamine may be applied preoperatively to help prevent postoperative postanesthesia nausea/vomiting with application 1 hour before surgery and removed within 24 to 36 hours. Transdermal scopolamine may cause drowsiness, dry mouth, and blurred vision. Using scopolamine with central nervous system depressants or alcohol may increase sedation. Scopolamine is also available in parenteral formulations for injection by various routes: intravenous, intramuscular, and subcutaneous. Scopolamine is available for ocular indications and in oral form. The contraindications that apply to atropine apply to scopolamine as well. Recommended dosages are given in the table on the previous page.

Pharmacokinetics: Scopolamine

Route	Onset of Action	Peak Plasma Concentration	Elimination Half-life	Duration of Action
IV	30-60 min	30-45 min	Variable	4 hr
Transdermal	4-5 hr	6 hr	Variable	72 hr

◆ tolterodine

Tolterodine (Detrol) is a muscarinic receptor blocker used for the treatment of urinary frequency, urgency, and urge incontinence caused by bladder (detrusor) overactivity. Another drug that is commonly used to treat these conditions is oxybutynin (profiled previously). Other older-generation drugs include propantheline, hyoscyamine, and the tricyclic antidepressant imipramine. These drugs are less commonly used today because of their antimuscarinic adverse effects, particularly dry mouth. Newer drugs for this purpose include solifenacin (Vesicare), darifenacin (Enablex), trospium (Sanctura), and fesoterodine (Toviaz). The newer drugs are associated with a much lower incidence of dry mouth, in part because of their pharmacologic specificity for the bladder as opposed to the salivary glands. The newest drug, Mirabegron (Myrbetriq), was approved for OAB. It is a beta$_3$ agonist and represents a new class of therapy for

this condition. Mirabegron does not have the same side effects as other drugs used to treat OAB because it is a beta$_3$ agonist, as opposed to being a muscarinic blocker. Mirabegron is described in Chapter 18.

Tolterodine is to be avoided in patients with angle-closure glaucoma or urinary retention. In patients with markedly decreased hepatic function or poor metabolizers taking drugs that inhibit cytochrome P-450 enzyme 3A4 (e.g., erythromycin or ketoconazole), the dose is reduced by half. Tolterodine is available only for oral use. Recommended dosages are given in the table on the previous page.

Pharmacokinetics: Tolterodine

Route	Onset of Action	Peak Plasma Concentration	Elimination Half-life	Duration of Action
PO	1 hr	1-2 hr	2-4 hr	5 hr

NURSING PROCESS

ASSESSMENT

The drugs known as *parasympatholytics, cholinergic blockers, cholinergic antagonists,* or *anticholinergics* (an older term) produce a number of physiologic effects that result from the blocking of cholinergic receptors. These effects include smooth muscle relaxation, decreased glandular secretion, and mydriasis (pupil dilation). Knowing the way these drugs work and the related physiology will assist you in the safe assessment and nursing care of patients taking these drugs. A thorough medical history; complete medication history with a listing of prescription drugs, over-the-counter drugs, and herbals; as well as a thorough head-to-toe examination will help you identify the presence of any contraindications, cautions, and/or potential drug interactions associated with the cholinergic-blocking drugs. The assessment data will help you document baseline findings and provide information for evaluating drug effectiveness. Lifespan considerations for the very young and/or older adult patient include the need for close assessment and monitoring. This is especially important because of the increased susceptibility of these age groups to the adverse effects of restlessness, irritability, disorientation, constipation, urinary retention, blurred vision (from pupil dilation), and tachycardia. If these drugs are taken for overactive bladder, assess for urinary frequency, urgency, as well as nocturia and incontinence. With *solifenacin (Vesicare),* assess urinary patterns and history of cardiac disease. In your assessment associated with *atropine* and other cholinergic blockers, check for allergies, glaucoma, certain eye conditions (e.g., adhesions in the iris and lens of the eye), gastroesophageal reflux disease, poor intestinal motility, obstructions of the GI and GU systems, and severe ulcerative colitis. These conditions and others may be exacerbated by the cholinergic blockers (see earlier in this chapter, as well as Chapters 18 to 20) and would be considered contraindications. Assess for associated cautions, contraindications, and drug interactions with *dicyclomine, glycopyrrolate,* and *oxybutynin.* Also, note any disorders of the bladder or GI tract. Apply the transdermal dosage form of *scopolamine* only after the order has been reviewed and the skin assessed.

Overactive Bladder

- In the U.S., an estimated 46 million adults aged 40 and older—or 1 in 3—report symptoms of overactive bladder (OAB). Approximately 30% of all men and 40% of all women in the U.S. live with OAB symptoms. Many individuals with OAB just learn to cope with the condition because of embarrassment about having the discussion with their health care provider or thinking it cannot be treated.
- Some questions to pose to the older adult patient regarding this condition are as follows:
  - Do you ever have a sudden and strong urge to urinate?
  - Do you urinate more than eight times in a 24-hour period?
  - Do you have to get up more than two times during the night to urinate?
  - Do you have "wetting" accidents?
  - Are these "wetting" accidents related to the uncontrollable urge to urinate?
  - NOTE: If the patient answers yes to some of these questions, the patient needs to be encouraged to contact his or her primary health care provider. Referral to a urologist may or may not be necessary.
- Various treatments for overactive bladder including behavioral therapy with lifestyle changes such as consuming less caffeine, alcohol, and spicy foods. Keep a daily food journal with a "bladder diary" to see if avoiding these foods helps with the frequent trips to the bathroom. Kegel exercises are encouraged to help relax your bladder muscle. These behavioral-type treatments may provide some help.
- Medications are also available and are very effective in treatment of OAB by relaxing the bladder muscle. These medications are available by various dosage routes such as oral, transdermal patch, or gel form.
- Solifenacin succinate (Vesicare), taken once daily, is indicated for treatment of all the major symptoms of overactive bladder, including urgency, frequency, and urge-related incontinence.
  - Oxybutynin (Ditropan) is used orally for OAB. There is a transdermal patch (Oxytrol), which is available over-the-counter. Tolterodine (Detrol) is also used for OAB.
  - A newer drug, mirabegron, works differently than other medications used, such as solifenacin succinate (Vesicare). Mirabegron is a beta$_3$ agonist and does not have the same side effects as the other drugs to treat OAB, which is very beneficial. See Chapter 18.
- Neuromodulation therapy is done through the delivery of harmless electrical impulses to nerves that may change how the nerves work and is used when medications or behavioral therapies are not successful.

Data from *Overactive bladder*, September 2014. Available at *www.mayoclinic.org/diseases-conditions/overactive-bladder/basics/treatment*. Accessed April 12, 2015.

NURSING DIAGNOSES

1. Constipation related to adverse effects of cholinergic-blocking drugs
2. Deficient knowledge related to lack of information about the therapeutic regimen, adverse effects, drug interactions, and precautions related to the use of cholinergic-blocking drugs
3. Risk for injury related to decreased sweating and loss of normal heat-regulating mechanisms due to the impact of the drug on the temperature-regulating mechanisms

PLANNING: OUTCOME IDENTIFICATION

1. Patient experiences/regains normal bowel patterns through measures such as increase in fluid (8 glasses/day) and fiber (40 g/day).
2. Patient demonstrates adequate knowledge about the use of the specific medication, adverse effects, and appropriate dosing at home.
3. Patient states measures to help prevent risk for injury from decreased impact in the ability to sweat such as avoiding hot climates, vigorous exercising (especially in heated or hot environments), saunas, and hot tubs.

IMPLEMENTATION

A preventive focus for nursing care is important to the effective use of *cholinergic-blocking drugs*, especially with regard to patient teaching about how to decrease the need for these medications. There are several nursing interventions that may maximize the therapeutic effects of these drugs and minimize the adverse effects. Some important nursing interventions include giving the drug at the same time each day and per the prescriber's orders, and giving the medication with adequate fluid intake (6 to 8 glasses of water daily).

Because drugs such as *atropine* and *glycopyrrolate* are compatible with some of the commonly used opioids (e.g., meperidine and morphine), they may be used in combination with these drugs and mixed in the same syringe for parenteral dosing. Checking for the compatibility of drugs combined in the same syringe is important with any medication. Always double-check compatibility for patient safety. If a cholinergic-blocking drug is given via the ophthalmic route, always check the concentration of the drug and, once it is given, apply light pressure with a tissue to the inner canthus of the eye for approximately 30 to 60 seconds. This helps to minimize the possibility of systemic absorption of the drug.

Atropine may be combined with other cholinergic-blocking drugs (e.g., *hyoscyamine*) for treatment of lower urinary tract discomfort or to help decrease GI and GU hypermotility, but give the drug via the correct route and with proper dosing as prescribed. The anticholinergic adverse effect of dry mouth may be managed with frequent mouth care, oral rinses, increase in fluids, and use of sugar-free gum or hard candy. *Solifenacin* is to be taken the same time every day and without regard to meals. *Oxybutynin* needs to be taken as directed either 1 hour before or 2 hours after meals, if tolerated. *Tolterodine* must be taken as directed and with food. Transdermal forms of these medications (e.g., *scopolamine*, *oxybutynin*) are to be applied to the skin only after the previous dosage form has been removed and the area gently cleansed of residual medication. Transdermal patches may be applied to any dry, nonhairy, nonirritated area. Rotation of transdermal sites is recommended to decrease skin irritation. Also associated with the cholinergic-blocking drugs are the adverse effects of constipation and inability to sweat or perspire. Because these may be significant to patients, include education on how to minimize these adverse effects. See the Patient-Centered Care: Patient Teaching section later in the chapter for more information on these specific drugs.

EVALUATION

Monitoring of goals and outcome criteria is a starting place for effective evaluation of therapy with these medications. In particular, therapeutic effects of *cholinergic-blocking drugs* include the following: (1) improved ability to carry out activities of daily living and fewer problems with tremors, salivation, and drooling in patients with Parkinson's disease; (2) decreased GI symptoms, such as hyperacidity, abdominal pain, and nausea and vomiting, with improved comfort; (3) decreased bladder hypermotility, with increased comfort and improved patterns of voiding with an increase in time between voidings; and (4) fewer bronchospasms with induction of anesthesia and fewer problems with thickened, viscous secretions in patients before, during, and after surgery. Monitor the patient for the occurrence of adverse effects such as constipation, tachycardia, palpitations, confusion, sedation, drowsiness, hallucinations, urinary retention, and decreased sweating leading to hot, dry skin. Toxic effects of *anticholinergics* include delirium, hallucinations, and cardiac dysrhythmias.

CASE STUDY

Patient-Centered Care: Transdermal Scopolamine

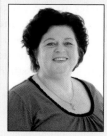

J., a 53-year-old schoolteacher, is going on a cruise to Alaska with her husband, L., for their thirtieth anniversary. She is very excited about the trip but is also worried because she gets "very seasick" whenever she is on a boat. She calls her doctor's office for a prescription for a medicine for motion sickness. Her physician prescribes transdermal scopolamine (Transderm-Scōp).

1. Before J. picks up the prescription, the nurse assesses for contraindications to scopolamine. What are the contraindications to the use of the scopolamine patch?
   The nurse provides patient education, and J. indicates that she understands how to use the patch. On the first day of the cruise, she applies the patch 4 hours before they board the ship.
2. That evening, J. and L. go to dinner. J. is feeling somewhat drowsy, but thirsty. The waiter asks if they would like to have champagne as part of the first-night-of-the-cruise celebration. How should J. respond?
3. The next morning, while out on the deck, L. and J. are taking pictures of the bright, snow-covered shoreline views. L. looks at J. and exclaims, "Look at your eyes! Is that a side effect of that patch?" What has L. noticed about J.'s blue eyes? What would you suggest for J. because of what L. has noticed?
4. Later that day, J. tells L., "I'm feeling great! I don't think I need this patch. I'm going to take it off, but I'll save it for later in case I get nauseated." Is this a good idea? Explain your answer.

For answers, see *http://evolve.elsevier.com/Lilley.*

PATIENT-CENTERED CARE: PATIENT TEACHING

- Medications need to be taken exactly as prescribed. Overdosage of anticholinergics may cause life-threatening problems, especially in the cardiovascular and central nervous systems.
- Anticholinergics may lead to dry mouth. Regular and thorough oral hygiene is required with brushing of teeth twice daily and dental flossing. Dry mouth may be minimized by forcing fluids, if not contraindicated, use of artificial saliva drops/gum, or sucking on sugar-free hard candy, as needed. Encourage regularly scheduled dental visits because of the risk for dental caries and gum disease with dry mouth. The use of water pick devices may stimulate gums and help prevent gum disease.
- Exercise must be done with caution and excessive sweating avoided because of drug-induced altered sweating. This may cause hyperthermia in the older adult patient or those with already altered sweating mechanisms.
- If there is sedation and/or blurred vision, the patient needs to avoid driving or engaging in activities that require quick decision making, alertness, or clear vision, such as operating heavy machinery, taking tests, and making important decisions. The adverse effects of sedation will decrease over time.
- Encourage the patient to wear dark or tinted glasses or sunglasses because of the increased sensitivity to light associated with these medications.
- The patient must understand the importance of always consulting the prescriber or other health care provider before taking any other medications, including prescription drugs, over-the-counter medications, herbals, and supplements.
- The older adult patient has existing age-related changes in body temperature–regulating mechanisms. With these medications, especially at high dosages, there is an increased risk for heat stroke or hyperthermia because of the drug's interference with the body's heat-regulating mechanisms. To prevent hyperthermia in this age group, encourage them to stay in shaded areas or inside in an air-conditioned or cooled environment when external temperatures are warm; remain well-hydrated with cool fluids; wear protective clothing and hats; avoid saunas, hot tubs, excessive heat, and strenuous exercise in warm environments; and keep portable fans on hand and maintain adequate ventilation in heated environments.
- All health care providers need to be informed about the treatment regimen, and a list of the patient's drugs must be given to all involved in the care of a patient taking anticholinergics or cholinergic blockers. The prescriber needs to be contacted if there is any unresolved constipation, palpitations, alterations in gait or balance, excessive dizziness, or inability to void.
- Constipation may be managed by the increased dietary intake of fluids and fiber and/or the use of over-the-counter fiber-containing supplements, such as psyllium products.

KEY POINTS

- *Cholinergic blockers, parasympatholytics, anticholinergics,* and *antimuscarinics* are all terms that refer to the drugs that block or inhibit the actions of acetylcholine in the parasympathetic nervous system.
- The use of these cholinergic blockers allows the sympathetic nervous system to dominate. These drugs are classified chemically as natural, semisynthetic, and synthetic cholinergic blockers. These drugs may be competitive antagonists (blockers) and compete with acetylcholine at the muscarinic receptors. In high dosages, they result in partial blocking actions at the nicotinic receptors.

NCLEX® EXAMINATION REVIEW QUESTIONS

1. The nurse is providing education about cholinergic-blocking drug therapy to an older adult patient. Which is an important point to emphasize for this patient?
   a. Avoid exposure to high temperatures.
   b. Limit liquid intake to avoid fluid overload.
   c. Begin an exercise program to avoid adverse effects.
   d. Stop the medication if excessive mouth dryness occurs.
2. The nurse is giving a cholinergic-blocking drug and will assess the patient for which contraindications to these drugs?
   a. Chronic bronchitis
   b. Peptic ulcer disease
   c. Irritable bowel syndrome
   d. Benign prostatic hyperplasia
3. When assessing for adverse effects of cholinergic-blocking drug therapy, the nurse would expect to find that the patient complains of which drug effect?
   a. Diaphoresis
   b. Dry mouth
   c. Diarrhea
   d. Urinary frequency
4. The nurse administering a cholinergic-blocking drug to a patient who is experiencing drug-induced extrapyramidal effects would assess for which therapeutic effect?
   a. Decreased muscle rigidity and tremors
   b. Increased heart rate
   c. Decreased bronchial secretions
   d. Decreased GI motility and peristalsis
5. During the assessment of a patient about to receive a cholinergic-blocking drug, the nurse will determine whether the patient is taking any drugs that may potentially interact with the anticholinergic, including:
   a. opioids, such as morphine sulfate.
   b. antibiotics, such as penicillin.
   c. tricyclic antidepressants, such as amitriptyline.
   d. anticonvulsants, such as phenobarbital.
6. A patient has been given a prescription for transdermal scopolamine patches (Transderm-Scōp) for motion sickness for use during a vacation cruise. The nurse will include which instructions? *(Select all that apply.)*
   a. "Apply the patch as soon as you board the ship."
   b. "Apply the patch 3 to 4 hours before boarding the ship."
   c. "The patch needs to be placed on a nonhairy area on your upper chest or upper arm."
   d. "The patch needs to be placed on a nonhairy area just behind your ear."
   e. "Change the patch every 3 days."
   f. "Rotate the application sites."
7. The preoperative order for an adult patient reads: "Give scopolamine, 0.7 mg IM on call for surgery." The medication is available in vials of 0.4 mg/mL. How many milliliters will the nurse administer for this dose? *(Record your answer using one decimal place.)*
8. The nurse is assessing a patient who has a prescription for dicyclomine (Bentyl). Which condition is considered a contraindication to this medication?
   a. GI atony
   b. Irritable bowel syndrome
   c. Overactive bladder
   d. Diabetes mellitus

1. a, 2. d, 3. b, 4. a, 5. c, 6. b, d, e, f, 7. 1.8 mL, 8. a.

CRITICAL THINKING AND PRIORITIZATION QUESTIONS

1. You are getting ready to administer atropine sulfate and an opioid, ordered as standard preoperative medications, to a 75-year-old woman who will be undergoing minor surgery. When you check her medical history, you see that she has a history of smoking and has angle-closure glaucoma. What is your priority action at this time regarding administration of the preoperative medications? Explain your answer.

2. In preparing a patient for emergency surgery, the order was to give 0.5 mg of atropine sulfate to the patient intravenously. The vial concentration is 1 mg/mL. In the haste of this emergency situation, 5 mL of the atropine solution is given. How much atropine did the patient receive? What is the nurse's priority action at this time?

For answers, see *http://evolve.elsevier.com/Lilley.*

EVOLVE WEBSITE

- Animations
- Answer Keys for Textbook Case Studies and Textbook Critical Thinking and Prioritization Questions
- Content Updates
- Key Points
- Review Questions
- Student Case Studies

Drugs Affecting the Cardiovascular and Renal Systems

Learning Strategies

STUDY TIME

When students learn a new topic for the first time, their brain looks for a connection to previous learning. If it finds a connection, then learning the content will be easier. In order to effectively learn a topic like pharmacology, students will have to spend a significant amount of their time studying. It is a good idea if students have a set routine and put aside a specific time to study. Many students find that if they review their lecture notes the same day as the class it helps them to remember the new concepts that were just introduced. You will need to find out what type of study schedule works best for you. You should not wait until just before a test or exam to study what you have been learning. A better plan is to work with the material frequently. This plan will enhance the connections formed in your brain as you review the material and help it become part of your long-term memory and learning.

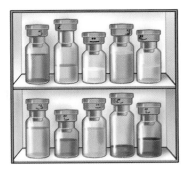

LEARNING STYLES

One of the best ways to study effectively is to understand the way you learn best, otherwise termed *learning styles*. As mentioned in the Introduction, everyone has a particular way that they learn best. Many references identify the learning styles as visual, auditory, and kinesthetic, while other sources define up to seven learning styles with inclusion of verbal (linguistic), logical (mathematical), solitary (intrapersonal), and social (interpersonal). There are several ways for you to find out your learning style(s). Textbooks and reference books are available, but the Internet/web-based resources provide a wealth of information. A few sites that may prove helpful include the following: *www.educationplanner.org/students/self-assessments/learning-styles-quiz.shtml* and *www.mindtools.com/ mnemlsty.html*. Self-assessment learning style tests are available within the Internet/web-based sites.

Here is a brief overview of each of the seven learning styles. The *visual* (spatial) learning style prefers using pictures, images, and spatial understanding such as using mind maps and working with pictures instead of words. The *aural-style* learner prefers sound and music including recordings, rhymes, and mnemonics and setting the learning of information to jingles. *Verbal* (linguistic) students learn best with both the spoken and written word including reading of content aloud, recording of and listening to lectures and to themselves, as well as participating in role playing. The *physical* (kinesthetic) style learner best comprehends/utilizes information with the use of their hands and through the sense of touch. These learners benefit from the use of physical objects as much as possible such as writing and drawing. *Logical* (mathematical) learners like to use logical reasoning and a systems approach. They like to find the reason behind the content and create/use lists of key points in their material. Students who fit the *social* (interpersonal) learning style prefer learning in groups or with other people. If this is your style, try role playing or working in groups as often as you can. The *solitary* (intrapersonal) style learns most effectively on their own and use self-study. They will align their goals with their personal beliefs and values (*www.edudemic.com/styles-of-learning*). Some of these seven learning styles will overlap, and you may find you learn more effectively with use of more than one learning style. There is no right or wrong way to learn. By finding your learning style, you can enhance the learning of content and get the most out of the learning experience.

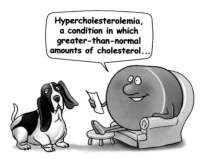

USE OF APPLICATIONS

Technology has come to play an important part in how students learn and study. As discussed previously, there are many applications available on smart phones and tablets that students can use to learn, study, and manage their time. You will want to start with your textbook and see what types of technology, learning strategies, and ancillary tools are offered as part of your textbook purchase. The student resources for this textbook includes interactive review questions, and downloadable files of the key points from each chapter to help you study for tests. For the visual and auditory learner, there are animations. Additionally, there are several types of practice questions, critical thinking questions, and case studies that are available in this textbook and online. These questions can be used as independent study or in a group situation. If you are a student who embraces technology, use your smart phone or tablet to conduct a search for applications (apps) to download and assist you in learning and/or quizzing yourself on various topics within pharmacology.

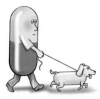

MNEMONICS

Additional learning strategies include the use of mnemonics, acronyms, and other memory aids. For the student who likes to search the Internet, there are a variety of mnemonics and acronyms that have been developed to help nursing students learn pharmacology. Some students learn best when studying with these strategies, and you can even develop your own. Others do not like using them. Try a few, and see if they help you. One mnemonic that helps students when learning the classifications of the cardiac drugs in this section are these phrases: All generic names of beta blocker end in "-olol" (e.g., propranolol); ACE inhibitors end in "-pril" (e.g., captopril); and angiotensin receptor blockers (ARBS) end in "-sartan" (e.g., losartan).

For the visual learner, there are books available using pictures and visual aids to help you to remember pharmacology terms, drug names, and the properties of certain drugs. Some aids even set the pharmacology information to the tune of nursery rhymes so the information seems familiar and sticks. Mosby's *Pharmacology Memory NoteCards* book published by Elsevier is a great workbook to use with your pharmacology textbook. It contains a wide variety of learning aids, mnemonics, illustrations, and humor, all aimed at making learning pharmacology easier and fun. This publication can also be downloaded, so you can have it on your mobile devices.

FLASH CARDS

Flash cards are another method of learning about pharmacology and medications. The kinesthetic learner learns best with these strategies. Students can make up their own flash cards listing important information about a particular drug they need to learn. Some students write out cards and use different colored inks for the various information, like green for drug indications and dosage, red for side effects, orange for contraindications, and blue for nursing implications. Students can use a program on their computer to make the flash cards and bring them up on their smart phone to study later. There are also Internet sites and mobile apps that have premade pharmacology flash cards you can use to quiz yourself.

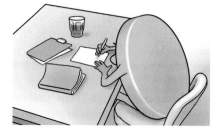

When you know how you learn the best, you can use those strategies to make the most of your time learning and studying pharmacology. Remember your textbook is a great place to start. Review the additional learning resources that are available from the publisher, and then you can seek out any of the other techniques mentioned in this section to help you successfully master your study time.

22

Antihypertensive Drugs

e http://evolve.elsevier.com/Lilley

When you reach the end of this chapter, you will be able to do the following:

1. Briefly discuss the normal anatomy and physiology of the autonomic nervous system, including the events that take place within the sympathetic and parasympathetic divisions as related to long-term and short-term control of blood pressure.
2. Define *hypertension*.
3. Compare primary and secondary hypertension and their related manifestations.
4. Describe the protocol for treating hypertension as detailed in the *Eighth Report of the Joint National Committee on Prevention, Detection, Evaluation, and Treatment of High Blood Pressure (JNC 8)*, including the rationale for its use.
5. List the criterion pressure values (in millimeters of mercury) for the hypertension categories of normal blood pressure, prehypertension, hypertension stage 1, and hypertension stage 2 as defined in *JNC 8*.
6. Using the most recent guidelines, compare the various drugs used in the pharmacologic management of hypertension with regard to mechanism of action, specific indications, adverse effects, toxic effects, cautions, drug interactions, contraindications, dosages, and routes of administration.
7. Discuss the rationale for the nonpharmacologic management of hypertension.
8. Develop a nursing care plan that includes all phases of the nursing process for patients receiving antihypertensive drugs.

DRUG PROFILES

bosentan, p. 353
♦captopril, p. 349
carvedilol, p. 347
♦clonidine, p. 347
doxazosin, p. 347
enalapril, p. 350
eplerenone, p. 353
♦hydralazine, p. 353

♦losartan, p. 351
nebivolol, p. 348
!sodium nitroprusside, p. 353
treprostinil, p. 353

♦ = *Key drug*
! = *High-alert drug*

KEY TERMS

Alpha₁ blockers Drugs that primarily cause arterial and venous dilation through their action on peripheral sympathetic neurons. (p. 345)

Antihypertensive drugs Medications used to treat hypertension. (p. 344)

Cardiac output The amount of blood ejected from the left ventricle. (p. 343)

Centrally acting adrenergic drugs Drugs that modify the function of the sympathetic nervous system in the brain by stimulating alpha₂ receptors. Alpha2 receptors are inhibitory in nature and thus have a reverse sympathetic effect and cause decreased blood pressure. (p. 345)

Essential hypertension Elevated systemic arterial pressure for which no cause can be found; also called *primary* or *idiopathic hypertension*. (p. 343)

Hypertension A common, often asymptomatic disorder in which systolic blood pressure persistently exceeds 150 mm Hg and/or diastolic pressure exceeds 90 mm Hg in patients over 60 years of age and 140/90 for patients younger than 60 and those who have chronic kidney disease or diabetes. (p. 343)

Orthostatic hypotension A common adverse effect of adrenergic-blocking drugs involving a sudden drop in blood pressure when a person changes position, especially when rising from a seated or horizontal position. (p. 346)

Prodrug A drug that is inactive in its given form and must be metabolized to its active form in the body, generally by the liver, to be effective. (p. 348)

Secondary hypertension High blood pressure caused by another disease such as renal, pulmonary, endocrine, or vascular disease. (p. 343)

ANATOMY, PHYSIOLOGY, AND PATHOPHYSIOLOGY OVERVIEW

Hypertension, defined as a persistent systolic blood pressure (SBP) of greater than 150 mm Hg and/or a diastolic blood pressure (DBP) greater than 90 mm Hg for patients 60 years of age or older and an SBP greater than 140 and DBP greater than 90 for patients younger than 60 years of age and those who have chronic kidney disease or diabetes. Hypertension affects approximately 70 million people in the United States and approximately 1 billion people worldwide, designating it as the most common disease state.

Hypertension is a major risk factor for coronary artery disease, cardiovascular disease (CVD), and death resulting from cardiovascular causes. It is the most important risk factor for stroke and heart failure, and it is also a major risk factor for renal failure and peripheral vascular disease. There is indisputable evidence regarding the relationship between blood pressure and risk for CVD; the higher the blood pressure, the greater the chance of developing CVD. For people 40 to 70 years of age, the risk for developing CVD doubles with each 20–mm Hg increase in systolic blood pressure or 10–mm Hg increase in diastolic pressure.

Blood pressure is determined by the product of **cardiac output** (4 to 8 L/min) and systemic vascular resistance (SVR). Cardiac output is the amount of blood that is ejected from the left ventricle and is measured in liters per minute. SVR is the resistance to blood flow that is determined by the diameter of the blood vessel and the vascular musculature. Numerous factors interact to regulate these two major variables and keep the blood pressure within normal limits. These are illustrated in Figure 22-1 and are the same factors that can cause high blood pressure (hypertension) and are the targets of action of many antihypertensive drugs.

The diagnosis and treatment of hypertension have varied considerably over the years. The Eighth Report of the Joint National Committee on Prevention, Detection, Evaluation, and Treatment of High Blood Pressure (*JNC 8*) was released in December 2013. This report provides treatment guidelines for hypertension assembled by two large expert panels based on a review of the latest clinical research publications on the disease. As with previous such reports, development of the *JNC 8* was sponsored by the National Heart, Lung, and Blood Institute of the National Institutes of Health. It should be noted that there is controversy among health care professional groups regarding the *JNC 8* definitions. However, this textbook adheres to *JNC 8* guidelines.

Hypertension can also be defined by its cause. When the specific cause of hypertension is unknown, it may be called **essential hypertension** (or idiopathic or primary hypertension). About 90% of cases of hypertension are of this type. **Secondary hypertension** accounts for the remainder. Secondary hypertension is most commonly the result of another disease such as pheochromocytoma (adrenal tumor), preeclampsia of pregnancy (a pregnancy complication involving acute hypertension, among other symptoms), renal artery disease, sleep apnea, thyroid disease, or parathyroid disease. It may also result from the use of certain medications. If the cause of secondary hypertension can be eliminated, blood pressure usually returns to normal. If untreated, hypertension can cause damage to end organs such as the heart, brain, kidneys, and eyes.

The goal of antihypertensive therapy is the reduction of cardiovascular and renal morbidity and mortality. According to the *JNC 8*, therapy should be started if blood pressure is at or greater than 150/90 for patients older than 60 years of age and 140/90 for patients younger than 60 and those who have chronic kidney disease or diabetes.

Significant advances have been made in both the ways to treat hypertension and in the understanding of the disease

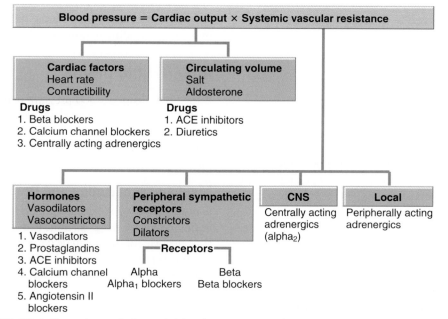

FIGURE 22-1 Normal regulation of blood pressure and corresponding medications. *ACE,* Angiotensin-converting enzyme; *CNS,* central nervous system.

process. Large numbers of clinical trials have shown that adequately treating hypertension can prevent or delay CVD. Over the past 40 years, the development of new antihypertensive medications has had an enormous impact on the quality of life of people with hypertension. Drug therapy for hypertension first became available in the early 1950s with the introduction of ganglionic-blocking drugs. However, unpleasant adverse effects and inconsistent therapeutic effects were common problems with these antihypertensive drugs. In 1953, the vasodilator hydralazine was introduced, and in 1958 the thiazide diuretics became available. Since that time, several additional drug classes have been developed.

PHARMACOLOGY OVERVIEW

Drug therapy for hypertension must be individualized. Important considerations in planning drug therapy are coexisting medical problems and what impact the drug therapy will have on the patient's quality of life. For example, sexual dysfunction in males is a common adverse effect of almost any antihypertensive drug and is the most common reason for nonadherence to drug therapy. Demographic factors, cultural implications, the ease of medication administration (e.g., a once-a-day dosing schedule or transdermal administration), and cost are other important considerations.

There are essentially seven main categories of pharmacologic drugs used to treat hypertension: diuretics, adrenergic drugs, vasodilators, angiotensin-converting enzyme (ACE) inhibitors, angiotensin receptor blockers (ARBs), calcium channel blockers (CCBs), and direct renin inhibitors. All of these antihypertensive drugs (with the exception of diuretics) have some vasodilatory action. Those drugs in the vasodilator category are also called *direct vasodilators*. Drugs in any of these classes may be used either alone or in combination. The various categories and subcategories of antihypertensive drugs are listed in Box 22-1. Calcium channel blockers are covered in detail in Chapter 23, and the diuretics are discussed in detail in Chapter 28. There is only one direct renin inhibitor, aliskiren (Tekturna), and it is not recommended as initial treatment of hypertension.

REVIEW OF AUTONOMIC NEUROTRANSMISSION

There are two divisions of the autonomic nervous system (ANS): the parasympathetic nervous system (PSNS) and sympathetic nervous system (SNS). Stimulation of the ANS is controlled by the neurotransmitters acetylcholine and norepinephrine. Receptors for both divisions of the ANS are located throughout the body in a variety of tissues. ANS physiology is reviewed in greater detail in Chapters 18 to 21. Receptors located between the postganglionic fiber and the effector cells (i.e., the postganglionic receptor) are called the *muscarinic* or *cholinergic* receptors in the PSNS. Receptors in the SNS are called *adrenergic* or *noradrenergic* receptors (i.e., alpha or beta receptors). Physiologic activity at muscarinic receptors is stimulated by acetylcholine and cholinergic agonist drugs (see Chapter 20) and is inhibited by cholinergic antagonists (anticholinergic

---

BOX 22-1   Categories and Subcategories of Antihypertensive Drugs

Adrenergic Drugs
- Centrally and peripherally acting adrenergic neuron blockers
- Centrally acting alpha$_2$ receptor agonists
- Peripherally acting alpha$_1$ receptor blockers
- Peripherally acting beta receptor blockers (beta blockers)
- Cardioselective (beta$_1$ receptor blockers)
- Nonselective (beta$_1$ and beta$_2$ receptor blockers)
- Peripherally acting dual alpha$_1$ and beta receptor blockers

Angiotensin-Converting Enzyme Inhibitors

Angiotensin II Receptor Blockers

Calcium Channel Blockers
- Benzothiazepines
- Dihydropyridines
- Phenylalkylamines

Diuretics
- Loop diuretics
- Potassium-sparing diuretics
- Thiazides and thiazide-like diuretics

Vasodilators
Act directly on vascular smooth muscle cells, *not* through alpha or beta receptors.

Direct Renin Inhibitors
- aliskiren

---

drugs; see Chapter 21). Similarly, physiologic activity at adrenergic receptors is stimulated by norepinephrine and epinephrine and adrenergic agonists (see Chapter 18) and inhibited by antiadrenergics (adrenergic blockers; i.e., alpha or beta receptor blockers) (see Chapter 19). Figure 22-2 shows how these various receptors are arranged in both the PSNS and SNS and indicates their corresponding neurotransmitters.

ADRENERGIC DRUGS

Adrenergic drugs are a large group of antihypertensive drugs, as shown in Box 22-1. The alpha blockers and combined alpha/beta blockers are described in detail in Chapter 19. The adrenergic drugs discussed here exert their antihypertensive action at different sites.

Mechanism of Action and Drug Effects

Five specific drug subcategories are included in the adrenergic antihypertensive drugs as indicated in Box 22-1. Each of these subcategories of drugs can be described as having central action (in the brain) or peripheral action (at the heart and blood vessels). These drugs include the adrenergic neuron blockers (central and peripheral), the alpha$_2$ receptor agonists (central), the alpha$_1$ receptor blockers (peripheral), the beta receptor blockers (peripheral), and the combination alpha$_1$ and beta receptor blockers (peripheral).

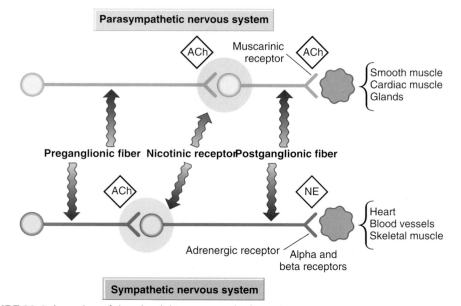

FIGURE 22-2 Location of the nicotinic receptors in the parasympathetic and sympathetic nervous systems. *ACh*, Acetylcholine; *NE*, norepinephrine.

Stimulation of the sympathetic nervous system (SNS) leads to an increase in heart rate and force of contraction, the constriction of blood vessels, and the release of renin from the kidney, resulting in hypertension. The **centrally acting adrenergic drugs** clonidine and methyldopa work by stimulating the alpha$_2$-adrenergic receptors in the brain. The alpha$_2$-adrenergic receptors are unique in that receptor stimulation actually reduces sympathetic outflow, in this case from the central nervous system (CNS). This results in a lack of norepinephrine production, which reduces blood pressure. Stimulation of the alpha$_2$-adrenergic receptors also affects the kidneys, reducing the activity of renin. Renin is the hormone and enzyme that converts the protein precursor angiotensinogen to the protein angiotensin I, the precursor of angiotensin II (AII), a potent vasoconstrictor that raises blood pressure.

In the periphery, the **alpha1 blockers** doxazosin, prazosin, and terazosin work by blocking the alpha$_1$-adrenergic receptors. When alpha$_1$-adrenergic receptors are stimulated by circulating norepinephrine, they produce increased blood pressure. Thus, when these receptors are blocked, blood pressure is decreased. The drug effects of the alpha$_1$ blockers are primarily related to their ability to dilate arteries and veins, which reduces peripheral vascular resistance and subsequently decreases blood pressure. This produces a marked decrease in the systemic and pulmonary venous pressures and an increase in cardiac output. The alpha$_1$ blockers also increase urinary flow rates and decrease outflow obstruction by preventing smooth muscle contractions in the bladder neck and urethra. This can be beneficial in cases of benign prostatic hyperplasia (BPH).

The beta blockers also act in the periphery and include propranolol, metoprolol, and atenolol as well as several other drugs. These drugs are discussed in more detail in Chapters 23 and 25 because they are also used for angina and conduction problems. Their antihypertensive effects are related to their reduction of the heart rate through beta$_1$ receptor blockade. Furthermore, beta blockers also cause a reduction in the secretion of the hormone renin (see the section on ACE inhibitors later in the chapter), which in turn reduces both AII-mediated vasoconstriction and aldosterone-mediated volume expansion. Long-term use of beta blockers also reduces peripheral vascular resistance.

Two dual-action alpha$_1$ and beta receptor blockers, labetalol and carvedilol, also act in the periphery at the heart and blood vessels. They have the dual antihypertensive effects of reduction in heart rate (beta$_1$ receptor blockade) and vasodilation (alpha$_1$ receptor blockade). Figure 22-3 illustrates the site and mechanism of action of the various antihypertensive drugs.

Indications

All of the drugs mentioned in this section are used primarily for the treatment of hypertension, either alone or in combination with other antihypertensive drugs. Various forms of glaucoma may also respond to treatment with some of these drugs. The alpha$_1$ blockers doxazosin, prazosin, and terazosin have been used to relieve the symptoms associated with BPH (see Chapter 19). They have also proved effective in the management of severe heart failure when used with cardiac glycosides (see Chapter 24) and diuretics (see Chapter 28).

Contraindications

Contraindications to the use of the adrenergic antihypertensive drugs include known drug allergy and may also include acute heart failure, concurrent use of monoamine oxidase inhibitors (see Chapter 16), peptic ulcer, and severe liver or kidney disease. Asthma may also be a contraindication to the use of any noncardioselective beta blocker (e.g., carvedilol).

Adverse Effects

The most common adverse effects of adrenergic drugs are bradycardia with reflex tachycardia, postural and postexercise hypotension, dry mouth, drowsiness, dizziness, depression,

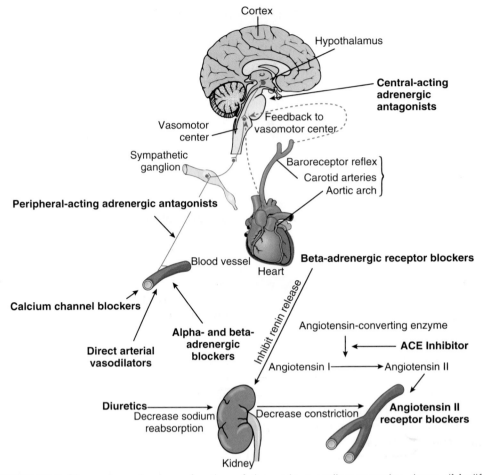

FIGURE 22-3 Site and mechanism of action of the various antihypertensive drugs. (Modified from Lewis SL, Dirksen SR, Heitkemper MM, et al: *Medical-surgical nursing: assessment and management of clinical problems,* ed 8, St Louis, 2011, Mosby.)

edema, constipation, and sexual dysfunction (e.g., impotence). Other effects include headache, sleep disturbances, nausea, rash, and palpitations. There is a high incidence of orthostatic hypotension (a sudden drop in blood pressure during changes in position) in patients taking alpha blockers. Orthostatic hypotension is commonly referred to as *postural hypotension*. A situation known as *first-dose syncope,* in which the hypotensive effect is severe enough to cause the patient to lose consciousness with even the first dose of medication, can occur. Educate the patient to change positions slowly.

In addition, the abrupt discontinuation of the centrally acting alpha₂ receptor agonists can result in rebound hypertension, characterized by a sudden and very high elevation of blood pressure. This may also be true for other antihypertensive drug classes, especially beta blockers. Nonselective blocking drugs are also commonly associated with bronchoconstriction as well as metabolic inhibition of glycogenolysis in the liver.

Any change in the dosing regimen for cardiovascular medications should be undertaken gradually and with appropriate patient monitoring and follow-up. Although the same is also true for most other classes of medications, abrupt dosage changes of cardiovascular medications, either up or down, can be especially hazardous for the patient. Some of these drugs can

also cause disruptions in blood count as well as in serum electrolyte levels and renal function. Periodic monitoring of white blood cell count, serum potassium, sodium and creatinine levels is necessary.

Interactions

Adrenergic drugs can cause additive CNS depression when taken with alcohol, benzodiazepines, and opioids. Other drug interactions that can occur with selected adrenergic drugs are summarized in Table 22-1. This list is merely representative and is not exhaustive. Always keep a drug information handbook available to check in cases in which a specific drug interaction is suspected.

Dosages

For dosage information on selected adrenergic antihypertensive drugs, see the table on the next page.

DRUG PROFILES

ALPHA₂-ADRENERGIC RECEPTOR STIMULATORS (AGONISTS)

Of the two alpha₂ receptor agonists—clonidine and methyldopa—clonidine is the most commonly used and is the

TABLE 22-1   Adrenergic Drugs: Drug Interactions

Drug	Interacts with	Mechanism	Result
clonidine	TCAs, MAOIs, appetite suppressants, amphetamines	Opposing actions	Decreased hypotensive effects
	Diuretics, nitrates, other antihypertensive drugs	Additive	Increased hypotensive effects
	Beta blockers	Additive	May potentiate bradycardia and increase the rebound hypertension in clonidine withdrawal

MAOIs, Monoamine oxidase inhibitors; *TCAs,* tricyclic antidepressants.

prototypical drug for this class. Methyldopa is commonly used to treat hypertension in pregnancy. However, these drugs are not typically prescribed as first-line antihypertensive drugs, because their use is associated with a high incidence of unwanted adverse effects such as orthostatic hypotension, fatigue, and dizziness. They may be used as adjunct drugs in the treatment of hypertension after other drugs have failed or may be used in conjunction with other antihypertensives such as diuretics.

◆ clonidine

Clonidine (Catapres) is used primarily for its ability to decrease blood pressure. It is also useful in the management of opioid withdrawal. It has a better safety profile than the other centrally acting adrenergics and has the advantage of being available in several dosage formulations, including both topical and oral preparations. When the patch dosage form is used, it is important to remove the old patch before applying a new one. Clonidine must not be discontinued abruptly, as this will lead to severe rebound hypertension. Its use is contraindicated in patients who have shown hypersensitivity reactions to it. Recommended dosages are given in the table on this page.

Pharmacokinetics: Clonidine

Route	Onset of Action	Peak Plasma Concentration	Elimination Half-life	Duration of Action
PO	30-60 min	3-5 hr	6-20 hr	8 hr

ALPHA₁ BLOCKERS

The alpha₁ blockers are doxazosin (Cardura), prazosin (Minipress), tamsulosin (Flomax), and terazosin (Hytrin). Their use is contraindicated in patients who have shown a hypersensitivity to them. They are classified as pregnancy category C drugs. They are available only as oral preparations. Tamsulosin is not used to control blood pressure but is indicated solely for symptomatic control of benign prostatic hyperplasia (BPH). This use is described further in Chapters 19 and 35.

doxazosin

Doxazosin (Cardura, Cardura XL) is a commonly used alpha₁ blocker. It reduces peripheral vascular resistance and blood pressure by dilating both arterial and venous blood vessels. It is available in immediate- and extended-release formulations. When the drug is released from the extended-release form, the matrix of the capsule is expelled in the stool. Educate patients that this will happen, and reassure that the active drug has been absorbed. Confusion over the presence of the capsule matrix could cause patients to take more than the prescribed dosage. Recommended dosages are given in the table on this page.

Pharmacokinetics: Doxazosin

Route	Onset of Action	Peak Plasma Concentration	Elimination Half-life	Duration of Action
PO	1-2 hr	2-3 hr	15-22 hr	Less than 24 hr

DUAL-ACTION ALPHA₁ AND BETA RECEPTOR BLOCKERS

carvedilol

Carvedilol (Coreg) is a widely used drug and is well tolerated by most patients. In addition to treatment of hypertension, it is also indicated for treatment of mild to moderate heart failure in conjunction with digoxin, diuretics, and ACE inhibitors. Contraindications include known drug allergy, cardiogenic

DOSAGES

Selected Antihypertensive Drugs: Adrenergic Agonists and Antagonists

Drug (Pregnancy Category)	Pharmacologic Class	Usual Dosage Range	Indications/Uses
carvedilol (Coreg, Coreg CR) (C)	Peripherally acting alpha₁, beta₁, and beta₂ receptor antagonist (blocker)	PO: 6.25-25 mg bid Coreg CR: 20-80 mg/day	Hypertension (also used in heart failure)
◆ clonidine (Catapres, Catapres-TTS) (C)	Centrally acting alpha₂ receptor agonist	PO: 0.2-0.6 mg/day in divided doses Transdermal patch: 0.1, 0.2, or 0.3 mg/24 hr, applied weekly	Hypertension
doxazosin (Cardura, Cardura XL) (C)	Peripherally acting alpha₁ receptor antagonist	PO: Initial dose 1 mg/day; may titrate up to maximum of 16 mg/day	Hypertension

shock, severe bradycardia or heart failure, bronchospastic conditions such as asthma, and various cardiac problems involving the conduction system. For dosage information, see the table on this page.

Pharmacokinetics: Carvedilol

Route	Onset of Action	Peak Plasma Concentration	Elimination Half-life	Duration of Action
PO	20-120 min	1-4 hr	6-8 hr	8-24 hr

BETA RECEPTOR BLOCKER
nebivolol

Nebivolol (Bystolic) is the newest beta blocker, released in 2008. It is a beta$_1$-selective beta blocker approved for use in hypertension. It is also used for the treatment of heart failure. Nebivolol is similar to other beta$_1$-selective blockers; however, in addition to blocking beta$_1$ receptors, it also produces vasodilatation, which results in a decrease in SVR. It is promoted as causing less sexual dysfunction. Like other beta blockers, it should not be stopped abruptly but must be tapered over 1 to 2 weeks.

ANGIOTENSIN-CONVERTING ENZYME (ACE) INHIBITORS

The ACE inhibitors are a large group of antihypertensive drugs. Currently, there are ten ACE inhibitors available for clinical use. In addition, various combination drug products are available in which a thiazide diuretic or a calcium channel blocker (CCB) is combined with an ACE inhibitor. Combination products tend to increase adherence since the patient is taking fewer drugs. The available ACE inhibitors are captopril (Capoten), benazepril (Lotensin), enalapril (Vasotec), fosinopril (Monopril), lisinopril (Prinivil), moexipril (Univasc), perindopril (Aceon), quinapril (Accupril), ramipril (Altace), and trandolapril (Mavik). These drugs are very safe and efficacious and are often used as first-line drugs in the treatment of both heart failure and hypertension. Some of the available drug combinations and dosing schedules for the various drugs that make up this large class of antihypertensives are summarized in Table 22-2. The ACE inhibitors as a class, are very similar to one another and differ in only a few of their chemical properties; however, there are some differences among them in their clinical properties.

Captopril has the shortest half-life and therefore must be dosed more frequently than any of the other ACE inhibitors. This may be an important drawback for patients with a history of nonadherence to their medication regimen. On the other hand, it may be best to start with a drug that has a short half-life in a patient who is critically ill, so that if problems arise they will be short-lived. Both captopril and enalapril can be dosed multiple times a day.

Captopril and lisinopril are the only two ACE inhibitors that are not prodrugs. A prodrug is a drug that is inactive in its administered form and must be metabolized to its active form in the body, generally by the liver, to be effective. This characteristic of captopril and lisinopril is an important advantage in treating a patient with liver dysfunction; all of the other ACE

TABLE 22-2	ACE Inhibitors	
Drug (Trade Name)	**Combination with Hydrochlorothiazide**	**Dosing Schedule**
benazepril (Lotensin)	Lotensin HCT	Once or twice a day
captopril (Capoten)	Capozide	Once or twice a day
enalapril (Vasotec)	Vaseretic	Once or twice a day
fosinopril (Monopril)	Monopril-HCTZ	Once or twice a day
lisinopril (Prinivil)	Prinzide	Once or twice a day
lisinopril (Zestril)	Zestoretic	Once or twice a day
moexipril (Univasc)	Uniretic	Once or twice a day
perindopril (Aceon)	None	Once or twice a day
quinapril (Accupril)	Accuretic	Once or twice a day
ramipril (Altace)	None	Once or twice a day
trandolapril (Mavik)	None	Once or twice a day

ACE, Angiotensin-converting enzyme.

inhibitors are prodrugs, and their transformation to active form is dependent upon liver function to reveal the active drug.

Enalapril is the only ACE inhibitor that is available in a parenteral preparation. All of the other ACE inhibitors, such as benazepril, fosinopril, lisinopril, quinapril, and ramipril, have long half-lives and long durations of action, which allows them to be given orally only once a day. A once-a-day medication regimen promotes better patient adherence.

All ACE inhibitors have detrimental effects on the unborn fetus and neonate. They are classified as pregnancy category C drugs for women in their first trimester and as pregnancy category D drugs for women in their second or third trimester. ACE inhibitors are to be used by pregnant women only if there are no safer alternatives.

Mechanism of Action and Drug Effects

The development of the ACE inhibitors was spurred by the discovery of the venom of a South American viper, which was found to inhibit kininase activity. Kininase is an enzyme that normally breaks down bradykinin, a potent vasodilator in the human body.

As their name implies, these drugs inhibit angiotensin-converting enzyme, which is responsible for converting Angiotensin I (AI) (formed through the action of renin) to angiotensin 2 (AII). AII is a potent vasoconstrictor and induces aldosterone secretion by the adrenal glands. Aldosterone stimulates sodium and water resorption, which can raise blood pressure. Together, these processes are referred to as the renin-angiotensin-aldosterone system. By inhibiting this process, blood pressure is lowered.

The primary effects of the ACE inhibitors are cardiovascular and renal. Their cardiovascular effects are due to their ability to reduce blood pressure by decreasing systemic vascular resistance (SVR). They do this by preventing the breakdown of the vasodilating substance bradykinin and substance P (another potent vasodilator), and preventing the formation of AII. These combined effects decrease afterload, or the resistance against which the left ventricle must pump to eject its volume of blood during contraction. The ACE inhibitors are beneficial in the treatment of heart failure because they prevent sodium and

TABLE 22-3 ACE Inhibitors: Therapeutic Effects

Body Substance	Effect in Body	Ace Inhibitor Action	Resulting Hemodynamic Effect
aldosterone	Causes sodium and water retention	Prevents its secretion	Diuresis = ↓ plasma volume = ↓ filling pressures or ↓ preload
angiotensin II	Potent vasoconstrictor	Prevents its formation	↓ SVR = ↓ afterload
bradykinin	Potent vasodilator	Prevents its breakdown	↓ SVR = ↓ afterload

↓, Decreased; *SVR*, systemic vascular resistance.

water resorption by inhibiting aldosterone secretion. This causes diuresis, which decreases blood volume and return to the heart. This in turn decreases preload, or the left ventricular end-diastolic volume, and the work required of the heart.

Indications

The therapeutic effects of the ACE inhibitors are related to their potent cardiovascular effects. They are excellent antihypertensives and adjunctive drugs for the treatment of heart failure. They may be used alone or in combination with other drugs such as diuretics in the treatment of hypertension or heart failure.

Because of their ability to decrease SVR (a measure of afterload) and preload, ACE inhibitors can stop the progression of left ventricular hypertrophy, which is sometimes seen after a myocardial infarction (MI). This pathologic process is known as *ventricular remodeling*. The ability of ACE inhibitors to prevent this is termed a *cardioprotective effect*. ACE inhibitors have been shown to decrease morbidity and mortality in patients with heart failure. They are considered the drugs of choice for hypertensive patients with heart failure. ACE inhibitors also have been shown to have a protective effect on the kidneys, because they reduce glomerular filtration pressure. For this reason, they are among the cardiovascular drugs of choice for diabetic patients. Numerous studies have shown that the ACE inhibitors reduce proteinuria, and they are considered by many to be standard therapy for diabetic patients to prevent the progression of diabetic nephropathy. The various therapeutic effects of the ACE inhibitors are listed in Table 22-3.

Contraindications

Contraindications to the use of ACE inhibitors include known drug allergy, especially a previous reaction of angioedema (e.g., laryngeal swelling) to an ACE inhibitor. Patients with a baseline potassium level of 5 mEq/L or higher may not be suitable candidates for ACE inhibitor therapy, because these drugs can promote hyperkalemia (see later discussion). All ACE inhibitors are contraindicated in lactating women, children, and in patients with bilateral renal artery stenosis.

Adverse Effects

Major CNS effects of the ACE inhibitors include fatigue, dizziness, mood changes, and headaches. A characteristic dry, nonproductive cough may occur that is reversible with discontinuation of the therapy. A first-dose hypotensive effect can cause a significant decline in blood pressure. Other adverse effects include loss of taste, hyperkalemia, angioedema, and renal impairment. In patients with severe heart failure whose renal function may depend on the activity of the renin-angiotensin-aldosterone system, treatment with ACE inhibitors may cause acute renal failure. ACE inhibitors promote potassium resorption in the kidney, although they promote sodium excretion due to their reduction of aldosterone secretion. For this reason, serum potassium levels must be monitored regularly. This is especially true when there is concurrent therapy with potassium-sparing diuretics, although many patients tolerate both types of drug therapy with no major problems. One rare, but potentially fatal, adverse effect is angioedema. Angioedema is a strong vascular reaction involving inflammation of submucosal tissues, which can progress to anaphylaxis.

Toxicity and Management of Overdose

The most pronounced symptom of an overdose of an ACE inhibitor is hypotension. Treatment is symptomatic and supportive and includes the administration of intravenous fluids to expand the blood volume. Hemodialysis is effective for the removal of captopril and lisinopril.

Interactions

Nonsteroidal antiinflammatory drugs (NSAIDs), such as ibuprofen, can reduce the antihypertensive effect of ACE inhibitors (see Chapter 44). The use of NSAIDs and ACE inhibitors may also predispose patients to the development of acute renal failure. Concurrent use of ACE inhibitors and other antihypertensives or diuretics can have hypotensive effects. Giving lithium and ACE inhibitors together can result in lithium toxicity. Potassium supplements and potassium-sparing diuretics, when administered with ACE inhibitors, may result in hyperkalemia. The monitoring of serum potassium levels becomes important in these cases.

Dosages

For dosage information on selected ACE inhibitors, see the table on this page.

DRUG PROFILES

◆ captopril

Captopril (Capoten) was the first available ACE inhibitor and is considered the prototypical drug for the class. Several large multicenter studies have shown its clinical efficacy in minimizing or preventing the left ventricular dilatation and dysfunction (also called *ventricular remodeling*) that can arise in the acute period after an MI and thereby improving the patient's chances of survival. It can also reduce the risk for heart failure in these patients. It has the shortest half-life of all of the currently available ACE inhibitors, and it must be given three or four times a day. Recommended dosages are given in the table on the next page.

DOSAGES

Selected Antihypertensive Drugs: ACE Inhibitors and Angiotensin II Receptor Blockers

Drug (Pregnancy Category)	Pharmacologic Class	Usual Adult Dosage Range	Indications
◆ captopril (Capoten) (C, first trimester; D, second and third trimesters)	ACE inhibitor	PO: 25-150 mg bid-tid	Hypertension, heart failure
enalapril (Vasotec) (C, first trimester; D, second and third trimesters)	ACE inhibitor	PO: 2.5-5 mg/day and increase to target dose of 10–40 mg/day as a single dose or in 2 equal doses	Hypertension
		PO: 2.5-20 mg bid	Heart failure
		IV: 0.625-1.25 mg every 6 hr over a 5-min period	Hypertension
◆ losartan (Cozaar) (C, first trimester; D, second and third trimesters)	Angiotensin II receptor blocker	PO: 25-100 mg as a single dose or divided bid	Hypertension

ACE, Angiotensin-converting enzyme.

Pharmacokinetics: Captopril

Route	Onset of Action	Peak Plasma Concentration	Elimination Half-life	Duration of Action
PO	15 min	1-2 hr	2 hr	2-6 hr

enalapril

Enalapril (Vasotec) is the only ACE inhibitor currently marketed that is available in both oral and parenteral preparations. The parenteral formulation (enalaprilat) is an active drug. It offers the hemodynamic benefit of inhibiting ACE activity in an acutely ill patient who cannot tolerate oral medications. The other benefit to intravenous enalapril is that it does not require cardiac monitoring as do the intravenous beta blockers and calcium channel blockers. The oral form of enalapril differs from captopril in that it is a prodrug, and the patient must have a functioning liver for the drug to be converted into its active form. As with captopril, it has been shown in many large studies to improve a patient's chances of survival after an MI and to reduce the incidence of heart failure. Recommended dosages are given in the table above.

Pharmacokinetics: Enalapril

Route	Onset of Action	Peak Plasma Concentration	Elimination Half-life	Duration of Action
PO	1 hr	4-6 hr	2 hr	12-24 hr
IV	15 min	1-4 hr	2 hr	4-6 hr

ANGIOTENSIN II RECEPTOR BLOCKERS

Angiotensin II receptor blockers (ARBs) are similar to the ACE inhibitors. The class includes losartan (Cozaar), eprosartan (Teveten), valsartan (Diovan), irbesartan (Avapro), candesartan (Atacand), olmesartan (Benicar), telmisartan (Micardis), and azilsartan (Edarbi).

Mechanism of Action and Drug Effects

The ARBs block the binding of AII to type 1 AII receptors. The ACE inhibitors such as enalapril block conversion of AI to AII.

For comparison, recall that ACE inhibitors block the breakdown of bradykinins and substance P, which accumulate and may cause adverse effects such as cough but might also contribute to the drugs' antihypertensive, cardiac, and nephroprotective effects. Bradykinins are potent vasodilators and help to reduce blood pressure by dilating arteries and decreasing SVR.

In contrast to ACE inhibitors, the ARBs affect primarily vascular smooth muscle and the adrenal gland. By selectively blocking the binding of AII to the type 1 AII receptors in these tissues, ARBs block vasoconstriction and the secretion of aldosterone. AII receptors have been found in other tissues throughout the body, but the effects of ARB blocking of these receptors is unknown.

Clinically, ACE inhibitors and ARBs appear to be equally effective for the treatment of hypertension. Both are well tolerated, but ARBs do not cause cough. There is evidence that ARBs are better tolerated and are associated with lower mortality after MI than ACE inhibitors. It is not yet clear whether ARBs are as effective as ACE inhibitors in treating heart failure (cardioprotective effects) or in protecting the kidneys, as in diabetes. Both types of drugs are contraindicated for use in the second or third trimester of pregnancy.

Indications

The therapeutic effects of ARBs are related to their potent vasodilating properties. They are excellent antihypertensives and adjunctive drugs for the treatment of heart failure. They may be used alone or in combination with other drugs such as diuretics in the treatment of hypertension or heart failure. The beneficial hemodynamic effect of ARBs is their ability to decrease SVR (a measure of afterload).

Contraindications

Contraindications to the use of ARBs are known drug allergy, pregnancy, and lactation. They need to be used cautiously in older adults and in patients with renal dysfunction. As with other antihypertensives, blood pressure and apical pulse rate need to be assessed before and during drug therapy.

TABLE 22-4   Angiotensin II Receptor Blockers: Drug Interactions

Drug	Mechanism	Result
NSAIDs	Decreased antihypertensive	Decreased effect of ARB and potential to cause renal failure
lithium	Inhibits lithium elimination	Increased lithium concentrations
rifampin	Increased metabolism	Decreased ARB effectiveness
Potassium supplements and potassium-sparing diuretics	Additive potassium-increasing effects	Possible hyperkalemia

ARB, Angiotensin II receptor blocker.

Adverse Effects

The most common adverse effects of ARBs are chest pain, fatigue, hypoglycemia, diarrhea, urinary tract infection, anemia, and weakness. Hyperkalemia and cough are less likely to occur than with the ACE inhibitors.

Toxicity and Management of Overdose

Overdose may manifest as hypotension and tachycardia; bradycardia occurs less often. Treatment is symptomatic and supportive, and includes the administration of intravenous fluids to expand the blood volume.

Interactions

The drugs that interact with ARBs, the mechanism responsible, and the result of the interaction are summarized in Table 22-4. In addition, as is the case with ACE inhibitors, ARBs can promote hyperkalemia, especially when taken concurrently with potassium supplements (although this occurs much less frequently than with ACE inhibitors). Monitoring of the serum potassium level is necessary for all patients.

Dosages

For dosage information on selected ARBs, see the table on the previous page.

DRUG PROFILE

♦losartan

Losartan (Cozaar) is beneficial in patients with hypertension and heart failure. The use of losartan is contraindicated in patients who are hypersensitive to any component of this product. It is to be used with caution in patients with renal or hepatic dysfunction and in patients with renal artery stenosis. Breastfeeding women must not take losartan, because it can cause serious adverse effects on the nursing infant. Recommended dosages are given in the table on the previous page.

Pharmacokinetics: Losartan

Route	Onset of Action	Peak Plasma Concentration	Elimination Half-life	Duration of Action
PO	1 hr	6 hr	6-9 hr	24 hr

CALCIUM CHANNEL BLOCKERS

Calcium channel blockers (CCBs) are discussed in detail in the chapters on antianginal drugs (see Chapter 23) and antidysrhythmic drugs (see Chapter 25). As a class, they are used for several indications and have many beneficial effects and relatively few adverse effects. Their primary use is for the treatment of hypertension and angina. Their effectiveness in treating hypertension is related to their ability to cause smooth muscle relaxation by blocking the binding of calcium to its receptors, which thereby prevents contraction. Because of their effectiveness and safety, they have been added to the list of first-line drugs for the treatment of hypertension. Amlodipine (Norvasc) is the CCB most commonly used for hypertension (see Chapter 23 for specifics). Calcium channel blockers are also effective antidysrhythmics (see Chapter 25). One specific CCB, nimodipine, can prevent the cerebral artery spasms that can occur after a subarachnoid hemorrhage. CCBs are also sometimes used in the treatment of Raynaud's disease and migraine headache. They are also used in combination with other drugs. Some examples are amlodipine/atorvastatin (Caduet), which is both an antihypertensive and a cholesterol-lowering drug (see Chapter 27); amlodipine/benazepril (Lotrel); amlodipine/olmesartan (Azar); and amlodipine/valsartan (Exforge).

DIURETICS

The diuretics are a highly effective class of antihypertensive drugs. They are listed as the current first-line antihypertensives in the *JNC 8* guidelines for the treatment of hypertension. They may be used as monotherapy (single-drug therapy) or in combination with drugs of other antihypertensive classes. Their primary therapeutic effect is decreasing the plasma and extracellular fluid volumes, which results in decreased preload. This leads to a decrease in cardiac output and total peripheral resistance, all of which decrease the workload of the heart. This large group of antihypertensives is discussed in detail in Chapter 28. The thiazide diuretics (e.g., hydrochlorothiazide) are the most commonly used diuretics for treatment of hypertension.

VASODILATORS

Vasodilators act directly on arteriolar and/or venous smooth muscle to cause relaxation. They do not work through adrenergic receptors. Vasodilator drugs include minoxidil, hydralazine (Apresoline), diazoxide (Hyperstat), and nitroprusside (Nitropress).

Mechanism of Action and Drug Effects

Direct-acting vasodilators are useful as antihypertensive drugs because of their ability to directly cause peripheral vasodilation. This results in a reduction in systemic vascular resistance (SVR). Vasodilators produce significant hypotension. Minoxidil (Rogaine) (in its topical form) is used to restore hair growth and is discussed in Chapter 56. Diazoxide, hydralazine, and minoxidil work primarily through arteriolar vasodilation, whereas nitroprusside has both arteriolar and venous effects.

Indications

All of the vasodilators can be used to treat hypertension, either alone or in combination with other antihypertensives. Sodium nitroprusside and intravenous diazoxide are reserved for the management of hypertensive emergencies, in which blood pressure is severely elevated.

Contraindications

Contraindications include known drug allergy and may also include hypotension, cerebral edema, head injury, acute MI, and coronary artery disease. They may also be contraindicated in cases of heart failure that is secondary to diastolic dysfunction.

Adverse Effects

Diazoxide has many undesirable adverse effects and is rarely used in clinical practice. Adverse effects of hydralazine include dizziness, headache, anxiety, tachycardia, edema, dyspnea, nausea, vomiting, diarrhea, hepatitis, systemic lupus erythematosus (SLE), vitamin B_6 deficiency, and rash. Minoxidil adverse effects include T-wave electrocardiographic changes, pericardial effusion or tamponade, angina, breast tenderness, rash, and thrombocytopenia. Adverse effects of sodium nitroprusside include bradycardia, decreased platelet aggregation, rash, hypothyroidism, hypotension, methemoglobinemia, and, rarely, cyanide toxicity. Cyanide ions are a by-product of nitroprusside metabolism. Cyanide and thiocyanate toxicity are seen clinically when nitroprusside is used at high dosages for long periods of time and/or in patients with renal insufficiency. When nitroprusside is combined with sodium thiosulfate, the potential for cyanide toxicity is greatly reduced.

Toxicity and Management of Overdose

Hydralazine toxicity or overdose produces hypotension, tachycardia, headache, and generalized skin flushing. Treatment is supportive and symptomatic and includes the administration of intravenous fluids, digitalization if needed, and the administration of beta blockers for the control of tachycardia.

The main symptom of sodium nitroprusside overdose or toxicity is severe hypotension. This drug is normally administered only to patients receiving intensive care. Excessive hypotension is usually avoidable. When it does occur, discontinuation of the infusion has an immediate effect because the drug is metabolized very rapidly (half-life of 10 minutes). The chemical structure of nitroprusside does contain cyanide groups, which are released upon its metabolism in the body and can result in cyanide or thiocyanate toxicity. This usually occurs clinically when the drug is used at high dosages for prolonged periods and/or in patients with renal failure. If cyanide or thiocyanate toxicity occurs, treatment can be administered using a standard cyanide antidote kit that includes sodium nitrite and sodium thiosulfate for injection and amyl nitrite for inhalation.

Interactions

The incidence of drug interactions is low for the direct-acting vasodilators as a class. Hydralazine can produce additive hypotensive effects when given with adrenergic or other antihypertensive drugs.

Dosages

For dosage information for selected vasodilator drugs, see the table on this page.

DOSAGES

Selected Antihypertensive Drugs: Vasodilators

Drug (Pregnancy Category)	Pharmacologic Class	Usual Adult Dosage Range	Indications
◆hydralazine (Apresoline) (C)	Direct-acting peripheral vasodilators	PO: 10-25 mg 2-4 times/day for 7 days, then increase to 50 mg bid-qid; titrate to effect to max dose of 300 mg/day IV: 10-20 mg/dose every 4 hr prn	Hypertension
!sodium nitroprusside (Nitropress) (C)		IV: 0.3-0.5 mcg/kg/min; titrate to desired effect; max of 10 mcg/kg/min	

DOSAGES

Miscellaneous Antihypertensive Drugs

Drug (Pregnancy Category)	Pharmacologic Class	Usual Adult Dosage Range	Indications
bosentan (Tracleer) (X)	Endothelin receptor antagonist	PO: 62.5 mg bid or 125 mg bid depending on weight	Pulmonary artery hypertension in patients with moderate to severe heart failure
eplerenone (Inspra) (B)	Aldosterone receptor antagonist	PO: Usual dosage range 25-50 mg daily to bid	Hypertension and post-MI status (to improve post-MI survival in patients with stable heart failure)
treprostinol (Remodulin) (B)	Vasodilator and platelet aggregation inhibitor	Continuous subcutaneous infusion: 1.25-2.5 ng/kg/min	Pulmonary artery hypertension in patients with severe heart failure

MI, Myocardial infarction.

DRUG PROFILES

♦ hydralazine

Hydralazine (Apresoline) is taken orally to treat routine cases of essential hypertension. It can also be given intravenously and is useful for patients who cannot tolerate oral therapy in the hospital or for hypertensive emergencies. Contraindications include drug allergy, coronary artery disease, and mitral valve dysfunction. A new combination drug product is a tablet that contains both 37.5 mg of hydralazine and 20 mg of the anti-anginal drug isosorbide dinitrate (see Chapter 23). This drug combination is known as BiDil, and it is specifically indicated as an adjunct for treatment of heart failure in African-American patients. This drug combination has been shown to improve patient survival and prolong time to hospitalization for heart failure in African-American patient populations.

Pharmacokinetics: Hydralazine

Route	Onset of Action	Peak Plasma Concentration	Elimination Half-life	Duration of Action
IV	5-20 min	30-45 min	2-8 hr	1-4 hr
PO	20-30 min	1-2 hr	2-8 hr	8 hr

! sodium nitroprusside

Sodium nitroprusside (Nitropress) is used in the intensive care setting for severe hypertensive emergencies and is titrated to effect by intravenous infusion. Its use is contraindicated in patients with a known hypersensitivity to the drug, severe heart failure, and known inadequate cerebral perfusion (especially during neurosurgical procedures). Recommended dosages are given in the table on the previous page.

Pharmacokinetics: Sodium Nitroprusside

Route	Onset of Action	Peak Plasma Concentration	Elimination Half-life	Duration of Action
IV	Less than 2 min	2-5 min	2 min	1-10 min

MISCELLANEOUS ANTIHYPERTENSIVE DRUGS

Eplerenone (Inspra) represents a new class of drugs called *selective aldosterone blockers* and is used for hypertension. Other miscellaneous drugs are used to treat pulmonary artery hypertension.

DRUG PROFILES

eplerenone

Eplerenone (Inspra) is currently the only drug in a new class of antihypertensive drugs called selective aldosterone blockers. It reduces blood pressure by blocking the actions of aldosterone at its corresponding receptors in the kidney, heart, blood vessels, and brain. Eplerenone is indicated for both routine treatment of hypertension and for post-MI heart failure. Its use is contraindicated in patients with known drug allergy, elevated serum potassium levels (higher than 5.5 mEq/L), or severe renal impairment and in those using a medication that inhibits the action of cytochrome P-450 enzyme 3A4. Many commonly used medications inhibit the action of this enzyme, including several antibiotic, antifungal, and antiviral drugs. Recommended dosages are given in the table on the previous page.

bosentan

Bosentan (Tracleer) works by blocking the receptors of the hormone endothelin. Normally this hormone acts to stimulate the narrowing of blood vessels by binding to endothelin receptors (ET_A and ET_B) in the endothelial (innermost) lining of blood vessels and in vascular smooth muscle. Bosentan reduces blood pressure by blocking this action. However, currently it is specifically indicated only for the treatment of pulmonary artery hypertension in patients with moderate to severe heart failure. It is available only through a limited distribution program directly from the manufacturer. Its use is contraindicated in patients with known drug allergy, pregnancy, or significant liver impairment, and in patients receiving concurrent drug therapy with cyclosporine or glyburide. Recommended dosages are given in the table on this page.

Other drugs used to treat pulmonary hypertension include epoprostenol, treprostinil, iloprost, ambrisentan, and macitentan. The erectile dysfunction drugs sildenafil and tadalafil are also used (see Chapter 35). Both of these drugs go by different trade names when used for pulmonary hypertension. Sildenafil, which is commonly known as Viagra, also has the trade name Revatio; and tadalafil, which is commonly known as Cialis, is called Adcirca when used for pulmonary hypertension.

treprostinil

Treprostinil (Remodulin) lowers blood pressure through a combined mechanism of action by dilating both pulmonary and systemic blood vessels and by inhibiting platelet aggregation. Like bosentan, it is indicated specifically for treatment of pulmonary artery hypertension in patients with moderate to severe heart failure. Its only current contraindication is known drug allergy. Prior to 2014 when an oral form of trepostinil (Orenitram) became available, it was given either by inhalation or infusion. Recommended dosages are given in the table on the previous page.

▌NURSING PROCESS

The National Institutes of Health (first issued in May 2003) has been instrumental in the switch from a stepped approach to a guideline-based approach to the diagnosis and treatment of hypertension. A complete description of the Joint National Committee (*JNC 8*) sponsored by the National Heart, Lung, and Blood Institute of the National Institutes of Health is presented in the pharmacology section. The nursing process discussion that follows provides both general and specific information related to the pharmacologic and nonpharmacologic treatment of all stages of hypertension.

▌ASSESSMENT

Before any *antihypertensive drug* is given to a patient, obtain a thorough health history and perform a head-to-toe physical assessment. Measure and document blood pressure, pulse rate, respirations, and pulse oximetry readings. An ECG may be ordered for baseline comparison requiring reporting of results to the prescriber. Monitor laboratory tests, including: (1) serum sodium, potassium, chloride, magnesium, and calcium levels; (2) CBC and platelet count; (3) renal function studies, including BUN, serum, and urinary creatinine levels; (4) C-reactive protein (CRP) to measure systemic inflammation; (4) cholesterol/lipid profiles; and (4) hepatic function studies, including serum levels of ALT and AST. Other cardiac-specific laboratory studies may be ordered for baseline comparative levels. These studies may include platelet function tests and cholesterol/lipid profiles. If a myocardial infarction is suspected, additional laboratory studies may include arterial blood gases (ABGs); erythrocyte sedimentation rate (ESR); and specific cardiac biomarkers/enzymes such as troponins (usually elevated within 4 to 6 hours after a heart attack and may be a reliable indicator up to 14 days after a heart attack), creatine phosphokinase–myocardial band (CPK-MB), LDH, and myoglobin levels. Laboratory tests will most likely be complemented by more sophisticated scans and imaging studies. Noninvasive ophthalmoscopic examination of the eye structures (e.g., optic nerve, optic disk, vessels) by a professionally trained health care practitioner (e.g., nurse practitioner, physician assistant, physician, ophthalmologist, optometrist) allows easy visualization of the structures impacted by hypertension. If hypertensive retinopathy is present, the examination will reveal narrowing of blood vessels in the eye, oozing of fluid from these blood vessels, spots on the retina, swelling of the macula and optic nerve, and/or bleeding in the back of the eye. These problems may be prevented by controlling the blood pressure or treating hypertension with appropriate follow-up once it is diagnosed. Additionally, assess for conditions, factors, or variables that may be underlying causes of a patient's hypertension, such as:

- Addison's disease
- Coarctation of the aorta
- Coronary heart disease
- Culture and race or ethnicity
- Cushing's disease
- Family history of hypertension
- Nicotine use
- Obesity
- Peripheral vascular disease
- Pheochromocytoma
- Preeclampsia of pregnancy
- Renal artery stenosis
- Renal or liver insufficiency
- Stressful lifestyle

Many of these factors demand very cautious use of *antihypertensive drugs*. Other cautions and contraindications include the use of these drugs in older adult patients and those with chronic illnesses because of further compromise of their physical condition due to uncontrolled or untreated hypertension or the adverse effects of antihypertensives (e.g., fluid loss, dehydration, electrolyte imbalances, hypotension). For a complete listing of adverse effects as well as drug interactions associated with antihypertensives, refer to the pharmacology section of this chapter.

Use of *alpha-adrenergic agonists* demands close assessment of the patient's blood pressure, pulse rate, and weight before and during treatment because of their strong vasodilating properties and subsequent hypotensive adverse effects. These drugs may also be associated with fluid retention and edema, so assess heart and breath sounds and intake and output, as well as dependent edema. The *alpha-adrenergic antagonists* need to be used cautiously because of the potential for hypotension-induced dizziness and syncope. The use of either of these groups of drugs requires close assessment of all parameters, especially in the older adult patient or other patients with preexisting dizziness or syncope, or a debilitated state. With *doxazosin*, first-dose orthostatic hypotension may occur within 2 to 6 hours; therefore, carefully assess blood pressures (supine and standing) and measure corresponding pulse rates before the first dose and 2 to 6 hours afterward, as well as with any subsequent increase in the dosage. When any antihypertensive drug is used, measure blood pressures and pulse rates (supine and standing), and assess for cautions, contraindications, and drug interactions. With *centrally acting alpha blockers*, also assess white blood cell counts, serum potassium and sodium levels, and level of protein in the urine (to identify proteinuria). Note the route of administration specified in the drug order because of concerns associated with different routes. For example, with clonidine transdermal patches, assess the skin for rash, redness, drainage, or broken integrity prior to application.

Review the *beta blockers* and their mechanisms of action before administering these drugs to a patient because of the risk for complications in certain patient populations. If the drug is a *nonselective beta blocker*, it blocks both beta$_1$ and beta$_2$ receptors and will have both cardiac and respiratory effects, whereas if a drug is only a *beta$_1$-blocking drug*, the cardiac system will be affected (pulse rate and blood pressure will decrease) but there will be no beta$_2$ effects. This limits any concern regarding respiratory problems (e.g., bronchoconstriction). Therefore, if a patient needs a beta blocker but has restrictive airway problems, a beta$_1$ blocker is recommended (to avoid bronchoconstriction). However, if there is no history of respiratory illness or concerns, the nonselective beta blockers may be very effective as antihypertensives. In addition, for patients with heart failure, understand that beta blockers also have a negative inotropic effect on the heart (decreased contractility); their use would lead to worsening of heart failure, which calls for a completely different class of antihypertensive drugs.

With the use of beta blockers, assess blood pressure and apical pulse rate immediately before each dose. If the systolic blood pressure is less than 90 mm Hg or the pulse rate is less than 60 beats/min, notify the prescriber because of the risk for adverse effects (e.g., hypotension, bradycardia). In such cases, the drug would usually be withheld, as ordered or per protocol. These blood pressure and pulse rate parameters are also applicable with use of other antihypertensives. Assess breath sounds and heart sounds before and during drug therapy.

With the use of *ACE inhibitors,* assess blood pressure, apical pulse rate, and respiratory status (because of the adverse effect of a dry, hacking, chronic cough). Take blood pressure readings immediately before initial and subsequent doses of the drug so that extreme fluctuations may be identified early. Assess serum potassium, sodium, and chloride levels, as ordered. Tests of baseline cardiac functioning will most likely be ordered prior to initiation of therapy. Because of the potential adverse effects of neutropenia and other blood disorders, assess complete blood count before and during therapy, as ordered. *Angiotensin receptor blockers (ARBs)* are to be used very cautiously in older adult patients and in patients with renal dysfunction because of their increased sensitivity to the drug's effects and increased risk for adverse effects.

Perform a baseline neurologic assessment with the use of *vasodilators,* with attention to level of consciousness and cognitive ability. Use these drugs with extreme caution with the older adult patient, because they are more sensitive to the drugs' blood pressure–lowering effects and may experience more problems with hypotension, dizziness, and syncope.

Assess for contraindications associated with *eplerenone (Inspra),* a drug from a new class of drugs *(selective aldosterone blockers),* such as elevated serum potassium levels (greater than 5.5 mEq/L) or severe renal impairment. This drug needs to be avoided in concurrent use of drugs that inhibit the action of cytochrome P-450 enzyme 3A4 such as antifungals, antivirals, and some antibiotic drugs. Assess baseline blood pressure readings.

In summary, many assessment parameters are similar for the various groups of *antihypertensives.* The difference in the level of assessment depends on the drug's specific mechanism of action, impact on blood pressure as well as the individual's response to the medication, and any preexisting illnesses or conditions. Other factors to be assessed in any patient receiving these drugs, as well as with most drugs, include the patient's cultural background (see Patient-Centered Care: Cultural Implications), racial or ethnic group, reading level, learning needs, developmental and cognitive status, financial status, mental health status, available support systems, and overall physical health. Encourage patients to learn how to assess and monitor themselves and their individual responses to drug therapy.

These findings are important to remember in the care of patients, whether they are in an inpatient setting; are being seen by a physician, physician's assistant, or nurse practitioner; or are being screened by a nurse in the community. The significance of these cultural-ethnic factors is that they allow a better understanding of the dynamics of pharmacologic treatment in hypertensive patients of different ethnic groups and also underscore the importance of a thorough nursing assessment that includes attention to cultural influences. These factors also allow an appreciation of individual responses to drug therapy and aid in achieving more successful treatment of the disease. These responses are often considered by health care providers in selecting first-line therapy.

NURSING DIAGNOSES

1. Ineffective peripheral tissue perfusion related to the impact of the hypertensive disease process and/or possible severe

---

⊕ PATIENT-CENTERED CARE: CULTURAL IMPLICATIONS

Antihypertensive Drug Therapy

The following are some important generalizations about demographics and the drugs used to treat hypertension:

- Both thiazide-type diuretics and calcium channel blockers (CCBs) are recommended as first-line therapy for management of hypertension in black patients.
- Asian patients receiving a CCB have been reported as achieving the highest rates of control of hypertension. ARBs and ACEIs appear to have tolerability and/or adherence advantages.
- The low use of diuretics in Asians may be related to the occurrence of serious side effects (i.e., hypokalemia, because of the usual low dietary intake of potassium in these individuals).
- As noted in Western hypertensive patients, many Asian patients will possibly require at least two antihypertensive medications to achieve blood pressure control. Use of single-pill combinations have shown to improve the convenience and simplicity of drug therapy regimens.
- Treatment with a thiazide diuretic, CCB, or ARB for isolated systolic hypertension is recommended as first-line therapy in the Taiwanese.
- Because of higher rates of cardiac morbidity in Hispanic Americans, researchers have suggested that ACEIs and ARBs may be useful in this population in protecting against end-organ damage secondary to hypertension.

Modified from Panel members appointed to the Eighth Joint National Committee (JNC 8), February 5, 2014. Available at *www.aafp.org/afp.* Accessed April 17, 2015; Park JB, Kario K, Wang J: Systolic hypertension: An increasing clinical challenge in Asia. *Hypertension Research* 38:227-236, 2015. Published online December 11, 2014. Accessed April 17, 2015; and Patel NK, Wood RC, Espino DV: Cultural considerations: Pharmacological and nonpharmacological means for improving blood pressure control among Hispanic patients. *International Journal of Hypertension,* 2012. Available at http://dx.doi.org/10.1155/2012/831016.

---

hypotensive adverse effects associated with antihypertensive drug therapy

2. Sexual dysfunction related to adverse effects of some antihypertensive drugs
3. Constipation related to the adverse effects of antihypertensive drugs
4. Noncompliance with drug therapy related to lack of familiarity with or acceptance of the disease process
5. Risk for injury (e.g., possible falls) related to possible antihypertensive drug–induced orthostatic hypotension with dizziness and syncope

PLANNING: OUTCOME IDENTIFICATION

Focus nursing goals for antihypertensive therapy on educating the patient, family, and/or caregiver about the critical importance of adequate management to prevent end-organ damage. Goals must include making sure the patient understands the nature of the disease, its symptoms and treatment, and the importance of adhering to the treatment regimen. The patient must also come to terms with the diagnosis as well as with the fact that there is no cure for the disease and treatment will be lifelong. Emphasize the influence of chronic illness and the importance of nonpharmacologic therapy, stress reduction, and follow-up care. Plan for ongoing assessment of blood pressure, weight, diet, exercise, smoking habits, alcohol intake, compliance with therapy, and sexual function in the patient receiving therapy for hypertension.

1. Patient regains control of blood pressure and adequate tissue perfusion through taking antihypertensive drug therapy, as prescribed, with the return of systolic blood pressure to 120 to 139 mmHg and/or diastolic pressure to 80 to 89 mmHg.
2. Patient openly discusses any difficulty in sexual functioning during antihypertensive therapy and implements suggestions/interventions shared by the prescriber with avoidance of abrupt discontinuation of drug therapy.
3. Patient experiences minimal changes in bowel elimination patterns through healthy lifestyle/dietary changes including increased fluids, increase in fruits/vegetables, and/or taking prescriber-suggested psyllium-based products.
4. Patient remains compliant with drug therapy with understanding of the importance of taking antihypertensive medication(s) exactly as prescribed, adverse effects to report to the prescriber, and avoidance of abrupt discontinuation.
5. Patient avoids injury to self by following instructions to maintain safety and minimize dizziness and syncope while on medication regimen by changing position slowly, carefully, and purposely and by keeping a daily journal with entries about diet, exercise, adverse effects, blood pressure readings, and daily weights.

IMPLEMENTATION

Nursing interventions may help patients achieve stable blood pressure while minimizing adverse effects during treatment with *antihypertensives*. Many patients have problems complying with treatment because the disease itself is silent or without symptoms. Because of this, some patients are unaware of their increased blood pressure or think that if they do not feel bad there is nothing wrong with them, which poses many problems for treatment. Also, the antihypertensives are often associated with multiple adverse effects that may impact patients' energy level, self-concept, and/or sexual integrity. These adverse effects may lead patients to abruptly stop taking the medication. Inform patients that any abrupt withdrawal is a serious concern because of the risk for developing rebound hypertension, which is a sudden and very high elevation of blood pressure. This places the patient at risk for a cerebrovascular accident or other cerebral or cardiac adverse events. It is important to understand that with *all* antihypertensives there is a risk for rebound hypertension (with abrupt withdrawal), and prevention of this through patient education is critical to patient safety. Other interventions related to each major group of drugs are discussed in the following paragraphs. See Patient-Centered Care: Patient Teaching later in the chapter for more information.

Because of the potential for drug-related orthostatic hypotensive effects, patients taking *alpha-adrenergic agonists* will need to monitor their blood pressure and pulse rate at home or have these parameters measured by a family member who has received instructions or by their health care provider. Blood

pressure machines found in grocery stores do not provide as accurate readings. *Alpha-adrenergic antagonist drugs* are associated with first-dose syncope, so, to avoid injury, advise patients to remain supine for the first dose of the drug. More than likely, these drugs will be prescribed to be given at bedtime to allow the patient to sleep through the drug's first-dose syncope effect. It may take 4 to 6 weeks for the drug to achieve its full therapeutic effects. Educate the patient about this delayed onset of action and bedtime dosing to avoid injury. The patient needs continued monitoring for dizziness, syncope, edema, and other adverse effects (e.g., shortness of breath, exacerbation of preexisting cardiac disorders). Diuretics may be ordered as adjunctive therapy to minimize the adverse effects of edema, but they may lead to more dizziness and electrolyte problems. *Centrally acting alpha blockers* require the same type of nursing interventions as other alpha blockers; however, as their name indicates, the mechanism of action of these drugs is central, so adverse effects are often more pronounced (e.g., hypotension, sedation, bradycardia, edema). See Patient-Centered Care: Patient Teaching later in the chapter for more information.

The *beta blockers* are either *nonselective* (block both beta$_1$ and beta$_2$ receptors; e.g., propranolol) or *cardioselective* (block mainly beta$_1$ receptors; e.g., atenolol). With any beta blocker, careful adherence to the drug regimen is critical to patient safety. Patients taking beta blockers may experience an exacerbation of respiratory diseases such as asthma, bronchospasm, and chronic obstructive pulmonary disease (because of increased bronchoconstriction due to beta$_2$ blocking) or an exacerbation of heart failure (because of the drug's negative inotropic effects, i.e., decreased contractility due to beta$_1$ blocking). Provide clear and concise instructions about reporting adverse effects and instructions for taking blood pressure and pulse rates. If a *beta$_1$ blocker* causes shortness of breath, it is most likely due to edema and/or exacerbation of heart failure. Any dizziness, postural hypotension, edema, constipation, or sexual dysfunction needs to be reported to the prescriber immediately. See Patient-Centered Care: Patient Teaching later in the chapter for more information.

ACE inhibitors must also be taken exactly as prescribed. If angioedema occurs, contact the prescriber immediately. If the drug must be discontinued, weaning is recommended (as with all antihypertensives) to avoid rebound hypertension. Monitor serum sodium and potassium levels during therapy. Serum potassium levels increase as an adverse effect of these drugs, resulting in hyperkalemia and possible complications. See the Safety: Laboratory Values Related to Drug Therapy box. Impaired taste may occur as an adverse effect and last up to 2 to 3 months after the drug has been discontinued. It is also important to educate the patient that it takes several weeks to see the full therapeutic effects and that potassium supplements are not needed with the ACE inhibitors because of the adverse effect of hyperkalemia.

Angiotensin receptor blockers (ARBs) must also be taken exactly as prescribed. They are often tolerated best with meals, as with many antihypertensives. The dosage must not be changed nor the medication discontinued except on the order of the prescriber. With ARBs, if the patient suffers from hypovolemia or hepatic dysfunction, the dosage may need to be reduced. A diuretic such as hydrochlorothiazide may be ordered in combination with an ARB for patients who have hypertension with left ventricular hypertrophy. *Losartan* is also an option for patients at risk for stroke and for those who are hypertensive and have left ventricular hypertrophy. Most importantly, with ARBs, report any unusual dyspnea, dizziness, or excessive fatigue to the prescriber immediately.

Nursing considerations for *vasodilators* are similar to those for other antihypertensives; however, the impact of the vasodilators on blood pressure may be more drastic, depending on the specific drug and dosage. *Hydralazine* given by injection may result in reduced blood pressure within 10 to 80 minutes after administration and requires that you closely monitor the patient. With hydralazine, systemic lupus erythematosus (SLE) may be an adverse effect if the patient is taking more than 200 mg/day orally. If signs and symptoms of SLE occur, such as photosensitivity, characteristic skin rashes, CNS changes, or various blood dyscrasias (hemolytic anemia, leukopenia, thrombocytopenia), discontinue the drug, contact the prescriber immediately, and continue to closely monitor the patient. Electrocardiographic changes, cardiovascular inadequacies, and hypotension may have pronounced effects on the patient's cardiac status, so *never* give the drug without adequate monitoring and frequent assessment. Always dilute *sodium nitroprusside* per the manufacturer's guidelines. Because this drug is a potent vasodilator, it may lead to extreme decreases in the patient's blood pressure. Severe drops in blood pressure may lead to irreversible ischemic injury and even death, so close monitoring is needed during drug administration. Remember that sodium nitroprusside is never to be infused at more than 10 minutes. If sodium nitroprusside does not control a patient's blood pressure after 10 minutes, the prescriber will most likely discontinue the drug.

Sodium nitroprusside is rarely used, but its toxicity is worthy of a brief discussion. In the clinical setting, cyanide and thiocyanate toxicity are seen when sodium nitroprusside is used at high dosages and for long periods and/or in patients with renal insufficiency. Prevention of cyanide toxicity begins with the infusion of an accurate dose and infusion time (see the pharmacology discussion). Prompt diagnosis and treatment of the cyanide toxicity is critical to patient safety and consists of discontinuing the administration of sodium nitroprusside and the possible infusion of sodium thiosulfate in sufficient quantity to convert the cyanide into thiocyanate. The medications necessary for this treatment are contained in commercially available cyanide antidote kits.

Calcium channel blockers (CCBs) and related nursing interventions are discussed only briefly here, because these drugs are covered in other chapters. These drugs are to be taken exactly as prescribed with a warning to the patient not to puncture, open, or crush the extended-release or sustained-release tablets and capsules. Be aware that CCBs are negative inotropic drugs (decrease cardiac contractility), and there may be more signs of heart failure because of this action. Monitoring of blood pressure and pulse rate before and during therapy will aid in prevention or early detection of any problems related to

SAFETY: LABORATORY VALUES RELATED TO DRUG THERAPY   QSEN

ACE Inhibitors

Laboratory Test	Normal Ranges	Rationale for Assessment
Serum creatinine and potassium levels	Serum Creatinine = 0.5-14 mg/dL Serum Potassium = 3.5-5.2 mEq/L Note: Laboratory values vary by health care institution.	ACE Inhibitors can cause renal impairment, which can be identified with serum creatinine. ACE Inhibitors can also cause hyperkalemia, and potassium levels need to be monitored.

the negative inotropic effects, negative chronotropic effects (decreased heart rate), and negative dromotropic effects (decreased conduction).

Remember always to base nursing interventions on a thorough assessment and plan of care that also includes consideration of the patient's cultural and ethnic group. This is particularly important with antihypertensives, because research studies have documented differences in responses to antihypertensives among different racial and ethnic groups. Some ethnic groups respond less favorably to certain drugs than to others. As for patients with any disease, patients with hypertension must be treated with respect and with an appreciation for a holistic approach to health care in which all physical, psychosocial, and spiritual needs are taken into consideration (see the Patient-Centered Care: Cultural Implications box). Remember that patient education is of critical importance and plays an important role in ensuring adherence to the drug regimen and in decreasing the incidence of problems related to these medications.

EVALUATION

Because patients with hypertension are at high risk for cardiovascular injury, it is critical for them to adhere to both their pharmacologic and nonpharmacologic treatment regimens. Monitoring patients for the adverse effects (e.g., orthostatic hypotension, dizziness, fatigue) and toxic effects of the various types of *antihypertensive drugs* helps to identify potentially life-threatening complications. The most important aspect of the evaluation process is collecting data and monitoring patients for evidence of controlled blood pressure. Blood pressure must be maintained at values lower than the parameters established by the Joint National Committee (see Box 22-1) or below the levels set by the Joint National Committee for "prehypertension," namely, a systolic blood pressure of 120 to 139 mm Hg and/or a diastolic blood pressure of 80 to 89 mm Hg. If compelling indications are present, such as diabetes mellitus or kidney disease, the blood pressure goal is often lower. Blood pressure needs to be monitored at periodic intervals. Patient education about self-monitoring is very important to the safe use of these drugs. Updated information on hypertension and its diagnosis, treatment, and evaluation is available at the National Heart, Lung, and Blood Institute website at *www.nhlbi.nih.gov*.

In addition to measuring blood pressure, the prescriber will examine the fundus of the patient's eye. Changes in the fundus have been found to be a more reliable indicator of the long-term effectiveness of treatment than blood pressure readings because of the changes in the vasculature of the eye caused by high blood pressure. Continually monitor the patient for the development of end-organ damage and for the presence of the specific problems that the medication can cause. Counsel and constantly monitor male patients receiving *antihypertensives* for complaints of sexual dysfunction. This is important because the patient may experience sexual dysfunction and, if the patient is not expecting it, may not report the problem and decide to stop taking the medication abruptly. Once an antihypertensive drug is stopped

abruptly, the patient is then placed at high risk for rebound hypertension and possible stroke or other complications. Communication is critical in these situations. Follow-up visits to the prescriber are important for monitoring these and other adverse effects and checking patient adherence to the drug regimen.

Therapeutic effects of antihypertensives in general include an improvement in blood pressure and in the disease process. Other therapeutic effects include a return to a normal baseline level of blood pressure with improved energy levels and decreased signs and symptoms of hypertension, such as less edema, improved breath sounds, no abnormal heart sounds, capillary refill in less than 5 seconds, and less shortness of breath. Monitor for the adverse effects discussed in the pharmacology section of this chapter as well as those described for each group of drugs earlier in the Nursing Process section.

QSEN | **EVIDENCE-BASED PRACTICE**

Effectiveness of Yoga for Hypertension: A Systematic Review and Meta-analysis

Type of Evidence

Several reviews regarding the potential benefits of yoga for reducing blood pressure control have been published, but the quality of studies identified is generally poor. Few reviews have focused on blood pressure control exclusively and with meta-analysis lacking. The degree to which blood pressure is decreased by yoga as compared to a comparison group is also unclear. This research paper attempts to address these gaps and present a systematic review and meta-analysis of controlled studies that look at the effects that practicing yoga has on systolic and diastolic blood pressure in those diagnosed with prehypertension and hypertension. Seventeen studies were examined for the effect of yoga on blood pressure control. The type of yoga intervention (postures, meditation, and breathing) was used as a subgroup.

Results of the Study

Yoga was associated with a small, yet significant, decline in both systolic and diastolic blood pressure. Yoga's effects on blood pressure was found to vary by type of yoga intervention and by comparison group but not by the duration of practice. The level of blood pressure control achieved by yoga was similar to that of lifestyle modifications (exercise, reduced sodium and alcohol intake) advocated by current guidelines. Larger reductions in blood pressure were observed when the analysis was restricted to studies using all three elements

of yoga practice (postures, meditation, and breathing). Additionally, yoga was associated with a significant decline of about 7.96 in systolic pressure and a 5.52 drop in diastolic pressure relative to no treatment but not compared to exercise in other forms. Overall, this is the first meta-analytic review on the effects of yoga on blood pressure. Strengths include the systematic literature search with multiple databases, while limitations include the fact that the style of yoga, qualifications of the instructors, practice environments, fitness level, and blood pressure assessment procedures were not assessed.

Link of Evidence to Nursing Practice

This study is the first meta-analysis examining the effects of yoga on blood pressure among those diagnosed with prehypertension and hypertension. Overall, yoga was associated with a modest decrease in blood pressure. The reductions in blood pressure may suggest that yoga offers an effective intervention for blood pressure reduction among this population. However, more studies with larger numbers of individuals are needed to further investigate the potential benefits of yoga in improving blood pressure in those with prehypertension and hypertension. A look at the impact of an optimal yoga program and its frequency of occurrence on blood pressure would be extremely beneficial. Nurses may be instrumental in conducting more research as well as recommending effective interventions for blood pressure control such as yoga.

Hagins M, States R, Selfe T, Innes K. Effectiveness of Yoga for Hypertension: Systematic Review and Meta-Analysis. *Evidence-Based Complementary and Alternative Medicine.* 2013 (2013) May 28. PubMed PMID: 23781266. Accessed April 18, 2014.

CASE STUDY

Patient-Centered Care: Drugs for Hypertension

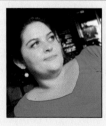

Hypertension was diagnosed in G., who is 30 years of age. Both her mother and sister have hypertension, and both were also in their thirties when it was diagnosed. G.'s most current blood pressure reading is 150/96 mm Hg, and for this reason the nurse practitioner has recommended therapy with captopril (Capoten), light exercise in the form of walking, and relaxation therapy. After 1 month of therapy, G.'s blood pressure is 145/86 mm Hg. Stress reduction has been the biggest obstacle in her treatment, because she is a lawyer with a prominent law firm and has found that her blood pressure is consistently elevated (160/100 mm Hg) whenever she measures it at work. At this follow-up visit, she

is also given a prescription for a diuretic to help with her blood pressure control. She plans to consult a therapist to work on stress-reduction techniques, and to begin exercising regularly.

1. What type of diuretic was probably prescribed for G. at this time? Explain your answer.
2. What possible adverse effects does G. need to be aware of while taking captopril?
3. G. tells you that she uses an over-the-counter pain reliever for occasional headaches. What potential interaction is of concern?
4. G. states that she and her husband are planning to start a family in 1 year. What will you, as her nurse, tell her about pregnancy and therapy with these drugs?

For answers, see *http://evolve.elsevier.com/Lilley*.

PATIENT-CENTERED CARE: PATIENT TEACHING

Antihypertensives in General

- Medications are to be taken exactly as ordered with avoidance of doubling up or omitting doses.
- Successful therapy requires adherence to the medication regimen as well as to any dietary restrictions (e.g., decreasing consumption of fatty or high-cholesterol foods).
- The patient needs to monitor stress levels and use biofeedback, imagery, and/or relaxation techniques or massage, as needed. Exercise, if approved by the prescriber, may also help in the management of hypertension and serves to relieve stress; supervised, prescribed exercise is usually ordered.
- Emphasize the importance of safety and the need to avoid smoking and excessive alcohol intake as well as excessive exercise, hot climates, saunas, hot tubs, and hot environments. Heat may precipitate vasodilation and lead to worsening of hypotension with the risk for fainting and injury to self.
- Frequent laboratory tests may be needed for the duration of therapy; emphasize the importance of keeping follow-up appointments to the patient.
- All medications must be kept out of the reach of children because of the potential for extreme toxicity. If a transdermal patch is used, instruct the patient on how to periodically check on its placement. There have been cases in which a patch that was placed on an adult later fell off and was accidentally picked up on the skin of a crawling infant, with severe consequences.
- Encourage the patient to wear a medical alert bracelet or necklace and to carry a medical identification card specifying his or her diagnosis, noting allergies, and listing all medications taken (e.g., prescribed drugs, over-the-counter medications, herbals, vitamins, and supplements). The same information must be kept in a visible location in the patient's car as well as in the patient's home (i.e., on the refrigerator) for emergency medical personnel.
- Emphasize the importance of recording blood pressure readings (and orthostatic blood pressure readings) and daily weights in a journal. Daily weights are to be done each morning, before breakfast, at the same time, and with the same amount of clothing. The patient must report to the prescriber an increase in weight by 2 pounds or more over a 24-hour period or 5 pounds or more in 1 week.
- Assess the patient's ability and comfort level in taking his or her own blood pressure and pulse rate. Monitor the patient's progress in the proper technique.
- Encourage the patient to inform all health care providers (e.g., dentist, surgeon) about his or her antihypertensive medication regimen.
- Careful, purposeful, and cautious changing of positions is encouraged because of the possible adverse effect of postural hypotension and associated risk for dizziness, lightheadedness, and possible fainting and falls.
- Instruct the patient to always keep an adequate supply of antihypertensive medications on hand, especially while traveling.

- Scheduling of periodic eye examinations is recommended every 6 months due to the need to evaluate treatment effectiveness because of the impact of hypertension on the vasculature of the eyes.
- With successful therapy, the patient's condition will improve; however, the patient must understand to never abruptly stop taking the medication just because he or she is feeling better. Lifelong therapy is usually required.
- Saliva substitutes, use of sugar-free hard candy/gum, and forcing fluids (unless contraindicated) may help with dry mouth. Forcing fluids and increasing dietary fiber may help with preventing constipation. Instruct the patient to contact the prescriber if constipation remains a problem.
- Sexual dysfunction may occur with antihypertensives. Encourage the patient to be open in reporting and discussing any problems or concerns. Inform the patient that, if this adverse effect occurs, options are available to help alleviate the problem, such as combination therapy that allows lower dosages of drugs to be used, as well as a change to other types of antihypertensives.
- Always reinforce the fact that these medications are never to be abruptly stopped because of the risk for severe hypertensive rebound.
- Inform the patient that antihypertensives may lead to depression and to report any change in emotional status to the prescriber.

Alpha-Adrenergic Agonists

- First-dose syncope is associated with alpha adrenergic agonists, so patients need to avoid conditions/situations/drugs that would exacerbate this.
- Caution the patient to be careful at first with driving and other activities requiring alertness. The patient may have to postpone driving and other activities until the drug-related drowsiness subsides.
- Instruct the patient to report any dizziness, palpitations, and orthostatic hypotension to the prescriber immediately.
- Because centrally acting alpha blockers may also affect the patient's sexual functioning (e.g., causing impotence or decreased libido), inform the patient of these possible adverse effects and advise the patient to contact the prescriber if these effects are problematic. Other treatment options may be indicated.
- Transdermal patches of clonidine are to be applied to non-hairy areas of the skin as ordered, and application sites rotated. All residual drug on the skin must be cleansed with a washcloth soaked in lukewarm water and the area thoroughly dried (avoid excess rubbing of site) before applying a new patch.

Beta Blockers

- Encourage the patient to move and change positions slowly to avoid possible dizziness, fainting, and falls. Instruct the patient to report a pulse rate lower than 60 beats/min, dizziness, or a systolic blood pressure of 90 mm Hg or lower to the prescriber.

- Prolonged sitting or standing and excessive physical exercise may also lead to exacerbation of hypotensive effects, so counsel the patient to avoid these activities or counteract them with healthy practices such as pumping the feet up and down while sitting.

- Heat may also exacerbate hypotensive effects of a beta blocker. Educate the patient to avoid saunas, hot tubs, and excessive heat, or syncope (fainting) may result.

KEY POINTS

- All antihypertensives in some way affect cardiac output. Cardiac output is the amount of blood ejected from the left ventricle and is measured in liters per minute.
- The major groups of antihypertensives are diuretics (see Chapter 28), alpha blockers, centrally acting alpha blockers, beta blockers, ACE inhibitors, vasodilators, CCBs, and ARBs.
- ACE inhibitors work by blocking a critical enzyme system responsible for the production of AII (angiotensin II; a potent vasoconstrictor). They (1) prevent vasoconstriction caused by AII, (2) prevent aldosterone secretion and therefore sodium and water resorption, and (3) prevent the breakdown of bradykinin (a potent vasodilator) by AII.
- ARBs work by blocking the binding of angiotensin at the receptors; the end result is a decrease in blood pressure.
- Calcium channel blockers may be used to treat angina, dysrhythmias, and hypertension and help to reduce blood pressure by causing smooth muscle relaxation and dilatation of blood vessels. If calcium is not present, then the smooth muscle of the blood vessels cannot contract.

- A thorough nursing assessment includes determining whether the patient has any underlying causes of hypertension, such as renal or liver dysfunction, a stressful lifestyle, Cushing's disease, Addison's disease, renal artery stenosis, peripheral vascular disease, or pheochromocytoma.
- Always assess for the presence of contraindications, cautions, and potential drug interactions before administering any of the antihypertensive drugs. Contraindications include a history of MI or chronic renal disease. Cautious use is recommended in patients with renal insufficiency or glaucoma. Drugs that interact with antihypertensive drugs include other antihypertensive drugs, anesthetics, and diuretics.
- Hypertension is managed by both pharmacologic and non-pharmacologic measures. Patients need to consume a diet low in fat, make any other necessary modifications in their diet (such as possibly decrease the intake of sodium and increase fiber intake), engage in regular supervised exercise, and reduce the amount of stress in their lives.

NCLEX® EXAMINATION REVIEW QUESTIONS

1. The nurse is administering antihypertensive drugs to older adult patients. The nurse knows that which adverse effect is of most concern for these patients?
   a. Dry mouth
   b. Hypotension
   c. Restlessness
   d. Constipation

2. When giving antihypertensive drugs, the nurse will consider giving the first dose at bedtime for which class of drugs?
   a. Alpha blockers such as doxazosin (Cardura)
   b. Diuretics such as furosemide (Lasix)
   c. ACE inhibitors such as captopril (Capoten)
   d. Vasodilators such as hydralazine (Apresoline)

3. A 46-year-old man started antihypertensive drug therapy 3 months earlier and is in the office for a follow-up visit. While the nurse is taking his blood pressure, he informs the nurse that he has had some problems with sexual intercourse. Which is the most appropriate response by the nurse?
   a. "Not to worry. Eventually, tolerance will develop."
   b. "The physician can work with you on changing the dose and/or drugs."
   c. "Sexual dysfunction happens with this therapy, and you will learn to accept it."
   d. "This is an unusual occurrence, but it is important to stay on your medications."

4. When a patient is being taught about the potential adverse effects of an ACE inhibitor, which of these effects should the

nurse mention as possibly occurring when this drug is taken to treat hypertension?
   a. Diarrhea
   b. Nausea
   c. Dry, nonproductive cough
   d. Sedation

5. A patient has a new prescription for an ACE inhibitor. During a review of the patient's list of current medications, which would cause concern for a possible interaction with this new prescription? (Select all that apply.)
   a. A benzodiazepine taken as needed for allergies
   b. A potassium supplement taken daily
   c. An oral anticoagulant taken daily
   d. An opioid used for occasional severe pain
   e. An NSAID taken as needed for headaches

6. The order reads: Give hydralazine (Apresoline) 0.75 mg/kg/day. The child weighs 16 pounds. How much hydralazine will be given? (Record your answer using two decimal places.)

7. The nurse is assessing a patient who will be starting antihypertensive therapy with an ACE inhibitor. Which condition, if present in the patient, would be a reason for cautious use?
   a. Asthma
   b. Rheumatoid arthritis
   c. Hyperthyroidism
   d. Renal insufficiency

1. b, 2. a, 3. b, 4. c, 5. b, e, 6. 5.45 mg/kg/day, 7. d.

CRITICAL THINKING AND PRIORITIZATION QUESTIONS

1. A 79-year-old woman has been admitted to the emergency department after experiencing severe headaches and "feeling faint." Upon admission, her blood pressure is measured as 286/190 mm Hg. A sodium nitroprusside infusion is started, and the nurse is monitoring the patient closely. After 8 minutes of infusion, the nurse notes that the patient's blood pressure suddenly drops to 100/60. What is the nurse's priority action at this time?

2. During a follow-up appointment, a 58-year-old man is pleased to hear that his blood pressure is 118/64 mm Hg. He says, "I've been hoping to hear this good news! Now I can stop taking these pills, right?" What is the nurse's best answer?

For answers, see *http://evolve.elsevier.com/Lilley*.

ⓔ EVOLVE WEBSITE

http://evolve.elsevier.com/Lilley
- Animations
- Answer Keys for Textbook Case Studies and Textbook Critical Thinking and Prioritization Questions
- Content Updates
- Key Points
- Review Questions
- Student Case Studies

Renal-ACES-50%.

23

Antianginal Drugs

http://evolve.elsevier.com/Lilley

When you reach the end of this chapter, you will be able to do the following:

1. Briefly describe the pathophysiology of myocardial ischemia and the subsequent occurrence of angina.
2. Describe the various factors that may precipitate angina as well as measures that decrease its occurrence.
3. Contrast the major classes of antianginal drugs (nitrates, calcium channel blockers, and beta blockers) with regard

to their mechanisms of action, dosage forms, routes of administration, cautions, contraindications, drug interactions, adverse effects, patient tolerance, and toxicity.

4. Develop a nursing care plan incorporating all phases of the nursing process related to the administration of antianginal drugs.

amlodipine, p. 370
♦atenolol, p. 367
♦diltiazem, p. 369
♦isosorbide dinitrate, p. 365
♦isosorbide mononitrate, p. 365
♦metoprolol, p. 368

♦nitroglycerin, p. 365
ranolazine, p. 370

_____
♦ = *Key drug*
! = *High-alert drug*

Angina pectoris Chest pain that occurs when the heart's supply of blood carrying oxygen is insufficient to meet the demands of the heart. (p. 363)

Atherosclerosis A common form of arteriosclerosis involving deposits of fatty, cholesterol-containing material (plaques) within arterial walls. (p. 363)

Chronic stable angina Chest pain that is primarily caused by atherosclerosis, which results in a long-term but relatively stable level of obstruction in one or more coronary arteries. (p. 363)

Coronary arteries Arteries that deliver oxygen to the heart muscle. (p. 363)

Coronary artery disease (CAD) Any one of the abnormal conditions that can affect the arteries of the heart and produce various pathologic effects, especially a reduced supply of oxygen and nutrients to the myocardium. (p. 363)

Ischemia Ischemia is damaged cells/tissue as the result of inadequate oxygen supply. (p. 363)

Ischemic heart disease Poor blood supply to the heart via the coronary arteries. (p. 363)

Myocardial infarction (MI) Necrosis of the myocardium following interruption of blood supply; it is almost always caused by atherosclerosis of the coronary arteries and is commonly called a *heart attack*. (p. 363)

Reflex tachycardia A rapid heartbeat caused by a variety of autonomic nervous system effects, such as blood pressure changes, fever, or emotional stress. (p. 364)

Unstable angina Early stage of progressive coronary artery disease. (p. 363)

Vasospastic angina Ischemia-induced myocardial chest pain caused by spasms of the coronary arteries; also referred to as *Prinzmetal* or *variant angina*. (p. 363)

362

OVERVIEW

The heart is a very efficient organ that pumps blood to all the tissues and organs of the body. It is very demanding in an aerobic sense because it requires a large supply of oxygen. There is a fine balance between oxygen supply and demand. The heart's much-needed oxygen supply is delivered to the heart muscle by means of the coronary arteries. When the heart's supply of blood carrying oxygen and energy-rich nutrients is insufficient to meet the demands of the heart, the heart muscle (or myocardium) aches. This is called angina pectoris, or chest pain. Angina pectoris results from a reduction in the oxygen supply/demand ratio. In order to alleviate the pain associated with angina, it is necessary to improve this ratio. This can be done either by increasing blood flow (which increases oxygen delivery or supply), or by decreasing oxygen demand (i.e., by decreasing myocardial oxygen consumption).

Damaged cells/tissue that is the result of inadequate oxygen supply is referred to as ischemia. When the heart is involved, the condition is called ischemic heart disease. Ischemic heart disease is the number-one killer in the United States today. The primary cause is a disease of the coronary arteries known as atherosclerosis (fatty plaque deposits in the arterial walls). When atherosclerotic plaques project from the walls into the lumens of these vessels, the vessels become narrow. The supply of oxygen and energy-rich nutrients needed for the heart is then decreased. This disorder is called coronary artery disease (CAD). An acute result of CAD and of ischemic heart disease is myocardial infarction (MI), or heart attack. An MI occurs when blood flow through the coronary arteries to the myocardium is completely blocked so that part of the heart muscle cannot receive any of the blood-borne nutrients (especially oxygen). If this process is not reversed immediately, that area of the heart will die and become necrotic (dead or nonfunctioning). Damage to a large enough area of the myocardium can be disabling or fatal.

The rate at which the heart pumps and the strength of each heartbeat (contractility) influence oxygen demands on the heart. There are many substances and situations that can increase heart rate and contractility and thus increase oxygen demand. These include caffeine, exercise, and stress, among others, and result in stimulation of the sympathetic nervous system, which leads to increased heart rate and contractility. In a patient with CAD who has an already overburdened heart, this stimulation can worsen the balance between myocardial oxygen supply and demand and result in angina. Some of the drugs used to treat angina are aimed at correcting the imbalance between myocardial oxygen supply and demand by decreasing heart rate and contractility.

The pain of angina is a result of the following process: Under ischemic conditions when the myocardium is deprived of oxygen, the heart shifts to anaerobic metabolism to meet its energy needs. One of the byproducts of anaerobic metabolism is lactic acid. Accumulation of lactic acid and other metabolic byproducts causes the pain receptors surrounding the heart to be stimulated, which produces the heart pain known as angina. This is the same pathophysiologic mechanism responsible for causing the soreness in skeletal muscles after vigorous exercise.

There are three classic types of chest pain, or angina pectoris. Chronic stable angina has atherosclerosis as its primary cause. Classic angina and effort angina are other names for it. Chronic stable angina can be triggered by exertion or other stress (e.g., cold, emotions). The nicotine in tobacco as well as alcohol, coffee, and other drugs that stimulate the sympathetic nervous system can also exacerbate it. The pain of chronic stable angina is commonly intense but subsides within 15 minutes of either rest or appropriate antianginal drug therapy. Unstable angina is usually the early stage of progressive coronary artery disease (CAD). It often ends in an MI in subsequent years. For this reason, unstable angina is also called preinfarction angina. Another term for this type of angina is crescendo angina, because the pain increases in severity, as does the frequency of attacks. In later stages, pain may even occur while the patient is at rest. Vasospastic angina results from spasms in the layer of smooth muscle that surrounds coronary arteries. In contrast to chronic stable angina, this type of pain often occurs at rest and without any precipitating cause. It does seem to follow a regular pattern, however, usually occurring at the same time of day. This type of angina is also called Prinzmetal angina or variant angina. Dysrhythmias and electrocardiogram (ECG) changes often accompany these different types of anginal attacks.

PHARMACOLOGY OVERVIEW

The three main classes of drugs used to treat angina pectoris are the nitrates and nitrites, the beta blockers, and the calcium channel blockers (CCBs). Their various therapeutic effects are summarized and compared in Table 23-1. There are three main therapeutic objectives of antianginal drug therapy: (1) minimize the frequency of attacks and decrease the duration and intensity of the anginal pain; (2) improve the patient's functional capacity with as few adverse effects as possible; and (3) prevent or delay the worst possible outcome, myocardial infarction. The overall goal of antianginal drug therapy is to increase blood flow to the ischemic myocardium, decrease myocardial oxygen demand, or both. Figure 23-1 illustrates how drug therapy works to alleviate angina.

NITRATES AND NITRITES

Nitrates have long been the mainstay for both the prophylaxis and treatment for angina and other cardiac problems. Today there are several chemical derivatives of the early precursors, all of which are organic nitrate esters. They are available in a wide variety of preparations, including sublingual and oral tablets; capsules; ointments; patches; a translingual spray; and intravenous solutions. The following are the rapid- and long-acting nitrates available for clinical use:

- Nitroglycerin (both rapid and long acting)
- Isosorbide dinitrate (both rapid and long acting)
- Isosorbide mononitrate (primarily long acting)

TABLE 23-1	Antianginal Drugs: Therapeutic Effects				
Therapeutic Effect	Nitrates	Beta Blockers*	Amlodipine	Verapamil	Diltiazem
Supply					
Blood flow	↑↑	↑	↑↑↑	↑↑↑	↑↑↑
Duration of diastole	0	↑↑↑	0/↑	↑↑↑	↑↑
Demand					
Preload†	↓↓	↑	↓/0	0	0/↓
Afterload	↓	0/↓	↓↓↓	↓↓	↓↓
Contractility	0	↓↓↓	↓	↓↓↓	↓↓
Heart rate	0/↑	↓↓↓	0/↓	↓↓	↓↓

↑, Increase; ↓, decrease; 0, little or no effect.
*In particular, those that are cardioselective and do not have intrinsic sympathomimetic activity.
†Preload is pressure in the heart caused by blood volume. The nitrates effectively move part of this blood out of the heart and into blood vessels, thereby decreasing preload or filling pressure.

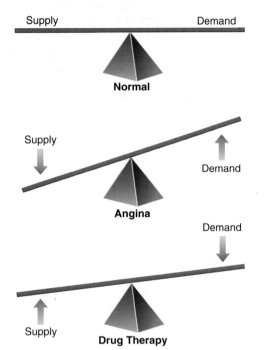
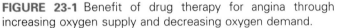

FIGURE 23-1 Benefit of drug therapy for angina through increasing oxygen supply and decreasing oxygen demand.

Mechanism of Action and Drug Effects

Medicinal nitrates and nitrites, more commonly referred to as *nitrates*, dilate all blood vessels. They predominantly affect venous vascular beds; however, they also have a dose-dependent arterial vasodilator effect. These vasodilatory effects are the result of relaxation of the smooth muscle cells that are part of the wall structure of veins and arteries. The nitrates have a potent dilating effect on the large and small coronary arteries. This causes redistribution of blood and oxygen to previously ischemic myocardial tissue and reduction of anginal symptoms. By causing venous dilation, the nitrates reduce venous return and, in turn, reduce the left ventricular end-diastolic volume

(or preload), which results in a lower left ventricular pressure. Left ventricular systolic wall tension is thus reduced, as is myocardial oxygen demand. These and other drug effects are summarized in Table 23-1.

Coronary arteries that have been narrowed by atherosclerosis can still be dilated as long as smooth muscle surrounding the coronary artery and the atherosclerotic plaque does not completely obstruct the arterial lumen. Exercise-induced spasms in atherosclerotic coronary arteries can also be reversed or prevented by administration of nitrates, which encourages healthy physical activity in patients.

Indications

The nitrates are used to treat stable, unstable, and vasospastic (Prinzmetal) angina. Long-acting dosage forms are used more for prevention of anginal episodes. Rapid-acting dosage forms, most often sublingual nitroglycerin tablets, or an intravenous drip in the hospital setting, are used to treat acute anginal attacks.

Contraindications

Contraindications to the use of nitrates include known drug allergy, as well as severe anemia, closed-angle glaucoma, hypotension, and severe head injury. Nitrates are also contraindicated with the use of the erectile dysfunction drugs sildenafil (Viagra), tadalafil (Cialis), and vardenafil (Levitra) (see Chapter 35).

Adverse Effects

Nitrates are well tolerated, and most adverse effects are usually transient and involve the cardiovascular system. The most common undesirable effect is headache, which generally diminishes soon after the start of therapy. Other cardiovascular effects include tachycardia and postural hypotension. If nitrate-induced vasodilation occurs too rapidly, the cardiovascular system overcompensates and increases the heart rate, a condition referred to as **reflex tachycardia**. This may occur with significant vasodilation that involves the systemic veins. There is a large shift in blood volume toward the systemic venous circulation and away from the heart. Baroreceptors (blood pressure receptors) in the heart then falsely sense that there has been a dramatic loss of blood volume. At this point, the heart begins beating more rapidly to move the apparently smaller volume of blood more quickly throughout the body, especially toward the vital organs (including the heart itself). However, the same baroreceptors soon sense that there has not been a loss of blood volume but that the volume of blood missing in the heart is now in the periphery (e.g., venous system), and the heart rate slows back to normal.

Topical nitrate dosage forms can produce various types of contact dermatitis (skin inflammation), but these are actually reactions to the dosage delivery system and not to the nitroglycerin itself; thus, it is not a true drug allergy. It is important for the nurse to document the type of allergic reaction, so that clinicians do not avoid this important drug class if the reaction is only a contact dermatitis.

Tolerance to the antianginal effects of nitrates can occur surprisingly quickly in some patients, especially those taking long-acting formulations or taking nitrates around the clock. In addition, cross-tolerance can arise when a patient receives more than one nitrate dosage form. To prevent this, a regular nitrate-free period is arranged to allow certain enzymatic pathways to replenish themselves. A common regimen with transdermal patches is to remove them at night for 8 hours and apply a new patch in the morning. This has been shown to prevent tolerance to the beneficial effects of nitrates. However, some studies have questioned the advisability of this practice.

Interactions

Nitrate antianginal drugs can produce additive hypotensive effects when taken in combination with alcohol, beta blockers, calcium channel blockers, phenothiazines, and erectile-dysfunction drugs such as sildenafil, tadalafil, and vardenafil. In fact, numerous deaths have been reported due to interactions with erectile-dysfunction drugs.

Dosages

The organic nitrates are available in an array of forms and doses. For dosage information, see the table on this page.

DRUG PROFILES

◆isosorbide dinitrate

Isosorbide dinitrate (Isordil) is an organic nitrate. It exerts the same effects as the other nitrates. When isosorbide dinitrate is metabolized in the liver, it is broken down into two active metabolites, both of which have the same therapeutic actions as isosorbide dinitrate itself. This drug is available in rapid-acting sublingual tablets, immediate-release tablets, and long-acting oral dosage forms.

Pharmacokinetics: Isosorbide Dinitrate

Route	Onset of Action	Peak Plasma Concentration	Elimination Half-life	Duration of Action
PO	1 hr	Unknown	3-5 hr	4-6 hr

DOSAGES

Selected Antianginal Nitrate Coronary Vasodilators

Drug (Pregnancy Category)	Usual Adult Dosage Range	Indications
◆isosorbide dinitrate (Isordil, Dilatrate-SR) (C)	PO: 10-40 mg bid-tid and 40-80 mg at 8 AM and 2 PM for SR formulations	Angina
◆isosorbide mononitrate (Imdur, Monoket) (C)	PO: 5-20 mg bid given 7 hr apart and 30-120 mg/day for SR formulations (Imdur)	
◆nitroglycerin (Nitro-Bid, Nitrostat, Nitrol, others) (C)	IV (continuous infusion): 5-200 mcg/min Ointment, 2%: 1- to 2-inch ribbon q8h Spray: 1-2 sprays sublingual every 5 min prn chest pain with a max of 3 doses within 15 min Sublingual: 1 tab under the tongue at first sign of chest pain; if pain not relieved after 2 doses, call 911; may repeat up to 3 tablets Patch: 0.1 to 0.8 mg/hr applied once daily for 12-14 hours, then remove	

SL, Sublingual; *SR,* sustained release.

◆isosorbide mononitrate

Isosorbide mononitrate (Imdur) is one of the two active metabolites of isosorbide dinitrate, but it has no active metabolites itself. Because of these qualities, it produces a more consistent, steady therapeutic response, with less variation in response within the same patient and between patients. It is available in both immediate- and sustained-release oral dosage forms but is most commonly used in the sustained-release form.

Pharmacokinetics: Isosorbide Mononitrate

Route	Onset of Action	Peak Plasma Concentration	Elimination Half-life	Duration of Action
PO	15-30 min	0.5-1 hr	5 hr	5-12 hr

◆nitroglycerin

Nitroglycerin is the prototypical nitrate and is manufactured by many pharmaceutical companies; therefore, it goes by many different trade names (e.g., Nitro-Bid, Nitrostat). It is often abbreviated as NTG or TNG. It has traditionally been the most important drug used in the symptomatic treatment of ischemic heart conditions such as angina. When given orally, nitroglycerin goes to the liver to be metabolized before it can become active in the body. During this process, a very large amount of the nitroglycerin is removed from the circulation. This is called a *large first-pass effect* (see Chapter 2). For this reason, nitroglycerin is administered by other routes to avoid the first-pass effect. Tablets administered by the sublingual route are used for the treatment of chest pain or angina of acute onset. They are also used for the prevention of angina when patients find themselves in situations likely to provoke an attack. Use of these routes is advantageous for relieving these acute conditions because the area under the tongue and inside the cheek is highly vascular. This means that the nitroglycerin is absorbed quickly and directly into the bloodstream, and hence its therapeutic effects occur rapidly. Sublingual nitroglycerin tablets must be stored in their original container, because exposure to air and moisture can inactivate the drug. Nitroglycerin also comes as a metered-dose aerosol that is sprayed under the tongue. Nitroglycerin is available in an intravenous form that is used for blood pressure control in hypertensive patients; for the treatment of ischemic pain, heart failure, and pulmonary edema associated with acute MI; and in hypertensive emergency situations. Oral and topical dosage formulations are used for the long-term prophylactic management of angina pectoris. The topical formulation offers the same advantages as the sublingual formulation in that it also bypasses the liver and the first-pass effect. This formulation allows for the continuous slow delivery of nitroglycerin, so that a steady dose of nitroglycerin is supplied to the patient. Patches are worn for 12-14 hours per day. See the Safety and Quality Improvement: Preventing Medication Errors box.

Pharmacokinetics: Nitroglycerin

Route	Onset of Action	Peak Plasma Concentration	Elimination Half-life	Duration of Action
Sublingual	2-3 min	Unknown	1-4 min	0.5-1 hr

BETA BLOCKERS

The beta-adrenergic blockers, more commonly referred to as *beta blockers*, have become the mainstay in the treatment of several cardiovascular diseases. These include angina, MI, hypertension (see Chapter 22), and dysrhythmias (see Chapter 25). Most available beta blockers demonstrate antianginal efficacy, although not all have been approved for this use. Those beta blockers approved as antianginal drugs are atenolol, metoprolol, nadolol, and propranolol.

Mechanism of Action and Drug Effects

The primary effects of the beta blockers are related to the cardiovascular system. As discussed in Chapters 19 and 22, the predominant beta-adrenergic receptors in the heart are the beta$_1$ receptors. Beta$_1$ receptors are located in the heart's conduction system and throughout the myocardium. The beta receptors are normally stimulated by the binding of the neurotransmitters epinephrine and norepinephrine. These catecholamines are released in greater quantities during times of exercise or other stress to stimulate the heart muscle to contract more strongly. At the normal heart rate of 60 to 80 beats/min, the heart spends 60% to 70% of its time in diastole. As the heart

Understanding Rate versus Dose

The Institute for Safe Medication Practices (ISMP) reported an incident in which a nitroglycerin intravenous drip was set to infuse at 60 mL/hr rather than 60 mcg/min. With the medication concentration used (50 mg/250 mL) the patient actually received 200 mcg/min instead of the ordered 60 mcg/min. Investigation of this incident revealed that the nurses were using a handwritten, nonstandard dosing table rather than one that corresponded to the available concentrations of premixed solutions in the hospital. According to the report, the patient became hypotensive but recovered.

It is crucial to understand the difference between "mL/hr" and "mcg/min" when programming infusion pumps; rates are not interchangeable with ordered doses! In addition, using standardized dosing charts that correspond to available concentrations of solutions is important. Some health care institutions also require double-checking of infusion pump settings before medication therapy is begun.

For more information, see Improvised dosing charts can cause errors, Nurse Advise-ERR 3(6):3, 2005. Available at *www.ismp.org/ newsletters/acutecare/articles/A4Q04Action.asp.* Accessed June 22, 2015.

rate increases during stress or exercise, the heart spends more time in systole and less time in diastole. The physiologic consequence is that the coronary arteries receive increasingly less blood, and eventually the myocardium becomes ischemic.

In an ischemic heart, the increased oxygen demand from increasing contractility (systole) also leads to increasing degrees of ischemia and chest pain. The physiologic act of systole requires energy in the form of adenosine triphosphate (ATP) and oxygen. Therefore, any decrease in the energy demands on the heart is beneficial for alleviating conditions such as angina. When beta blockers block the beta receptors, the rate at which the pacemaker (sinoatrial [SA] node) fires decreases, and the time it takes for the node to recover increases. The beta blockers also slow conduction through the atrioventricular (AV) node and reduce myocardial contractility (negative inotropic effect). Both of these effects serve to slow the heart rate (negative chronotropic effect). These effects reduce myocardial oxygen demand, which aids in the treatment of angina by reducing the workload of the heart. Slowing the heart rate is also beneficial in patients with ischemic heart disease, because the coronary arteries have more diastolic time to fill with oxygen- and nutrient-rich blood and deliver these substances to the myocardial tissues.

The beta blockers also have many therapeutic effects after an MI. Following an MI, there are high levels of circulating catecholamines (norepinephrine and epinephrine). These catecholamines will produce harmful consequences if their actions go unopposed. They cause the heart rate to increase, which leads to a further imbalance in the supply-and-demand ratio, and they irritate the conduction system of the heart, which can result in potentially fatal dysrhythmias. The beta blockers block all of these harmful effects, and their use has been shown to improve the chances for survival in patients after MI. Unless strongly contraindicated, beta blockers are given to all patients in the acute stages after an MI.

The beta blockers also suppress the activity of the hormone renin, which is the first step in the renin-aldosterone-angiotensin system. Renin is a potent vasoconstrictor released by the kidneys when they sense that they are not being adequately perfused. When beta blockers inhibit the release of renin, blood vessels to and in the kidney dilate, causing reduced blood pressure (see Chapter 22).

Indications

The beta blockers are most effective in the treatment of exertional angina (i.e., that caused by exercise). This is because the beta blockers blunt the usual physiologic effects of an increase in heart rate and systolic blood pressure that occur during exercise or stress, thereby decreasing the myocardial oxygen demand. For an individual with significant angina, "exercise" may simply be carrying out the activities of daily living, such as bathing, dressing, cooking, or housekeeping. Performing such activities with significant angina can become a major stressor. The beta blockers are also approved for the treatment of MI, hypertension (see Chapter 22), cardiac dysrhythmias (see Chapter 25), and essential tremor. Some uses that are common but are not U.S. Food and Drug Administration (FDA) approved are treatment of migraine headache and, in low dosages, even treatment of the tachycardia associated with stage fright.

Contraindications

There are a number of contraindications to the use of beta blockers, including systolic heart failure and serious conduction disturbances, because of the effects of beta blockade on heart rate and myocardial contractility. These drugs should be used with caution in patients with bronchial asthma, because any level of blockade of beta$_2$ receptors can promote bronchoconstriction. These contraindications are relative rather than absolute and depend on patient-specific risks and expected benefits of this drug therapy. Other relative contraindications include diabetes mellitus (due to masking of hypoglycemia-induced tachycardia) and peripheral vascular disease (the drug may further compromise cerebral or peripheral blood flow).

Adverse Effects

The adverse effects of the beta blockers result from their ability to block beta-adrenergic receptors (beta$_1$ and beta$_2$ receptors) in various areas of the body. Blocking of beta$_1$ receptors may lead to a decrease in heart rate, cardiac output, and cardiac contractility. Blocking of beta$_2$ receptors may result in bronchoconstriction and increased airway resistance in patients with asthma or chronic obstructive pulmonary disease. Beta blockers may lead to cardiac rhythm problems, decreased SA and AV nodal conduction, a decrease in systolic and diastolic blood pressures, and decreased renin release from the kidneys. Beta blockers can mask the tachycardia associated with hypoglycemia, and diabetic patients may not be able to tell when their blood sugar falls too low. The beta blockers can also cause both hypoglycemia and hyperglycemia, which is of particular concern in diabetic patients. Fatigue, insomnia, and weakness may occur because of the negative effects on the cardiac and

central nervous systems. Other common beta blocker–related adverse effects are listed in Table 23-2.

Interactions

There are many important drug interactions that involve the beta blockers. The more common and important of these are listed in Table 23-3.

Dosages

For dosage information on selected beta blockers, see the table on the next page.

DRUG PROFILES

Beta blockers are the mainstay in the treatment of a wide range of cardiovascular diseases, mainly hypertension, angina, and the acute stages of MI. The three most commonly used beta blockers are carvedilol, metoprolol, and atenolol. Carvedilol (Coreg) is not indicated for angina per se, but it is instead indicated for heart failure, essential hypertension, and left ventricular dysfunction. The newest beta blocker, nebivolol (Bystolic), is used to treat hypertension. Atenolol, metoprolol, nadolol, and propranolol all are indicated for angina. The drug profile for carvedilol appears in Chapter 19.

♦ atenolol

Atenolol (Tenormin) is a cardioselective beta$_1$-adrenergic receptor blocker and is indicated for the prophylactic treatment of angina pectoris. Use of atenolol after MI has been shown to decrease mortality. It was formerly available in an injectable form, but it is now only available in oral form.

TABLE 23-2 Beta Blockers: Adverse Effects

Body System	Adverse Effects
Cardiovascular	Bradycardia, hypotension, atrioventricular block
Central nervous	Dizziness, fatigue, depression, lethargy
Metabolic	Delay hypoglycemia recovery, mask symptoms of hypoglycemia, hyperlipidemia
Other	Wheezing, dyspnea, impotence

TABLE 23-3 Beta Blockers: Common Drug Interactions

Interacting Drug	Mechanism	Result
Diuretics and antihypertensives	Additive effects	Hypotension
Calcium channel blockers (diltiazem, verapamil)	Additive atrioventricular node suppression	Hypotension, bradycardia, heart block
Insulin and oral antidiabetic drugs	Masking of hypoglycemic effects	Unrecognized hypoglycemia

DOSAGES

Selected Beta₁-Adrenergic–Blocking Drugs

Drug (Pregnancy Category)	Pharmacologic Class	Usual Adult Dosage Range	Indications
◆atenolol (Tenormin) (C)	} Beta₁ blocker	PO: 50-200 mg/day	} Angina
◆metoprolol (Lopressor, Toprol-XL) (C)		PO: IR: 100-400 mg/day in 2 divided doses ER: 100-400 mg daily	

Pharmacokinetics: Atenolol

Route	Onset of Action	Peak Plasma Concentration	Elimination Half-life	Duration of Action
PO	1 hr	2-4 hr	6-7 hr	24 hr

◆ metoprolol

Metoprolol (Lopressor, Toprol-XL) is also a cardioselective beta₁-adrenergic receptor blocker that is used for the prophylactic treatment of angina and has many of the same characteristics as atenolol. It has shown similar efficacy in reducing mortality in patients after MI and in treating angina. It is available in both oral (immediate-release and long-acting) and parenteral (injectable) forms. Intravenous metoprolol is commonly administered to hospitalized patients after an MI and is used for treatment of hypertension in patients unable to take oral medicine.

Pharmacokinetics: Metoprolol

Route	Onset of Action	Peak Plasma Concentration	Elimination Half-life	Duration of Action
IV	1 min	20 min	3-8 hr	5-8 hr
PO	1 hr	2-4 hr	3-8 hr	10-20 hr

CALCIUM CHANNEL BLOCKERS

There are three chemical classes of calcium channel blockers (CCBs): phenylalkylamines, benzothiazepines, and dihydropyridines, commonly represented by verapamil, diltiazem, and amlodipine, respectively (Table 23-4). Although they all block calcium channels, their chemical structures and therefore their mechanisms of action differ slightly. More than nine CCBs are available today. Those that are used for the treatment of chronic stable angina are amlodipine, diltiazem, nicardipine, nifedipine, and verapamil.

Mechanism of Action and Drug Effects

Calcium plays an important role in the excitation-contraction coupling process that occurs in the heart and vascular smooth muscle cells, as well as in skeletal muscle. Preventing calcium from entering into this process prevents muscle contraction and promotes muscle relaxation. Relaxation of the smooth muscles that surround the coronary arteries causes them to dilate. This dilation increases blood flow to the ischemic heart, which in

TABLE 23-4   Classification of Calcium Channel Blockers

Generic Name	Trade Name	Available Routes
Benzothiazepines		
diltiazem	Cardizem, Dilacor, Tiazac, Dilacor XR, Cartia XT, Matzim LA, Taztia XT, Diltia XT	PO/IV
Dihydropyridines		
amlodipine	Norvasc	PO
felodipine	Plendil	PO
isradipine	DynaCirc	PO
nicardipine	Cardene	PO/IV
nifedipine	Adalat, Procardia	PO
nimodipine	Nimotop	PO
Phenylalkylamines		
verapamil	Calan, Isoptin, Verelan	PO/IV

turn increases the oxygen supply and helps shift the supply/demand ratio back to normal. Dilation also occurs in the arteries throughout the body, which results in a decrease in the force (systemic vascular resistance) against which the heart must exert itself when delivering blood to the body (afterload). Decreasing the afterload reduces the workload of the heart and therefore reduces myocardial oxygen demand. This is the primary antianginal effect of the dihydropyridine CCBs such as amlodipine and nifedipine. These drugs have a less negative inotropic effect than do verapamil and diltiazem.

Another cardiovascular effect of the CCBs is depression of the automaticity of and conduction through the SA and AV nodes. For this reason, they are useful in treating cardiac dysrhythmias (see Chapter 25). Finally, the CCBs reduce myocardial contractility and peripheral and coronary artery tone. Verapamil and diltiazem also decrease heart rate. Their strongest antianginal properties are secondary to their effects on myocardial contractility and the smooth muscle tone of peripheral and coronary arteries.

Indications

The therapeutic benefits of the CCBs are numerous. Because of their very acceptable adverse effect and safety profiles, they are considered first-line drugs for the treatment of such conditions as angina, hypertension, and supraventricular tachycardia. They are often effective for the treatment of coronary artery spasms (vasospastic or Prinzmetal angina). However, they may not be as effective as the beta blockers in blunting exercise-induced elevations in heart rate and blood pressure. CCBs are also used for the short-term management of atrial fibrillation and flutter (see Chapter 25), migraine headaches (see Chapter 13), and Raynaud's disease (a type of peripheral vascular disease). The dihydropyridine CCB nimodipine is indicated solely for cerebral artery spasms associated with aneurysm rupture.

Contraindications

Contraindications include known drug allergy, acute MI, second- or third-degree AV block (unless the patient has a pacemaker), and hypotension.

Adverse Effects

The adverse effects of the CCBs are limited and primarily relate to overexpression of their therapeutic effects. The most common adverse effects are listed in Table 23-5. Historically, immediate-release nifedipine was used to lower blood pressure in acute hypertensive emergencies (the capsule was punctured and given sublingually). However, negative outcomes were reported with the rapid, dramatic reduction in blood pressure. For this reason, only the extended-release form of nifedipine is used today. (The exception is the use of immediate-release nifedipine for the treatment of premature labor.) Medication errors have occurred when a nurse drew up the contents of the capsule to be given sublingually, but inadvertently gave it intravenously. For this reason, the Institute for Safe Medication Practices recommends that the contents be drawn up into an oral syringe by the pharmacy.

Interactions

Important drug interactions are listed in Table 23-6. A particular food interaction of note is the interaction with grapefruit juice, which can reduce the metabolism of the CCBs, especially nifedipine.

Dosages

For dosage information on selected CCBs, see the table on this page.

DRUG PROFILES

◆ diltiazem

Diltiazem (Cardizem, Dilacor, Tiazac, others) is the only benzothiazepine CCB. It has a particular affinity for the cardiac conduction system and is very effective for the treatment of angina pectoris resulting from coronary insufficiency and hypertension. It is one of the few CCBs that are also available in parenteral form, for which it is used in the treatment of atrial fibrillation and flutter along with paroxysmal supraventricular tachycardia (see Chapter 25). Verapamil is another CCB with similar indications. Several sustained-delivery formulations of diltiazem are available, which can be confused with each other. For example, there is Cardizem SR, which is taken twice a day, and Cardizem CD, which is taken once a day. In addition to other brands of these two dosage forms, the drug is also available in several strengths of immediate-release capsule as well as in intravenous form.

TABLE 23-5 Calcium Channel Blockers: Adverse Effects

Body System	Adverse Effects
Cardiovascular	Hypotension, palpitations, tachycardia or bradycardia
Gastrointestinal	Constipation, nausea
Other	Dyspnea, rash, flushing, peripheral edema

TABLE 23-6 Calcium Channel Blockers: Common Drug Interactions

Interacting Drug	Mechanism	Result
Beta blockers	Additive effects	Bradycardia and atrioventricular block
digoxin	Interference with drug elimination	Possible increased digoxin levels
amiodarone	Decreased metabolism	Bradycardia and decreased cardiac output
Azole antifungals, clarithromycin, erythromycin, HIV drugs	Decreased metabolism	Elevated levels and effects of calcium channel blockers
Statins	Inhibited statin metabolism	Increased risk for statin toxicity
Cyclosporine	Decreased metabolism of either drug	Possible toxicity of either drug

DOSAGES

Selected Calcium Channel–Blocking Drugs

Drug (Pregnancy Category)	Usual Adult Dosage Range	Indications
amlodipine (Norvasc) (C)	PO: 5-10 mg/day	
◆ diltiazem (Cardizem, Dilacor XR, Tiazac, Cartia XT, Diltia XT, Matzim LA, Taztia XT) (C)	PO: IR: Initial dose 30 mg qid; range of 120-360 mg divided in 3-4 doses ER: 120-320 mg/day; max dose varies with specific products	} Angina

Pharmacokinetics: Diltiazem

Route	Onset of Action	Peak Plasma Concentration	Elimination Half-life	Duration of Action
PO	0.5-1 hr	2-3 hr	3.5-9 hr	4-12 hr

amlodipine

Amlodipine (Norvasc) is currently the most popular CCB of the dihydropyridine subclass. It is indicated for both angina and hypertension and is available only for oral use.

Pharmacokinetics: Amlodipine

Route	Onset of Action	Peak Plasma Concentration	Elimination Half-life	Duration of Action
PO	30-50 min	6-12 hr	30-50 hr	24 hr

MISCELLANEOUS ANTIANGINAL DRUG

DRUG PROFILE

ranolazine

Ranolazine (Ranexa) is the newest antianginal drug, approved by the FDA in 2006 for chronic angina. Its mechanism of action is unknown. Unlike other antianginal drugs, its antianginal and antiischemic effects do not involve reductions in heart rate or blood pressure. Ranolazine is known to prolong the QT interval on the ECG. For this reason, this drug is reserved for patients who have failed to benefit from other antianginal drug therapy. In fact, ranolazine is contraindicated in patients with preexisting QT prolongation or hepatic impairment, in those taking other QT-prolonging drugs (see Chapter 25), and in patients taking moderately potent cytochrome P-450 enzyme 3A4 inhibitors such as diltiazem. Other significant drug interactions include interactions with ketoconazole and verapamil, both of which can raise ranolazine levels. Ranolazine can also raise digoxin levels. The drug is available only for oral use.

SUMMARY OF ANTIANGINAL PHARMACOLOGY

In patients with coronary artery disease, clinical symptoms result from a lack of or inadequate delivery of blood carrying oxygen and nutrients to the heart, which results in ischemic heart disease. Antianginal drugs such as nitrates, nitrites, beta blockers, and calcium channel blockers are used to reduce ischemia by increasing the delivery of oxygen-rich blood to cardiac tissues or by reducing oxygen consumption by the coronary vessels. Either of these mechanisms can reduce ischemia and lead to a decrease in anginal pain. Nitrates and nitrites work mainly by decreasing venous return to the heart (preload) and decreasing systemic vascular resistance (afterload). Calcium channel blockers decrease calcium influx into the smooth muscle, causing vascular relaxation. This either reverses or prevents the spasms of coronary vessels that cause the anginal pain associated with Prinzmetal or chronic angina. Beta blockers help by slowing the heart rate and decreasing contractility, thereby decreasing oxygen demands. Although these groups of

Not only are the pharmacokinetic properties of the nitrates very interesting, but knowledge of these specific properties is critical to safe and accurate nursing care. Moreover, the patient's understanding of nitrate pharmacokinetics is important because the level of the patient's knowledge may strongly influence adherence to the drug regimen and the effectiveness of treatment for angina. The pharmacokinetics differ for the various dosage forms of nitroglycerin and include the following:

Intravenous infusion: Onset of action 1 to 2 minutes (fastest of all dosage forms), peak action not applicable, duration of action 3 to 5 minutes

Sublingual tablet: Onset of action 2 to 3 minutes, peak action unknown, duration of action 0.5 to 1 hour

Immediate-release tablet: Onset of action 1 hour, peak action unknown, duration of action 4 to 6 hours

Transdermal patch: Onset 30 to 60 minutes, peak action 1 to 3 hours, duration of action 8 to 12 hours

If the goal of treatment is to abort or treat a sudden attack of angina, then *rapid* onset of action is needed, so the clinical decision (by the prescriber) would be to order either intravenous infusion, sublingual tablet, and/or translingual spray, which has a similar onset time. These dosage forms have pharmacokinetics that allow quick entry of the drug into the bloodstream and lead to more rapid vasodilation. This provides more oxygenated blood to the myocardium and aborts acute attacks. If symptoms persist, more drastic medical management would be indicated. The patient may also use the quick-onset nitroglycerin dosage forms before engaging in activities known to provoke angina, such as increased physical activity, sexual intercourse, or other forms of physical exertion. If the purpose of treatment is maintenance therapy, the nitrate form must have other pharmacokinetic properties, such as a longer duration of action to provide protection against angina; a longer onset of action is acceptable because stopping an attack is not needed in this situation. Use of ointments, transdermal patches, or extended-release preparations would be appropriate in such cases. If an acute episode of angina occurs while the patient is taking maintenance therapy, a dosage form with a rapid onset of action is indicated (as ordered). It is easy to see that thorough knowledge of a drug and its pharmacokinetics allows for safe and sound decisions about drug therapy for patients with angina.

drugs have similar clinical effects, the nursing process required for each is somewhat specific because of the characteristics and effects of the drugs and the indications for and contraindications to their use.

NURSING PROCESS

ASSESSMENT

Before *antianginal* drugs are administered, obtain a thorough past and present medical-health history and medication history (e.g., listing of all prescription drugs, over-the-counter products, herbals, vitamins, and supplements being taken) and document the findings. Measure weight, height, and vital signs, with attention to supine, sitting, and standing blood pressures. Report a systolic blood pressure reading of less than 90 mm Hg to the prescriber before administering a dose of any of these drugs. With use of any drugs affecting blood pressure or pulse rate, such as *antianginals*, take the apical pulse rate for 1 full minute. If the pulse rate is 60 beats/min or less or 100 beats/min or greater (reflex tachycardia is an adverse effect), contact the prescriber for further instructions. In addition to rate, assess the quality and rhythm of the heartbeat and document prior to the administration of antianginal drugs. If the patient is experiencing any chest pain, include in your assessment description of onset, character (e.g., sharp, dull, piercing, squeezing, radiating), intensity, location, duration, precipitating factors (e.g., physical exertion, exercise, eating, stress, sexual intercourse), alleviating factors, and presence of nausea or vomiting. The prescriber may order an ECG. Promptly review the results, and inform the prescriber of the results. Thoroughly assess for any contraindications, cautions, and drug interactions prior to giving these drugs. Significant interactions include alcohol, beta blockers, calcium channel blockers, phenothiazines, and erectile-dysfunction drugs such as sildenafil, tadalafil, and vardenafil. Taking these drugs with *nitrates* will result in worsening of hypotensive responses, paradoxical bradycardia, and a resultant increase in angina, with a subsequent significant risk for cardiac or cerebrovascular complications due to the decreased perfusion. Older adult patients often have difficulty with blood pressure control because of the occurrence of normal age-related periods of hypotension, and the use of antianginals may lead to worsening of hypotensive responses. If patients are taking nitrates on a long-term basis, it is important to assess continued therapeutic responses because of the development of tolerance to the drug's effects. During assessment and initiation of drug therapy, it is critical to patient safety to notify the prescriber of any increased angina, because another antianginal or vasodilating drug may be needed.

Concerns arise with the use of *nonselective beta blockers* and *beta₂ blockers* (as vasodilators) in patients with bronchospastic disease because of the drug-related effects of bronchoconstriction and increased airway resistance, which results in the adverse effects of wheezing and dyspnea. Therefore, if asthma or other respiratory problems are present, beta blockers would not be indicated because bronchoconstriction could be exacerbated. In addition, there are also concerns about the use of beta blockers in patients with peripheral vascular disease, hypotension, hyperglycemia or hypoglycemia (see pharmacology discussion), and bradycardia. Nonselective beta blockers may also exacerbate preexisting heart failure. Assessment for edema is important in patients with cardiac risk factors. If weight gain is of 2 pounds or more in 24 hours or 5 pounds or more in 1 week, notify the prescriber immediately. Assess for significant drug interactions, including the use of other antihypertensives, calcium channel blockers, and oral antidiabetic drugs (see Table 23-3 for more information).

In patients taking *calcium channel blockers (CCBs),* assess for possible drug-food interactions, including grapefruit. Grapefruit juice reduces the metabolism of *nifedipine,* leading to possible toxicity; grapefruit must be avoided. Another area to be thoroughly assessed is that of the dosage form of nifedipine, which is available in extended- and immediate-release forms. Therefore, follow the orders for administration of nifedipine carefully, and closely monitor the patient (e.g., vital

signs). *Diltiazem (Cardizem)* is available in several sustained-delivery forms; closely assess the order to avoid medication error. Cautious use is important in patients with a history of hypotension, palpitations, tachycardia/bradycardia, constipation, dyspnea, and edema. Significant drug interactions are included in Table 23-6.

Assess patients taking *ranolazine (Ranexa),* one of the newest antianginal drugs, for liver dysfunction through specific liver function testing prior to taking the medication. Additionally, assess for other medications the patient is taking, with an emphasis on medications that prolong the QT interval for which an ECG may also be ordered. Other medications to be concerned about include those that inhibit cytochrome P450, such as diltiazem.

NURSING DIAGNOSES

1. Decreased cardiac output related to the pathology of coronary artery disease
2. Deficient knowledge related to first-time use of antianginal drugs and a new diagnosis of coronary artery disease
3. Risk for injury to self related to possible adverse drug effect of hypotension with subsequent dizziness and/or syncope/falls

PLANNING: OUTCOME IDENTIFICATION

1. Patient exhibits therapeutic effects of antianginal drug therapy, such as improved cardiac output, with fewer episodes of chest pain while carrying out activities of daily living and/or prescribed, supervised exercise.
2. Patient demonstrates increased knowledge about disease process and drug therapy by stating rationale for antianginal drug therapy and its adequate dosing schedule.
3. Patient remains free from injury while receiving antianginal drug therapy through implementing safety measures such as changing positions slowly, moving legs while standing, increasing fluid intake, and removing safety barriers in the home setting.

IMPLEMENTATION

Always review and/or record the patient's vital signs and description of chest pain for the duration of therapy. Take into account the following dosage forms and routes of administration: (1) *For any dosage form:* Administer the drug while the patient is seated to avoid falls or injury from drug-induced hypotension. This hypotension may last for up to 30 minutes after dosing of the drug. When administering *nitrates,* monitor the patient's chest pain, and have the patient rate the pain on a scale of 1 to 10 before, during, and after therapy. Monitor the patient's response to drug therapy by measuring the patient's blood pressure and pulse rate and assessing for the presence of headache, dizziness, and/or lightheadedness. When the patient is in a supine position, an appropriate dose of a nitrate will produce a clinical response of a decrease in blood pressure of about 10 mm Hg and/or an increase in heart rate of 10 beats/

CASE STUDY

Patient-Centered Care: Nitroglycerin for Angina

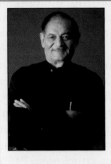

M.S., a 68-year-old accountant, has been diagnosed with coronary artery disease (CAD) after experiencing chest pain at times when he jogs. After undergoing a thorough physical examination, including cardiac catheterization, he is given a prescription for extended-release nitroglycerin capsules, 6.5 mg, three times a day. He also has a prescription for 0.4-mg sublingual nitroglycerin tablets to take as needed for chest pain.

1. What type of angina is M.S. experiencing, and what are the therapeutic goals of the drug therapy he has received?

M.S. asks you, "Why do I have two prescriptions for the same drug? It doesn't make sense to me!"

2. What is the best answer to the patient's question?

3. Two days after he begins the nitroglycerin, M.S. calls the office and says, "I'm having awful headaches. What is wrong?" What is the best explanation, and what can he do about the headaches?

After 1 month, M.S. is switched from the extended-release capsules to a transdermal nitroglycerin patch. He says that he is glad he does not have to remember to "take those pills" three times a day. However, 2 months later, he calls and says, "I don't think this patch is working. I'm having more episodes of chest pain now when I jog."

4. What could be the explanation for this, and what can be done?

For answers, see *http://evolve.elsevier.com/Lilley.*

---

min. However, the following parameters are alerts that there may be a problem with the patient and to contact the prescriber: a systolic blood pressure of 90 mm Hg or less and/or a pulse rate of 60 beats/min or less or a pulse rate greater than 100 beats/min. (2) *For oral dosage forms:* Counsel the patient that these forms are to be taken as ordered before meals and with at least 6 ounces of water. Extended-release preparations must not be crushed, chewed, or altered in any way. Acetaminophen may be given if there is a drug-related headache and if not contraindicated. (3) *For sublingual forms:* Advise the patient to place the tablet under the tongue as directed and *not* to swallow until the drug is completely dissolved. Metered-dose aerosol sprays are applied onto or under the tongue (see the dosages table on p. 365). Instruct the patient to keep *nitrates* in their original packaging or container (e.g., sublingual tablets come in a small amber-colored glass container with a metal lid). Exposure to light, plastic, cotton filler, and moisture must be avoided. (4) *For ointment:* Use the proper dosing paper supplied by the drug company to apply a thin layer on clean, dry, hairless skin of the upper arms or body. Avoid areas below the knees and elbows. Do not apply the ointment with the fingers unless a glove is worn to avoid contact with the skin and subsequent absorption. A tongue depressor may also be used, but in most situations the ointment may be squeezed directly from the tube onto the proper dosing paper. Once the ointment is in place, do *not* rub it into the skin; cover the area with an occlusive dressing if not provided (e.g., plastic wrap). Rotate application sites, and

remove all residual from the previous dose of ointment gently with soap and water and pat the area dry. (5) *For transdermal forms:* Apply patches to a clean, residue-free, hairless area, and rotate sites. If cardioversion or use of an automated electrical defibrillator is required, remove the transdermal patch to avoid burning of the skin and damage to the defibrillator paddles. Before a new patch is applied, locate and remove the old patch and clean the skin of any residual drug. Carefully dispose of used, unneeded, or defective transdermal patches of any medication as indicated by health care institution policy or per discharge instructions. It is important to follow any packaging insert instructions and/or health care institution policy because transdermal patches delivering potent medications need to be flushed down the toilet to avoid possible contact of residual drug by babies, children, pets, and even adults (see Chapter 9). For more information visit *www.nlm.nih.gov/medlineplus/druginfo/meds/a601085.html.* (6) *For intravenous forms:* Intravenous dosing is for use in emergency situations only and in settings that provide close automatic monitoring of the blood pressure and pulse as well as constant ECG monitoring. Intravenous administration of nitrates may lead to sudden and severe hypotension, cardiovascular collapse, and shock. Always check for incompatibilities and proper diluent. Only give intravenous solutions through an infusion pump and as ordered. Intravenous dosage forms are available as ready-to-use injectable doses and are administered using *specific nonpolyvinylchloride* (non-PVC) plastic intravenous bags and tubing. The non-PVC infusion kits are used to avoid absorption or uptake of the nitrate by the intravenous tubing and bag. This prevents decomposition of the nitrate with breakdown into cyanide when the drug is exposed to light. Intravenous forms of *nitroglycerin* are stable for about 96 hours after preparation. If parenteral solutions are not clear and are discolored, discard the solution.

With *isosorbide*, tablets are best taken on an empty stomach; however, if the patient complains of headache or gastrointestinal upset, the medicine needs to be taken with meals. Oral tablets of isosorbide can be crushed; however, the sublingual and extended-release forms are *not* to be crushed or chewed. As with sublingual nitroglycerin, instruct the patient not to swallow the medication until it is completely dissolved. If dizziness or lightheadedness occurs, assist the patient and encourage him or her to change positions slowly. Closely monitor the patient's blood pressure, including orthostatic blood pressures. Document the occurrence of anginal episodes, their character, precipitating factors, severity, and frequency noted.

Beta blockers need to be given as ordered and may be taken with or without food. Abrupt withdrawal must be avoided. Daily weights need to be recorded every day at the same time and with the patient wearing the same amount of clothing. If there is a weight gain of 2 pounds or more in 24 hours or 5 pounds or more in 1 week, contact the prescriber immediately. When these drugs are used, take measures to reduce the incidence of orthostatic hypotension, such as advising the patient to dangle the legs on the side of the bed before standing and to move slowly and purposefully. Instruct the patient to contact the prescriber immediately if any excessive or intolerable dizziness, fatigue/lethargy, wheezing, or dyspnea occurs (see Chapter 19 for further discussion).

Calcium channel blockers (CCBs) are to be taken as ordered and without sudden withdrawal. Abrupt withdrawal can precipitate rebound hypertension and worsening of tissue ischemia. Weight needs to be measured daily (see later discussion). Constantly monitor the patient for edema and shortness of breath. Instruct the patient to move and change positions slowly and cautiously to prevent syncope. Constipation may be prevented by increasing fluids and fiber in the diet. If the patient experiences palpitations, pronounced dizziness, nausea, or dyspnea, contact the prescriber immediately. Intravenous administration of any CCB requires the use of an infusion pump and careful monitoring (see Chapter 25).

Patients taking any of the *vasodilators* must avoid alcohol, saunas, hot tubs, hot showers, and hot weather or a hot environment. These conditions will exacerbate vasodilation and increase the occurrence of orthostatic hypotension, increasing the risk for dizziness, syncope, and falls. Caution the patient that with certain sustained-release forms of medication, the wax matrix may appear in the stool. Advise patients that the passing of the wax matrix occurs after the drug has been absorbed and that, even though the matrix is visible, it is of no concern. Instruct the patient on how to self-monitor blood pressure and pulse rate, as well as how to document the findings in a journal so that the information can be shared with health care providers. The journal can also list daily weights, response to the medication regimen, and any adverse effects. See Patient-Centered Care: Patient Teaching below for more information.

EVALUATION

Carefully monitor patients taking *antianginals* for the occurrence of an allergic reaction, which may be manifested by dyspnea, swelling of the face, or hives. Include in your evaluation a review for accomplishment of goals and outcomes, such as appropriate decrease in blood pressure, increase in cardiac output and tissue perfusion with decrease in angina, and a gradual increase in activity and performance of activities of daily living without exacerbation of anginal episodes. In addition, monitor the patient for adverse reactions such as headache, lightheadedness, dizziness, and decreased blood pressure, which may indicate the need to decrease the dosage. If the patient is receiving intravenous *nitroglycerin*, evaluate for excessive drops in blood pressure, worsening of angina, and significant changes in pulse rate (less than 60 beats/min or greater than 100 beats/min), and contact the prescriber immediately.

PATIENT-CENTERED CARE: PATIENT TEACHING

Nitroglycerin

- Emphasize the importance of keeping a daily journal with documentation of how the patient feels and number of anginal episodes, noting their intensity, frequency, duration, and character, as well as precipitating and/or relieving factors. Any evidence of possible tolerance to the medication is important to note and report to the prescriber.
- *Capsules* or *extended-release* dosage forms are never to be chewed, crushed, or altered in any way.
- Instruct the patient taking *aerosol* (spray) dosage forms not to shake the canister before lingual spraying and to avoid inhaling or swallowing the lingual aerosol until the drug is dispersed. With *sublingual* forms, the medication must be taken at the first sign of chest pain and not delayed until the pain is severe. The patient needs to sit or lie down and take one sublingual tablet. According to current guidelines, if the chest pain or discomfort is not relieved in 5 minutes, after *one* dose, the patient (or family member) must call 911 immediately. The patient can take one more tablet while awaiting emergency care and a third tablet 5 minutes later, but no more than three tablets total. These guidelines reflect the fact that angina pain that does not respond to nitroglycerin may indicate a myocardial infarction. The sublingual dose is to be placed under the tongue, and the patient must avoid swallowing until the tablet is dissolved. Instruct the patient not to eat or drink until the drug has completely dissolved.
- Educate the patient about the best place to store the medication, such as keeping medicine away from moisture, light, heat, and cotton filler material. The *sublingual* dosage form of nitroglycerin needs to be kept in its original amber-colored glass container with metal lid to avoid loss of potency from exposure to heat, light, moisture, and cotton filler.
- Potency of the sublingual nitroglycerin is noted if there is burning or stinging once the medication is placed under the tongue; if the medication does not burn, then the drug has lost its potency, and a new prescription must be obtained.
- It is important to emphasize that the medication is potent only for 3 to 6 months. Remind the patient to always have a fresh supply of the drug on hand, to plan ahead if traveling, and (no matter the dosage form) to sit or lie down when taking the medication to avoid falls secondary to a drop in blood pressure.
- With *all forms of nitrates,* educate the patient about adverse effects such as flushing of the face, dizziness, fainting, brief throbbing headache, increase in heart rate, and lightheadedness. Headaches associated with nitrates last approximately 20 minutes (with sublingual forms) and may be managed with acetaminophen. If headaches are bothersome when an oral dosage form is used, the drug may be taken with meals, and the patient must contact the prescriber if adverse effects continue. Blurred vision, dry mouth, or severe headaches may indicate drug overdose and require immediate medical attention. While taking an antianginal, the patient must avoid alcohol, hot environmental temperatures, saunas, hot tubs, and excessive exertion. These increase vasodilation with subsequent worsening of hypotension, which possibly can lead to syncope (fainting) and/or other cardiac events.

- In many situations, the prescriber specifies that nitroglycerin be taken *before* stressful activities or events such as emotional situations, consumption of large meals, smoking, or sudden increase in activity (e.g., sexual intercourse). The patient needs to follow the prescriber's directions regarding prophylactic dosing very closely.
- With *ointment* forms, remind the patient to use the appropriate dosage paper for application of the ointment and not to use the fingers to apply the medicine. The medication can be pressed evenly and directly from the tube onto the printed dosing line on the paper. Instruct the patient to squeeze a thin line of ointment onto the paper and follow instructions regarding its application, such as measuring and applying ½ inch of ointment. An occlusive covering must be used, such as applying a piece of plastic wrap taped around the edges to adhere the dose to the skin. Only clean, nonirritated, and nonhairy areas free of residual medication are to be used for these ointments.
- With *transdermal nitrate* use, the patient must apply the patch at the same time each day and be sure to have only one patch in place at a time, cleansing all residue off the skin before applying a new patch. Advise the patient to avoid skinfolds, hairy areas, and any area distal to the knees or elbows as application sites. A transdermal patch must never be applied to irritated or open skin, and if the patch becomes loose, the patient needs to remove it and gently wash off the residue with lukewarm soap and water, *pat* the area dry, and place another patch in another area. Encourage rotation of sites to prevent irritation (with ointments, too). The prescriber may order the removal of the patch for an 8-hour period on specific days to help decrease or prevent drug tolerance, which may develop over time. Emphasize all instructions with both written and verbal instructions.

Isosorbide Dinitrate or Isosorbide Mononitrate

- Educate the patient about the basic differences in oral nitrates (e.g., the mononitrate form is well absorbed after oral dosing; the dinitrate form is poorly absorbed, but its metabolite, isosorbide mononitrate, is active and well absorbed). It is important that the patient know that these drugs are *not interchangeable.*
- Inform the patient to take the medication exactly as ordered with emphasis on the need to lie down when doses are taken to avoid injury from the sudden drop in blood pressure. The sudden drop in blood pressure may lead to dizziness, lightheadedness, and fainting.
- Isosorbide dinitrate is generally given three times a day with a 12-hour drug-free interval, such as dosing at 0700, 1300, and 1900. The 12-hour drug-free interval helps prevent the development of tolerance.
- Oral dosage forms are not to be altered in any way and must be taken with 6 to 8 ounces of water.
- The patient must be cautious while taking these drugs and encouraged to rise slowly and move the legs around before standing up from a lying or sitting position to help prevent dizziness, possible fainting, and falls. The avoidance of alcohol, heat, and saunas must be emphasized because these factors exacerbate the hypotensive effects of the drug and may result in bodily harm/injury.
- Advise the patient that these and other antianginals are not to be stopped abruptly.

KEY POINTS

- Angina pectoris (chest pain) occurs because of a mismatch between the oxygen supply and oxygen demand, with either too high a demand for oxygen or too little oxygen delivery.
- The heart is a very aerobic (oxygen-requiring) muscle, and when it does not receive enough oxygen, pain (angina) occurs. When the coronary arteries that deliver oxygen to the heart muscle become blocked, a heart attack or MI occurs.
- Coronary artery disease is an abnormal condition of the arteries (blood vessels) that deliver oxygen to the heart muscle. These arteries may become narrowed, which results in reduced flow of oxygen and nutrients to the myocardium.
- Nitrates, CCBs, and beta blockers may be used to treat the symptoms of angina.
- Nitroglycerin is the prototypical nitrate. Nitrates dilate constricted coronary arteries, helping to increase the supply of oxygen and nutrients to the heart muscle. Nitrates also dilate all other blood vessels. The venous dilation results in a decrease in blood return to the heart (decreased preload), whereas the arterial dilation results in a decrease of peripheral resistance (decreased afterload—that is, the pressure or force against which the left ventricle must pump). Isosorbide dinitrates were the first group of oral drugs used to treat angina; isosorbide mononitrates are new and improved nitrates used for angina therapy. Beta blockers are also used to relieve angina and do so by decreasing the heart rate, reducing workload on the heart, and decreasing oxygen demand.
- Dosage forms for nitrates include conventional tablets, translingual spray, controlled-release and sustained-release capsules, transdermal patch, topical ointment, and intravenous injection.
- Quick-onset nitrates are used to treat acute anginal attacks, while longer-onset nitrates are used for prophylaxis.
- Instruct patients to always keep a fresh supply of sublingual nitroglycerin on their person and in their home, because the drug is only stable for 3 to 6 months.
- CCBs and beta blockers may be associated with the adverse effects of postural hypotension, dizziness, headache, and edema. The nonselective beta blockers may exacerbate congestive heart failure, problems related to respiratory bronchospasm, and hypoglycemia. Check the patient's pulse rate before drug administration, and if it is 60 beats/min or lower, contact the prescriber for further instructions.

Sodium Nitroprusside –10 min

NCLEX® EXAMINATION REVIEW QUESTIONS

1. A patient has a new prescription for transdermal nitroglycerin patches. The nurse teaches the patient that these patches are most appropriately used for which reason?
   a. To relieve exertional angina
   b. To prevent palpitations
   c. To prevent the occurrence of angina
   d. To stop an episode of angina

2. A nurse with adequate knowledge about the administration of intravenous nitroglycerin will recognize that which statement is correct?
   a. The intravenous form is given by IV push injection.
   b. Because the intravenous forms are short-lived, the dosing must be every 2 hours.
   c. Intravenous nitroglycerin must be protected from exposure to light through use of special tubing.
   d. Intravenous nitroglycerin can be given via gravity drip infusions.

3. Which statement by the patient reflects the need for additional patient education about the calcium channel blocker diltiazem (Cardizem)?
   a. "I can take this drug to stop an attack of angina."
   b. "I understand that food and antacids alter the absorption of this oral drug."
   c. "When the long-acting forms are taken, the drug cannot be crushed."
   d. "This drug may cause my blood pressure to drop, so I need to be careful when getting up."

4. While assessing a patient with angina who is to start beta blocker therapy, the nurse is aware that the presence of which condition may be a problem if these drugs are used?
   a. Hypertension
   b. Essential tremors
   c. Exertional angina
   d. Asthma

5. A 68-year-old male patient has been taking the nitrate isosorbide dinitrate (Isordil) for 2 years for angina. He recently has been experiencing erectile dysfunction and wants a prescription for sildenafil (Viagra). Which response would the nurse most likely hear from the prescriber?

   a. "He will have to be switched to isosorbide mononitrate if he wants to take sildenafil."
   b. "Taking sildenafil with the nitrate may result in severe hypotension, so a contraindication exists."
   c. "I'll write a prescription, but if he uses it, he needs to stop taking the isosorbide for one dose."
   d. "These drugs are compatible with each other, and so I'll write a prescription."

6. The nurse is reviewing drug interactions with a male patient who has a prescription for isosorbide dinitrate (Isordil) as treatment for angina symptoms. Which substances listed below could potentially result in a drug interaction? *(Select all that apply.)*
   a. A glass of wine
   b. Thyroid replacement hormone
   c. tadalafil (Cialis), an erectile dysfunction drug
   d. metformin (Glucophage), an antidiabetic drug
   e. carvedilol (Coreg), a beta blocker

7. The order reads, "Give metoprolol (Lopressor) 300 mg/day PO in 2 divided doses." The tablets are available in 50-mg strength. How many tablets will the patient receive per dose?

8. A patient with angina has been given a prescription for a calcium channel blocker. The nurse knows that this class of drugs is used to treat which type of angina?
   a. Effort
   b. Unstable
   c. Crescendo
   d. Vasospastic

1. c, 2. c, 3. a, 4. d, 5. b, 6. a, c, e, 7. 3 tablets per dose (150 mg per dose), 8. d.

CRITICAL THINKING AND PRIORITIZATION QUESTIONS

1. Mrs. A. has been shoveling snow all morning. As you work on the snow in your yard, you see her suddenly sit down in her driveway. When you go over to check on her, she says that she has nitroglycerin tablets in her jacket pocket but she forgot how to take them. What is your priority action at this time?

2. Your patient has been switched from oral nitroglycerin capsules to a transdermal form. What are the priorities for patient teaching regarding transdermal nitroglycerin therapy?

For answers, see *http://evolve.elsevier.com/Lilley.*

EVOLVE WEBSITE

http://evolve.elsevier.com/Lilley
- Animations
- Answer Keys for Textbook Case Studies and Textbook Critical Thinking and Prioritization Questions
- Content Updates
- Key Points
- Review Questions
- Student Case Studies

Heart Failure Drugs

e http://evolve.elsevier.com/Lilley

OBJECTIVES

When you reach the end of this chapter, you will be able to do the following:

1. Differentiate between the terms *inotropic, chronotropic,* and *dromotropic.*
2. Briefly discuss the pathophysiology of heart failure.
3. Identify the approach to treatment of heart failure as outlined by the American Heart Association and American College of Cardiology Guidelines for the Diagnosis and Management of Heart Failure in Adults (last updated in 2013).
4. Compare the mechanisms of action, pharmacokinetics, indications, dosages, dosage forms, routes of administration, cautions, contraindications, adverse effects, and toxicity of the following drugs used in treatment of heart failure: lisinopril, valsartan, carvedilol, metoprolol,

dobutamine, nesiritide, hydralazine/isosorbide dinitrate, milrinone, and digoxin.
5. Briefly discuss the process of rapid versus slow digitalization as well as the use of the antidote digoxin immune Fab.
6. Identify significant drug-drug, drug–laboratory test, and drug-food interactions associated with digoxin and other heart failure drugs.
7. Develop a nursing care plan that includes all phases of the nursing process for patients undergoing treatment for heart failure and that reflects the American Heart Association and American College of Cardiology Guidelines for the Diagnosis and Management of Heart Failure in Adults.

DRUG PROFILES

♦ digoxin, p. 383
digoxin immune Fab, p. 383
♦ dobutamine, p. 380
hydralazine/isosorbide dinitrate, p. 379
♦ lisinopril, p. 379
♦ milrinone, p. 381

♦ nesiritide, p. 380
♦ valsartan, p. 379

_____
♦ = *Key drug*
! = *High-alert drug*

KEY TERMS

Atrial fibrillation A common cardiac dysrhythmia with atrial contractions that are so rapid they prevent full repolarization of myocardial fibers between heartbeats. (p. 381)

Automaticity A property of specialized excitable tissue in the heart that allows self-activation through the spontaneous development of an action potential, such as in the pacemaker cells of the heart. (p. 379)

Chronotropic drugs Drugs that influence the rate of the heartbeat. (p. 377)

Dromotropic drugs Drugs that influence the conduction of electrical impulses within tissues. (p. 377)

Ejection fraction The proportion of blood that is ejected during each ventricular contraction compared with the total ventricular filling volume. (p. 377)

Heart failure An abnormal condition in which the heart cannot pump enough blood to keep up with the body's demand. It is often the result of myocardial infarction, ischemic heart disease, or cardiomyopathy. (p. 377)

Inotropic drugs Drugs that influence the force of muscular contractions, particularly contraction of the heart muscle. (p. 377)

Left ventricular end-diastolic volume The total amount of blood in the ventricle immediately before it contracts, or the preload. (p. 377)

Refractory period The period during which a *pulse generator* (e.g., the *sinoatrial node* of the heart) is unresponsive to an electrical input signal, and during which it is impossible for the myocardium to respond. This is the period during which the cardiac cell is readjusting its sodium and potassium levels and cannot be depolarized again. (p. 381)

OVERVIEW

Heart failure is not a specific disease per se but rather a clinical syndrome caused by numerous different cardiac disorders. It is a complex syndrome resulting from any functional or structural impairment to the heart, specifically ejection of blood or ventricular filling. More than 6.1 million people in the United States have heart failure. It is one of the most common causes for hospitalization in the United States, estimated to result in more than 3.9 million hospitalizations annually. The most common manifestations of heart failure are dyspnea, fatigue, fluid retention, and/or pulmonary edema. There is no single diagnostic test for heart failure, because it is a clinical diagnosis based on careful physical examination and history. The findings of one of the largest and most frequently cited studies involving patients with heart failure, the Framingham study, show that the 5-year survival rate in patients with heart failure is approximately 50%. The best way to prevent heart failure is to control risk factors associated with heart failure including hypertension, coronary artery disease, obesity, and diabetes.

Heart failure is a pathologic state in which the heart is unable to pump blood in sufficient amounts from the ventricles (i.e., cardiac output is insufficient) to meet the body's metabolic needs, or can do so only at elevated filling pressures. The signs and symptoms typically associated with this insufficiency make up the syndrome of heart failure. Initially, the patient is asymptomatic. As the disease progresses, so do the symptoms. Failure of the ventricle(s) to eject blood efficiently results in fluid volume overload, chamber dilation, and elevated intracardiac pressure. This syndrome can affect the left ventricle, the right ventricle, or both ventricles simultaneously. Left ventricular or "left-sided" heart failure often leads to pulmonary edema, coughing, shortness of breath, and dyspnea. Right ventricular heart failure typically involves systemic venous congestion, pedal edema, jugular venous distension, ascites, and hepatic congestion. Both syndromes occur due to increased hydrostatic pressure from the ventricles into the pulmonary and/or systemic circulation.

More specifically, heart failure occurs due to a reduced ratio of **ejection fraction** to **left ventricular end-diastolic volume.** The ejection fraction is the amount of blood ejected with each contraction, whereas the left ventricular end-diastolic volume is the total amount of blood in the ventricle just before contraction. The ejection fraction is an index of left ventricular function, and the normal value is approximately 65% (0.65) of the total volume in the ventricle.

When a person has heart failure, the heart cannot then meet the increased demands, and blood supply to certain organs is reduced. The organs that are most dependent on blood supply, the brain and heart, are the last to be deprived of blood. The kidney is relatively less dependent on blood supply and has its blood supply shunted away from it. This can lead to acute or chronic renal failure. It also contributes to conditions such as pulmonary edema, shortness of breath, and peripheral edema.

The physical defects causing heart failure are of two types: (1) a myocardial defect such as myocardial infarction or valve insufficiency, which leads to inadequate cardiac contractility

BOX 24-1   Myocardial Deficiency and Increased Ventricular Workload: Common Causes

Myocardial Deficiency	Increased Workload
Inadequate Contractility	***Pressure Overload***
Myocardial infarction	Pulmonary hypertension
Coronary artery disease	Systemic hypertension
Cardiomyopathy	Outflow obstruction
Valvular insufficiency	
	Volume Overload
Inadequate Filling	Hypervolemia
Atrial fibrillation	Congenital abnormalities
Infection	Anemia
Tamponade	Thyroid disease
Ischemia	Infection
	Diabetes

and ventricular filling; and (2) a defect outside the myocardium (e.g., coronary artery disease, pulmonary hypertension, or diabetes), which results in an overload on an otherwise normal heart. Either or both of these defects may be present in a given patient. These and other common causes of myocardial deficiency and systemic defects are listed in Box 24-1.

The emphasis of this chapter is on systolic dysfunction or inadequate ventricular contractions (systole) during the pumping of the heart. Less common, but still important, is diastolic dysfunction or inadequate ventricular filling during ventricular relaxation (diastole). This condition is most commonly associated with left ventricular hypertrophy secondary to chronic hypertension. However, it may also result from cardiomyopathy (e.g., virus induced), pericardial disease, and diabetes.

Heart failure can be stratified into classes using the older New York Heart Association's (NHYA) functional classification or the more recent American College of Cardiology Foundation/ American Heart Association (ACCF/AHA) stages of heart failure. Both methods provide useful information about the presence and severity of heart failure. The NYHA classes focus on the symptomatic status of the disease, whereas the ACCF/AHA stages emphasize the progression of the disease. See Box 24-2 for the specifics of each staging method. Drug therapy is individualized based on the patient's class or stage of heart failure.

PHARMACOLOGY OVERVIEW

Drugs that increase the force of myocardial contraction are called positive **inotropic drugs,** and they have a role in the treatment of failing heart muscle. Negative inotropic drugs reduce the force of contraction. Drugs that increase the rate at which the heart beats are called positive **chronotropic drugs.** Negative chronotropic drugs do the opposite. Drugs may also affect how quickly electrical impulses travel through the conduction system of the heart (the sinoatrial [SA] node, atrioventricular [AV] node, bundle of His, and Purkinje fibers) (Figure 24-1). Drugs that accelerate conduction are referred to as positive **dromotropic drugs.** Negative dromotropic drugs do

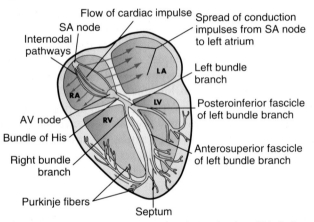

FIGURE 24-1 Conduction system of the heart. *AV,* Atrioventricular; *LA,* left atrium; *LV,* left ventricle; *RA,* right atrium; *RV,* right ventricle; *SA,* sinoatrial. (Modified from Kinney MR, Packa DR: *Andreoli's comprehensive cardiac care,* ed 8, St Louis, 1996, Mosby; Lewis SM, Dirksen SR, Heitkemper MM, et al: *Medical-surgical nursing: assessment and management of clinical problems,* ed 7, St Louis, 2007, Mosby.)

the opposite. This chapter focuses on the positive inotropic drugs, phosphodiesterase inhibitors and cardiac glycosides, and B-type natriuretic peptides. Although several other drugs are used in the treatment of heart failure, they are discussed in detail in other chapters; for example, angiotensin-converting enzyme (ACE) inhibitors and angiotensin receptor blockers (ARBs) are covered in Chapter 22; beta blockers are discussed in Chapters 19, 22, and 23; and diuretics are discussed in Chapter 28. These drugs are mentioned in this chapter as well, but for specifics, refer to the indicated chapters. In April 2015, the Food and Drug Administration (FDA) approved a new, first-in-class drug called ivabradine (Corlanor). Ivabradine is a hyperpolarization-activation cyclic nucleotide-gated channel blocker indicated to reduce the risk of hospitalization for

worsening heart failure. It works by blocking the I_f currents in the sinus node and lowers the heart rate and the amount of work the heart needs to do.

The treatment of heart failure has changed dramatically over the past decade. Digoxin used to be the mainstay in heart failure treatment, but because of adverse effects and drug interactions, it has been replaced by other drugs. According to the latest American Heart Association and American College of Cardiology Guidelines for the Diagnosis and Management of Heart Failure in Adults (2005, updated in 2013), the approach to the treatment of chronic heart failure revolves around reducing the effects of the renin-angiotensin-aldosterone system and the sympathetic nervous system. Therefore, the drugs of choice at the start of therapy are the ACE inhibitors (lisinopril, enalapril, captopril, and others) or ARBs (valsartan, candesartan, losartan, and others) and certain beta blockers (metoprolol, a cardioselective beta blocker; carvedilol, a nonspecific beta blocker). Loop diuretics (furosemide) are used to reduce the symptoms of heart failure secondary to fluid overload, and the aldosterone inhibitors (spironolactone, eplerenone) are added as the heart failure progresses. Only after these drugs are used is digoxin added. Dobutamine, a positive inotropic drug, has also been used to treat heart failure. In 2005, a combination drug containing hydralazine and isosorbide dinitrate became the first drug approved for a specific ethnic group. Hydralazine/isosorbide dinitrate (BiDil) was approved specifically for use in the African-American population.

ANGIOTENSIN-CONVERTING ENZYME INHIBITORS

The angiotensin-converting enzyme (ACE) inhibitors are a class of drugs that, as their name implies, inhibit angiotensin-converting enzyme, which is responsible for converting angiotensin I (formed through the action of renin) to angiotensin II. Angiotensin II is a potent vasoconstrictor and induces aldosterone secretion by the adrenal glands. Aldosterone stimulates sodium and water resorption, which can raise blood pressure. Together, these processes are referred to as the *renin-angiotensin-aldosterone system*. The ACE inhibitors are beneficial in the treatment of heart failure because they prevent sodium and water resorption by inhibiting aldosterone secretion. This causes diuresis, which decreases blood volume and blood return to the heart. This in turn decreases preload, or the left ventricular end-diastolic volume, and the work required of the heart.

Numerous ACE inhibitors are available, including lisinopril, enalapril, fosinopril, quinapril, captopril, ramipril, trandolapril, and perindopril. These drugs are all very similar, and lisinopril will be used as the class representative.

DRUG PROFILE

♦ lisinopril

Lisinopril (Prinivil, Zestril) is a commonly used ACE inhibitor and is available in a generic form. It is used for hypertension, heart failure, and acute myocardial infarction. Like all ACE inhibitors, it is classified as a category C drug for women in the first trimester of pregnancy and a category D drug for women in the second and third trimesters; it can cause fetal death when used in the last two trimesters. Hyperkalemia may occur with any ACE inhibitor, and potassium supplementation or potassium-sparing diuretics need to be used with caution. Like all ACE inhibitors, lisinopril can cause a dry cough, which will not harm the patient but is annoying. Lisinopril (and all ACE inhibitors) may be associated with a decrease in renal function and hyperkalemia. For drug interactions, see Chapter 22.

Pharmacokinetics: Lisinopril

Route	Onset of Action	Peak Plasma Concentration	Elimination Half-life	Duration of Action
PO	1 hr	6 hr	11-12 hr	24 hr

ANGIOTENSIN II RECEPTOR BLOCKERS

The therapeutic effects of angiotensin II receptor blockers (ARBs) in heart failure are related to their potent vasodilating properties. They may be used alone or in combination with other drugs such as diuretics in the treatment of hypertension or heart failure. The beneficial hemodynamic effect of ARBs is their ability to decrease systemic vascular resistance (a measure of afterload). Seven ARBs are currently available: valsartan (Diovan), candesartan (Atacand), eprosartan (Teveten), irbesartan (Avapro), telmisartan (Micardis), olmesartan (Benicar), and losartan (Cozaar). All of the ARBs are similar in action. Valsartan will be used as the class representative. In 2015, a new drug, Entreso (sacubitril/valsartan) was approved. Sacubitril is a neprilysin inhibitor that blocks the degradation of vasoactive peptides by inhibiting the neprilysin enzyme. Sacubitril is combined with valsartan, an ARB.

DRUG PROFILE

♦ valsartan

Valsartan (Diovan) is a commonly used ARB. Like all ARBs, it is a pregnancy category D drug. Valsartan shares many of the same adverse effects as lisinopril, profiled earlier. The ARBs are not as likely to cause the cough associated with the ACE inhibitors, nor are they as likely to cause hyperkalemia. For drug interactions, see Chapter 22.

Pharmacokinetics: Valsartan

Route	Onset of Action	Peak Plasma Concentration	Elimination Half-life	Duration of Action
PO	2 hr	Unknown	6 hr	12 hr

BETA BLOCKERS

Beta blockers (also discussed in Chapters 19, 22, and 23) work by reducing or blocking sympathetic nervous system stimulation to the heart and the heart's conduction system. By doing this, beta blockers prevent catecholamine-mediated actions on the heart. This is known as a *cardioprotective* quality of beta blockers. The resulting cardiovascular effects include reduced heart rate, delayed AV node conduction, reduced myocardial contractility, and decreased myocardial **automaticity**. Metoprolol is the beta blocker most commonly used to treat heart failure. Metoprolol is available as an immediate-release and a sustained-release product, as well as an intravenous formulation.

Carvedilol (Coreg) has many effects, including acting as a nonselective beta blocker, an alpha₁ blocker, and possibly a calcium channel blocker and antioxidant. It is used primarily in the treatment of heart failure but is also beneficial for hypertension and angina. It has been shown to slow the progression of heart failure and to decrease the frequency of hospitalization in patients with mild to moderate (class II or III) heart failure. Carvedilol is available only for oral use.

ALDOSTERONE ANTAGONISTS

Aldosterone antagonists spironolactone and eplerenone are useful in severe stages of heart failure. Activation of the renin-angiotensin-aldosterone system causes increased levels of aldosterone, which causes retention of sodium and water, leading to edema that can worsen heart failure. Spironolactone (Aldactone) is a potassium-sparing diuretic and is discussed in detail in Chapter 28. It also acts as an aldosterone antagonist, which has been shown to reduce the symptoms of heart failure. Eplerenone (Inspra) is a *selective aldosterone blocker*, blocking aldosterone at its receptors in the kidney, heart, blood vessels, and brain. It is discussed in detail in Chapter 22.

MISCELLANEOUS HEART FAILURE DRUGS

DRUG PROFILES

hydralazine/isosorbide dinitrate

Hydralazine/isosorbide dinitrate (BiDil) was the first drug approved for a specific ethnic group, namely African Americans. This combination of two older drugs contains 37.5 mg of hydralazine and 20 mg of isosorbide dinitrate. The individual drugs are discussed in detail in Chapter 22 (hydralazine) and Chapter 23 (isosorbide).

◆dobutamine

Dobutamine (generic, formerly Dobutrex) is a beta$_1$-selective vasoactive adrenergic drug that is structurally similar to the naturally occurring catecholamine dopamine. Through stimulation of the beta$_1$ receptors on heart muscle (myocardium), it increases cardiac output by increasing contractility (positive inotropy), which increases the stroke volume, especially in patients with heart failure. Dobutamine is available only as an intravenous drug and is given by continuous infusion. See Chapter 18 for further discussion on this drug.

B-TYPE NATRIURETIC PEPTIDE

The newest class of medications for heart failure, the B-type natriuretic peptides, currently includes only one drug, nesiritide.

DRUG PROFILE

◆nesiritide

Nesiritide (Natrecor) is classified as a synthetic version of *human B-type natriuretic peptide*. B-type natriuretic peptide (BNP) is a substance secreted from the ventricles of the heart in response to changes in pressure that occur when heart failure develops. The level of BNP in the blood increases when heart failure symptoms worsen. Nesiritide is a synthetic b-type natriuretic hormone that has vasodilating effects on both arteries and veins. This vasodilation takes place in the heart itself and throughout the body. The effects of nesiritide have been shown to include diuresis (urinary fluid loss), *natriuresis* (urinary sodium loss), and vasodilation. These properties lead to an indirect increase in cardiac output and suppression of neurohormonal systems such as the renin-angiotensin system.

Nesiritide is used in the intensive care setting as a final effort to treat severe, life-threatening heart failure, often in combination with several other cardiostimulatory medications. Due to worsened renal function and mortality reported, it is no longer recommended to be used as a first-line drug for heart failure. Its only current contraindication is known drug allergy, although it is not recommended for use in patients with low cardiac filling pressures. Adverse effects include hypotension, cardiac dysrhythmias, insomnia, headache, and abdominal pain. Currently identified drug interactions include additive hypotensive effects with coadministration of ACE inhibitors and diuretics. This drug is available only in injectable form.

Pharmacokinetics: Nesiritide

Route	Onset of Action	Peak Plasma Concentration	Elimination Half-life	Duration of Action
IV	15 min	1 hr	18 min	1 to several hr

PHOSPHODIESTERASE INHIBITORS

As the name implies, phosphodiesterase inhibitors (PDIs) are a group of inotropic drugs that work by inhibiting the

DOSAGES

Selected Drugs for Heart Failure

Drug (Pregnancy Category)	Pharmacologic Class	Usual Adult Dosage Range	Indications
◆digoxin (Lanoxin) (C)	Digitalis cardiac glycoside	PO/IV: Loading dose: PO 10-15 mcg/kg or IV 8-12 mcg/kg divided into 3 doses; usual oral maintenance dose: 0.125-0.25 mg/day	Heart failure, supraventricular dysrhythmias
◆milrinone (Primacor) (C)	Phosphodiesterase inhibitor	IV loading dose: 50 mcg/kg IV continuous infusion dose: 0.375-0.75 mcg/kg/min	Heart failure

action of an enzyme called *phosphodiesterase*. Only one drug in this category is available in the United States: milrinone (Primacor).

Mechanism of Action and Drug Effects

The mechanism of action of PDIs differs from other inotropic drugs such as digoxin and the catecholamines. They share a similar pharmacologic action with methylxanthines such as theophylline (see Chapter 37). Both types of drug inhibit the action of phosphodiesterase, which results in an increase in intracellular cyclic adenosine monophosphate (cAMP). However, milrinone is more specific for phosphodiesterase type III, which is common in the heart and vascular smooth muscles.

The beneficial effects of milrinone come from the intracellular increase in cAMP, which results in two beneficial effects in a patient with heart failure: a positive inotropic response and vasodilation. For this reason, this class of drugs may also be referred to as *inodilators* (inotropics and dilators). Milrinone has a 10 to 100 times greater affinity for smooth muscle fibers surrounding pulmonary and systemic blood vessels than they do for cardiac muscle. This suggests that the primary beneficial effects of inodilators come from their vasodilating effects, which cause a reduction in the force against which the heart must pump to eject its volume of blood.

Finally, inhibition of phosphodiesterase results in the availability of more calcium for myocardial muscle contraction. This leads to an increase in the force of contraction (i.e., positive inotropic action). The increased calcium present in heart muscle is taken back up into its storage sites at a much faster rate than normal. As a result, the heart muscle relaxes more than normal and is also more compliant. In summary, PDIs have positive inotropic and vasodilatory effects. They may also increase heart rate in some instances and therefore may also have positive chronotropic effects as well.

Indications

Phosphodiesterase inhibitors (PDIs) are primarily used in the intensive care unit setting for the short-term management of acute heart failure. PDIs are not recommended for long-term infusion.

Contraindications

Contraindications to the use of PDIs include known drug allergy and may include the presence of severe aortic or pulmonary valvular disease and heart failure resulting from diastolic dysfunction.

Adverse Effects

The primary adverse effect seen with milrinone therapy is dysrhythmia. Milrinone-induced dysrhythmias are mainly ventricular. Ventricular dysrhythmias occur in approximately 12% of patients treated with this drug. Some other adverse effects associated with milrinone therapy are hypotension, angina (chest pain), hypokalemia, tremor, and thrombocytopenia.

Toxicity and Management of Overdose

No specific antidote exists for an overdose of milrinone. Hypotension secondary to vasodilation is the primary effect seen with excessive dosages. The recommendation is to reduce the dosage or temporarily discontinue the drug if excessive hypotension occurs. This is to be done until the patient's condition has stabilized. Initiation of general measures for circulatory support is also recommended.

Interactions

Concurrent administration of diuretics may cause significant hypovolemia and reduced cardiac filling pressure. Additive inotropic effects may be seen with coadministration of digoxin. Furosemide must not be injected into intravenous lines with milrinone because it will precipitate immediately.

Dosages

For dosage information, see the table on the previous page.

DRUG PROFILE

♦ milrinone

Milrinone (Primacor) is the only available PDI. Milrinone is also referred to as an *inodilator* because it exerts both a positive inotropic effect and a vasodilatory effect. Milrinone is contraindicated in cases of known drug allergy. Adverse effects include cardiac dysrhythmias, headache, hypokalemia, tremor, thrombocytopenia, and elevated liver enzyme levels. Interacting drugs include diuretics (additive hypotensive effects) and digoxin (additive inotropic effects). Milrinone is available only in injectable form. Recommended dosages are given in the table on the previous page.

Pharmacokinetics: Milrinone

Route	Onset of Action	Peak Plasma Concentration	Elimination Half-life	Duration of Action
IV	5-15 min	Immediate	2-3 hr	8-10 hr

CARDIAC GLYCOSIDES

Cardiac glycosides are one of the oldest groups of cardiac drugs. Not only do they have beneficial effects on the failing heart, but they also help control the ventricular response to atrial fibrillation. They were originally obtained from either the *Digitalis purpurea* or *Digitalis lanata* plant, both commonly known as foxglove. For this reason, cardiac glycosides are sometimes referred to as *digitalis glycosides.* Cardiac glycosides were the mainstay of therapy for heart failure for more than 200 years; however, they are no longer used as first-line drugs. Digoxin is the only cardiac glycoside currently available in the United States. Although digoxin is a powerful positive inotropic drug, it has not been shown to reduce mortality.

Mechanism of Action and Drug Effects

The beneficial effect of digoxin is thought to be an increase in myocardial contractility—known as a *positive inotropic effect.* This occurs secondarily to the inhibition of the sodium-potassium adenosine triphosphatase pump. When the action of this enzyme-complex is inhibited, the cellular sodium and calcium concentrations increase. The overall result is enhanced myocardial contractility. Digoxin also augments cholinergic (or parasympathetic) stimulation via the vagus nerve of the parasympathetic nervous system. This is more commonly referred to as *vagal tone* and results in increased diastolic filling between heartbeats secondary to reduced heart rate. Vagal tone is also believed to sensitize cardiac baroreceptors, which reduces sympathetic stimulation from the central nervous system. All of these processes further enhance cardiac efficiency and output.

Digoxin changes the electrical conduction properties of the heart, and this markedly affects the conduction system and cardiac automaticity. Digoxin decreases the velocity (rate) of electrical conduction and prolongs the refractory period in the conduction system. The particular site in the conduction system where this occurs is the area between the atria and the ventricles (SA node to AV node). The cardiac cells remain in a state of depolarization longer and are unable to start another electrical impulse, which also reduces heart rate and improves cardiac efficiency.

The following is a summary of the inotropic, chronotropic, dromotropic, and other effects produced by digoxin:

- Positive inotropic effect—an increase in the force and velocity of myocardial contraction without a corresponding increase in oxygen consumption
- Negative chronotropic effect—reduced heart rate
- Negative dromotropic effect—decreased automaticity at the SA node, decreased AV nodal conduction, reduced conductivity at the bundle of His, and prolongation of the atrial and ventricular refractory periods
- Increase in stroke volume
- Reduction in heart size during diastole
- Decrease in venous blood pressure and vein engorgement
- Increase in coronary circulation
- Promotion of tissue perfusion and diuresis as a result of improved blood circulation

TABLE 24-1 Digoxin: Common Adverse Effects

Body System	Adverse Effects
Cardiovascular	Bradycardia or tachycardia; hypotension
Central nervous	Headache, fatigue, confusion, convulsions
Eye	Colored vision (i.e., green, yellow, or purple), halo vision
Gastrointestinal	Anorexia, nausea, vomiting, diarrhea

Normal therapeutic level = 0.5 to 2 ng/mL.

TABLE 24-2 Conditions Predisposing to Digitalis Toxicity

Condition/ Disease	Significance
Use of cardiac pacemaker	A patient with this device may exhibit digitalis toxicity at lower dosages than usual.
Hypokalemia or hypomagnesemia	The patient's risk for serious dysrhythmias is increased, and the patient is more susceptible to digitalis toxicity.
Hypercalcemia	The patient is at higher risk for experiencing sinus bradycardia, dysrhythmias, and heart block.
Atrioventricular block	Heart block may worsen with increasing levels of digitalis.
Dysrhythmias	Dysrhythmias may occur that did not exist before digitalis use and thus could be related to digitalis toxicity.
Hypothyroidism, respiratory disease, or renal disease	Patients with these disorders require lower dosages because they cause delayed renal drug excretion.
Advanced age	Because of decreased renal function and the resultant diminished drug excretion along with decreased body mass in this patient population, a lower dosage than usual is needed to prevent toxicity.
Ventricular fibrillation	Ventricular rate may actually increase with digitalis use.

- Decrease in exertional and paroxysmal nocturnal dyspnea, cough, and cyanosis
- Improved symptom control, quality of life, and exercise tolerance, but no apparent reduction in mortality

Indications

Digoxin is primarily used in the treatment of systolic heart failure and atrial fibrillation. However, the latest heart failure treatment guidelines recommend that it be used as an adjunct to drugs of other classes, including beta blockers, diuretics, ACE inhibitors, and ARBs in selected patients.

Contraindications

Contraindications to the use of digoxin include known drug allergy and may include second- or third-degree heart block, ventricular fibrillation, and heart failure resulting from diastolic dysfunction. However, digoxin may be used to treat some of these conditions, if recommended by a seasoned cardiologist, depending on the given clinical situation.

Adverse Effects

The common undesirable effects associated with digoxin use are cardiovascular, central nervous system, ocular, and gastrointestinal effects. These are outlined in Table 24-1.

Toxicity and Management of Overdose

Digoxin has a low therapeutic index (see Chapter 2). Digoxin levels are monitored when the patient first starts taking the drug. However, once the drug reaches steady state, monitoring is usually necessary only if there is suspicion of toxicity, noncompliance, or deteriorating renal function. Normal therapeutic levels for digoxin are 0.5 to 2 ng/mL. Low potassium or magnesium levels may increase the potential for digoxin toxicity. Therefore, frequent monitoring of serum electrolytes is also important. A decrease in renal function is a common cause of digoxin toxicity, because digoxin is excreted almost exclusively via the kidneys. Signs and symptoms of digoxin toxicity include bradycardia, headache, dizziness, confusion, nausea, and visual disturbances (blurred vision or yellow vision). With toxicity, ECG findings may include heart block, atrial tachycardia with block, or ventricular dysrhythmias. Predisposing factors to digoxin toxicity are listed in Table 24-2.

The treatment strategies for digoxin toxicity depend on the severity of the symptoms. These strategies can range from simply withholding the next dose to instituting more aggressive therapies.

When significant toxicity develops as a result of digoxin therapy, the administration of digoxin immune Fab may be indicated. Digoxin immune Fab is an antibody that recognizes digoxin as an antigen and forms an antigen-antibody complex with the drug, thus inactivating the free digoxin. Digoxin immune Fab therapy is indicated only for the following:
- Hyperkalemia (serum potassium level higher than 5 mEq/L) in a patient with digoxin toxicity
- Life-threatening cardiac dysrhythmias, sustained ventricular tachycardia or fibrillation, and severe sinus bradycardia or heart block unresponsive to atropine treatment or cardiac pacing
- Life-threatening digoxin overdose: more than 10 mg digoxin in adults; more than 4 mg digoxin in children

Interactions

A wide variety of significant drug interactions are possible with digoxin. Common examples are given in Table 24-3. The most important drug-drug interactions occurring with digoxin are interactions with amiodarone, quinidine, and verapamil. These three drugs can increase digoxin levels by 50%. When large amounts of bran are ingested, the absorption of oral digoxin may be decreased. Certain herbal supplements may interact with digoxin; for example, ginseng may increase digoxin levels, hawthorn may potentiate the effects of digoxin, licorice may

TABLE 24-3   Digoxin: Drug Interactions

Interacting Drug	Mechanism	Result
Antidysrhythmics calcium (IV)	Increase cardiac irritability	Increased digoxin toxicity
cholestyramine colestipol sucralfate	Decrease oral absorption	Reduced therapeutic effect
Beta blockers	Block beta$_1$ receptors in the heart	Enhanced bradycardic effect of digoxin
Calcium channel blockers	Block calcium channels in the myocardium	Enhanced bradycardic and negative inotropic effects of digoxin
verapamil quinidine amiodarone dronedarone cyclosporine Azole antifungals	Decrease clearance	Digoxin levels increased by 50%; digoxin dose should be reduced by 50%

increase the risk for cardiac toxicity due to potassium loss, and St. John's wort may reduce digoxin levels. Drugs that lower serum potassium or magnesium levels can predispose patients to digoxin toxicity.

Dosages

For dosage information, see the table on p. 380. Also see the Safety and Quality Improvement: Preventing Medication Errors box on this page.

DRUG PROFILES

◆ digoxin

Digoxin (Lanoxin) is indicated for the treatment of heart failure and atrial fibrillation and flutter. Digoxin use is contraindicated in patients who have shown a hypersensitivity to it and in those with ventricular tachycardia and fibrillation. Normal therapeutic drug levels of digoxin are between 0.5 and 2 ng/mL. However, levels higher than 2 ng/mL are used for the treatment of atrial fibrillation. Digoxin is available in oral and injectable forms. Because of digoxin's fairly long duration of action and half-life, a loading, or "digitalizing," dose is often given to bring serum levels of the drug up to a desirable therapeutic level more quickly. Recommended digitalizing doses and the daily oral and intravenous adult dosages are given in the table on p. 380.

Pharmacokinetics: Digoxin

Route	Onset of Action	Peak Plasma Concentration	Elimination Half-life	Duration of Action
PO	1-2 hr	2-8 hr	35-48 hr	3-4 days
IV	5-30 min	1-4 hr	35-48 hr	3-4 days

digoxin immune Fab

Digoxin immune Fab (Digifab) is the antidote for severe digoxin overdose and is indicated for the reversal of life-threatening cardiotoxic effects. Use of digoxin immune Fab is

contraindicated in patients who have shown a hypersensitivity to it. It is available only in parenteral form. It is dosed based on the patient's serum digoxin level in conjunction with his or her weight. The recommended dosages vary according to the amount of cardiac glycoside ingested. One vial binds 0.5 mg of digoxin. It is important to bear in mind that after digoxin immune Fab is given, all subsequent measurements of serum digoxin level will be elevated for days to weeks. Therefore, after its administration, the clinical signs and symptoms of digoxin toxicity, rather than the digoxin serum levels, are the primary focus in monitoring for the effectiveness of reversal therapy.

Pharmacokinetics: Digoxin Immune Fab

Route	Onset of Action	Peak Plasma Concentration	Elimination Half-life	Duration of Action
IV	Immediate	Immediate	14-20 hr	Days to weeks

⚡ SAFETY AND QUALITY IMPROVEMENT: PREVENTING MEDICATION ERRORS

The Importance of Decimal Points

Incorrect decimal placement can be lethal when calculating digoxin dosages! According to the Institute for Safe Medication Practices (ISMP), trailing zeros are *not* to be used after decimal points. In the case of digoxin, if a "1 mg" dose is ordered and is written as "1.0 mg," the order could be misread as "10 mg," and the patient would receive 10 times the ordered dose.

The ISMP also recommends that leading zeroes be used if a dose is less than a whole number. For example, ".25 mg" can look like "25 mg," which is 100 times the ordered dose. Instead, the order must be written as "0.25 mg" to avoid any errors.

Of course, such an error hopefully would be caught when the nurse realizes how many 250-mcg digoxin tablets it would take to give a "25 mg" dose, or how many milliliters would be needed for an intravenous dose. However, such errors have occurred. Consider what would happen if a digoxin overdose leads to digoxin toxicity and the serious effects this would have on the patient!

Data from Institute for Safe Medication Practices: ISMP's list of error-prone abbreviations, symbols, and dose designations. (2013). Available at *www.ismp.org/tools/errorproneabbreviations.pdf.* Accessed July 12, 2015.

NURSING PROCESS

ASSESSMENT

Before a drug used to treat heart failure is given, perform a thorough assessment, including assessment of the patient's past and present medical history, drug allergies, and family medical history with emphasis on any history of cardiac, hypertensive, or renal diseases. Your review may yield findings that either dictate very cautious use of the drug or may even represent contraindications to its use. Assess the following clinical parameters and other data:
- Blood pressure
- Pulse rate—both apical and radial, measured for 1 full minute
- Peripheral pulse location and grading of strength

- Capillary refill time
- Presence or absence of edema
- Heart sounds
- Breath sounds
- Weight
- Intake and output amounts
- Serum laboratory values such as potassium, sodium, magnesium, and calcium levels
- Electrocardiogram
- Results of renal function tests, including BUN and creatinine levels
- Results of liver function tests such as AST, ALT, CPK, LDH, and ALP levels
- Medication history and profile, including all prescription drugs, over-the-counter drugs, herbals, and nutritional supplements taken; for example, herbal products (e.g., Siberian ginseng) may increase digitalis drug levels; consumption of large amounts of bran with digoxin will decrease the drug's absorption
- Dietary habits and all meals and snacks consumed over the previous 24 hours
- Smoking history
- Alcohol intake

ACE inhibitors, such as *lisinopril,* require thorough assessment of cautions, contraindications, and drug interactions (see Chapter 22). Hyperkalemia is an adverse effect; therefore, assess serum potassium levels before giving these drugs, and administer potassium supplementation and/or potassium-sparing diuretics as prescribed and with caution. Assess respiratory history, specifically any previous problems of cough. ACE inhibitors may cause a dry cough, which is not harmful but may be annoying. Patients may be switched to an *ARB,* such as valsartan (see Chapter 22), if the cough becomes problematic for the patient.

As mentioned earlier, *metoprolol* is the *beta blocker* most commonly used to treat heart failure. *Carvedilol* also has many therapeutic effects (see Chapters 19, 22, and 23 for a detailed discussion) and is commonly added to existing regimens of digoxin, furosemide (loop diuretic), and ACE inhibitors in the management of heart failure. Related assessment information for alpha- and beta-blocking drugs may be found in Chapter 19. *Dobutamine,* a beta$_1$-selective adrenergic, is also used to treat heart failure and is discussed further in Chapter 18. The status of the patient's veins is important to assess when this drug is indicated because it is only given intravenously.

Aldosterone antagonists, such as *spironolactone* and *eplerenone,* require close assessment of heart and breath sounds as well as for the occurrence of edema, which is a known adverse effect (see Chapter 22 for more information). *Hydralazine/isosorbide dinitrate* is used mainly in African-American patients and is discussed further in Chapter 22.

The newest class of medications for heart failure, the *B-type natriuretic peptides,* includes the drug *nesiritide.* Carefully assess all body functions, especially cardiac function, with attention to heart sounds, blood pressure, pulse rate, and the presence of any cardiac dysrhythmias, hypotension, insomnia, and headache. These may be exacerbated with the use of this drug. See previous discussion for other cautions, contraindications, and drug interactions.

With any medication regimen, it is always important to assess support systems at home, because safe and effective therapy depends on close observation, monitoring of appropriate parameters (e.g., daily weight), attention to patient complaints, and evaluation of how the patient is feeling and functioning. With *milrinone,* a *phosphodiesterase inhibitor,* closely monitor cardiac status, which is critical to patient safety. These patients are usually in an ICU setting and require frequent assessment of heart sounds, vital signs, and any evidence of ventricular dysrhythmias on ECG readings. Assess also for any history of angina, hypotension, and hypokalemia, which may all be exacerbated with this drug. Significant drug interactions include parenteral furosemide that precipitates immediately if milrinone is present in the IV lines.

Before giving *digoxin,* closely monitor serum electrolytes. Specifically, assess potassium levels because low levels or hypokalemia may precipitate digoxin toxicity. Hypokalemia is manifested by muscle weakness, confusion, lethargy, anorexia, nausea, and changes in the ECG. Low levels of magnesium or hypomagnesemia may also precipitate digoxin toxicity. Hypomagnesemia is manifested by agitation, twitching, hyperactive reflexes, nausea, vomiting, and ECG changes. You also need to closely assess digoxin levels once it has been administered because of the narrow range between the therapeutic and toxic levels of digoxin (also called a *low therapeutic index;* see Chapter 2). Measure and document a baseline weight before therapy begins as well as during therapy. Perform a careful assessment of the following: (1) Neurologic system: Note any history of headaches, fatigue, confusion, and/or seizures; assess level of alertness and orientation to person, place, and time; (2) Gastrointestinal system: Document any changes in appetite (decreased) and/or complaints of diarrhea, nausea, or vomiting; (3) Cardiac system: Note the history of any irregularities or other cardiac manifestations; assess pulse for rate lower than 60 beats/min or higher than 100 beats/min; assess baseline blood pressure, and note any hypotension or hypertension. Auscultate heart sounds for any extra or abnormal heart sounds and note any abnormal ECG findings (if this test is ordered); and (4) Visual and sensory system: Document baseline vision as well as any changes in vision, such as green, yellow, or purple halo surrounding the peripheral field of vision. See Table 24-1 for more information on adverse effects of *digoxin.* Also assess for any cautions, contraindications, and drug interactions (see Table 24-2).

NURSING DIAGNOSES

1. Ineffective peripheral tissue perfusion related to the pathophysiologic influence of heart failure
2. Deficient knowledge related to lack of information and experience with heart failure as well as the first-time use of drugs indicated for heart failure
3. Noncompliance with therapy regimen related to lack of information about the disease process as well as the drug(s) and adverse effects

PATIENT-CENTERED CARE: LIFESPAN CONSIDERATIONS FOR THE PEDIATRIC PATIENT

Heart Failure

The cause, symptoms, treatment, and prognosis of heart failure in children vary depending on age. In infants, the cause of heart failure is generally due to holes in the heart or other structural problems. In older children, the structure of the heart may be normal but the heart muscle may be weakened. Symptoms of heart failure differ depending on age and become worse with age because the heart must keep up with increased oxygen demands and energy demands (with increased growth).

- Symptoms may include poor growth, difficulty in feeding, and tachypnea; in older children, inability to tolerate exercise and other activities, the need to rest more often, and dyspnea with minimal exertion occur more frequently.
- Treatment is generally age- and cause-specific. For septal defects, surgery or medication may be indicated. For more complex problems, surgery may be needed within the first few weeks of life.
- For some congenital heart disease patients, a heart transplant may be the only option. In older children with weakened heart muscle, medication may help decrease the workload of the heart and give it time to heal, but transplants may eventually be required.
- Drug therapy may include furosemide (a loop diuretic), angiotensin-converting enzyme inhibitors, beta blockers, and sometimes digoxin to help improve heart-pumping efficiency.
- Correct calculation of dosages for any of the medications used is very important to safe and cautious nursing care. A placement error of one decimal point placement will result in a tenfold dosage error, which could be fatal.
- Digoxin toxicity is manifested in children by nausea, vomiting, bradycardia, anorexia, and dysrhythmias.
- The prescriber must be notified immediately if any of the following develop or worsen: fatigue, sudden weight gain (2 pounds or more in 24 hours), palpitations, tachycardia or bradycardia, and/or respiratory distress.

Modified from Cincinnati Children's Hospital Medical Center: Signs and symptoms: congestive heart failure, 2013. Available at *www.cincinnatichildrens.org/health/c/chf.* Accessed April 17, 2015.

PLANNING: OUTCOME IDENTIFICATION

1. Patient exhibits improved cardiac output/tissue perfusion once drug therapy is initiated with strong peripheral pulses; pink, warm extremities; and improved tolerance of activities of daily living (ADLs).
2. Patient demonstrates sufficient knowledge about the disease process and its treatment, stating the importance of the need for lifelong treatment/lifestyle changes, constant monitoring by the health care provider, and stating action, adverse effects, and toxic effects of therapy.
3. Patient remains compliant with drug therapy regimen with improved heart function, heart rate, and heart rhythm.

IMPLEMENTATION

Nursing interventions associated with the use of *ACE inhibitors, ARBs, beta blockers,* and *adrenergic drugs* are discussed further in Chapters 18, 19, and 22. *Hydralazine/isosorbide dinitrate* must be used with extreme caution because of the associated syncope. If this occurs, the drug will most likely be discontinued. Monitor blood pressure and other vital signs, especially the first few doses of *hydralazine/isosorbide dinitrate* (because of the syncope).

When administering the *b-type natriuretic peptide nesiritide,* give the drug as ordered and with extreme caution. Nesiritide is strictly used in an intensive care setting in very ill patients who are experiencing acute decompensated heart failure and receiving continuous cardiac monitoring. While the drug is being administered intravenously, monitor the patient for associated severe adverse effects, such as hypotension, dysrhythmias, headache, and abdominal pain. If possible, avoid co-administration of drugs that decrease the patient's blood pressure, such as ACE inhibitors and diuretics.

Always check for compatibility of solutions when giving the *phosphodiesterase inhibitor milrinone.* Record intake and output, heart rate, blood pressure, daily weight, and respiration rate. Continue to assess heart and breath sounds. Report any evidence of hypokalemia to the prescriber immediately, and monitor the patient closely (vital signs). When heart failure drugs such as digoxin, milrinone, and digoxin immune Fab are administered parenterally, use an infusion pump unless otherwise prescribed.

Before administering any dose of the *cardiac glycoside digoxin,* check the serum potassium and magnesium levels to be sure they are within normal limits to help limit/prevent toxicity. Always measure the patient's apical pulse rate (auscultate the apical heart rate, found at the point of maximal impulse (PMI) located at the fifth left midclavicular intercostal space) for 1 full minute. If the pulse rate is 60 beats/min or lower, or if it is higher than 100 beats/min, you will generally withhold the dose and notify the prescriber of the problem immediately. Although withholding of the dose is usually indicated, health care facilities and prescribers often have their own protocols that apply to individual patients. In addition, contact the prescriber if the patient experiences any of the following signs and symptoms of digoxin toxicity: headache, dizziness, confusion, nausea, and visual disturbances (yellow-green halo or blurred vision). ECG findings in a patient with digoxin toxicity would show heart block, atrial tachycardia with block, or ventricular dysrhythmias. Remember that most health care institutions and/or nursing units follow protocol or policy with regard to the cardiac glycoside digoxin and its administration.

Other nursing interventions include checking the dosage form and prescribed amounts and the prescriber's order carefully to make sure that the correct drug dosage has been dispensed (e.g., 0.125 or 0.25 mg). Oral digoxin may be administered with meals but not with foods high in fiber (bran), because the fiber will bind to the digitalis and lead to altered absorption/bioavailability of the drug. If the medication is to be given intravenously, the following interventions are critical to patient safety: infuse undiluted intravenous forms at around 0.25 mg/min or over longer than a 5-minute period, or as per health care institution protocol. The administration of intramuscular forms of cardiac glycosides is extremely painful and is not indicated or recommended and may lead to tissue necrosis and erratic absorption. *Digoxin* is incompatible with many other medications in solution or syringe, so always double-check compatibility before parenteral administration.

Consider the interventions for patients undergoing digitalization separately from other drugs. Again, although digitalization is not commonly used in contemporary practice, it may still be performed in some areas of practice for the management of heart failure. Rapid digitalization (to achieve faster onset of action) is generally reserved for patients who have heart failure and are in acute distress. Such patients are hospitalized because digitalis toxicities can appear quickly (in this setting) and are directly correlated with the high drug concentrations used. If the patient undergoing rapid digitalization exhibits any of the manifestations of toxicity, contact the prescriber immediately. Continuously observe these patients, with frequent measurement of vital signs and serum drug as well as serum potassium levels. Slow digitalization (rarely used) is generally performed on an outpatient basis in patients with heart failure who are not in acute distress. In this situation, it takes longer for toxic effects to appear (depending on the drug's half-life) than with rapid digitalization. The main advantages of slow digitalization are that it can be performed on an outpatient basis, oral dosage forms can be used, and it is safer than rapid digitalization. The disadvantages are that it takes longer for the therapeutic effects to occur, and the symptoms of toxicity are more gradual in onset and therefore more insidious.

If toxicity occurs and digoxin rises to a life-threatening level, administer the antidote, *digoxin immune Fab*, as ordered. It is given parenterally over 30 minutes, and in some scenarios it is given as an intravenous bolus (e.g., if cardiac arrest is imminent). All vials of the drug need to be refrigerated. The drug is stable for 4 hours after being mixed; use it immediately, and if not used within 4 hours, discard the drug. One vial of digoxin immune Fab binds 0.5 mg of digoxin. Check compatible solutions for dilution prior to infusion of the antidote. Closely monitor blood pressure, apical pulse rate and rhythm, electrocardiogram, and serum potassium levels, and record the findings. Document baseline data, and begin observing closely for changes in assessment findings such as changes in muscle strength, occurrence of tremors and muscle cramping, changes in mental status, irregular cardiac rhythms (from hypokalemia), confusion, thirst, and cold clammy skin (from

hyponatremia). If the treatment does reduce the toxicity, these problems will improve considerably compared with the patient's baseline.

EVALUATION

Monitoring patients after the administration of drugs to improve heart contractility, or *positive inotropic drugs*, is critical for identifying therapeutic effects and adverse effects. Because positive inotropic drugs increase the force of myocardial contractility and alter electrophysiologic properties, leading to a decrease in heart rate (negative chronotropic effect) and a decrease in AV node conduction properties (negative dromotropic effect), the therapeutic effects of these drugs include the following: increased urinary output, decreased edema, decreased dyspnea and crackles, decreased fatigue, resolution of paroxysmal nocturnal dyspnea, and improvement in peripheral pulses, skin color, and skin temperature.

For patients taking *lisinopril, valsartan, metoprolol, dobutamine, nesiritide,* and *hydralazine/isosorbide dinitrate,* therapeutic effects include improvement in symptoms of heart failure and improved cardiac function. Evaluation must also include monitoring for the adverse effects of these medications (see the pharmacology discussion).

Therapeutic effects of *milrinone* include an improvement in cardiac function with a corresponding improvement in the patient's heart failure. Monitor for the adverse effects of hypotension, dysrhythmias, headache, ventricular fibrillation, chest pain, and hypokalemia. Evaluate patients taking milrinone for significant hypotension. If hypotension occurs, contact the prescriber; discontinue the infusion or decrease the rate while waiting to hear from the prescriber or per health care institution protocol, and continue to monitor the patient's vital signs frequently.

While monitoring for the therapeutic effects of *digoxin,* assess the patient for the development of toxicity because of the drug's low therapeutic index. Toxic effects associated with digoxin may include nausea, vomiting, and anorexia. Monitoring laboratory values such as serum creatinine, potassium, calcium, sodium, and chloride levels—as well as watching the serum levels of digoxin (normal levels between 0.5 and 2 ng/mL)—is important to ensure safe and efficacious treatment.

CASE STUDY

Patient-Centered Care: Phosphodiesterase Inhibitor for Heart Failure

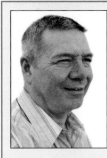

J., a 58-year-old retired bus driver, has been in the hospital for 1 week for treatment of heart failure. He had a myocardial infarction 1 year earlier and tells the nurse that he "hasn't felt well for weeks." He is currently receiving carvedilol, lisinopril, furosemide, and potassium supplements (all orally), but he has had little improvement.

Today during morning rounds, the nurse notes that J. is having increased difficulty with breathing, and his heart rate is up to 120 beats/min. His weight has increased from 72 to 76 kg overnight, and his lower legs and ankles show edema rated as 3+. Crackles are heard over both lungs, and his pulse oximetry reading is 91% (down from 98% earlier). In addition, J. is very restless. Oxygen is started, a Foley catheter is inserted, and J. is transferred to the intensive care unit.

After examining J., Dr. H. revises J.'s medication orders as follows:
Change furosemide to 60 mg intravenously twice a day
Continue carvedilol and lisinopril
Start an infusion of milrinone as follows:
  Loading dose: 50 mcg/kg over 10 minutes, followed by an infusion of 0.5 mcg/kg/min

1. Describe the drug effects of the medications J. is receiving for the heart failure.
2. What laboratory values will you need to monitor while J. is receiving the milrinone?

The charge nurse is in J.'s room when another nurse comes in to give J. the intravenous dose of furosemide. As the nurse reaches for the tubing of the milrinone infusion to administer the diuretic, the charge nurse gently stops the nurse from giving the medication. Out in the hallway, the charge nurse speaks to the nurse.

3. What was the potential problem?

The next morning, J.'s breathing is better, his lungs are clearer, and his peripheral edema is now evaluated as trace edema. However, he complains of feeling his heart "skip" more than usual.

4. Is there a concern? What will the nurse need to do at this point?

After 4 days, J.'s condition has improved greatly. The milrinone was stopped, he was transferred to a regular room, and today he is ready to go home.

5. In addition to receiving education regarding his medications, what should J. be taught to monitor while recovering at home?

For answers, see *http://evolve.elsevier.com/Lilley*.

PATIENT-CENTERED CARE: PATIENT TEACHING

- Hydralazine/isosorbide dinitrate may cause syncope. Explain to the patient that changing positions carefully and slowly is needed to prevent falls.
- Instruct the patient on how to take the radial pulse before each dose of digoxin or as indicated. Daily weights are important and need to be done at the same time every morning and with the exact amount of clothing. For the older adult patient or the physically or mentally challenged patient, it is important that home health care personnel or a heart failure/hospital-based clinic supervise the medication regimen. This is important because these individuals are at risk for adverse effects, toxicity, and drug interactions. If the pulse rate is below 60 beats/min or is erratic, if the pulse rate is 100 beats/min or higher, or if there is anorexia, nausea, or vomiting, the health care provider must be contacted. Emphasize the importance of the patient reporting any palpitations or a feeling that the heart is racing, change in heart rate and/or irregular heart rate, the occurrence of dizziness or fainting, any changes in vision, and weight gain (2 pounds or more in 24 hours or 5 pounds or more in 1 week).
- Advise the patient to keep a daily journal with notation of medications, daily weights, dietary intake and appetite, any adverse effects or changes in condition, and a rating of how the he or she is feeling day to day.
- Instruct the patient to wear a medical alert bracelet or necklace and to keep a current medication and medical history

card on his or her person at all times that lists allergies, medical diagnosis, and medications. Medical information and lists of medications need to be updated frequently or with each visit to the prescriber.
- Digoxin is usually taken once a day. Encourage the patient to take it at the same time every day. If a dose is missed, the patient may take the omitted dose if no more than 12 hours have passed from the time the drug was to have been taken. Instruct the patient that if more than 12 hours have passed since the missed dose, the patient should *not* skip that dose, *not* double up on the next digoxin dose, and contact the prescriber immediately for further instructions.
- Instruct the patient to *never* abruptly stop any of the medications being taken for heart failure. If problems occur, advise the patient to always contact the prescriber.
- If potassium-depleting diuretics are being taken as part of the therapy, encourage the patient to consume foods high in potassium and to report any weakness, fatigue, or lethargy. In addition, any worsening of dizziness or dyspnea or the occurrence of any unusual problems should be reported immediately.
- With medication regimens for heart failure, most patients are encouraged to avoid using antacids or eating ice cream, milk products, yogurt, cheese (dairy products), or bran for 2 hours before or 2 hours after taking medication to avoid interference with the absorption of the oral dosage forms of these medications.

KEY POINTS

- Inotropic drugs affect the force of myocardial contraction; positive inotropics (e.g., digoxin) increase the force of contractions, and negative inotropics (e.g., beta blockers, calcium channel blockers) decrease myocardial contractility.
- Chronotropics affect heart rate per minute, with positive chronotropics increasing the heart rate and negative chronotropics decreasing the heart rate.
- Dromotropic drugs affect the conduction of electrical impulses through the heart; positive dromotropic drugs increase the speed of electrical impulses through the heart, whereas negative dromotropic drugs have the opposite effect.
- Drugs used for the initiation of therapy for heart failure include ACE inhibitors (lisinopril, enalapril, captopril, and others) or ARBs (valsartan, candesartan, losartan, and others) and certain beta blockers (metoprolol, a cardioselective beta blocker; carvedilol, a nonspecific beta blocker).
- Be aware of the important physiologic concepts such as ejection fraction. A patient's ejection fraction reflects the contractility of the heart, and ejection fraction decreases as heart failure worsens because the heart is failing to pump effectively. The normal ejection fraction is approximately 65% (0.65) of the total volume in the ventricle.
- Recognize that hypotension, dysrhythmias, and thrombocytopenia are major adverse effects of milrinone.
- Keep informed of the contraindications to the use of digoxin, which include a history of allergy to the digitalis medications, ventricular tachycardia and fibrillations, and AV block.

NCLEX® EXAMINATION REVIEW QUESTIONS

1. When teaching the patient about the signs and symptoms of cardiac glycoside toxicity, the nurse should alert the patient to watch for
   a. visual changes such as photophobia.
   b. flickering lights or halos around lights.
   c. dizziness when standing up.
   d. increased urine output.
2. During assessment of a patient who is receiving digoxin, the nurse monitors for findings that would indicate an increased possibility of toxicity, such as:
   a. apical pulse rate of 62 beats/min.
   b. digoxin level of 1.5 ng/mL.
   c. serum potassium level of 2.0 mEq/L.
   d. serum calcium level of 9.9 mEq/L.
3. When monitoring a patient who is receiving an intravenous infusion of nesiritide (Natrecor), the nurse will look for which adverse effect?
   a. Dysrhythmia
   b. Proteinuria
   c. Hyperglycemia
   d. Hypertension
4. A patient is taking a beta blocker as part of the treatment plan for heart failure. The nurse knows that the purpose of the beta blocker for this patient is to
   a. increase urine output.
   b. prevent stimulation of the heart by catecholamines.
   c. increase the contractility of the heart muscle.
   d. cause peripheral vasodilation.
5. The nurse is assessing a patient who is receiving a milrinone infusion and checks the patient's cardiac rhythm on the heart monitor. What adverse cardiac effect is most likely to occur in a patient who is receiving intravenous milrinone?

   a. Tachycardia
   b. Bradycardia
   c. Atrial fibrillation
   d. Ventricular dysrhythmia
6. The nurse is administering an intravenous infusion of a phosphodiesterase inhibitor to a patient who has heart failure. The nurse will evaluate the patient for which therapeutic effects? *(Select all that apply.)*
   a. Positive inotropic effects
   b. Vasodilation
   c. Decreased heart rate
   d. Increased blood pressure
   e. Positive chronotropic effects
7. The medication order for a 5-year-old patient reads: "Give digoxin elixir, 15 mcg/kg, PO now." The child weighs 20 kg. How many milligrams will this patient receive?
8. A patient with heart failure will be starting the beta blocker metoprolol (Lopressor). The nurse will monitor for which expected cardiovascular effects? *(Select all that apply.)*
   a. Increased heart rate
   b. Increased myocardial contractility
   c. Delayed AV node conduction
   d. Reduced heart rate
   e. Decreased myocardial automaticity

1. b, 2. c, 3. a, 4. b, 5. d, 6. a, b, e, 7. 0.3 mg, 8. c, d, e.

CRITICAL THINKING AND PRIORITIZATION QUESTIONS

1. A nurse administered 125 mg of digoxin instead of 0.125 mg of digoxin intravenously. The patient has developed a severe heart block dysrhythmia, and the slow heart rate has not responded to administration of atropine and other measures. The nurse stays with the patient while the charge nurse notifies the cardiologist. What will be the priority in this situation? What will the nurse expect to give next? How could this situation have been prevented?

2. A patient is receiving an angiotensin-converting enzyme (ACE) inhibitor, a diuretic, and a beta blocker as treatment for heart failure. He has a history of hypothyroidism, which is controlled by thyroid replacement hormones, and chronic bronchitis. He states that he stopped smoking 1 year ago after smoking two packs a day for 30 years. This morning he complains of a dry cough but says he does not feel short of breath, even when getting up to go to the bathroom. He is unable to produce any sputum. When the nurse listens to his lungs, his breath sounds are clear except for very few scattered rhonchi bilaterally. His weight is the same as yesterday's weight, and his ankles show only trace edema (2 days ago he had 2+ edema on the edema scale). His temperature is 98.4° F (36.9° C), his pulse is 88 beats/min, and his blood pressure is 124/86 mm Hg. He says to the nurse, "This cough is awful! I am so afraid that my heart failure is getting worse or that I'm getting pneumonia!" What is the nurse's priority action at this time?

For answers, see *http://evolve.elsevier.com/Lilley*.

(e) EVOLVE WEBSITE

http://evolve.elsevier.com/Lilley
- Animations
- Answer Keys for Textbook Case Studies and Textbook Critical Thinking and Prioritization Questions

- Content Updates
- Key Points
- Review Questions
- Student Case Studies

Antidysrhythmic Drugs

http://evolve.elsevier.com/Lilley

OBJECTIVES

When you reach the end of this chapter, you will be able to do the following:

1. Describe the anatomy and physiology of the heart as well as cardiac electrophysiology, including normal conduction patterns, rate, and rhythm.
2. Briefly discuss the various disorders of cardiac electrophysiology and consequences to the patient.
3. Define the terms *dysrhythmia* and *arrhythmia.*
4. Identify the various causes of abnormal heart rhythms and their impact on the patient's health and activities of daily living.
5. Identify the most commonly encountered dysrhythmias.
6. Compare the various dysrhythmias with regard to their basic characteristics, impact on the structures of the heart, and related symptoms.
7. Contrast the various classes of antidysrhythmic drugs, citing prototypes in each class and describing their mechanisms of action, indications, routes of administration, dosing, any related drug protocols, adverse effects, cautions, contraindications, drug interactions, and any toxic reactions.
8. Develop a nursing care plan that includes all phases of the nursing process for patients receiving each class of antidysrhythmic drug.

DRUG PROFILES

adenosine, p. 405
◆!amiodarone, p. 403
◆atenolol, p. 402
◆diltiazem, p. 405
◆dofetilide, p. 404
!esmolol, p. 402
flecainide, p. 401
ibutilide, p. 404
◆!lidocaine, p. 401

◆metoprolol, p. 403
procainamide, p. 400
propafenone, p. 402
◆quinidine, p. 401
◆sotalol, p. 404
◆verapamil, p. 405

_____
◆ = *Key drug*
! = *High-alert drug*

KEY TERMS

Action potential Electrical activity that consists of a series of polarizations and depolarizations that travel across the cell membrane of a nerve fiber during transmission of a nerve impulse and across the cell membranes of a muscle cell during contraction. (p. 392)

Action potential duration The interval beginning with baseline (resting) membrane potential followed by depolarization and ending with repolarization to baseline membrane potential. (p. 393)

Arrhythmia Technically "no rhythm," meaning absence of heart rhythm (i.e., no heartbeat at all). More commonly used in clinical practice to refer to any variation from the normal rhythm of the heart. A synonymous term is *dysrhythmia,* which is the primary term used in this textbook. (p. 391)

Cardiac Arrhythmia Suppression Trial (CAST) A major research study conducted to investigate the possibility of eliminating sudden cardiac death in patients with asymptomatic ectopy after a myocardial infarction. (p. 401)

Depolarization The movement of positive and negative ions on either side of a cell membrane across the membrane in a direction that brings the net charge to zero. (p. 392)

Dysrhythmia Any disturbance or abnormality in heart rhythm. (p. 391)

Effective refractory period The period after the firing of an impulse during which a cell may respond to a stimulus but the response will not be passed along or continued as another impulse. (p. 393)

Internodal pathways (Bachmann bundle) Special pathways in the atria that carry electrical impulses generated by the sinoatrial node. These impulses cause the heart to beat. (p. 393)

Relative refractory period The time after generation of an action potential during which a nerve fiber will show a (reduced) response only to a strong stimulus. (p. 393)

Resting membrane potential (RMP) The voltage that exists when the cell membranes of heart muscle (or other muscle or nerve cells) are at rest. (p. 391)

Sodium-potassium adenosine triphosphatase (ATPase) pump A mechanism for transporting sodium and potassium ions across the cell membrane against an opposing concentration gradient. Energy for this transport is obtained from the hydrolysis of adenosine triphosphate (ATP) by means of the enzyme ATPase. (p. 391)

Sudden cardiac death Unexpected, fatal cardiac arrest. (p. 402)

Threshold potential The critical state of electrical tension required for spontaneous depolarization of a cell membrane. (p. 393)

Torsades de pointes A rare ventricular arrhythmia that is associated with long QT interval and can degenerate into ventricular fibrillation and sudden death without medical intervention; often simply referred to as *torsades*. (p. 396)

Vaughan Williams classification The system most commonly used to classify antidysrhythmic drugs. (p. 396)

DYSRHYTHMIAS AND NORMAL CARDIAC ELECTROPHYSIOLOGY

A **dysrhythmia** is any deviation from the normal rhythm of the heart. The term **arrhythmia** (literally "no rhythm") implies asystole, or no heartbeat at all. Thus, the more accurate term for an irregular heart rhythm is *dysrhythmia*. However, *arrhythmia* is commonly used in clinical practice. Dysrhythmias can develop in association with many conditions, such as after a myocardial infarction (MI), cardiac surgery, or as the result of coronary artery disease. Dysrhythmias are usually serious and may require treatment with an antidysrhythmic drug or nonpharmacologic therapies; however, not all dysrhythmias require medical treatment.

Disturbances in cardiac rhythm are the result of abnormally functioning cardiac cells. Thus, an understanding of the mechanism responsible for dysrhythmias first requires review of the electrical properties of these cells. Figure 24-1 on p. 378 shows the overall anatomy of the conduction system of the heart. Figure 25-1 illustrates some of the properties of this system from the standpoint of a single cardiac cell. Inside a resting cardiac cell, a net negative charge exists relative to the outside of the cell. This difference in the electronegative charge exists in all types of cardiac cells and is referred to as the **resting membrane potential (RMP)**. The RMP results from an uneven distribution of ions (e.g., sodium, potassium, and calcium) across the cell membrane. This is known as *polarization*. Each ion moves through its own specific channel, which is a specialized protein molecule that sits across the cell membrane. These proteins work continuously to restore the specific intracellular and extracellular concentrations of each ion. At RMP, the ionic concentration gradient (distribution) is such that potassium ions are more highly concentrated intracellularly, whereas sodium and calcium ions are more highly concentrated extracellularly. For this reason, potassium is generally thought of as an intracellular ion, whereas sodium and calcium are generally thought of as extracellular ions. Negatively charged intracellular and extracellular ions such as chloride (Cl⁻) and bicarbonate (HCO₃⁻) also contribute to this uneven distribution of ions, which is known as a *polarized* state. This polarized distribution of ions is maintained by the **sodium-potassium adenosine triphosphatase (ATPase) pump**, an energy-requiring ionic pump.

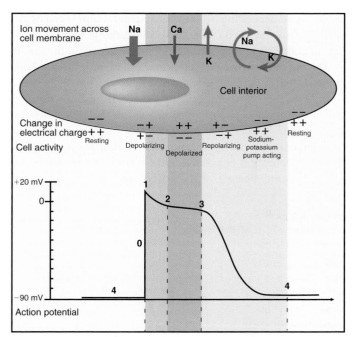

FIGURE 25-1 Phases of the action potential of a cardiac cell. In resting phase (4), the cell membrane is polarized. The cell's interior has a net negative charge, and the membrane is more permeable to potassium ions (K) than to sodium ions (Na). When the cell is stimulated and begins to depolarize (0), sodium ions enter the cell, potassium leaves the cell, calcium (Ca) channels open, and sodium channels close. In its depolarized phase (1), the cell's interior has a net positive charge. In the plateau phase (2), calcium and other positive ions enter the cell and potassium permeability declines, which lengthens the action potential. Then (3), calcium channels close and sodium is pulled from the cell by the sodium-potassium pump. The cell's interior then returns to its polarized, negatively charged state (4). (From Monahan FD: *Phipps' medical-surgical nursing: health and illness perspectives,* ed 8, St Louis, 2007, Mosby.)

The energy that drives this pump comes from molecules of adenosine triphosphate (ATP), which are a major source of energy in cellular metabolism.

Cardiac cells become excited when there is a change in the baseline distribution of ions across their membranes (RMP) that leads to the propagation of an electrical impulse. This change is known as an action potential. Action potentials occur in a continuous and regular manner in the cells of the cardiac conduction system, such as the sinoatrial node (SA), atrioventricular node (AV), and His-Purkinje system. All of these tissues have the property of spontaneous electrical excitability known as *automaticity*. This excited state creates action potentials, which in turn generate electrical impulses that travel through the myocardium ultimately to create the heartbeat via contraction of cardiac muscle fibers.

An action potential has five phases. Phase 0 is also called the *upstroke* because it appears as an upward line on the graph of an action potential, as shown in Figure 25-2, *A* and *B*. Both of these figures graphically illustrate the cycle of electrical changes that create an action potential. Note the variation in the shape of the curve depending on the relative conduction speed of the specific tissue involved (SA node versus Purkinje fiber). A faster rate of conduction corresponds to a steeper slope on the graph.

During phase 0, the resting cardiac cell membrane suddenly becomes highly permeable to sodium ions, which rush from the outside of the cell membrane to the inside (influx) through what are known as *fast channels* or *sodium channels*. This disruption of the earlier polarized state of the membrane is known as depolarization. Depolarization can be thought of as a temporary equalization of positive and negative charges across the cell membrane. Phase 1 of the action potential begins a rapid

process of repolarization that continues through phases 2 and 3 to phase 4, which is the RMP. In phase 1, the sodium channels close and the concentrations of each ion begin to move back toward their ion-specific RMP levels. During phase 2, calcium influx occurs through the slow channels or calcium channels. They are called *slow channels* because the calcium influx occurs relatively more slowly than the earlier sodium influx. Potassium ions then flow from inside of the cell to outside (efflux) through specific potassium channels. This is done to offset the elevated positive charge caused by the influx of sodium and calcium ions. In the case of the Purkinje fibers, this causes a partial plateau (flattening on the graph) during which the overall membrane potential changes only slightly, as seen in Figure 25-2, *B*. In phase 3, the ionic flow patterns of phases 0 to 2 are changed by the sodium-potassium ATPase pump (or, more simply, the *sodium pump*). This reestablishes the baseline polarized state by restoring both intracellular and extracellular concentrations of sodium, potassium, and calcium (see Figure 25-1). As a result, the cell membrane is ultimately repolarized to its baseline level or RMP (phase 4). Note that this entire process occurs over roughly 400 milliseconds—that is, four hundred thousandths (less than one half) of 1 second.

There is some variation in this time period between different parts of the conduction system. As an example, Figure 25-3 illustrates the pattern of movement of sodium, potassium, and calcium ions into and out of a Purkinje cell during the four

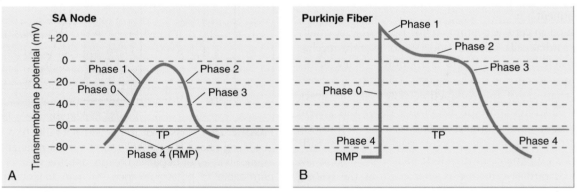

FIGURE 25-2 Action potentials. *RMP,* Resting membrane potential; *SA,* sinoatrial; *TP,* threshold potential.

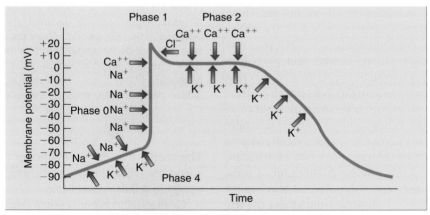

FIGURE 25-3 Purkinje fiber action potential.

phases of the action potential. Note that there are several differences in the action potentials of SA nodal cells and Purkinje cells. The level of the RMP for a given type of cell is an important determinant of the rate of its impulse conduction to other cells. The less negative (i.e., the closer to zero) the RMP at the onset of phase 0 of the action potential, the slower the upstroke velocity of phase 0. The slope of phase 0 is directly related to the impulse velocity. An upstroke with a steeper slope indicates faster conduction velocity. Thus, in Purkinje cells, electrical conduction is relatively fast, and therefore electrical impulses are conducted quickly. These cells are referred to as *fast-response cells,* or *fast-channel cells.* Purkinje fibers can therefore be thought of as fast-channel tissue. Many antidysrhythmic drugs affect the RMP and sodium channels, which in turn influences the rate of impulse conduction.

In contrast to Purkinje fibers, the cells of the SA node have a slower upstroke velocity, or a slower phase 0. This is illustrated in Figure 25-2, *A,* as an upstroke curve that is less steep, which indicates a relatively slower rate of electrical conduction in these cells.

AV nodal cells are comparable to SA nodal cells in this regard. This slower upstroke in the SA and AV nodes is primarily dependent on the entry of calcium ions through the slow channels or calcium channels. This means that nodal action potentials are affected by calcium influx as early as phase 0. The nodes are therefore called *slow-channel tissue,* and conduction is slower than that in other parts of the conduction system. Drugs that affect calcium ion movement into or out of these cells (e.g., calcium channel blockers) tend to have significant effects on the SA and AV nodal conduction rates.

The interval between phase 0 and phase 4 is called the **action potential duration** (Figure 25-4). The period between phase 0 and midway through phase 3 is called the absolute or **effective refractory period.** During the effective refractory period, the cardiac cell cannot be restimulated to depolarize and generate another action potential. During the remainder of phase 3 and until the return to the RMP (phase 4), the cardiac cell *can* be depolarized again if it receives a powerful enough impulse (such as one induced by drug therapy or supplied by an electrical pacemaker). This period is referred to as the **relative refractory period.** Figure 25-4 illustrates these various aspects of an action

potential. Again, the actual shape of the action potential curve varies in different parts of the conduction system.

The RMP of certain cardiac cells gradually decreases (becomes less negative) over time in ongoing cycles. This is due to small changes in the flux of sodium and potassium ions. Depolarization eventually occurs when a certain critical voltage is reached (**threshold potential**). This process of spontaneous depolarization is referred to as *automaticity,* or *pacemaker activity.* It is normal when it occurs in the SA node (see Figure 24-1 on p. 378). When spontaneous depolarizations occur elsewhere, however, dysrhythmias often result.

The SA node, the AV node, and His-Purkinje cells all possess the property of automaticity. The SA node is the natural pacemaker of the heart because it spontaneously depolarizes the most frequently. The SA node has an intrinsic rate of 60 to 100 depolarizations or beats per minute; that of the AV node is 40 to 60 beats per minute; and that of the ventricular Purkinje fibers is 40 or fewer beats per minute. The action potentials and other properties in different areas of the heart are compared in Table 25-1.

As the pacemaker of the heart, the SA node, which is located near the top of the right atrium, generates the electrical impulse that ultimately produces the heartbeat. First, however, this impulse travels through the atria via specialized pathways called the **internodal pathways** (**Bachmann bundle**). This causes the atrial myocardial fibers to contract, which creates the first heart sound. Next, the impulse reaches the AV node, which is located near the bottom of the right atrium. The AV node slows this very fast moving electrical impulse just long enough to allow the ventricles to fill with blood. If the AV node did not slow the impulse in this way, ventricular contraction would overlap that of the atria, which would result in a smaller volume of ejected ventricular blood and reduced cardiac output.

Next, the AV nodal cells generate an electrical impulse that passes into the bundle of His (or His bundle). The bundle of His is a band of cardiac muscle fibers located between the right and left ventricles in what is called the *ventricular septum* (wall between the ventricles). The bundle of His distributes the impulse into both ventricles via the right and left bundle branches. Each branch terminates in the Purkinje fibers that are located in the myocardium of the ventricles. Stimulation of the

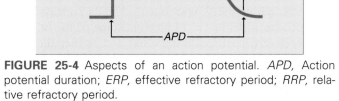

FIGURE 25-4 Aspects of an action potential. *APD,* Action potential duration; *ERP,* effective refractory period; *RRP,* relative refractory period.

			Threshold	**Conduction**
	Action	**Speed Of**	**Potential**	**Velocity**
Tissue	**Potential**	**Response**	**(mV)**	**(m/sec)**
SA node	⋀	Slow	260	Less than 0.05
Atrium	⋏	Fast	290	1
AV node	⋀	Slow	260	Less than 0.05
His-Purkinje system	⋏	Fast	295	3
Ventricle	⋏	Fast	290	1

TABLE 25-1   Comparison of Action Potentials in Different Cardiac Tissue

AV, Atrioventricular; *SA,* sinoatrial.

Purkinje fibers causes ventricular contraction and ejection of blood from the ventricles. Blood from the right ventricle is pumped into the pulmonary circulation, whereas blood from the left ventricle is pumped into the systemic circulation to supply the rest of the body. The bundle of His and Purkinje fibers are so named for the medical scientists who first identified them. Together, they are often referred to in the literature as the *His-Purkinje system.* Any abnormality in cardiac automaticity or impulse conduction often results in some type of dysrhythmia.

Electrocardiography

The electrophysiologic cardiac events described thus far in this chapter correspond more simply to the tracings of an electrocardiogram, abbreviated as ECG or EKG (Figure 25-5). The P wave corresponds to spontaneous impulse generation in the SA node followed immediately by depolarization of atrial myocardial fibers and their muscular contraction. This normally determines the heart rate. It is affected by the balance between sympathetic and parasympathetic nervous system tone, the intrinsic automaticity of the SA nodal tissue, the mechanical stretch of atrial fibers due to incoming blood volume, and cardiac drugs. The QRS complex (or QRS interval) corresponds to depolarization and contraction of ventricular fibers. The J point marks the start of the ST segment, which corresponds to the beginning of ventricular repolarization. The T wave corresponds to completion of the repolarization of these ventricular fibers. As an analogy, depolarization can be thought of as discharge or contraction of cardiac muscle fibers, whereas repolarization can be thought of as a relaxation of muscle fibers to prepare for the next contraction (heartbeat). Note that the repolarization of the atrial fibers is obscured on the ECG tracing by the QRS complex and thus has no corresponding deflection in the tracing. The U wave is not always present, and its physiologic basis is uncertain. When the U wave occurs, it is generally correlated with electrophysiologic events such as repolarization

of Purkinje fibers. These events may be a source of dysrhythmias caused by a triggered automaticity. Prominent U waves are often associated with sinus bradycardia, hypokalemia, use of quinidine and other class Ia antidysrhythmics, and hyperthyroidism. Abnormal U waves (inverted) are associated with serious conditions such as MI, acute angina, coronary artery spasms, and ischemic heart disease. The PR and QT intervals and the ST segment are parts of the ECG tracing that are often altered by disease or by the adverse effects of certain types of drug therapy or drug interactions, as discussed in later sections of this chapter.

Common Dysrhythmias

A variety of cardiac dysrhythmias are recognized. Some are easier to treat than others using drug therapy and/or interventional cardiology procedures such as pacemaker implantation, catheter ablation, cardioversion, and implantation of cardioverters-defibrillators. Dysrhythmias are subdivided into several broad categories depending on their anatomic site of origin in the heart. Supraventricular dysrhythmias originate above the ventricles in the SA or AV node or atrial myocardium. Ventricular dysrhythmias originate below the AV node in the His-Purkinje system or ventricular myocardium. Dysrhythmias that originate outside the conduction system (i.e., in atrial or ventricular cells) are known as *ectopic,* and their specific points of origin are called *ectopic foci* (*foci* is the plural of the Latin-derived word *focus*). Conduction blocks are dysrhythmias that involve disruption of impulse conduction between the atria and ventricles through the AV node, directly affecting ventricular function. They may also originate in the His-Purkinje system. Less commonly, impulse conduction between the SA and AV node is affected. Several of the most common dysrhythmias are described in Table 25-2, and corresponding ECG tracings are provided. They are also described further in the following text.

Atrial fibrillation is a common supraventricular dysrhythmia. It is characterized by rapid atrial contractions that incompletely pump blood into the ventricles. Atrial fibrillation is notable in that it predisposes the patient to stroke. This is due to the fact that the blood tends to stagnate in the incompletely emptied atria and is therefore more likely to clot. If such blood clots manage to make their way into the left ventricle, they may be embolized to the brain and cause a stroke. Patients with ongoing atrial fibrillation are often given aspirin or anticoagulant therapy to reduce the likelihood of stroke. The 2014 American College of Cardiology/American Heart Association guidelines downplay the use of aspirin and support the use of oral anticoagulants.

AV nodal reentrant tachycardia (AVNRT) is a conduction disorder that often gives rise to a dysrhythmia known as *paroxysmal supraventricular tachycardia (PSVT).* (The word *paroxysmal* means "sudden.") AVNRT occurs when electrical impulse transmission from the AV node into the His-Purkinje system of the ventricles is disrupted. As a result, some of the impulses circle backward (retrograde impulses) and reenter the atrial tissues to produce a tachycardic response. In Wolff-Parkinson-White syndrome, ectopic impulses that begin near the AV node actually bypass the AV node and reach the His-Purkinje system

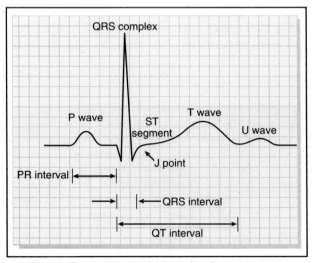

FIGURE 25-5 The waves and intervals of a normal electrocardiogram. (From Goldberger AL: *Clinical electrocardiography: a simplified approach,* ed 7, St Louis, 2006, Mosby.)

TABLE 25-2 Common Dysrhythmias

Dysrhythmia	Description and ECG Tracing
Atrial flutter (AF)	Often progresses to atrial fibrillation (F = flutter waves)
Atrial fibrillation (AF)	Rapid, ineffective atrial contractions (f = fibrillation waves)
Paroxysmal supraventricular tachycardia (PSVT)	Heart rate of 180-200 beats/min or higher
Premature ventricular contractions (PVCs)	Contractions generated by impulses arising from ectopic foci within ventricular myocardium
Nonsustained ventricular tachycardia (NSVT)	Relatively brief period (20 sec or less) in which ventricles contract rapidly on their own as well as in response to AV impulses
Sustained ventricular tachycardia (SVT)	Same as above but more prolonged

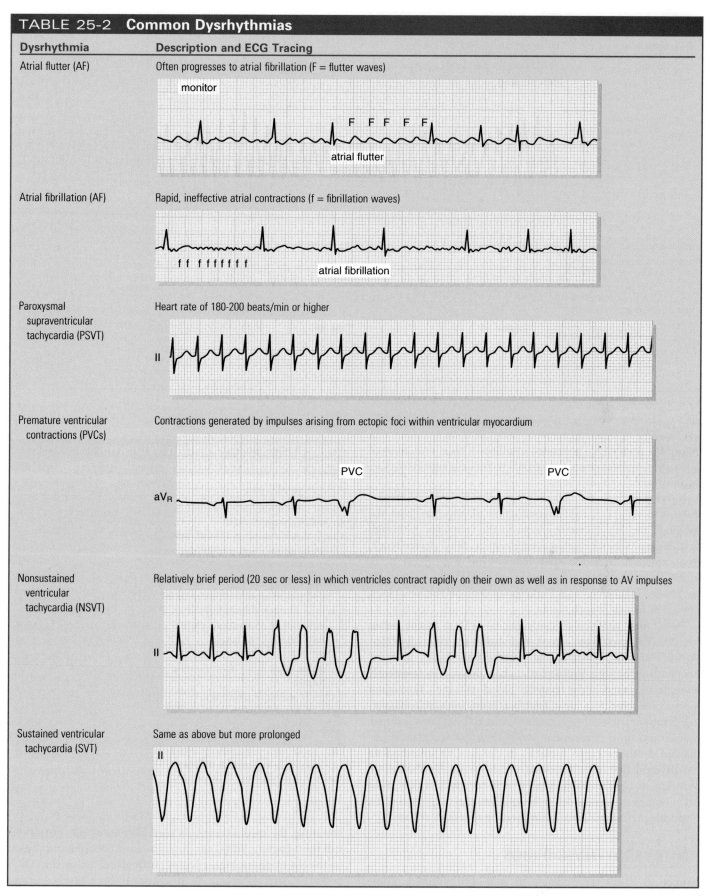

Continued

TABLE 25-2	Common Dysrhythmias—cont'd
Dysrhythmia	**Description and ECG Tracing**
Torsades de pointes (TdP)	Rapid ventricular tachycardia preceded by QT interval prolongation (often progresses to ventricular fibrillation) Monitor lead
Ventricular fibrillation (VF)	Rapid, ineffective ventricular contractions (fatal if not reversed)

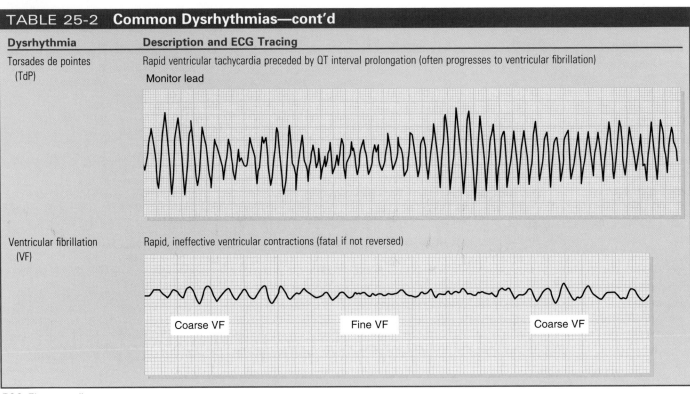

Coarse VF   Fine VF   Coarse VF

ECG, Electrocardiogram.

before the normal AV-generated impulses. This is one cause of ventricular tachycardia, although it is technically supraventricular in origin.

Varying degrees of AV block (often called *heart block*) involve different levels of disrupted conduction of impulses from the AV node and His-Purkinje system to the ventricles. Although first-degree AV block is often asymptomatic, third-degree block, or complete heart block, often requires use of a cardiac pacemaker to ensure adequate ventricular function. There can also be blocks within the His-Purkinje system of the ventricles, known as *bundle branch blocks.*

Premature ventricular contractions (PVCs) occur when impulses originate from ectopic foci within the ventricles (His-Purkinje system). PVCs probably occur periodically in many people; they become problematic when they occur frequently enough to compromise systolic blood volume. *Ventricular tachycardia* refers to a rapid heartbeat from impulses originating in the ventricles. It can be nonsustained (brief) or sustained, requiring definitive treatment. Worsening ventricular tachycardia can deteriorate into torsades de pointes, an intermediate dysrhythmia that often deteriorates into ventricular fibrillation. Ventricular fibrillation is fatal if not reversed, which most often requires electrical defibrillation. Torsades de pointes often responds preferentially to intravenous magnesium sulfate.

ANTIDYSRHYTHMIC DRUGS

Numerous drugs are available to treat dysrhythmias. These drugs are categorized according to where and how they affect cardiac cells. Although other classifications are described in the

TABLE 25-3 Vaughan Williams Classification of Antidysrhythmic Drugs	
Functional Class	**Drugs**
Class I: membrane-stabilizing drugs; fast sodium channel blockers	
Ia: ↑ blockade of sodium channel, delay repolarization, ↑ action potential duration	Quinidine, disopyramide, procainamide
Ib: ↑ blockade of sodium channel, accelerate repolarization, ± action potential duration	Lidocaine, phenytoin
Ic: ↑↑↑ blockade of sodium channel, ± repolarization; also suppress reentry	Flecainide, propafenone
Class II: beta-blocking drugs	All beta blockers
Class III: drugs whose principal effect on cardiac tissue is to ↑ action potential duration	Amiodarone, dronedarone, sotalol,* ibutilide, dofetilide
Class IV: calcium channel blockers	Verapamil, diltiazem
Other: antidysrhythmic drugs that have the properties of several classes and therefore cannot be placed in one particular class	Digoxin, adenosine

↑, Increase; ±, increase or decrease.
*Sotalol also has class II properties.

literature, the most commonly used system for this purpose is still the Vaughan Williams classification. This system is based on the electrophysiologic effect of particular drugs on the action potential. This approach identifies four major classes of drugs: I (including Ia, Ib, and Ic), II, III, and IV. The various drugs in these four classes are listed in Table 25-3.

TABLE 25-4 Antidysrhythmic Drugs: Mechanisms of Action

	VAUGHAN WILLIAMS CLASS			
	I	II	III	IV
Action	Blocks sodium channels, affects phase 0	Decreases spontaneous depolarization, affects phase 4	Prolongs action potential duration	Blocks slow calcium channels
Tissue	Fast	Slow	Fast	Slow
Effect on action potential				

There is currently a gradual trend away from the use of class Ia drugs. The formerly available class Ic drug encainide was removed from the market after research indicated a high risk for fatal cardiac dysrhythmias. The role of class II drugs (beta blockers) continues to grow in the field of cardiology, including in the management of dysrhythmias. Class III drugs have emerged as among the most widely used antidysrhythmics at this time. The class IV drugs (calcium channel blockers) have limited usefulness in treating tachydysrhythmias (dysrhythmias involving tachycardia), unlike most of the other classes. Digoxin, the cardiac glycoside discussed in Chapter 24, still has a place in dysrhythmia management, especially in the prevention of dangerous ventricular tachydysrhythmias secondary to atrial fibrillation.

Mechanism of Action and Drug Effects

Antidysrhythmic drugs work by correcting abnormal cardiac electrophysiologic function. Class I drugs are membrane-stabilizing drugs and exert their actions on the sodium (fast) channels. There are some slight differences in the actions of the drugs in this class, so they are divided into three subclasses. These subclasses are class Ia, Ib, and Ic drugs. The subclasses are based on the magnitude of the effects each drug has on phase 0, the action potential duration, and the effective refractory period. Class Ia drugs (quinidine, procainamide, and disopyramide) block the sodium channels; more specifically, they delay repolarization and increase the action potential duration. Class Ib drugs (phenytoin, lidocaine) also block the sodium channels, but unlike class Ia drugs, they accelerate repolarization and decrease the action potential duration. Phenytoin is more commonly used as an anticonvulsant (see Chapter 14) than as an antidysrhythmic drug. Class Ic drugs (flecainide, propafenone) have a more pronounced effect on the blockade of sodium channels but have little effect on repolarization or the action potential duration.

Class II drugs are the beta-adrenergic blockers (beta blockers; see Chapter 19), and they are commonly used as antihypertensives (see Chapter 22) and antianginal drugs (see Chapter 23). They work by blocking sympathetic nervous system stimulation to the heart and, as a result, the transmission of impulses in the heart's conduction system. This results in depression of phase 4 depolarization. These drugs mostly affect slower-conducting cardiac tissues.

Class III drugs (amiodarone, dronedarone, sotalol, ibutilide, and dofetilide) increase the action potential duration by prolonging repolarization in phase 3. They affect fast tissue and are most commonly used to manage dysrhythmias that are difficult to treat. They are usually reserved for patients for whom other therapies have failed. Sotalol actually has properties of both class II and class III drugs, and it may be listed as a member of either one or the other class, depending on the specific reference used.

Class IV drugs are the calcium channel blockers, which, like beta blockers, are also used as both antihypertensives (see Chapter 22) and antianginal drugs (see Chapter 23). As their name implies, they work specifically by inhibiting the calcium channels, which reduces the influx of calcium ions during action potentials. This results in depression of phase 4 depolarization. Diltiazem and verapamil are the calcium channel blockers most commonly used to treat cardiac dysrhythmias.

The mechanisms of action of the major classes of antidysrhythmics are summarized in Table 25-4. The effects of the various classes of antidysrhythmic drugs are presented in Box 25-1.

Indications

Antidysrhythmic drugs are effective in treating a variety of cardiac dysrhythmias. The antidysrhythmic drugs and the most common indications for their use are listed in Table 25-5.

Contraindications

As with all drugs, contraindications to the use of antidysrhythmic drugs include known drug allergy to a specific product. Other contraindications may include second- or third-degree AV block, bundle branch block, cardiogenic shock, sick sinus syndrome, and any other ECG changes depending on the clinical judgment of a cardiologist. The concurrent use of certain drugs that interact with antidysrhythmics must also considered. Antidysrhythmic drugs can potentially worsen existing dysrhythmias (also termed *dysrhythmogenic*). The risk is greater in patients with structural heart damage (e.g., after MI). In patients with AV block and bundle branch block, there is a danger of drug-induced ventricular failure if a drug further compromises the already existing AV conduction delays.

Adverse Effects

Adverse effects common to most antidysrhythmics include hypersensitivity reactions, nausea, vomiting, and diarrhea. Other common effects include dizziness, headache, and blurred vision. In addition, many antidysrhythmics are themselves

BOX 25-1 Effects of Antidysrhythmic Drugs

Class Ia (Disopyramide, Procainamide, Quinidine)
- Depress myocardial excitability
- Prolong the effective refractory period
- Eliminate or reduce ectopic foci stimulation
- Decrease inotropic effect
- Have anticholinergic (vagolytic) activity

Class Ib (Lidocaine, Phenytoin)
- Decrease myocardial excitability in the ventricles
- Eliminate or reduce ectopic foci stimulation in the ventricles
- Have minimal effect on the SA node and automaticity
- Have minimal effect on the AV node and conduction
- Have minimal anticholinergic (vagolytic) activity

Class Ic (Flecainide, Propafenone)
- Produce dose-related depression of cardiac conduction, especially in the bundle of His–Purkinje system
- Have minimal effect on atrial conduction
- Eliminate or reduce ectopic foci stimulation in the ventricles
- Have minimal anticholinergic (vagolytic) activity
- Flecainide use now reserved for the most serious dysrhythmias

Class II (Beta Blockers [e.g., Atenolol, Esmolol, Metoprolol])
- Block beta-adrenergic cardiac stimulation
- Reduce SA nodal activity
- Eliminate or reduce atrial ectopic foci stimulation
- Reduce ventricular contraction rate
- Reduce cardiac output and blood pressure

Class III (Amiodarone, Dronedarone, Sotalol,* Ibutilide, Dofetilide)
- Prolong the effective refractory period
- Prolong the myocardial action potential
- Block both alpha- and beta-adrenergic cardiac stimulation

Class IV (Diltiazem, Verapamil)
- Prolong AV nodal effective refractory period
- Reduce AV nodal conduction
- Reduce rapid ventricular conduction caused by atrial flutter

AV, Atrioventricular; *SA,* sinoatrial.
*Sotalol also has class II properties.

TABLE 25-5 Antidysrhythmic Drugs: Indications

Drug Class	Indications
Class Ia disopyramide procainamide quinidine	Atrial fibrillation, premature atrial contractions, premature ventricular contractions, ventricular tachycardia, Wolff-Parkinson-White syndrome
Class Ib lidocaine	Ventricular dysrhythmias only (premature ventricular contractions, ventricular tachycardia, ventricular fibrillation)
phenytoin	Atrial and ventricular tachydysrhythmias caused by digitalis toxicity, long QT syndrome
Class Ic flecainide propafenone	Ventricular tachycardia and supraventricular tachycardia dysrhythmias, atrial fibrillation and flutter, Wolff-Parkinson-White syndrome
Class II *Beta Blockers* atenolol esmolol metoprolol	Both supraventricular and ventricular dysrhythmias (act as general myocardial depressants)
Class III amiodarone dronedarone dofetilide ibutilide sotalol*	Life-threatening ventricular tachycardia or fibrillation Atrial fibrillation or flutter resistant to other drug therapy
Class IV *Calcium Channel Blockers* diltiazem verapamil	Paroxysmal supraventricular tachycardia; rate control for atrial fibrillation and flutter

*Sotalol also has class II properties.

capable of producing new dysrhythmias (prodysrhythmic effect). Prolongation of the QT interval is a potentially severe adverse effect shared by many antidysrhythmics. The concern with QT prolongation is the potential for induction of torsades de pointes. As with any drug class, there are also cases of unpredictable or idiosyncratic (see Chapter 2) adverse effects that are not related to drug concentration in the body. Table 25-6 summarizes the most commonly reported adverse effects by specific drug.

Toxicity and Management of Overdose

The main toxic effects of the antidysrhythmics involve the heart, circulation, and central nervous system (CNS). Specific antidotes are not available, and the management of an overdose involves maintaining adequate circulation and respiration using general support measures and providing any required symptomatic treatment.

Interactions

Antidysrhythmics can interact with many different categories of drugs. The most serious drug interactions are those that can result in dysrhythmias, hypotension or hypertension, respiratory distress, or excessive therapeutic or toxic drug effects. One particular interaction common to many antidysrhythmics is the potentiation of anticoagulant activity with warfarin (Coumadin) (see Chapter 26). Because many patients receiving antidysrhythmic therapy also need warfarin, the international normalized ratio (INR) must be closely monitored and necessary adjustments made to the warfarin dosage. This is especially true with amiodarone. The INR will increase by 50% in almost 100% of patients receiving amiodarone and warfarin. Grapefruit juice can also inhibit the metabolism of several antidysrhythmics such as amiodarone, disopyramide, and quinidine. Other common interactions are summarized in Table 25-7.

TABLE 25-6   Antidysrhythmic Drugs: Common Adverse Effects

Class	Drug	Adverse Effects
Ia	procainamide	Hypotension, rash, diarrhea, nausea, vomiting, agranulocytosis, SLE-like syndrome
	quinidine	Hypotension, QT prolongation, lightheadedness, diarrhea, bitter taste, anorexia, blurred vision, tinnitus, angina
Ib	lidocaine	Bradycardia, dysrhythmia, hypotension, anxiety, metallic taste
	phenytoin	Hypotension, bradycardia, thrombophlebitis, hypertrichosis, gingival hyperplasia
Ic	flecainide	Dizziness, visual disturbances, dyspnea, palpitations, nausea, vomiting, diarrhea, weakness
	propafenone	Prodysrhythmic effect, angina, tachycardia, syncope, AV block, dizziness, fatigue, dyspnea
II	Beta blockers	Bradycardia, hypotension, dizziness, fatigue, AV block, heart failure, wheezing, dry mouth, impotence, altered blood glucose levels
III	amiodarone	Pulmonary toxicity, thyroid disorders, bradycardia, hypotension, SA node dysfunction, AV block, ataxia, QT prolongation, torsades de pointes, vomiting, constipation, photosensitivity, abnormal liver function test results, jaundice, visual disturbances, hyperglycemia or hypoglycemia, dermatologic reactions including rash, toxic epidermal necrolysis, vasculitis, blue-gray coloring of the skin (face, arms, neck)
	dofetilide	Headache, insomnia, ventricular tachycardia, chest pain, torsades de pointes, rash, back pain, nausea, diarrhea
	ibutilide	Nonsustained ventricular tachycardia, ventricular extrasystoles, tachycardia, hypotension, AV block, headache, nausea
	sotalol*	Bradycardia, chest pain, palpitations, fatigue, dizziness, lightheadedness, weakness, dyspnea
	Calcium channel blockers	Constipation, bradycardia, heart block, hypotension, dizziness, dyspnea

AV, Atroventricular; SA, sinoatrial; SLE systemic lupus erythematosus.
*Sotalol also has class II properties.

TABLE 25-7   Selected Antidysrhythmic Drugs: Common Drug Interactions

Drug (Class)	Interacting Drugs	Effects*
quinidine (Ia)	Amiodarone, dronedarone, amitriptyline, erythromycin, haloperidol, sotalol, moxifloxacin	Additive QT prolongation
	Digoxin	Increase in digoxin levels by 50%
	HMG-CoA reductase inhibitors (statins)	Increased statin levels and toxicity
lidocaine (Ib)	Amiodarone, azole antifungals, beta blockers, erythromycin, verapamil, cimetidine, tolvaptan	Increased serum levels of lidocaine
propafenone (Ic)	Cimetidine, quinidine, conivaptan, pimozide	Increased propafenone levels; use is contraindicated
	Digoxin, warfarin, beta blockers	Increase in level of interacting drugs
	Class Ia and III antidysrhythmics, erythromycin	Prolonged QT interval
amiodarone (III)	Azole antifungals, clarithromycin, erythromycin, haloperidol, moxifloxacin, quinidine, procainamide	Prolonged QT interval
	Digoxin, diltiazem, verapamil, beta blockers	AV block
	Warfarin, digoxin	Increase in INR by 50% in almost 100% of patients, increase in digoxin levels by 50%
	Cyclosporine	Increased cyclosporine levels and toxicity
	HMG-CoA reductase inhibitors (statins)	Increased statin levels and toxicity
dofetilide (III)	Cimetidine, verapamil, hydrochlorothiazide (HCTZ), ketoconazole, trimethoprim	Increased dofetilide concentrations; use is contraindicated
	Bepridil, clarithromycin, erythromycin, tricyclic antidepressants, phenothiazines, moxifloxacin	Prolonged QT interval
sotalol (III)†	Calcium channel blockers	Additive effects on AV conduction, bradycardia
	Class I antidysrhythmics, erythromycin, bepridil, moxifloxacin, amiodarone	Prolonged QT interval, bradycardia
verapamil, diltiazem (IV)	Amiodarone, beta blockers, flecainide, digoxin	Bradycardia, decreased cardiac output, hypotension
	Azole antifungals, clarithromycin, erythromycin, isoniazid, HIV drugs	Increased verapamil effects
	HMG-CoA reductase inhibitors (statins)	Increased statin levels and toxicity

AV, Atrioventricular; HMG-CoA, hydroxymethylglutaryl-coenzyme A; INR, international normalized ratio.
*Note that enhanced activity of any antidysrhythmic drug may reach the level of drug toxicity, including potentially fatal cardiac dysrhythmias.
†Sotalol also has class II properties.

To explain the mechanism for each interaction is beyond the scope of this textbook. Readers needing more detailed information are encouraged to consult other appropriate references.

Dosages

For dosage information on selected antidysrhythmic drugs, see the table on this page.

DRUG PROFILES

The four classes of antidysrhythmics produce a variety of effects on the action potential of the cardiac cell and exert a major influence on cardiac electrophysiologic function. The diversity of therapeutic and adverse effects pose a special challenge to ensuring the safe and efficacious use of these drugs.

CLASS Ia DRUGS

Class Ia drugs are considered membrane-stabilizing drugs because they possess local anesthetic properties. They stabilize the membrane and have depressant effects on phase 0 of the action potential. These drugs include procainamide, quinidine, and disopyramide.

procainamide

The electrophysiologic effect of procainamide (Pronestyl) is similar to that of quinidine. Procainamide is useful in the management of atrial and ventricular tachydysrhythmias, although it is not used frequently. Procainamide is chemically related to the local anesthetic procaine. Significant adverse effects include ventricular dysrhythmias and blood disorders. It can cause a systemic lupus erythematosus–like syndrome, which occurs in about 30% of patients on long-term therapy.

It can also cause gastrointestinal effects such as nausea, vomiting, and diarrhea. Other adverse effects include fever, leukopenia, maculopapular rash, flushing, and torsades de pointes resulting from prolongation of the QT interval. Box 25-2 lists selected drugs known to prolong the QT interval. Use of procainamide is contraindicated in patients with a known hypersensitivity to it and in those with heart block and

DOSAGES

Selected Antidysrhythmic Drugs

Drug Name (Pregnancy Category)	Pharmacologic Class	Usual Adult Dosage Range
Class I		
◆ quinidine (Quinidex [sulfate], Quinaglute, Dura-Tab [gluconate]) (C)	Class Ia antidysrhythmic	Gluconate: PO: 324-648 mg every 8-12 hr Sulfate: PO: ER: 300-600 mg every 8-12 hr
◆ ! lidocaine (Xylocaine) (B)	Class Ib antidysrhythmic	IV: Bolus dose 1-1.5 mg/kg every 3-5 minutes; may repeat until effect; max dose 300 mg total bolus in 1 hr
propafenone (Rythmol) (C)	Class Ic antidysrhythmic	PO: ER: 225-425 mg every 12 hr
Class II		
! esmolol (Brevibloc) (D)	Beta$_1$ blocker (class II antidysrhythmic)	IV: 500 mcg/kg loading dose over 1 min; follow with 50 mcg/kg/min
Class III		
◆ ! amiodarone (Cordarone) (D)	Class III antidysrhythmic	IV: 150 mg over 10 min, then 360 mg over 6 hr, then 540 mg over 18 hr, then decrease to 0.5 mg/min PO: Usual maintenance dose 200-600 mg/day
◆ dofetilide (Tikosyn) (C)	Class III antidysrhythmic	PO: 125-500 mcg bid (note dose is individualized)
ibutilide (Corvert) (C)	Class III antidysrhythmic	IV: 1-mg infusion over 10 min (if less than 60 kg, then 0.1 mg/kg)
◆ sotalol* (Betapace) (B)	Class III antidysrhythmic	PO: 80-160 mg bid
Class IV		
◆ diltiazem (Cardizem)	Calcium channel blocker (class IV antidysrhythmic)	IV: Bolus dose 0.25 mg/kg over 2 min; second dose 0.35 mg/kg over 2 min after 15 min as needed, then 5-15 mg/hr by infusion for up to 24 hr Oral: 120-480 mg/day depending on form used
◆ verapamil (Calan, Isoptin, Verelan) (C)	Calcium channel blocker (class IV antidysrhythmic)	PO: 240-480 mg/day in divided doses IV: 2.5-10 mg bolus over 2 min; repeat dose of 5-10 mg
Unclassified		
adenosine (Adenocard) (C)	Unclassified antidysrhythmic	IV: 6-mg bolus over 1-2 sec; second rapid bolus of 12 mg as needed, which may be repeated a second time as needed

*Sotalol also has class II properties.

BOX 25-2　Selected Drugs That Prolong the QT Interval*

Antidysrhythmics: amiodarone, procainamide, quinidine, dofetilide, bepridil, sotalol, flecainide

Antibiotics: azithromycin, clarithromycin, erythromycin, levofloxacin, moxifloxacin, telithromycin

Anticancer: tamoxifen, sunitinib

Antifungals: fluconazole, itraconazole, ketoconazole, voriconazole

Antidepressants: amitriptyline, imipramine, fluvoxamine, nefazodone, doxepin, imipramine, sertraline, venlafaxine, citalopram, amoxapine, nortriptyline, trimipramine

Antinausea: dolasetron, droperidol, ondansetron, granisetron

Antipsychotics: haldoperidol, pimozide, thioridazine, chlorpromazine, risperidone, clozapine, quetiapine

Bronchodilators: albuterol, levalbuterol, salmeterol, ephedrine, metaproterenol, terbutaline

Calcium channel blockers: diltiazem, verapamil

Miscellaneous: cocaine, foscarnet, galantamine, indapamide, lithium, midodrine, tacrolimus, tolterodine, amantadine, felbmate, fosphenytoin, methadone, octreotide, solifenacin, vardenafil, tizanidine

Protease Inhibitors: indinavir, saquinavir, nelfinavir, ritonavir

*This list is not all-inclusive; rather, only selected agents are listed. Further information can be found at *www.qtdrugs.org*.

systemic lupus erythematosus. It is available in both oral and injectable forms.

Pharmacokinetics: Procainamide

Route	Onset of Action	Peak Plasma Concentration	Elimination Half-life	Duration of Action
IV/IM	10-30 min	10-60 min	3 hr	3 hr
PO	0.5-1 hr	1-2 hr	3 hr	3-8 hr

♦ quinidine

Quinidine (Quinidex) has both a direct action on the electrical activity of the heart and an indirect (anticholinergic) effect. Significant QT adverse effects of the drug include cardiac asystole and ventricular ectopic beats. Quinidine can cause cinchonism. Symptoms of mild cinchonism include tinnitus, loss of hearing, slight blurring of vision, and gastrointestinal upset. Contraindications to the use of the drug include hypersensitivity, thrombocytopenic purpura resulting from previous therapy, AV block, intraventricular conduction defects, and torsades de pointes. Quinidine is available in both oral and parenteral (injectable) forms and in three different salt forms. The oral preparations include sulfate and gluconate salts.

Pharmacokinetics: Quinidine

Route	Onset of Action	Peak Plasma Concentration	Elimination Half-life	Duration of Action
PO	1-3 hr	0.5-6 hr	6-7 hr	6-12 hr

CLASS Ib DRUGS

Class Ib drugs share many characteristics with class Ia drugs but act preferentially on ischemic myocardial tissue. They have little effect on conduction velocity in normal tissue. Class Ib drugs have a weak depressive effect on phase 0 depolarization, the action potential duration, and the effective refractory period. They include lidocaine and phenytoin.

♦ ! lidocaine

Lidocaine (Xylocaine) is the prototypical Ib drug. It is effective for the treatment of ventricular dysrhythmias, but it can only be administered intravenously because it has an extensive first-pass effect (i.e., when it is taken orally, the liver metabolizes most of it to inactive metabolites). Because of its extensive hepatic metabolism, dosage reduction by 50% is recommended for patients with liver failure or cirrhosis. Dosage reductions may also be necessary in patients with renal impairment because of extensive excretion of the drug and its metabolites by the kidney.

Lidocaine exerts its effects on the conduction system of the heart by making it difficult for the ventricles to develop a dysrhythmia. This action is known as *raising the ventricular fibrillation threshold*. It occurs by decreasing the sensitivity of the cardiac cell membrane to impulses and decreasing the cell's ability to depolarize on its own (decreasing automaticity). Many of these effects are accomplished by blocking the fast sodium channels.

Significant adverse effects include CNS toxic effects such as twitching, convulsions, and confusion; respiratory depression or arrest; and the cardiovascular effects of hypotension, bradycardia, and dysrhythmias. Use of the drug is contraindicated in patients who are hypersensitive to it, who have severe SA or AV intraventricular block, or who have Stokes-Adams or Wolff-Parkinson-White syndrome. Lidocaine is available only in parenteral form for intramuscular or intravenous administration. Lidocaine is commonly used as a local anesthetic (see Chapter 11); a transdermal form is also available for analgesia (see Chapter 10).

Pharmacokinetics: Lidocaine

Route	Onset of Action	Peak Plasma Concentration	Elimination Half-life	Duration of Action
IV	2-15 min	5-10 min	8 min	20 min-1.5 hr

CLASS Ic DRUGS

Class Ic drugs (flecainide, propafenone) produce a more pronounced blockade of the sodium channel than class Ia and Ib drugs but have little effect on repolarization or the action potential duration. These drugs significantly slow conduction in the atria, AV node, and ventricles. Because of their marked effect on conduction, class Ic drugs strongly suppress PVCs, reducing or eliminating them in a large number of patients.

flecainide

Flecainide (Tambocor) is a chemical analogue of procainamide. Historically, health care professionals have been hesitant to prescribe flecainide because of the findings of a large multicenter study called the Cardiac Arrhythmia Suppression Trial (CAST). This study showed that mortality and nonfatal cardiac arrest rates in patients treated with flecainide were actually comparable to or higher than those seen in patients who received the placebo. Because of these findings, the U.S. Food and Drug Administration (FDA) required that the labeling of flecainide be revised to indicate that its use is to be limited to the treatment of documented life-threatening ventricular dysrhythmias. However, since the findings of the CAST were initially published in 1992, there have been numerous studies showing that flecainide is safe and effective for the treatment of atrial fibrillation. In fact, according to the most current practice guidelines, flecainide is considered a first-line drug in the treatment of atrial fibrillation.

Flecainide is better tolerated than quinidine or procainamide. It has a negative inotropic effect and depresses left ventricular function. Less serious but more common noncardiac adverse effects include dizziness, visual disturbances, and dyspnea. Contraindications to its use include hypersensitivity, cardiogenic shock, second- or third-degree AV block, and non–life-threatening dysrhythmias. Flecainide is available only for oral use.

Pharmacokinetics: Flecainide

Route	Onset of Action	Peak Plasma Concentration	Elimination Half-life	Duration of Action
PO	3 hr	1.5-3 hr	11-12 hr	12-27 hr

propafenone

Propafenone (Rythmol) is similar in action to flecainide. It reduces the fast inward sodium current in Purkinje fibers and to a lesser extent in myocardial fibers. Unlike other class I drugs, propafenone has mild beta-blocking effects. This may contribute to its overall effects on the conduction system. It is also believed to have calcium channel–blocking effects, which may contribute to its mild negative inotropic effects.

Until recently, propafenone's use was limited to the treatment of documented life-threatening ventricular dysrhythmias, as was flecainide. Recent findings suggest that it has benefit in the treatment of atrial fibrillation as well. Treatment is started while the patient is in the hospital. Unlike flecainide, however, propafenone can be given to patients with depressed left ventricular function and may be a better drug than disopyramide, procainamide, and quinidine in these patients. Propafenone must be used with caution in patients with heart failure, because it has some beta-blocking properties and dose-dependent negative inotropic effects.

Propafenone is generally well tolerated. The most commonly reported adverse reaction is dizziness. Patients may also complain of a metallic taste, constipation, and headache, along with nausea and vomiting. These gastrointestinal adverse effects may be reduced by taking propafenone with food. Propafenone use is contraindicated in patients with a known hypersensitivity to it and in those with bradycardia, bronchial asthma, significant hypotension, uncontrolled heart failure, cardiogenic shock, and various conduction disorders. It is available only for oral use.

Pharmacokinetics: Propafenone

Route	Onset of Action	Peak Plasma Concentration	Elimination Half-life	Duration of Action
PO	2 hr	3-5 hr	2-10 hr	Unknown

CLASS II DRUGS

Class II antidysrhythmics are also known as beta blockers (see Chapter 19). They work by blocking sympathetic nervous system stimulation to the heart and the heart's conduction system. By doing this, beta blockers prevent catecholamine-mediated actions on the heart. This is known as a *cardioprotective* quality of beta blockers. The resulting cardiovascular effects include a reduced heart rate, delayed AV node conduction, reduced myocardial contractility, and decreased myocardial automaticity. The pharmacologic effects of the beta blockers are especially beneficial after an MI. Following an MI, many catecholamines are released that make the heart hyperirritable and predisposed to many types of dysrhythmias. Beta blockers offer protection from these potentially very dangerous complications. Several studies have demonstrated a significant reduction (on the average of 25%) in the incidence of sudden cardiac death after MI in patients treated with beta blockers on an ongoing basis.

Although there are several beta blockers, only a few are commonly used as antidysrhythmics. Those currently approved by the FDA for this purpose are acebutolol, esmolol, propranolol, and sotalol (which has both class II and class III properties); however, other beta blockers are commony used. Selected drugs are described here. The class II drugs are classified as pregnancy category C drugs, excepting acebutolol, pindolol, and sotalol, which are all category B drugs.

◆atenolol

Atenolol (Tenormin) is a cardioselective beta blocker, which means that it preferentially blocks the beta$_1$-adrenergic receptors that are located primarily in the heart. Noncardioselective beta blockers block not only the beta$_1$-adrenergic receptors in the heart but also the beta$_2$-adrenergic receptors in the lungs and therefore can exacerbate preexisting asthma or chronic obstructive pulmonary disease. In addition to having class II antidysrhythmic properties, atenolol is useful in the treatment of hypertension and angina. Its use is contraindicated in patients with severe bradycardia, second- or third-degree heart block, heart failure, cardiogenic shock, or a known hypersensitivity to it. This drug is available in oral form.

Pharmacokinetics: Atenolol

Route	Onset of Action	Peak Plasma Concentration	Elimination Half-life	Duration of Action
PO	1 hr	2-4 hr	6-7 hr	24 hr

!esmolol

Esmolol (Brevibloc) is an ultra–short-acting beta blocker with pharmacologic and electrophysiologic effects on the heart's conduction system similar to those of atenolol. Esmolol is also a cardioselective beta blocker that preferentially blocks the beta$_1$-adrenergic receptors in the heart. It is used in the acute treatment of supraventricular tachydysrhythmias or dysrhythmias that originate above the ventricles. It is also used to control hypertension and tachydysrhythmias that develop after an acute MI. Use of esmolol is contraindicated in patients with a known hypersensitivity to it or those with severe bradycardia, second- or third-degree heart block, heart failure, cardiogenic shock, or severe asthma. It is available only in injectable form and is most commonly used in anesthesia.

Pharmacokinetics: Esmolol

Route	Onset of Action	Peak Plasma Concentration	Elimination Half-life	Duration of Action
IV	Immediate	6 min	9 min	15-20 min

◆ metoprolol

Metoprolol (Lopressor) is another cardioselective beta blocker commonly given after an MI to reduce the risk for sudden cardiac death. It is also used in the treatment of hypertension and angina. The contraindications to metoprolol use are the same as those for the use of atenolol and esmolol. It is available in both oral and injectable forms.

Pharmacokinetics: Metoprolol

Route	Onset of Action	Peak Plasma Concentration	Elimination Half-life	Duration of Action
IV	1 min	20 min	3-8 hr	5-8 hr
PO	1 hr	2-4 hr	3-8 hr	10-20 hr

CLASS III DRUGS

Class III drugs consist of amiodarone, dronedarone, sotalol (which also has class II properties), ibutilide, and dofetilide. Amiodarone controls dysrhythmias by inhibiting repolarization and markedly prolonging refractoriness and the action potential duration. Ibutilide and dofetilide are both indicated for conversion of atrial fibrillation or flutter to a normal sinus rhythm. Amiodarone is indicated for the management of life-threatening ventricular tachycardia or ventricular fibrillation that is resistant to other drug therapy. This drug has also been very effective in the treatment of sustained ventricular tachycardias. Amiodarone has recently been used more frequently to treat atrial dysrhythmias as well.

Dronedarone (Multaq) is the newest antidysrhythmic drug. It is very similar to amiodarone and is thought to have less potential for causing the classic amiodarone adverse effects and less potential for drug interactions. However, as with any newly marketed drug, the true incidence of toxicity is not known until it is used in numerous patients. In 2011, the FDA issued an advisory regarding the potential for hepatotoxicity related to dronedarone. Later that year, they also issued a safety communication regarding an increased risk for death and serious cardiovascular events associated with its use.

◆!amiodarone

Amiodarone (Cordarone, Pacerone) markedly prolongs the action potential duration and the effective refractory period in all cardiac tissues. Besides exerting these dramatic effects, it is also known to block both the alpha- and beta-adrenergic receptors of the sympathetic nervous system. Clinically it is one of the most effective antidysrhythmic drugs for controlling supraventricular and ventricular dysrhythmias. It is indicated for the management of sustained ventricular tachycardia, ventricular fibrillation, and nonsustained ventricular tachycardia. It is reported to be effective in 40% to 60% of all patients with ventricular tachycardia. It is the drug of choice for ventricular dysrhythmias according to the Advanced Cardiac Life Support guidelines. Recently it has shown promise in the management of atrial dysrhythmias that are difficult to treat with other less toxic drugs.

Amiodarone has many unwanted adverse effects, and these can be attributed to its chemical properties. Amiodarone is very *lipophilic,* or fat loving. Therefore, it can penetrate and concentrate in the adipose tissue of any organ in the body. It also has iodine in its chemical structure. One organ that sequesters iodine from the diet is the thyroid gland. As a result, amiodarone can cause either hypothyroidism or hyperthyroidism. The package insert for amiodarone lists iodine allergy as a contraindication. However, evidence for avoiding amiodarone in patients with iodine hypersensitivity is extremely limited and does not appear to support its contraindication in patients with severe dysrhythmias.

Adverse reactions occur in approximately 75% of patients treated with this drug, but the incidence is higher and the severity greater with higher dosages (those exceeding 400 mg/day) and prolonged therapy. One of the most common adverse effects is corneal microdeposits, which may cause visual halos, photophobia, and dry eyes. This occurs in virtually all adults who take the drug for longer than 6 months. Photosensitivity is also very common, reported in 10% to 75% of patients taking amiodarone.

The most serious adverse effect is pulmonary toxicity, which is fatal in about 10% of patients and involves a clinical syndrome of progressive dyspnea and cough accompanied by damage to the alveoli. The result can be pulmonary fibrosis. Another serious complication of amiodarone therapy is that it not only may treat the dysrhythmias but also may provoke them.

Amiodarone has an exceptionally long half-life, approaching many days. As a result, the therapeutic as well as any adverse effects of amiodarone may linger long after the drug has been discontinued. In fact, it may take as long as 2 to 3 months after the drug has been stopped for some adverse effects to subside. Therapy is usually started in the hospital and is closely monitored until the patient's serum levels are within a therapeutic range.

Amiodarone has two very significant drug interactions, namely with digoxin and warfarin. It is reported that digoxin levels will increase by 50% and that the INR will increase by 50% in 100% of patients taking these drugs in combination with amiodarone. When amiodarone is started in patients who

TABLE 25-8 Recommendations for Oral Dosage After Intravenous Infusion of Amiodarone

Duration of Amiodarone IV Infusion	Initial Daily Dose of Oral Amiodarone
Less than 1 wk	800-1600 mg
1-3 wk	600-800 mg
More than 3 wk	400 mg

are already taking one of these drugs, the dose of digoxin or warfarin is recommended to be reduced by 50% at the start of amiodarone therapy.

Use of amiodarone is contraindicated in patients who have a known hypersensitivity to it and in those with severe sinus bradycardia or second- or third-degree heart block. For cases in which the patient is maintained on long-term oral amiodarone therapy after intravenous amiodarone administration is discontinued, recommended conversions are available (Table 25-8). This drug is marketed in both oral and injectable forms.

Pharmacokinetics: Amiodarone

Route	Onset of Action	Peak Plasma Concentration	Elimination Half-life	Duration of Action
PO	1-3 wk	2-10 hr	15-100 days	10-150 days

ibutilide

Ibutilide (Corvert) is a class III antidysrhythmic drug. Unlike the other two class III antidysrhythmics, ibutilide is indicated for atrial dysrhythmias. Atrial fibrillation and atrial flutter cause irregular contractions of the heart and can lead to serious conditions such as decreased cardiac output, heart failure, low blood pressure, and stroke. Although other pharmacologic therapies are used to treat atrial fibrillation and flutter, ibutilide and dofetilide are the only drugs available for rapid conversion of these two conditions to normal sinus rhythm. The only other treatment that can produce rapid conversion is electrical cardioversion. Although it is effective, electrical cardioversion carries the risk, expense, and inconvenience of both the procedure itself and the anesthesia it requires.

Ibutilide is dosed based on patient weight. Use of ibutilide is contraindicated in patients who have previously demonstrated hypersensitivity to it. As with other antidysrhythmic drugs, ibutilide is to be used with caution, because it can itself produce dysrhythmias, most significantly ventricular tachycardia and torsades de pointes. Class Ia antidysrhythmic drugs (e.g., disopyramide, quinidine, and procainamide) and other class III drugs (e.g., amiodarone and sotalol) are not to be administered with ibutilide, nor are they to be given within 4 hours after infusion of ibutilide because of their potential to prolong refractoriness. Ibutilide is available only in injectable form.

Pharmacokinetics: Ibutilide

Route	Onset of Action	Peak Plasma Concentration	Elimination Half-life	Duration of Action
IV	10 min	30 min	6 hr	4 hr

♦ dofetilide

Dofetilide (Tikosyn) is one of the newer antidysrhythmic drugs. Because dofetilide can cause serious toxicity, specifically torsades de pointes, only physicians who have received special training are allowed to prescribe it. Dofetilide therapy must be initiated in the hospital, and the patient must have continuous ECG monitoring for the first 3 days. Any dosage adjustment or re-initiation of therapy also requires hospitalization.

Dofetilide is contraindicated in patients with a known hypersensitivity to it, as well as patients with congenital or acquired long QT intervals or in whom the QT interval is longer than 440 msec. It is also contraindicated in patients with severe renal impairment and in those taking the following drugs: verapamil, cimetidine, hydrochlorothiazide, trimethoprim, itraconazole, ketoconazole, prochlorperazine, and megestrol. Other drugs that can prolong the QT interval must be used with great caution during dofetilide therapy. Dofetilide is also contraindicated in patients with hypokalemia and/or hypomagnesemia, because these two states predispose patients to toxicity.

The most common adverse effects are torsades de pointes, supraventricular dysrhythmias, headache, dizziness, and chest pain.

Pharmacokinetics: Dofetilide

Route	Onset of Action	Peak Plasma Concentration	Elimination Half-life	Duration of Action
PO	1 hr	2-3 hr	10 hr	12 hr

♦ sotalol

Sotalol (Betapace) is a selective beta blocker that is used to treat dysrhythmias. It is unique in that it possesses antidysrhythmic properties similar to those of the class III drugs (such as amiodarone) while simultaneously exerting beta blocker or class II effects on the conduction system of the heart. In addition, sotalol has prodysrhythmic properties similar to those of the class Ic drugs. This means that while patients are taking sotalol, it can cause serious dysrhythmias such as torsades de pointes or a new ventricular tachycardia or fibrillation. Like flecainide and propafenone, sotalol was historically reserved for the treatment of documented life-threatening ventricular dysrhythmias such as sustained ventricular tachycardia. However, recent data indicate it to be safe.

Contraindications to sotalol use include a known hypersensitivity to it, bronchial asthma, cardiogenic shock, and sinus bradycardia. Sotalol is available only in oral form.

Pharmacokinetics: Sotalol

Route	Onset of Action	Peak Plasma Concentration	Elimination Half-life	Duration of Action
PO	1-2 hr	2.5-4 hr	12 hr	8-16 hr

CLASS IV DRUGS

Class IV antidysrhythmic drugs are calcium channel blockers. Although more than nine such drugs are currently available, only a few are commonly used as antidysrhythmics. Besides being effective antidysrhythmics, calcium channel blockers are useful in the treatment of hypertension (see Chapter 22) and angina (see Chapter 23). Verapamil and diltiazem are the two calcium channel blockers most commonly used for treating dysrhythmias, specifically those that arise above the ventricles (PSVT) and for controlling the ventricular response to atrial fibrillation and flutter by slowing conduction and prolonging refractoriness of the AV node (i.e., preventing the ventricles from beating as fast as the atria).

These drugs block the slow inward flow of calcium ions into the slow (calcium) channels in cardiac conduction tissue. The conduction effects of these drugs are limited to the atria and the AV node, where conduction is prolonged and the tissues are made more refractory to stimulation. These drugs have little effect on the ventricular tissues.

♦ diltiazem

Diltiazem (Cardizem, others) is primarily indicated for the temporary control of a rapid ventricular response in patients with atrial fibrillation or flutter and PSVT. Its use is contraindicated in patients with a known hypersensitivity, acute MI, pulmonary congestion, Wolff-Parkinson-White syndrome, severe hypotension, cardiogenic shock, sick sinus syndrome, or second- or third-degree AV block. Diltiazem is available in both oral and parenteral forms.

Pharmacokinetics: Diltiazem

Route	Onset of Action	Peak Plasma Concentration	Elimination Half-life	Duration of Action
PO	0.5-1 hr	2-3 hr	3.5-9 hr	4-12 hr

♦ verapamil

Verapamil (Calan, others) has actions similar to those of diltiazem in that it also inhibits calcium ion influx across the slow calcium channels in cardiac conduction tissue. This results in dramatic effects on the AV node. Verapamil is used to prevent and convert recurrent PSVT and to control ventricular response in atrial flutter or fibrillation. It can also temporarily control a rapid ventricular response to these frequent atrial stimulations, usually decreasing the heart rate by at least 20%. Verapamil is not only used for the management of various dysrhythmias but is also used to treat angina, hypertension, and hypertrophic cardiomyopathy. The contraindications that apply to diltiazem apply to verapamil as well. It is also available in both oral and parenteral forms.

Pharmacokinetics: Verapamil

Route	Onset of Action	Peak Plasma Concentration	Elimination Half-life	Duration of Action
PO	1-2 hr	3 hr	4.5-12 hr	6-8 hr

UNCLASSIFIED ANTIDYSRHYTHMIC
adenosine

Adenosine (Adenocard) is an unclassified antidysrhythmic drug. It slows the electrical conduction time through the AV node and is indicated for the conversion of PSVT to sinus rhythm. It is particularly useful when the PSVT has failed to respond to verapamil or when the patient has coexisting conditions such as heart failure, hypotension, or left ventricular dysfunction that limit the use of verapamil. Its use is contraindicated in patients with second- or third-degree heart block, sick sinus syndrome, atrial flutter or fibrillation, or ventricular tachycardia, as well as in those with a known hypersensitivity to it. It has an extremely short half-life of less than 10 seconds. For this reason, it is administered only intravenously and only as a fast intravenous push. It commonly causes asystole for a period of seconds. All other adverse effects are minimal because of its very short duration of action. Adenosine is available only in parenteral form.

Pharmacokinetics: Adenosine

Route	Onset of Action	Peak Plasma Concentration	Elimination Half-life	Duration of Action
IV	Immediate	Immediate	Less than 10 sec	Very brief

⚡ SAFETY AND QUALITY IMPROVEMENT: PREVENTING MEDICATION ERRORS   `QSEN`

Look-Alike/Sound-Alike Drugs: Cardene and Cardizem

The Institute for Safe Medication Practices (ISMP) has received reports of mixups between Cardizem (a trade name for diltiazem) and Cardene (a trade name for nicardipine). Both of these drugs are calcium channel blockers and are used for hypertension and angina. Intravenous diltiazem is also used for treatment of atrial fibrillation/flutter and paroxysmal supraventricular tachycardia. In one reported case, a nurse prepared and administered a Cardene infusion when Cardizem was ordered; in another case, the nurse hung the correct drug on the smart pump (Cardene) but programmed the pump to infuse Cardizem. The patient received the correct drug but it did not infuse at the correct rate. It is essential follow the Nine Rights and ensure that the correct drug is infusing at the correct dose.

For more information, see the ISMP Quarterly Action Agenda (October to December 2013). Available at *www.ismp.org*.

█ NURSING PROCESS

█ ASSESSMENT

Before administering any *antidysrhythmic* to a patient, perform a thorough nursing assessment with a head-to-toe physical assessment, complete medical history, and medication profile. Assess for contraindications, cautions, and drug interactions. Assess and record the patient's gender and race-ethnicity (see the Evidence-Based Practice box on p. 407). Review any baseline ECGs, and interpret the results while also measuring vital signs with attention to blood pressure, postural blood pressures, as well as heart sounds and pulse rate, rhythm, and quality. Assess for signs and symptoms associated with decreased cardiac functioning (as a result of a dysrhythmia and decrease in cardiac output) such as apical-radial pulse deficits, jugular neck vein distension, edema, prolonged capillary refill (longer than 5 seconds), decreased urinary output, activity intolerance, chest pain or pressure, dyspnea, and fatigue. Document baseline and any changes in level of alertness, increase in anxiety levels, and/or restlessness, which may indicate hypoxia. Laboratory studies that are usually prescribed include hepatic (AST/ALT levels) and renal (BUN, creatinine levels) function tests. Abnormal hepatic and renal function indicate the possibility of a decreased ability to metabolize and excrete the drugs, leading to adverse effects and possible toxicity. With altered functioning, the prescriber may need to decrease the dosage of medication to prevent toxicity.

Assess for drug interactions with *antidysrhythmics* (see Table 25-7). Additionally, assess for other possible interactions such as with grapefruit juice. Grapefruit juice inhibits metabolism by cytochrome P-450 3A4 hepatic enzymes (see Chapter 2 for a more in-depth discussion of this topic). The interaction of grapefruit juice with *amiodarone, disopyramide,* and *quinidine* leads to an increased risk for toxicity and cinchonism (see Table 25-7).

With the use of *lidocaine,* assess the cardiovascular system, with attention to heart rate and blood pressure. With amiodarone, assess for respiratory, thyroid, hepatic, dermatologic, and/or hypertensive conditions due to possible drug-related pulmonary toxicity, exacerbation of thyroid disorders, abnormal liver function tests, and rash. Assess for drug interactions (see Table 25-7) as well as contraindications and cautions.

QSEN TEAMWORK AND COLLABORATION: PHARMACOKINETIC BRIDGE TO NURSING PRACTICE

A study of long-term oral amiodarone therapy for the treatment of dysrhythmias provides a different perspective on pharmacokinetics. To aid in evaluating the complex pharmacokinetic properties of amiodarone and developing an optimal dosing schedule for the drug in long-term oral drug therapy, serum concentrations of the drug and its metabolite, desethylamiodarone, were monitored in 345 Japanese patients receiving amiodarone. Serum concentrations of the drug and its metabolite were determined by an analysis called *chromatography.* In 245 participants who took fixed maintenance dosages of the drug for 6 months, there were small variations in the ratio of the serum level of the actual drug to the serum level of its metabolite. (The concept of metabolism as it relates to pharmacokinetics is discussed in Chapter 2.) Other pharmacokinetic properties of amiodarone included a slightly higher average clearance in women than in men, even though there were no differences between men and women with regard to age, dosage, or duration of action of the dose. Japanese patients showed little variation in the pharmacokinetics of the drug. From this study, one can see how important it is to understand basic pharmacokinetic parameters (e.g., dosing, clearance, drug metabolism, serum concentrations) and to recognize that they are very critical components of drug therapy and the nursing process. It is also important to note that culture, gender, age, and racial or ethnic group have an impact on how each person responds to a drug and how each drug may vary in its action.

Shiga T, Tanaka T, Irie S, Hagiwara N, Kasanuki H: Pharmacokinetics of intravenous amiodarone and its electrocardiographic effects on healthy Japanese subjects. *Heart and Vessels,* 26(3):274-281, 2011.

NURSING DIAGNOSES

1. Decreased cardiac output related to the pathology of the dysrhythmia

Patient-Centered Care: Antidysrhythmic Medications

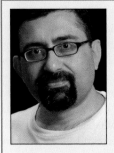

A 46-year-old patient, A.F., is admitted to the progressive care unit (PCU) after going to the hospital with complaints of chest pain. He has been on warfarin for several months due to a history of deep vein thrombosis. In the PCU, A.F.'s heart monitor indicates increased episodes of premature ventricular contractions (PVCs). Just now, the monitor technician calls the nurse to report a 20-second episode of ventricular tachycardia (VT). When the nurse goes to check A.F., he has another 10-second episode of VT. A.F. has no complaints except for feeling some lightheadedness. His blood pressure is 108/62, and his monitor shows sinus rhythm, rate 72 with frequent PVCs. The nurse notifies the on-call physician and receives orders for an amiodarone (Cordarone) infusion.

1. What is the purpose of the amiodarone infusion?

    Two days later, subsequent testing has ruled out pulmonary embolism and coronary artery blockage, and the physician orders the infusion to be discontinued and oral amiodarone to be started.

2. What dose of oral amiodarone will the nurse expect to be ordered? Explain your answer.

3. A.F. has been ill for some time and tells the nurse, "I cannot wait to get to my beach house and relax outside by the ocean. I'm sure the fresh air will be good for me." What is the priority for patient teaching at this time?

    The nurse reviews the prescriptions with A.F. and notes that there is a prescription for warfarin. A.F. states, "This dose is lower than what I was taking. Why is that?"

4. What will the nurse explain to A.F. about the warfarin?

For answers, see *http://evolve.elsevier.com/Lilley.*

2. Ineffective peripheral tissue perfusion related to the physiologic impact of the dysrhythmia
3. Deficient knowledge related to lack of experience with medication therapy

PLANNING: OUTCOME IDENTIFICATION

1. Patient experiences improved cardiac output with control of dysrhythmia.
2. Patient experiences improved peripheral perfusion/circulation with strong, regular bilateral peripheral pulses and warm, pink extremities.
3. Patient demonstrates adequate knowledge about the therapeutic effects and adverse effects of medication therapy.

IMPLEMENTATION

When *antidysrhythmics* are administered, monitor vital signs, especially pulse rate and blood pressure; if pulse rate is lower than 60 beats/min, notify the prescriber. During the initiation of therapy, closely monitor the electrocardiogram and vital signs because of possible prolongation of the patient's QT interval by more than 50%. The end result may be the occurrence of a variety of conduction disturbances. Advise the patient that oral dosage forms are generally better tolerated if taken with food and fluids to help minimize gastrointestinal upset, unless otherwise ordered. *Quinidine* comes in different salt forms, and these various forms are not interchangeable. During treatment with quinidine (or with any of the antidysrhythmics), immediately report the patient's complaint of angina, hypotension, lightheadedness, loss of appetite, tinnitus, or diarrhea to the prescriber. It is recommended that an infusion pump be used for intravenous dosing of any of the classes of antidysrhythmics, with proper solution and dilution.

With *lidocaine*, vials of clear solution are labeled as either for cardiac or not for cardiac use. This is important to remember when reading the vial's label so that the wrong drug is not given. It is also important to remember that lidocaine solutions need to be used with extreme caution and that it is the plain solution that is used to treat various cardiac conditions. Parenteral solutions of these drugs are usually stable only for 24 hours. Lidocaine is also used as an anesthetic, and so the different concentrations of the drug need to double-checked—if not triple-checked. In addition, lidocaine comes in a solution with epinephrine, a potent vasoconstrictor. This combined solution is indicated when the surgeon or physician is suturing or repairing wounds, with the lidocaine acting as an anesthetic and the epinephrine causing vasoconstriction of the local blood vessels and helping to control bleeding of the area, or in dental or oral situations. The solution with epinephrine must *never* be used intravenously and is only to be used as a topical anesthetic! With lidocaine, document vital signs prior to initiation of and during therapy. Often patients are in a cardiac step-down unit, telemetry unit, or intensive care setting when receiving this drug, and so closely monitor the ECG.

Amiodarone may lead to gastrointestinal upset, which may be prevented or decreased by taking the drug with food or a snack. Photosensitivity (sunburn and other exaggerated skin reactions to the sunlight) and photophobia (light sensitivity) are other concerns with this drug. With photosensitivity, protective clothing/hat and sunscreen are needed. Emphasize protection of the eyes, with wearing of sunglasses and/or tinted contact lenses, to patients taking this medication. Recommend consumption of a high-fiber diet and forcing of fluids to minimize the constipation that is a common adverse effect. When beta blockers are used with an *antidysrhythmic*, any shortness of breath, weight gain, changes in baseline blood glucose levels,

or excess fatigue (see Chapters 19 and 25) must be reported to the prescriber immediately.

Beta blockers, diltiazem, and *verapamil* may all be used to manage abnormal rhythms and are to be given only after checking and documenting pulse rates and blood pressures. Contact the prescriber and withhold the drug—if supported by health care institution policy and the prescriber's guidelines—if the pulse rate is 60 beats/min or lower or 100 beats/min or higher and/or the systolic blood pressure is 90 mm Hg or lower.

With the use of *dofetilide*, continually monitor the patient for any changes in the ECG, especially over the first few days of treatment. This drug requires specialized monitoring once ordered by the prescriber, who must have received special prescription training. Encourage the patient to report any difficulty such as chest pain, nausea, or diarrhea to the prescriber immediately. If a dosage amount requires adjustment, hospitalization may be necessary.

EVALUATION

Patients receiving any of the antidysrhythmic drugs need to be monitored closely for therapeutic effects as well as adverse effects and toxicities. The various drugs within *class I* through *class IV antidysrhythmics* have many overlapping therapeutic effects, including conversion to a regular heart rate/rhythm and regularity. The net effect is enhanced cardiac output as noted by improvement in vital signs, skin color/temperature, urinary output, and overall well-being. Other therapeutic effects include decreased chest discomfort and decreased fatigue. The adverse effects and toxicities vary depending on the specific drug and its corresponding pharmacological action and properties. A complete listing of adverse effects is included in Table 25-6, but some of the more common adverse effects for the *class I antidysrhythmics* include hypotension, rash, and diarrhea. *Class II* drugs (beta blockers) may result in bradycardia, AV block, heart failure, and changes in blood glucose levels. *Amiodarone,* a *class III* drug, may lead to pulmonary toxicity, thyroid disorders, and decreases in blood pressure and pulse rate. *Class IV* drugs or *calcium channel blockers* are associated with heart block, hypotension, and constipation.

QSEN EVIDENCE-BASED PRACTICE

Women versus Men with Chronic Atrial Fibrillation: Insights from the Standard versus Atrial Fibrillation spEcific managemenT studY (SAFETY)

Review
Gender-based differences exist clinically with cardiovascular disease (CVD), including atrial fibrillation (AF), and are being further identified as having significant influence on the outcomes of these patients. Diagnosis, management, evaluation, and prevention of all forms of CVD in women continues to be a tremendous challenge ranging from a burden perspective to developing a "robust" evidence base for those affected. CVD remains the single largest cause of death in women and is typically different from their male counterparts. To research this disease process and affected populations requires very astute interpretation of key clinical trials of new treatment strategies, but with females

remaining the minority. Gender-based differences in the pattern and outcomes of the presentation of CVD remain complex, with anatomic, physiologic, and genetic factors to health behavior differences; delays in the response to symptoms; and underuse of gold-standard testing and treatments. Remember, too, that the "typical" cardiac picture is based on the white middle-aged male with misconceptions about health care providers. These factors are also evident in atrial fibrillation (AF) and lead to inaccurate diagnosis and delay of treatment in women. Atrial fibrillation is the most common cardiac dysrhythmia. This study looked at the applicant of a systematic approach to identification of risk and optimizing management of those hospitalized patients with chronic forms of AF

Continued

Women versus Men with Chronic Atrial Fibrillation: Insights from the Standard versus Atrial Fibrillation spEcific managemenT studY (SAFETY)—cont'd

and undertaking the Standard versus Atrial Fibrillation spEcific management studY (SAFETY). The researchers also hypothesized that there would be gender-based differences in clinical presentation, thromboembolic risk, and therapeutic management for those patients recruited into SAFETY.

Type of Evidence

Some 335 participants, as hospital inpatients with chronic AF, were recruited from three tertiary hospitals in Australia. Patients were randomized to either usual postdischarge care or a home-based, multidisciplinary, AF-specific intervention group designed to decrease morbidity and mortality. Patients who were approached were 45 years of age or older; living independently; English-speaking; diagnosed with recurrent paroxysmal, persistent, or permanent AP; and able to provide written informed consent. There were several exclusions to the study, and basic socio-demographic information was collected. Questionnaires were focused at lifestyle (intake of alcohol, cigarette smoking, exercise, sleep habits), health-related quality of life, presence/absence of depression, cognitive functioning, and a comprehensive profile of the patient's experience with AF (see article for more information). A multicenter, randomized, controlled trial of a specific AF management intervention versus usual care was used.

Approximately 2400 patients with AF were screened, and 335 recruited into SAFETY: 48.1% were female and about 5 years older than their male counterparts. Female patients were found to have a higher thromboembolic risk with similar treatment regimens as the male patients. Comorbidities for females included thyroid dysfunction, depression, renal dysfunction, and obesity. Male patients presented more with coronary artery disease and/or chronic obstructive pulmonary disease.

Results of the Study

SAFETY represents one of the largest studies of its kind, and there was much difference noted in the typical demographic data as well as in the presenting clinical profile (of AF). In this particular study, female patients were typically older than the male patients, were more socially isolated, and were less educated. The female patients were also found to have a higher symptom burden,

were more likely to be treated with diuretics, and had an increased prevalence of hypertension, while the male patients had a higher prevalence of coronary artery disease. The identification of gender-related diversity may possibly reflect different pathways of development and/or promotion of AF. From the current data, the pathway to AF in men was related to coronary artery and/or ischemic heart disease. For the women, AF was more commonly associated with the comorbidity conditions of hypertension, obesity, and thyroid and renal dysfunction. There were several limitations (see article), but despite them (limitations) these data have important clinical implications. Findings from this study support the fact that gender differences must be recognized as valid stratifying features for treatment/prevention of poorer health outcomes in this patient group. It was found in this study that women experience AF differently than their male counterparts with consideration of the possible influence of estrogen therapy as well as electrophysiologic differences in atrial tissue.

Link of Evidence to Nursing Practice

The findings of this study hold significance to the gender variability in AF presentation and management. Therefore, more specific research about the prescription of gender-specific, evidence-based treatment strategies is needed. Educational factors may be that future research needs to also look at the fact that if women are typically less educated, then their patient teaching plans must be optimized. The higher symptom burden in women suggested in this study may well be the focus of another research study on the need for increased education about symptom recognition, clinical impact, early detection, and proper management prior to clinical deterioration. More research is also needed about creating a "picture" of the physiology behind gender-specific differences in patients with AF. More research is also needed on the inclusion and integration of the above factors/differences in the development and implementation of an AF-specific disease management. Nurses need to continue research in this area and encourage health care providers to be consistent in their attempt to individualize and optimize the management of patients with AF with the outcome of reduction of potential morbidity and mortality.

From Ball J, Carrington MJ, Wood KA and the SAFETY investigators: Women versus Men with chronic atrial fibrillation: insights from the Standard versus Atrial Fibrillation spEcific managemenT studY (SAFETY). *PLoS One* 8(5):e65795, 2013. Accessed April 25, 2014.

PATIENT-CENTERED CARE: PATIENT TEACHING

- Instruct patients not to crush or chew any oral dosage form that is identified as sustained-release, and not to alter the original dosage form of the drug in any way.
- Some dosage forms are delivered in a sustained-released tablet or capsule that may be composed of a wax matrix, and this matrix may be visible in the patient's stool. This extended-release dosage form provides for a slow release of the medicine, and the wax substance may then be passed out of the body through the stool. Advise patients that the passing of the matrix through the stool occurs after the drug has been absorbed, and although the matrix is often visible to the naked eye, it is of no major concern.
- If the use of an oral preparation is associated with continual and moderate or severe gastrointestinal upset, encourage the patient to take the drug with food and to contact the prescriber if nausea and vomiting worsen.

- If an antacid is needed, it is to be taken either 2 hours before or 2 hours after the drug to avoid interference with drug absorption.
- Recommend a well-balanced diet without an excess of alkaline ash foods (e.g., citrus fruits, vegetables, and milk). Encourage an increase in fluid intake of up to 8 glasses of water per day, unless contraindicated.
- Educate the patient to limit or avoid caffeine intake. Caffeine-containing foods and beverages include coffee (decaffeinated contains 2 to 4 mg caffeine per 8 ounces versus caffeinated 65 to 120 mg per 8 ounces), tea, some soft drinks, chocolate, and high-energy drinks.
- Instruct the patient to take medications exactly as prescribed without doubling up or omitting doses. If the patient forgets a dose or is ill and cannot take a dose, contact the prescriber for further instructions.

- Provide written and verbal instructions and demonstrations on measuring pulse and blood pressure. The local fire department and/or rescue station will usually take blood pressure and pulse rates, if needed.
- Journaling is important to document how the patient feels each day. Advise the patient to record in the journal any worsening or improvement of symptoms, adverse effects, daily weights, activity tolerance, blood pressure readings, and pulse rate.
- Daily weights need to be measured at the same time every day and with the same amount of clothing.
- Contact the prescriber immediately if there is a weight gain of 2 pounds or more in 24 hours or 5 pounds or more in 1 week.
- Inform the patient that changing positions purposefully and with caution is important because of the common adverse effect of postural hypotension. Moving too quickly may lead to dizziness, syncope, and subsequent injury or falls.
- At the beginning of therapy and after any dosage increase, encourage the patient to avoid driving and other hazardous activities until sedating adverse effects have resolved.
- Dry mouth may be helped by frequent mouth care, drinking fluids, sucking on sugarless gum or candy, and/or eating ice chips. Artificial saliva and special toothpaste made specifically for dry mouth and its management is available over the counter. Encourage frequent dental visits.
- Counsel the patient to avoid exertion, hot temperatures, saunas, and hot tubs because of heat-induced vasodilation,

leading to postural hypotension with dizziness and/or syncope and a subsequent risk for falls or injury. Alcohol intake may also lead to vasodilation and subsequent dizziness and syncope.
- Instruct the patient to carry a medical alert identification card on his or her person at all times. Medical alert jewelry is also available to provide information on medical diagnoses, allergies, and medications.
- Instruct the patient to report immediately to the prescriber any dizziness, shortness of breath, chest pain, and/or worsening of symptoms or occurrence of new symptoms.
- The patient must *never* stop taking these medications without specific instructions to do so; an abrupt discontinuation of these drugs may lead to severe or life-threatening complications.
- With amiodarone, photosensitivity is an adverse effect; advise the patient to avoid sun exposure and to wear sun-protective clothing and dark glasses when outside. Sunscreens are ineffective because they do not block ultraviolet B light, to which the patient may react while taking this medication. Instead, barrier sunblocks, such as zinc or titanium chloride, are recommended.
- With amiodarone, instruct the patient to immediately report any blue-gray discoloration of the skin (often after 1 year, and especially on the face, neck, and arms) as well as any jaundice, unusual rash or skin reactions, nausea, vomiting, or dizziness.

KEY POINTS

- The SA node, AV node, and His-Purkinje system are all areas in which there is automaticity (cells can depolarize spontaneously). The SA node is the pacemaker because it can spontaneously depolarize easier and faster than the other areas.
- Any disturbance or abnormality in the normal pattern of the heartbeat and pulse rate is termed a *dysrhythmia*.
- Antidysrhythmic drugs are used to correct dysrhythmias; however, they may also cause dysrhythmias, and for this reason are said to be *prodysrhythmic*. The Vaughan Williams classification is the system most commonly used to categorize antidysrhythmic drugs. It classifies drugs into the following groups according to where and how they affect cardiac cells and what their mechanisms of action is:
  - *Class I:* membrane-stabilizing drugs (e.g., class Ia, quinidine; class Ib, lidocaine; class Ic, flecainide)

  - *Class II:* beta-adrenergic blockers that depress phase 4 depolarization (e.g., atenolol)
  - *Class III:* drugs that prolong repolarization in phase 3 (e.g., amiodarone and dofetilide)
  - *Class IV:* calcium channel blockers that depress phase 4 depolarization (e.g., verapamil)
- Nursing actions for the various antidysrhythmics include skillful nursing assessment and close monitoring of heart rate, blood pressure, heart rhythms, general well-being, skin color, temperature, and heart and breath sounds.
- The therapeutic responses to antidysrhythmics include a decrease in blood pressure in hypertensive patients, a decrease in edema, and restoration of a regular pulse rate or a pulse rate without major irregularities or with improved regularity compared with the irregularity that existed before therapy.

NCLEX® EXAMINATION REVIEW QUESTIONS

1. A patient with a rapid, irregular heart rhythm is being treated in the emergency department with adenosine. During administration of this drug, the nurse will be prepared to monitor the patient for which effect?
   a. Nausea and vomiting
   b. Transitory asystole
   c. Muscle tetany
   d. Hypertension

2. When assessing a patient who has been taking amiodarone for 6 months, the nurse monitors for which potential adverse effect?
   a. Hyperglycemia
   b. Dysphagia
   c. Photophobia
   d. Urticaria

3. The nurse is assessing a patient who has been taking quinidine and asks about adverse effects. An adverse effect associated with the use of this drug includes:
   a. muscle pain.
   b. tinnitus.
   c. chest pain.
   d. excessive thirst.

4. A patient calls the family practice office to report that he has seen his pills in his stools when he has a bowel movement. How will the nurse respond?
   a. "The pills are not being digested properly. You need to take them on an empty stomach."
   b. "The pills are not being digested properly. You need to take them with food."
   c. "What you are seeing is the wax matrix that contained the medication, but the drug has been absorbed."
   d. "This indicates that you are not tolerating this medication and will need to switch to a different form."

5. The nurse is administering lidocaine and considers which condition, if present in the patient, a caution for the use of this drug?
   a. Tachycardia
   b. Hypertension
   c. Ventricular dysrhythmias
   d. Renal dysfunction

6. When the nurse is teaching a patient about taking an antidysrhythmic drug, which statements by the nurse are correct? *(Select all that apply.)*
   a. "Take the medication with an antacid if stomach upset occurs."
   b. "Do not chew sustained-release capsules."

   c. "If weight gain of 5 pounds within 1 week occurs, notify your physician at the next office visit."
   d. "If you experience severe adverse effects, stop the drug and notify your physician."
   e. "You may take the medication with food if stomach upset occurs."

7. A patient is in the emergency department with new-onset rapid-rate atrial fibrillation. The nurse is about to add a continuous infusion of diltiazem (Cardizem) at 5 mg/hr, but must first give a bolus of 0.25 mg/kg over 2 minutes. The patient weighs 220 pounds. The medication comes in a vial of 5 mg/mL. How many milligrams will the patient receive, and how many milliliters will the nurse draw up for this dose?

8. A patient is in the clinic for a follow-up visit. He has been taking amiodarone (Cordarone) for almost 1 year, and today he tells the nurse, "I am noticing some blue color around my face, neck, and upper arms. Is that normal?" Which is the nurse's correct response?
   a. "This is an expected side effect and should go away soon."
   b. "This is a harmless effect. As long as the medication is working, we'll just monitor your skin."
   c. "This can happen with amiodarone. I will let your doctor know about it right away."
   d. "How much sun exposure have you had recently?"

1. b, 2. c, 3. b, 4. c, 5. d, 6. b, e, 7. 25 mg, 5 mL, 8. c.

CRITICAL THINKING AND PRIORITIZATION QUESTIONS

1. A patient who was admitted to the hospital for treatment of atrial fibrillation is about to go home with a new prescription for diltiazem (Cardizem). As the nurse goes over the patient's medication list, the patient complains, "I'm feeling very tired. And when I stand up, I can hardly walk because I'm so dizzy." What is the nurse's priority action at this time?

2. A patient has been admitted to the emergency department and is experiencing PSVT that has not responded to

treatment with calcium channel blockers. Immediately after the patient receives a dose of adenosine (Adenocard) by intravenous push, the monitor shows asystole. What is the nurse's priority action in response to the asystole?

For answers, see *http://evolve.elsevier.com/Lilley.*

ⓔ EVOLVE WEBSITE

http://evolve.elsevier.com/Lilley
- Animations
- Answer Keys for Textbook Case Studies and Textbook Critical Thinking and Prioritization Questions

- Content Updates
- Key Points
- Review Questions
- Student Case Studies

Coagulation Modifier Drugs

http://evolve.elsevier.com/Lilley

OBJECTIVES

When you reach the end of this chapter, you will be able to do the following:

1. Briefly review the coagulation process and the impact of coagulation modifiers, including anticoagulants, antiplatelets, thrombolytics, and antifibrinolytics.
2. Compare the mechanisms of action, indications, cautions, contraindications, drug interactions, adverse effects, routes of administration, and dosages of the various anticoagulants, antiplatelets, thrombolytics, and antifibrinolytics.
3. Discuss the administration procedures and techniques as well as related standards of care for the various coagulation modifiers.
4. Identify any available antidotes for the coagulation modifiers.
5. Compare the laboratory tests used in conjunction with treatment with the various coagulation modifiers and their implications for therapeutic use of these drugs and monitoring for adverse reactions.
6. Develop a nursing care plan that includes all phases of the nursing process for patients receiving anticoagulants, antiplatelets, thrombolytics, and antifibrinolytics.

DRUG PROFILES

♦! alteplase, p. 424
aminocaproic acid, p. 426
! argatroban, p. 417
♦ aspirin, p. 422
♦ clopidogrel, p. 423
♦! dabigatran, p. 417
desmopressin, p. 426
♦! enoxaparin, p. 418

♦! eptifibatide, p. 423
♦! fondaparinux, p. 418
♦! heparin, p. 419
♦! rivaroxaban, p. 419
♦! warfarin, p. 419

_____

♦ = *Key drug*
! = *High-alert drug*

KEY TERMS

Anticoagulants Substances that prevent or delay coagulation of the blood. (p. 414)

Antifibrinolytic drugs Drugs that prevent the lysis of fibrin and in doing so promote clot formation. (p. 414)

Antiplatelet drugs Substances that prevent platelet plugs from forming. (p. 414)

Antithrombin III A substance that inactivates ("turns off") three major activating factors of the clotting cascade: activated factor II (thrombin), activated factor X, and activated factor IX. (p. 414)

Clot Insoluble solid elements of blood (e.g., cells, fibrin threads) that have chemically separated from the liquid (plasma) component of the blood. (p. 412)

Coagulation The process of blood clotting. More specifically, the sequential process by which the multiple coagulation factors of the blood interact in the *coagulation* cascade, ultimately forming an insoluble fibrin clot. (p. 412)

Coagulation cascade The series of steps beginning with the *intrinsic* or *extrinsic* pathways of coagulation and proceeding through the formation of a *fibrin clot*. (p. 412)

Deep vein thrombosis (DVT) The formation of a thrombus in one of the deep veins of the body. The deep veins most commonly affected are the iliac and femoral veins. (p. 414)

Embolus A blood clot *(thrombus)* that has been dislodged from the wall of a blood vessel and is traveling throughout the bloodstream. Emboli that lodge in critical blood vessels can result in ischemic injury to a vital organ (e.g., heart, lung, brain) and result in disability or death. (p. 412)

Enzyme A protein molecule that catalyzes chemical reactions of other substances without being altered or destroyed in the process. (p. 417)

Fibrin A stringy, insoluble protein produced by the action of thrombin on fibrinogen during the clotting process; a major component of blood *clots* or *thrombi* (see *thrombus*). (p. 412)

Fibrin specificity The property of some thrombolytic drugs of activating the conversion of plasminogen to plasmin only in the presence of established clots having fibrin threads rather than inducing systemic plasminogen activation throughout the body. (p. 424)

Fibrinogen A plasma protein that is converted into fibrin by thrombin in the presence of calcium ions. (p. 420)

Fibrinolysis The continual process of fibrin decomposition produced by the actions of the enzymatic protein fibrinolysin. It is the normal mechanism for removing small fibrin clots and is stimulated by anoxia, inflammatory reactions, and other kinds of stress. (p. 412)

Fibrinolytic system An area of the circulatory system undergoing fibrinolysis. (p. 412)

Hemophilia A rare, inherited blood disorder in which the blood does not clot normally. (p. 413)

Hemorheologic drugs Drugs that alter the function of platelets without compromising their blood-clotting properties. (p. 414)

Hemostasis The arrest of bleeding, either by the physiologic properties of vasoconstriction and coagulation or by mechanical, surgical, or pharmacologic means. (p. 412)

Hemostatic Referring to any procedure, device, or substance that arrests the flow of blood. (p. 414)

Plasmin The enzymatic protein that breaks down fibrin into fibrin degradation products; it is derived from plasminogen. (p. 412)

Plasminogen A plasma protein that is converted to plasmin. (p. 412)

Pulmonary embolism The blockage of a pulmonary artery by foreign matter such as fat, air, a tumor, or a thrombus (which usually arises from a peripheral vein). (p. 414)

Stroke Occlusion of the blood vessels of the brain by an embolus, thrombus, or cerebrovascular hemorrhage, resulting in ischemia of the brain tissue. (p. 414)

Thromboembolic events Events in which a blood vessel is blocked by an embolus carried in the bloodstream from the site of its formation. The tissue supplied by an obstructed artery may tingle and become cold, numb, cyanotic, and eventually necrotic (dead). (p. 414)

Thrombolytic drugs Drugs that dissolve thrombi by functioning similarly to *tissue plasminogen activator*. (p. 414)

Thrombus The technical term for a blood clot (plural: *thrombi*); an aggregation of platelets, fibrin, clotting factors, and the cellular elements of the blood that is attached to the interior wall of a vein or artery, sometimes occluding the vessel lumen. (p. 412)

Tissue plasminogen activator A naturally occurring plasminogen activator secreted by vascular endothelial cells in the walls of blood vessels. Thrombolytic drugs are based on this blood component. (p. 412)

OVERVIEW

Hemostasis is a general term for any process that stops bleeding. This can be accomplished by mechanical means (e.g., compression to the bleeding site) or surgical means (e.g., surgical clamping or cauterization of a blood vessel). When hemostasis occurs due to physiologic clotting of blood, it is called **coagulation**, which is the process of blood clot formation. The technical term for a blood clot is a **thrombus**. A thrombus that moves through blood vessels is called an **embolus**. Normal hemostasis involves the complex interaction of substances that promote **clot** formation and substances that either inhibit coagulation or dissolve the formed clot. Substances that promote coagulation include platelets, von Willebrand factor, activated clotting factors, and tissue thromboplastin. Substances that inhibit coagulation include prostacyclin, antithrombin III, and proteins C and S. In addition, **tissue plasminogen activator** is a natural substance that dissolves clots that are already formed.

The coagulation system is illustrated in Figures 26-1 and 26-2. It is called a *cascade* (or **coagulation cascade**) because each activated clotting factor serves as a catalyst that amplifies the next reaction. The result is a large concentration of a clot-forming substance called **fibrin**. The coagulation cascade is typically divided into the intrinsic and extrinsic pathways, and these pathways are activated by different types of injury. When

blood vessels are damaged by penetration from the outside (e.g., knife or bullet wound), thromboplastin, a substance contained in the walls of blood vessels, is released. This initiates the extrinsic pathway by activating factors VII and X (see Figure 26-1). The components of the intrinsic pathway are present in the blood in their inactive forms (see Figure 26-2). The intrinsic pathway is activated when factor XII comes in contact with exposed collagen on the inside of damaged blood vessels. Figures 26-1 and 26-2 illustrate the steps that occur in the extrinsic and intrinsic pathways, respectively, and the coagulation factors involved. They also illustrate the site of action of two commonly used anticoagulant drugs: warfarin and heparin.

Once a clot is formed and fibrin is present, the **fibrinolytic system** is activated. This system initiates the breakdown of clots and serves to balance the clotting process. **Fibrinolysis** is the reverse of the clotting process. It is the mechanism by which formed thrombi are lysed (broken down) to prevent excessive clot formation and blood vessel blockage. Fibrin in the clot binds to a circulating protein known as **plasminogen**. This binding converts plasminogen to plasmin. **Plasmin** is the enzymatic protein that eventually breaks down the fibrin thrombus into fibrin degradation products. This keeps the thrombus localized to prevent it from becoming an embolus that can travel to obstruct a major blood vessel in the lung, heart, or brain. Figure 26-3 illustrates the fibrinolytic system.

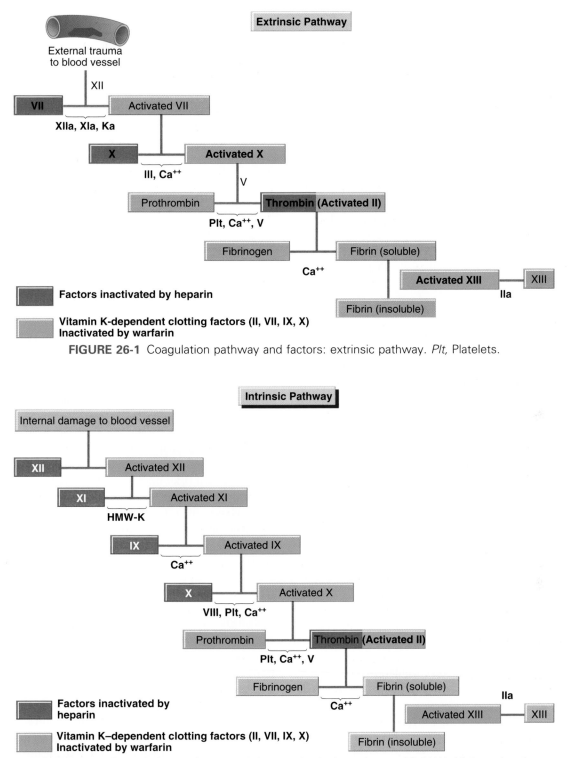

FIGURE 26-1 Coagulation pathway and factors: extrinsic pathway. *Plt,* Platelets.

FIGURE 26-2 Coagulation pathway and factors: intrinsic pathway. *HMW-K,* High–molecular-weight kininogen; *Plt,* platelets.

Hemophilia is a rare genetic disorder in which the previously mentioned natural coagulation and hemostasis factors are limited or absent. Hemophilia is categorized into two main types depending on which of the coagulation factors is absent (factor VII, factor VIII, and/or factor IX). Patients with hemophilia can bleed to death if coagulation factors are not given.

PHARMACOLOGY OVERVIEW

Drugs that affect coagulation are some of the most dangerous drugs used today, and numerous factors can affect their action. These drugs are among the most commonly associated with adverse drug reactions. The Joint Commission, a hospital accreditation agency, has made safe use of these drugs a National

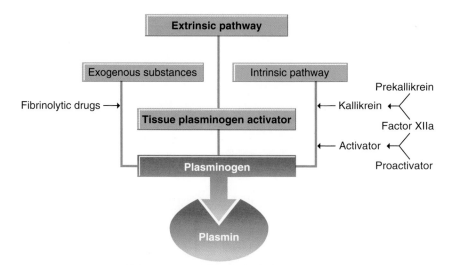

FIGURE 26-3 The fibrinolytic system.

Patient Safety Goal. This goal requires hospitals to take steps to prevent adverse events associated with these drugs. Further information on this national patient safety goal may be found at *www.jointcommission.org/standards_information/npsgs.aspx.*

The drugs discussed in this chapter aid the body in reversing or achieving hemostasis, and they can be broken down into several main categories based on their actions. Anticoagulants inhibit the action or formation of clotting factors and therefore prevent clots from forming. Antiplatelet drugs prevent platelet plugs from forming by inhibiting platelet aggregation, which can be beneficial in preventing heart attacks and strokes. Hemorheologic drugs alter platelet function without preventing the platelets from working. Sometimes clots form and totally block a blood vessel. When this happens in one of the coronary arteries, a heart attack occurs, and the clot must be lysed to prevent or minimize damage to the myocardial muscle. Thrombolytic drugs lyse (break down) clots, or thrombi, that have already formed. This is a unique difference between thrombolytics and anticoagulants, which can only prevent the formation of a clot. Antifibrinolytic drugs, also known as hemostatic drugs, have the opposite effect of these other classes of drugs; they actually promote blood coagulation. The various drugs in each category of coagulation modifiers are listed in Table 26-1.

ANTICOAGULANTS

Drugs that prevent the formation of a clot by inhibiting certain clotting factors are called *anticoagulants.* These drugs have no direct effect on a blood clot that has already formed. They prevent intravascular thrombosis by decreasing blood coagulability. Their uses vary from preventing clot formation to preventing the extension of an established clot, or a thrombus.

Once a clot forms on the wall of a blood vessel, it may dislodge and travel through the bloodstream. This is referred to as an *embolus.* If it lodges in a coronary artery, it causes a myocardial infarction (MI); if it obstructs a brain vessel, it causes a stroke; if it goes to the lungs, it is a pulmonary embolism (PE); and if it goes to a vein in the leg, it is a deep vein thrombosis (DVT). Collectively, these complications are called thromboembolic events, because they involve a thrombus that becomes an embolus and causes an adverse cardiovascular "event." Anticoagulants can prevent these from occurring if used in the correct manner. Both orally and parenterally administered anticoagulants are available, and each drug has a slightly different mechanism of action and indications. All anticoagulants have their own risks, mainly causing bleeding. The mechanisms of action of the anticoagulants vary depending on the drug. Drug classes of anticoagulants include older drugs such as unfractionated heparin and warfarin. There are also several newer drug classes, including low–molecular-weight heparins (LMWHs), direct thrombin inhibitors, and selective factor Xa inhibitors. For dosage information on anticoagulants, see the table on p. 418.

Mechanism of Action and Drug Effects

Anticoagulants are also called *antithrombotic drugs* because they work to prevent the formation of a clot or thrombus, a condition known as *thrombosis.* All anticoagulants work in the clotting cascade but do so at different points. As shown in Figures 26-1 and 26-2, heparin works by binding to a substance called antithrombin III, which turns off three main activating factors: activated factor II (also called *thrombin*), activated factor X, and activated factor IX. (Factors XI and XII are also inactivated but do not play as important a role as the other three factors.) Of these, thrombin is the most sensitive to the actions of heparin. Antithrombin III is the major natural inhibitor of thrombin in the blood. The overall effect of heparin is that it turns off the coagulation pathway and prevents clots from forming. However, it cannot lyse a clot. The drug name *heparin* usually refers to unfractionated heparin, which is a relatively large molecule and is derived from animal sources. In contrast, low–molecular-weight heparins are synthetic and have a smaller molecular structure. These include enoxaparin (Lovenox) and dalteparin

TABLE 26-1 Coagulation Modifiers: Comparison of Drug Subclasses

Type of Coagulation Modifier and Mechanism of Action	Drug Class	Individual Drugs
Prevent Clot Formation		
Anticoagulant		
Inhibit clotting factors IIa (thrombin) and Xa	Heparins	Unfractionated heparin ("heparin") and low–molecular-weight heparins (enoxaparin [Lovenox], dalteparin [Fragmin])
Inhibit vitamin K–dependent clotting factors II, VII, IX, and X	Coumarins	Warfarin (Coumadin)
Inhibit thrombin (factor IIa)	Direct thrombin inhibitors	Human antithrombin III (Thrombate), lepirudin (Refludan), argatroban (Argatroban), bivalirudin (Angiomax), dabigatran (Pradaxa)
Inhibit factor Xa	Selective factor Xa inhibitor	Fondaparinux (Arixtra), rivaroxaban (Xarelto), apixaban (Eliquis)
Antiplatelet Drugs		
Interfere with platelet function	Aggregation inhibitors	Cilostazol (Pletal), clopidogrel (Plavix), prasugrel (Effient)
	Aggregation inhibitors/ vasodilators	Treprostinil (Remodulin)
	Glycoprotein IIb/IIIa inhibitors	Abciximab (ReoPro), eptifibatide (Integrilin), tirofiban (Aggrastat)
	Miscellaneous	Anagrelide (Agrylin), dipyridamole (Persantine), vorapaxar (Zontivity)
Lyse a Preformed Clot		
Thrombolytics		
Dissolve thrombi	Tissue plasminogen activators	Alteplase (Activase, Cathflo Activase), reteplase (Retavase), tenecteplase (TNKase)
Promote Clot Formation		
Antifibrinolytics		
Prevent lysis of fibrin	Systemic hemostatics	Aminocaproic acid (Amicar), tranexamic acid (Cyklokapron)
Reduce Blood Viscosity	Hemorheologic (Trental)	Pentoxifylline
Reversal Drugs	Heparin antagonist	Protamine sulfate
	Warfarin antagonist	Vitamin K

(Fragmin). Both drugs work similarly to heparin. Heparin primarily binds to activated factors II, X, and IX, whereas the LMWHs differ from heparin in that they are much more specific for activated factor X (Xa) than for activated factor II (IIa, or thrombin). This property gives LMWHs a much more predictable anticoagulant response. As a result, frequent laboratory monitoring of bleeding times using tests such as activated partial thromboplastin time (aPTT), which is imperative with unfractionated heparin, is not required with LMWHs. When heparin is used for flushing catheters (10 to 100 units/mL), no monitoring is needed.

Warfarin (Coumadin) works by inhibiting vitamin K synthesis by bacteria in the gastrointestinal tract. This, in turn, inhibits production of clotting factors II, VII, IX, and X. These four factors are normally synthesized in the liver and are known as *vitamin K–dependent clotting factors*. As with heparin, the final effect is the prevention of clot formation. Figures 26-1 and 26-2 show where in the clotting cascade this occurs.

Fondaparinux (Arixtra) inhibits thrombosis by its specific action against factor Xa alone. Rivaroxaban (Xarelto), apixaban (Eliquis), and edoxaban (Savaysa) are new oral-acting factor Xa inhibitors. There are also currently five antithrombin drugs that

inhibit the thrombin molecules directly, one natural and four synthetic. The natural drug is human antithrombin III (Thrombate), which is isolated from the plasma of human donors. The synthetic drugs are lepirudin (Refludan), argatroban (Argatroban), bivalirudin (Angiomax), and dabigatran (Pradaxa). Dabigatran is a new oral direct thrombin inhibitor that was approved in 2010. All of these drugs work similarly to inhibit thrombus formation by inhibiting thrombin.

Indications

The ability of anticoagulants to prevent clot formation is of benefit in certain settings in which there is a high likelihood of clot formation. These include MI, unstable angina, atrial fibrillation, use of indwelling devices such as mechanical heart valves, and conditions in which blood flow may be slowed and blood may pool, such as major orthopedic surgery or prolonged periods of immobilization like hospitalization or even long plane rides. The ultimate consequence of a clot can be a stroke or a heart attack, DVT, or PE; therefore, the prevention of these serious events is the ultimate benefit of these drugs. Anticoagulants are used for both prevention and treatment of clots. Patients at risk for clots are given DVT prophylaxis while in the hospital and after major surgery. LMWHs, especially enoxaparin, are also routinely used as anticoagulant bridge therapy in situations in which a patient must stop warfarin for surgery or other invasive medical procedures. The term *bridge therapy* refers to the fact that enoxaparin acts as a bridge to provide anticoagulation while the patient must be off of his or her warfarin therapy.

Contraindications

Contraindications to the use of anticoagulants are similar for all of the different drugs. They include known drug allergy, any acute bleeding process, or high risk for such an occurrence. Warfarin is strongly contraindicated in pregnancy, whereas the other anticoagulants are rated in lower pregnancy categories (B or C). LMWHs are contraindicated in patients with an indwelling epidural catheter; they can be given 2 hours after the epidural is removed. This is very important to remember, because giving an LMWH with an epidural has been associated with epidural hematoma.

Adverse Effects

Bleeding is the main complication of anticoagulation therapy, and the risk increases with increasing dosages. Bleeding may be localized (e.g., hematoma at the site of injection) or systemic. It also depends on the nature of the patient's underlying clinical disorder and is increased in patients taking high doses of aspirin or other drugs that impair platelet function. One particularly notable adverse effect of heparin is *heparin-induced thrombocytopenia (HIT)*. There are two types of HIT. Type I is characterized by a more gradual reduction in platelets. In this type, heparin therapy can generally be continued. In contrast, in type II HIT there is an acute fall in the number of platelets (more than 50% reduction from baseline). Heparin therapy must be discontinued in patients with type II HIT. The greatest risk to the patient with HIT is the paradoxical occurrence of thrombosis, something that heparin normally prevents or alleviates. Thrombosis that occurs in the presence of HIT can be fatal. The incidence of this disorder ranges from 5% to 15%. The direct thrombin inhibitors lepirudin and argatroban are both specifically indicated for treatment of HIT. Warfarin can cause skin necrosis and "purple toes" syndrome. Other adverse effects are listed in Table 26-2.

TABLE 26-2 Anticoagulants: Common Adverse Effects

Drug Subclass	Adverse Effects
Heparins (unfractionated heparin, low–molecular-weight heparin)	Bleeding, hematoma, anemia, thrombocytopenia
Direct thrombin inhibitors (lepirudin, argatroban, bivalirudin, dabigatran)	Bleeding, dizziness, shortness of breath, fever, urticaria
Selective factor Xa inhibitor (fondaparinux, rivaroxaban)	Bleeding, hematoma, dizziness, rash, gastrointestinal distress, anemia
warfarin (Coumadin)	Bleeding, lethargy, muscle pain, purple toes

Toxicity and Management of Overdose

Treatment of the toxic effects of anticoagulants is aimed at reversing the underlying cause. Although the toxic effects of all anticoagulants are hemorrhagic in nature, the management is different for each drug. Symptoms include hematuria, melena (blood in the stool), petechiae, ecchymoses, and gum or mucous membrane bleeding. In the event of bleeding, the drug is to be stopped immediately. In the case of heparin, stopping the drug alone may be enough to reverse the toxic effects because of the drug's short half-life (1 to 2 hours). In severe cases or when large doses have been given intentionally (i.e., during cardiopulmonary bypass for heart surgery), IV injection of protamine sulfate is indicated. Protamine is a specific heparin antidote and forms a complex with heparin, completely reversing its anticoagulant properties. This occurs in as few as 5 minutes. In general, 1 mg of protamine can reverse the effects of 100 units of heparin. Protamine may also be used to reverse the effects of LMWHs. A 1-mg dose of protamine is administered for each milligram of LMWH given, (e.g., 1 mg protamine for 1 mg enoxaparin). If the heparin overdose has resulted in a large blood loss, replacement with packed red blood cells may be necessary.

In the event of warfarin toxicity or overdose, the first step is to discontinue the warfarin. As with heparin, the toxicity associated with warfarin is an extension of its therapeutic effects on the clotting cascade. However, because warfarin inactivates the vitamin K–dependent clotting factors and because these clotting factors are synthesized in the liver, it may take 36 to 42 hours before the liver can resynthesize enough clotting factors to reverse the warfarin effects. Giving vitamin K_1 (phytonadione) can hasten the return to normal coagulation. The dose and route of administration of the vitamin K depend on the clinical situation and its acuity (i.e., how quickly the warfarin-induced effects must be reversed and whether the patient is having significant bleeding). High doses of vitamin K (10 mg) given IV will reverse the anticoagulation within 6 hours. Current recommendations are to use the lowest amount of vitamin K possible, based on the clinical situation. This is because once vitamin K is given, warfarin resistance will occur for up to 7 days; thus the patient cannot be anticoagulated by warfarin during this period. In such cases, either heparin or an LMWH may need to be added to provide adequate anticoagulation. In acute situations in which bleeding is severe, it may be necessary to administer transfusions of human plasma or clotting factor concentrates. There are two prothrombin complex concentrate products (Kcentra and Profiline) that can be used for life-threatening bleeding from warfarin. They also can be used to reverse bleeding seen with the new oral antiXa products. Depending on the clinical situation, oral vitamin K is usually the preferred route. However, when the international normalized ratio (INR) is very elevated and/or the patient is bleeding, vitamin K is given IV. There is a risk for anaphylaxis when it is given by the IV route; the risk is diminished by diluting it and giving it over 30 minutes.

Interactions

Drug interactions involving the oral anticoagulants are profound and complicated. The main interaction mechanisms

TABLE 26-3 Anticoagulants: Drug Interactions

Drug	Mechanism	Result
Warfarin		
acetaminophen (high doses), amiodarone, bumetanide, furosemide	Displacement from inactive protein-binding sites	Increased anticoagulant effect
aspirin, other NSAIDs, broad-spectrum antibiotics	Decreased platelet activity	Increased anticoagulant effect
Barbiturates, carbamazepine, rifampin, phenytoin	Enzyme induction	Decreased anticoagulant effect
amiodarone, cimetidine, ciprofloxacin, erythromycin, ketoconazole, metronidazole, omeprazole, sulfonamides, macrolides, HMG-CoA reductase inhibitors (statins)	Enzyme inhibition	Increased anticoagulant effect
cholestyramine, sucralfate	Impaired warfarin absorption	Decreased effectiveness
Herbal therapies: dong quai, garlic, ginkgo	Unknown; case reports of increased INR	Increased bleeding risk from warfarin
St. John's wort	Unknown	Decreased effectiveness
Heparin		
aspirin, other NSAIDs	Decreased platelet activity	Increased bleeding risk
Oral anticoagulants, antiplatelet drugs, thrombolytics	Additive	Increased anticoagulant effect
Antiplatelets		
aspirin, NSAIDs	Decreased platelet activity	Increased bleeding risk
rifampin	Increased effects	Increased bleeding risk
warfarin, heparin, thrombolytics	Additive	Increased bleeding risk
Herbal therapies: garlic, ginkgo, kava	Platelet antagonism	Increased bleeding risk

HMG-CoA, Hydroxymethylglutaryl–coenzyme A; *INR,* international normalized ratio; *NSAIDs,* nonsteroidal antiinflammatory drugs.

responsible for increasing anticoagulant activity include the following:

- **Enzyme** inhibition of metabolism
- Displacement of the drug from inactive protein-binding sites
- Decrease in vitamin K absorption or synthesis by the bacterial flora of the large intestine
- Alteration in the platelet count or activity

The drugs that interact with warfarin and heparin are listed in Table 26-3. More specifics on significant drug interactions are discussed under the drug profiles. Although both aspirin and warfarin increase the risk for bleeding when given with heparin, they are commonly given together in clinical practice. In fact, when a patient is placed on IV heparin, it is recommended that warfarin be started at the same time. Recommendations are to continue overlap therapy of the heparin and warfarin for at least 5 days; the heparin is stopped after 5 days when the INR is above 2.

Dosages

For dosage information on selected anticoagulants, see the table on the next page.

DRUG PROFILES

Of the anticoagulants, warfarin, dabigatran, rivaroxaban, apixaban, and edoxaban are used orally. The rest are given by IV and/or subcutaneous injection only. Intramuscular (IM) injection of these drugs is contraindicated due to their propensity to cause large hematomas at the site of injection.

◆!argatroban

Argatroban, which has the same trade name, is a synthetic direct thrombin inhibitor. It is indicated both for treatment of active HIT and for *percutaneous coronary intervention* procedures in patients at risk for HIT (i.e., those with a history of the disorder). It is given only by the IV route. A lower dosage must be used in patients with severe hepatic dysfunction.

Pharmacokinetics: Argatroban

Route	Onset of Action	Peak Plasma Concentration	Elimination Half-life	Duration of Action
IV	Immediate	1-3 hr	30-50 min	Dependent on infusion duration

◆!dabigatran

Dabigatran (Pradaxa) is the first oral direct thrombin inhibitor that is approved for prevention of strokes and thrombosis in patients with nonvalvular atrial fibrillation. Dabigatran is a prodrug that becomes activated in the liver. It specifically and reversibly binds to both free and clot-bound thrombin. Dabigatran is excreted extensively in the kidneys, and the dose is dependent upon renal function. The most common and serious side effect is bleeding, with an increased in GI bleeding as compared to warfarin. No coagulation monitoring is required for dabigatran. Drug interactions include phenytoin, carbamazepine, rifampin, and St. John's wort (which cause a decreased effect) and strong CYP3A4 inhibitors such as amiodarone, quinidine, erythromycin, verapamil, azole antifungals, and HIV protease inhibitors (which cause an increased effect). Other anticoagulants are not to be given with dabigatran. Information about storage and handling is discussed in the Nursing Process section later in the chapter.

Pharmacokinetics: Dabigatran

Route	Onset of Action	Peak Plasma Concentration	Elimination Half-life	Duration of Action
PO	2-3 hr	2 hr	12-17 hr	12 hr

◆!enoxaparin

Enoxaparin (Lovenox) is the prototypical LMWH and is obtained by enzymatically cleaving large unfractionated heparin molecules into small fragments. These smaller fragments of heparin have a greater affinity for factor Xa than for factor IIa and have a higher degree of bioavailability and a longer elimination half-life than unfractionated heparin. Laboratory monitoring, as done with heparin therapy, is not necessary when enoxaparin is given because of its greater affinity for factor Xa. It is available only in injectable form. Dalteparin is another anticoagulant with comparable pharmacology and indications. Enoxaparin is the most frequently used LMWH and is commonly given for both prophylaxis and treatment. All LMWHs have a distinct advantage over heparin in that they do not require any laboratory monitoring and can be given at home. A potentially deadly medication error is to give heparin

in combination with enoxaparin (or any LMWH, dabigatran, rivaroxaban, or apixaban). Always double-check that enoxaparin and other anticoagulants are never given to the same patient. One exception, however, is that enoxaparin is often used with oral warfarin as overlap treatment for pulmonary embolus or deep vein thrombosis.

Enoxaparin is available in prefilled syringes in a range of dosage forms and strengths, for example 40 mg in 0.4 mL. Prefilled syringes and graduated prefilled syringes are for one-time use only and are available with systems that shield the needle after injection. The air bubble should not be expelled from prefilled syringes, as this is designed to remain next to the plunger to ensure the whole dose is administered.

Pharmacokinetics: Enoxaparin

Route	Onset of Action	Peak Plasma Concentration	Elimination Half-life	Duration of Action
Subcut	3-5 hr	4-5 hr	4-5 hr	12 hr

◆!fondaparinux

Fondaparinux (Arixtra) is a selective inhibitor of factor Xa, which is indicated for prophylaxis or treatment of DVT or PE. In 2009, the FDA required changes in the prescribing information to highlight potential adverse reactions and contraindications. It is contraindicated with known allergy or in patients

DOSAGES

Selected Anticoagulant Drugs

Drug (Pregnancy Category)	Pharmacologic Class	Usual Adult Dosage Range	Indications/Uses
!argatroban (Argatroban) (B)	Synthetic direct thrombin inhibitor	IV: 2 mcg/kg/min until aPTT in desired range	Thromboprevention and treatment of HIT and with PCI in patients at risk for HIT
◆!dabigatran (Pradaxa) (C)	Synthetic direct thrombin inhibitor	PO: 75-150 mg bid (depending on renal function)	Prevention of strokes and thrombosis in patients with nonvalvular atrial fibrillation
◆!enoxaparin (Lovenox) (B)	LMWH	Prophylaxis: Subcut: 30 mg every 12 hr or 40 mg/day Treatment: 1 mg/kg every 12 hr or 1.5 mg/kg/day	Prevention and treatment of thromboembolic and ischemic processes in unstable angina and postoperative and post-MI situations
◆!fondaparinux (Arixtra) (B)	Factor Xa inhibitor	Prophylaxis: 2.5 mg subcut daily Treatment: Less than 50 kg: 5 mg daily 50-100 kg: 7.5 mg daily Over 100 kg: 10 mg daily	Prevention and treatment of DVT and PE
◆!heparin (generic only) (C)	Natural anticoagulant	Prophylaxis: Subcut: 5000 units every 8-12 hr Treatment: IV infusion: 80 unit/kg bolus, then 18 units/kg/hr (depending on indication) aPTT determines maintenance dosage	Thrombosis/embolism, coagulopathies (e.g., DIC), DVT and PE prophylaxis, clotting prevention (e.g., open heart surgery, dialysis)
◆!rivaroxaban (Xarelto) (C)	Oral Xa inhibitor	15-30 mg daily depending on indication	DVT/PE treatment, DVT prophylaxis, stroke prevention in nonvavular atrial fibrillation, postoperative DVT prophylaxis
◆!warfarin (X)	Coumarin anticoagulant	INR determines maintenance dosage, usually 1-10 mg/day orally	Thromboprevention and treatment of DVT, PE, atrial fibrillation, post-MI status

aPTT, Activated partial thromboplastin time; *DIC*, disseminated intravascular coagulation; *DVT*, deep vein thrombosis; *HIT*, heparin-induced thrombocytopenia; *INR*, international normalized ratio; *LMWH*, low–molecular-weight heparin; *MI*, myocardial infarction; *PCI*, percutaneous coronary intervention; *PE*, pulmonary embolism.

with a creatinine clearance less than 30 mL/min or a body weight of less than 50 kg. Bleeding is the most common and serious adverse reaction. Thrombocytopenia has also been reported, and therapy should be stopped if platelet count falls below 100,000 platelets per microliter. It should not be given for at least 6 to 8 hours after surgery and should be used with caution in conjunction with warfarin. Other side effects include anemia, increased wound drainage, postoperative hemorrhage, hematoma, confusion, urinary tract infection, hypotension, dizziness, and hypokalemia. There is no antidote for fondaparinux, and its effect cannot be measured by standard anticoagulant tests. Fondaparinux is given only by subcutaneous injection. Fondaparinux has a black box warning regarding potential spinal hematomas if the patient has an epidural catheter.

Pharmacokinetics: Fondaparinux

Route	Onset of Action	Peak Plasma Concentration	Elimination Half-life	Duration of Action
Subcut	2 hr	2-3 hr	17-21 hr	24 hr

◆!heparin

Heparin is a natural anticoagulant obtained from the lungs or intestinal mucosa of pigs. One brand name for some of the commonly used heparin products is Hep-Lock. This brand name refers only to small vials of heparin IV flush solutions used to maintain the patency of heparin-lock IV insertion sites. Because of the risk for the development of HIT, most health care institutions routinely use normal saline (0.9% sodium chloride) as a flush for heparin-lock IV ports and have moved away from using heparin flush solutions for this purpose. Heparin flushes are still used for central catheters. When used for flushing purposes, there is no need for monitoring.

Heparin is commonly used for DVT prophylaxis in a dose of 5000 units two or three times a day given subcutaneously, and it does not need to be monitored when used for prophylaxis. When heparin is used therapeutically (for treatment), it is given by continuous IV infusion. Most hospitals have weight-based protocols for heparin administration. Because the dosage is based on the patient's weight in kilograms, ensure that the appropriate weight is recorded and that only kilograms are used, and not pounds. A potential double-dose medication error can occur if pounds and kilograms are mixed. This is also true for enoxaparin, because it is dosed on body weight when used therapeutically. When heparin is given by IV infusion, monitoring by frequent measurement of aPTT (usually every 6 hours until therapeutic effects are seen) is necessary.

Other drugs that affect the coagulation cascade can have additive effects with heparin, which may lead to bleeding. Even though warfarin can cause additive effects, it is combined with IV heparin therapy. In fact, it is usually started within the first day or two of heparin infusion.

Heparin is available only in injectable form in multiple strengths ranging from 10 to 40,000 units/mL. The vials of different strengths of heparin are very similar and look very much alike. In fact, several newborns have died when a vial of more concentrated heparin was mistaken for a more dilute solution.

Take great care in checking and double-checking the concentration of heparin before administering it.

Pharmacokinetics: Heparin

Route	Onset of Action	Peak Plasma Concentration	Elimination Half-life	Duration of Action
IV	Immediate	Immediate	1-2 hr	Dependent on infusion duration
Subcut	20-30 min	2-4 hr	1-2 hr	8-12 hr

◆!rivaroxaban

Rivaroxaban (Xarelto) is the first oral factor Xa inhibitor. It is approved for prevention of strokes in patients with nonvalvular atrial fibrillation, postoperative thromboprophylaxis with knee and hip replacement surgery, and treatment of DVT and PE. Doses of rivaroxaban differ for each indication and must be adjusted for renal dysfunction. Contraindications include known drug allergy and active bleeding. All of the oral factor Xa inhibitors have black box warnings regarding potential spinal hematomas if the patient has an epidural catheter and regarding the risk for thrombosis if they are discontinued abruptly.

The most frequent adverse effects include peripheral edema, dizziness, headache, bruising, diarrhea, hematuria, and bleeding. Drug interactions include a decreased effect seen with phenytoin, carbamazepine, rifampin, and St. John's wort. An increased effect is seen with strong CYP3A4 inhibitors (amiodarone, erythromycin, ketoconazole, HIV drugs, diltiazem, verapamil) and grapefruit juice. Apixaban (Eliquis) and edoxaban (Savaysa) are similar drugs with similar drug interactions and side effects. No routine monitoring is required for either drug, and they may falsely elevate INR. Rivaroxaban or apixaban are not to be given with any other anticoagulant.

Pharmacokinetics: Rivaroxaban

Route	Onset of Action	Peak Plasma Concentration	Elimination Half-life	Duration of Action
PO	2 hr	2-4 hr	5-13 hr	NA

◆!warfarin

Warfarin sodium (Coumadin) is a pharmaceutical derivative of the natural plant anticoagulant known as *coumarin*. Warfarin is the most commonly prescribed oral anticoagulant and is available oral and IV; however, it is used almost exclusively in the oral form. Use of this drug requires careful monitoring of the prothrombin time/international normalized ratio (PT/INR), which is a standardized measure of the degree to which a patient's blood coagulability has been reduced by the drug. A normal INR (without warfarin) is 1 whereas a therapeutic INR (with warfarin) ranges from 2 to 3.5, depending on the indication for use of the drug (e.g., atrial fibrillation, thromboprevention, prosthetic heart valve). Patients older than 65 years of age may have a lower INR threshold for bleeding complications and may need to be monitored accordingly. Recently, it has been shown that about one third of patients receiving warfarin metabolize it differently than expected, based on variations in certain genes, *CYP2CP* and *VKORC1*. Genetic testing for these genes is helpful in determining the appropriate initial dosage of warfarin. The maintenance dosage is still determined by the INR.

Warfarin has significant interactions with many drugs, including amiodarone, fluconazole, erythromycin, metronidazole, sulfonamide antibiotics, and cimetidine. Although many more drugs can interact with warfarin, the aforementioned are by far the most common. Combining warfarin and amiodarone will lead to a 50% increase in the INR. When amiodarone is added to warfarin therapy, it is recommended that the warfarin dose be cut in half.

Because warfarin inhibits vitamin K–dependent clotting factors, foods that are high in vitamin K may reduce warfarin's ability to prevent clots. Common foods rich in vitamin K include leafy green vegetables (e.g., kale, spinach, collard greens). The most important aspect of these food-drug interactions is consistency in diet. Educate patients to maintain consistency in their intake of leafy green vegetables. Many patients are under the misconception that they must avoid all leafy green vegetables. However, this is not true. Once their maintenance warfarin dose is established, patients may still eat greens, but they need to be consistent in their intake of green vegetables, because increasing or decreasing their intake can affect the INR. Herbal products that interact with warfarin and result in increased risk for bleeding include dong quai, garlic, and ginkgo. St. John's wort decreases warfarin's effect.

Pharmacokinetics: Warfarin

Route	Onset of Action	Peak Plasma Concentration	Elimination Half-life	Duration of Action
PO	24-72 hr	4 hr	0.5-3 days	2-5 days

ANTIPLATELET DRUGS

Another class of coagulation modifiers that prevent clot formation is the antiplatelet drugs. Remember, the anticoagulants work in the clotting cascade. In contrast, antiplatelet drugs work to prevent platelet adhesion at the site of blood vessel injury, which actually occurs before the clotting cascade.

Platelets normally flow through blood vessels without adhering to their surfaces. Blood vessels can be injured by a disruption of blood flow, trauma, or the rupture of plaque from a vessel wall. When such events occur, substances such as collagen and fibronectin, which are present in the walls of blood vessels, become exposed. Collagen is a potent stimulator of platelet adhesion, as is a prevalent component of the platelet membranes called *glycoprotein IIb/IIIa (GP IIb/IIIa)*. Once platelet adhesion occurs, stimulators (adenosine diphosphate [ADP], thrombin, thromboxane A$_2$ [TXA$_2$], and prostaglandin H$_2$) are released from the activated platelets. These cause the platelets to *aggregate* (accumulate) at the site of injury. Once at the site of vessel injury, the platelets change shape and release their contents, which include ADP, serotonin, and platelet factor IV. The hemostatic function of these substances is twofold. First,

they act as platelet recruiters, attracting additional platelets to the site of injury; second, they are potent vasoconstrictors. Vasoconstriction limits blood flow to the damaged blood vessel to reduce blood loss. A platelet plug that has formed at a site of vessel injury is not stable and can be dislodged. The clotting cascade is then stimulated to form a more permanent *fibrin* plug (blood clot). The role of platelets and their relationship to the clotting cascade are illustrated in Figure 26-4.

Mechanism of Action and Drug Effects

Many of the antiplatelet drugs affect the *cyclooxygenase* pathway, which is one of the common final enzymatic pathways in the complex *arachidonic acid* pathway that operates within platelets and on blood vessel walls. This pathway, as it functions in both platelets and blood vessel walls, is illustrated in Figure 26-5.

Aspirin is widely used for its analgesic, antiinflammatory, and antipyretic (antifever) properties (see Chapter 44). Aspirin also has antiplatelet effects. Aspirin inhibits cyclooxygenase in the platelet irreversibly so that the platelet cannot regenerate this enzyme. Therefore, the effects of aspirin last the lifespan of a platelet, or 7 days. This irreversible inhibition of cyclooxygenase in the platelet prevents the formation of TXA$_2$, a substance that causes blood vessels to constrict and platelets to aggregate. Thus, by preventing TXA$_2$ formation, aspirin prevents these actions, which results in dilation of the blood vessels and prevention of platelets from aggregating or forming a clot.

Dipyridamole, another antiplatelet drug, also works to inhibit platelet aggregation by preventing the release of ADP, platelet factor IV, and TXA$_2$, all substances that stimulate platelets to aggregate or form a clot. Figure 26-4 shows how these substances accomplish this. Dipyridamole may also directly stimulate the release of prostacyclin and inhibit the formation of TXA$_2$ (see Figure 26-5).

Clopidogrel is a drug that belongs to the class of antiplatelet drugs called the *ADP inhibitors*. Its use has largely superseded that of the original ADP inhibitor ticlopidine. Its works by altering the platelet membrane so that it can no longer receive the signal to aggregate and form a clot. This signal is in the form of fibrinogen molecules, which attach to glycoprotein receptors (GP IIb/IIIa) on the surface of the platelet. Clopidogrel inhibits the activation of this receptor. The combination of aspirin and clopidogrel has been shown to be effective in patients with known cardiovascular disease, but not in patients who only have risk factors. Prasugrel (Effient) is a newer antiplatelet drug that is similar to clopidogrel and is used primarily after interventional cardiac procedures and for patients who do not respond to clopidogrel. Ticagrelor (Brilinta) is similar to clopidogrel and prasugrel. It is indicated for patients with acute coronary syndrome. It must be avoided in patients taking more than 100 mg of aspirin daily.

Pentoxifylline, another antiplatelet drug, is a methylxanthine derivative with properties similar to those of other methylxanthines, such as caffeine and theophylline (see Chapter 37). It was one of the earliest antiplatelet drugs but is now much less commonly used. It reduces the viscosity of blood by increasing the flexibility of red blood cells and reducing the aggregation of platelets. It is sometimes referred to as a *hemorheologic* drug,

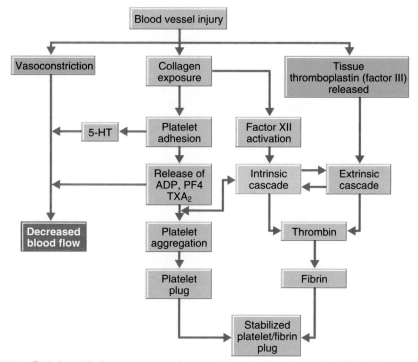

FIGURE 26-4 Relationship between platelets and the clotting cascade. *ADP,* Adenosine diphosphate; *5-HT,* serotonin; *PF4,* platelet factor IV; *TXA₂,* thromboxane A₂.

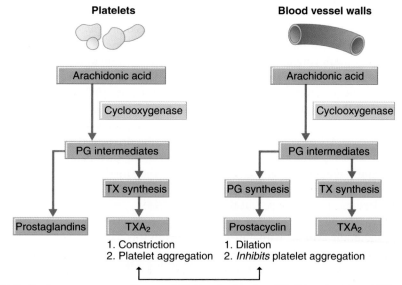

FIGURE 26-5 Cyclooxygenase pathway. *PG,* Prostaglandin; *TX,* thromboxane; *TXA₂,* thromboxane A₂.

or a drug that alters the fluid dynamics of the blood. The antiplatelet effects of pentoxifylline are attributed to its inhibition of ADP, serotonin, and platelet factor IV (see Figure 26-4). Pentoxifylline also stimulates the synthesis and release of prostacyclin from blood vessels (see Figure 26-5). In addition, it may have effects on the fibrinolytic system by raising the plasma concentrations of tissue plasminogen activator (see Figure 26-3).

Cilostazol is another antiplatelet drug, which works through inhibition of type 3 phosphodiesterase in the platelets and primarily lower-extremity blood vessels. Its effects are to reduce platelet aggregation and promote vasodilation.

In 2014, the FDA approved vorapaxar (Zontivity), a novel antiplatelet drug and the first in its class. Vorapaxar is an antagonist of protease-activated receptor-1 (PAR-1), which inhibits the action of thrombin on the platelet.

The final class of antiplatelet drugs is the GP IIb/IIIa inhibitors. They work by blocking the receptor protein by the same name that occurs in the platelet wall membranes. This protein plays a role in promoting the aggregation of platelets in preparation for fibrin clot formation. There are currently three available drugs in this class: tirofiban (Aggrastat), eptifibatide (Integrilin), and abciximab (ReoPro). The GP IIb/IIIa inhibitors are available only for IV infusion.

Indications

The therapeutic effects of the antiplatelet drugs depend on the particular drug. Aspirin is officially recommended for stroke prevention by the American Stroke Society in daily doses of 50 to 325 mg. (However, in clinical practice, dosages may vary.) Clopidogrel and others in its class are given to reduce the risk for thrombotic stroke, and for prophylaxis against transient ischemic attacks (TIAs), as well for post-MI prevention of thrombosis. Dipyridamole is used to decrease platelet aggregation in various other thromboembolic disorders. The GP IIb/IIIa inhibitors are used to treat acute unstable angina and MI, and are given during percutaneous coronary intervention procedures, such as angioplasty. Their purpose is to prevent the formation of thrombi. This is known as *thromboprevention*. This treatment approach is based on the fact that *prevention* of thrombus formation is easier and less risky overall from a pharmacologic standpoint than is lysing a formed thrombus. Pentoxifylline is indicated for peripheral vascular disease, whereas cilostazol is indicated specifically for *intermittent claudication* (pain and cramping in the calf muscles associated with walking). Cilostazol has been shown to be superior to pentoxifylline in improving exercise tolerance in older adult patients.

Vorapaxar (Zontivity), a novel antiplatelet drug and the first in its class, is an antagonist of protease-activated receptor-1 (PAR-1), which inhibits the action of thrombin on the platelet. It is indicated to reduce thrombotic cardiovascular events, MI, and stroke in patients with a history of MI or with peripheral arterial disease. It is available as a 2.08-mg tablet and is given once daily in combination with aspirin and/or clopidogrel. It is contraindicated in patients with history of stroke, TIA, intracranial hemorrhage, and active bleeding. The major risk of this drug is bleeding, and it is not recommended for patients with hepatic or renal impairment. It should be avoided with anticoagulants, NSAIDS, and strong inhibitors or inducers of CYP3A4 (see Chapter 2). Other side effects include depression, skin rash, and anemia. It is classified as a pregnancy category B drug.

Contraindications

Contraindications to the use of antiplatelet drugs include known drug allergy to a specific product, thrombocytopenia, active bleeding, leukemia, traumatic injury, gastrointestinal ulcer, vitamin K deficiency, and recent stroke.

Adverse Effects

The potential adverse effects of the various antiplatelet drugs can be serious, and they all pose a risk for inducing a serious bleeding episode. The most common adverse effects are listed in Table 26-4.

TABLE 26-4 **Selected Antiplatelet Drugs: Adverse Effects**

Body System	Adverse Effects
Aspirin	
Central nervous	Drowsiness, dizziness, confusion, flushing
Gastrointestinal	Nausea, vomiting, gastrointestinal bleeding
Hematologic	Thrombocytopenia, agranulocytosis, leukopenia, neutropenia, hemolytic anemia, bleeding
Clopidogrel	
Cardiovascular	Chest pain, edema
Central nervous	Flulike symptoms, headache, dizziness, fatigue
Gastrointestinal	Abdominal pain, diarrhea, nausea
Miscellaneous	Epistaxis, rash, and pruritus (itching)
Glycoprotein IIb/IIIa Inhibitors	
Cardiovascular	Bradycardia, hypotension, edema
Central nervous	Dizziness
Hematologic	Bleeding, thrombocytopenia

Interactions

The use of dipyridamole with clopidogrel, aspirin, and/or other nonsteroidal antiinflammatory drugs (NSAIDs) produces additive antiplatelet activity and increased bleeding potential. The combined use of steroids or nonaspirin NSAIDs with aspirin can increase the ulcerogenic effects of aspirin. The combined use of aspirin and heparin with GP IIb/IIIa inhibitors also further enhances antiplatelet activity and increases the likelihood of a serious bleeding episode. In spite of all of these interactions, it is not uncommon to see patients taking daily maintenance doses of aspirin for thrombopreventive purposes, sometimes in combination with other antiplatelet drugs. The most commonly used dose is the "baby aspirin" dose of 81 mg (the standard adult dose is 325 mg). Even though GP IIb/IIIa and heparin have additive therapeutic effects when given concurrently and are listed as interacting drugs, it is very common to see both used together. However, the therapeutic goal of heparin, and thus the dose, is lower when used with a GP IIb/IIIa inhibitor.

Dosages

For dosage information on selected antiplatelet drugs, see the table on this page.

DRUG PROFILES

Antiplatelet drugs are extremely useful in the management of thromboembolic disorders. Each has unique pharmacologic properties, and therefore they all are somewhat different from one another.

♦ aspirin

Aspirin is available in many combinations with other prescription and nonprescription drugs and goes by many product names. One unique contraindication for aspirin is flulike symptoms in children and teenagers. The use of aspirin in this situation is associated with the occurrence of Reye's syndrome, a rare, acute, and sometimes fatal condition involving hepatic and central nervous system damage (see Chapter 44). There is also

DOSAGES

Selected Antiplatelet Drugs

Drug (Pregnancy Category)	Pharmacologic Class	Usual Adult Dosage Range	Indications/Uses
◆ aspirin (C/D)	Salicylate antiplatelet	PO: 81-325 mg once daily	MI prophylaxis
		PO: 50-325 mg once daily	TIA prophylaxis
◆ clopidogrel (Plavix) (B)	ADP inhibitor	PO: 75 mg once daily	Reduction of atherosclerotic events; acute coronary syndrome without ST segment elevation
◆!eptifibatide (Integrilin) (B)*	GP IIb/IIIa inhibitor	IV: Single bolus followed by continuous infusion	Unstable angina, MI, percutaneous coronary procedures

ADP, Adenosine diphosphate; *GP*, glycoprotein; *MI*, myocardial infarction; *TIA*, transient ischemic attack.
*See table in package insert for specific dose.

allergic cross-reactivity between aspirin and other NSAIDs. Patients with documented aspirin allergy must not receive NSAIDs. Aspirin is available in both oral and rectal forms. A combination form of aspirin and dipyridamole (Aggrenox) is used for antiplatelet purposes.

Pharmacokinetics: Aspirin

Route	Onset of Action	Peak Plasma Concentration	Elimination Half-life	Duration of Action
PO	15-30 min	0.25-2 hr	2-3 hr	4-6 hr

◆ clopidogrel

Clopidogrel (Plavix) is currently the most widely used ADP inhibitor on the market. It is available only for oral use. Prasugrel (Effient) and ticagrelor (Brilinta) are similar to clopidogrel. Clopidogrel has a black box warning for patients with certain genetic abnormalities, who may have a higher rate of cardiovascular events due to reduced conversion to its active metabolite. Clopidogrel's effectiveness may be reduced by amiodarone, calcium channel blockers, NSAIDS, and proton pump inhibitors (see Chapter 50).

Pharmacokinetics: Clopidogrel

Route	Onset of Action	Peak Plasma Concentration	Elimination Half-life	Duration of Action
PO	1-2 hr	1 hr	8 hr	7-10 days

◆!eptifibatide

Eptifibatide (Integrilin) is a GP IIb/IIIa inhibitor, along with tirofiban (Aggrastat) and abciximab (ReoPro). These drugs are usually administered in intensive care or cardiac catheterization laboratory settings, where continuous cardiovascular monitoring is the norm. All are available only for IV use.

Pharmacokinetics: Eptifibatide

Route	Onset of Action	Peak Plasma Concentration	Elimination Half-life	Duration of Action
IV	1 hr	Unknown	2-2.5 hr	4 hr

THROMBOLYTIC DRUGS

Thrombolytics are coagulation modifiers that lyse thrombi in the blood vessels that supply the heart with blood, the coronary arteries. This reestablishes blood flow to the blood-starved heart muscle. If the blood flow is reestablished early, the heart muscle and left ventricular function can be saved. If blood flow is not reestablished early, the affected area of the heart muscle becomes ischemic, and eventually necrotic and nonfunctional.

Thrombolytic therapy made its debut in 1933 when a substance that broke down fibrin clots was isolated from a patient's blood. This substance was found to be produced by *beta-hemolytic streptococci (group A)*, and the substance was eventually called *streptokinase*.

Streptokinase was first used in 1947 to dissolve a clotted hemothorax, but it was not until 1958 that it was given to a patient with an acute MI. In 1960, a naturally occurring human plasminogen activator called *urokinase,* became available. In the 1980s, the underlying cause of acute MI was determined to be due to coronary artery occlusion. This marked the start of rapid growth in the use of thrombolytic drugs for the early treatment of acute MI. Since that time, several new thrombolytics have become available for this and other clinical uses. Several large landmark thrombolytic research studies showed that early thrombolytic therapy could bring about a 50% reduction in mortality, a reduction in the infarct size, an improvement in left ventricular function, and a reduction in the incidence and severity of congestive heart failure. However, the use of thrombolytics has almost completely been replaced by interventional cardiologic procedures, such as percutaneous coronary intervention. Thrombolytics are still a viable option in hospitals that do not offer percutaneous coronary intervention. Currently available thrombolytic drugs include t-PAs (anistreplase [Eminase], alteplase [Activase], reteplase [Retavase], and tenecteplase [TNKase]). For dosage information on thrombolytics, see the table on the next page.

Mechanism of Action and Drug Effects

There is a fine balance between the formation and dissolution of a clot. The coagulation system is responsible for forming clots, whereas the fibrinolytic system is responsible for dissolving clots. The natural fibrinolytic system within the blood takes several days to break down a clot (thrombus). This is of little value in the case of a clotted blood vessel that supplies blood to the heart muscle. Thrombolytics accomplish this by activating the conversion of plasminogen to plasmin, which breaks down, or lyses, the thrombus (see Figure 26-3). Plasmin is a proteolytic enzyme, which means that it breaks down proteins. It is a relatively nonspecific enzyme that is capable of degrading proteins such as fibrin, fibrinogen, and other procoagulant proteins like factors V, VIII, and XII. In other words, the substances that form clots are destroyed by plasmin. Essentially, thrombolytic drugs work by mimicking the body's own process of clot destruction. Although the individual thrombolytic drugs are somewhat diverse in their actions, they all have this common result.

Streptokinase, the original thrombolytic enzyme, and the naturally occurring urokinase have been removed from the U.S. market, primarily due to their adverse effects—namely, they were not fibrin specific. The newer thrombolytics have chemical specificity for fibrin threads (fibrin specificity) and work primarily at the site of a clot. They still carry some bleeding risk, but much less than that of the thrombolytic enzymes.

Tissue plasminogen activator is a naturally occurring plasminogen activator secreted by vascular endothelial cells (the walls of blood vessels). The amount secreted naturally is not sufficient to dissolve a coronary thrombus quickly enough to restore circulation to the heart and save the heart muscle. Recombinant DNA techniques are now used to produce t-PA, and thus it can be administered in quantities sufficient to dissolve a coronary thrombus quickly. It is fibrin specific (clot specific); that is, only the fibrin clot stimulates t-PA to convert plasminogen to plasmin. Therefore, it has a lower propensity to induce a systemic thrombolytic state, compared to the thrombolytic enzymes.

Indications

The purpose of all the thrombolytic drugs is to activate the conversion of plasminogen to plasmin, the enzyme that breaks down a thrombus. The presence of a thrombus that interferes significantly with normal blood flow on either the venous or the arterial side of the circulation is an indication for the use of thrombolytic therapy. The indications for thrombolytic therapy

include acute MI, arterial thrombosis, DVT, occlusion of shunts or catheters, pulmonary embolism, and acute ischemic stroke.

Contraindications

Contraindications to the use of thrombolytic drugs include known drug allergy to the specific product and any preservatives, and concurrent use of other drugs that alter clotting.

Adverse Effects

The most common undesirable effect of thrombolytic therapy is internal, intracranial, and superficial bleeding. Other problems include hypersensitivity, anaphylactoid reactions, nausea, vomiting, and hypotension. These drugs can also induce cardiac dysrhythmias.

Toxicity and Management of Overdose

Acute toxicity primarily causes an extension of the adverse effects of the thrombolytic drug. Treatment is symptomatic and supportive, because thrombolytic drugs have a relatively short half-life and no specific antidotes.

Interactions

The most common effect of drug interactions is an increased bleeding tendency resulting from the concurrent use of anticoagulants, antiplatelets, or other drugs that affect platelet function.

A laboratory test interaction that can occur with thrombolytic drugs is a reduction in the plasminogen and fibrinogen levels.

Dosages

For dosage information on alteplase, see the table on this page.

DRUG PROFILE

All thrombolytic drugs exert their effects by activating plasminogen and converting it to plasmin, which is capable of digesting fibrin, a major component of clots.

♦!alteplase

Alteplase (Activase) is a pharmaceutically available t-PA made through recombinant DNA techniques. It is fibrin specific and therefore does not produce a systemic lytic state. In addition, because it is present in the human body in a natural state, its

DOSAGES

Selected Thrombolytic Drugs

Drug (Pregnancy Category)	Pharmacologic Class	Usual Adult Dosage Range	Indications
♦!alteplase (Activase) (C)	Tissue plasminogen activator	IV: For adults >67 kg: 100 mg over 90 min given as a 15-mg IV bolus, then 50 mg over 30 min, then 35 mg over 60 min	Acute myocardial infarction
		IV: 0.9 mg/kg (total dose not to exceed 90 mg); 10% given as an IV bolus over 1 min, remainder over 60 min; must be given within 3 hr of onset of symptoms	Acute ischemic stroke

administration for therapeutic use does not induce an antigen-antibody reaction. Therefore, it can be re-administered immediately in the event of reinfarction. The drug t-PA has a very short half-life of 5 minutes. It is believed to open the clogged artery rapidly, but its action is short-lived. Therefore, it is given with heparin to prevent reocclusion of the affected blood vessel. Alteplase is available only in parenteral form. There is also a smaller dosage form known as Cathflo Activase that is used to flush clogged IV or arterial lines. Tenecteplase (TNKase) is a newer form of alteplase that is given by IV push after MI. Alteplase is also used for ischemic stroke.

Pharmacokinetics: Alteplase

Route	Onset of Action	Peak Plasma Concentration	Elimination Half-life	Duration of Action
IV	30 min	60 min	26-50 min	Dependent on infusion duration

ANTIFIBRINOLYTIC DRUGS

The individual antifibrinolytic drugs have varying mechanisms of action, but all prevent the lysis of fibrin. Fibrin is the substance that helps make a platelet plug insoluble and anchors the clot to the damaged blood vessel (see Figures 26-1 and 26-2). The term *antifibrinolytic* refers to what these drugs do, which is to prevent the lysis of fibrin; in doing so, they actually *promote* clot formation. For this reason, they are also called *hemostatic* drugs. Their effects are opposite to those of anticoagulant and antiplatelet drugs, which *prevent* clot formation. Three synthetic antifibrinolytics are available—aminocaproic acid, tranexamic acid, and desmopressin. Dosages, indications, and other information appear in the associated dosages table. There are also hemostatic drugs that are used *topically* (on the skin or tissue surface) in surgical settings to stop excessive bleeding. These include topical thrombin, microfibrillar collagen, absorbable gelatin, and oxidized cellulose.

Although not technically antifibrinolytic drugs, there are three drugs used for the treatment of hemophilia. These are produced by recombinant DNA technology, which eliminates the risk associated with obtaining them from human blood. Products currently available include rVII, rVIII, and rIX. As mentioned earlier, factors VII, VIII, and IX are important in the coagulation pathway. Warfarin also inhibits these factors. These products are used in patients with hemophilia and are also used in patients with severe bleeding due to warfarin therapy.

Mechanism of Action and Drug Effects

The antifibrinolytic drugs vary in several ways. The various antifibrinolytic drugs and their proposed mechanisms of action are described in Table 26-5.

The drug effects of the antifibrinolytics are very specific and limited. They do not have many effects outside of their hematologic ones. Aminocaproic acid and tranexamic acid inhibit the breakdown of fibrin, which prevents the destruction of the formed platelet clot. Desmopressin causes a dose-dependent increase in the concentration of plasma factor VIII

TABLE 26-5   Antifibrinolytics: Mechanisms of Action

Antifibrinolytic Drug	Mechanism of Action
aminocaproic acid (Amicar) and tranexamic acid (Cyklokapron)	Form a reversible complex with plasminogen and plasmin. By binding to the lysine-binding site of plasminogen, these drugs displace plasminogen from the surface of fibrin. This prevents plasmin from lysing the fibrin clot. Therefore, these drugs can work only if a clot has formed.
desmopressin (DDAVP)	Works by increasing the level of factor VII (von Willebrand factor), which anchors platelets to damaged vessels via the glycoprotein Ib platelet receptor. It appears that desmopressin acts as a general endothelial stimulant, promoting the release of factor VIII, prostaglandin I2, and plasminogen activator.

(von Willebrand factor), along with an increase in the plasma concentration of tissue plasminogen activator. The overall effect of this is increased platelet aggregation and clot formation. This drug is also an analogue of antidiuretic hormone and is discussed further in Chapter 30.

Indications

Antifibrinolytics are useful in both the prevention and treatment of excessive bleeding resulting from systemic hyperfibrinolysis or surgical complications. They have also proved successful in arresting excessive oozing from surgical sites such as chest tubes as well as in reducing the total blood loss and the duration of bleeding in the postoperative period.

Desmopressin may also be used in patients who have hemophilia A or type I von Willebrand disease. Recombinant factors VII, VIII, and IX are used to treat hemophilia or to stop the bleeding from excessive warfarin therapy.

Contraindications

Contraindications to the use of antifibrinolytic drugs include known drug allergy to a specific product and disseminated intravascular coagulation, which could be worsened by these drugs.

Adverse Effects

The adverse effects of antifibrinolytic drugs occur uncommonly and are mild. However, there have been rare reports of these drugs causing thrombotic events, such as acute cerebrovascular thrombosis and acute MI. The common adverse effects of antifibrinolytics are listed in Table 26-6.

Interactions

When drugs such as estrogens or oral contraceptives are used concurrently with aminocaproic acid or tranexamic acid, additive effects may occur, resulting in increased coagulation. Few specific interactions have been reported for desmopressin,

TABLE 26-6   Antifibrinolytics: Adverse Effects

Body System	Adverse Effects
Cardiovascular	Dysrhythmias, orthostatic hypotension, bradycardia
Central nervous	Headache, dizziness, fatigue, hallucinations, convulsions
Gastrointestinal	Nausea, vomiting, abdominal cramps, diarrhea

although use caution when giving to patients receiving lithium, large doses of epinephrine, heparin, or alcohol. Drugs such as chlorpropamide and fludrocortisone may potentiate the antidiuretic response, which may lead to edema.

Dosages

For dosage information on aminocaproic acid and desmopressin, see the table on this page.

DRUG PROFILES

aminocaproic acid

Aminocaproic acid (Amicar) is a synthetic antifibrinolytic drug used to prevent and control the excessive bleeding that can result from surgery or overactivity of the fibrinolytic system. It is available in both oral and parenteral preparations.

Pharmacokinetics: Aminocaproic Acid

Route	Onset of Action	Peak Plasma Concentration	Elimination Half-life	Duration of Action
IV	Unknown	1.2 hr	2 hr	3 hr

desmopressin

Desmopressin (DDAVP) is a synthetic polypeptide. It is structurally very similar to vasopressin, which is antidiuretic hormone, the natural human posterior pituitary hormone (see Chapter 30). Because of these physical characteristics, it is most often used to increase the resorption of water by the collecting ducts in the kidneys to prevent or control polydipsia, polyuria, and dehydration in patients with diabetes insipidus due to a deficiency of endogenous posterior pituitary vasopressin or in patients with polyuria and polydipsia resulting from trauma or surgery in the pituitary region.

Desmopressin also causes a dose-dependent increase in plasma factor VIII (von Willebrand factor), along with an increase in tissue plasminogen activator, which results in increased platelet aggregation and clot formation; thus it is often used to stop bleeding. Desmopressin is contraindicated in patients with a known hypersensitivity to it and in those with nephrogenic diabetes insipidus. It is available in both injectable and intranasal dosage forms. Desmopressin nasal spray is used for primary nocturnal enuresis.

Pharmacokinetics: Desmopressin

Route	Onset of Action	Peak Plasma Concentration	Elimination Half-life	Duration of Action
IV	15-30 min	1-2 hr	2 hr	Unknown

NURSING PROCESS

Coagulation modifiers have a variety of uses, including the following: (1) prevention or elimination of clotting in a peripherally inserted catheter (PIC, or PICC—a peripherally inserted central catheter), (2) maintenance of patency (without clotting) of central venous catheters, (3) clot prevention in coronary artery bypass grafting, (4) prevention of clotting after major vessel injury, (5) treatment of thrombophlebitis to prevent venous and/or arterial thromboembolism, and (6) prevention of clotting with use of prosthetics (e.g., heart valve replacements) and in atrial fibrillation. The drugs that are used for these different indications are varied in their mechanisms of action, and the related general and specific nursing process issues will be discussed.

ASSESSMENT

A thorough nursing assessment and health history must be initiated before the use of all *coagulation-modifying* drugs. This includes the following: any drug or food allergies, current and past medical issues as well as any underlying systemic or autoimmune disease processes, family health history, dietary habits, changes in body weight, ability to perform activities of daily living, level of exercise and/or degree of sedentary lifestyle, exercise tolerance, employment activities, success of previous treatment regimens, blood pressure, pulse rate, respirations, body

DOSAGES

Selected Antifibrinolytic Drugs

Drug (Pregnancy Category)	Pharmacologic Class	Usual Adult Dosage Range	Indications/Uses
aminocaproic acid (Amicar) (C)	Hemostatic	IV infusion: 4-5 g during first hour, then 1 g at 1-hr intervals up to a daily max of 30 g	Excessive bleeding caused by systemic hyperfibrinolysis or urinary fibrinolysis
desmopressin (DDAVP) (B)	Synthetic posterior pituitary hormone	IV: 0.3 mcg/kg infused over 15-30 min; preoperative use: drug is administered 30 min before surgery	Surgical and postoperative hemostasis and management of bleeding in patients with hemophilia A or type I von Willebrand disease

weight, height, dietary intake, and fluid intake. A medication history is also needed and must include a listing of all drugs the patient takes on a daily or other routine basis such as prescription drugs, over-the-counter medications, herbal products, dietary supplements, and intake of nicotine, alcohol, and illegal substances. Perform a thorough patient assessment to also identify the presence of the following risk factors for clot development: immobility; history of limited activity or prolonged bed rest (e.g., generally for longer than 3 to 5 days); dehydration; obesity; smoking; congestive heart failure; mitral or aortic stenosis; coronary heart disease with documented atherosclerosis or arteriosclerosis; peripheral vascular disease; pelvic, gynecologic-genitourinary, abdominal, orthopedic, or vascular major surgery; heart valve incompetency and/or replacement; history of thrombophlebitis, deep vein thrombosis (DVT), or thromboembolism, including pulmonary embolism, myocardial infarct, and atrial fibrillation; edema of the periphery; trauma to the lower extremities; use of oral contraceptives; and/or recent extended airline travel time. If the patient has a history of clotting disorders and/or thromboembolism, assess and document the following: presenting signs and symptoms of thrombophlebitis of the leg such as calf edema; pain, warmth, or redness directly over the vessel (more indicative of a superficial clot); increased diameter of the calf of the affected leg; pain upon gentle compression of the calf muscle against the tibial bone; and presenting signs and symptoms of pulmonary embolism such as chest pain, cough, dyspnea, tachypnea, drop in oxygen saturation (by oximetry or blood gas measurement), hemoptysis, tachycardia, drop in blood pressure, and possible shock. The use of Homan's sign is no longer recommended for assessment/evaluation of DVT of the leg due to its lack of reliability. All contraindications, cautions, and drug interactions also need to be assessed (see pharmacology discussion) and documented. The health care provider will order specific diagnostic testing if DVT is suspected.

Because of the effects of *anticoagulants,* it is also important to assess the skin, oral mucous membranes, gums, urine, and stool for any evidence of bleeding. Assess for any blood in the urine or stool, easy bruising, excessive bleeding from toothbrushing or shaving, or unexplained nosebleeds while receiving these medications. Laboratory tests performed before and during therapy with these drugs usually include, but are not limited to, baseline complete blood counts, hemoglobin level, hematocrit, lipoprotein fractionation, triglyceride and cholesterol levels, various clotting studies, and liver function tests. The serum laboratory tests that are usually ordered with anticoagulant therapy are presented in the Safety: Laboratory Values Related to Drug Therapy box.

With *heparin* and *LMWHs,* it is critical to patient safety to continually assess the skin to identify potential subcutaneous injection sites. For these injection sites, *avoid* any area within 2 inches of the umbilicus, open wounds, scars, open or abraded areas, incisions, drainage tubes, stomas, or areas of bruising or oozing. These sites would be at higher risk for further tissue damage with injection of the anticoagulant. Appropriate sites for injection of subcutaneous heparin and LMWHs include the upper, outer area of the arms, the thigh, and the subcutaneous fatty area across the lower abdomen and between the iliac crests (see Chapter 9 for more information).

With use of the *parenteral anticoagulant heparin,* to ensure patient safety and prevent injury, assess for allergies, contraindications, cautions, and drug interactions (see pharmacology discussion). Severe hypertension, ulcer disease, ulcerative colitis, aneurysms, malignant hypertension, alcoholism, and head injuries are all conditions in which a bleed is potential and possibly precipitated by parenteral anticoagulation. An important caution for heparin use is pregnancy or lactation; however, if there is a need for an anticoagulant during pregnancy, heparin is the drug of choice, not *warfarin.* Other information is presented in Table 26-1.

It is crucial to patient safety to remember that heparin is *not* interchangeable unit for unit with drugs in another class of anticoagulants, the LMWHs. It is important to know that heparin sodium contains benzyl alcohol; therefore, assess for allergy to this additional component. Although the use of *LMWHs* leads to fewer adverse reactions in some patients, these drugs are still associated with specific contraindications, cautions, and drug interactions (see previous discussion). When assessing the medication profile, remember that a potentially deadly medication error is to give heparin in combination with *enoxaparin* (or any LMWH). Always double-check that enoxaparin and heparin are *never* given to the patient simultaneously! The same assessment parameters discussed earlier for heparin are also appropriate for LMWHs. In addition, LMWHs contain sulfites and benzyl alcohol, and so assess the patient for allergies to these substances. It is important to note again that the LMWHs differ from standard heparin and also from each other and, for this reason, they are not interchangeable. LMWHs may be used for outpatient anticoagulant therapy because these drugs usually require less close monitoring than standard heparin. Assess the results of clotting studies prior to therapy.

The *oral anticoagulant warfarin* and its related contraindications, cautions, and drug interactions have been discussed earlier in this chapter. All of the previously mentioned assessment parameters are also applicable to warfarin. Because of the drug's action, withdraw warfarin (as with all drugs altering bleeding/clotting)—as ordered—before the patient undergoes any dental procedures or if there is any evidence of tissue necrosis, gangrene, diarrhea, intestinal flora imbalances, or steatorrhea. Important to emphasize with this drug is the fact that warfarin is indicated for prophylaxis and long-term treatment of a variety of thromboembolic disorders (see previous pharmacology discussion), and constant and skillful assessment of the patient and clotting results is required. Most prescribers use standard protocols for warfarin to assist in dosing the drug based on PT/INR (the standardized measures of blood coagulability). The most common starting dosage is 5 mg daily. However, the dose can range from 1 to 10 mg, depending on individual patient response. In most situations, the dosage for adults is between 1 and 5 mg orally every day. In addition, it is important to understand the pharmacokinetics of warfarin, because if a patient is placed on IV heparin and warfarin has been prescribed, it takes several days for the warfarin to have a therapeutic effect (see drug profile). Current recommendations are to continue overlap therapy of the heparin and warfarin for at least 5 days; the heparin is stopped after 5 days when the INR is above 2.

The new oral-acting *factor Xa inhibitors, rivaroxaban (Xarelto)* and *apixaban (Eliquis)*, carry the same assessment information as stated with other *anticoagulants*. Make sure to assess contraindications, cautions, and drug interactions (see the pharmacology discussion). A specific concern is to avoid the concurrent administration of these drugs with *heparin, LMWH,* and other *anticoagulants*.

Dabigatran (Pradaxa), although an anticoagulant, is the first oral *direct thrombin inhibitor*. Additional assessment parameters include renal function studies. No coagulation monitoring is needed for this drug. Assess for drug interactions with phenytoin and amiodarone. With *fondaparinux (Arixtra)*, carefully assess renal function. As with dabigatran, its effect cannot be measured by standard anticoagulant tests. Liver function tests need to be assessed prior to the use of *argatroban*.

With *antiplatelet* drugs, obtain a thorough nursing history, medication history, and physical assessment before beginning drug therapy. Possible drug interactions, cautions, and contraindications have been discussed, but close assessment of any bleeding is most important to patient safety. Because *aspirin, NSAIDs,* and other *antiplatelet drugs* alter bleeding times, withhold these drugs as ordered for 5 to 7 days before the patient undergoes surgical procedures. Specific guidelines are generally given by the prescriber to avoid the concurrent use of other *anticoagulants, antiplatelets,* and *fibrinolytics*. See Chapter 44 for more information on aspirin. Perform a baseline cardiovascular assessment with *clopidogrel*, and document any preexisting chest pain, edema, headache, dizziness, epistaxis, or flulike symptoms. Laboratory values usually include complete blood count, hemoglobin level and hematocrit, platelet counts, and PT and INR values. These laboratory values provide baseline levels with which therapy values can be compared. If platelet counts are at or fall below 80,000 cells/mm^3, notify the prescriber; antiplatelet therapy most likely will not be initiated (or will be discontinued).

In addition, it is important to patient safety to reemphasize the fact that aspirin is not to be used in children and teenagers, in patients with any bleeding disorder, in pregnant or lactating women, or in patients with vitamin K deficiency or peptic ulcer disease. These are situations in which major consequences could occur if *aspirin* were used; for example, Reye's syndrome in children and teenagers, teratogenic effects in pregnant women, and ulcers or bleeding tendencies in patients with vitamin K deficiency or peptic ulcer disease. Know how each drug works in the body so that a sound knowledge base exists for critical thinking and decision making; for example, the decision to call the prescriber and not to administer two antiplatelet drugs at the same time or not to give a *thrombolytic drug* with heparin, warfarin, aspirin, or NSAIDs. This type of critical drug information is very important to make sure the patient receives the safest and most appropriate care during all phases of the nursing process.

One of the newer *antiplatelet drugs, vorapaxar (Zontivity)*, inhibits the action of thrombin on the platelet and is contraindicated in those with a history of stroke, TIA, intracranial hemorrhage, and active bleeding. These conditions must be assessed for prior to administering the drug. Additionally, assess hepatic and renal functioning because it is also contraindicated in these patients. Perform a thorough medication profile because *vorapaxar* is not to be used with drugs that are strong inhibitors/inducers of CYP3A4 (see Chapter 2) and must be avoided with concurrent use of NSAIDs and *anticoagulants*.

The *GP IIb/IIIa inhibitors* (e.g., *eptifibatide, tirofiban, abciximab*) require the same baseline assessment information (e.g., vital signs, medical history, history of chest pain or cardiac disease, complete blood counts, hemoglobin level, hematocrit, renal function tests, platelet counts) as well as assessment for any edema, bradycardia, and/or leg pain. Before or during therapy, if the platelet count is below 90,000/mm^3, contact the prescriber for further orders.

Thrombolytics require similar assessments, including attention to baseline complete blood counts and results of clotting studies. Additional concerns include a history of hypotension and cardiac dysrhythmias. The use of *alteplase* and other thrombolytics always carries major concerns/cautions, contraindications, and drug interactions (see previous pharmacology discussion). Constantly assess any arterial punctures, venous cut-down sites, peripherally inserted central catheter sites, and central infusion ports or sites for bleeding. Do not use IM injections in any situation, as they pose problems with bleeding. As with any drugs that alter clotting and platelet activity, the thrombolytics are associated with the risk for bleeding from wounds or from the gastrointestinal, genitourinary, or respiratory tract, so assess any drainage, urine, stool, emesis, sputum, and secretions for the presence of blood.

Antifibrinolytics require the same skillful assessment of baseline parameters and laboratory testing; however, there are additional concerns for patients with dysrhythmias, hypotension, bradycardia, convulsive disorders, nausea, vomiting, abdominal pain, and diarrhea. These are possible adverse effects and situations in which the prescriber may need to decrease the dosage of medication.

NURSING DIAGNOSES

1. Deficient knowledge related to the new medication regimen and the need for altered lifestyle
2. Risk for ineffective cerebral tissue perfusion related to the clotting disorder, such as thrombus and subsequent embolus formation
3. Risk for injury related to possible adverse reactions to drugs altering blood clotting

PLANNING: OUTCOME IDENTIFICATION

1. Patient demonstrates adequate knowledge regarding medication therapy and its potential adverse effects as well as the need for lifestyle changes.

2. Patient exhibits improved blood flow/tissue perfusion as a result of the therapeutic effects of the anticoagulant with intact alertness, orientation, and stable neurologic status.

3. Patient remains free from injury such as bleeding and bruising resulting from the medication being taken.

IMPLEMENTATION

Routinely monitor vital signs, heart sounds, peripheral pulses, and neurologic status in all patients before, during, and immediately after *anticoagulant therapy*. The various laboratory values to be monitored are presented in the Safety: Laboratory Values Related to Drug Therapy box. If there is any change in pulse rate or rhythm, blood pressure, or level of consciousness, and/or unexplained restlessness occurs, contact the prescriber immediately. These changes may indicate bleeding or hemorrhage.

Knowledge of the proper techniques of administration is crucial for the safe and effective use of *heparin* and the *LMWHs* (see Box 26-1 for other dosing and route information). *Heparin* may be given by the subcutaneous or IV routes, but *not* IM. You can easily avoid inadvertent IM injection if you use only subcutaneous syringes to withdraw and administer the heparin.

The 25- to 28-gauge, ½-inch (1.5 cm) needle is often prepackaged with the syringe. No major harm would result if a subcutaneous dose were inadvertently administered IV. If rapid anticoagulation is needed, IV heparin by continuous or intermittent infusion may be prescribed. Whether the drug is given by IV infusion or subcutaneous injection, monitor daily clotting study results, and perform these studies as ordered for therapeutic doses (monitoring is not done for prophylactic treatment).

The drug effects of heparin can be reversed with the IV administration of protamine sulfate. With subcutaneous heparin, several doses of protamine sulfate may be needed to reverse the anticoagulant effect because of the variable rates of absorption of this dosage form. See Box 26-1 for the procedure for intermittent or continuous IV administration of heparin.

Administer *LMWHs* by subcutaneous injection deep into the injection site (see previous discussion) using the same techniques as for heparin. Rotate sites frequently. Avoid aspiration with subcutaneous injections to prevent hematoma formation and tissue injury. To avoid bruising, do not massage the site after the injection. Prefilled syringes of LMWHs are available for inpatient use and for at-home treatment. See Chapter 9 for detailed information about administering subcutaneous

---

BOX 26-1 Anticoagulation Therapy and Related Nursing Considerations

Subcutaneous Heparin and Low–Molecular-Weight Heparin Injections

- After thoroughly checking the prescriber's order, assess the patient for any allergies, contraindications, cautions, or drug interactions.
- Always begin by performing hand hygiene, and maintain Standard Precautions. Gloves must be worn. Prefilled syringes are available. When the medication is not available in a prefilled or premeasured syringe, use a ½- to ⅝-inch, 25- to 28-gauge needle. Check the site for bleeding or bruising, and *do not massage/ rub the site* before or after the injection. *Do not aspirate* before injecting to prevent hematoma formation. See Chapter 9 for more information on the technique associated with heparin and LMWH injections.
- Make sure the patient is comfortable, and then remove gloves and wash hands. Document the medication given on the medication record, and monitor the patient for a therapeutic response as well as for adverse reactions.

Intravenous Heparin Administration

- Always double-check the specific prescriber's order for dosage and rate of infusion before beginning therapy. Always follow the "Nine Rights" of medication administration to prevent overdosing or erroneous dosing. Make sure the proper diluent is used. Check the compatibility of solutions or other drugs before beginning the infusion.
- For continuous intravenous (IV) administration of heparin, an IV pump must be used to ensure a precise rate of infusion.
- Continuous dosing is preferred over intermittent dosing because continuous dosing helps maintain blood levels of the drug and because intermittent IV dosing is associated with a higher risk for bleeding abnormalities.
- Treatment by continuous IV infusion generally begins with a loading dose and is followed by a maintenance dose. Be aware that dosage adjustments are made exactly as ordered. The patient's activated partial thromboplastin time (aPTT) and/or results of other related clotting studies are used as parameters for dosing of standard heparin.
- For intermittent infusions, a heparin lock was used in the past. Heparin locks are now referred to as *intermittent infusion locks* or *saline locks*

(because the locks are flushed with isotonic saline and not with heparin). The exception is with PICC lines and central lines in which heparin is still used as a flush.

- Intermittent infusions of heparin are usually ordered to be given every 4 to 6 hours because of heparin's short half-life. Needleless systems are used for intermittent infusions and all other types of IV infusions.
- Regardless of the type of IV infusion (e.g., intermittent or continuous IV infusion), it is crucial to check the site to determine whether infiltration has occurred so that hematoma formation may be prevented. If infiltration is suspected, remove the lock and replace at a new site before the next scheduled infusion. Document appropriately.
- The therapeutic dosage of heparin is guided by aPTT with a targeted level of 1.5 to 2.5 times the control (normal) value. The aPTT is measured within 24 hours of beginning therapy, 24 to 48 hours after therapy starts, and 1 to 2 times weekly for about 3 to 4 weeks on average. With long-term therapy, aPTT is monitored 1 to 2 times per month.

Oral Anticoagulant Administration

- It is important to recheck the prescriber's orders and the patient's medication and medical history before administering any coagulation modifying drug. Always check to make sure the patient has no known hypersensitivity to the drug.
- Scored tablets may be crushed and may be given with or without food.
- Many more drugs can interact with oral anticoagulants than with heparin, especially those that are highly protein bound (see Table 26-3). Always check the patient's medication list before initiating therapy with warfarin.
- Dosages of warfarin are calculated based on international normalized ratio (INR) blood values. INRs are also used to monitor the effectiveness of therapy. Remember, however, that dosing is highly individualized!
- Oral anticoagulants are to be administered at the same time every day to maintain steady blood levels.
- Document the dose, time of administration, and any other pertinent facts with these and all other medications.

CASE STUDY

Safety: What Went Wrong? Heparin Therapy

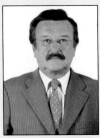

In the past 2 years, Mr. L., a 56-year-old architect, has experienced three episodes of deep vein thrombosis. All occurred without complications, and all were treated successfully with anticoagulant therapy and bed rest. He now arrives at the urgent care center because of increased pain and swelling in his left calf that has lasted for the past 3 days. On admission to the hospital for anticoagulant therapy, Mr. L. receives a bolus of 5000 units of heparin and is started on a continuous heparin infusion.

1. What nursing actions must be implemented to ensure the accuracy and safety of the continuous heparin infusion?
2. What patient findings would indicate a therapeutic response to the heparin therapy?

   During Mr. L.'s hospital stay, the physician orders an extra bolus of 10,000 units of heparin, IV push, because the results of Mr. L.'s laboratory tests indicate that his activated partial thromboplastin time (aPTT) is not at a therapeutic level. After giving the dose, the nurse notices that a dose of 50,000 units was given instead of 10,000 units.
3. What will the nurse do first, and what subsequent orders will the nurse prepare to carry out?
4. What went wrong? How could this error have been prevented?

For answers, see *http://www.elsevier.com/Lilley*.

injections and specifically *heparin* and *LMWH* injections. Solutions may be clear to pale yellow. The usual length of therapy is approximately 5 to 10 days, and it is important to constantly be aware of any bleeding problems while the patient is taking this or other *clotting-altering drugs*. Complete blood counts, platelet counts, and stool tests for occult blood are tests that will probably be performed during therapy for monitoring purposes. Tests for occult blood in the stool can be done simply if occult blood test paper and developer are available. Blood in the stool may occur as an adverse effect of LMWHs or any clotting-altering drug.

When the *oral anticoagulant warfarin* is prescribed, therapy is often initiated while the patient is still receiving heparin. This overlapping is done purposefully to allow time for the blood levels of warfarin to rise, so that when the heparin is eventually discontinued, therapeutic anticoagulation levels of warfarin will have been achieved. Recommendations for overlapping therapy of heparin and warfarin are for at least 5 days; the *heparin* is stopped after 5 days when the INR is above 2 (see pharmacology discussion). Monitoring results of the various clotting studies is still of utmost priority, as is watching for any clotting or bleeding problems. The administration procedures for warfarin are outlined in Box 26-1.

For conversion from heparin to an oral anticoagulant such as warfarin, the dose of the oral drug is the usual initial dosage amount, with the prescriber using the PT/INR levels to determine the next appropriate dosage of warfarin. Once there is continuous therapeutic anticoagulation coverage and warfarin has reached therapeutic levels, the heparin or LMWH may be discontinued without tapering. If uncontrolled bleeding occurs with any of these medications, take action to control bleeding,

institute emergency measures to stabilize the patient's condition, and contact the prescriber immediately.

The anticoagulant *dabigatran (Pradaxa)* is given orally. Important safety information about dabigatran (Pradaxa) from the U.S. Food and Drug Administration (FDA) includes that it is to be stored in and dispensed from its original bottle. This is important because if not stored properly and with the desiccant-drying agent (which absorbs moisture) in the packaging cap, the substance in the drug is easily broken down and a loss of potency occurs. This would result in less therapeutic effectiveness. This storage information is not widely disseminated and so it is important to be aware of these precautions. Additionally, the FDA is also alerting consumers that even though the label says to discard the drug after 30 days of opening the original container, recent data suggest that it can maintain its potency for up to 60 days if the cap is closed tightly after each use and the bottle is kept away from excessive moisture, heat, and/or cold. More information is to be released from the FDA once they complete further review of this product. The FDA suggests that Pradaxa be kept in the original bottle or blister package; not stored or placed in any other type of container; opened one bottle at a time; closed tightly after the capsule is removed; not used after 60 days; and have the blister package opened at time of use and not have the blister punctured prior to the use/administration of the drug. For more information, see *www.consumermedsafety.org/alerts*. *Fondaparinux (Aristra)* is given subcutaneously and, as with dabigatran, has no standard anticoagulant tests for monitoring.

There are antidotes available to counter the toxic effects of *anticoagulants*. The antidote to hemorrhage or uncontrolled bleeding resulting from heparin or LMWH therapy is protamine sulfate. For heparin, 1 mg of protamine sulfate given intravenously neutralizes 100 units of heparin. For the LMWHs, 1 mg of protamine sulfate neutralizes 1 mg of each LMWH given. It is important to note that too-rapid an infusion may lead to acute hypotensive episodes, bradycardia, dyspnea, and transient feelings of warmth and flushing. If the heparin overdose has resulted in a large blood loss, replacement with packed red blood cells may be necessary.

The aPTT ranges and hematocrit levels are generally used as ordered to monitor bleeding, clotting, and risk for bleeding. Always monitor the patient, especially for any changes in blood pressure and pulse rate. The antidote to oral anticoagulant (warfarin sodium) therapy is vitamin K. See the pharmacology section for more discussion on dosing and reversibility of vitamin K on the effects of warfarin. When given IV, vitamin K may lead to anaphylaxis with resultant dyspnea, dizziness, rapid or weak pulse, chest pain, and hypotension, which may progress to shock and cardiac arrest. Always check health care institution policy and the prescriber's order on the specific dosage and route of administration. Continual monitoring of the patient's vital signs, cardiac parameters, and bleeding times and other clotting study results are very important.

Constantly monitor the patient being treated with *antiplatelet drugs* (or any *clotting-altering drug*) for signs and symptoms of bleeding during and after their use, including epistaxis, hematuria, hematemesis, easy or excessive bruising, blood in the stools, and bleeding of the gums. If invasive procedures must be performed or injections given, apply appropriate pressure to bleeding sites, and closely watch all areas of venous or arterial catheter insertion for bleeding. Advise patients to take extended-release dosage forms in their entirety and without chewing or crushing. Enteric-coated *aspirin* is best taken with 6 to 8 ounces of water and with food to help decrease gastrointestinal upset. To avoid irritation to the esophagus, instruct the patient to remain upright and not lie down for up to 30 minutes after the dose of aspirin. If the aspirin has a strong, vinegar-like odor, discard the drug. Interventions with clopidogrel therapy are similar to those for aspirin. Advise the patient to report the following if they occur: aches in the joints, back pain, dizziness, severe headache, dyspepsia, flulike signs and symptoms, and epigastric pain. These drugs are often discontinued for 7 days prior to surgery, as ordered. However, some surgical procedures (e.g., cardiovascular surgery) may warrant that the patient remain in an anticoagulated state intraoperatively.

Oral forms of *dipyridamole*, another *anticoagulant*, are recommended to be taken on an empty stomach; however, if this is not tolerated, the patient can take the drug with food. If nausea occurs, cola, unsalted crackers, or dry toast may help to alleviate this adverse effect. In addition, it may take up to 2 to 3 months of continuous therapy for the drug to reach therapeutic levels. Encourage patients to change positions slowly and to take their time in going from lying to sitting to standing because of the adverse effects of dizziness and postural hypotension with *antiplatelet drugs*. *Vorapaxar* is given orally once daily and in combination with *aspirin* and/or *clopidogrel*.

Nursing considerations associated with the *GP IIb/IIIa inhibitors*, such as *abciximab, eptifibatide,* and *tirofiban*, include some similar, yet different, nursing actions. Close monitoring of all vital signs, electrocardiogram readings, peripheral pulses, heart sounds, skin color, and temperature are an important part of nursing care during and after the use of these drugs. Because these drugs are used in combination with *heparin* to treat individuals suspected of having acute coronary syndrome or those undergoing percutaneous transluminal coronary angioplasty (PTCA), there is always concern for the stability of the patient as well as a high risk for serious bleeding and/or extension of an acute MI. The patient in this situation is at risk for other medical complications, and this risk may be intensified by the drug. Avoid further invasive procedures while the patient is taking these drugs to help prevent bleeding. If invasive procedures are required, constantly monitor for bleeding and measure all vital parameters before, during, and after the procedure. Protect IV tirofiban from light. Discard any unused solutions 24 hours after an infusion has been started. Do NOT give any other drugs with this drug except for heparin, which may be administered through the same IV line. For PCTA, abciximab can be given by bolus or by continuous infusion; closely monitor infusion rates. Manufacturer guidelines call for the use of a sterile, nonpyrogenic, low–protein-binding 0.2- or 0.22-micron filter, and while the vascular shield is in position, keep the patient on complete bed rest with the head of the bed elevated 30 degrees. Maintain the affected extremity in a straight position, and constantly monitor peripheral pulses and the color and temperature of the distal extremities. Once the sheath is removed, apply pressure to the femoral artery for at least 30

minutes, either by manual or mechanical pressure. Apply a pressure dressing once bleeding has stopped. Closely monitor the site for any oozing or bleeding.

If serious bleeding occurs, discontinue the GP IIb/IIIa inhibitor and heparin (the usual protocol for PTCA) immediately, monitor the patient closely, and notify the prescriber immediately for initiation of emergency treatment. Always move and handle these patients with caution, and avoid unnecessary trauma because of the risk for hematoma formation or bleeding. Do *not* take blood pressures in the lower extremities, but keep a close and constant watch on the patient's blood pressure (for hypotension) and pulse rate (for tachycardia). Also closely monitor the patient for any complaints of abdominal or back pain, severe headache, and any other signs or symptoms of hemorrhage. When adhesive or sticky tape is removed, take care to avoid tearing or ripping the skin, which would lead to tissue trauma and further risk for bleeding. Monitor aPTT levels after the procedure, and observe for bleeding, with attention to IM injection sites, arterial or venous puncture sites, and bleeding from nasogastric tubes and/or urinary catheters. Avoid such invasive procedures, if at all possible, during and immediately after the angioplasty.

Nursing considerations related to *thrombolytics* are very similar to those for the other drugs already discussed. Specifically, carry out the preparation for their IV administration per manufacturer guidelines and per protocol. Avoid invasive procedures during the use of these drugs. Avoid simultaneous use of anticoagulants or antiplatelets. Frequently monitor IV infusion sites for bleeding, redness, and pain. IM injections of other drugs are contraindicated to prevent tissue damage and bleeding. Report any bleeding from gums or mucous membranes or the occurrence of epistaxis or increased pulse (higher than 100 beats/min) to the prescriber immediately, and frequently monitor all vital signs. Other nursing considerations include monitoring for hypotension, restlessness, and a decrease in hemoglobin level or hematocrit, which are to be reported to the prescriber immediately (indicating possible shock). Advise patients to report pink, red, or cloudy urine; black, tarry stools or frank red blood in the stools; abdominal or chest pain; dizziness; or severe headache. Continually monitor the INR, aPTT, platelet counts, and fibrinogen levels, beginning no later than 2 to 3 hours after the administration of *thrombolytics*. Measure the patient's fibrinogen level to check for the occurrence of fibrinolysis. With the breakdown of fibrin (or fibrinolysis), INR will increase and aPTT will be prolonged. If bleeding occurs, the prescriber will most likely discontinue the drug and replace fibrinogen through infusions of whole blood plasma or cryoprecipitate. The *antifibrinolytics aminocaproic acid* and/or *tranexamic acid* may also be given. See Patient-Centered Care: Patient Teaching later in the chapter.

With *antifibrinolytics*, it is important to understand the reasons for the use of these drugs, such as to stop bleeding from overdosages of thrombolytic drugs or to control bleeding during cardiac surgery. Aminocaproic acid and tranexamic acid are usually given IV until bleeding is controlled. Because of the possibility of drug-induced internal, intracranial, and superficial bleeding, closely monitor the patient, and notify the prescriber immediately if there is any change in motor strength or level of consciousness. You must apply your knowledge of certain adverse effects of drugs like these to prevent complications, maintain safety, and return the patient to a healthier state. It is also important to monitor heart rate and blood pressure with attention to the quality and strength of peripheral pulses. For the patient with hemophilia, *tranexamic acid* may be used to help decrease bleeding from dental extractions.

EVALUATION

Monitoring for the therapeutic and adverse effects of *coagulation modifier drugs* is crucial for safe administration. Because these drugs are used for a variety of purposes, therapeutic responses vary. Some of the therapeutic effects include decreased chest pain and a decrease in dizziness, as well as in other neurologic symptoms. Adverse effects of *anticoagulants* include bleeding and hematoma formation *(heparin)*; thrombocytopenia *(heparin and LMWHs)*; bleeding, dizziness, shortness of breath, and fever *(direct thrombin inhibitors)*; bleeding, hematoma, dizziness, and gastrointestinal distress *(selective factor Xa inhibitors)*; and bleeding, lethargy, and muscle pain *(warfarin)*. Early signs of drug overdose for any of the clotting-altering drugs (i.e., anticoagulants) include bleeding of the gums while brushing the teeth, unexplained nosebleeds or bruising, and heavier-than-usual menstrual bleeding. Abdominal pain, back pain, bloody or tarry stools, bloody urine, constipation, blood in the sputum, severe or continuous headaches, and the vomiting of frank red blood or a coffee ground–like substance (old blood) are all possible indications of internal bleeding.

Therapeutic effects of *clopidogrel* and other *antiplatelet drugs* include a decrease in the occurrence of clotting events such as TIA and stroke. Some of the adverse effects of *aspirin*, as an *antiplatelet drug*, include dizziness, confusion, nausea, vomiting, gastrointestinal bleeding. Adverse effects of clopidogrel may include chest pain, edema, headache, dizziness, and

epistaxis. See Table 26-4 for a more complete listing of adverse effects associated with antiplatelet drugs. With vorapaxar, evaluate for the adverse effects of bleeding, depression, skin rash, and anemia. Therapeutic levels of *anticoagulants* and other clotting-altering drugs or coagulation modifier drugs are also monitored by laboratory studies such as aPTT, PT, and INR, which are described in the Safety: Laboratory Values Related to Drug Therapy box. Remember, however, that aPTT levels are measured with *heparin*, whereas PT and INR are measured with *warfarin*. Once the level of the particular drug stabilizes and maintenance therapy is ongoing, the clotting studies may be performed at 1- to 4-week intervals, depending on the specific drug, the patient's response, and the patient's overall physical condition. If a heparin or LMWH overdose occurs, the antidote is protamine sulfate, whereas vitamin K, or phytonadione, is the antidote to oral anticoagulant overdose.

Continuous monitoring of the patient for the signs and symptoms of internal or external bleeding is critical during both the initiation and maintenance of therapy. Therapeutic effects of *thrombolytics* include improvement in cardiac status during an acute MI, improved blood flow from resolution of DVT, and improved neurologic status. Adverse effects include bleeding, hypotension, and cardiac dysrhythmias. Therapeutic effects of *antifibrinolytics* include the arrest of oozing of blood from a surgical site or a decrease in blood loss. Adverse effects associated with the *antifibrinolytics* are listed in Table 26-6. Because of the complexity and life-threatening nature of the conditions for which these drugs are used, continually monitor and reevaluate the patient's response to the treatment, document this response accordingly, and always keep goals and outcome criteria within the plan of care to serve as a benchmark. From the evaluation phase, the patient will hopefully emerge experiencing full therapeutic effects and minimal adverse and/or toxic effects related to drug therapy.

SAFETY: LABORATORY VALUES RELATED TO DRUG THERAPY

Anticoagulants

Laboratory Test	Normal Ranges	Rationale for Assessment
Activated partial thromboplastin time (aPTT), partial thromboplastin time (PTT)*	With heparin therapy, aPTT values need to fall between 1.5 and 2.5 times the control or baseline value. Normal control values are 25 to 35 seconds (sec). Target therapeutic level of anticoagulation is between 45 and 70 sec.	Therapeutic levels of aPTT indicate decreased levels of clotting factors and subsequent clotting activity. It is used to monitor heparin therapy. With continuous IV infusions of heparin, blood samples for aPTT testing are drawn 4-6 hours after starting heparin or after any dose adjustment. Monitoring of aPTT is not done for prophylactic doses (i.e., 5000 units every 12 hours subcut).
Prothrombin time (PT)	The normal control PT value ranges from 11 to 13 sec; target therapeutic level of anticoagulation is 1.5 times the control value, or about 18 sec.	Prothrombin is a vitamin K–dependent protein and a major component of the clotting process. It reflects clotting activity and is used to monitor the effectiveness of warfarin therapy. PT values vary for each laboratory center and are based on the specifics of the testing procedure.
International normalized ratio (INR)	Target levels of INR range from 2 to 3 or an average of 2.5. For individuals taking warfarin for treatment of recurring systemic clots or emboli and those with mechanical heart valves, the target INR may be 2.5 to 3.5, with a middle value of 3.	INR determination is a routine test to evaluate coagulation while patients are taking warfarin. When the therapy is initiated, the INR and PT are measured daily until a stable daily dose is reached (the dose maintains the PT and INR within therapeutic ranges and does not cause bleeding). INR values actually reflect the dose of warfarin given 36 to 72 hr prior to the testing. Advantages of INR testing include the fact that there is more consistency among laboratories and a more consistent warfarin dosage is achieved. Some laboratories report INR and PT together.

*These terms are used interchangeably.

PATIENT-CENTERED CARE: PATIENT TEACHING

- Emphasize the rationale for use of the coagulation-modifying drugs to prevent serious complications related to clotting, such as strokes, heart attacks, clot formation (deep vein thrombosis of the legs) with heart valve replacements, and mini-strokes/TIAs (transient ischemic attacks) and the need for frequent and close monitoring.

- Educate the patient that a healthy lifestyle is an important part of therapy and will most likely include eating the right foods, weight reduction if needed, smoking cessation, control of blood pressure, and stress reduction. Advise the patient to provide a listing of all medications to all possible prescribers (e.g., dentists).

- Direct the patient to take all of the clotting-altering drugs exactly as prescribed because too little of the drug may lead to clot formation and too much of the drug may lead to bleeding. Regular follow-up appointments are an important part of patient care, with frequent blood tests to monitor for therapeutic effects and adverse effects of the medication. The results of the blood tests will help the prescriber determine the proper dosage.

- The patient must carry an identification card or wear a medical alert bracelet or necklace at all times stating allergies, medical diagnosis, list of drugs, prescriber's name and phone number, as well as an emergency contact name and number.

- Home therapy with parenteral anticoagulants may require injections for a period of time, and LMWHs are generally used. If there is a switch from heparin to warfarin (Coumadin), there will be an overlap period of at least 5 days during which both drugs are taken to allow therapeutic levels of the oral warfarin to be reached before the heparin is discontinued. This process may occur in the hospital or at home. Provide complete and thorough instructions to the patient, and use return demonstrations to evaluate learning (see Chapter 9).

- Advise the patient to report to the prescriber any unusual bleeding from anywhere on the body or the occurrence of a severe headache, blurred vision, vomiting of blood, dizziness, fainting, fever, muscular or limb weakness, rash, nosebleeds, or excessive vaginal or menstrual bleeding.

- Emphasize the rationale for use of warfarin and that it works by inhibiting vitamin K–dependent clotting factors. With warfarin, foods high in vitamin K may reduce the drug's ability to prevent clots. Increasing and/or decreasing the intake of these vitamin K–containing foods can affect clotting and thus the INR. The average daily allowance for vitamin K is 120 mcg for adult men and 90 mcg for adult women. The most important aspect of these food-drug interactions is consistency in diet and keeping the intake of vitamin K about the same each day. While eating small amounts of foods that are rich in vitamin K should not cause a problem, it is still recommended to avoid large amounts of kale, spinach, Brussels sprouts, collard/mustard greens, lettuce, chard, and green tea. The "right" amount of vitamin K is the amount consumed with a fixed dose of warfarin to produce an INR within the patient's target range

time and time again. Beverages that may increase the effect of warfarin and are to be avoided include cranberry juice and alcohol. Herbal products that interact with warfarin and result in increased risk for bleeding include dong quai, garlic, and ginkgo. St. John's wort decreases warfarin's effect. The safest guideline is to avoid dietary supplements unless the prescriber approves. (Sources of information include: *www.ptinr.com/warfarin-you/dietary-food-beverage/vitamin-k-how-much-too-much*, *www.mayoclinic.org/diseases-conditions/thrombophlebitis/expert-answers/warfarin/*, and *www.cc.nih.gov/ccc/patient_education/drug_nutrient/coumadin1.pdf*).

- With dabigatran (Pradaxa), educate the patient to protect the original bottle from moisture. Once a bottle is opened, it must be used within 60 days; this needs to be written on the bottle/label with the date of expiration. Instruct the patient to remove only 1 capsule from the opened bottle at the time of use and that the bottle needs to be immediately and tightly closed. Encourage the patient to take the medication with food if dyspepsia occurs. These capsules are *not* to be repackaged or placed in other pillboxes/organizers. For more information, visit *www.pradaxapro.com*.

- Vorapaxar is administered orally once a day. Be sure to educate the patient about the contraindications of use with NSAIDS, anticoagulants, and strong inhibitors/inducers of CYP3A4.

- Journal keeping by the patient with daily notation of how the patient is feeling as well as how the patient is tolerating the medication and any adverse effects is beneficial to ensure safe, effective treatment.

- To reduce risk factors for cardiovascular disease, the prescriber may recommend consumption of a low-fat, low-cholesterol diet; cholesterol-lowering drug therapy; weight reduction; control of blood pressure if hypertension is present; avoidance of smoking; management of stress; and regular exercise.

- Teach the patient about clot-preventive measures, including situations to minimize sluggish circulation (e.g., avoid tight-fitting clothing, minimize sitting for prolonged periods of time, avoid crossing the legs at the knees and wearing of tight-fitting socks/stockings, avoid prolonged bed rest, make stops during long trips to walk around every 1 to 2 hours, keep well hydrated).

- When taking any of the anticoagulants (oral drugs and/or heparin or LMWHs) or clotting-altering drugs, encourage the patient to avoid brushing the teeth with a hard-bristled toothbrush, shaving with a straight razor, and/or engaging in any activity that would increase the risk for tissue injury. Always caution the patient when shaving, nail trimming, gardening, and/or participating in rough or contact sports.

- Capsicum (red pepper), feverfew, garlic, ginger, ginkgo, and St. John's wort are some herbals that have potential interactions, especially with warfarin. Educate the patient about these and other interactions.

- Report any decrease in urine output; constant ringing in the ears; swelling of the feet, ankles, or legs; dark urine; clay-colored stools; abdominal pain; rash (use needs to be discontinued as ordered if rash occurs); and/or blurred vision to the prescriber immediately.
- If doses of medications are omitted, advise the patient to contact the prescriber for further instructions.
- Oral dosage forms of any of these medications are to be taken with at least 8 ounces of water and/or with food to help minimize stomach upset.
- Keep all medication containers out of the reach of children, and use childproof tops. All syringes, needles, and other equipment must be kept out of the reach of children and other individuals as well.

KEY POINTS

- Coagulation modifiers work by preventing/promoting clot formation, lysing a preformed clot, and/or reversing the action of anticoagulants. Coagulation modifiers include anticoagulants, antiplatelets, thrombolytics, antifibrinolytics, and reversal drugs.
- Warfarin prevents clot formation by inhibiting vitamin K–dependent clotting factors (factors II, VII, IX, and X) and is used prophylactically to prevent clots from forming; it cannot lyse preformed clots.
- The degree of anticoagulation (for any of these medications) is monitored by the PT.
- Heparin, given IV or subcutaneously, prevents clot formation by binding to antithrombin III, which turns off certain activating factors. The overall effect is to inactivate the coagulation pathway and prevent clots from forming. Heparin does not lyse (break down) a clot. Antiplatelet drugs prevent clot formation by preventing platelet involvement in clot formation.

- Thrombolytics are able to break down or lyse preformed clots in blood vessels such as those that supply the heart with blood. Therapeutic effects for which to monitor include improved tissue perfusion, decreased chest pain, and prevention of further myocardial damage. The therapeutic effects of most coagulation modifier drugs include improved circulation, improved tissue perfusion, decreased pain, and prevention of further tissue damage. Before giving these drugs, a thorough physical assessment must be performed as well as checking of pertinent laboratory values (e.g., INR, aPTT, PT).
- Antifibrinolytics prevent the lysis of fibrin, thus promoting clot formation, and have an effect opposite to that of the anticoagulants. Nursing care is very individualized and is based on the characteristics of the patient, thorough assessment data, existing medical conditions, and the specific drug.

NCLEX® EXAMINATION REVIEW QUESTIONS

1. The nurse is monitoring a patient who is receiving antithrombolytic therapy in the emergency department because of a possible MI. Which adverse effect would be of the greatest concern at this time?
   a. Dizziness
   b. Blood pressure of 130/98 mm Hg
   c. Slight bloody oozing from the IV insertion site
   d. Irregular heart rhythm
2. A patient is receiving instructions regarding warfarin therapy and asks the nurse about what medications she can take for headaches. The nurse will tell her to avoid which type of medication?
   a. Opioids
   b. acetaminophen (Tylenol)
   c. NSAIDs
   d. There are no restrictions while taking warfarin.
3. The nurse is teaching a patient about self-administration of enoxaparin (Lovenox). Which statement will be included in this teaching session?
   a. "We will need to teach a family member how to give this drug in your arm."
   b. "This drug is given in the folds of your abdomen, but at least 2 inches away from your navel."
   c. "This drug needs to be taken at the same time every day with a full glass of water."
   d. "Be sure to massage the injection site thoroughly after giving the drug."

4. A patient is receiving dabigatran (Pradaxa), 150 mg twice daily, as part of treatment for atrial fibrillation. Which condition, if present, would be a concern if the patient were to receive this dose?
   a. Asthma
   b. Elevated liver enzymes
   c. Renal impairment
   d. History of myocardial infarction
5. A patient has received a double dose of heparin during surgery and is bleeding through the incision site. While the surgeons are working to stop the bleeding at the incision site, the nurse will prepare to take what action at this time?
   a. Give IV vitamin K as an antidote.
   b. Give IV protamine sulfate as an antidote.
   c. Call the blood bank for an immediate platelet transfusion.
   d. Obtain an order for packed red blood cells.
6. A patient is starting warfarin (Coumadin) therapy as part of treatment for atrial fibrillation. The nurse will follow which principles of warfarin therapy? *(Select all that apply.)*
   a. Teach proper subcutaneous administration.
   b. Administer the oral dose at the same time every day.
   c. Assess carefully for excessive bruising or unusual bleeding.
   d. Monitor laboratory results for a target INR of 2 to 3.
   e. Monitor laboratory results for a therapeutic aPTT value of 1.5 to 2.5 times the control value.

7. The order for enoxaparin (Lovenox) reads: Give 1 mg/kg subcut every 12 hours. The patient weighs 242 lb, and the medication is available in an injection form of 120 mg/0.8 mL. How many milligrams will this patient receive? How many milliliters will the nurse draw up for the injection? *(Round to hundredths.)*

8. The nurse is assessing a patient who has a new prescription for vorapaxar (Zontivity). Which of these conditions are considered contraindications to the use of vorapaxar? *(Select all that apply.)*

a. Impaired renal function
b. Impaired liver function
c. History of myocardial infarction
d. Peripheral artery disease
e. History of stroke

1. d, 2. c, 3. b, 4. c, 5. b, 6. b, c, d, 7. 110 mg; 0.73 mL, 8. a, b, e

CRITICAL THINKING AND PRIORITIZATION QUESTIONS

1. After a patient undergoes total hip replacement, the nurse reviews the new postoperative orders and notes an order for dalteparin (Fragmin) 2500 international units subcutaneously 6 hours after surgery, then 5000 international units daily for 7 days. When assessing the patient before administering the drug, the nurse sees that the patient has an epidural catheter for administration of pain medication. What is the nurse's priority action regarding the administration of the dalteparin?

2. A patient is going home and will be taking warfarin (Coumadin). While discussing his medications just before his discharge to home, the patient says, "I want to get back to taking my vitamins with gingko. They really help my memory." What is the priority as the nurse answers the patient's question?

For answers, see *http://evolve.elsevier.com/Lilley.*

ⓔ EVOLVE WEBSITE

http://evolve.elsevier.com/Lilley
- Animations
- Answer Keys for Textbook Case Studies and Textbook Critical Thinking and Prioritization Questions

- Content Updates
- Key Points
- Review Questions
- Student Case Studies

Antilipemic Drugs

http://evolve.elsevier.com/Lilley

OBJECTIVES

When you reach the end of this chapter, you will be able to do the following:

1. Explain the pathology of primary and secondary hyperlipidemia, including causes and risk factors.
2. Discuss the different types of lipoproteins and their role in cardiovascular diseases and in hyperlipidemia.
3. List the overall drug classes and specific drugs that are used to treat hyperlipidemia.
4. Compare the various drugs used to treat hyperlipidemia with regard to the rationale for treatment, indications, mechanisms of action, dosages, routes of administration, adverse effects, toxicity, cautions, contraindications, and associated drug interactions.
5. Develop a nursing care plan that includes all phases of the nursing process for patients receiving antilipemic drugs.

DRUG PROFILES

♦ atorvastatin, p. 442
♦ cholestyramine, p. 443
ezetimibe, p. 445
gemfibrozil, p. 445
♦ niacin, p. 444
♦ simvastatin, p. 442

♦ = *Key drug*
! = *High-alert drug*

KEY TERMS

Antilipemic drugs Drugs that reduce lipid levels. (p. 437)
Apolipoproteins The protein components of lipoproteins. (p. 437)
Cholesterol A fat-soluble steroid found in animal fats, oils, and egg yolk and widely distributed in the body, especially in the bile, blood, brain tissue, liver, kidneys, adrenal glands, and myelin sheaths of nerve fibers. (p. 437)
Chylomicrons Microscopic droplets made up of fat and protein that are produced by cells in the small intestine and released into the bloodstream. Their main purpose is to carry fats to the tissues throughout the body, primarily the liver. Chylomicrons consist of about 90% triglycerides and small amounts of cholesterol, phospholipids, and proteins. (p. 437)
Exogenous lipids Lipids originating outside the body or an organ (e.g., dietary fats). (p. 437)
Foam cells The characteristic initial lesion of atherosclerosis, also known as a *fatty streak*. (p. 438)
Hydroxymethylglutaryl–coenzyme A (HMG-CoA) reductase inhibitors A class of cholesterol-lowering drugs that work

by inhibiting the rate-limiting step in cholesterol synthesis; also commonly referred to as *statins*. (p. 440)
Hypercholesterolemia A condition in which higher than normal amounts of cholesterol are present in the blood. High levels of cholesterol and other lipids may lead to the development of atherosclerosis and serious illnesses such as coronary heart disease. (p. 438)
Lipoprotein A conjugated protein synthesized in the liver that contains varying amounts of triglycerides, cholesterol, phospholipids, and protein; classified according to its composition and density. (p. 437)
Statins A class of cholesterol-lowering drugs that are more formally known as *HMG-CoA reductase inhibitors*. (p. 440)
Triglycerides Compounds that consist of fatty acids and a type of alcohol known as *glycerol*. Triglycerides make up most animal and vegetable fats and are the principal lipids in the blood, where they circulate bound to a protein, forming high-density and low-density lipoproteins (HDLs and LDLs). (p. 437)

OVERVIEW

Key to understanding the use of antilipemic drugs is a working knowledge of the pathology of lipid abnormalities and their contribution to coronary heart disease (CHD). It is also important to understand, at the cellular level, the transporting and use of cholesterol and triglycerides in the human body. Lipoproteins, apolipoproteins, receptors, and enzyme systems are all integral parts of these processes.

LIPIDS AND LIPID ABNORMALITIES

Primary Forms of Lipids

Triglycerides and cholesterol are the two primary forms of lipids in the blood. Triglycerides function as an energy source and are stored in adipose (fat) tissue. Cholesterol is primarily used to make steroid hormones, cell membranes, and bile acids. Triglycerides and cholesterol are both water-insoluble fats that must be bound to specialized lipid-carrying proteins called apolipoproteins. The combination of triglycerides and cholesterol with an apolipoprotein is referred to as a lipoprotein.

TABLE 27-1 **Lipoprotein Classification**		
Lipid Content	**Lipoprotein Classification**	**Protein Content**
Most	Chylomicron	Least
↓	VLDL	↑
	LDL	
	IDL	
Least	HDL	Most

HDL, High-density lipoprotein; *IDL*, intermediate-density lipoprotein; *LDL*, low-density lipoprotein; *VLDL*, very–low-density lipoprotein.

SAFETY: HERBAL THERAPIES AND DIETARY SUPPLEMENTS   QSEN

Flax

Overview
Flax is a flowering annual found in Europe, Canada, and the United States. Both the seed and the oil of the plant are used medicinally.

Common Uses
Atherosclerosis, hypercholesterolemia, hypertriglyceridemia, gastrointestinal distress (especially constipation), menopausal symptoms, and bladder inflammation, among other uses

Adverse Effects
Diarrhea, allergic reactions

Potential Drug Interactions
Antidiabetic drugs and anticoagulant drugs

Contraindications
Not recommended during pregnancy

Lipoproteins transport lipids via the blood. The various types of lipoproteins are classified according to their density and the type of apolipoproteins they contain. The lipoproteins and their classifications are presented in Table 27-1.

Cholesterol Homeostasis

Cholesterol homeostasis involves a complex array of biochemical factors. Figure 27-1 summarizes the major concepts. Fats are taken into the body through the diet and are broken down in the small intestine to form triglycerides. Triglycerides are then incorporated into chylomicrons in the cells of the intestinal

QSEN **SAFETY: HERBAL THERAPIES AND DIETARY SUPPLEMENTS**

Garlic (Allium sativum)

Overview
Garlic obtains its pharmacologic effects from the active ingredient allicin.

Common Uses
Antispasmodic, antiseptic, antibacterial and antiviral, antihypertensive, antiplatelet, lipid reducer

Adverse Effects
Dermatitis, vomiting, diarrhea, anorexia, flatulence, antiplatelet activity

Potential Drug Interactions
May interact with warfarin, diazepam, protease inhibitors. Use with nonsteroidal antiinflammatory drugs may enhance bleeding. Possible interference with hypoglycemic therapy.

Contraindications
Contraindicated in patients who will undergo surgery within 2 weeks and in patients with human immunodeficiency virus infection or diabetes.

wall and are absorbed into the lymphatic system. The primary purpose of chylomicrons is to transport lipids obtained from dietary sources (exogenous lipids) from the intestines to the liver to be used to make steroid hormones, lipid structural components for peripheral body cells, and bile acids.

The liver is the major organ where lipid metabolism occurs. The liver produces very–low-density lipoprotein (VLDL) from both endogenous and exogenous sources. The major role of VLDL is the transport of endogenous lipids to peripheral cells. Once VLDL is circulating, it is enzymatically cleaved by lipoprotein lipase and then loses triglycerides. This creates intermediate-density lipoprotein (IDL), which is soon also cleaved by lipoprotein lipase to create low-density lipoprotein (LDL). Cholesterol is almost all that remains in LDL after this process. Any tissues that require LDL, such as endocrine cells, have LDL receptors. LDL and about half of IDL are reabsorbed from the circulation into the liver by means of LDL receptors on the liver.

High-density lipoprotein (HDL) is produced in the liver and intestines and is also formed when chylomicrons are broken down. Lipids that are not used by peripheral cells are transferred as cholesterol esters to HDL. HDL then transfers the cholesterol esters to IDL to be returned to the liver. HDL is responsible for the "recycling" of cholesterol. HDL is sometimes

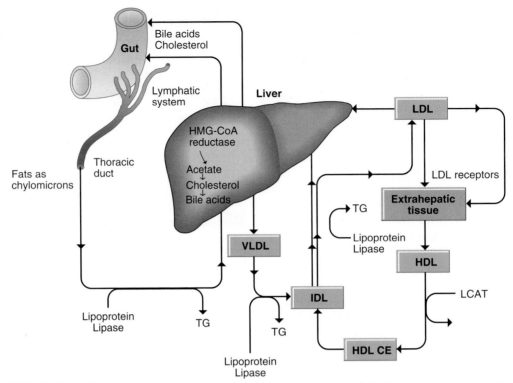

FIGURE 27-1 Cholesterol homeostasis. *CE,* Cholesterol ester; *HDL,* high-density lipoprotein; *HMG-CoA,* hydroxymethylglutaryl–coenzyme A; *IDL,* intermediate-density lipoprotein; *LCAT,* lecithin cholesterol acetyltransferase; *LDL,* low-density lipoprotein; *TG,* triglyceride; *VLDL,* very–low-density lipoprotein.

referred to as the *good lipid* (or good cholesterol) because it is believed to be cardioprotective.

If the liver has an excess amount of cholesterol, the number of LDL receptors on the liver decreases, which results in an accumulation of LDL in the blood. One explanation for **hypercholesterolemia** (cholesterol in the blood), therefore, is down-regulation (reduced production) of hepatic LDL receptors. A major function of the liver is to manufacture cholesterol, a process that requires acetyl coenzyme A (CoA) reductase. Inhibition of this enzyme thus results in decreased cholesterol production by the liver.

ATHEROSCLEROTIC PLAQUE FORMATION

Lipids and lipoproteins participate in the formation of atherosclerotic plaque, which subsequently leads to the development of CHD. When serum cholesterol levels are elevated, circulating monocytes adhere to the smooth endothelial surfaces of the coronary vasculature. These monocytes burrow into the next layer of the blood vessel (subendothelial tissue) and change into macrophage cells, which then take up cholesterol from circulating lipoproteins until they become filled with fat. Soon they become what are known as **foam cells,** the characteristic precursor lesion of atherosclerosis, also known as a *fatty streak.* Once this process is established, it is usually present throughout the coronary and systemic circulation.

CHOLESTEROL AND CORONARY HEART DISEASE

Numerous epidemiologic trials have shown that as blood cholesterol levels increase, the incidence of death and disability related to CHD also increases. The risk for CHD in patients with cholesterol levels of 300 mg/dL is three to four times greater than that in patients with levels of less than 200 mg/dL.

Statistics show that half of all Americans, both male and female, will die of a heart attack. Thus, the goals of treatment are two-pronged: primary prevention of cardiac events in patients with risk factors and secondary prevention of subsequent cardiac events in patients who have previously experienced a cardiac event (e.g., myocardial infarction). The benefits of cholesterol reduction for primary prevention have been illustrated in a number of trials. Results of some of the larger investigations support the view that, in patients with known risk factors for CHD, therapy with an antilipemic drug can reduce the occurrence of CHD. Drug therapy can also reduce first-time heart attack and death caused by heart disease. Benefits of cholesterol reduction for secondary prevention have been illustrated in a variety of trials as well. In patients with documented CHD, treatment with a cholesterol-lowering drug has many positive outcomes; decreased coronary events, regression of coronary atherosclerotic lesions, and prolonged survival.

Measures taken early in life to reduce and maintain cholesterol levels in a desirable range can have a dramatic effect in terms of preventing CHD. These include lifestyle modifications related to diet, weight, and activity level. Diets lower in saturated fat and higher in fiber and plant chemicals known as *sterols* and *stanols,* and possibly the substitution of soy-based proteins for animal proteins, appear to promote healthier lipid profiles. These are among the dietary recommendations made by the National Cholesterol Education Program (NCEP) Adult Treatment Panel III (ATP III) of the National Institutes of Health (For the full report, see *www.nhlbi.nih.gov/guidelines/ cholesterol/atp3full.pdf*). The consumption of fatty fish or dietary supplements containing omega-3 fatty acids appears to have beneficial effects on triglyceride and HDL levels and is currently recommended by the American Heart Association (AHA). The AHA also strongly emphasizes the substantial therapeutic benefits of even modest weight reduction and exercise in both improvement of lipid profiles and reduction of the likelihood of heart disease.

SAFETY: HERBAL THERAPIES AND DIETARY SUPPLEMENTS

QSEN

Omega-3 Fatty Acids

Overview
Omega-3 fatty acids are essential fatty acids, most commonly supplied as fish oil products. Several over-the-counter products are available, as well as a prescription product, known as Lovaza. (See the Safety and Quality Improvement: Preventing Medication Errors box.)

Common Uses
Cholesterol reduction

Adverse Effects
Rash, burping, allergic reactions, possible increase in total cholesterol or LDL levels in those patients with a combined hyperlipidemia, weight gain

Potential Drug Interactions
Anticoagulant drugs: May prolong bleeding time. There is a theoretical risk of increased bleeding with anticoagulant drugs, but the studies to date are inconclusive.

Contraindications
Pregnancy (more information is needed), allergy to fish oil

HYPERLIPIDEMIAS AND TREATMENT GUIDELINES

The decision to prescribe antilipemic drugs as an adjunct to dietary therapy in patients with an elevated cholesterol level is based on the patient's clinical profile. This includes the patient's age, sex, menopausal status for women, family history, and response to dietary treatment, as well as the presence of risk factors (other than hyperlipidemia) for premature CHD and the cause, duration, and phenotypic pattern of the patient's hyperlipidemia.

BOX 27-1 Patient Groups to Be Treated with Statin

Patients with...
- Clinical atherosclerotic cardiovascular disease (CVD)
- LDL cholesterol levels ≥190 mg/dL
- Diabetes who are 40 to 75 years of age with LDL levels 70 to 189 mg/dL and no evidence of CVD
- No evidence of CVD or diabetes but who have LDL levels between 70 and 189 mg/dL and a 10-year risk for CVD ≥7.5%

From Stone NJ, Robinson JG, Lichtenstein AH, et al; American College of Cardiology/American Heart Association Task Force on Practice Guidelines. 2013 ACC/AHA Guideline on the Treatment of Blood Cholesterol to Reduce Atherosclerotic Cardiovascular Risk in Adults: a report of the American College of Cardiology/American Heart Association Task Force on Practice Guidelines. *J Am Coll Cardiol* 63(25 Pt B):2889-2934, 2014.

TABLE 27-2 Types of Hyperlipidemia

| Phenotype | LIPID COMPOSITION | | |
	Lipoprotein Elevated	Cholesterol (mg/dL)	Triglyceride
I	Chylomicrons	Greater than or equal to 300	Greater than 3000
IIa	LDL	Greater than 300	Normal ≃ 148
IIb	LDL, VLDL	Greater than 300	Normal ≃ 148
III	IDL	Greater than 400	Greater than 600 (1-3 times higher than cholesterol)
IV	VLDL	Normal or mildly elevated approximately equal to 250	Greater than 400
V	VLDL, chylomicrons	Greater than 300	Greater than 2000

≃, Approximately equal to; *IDL,* intermediate-density lipoprotein; *LDL,* low-density lipoprotein; *VLDL,* very–low-density lipoprotein.

The major source of guidance for antilipemic treatment in the United States is the ACC/AHA Guideline on the Treatment of Blood Cholesterol to Reduce Atherosclerotic Cardiovascular Risk in Adults. These guidelines, updated in 2013, are from the American College of Cardiology and the American Heart Association in conjunction with the National Heart, Lung, and Blood Institute. The guidelines no longer recommend specific LDL and non-HDL targets; rather they identify four groups of primary- and secondary-prevention patients on whom physicians should focus their efforts. Box 27-1 lists the four major patient groups who should be treated with drug therapy (statins).

When the decision to institute drug therapy has been made, the choice of drug is determined by the specific lipid profile of the patient. Five patterns or phenotypes of hyperlipidemia have

BOX 27-2   Metabolic Syndrome: Identifying Features

- Waist circumference greater than 40 inches in men or 35 inches in women
- Serum triglyceride level of 150 mg/dL or more
- High-density lipoprotein cholesterol level of less than 40 mg/dL in men or less than 50 mg/dL in women
- Blood pressure of 130/85 mm Hg or higher
- Fasting serum glucose level higher than 100 mg/dL

TABLE 27-3   Intensity of Statin Therapy

High-Intensity	Moderate-Intensity	Low-Intensity
Lowers LDL-C on average by approximately 50%	*Lowers LDL-C on average by approximately 30% to <50%*	*Lowers LDL-C by less than 30%*
Atorvastatin 40-80 mg	Atorvastatin 10 mg	Pravastatin 10-20 mg
Rosuvastatin 20 mg	Rosuvastatin 10 mg	Lovastatin 20 mg
	Simvastatin 20-40 mg	
	Pravastatin 40 mg	
	Lovastatin 40 mg	
	Fluvastatin 40 mg bid	

Data from Stone NJ, Robinson JG, Lichtenstein AH, et al; American College of Cardiology/American Heart Association Task Force on Practice Guidelines. 2013 ACC/AHA Guideline on the Treatment of Blood Cholesterol to Reduce Atherosclerotic Cardiovascular Risk in Adults: a report of the American College of Cardiology/American Heart Association Task Force on Practice Guidelines. *J Am Coll Cardiol* 63(25 Pt B):2889-2934, 2014.

been identified, and these are defined by the plasma (serum) concentrations of total cholesterol, triglycerides, and lipoprotein fractions (i.e., HDL, LDL, IDL, VLDL). The various types of hyperlipidemia are listed in Table 27-2. The process of characterizing a patient's specific lipid profile in this way is referred to as *phenotyping*.

Metabolic syndrome is a set of risk factors associated with development of CVD, including obesity, hypertriglyceridemia, and low HDL level. Box 27-2 lists the identifying features of metabolic syndrome.

There are currently four established classes of drugs used to treat dyslipidemia: hydroxymethylglutaryl–coenzyme A (HMG-CoA) reductase inhibitors (statins), bile acid sequestrants, the B vitamin niacin (vitamin B₃, also known as *nicotinic acid*), and the fibric acid derivatives (fibrates). In addition, a cholesterol absorption inhibitor, ezetimibe (Zetia), is also available. Vytorin is an example of a combination tablet that contains both the statin drug simvastatin and ezetimibe. Mipomersen was recently approved as a once-weekly subcutaneous injection, as an adjunct to maximally tolerated lipid-lowering medications and diet for the treatment of patients with homozygous familial hypercholesterolemia. Lomitapide (Juxtapid), a microsomal triglyceride transfer protein inhibitor, was also recently approved. A new class of lipid-lowering drugs called proprotein convertase subtilisn kexin 9 (PCSK9) inhibitors are in development. No drugs in this new class are available at the time of this printing.

HYDROXYMETHYLGLUTARYL–COENZYME A REDUCTASE (HMG-COA REDUCTASE) INHIBITORS

HMG-CoA reductase is the rate-limiting enzyme in cholesterol synthesis. The hydroxymethylglutaryl–coenzyme A (HMG-CoA) reductase inhibitors competitively inhibit HMG-CoA reductase, and they are the most potent of the drugs available for reducing plasma concentrations of LDL cholesterol. Lovastatin was the first drug in this class to be approved for use, which occurred in 1987. Since that time, six other HMG-CoA reductase inhibitors have become available on the U.S. market: pravastatin, simvastatin, atorvastatin, fluvastatin, rosuvastatin, and pitavastatin. Because of the shared suffix of their generic names, these drugs are often collectively referred to as *statins*.

Lipid levels may not be lowered to their maximum extent until 6 to 8 weeks after the start of therapy. Few direct comparisons of the statins have been reported in the literature. The following doses of drugs are considered to be "therapeutically equivalent," meaning they produce the same therapeutic effect: simvastatin 20 mg, pravastatin 40 mg, lovastatin 40 mg, atorvastatin 10 mg, fluvastatin 80 mg, rosuvastatin 5 mg, and pitavastatin 2 mg. The 2013 ACC/AHA Guideline on the Treatment of Blood Cholesterol to Reduce Atherosclerotic Cardiovascular Risk in Adults categorizes statin therapy into high-, moderate-, and low-intensity, and these are listed in Table 27-3.

Mechanism of Action and Drug Effects

Statins lower the blood cholesterol level by decreasing the rate of cholesterol production. The liver requires HMG-CoA reductase to produce cholesterol. The statins inhibit this enzyme, thereby decreasing cholesterol production. When less cholesterol is produced, the liver increases the number of LDL receptors to recycle LDL from the circulation back into the liver, where it is needed for the synthesis of other required substances such as steroids, bile acids, and cell membranes.

Indications

The statins are recommended as first-line drug therapy for hypercholesterolemia (especially elevated levels of LDL cholesterol), the most common and dangerous form of dyslipidemia. More specifically, they are indicated for the treatment of type IIa and IIb hyperlipidemia and have been shown to reduce the plasma concentrations of LDL cholesterol by up to 50%. Their cholesterol-lowering properties are dose dependent; that is, the larger the dose, the greater the cholesterol-lowering effects. A 10% to 30% decrease in the concentrations of plasma triglycerides has also been observed in patients receiving these drugs. There is an overall tendency for the HDL cholesterol level to increase by 2% to 15%, a known beneficial factor that reduces risk (i.e., a negative risk factor) for cardiovascular disease.

These drugs appear to be equally effective in their ability to reduce LDL cholesterol concentrations. However, simvastatin, atorvastatin, and pitavastatin are more potent on a milligram basis. Atorvastatin appears to be more effective in lowering triglyceride levels than other HMG-CoA reductase inhibitors. Combined drug therapy with more than one class of antilipemic drug may be necessary for desired results. The statins are often combined with niacin or fibrates for this purpose, though this combination can increase the risk for adverse drug effects (see Adverse Effects).

Contraindications

Contraindications to the use of HMG-CoA reductase inhibitors (statins) include known drug allergy and pregnancy. Other contraindications may include liver disease or elevation of liver enzyme levels.

QSEN ⚡ SAFETY AND QUALITY IMPROVEMENT: PREVENTING MEDICATION ERRORS

Problems with Look-Alike/Sound-Alike Names: Why Omacar Changed to Lovaza

In 2006, the Institute for Safe Medication Practices (ISMP) received a report about problems that were occurring because of the look-alike, sound-alike names of Omacar, a new formulation of omega-3 fatty acids and Amicar (aminocaproic acid, see Chapter 26), an antifibrinolytic drug that has been available for years. In one case, a pharmacist misunderstood a telephone order for Omacar, 1 g twice a day as Amicar, 1 g twice a day. However, the astute patient read the drug information sheet before taking the new drug and called the pharmacist to say that he was expecting a drug to reduce triglyceride levels. As a result of this and other reports, the Food and Drug Administration (FDA) worked with the manufacturer for ways to reduce errors. In 2007, the manufacturer of Omacar agreed to change the name to Lovaza.

If the patient who needed a drug to reduce triglyceride levels had taken the Amicar, the patient would have been at high risk for thrombosis, along with other possible adverse reactions. If the patient who needed Amicar for hemostatis took Omacar instead, the result could be significant bleeding conditions.

For more information, see *www.fda.gov/downloads/safety/fdapatient safetynews/ucm417829.pdf* and *www.ismp.org/newsletters/ acutecare/archives/July07.asp*. Accessed July 12, 2015.

Adverse Effects

The HMG-CoA reductase inhibitors are generally well tolerated, and significant adverse effects are fairly uncommon. Abdominal pain, rash, and headache are most common; other effects are listed in Table 27-4. Elevations in liver enzyme levels may occur. Dose-dependent elevations in liver enzyme levels to values of more than three times the upper limit of normal have been noted in patients taking HMG-CoA reductase inhibitors. Serum creatine phosphokinase (CPK) concentrations may be increased to more than 10 times the normal level in patients receiving these drugs. Most of these patients have remained asymptomatic, however.

TABLE 27-4   HMG-CoA Reductase Inhibitors: Adverse Effects

Body System	Adverse Effects
Central nervous	Headache, dizziness, blurred vision, fatigue, insomnia
Gastrointestinal	Constipation, diarrhea, nausea
Other	Myalgias, skin rashes

TABLE 27-5   HMG-CoA Reductase Inhibitors: Drug Interactions

Drug	Mechanism	Effect
warfarin	Inhibit warfarin metabolism	Increased risk for bleeding
erythromycin, azole antifungals, quinidine, verapamil, amiodarone, grapefruit juice, HIV and hepatitis C protease inhibitors, cyclosporine, clarithromycin, diltiazem, amlodipine	Inhibit statin metabolism	Increased risk for myopathy
gemfibrozil	Potentiation	Increased risk for myopathy

A clinically important adverse effect is myopathy (muscle pain), which may progress to a serious condition known as *rhabdomyolysis*. Rhabdomyolysis is the breakdown of muscle protein accompanied by myoglobinuria, which is the urinary elimination of the muscle protein myoglobin. This can lead to acute renal failure and even death. It appears to be dose dependent and is more common in patients receiving a statin in combination with cyclosporine, gemfibrozil (a fibrate), or erythromycin. When recognized reasonably early, rhabdomyolysis is usually reversible with discontinuation of the statin drug. Risk factors for myopathy include: age older than 65 years, hypothyroidism, renal insufficiency, and drug interactions. Instruct patients to immediately report any signs of toxicity, including muscle soreness or changes in urine color.

Toxicity and Management of Overdose

Very limited data are available on the nature of toxicity and overdose in patients taking HMG-CoA reductase inhibitors. Treatment, if needed, is supportive and based on presenting symptoms.

Interactions

Drug interactions with the HMG-CoA reductase inhibitors are listed in Table 27-5. They are to be used cautiously in patients taking oral anticoagulants. In addition, the coadministration of the statins with drugs that are metabolized by cytochrome P-450 enzyme 3A4 (CYP3A4) (see Chapter 2), such as erythromycin, azole antifungals, verapamil, diltiazem, HIV and hepatitis C protease inhibitors, amiodarone, and grapefruit juice, may lead to the development of rhabdomyolysis. Patients are advised to limit grapefruit juice to less than 1 quart daily.

DOSAGES

Selected Antilipemic Drugs

Drug (Pregnancy Category)	Pharmacologic Class	Usual Adult Dosage Range	Indications
◆ atorvastatin (Lipitor) (X)	HMG-CoA reductase inhibitor	PO: 10-80 mg/day	
◆ cholestyramine (Questran) (C)	Bile acid sequestrant	PO: 4-16 g/day; give all other drugs 1 hr before or 4-6 hr after cholestyramine	
ezetimibe (Zetia) (C)	Cholesterol absorption inhibitor	PO: 10 mg once daily	Hyperlipidemia
gemfibrozil (Lopid) (C)	Fibric acid derivative	PO: 600 mg bid 30 min ac in AM and PM	
◆ niacin (nicotinic acid, vitamin B$_3$) (A; C if dose exceeds RDA)	B vitamin	ER: 500-2000 mg/day	
◆ simvastatin (Zocor) (X)	HMG-CoA reductase inhibitor	PO: 5-40 mg daily	

HMG-CoA, Hydroxymethylglutaryl–coenzyme A; *RDA,* recommended daily allowance.

Components in grapefruit juice inactivate the enzyme CYP3A4, which plays a key role in statin metabolism. The presence of grapefruit juice results in sustained levels of unmetabolized statin drug, which increases the risk for major drug toxicity (e.g., rhabdomyolysis). Pravastatin and fluvastatin inhibit CYP3A4 to a much smaller degree than the other statins, whereas lovastatin and simvastatin are the most potent inhibitors of this enzyme. The use of gemfibrozil and statins together is not recommended due to increased risk for rhabdomyolysis.

Laboratory Test Interactions

Laboratory interactions that can occur include abnormal liver function tests.

Dosages

For dosage information on atorvastatin, see the table above.

DRUG PROFILES

The HMG-CoA reductase inhibitors, or statins as they are commonly called, are all potent inhibitors of HMG-CoA reductase, the enzyme that catalyzes the rate-limiting step in the synthesis of cholesterol. Seven statins are currently on the market in the United States: atorvastatin (Lipitor), fluvastatin (Lescol), lovastatin (Mevacor), pravastatin (Pravachol), simvastatin (Zocor), rosuvastatin (Crestor), and pitavastatin (Livalo). There are some minor differences between drugs in this class of antilipemics; the most dramatic difference is that of potency. All statins are prescription-only drugs and are contraindicated in those with active liver dysfunction or elevated serum transaminase levels of unknown cause. They are classified as pregnancy category X drugs and are to be avoided during pregnancy and lactation. There is little evidence to recommend one drug over another. However, in terms of drug interactions, lovastatin and simvastatin are the statins most commonly involved.

◆ atorvastatin

Atorvastatin (Lipitor) has become one of the most commonly used drugs in this class of cholesterol-lowering drugs. It is used to lower total and LDL cholesterol levels as well as triglyceride levels. Atorvastatin has also been shown to raise levels of "good" cholesterol, the HDL component. All statins are dosed once daily, usually with the evening meal or at bedtime. Bedtime dosing provides peak drug levels in a time frame that correlates better with the natural *diurnal* (daytime) rhythm of cholesterol production in the body. It is classified as a pregnancy category X drug.

Pharmacokinetics: Atorvastatin

Route	Onset of Action	Peak Plasma Concentration	Elimination Half-life	Duration of Action
PO	0.5 hr	1-2 hr	7-14 hr	Unknown

◆ simvastatin

Simvastatin (Zocor) was the one of the first statins to become generic and is one of the most commonly used drugs in this class. As with all statins, it is used primarily to lower total and LDL cholesterol levels as well as triglyceride levels. It can also modestly raise levels of HDL, the "good" cholesterol. It is classified as a pregnancy category X drug. Drug interactions can be significant with simvastatin. The FDA imposed prescribing restrictions on simvastatin, stating "Physicians should limit using the 80-mg dose unless the patient has already been taking the drug for 12 months and there is no evidence of myopathy. Simvastatin 80 mg should not be started in new patients, including patients already taking lower doses of the drug." In addition, simvastatin is not to be used with certain other drugs including itraconazole, ketoconazole, posaconazole, erythromycin, clarithromycin, HIV protease inhibitors, nefazodone, femfibrozil, cyclosporine, and danazol. In patients taking verapamil and diltiazem, the dose of simvastatin is not to exceed 10 mg. In patients taking amiodarone, amlodipine, and ranolazine, the dose is not to exceed 20 mg.

Pharmacokinetics: Simvastatin

Route	Onset of Action	Peak Plasma Concentration	Elimination Half-life	Duration of Action
PO	3 days	1.3-2.4 hr	Unknown	Unknown

BILE ACID SEQUESTRANTS

Bile acid sequestrants, also called *bile acid–binding resins* and *ion-exchange resins,* include cholestyramine, colestipol, and colesevelam. The first two of these drugs have been used widely for more than 20 years and have been evaluated extensively in well-controlled clinical trials. They have proven efficacy, but their powdered forms are somewhat inconvenient to use. Colestipol is also available in tablet form. Colesevelam has a similar mechanism of action and is available only in tablet form. These drugs are considered second-line drugs after the more potent statins. They are suitable alternatives for patients intolerant of the statins. Generally these drugs lower the plasma concentrations of LDL cholesterol by 15% to 30%. They also increase the HDL cholesterol level by 3% to 8% and increase hepatic triglyceride and VLDL production, which may result in a 10% to 50% increase in the triglyceride level.

Mechanism of Action and Drug Effects

Bile acid sequestrants bind bile and prevent the resorption of the bile acids from the small intestine. An insoluble bile acid and resin (drug) complex is formed and then excreted in the bowel movement. Bile acids are necessary for the absorption of cholesterol from the small intestine and are also synthesized from cholesterol by the liver. This is one natural way that the liver excretes cholesterol from the body. The more that bile acids are excreted in the feces, the more the liver converts cholesterol to bile acids. This reduces the level of cholesterol in the liver and thus in the circulation as well. The liver then attempts to compensate for the loss of cholesterol by increasing the number of LDL receptors on its surface. Circulating LDL molecules bind to these receptors to be taken up into the liver, which has the benefit of reducing circulating LDL in the bloodstream.

Indications

Bile acid sequestrants may be used as primary or adjunct drug therapy in the management of type II hyperlipoproteinemia. A common strategy is to use them along with statins for an additive drug effect in reducing LDL cholesterol levels. In addition, cholestyramine is used to relieve the pruritus associated with partial biliary obstruction. Colesevelam may be better tolerated by higher-risk patients who are intolerant of other antilipemic therapy, including organ transplant recipients and those with serious liver or kidney disease.

Contraindications

Contraindications to the use of bile acid sequestrants include known drug allergy, biliary or bowel obstruction, and phenylketonuria (PKU).

Adverse Effects

The adverse effects of colestipol, cholestyramine, and colesevelam are similar; however, colesevelam is reported to have fewer gastrointestinal adverse effects and drug interactions. Constipation is a common problem and may be accompanied by heartburn, nausea, belching, and bloating. These adverse effects tend to disappear over time. Patients may require education and support to help them deal with the gastrointestinal effects and comply with the medication regimen. It is important that therapy be initiated with low dosages and that patients be instructed to take the drugs with meals to reduce the adverse

effects. Increasing dietary fiber intake or taking a fiber supplement such as psyllium (Metamucil and others), as well as increasing fluid intake, may relieve constipation and bloating. These drugs may also cause mild increases in triglyceride levels. The most common adverse effects of the bile acid sequestrants are listed in Table 27-6.

Toxicity and Management of Overdose

Because the bile acid sequestrants are not absorbed, an overdose can cause obstruction of the gastrointestinal tract. Therefore, treatment of an overdose involves restoring gut motility.

Interactions

The significant drug interactions associated with the use of bile acid sequestrants are limited to effects on the absorption of concurrently administered drugs. All drugs must be taken at least 1 hour before or 4 to 6 hours after the administration of bile acid sequestrants. In addition, high doses of a bile acid sequestrant decrease the absorption of fat-soluble vitamins (A, D, E, and K).

Dosages

For dosage information on a selected bile acid sequestrant, see the table on the previous page.

DRUG PROFILE

The bile acid sequestrants cholestyramine, colestipol, and colesevelam are indicated for the treatment of type IIa and IIb hyperlipidemia. They lower the cholesterol level, in particular the LDL cholesterol level, by increasing the destruction of LDL. Because of the high incidence of gastrointestinal adverse effects, adherence to the prescribed dosage schedules is often poor. However, educating patients about the purpose and expected adverse effects of therapy can foster improved adherence. Warn patients not to take bile acid sequestrants at the same time as other drugs because of reduced absorption. Other drugs must be taken at least 1 hour before or 4 to 6 hours after the bile sequestrant. This requirement cannot be overemphasized.

◆ cholestyramine

Cholestyramine (Questran) is a prescription-only drug that is contraindicated in patients with a known hypersensitivity to it and in those who have complete biliary obstruction or PKU. It may interfere with the distribution of proper amounts of fat-soluble vitamins to the fetus or nursing infant of a pregnant or nursing woman taking the drug. Cholestyramine is now being used for its constipating effect, often given as needed for loose bowel movements. Cholestyramine is available as a dry powder and poses a choking hazard if not diluted before administering.

TABLE 27-6 Bile Acid Sequestrants: Adverse Effects	
Body System	**Adverse Effects**
Gastrointestinal	Constipation, nausea, belching, bloating
Other	Headache, tinnitus, burnt odor of urine

NIACIN

Niacin, or nicotinic acid, is not only a unique lipid-lowering drug, it is also a vitamin. Much larger doses of the drug are required for its lipid-lowering effects than are commonly given when it is used as a vitamin. Niacin is a B vitamin, specifically vitamin B_3. It is an effective and inexpensive medication that exerts favorable effects on the plasma concentrations of all lipoproteins. Niacin may be given in combination with other antilipemic drugs to enhance the lipid-lowering effects. The most recent guidelines do not recommend routine use of niacin as first-line therapy.

Mechanism of Action and Drug Effects

Although the exact mechanism of action of niacin is unknown, its action is believed to be related to its ability to inhibit lipolysis in adipose tissue, decrease esterification of triglycerides in the liver, and increase the activity of lipoprotein lipase. The drug effects are primarily limited to reduction of the metabolism or catabolism of cholesterol and triglycerides. In large doses, it may produce vasodilatation that is limited to the cutaneous vessels. This effect seems to be induced by prostaglandins. Niacin also causes the release of histamine, which results in an increase in gastric motility and acid secretion. Niacin may also stimulate the fibrinolytic system to break down fibrin clots.

Indications

Niacin is used to lower lipid levels, including triglyceride, total serum cholesterol, and LDL cholesterol levels. It also increases HDL cholesterol levels. Niacin may also lower the levels of lipoprotein(a), except in patients with severe hypertriglyceridemia. It can be used in the treatment of type IIa, IIb, III, IV, and V hyperlipidemia. Niacin's effects on triglyceride levels begin to be noticed after 1 to 4 days of therapy, with the maximum effects seen after 3 to 5 weeks of continuous therapy. However, recent data indicate that niacin has no effect on cardiovascular outcomes in patients taking statins, but is associated with numerous adverse effects.

Contraindications

Contraindications to the use of niacin include known drug allergy and may include liver disease, peptic ulcer, and the presence of any active hemorrhagic process.

Adverse Effects

Niacin can cause flushing, pruritus, and gastrointestinal distress. Small doses of aspirin or nonsteroidal antiinflammatory drugs (NSAIDs) may be taken 30 minutes before the niacin dose to minimize the cutaneous flushing. These undesirable effects can also be minimized by starting patients on a low initial dosage and increasing it gradually, and by having patients take the drug with meals. The most common adverse effects associated with niacin therapy are listed in Table 27-7.

Interactions

Drug interactions associated with niacin are minimal. However, when niacin is taken with an HMG-CoA reductase inhibitor, the likelihood of myopathy development is increased.

TABLE 27-7	Niacin (Nicotinic Acid): Adverse Effects	
Body System	**Adverse Effects**
Gastrointestinal	Abdominal discomfort
Integumentary	Cutaneous flushing, pruritus
Other	Blurred vision, glucose intolerance, hepatotoxicity

Dosages

For dosage information on niacin, see the table on p. 442.

DRUG PROFILE

♦ niacin

Used alone or in combination with other lipid-lowering drugs, niacin (nicotinic acid, vitamin B_3) (Nicobid) is an inexpensive medication that may have effects on LDL cholesterol, triglyceride, and HDL cholesterol levels. Drug therapy is usually initiated at a small daily dose taken with or after meals to minimize the adverse effects. Liver dysfunction has been observed in individuals taking sustained-release forms of niacin, but not immediate-release forms. Extended-release dosage forms, which dissolve more slowly than the immediate-release but faster than the sustained-release forms, appear to have better adverse effect profiles, including less hepatotoxicity and flushing of the skin. Niacin is contraindicated in patients with a known hypersensitivity to it; in those with peptic ulcer, hepatic disease, or hemorrhage; and in lactating women. It is also not recommended for patients with gout. Niacin is available over the counter and by prescription.

Pharmacokinetics: Niacin

Route	Onset of Action	Peak Plasma Concentration	Elimination Half-life	Duration of Action
PO	Rapid	30-60 min	45 min	Unknown

FIBRIC ACID DERIVATIVES

Current fibric acid derivatives include gemfibrozil and fenofibrate. These drugs primarily affect the triglyceride levels but may also lower the total cholesterol and LDL cholesterol levels and raise the HDL cholesterol level. They are often collectively referred to as *fibrates*.

Mechanism of Action and Drug Effects

Fibrates work by activating lipoprotein lipase, an enzyme responsible for the breakdown of cholesterol. This enzyme cleaves off a triglyceride molecule from VLDL or LDL, leaving behind lipoproteins. Fibric acid derivatives also suppress the release of free fatty acid from adipose tissue, inhibit the synthesis of triglycerides in the liver, and increase the secretion of cholesterol into bile. They have been shown to reduce triglyceride levels and serum VLDL and LDL concentrations. Independent of their lipid-lowering actions, fibric acid derivatives can also induce changes in blood coagulation. This involves a tendency toward a decrease in platelet adhesiveness. They can also increase plasma fibrinolysis, the process that causes clots to be broken down.

Indications

The fibric acid derivatives gemfibrozil and fenofibrate decrease the triglyceride level and increase the HDL cholesterol level by as much as 25%. Both decrease the LDL concentrations in patients with type IIa and IIb hyperlipidemia but increase the LDL levels in patients with type IV and V hyperlipidemia. They are indicated for the treatment of type III, IV, and V hyperlipidemia, and in some cases the type IIb form, although other classes of antilipemics are usually tried first. The latest guidelines no longer recommend routine use of fibrates as first-line drugs.

Contraindications

Contraindications to the use of fibrates include known drug allergy and may include severe liver or kidney disease, cirrhosis, and gallbladder disease.

Adverse Effects

The most common adverse effects of the fibric acid derivatives are abdominal discomfort, diarrhea, nausea, headache, blurred vision, increased risk for gallstones, and prolonged pro-thrombin time. Liver function tests may also show increased enzyme levels. The more common adverse effects are listed in Table 27-8.

Toxicity and Management of Overdose

The management of fibrate overdose, which is uncommon, is supportive care based on presenting symptoms.

Interactions

Gemfibrozil can enhance the action of oral anticoagulants, thus careful adjustment of the dosage of warfarin is required. The risk for myositis, myalgias, and rhabdomyolysis is increased when either gemfibrozil or fenofibrate is given with a statin. Combining gemfibrozil with a statin is generally not recommended due to an increased risk for rhabdomyolysis. Laboratory test interactions that can occur in patients taking gemfibrozil include a decrease in the hemoglobin level, hematocrit value, and white blood cell count. In addition, the aspartate aminotransferase level, activated clotting time, lactate dehydrogenase level, and bilirubin level can be increased.

Fenofibrate may raise the blood level of ezetimibe if the two are taken concurrently.

TABLE 27-8 Fibric Acid Derivatives: Adverse Effects

Body System	Adverse Effects
Gastrointestinal	Nausea, vomiting, diarrhea, gallstones
Genitourinary	Impotence, decreased urine output, hematuria
Other	Drowsiness, dizziness, rash, pruritus, vertigo

Dosages

For dosage information on gemfibrozil, see the table on p. 442.

DRUG PROFILES

The fibric acid derivatives gemfibrozil and fenofibrate are prescription-only drugs and are the only two drugs available in this class. They are both classified as pregnancy category C drugs and are contraindicated in patients with a known hypersensitivity, preexisting gallbladder disease, significant hepatic or renal dysfunction, and primary biliary cirrhosis. Both drugs decrease the triglyceride levels and increase the HDL levels by as much as 25%. They are good drugs for the treatment of mixed hyperlipidemias.

gemfibrozil

Gemfibrozil (Lopid) is a fibric acid derivative that decreases the synthesis of apolipoprotein B and lowers the VLDL level. It can also increase the HDL level. It is effective for lowering plasma triglyceride levels Gemfibrozil is indicated for the treatment of type IV and V hyperlipidemia, and, in some cases, the type IIb form. Recommended dosages are given in the table on p. 442.

Pharmacokinetics: Gemfibrozil

Route	Onset of Action	Peak Plasma Concentration	Elimination Half-life	Duration of Action
PO	Several days	1-2 hr	1.3-1.5 hr	Unknown

MISCELLANEOUS ANTILIPEMIC DRUG

CHOLESTEROL ABSORPTION INHIBITOR

ezetimibe

Ezetimibe (Zetia) is currently the only cholesterol absorption inhibitor available. Ezetimibe has a novel mechanism of action in that it selectively inhibits absorption of cholesterol and related sterols in the small intestine. The result is a reduction in several blood lipid parameters: total cholesterol level, LDL cholesterol level, apolipoprotein B level, and triglyceride level. Serum levels of HDL cholesterol, the so-called *good* cholesterol, have been shown to increase with the use of ezetimibe. Beneficial effects of ezetimibe appear to be further enhanced when given with a statin drug. Ezetimibe may also be used as monotherapy. In 2011, the FDA expanded the use of ezetimibe in patients with moderate to severe chronic kidney disease, as studies showed it was effective in reducing the risk for vascular events in such patients.

Ezetimibe levels are increased by the fibric acid derivatives (fibrates). It is not known whether this is harmful, but concurrent use of ezetimibe and fibrates is not recommended. The use of ezetimibe with bile acid sequestrants has been shown to reduce the serum level of ezetimibe by 55% to 80%. Ezetimibe is contraindicated in those with a known hypersensitivity to it and in those with active liver disease or unexplained elevations in serum liver enzyme levels. It may be taken with or without food, and for patient convenience it may be dosed at the same time as a statin drug, if prescribed.

Pharmacokinetics: Ezetimibe

Route	Onset of Action	Peak Plasma Concentration	Elimination Half-life	Duration of Action
PO	Unknown	4-12 hr	22 hr	Unknown

NURSING PROCESS

ASSESSMENT

Before administering any *antilipemic* drug, obtain a thorough health and medication history with a listing of allergies and any prescription drugs, over-the-counter drugs, herbals, or supplements the patient is taking. Assess and document the patient's food intake over several weeks, dietary patterns, exercise program and frequency, weight, height, and vital signs. Also assess and document the patient's use of tobacco, alcohol, and/or social drugs, along with information about frequency, amount, and duration of use. Some lipid disorders are hereditary; therefore, assess the patient's family history. Assess for the presence of any positive risk factors for the detection of cholesterol disorders and other coronary heart disease (CHD) including the following: prior coronary heart disease, peripheral heart disease, stroke, age, gender, family history, cigarette smoking, high blood pressure, diabetes mellitus, obesity, and physical inactivity. (See coronary heart disease risk factors at *www.nhlbi.nih.gov.*)

Continue with an assessment of any cautions, contraindications, and potential drug interactions prior to use of any antilipemics. Assess serum lipid values and lipoprotein levels (see the Safety: Laboratory Values Related to Drug Therapy box on p. 448). With the use of *cholestyramine*, which contains aspartame, it is of particular interest to know if there is a history of PKU. Patients with PKU cannot properly process the amino acid phenylalanine, a component of protein. It is known that high levels of phenylalanine lead to behavioral, cognitive, and learning dysfunction as early as 3 weeks of age in such patients. Dietary restrictions must continue throughout life. Adult patients require monthly testing of phenylalanine levels. Because of the aspartame in cholestyramine, another class of antilipemics would be indicated, as ordered, to prevent further complications from this disorder.

HMG-CoA reductase inhibitors (the *statins*) are not to be used in patients with liver disease or who have increased liver enzymes. Other contraindications, cautions, and drug interactions have been previously discussed in the pharmacology section of this chapter. With the use of the statins and all antilipemics, assess the patient's intake of alcohol, including the amount consumed and the period of time that alcohol has been used, because of the potential for liver dysfunction associated with the majority of *antilipemics*. The statins may have more adverse effects on an already damaged liver. Monitor levels of liver enzymes that are indicative of liver function, including AST, CPK, and/or ALT. Review lipid and lipoprotein levels before, during, and after drug therapy with the statins as well as with other antilipemic drugs. Assess the patient for any musculoskeletal problems or complaints due to the possible adverse effect of myopathy. If AST or ALT blood levels increase or signs and symptoms of myopathy or rhabdomyolysis occur

(i.e., muscle soreness, changes in urine color, fever, malaise, nausea, or vomiting), the prescriber will most likely discontinue the drug. It is always important to assess for cultural practices because of the impact of one's beliefs on dietary restrictions. Cultural practices may also include herbal or homeopathic therapies that may pose as contraindications to use of statins and other antilipemics.

Use of *bile acid sequestrants* requires careful assessment of possible contraindications such as a patient history of biliary or bowel obstructions and PKU. Drug interactions are numerous (see previous discussion) because of the decreased absorption of drugs by the bile acid sequestrants. With *niacin*, patient assessment includes noting contraindications such as liver disease, peptic ulcer disease, gout, and any active bleeding. Liver function studies are usually ordered for baseline and comparative levels with the majority of antilipemics. *Fibric acid derivatives* are not used in patients with liver, kidney, or gallbladder disease, and so assessment for these disorders is critical to patient safety. With *ezetimibe* (*Zetia*), assess for liver disease and liver enzyme elevation before initiation of therapy.

NURSING DIAGNOSES

1. Imbalanced nutrition, less than body requirements, related to poor dietary habits
2. Deficient knowledge related to a lack of information about the disease, related complications, and lack of information about drug therapy
3. Risk for impaired liver function related to potential adverse and toxic effects of drug therapy

CASE STUDY

Patient-Centered Care: Antilipemic Drug Therapy

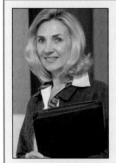

S.P., a 49-year-old mayor, lives a busy life but manages to exercise regularly and tries to follow a healthy lifestyle, including watching her diet. She is a nonsmoker and is not overweight. Recently S.P. had a medical checkup and, to her surprise, was told that her LDL levels are elevated at 220 mg/dL. She has no history of diabetes mellitus, and her blood pressure is within normal limits. Her nurse practitioner has recommended that she start the HMG-CoA reductase inhibitor (statin) drug atorvastatin (Lipitor) at a dosage of 20 mg every evening.

1. S.P. says, "Isn't there something else I can do instead of taking this medicine? I really don't like taking pills." What alternatives may be available to her?

    After 4 months, S.P.'s lipid levels are not improved. The nurse practitioner discusses with S.P. the consequences of not improving her lipid levels. S.P. agrees to try the statin drug and schedules a follow-up appointment for 3 months.

2. After 2 months, S.P. wakes up with some pain in her legs and feels extremely tired. She thinks she is suffering the effects of a new workout program that she started the previous day. But when she goes to work, the pain gets worse, and she calls the office nurse to describe her symptoms. What could be happening?

3. S.P. asks whether she will just be switched to another "statin" drug. How will the nurse respond?

For answers see *http://evolve.elsevier.com/Lilley.*

PLANNING: OUTCOME IDENTIFICATION

1. Patient states the importance of dietary restrictions with emphasis on low-fat, low-cholesterol, high-fiber, and low-calorie (if appropriate) diet as prescribed.
2. Patient demonstrates adequate knowledge about disease process, rationale for the need of lifelong drug therapy, and associated adverse effects.
3. Patient demonstrates knowledge of the risk for liver dysfunction associated with antilipemic therapy with identification of conditions that may arise for which the prescriber must be notified, such as jaundice and abdominal pain.

IMPLEMENTATION

Patients who are taking *antilipemics* for a long period may have altered levels of the fat-soluble vitamins and may then require supplementation of vitamins A, D, and K. Antilipemics may also cause problems with the liver and biliary systems and may cause gastrointestinal tract problems such as constipation. Appropriate actions need to be taken to avoid or minimize constipation, such as increasing intake of fiber and fluids. Monitoring the results of blood studies per the prescriber's instructions often includes reviewing levels of serum transaminases and results of other tests of liver function. Several omega-3 fatty acids that are essential fatty acids and available include prescription products *Lovaza* and *Epanova* (see pharmacology discussion; also see the Safety and Quality Improvement: Preventing Medication Errors Box on p. 441 for information about Lovaza). With the *HMG-CoA reductase inhibitors* or *statin* drugs, serum levels of the aforementioned components are often measured every 6 to 8 weeks for the first 6 months of statin therapy and then every 3 to 6 months, depending on the prescriber and the patient situation. If a lipid profile is ordered, instruct the patient to fast for 12 to 14 hours before the blood sample is drawn. Also, inform patients of the desired laboratory levels to achieve. Because severe cardiovascular diseases and cerebral vascular accidents (also known as *strokes*) are associated with very high cholesterol levels, it is critical to the maintenance of health and the prevention of complications that the patient continue with any prescribed nonpharmacologic and/or pharmacologic therapies, regardless of the specific antilipemic used. Another aspect to consider when administering these medications, specifically *simvastatin (Zocor)*, is dosage amount. The FDA has imposed prescribing restrictions on simvastatin 80-mg dosage forms (see pharmacology discussion). The FDA also recommends that the 80-mg dose of simvastatin "not be started in new patients, including patients already taking lower doses of the drug." There are additional concerns about simvastatin and other medications that have been discussed in the pharmacology section of this chapter.

Bile acid sequestrants often come in powder form and must be mixed thoroughly with food or fluids (at least 4 to 6 ounces of fluid). The powder may not mix completely at first, but patients need to be sure to mix the dose as much as possible and then dilute any undissolved portion with additional fluid. The powder needs to be dissolved for at least 1 full minute. Powder and/or granule dosage forms are *never* to be taken in dry form. It is important that *colestipol* and any of these drugs be taken 1 hour before or 4 to 6 hours after any other oral medication or meals because of the high risk for drug-drug and drug-food interactions. Bile acid sequestrants do interfere with the absorption of other medications. Colestipol is also available in tablet form. *Cholestyramine* is to be taken just before meals or with meals. *Never* give this drug to a patient with phenylketonuria (PKU) because cholestyramine contains aspartame (see previous discussion). Aspartame, an artificial sweetener, breaks down into phenylalanine and so is to be avoided in patients with PKU. Colestipol may cause constipation that may be prevented with high fiber and an increase in fluid intake.

With *niacin*, flushing of the face may occur; educate the patient on this adverse effect. To minimize gastrointestinal upset, advise the patient to take this medication with meals. Of the different dosage forms available, the extended-release dosage forms, which dissolve more slowly than the immediate-release forms but faster than the sustained-release forms, appear to be associated with less flushing of the skin. Other actions that may help to minimize flushing of the skin include titrating the drug dosage or taking a small dose of aspirin or NSAIDs 30 minutes before the niacin is taken, but only as ordered or recommended by the prescriber. Educate patients that *fibric acid derivatives* are to be taken as prescribed. Liver and kidney function tests and prothrombin times may be frequently monitored with these drugs. *The cholesterol absorption inhibitor ezetimibe (Zetia)* may be taken with or without food and may be taken with statin drugs.

EVALUATION

Evaluation of goals and outcome criteria is the best place to begin when trying to evaluate for the therapeutic versus adverse effects of these medications. In addition, cholesterol and triglyceride levels are used to monitor the patient's response to the medication regimen. For normal ranges of cholesterol, triglyceride, and lipids, (see the Safety: Laboratory Values Related to Drug Therapy box on the next page). While taking *antilipemics*, patients remain on a low-fat, low-cholesterol diet as an integrated part of a change in lifestyle. Monitor patients receiving antilipemic drugs for therapeutic and adverse effects during their therapy. The therapeutic effects of both nonpharmacologic and pharmacologic measures are evidenced by a decrease in cholesterol and triglyceride levels to within normal ranges (see previous serum laboratory values). Nonpharmacologic measures include a low-fat, low-cholesterol diet; supervised, moderate exercise; weight loss; cessation of smoking and drinking; and relaxation therapy. Adverse effects for which to monitor include gastrointestinal upset, increased liver enzyme levels, hepatomegaly, myalgias, and other effects mentioned earlier in the chapter. Closely monitor patients' renal and liver function before and throughout treatment to detect the development of liver or renal dysfunction.

QSEN EVIDENCE-BASED PRACTICE

Predictors of Statin Adherence, Switching, and Discontinuation in the USAGE Survey: Understanding the Use of Statins in America and Gaps in Patient Education

Review

After implementation of therapeutic lifestyle changes, statins are the first-line treatment in decreasing the elevation of low-density lipoprotein in cholesterol (LDL-C). Randomized clinical trials and epidemiological studies have shown that statins decrease the rates of myocardial infarction, stroke, as well as revascularization procedures. Statins have also been found to reduce the rate of cardiovascular and all-cause mortality in patients considered high-risk. The Understanding Statin Use in America and Gaps in Patient Education (USAGE) Survey was conducted to characterize current as well as former statin users, identify reasons for stopping use or switching of statins, and identify those factors associated with adherence.

Type of Evidence

USAGE is a cross-sectional, self-administered Internet-based survey to some 10,138 U.S. adults between September and October 2011. The following individuals who were statin users were identified and compared: adherent non-switchers, adherent switchers, nonadherent switchers, and discontinuers.

Results of the Study

A majority of the participants (82.5%) were current statin users who adhered with their prescribed statin regimen. Approximately 12% of former statin users identified the side effect of muscle pain as the primary reason for discontinuation (60%). The next reason for discontinuation in this same group was cost

(16%) followed by perceived lack of efficacy (13%). This study also found that individuals at risk for nonadherence included those with low household income, those experiencing muscle pain as a side effect while taking statins, and those taking medication for cardiovascular disease.

Link of Evidence to Nursing Practice

The fact that patients are not adherent to statin therapy is well-documented. Statin-related muscle side effects are common and do contribute significantly to the rates of discontinuation, switching, and nonadherence. As professional nurses, we can provide thorough patient teaching and communication about the side effects—but more importantly—the benefits of long-term statin use. Long-term adherence to statins has been associated with a greater cardiovascular disease risk reduction as compared to those individuals with poor adherence. Providing adequate opportunities for questioning and repeat educational sessions may help to improve the understanding of the need/benefit of statins with a subsequent increase in adherence and patient outcomes. More research on the at-risk, nonadherence populations, with a look at more effective means of education and improving patient-health care provider communication about drug therapy, may prove to be beneficial to rates of adherence. As professional nurses, we need to continue to use every opportunity to improve patient education/counseling about statin therapy, rationale for use, side effects, and the importance of adherence. The most effective, powerful tool we can provide to patients is that of education.

From Wei MY, Ito MK, Cohen JD, et al: Predictors of statin adherence, switching, and discontinuation in the USAGE survey: Understanding the use of statins in America and gaps in patient education. *J Clin Lipidol* 7(5), 472-483, 2013.

QSEN ⚡ SAFETY: LABORATORY VALUES RELATED TO DRUG THERAPY

Coronary Heart Disease

Laboratory Test	Normal Ranges*	Rationale for Assessment
Serum lipid panel with cholesterol, triglycerides, and various lipids	Serum cholesterol level: less than or equal to 200 mg/dL Triglyceride level: less than 150 mg/dL Low-density lipoprotein (LDL) cholesterol level: less than 100 mg/dL High-density lipoprotein (HDL) cholesterol level: greater than or equal to 60 mg/dL Very–low-density lipoprotein (VLDL) level: less than 130 mg/dL	A lipid panel is a serum test that measures the levels of lipids, fats, and fatty substances used as a source of energy in the body. Lipids include cholesterol, triglycerides, HDL, and LDL. When a lipid panel is ordered, the levels of all of the following are reported: total cholesterol, triglycerides, HDL, LDL, VLDL, ratio of total cholesterol to HDL, and ratio of LDL to HDL. Lipid levels are important to health status and are indicators of health; if there are abnormalities (e.g., high cholesterol, triglyceride, VLDL, and LDL levels and low HDL level), the individual is at increased risk for heart disease and stroke. Dietary and other lifestyle changes may be implemented to help decrease the levels of "bad" cholesterols (LDL and VLDL) and elevate the levels of "good" cholesterol (HDL).

*The values in this table are from the National Cholesterol Education Program of the National Institutes of Health.

▌ PATIENT-CENTERED CARE: PATIENT TEACHING

- Notify the prescriber if there are any new or troublesome symptoms or if there is persistent gastrointestinal upset, constipation, gas, bloating, heartburn, nausea, vomiting, abnormal or unusual bleeding, or yellow discoloration of the skin. Another symptom to report is muscle aches and pain.
- Advise the patient to keep these and all medications out of the reach of children and protected with childproof lids.
- Emphasize the importance of keeping a daily journal of fluid intake and dietary practices.

- Encourage a diet that is plentiful in raw vegetables, fruit, and bran. Increasing intake of fluids (up to 3000 mL/day unless contraindicated) may also help prevent the constipation associated with these medications.
- Advise the patient to inform health care providers about all medications he or she is taking, including antilipemics. These drugs are highly protein bound and are therefore associated with many drug interactions, including drugs that a dentist may prescribe. In addition, these drugs may alter

clotting if taken on a long-term basis. This information is also important for the patient to share with the dentist.

- Educate patients that exercise is to be done in moderation and often with supervision as indicated.
- Alert the patient to concerns regarding the use of 80-mg doses of simvastatin.
- When taking an HMG-CoA reductase inhibitor or statin drug, it is best taken with at least 6 to 8 ounces of water or with meals to help minimize gastric upset. It takes several weeks before therapeutic results are seen. Monitor liver and renal function laboratory studies every 3 to 6 months, as prescribed.
- Drug and food interactions associated with the statin drugs that must be avoided include oral anticoagulants, erythromycin, verapamil, some antifungal drugs, and grapefruit juice.
- With the HMG-CoA reductase inhibitors or statin drugs, any muscle soreness, change in color of the urine, fever, nausea, vomiting, and/or malaise must be reported to the prescriber immediately.
- If taking a bile acid sequestrant, advise the patient to take the medication with meals to decrease gastrointestinal upset. Other drugs must be taken 1 hour before or 4 to 6 hours after taking a bile acid sequestrant.
- Niacin is contraindicated in those with liver disease, peptic ulcer disease, gout, or active bleeding. Instruct patients to take niacin with meals to decrease gastrointestinal upset.

KEY POINTS

- There are two primary forms of lipids: triglycerides and cholesterol. Triglycerides function as an energy source and are stored in adipose (fat) tissue. Cholesterol is primarily used to make steroid hormones, cell membranes, and bile acids.
- Lipids and lipoproteins participate in the formation of atherosclerotic plaque, which leads to CHD, and it is important to understand the pathology of this disease process so that appropriate patient education may be delivered.
- When plaque forms in the blood vessels that supply the heart with needed oxygen and nutrients, the lumens of these blood vessels will eventually decrease in size and the amount of oxygen and nutrients that can reach the heart (and major organs) will be reduced.
- Antilipemic drugs are used to lower the high levels of lipids in the blood (triglycerides and cholesterol).
- The major classes of antilipemics include HMG-CoA reductase inhibitors, bile acid sequestrants, niacin, fibric acid derivatives, and cholesterol absorption inhibitors, with each having their own mechanism of action.
- While taking a history, it is important to assess the patient for any possible cautions, contraindications, and drug interactions.
- Fat-soluble vitamins may need to be prescribed for patients taking these medications for long periods because the antilipemics have long-term effects on the liver's production of these vitamins.
- Monitoring for adverse effects of the antilipemics includes periodic liver and renal function studies.
- The statins have gained much attention for their adverse effects of muscle aches and pain due to breakdown of muscle tissue. Some patients experience irreversible renal damage and severe pain and may have to alter dosages or change drugs as ordered by the prescriber.

NCLEX® EXAMINATION REVIEW QUESTIONS

1. A nurse administering niacin would implement which action to help to reduce adverse effects?
   a. Give the medication with grapefruit juice.
   b. Administer a small dose of aspirin or an NSAID 30 minutes before the niacin dose.
   c. Administer the medication on an empty stomach.
   d. Have the patient increase dietary fiber intake.
2. When administering niacin, the nurse needs to monitor for which adverse effect?
   a. Cutaneous flushing
   b. Muscle pain
   c. Headache
   d. Constipation
3. Which point will the nurse emphasize to a patient who is taking an antilipemic medication in the "statin" class?
   a. The drug needs to be taken on an empty stomach before meals.
   b. A low-fat diet is not necessary while taking these medications.
   c. It is important to report muscle pain immediately.
   d. Improved cholesterol levels will be evident within 2 weeks.
4. A patient is being assessed before a newly ordered antilipemic medication is given. Which condition would be a potential contraindication?
   a. Diabetes insipidus
   b. Pulmonary fibrosis
   c. Liver cirrhosis
   d. Myocardial infarction

5. A patient is currently taking a statin. The nurse considers that the patient may have a higher risk for developing rhabdomyolysis when also taking which product?
   a. NSAIDs
   b. A fibric acid derivative
   c. Orange juice
   d. Fat-soluble vitamins
6. The nurse is administering cholestyramine (Questran), a bile acid sequestrant. Which nursing intervention(s) is appropriate? *(Select all that apply.)*
   a. Administering the drug on an empty stomach
   b. Administering the drug with meals
   c. Instructing the patient to follow a low-fiber diet while taking this drug
   d. Instructing the patient to take a fiber supplement while taking this drug
   e. Increasing fluid intake
   f. Not administering this drug at the same time as other drugs

7. The medication order reads: niacin, 500 mg PO, every evening. The medication is available in 250-mg tablets. How many tablets will the patient receive per dose?
8. A patient has been taking simvastatin (Zocor) for 6 months. Today he received a call that he needs to come to the office for a "laboratory check." The nurse expects which laboratory studies to be ordered at this time? *(Select all that apply.)*
   a. PT/INR
   b. Total cholesterol
   c. Triglyceride
   d. Liver function studies
   e. Complete blood count
   f. HDL and LDL levels

1. b, 2. a, 3. c, 4. c, 5. b, 6. b, d, e, f, 7. 2 tablets, 8. b, c, d, f

CRITICAL THINKING AND PRIORITIZATION QUESTIONS

1. A patient has started taking niacin (nicotinic acid) as part of treatment for high cholesterol levels. After the first dose, he tells the nurse that he feels "hot" and that his face and neck are flushed. He says that he thinks he is having an allergic reaction. What is the nurse's priority action at this time?
2. While reviewing instructions for a newly prescribed antilipemic drug, a patient informs the nurse that he "hates to mix powdered medicines" and plans to take his cholestyramine (Questran) powder dry. What is the nurse's best response to this patient's comment?

For answers, see *http://evolve.elsevier.com/Lilley*.

ⓔ EVOLVE WEBSITE

Diuretic Drugs

http://evolve.elsevier.com/Lilley

OBJECTIVES

When you reach the end of this chapter, you will be able to do the following:

1. Describe the normal anatomy and physiology of the renal system.
2. Briefly discuss the impact of the renal system on blood pressure regulation.
3. Describe how diuretics work in the kidneys and how they lower blood pressure.
4. Distinguish among the different classes of diuretics with regard to mechanisms of action, indications, dosages, routes of administration, adverse effects, toxicity, cautions, contraindications, and drug interactions.
5. Develop a nursing care plan that includes all phases of the nursing process for patients receiving diuretics.

DRUG PROFILES

acetazolamide, p. 453
♦ furosemide, p. 455
♦ hydrochlorothiazide, p. 458
♦ mannitol, p. 456
metolazone, p. 459

♦ spironolactone, p. 457
triamterene, p. 457

_____
♦ = *Key drug*
! = *High-alert drug*

KEY TERMS

Afferent arterioles The small blood vessels approaching the glomerulus (proximal part of the nephron). (p. 452)

Aldosterone A mineralocorticoid steroid hormone produced by the adrenal cortex that regulates sodium and water balance. (p. 452)

Ascites Intraperitoneal accumulation of fluid (defined as a volume of 500 mL or more) containing large amounts of protein and electrolytes. (p. 455)

Collecting duct The most distal part of the nephron between the distal convoluted tubule and the ureters, which lead to the urinary bladder. (p. 452)

Distal convoluted tubule The part of the nephron immediately distal to the ascending loop of Henle and proximal to the collecting duct. (p. 452)

Diuretics Drugs or other substances that promote the formation and excretion of urine. (p. 452)

Efferent arterioles The small blood vessels exiting the glomerulus. At this point blood has completed its filtration in the glomerulus. (p. 452)

Filtrate The material that passes through a filter. In the kidney, the filter is the glomerulus and the filtrate is the material extracted from the blood (normally liquid) that becomes urine. (p. 452)

Glomerular capsule The open, rounded, and most proximal part of the proximal convoluted tubule that surrounds the glomerulus and receives the filtrate from the blood. (p. 452)

Glomerular filtration rate (GFR) An estimate of the volume of blood that passes through the glomeruli of the kidney per minute. (p. 452)

Glomerulus The cluster of kidney capillaries that marks the beginning of the nephron and is immediately proximal to the proximal convoluted tubule. (p. 452)

Loop of Henle The part of the nephron between the proximal and distal convoluted tubules. (p. 452)

Nephron The functional filtration unit of the kidney, consisting of (in anatomic order from proximal to distal) the glomerulus, proximal convoluted tubule, loop of Henle, distal convoluted tubule, and collecting duct, which empties urine into the ureters. (p. 452)

Open-angle glaucoma A condition in which pressure is elevated in the eye because of obstruction of the outflow of aqueous humor. (p. 453)

Proximal convoluted (twisted) tubule The part of the nephron that is immediately distal to the glomerulus and proximal to the loop of Henle. (p. 452)

OVERVIEW

Diuretics are drugs that accelerate the rate of urine formation via a variety of mechanisms. The result is the removal of sodium and water from the body. Diuretics were discovered by accident when it was noticed that a mercury-based antibiotic had a very potent diuretic effect. All the major classes of diuretic drugs in use today were developed between 1950 and 1970, and they remain among the most commonly prescribed drugs in the world.

The Eighth Report of the Joint National Committee on Prevention, Detection, Evaluation, and Treatment of High Blood Pressure reaffirmed the role of diuretics, especially the thiazides, as one of the first-line drugs in the treatment of hypertension. The hypotensive activity of diuretics is due to many different mechanisms. They cause direct arteriolar dilation, which decreases peripheral vascular resistance. They also reduce extracellular fluid volume, plasma volume, and cardiac output, which may account for the decrease in blood pressure. They have long been the mainstay of therapy not only for hypertension but also for heart failure. Two of their advantages are their relatively low cost and their favorable safety profile. The main problem with their use is the metabolic adverse effects that can result from excessive fluid and electrolyte loss. These effects are usually dose related and are controllable with dosage *titration* (careful adjustment).

This chapter reviews the essential properties and actions of the following important classes of diuretic drugs: carbonic anhydrase inhibitors, loop diuretics, osmotic diuretics, potassium-sparing diuretics, and thiazide and thiazide-like diuretics. All diuretics work primarily in the kidney.

The kidney plays a very important role in the day-to-day functioning of the body. It filters out toxic waste products from the blood while simultaneously conserving essential substances. This delicate balance between elimination of toxins and retention of essential chemicals is maintained by the nephron. The nephron is the main structural unit of the kidney, and each kidney contains approximately 1 million nephrons. Diuretics exert their effect in the nephron. The initial filtering of the blood takes place in the glomerulus, a cluster of capillaries surrounded by the glomerular capsule. The rate at which this filtering occurs is referred to as the glomerular filtration rate (GFR), and it is used as a gauge of how well the kidneys are functioning. The GFR can be estimated mathematically by calculating creatinine clearance. This is typically calculated by hospital pharmacists and is used to adjust drugs based on the patient's renal function.

The GFR, which can also be thought of as the rate at which blood flows into and out of the glomerulus, is regulated by the small blood vessels approaching the glomerulus (afferent arterioles) and the small blood vessels exiting the glomerulus (efferent arterioles). A mnemonic (memory aid) for remembering which arteriole is which is "A for *approach* and *afferent*" and "E for *exit* and *efferent.*" Alterations in blood flow such as those that occur in a patient in shock can therefore have a dramatic effect on kidney (renal) function. Diuretics may have diminished effects in situations of low blood flow,

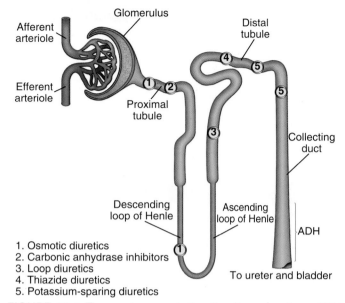

1. Osmotic diuretics
2. Carbonic anhydrase inhibitors
3. Loop diuretics
4. Thiazide diuretics
5. Potassium-sparing diuretics

FIGURE 28-1 The nephron and diuretic sites of action. *ADH,* Antidiuretic hormone.

because the kidney receives less blood, and therefore less diuretic reaches the site of action.

The proximal convoluted (twisted) tubule or, more simply, the *proximal tubule,* follows the glomerulus anatomically and returns 60% to 70% of the sodium and water from the filtered fluid back into the bloodstream. Blood vessels surround the nephrons and allow substances to be directly resorbed from or secreted into the bloodstream. This process is one of active transport that requires energy in the form of adenosine triphosphate (ATP) molecules. The active transport of sodium and potassium ions back into the blood causes the passive resorption of chloride and water. The chloride ions (Cl^-) and water passively follow the sodium ions (Na^+) and, to a lesser extent, potassium ions (K^+) by osmosis. Another 20% to 25% of sodium is resorbed back into the bloodstream in the ascending loop of Henle. Chloride is actively resorbed in the loop of Henle, and sodium passively follows.

The remaining 5% to 10% of sodium resorption takes place in the distal convoluted tubule, often called the *distal tubule,* which anatomically follows the ascending loop of Henle. In the distal tubule, sodium is actively filtered in exchange for potassium or hydrogen ions, a process regulated by the hormone aldosterone. The collecting duct is the final common pathway for the filtrate that started in the glomerulus. It is here that antidiuretic hormone acts to increase the absorption of water back into the bloodstream, thereby preventing it from being lost in the urine. The entire nephron, along with the sites of action of the different classes of diuretics, is shown in Figure 28-1.

PHARMACOLOGY OVERVIEW

Diuretics are classified according to their sites of action within the nephron, their chemical structure, and their diuretic potency. The sites of action of the various diuretics are determined by the way in which they affect the various solute

TABLE 28-1 Classification of Diuretics

Class	Drugs
Carbonic anhydrase inhibitors	Acetazolamide
Loop diuretics	Bumetanide, ethacrynic acid, furosemide, torsemide
Osmotic diuretics	Mannitol
Potassium-sparing diuretics	Amiloride, spironolactone, triamterene
Thiazide and thiazide-like diuretics	Chlorthalidone, chlorothiazide, hydrochlorothiazide, indapamide, metolazone

(electrolyte) and water transport systems located along the nephron (see Figure 28-1). The commonly used classes of drugs and the individual drugs in these classes are listed in Table 28-1. The most potent diuretics are the loop diuretics, followed by mannitol, metolazone (a thiazide-like diuretic), the thiazides, and the potassium-sparing diuretics. The potency of diuretics is a function of where they work in the nephron to inhibit sodium and water resorption. The more sodium and water they inhibit from resorption, the greater the amount of diuresis and therefore the greater the potency.

CARBONIC ANHYDRASE INHIBITORS

Carbonic anhydrase inhibitors (CAIs) are chemical derivatives of sulfonamide antibiotics. As their name implies, CAIs inhibit the activity of the enzyme carbonic anhydrase, which is found in the kidneys, eyes, and other parts of the body. The CAIs work at the location of the carbonic anhydrase enzyme system along the nephron, primarily in the proximal tubule. Acetazolamide is the CAI most commonly used today.

Mechanism of Action and Drug Effects

The carbonic anhydrase system in the kidney is located just distal to the glomerulus in the proximal tubules, where roughly two thirds of all sodium and water is resorbed into the blood. In the proximal tubules, there is an active transport system that exchanges sodium for hydrogen ions. For sodium and water to be resorbed back into the blood, hydrogen must be exchanged for it. Without hydrogen, this cannot occur, and the sodium and water will be eliminated with the urine. Carbonic anhydrase makes hydrogen ions available for this exchange. When its actions are inhibited by a CAI, such as acetazolamide, little sodium and water can be resorbed into the blood and they are eliminated with the urine. The CAIs reduce the formation of hydrogen (H^+) and bicarbonate (HCO_3^-) ions from carbon dioxide and water through the noncompetitive, reversible inhibition of carbonic anhydrase activity. This results in a reduction in the availability of the ions, mainly hydrogen, for use by active transport systems.

The reduction in the formation of bicarbonate and hydrogen ions can have effects on other parts of the body. CAIs can induce respiratory and metabolic acidosis. Both respiratory and metabolic acidosis can increase oxygenation during hypoxia by increasing ventilation, cerebral blood flow, and the dissociation of oxygen from oxyhemoglobin. These actions are usually beneficial to the patient. An undesirable effect of CAIs is elevation of the blood glucose level and glycosuria in diabetic patients. This may be due in part to CAI-enhanced potassium loss through the urine.

Indications

Therapeutic uses of CAIs include the treatment of glaucoma, edema, and high-altitude sickness.

CAIs are used as adjunct drugs in the long-term management of open-angle glaucoma that cannot be controlled by topical miotic drugs or epinephrine derivatives alone (see Chapter 57). Glaucoma is caused by the obstruction of the outflow of aqueous humor. When CAIs are given, an increase in the outflow of aqueous humor results. They are also used short term in conjunction with miotics to lower intraocular pressure in preparation for ocular surgery and as an adjunct in the treatment of secondary glaucoma.

Acetazolamide is also used to manage edema secondary to heart failure that has become resistant to other diuretics. However, as a class, CAIs are much less potent diuretics than loop diuretics or thiazides, and because of the metabolic acidosis they induce, their effectiveness diminishes in 2 to 4 days.

Acetazolamide is also effective in both the prevention and treatment of the symptoms of high-altitude sickness. These symptoms include headache, nausea, shortness of breath, dizziness, drowsiness, and fatigue.

Contraindications

Contraindications to the use of CAIs include known drug allergy, hyponatremia, hypokalemia, severe renal or hepatic dysfunction, adrenal gland insufficiency, and cirrhosis.

Adverse Effects

Common undesirable effects of CAIs are metabolic abnormalities such as acidosis and hypokalemia. Drowsiness, anorexia, paresthesias, hematuria, urticaria, photosensitivity, and melena (blood in the stool) can also occur.

Interactions

Because CAIs can cause hypokalemia, an increase in digoxin toxicity may occur when they are combined with digoxin. Use with corticosteroids may also cause hypokalemia. The effects of amphetamines, carbamazepine, cyclosporine, phenytoin, and quinidine may be increased when these drugs are taken concurrently with CAIs.

Dosages

The usual dose of acetazolamide is 250 to 500 mg per day, which may be given orally or IV.

DRUG PROFILE

acetazolamide

Use of acetazolamide (Diamox) is contraindicated in patients who have shown a hypersensitivity to it as well as in those with significant liver or kidney dysfunction, low serum potassium or sodium levels, acidosis, or adrenal gland failure. Acetazolamide is available in both oral and parenteral forms. It is classified as a pregnancy category C drug.

Pharmacokinetics: Acetazolamide

Route	Onset of Action	Peak Plasma Concentration	Elimination Half-life	Duration of Action
PO	1 hr	2-4 hr	10-15 hr	8-12 hr

LOOP DIURETICS

Loop diuretics (bumetanide, ethacrynic acid, furosemide, and torsemide) are very potent diuretics. Bumetanide, furosemide, and torsemide are chemically related to the sulfonamide antibiotics. Because they are structurally related to the sulfonamides, they are often listed as contraindicated in sulfa-allergic patients. However, analysis of the literature indicates that cross-reaction is unlikely to occur. Loop diuretics are commonly given to patients with sulfa allergy with no problems; however, it is prudent to always be aware of the potential of allergy.

Mechanism of Action and Drug Effects

Loop diuretics have renal, cardiovascular, and metabolic effects. These drugs act primarily along the thick ascending limb of the loop of Henle, blocking chloride and, secondarily, sodium resorption. They are also thought to activate renal prostaglandins, which results in dilation of the blood vessels of the kidneys, the lungs, and the rest of the body (i.e., reduction in renal, pulmonary, and systemic vascular resistance). The hemodynamic effects of loop diuretics are a reduction in both the preload and central venous pressures (which are the filling pressures of the ventricles). These actions make them useful in the treatment of the edema associated with heart failure, hepatic cirrhosis, and renal disease.

Loop diuretics are particularly useful when rapid diuresis is needed, because of their rapid onset of action. The diuretic effect lasts at least 2 hours. Loop diuretics have a distinct advantage over thiazide diuretics in that their diuretic action continues even when creatinine clearance decreases below 25 mL/min. This means that even when kidney function diminishes, loop diuretics can still work. Because of their potent diuretic effect and the duration of action, loop diuretics are usually effective when given in a single daily dose. This allows the renal tubule time to partially compensate for the potassium depletion and other electrolyte derangements that often accompany around-the-clock diuretic therapy. Despite this, the major adverse effect of loop diuretics is electrolyte disturbances. Prolonged administration of high dosages can rarely result in ototoxicity.

Summary of Major Drug Effects of Loop Diuretics

Loop diuretics produce a potent diuresis and subsequent loss of fluid. The resulting decreased fluid volume leads to a decreased return of blood to the heart, or decreased filling pressures. This has the following cardiovascular effects:
- Reduces blood pressure
- Reduces pulmonary vascular resistance
- Reduces systemic vascular resistance

TABLE 28-2 Loop Diuretics: Common Adverse Effects

Body System	Adverse Effects
Central nervous	Dizziness, headache, tinnitus, blurred vision
Gastrointestinal	Nausea, vomiting, diarrhea
Hematologic	Agranulocytosis, thrombocytopenia, neutropenia
Metabolic	Hypokalemia, hyperglycemia, hyperuricemia

- Reduces central venous pressure
- Reduces left ventricular end-diastolic pressure

The metabolic effects of the loop diuretics are secondary to the electrolyte losses resulting from the potent diuresis. Major electrolyte losses include loss of sodium and potassium and, to a lesser extent, calcium. Changes in the plasma levels of insulin, glucagon, and growth hormone have also been observed in association with loop diuretic therapy.

Indications

Loop diuretics are used to manage the edema associated with heart failure and hepatic or renal disease, to control hypertension, and to increase the renal excretion of calcium in patients with hypercalcemia.

Contraindications

Contraindications to the use of loop diuretics include known drug allergy, hepatic coma, and severe electrolyte loss. Although allergy to sulfonamide antibiotics is listed as a contraindication, analysis of the literature indicates that cross-reaction with the loop diuretics is unlikely to occur. Loop diuretics are commonly given to such patients in clinical practice.

Adverse Effects

Common undesirable effects of the loop diuretics are listed in Table 28-2. Hypokalemia is of serious clinical importance. To prevent hypokalemia, patients often receive potassium supplements along with furosemide. Furosemide can produce erythema multiforme, exfoliative dermatitis, photosensitivity, and in rare cases aplastic anemia. Torsemide may rarely cause blood disorders, including thrombocytopenia, agranulocytosis, leukopenia, and neutropenia. It may also cause a severe skin disorder called Stevens-Johnson syndrome.

Toxicity and Management of Overdose

Electrolyte loss and dehydration, which can result in circulatory failure, are the main toxic effects of loop diuretics that require attention. Treatment involves electrolyte and fluid replacement.

Interactions

Loop diuretics exhibit both neurotoxic and nephrotoxic properties, and they produce additive effects when given in combination with drugs that have similar toxicities. The drug interactions are summarized in Table 28-3.

Loop diuretics also affect certain laboratory results. They cause increases in the serum levels of uric acid, glucose, alanine

TABLE 28-3   Loop Diuretics: Common Drug Interactions

Interacting Drug	Mechanism	Results
Aminoglycosides vancomycin	Additive effect	Increased neurotoxicity, especially ototoxicity
Corticosteroids digoxin	Hypokalemia	Additive hypokalemia Increased digoxin toxicity
lithium	Decrease in renal excretion	Increased lithium toxicity
NSAIDs	Inhibition of renal prostaglandins	Decreased diuretic activity
Antidiabetic drugs	Antagonism	Decreased effectiveness of antidiabetic drugs (hyperglycemia)

NSAIDs, Nonsteroidal antiinflammatory drugs.

aminotransferase, and aspartate aminotransferase. Their combined use with a thiazide (especially metolazone) results in the blockade of sodium and water resorption at multiple sites in the nephron, a property referred to as *sequential nephron blockade,* which increases their effects. Nonsteroidal antiinflammatory drugs (NSAIDs) may diminish the reduction in vascular resistance induced by loop diuretics because these two drug classes have opposite effects on prostaglandin activity.

Dosages

For dosage information on loop diuretics, see the table on this page.

DRUG PROFILE

The currently available loop diuretics are bumetanide, ethacrynic acid, furosemide, and torsemide. Ethacrynic acid is rarely used clinically. As a class they are very potent diuretics, but potency varies for the different drugs. The equipotent doses of the drugs are as follows:

Bumetanide	Ethacrynic Acid	Furosemide	Torsemide
1 mg	50 mg	40 mg	10-20 mg

♦ furosemide

Furosemide (Lasix) is by far the most commonly used loop diuretic in clinical practice and the prototypical drug in this class. It has all the therapeutic and adverse effects of the loop diuretics mentioned earlier. It is used in the management of pulmonary edema and the edema associated with heart failure, liver disease, nephrotic syndrome, and ascites. It has also been used in the treatment of hypertension, usually that caused by heart failure.

Furosemide use is contraindicated in patients who have shown hypersensitivity to it or to the sulfonamides (see previous discussion regarding sulfonamide allergy) and in patients with anuria, hypovolemia, or electrolyte depletion. It is available in oral form as a solution, tablets, and an injectable form. It is classified as a pregnancy category C drug. Recommended dosages are given in the table below.

Pharmacokinetics: Furosemide

Route	Onset of Action	Peak Plasma Concentration	Elimination Half-life	Duration of Action
IV	5 min	15 min	1-2 hr	2 hr
PO	30-60 min	1-2 hr	1-2 hr	6-8 hr

OSMOTIC DIURETICS

The osmotic diuretics include mannitol, urea, organic acids, and glucose. Mannitol, a nonabsorbable solute, is the most commonly used of these drugs.

Mechanism of Action and Drug Effects

Mannitol works along the entire nephron. Its major site of action, however, is the proximal tubule and descending limb of the loop of Henle. Because it is nonabsorbable, it increases osmotic pressure in the glomerular filtrate, which in turn pulls fluid, primarily water, into the renal tubules from the surrounding tissues. This process also inhibits the tubular resorption of water and solutes, which produces a rapid diuresis. Ultimately, this reduces cellular edema and increases urine production, causing diuresis. However, it produces only a slight loss of electrolytes, especially sodium. Therefore, mannitol is not indicated for patients with peripheral edema because it does not promote sufficient sodium excretion.

Mannitol may induce vasodilation and in doing so increase both glomerular filtration and renal plasma flow. This makes it an excellent drug for preventing kidney damage during acute renal failure. It is also often used to reduce intracranial pressure

DOSAGES

Selected Loop Diuretics and Osmotic Diuretics

Drug	Pharmacologic Class	Usual Adult Dosage Range	Indications
♦ furosemide (Lasix)	Loop diuretic	IM/IV: 20-40 mg/dose PO: 20-120 mg/day	Heart failure, hypertension, renal failure, pulmonary edema, cirrhosis
♦ mannitol (Osmitrol)	Osmotic diuretic	Dose varies widely depending on indication	High intraocular or intracranial pressure

and cerebral edema resulting from head trauma. In addition, mannitol treatment may be tried when elevated intraocular pressure is unresponsive to other drug therapies.

QSEN 👪 **PATIENT-CENTERED CARE: LIFESPAN CONSIDERATIONS FOR THE PEDIATRIC PATIENT**

Diuretics

- Calculate pediatric dosages of diuretic medications carefully, regardless of whether the patient is in the hospital or in the home setting. Measure and record weight daily at the same time every day. This is important because pediatric patients are at greater risk for adverse effects and toxicity and, as such, need more cautious daily assessment to avoid exaggerated fluid and/or electrolyte loss, hypotension, and shock.
- The half-life of furosemide is increased in neonates, so the interval between doses may need to be lengthened, as ordered by the prescriber.
- The oral forms of diuretics may be taken with food or milk. Make sure to administer early in the day and at the same time every day, as prescribed.
- Lengthy exposure to either heat or sun must be avoided because it may precipitate heat stroke, exhaustion, and fluid volume loss in pediatric patients (taking diuretics).
- Thiazide diuretics cross the placenta and pass through to the fetus. Small amounts are distributed in breast milk; thus, breastfeeding is not advised for mothers who are taking these drugs.
- Alterations in laboratory test results that may be caused by diuretics include an increase in serum levels of calcium, glucose, and uric acid. Loop diuretics may interfere with BUN, chloride, magnesium, potassium, and sodium levels; therefore, perform frequent monitoring.

Indications

Mannitol is used in the treatment of patients in the early, oliguric phase of acute renal failure. For it to be effective in this setting, however, enough renal blood flow and glomerular filtration must still remain to enable the drug to reach the renal tubules. It can also be used to promote the excretion of toxic substances, reduce intracranial pressure, and treat cerebral edema.

Contraindications

Contraindications to the use of mannitol normally include known drug allergy, severe renal disease, pulmonary edema (loop diuretics are used instead), and active intracranial bleeding.

Adverse Effects

Significant undesirable effects of mannitol include convulsions, thrombophlebitis, and pulmonary congestion.

Interactions

There are no drugs that interact significantly with mannitol.

Dosages

For dosage information on mannitol, see the table on the previous page.

DRUG PROFILE

◆ mannitol

Mannitol (Osmitrol) is the prototypical osmotic diuretic. Its use is contraindicated in patients with a known hypersensitivity to it as well as in those with anuria, severe dehydration, pulmonary congestion, or cerebral hemorrhage. Treatment is terminated if severe cardiac or renal impairment develops after the initiation of therapy. It is available only in parenteral form as 5%, 10%, 15%, 20%, and 25% solutions for intravenous injection. The volume infused differs based on the concentration of mannitol provided, and the nurse may need to calculate the volume to be used. It is recommended to double-check calculations. Mannitol may crystallize when exposed to low temperatures. This is more likely to occur when concentrations exceed 15%. Because of this, mannitol is always administered intravenously through a filter, and vials of the drug are often stored in a warmer. Before administering mannitol, visually inspect the mannitol container for precipitants. Mannitol is classified as a pregnancy category C drug. Recommended dosages are given in the table on the previous page.

Pharmacokinetics: Mannitol

Route	Onset of Action	Peak Plasma Concentration	Elimination Half-life	Duration of Action
IV	0.5-1 hr	0.25-2 hr	1.5 hr	6-8 hr

POTASSIUM-SPARING DIURETICS

The currently available potassium-sparing diuretics are amiloride, spironolactone, and triamterene. These diuretics are also referred to as *aldosterone-inhibiting diuretics* because they block the aldosterone receptors. Spironolactone is a competitive antagonist of aldosterone, and for this reason it causes sodium and water to be excreted while potassium is retained. It is the most commonly used of the three drugs.

Mechanism of Action and Drug Effects

Potassium-sparing diuretics work in the collecting ducts and distal convoluted tubules, where they interfere with sodium-potassium exchange. Spironolactone competitively binds to aldosterone receptors and therefore blocks the resorption of sodium and water that is induced by aldosterone secretion. These receptors are found primarily in the distal tubule. Amiloride and triamterene do not bind to aldosterone receptors. However, they inhibit both aldosterone-induced and basal sodium resorption, working in both the distal tubule and collecting ducts. They are often prescribed for children with heart failure, because pediatric cardiac problems are frequently accompanied by an excess secretion of aldosterone.

The potassium-sparing diuretics are relatively weak compared with the thiazide and loop diuretics. When diuresis is needed, they are used as adjuncts to thiazide treatment. This combination is beneficial in two respects. First, the drugs have synergistic diuretic effects; second, the two drugs counteract the adverse metabolic effects of one another. The thiazide diuretics cause potassium, magnesium, and chloride to be lost in the urine, and the potassium-sparing diuretics counteract this by elevating the potassium and chloride levels.

Indications

Therapeutic applications of the potassium-sparing diuretics vary depending on the particular drug. Spironolactone and triamterene are used to treat hyperaldosteronism and hypertension and to reverse the potassium loss caused by the potassium-wasting (e.g., loop, thiazide) diuretics. One common feature of heart failure is a hyperactive renin-angiotensin-aldosterone system. Research has identified this hyperactivity as a causative factor in permanent ventricular myocardial wall damage, known as *remodeling,* following myocardial infarction. Various clinical trials have demonstrated a cardioprotective benefit of spironolactone in preventing this remodeling process, due to its aldosterone-inhibiting activity. The uses for amiloride are similar to those for spironolactone and triamterene, but amiloride is less effective in the long term. It may be more effective than spironolactone or triamterene in the treatment of metabolic alkalosis, however. It is primarily used in the management of heart failure. As with certain other classes of diuretics, potassium-sparing diuretics may also be indicated in cases of heart failure due to diastolic dysfunction.

Contraindications

Contraindications to the use of potassium-sparing diuretics include known drug allergy, hyperkalemia (i.e., serum potassium level exceeding 5.5 mEq/L), and severe renal failure or anuria. Triamterene use may also be contraindicated in cases of severe hepatic failure.

Adverse Effects

Potassium-sparing diuretics have several common undesirable effects, which are listed in Table 28-4. There are also significant adverse effects that are specific to individual drugs. Spironolactone can cause gynecomastia, amenorrhea, irregular menses, and postmenopausal bleeding. Triamterene may reduce folic acid levels and cause the formation of kidney stones and urinary casts. It may also precipitate megaloblastic anemia. However, adverse effects from triamterene are rare. Hyperkalemia may occur when potassium-sparing diuretics are used in combination with each other and/or with other potassium-sparing drugs such as angiotensin-converting enzyme (ACE) inhibitors (see Chapter 22, as well as the Interactions section to follow).

Interactions

Concurrent use of potassium-sparing diuretics and lithium, ACE inhibitors, or potassium supplements can result in significant drug interactions. The administration of ACE inhibitors or potassium supplements in combination with potassium-sparing diuretics can result in hyperkalemia. When lithium and potassium-sparing diuretics are given together, lithium toxicity can result. NSAIDs can inhibit renal prostaglandins, which decreases blood flow to the kidneys and therefore decreases the delivery of diuretic drugs to this site of action. This in turn can lead to a diminished diuretic response.

Dosages

For dosage information on potassium-sparing diuretics, see the table on this page.

DOSAGES

Selected Potassium-Sparing Diuretic Drugs

Drug	Usual Adult Dosage Range	Indications
amiloride (Midamor)	PO: 5-20 mg/day	Edema, heart failure (as an adjunct to loop diuretics)
♦ spironolactone (Aldactone)	PO: 25-200 mg/day; given once or divided twice daily	Edema, hypertension, heart failure, ascites
triamterene (Dyrenium)	PO: 50-100 mg bid; do not exceed 300 mg/day	

DRUG PROFILES

♦ spironolactone

Spironolactone (Aldactone) is a synthetic steroid that blocks aldosterone receptors. It is used in high dosages for the treatment of ascites, a condition commonly associated with cirrhosis of the liver. Monitor serum potassium levels frequently in patients who have impaired renal function or who are currently taking potassium supplements, because hyperkalemia is a common complication of spironolactone therapy. It is the potassium-sparing diuretic most commonly prescribed for children who have heart failure. Recently spironolactone has been shown to reduce morbidity and mortality in patients with severe heart failure when added to standard therapy. Of the three commonly used potassium-sparing diuretics, spironolactone has the greatest antihypertensive activity. It is available only in oral form. It also is available in combination with hydrochlorothiazide. Spironolactone is classified as a pregnancy category D drug. Recommended dosages are given in the table on this page.

Pharmacokinetics: Spironolactone

Route	Onset of Action	Peak Plasma Concentration	Elimination Half-life	Duration of Action
PO	1-3 days	2-3 days	13-24 hr	2-3 days

triamterene

The pharmacologic properties of triamterene (Dyrenium) are similar to those of amiloride. Like amiloride, triamterene acts

TABLE 28-4 Potassium-Sparing Diuretics: Common Adverse Effects

Body System	Adverse Effects
Central nervous	Dizziness, headache
Gastrointestinal	Cramps, nausea, vomiting, diarrhea
Other	Urinary frequency, weakness, hyperkalemia

directly on the distal renal tubule of the nephron to depress the resorption of sodium and the excretion of potassium and hydrogen. It has little or no antihypertensive effect. Triamterene is available only in oral form and is also available in combination with hydrochlorothiazide. It is classified as a pregnancy category D drug. Recommended dosages are given in the table on this page.

Pharmacokinetics: Triamterene

Route	Onset of Action	Peak Plasma Concentration	Elimination Half-life	Duration of Action
PO	2-3 hr	6-8 hr	2-3 hr	12-16 hr

THIAZIDES AND THIAZIDE-LIKE DIURETICS

Thiazide and thiazide-like diuretics are considered equivalent in their effects. Thiazide diuretics, like several of the loop diuretics, are benzothiadiazines, chemical derivatives of sulfonamide antibiotics. The thiazide diuretics include chlorothiazide and hydrochlorothiazide. Hydrochlorothiazide is the most commonly prescribed and the least expensive of the thiazide diuretics. Hydrochlorothiazide is included in numerous combination products with antihypertensive drugs. The thiazide-like diuretics are very similar to the thiazides and include chlorthalidone, indapamide, and metolazone. Metolazone may be more effective than other drugs in this class in the treatment of patients with renal dysfunction.

Mechanism of Action and Drug Effects

The primary site of action of thiazides and thiazide-like diuretics is the distal convoluted tubule, where they inhibit the resorption of sodium, potassium, and chloride. This results in osmotic water loss. Thiazides also cause direct relaxation of the arterioles (small blood vessels), which reduces peripheral vascular resistance (afterload). Decreased preload (filling pressures) and decreased afterload (the force the ventricles must overcome to eject the volume of blood they contain) are beneficial hemodynamic effects. This makes them very effective for the treatment of both heart failure and hypertension.

As renal function decreases, the efficacy of thiazides diminishes, because delivery of the drug to the site of activity is impaired. Thiazides are not to be used if creatinine clearance is less than 30 to 50 mL/min. Normal creatinine clearance is 125 mL/min, depending on age of the patient. However, metolazone remains effective to a creatinine clearance of 10 mL/min, and thus is used in cases of renal failure. The major adverse effects of the drugs stem from the electrolyte disturbances they produce. They are noted for precipitating hypokalemia and hypercalcemia, as well as metabolic disturbances such as hyperlipidemia, hyperglycemia, and hyperuricemia.

Indications

The thiazide and thiazide-like diuretics are used in the treatment of edema of various origins, idiopathic hypercalciuria, and diabetes insipidus, in addition to hypertension. They are also used as adjunct drugs in the management of heart failure

TABLE 28-5 Thiazide and Thiazide-Like Diuretics: Potential Adverse Effects

Body System	Adverse Effects
Central nervous	Dizziness, headache, blurred vision
Gastrointestinal	Anorexia, nausea, vomiting, diarrhea
Genitourinary	Impotence
Hematologic	Jaundice, leukopenia, agranulocytosis
Integumentary	Urticaria, photosensitivity
Metabolic	Hypokalemia, hyperglycemia, hyperuricemia, hypochloremic alkalosis

and hepatic cirrhosis. Any of these drugs can be used either as monotherapy or in combination with other drugs. As with certain other classes of diuretics, they may also be indicated in cases of heart failure due to diastolic dysfunction.

Contraindications

Contraindications to the use of thiazides and thiazide-like diuretics include known drug allergy, hepatic coma (metolazone), anuria, and severe renal failure.

Adverse Effects

Major adverse effects of the thiazide and thiazide-like diuretics relate to the electrolyte and metabolic disturbances they cause—mainly reduced potassium levels and elevated levels of calcium, lipids, glucose, and uric acid. Other effects, such as gastrointestinal disturbances, skin rashes, photosensitivity, thrombocytopenia, pancreatitis, and cholecystitis, are less common. Dizziness and vertigo are common adverse effects of metolazone therapy and are attributed to sudden shifts in the plasma volume brought about by the drug. Headache, impotence, and decreased libido are other important adverse effects of these drugs. Many of these adverse effects are dose related and are seen at higher doses, especially those above 25 mg. The more common adverse effects of the thiazide and thiazide-like diuretics are listed in Table 28-5.

Toxicity and Management of Overdose

An overdose of these drugs can lead to an electrolyte imbalance resulting from hypokalemia. Symptoms include anorexia, nausea, lethargy, muscle weakness, mental confusion, and hypotension. Treatment involves electrolyte replacement.

Interactions

Thiazides and related drugs interact with corticosteroids, diazoxide, digitalis, and oral hypoglycemics. The mechanisms and results of these interactions are summarized in Table 28-6.

Dosages

For dosage information on thiazides and thiazide-like diuretics, see the table on the next page.

DRUG PROFILES

♦hydrochlorothiazide

Hydrochlorothiazide (HydroDIURIL), which is considered the prototypical thiazide diuretic, is a very commonly prescribed

TABLE 28-6   Thiazide and Thiazide-Like Diuretics: Common Drug Interactions

Interacting Drug	Mechanism	Results
Antidiabetic drugs	Antagonism	Reduced therapeutic hypoglycemic effect (i.e., increased blood glucose levels)
Corticosteroids	Additive effect	Hypokalemia
digoxin	Hypokalemia	Increased digoxin toxicity
lithium	Decreased clearance	Increased lithium toxicity
NSAIDs	Inhibition of renal prostaglandins	Decreased diuretic activity

NSAIDs, Nonsteroidal antiinflammatory drugs.

and inexpensive thiazide diuretic. It is also a very safe and effective diuretic. Hydrochlorothiazide is used in combination with many other drugs, including methyldopa, propranolol, spironolactone, triamterene, hydralazine, ACE inhibitors, beta blockers, and labetalol. Dosages exceeding 50 mg/day rarely produce additional clinical results and may only increase drug toxicity. This property is known as a *ceiling effect.* However, doses up to 100 mg/day are not uncommon.

Hydrochlorothiazide is available only in oral form. It is classified as a pregnancy category B drug. Recommended dosages are given in the table below.

Pharmacokinetics: Hydrochlorothiazide

Route	Onset of Action	Peak Plasma Concentration	Elimination Half-life	Duration of Action
PO	2 hr	4-6 hr	5-15 hr	6-12 hr

metolazone

Metolazone (Zaroxolyn) is a thiazide-like diuretic that appears to be more potent than the thiazide diuretics. This greater potency becomes important in patients with renal dysfunction. It remains effective to a creatinine clearance as low as 10 mL/min. It may also be given in combination with loop diuretics to produce diuresis in patients with moderate to severe symptoms of heart failure. Metolazone is more efficacious when given 30 minutes before loop diuretics. It is available only in oral form.

Metolazone is classified as a pregnancy category B drug. Recommended dosages are given in the table on this page.

Pharmacokinetics: Metolazone

Route	Onset of Action	Peak Plasma Concentration	Elimination Half-life	Duration of Action
PO	1 hr	1-2 hr	6-20 hr	24 hr

NURSING PROCESS

ASSESSMENT

Before giving a patient any type of *diuretic,* obtain a complete and thorough patient and medication history. Perform a physical assessment and document all findings, with emphasis on the body systems affected by the disease process or indication for the diuretic as well as by potential drug-related adverse effects. This would most likely include baseline assessment of breath sounds, heart sounds, neurologic status, as well as checking skin turgor (for edema), moisture levels of mucus membranes, and capillary refill. Because fluid volume levels and electrolyte concentrations are affected by diuretics, assess and document vital signs, weights, and intake/output measurements. These parameters are especially important as a reflection of the patient's fluid volume status. Assess postural blood pressures (e.g., lying, sitting, standing) before and during drug therapy because of diuretic-induced fluid volume loss possibly precipitating postural or orthostatic hypotension. Postural or orthostatic hypotension is a drop in blood pressure of 20 mm Hg or more upon standing.

In addition, assess specific laboratory values associated with renal and hepatic functioning; for example, BUN level (normal range, 8 to 25 mg/100 mL) and creatinine level (normal range, 0.6 to 1.5 mg/100 mL) for renal function, and ALP (normal range, 13 to 39 units/L), AST (normal range, 8 to 46 units/L in males, 7 to 34 units/L in females), and LDH (normal range, 45 to 90 units/L) for hepatic function. It is important to note, however, that normal ranges of these laboratory values may vary somewhat among health care institutions or laboratories. Serum electrolyte levels are also critical to assess before and during diuretic therapy because of the subsequent loss of electrolytes through the urine. Specifically, obtain and document serum potassium, sodium, chloride, magnesium, calcium, uric

DOSAGES

Selected Thiazide and Thiazide-Like Diuretic Drugs

Drug	Pharmacologic Class	Usual Dosage Range	Indications
◆ hydrochlorothiazide (HydroDIURIL)	Thiazide diuretic	**Adult** 25-200 mg/day, usually divided **Older Adult** 12.5-25 mg/day	Edema, heart failure (as an adjunct to loop diuretics)
metolazone (Zaroxolyn)	Thiazide-like diuretic	**Adult** PO: 2.5-20 mg/day	

acid, and creatinine levels, as ordered. Arterial blood gas levels may also be ordered.

Carbonic anhydrase inhibitors require close assessment of sodium and potassium levels. These drugs are not to be used in patients with a history of renal or liver dysfunction. As with any *diuretic* resulting in potassium loss (excluding potassium-sparing diuretics), if these drugs are given concurrently with digoxin, there is increased risk for digoxin toxicity because of the hypokalemia.

Loop diuretics are more potent than thiazide diuretics, combination products, and potassium-sparing diuretics. These drugs may pose more problems for the older adult patient or those with severe electrolyte loss and liver failure. An additional and significant concern for patients taking loop diuretics is their interaction with other medications that are neurotoxic or ototoxic (see Table 28-3). Cross-sensitivity has been documented in patients who are allergic to sulfonamide antibiotics (see pharmacology discussion). Loop diuretics may also cause severe skin reactions (i.e., exfoliative dermatitis with *furosemide*, Steven Johnsons syndrome with *torsemide*), so a thorough assessment of the patient's skin prior to administration is important. With torsemide, assess baseline complete blood counts and clotting studies, if ordered, because of the adverse effects of leukopenia, neutropenia, and thrombocytopenia. Additionally, with loop diuretics, potential drug-laboratory value interactions include increased serum uric acid and glucose levels.

With *potassium-sparing diuretics*, hyperkalemia may be an adverse effect; therefore, assess the patient's serum levels of potassium. Additionally, because of the potassium-sparing effect, contraindications include drugs or conditions that may result in hyperkalemia. Thus, potassium supplements, ACE inhibitors, and severe renal failure are contraindications.

QSEN **PATIENT-CENTERED CARE: LIFESPAN CONSIDERATIONS FOR THE OLDER ADULT PATIENT**

Diuretic Therapy

- Before and during diuretic drug therapy, measure the patient's height, weight, intake and output, blood pressure, pulse rate, respiratory rate, and temperature. Assess breath and heart sounds. Assess and document any edematous areas. Monitor serum sodium, potassium, and chloride levels.
- Emphasize to the older adult patient that diuretics need to be taken at the same time every day. These drugs are generally ordered to be taken in the morning to help prevent nocturia (voiding at night), which can result in lack of sleep. More importantly, nocturia can lead to injury if the individual needs to get out of bed to void, becomes dizzy and/or confused, and falls. A bedside commode may be used to decrease the risk for injury.
- If the older adult patient is living alone and has minimal to no assistance with the medication regimen, visits from a home health aide or other health care professional may help ensure safety, efficacy, and compliance not only in taking the medication but also in following all aspects of the therapeutic regimen.
- Exercise caution in administering diuretics to the older adult patient, because they are more sensitive to the therapeutic effects of these drugs (often reacting to smaller dosages of medication than are required by other patients) and are also more likely to experience the adverse effects of diuretics such as dehydration, electrolyte loss, dizziness, and syncope.

- Encourage the patient to change positions slowly because of the risk for orthostatic hypotension and subsequent falls and injury. Emphasize the importance of keeping a daily journal with weight, blood pressure, and overall well-being.
- Advise patients to carry a card containing a brief medical history, blood pressure readings, names and telephone numbers of contact persons, and a list of medications to ensure safety and minimize complications. The card can be formatted so that it may fit in a wallet. A copy may also be placed in the kitchen on the refrigerator door or in another visible location so that it will be easily available to emergency personnel. Copies of the card may be given to the caregiver(s), family members, significant others, prescribers, dentist, and relevant health care personnel. The card then needs to be updated at regular intervals by the patient or another adult, caregiver, or prescriber involved in the patient's care. Such a card can be made easily using standard card stock or an index card. It can be placed in a wallet sleeve and information entered using an erasable pen or pencil. The following sample shows suggested headings and content for such a card:

Name: _____ Age: ___ Allergies (drug/food): _____ Medical history (place X to the right of all that apply; write in any not listed): Anemia__ Asthma__ Bleeding problems__ Blood clots__ Breathing problems__ Cancer__ Depression__ Diabetes__ Difficulty swallowing__ Heart problems__ High blood pressure__ Low blood pressure__ Nerve problems__ Pacemaker or defibrillator device__ Recent weight gain__ Recent weight loss__ Stroke__ Thyroid problems__ Others: _____
Surgery (list all with date, type of surgery, purpose, any complications): _____

Prosthetics used: _____ Dentures/dental problems: _____ Assistive devices: Glasses__ Hearing aids__ Mobility assistance _____
Contact names and phone numbers: _____

Current medications (prescription drugs; over-the-counter drugs; herbals, vitamins, others):
Name(s) _____
Dosage(s) _____
Frequency of doses _____
Why taking the drug? _____

Lithium toxicity may occur if given with these *diuretics* because of the hyperkalemia. See the pharmacology section of this chapter for further discussion of additional cautions, contraindications, and drug interactions associated with diuretic use.

NURSING DIAGNOSES

1. Decreased cardiac output related to drug effects and adverse effects of diuretics (e.g., fluid and electrolyte loss)
2. Deficient fluid volume related to drug effects and adverse effects of diuretics
3. Risk for injury related to postural hypotension and dizziness

PLANNING: OUTCOME IDENTIFICATION

1. Patient regains and maintains balanced cardiac output with vital signs, adequate intake, and output within normal limits (pulse between 60 and 100 beats/min; blood pressure 120/80 mm Hg or within normal parameters; urine output 30 mL/hr or higher) and intact pedal pulses.
2. Patient regains and maintains balanced fluid volume status with firm turgor and normal limits for urine specific gravity and serum electrolytes.
3. Patient remains free from injury while taking diuretic with adequate fluid intake while avoiding hypotensive episodes.

IMPLEMENTATION

Measure and record blood pressure, pulse rate, intake and output, and daily weights during *diuretic* therapy. Changes from the initial baseline assessment data that alert you to possible problems with the drug therapy include the presence of dizziness, fainting, lightheadedness on standing or changing positions, weakness, fatigue, tremor, muscle cramping, changes in mental status, or cold, clammy skin. Diuretic therapy may also precipitate cardiac irregularities or palpitations; therefore, continue to monitor heart rate and rhythm. Fluid loss from the action of the diuretic may lead to the adverse effect of constipation, so preventive measures are needed, such as increased intake of fluids and fiber (unless contraindicated) and/or the use of natural bulk-forming products. If constipation continues, the prescriber may need to provide alternatives to psyllium-based bulk-forming laxatives. Always give diuretics exactly as directed but with consideration of the patient's age and related needs. Dosing and timing of the drugs are often very important to enhance therapeutic effects and minimize adverse effects. Because diuretics taken late in the afternoon or evening may lead to nocturia (urination at night) and subsequent loss of

sleep, these medications are usually scheduled for morning dosing. Safety concerns exist with nocturia, especially in the older adult patient, because possible confusion and dizziness associated with getting up in the middle of the night may create the potential for falls and injury.

Loop diuretics (if taken at high dosages as ordered) may put patients at greater risk for fluid volume and electrolyte depletion (e.g., hypokalemia, hyponatremia, dehydration). Monitoring of therapy includes frequent assessment of blood pressure and pulse rate, including orthostatic blood pressures and pulse rates (supine and standing), hydration status, and capillary refill, as well as daily measurement of weight. Acute hypotensive episodes may occur with higher dosages of loop diuretics and precipitate syncope and falls; therefore, educate the patient about safety measures to prevent falls. Hypokalemia is the most commonly encountered electrolyte imbalance and may be very dangerous. Symptoms include anorexia, nausea, lethargy, muscle weakness, mental confusion, and hypotension. If intravenous dosage forms are given, it is crucial to check for proper diluents, drug incompatibilities, and intactness of the intravenous site. Double-check rates of infusion and use an infusion pump as deemed necessary.

With *potassium-sparing diuretics,* potassium is reabsorbed and not excreted (as previously discussed), and the problem that may occur is hyperkalemia rather than hypokalemia. Signs and symptoms of hyperkalemia include nausea, vomiting, and diarrhea (see Chapter 29), with toxic levels manifested by cardiac rhythm abnormalities. Any of the signs and symptoms of hyperkalemia need to be reported immediately. See Patient-Centered Care: Patient Teaching later in the chapter for more information.

EVALUATION

The therapeutic effects of *diuretics* include the resolution of or reduction in edema, fluid volume overload, heart failure, or hypertension, or a return to normal intraocular pressures (if used for that purpose, as with the *CAIs*). Monitor the patient for the occurrence of adverse reactions to the diuretics, such as hypotension (from volume loss), electrolyte imbalances, metabolic acidosis (arterial blood gas values may need to be measured), drowsiness (with *CAIs*), hypokalemia, tachycardia (less significant with *mannitol*), and hyperkalemia (*potassium-sparing diuretics*). Hypokalemia may be manifested by anorexia, nausea, lethargy, muscle weakness, mental confusion, and hypotension. With *potassium-sparing diuretics*, monitor for the adverse effect of hyperkalemia manifested by nausea, vomiting, and diarrhea (see Chapter 29). Cardiac rhythm abnormalities may occur with severe hyperkalemia. Review all goals and outcome criteria in the evaluation process.

CASE STUDY

Patient-Centered Care: Hydrochlorothiazide Therapy

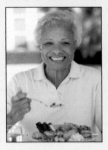

Dr. G., a 62-year-old university professor, has been diagnosed with primary hypertension and will be taking 50 mg of hydrochlorothiazide (HCTZ) daily. There is no evidence of renal insufficiency or cardiac damage at this time, nor is there evidence of retinopathy or other signs and symptoms of end-organ disease. She is anxious because the fall semester is starting and she has a heavy teaching load but is willing to take the steps needed for better health.

At her 1-month follow-up appointment, Dr. G. complains of "feeling so tired" and asks whether the medication causes sleepiness. When questioned, she says that she takes the HCTZ at dinnertime because she is afraid it will "interfere with her classes."

1. What do you suspect is happening with Dr. G., and what would you recommend?
2. During this follow-up appointment, you ask Dr. G. if she is eating foods high in potassium. She looks embarrassed and answers, "I lost that pamphlet about the foods with potassium, but I try to drink orange juice every day." What foods should she eat for the potassium content?
3. The report on Dr. G.'s potassium levels comes back from the laboratory, and the results are 3.4 mEq/L. She asks, "Am I going to be put on a potassium pill too?" What is your answer?
4. Six months later, Dr. G. is diagnosed with type 2 diabetes mellitus and is started on oral hypoglycemic therapy. What will you teach her about managing her diabetes while taking the HCTZ?

For answers see *http://evolve.elsevier.com/Lilley.*

PATIENT-CENTERED CARE: PATIENT TEACHING

- Patients taking diuretics need to maintain proper nutritional intake and fluid volume and eat potassium-rich foods, except when contraindicated or when potassium-sparing diuretics are used. Foods high in potassium include bananas, oranges, apricots, dates, raisins, broccoli, green beans, potatoes, tomatoes, meats, fish, wheat bread, and legumes.
- Potassium supplementation may be recommended by a prescriber, depending on the symptoms the patient presents and the serum levels. Normal serum potassium levels are 3.5 to 5 mEq/L (see Chapter 29).
- Frequent laboratory tests may be indicated at the beginning of and during therapy with diuretics. These tests may include measurement of electrolytes, uric acid, and blood gases.
- Encourage patients to change positions slowly and to rise slowly after sitting or lying to prevent dizziness and possible fainting (syncope).
- Forcing of fluids may be needed (if not contraindicated) to prevent dehydration and minimize constipation. Increased consumption of fiber may also help with constipation.
- Any unusual adverse effects or problems, such as excessive dizziness, syncope, weakness, or muscle aches, need to be reported immediately to the prescriber.
- Advise the patient to keep a daily journal; entries should include weight, how the patient feels each day, dosage of diuretic, and any other important information related to the diagnosis and medical treatment.
- Educate the patient about the signs and symptoms of hypokalemia, such as anorexia, nausea, lethargy, muscle weakness, mental confusion, and hypotension. In addition, emphasize the importance of being cautious with hot climates, excessive sweating, fever, and the use of saunas or hot tubs. Heat raises core body temperature and causes further loss of potassium, sodium, and water through sweat, which may increase the risk for more problems with hypotension and fluid-electrolyte imbalances. Fluid volume and electrolyte loss may also occur with vomiting and diarrhea.
- If the patient is taking a diuretic along with digoxin, educate the patient, family members, and anyone involved in the patient's care about how to monitor pulse rate. The warning signs and symptoms of digoxin toxicity include headache, dizziness, confusion, nausea, visual disturbances, and bradycardia. A pulse rate of 60 beats/min or lower is often used as a guideline, but always check health care institutiona policy or guidelines.
- Educate patients with diabetes who are also taking thiazide and/or loop diuretics about the need for close monitoring of blood glucose levels.

KEY POINTS

- The five main types of diuretics are CAIs, loop, osmotic, potassium-sparing, and thiazide and thiazide-like diuretics.
- The loop, potassium-sparing, and thiazide diuretics are the most commonly used. Remember that the loop diuretics are more potent than the thiazides, combination diuretics, and potassium-sparing diuretics.
- It is important to have a thorough knowledge of renal anatomy and physiology and how it relates to the action of the various diuretics; for example, if a loop diuretic is given, its site of action is the loop of Henle and it causes the excretion of sodium, potassium, and chloride into the urine.
- Methods for monitoring excess and deficit fluid volume states include assessment of skin and mucous membranes, blood pressure, pulse rate, intake and output, and daily weights.
- With diuretics, always be concerned about the more vulnerable patient populations, such as the older adult patient, those with chronic illnesses, and patients with altered renal or liver function.

NCLEX® EXAMINATION REVIEW QUESTIONS

1. The nurse is reviewing the medications that have been ordered for a patient for whom a loop diuretic has just been prescribed. The loop diuretic may have a possible interaction with which of the following?
   a. Vitamin D
   b. warfarin
   c. Penicillins
   d. NSAIDs

2. When monitoring laboratory test results for patients receiving loop and thiazide diuretics, the nurse knows to look for
   a. decreased serum levels of potassium.
   b. increased serum levels of calcium.
   c. decreased serum levels of glucose.
   d. increased serum levels of sodium.

3. When the nurse is checking the laboratory data for a patient taking spironolactone (Aldactone), which result would be a potential concern?
   a. Serum sodium level of 140 mEq/L
   b. Serum calcium level of 10.2 mg/dL
   c. Serum potassium level of 5.8 mEq/L
   d. Serum magnesium level of 2.0 mg/dL

4. Which statement needs to be included when the nurse provides patient education for a patient with heart failure who is taking daily doses of spironolactone (Aldactone)?
   a. "Be sure to eat foods that are high in potassium."
   b. "Avoid foods that are high in potassium."
   c. "Avoid grapefruit juice while taking this medication."
   d. "A low-fiber diet will help prevent adverse effects of this medication."

5. A patient with diabetes has a new prescription for a thiazide diuretic. Which statement will the nurse include when teaching the patient about the thiazide drug?
   a. "There is nothing for you to be concerned about when you are taking the thiazide diuretic."
   b. "Be sure to avoid foods that are high in potassium."
   c. "You need to take the thiazide at night to avoid interactions with the diabetes medicine."
   d. "Monitor your blood glucose level closely, because the thiazide diuretic may cause the levels to increase."

6. An older adult patient has been discharged following treatment for a mild case of heart failure. He will be taking a loop diuretic. Which instruction(s) from the nurse are appropriate? *(Select all that apply.)*
   a. "Take the diuretic at the same time each morning."
   b. "Take the diuretic only if you notice swelling in your feet."
   c. "Be sure to stand up slowly because the medicine may make you feel dizzy if you stand up quickly."
   d. "Drink at least 8 glasses of water each day."
   e. "Here is a list of foods that are high in potassium; you need to avoid these."
   f. "Please call your doctor immediately if you notice muscle weakness or increased dizziness."

7. The order reads: Give mannitol 0.5 g/kg IV now, over 2 hours. The patient weighs 165 lb, and you have a 100-mL vial of 20% mannitol. How many grams will the patient receive? How many milliliters of mannitol will you prepare for this infusion?

8. A patient is taking an aminoglycoside antibiotic for pneumonia, and will also be taking the loop diuretic furosemide (Lasix) due to fluid overload. The nurse will monitor carefully for which potential effect from the interaction of these two drugs?
   a. Nephrotoxicity
   b. Ototoxicity
   c. Pulmonary fibrosis
   d. Hepatotoxicity

1. d, 2. a, 3. c, 4. b, 5. d, 6. a, c, f, 7. 37.5 g, 187.5 mL, 8. b.

CRITICAL THINKING AND PRIORITIZATION QUESTIONS

1. A patient has been given a new order for spironolactone (Aldactone), 50 mg daily. While reviewing the patient's orders, the nurse notes that the patient has an existing order for potassium chloride (K-Dur), 20 mEq daily. The patient's potassium level is 3.9 mEq/L. What is the nurse's priority action at this time?

2. The nurse is administering a thiazide diuretic to a patient who has been receiving digoxin for several months as part of treatment for a cardiac dysrhythmia. What is the priority for regular assessment, considering the use of these two drugs together?

For answers see *http://evolve.elsevier.com/Lilley*.

EVOLVE WEBSITE

http://evolve.elsevier.com/Lilley
- Animations
- Answer Keys for Textbook Case Studies and Textbook Critical Thinking and Prioritization Questions

- Content Updates
- Key Points
- Review Questions
- Student Case Studies

29

Fluids and Electrolytes

ⓔ http://evolve.elsevier.com/Lilley

OBJECTIVES

When you reach the end of this chapter, you will be able to do the following:

1. Review the function of fluid volume and compartments within the body as well as the role of each of the major electrolytes in maintaining homeostasis.
2. Identify the various electrolytes, and give normal serum values for each.
3. Briefly discuss the various fluid and electrolyte disorders that commonly occur in the body with attention to fluid volume and/or electrolyte deficits and excesses.
4. Identify the fluid and electrolyte solutions commonly used to correct states of deficiency or excess.
5. Discuss the mechanisms of action, indications, dosages, routes of administration, contraindications, cautions, adverse effects, toxicity, and drug interactions of the various fluid and electrolyte solutions.
6. Compare the various solutions used to expand and/or decrease a patient's fluid volume and electrolytes with regard to how they work, why they are used, and specific antidotes available to counter any toxic effects.
7. Develop a nursing care plan that includes all phases of the nursing process for patients receiving fluid and electrolyte solutions.

DRUG PROFILES

albumin, p. 469
conivaptan, p. 473
dextran, p. 469
fresh frozen plasma, p. 470
packed red blood cells, p. 470
!potassium, p. 472

sodium chloride, p. 473
sodium polystyrene sulfonate (potassium exchange resin), p. 472

_____

♦ = *Key drug*
! = *High-alert drug*

KEY TERMS

Blood The fluid that circulates through the heart, arteries, capillaries, and veins, carrying nutriment and oxygen to the body cells. It consists of plasma, its liquid component, plus three major solid components: erythrocytes (red blood cells or RBCs), leukocytes (white blood cells or WBCs), and platelets. (p. 465)

Colloids Protein substances that increase the colloid oncotic pressure. (p. 468)

Colloid oncotic pressure Another name for oncotic pressure. It is a form of osmotic pressure exerted by protein in blood plasma that tends to pull water into the circulatory system. (p. 466)

Crystalloids Substances in a solution that diffuse through a semipermeable membrane. (p. 467)

Dehydration Excessive loss of water from the body tissues. It is accompanied by an imbalance in the concentrations of electrolytes, particularly sodium, potassium, and chloride. (p. 466)

Edema The abnormal accumulation of fluid in interstitial spaces. (p. 465)

Extracellular fluid (ECF) That portion of the body fluid comprising the interstitial fluid and intravascular fluid. (p. 465)

Gradient A difference in the concentration of a substance on two sides of a permeable barrier. (p. 467)

Homeostasis The tendency of a cell or organism to maintain equilibrium by regulating its internal environment and adjusting its physiologic processes. (p. 465)

Hyperkalemia An abnormally high potassium concentration in the blood, most often due to defective renal excretion but also caused by excessive dietary potassium or certain drugs, such as potassium-sparing diuretics or ACE inhibitors and other causes such as acidosis. (p. 471)

Hypernatremia An abnormally high sodium concentration in the blood; may be due to defective renal excretion but is more commonly caused by excessive dietary sodium or replacement therapy or loss of water. (p. 472)

KEY TERMS—cont'd

Hypokalemia A condition in which there is an inadequate amount of potassium in the bloodstream; possible causes include diarrhea, diuretic use, and others. (p. 471)

Hyponatremia A condition in which there is an inadequate amount of sodium in the bloodstream, caused by inadequate excretion of water or by excessive water intake. (p. 472)

Interstitial fluid (ISF) The extracellular fluid that fills in the spaces between most of the cells of the body. (p. 465)

Intracellular fluid (ICF) The fluid located within cell membranes throughout most of the body. It contains dissolved solutes that are essential to maintaining electrolyte balance and healthy metabolism. (p. 465)

Intravascular fluid (IVF) The fluid inside blood vessels. (p. 465)

Isotonic Having the same concentration of solutes as another solution and hence exerting the same osmotic pressure as that solution, such as an isotonic saline solution that

contains an amount of salt equal to that found in the intracellular and extracellular fluid. (p. 466)

Osmotic pressure The pressure produced by a solution necessary to prevent the osmotic passage of solvent into it when the solution and solvent are separated by a semipermeable membrane. (p. 466)

Plasma The watery, straw-colored fluid component of lymph and blood in which the leukocytes, erythrocytes, and platelets are suspended. (p. 465)

Serum The clear, cell-free portion of the blood from which fibrinogen has also been separated during the clotting process, as typically carried out with a laboratory sample. (p. 467)

Solute A substance that is dissolved in another substance. (p. 465)

Transcellular fluid The fluid that is contained within specialized body compartments such as cerebrospinal, pleural, and synovial cavities. (p. 465)

OVERVIEW

Fluid and electrolyte management is one of the cornerstones of patient care. Most disease processes, tissue injuries, and surgical procedures greatly influence the physiologic status of fluids and electrolytes in the body. Body fluids provide transportation of nutrients to cells and carry waste products away from cells. Understanding fluid and electrolyte management requires knowledge of the extent and composition of the various body fluid compartments.

Approximately 60% of the adult human body weight is composed of water. This is referred to as the *total body water (TBW)*. The percent of body water is higher in infants and lower in older adults. Both populations are more sensitive to fluid imbalances than the adult. Total body water is distributed in two main compartments: intracellular fluid (ICF) and extracellular fluid (ECF). Extracellular fluid is further divided into interstitial fluid (ISF) and intravascular fluid (IVF). This distribution is illustrated in Figure 29-1.

Fluid contained within the cells is called intracellular fluid (ICF), and it contains solutes such as electrolytes and glucose. Extracellular fluid (ECF) is the fluid outside the cells. It

functions to transport nutrients to cells as well as transport waste products away from cells. ECF is further broken down into intravascular fluid (contained within blood vessels) and interstitial fluid (surrounding the cell). Intravascular refers to the volume of blood in the circulatory system and contains protein-rich plasma and large amounts of albumin. In contrast, interstitial fluid (ISF) contains little or no protein. ISF is further broken down to transcellular fluid, which is contained within specialized body compartments such as the synovial, cerebrospinal, and pleural cavities.

Water existing within the human body is critical not only due to its vast quantity, but it also serves as a solvent to dissolve solutes and acts as a medium for metabolic reactions. Throughout the body, water is freely exchanged among all fluid compartments and is retained in a relatively constant amount. Internal control mechanisms responsible for maintaining fluid balance include thirst, antidiuretic hormone, and aldosterone. Movement into and out of cells is carried out through the following processes: diffusion, filtration, active transport, and osmosis.

The goal of fluid and electrolyte balance is to maintain homeostasis, where fluid intake is equal to fluid output. Fluid intake comes from liquids, solid foods, IV fluid, or parenteral fluid. Fluid loss (output) comes primarily from the kidney, and can also be from emesis or feces. Insensible losses (those that can't be measured) come from the skin, lungs, and GI tract. Other measurable loss can be from fistulas, drains, or GI suction. All measurable sources of intake and output are important to document in the hospitalized patient. A sudden change in weight is a strong indicator of fluid balance. If the amount of water gained exceeds the amount of water lost, the end result is overhydration. Such fluid excesses often accumulate in interstitial spaces, such as in the pericardial sac, joint capsules, and lower extremities. This is referred to as edema. In contrast, if the quantity of water lost exceeds that gained, a water deficit,

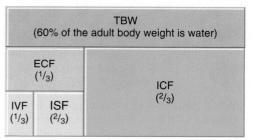

FIGURE 29-1 Distribution of total body water (TBW). *ECF,* Extracellular fluid; *ICF,* intracellular fluid; *ISF,* interstitial fluid; *IVF,* intravascular volume.

or dehydration, occurs. Death often occurs when 20% to 25% of TBW is lost.

Dehydration leads to a disturbance in the balance between the amount of fluid in the extracellular compartment and that in the intracellular compartment. Sodium is the principle extracellular electrolyte and plays a primary role in maintaining water concentration. In the initial stages of dehydration, water is lost first from the extracellular compartments. The amount of further fluid losses, colloid oncotic pressure changes, or both determines the type of clinical dehydration that develops (Table 29-1). Clinical conditions that can result in dehydration and fluid loss, as well as the symptoms of dehydration and fluid loss, are presented in Table 29-2. When fluid that has been lost must be replaced, there are three categories of agents that can be used to accomplish this: crystalloids, colloids, and blood products. The clinical situation dictates which category of agents is most appropriate.

Tonicity and *osmolality* are similar terms that are often used interchangeably, albeit they are not the exactly the same chemically speaking. Osmolality is used in reference to body fluids and is the concentration of particles in a solution. Normal osmolality of body fluids is between 290 and 310 mOsm/kg. Tonicity is used in reference to intravenous (IV) fluids and is the

measurement of the concentration of IV fluids as compared with the osmolality of body fluids. Tonicity can also be defined as the measure of osmotic pressure. The tonicity of IV solutions can be considered isotonic, hypotonic, or hypertonic. Isotonic means that the osmotic pressures inside and outside of the blood cell are the same. Hypotonic means that the solution outside the cell has a lower osmotic pressure than inside the cell. Hypertonic means the solution outside the blood cell has a higher osmotic pressure than inside the cell. Giving an isotonic solution such as normal saline (0.9% NaCl) or lactated Ringer's solution causes no net fluid movement. Administering a hypotonic solution (0.45% NaCl) causes fluid to move out of the vein and into the tissues and cells. Injecting a hypertonic solution (3% NaCl) causes fluid to move from the ISF into the veins. This is depicted in Figure 29-2.

Acid-base balance is also important to normal bodily functions and is regulated by the respiratory system and the kidney. An *acid* is a substance that can donate or release hydrogen ions, such as carbonic acid or hydrochloric acid. A *base* is a substance that can accept hydrogen ions, such as bicarbonate. The *pH* is a measure of the degree of acidosis and alkalinity and is inversely related to hydrogen ion concentration. For example, when hydrogen ion concentration increases, the pH decreases and leads to acidity. As the hydrogen ion concentration decreases, the pH increases, leading to more alkalinity. With the normal pH ranging from 7.35 to 7.45, acidosis occurs when pH falls below 7.35. Conversely, alkalosis occurs when the pH rises above 7.45.

Regulation of the acid-base balance requires healthy functioning of the respiratory and renal systems. The respiratory system compensates for metabolic problems and pH imbalances by regulation of CO_2. In acidosis, CO_2 can be exhaled to try to normalize the lower pH; in alkalosis, carbon dioxide will be retained by the respiratory system to try and elevate the pH. The kidney also compensates by reabsorbing and generating bicarbonate and excreting hydrogen ions in acidosis to normalize the low pH. Conversely, the kidney can excrete bicarbonate and retain hydrogen ions to normalize the high pH seen with alkalosis. The influence of the respiratory system is determined by an arterial blood gas (ABG) test. The influence of the body

TABLE 29-1	Types of Dehydration
Type of Dehydration	**Characteristics**
Hypertonic	Occurs when water loss is greater than sodium loss, which results in a concentration of solutes outside the cells and causes the fluid inside the cells to move to the extracellular space, thus dehydrating the cells. Example: Elevated temperature resulting in perspiration.
Hypotonic	Occurs when sodium loss is greater than water loss, which results in higher concentrations of solute inside the cells and causes fluid to be pulled from outside the cells (plasma and interstitial spaces) into the cells. Examples: Renal insufficiency and inadequate aldosterone secretion.
Isotonic	Caused by a loss of both sodium and water from the body, which results in a decrease in the volume of extracellular fluid. Examples: Diarrhea and vomiting.

TABLE 29-2	Conditions Leading to Fluid Loss or Dehydration and Associated Corresponding Symptoms*
Condition	**Associated Symptoms**
Bleeding	Tachycardia and hypotension
Bowel obstruction	Reduced perspiration and mucous secretions
Diarrhea	Reduced urine output (oliguria)
Fever	Dry skin and mucous membranes
Vomiting	Reduced lacrimal (tears) and salivary secretions

*There may be overlap involving more than one of the symptoms depending on the patient's specific condition.

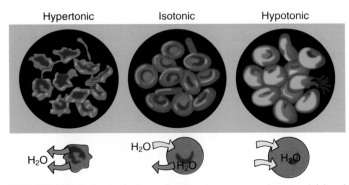

FIGURE 29-2 A depiction of what happens when red blood cells are exposed to different fluids. Isotonic solutions cause no net fluid movement. Hypertonic solutions cause water to move out of the cells and can cause the cells to shrink. Hypotonic solutions cause water to move into the cells, which can cause them to burst.

on acid-base balance is determined by a blood test, which measures total body CO_2 and is usually represented as HCO_3. Both are used in determining and treating acid-base disorders. Detailed determination and treatment of acid-base balance is complex and beyond the scope of this textbook. Certain drugs, such as the diuretic acetazolamide (see Chapter 28) and sodium bicarbonate (tablets or injection), can be used to correct metabolic acid-base disturbances.

CRYSTALLOIDS

Crystalloids are fluids given by intravenous (IV) injection that supply water and sodium to maintain the osmotic gradient between the extravascular and intravascular compartments. Their plasma volume–expanding capacity is related to their sodium concentration. Serum is a term closely related to plasma. The most commonly used crystalloids are normal saline (0.9% NaCl) and lactated Ringer's solution.

Mechanism of Action and Drug Effects

Crystalloid solutions contain fluids and electrolytes that are normally found in the body. They do not contain proteins (colloids), which are necessary to maintain the colloid oncotic pressure and prevent water from leaving the plasma compartment. In fact, the administration of large quantities of crystalloid solutions for fluid resuscitation decreases the colloid oncotic pressure, due to a dilutional effect. Crystalloids are distributed faster into the interstitial and intracellular compartments than colloids. This makes crystalloids better for treating dehydration than for expanding the plasma volume alone.

Indications

Crystalloid solutions are most commonly used as maintenance fluids. They are used to compensate for insensible fluid losses, to replace fluids, and to manage specific fluid and electrolyte disturbances. Crystalloids also promote urinary flow. They are much less expensive than colloids and blood products. In addition, there is no risk for viral transmission or anaphylaxis and no alteration in the coagulation profile associated with their use, unlike with blood products. The choice of whether to use a crystalloid or a colloid depends on the severity of the condition. Common indications for either crystalloid or colloid replacement therapy include:

- Acute liver failure
- Burns
- Cardiopulmonary bypass
- Hypoproteinemia
- Renal dialysis
- Shock

Contraindications to the use of crystalloids include known drug allergy to a specific product and hypervolemia, and may include severe electrolyte disturbance, depending on the type of crystalloid used.

Adverse Effects

Crystalloids are a very safe and effective means of replacing needed fluid. They do, however, have some unwanted effects.

Because they contain no large particles, such as proteins, they do not stay within the blood vessels and can leak out of the plasma into the tissues and cells. This may result in edema anywhere in the body. Peripheral edema and pulmonary edema are two common examples. Crystalloids also dilute the proteins that are in the plasma, which further reduces the colloid oncotic pressure. To be effective, large volumes (liters of fluid) are usually required. As a result, prolonged infusions may cause fluid overload. Another disadvantage of crystalloids is that their effects are relatively short-lived.

Interactions

Interactions with crystalloid solutions are rare because they are very similar if not identical to normal physiologic substances.

Dosage

The dose of crystalloids is determined by the specific condition being treated.

DRUG PROFILE

The most commonly used crystalloid solutions are normal saline (NS or 0.9% sodium chloride) and lactated Ringer's solution. Sodium chloride is also discussed briefly in the section on electrolytes and in the Nursing Process section under electrolytes.

sodium chloride

Sodium chloride (NaCl) is available in several concentrations, the most common being 0.9%. This is the physiologically normal concentration of sodium chloride (isotonic), and it is referred to as *normal saline* (NS). Concentrations considered hypotonic are 0.45% ("half-normal") and 0.25% ("quarter-normal"). Hypertonic saline (a high-alert solution) is available as 3% and 5%. These solutions have different indications and are used in different situations, depending on how urgently fluid volume restoration is needed and/or the extent of the sodium loss. Normal saline contains 154 mEq of sodium per liter.

Sodium chloride is a physiologic electrolyte that is present throughout the body's water. Thus, there are no hypersensitivity reactions to it. It is safe to administer it during any stage of pregnancy, but it is contraindicated in patients with hypernatremia and/or hyperchloremia. Hypertonic saline injections (3% and 5%) are contraindicated in the presence of increased, normal, or only slightly decreased sodium concentrations. Hypertonic saline is considered a high-risk drug because deaths have occurred when it is infused inappropriately. Correcting sodium too rapidly with hypertonic saline can lead to *osmotic demyelination syndrome*, which is potentially fatal. Conversely, infusing very low hypotonic saline (0.25% NaCl) is not recommended because it can cause hemolysis of the red blood cells. Sodium chloride is also available as a 650-mg tablet.

The dose of sodium chloride administered depends on the clinical situation. Generally speaking, the amount of 0.9% NaCl that is needed to increase intravascular or plasma volume by 1000 mL is 5000 to 6000 mL. By contrast, the amount of albumin, which is a colloid solution, (discussed later) needed to increase intravascular volume by the same 1000 mL is only 500 mL. Table 29-3 provides other examples.

TABLE 29-3 Crystalloids and Colloids: Dosing Guidelines

	CRYSTALLOIDS AND COLLOIDS			
	0.9% Saline	3% Saline*	5% Colloid†	25% Colloid‡
To Raise Plasma Volume by 1 L, Administer				
	5-6 L	1.5-2 L	1 L	0.5 L
Compartment to Which Fluid Is Distributed				
Plasma	25%	25%	100%	200%-300%
Interstitial space	75%	75%	0	Decreased fluid levels
Intracellular space	0	0	0	Decreased fluid levels

*Hypertonic saline is a high-risk drug and should not be given faster than 100 mL/hr for short periods. Frequent monitoring of serum levels is required.

†Iso-oncotic solutions such as 5% albumin, dextran 70, and hetastarch.

‡Hyperoncotic solutions such as 25% albumin.

TABLE 29-4 Commonly Used Colloids

	COMPOSITION (MEQ/L)			
Product	Na	Cl	Volume (mL)	Cost*
Dextran 70†	154	154	500	1
Dextran 40†	154	154	500	2
Hetastarch	154	154	500	5
5% Albumin	145	145	500	10
25% Albumin	145	145	100	10

Cl, Chloride; *Na*, sodium.

*Relative cost compared with the cost of dextran 70.

†Dextran is available in NaCl, which has 154 mEq/L of both Na and Cl. It is also available in 5% dextrose in water, which contains no Na or Cl.

COLLOIDS

Colloids are substances that increase the colloid oncotic pressure and move fluid from the interstitial compartment to the plasma compartment by pulling the fluid into the blood vessels. Normally, this task is performed by the three blood proteins: albumin, globulin, and fibrinogen. The total body protein level needs to be in the range of 7.4 g/dL. If this level falls below 5.3 g/dL, fluid shifts out of blood vessels into the tissues. When this happens, colloid replacement therapy is used to reverse this process by increasing the colloid oncotic pressure. Colloid oncotic pressure decreases with age and malnutrition. Commonly used colloids include albumin, dextran, and hetastarch. Information on the composition of these colloids can be found in Table 29-4.

Mechanism of Action and Drug Effects

The mechanism of action of colloids is related to their ability to increase the colloid oncotic pressure. Because the colloids cannot pass into the extravascular space, there is a higher

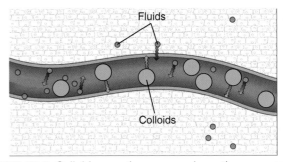

FIGURE 29-3 Colloid osmotic pressure (oncotic pressure). As shown, the colloids inside the blood vessel are too large to pass through the vessel wall. The resulting oncotic pressure exerted by the colloids draws fluid from the surrounding tissues and other extravascular spaces into the blood vessels and also keeps fluid inside the blood vessel.

concentration of colloid solutes (solid particles) inside the blood vessels (intravascular space) than outside the blood vessels. Fluid thus moves from the extravascular space into the blood vessels in an attempt to make it isotonic. See Figure 29-3. As such, colloids increase the blood volume, and they are sometimes called *plasma expanders*. They also make up part of the total plasma volume.

Colloids increase the colloid oncotic pressure and move fluid from outside the blood vessels to inside the blood vessels. They can maintain the colloid oncotic pressure for several hours. They are naturally occurring products and consist of proteins (albumin), carbohydrates (dextrans or starches), fats (lipid emulsion), and animal collagen (gelatin). Usually they contain a combination of both small and large particles. The small particles are eliminated quickly and promote diuresis and perfusion of the kidneys; the larger particles maintain the plasma volume. Albumin is the one exception in that it contains particles that are all the same size.

Indications

Colloids are used to treat a wide variety of conditions including shock and burns, or whenever the patient requires plasma volume expansion. Clinically, colloids are superior to crystalloids because of their ability to maintain the plasma volume for a longer time. However, colloids are significantly more expensive and are more likely to promote bleeding. Colloids are less likely than crystalloids to cause edema because of the larger volumes of crystalloids needed to achieve the desired clinical effect. Crystalloids are better than colloids for emergency short-term plasma volume expansion.

Contraindications

Contraindications to the use of colloids include known drug allergy to a specific product and hypervolemia, and may include severe electrolyte disturbance.

Adverse Effects

Colloids are relatively safe agents, although there are some disadvantages to their use. They have no oxygen-carrying ability and contain no clotting factors, unlike blood products. Because of this, they can alter the coagulation system through a dilutional effect, which results in impaired coagulation and possibly bleeding. Rarely, dextran therapy causes anaphylaxis or renal failure.

Interactions

No drug interactions occur with colloids.

Dosages

For dosage information on colloids, see Table 29-3.

DRUG PROFILES

The specific colloid used for replacement therapy varies from institution to institution. The three most commonly used are 5% albumin, dextran 40, and hetastarch. They all have a very rapid onset of action as well as a long duration of action. They are metabolized in the liver and excreted by the kidneys. Albumin is the one exception; it is metabolized by the reticuloendothelial system and excreted by the kidneys and the intestines. Hetastarch is a synthetic colloid with properties similar to those of albumin and dextran.

albumin

Albumin is a natural protein that is normally produced by the liver. It is responsible for generating approximately 70% of the colloid oncotic pressure. Human albumin is a sterile solution of serum albumin that is prepared from pooled blood, plasma, serum, or placentas obtained from healthy human donors. It is pasteurized to destroy any contaminants. Unfortunately, because it is derived from human donors, the supply is limited.

Albumin is contraindicated in patients with a known hypersensitivity to it and in those with heart failure, severe anemia, or renal insufficiency. Albumin is available only in parenteral form in concentrations of 5% and 25%. It is classified as a pregnancy category C drug. See Table 29-3 for dosing guidelines.

Pharmacokinetics: Albumin

Route	Onset of Action	Peak Plasma Concentration	Elimination Half-life	Duration of Action
IV	Less than 1 min	Unknown	16 hr	Less than 24 hr

dextran

Dextran is a solution of glucose. It is available in three concentrations, dextran 40 and the more concentrated dextran 70 and dextran 75, and it has a molecular weight similar to that of albumin. Dextran 40 is the more commonly used of the two. It has actions similar to those of human albumin in that it expands the plasma volume by drawing fluid from the interstitial space to the intravascular space.

Dextran is contraindicated in patients with a known hypersensitivity to it and in those with heart failure, renal insufficiency, and extreme dehydration. It is available only in parenteral form mixed in either a 5% dextrose solution or a 0.9% sodium chloride solution. It is classified as a pregnancy category C drug. See Table 29-3 for dosing guidelines.

Pharmacokinetics: Dextran

Route	Onset of Action	Peak Plasma Concentration	Elimination Half-life	Duration of Action
IV	5 min	Unknown	2-6 hr	4-6 hr

BLOOD PRODUCTS

Blood products can be thought of as biologic drugs. They augment the plasma volume. Red blood cell (RBC)–containing products can also improve tissue oxygenation. Blood products are significantly more expensive than crystalloids and colloids and are less available because they are natural products and require human donors. They are most often indicated when a patient has lost 25% or more blood volume.

Mechanism of Action and Drug Effects

The mechanism of action of blood products is related to their ability to increase the colloid oncotic pressure, and hence the plasma volume. They do so in the same manner as colloids and hypertonic crystalloids, by pulling fluid from the extravascular space to the intravascular space. Because of this they are also considered plasma expanders. RBC products also have the ability to carry oxygen. They can maintain the colloid oncotic pressure for several hours to days. Because they come from human donors, they have all the benefits (and hazards) that human blood products have. They are administered when a person's body is deficient in these products.

Indications

Blood products are used to treat a wide variety of clinical conditions, and the blood product used depends on the specific indication. The available blood products and the specific conditions they are used to treat are listed in Table 29-5.

TABLE 29-5	**Blood Products: Indications**
Blood Product	**Indication**
Cryoprecipitate and PPF	To manage acute bleeding (over 50% blood loss slowly or 20% rapidly)
FFP	To increase clotting factor levels
PRBCs	To increase oxygen-carrying capacity in patients with anemia, in patients with substantial hemoglobin deficits, and in patients who have lost up to 25% of their total blood volume
Whole blood	Same as for PRBCs, except that whole blood is more beneficial in cases of extreme (over 25%) loss of blood volume because whole blood also contains plasma and plasma proteins, the chief osmotic component, which help draw fluid back into blood vessels from surrounding tissues

FFP, Fresh frozen plasma; *PPF,* plasma protein fraction; *PRBCs,* packed red blood cells.

Contraindications

There are no absolute contraindications to the use of blood products. However, because there is a risk for transfer of infectious disease, although remote, their use needs to be based on careful clinical evaluation of the patient's condition.

Adverse Effects

Blood products can produce undesirable effects, some potentially serious. Because these products come from other humans, they can be incompatible with the recipient's immune system. These incompatibilities are tested for before their administration by determining the respective blood types of the donor and recipient and by performing cross-matching tests to screen for incompatibility between selected blood proteins. This helps reduce the likelihood that the recipient will reject the blood product, which would precipitate transfusion reactions and anaphylaxis. These products can also transmit pathogens (hepatitis and HIV, or human immunodeficiency virus) from the donor to the recipient. Various preparation techniques are now used to reduce the risk for pathogen transmission, and these have resulted in a drastic reduction in the incidence of such problems.

Interactions

As with crystalloids and colloids, blood products are very similar if not identical to normal physiologic substances; therefore, they are involved in very few interactions. Calcium and aspirin, which normally affect coagulation, may interact with these substances when infused in the body in much the same way that they interact with the body's own blood components. Blood must not be administered with any solution other than normal saline.

Dosages

Table 29-6 provides dosage information on blood products.

DRUG PROFILES

Packed red blood cells (PRBCs) and fresh frozen plasma (FFP) are among the most commonly used blood products. All of the

TABLE 29-6 Suggested Guidelines for Blood Products: Management of Bleeding

Amount of Blood Loss	Fluid of Choice
20% or less (slow loss)	Crystalloids
20%-50% (slow loss)	Nonprotein plasma expanders (dextran and hetastarch)
Over 50% (slow loss) or 20% (acutely)	Whole blood or PRBCs, and/or PPF and FFP
80% or more	As above, but for every 5 units of blood given, administer 1 to 2 units of FFP and 1 to 2 units of platelets to prevent the hemodilution of clotting factors and bleeding

FFP, Fresh frozen plasma; *PPF,* plasma protein fraction; *PRBCs,* packed red blood cells.

blood products are derived from pooled blood from human donors. Other less commonly used, but still important, blood products are whole blood, plasma protein fraction, cryoprecipitate, and platelets.

packed red blood cells

Packed red blood cells (PRBCs) are obtained by the centrifugation of whole blood and the separation of RBCs from plasma and the other cellular elements. The advantage of PRBCs is that their oxygen-carrying capacity is better than that of the other blood products, and they are less likely to cause cardiac fluid overload. Their disadvantages include high cost, limited shelf life, and fluctuating availability, as well as their ability to transmit viruses, trigger allergic reactions, and cause bleeding abnormalities. The suggested guidelines for use are given in Table 29-6.

fresh frozen plasma

Fresh frozen plasma (FFP) is obtained by centrifuging whole blood and thereby removing the cellular elements. The resulting plasma is then frozen. FFP is not recommended for routine fluid resuscitation, but it may be used as an adjunct to massive blood transfusion in the treatment of patients with underlying coagulation disorders. The plasma-expanding capability of FFP is similar to that of dextran but slightly less than that of hetastarch. The disadvantage of FFP use is that it can transmit pathogens. The suggested guidelines for use are given in Table 29-6.

PHYSIOLOGY OF ELECTROLYTE BALANCE

Electrolytes are solutes that work in conjunction with fluids to keep the body in balance. They are measured in millequivalent (mEq) units. Electrolytes are either positively charged (cations) or negatively charged (anions). The positively charged cations include sodium (Na^+), potassium (K^+), calcium (Ca^{++}), and magnesium (Mg^{++}). The negatively charged anions include chloride (Cl^-), phosphate (PO_4^-), and bicarbonate (HCO_3^-). Electrolytes are involved in nerve impulse transmission, muscle contraction, regulation of water distribution, blood clotting, enzyme reactions, and acid-base balance. Sodium (Na^+) and chloride (Cl^-) are the principal electrolytes in the extracellular fluid, whereas potassium (K^+) is the major electrolyte in the intracellular fluid. Other important electrolytes are calcium, magnesium, and phosphorus. Electrolytes are controlled by the renin-angiotensin-aldosterone system, antidiuretic hormone system, and sympathetic nervous system. When these neuroendocrine systems are out of balance, adverse electrolyte imbalances commonly result. Patients who receive diuretics (see Chapter 28) are at risk for electrolyte abnormalities.

POTASSIUM

Potassium is the most abundant electrolyte inside cells (the intracellular fluid), where the normal concentration is approximately 150 mEq/L. Approximately 95% of the potassium in the body is intracellular. In contrast, the amount of potassium outside the cells in the plasma ranges from 3.5 to 5 mEq/L. The ratio of intracellular to extracellular potassium is important. Small changes in the extracellular potassium level can lead to serious unwanted effects on the neuromuscular and cardiovascular systems.

Potassium is obtained from a variety of foods, the most common being fruit and juices, vegetables, fish, and meats. The average daily diet usually provides 35 to 100 mEq of potassium, which is well above the required daily amount. Excess dietary potassium is usually excreted by the kidneys in the urine.

Hypokalemia (a deficiency of potassium) is defined as a serum potassium level of less than 3.5 mEq/L. Hypokalemia can result from decreased intake, shifting of potassium into cells, increased renal excretion, and other losses such as diarrhea, vomiting, or tube drainage. Certain medications can also cause hypokalemia including diuretics, steroids, beta blockers, and aminoglycoside antibiotics. Early symptoms of hypokalemia include hypotension, lethargy, mental confusion, muscle weakness, and nausea. Late symptoms of hypokalemia include cardiac irregularities, neuropathies, and paralytic ileus. A low serum potassium level can increase the toxicity associated with digoxin, which can precipitate serious ventricular dysrhythmias. Treatment involves both identifying and treating the cause and restoring the serum potassium levels to normal (higher than 3.5 mEq/L). For mild hypokalemia, the consumption of potassium-rich foods is usually sufficient. Clinically significant hypokalemia requires the oral or parenteral administration of a potassium supplement.

Hyperkalemia is the term for an excessive serum potassium level and is defined as a serum potassium level exceeding 5.5 mEq/L. Hyperkalemia can result from increased potassium intake, reduced renal excretion of potassium or redistribution of potassium from the intracellular to the extracellular compartment following burns, or rhabdomyolysis. Symptoms of hyperkalemia include generalized fatigue, weakness, paresthesia, palpitations, and paralysis. Clinical manifestations of hyperkalemia are generally related to the heart. Severe hyperkalemia (>7 mEq/L) can precipitate ventricular fibrillation and cardiac arrest.

Mechanism of Action and Drug Effects

The importance of potassium as the primary intracellular electrolyte is highlighted by the number of life-sustaining physiologic functions it is involved in. Muscle contraction, the transmission of nerve impulses, and the regulation of heartbeats (the pacemaker function of the heart) are just a few of these functions. Potassium is also essential for the maintenance of acid-base balance, isotonicity, and the electrodynamic characteristics of the cell. It plays a role in many enzymatic reactions, and it is an essential component in gastric secretion, renal function, tissue synthesis, and carbohydrate metabolism.

Indications

Potassium replacement therapy is indicated in the treatment or prevention of potassium depletion. Potassium salts commonly used for this purpose include potassium chloride, potassium phosphate, and potassium acetate. The chloride is required to correct the hypochloremia (low level of chloride in the blood) that commonly accompanies potassium deficiency, and the phosphate is used to correct hypophosphatemia. The acetate salt may be used to raise the blood pH in acidotic conditions.

Contraindications

Contraindications to potassium replacement products include known allergy to a specific drug product, hyperkalemia from any cause, severe renal disease, acute dehydration, untreated Addison's disease, severe hemolytic disease, and conditions involving extensive tissue breakdown (e.g., multiple trauma, severe burns).

Adverse Effects

The adverse effects of oral potassium are primarily limited to the gastrointestinal (GI) tract, including diarrhea, nausea, and vomiting. More significant effects include GI bleeding and ulceration. The parenteral administration of potassium usually produces pain at the injection site. Cases of phlebitis have been associated with IV administration. The generally accepted maximum concentration for peripheral infusion is 20 to 40 mEq/L and up to 60 mEq/L for a central line. Excessive administration of potassium salts can lead to hyperkalemia and toxic effects. If IV potassium is administered too rapidly, cardiac arrest may occur. IV potassium must not be given faster than 10 mEq/hr to patients who are not on cardiac monitors. For critically ill patients on cardiac monitors, rates of 20 mEq/hr or more may be used.

Toxicity and Management of Overdose

The toxic effects of potassium are the result of hyperkalemia. Symptoms include muscle weakness, paresthesia, paralysis, cardiac rhythm irregularities that can result in ventricular fibrillation, and cardiac arrest. The treatment instituted depends on the degree of the hyperkalemia and ranges from reversal of life-threatening problems to simple dietary restrictions. In the event of severe hyperkalemia, the IV administration of dextrose and insulin, sodium bicarbonate, and calcium gluconate or chloride is often required. These drugs correct severe hyperkalemia by causing a rapid intracellular shift of potassium ions, which reduces the serum potassium concentration. Such interventions are often followed with orally or rectally administered sodium polystyrene sulfonate (Kayexalate) or hemodialysis to eliminate the extra potassium from the body. Less critical levels can be reduced with dietary restrictions.

Interactions

Concurrent use of potassium-sparing diuretics and ACE inhibitors can produce a hyperkalemic state. Concurrent use of non–potassium-sparing diuretics, amphotericin B, and mineralocorticoids can produce a hypokalemic state.

Dosages

Fluid and electrolyte therapy involves replacing any deficits or losses and/or providing maintenance levels for specific patient requirements. Accordingly, specific dosage amounts of fluids or electrolytes depend on several clinical factors, including the following:

- Specific patient losses
- Efficacy of patient physiologic systems involved in fluid and electrolyte metabolism, especially adrenal, cardiovascular, and kidney functions
- Current drug therapy for pathologic conditions that complicate the amount and duration of replacement
- Selection of oral or parenteral replacement formulations

Suggested dosage guidelines for potassium with subsequent adjustments are 10 to 20 mEq administered orally several times a day or parenteral administration of 30 to 60 mEq every 24 hours.

DRUG PROFILES

!potassium

Potassium supplements are administered either to prevent or to treat potassium depletion. The acetate, bicarbonate, chloride, citrate, and gluconate salts of potassium are available for oral administration, including tablets, solutions, elixirs, and powders for solution. The parenteral salt forms of potassium for IV administration are acetate, chloride, and phosphate. The dosage of potassium supplements is usually expressed in milliequivalents (mEq) of potassium and depends on the requirements of the individual patient. Different salt forms of potassium deliver varying milliequivalent amounts of potassium. It is classified as a pregnancy category A drug.

Pharmacokinetics: Potassium

Route	Onset of Action	Peak Plasma Concentration	Elimination Half-life	Duration of Action
IV	Immediate	Rapid	Variable	Variable

sodium polystyrene sulfonate (potassium exchange resin)

Sodium polystyrene sulfonate (Kayexalate) is known as a *cation exchange resin* and is used to treat hyperkalemia. It is usually administered orally via nasogastric tube or as an enema. It works in the intestine, where potassium ions from the body are exchanged for sodium ions in the resin. Although the drug effects in each case are unpredictable, approximately 1 mEq of potassium is lost from the body per gram of resin administered. It can cause disturbances in electrolytes other than potassium, such as calcium and magnesium. For this reason, patients' electrolytes are closely monitored during treatment with sodium polystyrene sulfonate. In 2011, the FDA required safety labeling changes to state that cases of intestinal or colonic necrosis and other serious GI adverse events (bleeding, ischemic colitis, perforation) had been reported. Kayexelate should not be used in patients who do not have normal bowel function and should be discontinued in patients who develop constipation. It should not be used concurrently with sorbitol. Concurrent use of sorbitol with kayexelate has been implicated in cases of intestinal colonic necrosis. This condition may be fatal. Other adverse effects include hypernatremia, hypokalemia, hypocalcemia, hypomagnesemia, nausea, and vomiting. Drug interactions include antacids and laxatives, which should be avoided. It is typically dosed in multiples of 15 to 30 grams until the desired effect on serum potassium occurs. Onset of action varies from 2 to 12 hours and is generally faster with the oral route than with rectal administration. It is available in 15 g/60 mL suspensions and in a powder for reconstitution. It is classified as a pregnancy category C drug.

SODIUM

Sodium is the counterpart of potassium, in that potassium is the principal cation inside cells, whereas sodium is the principal cation outside cells. The normal concentration of sodium outside cells is 135 to 145 mEq/L, and it is maintained through the dietary intake of sodium in the form of sodium chloride, which is obtained from salt, fish, meats, and other foods flavored, seasoned, or preserved with salt. Serum sodium concentration and serum osmolarity are maintained under tight control involving thirst, secretion of antidiuretic hormone (ADH), and renal mechanisms.

Hyponatremia is a condition of sodium loss or deficiency and occurs when the serum levels decrease to less than 135 mEq/L. It is manifested by lethargy, hypotension, stomach cramps, vomiting, diarrhea, and seizures. There are three types of hyponatremia and can be categorized as follows:

- Hypovolemic hyponatremia (when the TBW is decreased, but the total sodium is decreased to a greater extent)
- Euvolemic hyponatremia (when the TBW is increased, but the total sodium remains normal)
- Hypervolemic hyponatremia (when the total sodium is increased, but the TBW is increased to a greater extent)

Causes of hyponatremia include pneumonia, CNS infection, trauma, cancer, congestive heart failure, liver failure, medications, poor dietary intake, excessive perspiration, prolonged diarrhea or vomiting, renal disorders, hypothyroidism, or adrenal insufficiency. Medications known to cause hyponatremia include diuretics, carbamazepine, amiodarone, and SSRIs. The syndrome of inappropriate antidiuretic hormone (SIADH) is another common cause of hyponatremia. Symptoms of hyponatremia include anorexia, confusion, lethargy, agitation, headache, and/or seizures.

Hypernatremia is the condition of sodium excess and occurs when the serum levels of sodium exceed 145 mEq/L. Hypernatremia generally indicates that there is a relative deficit of TBW in relation to total body sodium. Causes of hypernatremia include water depletion, shifting of water into cells, or sodium overload. Symptoms of hypernatremia include anorexia, restlessness, lethargy, muscle weakness, and nausea. Severe neurologic symptoms can occur due to shifts of water from the brain intracellular to extracellular spaces.

Mechanism of Action and Drug Effects

Sodium is the major cation in extracellular fluid and is involved in the control of water distribution, fluid and electrolyte balance, and osmotic pressure of body fluids. Sodium also participates along with both chloride and bicarbonate in the regulation of acid-base balance. Chloride, the major extracellular anion (negatively charged substance), closely complements the physiologic action of sodium.

Indications

Sodium is primarily administered for the treatment or prevention of sodium depletion. Sodium chloride is the primary salt used for this purpose. Mild hyponatremia is usually treated with oral administration of sodium chloride tablets and/or fluid restriction. Pronounced sodium depletion is treated with IV normal saline or lactated Ringer's solution. These drugs were discussed earlier in this chapter.

Hypertonic saline (3% NaCl) is sometimes used to correct severe hyponatremia. It is considered a high-risk drug because giving it too rapidly or in too high of a dose can cause a syndrome known as *central pontine myelinolysis,* also known as *osmotic demyelination syndrome.* This can cause irreversible brainstem damage.

A new class of drugs for the treatment of euvolemic (normal fluid volume) hyponatremia is the dual arginine vasopressin (AVP) V1A and V2 receptor antagonists. These drugs are conivaptan (Vaprisol) and tolvaptan (Samsca). This class of drugs is often referred to as *vaptans.* Specific information on conivaptan is listed under its drug profile.

Contraindications

The only usual contraindications to the use of sodium replacement products are known drug allergy to a specific product and hypernatremia.

Adverse Effects

The oral administration of sodium chloride can cause gastric upset consisting of nausea, vomiting, and cramps. Venous phlebitis can be a consequence of its parenteral administration.

Interactions

Sodium is not known to interact significantly with any drugs with the exception of the antibiotic called quinapristin/dalfoprisitn (Synercid)

Dosages

Fluid and electrolyte therapy involves replacing any deficit losses and/or providing maintenance levels for specific patient requirements. Accordingly, specific dosage amounts vary based on the patient's situation.

DRUG PROFILES

sodium chloride

Sodium chloride is primarily used as a replacement electrolyte for either the prevention or treatment of sodium loss. It is also used as a diluent for the infusion of compatible drugs and in the assessment of kidney function after a fluid challenge. Sodium chloride is contraindicated in patients who are hypersensitive to it. It is available in many IV preparations and in oral form as 650-mg tablets. It is classified as a pregnancy category C drug.

Pharmacokinetics: Sodium Chloride

Route	Onset of Action	Peak Plasma Concentration	Elimination Half-life	Duration of Action
IV	Immediate	Rapid	Unknown	Variable

conivaptan

Conivaptan (Vaprisol) is a nonpeptide dual arginine vasopressin (AVP) V1A and V2 receptor antagonist. It inhibits the effects of arginine vasopressin, also known as *antidiuretic hormone,* on receptors in the kidneys. It is specifically indicated for the treatment of hospitalized patients with euvolemic hyponatremia, or low serum sodium levels at normal water volumes. Conivaptan is available for IV infusion. Adverse events associated with the use of conivaptan may include infusion site reactions (e.g., phlebitis, pain), thirst, headache, hypokalemia, vomiting, diarrhea, and polyuria. Closely monitor serum sodium levels during treatment, as overly rapid increases in serum sodium levels have been associated with potentially permanent adverse events, including osmotic demyelination syndrome. Several potential drug-drug interactions have been identified. Conivaptan is metabolized by the hepatic enzyme CYP3A4; coadministration of drugs that inhibit this enzyme (including but not limited to ketoconazole, itraconazole, clarithromycin, ritonavir, and indinavir) may increase serum levels. Tolvaptan (Samsca) is an oral version of conivaptan. It is available in 15-mg and 30-mg tablets.

Pharmacokinetics: Conivaptan

Route	Onset of Action	Peak Plasma Concentration	Elimination Half-life	Duration of Action
IV	Immediate	Rapid	6.7-8.6 hr	12 hr after infusion is stopped

NURSING PROCESS

ASSESSMENT

For fluid replacement, each patient has various needs. Any medications or solutions ordered must be given exactly as prescribed and without substitution. However, never take the prescriber's order at face value without confirming any medication order against authoritative resources (e.g., current drug reference guides, *Physician's Desk Reference,* nursing pharmacology textbook, manufacturer's drug insert) or speaking with a pharmacist. Remember that you are responsible for making sure that the drug therapy administration process—beginning with the assessment phase of the nursing process and through to evaluation—is accurate, safe, and meets professional standards of care.

To assist in the development of a thorough assessment, a brief review of the various solutions is needed. With isotonic solutions, such as *0.9% NaCl* or *lactated Ringer's* solution, there is no net fluid movement from the vein into the tissues/cells. These isotonic solutions (e.g., 0.9% NaCl [normal saline] and lactated Ringer's solution) are customarily used to augment extracellular volume in patients experiencing blood loss and/or severe vomiting. Isotonic NaCl is also used as diluting fluid for blood transfusions because D_5W results in hemolysis of red blood cells (in transfusions). Parenterally administered hydrating and hypotonic solutions, such as *0.45% NaCl*, are indicated for the prevention and/or treatment of dehydration. When giving these fluids, there is movement of fluid from the vein into the tissues and cells. Hypertonic solutions (e.g., *3% or 5% NaCl* and $D_{10}W$) result in movement of fluids from the ISF into the veins and are used for replacement of fluids and electrolytes in specific situations (see pharmacology discussion).

Because of the potential risks related to the use of these solutions, they are rarely administered outside of the hospital setting. After verifying all prescriber orders and checking for accuracy and completeness (as with all drugs), assess the solution or product, the patient, and the IV site (if applicable). Assess the following for IV infusions of fluids and/or electrolytes: the solution to be infused, infusion equipment, infusion rate of the solution, concentration of the parenteral solution, related mathematical calculations, laboratory values (e.g., serum sodium, chloride, and potassium levels), and parenteral compatibilities. More specific assessment of the patient who is to receive a parenteral replacement solution needs to focus on gathering information about the patient's medical history, including diseases of the GI, renal, cardiac, and/or hepatic systems. Obtain a medication history, including a list of prescription drugs, over-the-counter medications, supplements, and herbals. Also take a dietary history including specific dietary habits and recall of all foods consumed during the previous 24 hours. Assess fluid volume and electrolyte status through laboratory testing, as prescribed, and measurement of urinary specific gravity, vital signs, and intake and output. Because the skin and mucous membranes reflect a patient's hydration status, be sure to assess skin turgor and/or rebound elasticity of skin over the top of the hand and other areas over the body. Document the findings as "immediate" rebound or "delayed" rebound. Count the number of seconds that the patient's skin stays in the "pinched-up" position, with normal return being immediately or within 3 to 5 seconds.

Potassium is presented first in the discussion of electrolytes. Its normal range in the serum is 3.5 to 5 mEq/L. Serum potassium levels below 3.5 mEq/L, or hypokalemia, may result in a variety of problems, such as cardiac irregularities and muscle weakness. Early symptoms of hypokalemia include hypotension, lethargy, mental confusion, muscle weakness, and nausea. Late symptoms of hypokalemia include cardiac irregularities, neuropathies, and paralytic ileus. Avoid potassium supplementation, or use with extreme caution in patients taking ACE inhibitors or potassium-sparing diuretics (such as spironolactone). These drugs are associated with adverse effects of hyperkalemia and, if given with potassium supplementation, could worsen hyperkalemia and possibly result in severe cardiac dysrhythmias. Other concerns regarding contraindications with potassium include severe renal disease, untreated Addison's disease, severe tissue trauma, and acute dehydration. Because oral potassium supplements are irritants and may be ulcerogenic, perform a thorough GI tract assessment. If oral potassium supplementation is prescribed and the patient has a history of ulcers or GI bleeding, contact the prescriber for further instructions because oral potassium dosage forms may exacerbate these conditions.

The range of serum potassium levels defined as normal often varies depending on the health care institution and/or the prescriber. For identification and treatment of hyperkalemia, the normal range of potassium must be established. Realize that potassium levels of 5.3 mEq/L may be identified as abnormally high by some laboratories, whereas other laboratories may categorize 5.0 mEq/L as being abnormally high. Be sure to check institutional policy and laboratory guidelines for normal ranges and report any elevations (or decreases) in serum potassium. Symptoms of hyperkalemia include fatigue, weakness, paresthesia, palpitations, and paralysis. A serum level exceeding 5.5 mEq/L is considered by most sources to be toxic and dangerous to the patient; report this finding to the prescriber immediately. With close monitoring of patients, the dangerous effects of hyperkalemia (i.e., cardiac dysrhythmias) will hopefully be prevented or at least identified early and treated appropriately to prevent potentially life-threatening complications.

Venous access is an important issue with parenteral potassium supplementation because the vein can be irritated if infiltration occurs or if the solution has not been mixed thoroughly. The following are some important considerations regarding assessment and peripheral venous access (for potassium, sodium, fluid, and any other type of medication given by the IV route): (1) Assess the overall condition of the veins prior to selecting a site. (2) Try to use distal veins first as the IV site. (3) Know the purpose of administering potassium and other electrolytes. (4) Calculate and set the rate, as ordered, for the infusion. (5) Know the anticipated duration of therapy. (6) Know the restrictions imposed by the patient's history. For example, in postmastectomy patients with lymph node dissection, the affected arm must not be used. The affected arm of a patient with a stroke must not be used. Limb circulation may be inadequate in these situations and lead to edema and other complications if used as a venous access site.

SAFETY: LABORATORY VALUES RELATED TO DRUG THERAPY   QSEN

Serum Potassium

Laboratory Test	Normal Ranges	Rationale for Assessment
Serum potassium	3.5-5 mEq/L	The main function of potassium is the regulation of water and electrolyte content in the cell. A decrease is generally considered to be a level less than 5.5 mEq/L. A serum level less than 3.5 mEq/L is known as *hypokalemia*, and a small decrease in potassium levels may have profound effects with lethargy, muscle weakness, hypotension, and cardiac dysrhythmias. A serum potassium level greater than 5 mEq/L is known as *hyperkalemia* and is manifested by muscle weakness, paresthesia, paralysis, and cardiac rhythm abnormalities.

Sodium is another electrolyte that is an ingredient in various IV replacement solutions. Hyponatremia, or serum sodium level below 135 mEq/L, if not resolved with dietary and/or oral intake, may need to be treated with parenteral infusions. Signs and symptoms of hyponatremia include lethargy, hypotension, stomach cramps, vomiting, and diarrhea. Carefully assess venous access sites because of possible irritation of the vein and subsequent phlebitis. If replacement to correct hyponatremic states is overzealous, the result may be hypernatremia with fluid overload, edema, and dyspnea. Assess baseline vital signs. Continually monitor vital signs, hydration status of the skin and mucous membranes, and level of consciousness for safe replacement and prevention of further complications. Contraindications to sodium replacement include elevated serum sodium levels, edema, and hypertension.

Hypernatremia also requires careful assessment. Manifestations of hypernatremia include red, flushed skin; dry, sticky mucous membranes; increased thirst; temperature elevation; water retention (edema); hypertension; and decreased or absent urination. Identifying any precipitating events, medical concerns, and risk-prone patient situations is important to finding early solutions for treatment. The populations at risk for hypernatremia include the older adult, those with renal and cardiovascular diseases, patients who are receiving sodium supplements or who have increased sodium intake, and those with decreased fluid intake. Perform an assessment of cautions, contraindications, and drug interactions.

When administering *albumin* and other *colloids* (e.g., *dextran*), assess for cautions, contraindications, and drug interactions. Contraindications include patients with heart failure, severe anemia, and renal insufficiency. The rationale is that these products cause fluids to shift from interstitial to intravascular spaces. This places more strain on the patient's cardiac and respiratory systems. Assess the patient's hematocrit, hemoglobin levels, and serum protein levels. Assess the patient's blood pressure, pulse rate, respiratory status, and intake and output. Document and report any abnormal assessment findings (e.g., dyspnea, edema) immediately.

Fluid infusions may also include the giving of *blood* or *blood components*. Obtain a thorough history regarding any transfusions received previously and the patient's response. Report any history of adverse reactions to blood transfusions or problems with *PRBCs* and/or *FFP* to the prescriber, and document the nature of these reactions. Assess the status of venous access areas. Monitor the patient's laboratory values such as hematocrit, hemoglobin, white blood cells [WBCs], red blood cells [RBCs], platelets, and clotting factors. Note baseline vital signs, blood pressure, pulse rate, respiratory rate, and temperature before infusing blood or blood products. Even the general appearance of the patient, energy levels, ability to carry out activities of daily living, and color of extremities are important to note. Assess for any potential drug interactions, specifically aspirin and calcium because these may potentially alter clotting. During the infusion of blood components, assess continually for the occurrence of fever and blood in the urine. Both of these findings are indicative of a reaction requiring immediate medical attention.

In summary, safety and caution are top priorities when patients receive any drug; *fluid* and *electrolyte replacement drugs* are no exception. Deficient and/or excess fluid and electrolyte levels may pose tremendous risks to patients. A thorough assessment is critical to patient safety. In addition, because so many patients receive therapies in the home setting, there is even more accountability and responsibility for performing skillful and thorough assessment before, during, and after therapy.

NURSING DIAGNOSES

1. Risk for falls related to fluid and electrolyte losses
2. Risk for imbalanced fluid volume related to drug-induced fluid and electrolyte deficits and/or excesses
3. Risk for injury related to complications of the transfusion or infusion of blood products, blood components, or related agents

PLANNING: OUTCOME IDENTIFICATION

1. Patient remains free from falls and injury through slow and purposeful motions and changing of positions.
2. Patient regains balanced fluid volume status with intake of at least 8 to 10 glasses of water per day, unless contraindicated.
3. Patient remains free from injury related to complications of blood product infusion through knowledge about the rationale for treatment and adverse effects.

IMPLEMENTATION

Continued monitoring of the patient during *fluid* and *electrolyte therapy* is crucial to ensure safe and effective treatment. It is also important to continue monitoring to identify adverse effects early and to prevent complications of overzealous treatment and/or undertreatment. During *fluid* and *replacement therapy* therapy, serum electrolyte levels need to remain within normal ranges, thus the need for close monitoring. Educate patients at risk for volume deficits (especially the older adult) about this risk and about the effect of a hot, humid environment on physiologic functioning and the danger of exacerbation by excessive perspiration. Water is at the crux of every metabolic reaction that occurs within the body, and deficits will negatively impact physiologic reactions and alter the composition of fluids and electrolytes. For any age group, staying hydrated at all times is a preventive measure.

With parenteral dosing, you must monitor infusion rates as well as the appearance of the fluid or solution (i.e., potassium and saline solutions are clear, whereas albumin is brown, clear, and viscous). Frequently monitor the IV site, as per health care institution policy and nursing standards of care, for evidence of infiltration (e.g., swelling, coolness of skin to the touch around IV site, no or decreased flow rate, and no blood return from IV catheter) or thrombophlebitis (e.g., swelling, redness, heat, and pain at IV site). Volume overload, drug toxicity, fever, infection, and emboli are other complications of IV therapy. With the administration of any of these drugs per the intravenous route, maintain a steady and even flow rate to prevent complications.

Use of an infusion pump may be appropriate or indicated. Ensure that infusion rates follow the prescriber's orders, and recheck all calculations for accuracy. Check the IV site, tubing, IV bag, and fluids or solutions as well as expiration dates. Always behave in a prudent, safe, and thorough manner when administering fluids and electrolyte solutions. Remember that older adult patients and/or pediatric patients have an increased sensitivity to *fluids* and *electrolytes.*

With the various intravenous (IV) solutions, knowing their osmolality and concentrations is important to their safe use. Administration of *isotonic solutions* (e.g., *0.9% sodium chloride*) requires constant monitoring during and after therapy with vital signs and observation for possible fluid overload, especially in those at risk, or those with heart failure. *Hypertonic solutions* are used rarely because of the risk for cellular dehydration and vascular volume overload. These solutions are also associated with phlebitis and spasm if IV infiltration and/or extravasation occur in the peripheral veins. Therefore, if ordered, these solutions are to be administered through a larger bore vein (e.g., central line) and with frequent and close monitoring of the patient's vital signs and cardiac status.

For the patient who is at risk for hypokalemia, provide educational materials and patient teaching to encourage consumption of certain foods high in potassium. The minimal daily requirement for potassium is between 40 and 50 mEq for adults and 2 to 3 mEq/kg of body weight for infants. Share a list of foods containing potassium with the patient. Two medium-sized bananas or an 8-ounce glass of orange juice contains 45 mEq; 20 large dried apricots contain 40 mEq; and a level teaspoon of salt substitute (KCl) contains 60 mEq of potassium. Conversely, if the patient is already hyperkalemic, advise the patient to avoid these food items (see Patient-Centered Care: Patient Teaching later in the chapter for more information). If potassium levels do not increase with dietary changes, supplementation may be needed. Oral preparations of *potassium,* rather than parenteral dosage forms, are preferred whenever possible. Prepare the oral dosage forms per the manufacturer's insert or per institutional policy and standard of care. Generally, oral forms of potassium need to be taken with food to minimize gastric distress or irritation. Prepare powder or effervescent forms according to package guidelines, and mix thoroughly with at least 4 to 6 ounces of fluid before administering the medication. Enteric-coated and sustained-release forms may still result in gastric upset and lead to ulcer development (ulcerogenic). With oral supplementation, the safest and most effective intervention is frequent and close monitoring for complaints of nausea, vomiting, abdominal pain, or bleeding (such as the occurrence of melena or blood in the stool and/or hematemesis or blood in the vomitus). If abnormalities are noted, continue to monitor vital signs and other parameters, and report findings to the prescriber immediately. Monitor serum levels of potassium during therapy as well.

Hyperkalemia is treated with *sodium polystyrene sulfonate* (*Kayexalate*). It is used only under very specific situations and under very close monitoring of the patient and his or her serum potassium, sodium, calcium, and magnesium levels (see the pharmacology discussion). If Kayexalate is given orally (or via nasogastric tube), elevate the head of the patient's bed to prevent aspiration. The FDA issued a warning in 2011 regarding cases of intestinal necrosis associated with the use of Kayexalate (see pharmacology discussion). Never give Kayexelate with sorbitol because of the connection of these two drugs with the potentially fatal condition of colonic intestinal necrosis. If oral *Kayexalate* is given, do not give it with antacids or laxatives. Administer each dose as a suspension in a small quantity of water for improved palatability. Follow directions regarding the amount of water to use; it generally ranges from 20 to 100 mL, depending on the dose. If given per the rectal route, a retention enema is used. Follow the medication orders carefully, and expect that more than one dose may be needed. The enema must be retained as long as possible and followed by a physician-prescribed cleansing enema. Usually an initial cleansing enema is prescribed, and then the resin solution is administered. If leakage occurs, elevating the patient's hips on a pillow or placing the patient in a knee-chest position may be helpful.

Potassium chloride is the salt customarily used for IV infusions. The concern and caution with potassium chloride use is to avoid overdosage, because it can lead to cardiac arrest. *IV dosage forms of potassium must always be given in a DILUTED form. There is no use or place for undiluted potassium because undiluted potassium is associated with cardiac arrest!* Therefore, parenteral forms of potassium need to be diluted properly. Nowadays, most pharmacies premix the infusion; however, it is still imperative to double-check the order, amount of diluent, and concentration of potassium to diluent. Never assume that what was premixed is 100% correct, because you are ultimately responsible for whatever you administer. Additionally, *only give diluted potassium when there is adequate urine output of at least 30 mL/hr.* Adequate renal function is needed to prevent toxicity. Toxicity or overdosage of potassium (hyperkalemia) is manifested by cardiac rhythm irregularities, muscle spasms, paresthesia, and possible cardiac arrest. Most institutional policy protocols recommend that IV solutions be given at concentrations of less than 40 mEq/L of potassium and at a rate not exceeding 20 mEq/hr. As previously discussed, IV potassium is to be given no faster than 10 mEq/hr to those patients not on cardiac monitoring. In patients who are critically ill and on cardiac monitors, a rate of 20 mEq/hr or more may be used. Avoid adding potassium chloride to an already existing IV solution because the exact concentration cannot be accurately calculated, and overdosage or toxicity may result. Make sure that all IV fluids are labeled appropriately and documented, as with any medication. If the IV fluid rate must be monitored very closely, an infusion pump may be used. *There is no place for IV push or IV bolus potassium replacement!* Treatment of severe hyperkalemia caused by IV administration is through use of IV sodium bicarbonate, calcium gluconate or chloride, or dextrose solution with insulin. These drugs work by leading to a rapid shifting of intracellular potassium ions thereby reducing the serum potassium concentration.

Replacement of *sodium* carries the same concern regarding dosing and route of administration. When the patient is only mildly depleted, an increase in oral intake of sodium needs to be tried. Food items high in sodium include catsup, mustard, cured meats, cheeses, potato chips, peanut butter, popcorn, and table salt. In some situations, salt tablets may be necessary. If the patient is given salt tablets, advise him or her to take plenty of fluids, up to 3000 mL/24 hr, unless contraindicated. If the sodium deficit requires IV replacement, venous access issues and drip rate are as important as with volume and potassium infusions (see previous discussion regarding IV infusion and IV sites). *Hypertonic saline (3% NaCl)* is sometimes used for severe hyponatremia but is considered to be a high risk due to the possible occurrence of osmotic demyelination syndrome. This occurs if the 3% NaCl is given too fast or in too high amounts. It results in irreversible brainstem damage. Other treatment of hyponatremia includes the use of either IV *conivaptan (Vaprisol)* or orally administered *tolvaptan (Samsca)*. These drugs are indicated for euvolemic hyponatremia (see pharmacology discussion). Administer these drugs as ordered while monitoring serum sodium levels. In patients with hyponatremia, it is important to follow treatment guidelines carefully and to remain very astute in the monitoring of these patients. If hyponatremia is acute and severe, or occurring within hours, there is water movement into the brain. Cerebral edema and neurologic symptoms may occur. These adaptations, however, make the brain more vulnerable to injury if chronic hyponatremia is corrected too rapidly. If overly rapid correction occurs, a condition termed *osmotic demeyelination syndrome (ODS)* may occur. ODS was formerly known as *central pontine myelinolysis* because it was thought to be a condition impacting the pons area of the brain.

Hypernatremia is treated with increased fluid intake and dietary restrictions, so you must provide thorough and complete patient education. Intravenous *dextrose in water (D_5W or $D_{10}W$)* may be indicated and helps by creating intravascular sodium dilution and enhanced urine volume output with sodium excretion. It is important to remember that an overly rapid correction of hypernatremia may also be dangerous because of the risk for brain edema during treatment. Therefore, a state of significant hypernatremia (and/or hyponatremia) must be carefully treated by a physician experienced in diagnosis and treatment of electrolyte imbalances. The most important lesson from this discussion is to be astute and cautious in the correction of hyponatremia and hypernatremia.

Always carry out IV infusion of *albumin* and other *colloids* slowly and cautiously. Carefully monitor the patient to prevent fluid overload and potential heart failure, especially in patients who are at particular risk. Fluid overload is evidenced by shortness of breath, crackles at the bases of the lungs, decreased pulse oximeter readings, edema of dependent areas, and increase in weight (see previous parameters). Determine serum hematocrit and hemoglobin values in advance of therapy—as well as during and after therapy—so that any dilutional effects can be determined. For example, if a patient has received albumin and other colloids too quickly, and hypervolemia results, the patient's hemoglobin and hematocrit may actually be decreased. This decrease would be caused by a dilutional effect because of too much volume in relation to the concentration of solutes. Clinically, the patient would appear to be anemic, but in fact the deficit would be attributable to the increase in volume. It is also important to remember that albumin is to be given at room temperature.

For infusion of *blood*, always check the expiration date of *blood* and/or *blood components* to make sure that the blood is not outdated. *Under NO circumstances is outdated blood to be used!* Policies at most hospitals and other health care institutions require that blood and blood products be double-checked by another registered nurse BEFORE the blood is hung and infused. This is important to prevent a mixup in blood types. Blood types must always be a major concern because of the possible complications that can occur, some life-threatening, if the wrong blood type is given or if the blood is given to the wrong person. The "Nine Rights" of medication administration remain critical in all that you do with medications, and administering blood is no exception.

When blood and blood products are infused, safety is of top priority, so it is important to frequently monitor and document all vital signs and related parameters before, during, and after administration of the blood product, component (e.g., *PRBCs, FFP*), or solution. A transfusion reaction would be manifested by the occurrence of the following: apprehension, restlessness, flushed skin, increased pulse and respirations, dyspnea, rash, joint or lower back pain, swelling, fever and chills (a febrile reaction beginning 1 hour after the start of administration and possibly lasting up to 10 hours), nausea, weakness, and jaundice. Report these signs and symptoms to the prescriber immediately, stop the blood or product (regardless of when the reaction occurs), and keep the IV line patent with isotonic NS solution infusing at a slow rate. Monitor patient and vital signs closely. Always follow the health care institution's protocol for transfusion reactions.

In summary, encourage patients receiving any type of fluid or electrolyte substance, colloid, or blood component to immediately report unusual adverse effects to their prescriber. Such complaints may include chest pain, dizziness, weakness, and shortness of breath.

▌EVALUATION

The therapeutic response to *fluid, electrolyte*, and *blood* or *blood component* therapy includes normalization of fluid volume and laboratory values, including RBC and WBC counts, hemoglobin level, hematocrit, and sodium and potassium levels. In addition to review of these laboratory values, evaluation of the patient's cardiac, respiratory, musculoskeletal, and GI functioning is also important. Therapeutic effects include improved energy levels and tolerance of activities of daily living. Skin color will improve, and there will be improved shortness of breath as well as minimal to no chest pain, weakness, or fatigue. Correct treatment of blood volume problems will be evidenced by a return of laboratory values to the normal range, improved vital signs, an increase in energy, and near-normal oxygen saturation levels. The therapeutic response to *albumin* therapy includes an elevation of blood pressure, decreased edema, and increased serum albumin levels. Frequently monitor for adverse effects of any of these drugs and/or solutions, and check for distended neck veins; shortness of breath; anxiety; insomnia; expiratory crackles; frothy, blood-tinged sputum; and cyanosis (indicative of fluid volume overload).

CASE STUDY

Safety: What Went Wrong? Fluid and Electrolyte Replacement

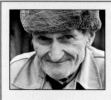

M.S., an 85-year-old retired engineer, seemed somewhat confused when his daughter came home from work. When she brings him to the emergency department, his blood pressure is 90/62 mm Hg, his heart rate is 114 beats/min, and his skin is dry but cool. His daughter says that he seems "much weaker" than usual, and he is unable to answer questions clearly. His daughter reports that he has "lost his appetite" lately and has not taken in much food or drink. The nurse starts an IV infusion of 0.9% sodium chloride (NS) at 100 mL/hr via a gravity drip infusion.

1. What do you think is M.S.'s main medical problem at this time?

    The emergency department is very busy, and when the nurse returns in 15 minutes, she is shocked to see that almost the entire 500-mL bag of NS has infused within 1 hour's time.

2. What went wrong? What will the nurse do first, and what will the nurse watch for at this time?

    Twenty-four hours after his admission, M.S. is much less confused and is able to move to a chair for lunch without much difficulty. He is receiving 5% dextrose/½ NS with 20 mEq of potassium chloride at a rate of 75 mL/hr via an infusion pump. His daughter notices that the area above the IV insertion site is red, and M.S. complains that the area is "very sore."

3. What went wrong? What needs to be done at this time?

For answers, see *http://evolve.elsevier.com/Lilley.*

PATIENT-CENTERED CARE: PATIENT TEACHING

- As needed, educate the patient about the difference in the signs and symptoms of hyponatremia and hypernatremia. Hyponatremia is manifested by lethargy, hypotension, stomach cramps, vomiting, diarrhea, and seizures. Some of the causes of hyponatremia include excessive perspiration, occurring during hot weather or physical work, and prolonged diarrhea or vomiting. The clinical presentation of hyponatremia/hypernatremia also depends on the associated fluid volume status.

- Hypernatremia is associated with symptoms of water retention (edema); hypertension; red, flushed skin; dry, sticky mucous membranes; increased thirst; temperature elevation; and decreased or absent urination. The most common cause is poor renal excretion as a result of kidney malfunction. Inadequate water consumption and dehydration are other causes.

- Educate the patient about the early symptoms of hypokalemia, such as hypotension, lethargy, mental confusion, nausea, and muscle weakness. Late symptoms include cardiac dysrhythmias (the patient may feel palpitations or shortness of breath), neuropathies, and paralytic ileus.

- Share the symptoms of hyperkalemia with the patient, including muscle weakness, paresthesia, paralysis, and cardiac rhythm abnormalities.

- Provide the patient with adequate and appropriate information about how to take oral potassium chloride. In the directions, include the fact that the powdered or liquid solutions require thorough mixing in at least 4 to 8 ounces of cold water/juice before drinking the mixture slowly. Encourage the patient to take oral doses with food or a snack, and tell patients taking potassium supplements to report to the prescriber immediately any GI upset or abdominal pain (indicative of gastric irritation from the oral potassium). Educate the patient about potential drug interactions such as potassium-sparing diuretics and ACE inhibitors because their concurrent use may produce hyperkalemia.

- Educate patients on foods high in potassium, including bananas, oranges, apricots, dates, raisins, broccoli, green beans, potatoes, tomatoes, meats, fish, wheat bread, and legumes.

- Advise patients that sustained-release potassium capsules and tablets must be swallowed whole and should not be crushed, chewed, or allowed to dissolve in the mouth.

- Encourage the patient to report any difficulty in swallowing, painful swallowing, or feeling that the capsule or tablet is getting stuck in the throat. Other serious adverse effects that need to be reported include vomiting of coffee ground–like material, stomach or abdominal pain or swelling, and black tarry stools.

- Educate the patient that extended-release dosage forms of potassium need to be taken in full. Each prescribed dose is to be taken with meals and a full glass of water. If the patient has difficulty swallowing the whole tablet, and if approved by the prescriber, the patient can break the tablet in half and take each half separately, drinking a half glass of water (4 ounces) with each half and taking the entire dose within a few minutes. The patient must take the full dose and not save partial dosages of potassium for later. Another option is to take the extended-release dosage form and place the whole tablet in 4 ounces of water. Instruct the patient to allow 2 minutes for the tablet to dissolve in the recommended 4 ounces of water, stir for 30 seconds, and then drink immediately. Adding 1 ounce of water to the glass, swirling it, and then drinking the residual will allow adequate dosing. Water is recommended as the fluid for mixing the extended-release dosage form. A straw may be used.

- Instruct the patient to dissolve effervescent potassium tablets, as directed. At least 3 ounces of cold water needs to be used per tablet. The patient needs to take the dose as soon as it is fully dissolved, sipping the mixture over 5 to 10 minutes and taking the dose after food to minimize GI upset.
- Educate the patient that salt substitutes contain potassium. Another alternative must be recommended if the patient is hyperkalemic.

- If receiving IV potassium, tell the patient to report any feelings of irritation (e.g., burning) at the IV site.
- Educate the patient about the safe use of salt tablets, and instruct him or her to take them as prescribed. Salt tablets must be taken with adequate fluid intake.

KEY POINTS

- Total body water (TBW) is divided into intracellular (inside the cell) and extracellular (outside the cell) compartments. Fluid volume outside the cells is either in the plasma (intravascular volume) or between the tissues, cells, or organs.
- Colloids are large protein particles that cannot leak out of the blood vessels. Because of their greater concentration inside blood vessels, fluid is pulled into the blood vessels. An example of a colloid is albumin. Administer albumin with caution because of the high risk for hypervolemia and possible heart failure. Monitor intake and output, weights, heart and breath sounds, and appropriate laboratory values.
- Blood products are the only fluids that are able to carry oxygen because they are the only fluids that contain hemoglobin. Patients will hopefully begin to show improved energy and increasing tolerance for activities of daily living as a result of the treatments with blood products. Pulse oximeter readings will also show improved readings.
- Dehydration may be hypotonic, resulting from the loss of salt; hypertonic, resulting from fever with perspiration; or isotonic, resulting from diarrhea or vomiting. Each form of dehydration is treated differently. Carefully assess intake and output as well as skin turgor, urine specific gravity, and blood levels of potassium, sodium, and chloride.
- Hypertonic solutions must be used very cautiously and given slowly because of the risk for hypervolemia from overzealous replacement.

- Early symptoms of hypokalemia include hypotension, lethargy, mental confusion, nausea, and muscle weakness. Late symptoms include cardiac dysrhythmias (the patient may feel palpitations or shortness of breath), neuropathies, and paralytic ileus.
- Symptoms of hyperkalemia include muscle weakness, paresthesia, paralysis, and cardiac rhythm abnormalities.
- Hyponatremia is manifested by lethargy, hypotension, stomach cramps, vomiting, diarrhea, and seizures. Hypernatremia is associated with symptoms of water retention but can be associated with normal fluid or even low fluid volume (edema); hypertension; red, flushed skin; dry, sticky mucous membranes; increased thirst; temperature elevation; and decreased or absent urination.
- Osmotic demyelination syndrome (previously called central pontine myelinolysis) may occur when there is rapid correction of chronic hyponatremia.
- With administration of blood products, measurement of vital signs and frequent monitoring of the patient before, during, and after infusions are critical to patient safety. Blood products must be given only with normal saline (0.9% sodium chloride), because the solution of D_5W results in hemolysis of red blood cells.

NCLEX® EXAMINATION REVIEW QUESTIONS

1. Which action by the nurse is most appropriate for the patient receiving an infusion of packed red blood cells?
   a. Flush the IV line with normal saline before the blood is added to the infusion.
   b. Flush the IV line with dextrose before the blood is added to the infusion.
   c. Check the patient's vital signs once the infusion is completed.
   d. Anticipate that flushed skin and fever are expected reactions to a blood transfusion.
2. When preparing an IV solution that contains potassium, the nurse knows that a contraindication to the potassium infusion would be
   a. diarrhea.
   b. serum sodium level of 145 mEq/L.
   c. serum potassium level of 5.6 mEq/L.
   d. dehydration.

3. When assessing a patient who is about to receive an albumin infusion, the nurse knows that a contraindication for albumin would be
   a. acute liver failure.
   b. heart failure.
   c. severe burns.
   d. fluid-volume deficit.
4. The nurse is preparing an infusion for a patient who has a deficiency in clotting factors. Which type of infusion is most appropriate?
   a. Albumin 5%
   b. Packed RBCs
   c. Whole blood
   d. Fresh frozen plasma

5. While monitoring a patient who is receiving an infusion of a crystalloid solution, the nurse will monitor for which potential problem?
   a. Bradycardia
   b. Hypotension
   c. Decreased skin turgor
   d. Fluid overload

6. The nurse is administering an IV solution that contains potassium chloride to a patient in the critical care unit who has a severely decreased serum potassium level. Which action(s) by the nurse are appropriate? *(Select all that apply.)*
   a. Administer the potassium by slow IV bolus.
   b. Administer the potassium at a rate no faster than 20 mEq/hr.
   c. Monitor the patient's cardiac rhythm with a heart monitor.
   d. Use an infusion pump for the administration of IV potassium chloride.
   e. Administer the potassium IV push.

7. The order reads: "Infuse 1000 mL of normal saline over the next 8 hours." The IV tubing has a drop factor of 15 gtt/mL. Calculate the mL/hour rate, and calculate the drops/minute setting for the IV tubing with this gravity infusion.

8. A patient is about to receive a dose of the nonprotein plasma expander dextran. The nurse knows that this product is indicated for which type of blood loss?
   a. Slow loss of 20% or less
   b. Slow loss of 20% to 50%
   c. Slow loss of over 50% or acute loss of 20%
   d. Loss of 80% or more

1. a. 2. c. 3. b. 4. d. 5. d. 6. b, c, d. 7. 125 mL/hr; 31 gtt/min, 8. b.

CRITICAL THINKING AND PRIORITIZATION QUESTIONS

1. After having vomiting and diarrhea from the flu for the previous 24 hours, a patient is admitted for treatment of dehydration. The nurse knows that the priority action is to administer which type of fluid? Explain your answer.

2. During a transfusion of packed red blood cells (PRBCs), the patient complains that his back is starting to "hurt" and he feels anxious. His temperature is 98.8°F (37.1°C). What is the nurse's priority action at this time?

For answers, see *http://evolve.elsevier.com/Lilley.*

ⓔ EVOLVE WEBSITE

http://evolve.elsevier.com/Lilley
- Animations
- Answer Keys for Textbook Case Studies and Textbook Critical Thinking and Prioritization Questions
- Content Updates
- Key Points
- Review Questions
- Student Case Studies

PART 5

Drugs Affecting the Endocrine and Reproductive Systems

Learning Strategies

STUDY GROUPS

Study groups can be a very successful way to learn and study pharmacology. When working with groups, you have the ability and advantage to get another person's perspective on a topic. Sometimes another student can explain something in a way that makes it easier for you to understand. A group working together can divide a lesson or assignment so everyone brings something to the table with everyone learning from one another. If you prefer to study alone, refer to Part 4.

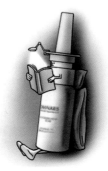

First, you need to find a study group that is compatible with your learning needs and availability. You also want to make sure that the students in your group will use the time together to actually study, discuss and quiz each other on the material, and not waste time engaging in social "chit chat." The majority of the time together needs to focus on the task at hand. If the group you joined does not meet your needs. do not hesitate to leave it and find a different group. When and where students meet for study group is also important. The environment needs to be conducive to learning for everyone in the group. Many collegiate/academic and public libraries have study rooms that students can use. Often there is a master sign-up sheet found with individuals at the front desk of the library. If the school cafeteria has a quiet section, then that may be another possible location for a study group. Students like to eat and study. A beneficial time to plan a study group would be right after or close to the time after the pharmacology lecture. This planning of time would allow everyone to review and discuss new information. If any information is not clearly understood, it can be cleared up prior to further studying.

CHAT ROOMS AND DISCUSSION GROUPS

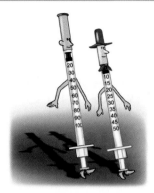

Because we live in such a mobile society and students lead busy lives, with school, raising families, and working, finding time for a study group can be difficult. In these instances, using chat rooms and discussion boards are a great alternative to face-to-face group meetings. Some social media sites allow for the formation of chat rooms where students can all log in to discuss their pharmacology content. These chat rooms need to be set up by the student and are usually free of charge. Feedback from other students from other schools can also be achieved in these social media sites. Chat rooms may be accessed from home, making group meetings/activities more convenient.

Many colleges and universities already incorporate online learning and learning management systems. The learning management systems go by various names and are usually used by instructors and professors to upload course content, assignments, and grades. These systems usually allow the capability to set up discussion boards. The discussion board facilitates group learning by allowing a forum for a student to post a question on a concept or topic that needs clarification and/or

reinforcement. Other students can go to the site and post an answer, add a question of their own, or share tips on learning, for example, posting a link to websites with useful mnemonics or other learning strategies. Discussion boards can be designed so the whole class participates or set up for small individual groups. Many of these sites can be controlled and monitored by the course instructors. Discussion groups can be accessed from anywhere that the student has an Internet connection.

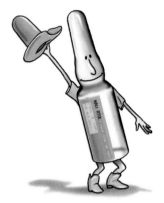

Study groups can be large or small. For best results, everyone should participate in the learning. You never know when a different perspective can mean the difference between the understanding or struggling with ideas or concepts. If you are the type of student who absolutely detests group studying and you feel you learn best by yourself, you should at least have a friend or partner to help you study for a test. Students who use the technique of "teaching another" find that it is very helpful. Only when you really understand a topic thoroughly can you teach it to someone else. So grab your notes with the key points, and teach the topic to a partner. Your partner will use your notes to make sure you have taught the topic completely. This activity also works well when studying for tests in the study groups.

Pituitary Drugs

http://evolve.elsevier.com/Lilley

OBJECTIVES

When you reach the end of this chapter, you will be able to do the following:

1. Describe the normal function of the anterior and posterior lobes of the pituitary gland and the impact of the pituitary gland on the human body.
2. Compare the various pituitary drugs with regard to their indications, mechanisms of action, dosages, routes of administration, adverse effects, cautions, contraindications, and drug interactions.
3. Develop a nursing care plan that includes all phases of the nursing process for patients receiving pituitary drugs, such as desmopressin, vasopressin, octreotide, and somatropin.

DRUG PROFILES

♦ **octreotide**, p. 486
♦ **somatropin**, p. 486
♦! **vasopressin**, p. 487

♦ = *Key drug*
! = *High-alert drug*

KEY TERMS

Hypothalamus The gland above and behind the pituitary gland and the optic chiasm. Both glands are suspended beneath the middle area of the bottom of the brain. The hypothalamus secretes the hormones vasopressin and oxytocin, which are stored in the posterior pituitary gland. The hypothalamus also secretes several hormone-releasing factors that stimulate the anterior pituitary gland to secrete a variety of hormones that control many bodily functions. (p. 483)

Negative feedback loop A system in which the production of one hormone is controlled by the levels of a second hormone in a way that reduces the output of the first hormone. A gland produces a hormone that stimulates a second gland to produce a second hormone. In response to the increased levels of the second hormone, the source gland of the first hormone reduces production of that hormone until blood levels of the second hormone fall below a certain minimum level needed; then the cycle begins again. (p. 484)

Neuroendocrine system The system that regulates the reactions to both internal and external stimuli and involves the integrated activities of the endocrine glands and nervous system. (p. 483)

Pituitary gland An endocrine gland that is suspended beneath the brain and supplies numerous hormones that control many vital processes. (p. 484)

ENDOCRINE SYSTEM

Maintenance of physiologic stability is the main goal of the endocrine system. The endocrine system must accomplish this task despite constant changes in the internal and external environments. Every cell and organ in the body comes under the influence of the endocrine system. It communicates with the nearly 50 million target cells in the body using a chemical "language" called *hormones*. Hormones are a large group of natural substances that cause highly specific physiologic effects in the cells of their target tissues. They are secreted into the bloodstream in response to the body's needs and travel through the blood to their site of action—the target cell.

For decades, the pituitary gland was believed to be the master gland that regulated and controlled the other endocrine glands. However, evidence now suggests that the central nervous system (CNS), specifically the **hypothalamus**, controls the pituitary gland. The hypothalamus and pituitary gland are now viewed as functioning together as an integrated unit, with the primary direction coming from the hypothalamus. For this reason, these structures are now commonly referred to as the **neuroendocrine system**. In fact, the endocrine system can be considered in much the same way as the CNS. Each is basically a system for signaling, and each operates in a stimulus-and-response manner. Together these two systems essentially govern all bodily functions.

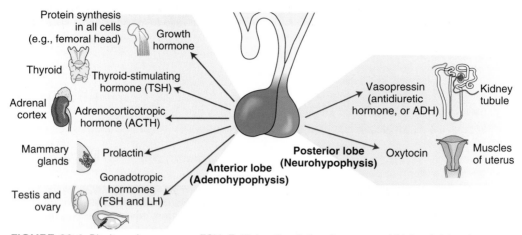

FIGURE 30-1 Pituitary hormones. *FSH,* Follicle-stimulating hormone; *LH,* luteinizing hormone. (Adapted from McKenry LM, Tessier E, Hogan MA: *Mosby's pharmacology in nursing,* ed 22, St Louis, 2006, Mosby.)

BOX 30-1 Hormones of the Anterior and Posterior Pituitary Gland

Anterior Pituitary Gland (Adenohypophysis)
Adrenocorticotropic hormone (ACTH)
Follicle-stimulating hormone (FSH)
Growth hormone (GH)
Luteinizing hormone (LH)
Prolactin (PH)
Thyroid-stimulating hormone (TSH)

Posterior Pituitary Gland (Neurohypophysis)
Antidiuretic hormone (ADH)
Oxytocin

The **pituitary gland** is made up of two distinct lobes—the anterior pituitary gland (adenohypophysis) and posterior pituitary gland (neurohypophysis). They are individually linked to and communicate with the hypothalamus, and each lobe secretes its own different set of hormones. These various hormones are listed in Box 30-1 and shown in Figure 30-1.

Hormones are either water- or lipid-soluble. The water-soluble hormones are protein-based substances such as the catecholamines norepinephrine and epinephrine. The lipid-soluble hormones consist of the steroid and thyroid hormones.

The activity of the endocrine system is regulated by a system of surveillance and signaling usually dictated by the body's ongoing needs. Hormone secretion is commonly regulated by a **negative feedback loop.** This is best explained using a fictional example: When gland X releases hormone X, this stimulates target cells to release hormone Y. When there is an excess of hormone Y, gland X senses this excess and decreases its release of hormone X.

PITUITARY DRUGS

A variety of drugs affect the pituitary gland. They are generally used either as replacement drug therapy to make up for a hormone deficiency or as diagnostic aids to determine the status of the patient's hormonal functions. The currently identified anterior and posterior pituitary hormones and the drugs that mimic or antagonize their actions are listed in Table 30-1.

The anterior pituitary drugs discussed in this chapter are cosyntropin, somatropin, and octreotide; the posterior pituitary drugs discussed in this chapter are vasopressin and desmopressin.

Mechanism of Action and Drug Effects

The mechanisms of action of the various pituitary drugs differ depending on the drug, but overall they either augment or antagonize the natural effects of the pituitary hormones. Exogenously administered corticotropin elicits all of the same pharmacologic responses as those elicited by endogenous corticotropin (also known as adrenocorticotropic hormone, or ACTH). Intravenous exogenous corticotropin is no longer manufactured; however, an intramuscular/subcutaneous injection, known as H.P. Acthar Gel, is available. The intravenous corticotropin has been replaced by cosyntropin (Cortrosyn). Cosyntropin travels to the adrenal cortex, located just above the kidney, and stimulates the secretion of cortisol (the drug form of which is hydrocortisone [Solu-Cortef]). Cortisol has many antiinflammatory effects, including reduction of inflammatory leukocyte functions and scar tissue formation. Cortisol also promotes renal retention of sodium, which can result in edema and hypertension.

The drugs that mimic growth hormone (GH) are somatropin and somatrem. These drugs promote growth by stimulating various anabolic (tissue-building) processes, liver glycogenolysis (to raise blood sugar levels), lipid mobilization from body fat stores, and retention of sodium, potassium, and phosphorus. Both drugs promote linear growth in children who lack normal amounts of the endogenous hormone.

Octreotide is a drug that antagonizes the effects of natural growth hormone (GH). It does so by inhibiting GH release. Octreotide is a synthetic polypeptide that is structurally and pharmacologically similar to GH release–inhibiting factor,

TABLE 30-1   Anterior and Posterior Pituitary Hormones and Drugs

Hormone	Function and Mimicking Drug
Anterior Pituitary Gland	
Adrenocorticotropic hormone (ACTH)	Targets adrenal gland; mediates adaptation to physical and emotional stress and starvation; redistributes body nutrients; promotes synthesis of adrenocortical hormones (glucocorticoids, mineralocorticoids, androgens); involved in skin pigmentation
	Cosyntropin: Used for diagnosis of adrenocortical insufficiency
Follicle-stimulating hormone (FSH)	Stimulates oogenesis and follicular growth in females and spermatogenesis in males
	Menotropins: Same pharmacologic effects as FSH; many of the other gonadotropins also stimulate FSH (see Chapter 34)
Growth hormone (GH)	Regulates anabolic processes related to growth and adaptation to stressors; promotes skeletal and muscle growth; increases protein synthesis; increases liver glycogenolysis; increases fat mobilization
	Somatropin, somatrem: Human GH for treatment of hypopituitary dwarfism
	Octreotide: A synthetic polypeptide structurally and pharmacologically similar to GH release–inhibiting factor; inhibits GH
Luteinizing hormone (LH)	Stimulates ovulation and estrogen release by ovaries in females; stimulates interstitial cells in males to promote spermatogenesis and testosterone secretion
	Pergonal and clomiphene: Increase LH levels and the chance of pregnancy
Prolactin	Targets mammary glands; stimulates lactogenesis and breast growth in females; purpose in males is poorly understood
	Bromocriptine: Inhibits action of prolactin and inhibits lactogenesis (see Chapter 15)
Thyroid-stimulating hormone (TSH)	Stimulates secretion of thyroid hormones T_3 and T_4 by the thyroid gland
	Thyrotropin: Increases production and secretion of thyroid hormones
Posterior Pituitary Gland	
Antidiuretic hormone (ADH)	Increases water resorption in distal tubules and collecting duct of nephron; concentrates urine; causes potent vasoconstriction
	Vasopressin: ADH; performs all the physiologic functions of ADH
	Desmopressin: A synthetic vasopressin
Oxytocin	Targets mammary glands; stimulates ejection of milk and contraction of uterine smooth muscle
	Pitocin: Has all the physiologic actions of oxytocin (see Chapter 34)

T_3, Triiodothyronine; T_4, thyroxine.

which is also called *somatostatin.* It also reduces plasma concentrations of vasoactive intestinal polypeptide (VIP), a protein secreted by a type of tumor known as a *VIPoma* that causes profuse watery diarrhea (see Chapter 46).

The drugs that affect the posterior pituitary gland, such as vasopressin and desmopressin, mimic the actions of the naturally occurring antidiuretic hormone (ADH). They increase water resorption in the distal tubules and collecting ducts of the nephrons, and they concentrate urine, reducing water excretion by up to 90%. Vasopressin is also a potent vasoconstrictor in larger doses and is therefore used in certain hypotensive emergencies, such as vasodilatory shock (septic shock). It is also used in the Advanced Cardiac Life Support (ACLS) guidelines for treatment of pulseless cardiac arrest. Vasopressin is also used to stop bleeding of esophageal varices. Desmopressin causes a dose-dependent increase in the plasma levels of factor VIII (antihemophilic factor), von Willebrand factor (acts closely with factor VIII), and tissue plasminogen activator. These properties make it useful in treating certain blood disorders. Desmopressin is also used for management of nocturnal enuresis. The drug form of oxytocin mimics the endogenous hormone, thus promoting uterine contractions (see Chapter 34).

Indications

Cosyntropin is used in the diagnosis of adrenocortical insufficiency. Upon diagnosis, the actual drug treatment generally involves replacement hormonal therapy using drug forms of the deficient corticosteroid hormones. These drugs are discussed in

more detail in Chapter 33. Somatropin and somatrem are human GH produced by recombinant technology. They are effective in stimulating skeletal growth in patients with an inadequate secretion of normal endogenous GH, such as those with hypopituitary dwarfism, and are also used for wasting associated with human immunodeficiency virus infection (HIV). Octreotide is useful in alleviating certain symptoms of carcinoid tumors stemming from the secretion of VIP, including severe diarrhea and flushing and potentially life-threatening hypotension associated with a carcinoid crisis. It is also used for the treatment of esophageal varices. Vasopressin and desmopressin are used to prevent or control polydipsia (excessive thirst), polyuria, and dehydration in patients with diabetes insipidus caused by a deficiency of endogenous ADH. Because of their vasoconstrictive properties, they are useful in the treatment of various types of bleeding, in particular gastrointestinal hemorrhage. Desmopressin is useful in the treatment of hemophilia A and type I von Willebrand's disease because of its effects on various blood-clotting factors.

Contraindications

Contraindications for the use of pituitary drugs vary with each individual drug and are listed in each of the drug profiles included in this chapter. Because even small amounts of these drugs can initiate major physiologic changes, they need to be used with special caution in patients with acute or chronic illnesses such as migraine headaches, epilepsy, and asthma.

TABLE 30-2 Octreotide: Common Adverse Effects

Body System	Adverse Effects
Central nervous	Fatigue, malaise, headache
Endocrine	Increase or decrease in blood glucose levels
Gastrointestinal	Diarrhea, nausea, vomiting
Respiratory	Dyspnea
Musculoskeletal	Arthralgia
Cardiovascular	Conduction abnormalities

TABLE 30-3 Desmopressin and Vasopressin: Common Adverse Effects

Body System	Adverse Effects
Cardiovascular	Increased blood pressure
Central nervous	Fever, vertigo, headache
Gastrointestinal	Nausea, heartburn, cramps
Genitourinary	Uterine cramping
Other	Nasal irritation and congestion, tremor, sweating

TABLE 30-4 Growth Hormone Analogues: Common Adverse Effects

Body System	Adverse Effects
Central nervous	Headache
Endocrine	Hyperglycemia, hypothyroidism
Genitourinary	Hypercalciuria
Other	Rash, urticaria, development of antibodies to growth hormone, inflammation at injection site, flulike syndrome

Adverse Effects

Most of the adverse effects of the pituitary drugs are specific to the individual drug. Those drugs possessing similar hormonal effects generally have similar adverse effects. The most common adverse effects of the pituitary drugs described here are listed in Tables 30-2, 30-3, and 30-4.

Interactions

Selected interactions involving pituitary drugs are summarized in Table 30-5.

Dosages

For dosage information on pituitary drugs, see the table on the next page.

DRUG PROFILES

◆ octreotide

Octreotide (Sandostatin) is useful in alleviating certain symptoms of carcinoid tumors stemming from the secretion of VIP, including severe diarrhea and flushing and potentially life-threatening hypotension associated with a carcinoid crisis. It is also used for the treatment of esophageal varices. It is contraindicated in patients who have a known hypersensitivity to it

TABLE 30-5 Pituitary Drugs: Selected Drug Interactions

Pituitary Drug	Interacting Drug	Potential Result
desmopressin	carbamazepine	Enhanced desmopressin effects
	lithium, alcohol, demeclocycline	Reduced desmopressin effects
octreotide	cyclosporine	Case report of transplant rejection
	thioridazine, ciprofloxacin	Prolongation of QT interval
somatropin	Glucocorticoids	Reduction of growth effects
vasopressin	carbamazepine, fludrocortisone	Enhanced antidiuretic effect
	demeclocycline, norepinephrine, lithium	Reduced antidiuretic effect

or any of its components. Octreotide may impair gallbladder function and needs to be used with caution in patients with renal impairment. It may affect glucose regulation, and severe hypoglycemia may occur in patients with type 1 diabetes. It may cause hyperglycemia in patients with type 2 diabetes or in patients without diabetes. Octreotide may enhance the toxic effects of drugs that prolong the QT interval. Ciprofloxacin may enhance the QT-prolonging effects of octreotide. Octreotide can be given intravenously (IV), intramuscularly (IM), or subcutaneously. It is classified as a pregnancy category B drug. Recommended dosages are given in the table on this page.

Pharmacokinetics: Octreotide

Route	Onset of Action	Peak Plasma Concentration	Elimination Half-life	Duration of Action
PO	Rapid	0.4-1 hr	1.7-1.9 hr	6-12 hr

◆ somatropin

Somatropin (Humatrope, Nutropin, Serostim, others) is a growth hormone that is indicated in the treatment of growth failure due to inadequate endogenous growth hormone secretion. It is also used for patients with HIV infection with wasting or cachexia in conjunction with antiviral therapy. It is classified as a pregnancy category B or C drug, depending on the manufacturer. Somatropin is contraindicated in patients with hypersensitivity to any component of the product and in children with closed growth plates, patients with tumors, and patients with acute illnesses. Adverse effects include headache, injection site reactions, muscle pain, hypoglycemia, or hyperglycemia. It is important not to shake the product. It is generally given subcutaneously; however, some manufactured products can be given intramuscularly. Check the specific prescribing information before administering.

Pharmacokinetics: Somatropin

Route	Onset of Action	Peak Plasma Concentration	Elimination Half-life	Duration of Action
Subcut or IM	Not available	2-6 hr	2-4 hr (subcut)	18-20 hr

DOSAGES

Selected Pituitary Drugs

Drug	Pharmacologic Class	Usual Dosage Range	Indications/Uses
◆ octreotide (Sandostatin), Sandostatin LAR Depot)	Somatostatin (GH inhibitor) analogue	**Adult*** IV/subcut: Initial dose of 50-100 mcg tid	Acromegaly
		IV/subcut: 100-600 mcg/day	Metastatic carcinoid tumor (to control flushing and diarrhea symptoms)
		IV/subcut: 150-750 mcg/day divided bid-qid	VIPoma
		IV: 50 mcg bolus, followed by 25-50 mcg/hr for 2-5 days	Esophageal varices
◆ somatropin (Humatrope, others)	Anterior pituitary hormone	**Pediatric** IM/subcut: 0.18-0.3 mg/kg/week	Growth hormone deficiency
◆❗vasopressin (Pitressin)	Natural or synthetic ADH	**Adult** IM/subcut: 5-10 units bid-qid	Diabetes insipidus
		Adult IV: 0.01-0.04 units/min	Vasodilatory shock (septic shock)

ADH, Antidiuretic hormone; *GH*, growth hormone; *VIPoma*, vasoactive intestinal peptide–producing tumor.
*Normally used only in adults.

◆❗vasopressin

Vasopressin (Pitressin) and desmopressin (DDAVP) are used to prevent or control polydipsia (excessive thirst), polyuria, and dehydration in patients with diabetes insipidus caused by a deficiency of endogenous ADH. Vasopressin is also used to control various types of bleeding (in particular gastrointestinal hemorrhage) and in pulseless arrest and vasodilatory shock. Desmopressin is also useful in the treatment of hemophilia A and type I von Willebrand's disease because of its effects on various blood-clotting factors. Vasopressin is contraindicated in patients with a known hypersensitivity to it. It is classified as a pregnancy category C drug. It should be used with caution in patients with seizure disorders, asthma, cardiovascular disease, and renal disease. IV infiltration may lead to severe vasoconstriction and localized tissue necrosis. Watch the IV site closely for any signs of infiltration, and use a central venous access device when possible. Vasopressin is available as a nasal spray or injection for IM or IV use. When used to treat septic shock, it is given by continuous IV infusion. Both drugs can be given via the nasal route. Vasopressin nasal is applied topically to nasal membranes and must not be inhaled. Desmopressin is given via nasal pump.

Pharmacokinetics: Vasopressin

Route	Onset of Action	Peak Plasma Concentration	Elimination Half-life	Duration of Action
IV	Rapid	1 hr	0.5 hr	2-8 hr

▎NURSING PROCESS

▎ASSESSMENT

Before administering any of the *pituitary drugs*, perform a thorough assessment and document the findings. Assess and record the patient's height, weight, and vital signs. Take a complete medication history, and note allergies, prescription drug use, and use of over-the-counter drugs, supplements, and herbals, and be attentive to any cautions, contraindications, and drug interactions. With *octreotide acetate*, the prescriber may order an electrocardiogram prior to use because of the adverse effect of conduction abnormalities. Assess baseline glucose levels, and note respiratory status with octreotide acetate use. Patients taking octreotide may require special dosing if they have decreased liver and kidney function; therefore, assess baseline liver and kidney function tests. It is also important to assess for sound-alike, look-alike drugs (SALAD) to prevent potential medication errors. Specifically, octreotide acetate, or *Sandostatin* and *Sandostatin LAR* are not to be confused with Sandimmune (cyclosporine) or Sandoglobulin (IV immune globulin).

With *desmopressin*, assess vital signs as well as a history of seizures, asthma, or cardiovascular disease. These conditions require cautious use with careful monitoring of vital signs, heart sounds, and breath sounds. For patients being treated for shock, if *vasopressin* is being used, close monitoring in an intensive care setting is needed with ECG, vital signs, and invasive monitoring methods such as arterial lines, central venous pressure lines, and/or arterial blood gases. With *growth hormones*, obtain baseline thyroid, glucose, and calcium levels, as prescribed, due to the potential side effects of hyperglycemia, hypothyroidism, and hypercalciuria. Specifically, use of *somatropin* requires attention to the growth, motor skills, height, and weight of the pediatric patient.

▎NURSING DIAGNOSES

1. Disturbed body image related to the specific disease process and/or drug adverse effects and their impact on the patient's physical characteristics
2. Acute pain related to gastrointestinal adverse effects associated with the use of various pituitary drugs

3. Deficient knowledge related to lack of information and experience with pituitary drug treatment

PLANNING: OUTCOME IDENTIFICATION

1. Patient maintains positive body image through verbalization of fears, anxieties, and concerns to health care professionals while receiving drug therapy.
2. Patient takes medications as prescribed thus experiencing minimal to no adverse effects of medication-induced gastrointestinal upset or epigastric distress.
3. Patient gains increased knowledge about drug therapy, remains compliant, and keeps follow-up appointments.

CASE STUDY

Patient-Centered Care: Octreotide for VIPoma-Related Diarrhea

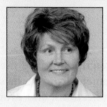

J.R., a 56-year-old beautician, has been diagnosed with a VIPoma (vasoactive intestinal peptide–producing tumor). She was scheduled for surgery but developed severe diarrhea. She has been hospitalized because she became dehydrated after 2 days of profuse, watery diarrhea. J.R. has not eaten for several days. In addition to having diarrhea, she is nauseated, has facial flushing, and has lost 5 pounds in 2 days. Intravenous fluid replacement with normal saline has been started, and she will be receiving octreotide (Sandostatin). She had her gallbladder removed 8 years ago but has no history of other illnesses.

1. How does the octreotide work to control the VIPoma-related diarrhea?
2. As J.R. begins therapy with octreotide, the nurse should continue to assess what parameters?
    After 2 days of treatment, the episodes of diarrhea have become less frequent. However, the nurse notes that J.R.'s blood glucose levels are elevated.
3. What is the best explanation for this elevation?

For answers, see *http://evolve.elsevier.com/Lilley.*

IMPLEMENTATION

Ocreatide acetate must be given as ordered with attention to the route of administration. To avoid giving the wrong medication, be careful not to confuse octreotide acetate injection with the injectable depot suspension dosage form. Use only clear solutions, and always check for incompatibilities. Make sure patients understand the importance of immediately reporting to the prescriber any abdominal distress such as diarrhea, nausea, or vomiting that is unmanageable. Stress the importance of follow-up appointments for laboratory testing during treatment with this drug. Monitor glucose levels during therapy, especially if patients are already diabetic, because octreotide acetate may precipitate alterations in blood glucose levels.

Administer *desmopressin* per the prescriber's orders because dosage and route may vary with the indication. Dosage forms include oral, IV, intranasal, and subcutaneous. For desmopressin and *somatropin*, rotate subcutaneous and/or intramuscular injection sites (see Chapter 9 for a description of injection sites and methods of administration). Mix injectable solutions by gently swirling the liquid, using only clear solutions. Intranasal use may lead to changes in the nasal mucosa with unpredictable drug absorption. If used in patients diagnosed with diabetes insipidus, fluid intake may be adjusted according to the predicted risk for water intoxication and sodium deficit. See Patient-Centered Care: Patient Teaching for more information on dosage administration.

Vasopressin is available as a nasal spray or as an intramuscular or intravenous injection. Always check the clarity of parenteral solutions before administering the medication. Discard the solution if there are visible particles or any fluid discoloration. Be alert to the adverse effects of elevated blood pressure, fever, nausea, or abdominal cramping. If these worsen or persist, notify the prescriber immediately.

EVALUATION

Once goals and outcome criteria have been reviewed, evaluate the therapeutic responses to these drugs. With *octreotide acetate*, therapeutic effects include improved symptoms related to carcinoid tumors, VIPoma, or esophageal varices. An improvement in diabetes insipidus, esophageal varices, or vasodilatory shock is expected with *vasopressin*. With *somatropin*, increased growth is expected for whom it is indicated. Evaluate for adverse effects including headache, muscle pain, and altered blood glucose levels. Adverse effects associated with *desmopressin* and vasopressin include increased blood pressure, fever, headache, abdominal cramps, and nausea. *Growth hormones* may lead to headache, hyperglycemia, hypothyroidism, hypercalciuria, and flulike syndrome.

PATIENT-CENTERED CARE: PATIENT TEACHING

• Carefully discuss routes and techniques of administration with the patient and anyone else involved in the patient's care. With pediatric patients, demonstrate the technique of administration to the family or caregiver before discharge. Evaluate comprehension with return demonstrations. Provide written instructions to the patient, if age-appropriate, but also to the parents or caregiver. Keeping a journal about how the drug is being tolerated may prove to be beneficial. As for any medication or illness, the patient should keep a medical alert bracelet, necklace, or wallet card on his or her person at all times.

• Intranasal dosage forms of desmopressin are to be given only after the nasal passages have been cleared. The pump must be primed prior to use. Instruct the patient to prime the nasal pump by pressing down the pump four times. The spray pump delivers 10 mcg of drug each time it is pressed. To administer a 10-mcg dose as ordered, place the spray nozzle in the nostril (for a child, have a parent/adult/

caregiver administer the dose) and press the spray pump once. If a higher dose has been prescribed, half the dose is to be administered in each nostril. The pump cannot deliver doses smaller than 10 mcg. Once completed, replace the cap on the bottle. The pump will stay primed for up to 1 week. After 1 week, the pump will require repriming. Carefully monitor the level of drug left in the pump so that there is always enough medication on hand. The pump may not have enough medication left after 25 doses (at 150 mcg per spray) or 50 doses (at 10 mcg per spray).

- Vasopressin is given topically to the nasal membranes and is not to be inhaled.
- Educate parents about the fact that children with endocrine disorders may have an increased risk for bone problems. Instruct parents that if they notice their child limping, this needs to be evaluated by the prescriber.
- Closely monitor the diabetic patient for changes in serum glucose levels if he or she is taking octreotide.
- Water intake amounts may need to be monitored closely in patients with diabetes insipidus. Exact amounts may be prescribed or determined for each patient.

KEY POINTS

- The pituitary gland is composed of two distinct lobes: anterior and posterior. Each lobe secretes its own set of hormones: *anterior:* thyroid-stimulating hormone (TSH), GH, ACTH, prolactin, follicle-stimulating hormone (FSH), luteinizing hormone; *posterior:* ADH, oxytocin.
- Pituitary drugs are used to either mimic or antagonize the action of endogenous pituitary hormones.
- Drugs that mimic the action of endogenous pituitary hormones include cosyntropin, somatropin, somatrem,

vasopressin, and desmopressin. A drug that antagonizes the actions of endogenous pituitary hormones is octreotide.
- In the assessment of patients receiving pituitary hormones, measure baseline vital signs, review blood glucose levels, and measure weight.
- For patients receiving somatropin, constantly monitor levels of thyroid hormones and growth hormones. Include measurement of vital signs, intake/output, and weight in the assessment.

NCLEX® EXAMINATION REVIEW QUESTIONS

1. A patient is experiencing severe diarrhea, flushing, and life-threatening hypotension associated with carcinoid crisis. The nurse will prepare to administer which drug?
   a. octreotide (Sandostatin)
   b. vasopressin (Pitressin)
   c. somatropin (Humatrope)
   d. cosyntropin (Cortrosyn)

2. A patient is suspected of having adrenocortical insufficiency. The nurse expects to administer which drug to aid in the diagnosis of this condition?
   a. octreotide (Sandostatin)
   b. vasopressin (Pitressin)
   c. somatropin (Humatrope)
   d. cosyntropin (Cortrosyn)

3. The nurse is reviewing the medication list for a patient who will be starting therapy with somatropin. Which type of drug would raise a concern that needs to be addressed before the patient starts the somatropin?
   a. Nonsteroidal antiinflammatory drug for arthritis
   b. Antidepressant drug
   c. Penicillin
   d. Glucocorticoid

4. A patient who is about to be given octreotide is also taking a diuretic, IV heparin, ciprofloxacin (Cipro), and an opioid as needed for pain. The nurse will monitor for what possible interaction?
   a. Hypokalemia due to an interaction with the diuretic
   b. Decreased anticoagulation due to an interaction with the heparin
   c. Prolongation of the QT interval due to an interaction with the ciprofloxacin
   d. Increased sedation if the opioid is given

5. When monitoring for the therapeutic effects of intranasal desmopressin (DDAVP) in a patient who has diabetes insipidus, which assessment finding will the nurse look for as an indication that the medication therapy is successful?
   a. Increased insulin levels
   b. Decreased diarrhea
   c. Improved nasal patency
   d. Decreased thirst

6. Which drugs have an action similar to that of the naturally occurring hormone ADH? *(Select all that apply.)*
   a. cosyntropin (Cortrosyn)
   b. desmopressin (DDAVP)
   c. somatropin (Humatrope)
   d. vasopressin (Pitressin)
   e. octreotide (Sandostatin)

7. The order reads: "Give octreotide (Sandostatin) 50 mcg subcut twice a day." The medication is available in an injectable form of 0.05 mg/mL. How many milliliters will the nurse draw up for the ordered dose?

8. The nurse is preparing to administer somatropin (Humatrope) and will monitor the patient for which adverse effects? *(Select all that apply)*
   a. Increased blood pressure
   b. Headache
   c. Flulike syndrome
   d. Nausea
   e. Hyperglycemia
   f. Fever

1. a, 2. d, 3. d, 4. c, 5. d, 6. b, d, 7. 1 mL, 8. b, c, e.

CRITICAL THINKING AND PRIORITIZATION QUESTIONS

1. When the nurse checks the insertion site of a patient who is receiving an IV infusion of vasopressin, the site is swollen and cool to the touch. What is the nurse's priority action at this time? Explain your answer.

2. A patient will be receiving intranasal desmopressin (DDAVP), and the nurse is teaching the patient how to self-administer the drug. After the nurse explains how the pump works and how to prime the pump, what is important for the nurse to tell the patient to do just before taking the medication?

For answers see *http://evolve.elsevier.com/Lilley.*

ⓔ EVOLVE WEBSITE

http://evolve.elsevier.com/Lilley
- Animations
- Answer Keys for Textbook Case Studies and Textbook Critical Thinking and Prioritization Questions

- Content Updates
- Key Points
- Review Questions
- Student Case Studies

Thyroid and Antithyroid Drugs

OBJECTIVES

When you reach the end of this chapter, you will be able to do the following:

1. Briefly describe the normal anatomy and physiology of the thyroid gland.
2. Discuss the various functions of the thyroid gland and related hormones.
3. Describe the differences in the diseases resulting from the hyposecretion and hypersecretion of thyroid gland hormones.
4. Identify the various drugs used to treat the hyposecretion and hypersecretion states of the thyroid gland.
5. Discuss the mechanisms of action, indications, dosages, routes of administration, contraindications, cautions, drug interactions, and adverse effects of the various drugs used to treat hypothyroidism and hyperthyroidism.
6. Develop a nursing care plan that includes all phases of the nursing process for patients receiving thyroid replacement therapy as well as for patients receiving antithyroid drugs.

DRUG PROFILES

- **levothyroxine, p. 493**
- **propylthiouracil, p. 495**

♦ = *Key drug*
! = *High-alert drug*

KEY TERMS

Euthyroid Referring to normal thyroid function. (p. 493)

Hyperthyroidism A condition characterized by excessive production of the thyroid hormones. A severe form of this disorder is called *thyrotoxicosis*. (p. 492)

Hypothyroidism A condition characterized by diminished production of the thyroid hormones. (p. 492)

Thyroid-stimulating hormone (TSH) An endogenous substance secreted by the pituitary gland that controls the release of thyroid gland hormones and is necessary for the growth and function of the thyroid gland (also called *thyrotropin*). (p. 492)

Thyroxine (T_4) The principle thyroid hormone that influences the metabolic rate. (p. 491)

Triiodothyronine (T_3) A secondary thyroid hormone that also affects body metabolism. (p. 491)

THYROID FUNCTION

The thyroid gland lies across the larynx in front of the thyroid cartilage ("Adam's apple"). Its lobes extend laterally on both sides of the front of the neck. It is responsible for the secretion of three hormones essential for the proper regulation of metabolism: thyroxine (T_4), triiodothyronine (T_3), and calcitonin (see Chapter 34). The thyroid gland is located close to and communicates with the parathyroid glands, which lie just above and behind it. The parathyroid glands are two pairs of bean-shaped glands. These glands are made up of encapsulated cells that are responsible for maintaining adequate levels of calcium in the extracellular fluid, primarily by mobilizing calcium from bone.

Thyroxine (T_4) and triiodothyronine (T_3) are produced in the thyroid gland through the coupling of iodine and the amino acid tyrosine. The iodide (I^-, which is the ionized form of iodine) needed for this process is acquired from the diet. One

mg of iodide is needed per week. This iodide is absorbed from the blood and then sequestered by the thyroid gland, where it is concentrated to 20 times its blood level. Here it is also converted to iodine (I_2), which is combined with tyrosine to make diiodotyrosine. The combination of two molecules of diiodotyrosine causes the formation of thyroxine, which therefore has four iodine molecules in its structure (T_4). Triiodothyronine is formed by the coupling of one molecule of diiodotyrosine with one molecule of monoiodotyrosine; thus it has three iodine molecules in its structure (T_3). The biologic potency of T_3 is about four times greater than that of T_4, but T_4 is present in much greater quantities. After the synthesis of these two thyroid hormones, they are stored in the follicles in the thyroid gland in a complex with thyroglobulin (a protein that contains tyrosine and an amino acid) called the *colloid*. When the thyroid gland is signaled to do so, the thyroglobulin–thyroid hormone complex is enzymatically broken down to release T_3 and T_4 into the circulation. This entire process is triggered by **thyroid-stimulating hormone (TSH),** also called *thyrotropin.* It is released from the anterior pituitary gland when blood levels of T_3 and T_4 are low.

The thyroid hormones are involved in a wide variety of processes. They regulate the basal metabolic rate and lipid and carbohydrate metabolism; are essential for normal growth and development; control the heat-regulating system (thermoregulatory center in the brain); and have various effects on the cardiovascular, endocrine, and neuromuscular systems. Therefore, hyperfunction or hypofunction of the thyroid gland can lead to a wide range of serious consequences.

PATHOPHYSIOLOGY OF HYPOTHYROIDISM

There are three types of **hypothyroidism.** Primary hypothyroidism stems from an abnormality in the thyroid gland itself. It occurs when the thyroid gland is not able to perform one of its many functions, such as releasing the thyroid hormones from their storage sites, coupling iodine with tyrosine, trapping iodide, converting iodide to iodine, or any combination of these defects. Primary hypothyroidism is the most common of the three types of hypothyroidism. Secondary hypothyroidism begins at the level of the pituitary gland and results from reduced secretion of thyroid stimulating hormone (TSH). TSH is needed to trigger the release of the T_3 and T_4 stored in the thyroid gland. Tertiary hypothyroidism is caused by a reduced level of the thyrotropin-releasing hormone from the hypothalamus. This reduced level, in turn, reduces TSH and thyroid hormone levels. Symptoms of hypothyroidism include cold intolerance, unintentional weight gain, depression, dry brittle hair and nails, and fatigue.

Hypothyroidism can also be classified by when it occurs in the lifespan. Hyposecretion of thyroid hormone during youth may lead to cretinism. Cretinism is characterized by low metabolic rate, retarded growth and sexual development, and possible mental retardation. Hyposecretion of thyroid hormone as an adult may lead to myxedema. Myxedema is a condition manifested by decreased metabolic rate, but it also involves loss of mental and physical stamina, weight gain, hair loss, firm edema, and yellow dullness of the skin.

Some forms of hypothyroidism may result in the formation of a goiter, which is an enlargement of the thyroid gland resulting from its overstimulation by elevated levels of TSH. The TSH level is elevated because there is little or no thyroid hormone in the circulation. Certain drugs can cause hypothyroidism, with amiodarone (see Chapter 25) being the most common. Interestingly, amiodarone can also cause hyperthyroidism.

PATHOPHYSIOLOGY OF HYPERTHYROIDISM

Excessive secretion of thyroid hormones, or **hyperthyroidism,** may be caused by several different diseases. Diseases known to cause hyperthyroidism include Graves' disease, which is the most common cause, and Plummer's disease (also known as *toxic nodular disease*), which is the least common cause. Thyroid storm is a severe and potentially life-threatening exacerbation

of the symptoms of hyperthyroidism that is usually induced by stress or infection.

Hyperthyroidism can affect multiple body systems, resulting in an overall increase in metabolism. Commonly reported symptoms are diarrhea, flushing, increased appetite, muscle weakness, fatigue, palpitations, irritability, nervousness, sleep disorders, heat intolerance, and altered menstrual flow.

THYROID REPLACEMENT DRUGS

Hypothyroidism is treated with thyroid hormone replacement using various thyroid preparations. These drugs can be either natural or synthetic in origin. The natural thyroid preparations are derived from the thyroid glands of animals such as cattle and hogs. Currently only one natural preparation is available in the United States, and it is called simply *thyroid* or *thyroid, desiccated. Desiccation* is the term for the drying process used to prepare this drug form. All natural preparations are standardized for their iodine content. The synthetic thyroid preparations are levothyroxine (T_4), liothyronine (T_3), and liotrix (which contains a combination of T_4 and T_3 in a 4:1 ratio). The approximate clinically equivalent doses of the drugs are given in Table 31-1. This information is useful for guiding dosage adjustments when a patient is switched from one thyroid hormone to another. Monitoring of serum TSH and free thyroid hormone levels are required to determine the appropriate dose of thyroid replacement drugs.

Mechanism of Action and Drug Effects

Thyroid drugs work in the same manner as the endogenous thyroid hormones, affecting many body systems. At the cellular level, they work to induce changes in the metabolic rate, including the rate of protein, carbohydrate, and lipid metabolism, and to increase oxygen consumption, body temperature, blood volume, and overall cellular growth and differentiation. They also stimulate the cardiovascular system by increasing the number of myocardial beta-adrenergic receptors. This, in turn, increases the sensitivity of the heart to catecholamines and ultimately increases cardiac output. In addition, thyroid hormones increase renal blood flow and the glomerular filtration rate, which results in a diuretic effect.

Indications

Thyroid preparations are given to replace what the thyroid gland itself cannot produce to achieve normal thyroid hormone

TABLE 31-1 **Thyroid Drugs: Clinically Equivalent Doses**	
Thyroid Drug	**Approximate Equivalent Dose**
Natural Thyroid Preparation	
thyroid	60-65 mg (1 grain)
Synthetic Thyroid Preparations	
levothyroxine	100 mcg or more
liothyronine	25 mcg
liotrix	50 mcg/12.5 mcg (T_4/T_3)

T_3, Triiodothyronine; T_4, thyroxine.

levels (**euthyroid** condition). Levothyroxine is the preferred thyroid drug because its hormonal content is standardized and its effect is predictable. Thyroid drugs can also be used for the diagnosis of suspected hyperthyroidism (as in a TSH-suppression test) and in the prevention or treatment of various types of goiters. They are also used for replacement hormonal therapy in patients whose thyroid glands have been surgically removed or destroyed by radioactive iodine in the treatment of thyroid cancer or hyperthyroidism. Hypothyroidism during pregnancy is treated with dosage adjustments every 4 weeks to maintain the TSH level at the lower end of the normal range. Fetal growth may be retarded if maternal hypothyroidism remains untreated during pregnancy.

Contraindications

Contraindications to thyroid preparations include known drug allergy, recent myocardial infarction, adrenal insufficiency, and hyperthyroidism.

Adverse Effects

The adverse effects of thyroid medications are usually the result of overdose. The most significant adverse effect is cardiac dysrhythmia with the risk for life-threatening or fatal irregularities. Other more common undesirable effects are listed in Table 31-2.

Interactions

Thyroid drugs may enhance the activity of oral anticoagulants, the dosages of which may need to be reduced. Cholestyramine binds to thyroid hormone in the gastrointestinal tract, which

possibly reduces the absorption of both drugs. See Table 31-3 for more drug interactions.

Dosages

For dosage information on the thyroid drugs, see the table below.

DRUG PROFILE

The most commonly used thyroid replacement drugs are the synthetic drugs levothyroxine and liotrix. Some patients experience better results with the animal-derived products. Although the thyroid drugs differ chemically, their therapeutic actions are all the same. Factors to be considered before the initiation of drug therapy with a thyroid drug include the desired ratio of T_3 to T_4, the cost, and the desired duration of effect. Thyroid hormone replacement drugs are classified as pregnancy category A drugs. They are all contraindicated in patients who have had a hypersensitivity reaction to them in the past and in those with adrenal insufficiency, previous myocardial infarction, or hyperthyroidism.

◆ levothyroxine

Levothyroxine (Levoxyl, Levothroid, Synthroid, others), or T_4, is the most commonly prescribed synthetic thyroid hormone and is generally considered the drug of choice. One advantage it has over the natural thyroid preparations is that it is chemically pure, being 100% T_4 (thyroxine); this makes its effects more predictable than other thyroid preparations. Its half-life is long enough that it only needs to be administered once a day. It is available in oral form and in parenteral form. It is classified as a pregnancy category A drug.

Switching between different brands of levothyroxine during treatment can destabilize the course of treatment. Thyroid

TABLE 31-2 Thyroid Drugs: Common Adverse Effects	
Body System	**Adverse Effects**
Cardiovascular	Tachycardia, palpitations, angina, dysrhythmias, hypertension
Central nervous	Insomnia, tremors, headache, anxiety
Gastrointestinal	Nausea, diarrhea, cramps
Other	Menstrual irregularities, weight loss, sweating, heat intolerance, fever

TABLE 31-3 Thyroid Drugs: Interactions	
Drug	**Action**
phenytoin and fosphenytoin	Reduced levothyroxine effectiveness
cholestyramine, antacids, calcium salts, iron, estrogen	Reduced levothyroxine effectiveness
warfarin	Increased warfarin effect

DOSAGES

Selected Thyroid Drugs

Drug (Pregnancy Category)	Pharmacologic Class	Usual Adult Dosage Range	Indications
◆ levothyroxine (Synthroid, Levoxyl, others) (A)	Synthetic thyroid hormone (T_4)	PO: 25-200 mcg/day IM/IV: 50% of oral dose	Hypothyroidism
		IV: 200-500 mcg in a single dose; repeat next day 100-300 mcg if necessary; continue 75-100 mcg/day until changed to oral dosing	Myxedema coma
thyroid, desiccated (Armour Thyroid, Westhroid)	Desiccated thyroid	PO: 30-120 mg/day	Hypothyroidism

function test results need to be monitored more carefully when switching products. Recommended dosages are given in the table on this page. Levothyroxine is dosed in micrograms. A common medication error is to write the intended dose in milligrams instead of micrograms. If not caught, this error would result in a thousand-fold overdose. Doses higher than 200 mcg need to be questioned in case this error has occurred. Levothyroxine is available in an intravenous form. The intravenous dose is generally 50% of the oral dose.

Pharmacokinetics: Levothyroxine

Route	Onset of Action	Peak Plasma Concentration	Elimination Half-life	Duration of Action
PO	3-5 days	24 hr	6-10 days	24 hr

QSEN ⚡ **SAFETY AND QUALITY IMPROVEMENT: PREVENTING MEDICATION ERRORS**

Giving IV Doses of Levothyroxine

Care must be taken when preparing IV doses of levothyroxine for infusions. The medication comes in vials for reconstitution, either in 200-mcg or 500-mcg vials. The vials must be reconstituted with 5 mL of 0.9% NaCl to provide a concentration of 40 mcg/mL (the 200-mcg vial) or 100 mcg/mL (the 500-mcg vial).

Errors have occurred when the final volume was miscalculated using 10 mL (the size of the vial), which yields an incorrect concentration of 50 mcg/mL. As a result, the patient received too much medication.

It is essential to remember that the vial must be diluted FIRST, and then the dose is calculated upon the concentration of the reconstituted medication, not the size of the vial.

Data from Institute for Safe Medication Practices (ISMP): ISMP Medication Safety Alert, Sept 6. 2000. Available at *www.ismp.org/Newsletters/acutecare/articles/20000906_2.asp.* Accessed June 25, 2015.

ANTITHYROID DRUGS

Treatment of hyperthyroidism is aimed at treating either the primary cause or the symptoms of the disease. Antithyroid drugs, iodides, ionic inhibitors, surgery, and radioactive isotopes of iodine are used to treat the underlying cause, and beta blockers are used to treat the symptoms. The focus of this discussion is on the antithyroid drugs called *thioamide derivatives,* namely methimazole and propylthiouracil. In addition to the thioamides, radioactive iodine (iodine-131) and potassium iodide may be used to treat hyperthyroidism. Radioactive iodine works by destroying the thyroid gland, in a process known as *ablation.* It is a commonly used treatment for both hyperthyroidism and thyroid cancer. Potassium iodide is also used as prophylaxis for radiation exposure (see Chapter 49).

Mechanism of Action and Drug Effects

Methimazole and propylthiouracil act by inhibiting the incorporation of iodine molecules into the amino acid tyrosine, a process required to make the precursors of T_3 and T_4. By doing so, these drugs impede the formation of thyroid hormone. Propylthiouracil has the added ability to inhibit the conversion of

T_4 to T_3 in the peripheral circulation. Neither drug can inactivate already existing thyroid hormone, however.

The drug effects of methimazole and propylthiouracil are primarily limited to the thyroid gland, and their overall effect is a decrease in the thyroid hormone level. Administration of these medications lowers the high levels of thyroid hormone, thereby normalizing the overall metabolic rate.

Indications

Antithyroid drugs are used to treat hyperthyroidism and to prevent the surge in thyroid hormones that occurs after the surgical treatment of or during radioactive iodine therapy for hyperthyroidism or thyroid cancer. In some types of hyperthyroidism, such as that seen in Graves' disease, the long-term administration of these drugs (for several years) may induce a spontaneous remission. Surgical resection of the thyroid gland (thyroidectomy) is often used both in patients who are intolerant of antithyroid drug therapy and in pregnant women, in whom both antithyroid drugs and radioactive iodine therapy are usually contraindicated.

Contraindications

The only usual contraindications to the use of the two antithyroid drugs is known drug allergy. Their use in pregnancy, although necessary, is somewhat controversial. Per the U.S. Food and Drug Administration (FDA), propylthiouracil is to be used during the first trimester only, and then methimazole is used for the remainder of the pregnancy. However, there are case reports of scalp abnormalities in the fetus when methimazole is used. The choice of how to treat pregnant patients is physician specific. Both drugs are classified as pregnancy category D drugs.

Adverse Effects

The most damaging or serious adverse effects of the antithyroid medications are liver and bone marrow toxicity. These and the more common adverse effects of methimazole and propylthiouracil are listed in Table 31-4.

Interactions

Drug interactions that occur with antithyroid drugs include additive leukopenic effects when they are taken in conjunction

TABLE 31-4 Antithyroid Drugs: Common Adverse Effects

Body System	Adverse Effects
Central nervous	Drowsiness, headache, vertigo, paresthesia
Gastrointestinal	Nausea, vomiting, diarrhea, hepatitis, loss of taste
Genitourinary	Smoky urine, decreased urine output
Hematologic	Agranulocytosis, leukopenia, thrombocytopenia, hypothrombinemia, lymphadenopathy, bleeding
Integumentary	Rash, pruritus
Musculoskeletal	Myalgia, arthralgia
Renal	Increased blood urea nitrogen and serum creatinine levels
Other	Enlarged thyroid gland, nephritis

with other bone marrow suppressants and an increase in the activity of oral anticoagulants.

Dosages

For dosage information on propylthiouracil, see the table on this page.

DOSAGES

Selected Antithyroid Drugs

Drug (Pregnancy Category)	Pharmacologic Class	Usual Adult Dosage Range	Indications
◆ propylthiouracil* (generic only) (D)	Antithyroid	100-150 mg/day	Hyperthyroidism
methimazole (Tapazole)	Antithyroid	5-15 mg/day	Hyperthyroidism

*Often abbreviated PTU.

DRUG PROFILE

◆ propylthiouracil

Propylthiouracil (PTU) is a thioamide antithyroid drug and is classified as a pregnancy category D drug. Approximately 2 weeks of therapy with propylthiouracil may be necessary before symptoms improve. It is available only in oral form as a 50-mg tablet. Methimazole is the only alternative drug in this class and is rarely used clinically. Recommended dosages are given in the table above.

Pharmacokinetics: Propylthiouracil

Route	Onset of Action	Peak Plasma Concentration	Elimination Half-life	Duration of Action
PO	Unknown	2 hr	1 hr	12-14 hr

NURSING PROCESS

ASSESSMENT

In assessing the patient taking *thyroid replacement drugs* for hypothyroidism, include baseline vital signs for comparative purposes. Assess levels of T_3, T_4, and TSH before and during drug therapy, as ordered. It is also important to thoroughly assess and document any past and present medical problems or concerns with a thorough physical assessment. Include in the assessment a thorough medication history including drug allergies as well as a list of all prescription drugs, over-the-counter drugs, herbals, and supplements. Assess also for cautions, contraindications, and drug interactions associated with the use of thyroid hormone. Review baseline vital signs, with particular attention to a history of cardiac dysrhythmias because of drug-related adverse effects of cardiac irregularities, which may be life-threatening. For the female patient, perform a thorough assessment of the reproductive system due to the impact of thyroid hormones (on this system).

It is also important to remember that certain thyroid replacement drugs may work faster than others because of their dosage form and properties (see the Teamwork and Collaboration: Pharmacokinetic Bridge to Nursing Practice box). Drug interactions that deserve emphasis because of their importance for patient safety and because they involve commonly used medications include interactions with oral anticoagulants (increased activity of the oral anticoagulants), digitalis glycosides (decrease in digitalis levels), cholestyramine, and oral hypoglycemic drugs. See Table 31-3 for a more detailed listing of drug interactions. If the patient is taking an oral anticoagulant, monitor blood levels of the anticoagulant closely. Lifespan considerations include increased sensitivity to the effects of thyroid replacement drugs in older adult patients. Individualization of drug therapy is important because different patients may respond very differently to the same drug and/or dosage.

For *antithyroid drugs,* such as *propylthiouracil* and *methimazole,* assess vital signs and for signs and symptoms of thyroid crisis, or what is often called thyroid storm. Thyroid storm is manifested by exacerbation of hyperthyroidism symptoms (see the pharmacology discussion) and is potentially life-threatening.

TEAMWORK AND COLLABORATION: PHARMACOKINETIC BRIDGE TO NURSING PRACTICE [QSEN]

Thyroid replacement drugs possess very specific pharmacokinetic characteristics, as do many drugs. You must understand the pharmacokinetics to think your way critically through clinical situations involving patients who are taking thyroid replacement drugs. For levothyroxine (Synthroid, Levothroid, Levoxyl), the pharmacokinetic characteristics include an onset of action of 3 to 5 days, peak plasma concentrations within 24 hours, elimination half-life of 6 to 10 days, and a duration of action of 24 hours. Due to the prolonged half-life of this drug, there is an increased risk for toxicity. Toxicity is manifested by the following: weight loss, tachycardia, nervousness, tremors, hypertension, headache, insomnia, menstrual irregularities, and cardiac irregularities or palpitations. Another important pharmacokinetic property is that the drug is protein bound. A highly protein-bound drug acts like a biologic sustained-release drug and remains in the body longer, with increased risk for more interactions with other highly protein-bound drugs as well as a greater potential for toxicity. This is yet another example of how important a current and thorough knowledge base about drugs—and specifically about their pharmacokinetics—is to their safe and efficient administration.

Assessing for thyroid storm also means assessing for precipitating causes, such as stress or infection. Related cautions and contraindications have been discussed previously, but some important drug interactions to reemphasize include the interactions with oral anticoagulants (which can cause an increase in anticoagulation and thus risk for bleeding) and any medications that may lead to bone marrow suppression or cause leukopenia (antithyroid drugs may cause additive effects or worsening of bone marrow suppression).

PATIENT-CENTERED CARE: LIFESPAN CONSIDERATIONS FOR THE OLDER ADULT PATIENT

Thyroid Hormones

- Older adult patients are much more sensitive to thyroid hormone replacement drugs (as they are to most drugs). They are also more likely to experience adverse reactions to thyroid hormones than are patients in any other age group.
- This age group of patients experience more negative consequences related to drug therapy because their hepatic and renal functioning is decreased.
- Thyroid hormone replacement requirements are approximately 25% lower in patients 60 years of age and older than in younger patients. Dosage in older adult patients may therefore need to be adjusted or titrated downward.
- Older adult patients must contact the prescriber immediately if they experience palpitations, chest pain, stumbling, falling, depression, incontinence, sweating, shortness of breath and/or aggravated heart disease, cold intolerance, or weight gain.
- Drug therapy for the older adult patient must be initiated with caution and with very individualized dosages. If higher dosages are necessary, increases must be made with the prescriber's guidance and done gradually.

NURSING DIAGNOSES

1. Noncompliance due to lack of experience/education regarding thyroid hormone replacement and the need for everyday self-administration.
2. Ineffective health management due to lack of experience/education about the use of thyroid medication
3. Risk for infection related to the bone marrow suppression caused by antithyroid medication

PLANNING: OUTCOME IDENTIFICATION

1. Patient remains compliant with daily administration of thyroid hormone replacement therapy.
2. Patient demonstrates improvement in health management behaviors by taking the medication as prescribed and reporting any adverse effects or signs for the need to reregulate the dosage.
3. Patient states ways of decreasing the risk for infection (i.e., proper dietary intake, adequate rest) while receiving antithyroid medication.

IMPLEMENTATION

When a *thyroid replacement drug* is administered, it is important that the drug be given at the same time every day to help maintain consistent blood levels of the drug. Emphasize to the patient that it is best to take this medication once daily, as prescribed. It is extremely important to take thyroid replacement medication in the morning and on an empty stomach, preferably at least 30 minutes before breakfast. Taking the medication in the afternoon/evening will lead to a subsequent increase in energy level and sleeplessness. Other significant instructions

include avoiding taking the thyroid replacement drug with vitamins or supplements containing iron and/or calcium within a 4-hour time frame. Antacids and OTC preparations with iodine must also be avoided. Encourage reading of labels of all prescribed and OTC medications. Iodized salt and iodine-rich foods, such as soybeans, tofu, turnips, high-iodine seafood, and some breads must also be avoided. Patients must also avoid interchanging brands because of possible differences in the bioequivalence of drugs from various manufacturers. If needed, patients may crush tablets. If the patient is scheduled to undergo radioactive iodine isotope studies, the thyroid replacement drug is usually discontinued about 4 weeks before the test, but only as prescribed. Older adult patients may require alteration of the dosage amount, with a decrease of up to 25% for patients 60 years of age and older.

CASE STUDY

Patient-Centered Care: Antithyroid Drug Therapy

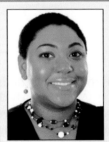

R.C., a 28-year-old woman, has been diagnosed with hyperthyroidism due to Graves' disease. Her health care provider has explained the proposed therapy with propylthiouracil to her and her husband. She has no other known health problems at this time.

1. What laboratory studies will be performed before drug therapy with propylthiouracil is started? Explain your answer.
2. R.C. asks, "What do I need to know while I'm taking this drug?" List pertinent patient teaching points.
3. After 1 month of therapy, R.C. comes into the health care provider's office for a follow-up visit. She is upset because a friend told her about a relative who had antithyroid therapy for cancer and said he was "radioactive." She is wondering if her medication has made her "radioactive." How will the nurse answer her question?
4. Six months later, R.C. calls the office and says, "I think I might be pregnant. What do I do about taking this drug?" What does the nurse need to tell her?

For answers, see *http://evolve.elsevier.com/Lilley.*

Educate the patient taking the antithyroid drug *propylthiouracil* about dosing the medication with meals to help decrease stomach upset. Any fever, sore throat, mouth ulcers or sores, or skin eruptions, as well as any unusual bleeding or bruising needs to be reported to the prescriber immediately. These symptoms may indicate problems of liver toxicity and/or bone marrow toxicity with possible leukopenia. Monitor liver function tests and CBC counts, as prescribed. Further educate patients to avoid the use of iodized salt or eating shellfish because of their potential for altering the drug's effectiveness. Advise patients to be aware of the signs and symptoms of hypothyroidism, including unexplained weight gain, loss of mental and physical stamina, hair loss, firm edema, and yellow dullness of the skin (indicative of myxedema or a decrease in metabolic rate). If these occur, patients must immediately report them to the prescriber.

EVALUATION

A therapeutic response to *thyroid replacement drugs* is manifested by the disappearance of the symptoms of hypothyroidism; the patient would demonstrate improved energy levels as well as improved mental and physical stamina. Adverse effects to monitor for include cardiac dysrhythmia (see Table 31-2), irritability, and increased anxiety. Clues that a patient is possibly receiving inadequate doses of the thyroid replacement drug include a return of the symptoms of hypothyroidism (see previous discussion). Routine follow-up appointments and serum laboratory testing is needed to adequately evaluate the effectiveness any hormonal replacement therapy.

A therapeutic response to *antithyroid medications* includes a return to normal status with little to no evidence of hyperthyroid. Adverse effects include the possibility of leukopenia, which may be manifested by fever, sore throat, lesions, or other signs of infection. Clues that a patient is not receiving adequate doses include continued signs and symptoms of hyperthyroidism (see previous discussion).

PATIENT-CENTERED CARE: PATIENT TEACHING

- Thyroid replacement drugs are best taken ½ to 1 hour before breakfast on an empty stomach to enhance their absorption orally and maintain consistent hormone levels. Sleeplessness may be prevented by taking this medication in the morning.
- These medications are not to be abruptly discontinued. Lifelong therapy is usually the norm.
- Emphasize to the patient the importance of keeping follow-up visits so the prescriber can monitor thyroid hormone levels, complete blood counts, and results of liver function studies.
- Brands of thyroid replacement drugs cannot be interchanged. Advise patients to always check that the pharmacy has provided the correct brand of thyroid replacement drug.
- Signs and symptoms associated with hypothyroidism include myxedema with decreased metabolic rate, loss of mental/physical stamina, weight gain, hair loss, firm edema, and yellow dullness of the skin. Share this information with the patient.
- Do not take thyroid replacement drug at the same time with vitamins and supplements.
- Take the drug with sufficient amounts of water, at least 6 to 8 ounces.
- Instruct the patient taking thyroid replacement drugs to immediately report any of the following to the prescriber: chest pain, weight loss, palpitations, tremors, sweating, nervousness, shortness of breath, or insomnia. These may indicate toxicity.

- Encourage the patient to keep a daily journal, with notations about how the patient is feeling, energy levels, appetite, and any adverse effects.
- Advise the patient that it may take several weeks to see the full therapeutic effects of thyroid drugs.
- Instruct the patient that all thyroid tablets must be protected from light.
- Signs and symptoms of hyperthyroidism include increased metabolic rate, diarrhea, flushing, increased appetite, muscle weakness, fatigue, palpitations, irritability, nervousness, sleep disorders, heat intolerance, and altered menstrual flow. Patients with this disorder and on drug therapy need to be aware of these signs and symptoms.
- Advise patients that antithyroid medications are better tolerated when taken with meals or a snack. These drugs must also be given at the same time every day to maintain consistent blood levels of the drug. They must never be withdrawn abruptly.
- Instruct patients taking thyroid or antithyroid drugs not to take any over-the-counter medications without first consulting with the prescriber or pharmacist and to read all drug labels thoroughly.
- Patients taking antithyroid medications must avoid eating foods high in iodine, such as tofu and other soy products, turnips, seafood, iodized salt, and some breads. These foods may interfere with the effectiveness of the antithyroid drug.

KEY POINTS

- T_4 and T_3 are the two hormones produced by the thyroid gland; thyroid hormones are made by iodination and coupling with the amino acid tyrosine.
- Thyroid hormone replacement is generally carried out carefully by the prescriber with frequent monitoring of serum levels until stabilization appears to have occurred. Monitor and review laboratory values to be sure that serum levels are within normal limits to avoid possible toxicity.
- Hyperthyroidism is caused by excessive secretion of thyroid hormone by the thyroid gland and may be caused by different diseases (Graves' disease, Plummer's disease, and multinodular disease) or drugs. Always assess and document important information about the patient's medical history appropriately.

- Patients receiving levothyroxine need to report the occurrence of excitability, irritability, or palpitations to the prescriber because these symptoms may indicate toxicity.
- Adverse effects associated with thyroid drugs include tachycardia, palpitations, angina, dysrhythmias, hypertension, insomnia, tremors, headache, anxiety, nausea, diarrhea, cramps, menstrual irregularities, weight loss, sweating, fever, and heat intolerance.
- Adverse effects associated with antithyroid drugs include drowsiness, headache, vertigo, nausea, vomiting, diarrhea, loss of taste, bleeding, leukopenia, rash, myalgia, and arthralgia.

NCLEX® EXAMINATION REVIEW QUESTIONS

1. When monitoring the laboratory values for a patient who is taking antithyroid drugs, the nurse knows to watch for
   a. increased platelet counts.
   b. increased white blood cell counts.
   c. increased blood urea nitrogen level.
   d. increased blood glucose levels.

2. The pharmacy has called a patient to notify her that the current brand of thyroid replacement hormone is on back order. The patient calls the clinic to ask what to do. Which is the best response by the nurse?
   a. "Go ahead and take the other brand that the pharmacy has available for now."
   b. "You can stop the medication until your current brand is available."
   c. "You can split the thyroid pills that you have left so that they will last longer."
   d. "Let me ask your prescriber what needs to be done; we will need to watch how you do if you switch brands."

3. The nurse is assessing a 64 year-old patient who will be starting thyroid replacement therapy. Which statement is true regarding the dosage of thyroid replacement hormones for the older adult?
   a. Thyroid hormone replacement requirements are approximately 25% lower for this age group.
   b. Older adults require higher dosages of thyroid replacement hormone for therapeutic effects.
   c. There is no difference in the dosage of thyroid replacement hormone in older adults versus younger adults.
   d. The dosage of thyroid hormone will depend upon the amount of iodine in the patient's diet.

4. To help with the insomnia associated with thyroid hormone replacement therapy, the nurse will teach the patient to
   a. take half the dose at lunchtime and the other half 2 hours later.
   b. use a sedative to assist with falling asleep.
   c. take the dose upon awakening in the morning.
   d. reduce the dosage as needed if sleep is impaired.

5. The nurse is teaching a patient who has a new prescription for the antithyroid drug propylthiouracil (PTU). Which statement by the nurse is correct?
   a. "There are no food restrictions while on this drug."
   b. "You need to avoid foods high in iodine, such as iodized salt, seafood, and soy products."
   c. "This drug is given to raise the thyroid hormone levels in your blood."
   d. "Take this drug in the morning on an empty stomach."

6. When teaching a patient who has a new prescription for thyroid hormone, the nurse will instruct the patient to notify the prescriber if which adverse effects are noted? (Select all that apply.)
   a. Palpitations
   b. Weight gain
   c. Angina
   d. Fatigue
   e. Cold intolerance

7. The nurse is giving an intravenous dose of levothyroxine (Synthroid). The order reads: "Give 0.1 mg IV push now." What is the ordered dose in micrograms?

8. The nurse knows that which laboratory tests are used to monitor thyroid hormone replacement therapy? (Select all that apply.)
   a. Serum TSH
   b. BUN
   c. CBC
   d. Free thyroid hormone levels
   e. Serum iodine levels

1. c, 2, d, 3, a, 4, c, 5, b, 6, a, c, 7, 100 mcg, 8, a, d.

CRITICAL THINKING AND PRIORITIZATION QUESTIONS

1. A patient has been taking thyroid drugs for about 16 months and has recently noted palpitations and some heat intolerance. What are the nurse's priority actions at this time?

2. A patient with a history of hypothyroidism is in her first trimester of pregnancy. She asks the nurse, "How often will they check my thyroid hormone levels? I'm very worried about how this will affect my baby." What is the nurse's best response?

For answers see *http://evolve.elsevier.com/Lilley*.

ⓔ EVOLVE WEBSITE

http://evolve.elsevier.com/Lilley
• Animations
• Answer Keys for Textbook Case Studies and Textbook Critical Thinking and Prioritization Questions
• Content Updates
• Key Points
• Review Questions
• Student Case Studies

Antidiabetic Drugs

http://evolve.elsevier.com/Lilley

OBJECTIVES

When you reach the end of this chapter, you will be able to do the following:

1. Discuss the normal functions of the pancreas.
2. Contrast age of onset, signs and symptoms, pharmacologic and nonpharmacologic treatment, incidence, and etiology of type 1 and type 2 diabetes mellitus.
3. Differentiate gestational diabetes from type 1 and type 2 diabetes mellitus.
4. Discuss the various factors influencing blood glucose level in nondiabetic individuals and in patients with diabetes mellitus.
5. Identify the various drugs used to manage type 1 and type 2 diabetes mellitus.
6. Discuss the mechanisms of action, indications, contraindications, cautions, drug interactions, and adverse effects of insulin, oral antidiabetic drugs, and injectable antidiabetic drugs.
7. Compare rapid-, short-, intermediate-, and long-acting insulins with regard to their onset of action, peak effects, and duration of action.
8. Compare the signs and symptoms of hypoglycemia and hyperglycemia and their related treatments.
9. Develop a nursing care plan that includes all phases of the nursing process for patients with type 1 or type 2 diabetes with a focus on drug therapies.

DRUG PROFILES

acarbose, p. 511
♦ ! glipizide, p. 511
♦ ! insulin glargine and ! insulin detemir, p. 507
♦ ! insulin isophane suspension (NPH), p. 507
♦ ! insulin lispro, p. 506
♦ liraglutide, p. 513
♦ metformin, p. 512

♦ pioglitazone, p. 512
♦ ! regular insulin, p. 507
♦ repaglinide, p. 512
♦ sitagliptin, p. 512

—————————
♦ = *Key drug*
! = *High-alert drug*

KEY TERMS

Diabetes mellitus A complex disorder of carbohydrate, fat, and protein metabolism resulting from the lack of insulin secretion by the beta cells of the pancreas or from defects of the insulin receptors; it is commonly referred to simply as *diabetes*. There are two major types of diabetes: type 1 and type 2. (p. 501)

Diabetic ketoacidosis (DKA) A severe metabolic complication of uncontrolled diabetes that, if untreated, leads to diabetic coma and death. (p. 503)

Gestational diabetes Diabetes that develops during pregnancy. It may resolve after pregnancy but may also be a precursor of type 2 diabetes in later life. (p. 503)

Glucagon A hormone produced by the alpha cells in the islets of Langerhans that stimulates the conversion of glycogen to glucose in the liver. (p. 500)

Glucose One of the simple sugars that serves as a major source of energy. It is found in foods (e.g., refined sweets) and also is the final breakdown product of complex carbohydrate metabolism in the body; it is commonly referred to as *dextrose*. (p. 500)

Glycogen A polysaccharide that is the major carbohydrate stored in animal cells. (p. 500)

Glycogenolysis The breakdown of glycogen to glucose. (p. 500)

Hemoglobin A1C (A1C) Hemoglobin molecules bound to glucose molecules; blood levels of hemoglobin A1C are used as a diagnostic measure of average daily blood glucose levels in the monitoring and diagnosing of diabetes; it is also called *glycosylated hemoglobin* and most commonly referred to as *A1C*. (p. 504)

Hyperglycemia A fasting blood glucose level of 126 mg/dL or higher or a nonfasting blood glucose level of 200 mg/dL or higher. (p. 500)

Hyperosmolar hyperglycemic syndrome (HHS) A metabolic complication of uncontrolled type 2 diabetes, similar in severity to diabetic ketoacidosis but without ketosis and acidosis. (p. 503)

Hypoglycemia A blood glucose level of less than 70 mg/dL, or above 50 mg/dL with signs and symptoms of hypoglycemia. (p. 514)

Insulin A naturally occurring hormone secreted by the beta cells of the islets of Langerhans in the pancreas in response to increased levels of glucose in the blood. (p. 500)

Ketones Organic chemical compounds produced through the oxidation of secondary alcohols (e.g., fat molecules), including dietary carbohydrates. (p. 500)

Polydipsia Chronic excessive intake of water; it is a common symptom of uncontrolled diabetes. (p. 500)

Polyphagia Excessive eating; it is a common symptom of uncontrolled diabetes. (p. 500)

Polyuria Increased frequency or volume of urinary output; it is a common symptom of diabetes. (p. 500)

Type 1 diabetes mellitus Diabetes mellitus that is a genetically determined autoimmune disorder characterized by a complete or nearly complete lack of insulin production; it most commonly arises in children or adolescents. (p. 502)

Type 2 diabetes mellitus A type of diabetes mellitus that most commonly presents in adults and is becoming more common in children and adolescents due to inactivity and weight gain. The disease may be controlled by lifestyle modifications, oral drug therapy, and/or insulin, but patients are not necessarily dependent on insulin therapy. (p. 503)

PANCREAS

The pancreas is a large, elongated organ that is located behind the stomach. It is both an exocrine gland (secreting digestive enzymes through the pancreatic duct) and an endocrine gland (secreting hormones directly into the bloodstream and not through a duct). The endocrine functions of the pancreas are the focus of this chapter. Two main hormones that are produced by the pancreas are **insulin** and **glucagon**. Both hormones play an important role in the regulation of glucose homeostasis, specifically the use, mobilization, and storage of glucose by the body. **Glucose** is one of the primary sources of energy for the cells of the body. It is also the simplest form of carbohydrate (sugar) found in the body and is often referred to as *dextrose*. There is a normal amount of glucose that circulates in the blood to meet requirements for quick energy. When the quantity of glucose in the blood is sufficient, the excess is stored as **glycogen** in the liver and, to a lesser extent, in skeletal muscle tissue, where it remains until the body needs it. Glucose is also stored in adipose tissue as triglyceride body fat. When more circulating glucose is needed, glycogen—primarily that stored in the liver—is converted back to glucose through a process called **glycogenolysis**. The hormone responsible for initiating this process is glucagon. Glucagon has only minimal effects on muscle glycogen and adipose tissue triglyceride stores.

Glucagon is a protein hormone that is released from the alpha cells of the islets of Langerhans in the pancreas. Insulin is secreted from the beta cells of these same islets. There is a continuous homeostatic balance in the body between the actions of insulin and those of glucagon. This natural balance serves to maintain optimal blood glucose levels, which normally range between 70 and 100 mg/dL. Because of the critical role of the pancreas in producing and maintaining these two hormones, the drastic measures of pancreatic or islet cell transplant are sometimes undertaken to treat type 1 diabetes that has not been successfully controlled by other means. Insulin serves

several important metabolic functions in the body. It stimulates carbohydrate metabolism in skeletal and cardiac muscle and in adipose tissue by facilitating the transport of glucose into these cells. In the liver, insulin facilitates the phosphorylation of glucose to glucose-6-phosphate, which is then converted to glycogen for storage. By causing glucose to be stored in the liver as glycogen, insulin keeps the kidney free of glucose. Without insulin, blood glucose levels rise; when the kidneys are unable to reabsorb this excess glucose, they excrete large amounts of glucose (a critical body nutrient and energy source), **ketones**, and other solutes into the urine. This loss of nutrient energy sources eventually leads to **polyphagia**, weight loss, and malnutrition. The presence of these solutes in the distal renal tubules and collecting ducts also draws large volumes of water into the urine through osmotic diuresis, which leads to **polyuria**, dehydration, and **polydipsia**.

Insulin also has a direct effect on fat metabolism. It stimulates lipogenesis and inhibits lipolysis and the release of fatty acids from adipose cells. In addition, insulin stimulates protein synthesis and promotes the intracellular shift of potassium and magnesium into the cells, thereby temporarily decreasing elevated blood concentrations of these electrolytes. Other substances such as cortisol, epinephrine, and growth hormone work synergistically with glucagon to counter the effects of insulin and cause increases in the blood glucose level.

PATHOPHYSIOLOGY OF DIABETES MELLITUS

Hyperglycemia is a state involving excessive concentrations of glucose in the blood and results when the normal counterbalancing actions of glucagon and insulin fail to maintain normal glucose homeostasis (i.e., serum levels of 70 to 100 mg/dL). It is important to note that the diagnostic definition of diabetes established by the American Diabetes Association (ADA) differs from that issued by the American College of Endocrinology. This textbook uses the ADA as a reference. Complications in

BOX 32-1 Criteria for Diagnosis of Diabetes

Fasting plasma glucose level of 126 mg/dL or higher, or A1C greater than 6.5%. "Fasting" is defined as no caloric intake for at least 8 hours.

OR

Symptoms of diabetes plus casual plasma glucose level of 200 mg/dL or higher. "Casual" means measured at any time of day without regard to time since last meal. The classic symptoms of hyperglycemia include polyuria, polydipsia, and unexplained weight loss.

OR

Two-hour plasma glucose level of 200 mg/dL or higher during an oral glucose tolerance test (OGTT). The glucose load should contain the equivalent of 75 gm of glucose dissolved in water. Note that the OGTT is not recommended for routine clinical use.

Any positive finding for the above assessments should be confirmed by repeat testing on a different day.

Data from American Diabetes Association: Standards of medical care in diabetes 2015. *Diabetes Care* 38(Suppl 1):S8-S16, 2015.

TABLE 32-1 Major Long-Term Consequences of Type 1 and Type 2 Diabetes

Pathology	Possible Consequences
Macrovascular (Atherosclerotic Plaque)	
Coronary arteries	Myocardial infarction
Cerebral arteries	Stroke
Peripheral vessels	Peripheral vascular disease (e.g., neuropathies [see below], foot ulcers, possible amputations)
Microvascular (Capillary Damage)	
Retinopathy (retinal damage)	Partial or complete blindness
Neuropathy (autonomic and somatic nerve damage, due to both metabolic alterations and compromised circulation)	Autonomic nerve damage: Example: diabetic gastroparesis, bladder dysfunction, unawareness of hypoglycemia, sexual dysfunction Somatic nerve damage: Example: diabetic foot ulcer and/or leg or foot amputation
Nephropathy (kidney damage)	Proteinuria (microalbuminuria), chronic renal failure (may require dialysis or kidney transplantation)

Data from American Diabetes Association: Standards of medical care in diabetes 2015, *Diabetes Care* 38(Suppl 1), 2015.

protein and fat metabolism (*dyslipidemia*; see Chapter 27) are also involved. The current key diagnostic criterion for diabetes mellitus is hyperglycemia with a fasting plasma glucose level of higher than 126 mg/dL or a hemoglobin A1C (A1C) level greater than or equal to 6.5%. Diagnostic indicators are described in more detail in Box 32-1.

Diabetes mellitus, more commonly referred to simply as *diabetes,* is primarily a disorder of carbohydrate metabolism that involves either a deficiency of insulin, a resistance of tissue (e.g., muscle, liver) to insulin, or both. Whatever the cause of the diabetes, the result is hyperglycemia. Uncontrolled hyperglycemia correlates strongly with serious long-term macrovascular and microvascular complications. Macrovascular complications are usually secondary to large vessel damage caused by deposition of atherosclerotic plaque. This compromises both central and peripheral circulation. In contrast, microvascular complications are secondary to damage to the capillary vessels, which impairs peripheral circulation and damages the eyes and kidneys. In addition, both autonomic and somatic nerve damage occur, caused primarily by the metabolic changes themselves and to a lesser degree by the compromised circulation. Table 32-1 lists the common long-term complications of diabetes.

Diabetes mellitus has been recognized since 1550 BC, when Egyptians wrote of a malady they called *honeyed urine.* The first step toward identifying the cause of diabetes mellitus occurred in 1788 when Thomas Cawley, an English physician, voiced his suspicion that the source of the illness lay in the pancreas. Not until the early 1920s was insulin isolated. Its discovery is considered one of the greatest triumphs of twentieth-century medicine, and its use in the treatment of diabetes mellitus has proved to be life saving for millions of people affected by the disease.

Diabetes mellitus actually is not a single disease, but a group of progressive diseases. For this reason, it is often regarded as a syndrome rather than a disease. In some cases, diabetes is caused by a relative or absolute lack of insulin that is believed to result from the destruction of beta cells in the pancreas. As a result,

insulin cannot be produced. However, hyperglycemia can also be caused by defects in insulin receptors that result in insulin resistance. The proteins that serve as insulin receptors are attached to the surface of cells in the liver, muscle, and adipose tissue. These receptor proteins are stimulated by insulin molecules to move glucose from blood to cells. When insulin receptors become defective, they no longer respond normally to insulin molecules. Although serum insulin and glucose levels are both elevated, they do not respond and transport glucose into the cell where it is needed. The result is that glucose molecules remain in the blood, rather than being used in the cell or stored in the tissues.

Two major types of diabetes mellitus are currently recognized and designated by the ADA: type 1 and type 2. Type 1 diabetes was previously called *insulin-dependent diabetes mellitus (IDDM)* or *juvenile-onset diabetes.* Type 2 diabetes was previously called *non–insulin-dependent diabetes mellitus (NIDDM)* or *adult-onset diabetes.* Obesity is one of the major risk factors for the development of type 2 diabetes. Nonwhite ethnic groups, including African Americans, Asian Americans, Hispanic Americans, and Native Americans, are all at higher risk for the disease than are whites.

The usual differences between type 1 and type 2 diabetes mellitus are listed in Table 32-2. Interestingly, approximately 10% of patients with type 2 diabetes have circulating antibodies that suggest an autoimmune origin for the disease. This condition is known as *latent autoimmune diabetes in adults (LADA)* and is basically a more slowly progressing form of type 1 diabetes.

The most common signs and symptoms of diabetes are elevated blood glucose level (fasting glucose level higher than

TABLE 32-2	Characteristics of Type 1 and Type 2 Diabetes	
Characteristic	**Type 1**	**Type 2**
Etiology	Autoimmune destruction of beta cells in the pancreas	Multifactorial genetic defects; strong association with obesity and insulin resistance resulting from a reduction in the number or activity of insulin receptors
Incidence	10% of cases	90% of cases
Onset	Juvenile onset, usually younger than 20 yr	Previously maturity onset, age older than 40 yr; now increasingly seen in younger adults and even adolescents—attributed to obesity epidemic
Endogenous insulin	Little or none	Normal or high levels in early disease; reduced later in disease
Insulin receptors	Normal	Decreased or defective
Body weight	Usually nonobese	Obese (80% of cases)
Treatment	Insulin	Weight loss, diet and exercise, and oral hypoglycemics; only about one third of all patients need insulin. Earlier use of insulin is associated with improved outcomes.

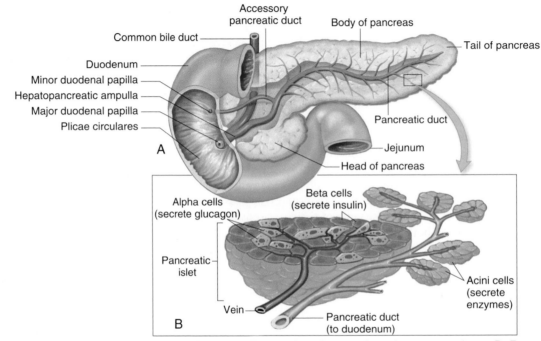

FIGURE 32-1 The pancreas. **A,** Pancreas dissected to show main and accessory ducts. **B,** Exocrine glandular cells (around small pancreatic ducts) and endocrine glandular cells of the pancreatic islets (adjacent to blood capillaries). Exocrine pancreatic cells secrete pancreatic enzymes, alpha endocrine cells secrete glucagon, and beta endocrine cells secrete insulin. (From Patton KT, Thibodeau GA: *Anatomy and physiology*, ed 7, St Louis, 2010, Mosby.)

126 mg/dL) and polyuria, polydipsia, polyphagia, glucosuria, weight loss, blurred vision, and fatigue.

TYPE 1 DIABETES MELLITUS

Type 1 diabetes mellitus is characterized by a lack of insulin production or by the production of defective insulin, which results in acute hyperglycemia. Affected patients require exogenous insulin to lower the blood glucose level and prevent diabetic complications. It is believed that a genetically determined autoimmune reaction gradually destroys the insulin-producing beta cells of the pancreatic islets of Langerhans (Figure 32-1). The preclinical phase of beta cell destruction may be prolonged, possibly lasting several years. At some critical point, a rapid transition from preclinical to clinical type 1 diabetes occurs. This transition is believed to be triggered by a specific event such as an acute illness or major emotional stress. Those stressors trigger the release of the counterregulatory hormones cortisol and epinephrine. These hormones then mobilize glucagon to release glucose from the storage sites in the liver. This further increases the already rising levels of glucose in the blood secondary to islet cell damage. At some point during this critical cascade of events, an autoimmune reaction may be initiated that destroys the insulin-producing beta cells of the pancreatic islets of Langerhans. The result is essentially a complete lack of endogenous insulin production by the pancreas, which necessitates long-term insulin replacement therapy. Fortunately, type 1 diabetes accounts for fewer than 10% of all diabetes cases.

Uncontrolled type 1 diabetes is often referred to as *brittle diabetes,* and these patients have large fluctuations in their blood glucose levels.

Acute Diabetic Complications: Diabetic Ketoacidosis and Hyperosmolar Hyperglycemic Syndrome

When blood glucose levels are high but no insulin is present to allow glucose to be used for energy production, the body may break down fatty acids for fuel, producing ketones as a metabolic by-product. If this occurs to a sufficient degree, diabetic ketoacidosis (DKA) may result. DKA is a complex multisystem complication of uncontrolled diabetes. Without treatment, DKA will lead to coma and death. DKA is characterized by extreme hyperglycemia, the presence of ketones in the serum, acidosis, dehydration, and electrolyte imbalances. Approximately 25% to 30% of patients with newly diagnosed type 1 diabetes mellitus present with DKA. Another complication of comparable severity that is also triggered by extreme hyperglycemia is hyperosmolar hyperglycemic syndrome (HHS). The most common precipitator of DKA and HHS is some type of physical or emotional stress. It was formerly believed that DKA occurred only in type 1 diabetes and HHS occurred only in type 2 diabetes. However, it is now recognized that both disorders can occur with diabetes of either type, and this overlap is increasingly common with the rapidly decreasing age of patients with type 2 diabetes.

Table 32-3 describes the subtle differences between DKA and HHS. Treatment for either complication involves fluid and electrolyte replacement as well as intravenous insulin therapy (more common for DKA).

TYPE 2 DIABETES MELLITUS

Type 2 diabetes mellitus is by far the most common form of diabetes, accounting for at least 90% of all cases of diabetes mellitus and affecting over 23 million people in the United States. Type 2 diabetes mellitus is caused by both insulin resistance and insulin deficiency, but there is no absolute lack of insulin as in type 1 diabetes. One of the normal roles of insulin is to facilitate the uptake of circulating glucose molecules into tissues to be used as energy. In type 2 diabetes, all of the main target tissues of insulin (i.e., muscle, liver, and adipose tissue) are hyporesponsive (resistant) to the effects of the hormone. Not only is the absolute number of insulin receptors in these tissues reduced, but their individual sensitivity and responsiveness to insulin is decreased as well. Therefore, it is possible for a patient with type 2 diabetes mellitus to have normal or even elevated levels of insulin yet still have high blood glucose levels. These processes also result in impaired postprandial (after a meal) glucose metabolism, which is another problematic feature of type 2 diabetes that contributes to the hazardous hyperglycemic state.

In addition to the reduction in the number and sensitivity of insulin receptors in type 2 diabetes, there is often reduced insulin secretion by the pancreas. This insulin deficiency results from a loss of the normal responsiveness of the beta cells in the pancreas to elevated blood glucose levels. When the beta cells do not recognize glucose, they do not secrete insulin, and the normal insulin-facilitated transport of glucose into cells of muscle, liver, and adipose tissue does not occur.

Type 2 diabetes is a multifaceted disorder. Although loss of blood glucose control is its primary hallmark, several other significant conditions are strongly associated with the disease. These include obesity, coronary heart disease, dyslipidemia, hypertension, microalbuminuria (spilling of protein into the urine), and an increased risk for thrombotic (blood clotting) events. These comorbidities are strongly associated with the development of type 2 diabetes and are collectively referred to as *metabolic syndrome* (also known as *insulin-resistance syndrome* and *syndrome X*). Roughly 80% of patients with diabetes are obese at the time of initial diagnosis. Obesity serves only to worsen the insulin resistance, because adipose tissue is often the site of a large proportion of the body's defective insulin receptors.

GESTATIONAL DIABETES

Gestational diabetes is a type of hyperglycemia that develops during pregnancy. Relatively uncommon, it occurs in about 2% to 10% of pregnancies. Many patients are well controlled with diet, but the use of insulin may be necessary to decrease the risk for birth defects, hypoglycemia in the newborn, and high birth weight. In most cases, gestational diabetes subsides after delivery. However, as many as 30% of patients who experience gestational diabetes are estimated to develop type 2 diabetes within 10 to 15 years.

TABLE 32-3	**Comparison of Features of Diabetic Ketoacidosis and Hyperosmolar Hyperglycemic Syndrome**	
Feature	**Diabetic Ketoacidosis**	**Hyperosmolar Hyperglycemic Syndrome**
Age of patient	Younger than 40 yr	Older than 40 yr
Duration of symptoms	Less than 2 days	More than 5 days
Serum glucose level	Lower than 600 mg/dL	Higher than 600 mg/dL
Serum Na level	Normal or low	Normal or high
Serum HCO3 level	Low	Normal
Ketone bodies	At least 4+	Less than 2+
pH	Low	Normal
Serum osmolality	Less than 320 mOsm/kg	Greater than 320 mOsm/kg
Prognosis	3% to 10% mortality	10% to 20% mortality or more
Subsequent course	Insulin therapy required in all cases	Insulin therapy not required in many cases after initial treatment

Adapted from Kitabchi AE, Umpierrez GE, Murphy MB, Kreisberg RA. Hyperglycemic crises in adult patients with diabetes: a consensus statement from the American Diabetes Association, *Diabetes Care* 29(12):2739-2748, 2006.

All pregnant women need to have blood glucose screenings at regular prenatal visits. Women who develop gestational diabetes need to be screened for lingering diabetes 6 to 8 weeks postpartum and be advised of their increased risk for recurrent diabetes and of the importance of regular medical checkups and weight control.

NONPHARMACOLOGIC TREATMENT INTERVENTIONS

Patients diagnosed with type 1 diabetes always require insulin therapy. For patients with new-onset type 2 diabetes, lifestyle changes should be initiated as a first step in treatment. Weight loss not only lowers the blood glucose and lipid levels of these patients, but it also reduces another common comorbidity, hypertension. Other recommended lifestyle changes include improved dietary habits (e.g., consumption of a diet higher in protein and lower in fat and carbohydrates), smoking cessation, reduced alcohol consumption, and regular physical exercise. Cigarette smoking doubles the risk for cardiovascular disease in diabetic patients, largely because of its effects on peripheral vascular circulation and respiratory function. In fact, smoking cessation would probably save far more lives than antihypertensive, antilipemic, and antidiabetic drug treatment combined!

GLYCEMIC GOAL OF TREATMENT

The glycemic goal recommended by the ADA for diabetic patients is a hemoglobin A1C (A1C) level of less than 7%. The A1C test measures the percentage of hemoglobin A that is irreversibly glycosylated. A1C is an indicator of glycemic control in a patient over the preceding 2 to 3 months (the average lifespan of a red blood cell) and is not affected by recent fluctuations in blood glucose levels. The ADA recommended a fasting blood glucose goal for diabetic patients of 80 to 130 mg/dL. A new term, *estimated average glucose (eAG)* is a mathematical conversion of the A1C into an average blood glucose level in the units of measure seen by patients on glucose meters for self-monitoring (mg/dL). Similar to A1C, eAG evaluates a patient's overall success at controlling glucose levels and helps patients understand the monitoring of their long-term treatment.

PHARMACOLOGY OVERVIEW

The major classes of drugs used to treat diabetes mellitus are the insulins and the oral antidiabetic drugs. Several new classes of injectable drugs with unique mechanisms of action have been developed that may be used in addition to insulins or oral antidiabetic drugs to treat resistant diabetes. All of these drugs are referred to as *antidiabetic drugs,* and they are aimed at producing a normoglycemic or euglycemic (normal blood glucose) state.

INSULINS

Insulin is required in patients with type 1 diabetes. Patients with type 2 diabetes are not generally prescribed insulin until other

measures (i.e., lifestyle changes and oral drug therapy) no longer provide adequate glycemic control. Currently insulin is synthesized in laboratories using recombinant deoxyribonucleic acid (DNA) technology and is referred to as *human insulin.* Insulin was originally isolated from cattle or pigs, but bovine (cow) and porcine (pig) insulins are associated with a higher incidence of allergic reactions and insulin resistance than human insulin and are no longer available in the U.S. market. The pharmacokinetic properties of insulin (onset of action, peak effect, and duration of action) can be altered by making various minor modifications to either the insulin molecule itself or the drug formulation (final product). This practice has led to the development of many different insulin preparations, including several combination insulin products that contain more than one type of insulin in the same solution. Further modifications can be accomplished by mixing compatible insulin preparations in the syringe before administration. The latest syringe compatibility data for insulin products are given in Table 32-4. Thoroughly educate patients regarding how, when, and if they can (or cannot) mix different types of insulin. Some combinations are chemically incompatible and can result in alteration of glycemic effects.

Mechanism of Action and Drug Effects

Exogenous insulin functions as a substitute for the endogenous hormone. It serves to replace the insulin that is either not made or is made defectively in a diabetic patient. The drug effects of exogenously administered insulin involve many body systems. They are the same as those of normal endogenous insulin. That is, exogenous insulin restores the patient's ability to metabolize carbohydrates, fats, and proteins; to store glucose in the liver; and to convert glycogen to fat stores. Unfortunately, exogenous insulin does not reverse defects in insulin receptor sensitivity. Insulin pumps are a very attractive way to administer insulin to

TABLE 32-4	Insulin Mixing Compatibilities
Type of Insulin	**Compatible with**
Regular insulin (Humulin R, Novolin R)	All insulins except glargine, and glulisine
Insulin glulisine (Apidra)	NPH only
Insulin lispro (Humalog), insulin aspart (NovoLog)	Regular, NPH insulins
Insulin detemir (Levemir)	Must be given alone
Insulin glargine (Lantus)	Must be given alone due to low pH of diluent
NPH 70% and regular insulin 30% (Humulin 70/30, Novolin 70/30)	Premixed; do not mix with other insulins
NPH 50% and regular insulin 50% (Humulin 50/50)	
Insulin aspart protamine suspension 75% and insulin aspart 25% (NovoLog Mix 75/25)	
Insulin lispro protamine suspension 75% and insulin lispro 25% (Humalog Mix 75/25)	

patients. The insulin pump provides an alternative to multiple daily subcutaneous injections and allows patients to match their insulin intake to their lifestyle. When an insulin pump is used, insulin is administered constantly over a 24-hour period, and the patient is then allowed to give bolus injections based on the amount of food ingested. Insulin pumps are described further in the Nursing Process section later in the chapter.

Indications

All insulin preparations can be used to treat both type 1 and type 2 diabetes, but each patient requires careful customization of the dosing regimen for optimal glycemic control. Additional therapeutic approaches such as lifestyle modifications (e.g., dietary and exercise habits) are also indicated and, for type 2 diabetes, oral drug therapy as well.

Contraindications

Contraindications to the use of all insulin products include known drug allergy to the specific product. Insulin is never to be administered to an already hypoglycemic patient. Blood glucose must always be tested prior to administration.

Adverse Effects

Hypoglycemia resulting from excessive insulin dosing can result in brain damage, shock, and possible death. This is the most immediate and serious adverse effect of insulin. Other adverse effects of insulin therapy include weight gain, lipodystrophy at the site of repeated injections, and in rare cases allergic reactions. Because weight gain is a common and often undesirable adverse effect, insulin therapy is usually delayed in type 2 patients until other agents and lifestyle changes have failed to bring the blood glucose to target levels.

Interactions

Drug interactions that can occur with the insulins are significant; they are listed in Table 32-5.

Dosages

For dosage information on the various insulin products, see the table on this page. The concentration of insulin is expressed as the number of units of insulin per milliliter. For example, U-100 insulin has 100 units in 1 milliliter. Insulin is usually given by subcutaneous injection or via a subcutaneous infusion pump.

DOSAGES

Selected Human-Based Insulin Products

Drug (Pregnancy Category)	Pharmacologic Class	Usual Dosage Range	Indications
Rapid Acting ◆ ! insulin lispro (Humalog) (B)	Human recombinant rapid-acting insulin analogue	Subcut: 0.5-1 unit/kg/day; doses are individualized to desired glycemic control; rapid-acting insulins are best given at least 15 min before a meal. May be given per sliding scale or as basal/bolus; may also be given via continuous subcutaneous infusion pump	
Short Acting ◆ ! regular insulin (Humulin R, Novolin R) (B)	Human recombinant short-acting insulin	Subcut: Same dosage as insulin lispro; subcut doses of regular insulin are best given 30 min before a meal. Regular insulin may also be given per sliding scale or basal/bolus and is the insulin usually given IV as a continuous infusion	Diabetes mellitus type 1 and type 2
Long Acting ◆ ! insulin glargine (Lantus) (C)	Human recombinant long-acting insulin analogue	Subcut only: 0.2 units/kg/day given once or twice daily (basal dosing)	

TABLE 32-5 Selected Drug Interactions with Antidiabetic Drugs

Drug	Interacting Drug	Mechanism	Result
insulin	Corticosteroids, estrogen, diuretics, thyroid drugs	Interferes with insulin	Increased blood glucose levels
	Nonselective beta blockers	Masks the tachycardia from hypoglycemia	Risk for not noticing hypoglycemic symptoms
	Hypoglycemic drugs	Additive effects	Additive hypoglycemia
metformin	Cimetidine	Inhibits metabolism	Increased metformin effects
	Diuretics, corticosteroids	Additive effects	Additive hypoglycemia
	Contrast media	Decreases excretion	Lactic acidosis
glipizide	Beta blockers, cimetidine, erythromycin, fluconazole, sulfonamide antibiotics, DPP4 inhibitors, garlic, ginger, ginseng	Enhanced effects	Increased hypoglycemia
	Carbamazepine, phenobarbital, phenytoin, rifampin	Increases metabolism	Decreased effectiveness

In emergency situations requiring prompt insulin action, regular insulin can be given intravenously. Insulin also is available as a U-500 (which is a high-alert medication). Great care must be taken with its use to ensure that the correct dose is administered. Many hospitals do not allow U-500 insulin because of the potential for errors.

Insulin Use in Special Populations

Two special patient populations for whom careful attention is required during insulin therapy are pediatric patients and pregnant women. Insulin dosages for both are calculated by weight as they are for the general adult population. The usual dosage range is 0.5 to 1 units/kg/day as a total daily dose. Be aware that there are a few important differences regarding the use of some insulin products in pediatric populations. The rapid-acting insulin lispro is approved for use in children older than 3 years of age. However, the combination lispro product Humalog 75/25, which contains 75% insulin lispro protamine (an intermediate-acting insulin) and 25% insulin lispro (a rapid-acting insulin), is not currently approved for use in children younger than 18 years of age. Children need age-appropriate education and supervision by health care professionals and parents, which includes a safe and gradual transfer of responsibility for self-management of their illness, as appropriate.

Pregnant women also require special care with regard to diabetes management. Although most of these mothers will return to a normal glycemic state after pregnancy, they are at risk for developing diabetes again in later life. All currently available oral and injectable antidiabetic drugs are classified as pregnancy category B or C drugs. Oral medications are generally not recommended for pregnant patients because of a lack of firm safety data. For this reason, insulin therapy is the only currently recommended drug therapy for pregnant women with diabetes. Roughly 15% of women who develop gestational diabetes require insulin therapy during pregnancy. Insulin does not normally cross the placenta. Effective glycemic control during pregnancy is essential because infants born to women with gestational diabetes have a twofold to threefold greater risk for congenital anomalies. In addition, the incidence of stillbirth is directly related to the degree of maternal hyperglycemia. Weight reduction is generally not advised for these women, because it can jeopardize fetal nutritional status. Women with gestational diabetes tend to have babies that weigh more, and these children may have low blood sugar in the postnatal period. Insulin is excreted into human milk. It is very important that insulin therapy and diet be well controlled for a nursing mother, because inadequate or excessive glycemic control may reduce milk production.

DRUG PROFILES

There are currently four major classes of insulin, as determined by their pharmacokinetic properties: rapid acting, short acting, intermediate acting, and long acting. The duration of action ranges from several hours to over 24 hours depending on the insulin class (Figure 32-2). The insulin dosage regimen for all diabetic patients is highly individualized and may consist of one or more classes of insulin administered at either fixed dosages

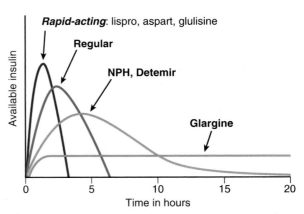

FIGURE 32-2 Comparison of the pharmacokinetics of various insulins. (From Messinger-Rapport BJ, Thomas DR, Gammack JK: Clinical update on nursing home medicine: 2008, *J Am Med Dir Assoc* 9(7):460-475, 2008.)

or variable dosages in response to self-measurements of blood glucose level or the number of grams of carbohydrate consumed. With the use of insulins, clarity, color, and appearance are important to understand for patient safety and for the prevention of adverse effects and complications. Several insulins are clear, colorless solutions. These include regular insulin, insulin lispro (Humalog), and insulin glargine (Lantus). Other insulins, such as NPH insulin (insulin isophane), are white opaque (cloudy) solutions. This issue is discussed further in the Implementation section under Nursing Process. Note that *all* insulins are considered high-alert medications.

RAPID-ACTING INSULINS
♦!insulin lispro

There are currently three insulin products that are classified as rapid acting: insulin lispro (Humalog), insulin aspart (NovoLog), and the most recently developed, insulin glulisine (Apidra). These have the most rapid onset of action (roughly 15 minutes) as well as a shorter duration of action than other insulin categories. The effect of insulin lispro is most like that of the endogenous insulin produced by the pancreas in response to a meal. After or during a meal, the glucose that is ingested stimulates the pancreas to secrete insulin. This insulin then facilitates the uptake of the excess glucose at hepatic insulin receptor sites for storage in the liver as glycogen. In people with diabetes, the insulin response to meals is often impaired; therefore, a rapid-acting insulin product is often used within 15 minutes of mealtime. This corresponds to the time required for the onset of action of these products. It is essential that patients with diabetes eat a meal after injection. Otherwise profound hypoglycemia may result.

In 2014, the FDA approved a new method of insulin delivery. Afrezza is a rapid-acting insulin that is inhaled. Because it is inhaled, it has a rapid onset of action, with a peak of 12 to 15 minutes and a short duration of action of 2 to 3 hours. It is administered within 20 minutes before each meal. It must be given in conjunction with long-acting insulins or oral diabetic agents (for type 2 diabetes). The most common side effects in clinical trials included hypoglycemia, cough, and throat pain. It must not be used in smokers or those with chronic lung diseases. Afrezza has a black-box warning regarding the risk for acute bronchospasms.

Pharmacokinetics: Insulin Lispro

Route	Onset of Action	Peak Plasma Concentration	Elimination Half-life	Duration of Action
Subcut	15 min	1-2 hr	80 min	3-5 hr

SHORT-ACTING INSULIN
◆! regular insulin

Regular insulin (Humulin R) is currently the only insulin that is classified as a short-acting insulin. Regular insulin can be given via intravenous bolus, intravenous infusion, or intramuscularly along with the most common route, subcutaneously. These routes, especially the intravenous infusion route, are often used in cases of DKA or coma associated with uncontrolled type 1 diabetes.

There are some differences between regular insulin and the newer rapid-acting drugs. The rapid acting insulins are considered human insulin analogues. This means that they are insulin molecules with synthetic alterations to their chemical structures that alter their onset or duration of action. They have a faster onset of action and a shorter time to peak plasma level, but they also have a shorter duration of action than does regular insulin. Regular insulin is made from human insulin sources using recombinant DNA technology.

Pharmacokinetics: Regular Insulin

Route	Onset of Action	Peak Plasma Concentration	Elimination Half-life	Duration of Action
Subcut	30-60 min	2.5 hr	Unknown	6-10 hr

INTERMEDIATE-ACTING INSULINS
◆! insulin isophane suspension (NPH)

Insulin isophane suspension (also known as *NPH insulin*) is the only available intermediate-acting insulin product. NPH is an acronym for *neutral protamine Hagedorn insulin,* the original name of this type of insulin. NPH insulin is a sterile suspension of zinc insulin crystals and protamine sulfate in buffered water for injection. The suspension appears cloudy or opaque. NPH insulin has a slower onset and longer duration of action than regular insulin, but not as long as the long-acting insulins. NPH insulin is often combined with regular insulin to reduce the number of insulin injections per day.

Pharmacokinetics: NPH insulin

Route	Onset of Action	Peak Plasma Concentration	Elimination Half-life	Duration of Action
Subcut	1-2 hr	4-8 hr	Unknown	10-18 hr

LONG-ACTING INSULINS
◆! insulin glargine and ! insulin detemir

Two long-acting insulin products are available: insulin glargine (Lantus) and insulin detemir (Levemir). Insulin detemir can be classified as an intermediate- or long-acting insulin, since it is given twice daily. However, in clinical practice it is considered long acting. Insulin glargine is normally a clear, colorless solution with a pH of 4.0. Once it is injected into subcutaneous tissue at physiologic pH, it forms microprecipitates that are slowly absorbed over the next 24 hours. It is a recombinant DNA–produced insulin analogue and is unique in that it provides a constant level of insulin in the body. This enhances its safety because blood levels do not rise and fall as with other insulins. Insulin glargine is usually dosed once daily, but the drug may be dosed every 12 hours, depending on the patient's glycemic response. Because insulin glargine provides a more prolonged, consistent blood glucose level, it is sometimes referred to as a *basal insulin.*

Insulin detemir has a different mechanism of action from insulin glargine, and the two insulins are not considered interchangeable. The duration of action of insulin detemir is dose dependent, so that lower doses require twice-daily dosing and higher doses may be given once daily.

Pharmacokinetics: Insulin Glargine

Route	Onset of Action	Peak Plasma Concentration	Elimination Half-life	Duration of Action
Subcut	1-2 hr	None	Unknown	24 hr

FIXED-COMBINATION INSULINS

Currently available fixed-combination insulin products include Humulin 70/30, Humulin 50/50, Novolin 70/30, Humalog Mix 75/25, Humalog 50/50, and NovoLog 70/30. Each of these products contains two different insulins; one intermediate-acting type and either one rapid-acting type (Humalog, NovoLog) or one short-acting type (Humulin). The numeric designations indicate the percentages of each of the two components in the product. For example, Novolin 70/30 has 70% intermediate-acting and 30% short-acting insulin. Notice that the numbers add up to 100 (percent). These products were developed to closely simulate the varying levels of endogenous insulin that occur normally in nondiabetic people. In most insulin regimens, patients take a combination of a rapid-acting insulin to deal with the surges in glucose that occur after meals and an intermediate- or long-acting insulin for the period between meals when glucose levels are lower. However, this requires the mixing and administration of different types of insulins. Fixed-combination products were developed in an attempt to simplify the dosing process. The insulin lispro protamine component of Humalog Mix 75/25 is a modified insulin lispro molecule with a longer duration of action. These combinations allow for twice daily dosing but often result in glycemic control that is not as tight as daily dosing with meals. Patients who cannot afford frequent glucose monitoring or who refuse more than two injections per day may insist on using a combination insulin with twice daily dosing.

BASAL-BOLUS AND SLIDING-SCALE INSULIN DOSING

Historically, sliding scale insulin was used to correct blood glucose levels. In this method, subcutaneous doses of rapid-acting (lispro or aspart) or short-acting (regular) insulin are adjusted according to blood glucose test results. This method was typically used in treating hospitalized diabetic patients, whose insulin requirements may vary drastically because of stress (e.g., infections, surgery, acute illness), inactivity, or variable caloric intake, including receipt of total parenteral nutrition (TPN), enteral nutrition, or time spent with a "nothing by mouth" (NPO) diet. When an individual is on a sliding-scale insulin regimen, blood glucose concentrations are determined several times a day (e.g., before meals and at bedtime) for patients on normal meal schedules, or every 4 to 6 hours around the clock for patients receiving TPN or enteral tube feedings. Subcutaneously administered regular or rapid insulin is then given in an amount that increases with the rise in blood glucose level. The disadvantage of sliding-scale dosing is that, because it delays insulin administration until hyperglycemia occurs, it does not meet basal insulin requirements and results in large swings in glucose control. Current research does not support the use of sliding scales or insulin without basal insulin, and many institutions are moving away from sliding-scale coverage. Nonetheless, sliding-scale dosing is still commonly used.

Basal-bolus insulin therapy is now the preferred method of treatment for hospitalized diabetic patients. Basal-bolus therapy is the attempt to mimic a healthy pancreas by delivering basal insulin constantly as a basal and then as needed as a bolus. The basal insulin is a long-acting insulin (insulin glargine) administered constantly to keep the blood glucose from fluctuating due to the normal release of glucose from the liver. Bolus insulin (insulin lispro or insulin aspart) mimics the burst secretions of the pancreas in response to increases in blood glucose levels. Bolus insulin is broken up into meal and correction boluses. Meal boluses are given to reduce blood glucose with the intake of carbohydrates. Correction boluses are any boluses taken to bring blood glucose back to normal. Blood glucose levels are monitored frequently when using basal-bolus insulin. This method of treatment is far superior to the traditional sliding scale. Still, patients who need to receive nothing by mouth for therapeutic or diagnostic reasons are not good candidates for basal insulin due to the risk for hypoglycemia and the unpredictability of insulin needed for glucose control while not eating.

ORAL ANTIDIABETIC DRUGS

Type 2 diabetes is a very complex illness. Effective treatment involves several elements, including lifestyle modifications, careful monitoring of blood glucose levels, and therapy with one or more drugs. In addition, the treatment of associated comorbid conditions (such as high cholesterol and high blood pressure) is a necessity that serves to further complicate the entire process.

The 2015 ADA Guidelines recommend that new-onset type 2 diabetes be treated with both lifestyle interventions and the oral biguanide drug metformin, if there are no contraindications to the drug. If lifestyle modifications and the maximum tolerated metformin dose do not achieve the recommended A1C goals after 3 to 6 months, additional treatment with a

second oral agent, a GLP-1 agonist (liraglutide, exenatide, abliglutide), or insulin is added to the regimen. Choice of pharmacologic therapy should be based on a patient-centered approach. Factors to be considered include efficacy, cost, side effects, comorbidities, effects on weight, hypoglycemia risk, and patient preference.

BIGUANIDE

Mechanism of Action and Drug Effects

Metformin is currently the only drug classified as a biguanide. It is considered a first-line drug and is the most commonly used oral drug for the treatment of type 2 diabetes. It is not used for type 1 diabetes. Metformin works by decreasing glucose production by the liver. It may also decrease intestinal absorption of glucose and improve insulin receptor sensitivity. This results in increased peripheral glucose uptake and use, and decreased hepatic production of triglycerides and cholesterol. Unlike sulfonylureas, metformin does not stimulate insulin secretion and therefore is not associated with weight gain and significant hypoglycemia when used alone.

Indications

The ADA guidelines recommend metformin as the initial oral antidiabetic drug for treatment of newly diagnosed type 2 diabetes if no contraindications exist. Because it may also cause moderate weight loss, it is particularly useful for the many patients with type 2 diabetes who are overweight or obese. Metformin may be used as monotherapy or in combination with other oral antidiabetic drugs if single-drug therapy is unsuccessful. For this reason, it is available in combination products containing either sulfonylureas, thiazolidinediones, or incretin mimetics. Metformin may also be combined with insulin. It is also used in prediabetic patients.

Contraindications

Metformin is contraindicated in patients with renal disease or renal dysfunction (serum creatinine level higher than 1.5 mg/dL in males or higher than 1.4 mg/dL in females). Because metformin is primarily excreted by the kidneys, it can accumulate in these individuals, increasing the risk for development of lactic acidosis. Other contraindications include alcoholism, metabolic acidosis, hepatic disease, heart failure, and other conditions that predispose to tissue hypoxia and increase the risk for lactic acidosis.

Adverse Effects

The most common adverse effects of metformin are gastrointestinal. Metformin can cause abdominal bloating, nausea, cramping, a feeling of fullness, and diarrhea, especially at the start of therapy. Some research attributes the weight loss experienced early in the course of treatment with these side effects. These effects are all usually self-limiting and can be lessened by starting with low dosages, titrating up slowly, and taking the medication with food. Less common adverse effects with metformin are a metallic taste, hypoglycemia, and a reduction in vitamin B_{12} levels after long-term use. Lactic acidosis is an

DOSAGES

Selected Oral Antidiabetic Drugs

Drug (Pregnancy Category)	Pharmacologic Class	Usual Dosage Range	Indications
acarbose (Precose) (B)	Alpha-glucosidase inhibitor	PO: 25-100 mg three times daily, taken with first bite of meal	
♦ liraglutide (Victoza) (C)	GLP-1 receptor agonist	Subcut: 0.6-1.8 mg daily	
♦! glipizide (Glucotrol, Glucotrol XL) (C)	Second-generation sulfonylurea	PO: IR: 2.5-20 mg/day (max daily dose 40 mg)	
! glimepiride (Amaryl) (C)	Second-generation sulfonylurea	PO: 1-4 mg daily (max daily dose 8 mg)	
♦ metformin (Glucophage, Glucophage XR) (B)	Biguanide	PO: IR: 500-1000 mg bid (max dose 2550 mg/day) PO: ER: 500-2000 mg/day (max dose 2000 mg/day)	
♦ pioglitazone (Actos) (C)	Thiazolidinedione	PO: 15-45 mg once daily	
♦ repaglinide (Prandin) (C)	Meglitinide	PO: 0.5-4 mg three times daily; best taken 15 min before a meal	
♦ sitagliptin (Januvia) (B)	DPP-IV Inhibitor	PO: 100 mg daily	Diabetes mellitus type 2
Combination Oral Drugs			
! glipizide/metformin (Metaglip) (C)	Combination sulfonylurea/biguanide	PO: 1-2 tablets once to twice daily	
pioglitazone/metformin (ACTOplus Met) (C)	Combination thiazolidinedione/biguanide	PO: 1 tablet once to three times daily	
sitagliptin/metformin (Janumet) (C)	Combination incretin mimetic/biguanide	PO: 1 tablet twice daily	
saxagliptin/metformin (Kombiglyze XR) (C)	Combination incretin mimetic/biguanide	PO: 1-2 tablets daily with evening meal	

extremely rare complication with metformin, but the risk increases with very high blood glucose levels and/or clinical conditions predisposing to hypoxemia. Lactic acidosis is lethal in up to 50% of cases. Symptoms of lactic acidosis include hyperventilation, cold and clammy skin, muscle pain, abdominal pain, dizziness, and irregular heartbeat.

Interactions

Drug interactions with metformin are listed in Table 32-5. In addition, the use of metformin with iodinated (iodine-containing) radiologic contrast media has been associated with both acute renal failure and lactic acidosis. For these reasons, metformin therapy is to be discontinued the day of the test and for at least 48 hours after the patient undergoes any radiologic study that requires the use of such contrast media.

Dosages

For dosage information on metformin, see the table above.

SULFONYLUREAS

Mechanism of Action and Drug Effects

The sulfonylureas are the oldest group of oral antidiabetic drugs. Those currently used are second-generation drugs and have a better potency and adverse effect profile than first-generation drugs (e.g., acetazolamide and tolbutamide), which are no longer used clinically. Second-generation drugs include glipizide (Glucotrol), glyburide (Diabeta), and glimepiride (Amaryl). Sulfonylureas bind to specific receptors on beta cells in the pancreas to stimulate the release of insulin. In addition, sulfonylureas appear to secondarily decrease the secretion of

glucagon. For this class of drugs to be effective, the patient must still have functioning beta cells in the pancreas. Thus, these drugs work best during the early stages of type 2 diabetes and are not used in type 1 diabetes.

Indications

Because they have different mechanisms of action, sulfonylureas can be used in conjunction with metformin and thiazolidinediones. Sulfonylureas should not be used in patients with advanced diabetes dependent on insulin administration, because the beta cells in such patients are no longer able to produce insulin. Once insulin is started, sulfonylurea medication is stopped.

Contraindications

Contraindications include hypoglycemia or conditions that can predispose to hypoglycemia, such as reduced caloric intake (e.g., NPO), ethanol use, or advanced age. There is a potential for cross-allergy in patients who are allergic to sulfonamide antibiotics. Although such an allergy is listed as a contraindication by the manufacturer, most clinicians will prescribe sulfonylureas for such patients. However, be aware of the potential for cross-allergy, and inform patients of the possibility.

Adverse Effects

The most common adverse effect of the sulfonylureas is hypoglycemia, the degree to which depends on the dose, eating habits, and presence of hepatic or renal disease. Another predictable adverse effect is weight gain because of the stimulation of insulin secretion. Other adverse effects include skin rash, nausea, epigastric fullness, and heartburn.

Interactions

Drug interactions with the second-generation sulfonylureas are listed in Table 32-5.

Dosages

For dosage information on sulfonylureas, see the table on the previous page.

GLINIDES

Mechanism of Action and Drug Effects

Repaglinide (Prandin) and nateglinide (Starlix) are currently the only two drugs in the glinide class. They are structurally different from the sulfonylureas but have a similar mechanism of action in that they also increase insulin secretion from the pancreas. However, they have a much shorter duration of action and must be given with each meal.

Indications

Like the sulfonylureas, the glinides are indicated for treatment of type 2 diabetes. They may be particularly useful for diabetic patients with high postprandial glucose levels who have low levels of circulating insulin. Glinides can be used along with metformin and thiazolidinediones, but not combined with sulfonylureas, because they share a similar mechanism of action.

Contraindications

Contraindications are similar to those for the sulfonylureas.

Adverse Effects

The most commonly reported adverse effect of the glinides is hypoglycemia, which can occur particularly if food is not eaten after a dose. Weight gain is also commonly reported.

Interactions

Drug interactions with the glinides are similar to those with the sulfonylureas.

Dosages

For dosage information on glinides, see the table on the previous page.

THIAZOLIDINEDIONES (GLITAZONES)

Mechanism of Action and Drug Effects

The third major drug category of oral treatment of type 2 diabetes mellitus is the thiazolidinediones, most commonly referred to as *glitazones*. This class of drugs acts by regulating genes involved in glucose and lipid metabolism. The first drug in this class to be used in the United States was troglitazone (Rezulin). In 2000, it was removed from the market because of concerns about liver toxicity.

Glitazones are referred to as *insulin-sensitizing drugs*. They work to decrease insulin resistance by enhancing the sensitivity of insulin receptors. These drugs are also known to directly stimulate peripheral glucose uptake and storage, as well as to inhibit glucose and triglyceride production in the liver. Because glitazones affect gene regulation, they have a slow onset of activity over several weeks, and maximal activity may not be evident for several months. Some amount of preservation of beta cell function has also been reported with glitazone administration, thereby slowing disease progression in type 2 diabetes.

Indications

Thiazolidinediones (glitazones) are indicated for the management of type 2 diabetes. They may also be combined with metformin or a sulfonylurea for a synergistic effect. Pioglitazone can be used with insulin.

Contraindications

Initiation of therapy with thiazolidinediones is contraindicated in patients with New York Heart Association class III or IV heart failure and are to be used with caution in patients with liver or kidney disease.

Adverse Effects

The glitazones have a black box warning indicating that they can cause or exacerbate heart failure and are not recommended for use in patients with symptomatic heart failure. The glitazones also commonly cause peripheral edema and weight gain. The weight gain may be due to both water retention and an increase in adipose tissue. Their use has also been associated with reduced bone mineral density and an increased risk for fractures.

Interactions

Pioglitazone is partly metabolized by cytochrome P-450 enzyme 3A4 (CYP3A4). Serum concentrations of pioglitazone may be increased if the drug is taken concurrently with a CYP3A4 inhibitor such as ketoconazole or erythromycin.

Dosages

For dosage information on thiazolidinediones, see the table on the previous page.

ALPHA-GLUCOSIDASE INHIBITORS

Mechanism of Action and Drug Effects

Less commonly used oral drugs are the alpha-glucosidase inhibitors, acarbose (Precose) and miglitol (Glyset). As the name implies, these drugs work by reversibly inhibiting the enzyme alpha-glucosidase that is found in the small intestine. This enzyme is responsible for the hydrolysis of oligosaccharides and disaccharides to glucose. When this enzyme is blocked, glucose absorption is delayed. The timing of administration of the alpha-glucosidase inhibitors is important, and they must be taken with food. When an alpha-glucosidase inhibitor is taken with a meal, excessive postprandial blood glucose elevation (a glucose "spike") can be prevented or reduced, making them impractical for directly lowering fasting blood glucose.

Indications

The alpha-glucosidase inhibitors are used to treat type 2 diabetes, usually in combination with another oral hypoglycemic drug. They may be particularly effective in controlling high postprandial glucose levels.

Contraindications

Because of their adverse gastrointestinal effects, alpha-glucosidase inhibitors are not recommended for use in patients with inflammatory bowel disease, malabsorption syndromes, or intestinal obstruction.

Adverse Effects

These drugs can cause a high incidence of flatulence, diarrhea, and abdominal pain. At high dosages, they may also elevate levels of hepatic enzymes (transaminases). Unlike sulfonylureas, they do not cause hypoglycemia or weight gain. In the rare instance that a patient develops hypoglycemia from these drugs, complex carbohydrates cannot be used because alpha-glucosidase is blocked; IV or oral glucose must be administered.

Interactions

The bioavailability of digoxin, ranitidine, and propranolol may be reduced when they are taken with alpha-glucosidase inhibitors.

Dosages

For dosage information on alpha-glucosidase inhibitors, see the table on p. 509.

DIPEPTIDYL PEPTIDASE IV (DPP-IV) INHIBITORS

Mechanism of Action and Drug Effects

Dipeptidyl peptidase-IV (DPP-IV) inhibitors work by delaying the breakdown of incretin hormones by inhibiting the enzyme DPP-IV. Incretin hormones are released throughout the day and are increased after a meal. When blood glucose concentrations are normal or high, the incretin hormones increase insulin synthesis and lower glucagon secretion. By inhibiting the enzyme responsible for incretin breakdown (DPP-IV), the DPP-IV inhibitors reduce fasting and postprandial glucose concentrations. Currently there are four DPP-IV inhibitors: sitagliptin (Januvia), saxagliptin (Onglyza), linagliptin (Tradjenta), and alogliptin (Nesina). There are several DPP-IV inhibitors currently under investigation. This class of drugs is commonly referred to as the *gliptins*.

Indications

The DPP-IV inhibitors are indicated as an adjunct to diet and exercise to improve glycemic control in adults with type 2 diabetes mellitus.

Contraindications

The DPP-IV inhibitors are contraindicated in patients with known drug allergy.

Adverse Effects

The most common effects are upper respiratory tract infection, headache, and diarrhea. Hypoglycemia can occur and is more common if used in conjunction with a sulfonylurea. Cases of pancreatitis have been reported.

Interactions

Sitagliptin may increase digoxin levels. Concurrent use of sulfonylureas and insulin may increase the risk for hypoglycemia. The metabolism of saxagliptin is inhibited by strong CYP4A inhibitors. Rifampin may decrease the efficacy of linagliptin.

Dosages

The recommended dosage of sitagliptin is 100 mg daily; saxagliptin is 5 mg daily; linagliptin is 5 mg daily, and alogliptin 25 mg daily.

DRUG PROFILES

acarbose

Acarbose (Precose) is one of the two currently available alpha-glucosidase inhibitors. The other drug in this drug category is miglitol (Glyset). These drugs work by blunting the elevation of blood glucose levels after a meal. To work optimally, they are to be taken with the first bite of each meal. They also may be taken along with sulfonylurea drugs or with metformin. Acarbose use is contraindicated in patients with a hypersensitivity to alpha-glucosidase inhibitors, DKA, cirrhosis, inflammatory bowel disease, colonic ulceration, partial intestinal obstruction, or chronic intestinal disease.

Pharmacokinetics: Acarbose

Route	Onset of Action	Peak Plasma Concentration	Elimination Half-life	Duration of Action
PO	1-1.5 hr	2 hr	2-3 hr	Unknown

♦!glipizide

Glipizide (Glucotrol) is a second-generation sulfonylurea drug. In contrast to another second-generation sulfonylurea, glimepiride, it has a very rapid onset and short duration of action, with no active metabolites. The rapid onset of action allows it to function much like the body normally does in response to meals when greater levels of insulin are required rapidly to deal with the increased glucose in the blood. When a patient with type 2 diabetes mellitus takes glipizide, it rapidly stimulates the pancreas to release insulin. This, in turn, facilitates the transport of excess glucose from the blood into the cells of the muscles, liver, and adipose tissues.

Glipizide use is contraindicated in cases of known drug allergy as well as in type 1 or brittle type 2 diabetes. Unlike most other oral antidiabetic drugs, it is not contraindicated in patients with severe renal failure. It works best if given 30 minutes before meals, usually before breakfast. This allows the timing of the insulin secretion induced by the glipizide to correspond with the elevation in blood glucose level induced by the meal in much the same way as endogenous insulin levels are raised in a person without diabetes. The extended-release dosage form of glipizide can be given once daily.

Pharmacokinetics: Glipizide

Route	Onset of Action	Peak Plasma Concentration	Elimination Half-life	Duration of Action
PO	1 hr	1-3 hr	2-5 hr	6-8 hr

◆ metformin

Metformin (Glucophage) is currently the only biguanide oral antidiabetic drug. It works by inhibiting hepatic glucose production and increasing the sensitivity of peripheral tissue to insulin. Because its mechanism of action differs from that of sulfonylurea drugs, it may be given along with these drugs.

Metformin use is contraindicated in patients with a known hypersensitivity to biguanides, hepatic or renal disease, alcoholism, or cardiopulmonary disease.

Pharmacokinetics: Metformin

Route	Onset of Action	Peak Plasma Concentration	Elimination Half-life	Duration of Action
PO	Less than 1 hr	1-3 hr	1.5-5 hr	24 hr

◆ pioglitazone

Pioglitazone (Actos) is classified as a glitazone or derivative. Pioglitazone is used alone or with a sulfonylurea, metformin, or insulin. It works by decreasing insulin resistance. It can worsen or precipitate heart failure. The safety of these drugs for use in pregnant women and children has not been established.

Pharmacokinetics: Pioglitazone

Route	Onset of Action	Peak Plasma Concentration	Elimination Half-life	Duration of Action
PO	Delayed	2 hr	3-7 hr	Unknown

◆ repaglinide

Repaglinide (Prandin) is one of two antidiabetic drugs classified as *glinides,* the other being nateglinide (Starlix). These drugs have a mechanism of action similar to that of the sulfonylureas in that they also stimulate the release of insulin from pancreatic beta cells. They are especially helpful in the treatment of patients who have erratic eating habits, because the drug dose is skipped when a meal is missed. Contraindications include known drug allergy.

Pharmacokinetics: Repaglinide

Route	Onset of Action	Peak Plasma Concentration	Elimination Half-life	Duration of Action
PO	15-60 min	1 hr	2-3 hr	4-6 hr

◆ sitagliptin

Sitagliptin (Januvia) was the first DPP-IV inhibitor approved. It is an oral drug that selectively inhibits the action of DPP-IV, thus increasing concentrations of the naturally occurring incretins GLP-1 and GIP. Sitagliptin is indicated for management of type 2 diabetes, either as monotherapy or in combination with metformin, a sulfonylurea, or a glitazone. Recent studies indicate it is safe and effective when added to insulin. Clinical trials have demonstrated A1C reductions of 0.6% to 0.8%, which is less than the reductions seen with traditional oral antidiabetic drugs. Significant hypoglycemia may occur when the drug is combined with a sulfonylurea. There have been no significant adverse effects. However, in September 2009, the FDA received postmarketing cases of acute pancreatitis and advised health care professionals to monitor patients closely for the development of pancreatitis after both initiation and dose increases. It is classified as a pregnancy category B drug. Other DPP-IV inhibitors include saxagliptin (Onglyza), linagliptin (Tradjenta), and alogliptin (Nesina).

Pharmacokinetics: Sitagliptin

Route	Onset of Action	Peak Plasma Concentration	Elimination Half-life	Duration of Action
PO	15-30 min	1 hr	12 hr	Unknown

INJECTABLE ANTIDIABETIC DRUGS

AMYLIN AGONISTS

Mechanism of Action and Drug Effects

Amylin is a natural hormone secreted by the beta cells of the pancreas along with insulin in response to food. It functions to decrease postprandial plasma glucose levels, which it accomplishes in the following three ways: (1) It slows gastric emptying; (2) suppresses glucagon secretion and hepatic glucose production; and (3) increases satiety (sense of having eaten enough).

When given before major meals, the amylin agonists work by mimicking the action of the natural hormone amylin.

Indications

Pramlintide (Symlin; pregnancy category C) is the only available amylin agonist. It is available only as a subcutaneous injection. It is indicated for use in patients with type 1 or type 2 diabetes receiving mealtime insulin who failed to achieve optimal glucose control with insulin. Pramlintide was the first drug approved for use in type 1 diabetes since insulin was discovered in the early twentieth century.

Contraindications

Pramlintide is contraindicated in patients with gastroparesis or those taking drugs that alter gastrointestinal motility.

Adverse Effects

Adverse effects include nausea, vomiting, anorexia, and headache.

Interactions

Pramlintide itself does not cause hypoglycemia, but if the patient is taking any preprandial rapid- or short-acting insulin product, the insulin dose usually needs to be reduced by 50%. It can delay the oral absorption of any drug taken at the same time and needs to be given at least 1 hour before other medications.

Dosages

Recommended dosage ranges are from 15 to 60 mcg for management of type 1 diabetes and 60 to 120 mcg for management of type 2 diabetes, taken before any major meal.

INCRETIN MIMETICS

Mechanism of Action and Drug Effects

Incretins are hormones released by the gastrointestinal tract in response to food. Incretins do the following: stimulate insulin secretion; reduce postprandial glucagon production; slow gastric emptying; and increase satiety.

The most important incretin hormones that have been identified so far are glucagon-like peptide 1 (GLP-1) and gastric inhibitory peptide (GIP). These hormones are rapidly deactivated by the enzyme DPP-IV. The incretin mimetics enhance glucose-dependent insulin secretion, suppress elevated glucagon secretion, and slow gastric emptying. Currently, there are four incretin mimetics: exenatide, (Byetta, Bydureon), dulaglutide, (Trulicity), liraglutide (Victoza), and albiglutide (Tanzeum), all of which are pregnancy category C.

Indications

Exenatide was approved by the FDA in 2005 as the first incretin mimetic drug. Exenatide is a long-acting analogue of GLP-1 that was initially derived from the salivary gland of the Gila monster. All incretin mimemtics are available only as a subcutaneous injection and indicated only for patients with type 2 diabetes who have been unable to achieve blood glucose control with metformin, a sulfonylurea, and/or a glitazone. Concomitant use with insulin is not routinely recommended; however, the combination is currently under investigation. Incretin mimetics are best given 60 minutes before a meal Dulaglutide and albiglutide are given only once a week, where as exenatide and liraglutide are given daily.

Contraindications

Contraindications include hypersensitivity to the drug or any component of the formulations; history or family history of medullary thyroid carcinoma and patients with multiple endocrine neoplasia syndrome type 2.

Adverse Effects

The incretin mimetics share a black box warning for the risk of developing thyroid C-cell tumors. Adverse effects include nausea, vomiting, and diarrhea. Rare cases of hemorrhagic or necrotizing pancreatitis have also been reported. Patients may experience weight loss of 5 to 10 pounds.

Interactions

The incretin mimetics can delay absorption of other orally administered drugs by slowing gastric emptying. In patients taking sulfonylurea drugs, the dose may need to be reduced if hypoglycemia appears.

Dosages

The usual starting dosage of exenatide is 5 mcg within 1 hour of both the morning and evening meals. If necessary, the dosage may be increased after 1 month to 10 mcg twice daily before meals. The dose of liraglutide is 0.6 mg titrated up to 1.2 or 1.8 mg daily. Dulaglutide is dosed as 0.75 mg once weekly and may be increased to 1.5 mg once weekly. Albiglutide is dosed at 30 mg once weekly and may be titrated to 50 mg weekly.

DRUG PROFILE

♦liraglutide

Liraglutide (Victoza) is an incretin mimetic drug. The incretin mimetics enhance glucose-dependent insulin secretion, suppress elevated glucagon secretion, and slow gastric emptying. Liraglutide is administered subcutaneously and is given once a day.

Pharmacokinetics: Liraglutide

Route	Onset of Action	Peak Plasma Concentration	Elimination Half-life	Duration of Action
Subcutaneous	3 minutes	8-12 hours	13 hours	24 hours

SODIUM GLUCOSE COTRANSORTER INHIBITORS (SGLT2 INHIBITORS)

Mechanism of Action and Drug Effects

Approximately 180 g of glucose is filtered by the kidney daily. Most of this glucose is reabsorbed into the circulation via sodium glucose–linked cotransporters (SGLTs). SGLTs transport sodium and glucose into cells using sodium/potassium ATPase pumps and are responsible for 90% of glucose reabsorption. Inhibition of SGLT2 leads to a decrease in blood glucose due to an increase in renal glucose excretion.

The SGLT2 inhibitors are a new class of oral drugs for the treatment of type 2 diabetes mellitus. They inhibit glucose reabsorption in the proximal renal tubules. They work independently of insulin to prevent glucose reabsorption, which results glycosuria. They may also increase insulin sensitivity and glucose uptake in the muscle cells and decrease gluconeogeneisis. Their use in clinical practice is associated with improved glycemic control, weight loss, and a low risk for hypoglycemia.

There are several SGLT2 inhibitors currently under development including ipragliflozin and tofogliflozin. Canagliflozin (Invokana), dapagliflozin (Farxiga), and empagliflozin (Jardiance) are the three that are currently FDA approved at the time of this writing. They are all classified as pregnancy category C drugs.

Indications

The SGLT2 inhibitors are indicated for type 2 diabetes mellitus. They can be used as monotherapy or can be used in combination with other drugs.

Contraindications

These drugs are contraindicated in diabetic ketoacidosis and in moderate to severe kidney impairment.

Adverse Effects

The most common adverse effects include genital yeast infections, urinary tract infections, and increased urination. The most serious adverse effects include hypotension, hypovolemia, hyperkalemia, and an increase in LDL cholesterol. In 2015, the FDA issued a class warning regarding the risk of ketoacidosis with the SGLT2 inhibitors.

Interactions

Rifampin can decrease effects of these drugs. Hypoglycemia can occur when used with other antidiabetic drugs.

Dosages

Canagliflozin (Invokana) is dosed as 100 to 300 mg daily. Dapafliflozin (Farxiga) is dosed as 5 to 10 mg daily. Empagliflozin (Jardiance) is dosed as 10 to 25 mg daily. All drugs are to be given in the morning and should not be used in patients with renal impairment.

GLUCOSE-ELEVATING DRUGS

Hypoglycemia is an abnormally low blood glucose level (generally below 70 mg/dL). When the cause is organic and the effects are mild, treatment usually consists of dietary modifications (a higher intake of protein and lower intake of carbohydrates) to prevent a rebound postprandial hypoglycemic effect. Hypoglycemia is also a common adverse effect of many antidiabetic drugs when their pharmacologic effects are greater than expected. Because the brain needs a constant amount of glucose to function, early symptoms of hypoglycemia include the central nervous system (CNS) manifestations of confusion, irritability, tremor, and sweating. Later symptoms include hypothermia and seizures. Without adequate restoration of normal blood and CNS glucose levels, coma and death will occur.

Oral forms of concentrated glucose are available for patients to use in the event of a hypoglycemic crisis. Dosage forms include rapidly dissolving buccal tablets and semisolid gel forms designed for oral use and rapid mucosal absorption. Table sugar, which is sucrose, will not produce as rapid an effect as the glucose products. This is because sucrose is a disaccharide (two-molecule) sugar that must first be digested in the body to yield glucose as a monosaccharide (one-molecule) by-product. In the hospital setting or when the patient is unconscious, intravenous glucose is an obvious option to treat hypoglycemia. Concentrations of up to 50% dextrose in water ($D_{50}W$) are most often used for this purpose.

In addition to oral and/or intravenous glucose, glucagon, a natural hormone secreted by the pancreas, is available as a subcutaneous injection to be given when a quick response to severe hypoglycemia is needed. Because glucagon injection may induce vomiting, roll an unconscious patient onto his or her side before injection. Glucagon is useful in the unconscious hypoglycemic patient without established intravenous access.

TEAMWORK AND COLLABORATION: PHARMACOKINETIC BRIDGE TO NURSING PRACTICE   **QSEN**

Continuous subcutaneous insulin infusion has been used in patients with type 1 diabetes for over a quarter of a century and is increasing. Provision of insulin therapy by continuous subcutaneous insulin infusion (CSII) is becoming an option for selected diabetic patients in an attempt to minimize the risks and complications of the disease. One previously used option for achieving tight control of blood glucose levels was multiple daily injections of insulin (MDI). With CSII, normal serum glucose levels are maintained by the continuous delivery of basal insulin, and then with food intake—primarily carbohydrate consumption—bolus doses of insulin are given. Use of an insulin pump (i.e., CSII) leads to a more rapid, consistent absorption of the drug and a reduction in the occurrence of hypoglycemia. Research has also shown that use of an insulin pump helps to decrease the occurrence of elevated prebreakfast serum glucose levels, often called the *dawn phenomenon* (referring to the dawn of the day). Because the insulin pump delivers insulin through the subcutaneous route and the infusion is a continuous one, fewer problems occur than with once- or twice-daily injections. Patients using CSII achieve mean serum glucose and A1C levels that remain somewhat lower than those associated with MDI, so that the risk for hypoglycemia is decreased. Understanding new and different drugs and their pharmacokinetic properties allows you to help patients achieve a better quality of life, minimize risks, and maximize wellness.

NURSING PROCESS

ASSESSMENT

Before administering any type of *antidiabetic drug*, assess the patient's knowledge about the disease and recommended treatment. Perform a complete head-to-toe physical assessment and nursing assessment, including a thorough medication history with attention to the patient's listing of all current medications including over-the-counter drugs, herbal products, and supplements. With *insulin*, as well as other antidiabetic drugs, review the appropriate laboratory test results (e.g., fasting blood glucose level, A1C level) for any abnormalities compared with baseline levels. Assess the prescriber's order for insulin, paying close attention to the use of the correct drug, route, type of insulin (i.e., *rapid-acting, short-acting, intermediate-acting, short-* and *intermediate-acting mixtures, long-acting*), and dosage. Assess the specific insulin, with attention to the specific pharmacokinetics such as onset of action, peak, and duration of action. Knowing this information prior to giving the insulin is key to patient safety because these drug properties actually define parameters within which reactions, adverse effects, or problems versus therapeutic effects potentially occur. If more than one insulin type is prescribed, mixing of insulins may be ordered. It is important for you to know the chemically compatible combinations (see Table 32-4) so as to avoid an undesirable altered glycemic effect. Additionally, with all insulin orders, perform a second check of the prepared insulin dosage against the medication order with another registered nurse, or perform per health care institution policy and document.

Assess blood glucose levels prior to administering insulin to avoid giving the drug to a patient who is already hypoglycemic. The 2015 ADA guidelines identify the current key diagnostic criterion for diabetes mellitus as hyperglycemia with a fasting plasma glucose level of higher than 126 mg/dL or a hemoglobin A1C level greater than 6.5% (see Box 32-1 for more detail on diagnostic indicators). Furthermore, the ADA recommends the following control criteria for the diabetic patient: fasting blood glucose within the range of 70 to 130 mg/dL and/or a hemoglobin A1C less than 7%. Keep in mind that allergic reactions are less likely to occur with *recombinant human insulins* because of their similarity with endogenous insulin; however, allergies may still occur and have to be considered in the assessment. Contraindications and cautions associated with *insulin* have been previously discussed. Significant drug interactions are presented in Table 32-5, but it is important to remember that the drugs that work against the effect of insulin include corticosteroids, thyroid drugs, and diuretics. Drugs that increase the hypoglycemic effects of insulin include alcohol, sulfa antibiotics, and salicylates. Assess the medication order for all insulins, especially the U-500 insulin. This dose must be administered with great caution. Contraindications with the use of *Afrezza*, a newer *rapid-acting insulin*, that is administered via inhaled dosage form, include individuals who smoke and those with chronic asthma and chronic obstructive pulmonary disease. Afrezza also carries a black-box warning about the risk for acute bronchospasms.

Oral antidiabetic drugs also require close assessment for contraindications, cautions, and drug interactions, so obtain a thorough medication and patient history. Make sure to know the patient's history because type 2 diabetes can be treated with oral antidiabetic drugs, most of which require functioning beta cells in the pancreas. Functioning beta cells are not present in type 1 diabetes. With *biguanides,* be aware that older adult or malnourished patients may react adversely to this group of drugs. Contraindications, cautions, and interactions for this drug class have been previously discussed, but it is important to patient safety to emphasize the interaction between *metformin* and the iodine-containing radiologic contrast media used for certain diagnostic purposes (e.g., computed tomography with contrast). This interaction is associated with an increased risk for acute renal failure and lactic acidosis. If the patient is taking metformin, closely assess and monitor for this scenario so that the metformin may be discontinued on the day of the test and for at least 48 hours afterward. See Table 32-5 for more drug interactions associated with the *oral antidiabetic drugs.*

With *sulfonylureas,* it is important to know baseline glucose levels as well as conditions that may predispose the patient to hypoglycemia, such as a drop in caloric intake, alcohol use, or advanced age. Assessment of allergic reaction to sulfonamide antibiotics is important, as well, because of a potential for cross-allergic reactions. With *glinides,* cautions, contraindications, and drug interactions are similar to those for sulfonylureas. The *thiazolidinediones (glitazones)* have a black box warning indicating they can cause or exacerbate heart failure and are not recommended for use in patients with symptomatic heart failure.

With *alpha-glucosidase inhibitors* (e.g., *acarbose, miglitol*), assess for contraindications, such as inflammatory bowel disease or malabsorption syndromes. With *second-generation sulfonylureas,* assess the patient's type of diabetes because these drugs are contraindicated in type 1 diabetes.

The *amylin mimetics,* such as *pramlintide,* are contraindicated in patients with gastroparesis or in patients who are taking medications that alter gastrointestinal (GI) motility. Assessing for the type of diabetes is important because pramlintide is indicated for both patients with type 1 or type 2 diabetes with particular mealtime needs and who are not able to achieve optimal blood glucose level control with insulin. *Exenatide,* an *incretin mimetic,* requires assessment of the patient's diagnosis because the drug is used for patients with type 2 diabetes and an inability to control blood glucose levels with *metformin,* a *sulfonylurea,* and/or a *glitazone.* It should not be used with insulin.

The newest class of oral drugs include *empagliflozin, ipragliflozin, canagliflozin,* and *dapagliflozin* and may be used alone or in combination with other drugs. Assess for contraindications such as impaired kidney function and diabetic ketoacidosis. Drug interactions include rifampin, which may lead to decreased drug effectiveness. Assess for use with other antidiabetic drugs because of possible hypoglycemia.

With diabetes mellitus, unstable serum glucose levels require immediate attention, so assess the patient for any signs and symptoms of hypoglycemia (e.g., acute onset of confusion, irritability, tremor, and sweating, with progression to possible hypothermia and seizures, and blood glucose level of less than 50 mg/dL) or of hyperglycemia (e.g., polyuria, polydipsia, polyphagia, glucosuria, weight loss, and fatigue, with a fasting blood glucose level of 126 mg/dL or higher or a nonfasting blood glucose level of 200 mg/dL or higher). Assessment is even more critical for a diabetic patient who is also under stress, has an infection or is ill, is pregnant or lactating, or is experiencing trauma or any serious change in health status. With treatment, diabetic patients are at risk for hypoglycemia with the potential danger of loss of consciousness; therefore, constantly assess serum glucose levels and neurologic status. Along with assessment of the therapeutic regimen and patient adherence to treatment, note any cultural factors, socioeconomic factors, and family support, and follow throughout therapy.

Glucose-elevating drugs are to be given only after thorough assessment of the patient's presenting clinical picture and a thorough collection of data, including laboratory values, medication and patient history, as well as a list of current medications. Assess for level of consciousness as well because *glucagon* injection may induce vomiting, and precautions must be implemented to prevent aspiration.

NURSING DIAGNOSES

1. Imbalanced nutrition, less than body requirements, related to the body's inability to use glucose (for type 1)
2. Ineffective family health management related to lack of experience with a significant daily treatment regimen of diabetes mellitus

CASE STUDY

Patient-Centered Care: Diabetes Mellitus: Lispro Insulin

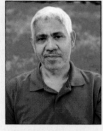 B.G., age 58, was diagnosed with type 2 adult-onset diabetes mellitus 10 years ago. Although he has type 2 diabetes mellitus, he has needed to take insulin for the last 2 years. He has been recovering, without complications, from a laparoscopic chole-cystectomy, but his blood glucose levels have shown some wide fluctuations over the past 24 hours. The physician has changed B.G.'s insulin from regular to lispro (Humalog) to see if it will provide better control of his blood glucose levels.

1. Before his surgery, B.G.'s hemoglobin A1C level was 9%. What does this value imply regarding his glycemic control?
2. While reviewing the instructions for the lispro insulin, B.G. states, "I took my regular insulin shots about 30 minutes before my meals. Hopefully I can keep that same routine." How will the nurse respond to this statement?
3. After his discharge, B.G. wakes up one morning feeling nauseated. He gives himself the lispro insulin injection, but then after eating breakfast he vomits and cannot keep any food down. What must he do at this time?

For answers, see *http://evolve.elsevier.com/Lilley.*

QSEN ⚡ **SAFETY AND QUALITY IMPROVEMENT: PREVENTING MEDICATION ERRORS**

Insulin Pens Are for Single-Patient Use Only

The Institute for Safe Medication Practices (ISMP) has received numerous reports of hospital staff using a single insulin pen for multiple patients. It is thought that there is a widespread misunderstanding that sterility can be maintained between patients by using a fresh, sterile needle on the pen device for each use. However, several studies have reported that the possibility of cross-contamination exists when a single pen is used for multiple patients.

This problem has been reported for several years, despite efforts to educate about the proper use of insulin pens. As a result, the ISMP has recommended that hospitals consider moving away from using these pens, which were originally designed for outpatient use. If they are used in the inpatient setting, insulin pens need to be labeled with a specific patient's information in a manner that does not cover the drug name.

For more information, see the Centers for Disease Control and Prevention's clinical reminder at *www.cdc.gov/injectionsafety/ clinical-reminders/insulin-pens.html.* Also see the Institute for Safe Medication Practices website at *www.ismp.org/newsletters/ acutecare/showarticle.aspx?id=41.* Accessed September 25, 2014.

---

3. Risk for injury related to unstable glucose levels with onset of possible signs and symptoms of diabetes mellitus

PLANNING: OUTCOME IDENTIFICATION

1. Patient maintains adequate, balanced nutrition while adhering to the diet recommended by the ADA or other dietary advisor per the orders of the prescriber or nutritional consultant.
2. Patient and family report increase in therapeutic regimen management as noted by support (by family), keeping all scheduled appointments with the prescriber to monitor therapeutic effectiveness, diet, and lifestyle change implementation and awareness for the complications of therapy.
3. Patient avoids injury by maintaining targeted goal (70 to 130 mg/dL and/or hemoglobin A1C less than 7%) of fasting blood glucose levels (fasting is considered to be no food/meals/snacks for at least 8 hours) with reporting of signs and symptoms of hyperglycemia or hypoglycemia.

IMPLEMENTATION

With any patient who is taking *insulin* (or *oral antidiabetic drugs*), always check serum glucose levels (and other related laboratory values, as ordered) before giving the drug so that accurate baseline glucose levels are obtained and documented. Do not shake *NPH* (cloudy) and *premixed insulin mixtures*, but roll between the hands before administering the prescribed dose. The rolling helps to avoid air in the syringe and inaccurate dose administration. Administer insulins at room temperature. Insulin may be stored at room temperature if used within 1 month; otherwise, refrigeration is needed. Refrigeration is also recommended in warm or hot climates and with any major changes in environmental temperatures from cold to hot. Never use expired or discolored insulin. Box 32-2 contains more information about the administration, handling, mixing, and storage of insulin.

Administer insulin subcutaneously at a 90-degree angle unless the patient is emaciated, in which case you may give the insulin at a 45-degree angle. Only *regular insulin* may be administered intravenously and is often used in intensive care settings. Only use insulin syringes for subcutaneous injections or when drawing up insulin dosage amounts. These syringes are easy to identify because of their orange caps and calibration in units, not milliliters. These syringes have preattached needles that are 29 gauge and ½ inch in length. When *insulins* are mixed (if ordered), withdraw the *regular* or *rapid-acting insulin* (unmodified and clear) first, followed by withdrawing the *intermediate-acting* or *NPH insulin* (modified and cloudy). Only do this after the appropriate amount of air has been injected into the vials. The amount of air to inject into the vials equals the prescribed number of units. Inject air into the intermediate-acting insulin vial first. Next, inject air into the regular or rapid- or short-acting insulin vial. This technique helps keep the intermediate-acting insulin from contaminating the rapid-acting insulin vial. This contamination would lead to a change in the *regular, short-acting, unmodified insulin* by the *NPH, intermediate-acting, modified insulin.* The net effect is an interference of the activity of the regular insulin (no longer considered modified), thus impacting its effect in the patient (see Table 32-4 and Chapter 9).

Understanding the action of the insulin and its related pharmacokinetics (e.g., onset, peak, duration) is critical for safe care and patient education. For example, it is important to know that the *rapid-acting insulins* (*insulin lispro, insulin aspart,* and *insulin glulisine*) have an onset of action of about 15 minutes and must be given at least 15 minutes before meals, compared with 30 minutes before meals for regular insulin or a short-acting

BOX 32-2   Administration, Handling, and Storage of Insulin

Dosages, Storage, Handling, and Mixing

1. Individualize insulin dosages, and monitor closely for adequate control of hypoglycemia and hyperglycemia. Follow guidelines for basal/bolus insulin therapy or sliding scale, depending on specific regimen identified in the hospital setting.

2. Adjust dosages, as ordered, to achieve the prescriber's specific fasting blood glucose level for the patient. Using the ADA 2012 guidelines, this would be a fasting blood glucose level of 70 to 130 mg/dL and/or hemoglobin A1C less than 7% for the diabetic patient.

3. Store insulin for current use at room temperature. Avoid extreme temperatures and exposure to sunlight, because the insulin's protein structure will be permanently denatured. Extra vials not in use may be kept in the refrigerator. Vials being used in high environmental temperatures need to be stored in the refrigerator, but never give cold insulin. Never freeze insulin. To maintain drug stability, only store insulin for up to 1 month at room temperature or up to 3 months in the refrigerator.

4. Discard unused vials if they have not been used for several weeks (or follow institutional policy). Do not use any insulin that does not have the proper clarity or color (e.g., clear for regular, cloudy for NPH).

5. Store prefilled insulin syringes in the refrigerator for up to 1 week.

6. Always check expiration dates of insulin and all equipment.

Administration

1. Administer insulin subcutaneously (see Chapter 9); however, regular insulin may be given intravenously in special situations (e.g., intravenous drip in patient with diabetic ketoacidosis; in postoperative patients) if ordered.

2. Roll the cloudy drug vial gently between the hands without shaking to avoid bubble formation in the vial, which may lead to inaccurate dosage withdrawal. Give freshly mixed insulins within 5 minutes of mixing to avoid binding of the solution and subsequent altered activity of the drugs.

3. Administer insulin at the recommended times, but always with meals or meal trays ready. Give insulin lispro and other rapid-acting insulins approximately at least 15 minutes before meals (it has a quicker onset of action) and only after monitoring the patient's fasting serum glucose level (as with all insulin administration). Give regular insulin (short-acting insulin) 30 minutes before meals, and NPH intermediate insulin 30 to 60 minutes before meals.

4. When giving regular and NPH insulin at the same time (if ordered), mix the two appropriately (see discussion of mixing insulins in the Implementation subsection under Nursing Process earlier in the chapter).

5. Administer insulin subcutaneously at a 90-degree angle. However, if the patient is emaciated, the injection may be given at a 45-degree angle. Only use insulin syringes (see text discussion and Chapter 9).

6. Instruct patients using insulin injections to rotate sites within the same general location for about 1 week before moving to a new location (e.g., all injections for a week in the upper right thigh before moving a little lower on the right thigh). This technique allows for better insulin absorption. Each injection site should be at least ½ to 1 inch away from the previous injection site. If this practice is followed, it will be approximately 6 weeks before the patient will have to rotate to a totally new area of the body. Note the following sites for subcutaneous insulin injections: thigh areas (front and back), outer areas of the upper arm (middle third of the upper arm between the shoulder and the elbow), and the abdominal area using the iliac crests as landmarks and using the fatty part of the abdomen, but not within 2 inches of the umbilicus or an incision/stoma (see Chapter 9).

7. Continuous subcutaneous insulin infusion and/or multiple daily injections may be ordered for tight glucose control.

---

insulin, which has an onset of action of 30 to 60 minutes. Additionally, if giving the newer insulin, *Afrezza,* it is given via inhaled dosage form. It is a *rapid-acting inhaled insulin* that is prescribed to give prior to meals or within 20 minutes of starting a meal. It is not a substitute for *long-acting insulin* and is to be used in combination with long-acting insulin in patients with type 1 diabetes. Because it is inhaled, it is absorbed quickly and peaks in the serum in about 15 to 20 minutes, with a duration of action of about 2 to 3 hours. It has not become common use at the time of writing this edition. If *lispro insulin* is to be mixed with *NPH (intermediate-acting) insulin,* give the *combination* 15 minutes before meals. Always double-check the prescriber's orders for clarification of the dosage and drug as well as of any change in dietary intake, such as a possible increase in carbohydrates and decrease in fat to avoid postprandial hypoglycemia. A meal high in fat can delay carbohydrate absorption while rapid-acting insulin is already in its peak action.

Regardless of the specific type of *recombinant human insulin* used, understanding the peak, onset, and duration of action of the *insulin* to be used (e.g., *rapid-acting* versus *short-acting* versus *intermediate-acting* versus *long-acting*) will help determine when food or meals are to be given. The *intermediate-acting insulin (NPH)* has an onset of action of 1 to 2 hours, so serve meals at least 30 to 45 minutes prior to its administration. Many combination products of rapid- and short-acting with intermediate-acting insulin are available; give these combination insulins 15 to 30 minutes before meals. In the hospital setting, be sure that meal trays have arrived on the unit before giving insulin to avoid time lapses and subsequent hypoglycemic episodes. Also be sure that other forms of allowed foods are available to the patient in case meals are delayed and insulin has already been administered. If *U-500* insulin is prescribed, a multilayered, multidisciplinary process is recommended to safeguard every step of the medication administration process. A two-pharmacist order-entry process may be used, with the pharmacist hand delivering the dose to the charge nurse and bedside nurse. Use of at least a three-time check of the medication order is also needed at this time.

Patients may require dosing by a sliding-scale or a basal-bolus method in a hospital setting. Sliding scale has historically been the method for administering subcutaneous regular insulin doses adjusted according to serum glucose test results. Although controversial (see previous pharmacology discussion), sliding-scale dosing may be used for hospitalized diabetic patients experiencing drastic changes in serum glucose levels due to physical and/or emotional stress, infections, surgery, acute illness, inactivity, or variable caloric intake, as well as for patients needing intensive insulin therapy or patients—even if nondiabetic—receiving total parenteral nutrition (TPN) with a high glucose concentration. When this insulin regimen is used, measure blood glucose levels several times per day (e.g., every

4 hours, every 6 hours, or at specified times such as 7 AM, 11 AM, 4 PM, and midnight) to obtain fasting and/or premeal blood glucose values. The newer method, basal-bolus *insulin* dosing, is now the preferred method of treatment for hospitalized diabetic patients; orders for the dosages and frequency will be issued by the prescriber. A *long-acting insulin (insulin glargine)* is used to mimic the basal secretion of a healthy pancreas and constant delivery of an amount of insulin, and then the bolus is used (*insulin lispro* or *insulin apart*) to control increases in daily blood glucose levels. Bolus insulin is divided into meal and correction boluses (see the pharmacology discussion). Monitor blood glucose levels frequently when using these methods.

Oral antidiabetic drugs are usually given at least 30 minutes before meals, as ordered. With any antidiabetic drug or insulin, it is important for both you and the patient to know what to do if symptoms of hypoglycemia occur—for example, the patient needs to take glucagon; eat glucose tablets or gel, corn syrup, or honey; drink fruit juice or a nondiet soft drink; or eat a small snack such as crackers or half a sandwich. If the patient receiving *metformin* is to undergo diagnostic studies with contrast dye, the prescriber will need to discontinue the drug prior to the procedure and restart it after the tests, but only after reevaluation of the patient's renal status. During therapy with metformin, the risk for lactic acidosis is possible, so it is important to monitor for and then report hyperventilation, cold and clammy skin, muscle pain, abdominal pain, dizziness, and irregular heartbeat. Some of the *sulfonylureas* are to be taken with breakfast; the *alpha-glucosidase inhibitors* are always taken with the first bite of each main meal, and the *thiazolidinediones* are given once daily or in two divided doses. Always check the exact timing of the dose against the prescriber's order and with consideration of the drug's onset of action.

It is critical to the safe and efficient use of oral antidiabetics to be sure that food will be or is being tolerated before the dose is given. If the oral drug is taken and no meal is consumed or it is consumed at a later time than usual, hypoglycemia may be problematic and result in negative health consequences and even unconsciousness. Because the *glitazones* (e.g., *rosiglitazone, pioglitazone*) may both cause moderate weight gain and edema, it is important to weigh the patient daily at the same time every day and in the same amount of clothing. Several combination oral antidiabetic drug products are available (see the pharmacology discussion) and need to be given exactly as prescribed. *Pramlintide* needs to be given before any major meal. *Exenatide* is given by subcutaneous injection in patients with type 2 diabetes and cannot be used with insulin. *Sitagliptin* is not to be used with insulin and may be taken with or without food. With use of the newer drugs *SGLT2 inhibitors*, administer as prescribed, which is usually in the morning prior to the first meal.

In special situations, such as when the patient has been ordered to have nothing by mouth (NPO status) and is taking either an oral antidiabetic drug or insulin, it is crucial to follow the prescriber's orders regarding drug administration. If there are no written orders about this situation, contact the prescriber for further instructions. If a patient is on NPO status but is receiving an intravenous solution of dextrose, the prescriber

may still order insulin, but always clarify this (with the prescriber). Contact the prescriber if a patient becomes ill and unable to take the usual dosage of an oral antidiabetic drug (or insulin). Encourage the patient to always wear a medical alert bracelet or necklace giving the diagnosis, list of medications, and emergency contact information.

It is also very important to stay informed and up to date about the latest research on diabetes and to keep patients and family members well informed. For example, as previously discussed in the pharmacology section, macrovascular and microvascular problems are now being recognized to occur at fasting blood glucose levels as low as 126 mg/dL. See the Evidence-Based Practice box on the next page for more information on specific nursing research.

In summary, there are many nursing considerations related to drug therapy in patients with diabetes mellitus. Patient education is also very important and needs to begin the moment the patient has entered into the health care system or upon diagnosis. Instruction that is tailored to the patient's educational level and that uses appropriate teaching-learning concepts and teaching aids is important to patient adherence with the treatment regimen. In addition, be sure that all necessary resources are made available to patients (e.g., financial assistance, visual assistance, dietary plans, daily menus, ADA information, transportation assistance, and Meals on Wheels and other community services). See Patient Centered Care: Patient Teaching on the next page for more information.

EVALUATION

It is important to understand current therapeutic guidelines. The prevailing key diagnostic criterion for diabetes mellitus is hyperglycemia with a fasting blood glucose level of 126 mg/dL or higher or a nonfasting blood glucose level of 200 mg/dL or higher; however, the therapeutic response to *insulin* and any of the *oral antidiabetic drugs* is a decrease in blood glucose to the level prescribed by the prescriber or to near-normal levels. Most often, fasting blood glucose levels are used to measure the degree of glycemic control. To provide a picture of the patient's adherence to the therapy regimen for the previous several months, the level of A1C is measured. This value reflects how well the patient has been doing with diet and drug therapy. Patients with diabetes need to be monitored frequently by their prescribers (as well as at home) to make sure they are adhering to the therapy regimen as evidenced by normalization of blood test results. It is important to monitor the patient for indications of hypoglycemia or hyperglycemia and insulin allergy as well. With *short-acting insulins* such as *lispro*, the onset of action is more rapid than with *regular insulin* and the duration of action is shorter, so monitor blood glucose levels very closely until the dosage is regulated and blood glucose is at the level the prescriber desires. If a patient is switched from one insulin or oral antidiabetic drug to another, advise the patient that glucose levels must be monitored very closely at home or by the prescriber. Always evaluate whether identified goals and outcome criteria are being met, and plan nursing care accordingly.

EVIDENCE-BASED PRACTICE

Sensor-Augmented Insulin Pump Therapy Trumps Multiple Daily Injections

Review

In patients with type 1 diabetes and poor glycemic control, a sensor-augmented insulin pump is significantly improving glycated hemoglobin levels as compared with regimens with multiple daily insulin injections. This research was presented at the American Diabetes Association 70th Scientific Session on June 29, 2010. Research has confirmed that the use of these pumps has demonstrated more effective control than the use of multiple daily injections.

Type of Evidence

Some 329 adults and 156 children were randomly assigned to either pump therapy with the MiniMed Paradigm REAL-Time system (Medtronic) or to continue with their regimen of multiple daily injections under close supervision for the duration of the study, which lasted for 1 year. Patients in the study received intensive diabetes management education and training including carbohydrate counting and the administration of correction doses of insulin. Once patients were randomized to insulin pump therapy, they were placed on it for 2 weeks. After they had become comfortable with the pump, the glucose sensor was added. This group used the insulin aspart, and the injection therapy group used both insulin aspart and insulin glargine. All patients were seen at 3, 6, 9, and 12 months and used CareLink, a diabetes-management software program. This program was used to relay the patients' glucose data to communicate with their health care providers from home. It is important to know that the sensor-augmented pump therapy uses the two technologies of an insulin pump and continuous glucose monitoring all in one system. This pump allows patients and their providers to monitor treatment and their response through Internet-based software. The patients needed to have computer access to participate in the study.

Results of the Study

At 1 year, the researchers found that the patients on pump therapy had hemoglobin A1C levels that were significantly lower than the injection-therapy group. The baseline mean glycated hemoglobin level, which was 8.3% in the two groups, decreased to 7.5% in the pump therapy group as compared to 8.1% in the injection therapy group. Among the adults, the absolute reduction in the mean glycated hemoglobin level was 1.0% ± 0.7% in the pump-therapy group and 0.4% ± 0.8% in the injection-therapy group. The between-group difference in the pump-therapy group was −0.6%. The occurrence of hypoglycemia and diabetic ketoacidosis was similar in both groups. There was no significant weight gain in adult or child participants.

Link of Evidence to Nursing Practice

This study has been identified as one of the longest and largest randomized controlled studies of sensor-augmented insulin pump therapy in type 1 diabetic patients. Another significant point to this study was the comparison of two therapeutic approaches. For nursing and for the care of diabetic patients, the impact of this study is important in that patients may be able to achieve better control of their diabetes with improved outcomes and safety. Having the positive results without the occurrence of increased hypoglycemia represents even larger breakthroughs in the care of these patients as well as the possibility of increased adherence to treatment. This study holds great promise in the treatment of type 1 diabetic patients and for evidenced-based nursing practice. The possibility of enhanced quality of life and prevention of complications in the treatment of patients with chronic illnesses, such as type 1 diabetes, is truly exciting and promising.

Reference: Bergenstal RM, Tamborlane WV, Ahmann A, et al: Effectiveness of sensor-augmented insulin-pump therapy in type 1 diabetes, *N Engl J Med* 363(4):311-320, 2010.

PATIENT-CENTERED CARE: PATIENT TEACHING

- Encourage the patient to keep medical alert jewelry or a medical alert card on his or her person at all times. In the home environment, all medical information must be kept in clear view on the refrigerator with pertinent information highlighted in some fashion.
- Provide instructions and demonstrations regarding the proper storage of insulin, equipment needed for administration, drawing up and/or mixing of insulins (if ordered), technique for insulin injections, and rotation of subcutaneous insulin injection sites. Be prepared to always provide opportunities for return demonstrations from the patient, including rotation of sites (See Chapter 9 for more information about insulin injections). Emphasize that insulin may be stored at room temperature unless the heat is extreme or the patient is traveling. Educate about the need to have serum glucose levels monitored, as prescribed. Emphasize instructions that are specific to the patient's particular glucometer. Stress the importance of exercise, hygiene, foot care, dietary plan, and weight control in the management of diabetes. Keeping a daily journal including information about daily dietary intake, serum glucose levels, and a description of how the patient is feeling and any complaints will be beneficial to those monitoring the patient's progress and/or compliance.

- Patients need thorough information about the anticipated costs of diabetes and a listing of financial resources. People with diagnosed diabetes, on average, have medical expenditures approximately 2.3 times higher than those individuals without diabetes or about $11,744 per year. Blood glucose monitoring may cost over $1 for each check. Expenses can add up quickly, especially for those who are economically and medical insurance disadvantaged. For more information, visit *www.diabetes.org/advocacy/news-events/cost-of -diabetes.html#sthash.51EqlTjK.dpuf*. A listing of financial and other resources is available at *http://diabetes.niddk .nih.gov/dm/pubs/financialhelp/#15* (accessed May 22, 2014). This list includes but is not limited to Medicare, SHIP (State Health Insurance Assistance Program), Social Security Administration, Medicaid, Bureau of Primary Health Care, Hill-Burton Act, Amputee Coalition of America, Easter Seals, and the U.S. Department of Agriculture's Women, Infants, and Children (WIC) program.
- Emphasize the importance of A1C monitoring. The American Diabetes Association recommends monitoring at least two times per year for patients with good glycemic control and every quarter for those who are not reaching target values, have changed their therapy, or are not compliant with their therapeutic regimen (Table 32-6).

TABLE 32-6   Diabetes Care: Correlation of Glycosylated Hemoglobin Levels with Mean Serum Glucose Levels

Hemoglobin A1C (%)	Mean Serum Glucose Level (mg/dL)
6	126
7	154
8	183
9	212
10	240
11	269
12	298

Data from American Diabetes Association: Standards of medical care in diabetes 2015, *Diabetes Care* 38(Suppl 1): 2015.

- Review lifestyle modifications, including weight control and glucose level maintenance with diet, exercise, and/or drug therapy. Make appropriate referrals so that the patient, family, and or significant others are educated thoroughly regarding the disease process and treatment recommendations. Family must be included and "on-board" to enhance compliance. Remember that patients with type 2 diabetes have a greater therapeutic response to diet and exercise and glucose level control as compared to patients with type 1 diabetes.

- A nutritional consult with specific menu planning may help the patient with changes in dietary intake (e.g., low-fat diet with 160 to 300 g of carbohydrates). The ADA encourages use of the "Create Your Plate" method of meal planning. The plate is divided into three sections using an imaginary line down the middle of the plate. One side of the plate provides for larger portions of nonstarchy vegetables. The other side of the plate is further divided into two equal sections that are filled with starchy foods and protein. Non-starchy vegetables include spinach, carrots, greens, bok choy, and broccoli; starchy foods include whole-grain breads, high-fiber cereal, oatmeal, cooked beans, and peas. The remaining small section is to be filled with protein such as chicken or turkey without the skin, tuna, and/or salmon. A serving of fruit and/or a serving of dairy is to be added.

- Advise the patient to avoid smoking and alcohol consumption (with oral antidiabetic drugs) and maintain strict adherence to dietary instructions. Instruct the patient to avoid skipping meals or skipping doses of insulin or oral antidiabetic drugs, and to contact the prescriber for further instructions when needed.

- Explain the difference between hypoglycemia and hyperglycemia (see earlier discussion for specific signs and symptoms), with emphasis on the treatment of each (e.g., having on hand quick sources of glucose, such as candy, sugar packets, over-the-counter glucose tablets, sugar cubes, honey, corn syrup, orange juice, or nondiet soda beverages for hypoglycemia, and having more insulin on hand for hyperglycemia, as ordered). Encourage the patient to keep quick dosage forms of glucose in possession at all times!

- Share with the patient information about situations or conditions that may lead to altered serum glucose levels, such as fever, illness, stress, increased activity/exercise, surgery, and emotional distress. Encourage the patient to contact the prescriber for any questions or concerns about maintaining glucose control.

- Educate the patient about the importance of knowing premeal serum glucose levels before taking insulin and the importance of timing meals related to the type of insulin.

- Emphasize the importance of having adequate supplies of insulin and equipment at all times and planning ahead for vacations. Instruct the patient to keep all medications and related equipment out of the reach of children. If needed, magnifying attachments are available for syringes and vials. Specialized syringes are available for those with impaired vision. Patients using these types of syringes learn to rely on the sound the syringe makes when a dosage is selected; for example, with the NovoLog pen, 5 clicks equals 5 units.

- Encourage the diabetic patient to report any yellow discoloration of the skin, dark urine, fever, sore throat, weakness, or unusual bleeding or easy bruising.

- With use of rapid-acting Afrezza, educate the patient about its inhaled dosing and that it peaks in 15 to 20 minutes so needs to be taken within 20 minutes prior to meals. It has a short duration of action of 2 to 3 hours. Educate the patient that it will not replace the need for injected long-acting insulin for those who need it. It is used in combination with long-acting insulin in patients with type 1 diabetes. Emphasize the side effects (identified in clinical trials) of hypoglycemia, cough, and throat pain or irritation. Once the drug has an established history of use, more data will become available.

- Emphasize the importance of the American Heart Association recommendations for diabetic patients, including 30 minutes of exercise daily with use of a treadmill, prolonged walking, swimming or aquatic aerobics, bicycling, rowing, chair exercises, arm exercises, and non–weight-bearing exercises. It is recommended to use a pedometer and to exercise for 150 minutes per week.

- Emphasize that therapy will be lifelong and that strict blood glucose control, drug therapy, and lifestyle changes are critical to reducing complications.

- Educate the patient about the need to monitor blood sugar before and after physical exercise to avoid hypoglycemia and adjusting insulin as needed/ordered/directed.

- Stress the need for strict foot care to the patient and those involved in the patient's care. Begin with the need for a daily basic assessment of the feet and toes to check for sores, lesions, cuts, bruises, ingrown toenails, and any other changes. Foot care is needed to enhance circulation and prevent infections. It may include soaking the feet daily or as ordered in lukewarm water (the temperature of the water must be checked), adequate drying of the feet, and then application of moisturizing lotion, and checking the feet and legs for abnormal changes in color (e.g., purplish or reddish discoloration), cool temperature of the feet to the touch, swelling of the extremities or feet, and the appearance of any drainage. Emphasize the importance of contacting the prescriber for further instructions if there is suspicion of any type of wound or alteration in skin integrity. Frequent pedicures and nail trimming by a podiatrist or other licensed, certified individual may be indicated.

- Some of the oral antidiabetic drugs cause photosensitivity. Instruct the patient on wearing protective sunscreen and proper clothing when exposed to the sun. Advise against the use of tanning beds.

KEY POINTS

- Insulin normally facilitates removal of glucose from the blood and its storage as glycogen in the liver.
- Type 1 diabetes mellitus was formerly known as *insulin-dependent diabetes* or *juvenile-onset diabetes*. Little or no endogenous insulin is produced by individuals with type 1 diabetes. It is much less common than type 2 diabetes and affects only about 10% of all diabetic patients. Patients with type 1 diabetes usually are not obese. Because insulin therapy is required for type 1 diabetics, type 1 patients who have the cognitive and financial ability need to be encouraged to consider adding an insulin pump with continuous glucose monitoring as part of their therapy.
- The primary treatment for type 1 diabetes mellitus is insulin therapy. Patients with type 2 diabetes are managed with lifestyle changes (dietary changes, exercise, smoking cessation) and oral drug therapy (one or more drugs). If normal blood glucose levels are not achieved after 2 to 3 months of lifestyle changes, treatment with oral antidiabetic drugs is often added to the regimen.
- Insulin was originally isolated from cattle and pigs, but bovine and porcine insulins are associated with a higher incidence of allergic reactions and insulin resistance than human insulin and are no longer available in the U.S. market.

- Complications associated with diabetes include retinopathy, neuropathy, nephropathy, hypertension, cardiovascular disease, and coronary artery disease. Annual screening with an ophthalmologist specializing in retinopathies is needed in the care of diabetic patients for screening purposes. Because of the renal complications (e.g., nephropathies), annual urinalysis screening and renal function studies are also recommended for diabetic patients.
- All rapid-acting, short-acting, and long-acting insulin preparations are clear solutions. Intermediate-acting insulins are cloudy solutions. Mixtures of short- and intermediate-acting insulins still look uniformly cloudy. The cloudy appearance of these mixtures is due to the presence of the intermediate-acting insulin. Insulin vials are to be rolled in the hands instead of shaken, when used.
- Always carefully check the exact timing of the dose of insulin or oral antidiabetic drug against the prescriber's order. Take into consideration the drug's pharmacokinetics, including onset, peak, and duration of action.
- Nursing care must be individualized with patient education focused on the patient's needs and learning abilities. Include pertinent and age-appropriate information on the disease process, drug therapy, and lifestyle modifications.

NCLEX® EXAMINATION REVIEW QUESTIONS

1. Which is the most appropriate timing regarding the nurse's administration of a rapid-acting insulin to a hospitalized patient?
   a. Give it 15 minutes before the patient begins a meal.
   b. Give it ½ hour before a meal.
   c. Give it 1 hour after a meal.
   d. The timing of the insulin injection does not matter with insulin lispro.

2. Which statement is appropriate for the nurse to include in patient teaching regarding type 2 diabetes?
   a. "Insulin injections are never used with type 2 diabetes."
   b. "You don't need to measure your blood glucose levels because you are not taking insulin injections."
   c. "A person with type 2 diabetes still has functioning beta cells in his or her pancreas."
   d. "Patients with type 2 diabetes usually have better control over their diabetes than those with type 1 diabetes."

3. The nurse monitoring a patient for a therapeutic response to oral antidiabetic drugs will look for
   a. fewer episodes of diabetic ketoacidosis (DKA).
   b. weight loss of 5 pounds.
   c. hemoglobin A1C levels of less than 7%.
   d. glucose levels of 150 mg/dL.

4. A patient with type 2 diabetes is scheduled for magnetic resonance imaging (MRI) with contrast dye. The nurse reviews the orders and notices that the patient is receiving metformin (Glucophage). Which action by the nurse is appropriate?
   a. Proceed with the MRI as scheduled.
   b. Notify the radiology department that the patient is receiving metformin.
   c. Expect to hold the metformin the day of the test and for 48 hours after the test is performed.
   d. Call the prescriber regarding holding the metformin for 2 days before the MRI is performed.

5. A patient with type 2 diabetes has a new prescription for repaglinide (Prandin). After 1 week, she calls the office to ask what to do, because she keeps missing meals. "I work right through lunch sometimes, and I'm not sure whether I need to take it. What do I need to do?" What is the nurse's best response?
   a. "You need to try not to skip meals, but if that happens, you will need to skip that dose of Prandin."
   b. "We will probably need to change your prescription to insulin injections because you can't eat meals on a regular basis."

   c. "Go ahead and take the pill when you first remember that you missed it."

   d. "Take both pills with the next meal, and try to eat a little extra to make up for what you missed at lunchtime."

6. When checking a patient's fingerstick blood glucose level, the nurse obtains a reading of 42 mg/dL. The patient is awake but states he feels a bit "cloudy-headed." After double-checking the patient's glucose level and getting the same reading, which action by the nurse is most appropriate?

   a. Administer two packets of table sugar.

   b. Administer oral glucose in the form of a semisolid gel.

   c. Administer 50% dextrose IV push.

   d. Administer the morning dose of lispro insulin.

7. A patient is taking metformin for new-onset type 2 diabetes mellitus. When reviewing potential adverse effects, the nurse will include information about: *(Select all that apply.)*

   a. Abdominal bloating

   b. Nausea

   c. Diarrhea

   d. Headache

   e. Weight gain

   f. Metallic taste

8. A patient who has a new diagnosis of type 2 diabetes asks the nurse about a new insulin that can be inhaled. "Is there a reason I can't take that drug?" Which condition, if present in the patient, would be a concern?

   a. Atrial fibrillation

   b. Chronic lung disease

   c. Hypothyroidism

   d. Rheumatoid arthritis

1. a, 2. c, 3. c, 4. c, 5. a, 6. b, 7. a, b, c, f, 8. b.

CRITICAL THINKING AND PRIORITIZATION QUESTIONS

1. A 25-year-old woman has been diagnosed with type 1 diabetes mellitus. She has been placed on a 1500-calorie diabetic diet and is to be started on insulin glargine. Today she has received teaching about her diet, about insulin injections, and about management of diabetes. She received the first dose of insulin glargine at 9 PM; the next morning she complained of feeling "dizzy." The nurse assesses that she is diaphoretic, weak, and pale, with a heart rate of 110 beats/min. What is the nurse's priority action at this time? What is the best explanation for these symptoms?

2. A patient with type 2 diabetes comes to the emergency department with an acute asthma attack and pneumonia. Her condition is stabilized, and she is admitted to the hospital to receive intravenous doses of antibiotics and corticosteroids. She says that, before this episode, she took oral drugs for diabetes and had her diabetes "under control," with fasting blood glucose levels ranging from 99 to 106 mg/dL on most mornings. However, the next morning, her fasting blood glucose level is 177 mg/dL, and her glucose levels remain elevated for the next few days. The patient is upset and declares, "I'm hardly eating anything extra. Why is my blood sugar so high?" What is the nurse's best answer to the patient's concerns?

For answers, see *http://evolve.elsevier.com/Lilley*.

Ⓔ EVOLVE WEBSITE

http://evolve.elsevier.com/Lilley

- Animations
- Answer Keys for Textbook Case Studies and Textbook Critical Thinking and Prioritization Questions

- Content Updates
- Key Points
- Review Questions
- Student Case Studies

Adrenal Drugs

http://evolve.elsevier.com/Lilley

OBJECTIVES

When you reach the end of this chapter, you will be able to do the following:

1. Discuss the normal anatomy, physiology, and related functions of the adrenal glands, including specific hormones released from the glands.
2. Briefly compare the hormones secreted by the adrenal medulla with those secreted by the adrenal cortex.
3. Contrast Cushing's syndrome, Addison's disease, and addisonian crisis.
4. Compare the glucocorticoids and mineralocorticoids with regard to the roles they perform in normal bodily

functions, the diseases that alter them, how they are used in pharmacotherapy, and their basic properties.

5. Contrast the mechanisms of action, indications, dosages, routes of administration, cautions, contraindications, drug interactions, and adverse effects of glucocorticoids, mineralocorticoids, and antiadrenal drugs.
6. Develop a nursing care plan that includes all phases of the nursing process for patients taking adrenal and antiadrenal drugs.

DRUG PROFILES

- ⬦ **fludrocortisone, p. 527**
- ⬦ **methylprednisolone, p. 528**
- ⬦ **prednisone, p. 527**

⬦ = *Key drug*
❗ = *High-alert drug*

KEY TERMS

Addison's disease A chronic disease associated with the hyposecretion of corticosteroids. (p. 524)

Adrenal cortex The outer portion of the adrenal gland. (p. 524)

Adrenal crisis An acute, life-threatening state of profound adrenocortical insufficiency requiring immediate medical management. It is characterized by glucocorticoid deficiency, a drop in extracellular fluid volume, hyponatremia, and hyperkalemia. (p. 529)

Adrenal medulla The inner portion of the adrenal gland. (p. 524)

Aldosterone A mineralocorticoid hormone produced by the adrenal cortex that acts on the renal tubule to regulate sodium and potassium balance in the blood. (p. 524)

Cortex The general anatomic term for the outer layers of a body organ or other structure. (p. 524)

Corticosteroids Any of the natural or synthetic adrenocortical hormones; those produced by the cortex of the adrenal gland (adrenocorticosteroids). (p. 524)

Cushing's syndrome A metabolic disorder characterized by abnormally increased secretion of the corticosteroids. (p. 524)

Epinephrine An endogenous hormone secreted into the bloodstream by the adrenal medulla; also a synthetic drug that is an adrenergic vasoconstrictor and also increases cardiac output. (p. 524)

Glucocorticoids A major group of corticosteroid hormones that regulate carbohydrate, protein, and lipid metabolism and inhibit the release of adrenocorticotropic hormone. (p. 524)

Hypothalamic-pituitary-adrenal (HPA) axis A negative feedback system involved in regulating the release of corticotropin-releasing hormone by the hypothalamus, adrenocorticotropic hormone (corticotropin) by the pituitary gland, and corticosteroids by the adrenal glands. Suppression of the HPA may lead to Addison's disease and possible adrenal crisis or addisonian crisis. This suppression results from chronic disease or exogenous sources, such as long-term glucocorticoid therapy. (p. 524)

Medulla An anatomic term for the most interior portions of an organ or structure. (p. 524)

Mineralocorticoids A major group of corticosteroid hormones that regulate electrolyte and water balance; in humans the primary mineralocorticoid is aldosterone. (p. 524)

Norepinephrine An adrenergic hormone, secreted by the adrenal medulla, that increases blood pressure by causing vasoconstriction but does not appreciably affect cardiac output; it is the immediate metabolic precursor to epinephrine. (p. 524)

ADRENAL SYSTEM

The adrenal gland is an endocrine organ that sits on top of the kidney like a cap. It is composed of two distinct parts called the adrenal cortex and the adrenal medulla; both are structurally and functionally different from one another. In general, the term cortex refers to the outer layers of various organs (e.g., cerebral cortex), whereas the term medulla refers to the most internal layers. The adrenal cortex composes roughly 80% to 90% of the entire adrenal gland; the remainder is the medulla. The adrenal cortex is made up of regular endocrine tissue (hormone driven). The adrenal medulla is made up of neurosecretory endocrine tissue (driven by both hormones and peripheral autonomic nerve impulses). Therefore, the adrenal gland actually functions as two different endocrine glands, each secreting different hormones.

The adrenal medulla secretes two important hormones, both of which are catecholamines. These are epinephrine, which accounts for about 80% of the secretion, and norepinephrine, which accounts for the other 20% (both are discussed in Chapter 18). Characteristics of the adrenal cortex and the adrenal medulla and the various hormones secreted by each are presented in Table 33-1.

The hormones secreted by the adrenal cortex are broadly referred to as corticosteroids. They arise from the cortex and are steroid hormones; that is, they have the steroid chemical structure. There are two types of corticosteroids: glucocorticoids and mineralocorticoids.

The mineralocorticoids get their name from the fact that they play an important role in regulating mineral salts (electrolytes) in the body. In humans, the only physiologically important mineralocorticoid is aldosterone. Its primary role is to maintain normal levels of sodium in the blood (sodium homeostasis) by causing sodium to be resorbed from the urine back into the blood in exchange for potassium and hydrogen ions. It not only regulates blood sodium levels but also influences the potassium levels in the blood and blood pH. The glucocorticoids predominantly affect the metabolism of carbohydrates and, to a lesser extent, fats and proteins. Cortisol is the major natural glucocorticoid.

The corticosteroids are necessary for many vital bodily functions. Some of the more important ones are listed in Box 33-1. Without these hormones, life-threatening consequences may arise.

Corticosteroids are synthesized as needed; the body does not store them as it does other hormones. The levels of these hormones are regulated by the hypothalamic-pituitary-adrenal (HPA) axis. As the name implies, this axis consists of a very organized system of communications between the adrenal gland, the pituitary gland, and the hypothalamus. As is the case for the other endocrine glands, it uses hormones as the messengers and a negative feedback mechanism as the controller and maintainer of the process. This feedback mechanism operates as follows: When the level of a particular corticosteroid is low, corticotropin-releasing hormone is released from the hypothalamus into the bloodstream and travels to the anterior pituitary gland, where it triggers the release of adrenocorticotropic hormone (ACTH; also called *corticotropin*). The ACTH is then transported in the blood to the adrenal cortex, where it stimulates the production of the corticosteroids. Corticosteroids are then released into the bloodstream. When they reach peak levels, a signal (negative feedback) is sent to the hypothalamus, and the HPA axis is inhibited until the level of corticosteroids again falls below physiologic threshold, whereupon the axis is stimulated once again.

The oversecretion (hypersecretion) of adrenocortical hormones can lead to a group of signs and symptoms called Cushing's syndrome. This hypersecretion of glucocorticoids results in the redistribution of body fat from the arms and legs to the face, shoulders, trunk, and abdomen, which leads to the characteristic "moon face." Such a glucocorticoid excess can be due to several causes, including ACTH-dependent adrenocortical hyperplasia or tumor, ectopic ACTH-secreting tumor, or excessive administration of steroids. The hypersecretion of aldosterone, or primary aldosteronism, leads to increased retention of water and sodium, which causes muscle weakness due to the potassium loss.

The undersecretion (hyposecretion) of adrenocortical hormones causes a condition known as Addison's disease. It is associated with decreased blood sodium and glucose levels,

TABLE 33-1	Adrenal Gland: Characteristics	
Type of Tissue	Type of Hormone Secreted	Hormones Secreted and Related Drugs
Adrenal Cortex		
Endocrine	Glucocorticoids	Adrenocorticotropic hormone, betamethasone, cortisone, dexamethasone, hydrocortisone, methylprednisolone, prednisolone, triamcinolone
	Mineralocorticoids	Aldosterone, desoxycorticosterone, fludrocortisone
Adrenal Medulla		
Neuroendocrine	Catecholamines	Epinephrine, norepinephrine

BOX 33-1 Adrenal Cortex Hormones: Biologic Functions

Glucocorticoids
Antiinflammatory actions
Carbohydrate and protein metabolism
Fat metabolism
Maintenance of normal blood pressure
Stress effects

Mineralocorticoids
Blood pressure control
Maintenance of serum potassium levels
Maintenance of pH levels in the blood
Sodium and water resorption

increased potassium levels, dehydration, and weight loss. The combination of a mineralocorticoid (fludrocortisone) and a glucocorticoid (prednisone) is used for treatment.

ADRENAL DRUGS

All of the naturally occurring corticosteroids are available as exogenous drugs. There are also higher-potency synthetic analogues. The adrenal glucocorticoids are an extremely large group of steroids and can be categorized in various ways. They can be classified by whether they are a natural or synthetic corticosteroid, by the method of administration (e.g., systemic, topical), by their salt- and water-retention potential (mineralocorticoid activity), by their duration of action (i.e., short-, intermediate-, or long-acting), or by some combination of these methods. The only corticosteroid drug with exclusive mineralocorticoid activity is fludrocortisone. Its uses are much more specific than those of the glucocorticoids. The currently available synthetic adrenal hormones and adrenal steroid inhibitors are listed in Table 33-2.

Mechanism of Action and Drug Effects

The action of the corticosteroids is related to their involvement in the synthesis of specific proteins. There are several steps to this process. Initially the steroid hormone binds to a receptor on the surface of a target cell to form a steroid-receptor complex, which is then transported through the cytoplasm to the nucleus of that target cell. Once inside the nucleus, the complex stimulates the cell's deoxyribonucleic acid (DNA) to produce messenger ribonucleic acid (mRNA), which is then used as a template for the synthesis of a specific protein. It is these proteins that exert specific effects.

Most of the corticosteroids exert their effects by modifying enzyme activity; therefore, their role is more intermediary than direct. The naturally occurring mineralocorticoid aldosterone affects electrolyte and fluid balance by acting on the distal renal tubule. It promotes sodium resorption from the nephron into the blood, which pulls water and fluid along with it. In doing so, it causes fluid and water retention, which leads to edema and hypertension. It also increases urinary excretion of potassium and hydrogen via the kidney.

The glucocorticoid drugs hydrocortisone (called *cortisol* in its naturally occurring form) and cortisone have some mineralocorticoid activity and therefore have some of the same effects as aldosterone (i.e., fluid and water retention). However, their main effect is the inhibition of inflammatory and immune responses. Glucocorticoids inhibit or help control the inflammatory response by stabilizing the cell membranes of inflammatory cells called *lysosomes,* decreasing the permeability of capillaries to the inflammatory cells, and decreasing the migration of white blood cells into already inflamed areas. They may lower fever by reducing the release of interleukin-1 from white blood cells. They also stimulate the *erythroid cells* that eventually become red blood cells. The glucocorticoids also promote the breakdown (catabolism) of protein, the production of glycogen in the liver (glycogenesis), and the redistribution of fat from peripheral to central areas of the body. In addition, they have the following effects on various bodily functions: increasing levels of blood sugar, increasing the breakdown of proteins to amino acids, inducing lipolysis, stimulating bone demineralization, and stabilizing mast cells.

Indications

All of the systemically administered glucocorticoids have a similar clinical efficacy but differ in their potency and duration of action and in the extent to which they cause salt and water retention (Table 33-3). These drugs have broad indications, including the following:
- Adrenocortical deficiency
- Adrenogenital syndrome
- Bacterial meningitis
- Cerebral edema
- Collagen diseases (e.g., systemic lupus erythematosus)
- Dermatologic diseases (e.g., exfoliative dermatitis, pemphigus)
- Endocrine disorders (thyroiditis)
- Gastrointestinal (GI) diseases (e.g., ulcerative colitis, regional enteritis)
- Exacerbations of chronic respiratory illnesses such as asthma and chronic obstructive pulmonary disease
- Hematologic disorders (reduce bleeding tendencies)
- Ophthalmic disorders (e.g., nonpyogenic inflammations)
- Organ transplantation (decrease immune response to prevent organ rejection)
- Leukemias and lymphomas (palliative management)
- Nephrotic syndrome (remission of proteinuria)
- Spinal cord injury

Glucocorticoids are also administered by inhalation for the control of steroid-responsive bronchospastic states. However,

TABLE 33-2 Available Synthetic Corticosteroids		
Type of Hormone	**Method of Administration**	**Individual Drugs**
Glucocorticoid	Topical	Alclometasone, betamethasone, clobetasol dexamethasone, fluocinolone, halobetasol hydrocortisone, mometasone, triamcinolone
	Systemic	Betamethasone, cortisone, dexamethasone, hydrocortisone, methylprednisolone, prednisolone, prednisone, triamcinolone
	Inhaled	Beclomethasone, dexamethasone, flunisolide, triamcinolone, fluticasone
	Nasal	Beclomethasone, dexamethasone, flunisolide, triamcinolone, fluticasone
Mineralocorticoid	Systemic	Fludrocortisone

TABLE 33-3   Systemic Glucocorticoids: A Comparison

Drug	Origin	Duration of Action	Equivalent Dose (mg)*	Salt and Water Retention Potential
betamethasone	Synthetic	Long	0.75	Very low
cortisone	Natural	Short	25	High
dexamethasone	Synthetic	Long	0.75	Very low
hydrocortisone	Natural	Short	20	High
methylprednisolone	Synthetic	Intermediate	4	Low
prednisolone	Synthetic	Intermediate	5	Low
prednisone	Synthetic	Intermediate	5	Low
triamcinolone	Synthetic	Intermediate	4	Very low

*Drugs with higher potency require smaller milligram doses than those with lower potency. This column lists the approximate dose equivalency between different drugs that is expected to achieve a comparable therapeutic effect.

TABLE 33-4   Corticosteroids: Common Adverse Effects

Body System	Adverse Effects
Cardiovascular	Heart failure, edema, hypertension—all due to electrolyte imbalances (e.g., hypokalemia, hypernatremia)
Central nervous	Convulsions, headache, vertigo, mood swings, psychic impairment, nervousness, insomnia
Endocrine	Growth suppression, Cushing's syndrome, menstrual irregularities, carbohydrate intolerance, hyperglycemia, hypothalamic-pituitary-adrenal axis suppression
Gastrointestinal	Peptic ulcers, pancreatitis, ulcerative esophagitis, abdominal distension
Integumentary	Fragile skin, petechiae, ecchymosis, facial erythema, poor wound healing, hirsutism, urticaria
Musculoskeletal	Muscle weakness, loss of muscle mass, osteoporosis
Ocular	Increased intraocular pressure, glaucoma, cataracts
Other	Weight gain

glucocorticoid inhalers are not used as rescue inhalers for acute bronchospasm. Nasally administered glucocorticoids are used to manage rhinitis and to prevent the recurrence of polyps after surgical removal (see Chapter 36). Topical steroids are used in the management of inflammation of the eye, ear, and skin. Prednisone is the most commonly used oral drug, followed by dexamethasone. Methylprednisolone is the most commonly used injectable glucocorticoid, followed by hydrocortisone and dexamethasone. Betamethasone is the drug of choice for women in premature labor to accelerate fetal lung maturation.

Contraindications

Contraindications to the administration of glucocorticoids include known drug allergy and may include cataracts, glaucoma, peptic ulcer disease, mental health problems, and diabetes mellitus. The adrenal drugs may intensify these diseases. For example, one common adverse effect seen in hospitalized patients is an increase in blood glucose levels, often requiring insulin. This is not to say that diabetic patients who require glucocorticoids should not receive them, but the potential for increases in blood glucose levels exists. Because of their immunosuppressant properties, glucocorticoids are often avoided in the presence of any serious infection, including septicemia, systemic fungal infections, and varicella. One exception is tuberculous meningitis, for which glucocorticoids may be used to prevent inflammatory central nervous system damage. Caution is emphasized in treating any patient with gastritis, reflux disease, or ulcer disease because of the potential of these drugs to cause gastric perforation, as well as any patient with cardiac, renal, and/or liver dysfunction because of the associated alterations in elimination.

Adverse Effects

The potent metabolic, physiologic, and pharmacologic effects of the corticosteroids can influence every body system, so these drugs can produce a wide variety of significant undesirable effects. The more common of these are summarized in

Table 33-4. Moon face is a very common adverse effect of long-term use. Two of the adverse effects most commonly seen in hospitalized patients are hyperglycemia and psychosis. The most serious adverse effect of glucocorticoids is adrenal (or HPA) suppression, which is discussed in the drug profiles. Glucocorticoids should be used with caution in patients with heart failure, due to their ability to cause fluid retention.

Interactions

Systemically administered corticosteroids can interact with many drugs:

- Non–potassium-sparing diuretics (e.g., thiazides, loop diuretics) can lead to severe hypocalcemia and hypokalemia.
- Aspirin, other nonsteroidal antiinflammatory drugs, and other ulcerogenic drugs produce additive GI effects and an increased chance for gastric ulcer development.
- Anticholinesterase drugs produce weakness in patients with myasthenia gravis.
- Corticosteroids can inhibit the immune response when given in combination with immunizing biologics.
- Corticosteroids can reduce the hypoglycemic effects of antidiabetic drugs and result in elevated blood glucose levels.

Many other drugs can interact with glucocorticoids, including thyroid hormones and antifungal drugs (such as fluconazole), which can decrease renal clearance of the adrenal drug. Barbiturates and hydantoins can increase the metabolism of prednisone and similar drugs. Increased effects from warfarin can be seen. Oral contraceptives can increase the half-life of adrenal drugs. Various other drug interactions may be possible between adrenal drugs and over-the-counter drugs and herbals.

Dosages

For dosage information on adrenal drugs, see the table on the next page.

DOSAGES

Selected Antiadrenal and Corticosteroid Drugs

Drug	Pharmacologic Class	Usual Adult Dosage Range	Indications
◆ fludrocortisone (Florinef)	Synthetic mineralocorticoid	PO: 0.05-0.2 mg every 24 hr	Addison's disease
◆ methylprednisolone (Solu-Medrol)	Systemic corticosteroid	IV: 10-250 mg every 6 hr	Wide variety of endocrine disorders (including adrenocortical insufficiency) and rheumatic, collagen, dermatologic, allergic, ophthalmic, respiratory, hematologic, neoplastic, GI, and nervous system disorders; edematous states
◆ prednisone (Deltasone, Sterapred, Liquid Pred, others)	Synthetic intermediate-acting glucocorticoid	PO: 5-60 mg/day	Same indications as for methylprednisolone

GI, Gastrointestinal.

DRUG PROFILES

CORTICOSTEROIDS

The systemic corticosteroids consist of 13 chemically different but pharmacologically similar hormones. They all exert varying degrees of glucocorticoid and mineralocorticoid effects. Their differences are due to slight changes in their chemical structures.

Corticosteroid drugs are classified as pregnancy category C drugs. They can be secreted in breast milk. Their use is contraindicated in patients who have exhibited hypersensitivity reactions to them in the past as well as in patients with fungal or bacterial infections. Short- or long-term use can lead to a condition known as *steroid psychosis*. One very important point about long-term use of steroids is that they must not be stopped abruptly. These drugs require a tapering of the daily dose, because the administration of these drugs causes the endogenous (body's own) production of the hormones to stop. This is referred to as *HPA* or *adrenal suppression*. This suppression can cause impaired stress response and place the patient at risk for developing hypoadrenal crisis (shock, circulatory collapse) in times of increased stress (i.e., surgery, trauma). Adrenal suppression can occur as early as 1 week after a corticosteroid is started. HPA suppression typically does not occur in patients taking prednisone 5 mg/day (or equivalent) or less. Tapering of daily doses allows the HPA axis the time to recover and to start stimulating the normal production of the endogenous hormones. Patients on long-term steroid therapy who are taking at least 10 mg/day (or equivalent) of prednisone and who undergo trauma or require surgery will need replacement doses of steroids (also known as *stress doses*).

◆ fludrocortisone

Fludrocortisone (Florinef) is the most commonly prescribed mineralocorticoid. It is used as partial replacement therapy for adrenocortical insufficiency in Addison's disease and in the treatment of salt-losing adrenogenital syndrome. It is contraindicated in cases of systemic fungal infection. Adverse effects generally relate to water retention and include heart failure, hypertension, and elevated intracerebral pressure (e.g.,

leading to seizures). Other potential adverse effects involve several body systems and include skin rash, menstrual irregularities, peptic ulcer, hyperglycemia, hypokalemia, muscle pain and weakness, compression bone fractures, glaucoma, and thrombophlebitis, among others. Drugs with which fludrocortisone interacts include barbiturates, hydantoins, and rifamycins (increased fludrocortisone clearance); estrogens (reduced fludrocortisone clearance); amphotericin B and thiazide and loop diuretics (hypokalemia); anticoagulants (enhanced anticoagulant activity); digoxin (increased risk for dysrhythmias due to fludrocortisone-induced hypokalemia); salicylates (reduced efficacy); and vaccines (increased risk for neurologic complications). Fortunately, adverse effects and serious drug interactions secondary to fludrocortisone therapy are uncommon due to the relatively small dosages of the drug that are normally prescribed. This drug is available only in oral form as a 0.1-mg tablet. It is classified as a pregnancy category C drug. Recommended dosages are given in the table above.

Pharmacokinetics: Fludrocortisone

Route	Onset of Action	Peak Plasma Concentration	Elimination Half-life	Duration of Action
PO	10-20 min	1.7 hr	18-36 hr	Unknown

◆ prednisone

Prednisone is one of the four intermediate-acting glucocorticoids; the others are methylprednisolone, prednisolone, and triamcinolone. These drugs have half-lives that are more than double those of the short-acting corticosteroids (2 to 5 hours), and therefore they have longer durations of action. Prednisone is the most commonly used oral glucocorticoid for antiinflammatory or immunosuppressant purposes. Along with methylprednisolone and prednisolone, it is also used to treat exacerbations of chronic respiratory illnesses. Prednisone has only minimal mineralocorticoid properties and therefore alone is inadequate for the management of adrenocortical insufficiency (Addison's disease).

Prednisolone, a prednisone metabolite, is also the liquid drug form of prednisone. Prednisone itself comes in solid form. It is classified as a pregnancy category C drug. Recommended dosages are given in the table on the previous page.

Pharmacokinetics: Prednisone

Route	Onset of Action	Peak Plasma Concentration	Elimination Half-life	Duration of Action
PO	Unknown	1-2 hr	18-36 hr	36 hr

◆ methylprednisolone

Methylprednisolone (Solu-Medrol) is the most commonly used injectable glucocorticoid drug. It is used primarily as an antiinflammatory or immunosuppressant drug. It is usually given intravenously. It is available in a long-acting (depot) formulation as well. Like prednisone, it is classified as a pregnancy category C drug. Most injectable formulations contain a preservative (benzyl alcohol) that cannot be given to children younger than 28 days of age.

Pharmacokinetics: Methylprednisolone

Route	Onset of Action	Peak Plasma Concentration	Elimination Half-life	Duration of Action
IV	Immediate	30 min	3-4 hr	24-36 hr

QSEN ⚡ **SAFETY AND QUALITY IMPROVEMENT: PREVENTING MEDICATION ERRORS**

Look-Alike/Sound-Alike Drugs: Solu-Cortef and Solu-Medrol

Be careful about sound-alike, look-alike drugs! Medication errors often occur when drug names are similar.

Solu-Cortef is a trade name for hydrocortisone; Solu-Medrol is a trade name for methylprednisolone. Both are commonly used glucocorticoids and are given intravenously. However, 4 mg of Solu-Medrol is equivalent to 20 mg of Solu-Cortef; therefore, Solu-Medrol is five times stronger than Solu-Cortef. Despite the similar names, these drugs are not interchangeable!

NURSING PROCESS

ASSESSMENT

Before administering any of the *adrenal* or *antiadrenal drugs,* perform a thorough physical assessment to determine the patient's baseline nutritional, hydration, and immune status. The patient's baseline weight, intake and output, vital signs (especially blood pressure ranges), and the patient's skin condition (noting bruising, fragility, turgor, and color) also need to be assessed and recorded. Baseline laboratory values that will most likely be ordered include serum sodium, serum potassium,

and serum glucose. These specific laboratory tests are important because of the potential drug-related adverse effects (see Table 33-4). For instance, serum potassium levels usually decrease and blood glucose levels increase when a *glucocorticoid* (e.g., *prednisone*) is given. Additionally, assess the patient's muscle strength and body stature. Assess any potential contraindications, cautions, and drug interactions with prescription drugs, over-the-counter drugs, and herbals.

For *adrenal drugs,* lifespan considerations include concern about their use during pregnancy and lactation. Growth suppression may occur in children who are receiving long-term adrenal drug therapy (e.g., *glucocorticoids*) if the epiphyseal plates of the long bones have not closed. However, there may be situations in which the benefits to the therapy outweigh the risks of the drug's adverse effects. Perform and document baseline height and weight measurements in pediatric patients. Older adult patients are more prone to adrenal suppression with prolonged adrenal drug therapy and may require dosage alterations by the prescriber to minimize the impact of the drug on muscle mass, blood pressure, and serum glucose and electrolyte levels. Adrenal drugs may exacerbate muscle weakness; produce fatigue; worsen or precipitate osteoporosis, peptic ulcer disease, glaucoma, and cataracts; and increase intraocular pressure. Additionally, because adrenal drugs are associated with the adverse effects of sodium retention, closely assess patients for exacerbation of any preexisting edema and/or cardiac disease.

NURSING DIAGNOSES

1. Disturbed body image related to the physiologic effects of diseases of the adrenal gland on the body or the cushingoid appearance caused by glucocorticoid therapy (e.g., prednisone)
2. Excess fluid volume related to the fluid retention associated with glucocorticoid and mineralocorticoid use
3. Risk for infection related to the antiinflammatory, immunosuppressive, metabolic, and dermatologic effects of long-term glucocorticoid therapy

PLANNING: OUTCOME IDENTIFICATION

1. Patient experiences minimal body image disturbances by openly verbalizing fears about changes to body and/or health status.
2. Patient maintains normal fluid volume status during glucocorticoid/mineralocorticoid therapy.
3. Patient remains free from infection during adrenal drug therapy.

IMPLEMENTATION

It is important for the patient to understand how *glucocorticoids* work in the body so that they may state and implement measures that maximize the drug's therapeutic effects and minimize adverse effects. Remember the following points when giving these drugs: (1) Hormone production by the adrenal gland is influenced by time of day and follows a diurnal (daily or

24-hour) pattern, with peak levels occurring early in the morning between 6 AM and 8 AM, a decrease during the day, and a lower peak in the late afternoon between 4 PM and 6 PM. (2) Cortisol levels increase in response to both emotional and physiologic stress. (3) Cortisol levels increase when endogenous levels decrease due to a physiologic negative feedback system. (4) When exogenous glucocorticoids are given, endogenous levels decrease; for endogenous production to resume, exogenous levels must be decreased gradually so that hormone output responds to the negative feedback system. (5) The best time to give exogenous glucocorticoids, if at all possible, is early in the morning (6 AM to 9 AM) to minimize the amount of adrenal suppression. It is important to remember, however, that the patient must not alter dosing or abruptly discontinue medication without consulting the prescriber.

CASE STUDY

Patient-Centered Care: Glucocorticoid Drug Therapy

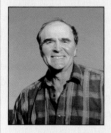

Mr. J., a 68-year-old farmer, has been in the hospital for 1 week because of an exacerbation of chronic emphysema, which was aggravated by dust from the fall harvesting. He has a history of diabetes mellitus type 2. He says that he stopped smoking "4 years ago" and tries to "watch what I eat." He has no history of drug allergies. He is receiving oxygen at 1 L/min through a nasal cannula. At this time, he is breathing more easily and hopes to be going home soon. His medication orders include the following, among others:

- metformin/glipizide (Metaglip) 500 mg/5 mg twice a day by mouth (PO)
- prednisone (Deltasone), 20 mg every morning PO
- albuterol (Ventolin) inhaler, 2 puffs every 4 hours

Mr. J. is complaining of a headache. When you check the medication sheet, you see two orders:

- acetaminophen (generic), 650 mg PO every 4 hours as needed for pain
- ibuprofen (generic), 200 mg PO every 6 hours as needed for pain

1. Which medication will you choose to give to Mr. J.? Explain your answer.

In the morning, while assessing Mr. J., you notice that he now has increased edema around his ankles, measured at 2+ bilaterally. When you listen to his lungs, you hear scattered rhonchi but no crackles, and his weight has increased since yesterday by 1.5 kg. When you call his physician, you receive orders for furosemide (Lasix) 40 mg intravenously now, then 20 mg every morning PO. When you check Mr. J.'s fasting fingerstick blood glucose level, the result is 236 mg/dL. Mr. J. is surprised at this result.

2. Considering Mr. J.'s medications, what could be contributing to this elevated glucose level? What other laboratory values need to be monitored closely during this time?

One week later, Mr. J. is discharged. His prednisone prescription contains instructions for tapering the dose over the next 2 weeks. You provide patient teaching for his medication management, and both Mr. and Mrs. J. demonstrate that they understand the information. However, 3 days later, Mr. J. is back in the emergency department with severe nausea, vomiting, and fatigue. His blood pressure is 92/56 mm Hg, and the results of his stat laboratory tests reflect hyponatremia and hyperkalemia. His wife says that she hates the way the "prednisone makes him look and feel," and she is not sure whether he was taking his medicine.

3. What do you expect happened to cause these symptoms?
4. What nursing diagnoses are appropriate for Mr. J.?

For answers, see *http://evolve.elsevier.com/Lilley.*

Prednisone, a synthetic glucocorticoid, and *fludrocortisone,* a synthetic *mineralocorticoid,* are given orally. It is recommended that oral dosage forms be given with a snack and/or a meal to help minimize GI upset. An order for an H_2 receptor antagonist or a proton pump inhibitor may be prescribed to minimize GI upset and to minimize ulcer formation because these drugs are ulcerogenic. Emphasize to patients the importance of avoiding alcohol, caffeine, and aspirin and other nonsteroidal antiinflammatory drugs to minimize gastric irritation and possible gastric bleeding from the compounding ulcerogenic effects. In long-term therapy, alternate-day dosing of glucocorticoids, if possible, will help minimize the adrenal suppression. Because of the immunosuppression with these drugs, monitor patients for flulike symptoms, sore throat, and fever. If an incision or wound is present, assess affected area for redness, edema, drainage, and approximation. *Methylprednisolone,* a systemic *corticosteroid,* is given intravenously. Mix all parenteral forms per manufacturer guidelines, with intravenous doses administered over the recommended time period and in the proper diluent.

With oral and all other forms of glucocorticoids that are given short and/or long term, abrupt withdrawal must be avoided. Abrupt withdrawal of adrenal drugs (e.g., prednisone, methylprednisolone) may lead to a sudden decrease in or no production of endogenous glucocorticoids, resulting in adrenal insufficiency. Signs and symptoms of partial or complete adrenal insufficiency or Addison's disease include fatigue, nausea, vomiting, and hypotension. If left untreated, this condition may lead to an adrenal crisis or a life-threatening state of profound adrenocortical insufficiency requiring immediate medical management. Signs and symptoms include a drop in extracellular fluid volume, hyponatremia, and hyperkalemia. This is also referred to as *addisonian crisis.*

Other adrenal drug dosage forms include those for intraarticular, intrabursal, intradermal, intralesional, and intrasynovial administration (see Table 33-3). Overuse of intraarticular injections must be avoided, and if a joint is injected with medication, the patient needs to rest that area for up to 48 hours after the injection is given. Application of cold packs over the injected area may be indicated for up to the first 24 hours to help minimize the discomfort associated with intraarticular injections. Topical dosage forms (e.g., for skin, eye, or inhalation into the bronchial tree) are also available and must be given exactly as ordered. For dermatologic use, clean and dry the skin before application. Wear gloves, and apply the medication with either a sterile tongue depressor or a cotton-tipped applicator. Use sterile technique if the skin is not intact. Nasally administered glucocorticoids (e.g., *beclomethasone*) must also be used exactly as ordered (see Chapter 36). Any written instructions that come with the product must be read and followed carefully. Before using the nasal sprays (see Chapter 9 for more information), the patient needs to first clear the nasal passages and then use the spray per instructions. After the nasal passages are cleared, the container is placed gently inside the nasal passage and the medication is released at the same time that the patient breathes in through the nose, one nasal passage at a time or as ordered. Instructions for use must be followed exactly.

Glucocorticoid inhalers (e.g., *beclomethasone, dexamethasone, flunisolide, triamcinolone, fluticasone*) are to be used strictly as ordered; explain the negative consequences of overuse to the patient. Use of these inhaled glucocorticoids may lead to fungal infections (candidiasis) of the oral mucosa and oral cavity, larynx, and pharynx. Therefore, the patient must rinse the mouth and oral mucous membranes with lukewarm water after each use to help prevent fungal overgrowth and further complications. In addition to fungal infections, hoarseness, throat irritation, and dry mouth are also possible adverse effects associated with the use of inhaled glucocorticoids. Occurrence of any of these conditions needs to be reported to the prescriber. See Chapter 9 and Patient-Centered Care: Patient Teaching for more information on inhaled dosage forms.

If a patient is receiving long-term maintenance glucocorticoid therapy and requires surgery, recognize the importance of reviewing the patient's medical records for laboratory values, cautions, contraindications, and drug interactions. If the preoperative orders do not include the maintenance dosage of glucocorticoid therapy, contact the surgeon and/or other prescriber and ensure that he or she is aware of the situation and the possible need for a rapid-acting *cortiocosteroid*. After surgery, the dosage of steroid may well be increased, with a gradual decrease in dosage over several days until the patient returns to baseline. In addition, you must be constantly aware of the decrease in wound healing in patients taking these drugs on a long-term basis.

In summary, because of their suppressed immune systems, patients taking corticosteroids need to avoid contact with people with known infections and report any fever, increased weakness and lethargy, or sore throat. Monitoring nutritional status, weight, fluid volume, electrolyte status, skin turgor, and glucose levels during therapy is very important to ensure safe and effective therapy. The prescriber needs to be notified if there is any edema, shortness of breath (possible heart failure), joint pain, fever, mood swings, or other unusual symptoms.

▌EVALUATION

A therapeutic response to *glucocorticoids* includes a resolution of the underlying manifestations of the disease or pathology, such as a decrease in inflammation, increased feeling of well-being, less pain and discomfort in the joints, decrease in lymphocytes, or other improvement in the condition for which the medication was ordered. Adverse effects include weight gain; increased blood pressure; sodium increase and potassium loss; mental status changes such as mood swings, psychic impairment, and nervousness; abdominal distension; ulcer-related symptoms; and changes in vision. Cushing's syndrome occurs with prolonged or frequent use of glucocorticoids and is characterized by moon face, obesity of the trunk area (often referred to as *belly fat*), increase in blood glucose and sodium levels, loss of serum potassium, wasting of muscle mass, buffalo hump, and other features previously discussed. Cataract formation and osteoporosis may also occur with long-term use. Rapid drops in cortisol levels (e.g., from abrupt withdrawal of medication) may lead to Addison's disease and addisonian crisis (see previous discussions).

▌ PATIENT-CENTERED CARE: PATIENT TEACHING

- Glucocorticoids are to be taken exactly as ordered and never abruptly discontinued. Contact the prescriber if there are situations that prevent proper dosing. Abrupt withdrawal may precipitate adrenal crisis or Addison's disease and/or possible addisonian crisis.
- If a once-a-day dose of glucocorticoids is missed, the patient needs to take the dose as soon as possible after remembering that the dose was missed. If the patient does *not* remember until close to the time for the next dose, then he or she is usually instructed to skip the dose and resume dosing on the next day without doubling up. If any questions arise, the patient needs to clarify with the prescriber. Educate the patient about the adverse effects of long-term therapy, such as changes in body appearance including acne, buffalo hump, obesity of the trunk area, moon face, and thinning of the extremities.
- With glucocorticoid therapy, emphasize the importance of bone health and ways to prevent falls due to the possibility of osteoporosis with long-term use. Foods high in vitamin D include cod liver oil (amount to be recommended by health care provider) and salmon. Foods high in calcium include milk, cheese, yogurt, and ice cream. Fortified dairy products are high in both vitamin D and calcium. The prescriber may suggest a daily supplement of oral calcium and vitamin D.

- Contact the prescriber immediately if any signs and symptoms of acute adrenal insufficiency appear, such as decreased serum sodium and glucose levels, increased potassium levels, dehydration, and weight loss.
- Fludrocortisone, a mineralocorticoid, is better tolerated if taken with food or milk to minimize GI upset. With any of the adrenal drugs, weight gain of 2 pounds or more in 24 hours or 5 pounds or more in 1 week needs to be reported to the prescriber immediately.
- Encourage the patient to keep a journal to document responses to treatment, blood pressure readings, daily weight measurements, mood changes, and any adverse effects.
- Emphasize the importance of follow-up appointments with the prescriber so that electrolyte levels and adverse effects may be monitored. Also, stress the importance of maintaining a low-sodium and high-potassium diet, if ordered.
- Encourage the patient to wear a medical alert identification bracelet or necklace with the diagnosis and a list of medications and allergies. A medical card with important relevant information needs to be kept on the person at all times and updated frequently.

KEY POINTS

- The adrenal gland is an endocrine organ that is located on top of the kidney and is composed of two distinct tissues: the adrenal cortex and the adrenal medulla. The adrenal medulla secretes two important hormones: epinephrine and norepinephrine; the adrenal cortex secretes two classes of hormones known as *corticosteroids:* glucocorticoids and mineralocorticoids.
- The biologic functions of glucocorticoids include antiinflammatory actions; maintenance of normal blood pressure; carbohydrate, protein, and fat metabolism; and stress effects. The biologic functions of mineralocorticoids include sodium and water resorption, blood pressure control, and maintenance of potassium levels and pH of the blood.
- Patients taking adrenal drugs may receive them by various routes, such as orally, intramuscularly, intravenously, intranasally, intraarticularly, and by inhalation.

- Glucocorticoid inhaled dosage forms are only to be used as prescribed and only after adequate patient education. Rinsing of the mouth after each use is needed to avoid oral fungal infections (oral candidiasis) and oral-pharyngeal irritation.
- Long-term or frequent glucocorticoid use produces increased levels of glucocorticoids, which can lead to Cushing's syndrome. Abrupt withdrawal of glucocorticoids leads to adrenal insufficiency and negative effects on the patient's homeostasis.
- With once-a-day dosing of these drugs, adrenal suppression from corticosteroid therapy can be minimized if the dose is given between 6 AM and 9 AM, but it needs to be given only as ordered.

NCLEX® EXAMINATION REVIEW QUESTIONS

1. When monitoring for a therapeutic response to prednisone, the nurse will look for which potential outcome?
   a. Increased lymphocyte levels
   b. Decreased inflammation
   c. Increased growth characteristics
   d. Decrease in Cushing's syndrome characteristics
2. The nurse has provided teaching about oral corticosteroid therapy to a patient. Which statement by the patient shows a need for more teaching?
   a. "I will report any fever or sore throat symptoms."
   b. "I will stay away from anyone who has a cold or infection."
   c. "I can stop this medication if I have severe adverse effects."
   d. "I will take this drug with food or milk."
3. During long-term corticosteroid therapy, the nurse will monitor the patient for Cushing's syndrome, which is manifested by
   a. weight loss.
   b. moon face.
   c. hypotension.
   d. thickened hair growth.
4. When teaching a patient who has been prescribed a daily dose of prednisone (Deltasone), the nurse knows that the patient will be told to take the medication at which time of day to help reduce adrenal suppression?
   a. In the morning
   b. At lunchtime
   c. At dinnertime
   d. At bedtime

5. Which teaching is appropriate for a patient who is taking an inhaled glucocorticoid for asthma?
   a. "Exhale while pushing in on the canister of the inhaler."
   b. "Blow your nose after taking the medication."
   c. "Rinse your mouth thoroughly after taking the medication."
   d. "Do not eat immediately after taking the medication."
6. During long-term corticosteroid therapy, the nurse will monitor the patient's laboratory results for adverse effects, such as: *(Select all that apply.)*
   a. Increased serum potassium levels
   b. Decreased serum potassium levels
   c. Increased sodium levels
   d. Decreased sodium levels
   e. Hyperglycemia
   f. Hypoglycemia
7. The order reads: "Give methylprednisolone (Solu-Medrol) 100 mg IV every 6 hours." The drug is available in vials of 80 mg/mL. How many mL will the nurse draw up for each dose?
8. A patient with acute adrenal insufficiency is to receive 300 mg/day of hydrocortisone (Solu-Cortef), divided into 3 doses every 8 hours. How many milligrams will the patient receive for each dose?

1. b, 2. c, 3. b, 4. a, 5. c, 6. b, c, e, 7. 1.25 mL, 8. 100 mg.

CRITICAL THINKING AND PRIORITIZATION QUESTIONS

1. A patient has been taking high doses of oral prednisone for 1 week due to an exacerbation of asthma symptoms. He is about to go home and is given a prescription for another week of prednisone (Deltasone) therapy, but with doses tapering downward before the medication is stopped. The patient asks, "Why do I need to bother with this drug if it's only for a week? Can't I just stop it now?" What is the priority when the nurse answers this patient's questions? Explain your answer.

2. A patient with type 2 diabetes mellitus will be receiving intravenous doses of methylprednisolone (Solu-Medrol) to prevent cerebral edema after a head injury from a fall. A nursing student is working with you as you prepare to give this medication. The student asks, "Isn't this drug going to cause problems for this patient? Should we be giving it?" What priority do you consider when answering the nursing student?

For answers see *http://evolve.elsevier.com/Lilley.*

ⓔ EVOLVE WEBSITE

http://evolve.elsevier.com/Lilley
- Animations
- Answer Keys for Textbook Case Studies and Textbook Critical Thinking and Prioritization Questions

- Content Updates
- Key Points
- Review Questions
- Student Case Studies

Women's Health Drugs

http://evolve.elsevier.com/Lilley

OBJECTIVES

When you reach the end of this chapter, you will be able to do the following:

1. Discuss the normal anatomy and physiology of the female reproductive system.
2. Describe the normal hormonally mediated feedback system that regulates the female reproductive system.
3. Briefly describe the variety of disorders affecting women's health and the drugs used to treat them.
4. Discuss the rationale for use, indications, adverse effects, cautions, contraindications, drug interactions, dosages, and routes of administration for estrogen, progestins, uterine motility–altering drugs, and osteoporosis drugs.
5. Develop a nursing care plan that includes all phases of the nursing process for patients receiving any of the drugs related to women's health (e.g., estrogens, progestins, uterine mobility–altering drugs, and osteoporosis drugs).

DRUG PROFILES

KEY TERMS

Chloasma Hyperpigmentation of the skin, characterized by brownish macules on the cheeks, forehead, lips, and/or neck; a common dermatologic adverse effect of female hormonal medications (also called *melasma*). (p. 537)

Corpus luteum The structure that forms on the surface of the ovary after every ovulation and acts as a short-lived endocrine organ that secretes progesterone. (p. 534)

Endocrine glands Glands that secrete one or more hormones directly into the blood. (p. 534)

Estrogens The term for a major class of female sex steroid hormones; of the estrogens, estradiol is responsible for most estrogenic physiologic activity. (p. 534)

Fallopian tubes The passages through which ova are carried from the ovary to the uterus. (p. 534)

Gonadotropin The hormone that stimulates the testes and ovaries. (p. 534)

Hormone replacement therapy (HRT) The term used to describe any replacement of natural body hormones with hormonal drug dosage forms. Most commonly, HRT refers to estrogen replacement therapy for treating symptoms associated with menopause-related estrogen deficiency. It is also referred to as simply hormone therapy. (p. 537)

Implantation The attachment to, penetration of, and embedding of the fertilized ovum in the lining of the uterine wall; it is one of the first stages of pregnancy. (p. 534)

Menarche The first menses in a young woman's life and the beginning of cyclic menstrual function. (p. 534)

Menopause The cessation of menses for 12 consecutive months that marks the end of a woman's childbearing capability. (p. 534)

Menses The normal flow of blood that occurs during menstruation. (p. 534)

Menstrual cycle The recurring cycle of changes in the endometrium in which the decidual layer is shed, regrows, proliferates, is maintained for several days, and is shed again at menstruation unless a pregnancy begins. Also referred to as the *uterine cycle*. (p. 534)

Osteoporosis A condition characterized by the progressive loss of bone density and thinning of bone tissue; it is associated with increased risk for fractures. (p. 541)

Ova Female reproductive or germ cells (singular: *ovum;* also called *eggs*). (p. 534)

Ovarian follicles The location of egg production and ovulation in the ovary; the follicle is the precursor to the corpus luteum. (p. 534)

Ovaries The pair of female gonads located on each side of the lower abdomen beside the uterus. They store the *ova* (eggs) and release ova during the ovulation phase of the menstrual cycle. (p. 534)

Ovulation The rupture of the ovarian follicle, which results in the release of an unfertilized ovum into the peritoneal cavity, from which it normally enters the fallopian tube. (p. 534)

Progesterone A sex hormone that is produced by the corpus luteum and serves to prepare the uterus for possible implantation. (p. 534)

Progestins Synthetic or natural substances that have properties similar to progesterone, but are not considered

to be the naturally occurring progesterone that is present in the human female body. (p. 538)

Puberty The period of life when the ability to reproduce begins. (p. 534)

Uterus The hollow, pear-shaped female organ in which the fertilized ovum is implanted (see *implantation*) and the fetus develops. (p. 534)

Vagina The part of the female genitalia that forms a canal from its external orifice through its vestibule to the uterine cervix. (p. 534)

FEMALE REPRODUCTIVE FUNCTIONS

The female reproductive system consists of the ovaries, fallopian tubes, uterus, vagina, and the external structure known as the *vulva*. The development of these primary sex structures, initiation of their subsequent reproductive functions (starting at puberty), and their maintenance are controlled by pituitary gonadotropin hormones and the female sex steroid hormones—estrogens and progesterone. Pituitary gonadotropins include follicle-stimulating hormone (FSH) and luteinizing hormone (LH). Both play a primary role in hormonal communication between the pituitary gland (see Chapter 30) and the ovaries in the continuous regulation of the menstrual cycle from month to month.

Estrogens are also responsible for stimulating the development of secondary female sex characteristics, including the breast, skin, bone development, and distribution of body fat and hair. Progesterone helps create optimal conditions for pregnancy in the endometrium just after ovulation and also promotes the start of menses in the absence of a fertilized ovum.

The ovaries (female gonads) are paired glands located on each side of the uterus. They function both as endocrine glands and as reproductive glands. As reproductive glands, they produce mature ova within ovarian follicles, which are then released into the space in the peritoneal cavity between the ovary and the fallopian tube. Fingerlike projections known as *fimbriae* lie adjacent to each ovary and catch the released ovum and guide it into the fallopian tube. Once inside the fallopian tube, the ovum is moved through its lumen to the uterus. Fertilization of the ovum, when it occurs, takes place in the fallopian tube.

As endocrine glands, the ovaries are responsible for producing the two sex steroid hormones, estrogen and progesterone. Chemically speaking, the estrogens and progestational hormones include several distinct substances. However, only two of these hormones occur in significant amounts, and have the greatest physiologic activity. These are the estrogen estradiol and the progestational hormone progesterone. Estradiol is the principal secretory product of the ovary and has several estrogenic effects. One of these effects is the regulation of gonadotropin (FSH and LH) secretion via negative feedback to the

pituitary gland. Others include promotion of the development of women's secondary sex characteristics, monthly endometrial growth, thickening of the vaginal mucosa, thinning of the cervical mucus, and growth of the ductal system of the breasts. Progesterone is the principle secretory product of the corpus luteum and has progestational effects. These include promotion of tissue growth and secretory activity in the endometrium following the estrogen-driven *proliferative phase* of the menstrual cycle. This important secretory process is required for endometrial egg implantation and maintenance of pregnancy. Other progestational effects include induction of menstruation when fertilization has not occurred and, during pregnancy, inhibition of uterine contractions, increase in the viscosity of cervical mucus (which protects the fetus from external contamination), and growth of the alveolar glands of the breasts.

The uterus consists of three layers: the outer protective *perimetrium*, the muscular *myometrium*, and the inner mucosal layer known as the *endometrium*. The myometrium provides the powerful smooth muscle contractions needed for childbirth. The endometrium is the site of the following: implantation of a fertilized ovum and development of the fetus; initiation of labor and birthing of the infant; and menstruation.

The vagina serves as a common passageway for birthing and menstrual flow. In addition, it is a receptacle for the penis during sexual intercourse and for the sperm after male ejaculation.

The menstrual cycle usually takes roughly 1 month to complete. Menstrual cycles begin during puberty with the first menses (menarche) and cease at menopause, which in most women occurs between 45 and 55 years of age. The hormonally controlled menstrual cycle consists of four distinct but interrelated phases that occur in overlapping sequence. Phase names correspond to activity in either the ovarian follicle or the endometrium (Table 34-1).

- **Phase 1:** the *menstruation phase* (uterine cycle), which initiates the cycle and lasts from 5 to 7 days.
- **Phase 2:** the *follicular phase* (ovarian cycle), during which a mature ovum develops from an ovarian follicle. This phase is also called the *proliferative* or *preovulatory phase* and is characterized by rising estrogen secretion from the ovary and LH secretion from the pituitary gland. It terminates on or about day 14 of the cycle.

- **Phase 3:** the *ovulation phase,* which involves release of the unfertilized ovum from the ovary. This process occurs over a roughly 24- to 48-hour period starting at about day 14. Both estrogen and LH levels peak near this time.

- **Phase 4:** the final phase of the cycle, called the *luteal* or *postovulatory phase.* It is also known as the *secretory phase.* It occurs when the corpus luteum forms from the ruptured ovarian follicle.

The corpus luteum is a mass of secretory cells on the surface of the ovary. Its primary function is to produce progesterone, which helps to optimize the endometrial mucosa for implantation of a fertilized ovum. The corpus luteum also serves as an initial source of the progesterone needed during early pregnancy. This function is later assumed by the developing placenta. If fertilization does not occur, the corpus luteum then degenerates causing a fall in progesterone levels. The menstrual cycle begins again on or about day 28.

Figure 34-1 illustrates the sequence of hormone secretions and related events that take place during the menstrual cycle.

TABLE 34-1	Phases of the Menstrual Cycle	
Phase	**Ovarian Follicle Activity**	**Endometrium Activity**
Phase 1	Menstruation	Menstruation
Phase 2	Follicular phase (preovulatory)	Proliferative phase
Phase 3	Ovulation	Ovulation
Phase 4	Luteal phase (postovulatory)	Secretory phase

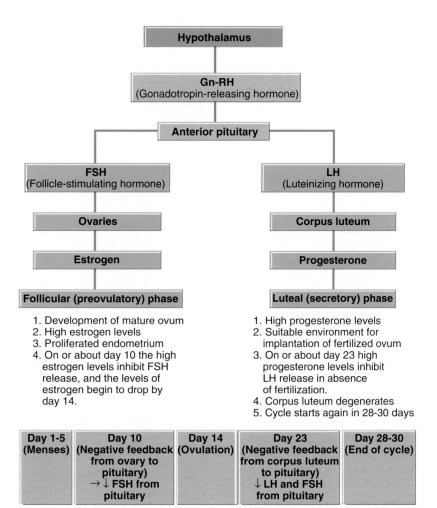

FIGURE 34-1 Hormonal activity during the monthly menstrual cycle. Gonadotropin-releasing hormone (Gn-RH) from the hypothalamus stimulates the pituitary gland, causing it to secrete follicle-stimulating hormone (FSH) early in the cycle (coinciding with the menses) and later luteinizing hormone (LH). FSH stimulates the ovaries to produce estrogen (primarily estradiol). Later in the cycle, the combined surges in the levels of estrogen, Gn-RH, FSH, and LH stimulate ovulation. The corpus luteum then secretes estrogen and progesterone, which provide negative feedback to the hypothalamus and pituitary gland to reduce Gn-RH, FSH, and LH secretions. If the ovum (egg) is not fertilized by a spermatozoon, levels of estrogen and progesterone then fall to their monthly lows, Gn-RH and FSH rise again, and the onset of menses begins a new cycle.

FEMALE SEX HORMONES

ESTROGENS

There are three major endogenous estrogens: estradiol, estrone, and estriol. All are synthesized from cholesterol in the ovarian follicles and have the basic chemical structure of a steroid, known as the *steroid nucleus*. For this reason, they are referred to as *steroid hormones*. Estradiol is the most active of the three and represents the end product of estrogen synthesis.

Exogenous estrogenic drugs, those used as drug therapy, were developed because most of the endogenous estrogens are inactive when taken orally. These synthetic drugs fall into two categories: steroidal and nonsteroidal. Nonsteroidal estrogen products are no longer available in the United States because major adverse effects occurred when one of them, diethylstilbestrol (DES), was used in obstetrics. Box 34-1 describes this important episode in medical history. The estrogenic drugs currently in use are as follows:

- Conjugated estrogens (Premarin)
- Esterified estrogens (Estratab)
- Estradiol transdermal (Estraderm, Climara, Vivelle)
- Estradiol cypionate (Depo-Estradiol, DepoGen)
- Estradiol valerate (Delestrogen)
- Ethinyl estradiol (Estinyl)
- Estradiol vaginal dosage forms (Vagifem, Estrace Vaginal Cream)
- Estrone (Estrone Aqueous)
- Estropipate (Ogen, Ortho-Est)

The most widely used estrogen product is an estrogen mixture known as *conjugated estrogens*. This mixture contains a combination of natural estrogen compounds equivalent to the average estrogen composition of the urine of pregnant mares, hence its brand name of Premarin. A non-animal source for this conjugated estrogen mixture is also available. Cenestin is composed of various conjugated estrogens obtained from soy and yam plants. This product was developed in response to consumer demand from women who wanted an alternative to an animal-derived product (see the Safety: Herbal Therapies and Dietary Supplements box on this page). Some women obtain other natural estrogen products from naturopathic prescribers.

Ethinyl estradiol is one of the more potent estrogens and is most commonly found in oral contraceptive drugs. Another commonly used form of estrogen is the patch formulation. Several patches exist, all of which are dosed differently, thus patient education is necessary to ensure proper use. The most commonly used patch is Climara (estradiol). Two new drugs have been recently approved. Duavee (conjugated estrogen/bazedoxifene) is approved for hot flashes associated with menopause and for osteoporosis. Duavee is a combination of conjugated estrogen and bazedoxifene, which is an estrogen agonist/antagonist. Ospemifene (Osphena) is an estrogen agonist/antagonist that is the first drug approved to treat moderate to severe dyspareunia (painful intercourse) in postmenopausal women.

Mechanism of Action and Drug Effects

The binding of estrogen to intracellular estrogen receptors stimulates the synthesis of nucleic acids (deoxyribonucleic acid [DNA] and ribonucleic acid [RNA]) and proteins, which are the building blocks for all living tissue. Estrogens are also required at puberty for the development and maintenance of the female reproductive system and the development of female secondary sex characteristics, a process known as *feminization*.

🍃 SAFETY: HERBAL THERAPIES AND DIETARY SUPPLEMENTS [QSEN]

Soy (Glycine max)

Overview
Soy is a bean commonly grown throughout the world. The isoflavones in soy are chemically similar to the female hormone estradiol. Some studies have shown soy to be useful in the prevention of menopausal symptoms in perimenopausal women. Estrasorb is a new form of estrogen therapy that is a soy-based emulsion applied like a lotion. Other studies have found that soy reduces both low-density lipoprotein and total cholesterol levels.

Common Uses
Reduction of cholesterol level, relief of menopause symptoms (alternative to hormonal therapy), osteoporosis prevention

Adverse Effects
Nausea, bloating, diarrhea, abdominal pain (ingested forms), and hypersensitivity reaction have been reported from soy. When Estrasorb is used, it has been found that estradiol is still present on the skin up to 8 hours after application and can transfer to men, which results in increased estradiol levels.

Potential Drug Interactions
Orally administered soy may interfere with thyroid hormone absorption (avoid concurrent use).

Contraindications
Allergy to soy products; Estrasorb shares the same contraindications as other estrogen products

---

BOX 34-1 Diethylstilbestrol

Between 1940 and 1971, an estimated 6 million mothers and their fetuses were exposed to diethylstilbestrol (DES). The drug was used to prevent reproductive problems such as miscarriage, premature delivery, intrauterine fetal death, and toxemia. This use resulted in significant complications of the reproductive system in both female and male offspring. Two large groups have been established to monitor these complications: the Registry for Research on Hormonal Transplacental Carcinogenesis and the National Cooperative Diethylstilbestrol Adenosis (DESAD) Project.

Estrogens produce their effects in estrogen-responsive tissues, which have a large number of estrogen receptors. These tissues include the female genital organs, the breasts, the pituitary gland, and the hypothalamus. At the time of puberty, the production of estrogen increases greatly. This causes initiation of the menses, breast development, redistribution of body fat, softening of the skin, and other feminizing changes.

BOX 34-2 Indications for Estrogen Therapy

- Atrophic vaginitis (shrinkage of the vagina and/or urethra)
- Hypogonadism
- Oral contraception (in combination with a progestin)
- Ovarian failure or castration (or removal of ovaries)
- Uterine bleeding
- Breast or prostate cancer (palliative treatment of advanced inoperable cases)
- Osteoporosis (treatment and prophylaxis)
- Vasomotor symptoms of menopause (e.g., hot flashes)

TABLE 34-2 Estrogens: Common Adverse Effects

Body System	Adverse Effects
Cardiovascular	Hypertension, thromboembolism, edema
Gastrointestinal	Nausea, vomiting, diarrhea, constipation
Genitourinary	Amenorrhea, breakthrough uterine bleeding
Dermatologic	Chloasma (facial skin discoloration; also called *melasma*), hirsutism, alopecia
Other	Tender breasts, fluid retention, headache

Indications

Estrogens are used in the treatment or prevention of a variety of disorders that result primarily from estrogen deficiency. These conditions are listed in Box 34-2. Hormone replacement therapy (HRT) to counter such estrogen deficiency is most commonly known for its benefits in treating menopausal symptoms (e.g., hot flashes).

Contraindications

Contraindications for estrogen administration include known drug allergy, any estrogen-dependent cancer, undiagnosed abnormal vaginal bleeding, pregnancy, and active thromboembolic disorder (e.g., stroke, thrombophlebitis) or a history of such a disorder.

Adverse Effects

The most serious adverse effects of the estrogens are thromboembolic events. The most common undesirable effect of estrogen use is nausea. Photosensitivity also may occur with estrogen therapy. One common dermatologic effect of note is chloasma. This and other adverse effects are listed in Table 34-2.

Interactions

Estrogens can decrease the activity of the oral anticoagulants, and the concurrent administration of rifampin and St. John's wort can decrease their estrogenic effect. Their use with tricyclic antidepressants may promote toxicity of the antidepressant. Smoking should be avoided during estrogen therapy, because this, too, can diminish the estrogenic effect and add to the risk for thrombosis.

Dosages

For dosage information on some of the many available estrogen products, see the table on this page.

DRUG PROFILE

◆estrogen

Estrogen is indicated for the treatment of many clinical conditions, primarily those resulting from estrogen deficiency (see Box 34-2). Many of these conditions occur around menopause, when the endogenous estradiol level is declining. Any estrogen capable of binding to the estrogen receptors in target organs can alleviate menopausal symptoms. As a general rule, the smallest dosage of estrogen that relieves the symptoms or prevents the condition is used.

Two studies that were performed as part of the Women's Health Initiative (WHI), a large research program sponsored by the National Institutes of Health, demonstrated the possible detrimental effects of estrogen and estrogen-progestin therapy.

Both studies attempted to determine the value of HRT, if any, in preventing diseases and conditions commonly affecting older women, including breast cancer, heart disease, stroke, and hip fracture. The WHI was launched in 1991 under the direction of the National Heart, Lung, and Blood Institute (NHLBI). In one of the WHI studies of HRT, research subjects who took a certain estrogen-progestin combination product were found to have an increased risk for breast cancer, heart disease, stroke, and blood clots, although their risk for hip fractures and colon cancer was reduced. These preliminary results were so alarming that this study of combined estrogen-progestin therapy was discontinued in 2002.

DOSAGES

Selected Estrogenic Drugs

Drug (Pregnancy Category)	Pharmacologic Class	Usual Dosage Range	Indications
◆conjugated estrogens (Cenestin, Premarin) (X) and esterified estrogens (Estratab, Menest) (X)	Estrogenic hormone mixture	PO: 0.3-1.25 mg/day	Atrophic vaginitis, vasomotor symptoms of menopause
estradiol (Estrace) (X)	Estrogenic hormone	PO: 1-2 mg daily	Vasomotor symptoms of menopause, ovarian failure
estradiol transdermal (Estraderm, FemPatch, Vivelle, Climara, Menostar) (X)	Estrogenic hormone	Transdermal: 1 patch applied once or twice weekly to lower abdomen (not breast); 0.025 to 0.1 mg (instructions may vary by product)	Vasomotor symptoms of menopause

A part of the WHI investigation focusing on cognitive function, the WHI Memory Study, also identified adverse cognitive effects in women receiving combination estrogen-progestin therapy. These patients showed an increased risk for developing dementia and demonstrated reduced performance on tests of cognitive function. A second HRT study was begun in which women who had undergone hysterectomy received estrogen alone without progestin. In March 2004, however, these participants were advised to stop taking their assigned medication, because the estrogen-only therapy appeared to be associated with an increased risk for stroke. The data also indicate that estrogen therapy had no effect on the rates of coronary heart disease or breast cancer but was associated with a reduced rate of hip fracture.

Since publication of the WHI studies, much confusion and controversy has arisen. One of the biggest challenges to the WHI study is that the majority of the women studied were at least 10 years postmenopause. Recent data have suggested that the use of estrogen in women who are younger is beneficial. Follow-up of the WHI study subjects began in 2010. The North American Menopause Society (NAMS) also updated its position statement in 2012 regarding estrogen use in perimenopausal and postmenopausal women. The updated recommendations support the initiation of HT (hormonal therapy) around the time of menopause to treat menopause-related symptoms and to treat or reduce the risk for certain disorders, such as osteoporosis or fractures. Hormone replacement is not recommended for women with histories of endometrial cancer. In women with breast cancer, estrogen therapy has not been proven safe and might raise recurrence risk. When hormone therapy is discontinued after several years of use, assess bone-mineral density and begin treatment if indicated. The reader is referred to the website of the North American Menopause Society at *www.menopause.org* for the latest position statements.

The pharmacologic effects of all estrogens are similar because there are only slight differences in their chemical structures. These differences yield drugs of different potencies, which in turn make them useful for a variety of indications. They also allow the drugs to be given by different routes of administration and at often highly customized dosages.

Fixed estrogen-progestin combination products have been developed over the years. Their use is commonly referred to as *continuous combined hormone replacement therapy.* The use of estrogen therapy alone has been associated with an increased risk for endometrial hyperplasia, a possible precursor of endometrial cancer. The addition of continuously administered progestin to an estrogen regimen reduces the incidence of endometrial hyperplasia associated with unopposed estrogen therapy. Examples of these fixed combinations are conjugated estrogens with medroxyprogesterone, norethindrone acetate with ethinyl estradiol, and estradiol with norethindrone.

PROGESTINS

Available progestational medications, or progestins, include both natural and synthetic drugs. Progesterone is the most active natural progestational hormone and is the primary progestin

component in most drug formulations. It is produced by the corpus luteum after each ovulation and during pregnancy by the placenta. In addition, there are two other major natural progestational hormones. The first is 17-hydroxyprogesterone, an inactive metabolite of progesterone. The second is pregnenolone, a chemical precursor to all steroid hormones that is synthesized from cholesterol in the ovary. Because orally administered progesterone is relatively inactive and parenterally administered progesterone causes local reactions and pain, chemical derivatives were developed. The following are some of the most commonly used progestins:

- Hydroxyprogesterone (Hylutin)
- Levonorgestrel (Plan B)
- Medroxyprogesterone (Provera, Depo-Provera)
- Megestrol (Megace)
- Norethindrone acetate (Aygestin)
- Norgestrel (Ovrette, Ovral)
- Progesterone (Prometrium)
- Etonogestrel implant (Implanon)

Mechanism of Action and Drug Effects

All of the progestin products produce the same physiologic responses as those produced by progesterone itself. These responses include induction of secretory changes in the endometrium, including diminished endometrial tissue proliferation; an increase in the basal body temperature; thickening of the vaginal mucosa; relaxation of uterine smooth muscle; stimulation of mammary alveolar tissue growth; feedback inhibition (negative feedback) of the release of pituitary gonadotropins (FSH and LH); and alterations in menstrual blood flow, especially in the presence of estrogen.

Indications

Progestins are useful in the treatment of functional uterine bleeding caused by a hormonal imbalance, fibroids, or uterine cancer; in the treatment of primary and secondary amenorrhea; in the adjunctive and palliative treatment of some cancers and endometriosis; and, alone or in combination with estrogens, in the prevention of conception. They may also be helpful in preventing a threatened miscarriage and alleviating the symptoms of premenstrual syndrome. Medroxyprogesterone is the one most commonly used. Norethindrone and norgestrel are commonly used alone or in combination with estrogens as contraceptives. Megestrol is commonly used as adjunct therapy in the treatment of breast and endometrial cancers. When estrogen replacement therapy is initiated after menopause, progestins are often included to decrease the endometrial proliferation that can be caused by unopposed estrogen in women with an intact uterus. Formulations of progesterone itself are also used to treat female infertility (see the dosages table on the next page).

Contraindications

Contraindications for progestin are similar to those for estrogens.

Adverse Effects

The most serious undesirable effects of progestin use include liver dysfunction and thromboembolic disorders such as

TABLE 34-3 Progestins: Common Adverse Effects

Body System	Adverse Effects
Gastrointestinal	Nausea, vomiting
Genitourinary	Amenorrhea, spotting
Other	Edema, weight gain or loss, rash, pyrexia, somnolence or insomnia, depression

Pharmacokinetics: Medroxyprogesterone (Depo-Provera)

Route	Onset of Action	Peak Plasma Concentration	Elimination Half-life	Duration of Action
IM	Unknown	2-7 hr	14.5 hr	3 mo

pulmonary embolism. The more common adverse effects are listed in Table 34-3.

Interactions

Progestins may increase the effects of benzodiazepines and voriconazole. Barbiturates, carbamazepine, phenytoin, rifampin, and St. John's wort, which are all enzyme inducers, may decrease the effectiveness of progestin.

Dosages

For recommended dosages of selected progestins, see the dosages table below.

DRUG PROFILES

♦ medroxyprogesterone

Medroxyprogesterone (Provera, Depo-Provera) inhibits the secretion of pituitary gonadotropins, which prevents follicular maturation and ovulation, stimulates the growth of mammary tissue, and has an antineoplastic action against endometrial cancer. Medroxyprogesterone is used to treat uterine bleeding, secondary amenorrhea, endometrial cancer, and renal cancer and is also used as a contraceptive. It is also sometimes used as adjunct therapy in certain types of cancer (see Chapter 46). Medroxyprogesterone is available in both oral and parenteral preparations. It is also available in a long-acting injection formulation called Depo-Provera.

Depo-Provera is used for birth control, and one shot protects the woman for 3 months. There is concern about its use in women younger than 25 years of age and use for longer than 2 years due to the potential for bone density loss.

megestrol

Megestrol (Megace) is a synthetic progestin that is very similar to progesterone. It is primarily used in the palliative management of recurrent, inoperable, or metastatic endometrial or breast cancer. Because it can cause appetite stimulation and weight gain, it is also used in the management of anorexia, cachexia, or unexplained substantial weight loss in patients with acquired immunodeficiency syndrome (AIDS) and in patients with cancer. It is available only for oral use.

Pharmacokinetics: Megestrol

Route	Onset of Action	Peak Plasma Concentration	Elimination Half-life	Duration of Action
PO	6-8 wk	1-3 hr	13-105 hr	4-10 mo

CONTRACEPTIVE DRUGS

Contraceptive drugs are used to prevent pregnancy. Contraceptive devices are nondrug methods of pregnancy prevention such as intrauterine devices, male and female condoms, cervical diaphragms, and others, which are beyond the scope of a pharmacology text. Patients must be informed of the fact that contraceptive drug therapy serves only to prevent pregnancy and does not protect them from sexually transmitted diseases, including human immunodeficiency virus (HIV) infection/AIDS. This includes spermicidal drugs such as over-the-counter (OTC) foams for intravaginal use.

Aside from sexual abstinence, oral contraceptives are the most effective form of birth control currently available. Estrogen-progestin combinations, often referred to as "the pill," are oral contraceptives that contain both estrogenic and progestational steroids. The most common estrogenic component is ethinyl estradiol, a semisynthetic steroidal estrogen. The most common progestin component is norethindrone.

DOSAGES

Selected Progestational Drugs

Drug (Pregnancy Category)	Pharmacologic Class	Usual Dosage Range	Indications
♦ medroxyprogesterone acetate (Provera, others) (X)	Progestin	PO: 2.5-10 mg/day for a set number of days or cyclically depending on indication	Amenorrhea, uterine bleeding, vasomotor symptoms of menopause
megestrol (Megace) (X)		PO: 400-800 mg/day	Severe weight loss in male and female patients with HIV/AIDS
		PO: 40-320 mg/day in divided doses	Endometrial/breast cancer

AIDS, Acquired immunodeficiency syndrome; *HIV*, human immunodeficiency virus (infection).

The currently available oral contraceptives may be *biphasic, triphasic,* or *monophasic,* in terms of the doses taken at different times of the menstrual cycle. The newest are the extended-cycle oral contraceptives. The biphasic drugs contain a fixed estrogen dose combined with a low progestin dose for the first 10 days and a higher dose for the rest of the cycle and are available in 21- or 28-day dosage packages. The triphasic oral contraceptives contain three different estrogen-progestin dose ratios that are administered sequentially during the cycle and are provided in 21- or 28-day dosage packages. The triphasic products most closely duplicate the normal hormonal levels of the female cycle. These contraceptives also come in monophasic forms, in which the estrogen and progestin doses are the same throughout the cycle. There are also oral contraceptives that are progestin-only drugs. The monophasic and triphasic oral contraceptives are the most numerous on the market and the most widely prescribed. The extended-cycle oral contraceptives differ from the traditional 21 days on, 7 days off pills by decreasing or eliminating the hormone-free dosing interval. Consecutive days of hormonal therapy may extend to 84 to 365 days. Reasons for switching to an extended-cycle product include improved efficacy in women who forget to restart the pill and patient preference to decrease the frequency of menstrual bleeding. Some patients (e.g., those with menstrual irregularities) may require special assistance in selecting drug products with their prescribers. Other important contraceptive medications are a long-acting injectable form of medroxyprogesterone, a transdermal contraceptive patch, implantable rods. and an intravaginal contraceptive ring.

Mechanism of Action and Drug Effects

Contraceptive drugs prevent ovulation by inhibiting the release of gonadotropins and by increasing uterine mucous viscosity, which results in (1) decreased sperm movement and fertilization of the ovum, and (2) possible inhibition of implantation (nidation) of a fertilized egg (zygote) into the endometrial lining.

Oral contraceptives have many of the same hormonal effects as those normally produced by endogenous estrogens and progesterone. The contraceptive effect results mainly from the suppression of the hypothalamic-pituitary system, which in turn prevents ovulation. Other incidental benefits to their use are that they improve menstrual cycle regularity and decrease blood loss during menstruation. A decreased incidence of functional ovarian cysts and ectopic pregnancies has also been associated with their use.

Indications

Oral contraceptive drugs are primarily used to prevent pregnancy. In addition, they are used to treat endometriosis and hypermenorrhea and to produce cyclic withdrawal bleeding in patients with amenorrhea. Occasionally combination oral contraceptives are used to provide postcoital emergency contraception. Emergency contraception pills are not effective if the woman is already pregnant (i.e., egg implantation has occurred). They should therefore be taken within 72 hours of unprotected intercourse with a follow-up dose 12 hours after the first dose. They are intended to prevent pregnancy after known or

TABLE 34-4   Oral Contraceptives: Common Adverse Effects

Body System	Adverse Effects
Cardiovascular	Hypertension, edema, thromboembolism, pulmonary embolism, myocardial infarction
Central nervous	Dizziness, headache, migraines, depression, stroke
Gastrointestinal	Nausea, vomiting, diarrhea, anorexia, cramps, constipation, increased weight
Genitourinary	Amenorrhea, cervical erosion, breakthrough bleeding, dysmenorrhea, breast changes

suspected contraceptive failure or unprotected intercourse. Preven, Plan B, and generics are used for this indication. One oral contraceptive of note is Seasonale (extended cycle), which includes both estrogen and progestin components. It is sold in packages containing 3 months' worth of medication, including 1 week's worth of nonhormonal tablets. This is because Seasonale reduces a woman's menstrual cycles to once every 3 months.

Contraindications

Contraindications to the use of oral contraceptives include known drug allergy to a specific product, pregnancy, and known high risk for or history of thromboembolic events such as myocardial infarction, venous thrombosis, pulmonary embolism, or stroke.

Adverse Effects

Common adverse effects associated with the use of oral contraceptives are listed in Table 34-4. Other effects include hypertension, thromboembolism, alterations in carbohydrate and lipid metabolism, increases in serum hormone concentrations, and alterations in serum metal and plasma protein levels. It is the estrogen component that appears to be the source of most of these metabolic effects.

Interactions

Several drugs and drug classes can potentially reduce the effectiveness of oral contraceptives, which can possibly result in an unintended pregnancy. Educate patients about the need to use alternative birth control methods for at least 1 month during and after taking any of the following drugs: antibiotics (especially penicillins and cephalosporins), barbiturates, isoniazid, and rifampin. The effectiveness of other drugs, such as anticonvulsants, beta blockers, hypnotics, antidiabetic drugs, warfarin, theophylline, tricyclic antidepressants, and vitamins, may be reduced when they are taken with oral contraceptives.

Dosages

For the recommended dosages of oral contraceptives, see the dosages table on the next page.

DRUG PROFILE

CONTRACEPTIVE DRUGS

The dosages table on the next page provides selected examples of the many contraceptive drugs available. All work in similar

DOSAGES

Selected Contraceptive Drugs

Drug (Pregnancy Category)	Pharmacologic Class	Usual Dosage Range
Oral Contraceptives		
norethindrone and ethinyl estradiol (Ortho-Novum, Necon, Jenest, others) (X)	Biphasic: fixed estrogen–variable progestin 21- or 28-day products	1 pill daily for either 21 or 28 days
norethindrone and ethinyl estradiol (Loestrin, Modicon, Necon, others) (X)	Monophasic: fixed estrogen-progestin combinations; 21- or 28-day products; 28-day products contain 7 inert tabs	
norethindrone and ethinyl estradiol (Ortho-Novum 7/7/7, Estrostep, Tri-Norinyl, others) (X)	Triphasic: 3 or 4 monthly phases of variable estrogen and progestin combinations; 21- or 28-day products; 28-day products contain 7 inert tabs	
levonorgestrel and ethinyl estradiol (Seasonale, Yaz, Lybrel, others) (X)	Extended-cycle products	
Injectable Contraceptives (Depot)		
medroxyprogesterone (Depo-Provera) (X)	Progestin-only injectable contraceptive	IM: 150 mg every 3 months
Transdermal Contraceptives		
norelgestromin and ethinyl estradiol (X)	Fixed-combination estrogen-progestin transdermal contraceptive	Transdermal patch: 1 patch applied weekly for 3 wk each month
Intravaginal Contraceptives		
etonogestrel–ethinyl estradiol vaginal ring (NuvaRing) (X)	Fixed-combination estrogen-progestin intravaginal contraceptive	1 ring inserted into vagina and left in place for 3 wk, followed by removal for 1 wk

fashion to prevent pregnancy. They are classified as pregnancy category X drugs by the U.S. Food and Drug Administration (FDA). Drugs that are intended for termination of pregnancy are known as *abortifacients* and are discussed later in this chapter.

DRUGS FOR OSTEOPOROSIS

Approximately 8 million women in the United States are currently affected by osteoporosis, or low bone mass with increased risk for fracture. Nearly 40% of U.S. women over 50 years of age will develop an osteoporotic fracture, and the annual costs to society equal nearly $11 billion. Risk factors for postmenopausal osteoporosis include white or Asian descent, slender body build, early estrogen deficiency, smoking, alcohol consumption, low-calcium diet, sedentary lifestyle, and family history of osteoporosis. Although osteoporosis is primarily a disorder that affects women, up to 20% of individuals with this condition are men.

Supplementation with calcium and vitamin D are thought to play a role in the prevention of this common bone disorder. Current recommendations are that women, especially those older than 60 years of age, *consider* taking calcium and vitamin D supplements for bone health.

Several drug classes are used for the treatment of existing osteoporosis: the bisphosphonates, the selective estrogen receptor modulators (SERMs), the hormones calcitonin and teripartide, and most recently, denosumab. Currently available bisphosphonates used for osteoporosis prevention and treatment include alendronate, ibandronate, risedronate, and the once-a-year injection zoledronic acid. Raloxifene and tamoxifen are the currently available SERMs. Tamoxifen is primarily

used in oncology settings and is discussed further in Chapter 46. Raloxifene is indicated for use in the prevention and treatment of osteoporosis. A drug form of the hormone calcitonin is also commonly used. Teripartide stimulates bone formation, while denosumab (Prolia) prevents bone resorption.

Mechanism of Action and Drug Effects

Bisphosphonates

The bisphosphonates work by inhibiting osteoclast-mediated bone resorption, which in turn indirectly enhances bone mineral density. *Osteoclasts* are bone cells that break down bone, causing calcium to be reabsorbed into the circulation; this resorption eventually leads to osteoporosis if not controlled or countered by adequate new bone formation. Strong clinical evidence indicates that bisphosphonates can reverse lost bone mass and reduce facture risk.

Selective Estrogen Receptor Modulators

Raloxifene helps prevent osteoporosis by stimulating estrogen receptors on bone and increasing bone density in a manner similar to that of the estrogens themselves.

Calcitonin

Like the natural thyroid hormone, calcitonin directly inhibits osteoclastic bone resorption.

Teriparatide

In contrast to the other therapies described thus far, which inhibit bone resorption, teriparatide is the first and currently the only drug available that acts by stimulating bone formation. It is a derivative of parathyroid hormone and works to treat osteoporosis by modulating the body's metabolism of calcium and phosphorus in a manner similar to that of the natural parathyroid hormone.

Denosumab

Denosumab (Prolia) is a monoclonal antibody that blocks osteoclast activation, thereby preventing bone resorption. It is given as a subcutaneous injection once every 6 months along with daily calcium and vitamin D. Denosumab is used in the treatment of osteoporosis and bone metastases.

Indications

Raloxifene is primarily used for the prevention of postmenopausal osteoporosis. The bisphosphonates are used in both the prevention and treatment of osteoporosis. Teriparatide is used primarily for the subset of osteoporosis patients at highest risk for fracture (e.g., those with prior fracture); calcitonin and denoxumab are used for treatment of osteoporosis.

Contraindications

Bisphosphonates

Contraindications to bisphosphonate use include known drug allergy, hypocalcemia, esophageal dysfunction, and the inability to sit or stand upright for at least 30 minutes after taking the medication.

Selective Estrogen Receptor Modulators (SERMs)

The use of SERMs is contraindicated in women with a known drug allergy, in women who are or may become pregnant, and in women with a venous thromboembolic disorder, including deep vein thrombosis, pulmonary embolism, and retinal vein thrombosis, or with a history of such a disorder.

Calcitonin

Contraindications to calcitonin use include known drug allergy or allergy to salmon (the drug is salmon derived).

Teriparatide

Contraindications to the use of teriparatide include known drug allergy.

Denosumab

Contraindications to the use of denosumab are hypocalcemia, renal impairment or failure, and infection.

Adverse Effects

The primary adverse effects of SERMs are hot flashes and leg cramps. They can increase the risk for venous thromboembolism and are teratogenic. Leukopenia may also occur and predispose the patient to various infections. The most common adverse effects of bisphosphonates are headache, gastrointestinal (GI) upset, and joint pain. However, the bisphosphonates are usually well tolerated. There is a risk for esophageal burns with these medications if they become lodged in the esophagus before reaching the stomach. For this reason, the patient must take these medications with a full glass of water and must remain sitting upright or standing for at least 30 minutes

afterward. Several case reports of osteonecrosis of the jaw in patients taking bisphosphonates have been released. The FDA issued a public health advisory in January 2008 alerting practitioners to the possible association between bisphosphonate use and the development of severe (possibly incapacitating) bone, muscle, and/or joint pain, as well as low energy fractures when taking bisphosphates for long periods. Common adverse effects of calcitonin include flushing of the face, nausea, diarrhea, and reduced appetite. Common adverse effects of teriparatide include chest pain, dizziness, hypercalcemia, nausea, and arthralgia. Infections occur more frequently in those taking denosumab.

Interactions

Cholestyramine decreases the absorption of raloxifene, and raloxifene can decrease the effects of warfarin. Calcium supplements and antacids can interfere with the absorption of the bisphosphonates, and therefore they need to be spaced 1 to 2 hours apart to avoid this interaction. Calcium supplements, although often needed by patients with osteoporosis, are also more likely to cause hypercalcemia in patients receiving calcitonin. Aspirin and other nonsteroidal antiinflammatory drugs (NSAIDs) have the potential for additive GI irritation if taken with bisphosphonates.

Dosages

For the recommended dosages of osteoporosis drugs, see the dosages table on this page.

DRUG PROFILES

♦ alendronate

Alendronate (Fosamax) is an oral bisphosphonate and the first nonestrogen nonhormonal option for preventing bone loss. This drug works by inhibiting and/or reversing osteoclast-mediated bone resorption. The bisphosphonates represent a major breakthrough in the treatment of osteoporosis. Alendronate is indicated for the prevention and treatment of osteoporosis in men and in postmenopausal women. It is also indicated for the treatment of glucocorticoid-induced osteoporosis in men and for the treatment of Paget disease in women.

Data show that alendronate therapy may reduce the risk for hip fracture by 51%, of spinal fracture by 47%, and of wrist fracture by 48%. Take precautions in patients with dysphagia, esophagitis, esophageal ulcer, or gastric ulcer, because the drug can be very irritating. Case reports of esophageal erosions have been published. It is recommended that alendronate be taken with an 8-ounce glass of water immediately upon arising in the morning and that the patient not lie down for at least 30 minutes after taking it. When patients whose condition has been stabilized on alendronate are hospitalized and cannot comply with these recommendations, the medication is often withheld. Alendronate has an extremely long half-life, therefore going several days without taking a dose will do little to reduce the therapeutic efficacy of the drug. There is debate on how long a woman should remain on bisphosphonate therapy, with most experts recommending roughly 5 years.

DOSAGES

Selected Drugs Used Specifically for Osteoporosis

Drug (Pregnancy Category)	Pharmacologic Class	Usual Dosage Range	Indications/Uses
◆ alendronate (Fosamax) (C)	Bisphosphonate	PO: 5 mg/day or 35 mg/wk	Osteoporosis prevention
		PO: 10 mg/day or 70 mg/wk	Osteoporosis treatment
calcitonin, salmon (Calcimar, Miacalcin, others) (C)	Calcitonin hormonal substitute derived from salmon	IM/subcut: 100 units every other day	Osteoporosis treatment
		Nasal spray: 1 spray/day	
raloxifene (Evista) (X)	Selective estrogen receptor modulator	PO: 60 mg/day	Osteoporosis prevention and treatment

Pharmacokinetics: Alendronate

Route	Onset of Action	Peak Plasma Concentration	Elimination Half-life	Duration of Action
PO	3 wk	Unknown	Longer than 10 yr due to storage in bone tissue	Unknown

raloxifene

Raloxifene (Evista) is a SERM. It is used primarily for the prevention of postmenopausal osteoporosis. Interestingly, raloxifene has positive effects on cholesterol level, but it is not normally used specifically for this purpose. It may not be the best choice for women near menopause, because use of the drug is associated with the adverse effect of hot flashes. It is available only for oral use.

Pharmacokinetics: Raloxifene

Route	Onset of Action	Peak Plasma Concentration	Elimination Half-life	Duration of Action
PO	8 wk	Unknown	28 hr	Unknown

calcitonin

Calcitonin, in its drug forms, is derived from salmon (fish) sources. Although it is available in both injectable form and nasal spray, the nasal spray (Miacalcin) is now more commonly used.

Pharmacokinetics: Calcitonin

Route	Onset of Action	Peak Plasma Concentration	Elimination Half-life	Duration of Action
Inhalation (nasal spray)	Unknown	30-40 min	43 min	Unknown

DRUGS RELATED TO PREGNANCY, LABOR, DELIVERY, AND THE POSTPARTUM PERIOD

FERTILITY DRUGS

Infertility in women is often the result of absence of ovulation (anovulation), which is normally due to various imbalances in female reproductive hormones. Such imbalances can occur at the level of the hypothalamus, the pituitary gland, the ovary, or any combination of these. Exogenous administration of estrogens or progestins may be used to fortify the blood levels of these hormones when ovarian output is inadequate. The use of drug forms of these hormones was described earlier in this chapter.

Hormone deficiencies at the hypothalamic and pituitary levels are often treated with gonadotropin ovarian stimulants. These drugs stimulate increased secretion of gonadotropin-releasing hormone (Gn-RH) from the hypothalamus, which then results in increased secretion of FSH and LH from the pituitary gland. These hormones, in turn, stimulate the development of ovarian follicles and ovulation. They also stimulate ovarian secretion of the estrogens and progestins that are part of the normal ovulatory cycle. Proper selection and dosage adjustment of fertility drugs requires the expertise of a fertility specialist. The various medical techniques used in the treatment of infertility, including drug therapy, are now collectively referred to as *assisted reproductive technology*. In vitro fertilization is a common procedure, during which a woman's ovum is fertilized with her partner's sperm in a laboratory and the fertilized ovum is then implanted into the woman's uterus. Infants born through the use of this technique used to be referred to as "test tube babies." The success of such fertilization techniques is aided by the use of medications described earlier. Representative examples of ovulation stimulants include the drugs clomiphene, menotropins, and choriogonadotropin alfa.

Mechanism of Action and Drug Effects

Clomiphene is a nonsteroidal ovulation stimulant that works by blocking estrogen receptors in the uterus and brain. This results in a false signal of low estrogen levels to the brain. The hypothalamus and pituitary gland then increase their production of Gn-RH (from the hypothalamus) and FSH and LH (from the pituitary gland), which stimulates the maturation of ovarian follicles. Ideally this leads to ovulation and increases the likelihood of conception.

Menotropins is the drug name for a standardized mixture of FSH and LH that is derived from the urine of postmenopausal women. The FSH component stimulates the development of ovarian follicles, which leads to ovulation. The LH component stimulates the development of the corpus luteum, which supplies female sex hormones (estrogens and progesterone) during the first trimester of pregnancy. Choriogonadotropin alfa is a recombinant form (i.e., developed using recombinant DNA technology) of the hormone human chorionic gonadotropin. This hormone is naturally produced by the placenta during pregnancy and can be isolated from the urine of pregnant women. It is an analogue of LH and can provide a substitute for the natural LH surge that promotes ovulation. It does this by binding to LH receptors in the ovary and stimulating the rupture of mature ovarian follicles and the subsequent development of the corpus luteum. Human chorionic gonadotropin also maintains the viability of the corpus luteum during early pregnancy. This is critical, because the corpus luteum provides the supply of estrogens and progesterone necessary to support the first trimester of pregnancy until the placenta assumes this role. Choriogonadotropin alfa is often given in a carefully timed fashion after FSH-active therapy such as menotropin or clomiphene therapy, when patient monitoring indicates sufficient maturation of ovarian follicles.

Indications

These drugs are used primarily for the promotion of ovulation in anovulatory female patients. They may also be used to promote spermatogenesis in infertile men. As mentioned previously, progesterone formulations are also used to treat female infertility.

Contraindications

Contraindications to the use of the ovarian stimulants include known drug allergy to a specific product and may also include primary ovarian failure, uncontrolled thyroid or adrenal dysfunction, liver disease, pituitary tumor, abnormal uterine bleeding, ovarian enlargement of uncertain cause, sex hormone–dependent tumors, and pregnancy.

Adverse Effects

The most common adverse effects of the ovulation stimulants are listed in Table 34-5.

Interactions

Few drugs interact with fertility drugs. The most notable are the tricyclic antidepressants, the butyrophenones (e.g., haloperidol), the phenothiazines (e.g., promethazine), and the antihypertensive drug methyldopa. When any of these drugs is taken with the fertility drugs, prolactin concentrations may be increased, which may impair fertility.

Dosages

For recommended dosages of clomiphene, see the dosages table on this page.

TABLE 34-5   Fertility Drugs: Most Common Adverse Effects

Body System	Adverse Effects
Cardiovascular	Tachycardia, deep vein thrombosis
Central nervous	Dizziness, headache, flushing, depression, restlessness, anxiety, nervousness, fatigue
Gastrointestinal	Nausea, bloating, constipation, vomiting
Other	Urticaria, ovarian hyperstimulation, multiple pregnancy (twins or more), blurred vision, diplopia, photophobia, breast pain

DRUG PROFILE

clomiphene

Clomiphene (Clomid) is primarily used to stimulate the production of pituitary gonadotropins, which in turn induces the maturation of the ovarian follicle and eventually ovulation. It is currently available only for oral use.

Pharmacokinetics: Clomiphene

Route	Onset of Action	Peak Plasma Concentration	Elimination Half-life	Duration of Action
PO	4-12 days	Unknown	5 days	30 days

UTERINE STIMULANTS

A variety of medications are used to alter the dynamics of uterine contractions either to promote or to prevent the start or progression of labor. In the immediate postpartum period, medications may be used to promote rapid shrinkage (involution) of the uterus to reduce the risk for postpartum hemorrhage.

Four types of drugs are used to stimulate uterine contractions: ergot derivatives, prostaglandins, the progesterone antagonist mifepristone (RU-486), and the hormone oxytocin. These drugs all act on the uterus, a highly muscular organ that has a complex network of smooth muscle fibers and a large blood supply. These drugs are often collectively referred to as *oxytocics*, after the naturally occurring hormone oxytocin, whose action they mimic. The uterus undergoes several changes during normal gestation and childbirth that at different times make it either resistant or susceptible to various hormones and drugs. Oxytocin is one of the two hormones secreted by the posterior lobe of the pituitary gland. The other is vasopressin, which is also known as *antidiuretic hormone* (see Chapter 30).

Mechanism of Action and Drug Effects

The uterus of a woman who is not pregnant is relatively insensitive to oxytocin, but during pregnancy the uterus becomes more sensitive to this hormone and is most sensitive at term (the end of gestation).

During childbirth, oxytocin stimulates uterine contraction, and during lactation it promotes the movement of milk from the mammary glands to the nipples. Another class of oxytocic drugs is the prostaglandins, natural hormones involved in regulating the network of smooth muscle fibers of the uterus. This network is known as the myometrium. The prostaglandins cause very potent contractions of the myometrium and may also play a role in the natural induction of labor. When the prostaglandin concentrations increase during the final few weeks of pregnancy, mild myometrial contractions, commonly known as Braxton Hicks contractions, are stimulated. The third major class of oxytocic drugs is the ergot alkaloids, which are also potent simulators of uterine muscle. These drugs increase the force and frequency of uterine contractions. One of the most politically charged prescription drug approvals ever made by the FDA was approval of the progesterone antagonist mifepristone (Mifeprex), also known as the "abortion pill." This

DOSAGES

Selected Fertility Drugs

Drug (Pregnancy Category)	Pharmacologic Class	Usual Dosage Range	Indications
clomiphene (Clomid, Serophene) (X)	Ovulation stimulant	PO: 50-100 mg daily for 5 days; repeatable cycle depending on response	Female infertility in selected patients

drug also stimulates uterine contractions and is used to induce elective termination of pregnancy.

Indications

Oxytocin is available in a synthetic injectable form (e.g., Pitocin). This drug is used to induce labor at or near full-term gestation and to enhance labor when uterine contractions are weak and ineffective. Oxytocin is also used to prevent or control uterine bleeding after delivery, to induce completion of an incomplete abortion (including miscarriages), and to promote milk ejection during lactation.

The prostaglandins may be used therapeutically to induce labor by softening the cervix (cervical ripening) and enhancing uterine muscle tone. They may also be used to stimulate the myometrium to induce abortion during the second trimester when the uterus is resistant to oxytocin. Examples of these drugs are dinoprostone and misoprostol. Misoprostol is an oral tablet and is also used as a stomach protectant (see Chapter 44). Misoprostol is used off-label for cervical ripening and is administered orally or intravaginally. It offers the advantage of costing pennies as opposed to the hundreds of dollars paid for dinoprostone. Misoprostol is widely used in third-world countries as well as throughout the United States.

Ergot alkaloids are used after delivery of the infant and placenta to prevent postpartum uterine atony (lack of muscle tone) and hemorrhage.

Mifepristone is used to induce abortion and is often given with the synthetic prostaglandin drug misoprostol for this purpose.

Contraindications

Contraindications to the use of labor-inducing uterine stimulants include known drug allergy to a specific product and may include pelvic inflammatory disease, cervical stenosis, uterine fibrosis, high-risk intrauterine fetal positions before delivery, placenta previa, hypertonic uterus, uterine prolapse, or any condition in which vaginal delivery is contraindicated (e.g., increased bleeding risk). Contraindications to the use of abortifacients include known drug allergy as well as the presence of an intrauterine device, ectopic pregnancy, concurrent anticoagulant therapy or bleeding disorder, inadequate access to emergency health care, or the inability to understand or comply with follow-up instructions.

TABLE 34-6 Oxytocic Drugs: Most Common Adverse Effects

Body System	Adverse Effects
Cardiovascular	Hypotension or hypertension, chest pain
Central nervous	Headache, dizziness, fainting
Gastrointestinal	Nausea, vomiting, diarrhea
Genitourinary	Vaginitis, vaginal pain, cramping
Other	Leg cramps, joint swelling, chills, fever, weakness, blurred vision

Adverse Effects

The most common undesirable effects of oxytocic drugs are listed in Table 34-6.

Interactions

Few clinically significant drug interactions occur with the oxytocic drugs. The most common and important of these involve sympathomimetic drugs. Combining drugs that produce vasoconstriction, such as sympathomimetics, with the oxytocic drugs can result in severe hypertension.

Dosages

For the recommended dosages of selected oxytocic drugs, see the dosages table on the next page.

DRUG PROFILES

◆ dinoprostone

Dinoprostone (Prostin E$_2$, Cervidil, Prepidil) is a synthetic derivative of the naturally occurring hormone prostaglandin E$_2$. It is used for the termination of pregnancy from the twelfth through the twentieth gestational week; for evacuation of uterine contents in the management of missed abortion or intrauterine fetal death up to 28 weeks of gestational age; and, most commonly, for ripening of an unfavorable cervix in pregnant women at or near term when there is a medical or obstetric need for labor induction. It is available only for vaginal use in various dosage forms.

Pharmacokinetics: Dinoprostone

Route	Onset of Action	Peak Plasma Concentration	Elimination Half-life	Duration of Action
Topical gel	Rapid	30-45 min	Unknown	Not available

◆ methylergonovine

The ergot alkaloid methylergonovine (Methergine) is used in the immediate postpartal period to enhance myometrial tone and reduce the likelihood of postpartum uterine hemorrhage. Its use is contraindicated in patients with a known hypersensitivity to ergot medications and in those with pelvic inflammatory disease. It must be used with caution in patients with hypertension. It is not to be used for augmentation of labor, before delivery of the placenta, during a spontaneous abortion, or given to patients with pregnancy-induced hypertension. Methylergonovine is available in both oral and injectable forms.

DOSAGES

Selected Uterine Stimulants

Drug (Pregnancy Category)*	Pharmacologic Class	Usual Dosage Range	Indications/Uses
◆ dinoprostone (Prostin E₂, Prepidil, Cervidil) (X)	Prostaglandin E₂ abortifacient and cervical-ripening drug	Cervical gel (Prepidil): 0.5 mg into cervical canal at 6-hr dosing intervals (max 1.5 mg/24 hr)	Cervical ripening for induction of labor
		Vaginal suppository (Cervidil): 10 mg into posterior vaginal fornix (space behind cervix) for 1 dose	Cervical ripening for induction of labor
◆ methylergonovine (Methergine) (X)	Oxytocic ergot alkaloid	IM/IV: 0.2 mg after delivery of placenta, repeatable at 2- to 4-hr intervals	Postpartum uterine atony and hemorrhage
		PO: 0.2 mg tid-qid for up to 7 days postpartum	
◆! oxytocin (Pitocin) (X)	Oxytocic hypothalamic hormone	IV infusion: 0.5-20 milliunits/min, titrated to effect	Labor induction
		IV infusion: 10-40 units in 1 L of D₅LR, titrated to effect	Postpartum uterine atony and hemorrhage
		IM: 10 units in a single dose after delivery of placenta	

D_5LR, Dextrose 5% in lactated Ringer's solution.

*Use of these medications is contraindicated in pregnancy (pregnancy category X) unless needed for the indications listed.

Pharmacokinetics: Methylergonovine

Route	Onset of Action	Peak Plasma Concentration	Elimination Half-life	Duration of Action
PO	5-15 min	30 min	2 hr	3 hr

◆! oxytocin

The drug oxytocin (Pitocin, Syntocinon) is the synthetic form of the endogenous hormone oxytocin and has all of its pharmacologic properties.

Pharmacokinetics: Oxytocin

Route	Onset of Action	Peak Plasma Concentration	Elimination Half-life	Duration of Action
IV	Immediate	Immediate	3-5 min	1 hr

DRUGS FOR PRETERM LABOR MANAGEMENT

Preterm labor is defined as substantial uterine contractions that could progress to delivery and occur prior to the 37th week of pregnancy. When contractions of the uterus begin before term, it may be desirable to stop labor, because premature birth increases the risk for neonatal death. Postponing delivery increases the likelihood of the infant's survival. However, this measure is generally employed only between weeks 20 to 37 of gestation, because spontaneous labor occurring before the twentieth week is commonly associated with a nonviable fetus and thus is usually not interrupted.

The nonpharmacologic treatment of premature labor includes bed rest, sedation, and hydration. Drugs given to inhibit labor and maintain the pregnancy are called *tocolytics*. Historically, terbutaline, a beta-adrenergic drug (see Chapter 18), was the drug of choice for preterm labor. It works by directly relaxing uterine smooth muscle. However, in 2011, the FDA stated that terbutaline should not be used to prevent preterm labor or for prolonged treatment due to maternal and fetal safety risks. Concentrated solutions of the electrolyte magnesium sulfate (a high-alert medication) have been used for this purpose. In 2013, The FDA issued a warning against the extended use of IV magnesium for preterm labor prevention. Magnesium sulfate is used in pregnancy-induced hypertension. Calcium gluconate must be readily available to reverse magnesium toxicity if it occurs.

The current recommendations for the management of preterm labor include the use of the nonsteroidal antiinflammatory agent, indomethacin (see Chapter 44), and the calcium channel blocker, nifedipine (see Chapter 23). Indomethacin is the most effective tocolytic currently available and works by inhibiting prostaglandin activity. Nifedipine inhibits myometrial activity by blocking calcium influx. When these treatments are ineffective and delivery is proceeding, corticosteroids (betamethasone or dexamethasone) (see Chapter 33) are given to the mother to promote lung maturity in the fetus between 24 and 34 weeks of gestation.

NURSING PROCESS

ASSESSMENT

In this section, *estrogenic* and *progestational drugs* are discussed first, followed by the major drug classes used in the treatment of osteoporosis. Next, information on *fertility drugs, uterine stimulants*, and *preterm labor management drugs* is discussed. Before initiating therapy with any of the *hormonal drugs* (e.g., *estrogens, progestins*) or other women's health–related drugs, obtain the patient's blood pressure and weight, and document the findings. Assess and document drug allergies, contraindications, cautions, and drug interactions. Include a thorough medication history, medical history, and menstrual history in your patient assessment. Note the results of the patient's last physical examination, provider-performed breast examination, and gynecologic examination as well.

TEAMWORK AND COLLABORATION: PHARMACOKINETIC BRIDGE TO NURSING PRACTICE

Estrasorb is a form of estrogen that is FDA approved to help ease the severity of postmenopausal hot flashes by increasing estrogen levels when these are found to be deficient in the patient. Estrasorb contains estradiol, which is identical to the estrogen produced in the woman's body. The absorption of the topical emulsion dosage form results in measurable levels of estradiol on the skin for up to 8 hours after application. It is important to fully understand this pharmacokinetic property, because the transfer of the drug to another individual may result. In fact, traces of Estrasorb have been found on other individuals from such transfer for up to a 2-day period. This transfer of medication to other individuals may be reduced by allowing the dosage form to fully dry and then covering it with clothing before having contact with another individual. Although no specific investigation of the tissue distribution of the estradiol absorbed from Estrasorb in humans has been conducted, it is known that the distribution of exogenous estrogens is similar to that of endogenous estrogens. The metabolism of exogenous estrogens is also similar to that of endogenous estrogens, with biotransformation taking place mainly in the liver and excretion in the urine. The specific dosage form of an emulsion is desirable because it may be applied easily, once daily to the thighs and/or calves. One dose is contained in two separate foil pouches, and patients need to be fully aware of the application instructions. For example, sunscreen products are not to be applied at the same time, because sunscreen reduces the absorption of Estrasorb.

Knowing the pharmacokinetic properties of Estrasorb is necessary for safe and efficient administration of the drug. It is also important to understand all the pharmacokinetic properties of this drug to be able to fully educate patients about the drug, its effect on the body, and the subsequent implications for its absorption, distribution, metabolism, and excretion.

Estrogen-only hormones are only to be given after the following disorders and conditions have been ruled out: estrogen-dependent cancer, undiagnosed abnormal vaginal bleeding, active thromboembolic disorders such as stroke or thrombophlebitis, or a history of these disorders. Include questions about breast examination, breast self-examination practices, and dates of last complete physical examination and Papanicolaou (Pap) smear in the assessment. It is important to assess for potential drug interactions such as with tricyclic antidepressants, which may reach toxic levels if given with estrogens. Advise patients to avoid smoking because of the risk for thrombosis. It has been documented that smoking also decreases the effectiveness of estrogen; hence, take a thorough smoking history. Question about the number of packs smoked per day and the number of years the patient has smoked. Other drug interactions to assess for include oral anticoagulants (decreased effectiveness) as well as rifampin and St. John's wort (decreased estrogen effectiveness). If being used for *hormonal replacement therapy* for menopausal symptoms, recent changes to older recommendations from the North American Menopause Society include the following: hormonal replacement is not recommended for women with histories of endometrial cancer; in women with breast cancer, estrogen therapy has not been proven safe and may raise recurrence risk. Therefore, perform a thorough assessment for history or diagnosis of endometrial

and/or breast cancer. Bone density may also be impacted once hormonal therapy is discontinued; further assessment is needed in these particular patients.

Assess the patient's knowledge about the use of *hormonal replacement drugs* (e.g., *estrogens, progestins*), whether for contraception or replacement therapy. Also assess the patient's readiness to learn, educational level, and degree of adherence to other medication regimens. The success of treatment with *oral contraceptives, hormone replacement drugs,* and other therapies depends heavily on the patient's understanding instructions. With *oral contraceptive drugs* (e.g., *combination estrogen-progestin drugs*), perform a pregnancy test and assess for history of vascular and/or thromboembolic disorders (such as myocardial infarction, venous thrombosis, stroke), malignancies of the reproductive tract, and abnormal vaginal bleeding. Closely monitor patients with the following: hypertension, migraine headaches, alterations in lipid and/or carbohydrate metabolism, fluid retention or edema, hair loss, amenorrhea, breakthrough vaginal/uterine bleeding, and uterine fibroids. The concern is for exacerbation of these conditions and the potential for subsequent complications. Closely monitor patients who smoke because of the increased risk for complications (increased risk for thrombosis) with estrogens. Assess for drug interactions, such as with drugs leading to decreased effectiveness of oral contraception, including antibiotics (especially penicillins and cephalosporins), barbiturates, isoniazid, and rifampin. Drugs that may have their therapeutic effects decreased if taken concurrently with oral contraceptives include antiepileptic drugs, beta blockers, hypnotics, antidiabetic drugs, warfarin, theophylline, tricyclic antidepressants, and vitamins. When combination oral contraceptives are used in emergency situations for postcoital conception, the same contraindications, cautions, and drug interactions apply, even if the drug is for one-time use.

The chemically derived progestins, such as *medroxyprogesterone* and *megestrol,* have the same contraindications as estrogens. Additionally, with progestins, assess for a history of liver/gallbladder disease, thrombophlebitis, and thromboembolic disorders due to possible adverse effects (see Table 34-3). Be mindful that a significant drug interaction occurs with the antidiabetic drugs. Look thoroughly at the patient's medical history in reference to the specific condition for which the progestin is ordered. Some of these include prevention of endometrial cancer caused by *estrogen therapy,* palliative management of recurrent endometrial or breast cancer, as well as management of anorexia and cachexia in those with AIDS or cancer.

With the osteoporosis drug class of *bisphosphonates,* there are many contraindications, cautions, and drug interactions. Assessment of the following is therefore important to patient safety: drug allergy, esophageal dysfunction, hypocalcemia, and the inability to sit or stand upright for at least 30 minutes after taking the medication. *Selective estrogen receptor modulators (SERMs)* are not to be used in patients who are or may become pregnant and in women with thromboembolic disorders including deep vein thrombosis. Assess for allergies to salmon with the use of *calcitonin* because the drug is derived from this fish. Drug interactions to assess for include ampicillin and cholestyramine because they decrease the absorption of raloxifene. *Raloxifene* also decreases the effects of warfarin. Assess patients for the drug interaction between *bisphosphonates* and calcium supplements and/or antacids (decreased absorption) as well as aspirin and NSAIDs (potential for additive GI irritation).

Use of *clomiphene* requires assessment of the patient's medical and medication history with attention to the patient's menstrual history. Medical history is critical, especially reproductive and uterine status, because use of the drug may result in multiple pregnancy (twins or more) and compromise maternal health status. Assess family stability and economic status because of the additional family and financial stressors associated with a multiple birth. Assess thoroughly for contraindications such as primary ovarian failure, adrenal and/or thyroid dysfunction, liver disease, and abnormal uterine bleeding. Assess also for potential drug interactions with tricyclic antidepressants, haloperidol, phenothiazines, and methyldopa (an antihypertensive drug). Fertility may be impaired if clomiphene is given with these drugs.

Before administering *uterine stimulants* (e.g., oxytocin, prostaglandins), assess and document the patient's blood pressure, pulse, and respiration. Determine the fetal heart rate and contraction-related fetal heart rates, and document the findings. Contraindications to the use of *uterine stimulants* in early pregnancy include the presence of an intrauterine device for birth control, ectopic pregnancy, use of anticoagulants, bleeding disorders, and inability to understand and then comply with instructions. Assess for the concurrent use of sympathomimetics because of enhanced vasoconstrictive effects possibly leading to severe hypertension. For labor and delivery, the patient's cervix must be ready for induction. (Consult a current maternal child health or obstetric nursing textbook for more information on the rating of the cervix.) Perform continuous monitoring of maternal blood pressure, pulse, contractions, and fluid status, as well as fetal heart rate. *Oxytocin* is *not* used during the first trimester except in some cases of spontaneous or induced abortion.

With the *ergot alkaloid methylergonovine maleate*, assess the medication order after vital signs and note that the first dose is given after delivery of the placenta to help stimulate the uterus to contract and decrease blood loss after delivery in special situations. Continue to assess blood pressure during the drug's administration. Assess for contraindications such as pregnancy, labor, liver/renal disease, cardiac disease, and pregnancy-induced hypertension. Assess for any history of seizures. If this drug is given to hypertensive women, it may precipitate seizures or a stroke. The use of *dinoprostone* or other *prostaglandin E₂* drugs is indicated in specific situations requiring termination of pregnancy. Question the patient about the presence of any contraindications, cautions, and drug interactions. *Misoprostol* is also used intravaginally as an "off-label" use for cervical ripening.

Terbutaline was formerly the drug of choice for the management of preterm labor but has been identified as having maternal and fetal risks. Instead, patients may receive *indomethacin* (see Chapter 44), *nifedipine* (see Chapter 23), or *magnesium*

sulfate. Take baseline maternal vital signs, and assess fetal heart rate prior to administering any drug indicated for preterm labor. Assess the maternal history for estimated gestation as these medications are generally used between weeks 20 to 37. Spontaneous labor before the twentieth week is commonly associated with a nonviable fetus, and the labor is not interrupted. With *indomethacin*, additional concerns to assess for include a history of coagulation disorders, chronic hypertension, heart failure, impaired liver function, and cardiovascular disease. With *nifedipine*, a history of hypotension and cardiovascular problems are contraindications.

⊕ **PATIENT-CENTERED CARE: CULTURAL IMPLICATIONS**   QSEN

Racial Disparities in Uterine and Endometrial Cancer

Approximately 54,870 new cases of cancer of the body of the uterus (uterine body or corpus) will be diagnosed in the United States for 2015, with approximately 11,000 deaths. These estimates include both endometrial cancers and uterine sarcomas. Endometrial cancer is rare in women under the age of 45 years, and about 3 out of 4 cases are found in women aged 55 and over. The average chance of a female being diagnosed this form of cancer during her lifetime is 1 in 37. There are over 600,000 female survivors of endometrial cancer. Endometrial cancer is slightly more common in white women; however, black women are more likely to die from it.

In 2012, the number of new cases of endometrial cancer was 25.1 per 100,000 women/year, with the number of deaths at 4.4 per 100,000 women/year. It is estimated that 2.8% of women will be diagnosed with endometrial cancer at some point in their lifespans (based on 2010-2012 data).

Studies from 2011 reported that following white women with the highest incidence of getting uterine cancer were black, Hispanic, Asian/Pacific Islander, and American Indian/Alaska Native women. Between 1999 and 2011, the rate of women dying from uterine cancer has varied depending on race and ethnicity. Black women were more likely to die of uterine cancer than any other group, followed by white, Hispanic, and Asian/Pacific Islander and American Indian/Alaska Native women (who were tied).

Sources: U.S. Mortality Files, National Center for Health Statistics, Division of Cancer Prevention and Control, Centers for Disease Control and Prevention. Available at *www.cdc.gov/cancer/uterine/statistics/race*. Updated August 27, 2014. Accessed July 4, 2015; and American Cancer Society. Available at *www.cancer.org*. Revised March, 2015. Accessed July 3, 2015.

▌NURSING DIAGNOSES

1. Decisional conflict related to the risks versus benefits of postmenopausal estrogen replacement therapy
2. Acute pain related to adverse effects and improper dosing of SERM
3. Noncompliance related to lack of information and experience with daily dosing of oral contraceptives

▌PLANNING: OUTCOME IDENTIFICATION

1. Patient makes informed decision regarding the safe self-use of estrogen replacement therapy.
2. Patient self-administers SERM as prescribed with minimal pain (epigastric).
3. Patient remains compliant with oral contraceptive therapy.

IMPLEMENTATION

When administering *estrogens,* directions need to be followed exactly. Provide precise and thorough instructions to patients when self-administration of the hormone is ordered. Oral dosage forms are best taken at the same time every day and with meals or a snack to minimize GI upset.

It is also important to understand the indication and rationale for the use of *estrogen* so that accurate facts about the drug are given to the patient. If *estradiol* is being given, vasomotor symptoms of menopause are generally the indication, and the drug is to be given daily at the same time. If the estradiol transdermal patch is given, it is to be applied as ordered, which is usually one patch applied once or twice weekly to the lower abdomen and not to the breast and chest areas. See Patient-Centered Care: Patient Teaching later in the chapter for more information.

Use of *progestins* is indicated for birth control, such as the use of *Depo-Provera* with one IM injection every 3 months. Depo-Provera, however, remains controversial in women of any reproductive age because of the associated bone density loss. Give these injections in deep muscle mass, and rotate sites. Oral forms of *medroxyprogesterone acetate* are used for amenorrhea and uterine bleeding and are to be taken exactly as ordered, such as for a specific number of days or cyclically. *Megestrol,* a synthetic *progestin,* is often indicted for palliative reasons or for management of anorexia, cachexia, or weight loss that is unexplained in AIDS patients. It is given orally as ordered and given to maximize appetite. It is recommended, however, that the lowest dosage possible of either *estrogens* and/or *progestins* be used and titrated as needed, but only as ordered.

Oral contraception is available in various formulations based on doses that are taken at different times of the menstrual cycle (see pharmacology discussion). Progestin-only oral contraceptive pills are taken daily. It is important for the patient to take this oral contraceptive at the same time every day so that effective hormone serum levels are maintained. Because use of the progestin-only pill leads to a higher incidence of ovulatory cycles, there is an increased rate and risk for contraceptive failure if not taken as per instructions. Be aware that this type of pill is usually prescribed for those women who cannot tolerate estrogens or for whom these hormones are contraindicated. Often it is more effective in women who are older than 35 years of age and women who are breastfeeding. *Combination estrogen-progestin* pills contain low doses of the hormones. *Biphasic* forms contain *fixed estrogen* and *variable progestin* for 21- or 28-day products. The low-dose *monophasic (fixed estrogen-progestin combination)* types are provided as 21 or 28 days of pills, with the 28-day products containing 7 inert tablets. Triphasic products offer 3 or 4 phases of variable estrogen and progestin combinations, and there are also new extended-cycle products available. Make sure the patient fully understands how to take the medication. Emphasize that the reduction in the level of estrogen has been associated with a decrease in adverse effects and a decrease in the risk for complications; however, more breakthrough bleeding may occur.

The success of therapy with *bisphosphonates* depends on providing thorough patient teaching and ensuring that the patient understands all aspects of the drug regimen. With oral bisphosphonates, emphasize the need to take the medication upon rising in the morning with a full glass (6 to 8 ounces) of water at least 30 minutes before the intake of any food, other fluids, or other medication. In addition, emphasize that the patient remain upright in either a standing or sitting position for approximately 30 minutes after taking the drug to help prevent esophageal erosion or irritation. Inform the patient taking the *SERM raloxifene* that the drug must be discontinued 72 hours before and during prolonged immobility. Therapy may be resumed, as ordered, once the patient becomes fully ambulatory. See Patient-Centered Care: Patient Teaching on the next page for more information.

Fertility drugs (e.g., *clomiphene*) are often self-administered. Provide specific instructions regarding how to administer the drug at home and how to monitor drug effectiveness to improve the success of treatment. Journal tracking of the medication regimen is helpful to those involved in the care of the infertile patient or couple. See Patient-Centered Care: Patient Teaching later in the chapter for more information.

With *tocolytics,* either *indomethacin (Indocin)* or *nifedipine (Procardia)* will be used. It is important to note, however, that *magnesium sulfate* may also be used. Follow the dosing and routes exactly as determined by the prescriber. Long-term dosing of indomethacin is not recommended due to birth defects. Nifedipine may lead to potentially life-threatening maternal-fetal problems. Discontinue both medications, as prescribed, once contractions cease. Monitor vital signs and fetal heart rates closely with these drugs. Placement of the patient in the left lateral recumbent position minimizes hypotension, increases renal blood flow, and increases blood flow to the fetus.

Administer *oxytocin* only as ordered, and strictly follow any instructions or protocols. The cervix must be ripe (see earlier discussion). *Prostaglandin E_2* may be instilled vaginally to help accomplish this if the mother's cervix is not ripe or at a Bishop score of 5 or higher. Because oxytocin has vasopressive and antidiuretic properties, the patient is at risk for hypertensive episodes as well as fluid retention; continuously monitor maternal blood pressure and pulse rate as well as fetal heart rate. Report any of the following to the prescriber immediately if they occur: strong contractions, edema, and any changes in fetal heart rate. Administer intravenous infusions (via infusion pump) of oxytocin with the proper dilutional fluid and at the proper rate. To minimize the adverse effects of the drug, intravenous piggyback dosing is often ordered so that the diluted oxytocin solution can be discontinued immediately if maternal and/or fetal decline occurs while an intravenous line with hydration is maintained. Doses are generally titrated as ordered and are based on the progress of labor and degree of fetal tolerance of the drug. If the labor progresses at 1 cm/hr, oxytocin may no longer be needed. This decision is made by the prescriber and on an individual basis. Generally speaking, if there are hypertensive responses or major changes in the maternal vital signs *or* if the fetal heart rate shows any indication of fetal intolerance of labor, contact the prescriber immediately.

Hyperstimulation may also occur. If contractions are more frequent than every 2 minutes and last longer than 1 minute (and are accompanied by changes in other parameters), stop the infusion of *oxytocin* and contact the prescriber immediately. If this does occur, place the patient in a side-lying position, maintain administration of intravenous fluids, give oxygen as ordered (generally via tight face mask at 10 to 12 L/min), and monitor the patient and fetus closely. If there is concern about overstimulation, discuss concerns with the prescriber and document actions thoroughly. When *misoprostol* is used, give orally or intravaginally for cervical ripening and only as ordered.

CASE STUDY

Patient-Centered Care: Bisphosphonate Drug Therapy for Osteoporosis

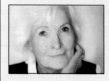 Mrs. S. is a relatively healthy 73-year-old retired clerk who has recently been diagnosed with postmenopausal osteoporosis. She has been prescribed treatment with ibandronate (Boniva), 150 mg each month. She has many questions, and you are reviewing the drug and its use with her.

1. Mrs. S. tells you that she likes to have breakfast, take her morning medicines, and then lie down on the couch to read the morning newspaper. She asks whether the ibandronate will fit into her routine. What will you tell her?
2. Mrs. S. calls the clinic to ask what to use for headaches. "I have several different types of headache pills, so aren't they all the same?" How will you respond?
3. A few months later, Mrs. S. comes in for a follow-up visit. She tells you that she is due for her next osteoporosis pill next week, but she has been having some jaw pain ever since she went to the dentist 2 weeks earlier to have a tooth pulled. She is worried that her osteoporosis has affected her jaw. What could be the reason for this pain? What do you think will be done about it?

For answers, see *http://evolve.elsevier.com/Lilley*.

Dinoprostone is given by vaginal suppository to patients who are 12 to 20 weeks pregnant and are seeking termination and/or to those in whom evacuation of the uterus is needed for the management of incomplete spontaneous abortion or intrauterine fetal death (up to 28 weeks). Give the drug exactly as ordered, and monitor the patient closely.

EVALUATION

Measure therapeutic responses to the various drugs discussed in this chapter by evaluating whether goals and outcome criteria have been met. Many drugs have been discussed, often with several indications for use; thus, the therapeutic response will be the occurrence of the indicated therapeutic effect. Monitor the patient for adverse effects and/or toxicity as well.

Therapeutic effects of *estrogens* may range from prevention of pregnancy to a decrease in menopausal symptoms to a reduction in the size of a tumor. Adverse effects of estrogens may include hypertension, thromboembolism, edema, amenorrhea, nausea, vomiting, facial skin discoloration, hirsutism, breast tenderness, and headache. Therapeutic responses to *progestins* include a decrease in abnormal uterine bleeding and the disappearance of menstrual disorders (e.g., amenorrhea). Some of the most common adverse effects of progestins include nausea, vomiting, amenorrhea, and weight gain. (See Table 34-3 for a more complete listing.) Adverse effects associated with *oral contraceptives* include hypertension, edema, thromboembolism, headache, migraines, depression, stroke, nausea, vomiting, amenorrhea, and breakthrough bleeding.

Therapeutic effects of *oxytocin* and other *uterine stimulants* include stimulation of labor and control of postpartum bleeding. Adverse effects may include hypotension or hypertension, chest pain, nausea, vomiting, blurred vision, and fainting. The primary therapeutic effect of tocolytics includes absence of preterm labor. Adverse effects of *tocolytics*, such as *indomethacin*, are discussed in Chapter 44.

The therapeutic effects of *fertility drugs* include successful conception. Some of the more common adverse reactions include tachycardia, deep vein thrombosis, headache, fatigue, nausea, vomiting, bloating, ovarian hyperstimulation, blurred vision, and photophobia. Therapeutic effects of *osteoporosis drugs* include increased bone density and prevention or management of osteoporosis. Some of the more common adverse effects of *SERMs* include hot flashes and leg cramps. These drugs also increase the risk of venous thromboembolism as well as an increased risk of various infecitons from leukopenia. *Bisphosphonates* are associated with the adverse effects of headache, GI upset, and joint pain. Monitor also for the increased risk for esophageal burns (producing pain and discomfort).

PATIENT-CENTERED CARE: PATIENT TEACHING

- Hormonal drugs are better tolerated if taken with food or milk to minimize GI upset.
- With the use of oral contraceptives as well as any form of hormonal replacement therapy (HRT) with estrogens and/or progestins, encourage the patient to openly discuss concerns about the medications. Assure the patient that, although risks may be associated with HRT, the prescriber will weigh each case individually and make a recommendation based on the benefits versus risks, but with the ultimate decision resting with the patient.

- With estrogens and progestins, advise the patient to report the following conditions to the prescriber immediately: hypertension, edema, thromboembolism, migraines, depression, and breakthrough bleeding.
- Instruct the patient to report a weight gain of 2 pounds or more in 24 hours or 5 pounds or more in 1 week, as well as any breakthrough bleeding or a change in menstrual flow.
- Instruct the patient to take oral contraceptives exactly as ordered and to keep all appointments for follow-up

examinations (e.g., pelvic examination, Pap smear, and practitioner-performed breast examination).

- Instruct the patient on the importance of and technique for monthly breast self-examinations during the ideal time— that is, 7 to 10 days after the start of menstruation or 2 to 5 days after menses ends. Stress the need for follow-up appointments and annual examinations by a health care provider.

- Hormones make the patient sensitive to sunlight and tanning beds. Emphasize that the patient must use appropriate sun protection at all times.

- If the patient is using a progesterone-only intravaginal gel with other gels, advise the patient to be sure to insert the other gels at least 6 hours before or after the progesterone-based product.

- Slow-release progesterone intrauterine devices are placed in the uterine cavity by a health care provider. Provide thorough education that inserts are left in place for 5 years (after insertion) and then must be replaced. Advise the patient to report abnormal uterine bleeding, cramping, abdominal pain, or amenorrhea immediately.

- Instruct the patient using an estrogen/progestin vaginal ring for contraception on what to expect with its insertion. Use of this contraceptive device requires thorough teaching and follow-up, including instruction on insertion and removal techniques and a return demonstration before the patient leaves the prescriber's office. Inform the patient that menstruation will follow in 2 to 3 days after the ring is removed and to replace the used ring in its foil pouch and discard it in the trash rather than flushing it down the commode.

- Oral contraceptive hormones must be taken at the same time every day and exactly as prescribed. If one dose is missed, advise the patient to take the dose as soon as it is remembered; however, if it is close to the next dose time, advise the patient not to double up and to use a backup form of contraception in these situations. Provide more specific instructions regarding the omission of more than one pill and/or 1 day's dose depending on the specific oral contraceptive drug prescribed. These specific instructions will most likely include the following: If the patient misses one "active" tablet in weeks 1, 2, or 3, the tablet needs to be taken as soon as she remembers. If the patient misses two "active" tablets in week 1 or week 2, the patient needs to take two tablets the day she remembers and two tablets the next day, and then continue taking one tablet a day until the pack is finished. The patient needs to be instructed to use a backup method of birth control such as condoms if she has sex in the 7 days after missing pills. If the patient misses two "active" tablets in the third week or misses three or more "active" tablets in a row, the patient needs to throw out the rest of the pack and start a new pack that same day. Instruct the patient to use a backup method of birth control if she has sex in the seven 7 days after missing pills.

- Stress the importance of using condoms with oral contraception to prevent sexually transmitted diseases.

- Emphasize to the patient that backup contraception (e.g., condom use) is needed when antibiotics, barbiturates, griseofulvin, isoniazid, rifampin, or St. John's wort is taken with oral contraceptives. These drugs and herbs diminish the effectiveness of oral contraception.

- Estrasorb is generally applied once daily to the thighs and calves, as ordered, with one dose provided in two separate pouches. Do not apply sunscreen and other lotions at the same time because they interfere with the drug. To reduce the chance of transfer of this medication to other individuals, allow the application areas to dry completely before covering them with clothing. The drug contained in this dosage form, estradiol, has been found to be present on the skin for up to 8 hours after application.

- Conjugated estrogens are used for menopausal symptoms and are given orally every day; however, other uses of these estrogens may require different doses and a different dosage schedule/regimen. Emphasize the expected adverse effects such as edema, nausea, diarrhea/constipation, breakthrough uterine bleeding, chloasma (facial skin discoloration), hirsutism, tender breasts, and headache. Encourage the patient to report the following conditions: elevated blood pressure, severe headache with changes in vision and vomiting, abdominal pain, and edema.

- Bisphosphonates (e.g., alendronate) are to be taken exactly as prescribed; that is, the drug is taken at least 30 minutes before the first morning beverage, food, or other medication and with at least 6 to 8 ounces of water. Emphasize the importance of remaining upright for at least 30 minutes after taking the medication to prevent esophageal and GI adverse effects. Esophageal irritation, dysphagia, severe heartburn, and retrosternal pain must be reported to the prescriber immediately to help prevent severe reactions.

- Patients taking bisphosphonates may also require supplemental calcium and vitamin D, as ordered by the prescriber.

- Educate the patient about making lifestyle changes as recommended, such as engaging in weight-bearing exercise (e.g., walking), stopping smoking, and limiting or eliminating alcohol intake. These measures will help encourage fewer adverse effects of oral contraception and/or drug therapy with hormones.

- Patients using the conjugated estrogen/bazedoxifene, Duavee, for hot flashes may experience side effects of nausea, diarrhea, upset stomach, and dizziness.

- Ospemifene (Osphena) is taken orally and needs to be taken with food once daily, as prescribed, to minimize GI upset. Talk regularly with your health care provider about the length of time of treatment.

KEY POINTS

- Three major estrogens are synthesized in the ovaries: estradiol (the principal estrogen), esterone, and estriol. Exogenous estrogens can be classified into two main groups: steroidal estrogens (e.g., conjugated estrogens, esterified estrogens, estradiol) and nonsteroidal estrogens (e.g., chlorotrianisene, dienestrol, diethylstilbestrol).
- Progestins have a variety of uses, including treatment of uterine bleeding and amenorrhea and adjunctive and palliative treatment of some cancers.
- Oral contraceptives containing a combination of estrogens and progestins are the most effective forms of reversible contraception currently available.
- Uterine stimulants (sometimes called *oxytocic drugs*) include ergot derivatives, prostaglandins, and oxytocin.
- Uterine relaxants (often called *tocolytic drugs*) are used to stop preterm labor and maintain pregnancy by halting uterine contractions.

- A thorough nursing assessment is necessary to ensure the safe and effective use of female reproductive drugs. Obtain information on the patient's past medical problems, history of menses and problems with the menstrual cycle, medications taken (prescribed and OTC), number of pregnancies and miscarriages, last menstrual period, and any related surgical or medical treatments.
- Two new estrogen-related products that have been recently approved include Duavee (conjugated estrogen/bazedoxifene) and Osphena (ospemifene). Duavee is indicated for hot flashes associated with menopause and for osteoporosis. Ospemifene (Osphena) is an estrogen agonist/antagonist that is the first drug approved to treat moderate to severe dyspareunia (painful intercourse) in postmenopausal women.

NCLEX® EXAMINATION REVIEW QUESTIONS

1. The nurse is assessing a patient who is to receive dinoprostone (Prostin E₂). Which condition would be a contraindication to the use of this drug?
   a. Pregnancy at 15 weeks' gestation
   b. GI upset or ulcer disease
   c. Ectopic pregnancy
   d. Incomplete abortion

2. When teaching a patient who is taking oral contraceptive therapy for the first time, the nurse relates that adverse effects may include which of the following?
   a. Dizziness
   b. Nausea
   c. Tingling in the extremities
   d. Polyuria

3. The nurse is reviewing the use of obstetric drugs. Which situation is an indication for an oxytocin (Pitocin) infusion?
   a. Termination of a pregnancy at 12 weeks
   b. Hypertonic uterus
   c. Cervical stenosis in a patient who is in labor
   d. Induction of labor at full term

4. The nurse has provided patient education regarding therapy with the SERM raloxifene (Evista). Which statement from the patient reflects a good understanding of the instruction?
   a. "When I take that long flight to Asia, I will need to stop taking this drug at least 3 days before I travel."
   b. "I can continue this drug even when traveling as long as I take it with a full glass of water each time."
   c. "After I take this drug, I must sit upright for at least 30 minutes."
   d. "One advantage of this drug is that it will reduce my hot flashes."

5. The nurse is discussing therapy with clomiphene (Clomid) with a husband and wife who are considering trying this drug as part of treatment for infertility. It is important that they be informed of which possible effect of this drug?
   a. Increased menstrual flow
   b. Increased menstrual cramping
   c. Multiple pregnancy (twins or more)
   d. Sedation

6. A patient calls the clinic because she realized she missed one dose of an oral contraceptive. Which statement from the nurse is appropriate? (*Select all that apply.*)
   a. "Go ahead and take the missed dose now, along with today's dose."
   b. "Don't worry, you are still protected from pregnancy."
   c. "Please come to the clinic for a reevaluation of your therapy."
   d. "Wait 7 days, and then start a new pack of pills."
   e. "You will need to use a backup form of contraception concurrently for 7 days."

7. The order reads: "Give calcitonin (Miacalcin) 50 international units subcut daily." The medication is available in a vial that contains 200 international units/mL. How many milliliters will the nurse draw up in the syringe for this dose?

8. A woman comes into the emergency department. She says that she is pregnant and that she is having contractions every 3 minutes but she is "not due yet." She is very upset. While assessing her vital signs and fetal heart tones, what is the most important question the nurse must ask the patient?
   a. "What were you doing when the contractions started?"
   b. "Are you preregistered at this hospital to give birth?"
   c. "How many weeks have you been pregnant?"
   d. "Have you felt the baby move today?"

1. c, 2. b, 3. d, 4. a, 5. c, 6. a, e, 7. 0.25 mL, 8. c.

CRITICAL THINKING AND PRIORITIZATION QUESTIONS

1. A patient in her first pregnancy has spent 14 hours in labor and has made little progress. She is becoming exhausted, and the uterine contractions have decreased in strength. She is now receiving an oxytocin (Pitocin) infusion. During this infusion, the nurse will perform many assessments. What are the priorities during the assessments?

2. The nurse is reviewing a cephalosporin prescription for a patient who has a severe sinus infection. The patient tells the nurse that she is taking a birth control pill and asks the nurse if there will be any problems with the antibiotic. What is the nurse's best answer?

For answers, see *http://evolve.elsevier.com/Lilley.*

ⓔ EVOLVE WEBSITE

http://evolve.elsevier.com/Lilley
- Animations
- Answer Keys for Textbook Case Studies and Textbook Critical Thinking and Prioritization Questions
- Content Updates
- Key Points
- Review Questions
- Student Case Studies

Men's Health Drugs

ⓔ http://evolve.elsevier.com/Lilley

OBJECTIVES

When you reach the end of this chapter, you will be able to do the following:

1. Discuss the normal anatomy, physiology, and functions of the male reproductive system.
2. Compare the various men's health drugs, with discussion of their rationale for use, dosages, and dosage forms.
3. Describe the mechanisms of action, dosages, adverse effects, cautions, contraindications, drug interactions, and routes of administration for the various men's health drugs.
4. Develop a nursing care plan that includes all phases of the nursing process for patients receiving men's health drugs for treatment of benign prostatic hyperplasia, sexual dysfunction, hormone deficiency, or prostate cancer.

DRUG PROFILES

finasteride, p. 558
♦sildenafil, p. 558
♦testosterone, p. 559

♦ = *Key drug*
❗ = *High-alert drug*

KEY TERMS

Anabolic activity Any metabolic activity that promotes the building up of body tissues, such as the activity produced by testosterone that causes the development of bone and muscle tissue; also called *anabolism*. (p. 554)

Androgenic activity The activity produced by testosterone that causes the development and maintenance of the male reproductive system and male secondary sex characteristics. (p. 554)

Androgens Male sex hormones responsible for mediating the development and maintenance of male sex characteristics. Chief among these are testosterone and its various biochemical precursors. (p. 554)

Benign prostatic hyperplasia (BPH) (also called *hypertrophy*) Nonmalignant (noncancerous) enlargement of the prostate gland. (p. 555)

Catabolism The opposite of anabolic activity; any metabolic activity that results in the breakdown of body tissues. Examples of conditions in which catabolism occurs are debilitating illnesses such as end-stage cancer and starvation. (p. 554)

Erythropoietic effect The effect of stimulating the production of red blood cells (erythropoiesis). (p. 555)

Prostate cancer A malignant tumor within the prostate gland. (p. 556)

Testosterone The main androgenic hormone. (p. 554)

MALE REPRODUCTIVE SYSTEM

The male reproductive system consists of several structures; two of these structures, the testes and seminiferous tubules, produce the primary male hormones. The *testes,* a pair of oval glands located in the scrotal sac, are the male gonads. The testes produce male sex hormones. The *seminiferous tubules,* which are channels in the testes, are the site of spermatogenesis, which is the process by which mature sperm cells are produced.

Androgens are the group of male sex hormones (primarily testosterone) that mediate the normal development and maintenance of the primary and secondary male sex characteristics. Secondary male sex characteristics include advanced development of the prostate, seminal vesicles (two glands adjacent to the prostate), penis, and scrotum, as well as male hair distribution, laryngeal enlargement, thickening of the vocal cords, and male body musculature and fat distribution. Androgens must be secreted in adequate amounts for these characteristics to appear. The most important androgen is testosterone, which is produced from clusters of interstitial cells located between the seminiferous tubules. Besides having androgenic activity, testosterone is also involved in the development of bone and muscle tissue; inhibition of protein catabolism (metabolic breakdown); and retention of nitrogen, phosphorus, potassium, and sodium. These functions contribute to its anabolic activity. The hormone initiates the synthesis of specific proteins needed for androgenic and anabolic activity by binding to chromatin (strands of deoxyribonucleic acid [DNA]) in the nuclei of interstitial cells. In addition, testosterone appears to have an erythropoietic effect in that it stimulates the production of red blood cells (see Chapter 54).

ANDROGENS AND OTHER DRUGS PERTAINING TO MEN'S HEALTH

Testosterone deficiency is treated with exogenous testosterone. There are several synthetic derivatives of testosterone that have improved pharmacokinetic and pharmacodynamic characteristics over the naturally occurring hormone. This is accomplished by combining various esters with testosterone, which prolongs the duration of action of the hormone. For example, testosterone propionate is formulated as an oily solution, and its hormonal effects last for 2 to 3 days; the effects of testosterone cypionate and testosterone enanthate in oil last for up to 2 to 4 weeks. Orally administered testosterone has very poor absorption, because most of the dose is metabolized and destroyed by the liver before it can reach the circulation (first-pass effect; see Chapter 2). To circumvent this problem, researchers developed methyltestosterone (Android) and fluoxymesterone (Halotestin). Both are synthetic dosage forms (tablets or capsules) designed to be effective following oral administration. Methyltestosterone is also available in a buccal tablet, which is dissolved in the buccal cavity (the space in the mouth between the cheek and teeth) and in an injectable form. Transdermal dosage forms of testosterone, including skin patches, gels, and underarm spray, have provided another way to circumvent the first-pass effect that occurs with oral administration of this hormone.

There are other chemical derivatives of testosterone known as *anabolic steroids*. These are synthetic drugs that closely resemble the natural hormone but possess high anabolic activity. Currently three anabolic steroid drug products are commercially available. These include oxymetholone (Anadrol-50), oxandrolone (Oxandrin), and nandrolone (Deca-Durabolin). Approved indications include its use as adjunctive therapy to promote weight gain following extensive surgery, trauma, chronic diseases, anemia, hereditary angioedema, and metastatic breast cancer. Anabolic steroids have a great potential for misuse by athletes, especially bodybuilders and weight lifters, because of their muscle-building properties. Improper use of these substances can have many serious consequences, such as sterility, cardiovascular diseases, and liver cancer. For this reason, anabolic steroids are currently classified as Schedule III controlled substances by the U.S. Drug Enforcement Administration. This classification implies that misuse of these drugs can lead to psychologic or physical dependence, or both.

Another synthetic androgen is danazol (Danocrine). Its labeled uses include treatment of hereditary angioedema, and, in women, endometriosis and fibrocystic breast disease.

Mechanism of Action and Drug Effects

The natural and synthetic androgens and the synthetic anabolic steroids have effects similar to those of the endogenous androgens. These include stimulation of the normal growth and development of the male sex organs (primary sex characteristics) and development and maintenance of the secondary sex characteristics. Androgens stimulate the synthesis of ribonucleic acid (RNA) at the cellular level, thereby promoting cellular growth and reproduction. They also retard the breakdown of amino acids. These properties contribute to an increased synthesis of body proteins, which aids in the formation and maintenance of muscle tissue. Another potent anabolic effect of androgens is the retention of nitrogen, also essential for protein synthesis. Nitrogen also promotes the storage of inorganic phosphorus, sulfate, sodium, and potassium, all of which have important metabolic roles, including protein synthesis, nerve impulse conduction, and muscular contractions. All of these effects result in weight gain and an increase in muscular strength. Finally, androgens also stimulate the production of erythropoietin by the kidney, which leads to enhanced erythropoiesis (red blood cell synthesis; see Chapter 54). The administration of exogenous androgens causes the release of endogenous testosterone to be inhibited as a result of the feedback inhibition of pituitary luteinizing hormone. Large doses of exogenous androgens may also suppress sperm production as a result of the feedback inhibition of pituitary follicle-stimulating hormone, which leads to infertility.

Androgen inhibitors block the effects of naturally occurring (endogenous) androgens. This is accomplished via inhibition of a specific enzyme, 5-alpha reductase. For this reason, these drugs are also called *5-alpha reductase inhibitors*. For unknown reasons, normal male physiology often results in an enlargement of the prostate known as benign prostatic hyperplasia (BPH). This process begins as early as 30 years of age and is present in at least 85% of men by 80 years of age. The most troubling symptom is usually varying degrees of obstructed urinary outflow. Although surgical treatment by *transurethral resection of the prostate (TURP)* is a common strategy, BPH is also often treatable with a 5-alpha reductase inhibitor. There are currently two such drugs: finasteride and dutasteride. Finasteride (Proscar), the prototypical drug for this class, works by inhibiting this enzyme, which normally converts testosterone to 5-alpha dihydrotestosterone (DHT). DHT is a more potent form of testosterone and is the principal androgen responsible for stimulating prostatic growth, as well as the expression of other male primary and secondary sex characteristics. Finasteride can dramatically lower the prostatic DHT concentrations, which helps to reduce the size of the prostate gland to ease the passage of urine. Fortunately, finasteride does not cause antiandrogen adverse effects that might be expected, such as loss of muscle strength, and fertility.

The effects of finasteride are limited primarily to the prostate, but this drug may also affect 5-alpha reductase–dependent processes elsewhere in the body, such as in the hair follicles, skin, and liver. Research has demonstrated that the pharmacologic inhibition of 5-alpha reductase prevents the thinning of hair caused by increased levels of DHT. It has been noted that men taking finasteride experience increased hair growth. Therefore, finasteride is also indicated for the treatment of male-pattern baldness under the trade name Propecia. Finasteride is indicated for the treatment of baldness only in men, not in women. Finasteride can be teratogenic in pregnant women, and its use in women of any age (pregnant or not) is not recommended. Women need to wear gloves when handling finasteride. Another medication, minoxidil (Rogaine), can be used topically to treat baldness in both men and women. It is discussed in more detail in Chapter 56.

Another class of drugs that may be used to help alleviate the symptoms of obstruction due to BPH are the alpha₁-adrenergic blockers. These drugs are discussed in greater detail in Chapter 19. The alpha₁-adrenergic blockers that are most commonly used for symptomatic relief of obstruction secondary to BPH are terazosin (Hytrin), doxazosin (Cardura), tamsulosin (Flomax), alfuzosin (Uroxatral), and silodosin (Rapaflo). Tamsulosin, alfuzosin, and silodosin appear to have a greater specificity for the alpha₁-receptors in the prostate and thus may cause less hypotension. These drugs have clinical effects of prostate shrinkage immediately, as opposed to the 5-alpha reductase inhibitors, which may take up to 6 months of continual therapy.

There are also two other classes of androgen inhibitors. The first includes the androgen receptor blockers flutamide (Eulexin), nilutamide (Nilandron), and bicalutamide (Casodex). These drugs work by blocking the activity of androgen hormones at the level of the receptors in target tissues (e.g., prostate). For this reason, these drugs are used in the treatment of prostate cancer (see Chapter 46). The second class is the gonadotropin-releasing hormone (Gn-RH) analogues, including leuprolide (Lupron), goserelin (Zoladex), and triptorelin (Trelstar). These drugs work by inhibiting the secretion of pituitary gonadotropin, which eventually leads to a decrease in testosterone production. Both androgen receptor blockers and Gn-RH analogues are used most commonly to treat prostate cancer and are discussed in further detail in Chapter 46.

Phosphodiesterase inhibitors are used in the treatment of erectile dysfunction. Sildenafil (Viagra) was the first oral drug approved for the treatment of erectile dysfunction. Sildenafil works by inhibiting the action of the enzyme phosphodiesterase. This in turn allows the buildup in the penis of the chemical cyclic guanosine monophosphate, which causes relaxation of the smooth muscle in the corpora cavernosa (erectile tubes) of the penis and permits the inflow of blood. Nitric oxide is also released inside the corpora cavernosa during sexual stimulation and contributes to the erectile effect. Two drugs that are similar but have a longer duration of action are vardenafil (Levitra) and tadalafil (Cialis). Collectively, these drugs are referred to as *erectile dysfunction drugs*. Sildenafil and tadalafil are also used to treat pulmonary hypertension (see Chapter 22) under different trade names. Avanafil (Stendra) is the newest phosodiesterase inhibitor approved for erectile dysfunction.

A second type of drug used to treat erectile dysfunction is the prostaglandin alprostadil (Caverject). This drug must be given by injecting it directly into the erectile tissue of the penis or pushing a suppository form of the drug into the urethra.

A list of all of the men's health drugs mentioned in this chapter appears in Box 35-1. More information on selected drugs can be found in the Drug Profiles section.

Indications

The primary use for androgens is as hormone replacement therapy. Indications for other types of drugs discussed in this chapter are listed in Table 35-1.

Contraindications

Contraindications to the use of androgenic drugs include known androgen-responsive tumors. Use of sildenafil, vardenafil,

---

QSEN ⊕ **PATIENT-CENTERED CARE: CULTURAL IMPLICATIONS**

Men's Health Concerns: Prostate Cancer and Its Occurrence and Mortality

Prostate cancer is the second common cancer and the second leading cause of cancer-related death in men in the United States. The American Cancer Society estimates that approximately 220,800 new cases of prostate cancer will be diagnosed in the United States during 2015. It is also estimated that 1 in 7 men will be diagnosed with prostate cancer during their lifetime. The older adult male, 65 years of age or older, is most likely affected with 6 cases in 10. The mean age is about 66. African-American men have the highest incidence of the cancer and at least twice the mortality rate of men as compared to other racial/ethnic groups. Incidence rates by race per 100,000 men are as follows (from cases diagnosed from 2007 to 2011): 147.8 per 100,000 for all races, 139.9 for whites, 223.9 for African Americans, 79.3 for Asians and Pacific Islanders, 71.5 for Native Americans and Alaska Natives, 122.6 for Hispanics, and 151.5 for non-Hispanics.

Data from Howlader N, Noone AM, Krapcho M, et al, eds: *SEER cancer statistics review, 1975-2008*, Bethesda, MD, 2011, National Cancer Institute. Available at *http://seer.cancer.gov/csr/1975_2008/*. Accessed May 25, 2011; National Cancer Institute at the National Institutes of Health: Prostate cancer, available at *www.cancer.gov/cancertopics/types/prostate*. Accessed May 2, 2015.

BOX 35-1   Currently Available Men's Health Drugs

Alpha₁-Adrenergic Blockers
doxazosin
tamsulosin
terazosin
alfuzosin

Anabolic Steroids
nandrolone
oxandrolone
oxymetholone

Other Androgens
danazol
fluoxymesterone
methyltestosterone
testosterone

Antiandrogens
bicalutamide
flutamide
nilutamide

5-Alpha Reductase Inhibitors
finasteride
dutasteride

Gonadotropin-Releasing Hormone Analogues
goserelin
leuprolide
triptorelin

Peripheral Vasodilator
minoxidil

Drugs for Erectile Dysfunction
avanafil
sildenafil
tadalafil
vardenafil
alprostadil

PATIENT-CENTERED CARE: LIFESPAN CONSIDERATIONS FOR THE OLDER ADULT PATIENT

Sildenafil: Use and Concerns

- One in 10 men in the world has erectile dysfunction (ED). The National Institutes of Health estimates that incidence increases with age as follows: About 4% of men in their 50s, 17% of men in their 60s, and approximately 47% of men older than 75 years of age.
- Causes of erectile dysfunction include aging, hypertension, diabetes mellitus, cigarette smoking, atherosclerosis, depression, nerve/spinal cord damage, side effects of medications, alcoholism and other substance abuse, and low testosterone levels.
- Treatment options include psychotherapy; lifestyle changes/modifications; oral PDE5 (phosphodiesterase) inhibitors including vardenafil (Levitra), tadalafil (Cialis), sildenafil (Viagra), and avanafil (Stendra); intraurethral and intracavernosal injections; vacuum devices; and surgery. Additionally, it is important for health care providers to try and avoid medications that may lead to impaired erectile function if at all possible.
- The older adult patient generally has one or more medical conditions (e.g. diabetes, renal disorders, hypertension, atherosclerosis) that lead to the use of polypharmacy and subsequent higher risk for the occurrence of erectile dysfunction.
- Sildenafil (Viagra) is a prescription medication that is commonly ordered to treat erectile dysfunction. Sildenafil is highly protein bound, which causes it to stay in the body longer and thus increases the possibility for drug interactions and toxicity.
- With the older adult patient, a decreased dosage of sildenafil and other erectile dysfunction medications may be indicated because of impaired liver/renal functioning.
- Adverse effects to be concerned about in any age male patient include headache, flushing, and dyspepsia. These would be exacerbated in the older adult patient.
- Sildenafil is to be used very cautiously in patients who have cardiac disease and angina, because these patients are at greater risk for complications. This is especially a concern for the patient taking nitrates (for cardiovascular disease) because of the severe hypotension that may occur.
- Discussing topics of a sexual nature may be comfortable for some patients but very anxiety producing for others. Be aware of cultural and gender differences in how individuals perceive their own sexuality and how they generally deal with sexual performance issues. Be respectful of each individual's beliefs and feelings and their sexual beliefs and practices. This requires knowledge, sensitivity, and objectivity.

TABLE 35-1 Men's Health Drugs: Indications	
Drug	**Indication**
danazol and stanozolol	Hereditary angioedema
Finasteride	Benign prostatic hyperplasia
	Male androgenetic alopecia
fluoxymesterone and methyltestosterone	Male hypogonadism, inoperable breast cancer
methyltestosterone	Postpubertal cryptorchidism
minoxidil	Hypertension
	Female and male androgenetic alopecia
oxandrolone	Weight gain
sildenafil, tadalafil, vardenafil, avanafil	Erectile dysfunction
testosterone	Primary or secondary hypogonadism

tadalafil, and avanafil is also contraindicated in men with major cardiovascular disorders, especially if they use nitrate medications such as nitroglycerin. Concurrent use of erectile dysfunction drugs and nitrates may cause severe hypotension, which may not respond to treatment. Use of finasteride is contraindicated in women (especially pregnant women) and children.

Adverse Effects

Although rare, some of the most devastating effects of androgenic steroids occur in the liver, where they cause the formation of multiple, randomly distributed blood-filled spaces or cavities, a condition known as *peliosis of the liver*. This condition is a possible consequence of the long-term administration of androgenic anabolic steroids and can be life-threatening if they rupture. Other serious hepatic effects are hepatic neoplasms (liver cancer), cholestatic hepatitis, jaundice, and abnormal liver function. Fluid retention is another adverse effect of androgens and may account for some of the weight gain seen. The serious adverse effects that can be caused by the androgens far outweigh the advantages to be gained from their use by those seeking improved athletic ability. Other less serious adverse effects of androgens are listed in Table 35-2. In 2014, the FDA issued a special alert regarding the use of testosterone and the risk for developing stroke and heart attack in men. Additionally, the FDA also is requiring manufacturers to place a warning on all testosterone products regarding the potential for developing thromboembolic disorders (i.e., deep vein thrombosis [DVT], pulmonary embolism [PE]).

Sildenafil, vardenafil, tadalafil, and avanafil appear to have relatively favorable adverse effect profiles. In patients with pre-existing cardiovascular disease, especially those taking nitrates (e.g., nitroglycerin, isosorbide mononitrate, or dinitrate), these drugs can lower blood pressure substantially, potentially leading to more serious adverse events. Headache, flushing, and dyspepsia are the most common adverse effects reported. *Priapism* or abnormally prolonged penile erection is a relatively uncommon, but possible, adverse effect of both the erectile dysfunction drugs and the androgens. This condition is a medical emergency and warrants urgent medical attention. It is simply due to an excessive therapeutic drug response. Phosphodiesterase inhibitors can also cause unexplained visual loss.

Finasteride has been reported to cause loss of libido, loss of erection, ejaculatory dysfunction, hypersensitivity reactions,

TABLE 35-2   Men's Health Drugs: Selected Adverse Effects

Drug Class	Adverse Effects
Alpha₁-adrenergic blockers	Tachycardia, hypotension, syncope, depression, drowsiness, rash, impotence, urinary frequency, dyspnea, visual changes, headache
Androgens (including anabolic steroids)	Headache; changes in libido; anxiety; depression; acne; male pattern baldness; hirsutism; nausea; abnormal liver function tests; priapism; elevated cholesterol level; risk for blood clots, stroke, and heart attack
5-Alpha reductase inhibitors	Reduced libido, hypotension, dizziness, drowsiness
Peripheral vasodilator (topical minoxidil)	With topical route, usually limited to localized dermatologic reactions, including erythema, dermatitis, eczema, pruritus
Drugs for erectile dysfunction	Dizziness, headache, muscular pain, chest pain, hypertension or hypotension, rash, dry mouth, nausea, vomiting, diarrhea, priapism

gynecomastia, and severe myopathy. The drug has also caused a 50% decrease in prostate-specific antigen (PSA) concentrations. Pregnant women must not handle crushed or broken tablets on a regular basis because of the possibility of topical absorption, which can lead to teratogenic effects.

Interactions

Androgens, when used with oral anticoagulants, can significantly increase or decrease anticoagulant activity (see Chapter 26). Concurrent use of androgens with cyclosporine (see Chapter 48) increases the risk for cyclosporine toxicity and is not recommended. Sildenafil, vardenafil, tadalafil, and avanafil may cause severe hypotension when given together with nitrates such as nitroglycerin, isosorbide mononitrate, or isosorbide dinitrate (see Chapter 23). Alpha blockers can cause additive hypotension when given with other drugs that lower blood pressure (see Chapter 22). Effects of tamsulosin may be increased when it is taken with azole antifungal drugs, erythromycin and clarithromycin (see Chapter 38), cardiac drugs such as propranolol and verapamil (see Chapters 19 and 25), and protease inhibitors (see Chapter 40).

Dosages

For dosage information on the men's health drugs, see the table on this page.

DRUG PROFILES

finasteride

Finasteride (Proscar) is available in two tablet forms of 1- and 5-mg strengths. The lower strength is indicated for androgenetic alopecia in men. The higher strength is indicated for BPH, with clinical effects of prostate shrinkage in approximately 3 to 6 months of continual therapy. A similar drug, dutasteride (Avodart), is also indicated for BPH and is currently available in 0.5-mg capsule form. Both drugs are contraindicated in patients who have a known hypersensitivity and in pregnant women and children. It is considered potentially dangerous for a pregnant woman even to handle crushed or broken tablets. Both drugs are classified as pregnancy category X. Recommended dosages are given in the table on this page.

Pharmacokinetics (finasteride)

Route	Onset of Action	Peak Plasma Concentration	Elimination Half-life	Duration of Action
PO	3-12 mo	8 hr	4-15 hr	Unknown

◆ sildenafil

Sildenafil (Viagra) is approved for the treatment of erectile dysfunction. Other erectile dysfunction drugs with longer durations of action include vardenafil, tadalafil, and avanafil.

DOSAGES

Selected Men's Health Drugs

Drug	Pharmacologic Class	Usual Dosage Range	Indications
finasteride (Propecia, Proscar)	5-Alpha reductase inhibitor	**Adult** PO: 1 mg daily (Propecia)	Androgenetic alopecia (baldness) (males only)
		PO: 5 mg daily (Proscar)	Benign prostatic hyperplasia
◆ sildenafil (Viagra)	Phosphodiesterase inhibitor	**Adult (males only)** PO: 25-100 mg 1 hr before intercourse, no more than once daily	Erectile dysfunction
◆ testosterone cypionate (Depo-Testosterone)	Androgenic hormone	**Adult and adolescent** IM: 50-400 mg every 2-4 wk	Delayed puberty or hypogonadism (in males)
◆ testosterone, transdermal (Androderm, AndroGel)	Androgenic hormone	**Adult and adolescent** Androderm patch (applied to skin of back, abdomen, upper arms, or thighs): 1-2 patches per day AndroGel 1% (applied to shoulders, arms, or abdominal skin): 1-3 actuations per day	Male hypogonadism

Sildenafil potentiates the physiologic sexual response, causing penile erection after sexual arousal by relaxing smooth muscle and increasing blood flow into the penis.

Sildenafil use is contraindicated in patients with a known hypersensitivity to it. Sildenafil can potentiate the hypotensive effects of nitrates, and its administration to patients who are using organic nitrates in any form, either regularly or intermittently, is therefore contraindicated. Recommended dosages are given in the table on the previous page.

Pharmacokinetics: Sildenafil

Route	Onset of Action	Peak Plasma Concentration	Elimination Half-life	Duration of Action
PO	0.5-1 hr	1 hr	4 hr	4-6 hr

◆testosterone

Testosterone (Androderm) is a naturally occurring anabolic steroid. It is used for primary and secondary hypogonadism but may also be used to treat oligospermia in men as well as inoperable breast cancer in women, where its purpose is to counteract tumor-enhancing estrogen activity. When it is used as hormone replacement therapy, a transdermal product is desirable. There are presently two transdermal patch formulations. They attempt to mimic the normal circadian variation in testosterone concentration seen in young healthy men, in whom the maximum testosterone levels occur in the early morning hours and the minimum concentrations occur in the evening. Of the two available transdermal delivery systems, Testoderm is always applied to the scrotal skin, whereas Androderm is always applied to skin elsewhere on the body and never to the scrotal skin. Axiron, a testosterone underarm spray, is also available. Educate patients to wash their hands and cover the area where testosterone is applied, as transfer to others can occur.

Testosterone use is contraindicated in patients with severe renal, cardiac, or hepatic disease; male breast cancer; prostate cancer; hypersensitivity; genital bleeding; as well as in pregnant or lactating women. Testosterone is considered a Schedule III controlled substance under the Anabolic Steroids Control Act. It is available as intramuscular injections, transdermal gel, transdermal patches, and even implantable pellets. In 2014, the FDA issued warnings regarding the risk for developing blood clots, stroke, or heart attack with the use of testosterone. It is classified as a pregnancy category X drug. Recommended dosages are given in the table on the previous page.

Pharmacokinetics: Testosterone Gel

Route	Onset of Action	Peak Plasma Concentration	Elimination Half-life	Duration of Action
Topical	30-60 min	2-4 hr	10-100 min	24 hrs

NURSING PROCESS

ASSESSMENT

For patients being treated for benign or malignant diseases of the male reproductive tract, thoroughly assess presenting

TEAMWORK AND COLLABORATION: PHARMACOKINETIC BRIDGE TO NURSING PRACTICE

Drugs used to manage erectile dysfunction (e.g., sildenafil) essentially work in the same way as the body to assist the male patient in achieving an erection. The related pharmacokinetics must be understood so that the drug is taken safely and effectively. Sildenafil is a rapidly absorbed drug with an onset of action within 1 hour, a peak plasma concentration within 1 hour, and a duration of action of up to 4 to 6 hours. If the drug is taken with a high-fat meal, absorption will be delayed, and it may take an additional 60 minutes for the drug to reach peak levels. This is yet another example of how specific drug pharmacokinetics may be affected by variables in a patient's everyday life, such as eating habits. Another pharmacokinetic consideration is that patients who are 65 years of age or older have reduced clearance of sildenafil and may experience increased plasma concentrations of free (or pharmacologically active) drug. This could possibly lead to drug accumulation and/or toxicity.

symptoms and obtain a complete history of past and present medical diseases or conditions. In addition, assess and document the patient's urinary elimination patterns and any difficulties. The health care provider usually performs a rectal examination to palpate for enlargement of the prostate or for other possible pathology. If enlargement exists, a serum prostate specific antigen (PSA) test will most likely be ordered. PSA levels may be increased in pathologic conditions such as prostate cancer. Monitor levels for baseline and comparative reasons. PSA levels are expected to decrease with effective therapeutic regimens. More recent research encourages the use of a PSA value of less than 2.5 or 3 ng/mL as the criterion for normal levels, especially for younger patients.

With *testosterone* and related drugs, assess the patient for liver disease because formation of blood-filled cavities may occur. This condition, also called peliosis, is associated with long-term therapy and may be life-threatening (see pharmacology discussion). Perform liver function studies (e.g., LDH, CPK, and bilirubin levels) as ordered to monitor for the possible adverse effect of abnormal liver function and jaundice. Because edema is also a problem with these drugs, assess and record baseline weights, intake and output, and history of any cardiovascular diseases. Another contraindication to assess for is that of a history of known androgen-responsive tumors.

Finasteride requires baseline assessment of urinary patterns with attention to frequency, urgency, and flow of urine with micturition. As the tissue responds to the drug and there is a reduction in the size of the prostate gland and thus improvement in the symptoms of BPH, urinary flow will be increased. With potentially teratogenic drugs such as finasteride, follow special handling precautions and advise any pregnant caregiver or partner to do the same. Finasteride is not to be given to women. Assessment of the patient's sexual functioning and libido is also important.

Before administering *drugs for erectile dysfunction*, perform a thorough nursing assessment including vital signs. Obtain and record a thorough medication history. Take a thorough cardiac history, and assess for contraindications with the use of *phosphodiesterase inhibitors* (e.g., *sildenafil, vardenafil [Levitra], tadalafil [Cialis]*), such as major cardiovascular disorders or the use of nitrate medications (nitroglycerin, isosorbide mononitrate, or dinitrate). The interaction between *erectile dysfunction drugs* and nitrates leads to severe hypotension.

NURSING DIAGNOSES

1. Decreased cardiac output related to drug interaction between erectile dysfunction drug and nitrates
2. Ineffective sexuality pattern related to the effects of treatment with androgen and/or therapy with phosphodiesterase inhibitors
3. Deficient knowledge related to lack of information about drug therapy and the disease process of BPH as well as drug interactions with finasteride

PLANNING: OUTCOME IDENTIFICATION

1. Patient maintains normal and adequate cardiac output during the course of drug therapy with taking of medications, as prescribed, and being proactive about possible drug actions and interactions.
2. Patient maintains or regains effective sexual patterns and functioning.
3. Patient displays adequate knowledge regarding disease process and rationale for recommended drug therapy.

IMPLEMENTATION

The therapeutic effects of *testosterone* are maximized when the drug is taken as ordered and at regular intervals so that steady levels are maintained. If the drug is being used for hypogonadism or induction of puberty, dosages may be managed differently, so that at the end of the growth spurt the patient is placed on maintenance dosages. Instruct patients to apply *Testoderm* transdermal patches as ordered, which is usually application to clean, dry scrotal skin that has been shaved for optimal skin contact. The dosage form is to be replaced as prescribed. Advise the patient to follow instructions for application and time of duration per the prescriber's orders. Educate patients that *Androderm* patches are to be applied to clean, dry skin on the back, abdomen, upper arms, or thighs; the scrotum and bony areas (shoulder, hip) are to be avoided with this particular drug. Be sure the proper patch is being used and that drugs are not confused. *AndroGel* is to be applied to shoulders, arms, or abdominal skin as ordered. If testosterone is being given intramuscularly, it is usually given every 2 to 4 weeks as prescribed. Mix the vial of medication thoroughly by agitating it before withdrawing the prescribed amount of medication.

Finasteride may be given orally without regard to meals. When used for treatment of the urinary symptoms of benign prostatic hypertrophy (BPH), *finasteride* and related drugs may be ordered for approximately 3 to 6 months with a reevaluation of the condition at that time. Advise the patient to protect the drug from exposure to light and heat. Due to the teratogenic effects of *finasteride*, emphasize that it must not be handled in any form by a pregnant woman. Recommend that female patients/caregivers and/or nurses/members of the health care team wear gloves when handling this medication.

✒ SAFETY: HERBAL THERAPIES AND DIETARY SUPPLEMENTS   [QSEN]

Saw Palmetto (Serenoa repens, Sabal serrulata)

Overview
Saw palmetto comes from a tree that is also known as the American dwarf palm. The therapeutically active part of the tree is its ripe fruit. Saw palmetto is believed to inhibit dihydrotestosterone and 5-alpha reductase. A prostatic-specific antigen test and digital rectal examination should be performed before initiation of treatment with saw palmetto for benign prostatic hyperplasia.

Common Uses
Diuretic, urinary antiseptic, treatment of benign prostatic hyperplasia, treatment of alopecia

Adverse Effects
Gastrointestinal upset, headache, back pain, dysuria

Potential Drug Interactions
Nonsteroidal antiinflammatory drugs, hormones such as estrogen replacement therapy and oral contraceptives, immunostimulants

Contraindications
None

It is recommended that women of any age do not take this medication. See the Safety: Herbal Therapies and Dietary Supplements box for a description of saw palmetto, an herbal supplement that is often taken to relieve symptoms of an enlarged prostate.

For patients taking *erectile dysfunction drugs*, alert them to the drug interaction–related serious adverse effect of severe drop in blood pressure if taken with nitrates. When taking *sildenafil, vardenafil,* or *tadalafil*, priapism may occur. Priapism is the abnormally prolonged erection of the penis and is considered a medical emergency. Immediate and urgent medical attention is needed. See Patient-Centered Care: Patient Teaching for more information.

EVALUATION

The therapeutic effects of drugs related to the male reproductive tract include improvement of the condition and/or signs and symptoms for which the patient is being treated, such as hypogonadism, sexual dysfunction, erectile dysfunction, and urinary elimination problems caused by BPH. The therapeutic effects of some drugs (e.g., *finasteride*) may not be seen for 3 to 6 months, so it is important to observe and monitor the patient for the intended effects of the drugs. In addition, evaluate for the adverse effects of these medications (see the pharmacology section for specific adverse effects). Always evaluate goals and outcome criteria to see if the patient's needs have been met.

CASE STUDY

Safety: What Went Wrong? Erectile Dysfunction Drugs

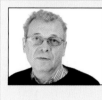

Mr. S., a 63-year-old college professor, is in the office for a yearly checkup. He feels he is generally healthy, and he does not take any medications. He does say that he has one problem that he wants to discuss with the prescriber. During his physical examination, he tells the prescriber, "I have something embarrassing to ask. I want to try one of those drugs that can help my sex life." The prescriber reassures Mr. S. that he does not need to be embarrassed to ask about this. The prescriber then assesses Mr. S.'s sexual difficulties. At the end of the examination and assessment, Mr. S. is given a prescription for sildenafil (Viagra).

1. What teaching is important for Mr. S. before he starts this medication?

    Eleven months later, Mr. S. is admitted to the emergency department with chest pains. After a thorough examination, including a cardiac catheterization, he is diagnosed with mild coronary artery disease and is started on isosorbide dinitrate, sustained-release, 40 mg every 12 hours. He is given a follow-up appointment with his physician in 1 week.

2. A week later, Mr. S. is back in the emergency department after falling in his bathroom one evening. He said he suddenly felt "so dizzy" and everything went black. What went wrong? What do you think could have caused this syncope?

3. One month later, Mr. S. comes to the office for the follow-up appointment and tells the nurse that he wants to try saw palmetto for his prostate health. He has a neighbor who takes it and has no problems with it, and he has noticed that he has had a slight increase in difficulty with urination. How will the nurse respond to Mr. S., and what assessments are needed at this time?

For answers, see *http://evolve.elsevier.com/Lilley.*

PATIENT-CENTERED CARE: PATIENT TEACHING

- With finasteride, provide education at the patient's educational level about the drug's therapeutic effects as well as adverse effects (see the pharmacology discussion for more information). Educate female family members, significant others, and caregivers who are pregnant or of childbearing age about the need to avoid exposure during handling of this drug, including *not* touching any broken or crushed tablets, which could result in exposure to the drug and the risk for teratogenic effects. Emphasize the need to wear gloves when handling the medication.
- Finasteride may be given orally without regard to meals. Instruct patients to protect the drug from exposure to light and heat.
- Sildenafil is usually prescribed to be taken about 1 hour before sexual activity. This drug, and other drugs for erectile dysfunction, should not be taken with nitrates. This interaction may lead to significant hypotensive consequences that could be life-threatening.
- Inform the patient that drug therapy for erectile dysfunction is not effective without sexual stimulation and arousal.
- With testosterone, educate the patient about all therapeutic and adverse effects. Emphasize the importance of follow-up appointments, which are crucial to evaluating the therapeutic effectiveness of this and other medications.
- Prolonged erections (i.e., longer than 4 hours) must be reported immediately to the appropriate health care provider and are considered to be a medical emergency.
- Testosterone is not to be withdrawn abruptly except under the supervision of the prescriber. Weaning is usually done over several weeks.

KEY POINTS

- The most commonly used drugs related to male health and the male reproductive tract are finasteride, sildenafil, and testosterone. It is important to know the way these drugs work and their adverse effects, contraindications, cautions, and drug interactions to ensure their safe and effective use.
- Testosterone is responsible for the development and maintenance of the male reproductive system and secondary sex characteristics. Oral testosterone has very poor pharmacokinetic and pharmacodynamic characteristics, and therefore it is recommended that testosterone be administered via injection (parenteral route) or a transdermal patch.
- Methyltestosterone was developed to circumvent the problems associated with the oral administration of testosterone.
- Finasteride is usually indicated to stop growth of the prostate in men with BPH and to treat men with androgenic alopecia.
- Warn patients taking drugs for erectile dysfunction (e.g., sildenafil) about potential adverse effects, such as hypotension, headache, and heartburn.
- There are major concerns about heart-related deaths associated with concurrent use of nitrates and drugs used for erectile dysfunction. Focus patient education on the prevention of drug interactions and related adverse effects and complications.

NCLEX® EXAMINATION REVIEW QUESTIONS

1. A patient has been taking finasteride (Proscar) for almost 1 year. The nurse knows that which is most important to evaluate at this time?
   a. Complete blood count
   b. PSA levels
   c. Blood pressure
   d. Fluid retention

2. The nurse is performing an assessment of a patient who is asking for a prescription for sildenafil (Viagra). Which finding would be a contraindication to its use?
   a. 65 years of age
   b. History of thyroid disease
   c. Medication list that includes nitrates
   d. Medication list that includes saw palmetto

3. During a counseling session for a group of teenage athletes, the use of androgenic steroids is discussed. The nurse will explain that which problem is a rare but devastating effect of androgenic steroid use?
   a. Peliosis of the liver
   b. Bradycardia
   c. Kidney failure
   d. Tachydysrhythmias

4. The nurse is teaching a patient about the possible adverse effect of priapism, which may occur when taking erectile dysfunction drugs. The nurse emphasizes that, if this occurs, the most important action is to
   a. stay in bed until the erection ceases.
   b. apply an ice pack for 30 minutes.
   c. turn toward his left side and rest.
   d. seek medical attention immediately.

5. A patient is asking about the use of saw palmetto for prostate health. The nurse tells him that drugs that interact with saw palmetto include:
   a. acetaminophen (Tylenol).
   b. nitrates.
   c. nonsteroidal antiinflammatory drugs.
   d. antihypertensive drugs.

6. When the Testoderm form of testosterone is ordered to treat hypogonadism in a teenage boy, which instructions by the nurse are correct? *(Select all that apply.)*
   a. Place the patch on clean, dry skin on the back, upper arms, abdomen, or thighs.
   b. Place the patch on clean, dry scrotal skin that has been shaved.
   c. Place the patch on clean, dry scrotal skin, but do not shave the skin first.
   d. Place the patch on any clean, dry, nonhairy area of the body.
   e. Remove the old patch before applying a new patch.

7. A 16-year-old male is to receive testosterone cypionate (Depo-Testosterone), 50 mg IM every 2 weeks. The medication is available in 100-mg/mL containers. How many mL will the nurse draw up in the syringe to administer for each dose?

8. The nurse is reviewing the medication list for a patient and notes that finasteride (Propecia) 1 mg daily is on the list. This drug is for which of these problems?
   a. Benign prostatic hypertrophy (BPH)
   b. Erectile dysfunction
   c. Alopecia in male patients
   d. Alopecia in male and female patients.

1. b, 2. c, 3. a, 4. d, 5. c, 6. b, 7. 0.5 mL per dose, 8. c.

CRITICAL THINKING AND PRIORITIZATION QUESTIONS

1. A male patient calls the office to ask about topical testosterone gel. This morning, he applied the daily dose to his upper arms and, without thinking, picked up his young granddaughter soon afterward. He is upset because he thinks this will harm his granddaughter. What is the nurse's priority action at this time?

2. During an office checkup, a patient tells you, "Ever since I started that pill for my prostate gland I'm having trouble with sex. I just don't have the interest anymore. Could it be the pill?" When you check his medical record, you see that he started taking dutasteride (Avodart), a 5-alpha reductase inhibitor, 3 months ago. What is the nurse's best response?

For answers, see *http://evolve.elsevier.com/Lilley*.

ⓔ EVOLVE WEBSITE

http://evolve.elsevier.com/Lilley
- Animations
- Answer Keys for Textbook Case Studies and Textbook Critical Thinking and Prioritization Questions

- Content Updates
- Key Points
- Review Questions
- Student Case Studies

PART 6

Drugs Affecting the Respiratory System

Learning Strategies

TIME MANAGEMENT

Time management is an extremely important task to master as a nursing student. You are embarking on a profession in which the learning, educational, and clinical preparation are all very intense. Additionally, the course work is heavy and time seems to always be running out. But take heart, many students have preceded you and made it to the other side. Those students will be the first ones to tell you they could not have done it without strict time management, writing out a schedule, and following it.

To be successful at time management, you need to start with a tool to keep you on task. One of the most commonly used tools is the school planner, or a calendar. You will want to get one that has enough space for each day to accommodate all the information you need to manage. If you are just juggling classes, a small planner will do. However, if you are a parent in charge of school-age kids and/or attending school and working, you will need a planner that easily accommodates all those important dates. The best way to be successful is to plan things out. If a pharmacology test falls on the day after your child's school play or after a long work weekend, you will need to see it in advance. The only way to "see it" is to plot it on a planner and often weeks or months at a time. Nothing makes failure inevitable like being unaware of upcoming work, projects, quizzes, tests, and/or exams and being caught unprepared. Students often make their planners as creative and functional as they can by using stickers, different-colored inks, and sticky notes, as well as organizing sections of information. Smart phones and tablets may also be used to help students manage their time and stay on task. Mobile devices have timers and/or alarms that students can set so they are certain to allow time to study or complete an assignment on time. But remember … planners and other scheduling devices need to be used daily and frequently to be effective!

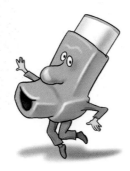

Upon beginning to use a planner, whether on a handwritten calendar or a smart device, start by filling in all deadlines for papers, assignments, and test dates. If you have a study group, put those hours down, too. Fill in your children's, spouse's, and your work schedule. When you have everything plotted, begin to look for conflicts or dates where school deadlines and home or work obligations overlap. Make plans immediately for what you need to do to be successful in your courses. Maybe you need to ask someone else to fill in for you at work. Time management means making difficult decisions, but these decisions will pay off in the long run.

Students find nursing school can be stressful, but preventing conflicts in their schedule before they happen reduces the stress and the feeling of being overwhelmed. When you have your life in the next 10 to 16 weeks laid out before you, it becomes easier to see when you can catch a break and get some down time. It doesn't seem quite so overwhelming when it is spread out. Sure, there may be a few weeks that look like they will be impossible, like during midterm and final exams, but knowing what to expect puts it all in perspective. Time management really means you are in control. If you do not plan it, it is easy for your time to begin to control you. You can be as detailed or as sketchy in your planner as you need to, but the important thing is to make it whatever you need to keep your life running as smoothly as possible. If you have to plot every chapter that you need to read, than plot it. If you only need the assignments and test dates recorded, then just record those. Don't forget to remember yourself if a holiday or day off falls on your planner. You need a break, and your family needs you too. Put the books aside for one day. Plan on it.

PRACTICE QUESTIONS

As you read the text, you'll need to ask yourself questions to make sure you are understanding the concept being presented. Use the chapter Key Points to formulate questions to check your understanding of the content. For example, from the Key Points in Chapter 13 on central nervous system stimulants, you can make the following questions: What are CNS stimulants? What are the three neurotransmitters CNS drugs mimic? What are the therapeutic uses for amphetamines, analeptics, and anorexiants? What symptoms need to be reported to a prescriber right away after the administration of a serotonin agonist? How do anorexiants work? What are contraindications for using anorexiants and CNS stimulants? Which group of patients should not receive SSRAs? How do amphetamines work? What is the purpose of journaling? When you answer your questions,

reinforcement of the key points of the chapter is occurring. Because you are learning pharmacology in relation to the nursing process, you will want to formulate questions along those lines, as well. What kind of assessment must I perform before administering this drug? What kind of teaching does the patient, family, and/or significant other(s) need? What side effects must I watch for? How will I know if the medication is working? Using these types of questions allows you to see the bigger picture of the role of drug therapy and the nursing process in nursing care.

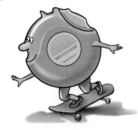

The practice questions provided in your textbook are one of the best gifts the authors have given to you. These questions allow you a chance to check your understanding of the content, the concepts, and the overall application of pharmacology to nursing. It is best to use them often when you are reading and as you work in your study groups. Do not just save them for when you are studying for a test. The authors have included NCLEX-style review questions online and at the end of each chapter. They have included critical thinking and prioritization questions as well as case studies in each chapter. These are the type of questions you will be expected to answer on the NCLEX® examination for licensure. Make sure you take time to not only understand why the answer is correct but what made the incorrect answers wrong. You want to understand the rationale behind the reasoning. Again it is all about making connections and really understanding the content. If you do not understand why an answer is correct, talk it out with your peers or question your instructor.

Antihistamines, Decongestants, Antitussives, and Expectorants

http://evolve.elsevier.com/Lilley

OBJECTIVES

When you reach the end of this chapter, you will be able to do the following:

1. Provide specific examples of the drugs categorized as antihistamines (both sedating and nonsedating), decongestants, antitussives, and expectorants.
2. Discuss the mechanisms of action, indications, contraindications, cautions, drug interactions, adverse effects, dosages, and route of administration for antihistamines, decongestants, antitussives, and expectorants.
3. Develop a nursing care plan that includes all phases of the nursing process for patients taking any of the antihistamines, decongestants, antitussives, and/or expectorants.

DRUG PROFILES

benzonatate, p. 573
codeine, p. 573
♦ dextromethorphan, p. 573
♦ diphenhydramine, p. 570
♦ guaifenesin, p. 574

♦ loratadine, p. 569
naphazoline, p. 572

_____
♦ = *Key drug*
! = *High-alert drug*

KEY TERMS

Adrenergics (sympathomimetics) Drugs that stimulate the sympathetic nerve fibers of the autonomic nervous system that use epinephrine or epinephrine-like substances as neurotransmitters. (p. 570)

Antagonists Drugs that exert an action opposite to that of another drug or compete for the same receptor sites. (p. 567)

Anticholinergics (parasympatholytics) Drugs that block the action of acetylcholine and similar substances at acetylcholine receptors, which results in inhibition of the transmission of parasympathetic nerve impulses. (p. 570)

Antigens Substances capable of inducing specific immune responses and reacting with the specific products of those responses, such as antibodies and specifically sensitized T lymphocytes. Antigens can be soluble (e.g., a foreign protein) or particulate or insoluble (e.g., a bacterial cell). (p. 567)

Antihistamines Substances capable of reducing the physiologic and pharmacologic effects of histamine. (p. 567)

Antitussive A drug that reduces coughing, often by inhibiting neural activity in the cough center of the central nervous system. (p. 572)

Corticosteroids Any of the hormones produced by the adrenal cortex, either in natural or synthetic drug form. They control many key processes in the body, such as carbohydrate and protein metabolism, the maintenance of serum glucose levels, electrolyte and water balance, and the functions of the cardiovascular system, skeletal muscle, kidneys, and other organs. (p. 570)

Decongestants Drugs that reduce congestion or swelling, especially of the upper or lower respiratory tract. (p. 570)

Empiric therapy A method of treating disease based on observations and experience, rather than a knowledge of the precise cause for the disorder. (p. 566)

Expectorants Drugs that increase the flow of fluid in the respiratory tract, usually by reducing the viscosity of secretions, and facilitate their removal by coughing. (p. 573)

Histamine antagonists Drugs that compete with histamine for binding sites on histamine receptors. (p. 567)

Influenza A highly contagious infection of the respiratory tract that is transmitted by airborne droplets. (p. 566)

Nonsedating antihistamines Medications that primarily work peripherally to block the actions of histamine and therefore do not generally have the central nervous system effects of many of the older antihistamines; also called *second-generation antihistamines* and *peripherally acting antihistamines*. (p. 569)

Reflex stimulation An irritation of the respiratory tract occurring in response to an irritation of the gastrointestinal tract. (p. 572)

KEY TERMS—cont'd

Rhinovirus Any of about 100 serologically distinct ribonucleic acid (RNA) viruses that cause about 40% of acute respiratory illnesses. (p. 566)

Sympathomimetic drugs A class of drugs whose effects mimic those resulting from the stimulation of the sympathetic nervous system. (p. 571)

Upper respiratory tract infection (URI) Any infectious disease of the upper respiratory tract, including the common cold, laryngitis, pharyngitis, rhinitis, sinusitis, and tonsillitis. (p. 566)

OVERVIEW

Common colds result from a viral infection, most often infection with a **rhinovirus** or an **influenza** virus. These viruses invade the tissues (mucosa) of the upper respiratory tract (nose, pharynx, and larynx) to cause an **upper respiratory tract infection (URI)**. The inflammatory response elicited by these viruses stimulates excessive mucus production. This fluid drips behind the nose, down the pharynx, and into the esophagus and lower respiratory tract, which leads to symptoms typical of a cold: sore throat, coughing, and upset stomach. Irritation of the nasal mucosa often triggers the sneeze reflex and also causes the release of several inflammatory and vasoactive substances, which results in dilation of the small blood vessels in the nasal sinuses and leads to nasal congestion. Treatment of the common symptoms of URI involves the combined use of antihistamines, nasal decongestants, antitussives, and expectorants.

In 2008, the U.S. Food and Drug Administration (FDA) issued recommendations that over-the-counter (OTC) cough and cold products not be given to children younger than 2 years of age. This followed numerous case reports of symptoms such as oversedation, seizures, tachycardia, and even death in toddlers. There is also evidence that such medications are simply not effective in small children, and parents are advised to consult their pediatrician on the best ways to manage these illnesses. A 2010 study showed a dramatic decrease in young children's emergency department visits since the FDA recommendation.

Many antihistamines, nasal decongestants, antitussives, and expectorants are available without prescription. However, these drugs can only relieve the symptoms of a URI. They can do nothing to eliminate the causative pathogen. Antiviral drugs are currently the only drugs that are effective; however, treatment with these mediations is often hampered by the fact that the viral cause cannot be readily identified. Because of this, the treatment rendered can only be based on what is believed to be the most likely cause, given the presenting clinical symptoms. Such treatment is called **empiric therapy**. Some patients seem to gain benefit from the use of herbal products and other supplements, such as vitamin C, to prevent the onset of cold signs and symptoms or at least to decrease their severity. Herbal products commonly used for colds are echinacea and goldenseal (see the Safety: Herbal Therapies and Dietary Supplements boxes on this page and the next). There is limited research data regarding the efficacy of herbal products, and some can have significant drug-drug or drug-disease interactions.

ANTIHISTAMINES

Histamine is a substance that performs many functions. It is involved in nerve impulse transmission in the central nervous system (CNS), dilation of capillaries, contraction of smooth muscle, stimulation of gastric secretion, and acceleration of the heart rate. There are two types of cellular receptors for histamine. Histamine 1 (H_1) receptors mediate smooth muscle contraction and dilation of capillaries; histamine 2 (H_2) receptors mediate acceleration of the heart rate and gastric acid secretion. The release of excessive amounts of histamine can lead to anaphylaxis and severe allergic symptoms and may result in any or all of the following physiologic changes:

- Constriction of smooth muscle, especially in the stomach and lungs
- Increase in body secretions

SAFETY: HERBAL THERAPIES AND DIETARY SUPPLEMENTS   QSEN
Echinacea (Echinacea)

Overview
The three species of echinacea used medicinally are *Echinacea angustifolia*, *Echinacea pallida*, and *Echinacea purpurea*. Echinacea has been shown in clinical trials to reduce cold symptoms and recovery time when taken early in the illness. This is believed to be due to its immunostimulant effects. At this time, there is no strong research evidence to warrant recommending the herb for urinary tract infections, wound healing, or prevention of colds; further study is needed to provide evidence of its therapeutic effects and indications.

Common Uses
Stimulation of the immune system, antisepsis, treatment of viral infections and influenza-like respiratory tract infections, promotion of wound healing, and chronic ulcerations

Adverse Effects
Dermatitis, upset stomach or vomiting, dizziness, headache, unpleasant taste

Potential Drug Interactions
Amiodarone, cyclosporine, phenytoin, methotrexate, ketoconazole, barbiturates; tolerance likely to develop if used for more than 8 weeks. Because some preparations have a high alcohol content, they may cause acetaldehyde syndrome with disulfiram (Antabuse) (see Chapter 17).

Contraindications
Contraindicated for patients with acquired immunodeficiency syndrome, tuberculosis, connective tissue diseases, multiple sclerosis

SAFETY: HERBAL THERAPIES AND DIETARY SUPPLEMENTS

Goldenseal (Hydrastis canadensis)

Overview

Goldenseal is found in wooded areas from the northeastern to midwestern United States. It is the dried root of the plant that is most commonly used. These components have been shown to have antibacterial, antifungal, and antiprotozoal activity. The alkaloid berberine has both anticholinergic and antihistaminic activity.

Common Uses

Treatment of upper respiratory tract infections, allergies, nasal congestion, and numerous genitourinary, skin, ophthalmic, and otic conditions

Adverse Effects

Gastrointestinal (GI) distress, emotional instability, mucosal ulceration (e.g., when used as a vaginal douche)

Potential Drug Interactions

Gastric acid suppressors (including antacids, histamine H_2 blockers [e.g., ranitidine], proton pump inhibitors [e.g., omeprazole]): reduced effectiveness due to acid-promoting effect of herb

Antihypertensives: reduced effectiveness due to vasoconstrictive activity of herb

Contraindications

Acute or chronic GI disorders; pregnancy (has uterine stimulant properties); should be used with caution by those with cardiovascular disease.

- Vasodilatation and increased capillary permeability, which results in the movement of fluid out of the blood vessels and into the tissues and thus causes a drop in blood pressure and edema

Antihistamines are drugs that directly compete with histamine for specific receptor sites. For this reason, they are also called **histamine antagonists.** Antihistamines that compete with histamine for the H_2 receptors are called H_2 **antagonists** or *H_2 blockers* and include cimetidine (Tagamet), ranitidine (Zantac), famotidine (Pepcid), and nizatidine (Axid). Because they act on the gastrointestinal (GI) system, they are discussed in detail in Chapter 50. This chapter focuses on the H_1 antagonists (also called *H_1 blockers*); they are the drugs commonly known as *antihistamines.* They are very useful drugs, because approximately 10% to 20% of the general population is sensitive to various environmental allergens. Histamine is a major inflammatory mediator in many allergic disorders, such as allergic rhinitis (e.g., hay fever; mold and dust allergies), anaphylaxis, angioedema, drug fevers, insect bite reactions, pruritus (itching), and urticaria (hives).

H_1 antagonists include drugs such as diphenhydramine (Benadryl), chlorpheniramine (generic), fexofenadine (Allegra), loratadine (Claritin), and cetirizine (Zyrtec). They are of greatest value in the treatment of nasal allergies, particularly seasonal hay fever. They are also given to relieve the symptoms of the common cold, such as sneezing and runny nose. In this regard they are palliative, not curative; that is, they can help alleviate the symptoms of a cold but can do nothing to destroy the virus causing it.

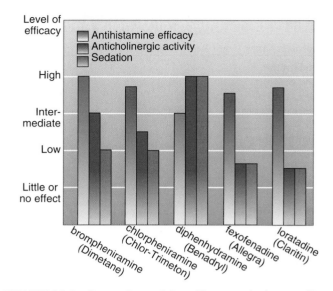

FIGURE 36-1 Comparison of the efficacy and adverse effects of selected antihistamines.

The clinical efficacy of the different antihistamines is very similar, although they have varying degrees of antihistaminic, anticholinergic, and sedating properties. The particular actions and indications for a particular antihistamine are determined by its specific chemical makeup. All antihistamines compete with histamine for the H_1 receptors in the smooth muscle surrounding blood vessels and bronchioles. They also affect the secretions of the lacrimal, salivary, and respiratory mucosal glands, which are the primary anticholinergic actions of antihistamines. These drugs differ from each other in their potency and adverse effects, especially in the degree of drowsiness they produce. The antihistaminic, anticholinergic, and sedative properties of some of the more commonly used antihistamines are summarized in Figure 36-1. Because of their antihistaminic properties, they are indicated for the treatment of allergies. They are also useful for the treatment of problems such as vertigo, motion sickness, insomnia, and cough. Several classes of antihistamines are listed in Table 36-1, along with their various anticholinergic and sedative effects.

Mechanism of Action and Drug Effects

During allergic reactions, histamine and other substances are released from mast cells, basophils, and other cells in response to **antigens** circulating in the blood. Histamine molecules then bind to and activate other cells in the nose, eyes, respiratory tract, GI tract, and skin, producing the characteristic allergic signs and symptoms. For example, in the respiratory tract, histamine causes extravascular smooth muscle (e.g., in the bronchial tree) to contract, whereas antihistamines cause it to relax. Also, histamine causes pruritus by stimulating nerve endings. Antihistamines can prevent or alleviate itching.

Circulating histamine molecules bind to histamine receptors on basophils and mast cells. This stimulates further release of histamine stored within these cells. Antihistamine drugs work by blocking the histamine receptors on the surfaces of basophils and mast cells, thereby preventing the release and actions of

TABLE 36-1 Effects of Various Antihistamines

Chemical Class	Anticholinergic Effects	Sedative Effects	Comments
Alkylamines			
brompheniramine	Moderate	Low	Cause less drowsiness and more CNS stimulation; suitable for
chlorpheniramine	Moderate	Low	daytime use.
dexchlorpheniramine	Moderate	Low	
Ethanolamines			
Clemastine	High	Moderate	Substantial anticholinergic effects; commonly cause sedation;
Diphenhydramine	High	High	drowsiness occurs in about 50% of patients; diphenhydramine and
Dimenhydrinate	High	High	dimenhydrinate also used as antiemetics.
Phenothiazine			
Promethazine	High	High	Drugs in this class are principally used as antipsychotics; promethazine is useful as an antihistamine and antiemetic.
Piperidines			
Cyproheptadine	Moderate	Low	Used in the treatment of motion sickness; hydroxyzine is used as a
Hydroxyzine	Moderate	Moderate	tranquilizer, sedative, antipruritic, and antiemetic.
Miscellaneous			
Fexofenadine	Low to none	Low to none	Very few adverse anticholinergic or sedative effects; almost
loratadine	Low	Low to none	exclusively antihistaminic effects; can be taken during the day because no sedative effects occur; they are longer acting and have fewer adverse effects than other classes.

TABLE 36-2 Antihistamines: Drug Effects

Body System	Histamine Effects	Antihistamine Effects
Cardiovascular (small blood vessels)	Dilates blood vessels, increases blood vessel permeability (allows substances to leak into tissues)	Reduces dilation of blood vessels and increased permeability
Immune (release of various substances commonly associated with allergic reactions)	Released from mast cells along with several other substances, which results in allergic reactions	Does not stabilize mast cells or prevent the release of histamine and other substances, but does bind to histamine receptors and prevent the actions of histamine
Smooth muscle (on exocrine glands)	Stimulates salivary, gastric, lacrimal, and bronchial secretions	Reduces salivary, gastric, lacrimal, and bronchial secretions

histamine stored within these cells. They do not push off histamine that is already bound to a receptor but compete with histamine for unoccupied receptors. Therefore, they are most beneficial when given early in a histamine-mediated reaction, before all of the free histamine molecules bind to cell membrane receptors. The binding of H_1 blockers to these receptors prevents the adverse consequences of histamine binding: vasodilation; increased GI, respiratory, salivary, and lacrimal secretions; and increased capillary permeability with resultant edema. The various drug effects of antihistamines are listed in Table 36-2.

Indications

Antihistamines are indicated for the management of nasal allergies, seasonal or perennial allergic rhinitis (e.g., hay fever), urticaria, and some of the typical symptoms of the common cold. They are also useful in the treatment of allergic reactions, motion sickness, Parkinson's disease (due to their anticholinergic effects), and vertigo. In addition, they are sometimes used as sleep aids.

Contraindications

Use of antihistamines is contraindicated in cases of known drug allergy. They are not to be used as the sole drug therapy during acute asthmatic attacks. In such cases, a rapidly acting bronchodilator such as albuterol, or in extreme cases epinephrine, is urgently needed. Other contraindications may include narrow-angle glaucoma, cardiac disease, kidney disease, hypertension, bronchial asthma, chronic obstructive pulmonary disease, peptic ulcer disease, seizure disorders, benign prostatic hyperplasia, and pregnancy. Fexofenadine is not recommended for those with renal impairment. Loratadine is not recommended for children younger than 2 years of age. Antihistamines should be used with caution in patients with impaired liver function or renal insufficiency, as well as in lactating mothers.

Adverse Effects

Drowsiness is usually the chief complaint of people who take antihistamines, but the sedative effects vary from class to class (see Table 36-1). Fortunately, sedative effects are much less common, although still possible, with the newer "nonsedating"

TABLE 36-3 Antihistamines: Reported Adverse Effects

Body System	Adverse Effects
Cardiovascular	Hypotension, palpitations, syncope
Central nervous	Sedation, dizziness, muscular weakness, paradoxical excitement, restlessness, nervousness, seizures
Gastrointestinal	Nausea, vomiting, diarrhea, constipation
Other	Dryness of mouth, nose, and throat; urinary retention; vertigo; visual disturbances; tinnitus; headache

TABLE 36-4 Antihistamines: Drug Interactions

Drug	Interacting Drug	Mechanism	Result
fexofenadine	Erythromycin and other CYP450 inhibitors	Inhibit metabolism	Increased fexofenadine levels
	Phenytoin	Increased metabolism	Decreased fexofenadine levels
loratadine	Ketoconazole, cimetidine, erythromycin	Inhibit metabolism	Increased loratadine levels
diphenhydramine, cetirizine	Alcohol, MAOIs, CNS depressants	Additive effects	Increased CNS depression

drugs. The anticholinergic (drying) effects of antihistamines can cause adverse effects such as dry mouth, changes in vision, difficulty urinating, and constipation. Reported adverse effects of the antihistamines are listed in Table 36-3.

Interactions

Drug interactions of antihistamines are listed in Table 36-4. An allergist will usually recommend discontinuation of antihistamine drug therapy at least 4 days prior to allergy testing.

Dosages

For dosage information on selected antihistamines, see the table on this page.

DRUG PROFILES

Although some antihistamines are prescription drugs, most are available over the counter. Antihistamines are available in many dosage forms to be administered orally, intramuscularly, intravenously, or topically.

NONSEDATING ANTIHISTAMINES

A major advance in antihistamine therapy occurred with the development of the nonsedating antihistamines loratadine, cetirizine, desloratadine, and fexofenadine. These drugs were developed to eliminate many of the unwanted adverse effects (mainly sedation) of the older antihistamines. They work peripherally to block the actions of histamine and therefore have significantly less of the CNS effects of many older antihistamines. For this reason, these drugs are also called *peripherally acting antihistamines* because they do not readily cross the blood-brain barrier, unlike their traditional counterparts. Another advantage of the nonsedating antihistamines is that they have longer durations of action, which allow for once-daily dosing. This increases patient adherence to therapy. The original nonsedating antihistamines terfenadine and astemizole were withdrawn from the U.S. market in the 1990s following the occurrence of several cases of fatal drug-induced cardiac dysrhythmias. Fexofenadine is the active metabolite of terfenadine but is not associated with such severe cardiac effects, nor are loratadine or cetirizine. All of the nonsedating antihistamines are available over-the-counter.

◆ loratadine

Loratadine (Claritin) is a nonsedating antihistamine and is taken once a day. It is structurally similar to cyproheptadine, but it does not readily distribute into the CNS, which diminishes the sedative effects associated with traditional antihistamines. However, at higher doses, central side effects such as drowsiness, headache, and fatigue can be seen. Loratadine is used to relieve the symptoms of seasonal allergic rhinitis (e.g., hay fever) as well as urticaria.

However, a drug containing its primary active metabolite, desloratadine is currently available only by prescription.

Drug allergy is the only contraindication to the use of loratadine. It should not be given with the following drugs:

DOSAGES

Selected Antihistamines

Drug (Pregnancy Category)	Pharmacologic Class	Usual Adult Dosage Range	Indications
Nonsedating Antihistamine			
◆ loratadine (Claritin) (B)	H_1 antihistamine	PO: 10 mg once daily	Allergic rhinitis, chronic urticaria
Traditional Antihistamine (More Commonly Associated with Sedation)			
◆ diphenhydramine (Benadryl) (B)	H_1 antihistamine	PO/IM/IV: 25-50 mg tid-qid 25-50 mg at bedtime as needed; for short-term use	Allergic disorders, motion sickness, PD symptoms Nighttime insomnia

PD, Parkinson's disease.

aclidinium, azelastine, ipratropium, orphenadrine, potassium chloride, tiotropium, and umeclidinium. The drug is available in oral form as a 10-mg tablet, as a 1-mg/mL syrup, as a 10-mg rapidly disintegrating tablet, and in a combination tablet with the decongestant pseudoephedrine. It is classified as a pregnancy category B drug. Recommended dosages are given in the table on the previous page.

Pharmacokinetics: Loratadine

Route	Onset of Action	Peak Plasma Concentration	Elimination Half-life	Duration of Action
PO	1-3 hr	8-12 hr	8-24 hr	24 hr

TRADITIONAL ANTIHISTAMINES

The traditional antihistamines are older drugs that work both peripherally and centrally. They also have anticholinergic effects, which in some cases make them more effective than nonsedating antihistamines. Some of the commonly used older drugs are brompheniramine, chlorpheniramine, dimenhydrinate, diphenhydramine, meclizine, and promethazine. They are used either alone or in combination with other drugs in the symptomatic relief of many disorders ranging from insomnia to motion sickness. Many patients respond to and tolerate the older drugs quite well, and because many are generically available, they are much less expensive. These drugs are available both OTC and by prescription.

◆ diphenhydramine

Diphenhydramine (Benadryl) is a traditional antihistamine that works both peripherally and centrally. It also has anticholinergic and sedative effects. It is used as a hypnotic drug because of its sedating effects. Its use is not advised in older adults, however, because of the "hangover" effect and increased potential for falls. Diphenhydramine is one of the most commonly used antihistamines, in part because of its excellent safety profile and efficacy. It has the greatest range of therapeutic indications of any antihistamine available. It is used for the relief or prevention of histamine-mediated allergies, motion sickness, the treatment of Parkinson's disease (due to its anticholinergic effects; see Chapter 15), and the promotion of sleep (see Chapter 12). It is also used in conjunction with epinephrine in the management of anaphylaxis and in the treatment of acute dystonic reactions.

Diphenhydramine is classified as a pregnancy category B drug, and its use is contraindicated in patients with a known hypersensitivity to it. It is to be used with caution in nursing mothers, neonates, and patients with lower respiratory tract symptoms. It is available in oral, parenteral, and topical preparations. In oral form, diphenhydramine is available as capsules, tablets, and liquid, as well as in several combination products that contain other cough and cold medications. It is also available as an injection. In topical form, diphenhydramine is available as a cream, gel, and spray. It also is available in combination with several other drugs that are commonly given topically, such as calamine, camphor, and zinc oxide. These combination preparations come in the form of aerosols, creams, gels, and lotions. Recommended dosages for the oral and injectable forms are given in the table on the previous page.

Pharmacokinetics: Diphenhydramine

Route	Onset of Action	Peak Plasma Concentration	Elimination Half-life	Duration of Action
PO	15-30 min	2-4 hr	2-7 hr	4 hr

DECONGESTANTS

Nasal congestion is due to excessive nasal secretions and inflamed and swollen nasal mucosa. The primary causes of nasal congestion are allergies and URIs, especially the common cold. There are three separate groups of nasal **decongestants**: **adrenergics (sympathomimetics)**, which are the largest group; **anticholinergics (parasympatholytics)**, which are somewhat less commonly used; and selected topical **corticosteroids** (intranasal steroids).

Decongestants can be taken orally to produce a systemic effect, inhaled, or can be administered topically to the nose. Each method of administration has its advantages and disadvantages. Drugs administered by the oral route produce prolonged decongestant effects, but the onset of action is more delayed and the effect less potent than for decongestants applied topically. However, the clinical problem of rebound congestion associated with topically administered drugs is nonexistent with oral dosage forms. Rebound congestion occurs with repeated use of inhaled decongestants because of the very rapid absorption of drug through mucous membranes followed by a more rapid decline in therapeutic activity. This rebound congestion can lead to overuse and dependence on the nasal spray, as patients take it frequently due to the rapid decline in activity. This is in contrast to oral dosage forms, which provide a more gradual increase and decline in pharmacologic activity due to the time required for GI absorption. Decongestants suitable for nasal inhalation include ephedrine, oxymetazoline, phenylephrine, and tetrahydrozoline.

Inhaled intranasal steroids and anticholinergic drugs are not associated with rebound congestion and are often used prophylactically to prevent nasal congestion in patients with chronic upper respiratory tract symptoms. Commonly used intranasal steroids include the following:

- beclomethasone dipropionate (Beconase)
- budesonide (Rhinocort)
- flunisolide (Nasalide)
- fluticasone (Flonase)
- triamcinolone (Nasacort)
- ciclesonide (Omnaris)

The only intranasal anticholinergic drug in use is ipratropium nasal spray (Atrovent

Mechanism of Action and Drug Effects

Nasal decongestants are most commonly used for their ability to shrink engorged nasal mucous membranes and relieve nasal stuffiness. Adrenergic drugs (e.g., ephedrine, oxymetazoline) accomplish this by constricting the small arterioles that supply the structures of the upper respiratory tract, primarily the blood vessels surrounding the nasal sinuses. When these blood vessels are stimulated by alpha-adrenergic drugs, they constrict. Once these blood vessels shrink, the nasal secretions in the swollen mucous membranes are better able to drain, either externally through the nostrils or internally through reabsorption into the bloodstream or lymphatic circulation. Because stimulation of the sympathetic nervous system produces the same effect, these drugs are also referred to as *sympathomimetics.*

Nasal steroids are aimed at the inflammatory response elicited by invading organisms (viruses and bacteria) or other antigens (e.g., allergens). The body responds to these antigens by producing inflammation in an effort to isolate or wall off the area and by attracting various cells of the immune system to consume and destroy the offending antigens. Steroids exert their antiinflammatory effect by causing these cells to be turned off or rendered unresponsive. The goal is *not* complete immunosuppression of the respiratory tract but rather to reduce the inflammatory symptoms to improve patient comfort and air exchange. The drug effects of intranasal steroids are discussed in more detail in Chapter 33.

Indications

Nasal decongestants reduce the nasal congestion associated with acute or chronic rhinitis, the common cold, sinusitis, and hay fever or other allergies. They may also be used to reduce swelling of the nasal passages and to facilitate visualization of the nasal and pharyngeal membranes before surgery or diagnostic procedures.

Contraindications

Contraindications to the use of decongestants include known drug allergy. Adrenergic drugs are contraindicated in narrow-angle glaucoma, uncontrolled cardiovascular disease, hypertension, diabetes, and hyperthyroidism. They are also contraindicated in situations in which the patient is unable to close his or her eyes (such as after a cerebrovascular accident), as well as in patients with a history of cerebrovascular accident or transient ischemic attacks, long-standing asthma, benign prostatic hyperplasia, or diabetes.

Adverse Effects

Adrenergic drugs are usually well tolerated. Possible adverse effects of these drugs include nervousness, insomnia, palpitations, and tremor. The most common adverse effects of intranasal steroids are localized and include mucosal irritation and dryness.

Although a topically applied adrenergic nasal decongestant can be absorbed into the bloodstream, the amount absorbed is usually too small to cause systemic effects at normal dosages. Excessive dosages of these medications are likely to cause systemic effects elsewhere in the body. These may include cardiovascular effects such as hypertension and palpitations and CNS effects such as headache, nervousness, and dizziness. These systemic effects are the result of alpha-adrenergic stimulation of the heart, blood vessels, and CNS.

Interactions

There are few significant drug interactions with nasal decongestants. Systemic sympathomimetic drugs and sympathomimetic nasal decongestants are likely to cause drug toxicity when given together. Monoamine oxidase inhibitors (MAOIs) may result in additive pressor effects (e.g., raising of the blood pressure) when given with sympathomimetic nasal decongestants. Other interacting drugs include methyldopa and urinary acidifiers and alkalinizers.

Dosages

For dosage information on naphazoline, see the table below.

DRUG PROFILE

Many of the decongestants are OTC drugs, but many of the corticosteroids are available only by prescription. There are two nasal steroids available over the counter, including Nasacort AQ (triamcinolone acetonide) and Flonase Allergy

DOSAGES

Selected Decongestant, Expectorant, and Antitussive Drugs

Drug (Pregnancy Category)	Pharmacologic Class	Usual Adult Dosage Range	Indications
naphazoline (Privine) (C)	Alpha-adrenergic vasoconstrictor	1 or 2 drops or sprays in each nostril q6h prn, usually for no more than 3-5 days	Nasal congestion
benzonatate (Tessalon Perles) (C)	Nonopioid antitussive	PO: 100-200 mg tid	Cough
codeine (as part of a combination product such as Tussar SF, Robitussin A-C, others) (C)	Opioid antitussive	PO: 10-20 mg every 4-6 hr; max 120 mg/24 hr	
♦ dextromethorphan (as part of a combination product such as Vicks Formula 44, Robitussin DM, others) (C)	Nonopioid antitussive	PO: 10-30 mg every 4-8 hr; max 120 mg/24 hr	
♦ guaifenesin (glyceryl guaiacolate) (Robitussin, Mucinex, others) (C)	Expectorant	PO: 100-400 mg every 4 hr; max 2400 mg/24 hr	Respiratory congestion, cough

Relief (fluticasone proprionate). Although nasal steroids are relatively safe, their use is also contraindicated in some circumstances, including in patients with nasal mucosal infections (because of their ability to depress the body's immune response as part of their antiinflammatory effect) or known drug allergy.

Many inhaled corticosteroids (e.g., beclomethasone, dexamethasone, flunisolide) are discussed in greater detail in Chapter 33. The adrenergic drugs (e.g., naphazoline) are discussed in this chapter. Both of these drug categories are generally first-line drugs for the treatment of chronic nasal congestion.

naphazoline

Naphazoline (Privine) is chemically and pharmacologically similar to the other sympathomimetic drugs oxymetazoline and tetrahydrozoline. During a cold, the blood vessels that surround the nasal sinus are dilated and engorged with plasma, white blood cells, mast cells, histamines, and many other blood components that are involved in fighting infections of the respiratory tract. This swelling, or dilation, blocks the nasal passages, which results in nasal congestion. When these drugs are administered intranasally, they cause dilated arterioles to constrict, which reduces nasal blood flow and congestion. Naphazoline is classified as a pregnancy category C drug and has the same contraindications as the other nasal decongestants. Naphazoline for nasal administration is available as a 0.05% solution and is meant to be instilled into each nostril. Recommended dosages are given in the table on this page.

Pharmacokinetics: Naphazoline

Route	Onset of Action	Peak Plasma Concentration	Elimination Half-life	Duration of Action
Intranasal	5-10 min	Unknown	Unknown	2-6 hr

ANTITUSSIVES

Coughing is a normal physiologic function and serves the purpose of removing potentially harmful foreign substances and excessive secretions from the respiratory tract. The cough reflex is stimulated when receptors in the bronchi, alveoli, and pleura (lining of the lungs) are stretched. This causes a signal to be sent to the cough center in the medulla of the brain, which in turn stimulates the cough. Most of the time coughing is a beneficial response; however, there are times when it is not useful and may even be harmful (e.g., after a surgical procedure such as hernia repair or in cases of nonproductive or "dry" cough). In these situations, the use of an antitussive drug may enhance patient comfort and reduce respiratory distress. There are two main categories of antitussive drugs: opioid and nonopioid.

Although all opioid drugs have antitussive effects, only codeine and hydrocodone are used as antitussives. Both drugs are effective in suppressing the cough reflex, and if they are taken in the prescribed manner, their use does not generally lead to dependency. These two drugs are commonly incorporated into various combination formulations with other respiratory drugs and are rarely used alone for the purpose of cough suppression.

Nonopioid antitussive drugs are less effective than opioid drugs and are available either alone or in combination with other drugs in an array of OTC cold and cough preparations. Dextromethorphan is the most widely used of the nonopioid antitussive drugs and is a derivative of the synthetic opioid levorphanol. Benzonatate is another nonopioid antitussive.

Mechanism of Action and Drug Effects

The opioid antitussives codeine and hydrocodone suppress the cough reflex through direct action on the cough center in the CNS (medulla). Opioid antitussives also provide analgesia and have a drying effect on the mucosa of the respiratory tract, which increases the viscosity of respiratory secretions. This helps to reduce symptoms such as runny nose and postnasal drip. The nonopioid cough suppressant dextromethorphan works in the same way. Because it is not an opioid, however, it does not have analgesic properties, nor does it cause CNS depression. Another nonopioid antitussive is benzonatate. Its mechanism of action is entirely different from that of the other drugs. Benzonatate suppresses the cough reflex by anesthetizing (numbing) the stretch receptor cells in the respiratory tract, which prevents reflex stimulation of the medullary cough center.

Indications

Although they have other properties, such as analgesic effects for the opioid drugs, antitussives are used primarily to stop the cough reflex when the cough is nonproductive and/or harmful.

Contraindications

The only absolute contraindication to the antitussives is known drug allergy. Relative contraindications include opioid dependency (for opioid antitussives) and high risk for respiratory depression. Patients with these conditions are often able to tolerate lower medication dosages and still experience some symptom relief.

Additional contraindications and cautions include the following:

- Benzonatate: no known contraindications but cautious use in those with productive cough
- Dextromethorphan: contraindications of hyperthyroidism, advanced cardiac and vessel disease, hypertension, glaucoma, and use of MAOIs within the past 14 days
- Diphenhydramine: see Antihistamines earlier in the chapter.
- Codeine and hydrocodone: contraindicated with alcohol use; cautious use required with CNS depression; anoxia, hypercapnia, and respiratory depression; increased intracranial pressure; impaired renal function; liver diseases; benign prostatic hyperplasia; and chronic obstructive pulmonary disease

Adverse Effects

The following are the common adverse effects of selected antitussive drugs:

- Benzonatate: dizziness, headache, sedation, nausea, constipation, pruritus, and nasal congestion

- Codeine and hydrocodone: sedation, nausea, vomiting, lightheadedness, and constipation
- Dextromethorphan: dizziness, drowsiness, and nausea
- Diphenhydramine: sedation, dry mouth, and other anticholinergic effects

Interactions

Very few drug interactions occur with benzonatate. Opioid antitussives (codeine and hydrocodone) may potentiate the effects of other opioids, general anesthetics, tranquilizers, sedatives and hypnotics, tricyclic antidepressants, alcohol, and other CNS depressants.

Dosages

For dosage information on selected antitussive drugs, see the table on p. 571.

DRUG PROFILES

Antitussives come in many oral dosage forms and are available both with and without a prescription. Most of the opioid antitussives are available only by prescription. Dextromethorphan is the most popular nonopioid antitussive available OTC.

benzonatate

Benzonatate (Tessalon Perles) is a nonopioid antitussive drug that is thought to work by anesthetizing or numbing the cough receptors. It is available in oral form as 100- and 200-mg capsules. Its use is contraindicated in patients with a known hypersensitivity to it. It is classified as a pregnancy category C drug. Recommended dosages are given in the table on p. 571.

Pharmacokinetics: Benzonatate

Route	Onset of Action	Peak Plasma Concentration	Elimination Half-life	Duration of Action
PO	15-20 min	Unknown	Unknown	3-8 hr

codeine

Codeine is a popular opioid antitussive drug. It is used in combination with many other respiratory medications to control coughs. Because it is an opioid, it is potentially addictive and can depress respirations as part of its CNS depressant effects. For this reason, codeine-containing cough suppressants are controlled substances. Many states allow persons over 18 years of age to purchase at least one oral liquid combination product without a prescription. However, most codeine antitussive products are obtained with a prescription. Codeine alone, without being combined with other drugs, is a Schedule II drug. Codeine-containing cough suppressants are Schedule V. They are available in many oral dosage forms: solutions, tablets, capsules, and suspensions. Their use is contraindicated in patients with a known hypersensitivity to opiates and in those who have respiratory depression, increased intracranial pressure, seizure disorders, or severe respiratory disorders. It is classified as a pregnancy category C drug. Recommended dosages are given in the table on p. 571.

Pharmacokinetics: Codeine

Route	Onset of Action	Peak Plasma Concentration	Elimination Half-life	Duration of Action
PO	15-30 min	34-45 min	2.5-4 hr	4-6 hr

♦ dextromethorphan

Dextromethorphan is a nonopioid antitussive that is available alone or in combination with many other cough and cold preparations. It is widely used because when used in recommended dosages, it is safe, nonaddicting, and does not cause respiratory or CNS depression. Unfortunately, dextromethorphan has become a popular drug of abuse and is discussed in detail in Chapter 17. Its use is contraindicated in cases of known drug allergy, asthma or emphysema, or persistent headache. Dextromethorphan is available as lozenges, solution, liquid-filled capsules, granules, tablets (chewable, extended-release, and film-coated), and extended-release suspension. It is classified as a pregnancy category C drug. Recommended dosages are given in the table on p. 571.

Pharmacokinetics: Dextromethorphan

Route	Onset of Action	Peak Plasma Concentration	Elimination Half-life	Duration of Action
PO	15-30 min	2.5 hr	Unknown	3-6 hr

EXPECTORANTS

Expectorants aid in the expectoration (i.e., coughing up and spitting out) of excessive mucus that has accumulated in the respiratory tract. They work by breaking down and thinning out the secretions. The clinical effectiveness of expectorants is somewhat questionable. Placebo-controlled clinical evaluations have failed to confirm that expectorants reduce the viscosity of sputum. Despite this, expectorants are popular drugs, are contained in most OTC cold and cough preparations, and provide symptom relief for many users. The most common expectorant in OTC products is guaifenesin.

Mechanism of Action and Drug Effects

Expectorants have one of two different mechanisms of action, depending on the drug. The first is reflex stimulation, in which loosening and thinning of respiratory tract secretions occurs in response to an irritation of the GI tract produced by the drug. Guaifenesin is the only such drug currently available. The second mechanism of action is direct stimulation of the secretory glands in the respiratory tract.

Indications

Expectorants are used for the relief of productive cough commonly associated with the common cold, bronchitis, laryngitis, pharyngitis, pertussis, influenza, and measles. They may also be used for the suppression of coughs caused by chronic paranasal sinusitis. By loosening and thinning sputum and the bronchial secretions, they may also indirectly diminish the tendency to cough.

Contraindications

Guaifenesin is contraindicated if drug allergy is present.

Adverse Effects

The adverse effects of expectorants are minimal. Guaifenesin may cause nausea, vomiting, and gastric irritation.

Interactions

There are no known significant interactions involving guaifenesin.

Dosages

For dosage information on guaifenesin, the only expectorant profiled, see the table on p. 571.

DRUG PROFILE

♦ guaifenesin

Guaifenesin (Mucinex) is a commonly used expectorant that is available in several different oral dosage forms: capsules, tablets, solutions, and granules. It is used in the symptomatic management of coughs of varying origin. It is beneficial in the treatment of productive coughs because it thins mucus in the respiratory tract that is difficult to cough up. There are few published pharmacokinetic data on guaifenesin, but its half-life is estimated to be approximately 1 hour. Immediate-release guaifenesin is dosed multiple times throughout the day. The sustained- release products are given once or twice a day. Although this drug remains popular, there is some evidence in the literature to suggest that it has no greater therapeutic activity than water in terms of loosening respiratory tract secretions. It is classified as a pregnancy category C drug. For dosage information on guaifenesin, see the table on p. 571.

NURSING PROCESS

ASSESSMENT

When the patient is receiving or taking drugs to treat symptoms related to the respiratory tract, first assess if the symptoms may be reflective of an allergic reaction. Obtaining the patient's medical history and medication profile, completing a thorough head-to-toe physical assessment, and taking a nursing history are critical to understanding possible causes, risks, or links to diseases or conditions such as allergy, a cold, or flu. For example, if an allergic reaction to a drug, food, or substance has occurred, the patient may be experiencing signs and symptoms such as hives, wheezing or bronchospasm, tachycardia, or hypotension (requiring immediate medical attention). However, if the cause is a cold or flu, the symptoms are different and treated completely differently. The drug of choice is then selected based on the type and severity of the symptoms.

Most *nonsedating antihistamines* (e.g., *fexofenadine, loratadine, cetirizine*) are contraindicated in those with known drug allergy. Remember with the *traditional* and *nontraditional antihistamines* that if allergy testing is to be performed, these medications are usually discontinued at least 4 days before the testing, but only on a prescriber's order and as directed. Assess for the following possible drug interactions that need to be avoided: fexofenadine given with erythromycin and other CYP450 inhibitors, leading to increased *antihistamine* levels; fexofenadine and phenytoin, leading to decreased fexofenadine levels; loratadine given with some antifungals, cimetidine, and erythromycin, leading to increased antihistamine levels; and diphenhydramine and cetirizine given with alcohol, MAOIs, and CNS depressants, leading to increased CNS depression.

Before administering the *traditional antihistamines* such as *diphenhydramine, chlorpheniramine,* or *brompheniramine,* ensure that the patient has no allergies to this group of medications, even though these drugs are used for allergic reactions. Assess contraindications, cautions, and drug interactions with these and all other drugs. Use of these antihistamines is of concern in patients who are experiencing an acute asthma attack and in those who have lower respiratory tract disease or are at risk for pneumonia. The rationale for not using these drugs in these situations is that antihistamines (and nonsedating antihistamines) dry up secretions; if the patient cannot expectorate the secretions, the secretions may become viscous (thick), occlude airways, and lead to atelectasis, infection, or occlusion of the bronchioles. It is also important to know that these drugs may lead to paradoxical reactions in older adults, with subsequent irritability as well as dizziness, confusion, sedation, and hypotension.

Use of *decongestants* requires assessment of contraindications, cautions, and drug interactions. Because decongestants are available in oral, nasal drop and spray, and eyedrop dosage forms, any condition that could affect the functional structures of the eye or nose may be a possible caution or contraindication. Decongestants may increase blood pressure and heart rate, so assess and document the patient's blood pressure, pulse, and other vital parameters. Because so many of these drugs are found in over-the-counter (OTC) cough and cold products and have been associated with numerous cases of oversedation, seizures, tachycardia, and even death, their use warrants extreme caution. Contraindications to the use of decongestants include known drug allergy, narrow-angle glaucoma, uncontrolled cardiovascular disease, hypertension, diabetes, and prostatitis. Topically applied *adrenergic nasal decongestants* may be absorbed into the circulation; however, the dosage amount absorbed is usually too small to cause systemic effects. If there are excessive dosages (e.g., excessive use or amounts), these may precipitate cardiovascular effects such as increase in blood pressure and CNS stimulation with headache, nervousness, or dizziness. Some drug interactions include the use of systemic *sympathomimetics* and sympathomimetic nasal decongestants with possible toxicity when given together. Other drug interactions to assess for with nasal decongestants include their use with MAOIs.

Inhaled intranasal steroids are contraindicated in situations in which the patient is experiencing a nasal mucosal infection or drug allergy. Chapter 33 discusses some of the inhaled *corticosteroids.* With the use of any decongestant, always perform a thorough assessment of signs and symptoms before and after use of these drugs. Include description of cough, secretions, and breath sounds in this assessment.

With *antitussive* therapy, assessment is tailored to the patient and the specific drug. Most of these drugs result in sedation, dizziness, and drowsiness, so assessment of the patient's safety is very important. Complete an assessment for allergies, contraindications, cautions, and drug interactions, and document the findings. In the respiratory assessment (as for all of the drugs in this chapter), include rate, rhythm and depth, as well as breath sounds, presence of cough, and description of cough and sputum if present. For individuals with chronic respiratory disease, the prescriber may order further studies to determine the safety of using these drugs without causing further respiratory concerns or depression. Pulse oximetry readings with measurement of vital signs may be used to provide more information. Assess for potential drug interactions including alcohol, MAOIs, and antihistamines. With use of *codeine* and *hydrocodone antitussives*, there are contraindications with alcohol and other opioid drugs; these drugs must be used cautiously with CNS depression, anoxia, hypercapnia, respiratory depression, and impaired renal function and in those with chronic obstructive pulmonary disease such as emphysema. With the *nonopioid antitussive dextromethorphan*, monitor its use carefully because it is a popular drug of abuse (see Chapter 17).

Expectorants are generally tolerated well, and the only contraindication is with known drug allergy. There are no known drug interactions to assess for with use of *guaifenesin (Mucinex)*.

CASE STUDY

Patient-Centered Care: Decongestants

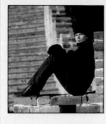

A 22-year-old college student has suffered with allergy symptoms since moving into his dormitory. When he calls the student health center, he is told to try an over-the-counter (OTC) nasal decongestant spray. He tries this and is excited about the relief he experiences at first, but 2 weeks later, he calls the student health center again. "I am congested all the time again, and I have to use the spray more and more to get any relief, but it does not last very long." He is upset because his symptoms are now worse.

1. What explanation do you have for the worsening symptoms?
2. What patient education is important when this type of drug is used?
3. What other over-the-counter drugs and nonpharmacologic measures could be suggested for this situation?

For answers, see *http://evolve.elsevier.com/Lilley*.

NURSING DIAGNOSES

1. Impaired gas exchange related to the disorder, condition, or disease affecting the respiratory system and various respiratory-related signs and symptoms
2. Ineffective airway clearance related to diminished ability to cough and/or a suppressed cough reflex (with antitussives)
3. Deficient knowledge related to the effective use of cold medications and other related products due to lack of information and patient teaching

---

PLANNING: OUTCOME IDENTIFICATION

1. Patient experiences improved gas exchange with drug therapy as noted with a return to normal breath sounds, respiratory rate, and rhythm.
2. Patient has improved airway clearance and relief of symptoms with minimal to no congestion, pain, or fever.
3. Patient displays improved knowledge about drug therapy and its therapeutic as well as adverse effects.

IMPLEMENTATION

If patients are receiving a *nonsedating antihistamine*, advise them to take the drug as directed. Reduced dosages may be needed for older adults or patients who have decreased renal function. The H_1 *receptor antagonist drugs* do not cross the blood-brain barrier as readily as do older antihistamines and are therefore less likely to cause sedation. They are generally very well tolerated with minimal adverse effects.

Instruct patients taking *traditional antihistamines* (e.g., *diphenhydramine*) to take the medications as prescribed. Most of these medications, including the OTC antihistamines, are best tolerated when taken with meals. Although food may slightly decrease absorption of these drugs, it has the benefit of minimizing the GI upset these drugs may cause. Encourage patients who experience dry mouth to chew or suck on candy (sugar-free if needed) or OTC throat, cough, or cold lozenges, or to chew gum, as well as to perform frequent mouth care to ease the dryness and related discomfort. Other OTC or prescribed cold or cough medications must not be taken with antihistamines unless they were previously approved or ordered by the prescriber because of the potential for serious drug interactions. Dosage amounts and routes may vary depending on whether the patient is an older adult, an adult, or younger than 12 years of age, so encourage proper dosing and usage. Monitor blood pressure and other vital signs as needed. Monitor older adults and children for any paradoxical reactions, which are common with these drugs.

Patients taking *decongestants* are generally using these drugs for nasal congestion. These drugs come in oral dosage forms, including sustained-release and chewable forms. Educate patients that all dosage forms are to be taken as instructed and with an increase in fluid intake of up to 3000 mL per day, unless contraindicated. The fluid helps to liquefy secretions, assists in breaking up thick secretions, and makes it easier to cough up secretions. Counsel patients to use nasal decongestant dosage forms exactly as ordered and with no increase in frequency. Excessive use of decongestant nasal sprays/drops may lead to rebound congestion. See Patient-Centered Care: Patient Teaching for further information.

With *antitussives*, instruct patients that the various dosage forms of the drugs are to be used exactly as ordered. Drowsiness or dizziness may occur with the use of antitussives; therefore, caution patients against driving a car or engaging in other activities that require mental alertness until they feel back to normal. If the antitussive contains codeine, the CNS depressant effects of the opiate may further depress breathing and respiratory effort. Other *antitussives*, such as *dextromethorphan*, as well as the *codeine-containing antitussives* are to be given at evenly spaced intervals so that the drug reaches a steady state.

EVALUATION

A therapeutic response to drugs given to treat respiratory conditions, such as *antihistamines, decongestants, antitussives,* and *expectorants,* includes resolution of the symptoms for which the drugs were originally prescribed or taken. These symptoms may include cough; nasal, sinus, or chest congestion; nasal, salivary, and lacrimal gland hypersecretion; motion sickness; sneezing; watery, red, or itchy eyes; itchy nose; allergic rhinitis; and allergic symptoms. Monitor for the adverse effects of excessive dry mouth, nose, and throat; urinary retention; drowsiness; oversedation; dizziness; paradoxical excitement; nervousness; restlessness; dysrhythmias; palpitations; nausea; diarrhea or constipation; and headache, depending on the drug prescribed.

PATIENT-CENTERED CARE: PATIENT TEACHING

- Provide the patient with education about the sedating effects of traditional antihistamines. The patient needs to avoid activities that require mental alertness until tolerance to sedation occurs or until he or she accurately judges that the drug has no impact on motor skills or responses to motor activities. Include a list of drugs the patient must avoid, such as alcohol and CNS depressants.
- With traditional and nonsedating antihistamines, a humidifier may be needed to help liquefy secretions, making expectoration of sputum easier. Encourage intake of fluids, unless contraindicated.
- Educate patients with upper or lower respiratory symptoms or disease processes of the impact of the environment on their symptoms or condition, and instruct patients to avoid dry air, smoke-filled environments, and allergens.
- Encourage the patient to always check for possible drug interactions because many OTC and prescription drugs could lead to adverse effects if taken concurrently with any of the antihistamines, decongestants, antitussives, or expectorants.
- Advise the patient to take the medication with a snack or meals to minimize GI upset.
- Advise the patient to immediately report to the prescriber any difficulty breathing, palpitations, or unusual adverse effects.

- Instruct the patient to take antitussives with caution and to report to the prescriber any fever, chest tightness, change in sputum from clear to colored, difficult or noisy breathing, activity intolerance, or weakness.
- With decongestants, emphasize the importance of only taking the medication as ordered and adhering to instructions regarding dose and frequency. Emphasize that frequent, long-term, or excessive use of decongestants (whether oral forms or nasal inhaled forms) may lead to rebound congestion in which the nasal passages become more congested as the effects of the drug wear off. When this occurs, the patient generally uses more of the drug, precipitating a vicious cycle with more congestion. Advise the patient to report to the prescriber any excessive dizziness, heart palpitations, weakness, sedation, or excessive irritability.
- Patients taking expectorants must avoid alcohol and products containing alcohol and should not use these medications for longer than 1 week. If cough or symptoms continue, the patient should contact the prescriber for further instructions or assessment. Encourage intake of fluids, unless contraindicated, to help thin secretions for easier expectoration.
- Decongestants and expectorants are recommended to treat cold symptoms, but the patient must report a fever of higher than 100.4° F (38° C), cough, or other symptoms lasting longer than 3 to 4 days.

KEY POINTS

- There are two types of histamine blockers: H_1 blockers and H_2 blockers. H_1 blockers are the drugs to which most people are referring when they use the term *antihistamine*. H_1 blockers prevent the harmful effects of histamine and are used to treat seasonal allergic rhinitis, anaphylaxis, reactions to insect bites, and so forth. H_2 blockers are used to treat gastric acid disorders, such as hyperacidity or ulcer disease.
- Educate the patient about the purposes of the medication regimen, the expected adverse effects, and any drug interactions. A list of all medications (prescription, over-the-counter, and herbal) needs to be provided to all health care providers.

- Decongestants work by causing constriction of the engorged and swollen blood vessels in the sinuses, which decreases pressure and allows mucous membranes to drain. It is important to understand the action of these drugs and know other important information such as significant adverse effects, including cardiac and CNS-stimulating effects.
- Nonopioid antitussive drugs may also cause sedation, drowsiness, or dizziness. Patients should not drive a car or engage in other activities that require mental alertness if these adverse effects occur. Codeine-containing antitussives may lead to CNS depression; these drugs are to be used cautiously and are not to be mixed with anything containing alcohol.

NCLEX® EXAMINATION REVIEW QUESTIONS

1. When assessing a patient who is to receive a decongestant, the nurse will recognize that a potential contraindication to this drug would be which condition?
   a. Glaucoma
   b. Fever
   c. Peptic ulcer disease
   d. Allergic rhinitis

2. When giving decongestants, the nurse must remember that these drugs have alpha-adrenergic–stimulating effects that may result in which effect?
   a. Fever
   b. Bradycardia
   c. Hypertension
   d. CNS depression

3. The nurse is reviewing a patient's medication orders for prn (as necessary) medications that can be given to a patient who has bronchitis with a productive cough. Which drug will the nurse choose?
   a. An antitussive
   b. An expectorant
   c. An antihistamine
   d. A decongestant

4. The nurse knows that an antitussive cough medication would be the best choice for which patient?
   a. A patient with a productive cough
   b. A patient with chronic paranasal sinusitis
   c. A patient who has had recent abdominal surgery
   d. A patient who has influenza

5. A patient is taking a decongestant to help reduce symptoms of a cold. The nurse will instruct the patient to observe for which possible symptom, which may indicate an adverse effect of this drug?
   a. Increased cough
   b. Dry mouth
   c. Slower heart rate
   d. Heart palpitations

6. The nurse is giving an antihistamine and will observe the patient for which side effects? (*Select all that apply.*)
   a. Hypertension
   b. Dizziness
   c. "Hangover" effect
   d. Drowsiness
   e. Tachycardia
   f. Dry mouth

7. The order for a 4-year-old patient reads: "Give guaifenesin, 80 mg PO, every 4 hours as needed for cough. Maximum of 600 mg/24 hours." The medication comes in a bottle that has 100 mg/5 mL. How many milliliters will the nurse give per dose?

8. The nurse notes in a patient's medication history that the patient is taking benzonatate (Tessalon Perles) as needed. Based on this finding, the nurse interprets that the patient has which problem?
   a. Cough
   b. Seasonal allergies
   c. Chronic rhinitis
   d. Motion sickness

1. a, 2. c, 3. b, 4. c, 5. d, 6. b, c, d, f, 7. 4 mL, 8. a.

CRITICAL THINKING AND PRIORITIZATION QUESTIONS

1. An older adult patient is discussing the use of guaifenesin with the nurse. He asks, "What else can I do to fight this terrible cold? I don't want to just take a pill." What is the nurse's best answer?

2. A patient is recovering from an emergency exploratory laparotomy because of an abdominal mass. He had a cold before his surgery and is now coughing up large amounts of whitish sputum. He is receiving intravenous fluids. He asks the nurse for something to make him stop coughing. The nurse reviews the medication sheet and sees both an expectorant and an antitussive ordered. Which medication would be the best choice at this time? Explain your answer.

For answers, see *http://evolve.elsevier.com/Lilley*.

ⓔ EVOLVE WEBSITE

http://evolve.elsevier.com/Lilley
- Animations
- Answer Keys for Textbook Case Studies and Textbook Critical Thinking and Prioritization Questions

- Content Updates
- Key Points
- Review Questions
- Student Case Studies

Respiratory Drugs

http://evolve.elsevier.com/Lilley

OBJECTIVES

When you reach the end of this chapter, you will be able to do the following:

1. Describe the anatomy and physiology of the respiratory system.
2. Discuss the impact of respiratory drugs on various lower and upper respiratory tract diseases and conditions.
3. List the classifications of drugs used to treat diseases and conditions of the respiratory system, and provide specific examples.
4. Discuss the mechanisms of action, indications, contraindications, cautions, drug interactions, dosages, routes of administration, adverse effects, and toxic effects of the bronchodilators and other respiratory drugs.
5. Develop a nursing care plan that includes all phases of the nursing process for patients who use bronchodilators and other respiratory drugs.

DRUG PROFILES

KEY TERMS

Allergen Any substance that evokes an allergic response. (p. 579)

Allergic asthma Bronchial asthma caused by hypersensitivity to an allergen or allergens. (p. 579)

Alveoli Microscopic sacs in the lungs where oxygen is exchanged for carbon dioxide; also called *air sacs.* (p. 579)

Antibodies Immunoglobulins produced by lymphocytes in response to bacteria, viruses, or other antigenic substances. (p. 579)

Antigen A substance (usually a protein) that causes the formation of an antibody and reacts specifically with that antibody. (p. 579)

Asthma attack The onset of wheezing together with difficulty breathing. (p. 579)

Bronchial asthma The general term for recurrent and reversible shortness of breath resulting from narrowing of the bronchi and bronchioles; it is often referred to simply as *asthma.* Key characteristics are inflammation, bronchial smooth muscle spasticity, and sputum production; inflammation is the most important. (p. 579)

Bronchodilators Medications that improve airflow by relaxing bronchial smooth muscle cells (e.g., xanthines, adrenergic agonists). (p. 581)

Chronic bronchitis Chronic inflammation and low-grade infection of the bronchi. (p. 579)

Emphysema A condition of the lungs characterized by enlargement of the air spaces distal to the bronchioles. (p. 579)

Immunoglobulins Proteins belonging to any of five structurally and antigenically distinct classes of antibodies present in the serum and external secretions of the body; they play a major role in immune responses; *immunoglobulin* is often abbreviated *Ig.* (p. 579)

Lower respiratory tract (LRT) The division of the respiratory system composed of organs located almost entirely within the chest. (p. 579)

Status asthmaticus A prolonged asthma attack. (p. 579)

Upper respiratory tract (URT) The division of the respiratory system composed of organs located outside the chest cavity (thorax). (p. 579)

OVERVIEW

The main function of the respiratory system is to deliver oxygen to, and remove carbon dioxide from, the cells of the body. To perform this deceptively simple task requires a very intricate system of tissues, muscles, and organs called the *respiratory system*. It consists of two divisions or tracts: the upper and lower respiratory tracts. The **upper respiratory tract (URT)** is composed of the structures that are located outside of the chest cavity or thorax. These are the nose, nasopharynx, oropharynx, laryngopharynx, and larynx. The **lower respiratory tract (LRT)** is located almost entirely within the thorax and is composed of the trachea, all segments of the bronchial tree, and the lungs. The URT and LRT have four main accessory structures that aid in their overall function. These are the oral cavity (mouth), the rib cage, the muscles of the rib cage (intercostal muscles), and the diaphragm. The upper and lower respiratory tracts together with the accessory structures make up the respiratory system. Elements of this system are in constant communication with each other as they perform the vital function of respiration and the exchange of oxygen for carbon dioxide.

Air is a mixture of many gases. During inhalation, oxygen molecules from the air diffuse across the semipermeable membranes of the **alveoli,** where they are exchanged for carbon dioxide molecules, which are then exhaled. The lungs also filter, warm, and humidify the air. Oxygen is then delivered to the cells by the blood vessels of the circulatory system, where the respiratory system transfers the oxygen it has extracted from inhaled air to the hemoglobin protein molecules contained within red blood cells. Also within the circulatory system, the cellular metabolic waste product carbon dioxide is collected from the tissues by the red blood cells. This waste is then transported back to the lungs via the circulatory system, where it diffuses back across the alveolar membranes and is then exhaled into the air. The respiratory system also plays a central role in speech, smell, and regulation of pH (acid-base balance).

PATHOPHYSIOLOGY OF DISEASES OF THE RESPIRATORY SYSTEM

Several diseases impair the function of the respiratory system. Those that affect the URT include colds, rhinitis, and hay fever. These conditions are discussed in Chapter 36. The major diseases that impair the function of the LRT include asthma, **emphysema,** and **chronic bronchitis**. All of these diseases have one feature in common; they all involve the obstruction of airflow through the airways. Chronic obstructive pulmonary disease (COPD) is the name applied collectively to emphysema and chronic bronchitis, because the obstruction is relatively constant. Asthma that is persistent and present most of the time despite treatment is also considered a COPD. Cystic fibrosis and infant respiratory distress syndrome are other disorders that affect the LRT.

Asthma

Bronchial asthma is defined as a recurrent and reversible shortness of breath and occurs when the airways of the lung (bronchi and bronchioles) become narrow as a result of bronchospasm, inflammation, and edema of the bronchial mucosa, and the production of viscous (sticky) mucus. This leads to an obstruction of the airflow in the airways and prevents carbon dioxide from leaving the air spaces and oxygen from getting in. Symptoms include wheezing and difficulty breathing. When an episode has a sudden and dramatic onset, it is referred to as an **asthma attack**. Most asthma attacks are short, and normal breathing is subsequently recovered. However, an asthma attack may be prolonged and may not respond to typical drug therapy. This is a condition known as **status asthmaticus** and requires hospitalization. The onset of asthma occurs before 10 years of age in 50% of patients and before 40 years of age in about 80% of patients.

There are different types of asthma: intrinsic (occurring in patients with no history of allergies), extrinsic (occurring in patients exposed to a known allergen), exercise induced, and drug induced. **Allergic asthma,** or extrinsic asthma, is caused by a hypersensitivity to an allergen or allergens in the environment. An **allergen** is any substance that elicits an allergic reaction. Examples include pollen, mold, dust, animal dander, and cigarette smoke, from either smoking or exposure to secondhand smoke. Examples of common food allergens include nuts, eggs, and corn. Exposure to the offending allergen in a patient with allergic asthma causes an immediate allergic reaction in the form of an asthma attack. This attack is mediated by antibodies already present in the patient's body that chemically recognize the allergen to be a foreign substance, or **antigen.** These **antibodies** are specialized immune system proteins known as **immunoglobulins.** The antibody involved with asthma is usually immunoglobulin E (IgE), which is one of the five types of antibodies in the body (the others are IgG, IgA, IgM, and IgD). On exposure to the allergen, the patient's body responds by mounting an immediate and potent antigen-antibody reaction (immune response). This reaction occurs on the surfaces of cells such as mast cells that are rich in histamines, leukotrienes, and other substances involved in the immune response. These substances are collectively known as inflammatory mediators, and they are released from the mast cells as part of the immune response. This in turn triggers the mucosal swelling and bronchoconstriction that are characteristic of an allergic asthma attack. The sequence of events that occurs in a patient with allergic asthma is shown in Box 37-1.

The specific cause of intrinsic, or idiopathic, asthma is unknown. It is not mediated by IgE, and there is often no family history of allergies. Certain factors have been noted to precipitate asthma attacks in these patients, including respiratory infections, stress, and cold weather. Patients with exercise-induced asthma have bronchospasm at the beginning of exercise, and symptoms stop when exercise is halted. Drug-induced asthma can be the result of different drugs including NSAIDs (see Chapter 44), beta blockers (see Chapters 22 and 24), sulfites, or certain foods. Patients with any type of asthma who know their suspected "triggers" are advised to avoid these triggers as much as is feasible. When it is not feasible or advisable to avoid a certain trigger (e.g., exercise), patients will require drug therapy.

BOX 37-1   Steps Involved in an Attack of Allergic Asthma

1. The offending allergen provokes the production of hypersensitive antibodies (most commonly immunoglobulin E [IgE]) that are specific to the allergen. This immunologic response initiates patient sensitivity.
2. The IgE antibodies collect on the surface of mast cells, thus sensitizing the patient to the allergen.
3. Subsequent allergen contact provokes the antigen-antibody reaction on the surface of mast cells.
4. Mast cell integrity is then violated, and these cells release chemical mediators stored in the cell. They also synthesize and then release other chemical mediators. These mediators include bradykinin, eosinophil chemotactic factor of anaphylaxis, histamine, prostaglandins, and slow-reacting substance of anaphylaxis (SRS-A).
5. The released chemical mediators, especially histamine and SRS-A, trigger bronchial constriction and an asthma attack.

BOX 37-2   Classifications of Drugs Used to Treat Asthma

Long-Term Control
Leukotriene receptor antagonists
Mast cell stabilizers
Inhaled corticosteroids
Anticholinergic agents
Long-acting beta$_2$ agonists (LABAs)
theophylline
Long-acting beta$_2$ agonists in combination with inhaled corticosteroids

Quick Relief
Intravenous systemic corticosteroids
Short-acting inhaled beta$_2$ agonists (rescue agents)

TABLE 37-1   Stepwise Therapy for the Management of Asthma

Step	Drug Classification
Step 1	Short-acting inhaled beta$_2$ agonist as needed
Step 2	Preferred: low-dose inhaled corticosteroid (ICS)
	Alternative: cromolyn, nedocromil, leukotriene receptor antagonist (LTRA), or theophylline
Step 3	Preferred: low-dose ICS and long-acting beta$_2$ agonist (LABA) or medium-dose ICS
	Alternative: low-dose ICS and either LTRA, theophylline, or zileuton
Step 4	Preferred: medium-dose ICS plus LABA
	Alternative: medium-dose ICS plus either LTRA, theophylline, or zileuton
Step 5	High-dose ICS and LABA, and consider omalizumab for patients with allergies
Step 6	High-dose ICS and LABA and oral corticosteroid, and consider omalizumab for patients with allergies

Adapted from National Institutes of Health: Expert Panel Report 3: Guidelines for the diagnosis and management of asthma, 2007, U.S. Department of Health and Human Services, available at *www.nhlbi.nih.gov/guidelines/asthma*. Accessed May 2, 2015.

The National Asthma Education and Prevention Panel (NAEPP) of the National Heart, Lung, and Blood Institute has maintained ongoing guidelines for the diagnosis and management of asthma since 1989. The current guideline revision was published in 2007. In general, these guidelines classify asthma medications as either for long-term symptom control or rapid symptom relief. The specific drugs in each classification are listed in Box 37-2. The guidelines advocate the use of a stepwise approach in the treatment of asthma. The particular steps and recommended drug classifications for treatment at each step are listed in Table 37-1. In 2014, international guidelines for severe asthma were published. These guidelines recommend higher than usual doses of inhaled corticosteroids for patients with severe asthma, however this book utilizes the NAEPP guidelines.

Chronic Bronchitis

Chronic bronchitis is a continuous inflammation and low-grade infection of the bronchi. Inflammation in the associated bronchioles (smaller bronchi) is responsible for most of the airflow obstruction. Chronic bronchitis involves the excessive secretion of mucus and certain pathologic changes in the bronchial structure. It is usually precipitated by prolonged exposure to bronchial irritants, the most common being cigarette smoke. Some patients acquire the disease because of other predisposing factors such as viral or bacterial pulmonary infections during childhood. Others causes include impairment of the ability to inactivate proteolytic (protein-destroying) enzymes, which then damage the airway mucosal tissues. Unknown genetic characteristics may be responsible as well.

Emphysema

Emphysema is a condition in which the air spaces enlarge as a result of the destruction of the alveolar walls. This appears to be caused by the effect of proteolytic enzymes released from leukocytes in response to alveolar inflammation. Because the alveolar walls are partially destroyed, the surface area available for oxygen and carbon dioxide exchange is reduced, which impairs effective respiration. As with chronic bronchitis, cigarette smoke appears to be the primary irritant responsible for the development of emphysema. There is also an associated genetic deficiency of the enzyme alpha$_1$-antitrypsin.

TREATMENT OF DISEASES OF THE LOWER RESPIRATORY TRACT

In the past, the treatment of asthma and other COPDs was focused primarily on the use of drugs that cause the airways to dilate. The emphasis of research has shifted from the bronchoconstriction component of the disease to the inflammatory component. This is reflected in the various medication classes used to treat COPDs, although bronchodilators still play an important role. A synopsis of the mechanisms of action of the various classes of antiasthmatic drugs is provided in Table 37-2. Figure 37-1 gives an overview of the various drugs used in asthma.

TABLE 37-2   Mechanisms of Antiasthmatic Drug Action

Antiasthmatic	Mechanism in Asthma Relief
Anticholinergics	Block cholinergic receptors, thus preventing the binding of cholinergic substances that cause bronchoconstriction and increase secretions
Leukotriene receptor antagonists	Modify or inhibit the activity of leukotrienes, which decreases arachidonic acid–induced inflammation and allergen-induced bronchoconstriction
Beta agonists and xanthine derivatives	Raise intracellular levels of cyclic adenosine monophosphate, which in turn produces smooth muscle relaxation and relaxes and dilates the constricted bronchi and bronchioles
Corticosteroids	Prevent the inflammation commonly provoked by the substances released from mast cells
Mast cell stabilizers (cromolyn and nedocromil)	Stabilize the cell membranes of the mast cells in which the antigen-antibody reactions take place, thereby preventing the release of substances such as histamine that cause constriction

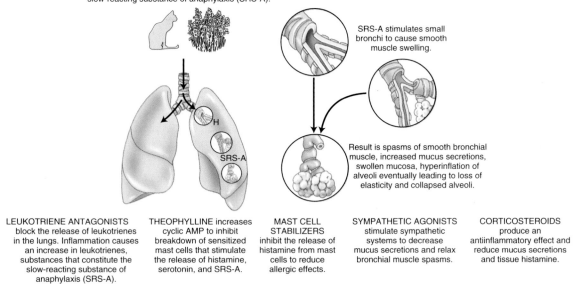

FIGURE 37-1 Overview of the effects of various antiasthmatic medications. (From McKenry LM, Tessier E, Hogan M: *Mosby's pharmacology in nursing*, ed 22, St Louis, 2006, Mosby.)

BRONCHODILATORS

Bronchodilators are an important part of the pharmacotherapy for all respiratory diseases. These drugs relax bronchial smooth muscle, which causes dilation of the bronchi and bronchioles that are narrowed as a result of the disease process. There are three classes of such drugs: beta adrenergic agonists, anticholinergics, and xanthine derivatives.

BETA-ADRENERGIC AGONISTS

The beta-adrenergic agonists are a group of drugs that are commonly used during the acute phase of an asthmatic attack to quickly reduce airway constriction and restore airflow to normal. They are agonists of the adrenergic receptors in the sympathetic nervous system. The beta and alpha adrenergic receptors are discussed in Chapters 18 and 19. The beta agonists imitate the effects of norepinephrine on beta receptors. For this reason, they are also called *sympathomimetic*

bronchodilators. The beta agonists are categorized by their onset of action. Short-acting beta agonist (SABA) inhalers include albuterol (Ventolin), levalbuterol (Xopenex), pirbuterol (Maxair), terbutaline (Brethine), and metaproterenol (Alupent). Long-acting beta agonist (LABA) inhalers include arformoterol (Brovana), formoterol (Foradil, Perforomist), and salmeterol (Serevent). The newest long-acting beta agonists are indacterol (Arcapta Neohaler); vilanterol in conjunction with fluticasone (Breo Ellipta); and vilanterol in conjunction with the anticholinergic umeclidinium (Anoro Ellipta). The term *Ellipta* refers to a new delivery system. Because the long-acting beta agonists (LABAs) have a longer onset of action, they must never be used for acute treatment. Patients must be taught to use the short-acting beta agonist (SABA) as rescue treatment.

Mechanism of Action and Drug Effects

The beta agonists relax and dilate airways by stimulating the beta$_2$-adrenergic receptors located throughout the lungs.

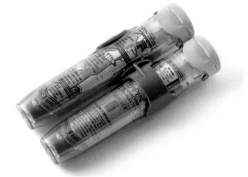

FIGURE 37-2 The EpiPen Auto-Injector (epinephrine) is used for immediate treatment of anaphylaxis (allergic emergencies). The EpiPen is given into the outer thigh, through the clothing. Anaphylactic emergencies also require emergency medical services in addition to the EpiPen. Additional information is available at *www.epipen.com*. (Copyright Mylan Specialty, L.P. Used with permission.)

TABLE 37-3 Beta Agonist Bronchodilators

Drug	Type	Trade Names	Administration
Short Acting			
albuterol	Beta₂	Proventil, Ventolin	PO, inhalation
ephedrine	Alpha/beta	None (various generic)	IM, IV, subcut
epinephrine	Alpha/beta	Adrenalin	Subcut, IM
levalbuterol	Beta₂	Xopenex	Inhalation
metaproterenol	Beta₁/beta₂	Alupent, Metaprel	PO, inhalation
pirbuterol	Beta₂	Maxair	Inhalation
terbutaline	Beta₂	Brethine	PO, subcut, inhalation
Long Acting			
salmeterol	Beta₂	Serevent, Serevent Diskus	Inhalation
formoterol	Beta₂	Foradil, Perforomist	Inhalation
arformoterol	Beta₂	Brovana	Inhalation

DOSAGES

Bronchodilators

Drug (Pregnancy Category)	Pharmacologic Class	Usual Adult Dosage Range	Indication
◆ albuterol (Proventil, Proventil Repetabs, Ventolin, others) (C)	Short-acting beta₂ agonist (SABA)	MDI: 2 puffs qid Inhalation nebulizer solution: 2.5 mg 3-4 times daily	Asthma
ipratropium (Atrovent) (B)	Anticholinergic	MDI: 2 puffs 4 times per day	Bronchospasm
◆ salmeterol* (Severent Diskus) (C)	Long-acting beta₂ agonist (LABA)	1 puff twice a day	Asthma, COPD

*Long-acting beta agonists are no longer recommended to be used alone; they need to be combined with an asthma-controlling medication such as an inhaled corticosteroid (e.g., Advair inhaler [fluticasone and salmeterol]).
MDI, metered-dose inhaler.

There are three subtypes of these drugs, based on their selectivity for beta₂ receptors:

1. Nonselective adrenergic drugs, which stimulate the beta, beta₁ (cardiac), and beta₂ (respiratory) receptors. Example: epinephrine. (NOTE: Epinephrine inhalers were taken off the market in 2012 because they did not comply with FDA requirements). Epinephrine is available as a prefilled syringe for self-administration by patients with severe allergic reactions and is called EpiPen (Figure 37-2).
2. Nonselective beta-adrenergic drugs, which stimulate both beta₁ and beta₂ receptors. Example: metaproterenol.
3. Selective beta₂ drugs, which primarily stimulate the beta₂ receptors. Example: albuterol.

These drugs can also be categorized according to their routes of administration as oral, injectable, or inhaled. The various beta agonist bronchodilators are listed in Table 37-3. The bronchioles are surrounded by smooth muscle. When the smooth muscle contracts, the airways are narrowed and the amount of oxygen and carbon dioxide exchanged is reduced. The action of beta agonist bronchodilators begins at the specific receptor stimulated and ends with the relaxation and dilation of the airways. However, many reactions must take place at the cellular level for bronchodilation to occur. When a beta₂-adrenergic receptor is stimulated by a beta agonist, adenylate cyclase is activated and produces cyclic adenosine monophosphate (cAMP). Adenylate cyclase is an enzyme needed to make cAMP. The increased levels of cAMP cause bronchial smooth muscles to relax, which results in bronchial dilation and increased airflow into and out of the lungs.

Nonselective adrenergic agonist drugs such as epinephrine also stimulate alpha-adrenergic receptors, causing constriction within the blood vessels. This vasoconstriction reduces the amount of edema or swelling in the mucous membranes and limits the quantity of secretions produced by these membranes. In addition, these drugs stimulate beta₁ receptors, which results in cardiovascular adverse effects such as an increase in heart rate, force of contraction, and blood pressure, as well as central nervous system (CNS) effects such as nervousness and tremor.

Drugs such as albuterol that predominantly stimulate the beta$_2$ receptors have more specific drug effects and cause less adverse effects. By primarily stimulating the beta$_2$-adrenergic receptors of the bronchial and vascular smooth muscles, they cause bronchodilation and may also have a dilating effect on the peripheral vasculature.

Indications

The primary therapeutic effect of the beta agonists is the prevention or relief of bronchospasm related to bronchial asthma, bronchitis, and other pulmonary diseases. However, they are also used for effects outside the respiratory system. Because some of these drugs have the ability to stimulate both beta$_1$- and alpha-adrenergic receptors, they may be used to treat hypotension and shock (see Chapter 18).

Contraindications

Contraindications include known drug allergy, uncontrolled hypertension or cardiac dysrhythmias, and high risk for stroke (because of the vasoconstrictive drug action).

Adverse Effects

Mixed alpha/beta agonists produce the most adverse effects because they are nonselective. These include insomnia, restlessness, anorexia, cardiac stimulation, hyperglycemia, tremor, and vascular headache. The adverse effects of the nonselective beta agonists are limited to beta-adrenergic effects, including cardiac stimulation, tremor, anginal pain, and vascular headache. The beta$_2$ drugs can cause both hypertension and hypotension, vascular headaches, and tremor. Overdose management may include careful administration of a beta blocker while the patient is under close observation due to the risk for bronchospasm. Because the half-life of most adrenergic agonists is relatively short, the patient may just be observed while the body eliminates the medication.

Interactions

When nonselective beta blockers are used with the beta agonist bronchodilators, the bronchodilation from the beta agonist is diminished. The use of beta agonists with monoamine oxidase inhibitors and other sympathomimetics is best avoided because of the enhanced risk for hypertension. Patients with diabetes may require an adjustment in the dosage of their hypoglycemic drugs, especially patients receiving epinephrine, because of the increase in blood glucose levels that can occur.

Dosages

For dosage information on selected beta agonists, see the table on this page.

DRUG PROFILES

◆ albuterol

Albuterol (Proventil HFA, Ventolin HFA, ProAir HFA) is a short-acting beta$_2$-specific bronchodilating beta agonist. Other similar drugs include bitolterol (Tornalate), levalbuterol (Xopenex), pirbuterol (Maxair), and terbutaline (Brethine). Albuterol is the most commonly used drug in this class. If albuterol is used too frequently, dose-related adverse effects may be seen, because albuterol loses its beta$_2$-specific actions, especially at larger dosages. As a consequence, the beta$_1$ receptors are stimulated, which causes nausea, increased anxiety, palpitations, tremors, and an increased heart rate.

Albuterol is available for both oral and inhalational use. Inhalational dosage forms include metered-dose inhalers (MDIs) as well as solutions for inhalation. The levorotatory isomeric form of albuterol, levalbuterol, is sometimes prescribed as an albuterol alternative for patients with certain risk factors (e.g., tachycardia, including tachycardia associated with albuterol treatment).

Pharmacokinetics: Albuterol

Route	Onset of Action	Peak Plasma Concentration	Elimination Half-life	Duration of Action
Inhalation	Immediate	10-25 min	3-4 hr	3-4 hr

◆ salmeterol

Salmeterol (Serevent Diskus) is a long-acting beta$_2$ agonist bronchodilator. Other long-acting inhalers include formoterol (Foradil, Perforomist), arformoterol (Brovana), and indacaterol (Arcapta Neohaler). The long-acting inhalers are never to be used for acute treatment. Salmeterol is used for the maintenance treatment of asthma and COPD and is used in conjunction with an inhaled corticosteroid. It is given twice daily for maintenance treatment only. In 2006, a large randomized clinical trial showed that use of salmeterol was associated with an increase in asthma-related deaths (when added to usual asthma therapy). The risk appears to be higher in African-American patients. All LABAs have a black box warning regarding this risk. Adverse effects include immediate hypersensitivity reactions, headache, hypertension, and neuromuscular and skeletal pain. Salmeterol should never be given more than twice daily nor should the maximum daily dose (one puff twice daily) be exceeded. It is available as a powder for inhalation either alone (Serevent Diskus) or combined with a corticosteroid (Advair). The long-acting inhalers, including salmeterol, are not to be used alone, but in combination with other drugs such as the inhaled corticosteroids. Advair (salmeterol and fluticasone) is a very popular inhaler for COPD. Symbicort, a newer inhaler consisting of the corticosteroid budesonide and the bronchodilator formoterol, is similar to Advair as is Dulera, which is a combination of formoterol and mometasone.

Pharmacokinetics: Salmeterol

Route	Onset of Action	Peak Plasma Concentration	Elimination Half-life	Duration of Action
Inhalation	Asthma: 30-48 min COPD: 2 hr	Asthma: 2-4 hr COPD: 3-4.5 hr	5.5 hr	12 hr

ANTICHOLINERGICS

Currently there are four anticholinergic drugs used in the treatment of COPD: ipratropium (Atrovent), tiotropium (Spiriva), aclidinium (Tudorza), and the combination product umeclidinium and vilanterol (Anoro Ellipta).

Mechanism of Action and Drug Effects

On the surface of the bronchial tree are receptors for acetylcholine (ACh), the neurotransmitter for the parasympathetic nervous system (PSNS). When the PSNS releases ACh from its nerve endings, it binds to the ACh receptors on the surface of the bronchial tree, which results in bronchial constriction and narrowing of the airways. Anticholinergic drugs block these ACh receptors to prevent bronchoconstriction. This indirectly causes airway relaxation and dilation. Anticholinergic agents also help reduce secretions in COPD patients.

Indications

Because their actions are slow and prolonged, anticholinergics are used for the prevention of bronchospasm associated with chronic bronchitis or emphysema and not for the management of acute symptoms.

Contraindications

The only usual contraindication to the use of bronchial anticholinergic drugs is known drug allergy, including allergy to atropine. In the past, an allergy to peanuts or soy was listed as a contraindication to ipratropium inhalers. This was related to the propellant used, and the new HFA inhalers have eliminated the concern. Thus, there is no contraindication using ipratropium in patients with peanut or soy allergies. Caution is necessary in patients with acute narrow-angle glaucoma and prostate enlargement.

Adverse Effects

The most commonly reported adverse effects of inhaled anticholinergics are related to their pharmacology and include dry mouth or throat, nasal congestion, heart palpitations, gastrointestinal (GI) distress, urinary retention, increased intraocular pressure, headache, coughing, and anxiety. Ipratropium is classified as a pregnancy category B drug; all others in this class are pregnancy category C.

Drug Interactions

Possible additive toxicity may occur when anticholinergic bronchodilators are taken with other anticholinergic drugs.

Dosages

For dosage information on anticholinergic drugs, see the table on p. 582.

DRUG PROFILE

ipratropium

Ipratropium (Atrovent) is the oldest anticholinergic bronchodilator. It is pharmacologically very similar to atropine (see Chapter 21). It is available both as a liquid aerosol for inhalation and as a multidose inhaler; both forms are usually dosed twice daily. Tiotropium (Spiriva) and aclidinium (Tudorza) are similar drugs. Spiriva is given once a day, whereas Tudorza is given twice daily. Many patients also benefit from taking both

a beta₂ agonist and an anticholinergic drug, with the most popular combination being albuterol and ipratropium. Although many patients receive the two drugs separately, two combination products are available containing both of these drugs: Combivent (an MDI) and DuoNeb (an inhalation solution).

Pharmacokinetics: Ipratropium

Route	Onset of Action	Peak Plasma Concentration	Elimination Half-life	Duration of Action
Inhalation	5-15 min	1-2 hr	1.6 hr	4-5 hr

DOSAGES

Theophylline Salts

Drug (Pregnancy Category)	Pharmacologic Class	Usual Adult Dosage Range	Indication
theophylline (Theo-Dur, others) (C)	Xanthine-derived bronchodilator	PO: 300-600 mg/day in 1-4 divided doses	Asthma

XANTHINE DERIVATIVES

The natural xanthines consist of the plant alkaloids caffeine, theobromine, and theophylline, but only theophylline and caffeine are currently used clinically. Synthetic xanthines include aminophylline and dyphylline. Caffeine, which is actually a metabolite of theophylline, has other uses described later in the chapter.

Mechanism of Action and Drug Effects

Xanthines cause bronchodilation by increasing the levels of the energy-producing substance cAMP. They do this by competitively inhibiting phosphodiesterase, the enzyme responsible for breaking down cAMP. In patients with COPD, cAMP plays an integral role in the maintenance of open airways. Higher intracellular levels of cAMP contribute to smooth muscle relaxation and also inhibit IgE-induced release of the chemical mediators that drive allergic reactions (histamine, slow-reacting substance of anaphylaxis, and others).

Theophylline is metabolized to caffeine in the body, whereas aminophylline is metabolized to theophylline. Theophylline and other xanthines stimulate the CNS, but to a lesser degree than caffeine. This stimulation of the CNS has the beneficial effect of acting directly on the medullary respiratory center to enhance respiratory drive. In large doses, theophylline may stimulate the cardiovascular system, which results in both an increased force of contraction (positive inotropy) and an increased heart rate (positive chronotropy). The increased force of contraction raises cardiac output and hence blood flow to the kidneys. This, in combination with the ability of the xanthines to dilate blood vessels in and around the kidney, increases the glomerular filtration rate, which produces a diuretic effect.

Indications

Xanthines are used to dilate the airways in patients with asthma, chronic bronchitis, or emphysema. They may be used in mild to moderate cases of acute asthma and as an adjunct drug in the management of COPD. Xanthines are now deemphasized because of their potential for drug interactions and the inter-patient variability in therapeutic drug levels in the blood. Because of their relatively slow onset of action, xanthines are used for the prevention of asthmatic symptoms and COPD, not for the relief of acute asthma attacks.

Caffeine is used without prescription as a CNS stimulant, or analeptic (see Chapter 13), to promote alertness (e.g., for long-duration driving or studying). It is also used as a cardiac stimulant in infants with bradycardia and for enhancement of respiratory drive in infants.

Contraindications

Contraindications to therapy with xanthine derivatives include known drug allergy, uncontrolled cardiac dysrhythmias, seizure disorders, hyperthyroidism, and peptic ulcers.

Adverse Effects

The common adverse effects of the xanthine derivatives include nausea, vomiting, and anorexia. Cardiac adverse effects include sinus tachycardia, extrasystole, palpitations, and ventricular dysrhythmias. Transient increased urination and hyperglycemia are other possible adverse effects. Overdose and other toxicity of xanthine derivatives are usually treated by the repeated administration of doses of activated charcoal.

Interactions

The use of xanthine derivatives with any of the following drugs causes an increase in the serum level: allopurinol, cimetidine, macrolide antibiotics (e.g., erythromycin), quinolones (e.g., ciprofloxacin), influenza vaccine, and oral contraceptives. Their use with sympathomimetics, or even caffeine, can produce additive cardiac and CNS stimulation. Rifampin increases the metabolism of theophylline, which results in decreased theophylline levels. St. John's wort enhances the metabolism of xanthine drugs; thus, higher dosages of theophylline may be needed. Cigarette smoking has a similar effect because of the enzyme-inducing effect of nicotine. Interacting foods include charcoal-broiled, high-protein, and low-carbohydrate foods. These foods may reduce serum levels of xanthines through various metabolic mechanisms.

Dosages

For dosage information on selected theophylline salts, see the table on this page.

DRUG PROFILE

theophylline

Theophylline is the most commonly used xanthine derivative, albeit not often used. It is available in oral, rectal, injectable (as aminophylline), and topical dosage forms. Besides theophylline, the other xanthine bronchodilator used clinically for the treatment of bronchoconstriction is aminophylline. Aminophylline is a prodrug of theophylline; it is metabolized to theophylline in the body. Aminophylline is sometimes given intravenously to patients with status asthmaticus who have not responded to fast-acting beta agonists such as epinephrine.

The beneficial effects of theophylline can be maximized by maintaining blood levels within a certain target range. If these levels become too high, unwanted adverse effects can occur. If the levels become too low, the patient receives little therapeutic benefit. Although the optimal level may vary from patient to patient, most standard references have suggested that the therapeutic range for theophylline blood level is 10 to 20 mcg/mL. However, most prescribers now advise levels between 5 and 15 mcg/mL. Laboratory monitoring of drug blood levels is common to ensure adequate dosage, especially in the hospital setting.

Pharmacokinetics: Theophylline

Route	Onset of Action	Peak Plasma Concentration	Elimination Half-life	Duration of Action
PO	Unknown	1-2 hr	7-9 hr	12 hr

NONBRONCHODILATING RESPIRATORY DRUGS

Bronchodilators (beta-adrenergic agonists, anticholinergics, and xanthines) are just one type of drug used to treat asthma, chronic bronchitis, and emphysema. There are also other drugs that are effective in suppressing the various underlying causes of some of these respiratory illnesses. These include leukotriene receptor antagonists (montelukast, zafirlukast, and zileuton) and corticosteroids (beclomethasone, budesonide, dexamethasone, flunisolide, fluticasone, ciclesonide, and triamcinolone). Another drug class known as *mast cell stabilizers* is now rarely used. However, these drugs are still listed in the national guidelines as *alternative* therapy and include cromolyn and nedocromil; they are sometimes used for exercise-induced asthma. As their class name implies, they work by stabilizing the cell membranes of mast cells to prevent the release of inflammatory mediators such as histamine.

LEUKOTRIENE RECEPTOR ANTAGONISTS

When they became available in the 1990s, the leukotriene receptor antagonists (LTRAs) were the first new class of asthma medications to be introduced in more than 20 years.

Before the development of LTRAs, most asthma treatments focused on relaxing the contraction of bronchial muscles with bronchodilators. More recently, researchers have begun to understand how asthma symptoms are caused by the immune system at the cellular level. A chain reaction starts when a trigger allergen, such as cat hair or dust, initiates a series of chemical reactions in the body. Several substances are produced, including a family of molecules known as *leukotrienes*. In people with asthma, leukotrienes cause inflammation, bronchoconstriction, and mucus production. This in turn leads to coughing, wheezing, and shortness of breath.

Mechanism of Action and Drug Effects

Currently two subclasses of LTRAs are available. These subclasses differ in the mechanism by which they block the inflammatory process in asthma. The first subclass of LTRAs acts by an indirect mechanism and inhibits the enzyme 5-lipoxygenase, which is necessary for leukotriene synthesis. Zileuton (Zyflo) is the only drug of this type currently available. Drugs in the second subclass of LTRAs act more directly by binding to the D_4 leukotriene receptor subtype in respiratory tract tissues and organs. These drugs include montelukast (Singulair) and zafirlukast (Accolate).

The drug effects of LTRAs are primarily limited to the lungs. As their name implies, LTRAs prevent leukotrienes from attaching to receptors located on circulating immune cells (e.g., lymphocytes in the blood) as well as local immune cells within the lungs (e.g., alveolar macrophages). This alleviates asthma symptoms in the lungs by reducing inflammation. They prevent smooth muscle contraction of the bronchial airways, decrease mucus secretion, and reduce vascular permeability (which reduces edema) through their reduction of leukotriene synthesis. Other antileukotriene effects of these drugs include prevention of the mobilization and migration of such cells as neutrophils and lymphocytes into the lungs. This also serves to reduce airway inflammation.

Indications

The LTRAs montelukast, zafirlukast, and zileuton are used for the prophylaxis and long-term treatment and prevention of asthma in adults and children 12 years of age and older. Because it is dosed once daily, montelukast is the most widely used of these drugs and has also been approved for treatment of allergic rhinitis, a condition discussed in Chapter 36. These drugs are not meant for the management of acute asthmatic attacks. Improvement with their use is typically seen in about 1 week.

Contraindications

Known drug allergy or other previous adverse drug reaction is the primary contraindication to the use of these drugs. Allergy to povidone, lactose, titanium dioxide, or cellulose derivatives is also important to note, because these are inactive ingredients in these drugs.

Adverse Effects

The adverse effects of LTRAs differ depending on the specific drug. The most commonly reported adverse effects of zileuton include headache, nausea, dizziness, and insomnia. The most common adverse effects of montelukast and zafirlukast include headache, nausea, and diarrhea.

Interactions

Montelukast has fewer drug interactions than zafirlukast or zileuton. Phenobarbital and rifampin, both of which are enzyme inducers, decrease montelukast concentrations. For information on the drugs that interact with zafirlukast and zileuton, see Table 37-4.

Dosages

For dosage information on montelukast, see the table on this page.

TABLE 37-4 Drug Interactions: Leukotriene Receptor Antagonists

Drug	Interacting Drugs	Mechanism	Result
montelukast (Singulair)	phenobarbital, rifampin	Increased metabolism	Decreased montelukast levels
zafirlukast (Accolate)	aspirin	Decreased clearance	Increased zafirlukast levels
	erythromycin	Decreased bioavailability	Decreased zafirlukast levels
	warfarin	Decreased clearance	Increased warfarin levels
zileuton (Zyflo)	propranolol	Decreased clearance	Increased propranolol levels
	theophylline	Decreased clearance	Increased theophylline levels
	warfarin	Decreased clearance	Increased warfarin levels

DOSAGES

Selected Antileukotriene Drug

Drug (Pregnancy Category)	Pharmacologic Class	Usual Adult Dosage Range	Indications
◆ montelukast (Singulair) (B)	Leukotriene receptor antagonist	10 mg daily in evening	Asthma (prophylaxis and maintenance treatment)

DRUG PROFILE

LTRAs are used primarily for oral prophylaxis and long-term treatment of asthma. The three drugs currently available are zileuton, zafirlukast, and montelukast. These drugs are not to be used for treatment of acute asthma attacks.

◆ **montelukast**

Montelukast (Singulair) belongs to the same subcategory of LTRAs as zafirlukast. Montelukast and zafirlukast work by blocking leukotriene D_4 receptors to augment the inflammatory response. Montelukast offers the advantage of being approved for use in children 2 years of age and older. It also has fewer adverse effects and drug interactions than zafirlukast. Use of montelukast is contraindicated in patients with a known hypersensitivity to it. It is available only for oral use. It is classified as a pregnancy category B drug. Recommended dosages are given in the table on this page.

Pharmacokinetics: Montelukast

Route	Onset of Action	Peak Plasma Concentration	Elimination Half-life	Duration of Action
PO	30 min	3-4 hr	2.7-5 hr	24 hr

CORTICOSTEROIDS

Corticosteroids, also known as *glucocorticoids,* are either naturally occurring or synthetic drugs used in the treatment of pulmonary diseases for their antiinflammatory effects. All have actions similar to those of the natural steroid hormone cortisol, which is chemically the same as the drug hydrocortisone. Synthetic steroids are more commonly used in drug therapy. They can be given by inhalation, orally, or even intravenously in severe cases of asthma. Corticosteroids administered by inhalation have an advantage over those administered orally in that their action is relatively limited to the topical site in the lungs. This generally limits, although does not totally prevent, systemic effects. The chemical structures of the corticosteroids given by inhalation have also been slightly altered to limit their systemic absorption from the respiratory tract. The corticosteroids administered by inhalation include the following:

- beclomethasone dipropionate (Beclovent)
- budesonide (Pulmicort Turbuhaler)
- dexamethasone sodium phosphate (Decadron Phosphate Respihaler)
- flunisolide (AeroBid)
- fluticasone (Flovent)
- triamcinolone acetonide (Azmacort)
- ciclesonide (Omnaris)

The systemic use of corticosteroids is described in Chapter 33. The systemic corticosteroids most commonly used for respiratory illness include prednisone (oral) and methylprednisolone (IV).

Mechanism of Action and Drug Effects

Although the exact mechanism of action of the corticosteroids has not been determined, it is thought that they have the dual effect of both reducing inflammation and enhancing the activity of beta agonists. The corticosteroids produce their antiinflammatory effects through a complex sequence of actions. The overall effect is to prevent various nonspecific inflammatory processes. Corticosteroids essentially work by stabilizing the membranes of cells that normally release bronchoconstricting substances. These cells include leukocytes, which is another name for white blood cells (WBCs). There are five different types of WBC, each with its own specific characteristics. The five types of WBC, their role in the inflammatory process, and the way in which corticosteroids inhibit their normal action, combat inflammation, and produce bronchodilation are summarized in Table 37-5. Inflammatory mediators are primarily released by lymphocytes in the circulation as well as by mast cells and alveolar macrophages. These latter two cell types are stationary (noncirculating) inflammatory cells that remain localized in the various tissues and organs of the respiratory tract.

Corticosteroids have also been shown to restore or increase the responsiveness of bronchial smooth muscle to beta-adrenergic receptor stimulation, which results in more pronounced stimulation of the beta$_2$ receptors by beta agonist drugs such as albuterol. It may take several weeks of continuous therapy before the full therapeutic effects of the corticosteroids are realized.

Indications

Inhaled corticosteroids are used for the primary treatment of bronchospastic disorders to control the inflammatory responses that are believed to be the cause of these disorders; they are indicated for persistent asthma. They are often used concurrently with the beta-adrenergic agonists. In respiratory illnesses, systemic corticosteroids are generally used only to treat acute exacerbations, or severe asthma. Their long-term use is associated with adverse effects (see later). When a rapid, pronounced antiinflammatory effect is needed, as in an acute exacerbation of asthma or other COPD, intravenous corticosteroids (e.g., methylprednisolone) are often used.

Contraindications

Drug allergy is the primary contraindication and is usually due to other ingredients in the drug formulation. These drugs

TABLE 37-5 White Blood Cells (Leukocytes)

WBC Type*	Role in Inflammation	Corticosteroid Effect
Granulocytes		
Neutrophils (65%)	Contain powerful lysosomes; release chemicals that destroy invading organisms and also attack other WBCs	Stabilize cell membranes so that inflammation-causing substances are not released
Eosinophils (2%-5%)	Function mainly in allergic reactions and protect against parasitic infections; ingest inflammatory chemicals and antigen-antibody complexes	Little effect if any
Basophils (0.5%-1%)	Contain histamine, an inflammation-causing substance, and heparin, an anticoagulant	Stabilize cell membranes so that histamine is not released
Agranulocytes		
Lymphocytes (25%)	Two types: T lymphocytes and B lymphocytes; T cells attack infecting microbial or cancerous cells; B cells produce antibodies against specific antigens	Decrease activity of the lymphocytes
Monocytes (3%-5%)	Produce macrophages, which can migrate out of the bloodstream to such places as mucous membranes, where they are capable of engulfing large bacteria or virus-infected cells	Inhibit macrophage accumulation in already inflamed areas, thus preventing more inflammation

*Value in parentheses is the percentage of all leukocytes represented by the given type.

are not intended as sole therapy for acute asthma attacks. Inhaled corticosteroids are contraindicated in patients who are hypersensitive to glucocorticoids, in patients whose sputum tests positive for *Candida* organisms, and in patients with systemic fungal infection, as the corticosteroids can suppress the immune system.

Adverse Effects

The main undesirable local effects of typical doses of inhaled corticosteroids in the respiratory system include pharyngeal irritation, coughing, dry mouth, and oral fungal infections. Instruct patients to rinse their mouths after use of an inhaled corticosteroid. Most of the drug effects of inhaled corticosteroids are limited to their topical site of action in the lungs. There is relatively little systemic absorption of the drugs when they are administered by inhalation at normal therapeutic dosages. However, the degree of systemic absorption is more likely to be increased in patients who require higher inhaled dosages. When there is significant systemic absorption, which is most likely with high-dose intravenous or oral administration, corticosteroids can affect any of the organ systems in the body. Some of these systemic drug effects include adrenocortical insufficiency, increased susceptibility to infection, fluid and electrolyte disturbances, endocrine effects, CNS effects (insomnia, nervousness, seizures), and dermatologic and connective tissue effects, including brittle skin, bone loss, osteoporosis, and Cushing's syndrome (see Chapter 33).

It is important to remember that when patients are switched to inhaled corticosteroids after receiving systemic corticosteroids, adrenal suppression (Addisonian crisis) may occur when the systemically administered corticosteroid is not tapered slowly. Patient deaths have been reported due to adrenal gland failure in such cases when the switch to inhaled corticosteroids is made quickly and the dosage of systemic corticosteroids is not reduced gradually. The patient who is dependent on systemic corticosteroids may need up to 1 year of recovery time after discontinuation of systemic therapy. There is evidence that bone growth is suppressed in children and adolescents taking corticosteroids. This suppression is more apparent in children receiving larger systemic (versus inhaled) dosages over longer treatment durations.

Interactions

Drug interactions are more likely to occur with systemic (versus inhaled) corticosteroids. These drugs may increase serum glucose levels, possibly requiring adjustments in dosages of antidiabetic drugs. Because of interactions related to metabolizing enzymes, they may also raise blood levels of the immunosuppressants cyclosporine and tacrolimus. Likewise, the antifungal drug itraconazole may reduce clearance of the steroids, whereas phenytoin, phenobarbital, and rifampin may enhance clearance. There is also greater risk for hypokalemia with concurrent use of potassium-depleting diuretics such as hydrochlorothiazide and furosemide.

Dosages

For dosage information on selected corticosteroids, see the table on this page.

DRUG PROFILES

fluticasone propionate

Fluticasone is administered intranasally (Flonase) (one inhalation in each nostril daily) and by oral inhalation (Flovent) (usually one inhalation by mouth twice daily). Fluticasone is also available in a combination formulation with the bronchodilator salmeterol (Advair). Advair is one of the most commonly used inhalers, but because it contains a long-acting beta agonist, it must never be used for acute treatment.

Pharmacokinetics: Fluticasone Propionate

Route	Onset of Action	Peak Plasma Concentration	Elimination Half-life	Duration of Action
Inhalation	Unknown	Unknown	3 hr	Up to 24 hr

methylprednisolone

Methylprednisolone is a systemic corticosteroid available in both oral (Medrol) and injectable (Solu-Medrol) forms.

Pharmacokinetics: Methylprednisolone

Route	Onset of Action	Peak Plasma Concentration	Elimination Half-life	Duration of Action
IV	Immediate	30 min	3-4 hr	24-36 hr

DOSAGES

Selected Corticosteroids

Drug (Pregnancy Category)	Pharmacologic Class	Usual Adult Dosage Range	Indications
fluticasone propionate (Flovent) (C)	Synthetic glucocorticoid	Flovent HFA MDI, 3 strengths available: 44 mcg, 110 mcg, 220 mcg; 2 puffs twice daily Flovent Discus inhalation powder, 2 strengths available; 100 mcg, 250 mcg/actuation; 1-2 puffs bid	Asthma (prophylaxis and maintenance treatment) Seasonal allergic rhinitis
methylprednisolone (Solu-Medrol injection, Medrol tablets) (C)	Synthetic glucocorticoid	40-80 mg/day in divided doses	Exacerbations of asthma or COPD

COPD, Chronic obstructive pulmonary disease; *MDI,* metered-dose inhaler.

CASE STUDY

Patient-Centered Care: Bronchodilators and Corticosteroids for COPD

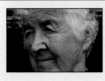

Ms. B. is a 73-year-old woman who worked in the local traffic tunnel for about 25 years and has had chronic obstructive pulmonary disease (COPD) for 10 years, caused by exposure to environmental pollutants while on the job and by cigarette smoking. She is now retired and is frequently admitted to the hospital for treatment of her condition. She quit smoking about 8 years ago. Ms. B. is now in the hospital for treatment of an acute exacerbation of her COPD and an upper respiratory tract infection. The physician has ordered the following: oxygen per nasal cannula at 2 L/min; methylprednisolone (Solu-Medrol) 125 mg IV push, then 80 mg IVPB every 6 hours; Advair 50 mcg/250 mcg, 1 dose every 12 hours; albuterol (Accuneb) 2.5 mg by nebulizer every 4 hours for 2 days, then every 4 hours as needed; piperacillin/tazobactam (Zosyn) antibiotic therapy, 3.375 g IV every 6 hours; measurement of intake and output; daily weight measurement; assessment of vital signs with breath sounds and pulse oximetry every 2 hours until stable; and chest physiotherapy twice a day and as needed.

1. What is in Advair, and what does the "50 mcg/250 mcg" mean? Explain the class and purposes of the drug(s) it contains.

Within 2 days, Ms. B's condition stabilizes, and the methylprednisolone dose is gradually reduced. After 1 week, the IV corticosteroid is discontinued and she is started on oral prednisone (generic) 40 mg daily. Her discharge medications include the following: prednisone (generic) 40 mg PO daily for 3 days, then taper and discontinue by reducing the dose by 5 mg daily (prescription calls for 5-mg tablets); Advair 50 mcg/250 mcg, 1 dose every 12 hours; albuterol (Proventil HFA) metered-dose inhaler, 90 mcg/spray, every 4 hours as needed.

2. What is the reason for tapering the methylprednisolone and prednisone before they are discontinued?
3. Ms. B states, "This is confusing! How do I know how many tablets to take? It's different each day!" What can you do to help her with the tapering dosage of prednisone?
4. While going over the medications, Ms. B asks you, "So which inhaler do I take if I feel short of breath? The Advair or the albuterol? Aren't they the same thing?" What is the nurse's best response?

For answers, see *http://evolve.elsevier.com/Lilley*.

PHOSPHODIESTERASE-4 INHIBITOR

In 2011, the FDA approved roflumilast (Daliresp), which is a selective inhibitor of the enzyme called *phosphodiesterase type 4 (PDE4)*. It is indicated to prevent coughing and excess mucus from worsening and to decrease the frequency of life-threatening COPD exacerbations. It is not intended to treat acute bronchospasm. The most commonly reported adverse effects include nausea, diarrhea, headache, insomnia, dizziness, weight loss, and psychiatric symptoms. The FDA requires a medication guide that informs patients of the potential risk for psychiatric adverse effects. Further information can be found at *www.daliresp.com*.

MONOCLONAL ANTIBODY ANTIASTHMATIC

Omalizumab (Xolair) is the newest antiasthmatic medication to become available. It is a monoclonal antibody that selectively binds to the immunoglobulin IgE, which in turn limits the release of mediators of the allergic response. Omalizumab is given by injection and has the potential for producing anaphylaxis. Patients receiving omalizumab must be monitored closely for hypersensitivity reactions.

NURSING PROCESS

ASSESSMENT

The net drug effect of *beta agonists, xanthine derivatives, anticholinergics, LTRAs,* and *corticosteroids* is improved airflow in airway passages and increased oxygen supply. With the use of these drugs, thoroughly assess their cautions, contraindications, and drug interactions. Additionally, perform a thorough assessment of the patient's skin color, temperature, respiration rate (at a rate of 12 to 24 breaths/min), respiration depth and rhythm, breath sounds, blood pressure, and pulse rate. Determine if the patient is having problems with cough, dyspnea, orthopnea, or hypoxia, or has other signs or symptoms of respiratory distress. If a cough is present, assess its character, frequency, and the presence or absence of sputum. If sputum is present, assess its color and consistency. Assess for the presence of any of the following: sternal retractions, cyanosis, restlessness, activity intolerance, cardiac irregularities, palpitations, hypertension, tachycardia, and use of accessory muscles to breathe. If present, these would indicate significant respiratory compromise. Determine the anterior-posterior diameter of the thorax. Note pulse oximetry levels to determine oxygen saturation levels.

Obtain a complete medication history that includes information about prescription and over-the-counter (OTC) drugs, herbal products, alternative therapies, use of nebulizers and/or humidifiers, use of a home air purifier, and presence of a heating and/or air conditioning system. Inquire about the condition of these systems as well as duct work in the home/living quarters. Collect information about environmental allergies, such as to dust, mold, pollen, and mildew, and seasonal allergies. Record any known food allergies. Note the characteristics of any respiratory symptoms (e.g., seasonally induced, exercise-induced, or stress-induced) and any family history of respiratory diseases. Identify any environmental exposures, such as to chemicals or irritants, as well as precipitating and alleviating factors for any respiratory symptoms and/or disease processes. Assess smoking habits, as smoking exacerbates respiratory symptoms and nicotine interacts with many respiratory drugs.

Cardiac status may be compromised due to respiratory distress and respiratory illnesses; therefore, closely assess the patient's blood pressure, pulse rate, and heart sounds. Further assess any additional prescribed testing such as electrocardiogram, blood gas analysis with specific attention to the patient's pH, oxygen, carbon dioxide, and serum bicarbonate levels. Assess nail beds for abnormalities (e.g., clubbing, cyanosis) and the area around the lips for cyanotic changes. Restlessness is often the first sign of hypoxia, so frequent assessment before, during, and after drug treatment is needed. If hypoxia is present, contact the prescriber immediately. If chest radiographs, scans, or magnetic resonance images have been ordered, review the findings. Along with a physical assessment, perform a psychosocial and emotional assessment, because anxiety, stress, and fear may only further compromise the patient's respiratory status and oxygen levels. Be sure to note the age of the patient because of increased drug sensitivity in the very young and the older adult patient.

For the *beta agonists* (e.g., *albuterol, salmeterol*), cautions, contraindications, and drug interactions associated with these drugs must be noted. The newest *long-acting beta agonist* drugs include *indacterol (Arcapta Neohaler); vilanterol* with a *corticosteroid, fluticasone (Breo Ellipta)*; and *vilanterol* with an *anticholinergic, umeclidinium (Anoro Ellipta)*. As mentioned previously in the pharmacology section, the term *Ellipta* refers to a new delivery system. Additionally, with these combinations/long-acting products, both medications need to be included in the nursing process. A respiratory assessment is needed to assess for allergies to any of the medications included in any of the dosage forms, including the inhaled forms. Assess for the contraindications in patients with dysrhythmias and those at risk for stroke. Assess the patient's intake of caffeine (e.g., chocolate, tea, coffee, candy, and sodas) and use of OTC medications containing caffeine (e.g., appetite suppressants, pain relievers). The intake of caffeine is important to determine, because of its sympathomimetic effects and possible potentiation of adverse effects along with albuterol and other beta agonists (e.g., restlessness, cardiac stimulation, tremor, hyperglycemia, and vascular headache; hypotension/hypertension with beta$_2$ drugs). Assess the patient's medication history because these drugs are not to be taken with monoamine oxidase inhibitors because of the enhanced risk for hypertension. Assess educational level and readiness to learn.

With use of the *nonselective adrenergic agonist drug EpiPen* (0.3 mg *epinephrine*) or *EpiPen Jr* (0.15 mg *epinephrine*) *Auto-Injectors*, assess for the main indication (which is emergency use with severe allergic reactions caused by allergens, exercise, and unknown triggers) and for those individuals who are considered at increased risk for these reactions.

In the past, the use of *anticholinergics* was associated with a concern for the use of nebulized *ipratropium bromide* in patients with allergy to soy lecithin, peanut oils, peanuts, soybeans, and other legumes, with reported cases of severe anaphylactic reactions. However, due to changes in the delivery mechanism of newer inhalers, this is no longer an issue of concern. In your assessments for patients taking anticholinergics, include any history of heart palpitations, GI distress, benign prostatic hyperplasia and/or urinary retention, and glaucoma due to the adverse effects of the drugs, leading to potentiation of these conditions or symptoms. Ipratropium and its aerosol forms

have been associated with bronchospasm, so assess for any pre-existing problems with the use of MDIs. If a combination product containing both *ipratropium* and *albuterol* is prescribed, perform an assessment appropriate to the use of both of these drugs.

In patients taking *xanthine derivatives* (e.g., *theophylline*), identify any contraindications and cautions. Perform a careful cardiovascular assessment, noting heart rate, blood pressure, and history of cardiac disease. This is important because of the adverse effects of sinus tachycardia and palpitations. GI reflux may also occur with these drugs. Assess bowel patterns and for preexisting disease, such as gastroesophageal reflux and/or ulcers. Because of possible drug-induced transient urinary frequency, conduct a baseline assessment of urinary patterns. Assessment needs to also include the patient's medication history to assess for possible drug interactions such as with allopurinol, cimetidine, erythromycin, ciprofloxacin, oral contraceptives, caffeine, and sympathomimetics. Perform a dietary assessment, including questions about consumption of a low-carbohydrate, high-protein diet and intake of charcoal-broiled meat. These dietary practices may lead to increased theophylline elimination and decrease the therapeutic levels of the drug. Note caffeine-containing foods, beverages, prescription drugs, OTC drugs, and herbals because of additional interactions.

With *LTRAs,* assess for contraindications, cautions, and drug interactions. Determine liver functioning because of specific concerns about the use of these drugs in patients with altered hepatic function. As with other medications, older adult patients are more sensitive to these drugs.

PATIENT-CENTERED-CARE: LIFESPAN CONSIDERATIONS FOR THE OLDER ADULT PATIENT

Xanthine Derivatives

- Administer xanthine derivatives cautiously with careful monitoring in the older adult because sensitivity to these drugs is increased in this patient population due to decreased drug metabolism.
- Assess for signs and symptoms of xanthine toxicity, which include nausea, vomiting, restlessness, insomnia, irritability, and tremors. Discriminating the cause of restlessness (e.g., hypoxia versus drug toxicity) is important to patient safety.
- Instruct older adult patients to never chew or crush sustained-released dosage forms and to remain aware of drug interactions, especially interactions with other asthma-related drugs/bronchodilators. Advise older adult patients to avoid omitting and/or doubling up on doses. If a dose is missed, instruct the patient to contact the prescriber for further instructions.
- Monitoring of serum levels during follow-up visits is important to avoid possible toxicity and ensure therapeutic blood levels.
- Lower dosages may be necessary initially in older adult patients, not only because of their increased sensitivity to the drug but also because of the possibility of decreased liver and renal functioning. Close monitoring for adverse effects and toxicity should be part of everyday therapy. Note and report any palpitations and increased blood pressure (from cardiovascular and central nervous system stimulation).

With use of *corticosteroids* (also known as *glucocorticoids* and/or *antiinflammatory adrenal drugs*), perform a baseline assessment of vital signs, breath sounds, and heart sounds.

Assessment for underlying adrenal disorders is important because of the adrenal suppression that occurs with the use of these medications. Age is important to consider because *corticosteroids* may be problematic for the pediatric patient if long-term therapy and/or high dosage amounts are used. The systemic impact on the pediatric patient is suppressed growth (see the Pharmacology section for further discussion). This suppressed growth is more apparent in children receiving larger systemic dosages, as opposed to inhaled dosage forms, and for over longer periods of time. As with the other drugs in this chapter, awareness of basic information about these drugs, especially their action, is very important for safe use and prevention of medication errors. For example, *glucocorticoids* are used for their antiinflammatory effects, *beta agonists* and *xanthines* for their bronchorelaxation/bronchodilating effects, and *anticholinergics* for their blockage of cholinergic receptors. Knowledge about mechanisms of action and indications helps to prevent or decrease medication errors and adverse effects. Assess for significant drug interactions, especially with systemic versus inhaled corticosteroids, including antidiabetic drugs, antifungals, phenytoin, phenobarbital, rifampin, and potassium-sparing diuretics. See Chapter 33 for more information on these *antiinflammatory adrenal drugs*.

With the *PDE4 inhibitors,* assess for presenting symptoms as well as any baseline psychiatric issues or disorders. Note that these drugs are not indicated for acute episodes of bronchospasms but are used to limit the release of mediators and prevent allergic response. *Omalizumab,* a *monoclonal antibody antiasthmatic drug,* requires additional assessment of known risks associated with certain malignancies. Taking a thorough nursing history will help identify any of these risks. Assess also for signs and symptoms of hypersensitivity due to an increased incidence with this classification of drugs.

QSEN ⚡ **SAFETY AND QUALITY IMPROVEMENT: PREVENTING MEDICATION ERRORS**

Oral Ingestion of Capsules for Inhalation Devices

Some inhalation products use capsules and a device that pierces the capsules to allow the powdered medication to be inhaled with a special inhaler. Two products, Foradil Aerolizer (formoterol fumarate inhalation powder) and Spiriva HandiHaler (tiotropium bromide inhalation powder) contain such capsules. Even though these capsules are packaged with inhaler devices, they closely resemble oral capsules. The U.S. Food and Drug Administration (FDA) has received reports that the capsules have been taken orally by patients, which can potentially result in adverse effects. If the capsules are swallowed instead of taken using the inhalation device, the medication's onset of action may be delayed, the efficacy is reduced, and as a result the patient receives inadequate drug delivery. The FDA has taken steps to work with the drug manufacturers to mark the packaging clearly. Be certain to instruct patients on the proper use and correct route of administration for these inhaled drugs to prevent their confusion with oral products.

Data from FDA. *www.fda.gov/downloads/drugs/drugsafety/ medicationerrors/ucm080689.pdf.* Accessed July 15, 2015.

NURSING DIAGNOSES

1. Impaired gas exchange related to pathophysiologic changes caused by respiratory disease

2. Fatigue related to the disease process and lack of oxygen saturation
3. Noncompliance with the medication regimen related to undesirable adverse effects of drug therapy

PLANNING: OUTCOME IDENTIFICATION

1. Patient experiences increased gas exchange due to drug and nondrug therapeutic regimen's impact on pathologic disease process.
2. Patient exhibits improved energy and less fatigue from minimizing oxygen demands.
3. Patient remains compliant with the drug and nondrug regimens and experiences maximal therapeutic benefits and minimal adverse effects.

IMPLEMENTATION

Nursing interventions that apply to patients with respiratory disease processes (e.g., COPD, asthma, other upper and lower respiratory tract disorders) include patient education and an emphasis on compliance and prevention, in addition to the specific actions related to the prescribed drug therapy. Emphasize measures that help to prevent, relieve, and/or decrease the manifestations of the disease. A resource that provides excellent information as well as photographs and slideshows can be found at *www.medicinenet.com*; within the search mode, type in the term *asthma*.

Bronchodilators and other respiratory drugs must be given exactly as prescribed and by the prescribed route (e.g., parenterally, orally, by intermittent positive pressure breathing, or by inhalation). Demonstrate the proper method for administering the inhaled forms of these drugs to the patient (see Chapter 9). Provide time for a return demonstration. Emphasize the importance of taking only the prescribed dose of the *beta agonists, anticholinergics, xanthines, LTRAs,* and *other respiratory drugs* because of the possible adverse effects, such as cardiac stimulation, hypertension or hypotension, vascular headaches, heart palpitations, GI distress, urinary retention, gastroesophageal reflux, dysrhythmias, nausea, and dizziness.

The use of MDIs requires coordination to inhale the medication correctly and to obtain approximately 10% of drug delivery to the lungs. If a second puff of the same drug is ordered, instruct the patient to wait 1 to 2 minutes between puffs. If a second type of inhaled drug is ordered, instruct the patient to wait 2 to 5 minutes between the medications or as prescribed. Use of a spacer device (holding chamber for an MDI) may be indicated to increase the amount of drug delivered. See the Teamwork and Collaboration: Legal and Ethical Principles box on the next page for information concerning the environmental hazards associated with chlorofluorocarbon (CFC) inhalers. Dry powder inhalers (DPIs) are small handheld devices that deliver a specific amount of dry micronized powder with each inhaled breath. The use of the spacer device may be beneficial to those having difficulty using metered-dose inhalers, whereas dry powder inhalers are breath-activated and may better suit patients with coordination issues. A nebulizer dosage form delivers small amounts of misted droplets of the drug to the lungs through a small mouthpiece or mask. Although a nebulizer may take a longer time to deliver the drug to the lungs than the inhalers, the nebulizer dosage form may be more effective for some patients. See Chapter 9 for more information on these dosage routes.

QSEN **TEAMWORK AND COLLABORATION: LEGAL AND ETHICAL PRINCIPLES**

Inhaled Medications and the Environment: Phase-out of Chlorofluorocarbon (CFC) Inhalers

The U.S. Food and Drug Administration phased-out all inhaler medical products containing chlorofluorocarbons (CFCs) on December 31, 2013. This traditional method of delivery or route of administration for inhalers has been phased out to comply with an international treaty to protect the ozone layer by phasing out the worldwide production of numerous substances including CFCs. CFCs were proven to contribute to ozone depletion. The phasing-out of inhaler products containing CFCs was a well-publicized process occurring over a period of years. More than 25 million people suffer from asthma, and an additional 15 million people diagnosed with COPD require treatment with an inhaled medication. CFCs were used as propellants to move the drug out of the inhalers so that patients could inhale the medication for access to the lungs. The FDA and EPA collaborated to "phase-out CFCs in inhalers for more than two decades with input from the public, advisory committees, manufacturers, and stakeholders." CFCs were replaced with propellants called hydrofluoroalkanes (HFAs). HFA inhalers may taste and feel different but are used in the same way as CFC inhalers and for the same FDA-approved uses while remaining environmentally safe. For more information, visit *www.fda.gov/Drugs/ResourcesForYou/Consumers/QuestionsAnswers/ucm077808.htm.*

Modified from the U.S. Food and Drug Administration: How to dispose of unused medications, *FDA Consumer Updates,* February 20, 2015. Available at *www.fda.gov/forconsumers/consumerupdates/ucm101653.htm.* Accessed March 13, 2015.

Beta agonists must be taken exactly as prescribed because overdosage may be life-threatening. Educate patients not to crush or chew oral sustained-release tablets and to take them with food to decrease gastrointestinal (GI) upset. Instructions for inhaled dosage forms are presented in Chapter 9. See Figure 37-2 for instructions for use of the *EpiPen Auto-Injector.* Reassess the respiratory status and breath sounds before, during, and after therapy with these drugs to determine therapeutic effectiveness.

Anticholinergic drugs used for respiratory diseases (e.g., *ipratropium*) are to be taken daily as ordered and with appropriate use of the MDI. See Patient-Centered Care: Patient Teaching on the next page for more information on the administration of these drugs. It is important that the patient waits from 1 to 2 minutes (or as prescribed) before inhaling the second dose of the drug to allow for maximal lung penetration. Emphasize the importance of rinsing the mouth with water immediately after use of any inhaled or nebulized drug to help prevent mucosal dryness and/or irritation dryness.

Xanthine derivatives are to be given exactly as prescribed. If they are prescribed to be administered parenterally, determine the correct diluent, compatibility, and rate of administration. Use intravenous infusion pumps to ensure dosage accuracy and help prevent toxicity. Too rapid an infusion may lead to profound hypotension with possible syncope, tachycardia, seizures, and even cardiac arrest. Oral forms are to be taken with food to decrease GI upset. To prevent a sudden increase in drug release with risk for toxicity as well as irritating effects on the gastric mucosa, instruct patients not to crush or chew timed-release preparations. Educate patients that suppository forms of the drug need to be refrigerated, and to notify the prescriber if rectal burning, itching, or irritation occurs. Continue to monitor the patient for respiratory status and improvement in baseline condition during drug therapy.

The *LTRAs,* specifically *zileuton, montelukast,* and *zafirlukast,* are given orally. Of most concern are the montelukast chewable tablets, which contain aspartame and approximately 0.842 mg of phenylamine per 5-mg tablet. Some patients may need to avoid these substances. Emphasize that these drugs are indicated for treatment of chronic, not acute, asthma attacks. Stress that these drugs are to be taken as ordered and on a continuous schedule, even if symptoms improve. Advise the patient to increase fluid intake (as with all the respiratory drugs) to help decrease the viscosity of secretions.

Inhaled *corticosteroids* (*glucocorticoids*) are yet another group of drugs that must be used as prescribed and with cautions regarding overuse. Advise the patient to take the medication as ordered every day, regardless of whether or not he or she is feeling better. Often these drugs (e.g., *flunisolide*) are used as maintenance drugs and are taken twice daily for maximal response. An inhaled beta$_2$ agonist may be used before the inhaled corticosteroid to provide bronchial relaxation/dilation before administration of the antiinflammatory drug. The bronchodilator inhaled drug is generally taken 2 to 5 minutes (or as ordered) before the corticosteroid aerosol. Stress the importance of keeping all equipment (inhalers or nebulizers) clean, cleaning and changing filters (nebulizers), and maintaining equipment in good working condition. Use of a spacer may be indicated, especially if success with inhalation is limited. Recommend rinsing the mouth immediately after use of the inhaler or nebulizer dosage forms of corticosteroids to help prevent overgrowth of oral fungi and subsequent development of oral candidiasis (thrush). Pediatric patients may need a prescriber's order to have these medications on hand, at school, and during athletic events or physical education. Peak flow meter use is also encouraged to help patients of all ages better regulate their disease. A peak flow meter is a handheld device used to monitor a patient's ability to breathe out air and reflects the airflow through the bronchi and thus the degree of obstruction in the airways. Encourage journaling to record peak flow levels, signs and symptoms of the disease, any improvement, and the occurrence of adverse effects associated with therapy. For pediatric patients, use of systemic forms of corticosteroids is a concern. Specifically in children, the use of systemic forms of these drugs may lead to suppression of the hypothalamic-pituitary-adrenal axis and subsequent growth stunting. However, the benefits are considerable when compared to the risks. Inhaled forms are often combined with short-term systemic therapy in pediatric patients. Continue to monitor the patient's condition during therapy with a focus on the respiratory, cardiac, and central nervous systems.

With *PDE4 inhibitor drugs*, educate the patient about the importance of reporting any change in psychiatric status to the prescriber immediately. The *monoclonal antibody antiasthmatic drug omalizumab* is to be taken exactly as ordered. Since it is given as a subcutaneous injection, instruct the patient in self-injection, or alert the patient that frequent visits to the prescriber, nurse, or other health care provider to receive the injection are necessary. This drug is usually given every 2 to 4 weeks. Omalizumab is not indicated for acute asthma attacks, and it may be used in conjunction with other acute-acting asthma medications. Closely monitor the patient for any allergic or hypersensitivity reactions.

▌EVALUATION

The therapeutic effects of any of the drugs used to improve the control of acute or chronic respiratory diseases and to treat or help prevent respiratory symptoms include the following: decreased dyspnea, wheezing, restlessness, and anxiety; improved respiratory patterns with return to normal rate and quality; improved oxygen saturation levels; improved activity tolerance and arterial blood gas levels; improved quality of life; and decreased severity and incidence of respiratory symptoms. The therapeutic effects of *bronchodilators* (e.g., *xanthines, beta agonists*) include decreased symptoms and increased ease of breathing. Blood levels of *theophylline* need to be between 5 and 15 mcg/mL and need to be frequently monitored. Peak flow meters are easy to use and help reveal early decreases in peak flow caused by bronchospasm. They also aid in monitoring treatment effectiveness. Other respiratory drugs produce therapeutic effects as related to the specific drug. Adverse effects for which to monitor during therapy include the following: *beta agonists*—headache, insomnia, cardiac stimulation, and tremor; *anticholinergics*—headache, GI distress, urinary retention, and increased intraocular pressure; *xanthines*—nausea, vomiting, and palpitations; *LTRAs*—nausea, headaches, and insomnia; and *corticosteroids*—adrenocortical insufficiency, increased susceptibility to infection, fluid and electrolyte disturbances, and insomnia. With *corticosteroids*, adrenal suppression may occur with high doses over an extended period of time. See the previous discussion for a complete listing of adverse effects.

▌PATIENT-CENTERED CARE: PATIENT TEACHING

Beta Agonists

- Educate the patient about any potential drug interactions.
- Educate about the action and duration of action of these medications, especially the long-acting beta agonists because they are NOT to be used for acute treatment!!
- Encourage patients with asthma, bronchitis, or COPD to avoid precipitating events such as exposure to conditions or situations that may lead to bronchoconstriction and/or worsening of the disorder (e.g., allergens, stress, smoking, and/or air pollutants).
- Provide instructions about the proper use and care of MDIs, dry powder inhalers, and other such devices. Dosage instructions must be closely adhered to in order to prevent toxicity. For specific information on general inhaler use and care, including the new HFA inhalers, see Chapter 9. Box 37-3 contains online references for specific types of inhaler

devices. Emphasize the importance of not overusing the medication due to the risk for rebound bronchospasm.

Xanthines

- Educate the patient about the interaction between smoking and xanthines (e.g., smoking decreases the blood concentrations of aminophylline and theophylline). Xanthines also interact with charcoal-broiled foods and may lead to decreased serum levels of xanthine drugs.
- Instruct patients about food and beverage items that contain caffeine (e.g., chocolate, coffee, cola, cocoa, tea), because their consumption can exacerbate CNS stimulation.
- Encourage the patient to take medications around the clock to maintain steady-state drug levels. Extended-released dosage forms and other oral dosage forms are not to be crushed or chewed. Advise the patient that any worsening of adverse effects, such as epigastric pain, nausea, vomiting, tremors, and headache, must be reported immediately.
- Encourage the patient to keep follow-up appointments because of the importance in monitoring therapeutic levels of medications and therapeutic effectiveness.
- Some patients may need to learn to take their own pulse rate. Demonstrate proper technique.

Anticholinergics

- Educate patients that ipratropium is used prophylactically to decrease the frequency and severity of asthma and must be taken as ordered and generally year round for therapeutic

BOX 37-3	Inhaler Instructions	
Inhaler Name	**Website Reference**
fluticasone furoate and vilanterol (Breo Ellipta)	www.mybreo.com
tiotropium bromide (Spiriva)	www.spiriva.com
fluticasone propionate and salmeterol (Advair)	www.advair.com
budesonide and formoterol (Symbicort)	www.mysymbicort.com
formoterol and mometasone (Dulera)	www.dulera.com
Indacaterol (Arcapta Neohaler)	www.arcapta.com

effectiveness. This drug must be avoided in patients with existing allergy to soybeans, peanuts, or other legumes.

- Encourage forcing fluids, unless contraindicated, to decrease the viscosity of secretions and increase the expectoration of sputum.
- When inhaled forms of these drugs (and other respiratory drugs) are used, instruct the patient to take the prescribed number of puffs of the inhaler. Educate the patient about how to properly use an MDI with or without a spacer, how to use a dry powder inhaler (DPI), and how to properly clean and store the equipment (see Chapter 9). Instruct the patient to wait 2 to 5 minutes (or as prescribed) before using additional different inhaled medications.

Leukotriene Receptor Antagonists

- Educate the patient about the action and purpose of LTRAs and how they work differently by preventing leukotriene formation and thus preventing/decreasing inflammation, bronchoconstriction, and mucus production. Emphasize that these drugs are indicated for prevention, not treatment, of acute asthmatic attacks. Instruct patients to take montelukast at night.

Corticosteroids (Glucocorticoids)

- In addition to adhering to the specified dose and frequency of these drugs, if inhaled forms are used, the patient must practice good oral hygiene (e.g., rinsing of the mouth) after the last inhalation. Rinsing the mouth with water is appropriate and necessary to prevent oral fungal infections. Instruct the patient about keeping the inhaler clean. Each HFA inhaler has different instructions for priming and cleaning, so reviewing the patient information instructions with each inhaler is important to patient safety. Corticosteroid inhalers (such as beclomethasone dipropionate HFA inhalation aerosol) need to be primed before using them for the first time or if they have not been used in in the last 10 days or longer. DO NOT wash the inhaler OR get any part of it wet! Clean the mouthpiece weekly with a clean, dry tissue or cloth. After you have finished with the inhaler, rinse your mouth with water (see Chapter 9). DISCARD inhaler by the date printed on the canister. Although the inhaler may not be completely empty at this time, inhalations AFTER this may not provide you with the proper amount and/or dosage of medication. Encourage patients to consult with their health care provider before the discard date regarding refills. DO NOT take extra doses or stop this medication without consulting your health care provider/prescriber. Instruct the patient to keep track of the doses left in the MDI. Many inhalers have built-in counters, but if not, the patient can do the following: Divide the number of doses in the canister by the number of puffs used per day. For example, assume that two puffs are taken four times a day, and the inhaler has a capacity of 200 inhalations. Two puffs four times a day equals eight inhalations per day. Eight divided into 200 yields 25; that is, the inhaler will last approximately 25 days. The MDI may then be marked with the date it will be empty and a refill obtained a few days before that date. Note that using extra doses will alter the refill date. Advise the patient to always check expiration dates.

- Stress the importance of journaling, which should include notation of how the patient feels, medications being taken, adverse effects, and precipitators/alleviators/symptoms of the asthma/illness.
- Counsel the patient to wear a medical alert bracelet or necklace at all times and to keep a medical card with the diagnoses and list of medications and allergies on his or her person at all times. Emergency contact persons and phone numbers must also be listed.
- With intranasal dosage forms, instruct the patient to clear nasal passages before administration. The patient needs to tilt his or her head slightly forward and insert the spray tip into one nostril and point toward the inflamed nasal turbinates. Instruct the patient to pump the medication into the nasal passage as the patient sniffs inward while holding the other nostril closed. This procedure may then be repeated in the other nostril. It is recommended to discard any unused portion after 3 months or by the expiration date.
- Educate the patient about the fact that excess levels of systemic corticosteroids may lead to Cushing's syndrome with symptoms such as moon face, acne, an increase in fat pads, and swelling. Although use of inhaled forms helps to minimize this problem, education about it remains important to patient safety. As noted previously, the risk for occurrence of these signs and symptoms is higher when these drugs are given systemically (e.g., oral or parenteral dosage forms).
- Educate the patient about the possibility of Addisonian crisis, which may occur if a systemic corticosteroid is abruptly discontinued. These drugs require weaning prior to discontinuation of the medication. Addisonian crisis may be manifested by nausea, shortness of breath, joint pain, weakness, and fatigue, and the patient must contact the prescriber immediately if these occur.
- Educate the patient about the importance of reporting to the prescriber any weight gain of 2 pounds or more in 24 hours or 5 pounds or more in 1 week.

Phosphodiesterase-4 Inhibitor

- Emphasize that the patient report any change in mood or emotions to the prescriber immediately.

Monoclonal Antibody Antiasthmatic Drugs

- Omalizumab is used for the treatment of moderate to severe asthma and not for aborting acute asthma attacks. The patient needs to provide return demonstrations of subcutaneous injection techniques. Instruct the patient to keep medications and needles, syringes, and other equipment out of the reach of children and to use puncture-proof needle waste containers. Each needle is used for only one injection.

KEY POINTS

- The beta agonists stimulate beta$_1$ and beta$_2$ receptors. The beta$_2$ agonists are specific for the lungs.
- Xanthines, such as theophylline, help to relax the smooth muscles of the bronchioles by inhibiting phosphodiesterase. Phosphodiesterase breaks down cAMP, which is needed to relax smooth muscles.
- Anticholinergic drugs are used for maintenance and not for relief of acute bronchospasm and work by blocking the bronchoconstrictive effects of ACh.
- Corticosteroids (e.g., beclomethasone, dexamethasone, flunisolide, triamcinolone) have many indications and work by stabilizing the membranes of cells that release harmful bronchoconstricting substances.
- The LTRAs, such as zileuton and zafirlukast, are given orally. Adverse effects include headache, dizziness, insomnia, and dyspepsia.
- Omalizumab, a monoclonal antibody antiasthmatic drug, works by preventing the release of mediators that lead to allergic responses. It is given for preventive purposes.

NCLEX® EXAMINATION REVIEW QUESTIONS

1. A patient who has a history of asthma is experiencing an acute episode of shortness of breath and needs to take a medication for immediate relief. The nurse will choose which medication that is appropriate for this situation?
   a. A beta agonist, such as albuterol
   b. A leukotriene receptor antagonist, such as montelukast
   c. A corticosteroid, such as fluticasone
   d. An anticholinergic, such as ipratropium

2. After a nebulizer treatment with the beta agonist albuterol, the patient complains of feeling a little "shaky," with slight tremors of the hands. The patient's heart rate is 98 beats/min, increased from the pretreatment rate of 88 beats/min. The nurse knows that this reaction is an
   a. expected adverse effect of the medication.
   b. allergic reaction to the medication.
   c. indication that he has received an overdose of the medication.
   d. idiosyncratic reaction to the medication.

3. A patient has been receiving an aminophylline (xanthine derivative) infusion for 24 hours. The nurse will assess for which adverse effect when assessing the patient during the infusion?
   a. CNS depression
   b. Sinus tachycardia
   c. Increased appetite
   d. Temporary urinary retention

4. During a teaching session for a patient who will be receiving a new prescription for the LTRA montelukast (Singulair), the nurse will tell the patient that the drug has which therapeutic effect?
   a. Improves the respiratory drive
   b. Loosens and removes thickened secretions
   c. Reduces inflammation in the airway
   d. Stimulates immediate bronchodilation

5. After the patient takes a dose of an inhaled corticosteroid, such as fluticasone (Flovent), what is the most important action the patient needs to do next?

   a. Hold the breath for 60 seconds.
   b. Rinse out the mouth with water.
   c. Follow the corticosteroid with a bronchodilator inhaler, if ordered.
   d. Repeat the dose in 15 minutes if the patient feels short of breath.

6. The nurse is teaching a patient about the inhaler Advair (salmeterol/fluticasone). Which statements by the patient indicate a correct understanding of this medication? *(Select all that apply.)*
   a. "I will rinse my mouth with water after each dose."
   b. "I need to use this inhaler whenever I feel short of breath, but not less than 4 hours between doses."
   c. "This medication is taken twice a day, every 12 hours."
   d. "I can take this inhaler if I get short of breath while exercising."
   e. "I will call my doctor if I notice white patches inside my mouth."

7. A patient who is taking a xanthine derivative for chronic bronchitis asks the nurse, "I miss my morning coffee. I can't wait to go home and have some." What is the nurse's best response?
   a. "I know how you feel. I'd miss my coffee too."
   b. "I can get some coffee for you. I'll be right back."
   c. "It's important not to take coffee or other caffeinated products with this medicine as it may cause an increased heart rate as well as other problems."
   d. "You've been on this medicine for a few days. I can call your prescriber to ask whether you can have some coffee."

8. The nurse is preparing to administer the elixir form of theophylline to a patient who has a PEG tube. The dose is 240 mg daily, and the medication is available in a concentration of 80 mg/15 mL. How many milliliters of medication will the nurse give per dose?

1. a, 2. a, 3. b, 4. c, 5. b, 6. a, c, e, 7. c, 8. 45 mL.

CRITICAL THINKING AND PRIORITIZATION QUESTIONS

1. A patient was prescribed an oral leukotriene receptor antagonist (LRTA) 1 month ago. At today's follow-up appointment, he tells the nurse, "I don't think this pill works. I took it when I was short of breath, but it did not help." What is the nurse's priority action when answering this patient's concerns?

2. A 13-year-old patient is taken to the school clinic because he started to have an asthma attack while running outside in the cold air. The school nurse has two metered-dose inhalers on file for him: fluticasone and albuterol. Which inhaler is the priority at this time? Explain your answer.

For answers, see *http://evolve.elsevier.com/Lilley.*

ⓔ EVOLVE WEBSITE

http://evolve.elsevier.com/Lilley

- Animations
- Answer Keys for Textbook Case Studies and Textbook Critical Thinking and Prioritization Questions
- Content Updates
- Key Points
- Review Questions
- Student Case Studies

PART 7

Antiinfective and Antiinflammatory Drugs

Learning Strategies

ACTIVE QUESTIONING

In Part 6, you were provided with a strategy for formulating practice questions from the Key Points to help you learn concepts as you read your textbook. Using practice questions is a form of active questioning. This technique not only assists you with comprehension as you read, but also helps to store the material in your long-term memory. Active questioning allows you to retrieve the information when you need it, while preparing for and when taking your tests.

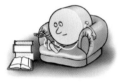

This simple mental picture helps students understand how their brain works and the best ways to build long-term memory and learning. Your brain can be compared to a file cabinet. As you learn and gain more knowledge, it is stored away in the correct file in your long-term memory, for easy retrieval at a later date. The more concepts you learn, the more files are constructed. To make sure the files remain intact, you need to recall the information on a regular basis and link that information to a connection, like one of your other courses or a previous life experience (see Part 8, Application of Pharmacology and Making Connections). Using the different learning strategies previously discussed along with active questioning assists in accomplishing this task. If information is not recalled on a regular basis, your brain considers the information to be short-term memory, and the file may empty out before you need it. Active questioning keeps the memory flowing and helps to move the information over to long-term memory.

Once you have read your assigned chapters, listened to lecture presentations, and participated in learning exercises during class, you will achieve a better understanding of the concepts. In addition, you will also have a clearer idea of the key points and nursing considerations that your instructor wants you to focus on in your lessons. Now you can use a different set of active questions to recall what you have learned.

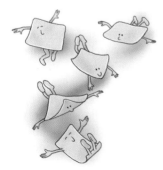

The questions you formulate now in preparation for your test are more concise and can further refine your knowledge. Some of the questions that you can use include the following:

- Compare _____ and _____ with regard to _____.
- Describe/explain _____ in your own words.
- How does _____ affect _____?
- How does _____ tie in with what you learned in previous chapters or lessons?
- What are the differences/similarities between _____ and _____?
- What are the implications of _____?
- Why is _____ important?

In these statements, fill in the blanks with any concept (e.g., drug classification, drug name, key term, or key point), which will test your comprehension and assure you have a deep understanding. Once you have that deeper understanding, then it will be easy to take it a step further and apply the information to a patient situation. Or you can use the following types of questions:

- How does _____ apply to the patient with _____ disease?
- What are the nursing implications of _____?
- What would happen to your patient if _____?

These questions can be used in your study group or for self-study. You can see how using questioning techniques can not only assist you in comprehending the lessons in your chapter, but also can help you apply the learning in anticipation of your tests. As always, remember you are not just learning the information to pass the test. This knowledge will be used in other courses and in your future practice as a nurse.

NCLEX® PRACTICE

In order to practice as a nurse, every student has to pass the NCLEX® (National Council Licensure Examination®). There are many resources available to practice test questions similar to those found on the NCLEX® examination. As mentioned in Part 6, the authors have included NCLEX® review questions at the end of each chapter in this textbook. There are also critical thinking and prioritization questions available for additional practice on the website *http://evolve.elsevier.com/Lilley*.

Critical thinking is the hallmark of nursing. In order for nurses to practice safely, they need to be able to effectively prioritize. The questions on the NCLEX® examination test both of these nursing skills. The questions on this examination are written at a higher level. As mentioned previously, you will not be asked questions at a knowledge or comprehension level. Instead, many of the test questions will be at the application or analysis level. This means that pure memorization of the concepts will not be useful. You will be expected to apply and analyze your knowledge about the concept. If you want to be successful on your NCLEX® examination, the more you practice these types of questions the better you will become. In turn, learning this skill will help you to be successful on your pharmacology examinations in the classroom.

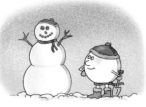

Here is an example of a test question written at the application level. It also requires you to prioritize your intervention by asking what will you do FIRST. In the following question, you are evaluating a patient's response to a medication:

The patient was given the first dose of lisinopril (Zestoril) for heart failure. The patient calls the nurse complaining of dizziness. Which intervention should the nurse take first?
a. Auscultate lungs sounds for crackles
b. Obtain a 12-lead electrocardiogram
c. Notify the health care provider
d. Obtain a blood pressure reading

To correctly answer this question, you need to understand that dizziness can be caused by many things. It can be a clinical manifestation of low blood pressure. In Chapter 22 on Antihypertensive Drugs, you learned that an adverse effect of ace inhibitors is the *first-dose hypotensive effect*, which can cause a significant drop in blood pressure. Therefore, to check if hypotension is the cause of the dizziness, the nurse will need to obtain a blood pressure. This type of question requires the student to not only learn about the drugs and their side effects but also to show that they can apply the nursing process and choose the correct intervention.

An excellent way to study for these types of questions is to work with your study group and ask each other questions that apply or analyze the concepts. Try to write your own questions to quiz the group. Use the chapter objectives and the key points at the end of the chapter to guide you. Remember to ask questions based on the nursing process since those types of questions will help you critically think and actively apply your knowledge. Complete the NCLEX® questions that are provided in your textbook and the online resources. This will provide you with practice answering the application and analysis type questions.

In addition to the NCLEX® questions available in your textbook and online, there are numerous NCLEX® review resources available for you to use. Most college and university libraries have these books available on their shelves or in their reference section for your use. Some of these review books have their questions ordered by topic, so you can practice answering questions according to the topic in your pharmacology book. Others have a single section on pharmacology. On your computer, using a search engine, like Google, can lead to many websites where you can practice answering questions about pharmacology. There are also applications for tablets and smart phones to practice answering pharmacology NCLEX® questions on the go.

Although your actual NCLEX® examination is a few years away, it does not hurt to keep practicing. The more you answer these types of questions, the easier they become.

Antibiotics Part 1

e http://evolve.elsevier.com/Lilley

OBJECTIVES

When you reach the end of this chapter, you will be able to do the following:

1. Discuss the general principles of antibiotic therapy.
2. Explain how antibiotics work to rid the body of infection.
3. Briefly compare the characteristics and uses of antiseptics and disinfectants.
4. List the most commonly used antiseptics and disinfectants.
5. Discuss any nursing-related considerations associated with the environmental use of antiseptics and disinfectants.
6. Discuss the pros and cons of antibiotic use with attention to the overuse or abuse of antibiotics and the development of drug resistance.
7. Classify the various antibiotics by general category, including sulfonamides, penicillins, cephalosporins, macrolides, and tetracyclines.
8. Discuss the mechanisms of action, indications, cautions, contraindications, routes of administration, and drug interactions for the sulfonamides, penicillins, cephalosporins, macrolides, and tetracyclines.
9. Identify drug-specific adverse effects and toxic effects of each of the antibiotic classes listed earlier, and cite measures to decrease their occurrence.
10. Briefly discuss superinfection, including its etiology and prevention.
11. Develop a nursing care plan that includes all phases of the nursing process for patients receiving drugs in each of the following classes of antibiotic: sulfonamides, penicillins, cephalosporins, macrolides, and tetracyclines.

DRUG PROFILES

♦ amoxicillin, p. 608
ampicillin, p. 608
♦ azithromycin and ♦ clarithromycin, p. 615
aztreonam, p. 613
♦ cefazolin, p. 610
cefepime, p. 612
♦ cefoxitin, p. 611
ceftaroline, p. 612
ceftazidime, p. 612
♦ ceftriaxone, p. 612
cefuroxime, p. 611
♦ cephalexin, p. 610

demeclocycline, p. 617
♦ doxycycline, p. 617
♦ erythromycin, p. 615
♦ imipenem/cilastatin, p. 612
nafcillin, p. 608
♦ penicillin G and penicillin V potassium, p. 608
sulfamethoxazole/trimethoprim (co-trimoxazole), p. 605
tigecycline, p. 617

_____

♦ = *Key drug*
! = *High-alert drug*

KEY TERMS

Antibiotic Having the ability to destroy or interfere with the development of a living organism. The term is used most commonly to refer to antibacterial drugs. (p. 600)

Antiseptic One of two types of topical antimicrobial agents; a chemical that inhibits the growth and reproduction of microorganisms without necessarily killing them. Antiseptics are also called *static agents*. (p. 601)

Bactericidal antibiotics Antibiotics that kill bacteria. (p. 606)

Bacteriostatic antibiotics Antibiotics that do not actually kill bacteria but rather inhibit their growth. (p. 604)

Beta-lactam The designation for a broad class of antibiotics that includes four subclasses: penicillins, cephalosporins, carbapenems, and monobactams; so named because of the beta-lactam ring that is part of the chemical structure of all drugs in this class. (p. 605)

Beta-lactamase Any of a group of enzymes produced by bacteria that catalyze the chemical opening of the crucial beta-lactam ring structures in beta-lactam antibiotics. (p. 606)

Beta-lactamase inhibitors Medications combined with certain penicillin drugs to block the effect of beta-lactamase enzymes. (p. 606)

Colonization The establishment and growth of microorganisms on the skin, open wounds, or mucous membranes, or in secretions without causing an infection. (p. 601)

Community-associated infection An infection that is acquired by persons who have not been hospitalized or had a medical procedure recently. (p. 601)

Definitive therapy The administration of antibiotics based on known results of culture and sensitivity testing identifying the pathogen causing infection. (p. 602)

Disinfectant One of two types of topical antimicrobial agents; a chemical applied to nonliving objects to kill microorganisms. Also called *cidal agents*. (p. 601)

Empiric therapy The administration of antibiotics based on the practitioner's judgment of the pathogens most likely to be causing an apparent infection; it involves the presumptive treatment of an infection to avoid treatment delay before specific culture information has been obtained. (p. 602)

Glucose-6-phosphate dehydrogenase (G6PD) deficiency An inherited disorder in which the red blood cells are partially or completely deficient in glucose-6-phosphate dehydrogenase, a critical enzyme in the metabolism of glucose. Certain medications can cause hemolytic anemia in patients with this disorder. This is an example of a host factor related to drug therapy. (p. 603)

Health care–associated infection An infection that is acquired during the course of receiving treatment for another condition in a health care institution. The infection is not present or incubating at the time of admission; also known as a *nosocomial infection*. (p. 601)

Host factors Factors that are unique to a particular patient that affect the patient's susceptibility to infection and response to various antibiotic drugs. Examples include a low neutrophil count or a lack of immunoglobulins in the blood that carry antibodies. (p. 603)

Infections Invasions and multiplications of microorganisms in body tissues. (p. 600)

Microorganisms Microscopic living organisms (also called *microbes*). (p. 600)

Prophylactic antibiotic therapy Antibiotics taken before anticipated exposure to an infectious organism in an effort to prevent the development of infection. (p. 602)

Pseudomembranous colitis A potentially-necrotizing inflammatory bowel condition that is often associated with antibiotic therapy; often caused by the bacteria *Clostridium difficile*. A more general term that is also used is *antibiotic-associated colitis*. (p. 602)

Slow acetylation A common genetic host factor in which the rate of metabolism of certain drugs is reduced. (p. 603)

Subtherapeutic Generally refers to blood levels below therapeutic levels due to insufficient dosing. Also refers to antibiotic treatment that is ineffective in treating a given infection. Possible causes include inappropriate drug therapy, insufficient drug dosing, and bacterial drug resistance. (p. 602)

Superinfection (1) An infection occurring during antimicrobial treatment for another infection, resulting from overgrowth of an organism not susceptible to the antibiotic used. (2) A secondary microbial infection that occurs in addition to an earlier primary infection, often due to weakening of the patient's immune system function by the first infection. (p. 602)

Teratogens Substances that can interfere with normal prenatal development and cause one or more developmental abnormalities in the fetus. (p. 603)

Therapeutic Referring to antibiotic therapy that is given in sufficient doses so that the concentration of the drug in the blood or other tissues renders it effective against specific bacterial pathogens. (p. 602)

MICROBIAL INFECTION

Microorganisms are everywhere, both in the external environment and in parts of the internal environment of our bodies. They can be harmful, or they can be beneficial under normal circumstances but become harmful when conditions are altered. A person is normally able to remain healthy and resistant to infectious microorganisms because of the existence of certain host defenses. These defenses include actual physical barriers, such as intact skin or the ciliated respiratory mucosa, or physiologic defenses, such as the gastric acid in the stomach and immune factors such as antibodies. Other defenses are the phagocytic cells (macrophages and polymorphonuclear neutrophils) that are part of the mononuclear phagocyte system.

Every known major class of microbes contains organisms that can infect humans. This includes bacteria, viruses, fungi, and protozoans. The focus of this chapter is common bacterial infections.

Recall from microbiology that bacteria may take a number of different shapes. This property of bacteria is called their morphology (Figure 38-1), and they are often grouped based on this property. Bacteria may also be grouped according to other common recognizable characteristics. One of the most important ways of categorizing different bacteria is on the basis of their response to the Gram stain procedure. Bacterial species that stain purple with Gram staining are classified as *gram-positive* organisms. Bacteria that stain red are classified as *gram-negative* organisms. This seemingly simple difference proves to be very significant in guiding the choice of antibiotic therapy.

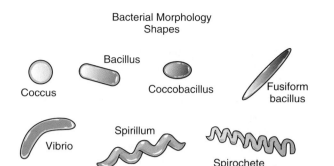

FIGURE 38-1 General morphology of bacteria. (From Murray PR, Rosenthal KS, Pfaller MA: *Medical microbiology*, ed 6, St Louis, 2009, Mosby.)

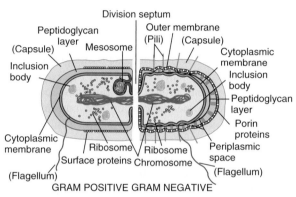

FIGURE 38-2 Gram-positive and gram-negative bacteria. A gram-positive bacterium has a thick layer of peptidoglycan *(left)*. A gram-negative bacterium has a thin peptidoglycan layer and an outer membrane *(right)*. Structures in parentheses are not found in all bacteria. (From Murray PR, Rosenthal KS, Pfaller MA: *Medical microbiology*, ed 6, St Louis, 2009, Mosby.)

Gram-positive organisms have a very thick cell wall, known as peptidoglycan, and they also have a thick outer capsule. Gram-negative organisms have a cell wall structure that is more complex, with a smaller outer capsule and peptidoglycan layer and two cell membranes: an outer and an inner membrane (Figure 38-2). These differences usually make gram-negative bacterial infections more difficult to treat, because the drug molecules have a harder time penetrating the more complex cell walls of gram-negative organisms.

When the normal host defenses are somehow compromised, that person becomes susceptible to infection. The microorganisms invade and multiply in the body tissues, and if the infective process overwhelms the body's defense system, the infection becomes clinically apparent. The patient usually manifests some of the following classic signs and symptoms of infection: fever, chills, sweats, redness, pain and swelling, fatigue, weight loss, increased white blood cell (WBC) count, and the formation of pus. Not all patients will exhibit signs of the infection. This is especially true in older adults and immunocompromised patients.

To help the body and its normal host defenses combat an infection, antibiotic therapy is often required. Antibiotics are most effective when their actions are combined with functioning bodily defense mechanisms. Oftentimes patients will become colonized with bacteria. Although bacteria are present in open wounds, in secretions, on mucous membranes, or on the skin, these patients do not have any overt signs of infection. Colonization does not require antibiotic treatment. However, it is not uncommon for these colonizations to be treated, which may be one way in which drug-resistant organisms emerge.

Health Care–Associated Infection

A community-associated infection is defined as an infection that is acquired by a person who has not recently (within the past year) been hospitalized or had a medical procedure (e.g., dialysis, surgery, catheterization). A health care–associated infection, previously known as a *nosocomial infection*, is defined as an infection that a patient acquires during the course of receiving treatment for another condition in a health care institution. The infection was not present or incubating at the time of admission but occurs greater than 48 hours after admission. Health care–associated infections are one of the top ten leading causes of death in the United States. They tend to be more difficult to treat because the causative microorganisms have been exposed to strong antibiotics in the past and are the most drug resistant and the most virulent. The particular organisms that cause health care–associated infections have changed over time, with methicillin-resistant *Staphylococcus aureus* (MRSA) now being the most common. Other serious pathogens include *Enterococcus, Klebsiella, Acinetobacter,* and *Pseudomonas aeruginosa.* Most of these microorganisms are now resistant to many of the commonly used antibiotics.

Health care–associated infections develop in over 700,000 patients per year. The cost of these infections is estimated to be $9.8 billion annually. The most common health care–associated infections include urinary tract infections (UTIs), surgical site infections, bloodstream infections, and pneumonia. Often they are acquired from various devices, such as mechanical ventilators, intravenous (IV) infusion lines, catheters, and dialysis equipment. Areas of the hospital associated with the greatest risk for acquiring a health care–associated infection are the critical care, dialysis, oncology, transplant, and burn units. This is because the host defenses of the patients in these areas are typically compromised, which makes them more vulnerable to infection. Over 70% of health care–associated infections are preventable. The most common mode of transmitting health care–associated infections is by direct contact. Handwashing is the single most important thing health care professionals can do to prevent the spread of these potentially deadly infections.

Other methods of reducing health care–associated infections include the use of disinfectants and antiseptics. A disinfectant is able to kill organisms and is used only on nonliving objects to destroy organisms that may be present. Disinfectants are sometimes called *cidal agents.* An antiseptic generally only inhibits the growth of microorganisms but does not necessarily kill them and is applied exclusively to living tissue. Antiseptics are also called *static agents.* The differences between antiseptics and disinfectants in a clinical sense are summarized in Table 38-1. Topical antimicrobial drugs and skin preparation drugs are discussed further in Chapter 56.

TABLE 38-1

TABLE 38-1 Antiseptics versus Disinfectants		
	Antiseptics	**Disinfectants**
Where used	Living tissue	Nonliving objects
Potency	Lower	Higher
Activity against organisms	Primarily inhibit growth of bacteria (bacteriostatic)	Kill bacteria (bactericidal)

PHARMACOLOGY OVERVIEW

The selection of antimicrobial drugs requires clinical judgment and detailed knowledge of pharmacologic and microbiologic factors. Antibiotics have three general uses: empiric therapy, definitive therapy, and prophylactic or preventive therapy. Antibiotic drug therapy begins with a clinical assessment of the patient to determine whether he or she has the common signs and symptoms of infection. The patient is assessed during and after antibiotic therapy to evaluate the effectiveness of the drug therapy, monitor for adverse drug effects, and make sure the infection is not recurring.

Often the signs and symptoms of an infection appear long before a causative organism can be identified. When this happens and the risk for life-threatening or severe complications is high (e.g., suspected acute meningitis), an antibiotic is given to the patient immediately. The antibiotic selected is one that can best kill the microorganisms known to be the most common causes of the infection. This is called empiric therapy. Before the start of empiric antibiotic therapy, specimens are obtained from suspected areas of infection to be cultured in an attempt to identify a causative organism. It must be emphasized that culture specimens must be obtained before drug therapy is initiated whenever possible. Otherwise, the presence of antibiotics in the tissues may result in misleading culture results. However, in some situations it is not possible to obtain a sample (especially sputum) in a reasonable amount of time, and antibiotic therapy is begun without a sample. If an organism is identified in the laboratory, it is then tested for susceptibility to various antibiotics. The results of these tests can confirm whether the empiric therapy chosen is appropriate for eradicating the organism identified. If not, therapy can be adjusted to optimize its efficacy against the specific infectious organism(s). Once the results of culture and sensitivity testing are available (usually in 48 to 72 hours), the antibiotic therapy is then tailored to treat the identified organism by using the most narrow-spectrum, least toxic drug based on sensitivity results. This is known as definitive therapy. *Broad-spectrum antibiotics* are those that are active against numerous organisms (gram-positive, gram-negative, and anaerobic). *Narrow-spectrum antibiotics* are effective against only a few organisms. Once the results of culture and sensitivity testing are available, it is always better to use an antibiotic that targets the specific organism identified (i.e., a narrow-spectrum antibiotic). Overuse of broad-spectrum antibiotics contributes to resistance. The goal of therapy is to use the most narrow-spectrum drug when possible based on sensitivity results.

Antibiotics are also given for prophylaxis. This is often the case when patients are scheduled to undergo a procedure (i.e., surgery) in which the likelihood of dangerous microbial contamination is high during or after the procedure. Prophylactic antibiotic therapy is used to prevent an infection. The risk for infection varies depending on the procedure being performed. For example, the risk for infection in a patient undergoing coronary artery bypass surgery (with standard preoperative cleansing of the body) is relatively low compared with that in a patient undergoing intraabdominal surgery for the treatment of injuries sustained in a motor vehicle accident. In the latter case, contamination with bacteria from the gastrointestinal (GI) tract is more likely to be present in the abdominal cavity. This would constitute a contaminated or "dirty" surgical field, and therefore the likelihood of clinically serious infection would be much higher. Antibiotic therapy would likely be required for a longer period after the procedure. To be effective, prophylactic antibiotics need to be given before the procedure, generally 30 minutes before the incision to ensure adequate tissue penetration. The Surgical Care Improvement Project (SCIP) is a national performance improvement project that provides hospitals with evidence-based recommendations on the administration of prophylactic antibiotics. More information can be found at *www.jointcommission.org/surgical_care_improvement_project/*.

To optimize antibiotic therapy, the patient is continuously monitored for both therapeutic efficacy and adverse drug effects. A therapeutic response to antibiotics is one in which there is a decrease in the specific signs and symptoms of infection compared with the baseline findings (e.g., fever, elevated WBC count, redness, inflammation, drainage, pain). Antibiotic therapy is said to be subtherapeutic when these signs and symptoms do not improve. This can result from use of an incorrect route of drug administration, inadequate drainage of an abscess, poor drug penetration to the infected area, insufficient serum levels of the drug, or bacterial resistance to the drug. Antibiotic therapy is considered toxic when the serum levels of the antibiotic are too high or when the patient has an allergic or other major adverse reaction to the drug. These reactions include rash, itching, hives, fever, chills, joint pain, difficulty breathing, or wheezing. Relatively minor adverse drug reactions such as nausea, vomiting, and diarrhea are quite common with antibiotic therapy and are usually not severe enough to require drug discontinuation.

Superinfection can occur when antibiotics reduce or completely eliminate the normal bacterial flora, which consist of certain bacteria and fungi that are needed to maintain normal function in various organs. When these bacteria or fungi are killed by antibiotics, other bacteria or fungi are permitted to take over and cause infection. An example of a superinfection caused by antibiotics is the development of a vaginal yeast infection when the normal vaginal bacterial flora is reduced by antibiotic therapy and yeast growth is no longer kept in balance. Antibiotic use is strongly associated with the potential for the development of diarrhea. Antibiotic-associated diarrhea is a common adverse effect of antibiotics. However, it becomes a serious superinfection when it causes antibiotic-associated colitis, also known as pseudomembranous colitis or simply *C. difficile* infection. This happens because antibiotics disrupt the normal gut flora and can cause an overgrowth of *Clostridium difficile.* The most common symptoms of *C. difficile* colitis are watery diarrhea, abdominal pain, and fever. Whenever a patient who was previously treated with antibiotics develops watery diarrhea, the patient needs to be tested for *C. difficile* infection. If the results are positive, the patient will need to be treated for this serious superinfection. Infections with *C. difficile* are increasingly becoming resistant to standard therapy. There is some evidence to suggest probiotics may help prevent *C. difficile* infections.

Another type of superinfection occurs when a second infection closely follows the initial infection and comes from an external source (as opposed to normal body flora). A common example is a case in which a patient who has a viral respiratory infection develops a secondary bacterial infection. This is likely due to weakening of the patient's immune system function by the primary viral infection. Although the viral infection will not respond to antibiotic therapy, antibiotics may be needed to treat the secondary bacterial infection. This situation calls for some diagnostic finesse on the part of the prescriber, who needs to avoid prescribing unnecessary antibiotics for a viral infection. The presence of colored sputum (e.g., green or yellow) may or may not be a sign of a bacterial superinfection during a viral respiratory illness. Patients will often expect to receive an antibiotic prescription even when they show no signs of a bacterial superinfection. From their perspective, they know they are "sick" and want "some medicine" to expedite their recovery from illness. This can create both diagnostic confusion and an emotional dilemma for the prescriber.

Over the decades, many easily treatable bacterial infections have become resistant to antibiotic therapy. One major cause of this phenomenon is considered to be the overprescribing of antibiotics, often in the clinical situations described earlier. Antibiotic resistance is now considered one of the world's most pressing public health problems. Another factor that contributes to this problem is the tendency of many patients not to complete their antibiotic regimen. Patients must be counseled to take the entire course of prescribed antibiotic drugs, even if they feel that they are no longer ill.

Food-drug and drug-drug interactions are common problems when antibiotics are taken and can affect the efficacy of the antibiotic therapy. One of the more common food-drug interactions is that between milk or cheese and tetracycline, which results in decreased GI absorption of tetracycline. An example of a drug-drug interaction is that between quinolone antibiotics and antacids or multivitamins with iron, which leads to decreased absorption of quinolones. This is especially important, as discussed later, because quinolone antibiotics are used orally to treat serious infections. If they are not absorbed, treatment failure is likely to ensue.

Other important factors that must be understood to use antibiotics appropriately are host-specific factors, or **host factors**. These are factors that pertain specifically to a given patient, and they can have an important bearing on the success or failure of antibiotic therapy. Some of these host factors are age, allergy history, kidney and liver function, pregnancy status, genetic characteristics, site of infection, and host defenses.

Age-related host factors are those that apply to patients at either end of the age spectrum. For example, infants and children may not be able to take certain antibiotics such as tetracyclines, which affect developing teeth or bones; quinolones, which may affect bone or cartilage development in children; and sulfonamides, which may displace bilirubin from albumin and precipitate kernicterus (hyperbilirubinemia) in neonates. The aging process affects the function of various organ systems. As people age, there is a gradual decline in the function of the kidneys and liver, the organs primarily responsible for metabolizing and eliminating antibiotics. Therefore, depending on the level of kidney or liver function of a given older adult, dosage adjustments may be necessary. Pharmacists often play a role in evaluating the dosages of antibiotics and other medications to ensure optimal dosing for a given patient's level of organ function.

A patient history of allergic reaction to an antibiotic is important in the selection of the most appropriate antibiotic. Penicillins and sulfonamides are two broad classes of antibiotic to which many people have allergic anaphylactic reactions. Symptoms of anaphylaxis include flushing, itching, hives, anxiety, fast irregular pulse, and throat and tongue swelling. The most dangerous such reaction is anaphylactic shock, in which a patient can suffocate from drug-induced respiratory arrest. Although this outcome is the most extreme, the potential for it does underscore the importance of consistently assessing patients for drug allergies and documenting any known allergies clearly in the medical record. All reported drug allergies are to be taken seriously and investigated further before a final decision is made about whether to administer a given drug. Many patients will say that they are "allergic" to a medication when in fact what they experienced was a common mild adverse effect such as stomach upset or nausea. Patients who report drug allergies need to be asked open-ended questions to elicit descriptions of prior allergic reactions so that the actual severity of the reaction can be assessed. The most common severe reactions to any medication that need to be noted in the patient's chart are any difficulty breathing; significant rash, hives, or other skin reaction; and severe GI intolerance. Although some antibiotics are ideally taken on an empty stomach, eating a small amount of food with the medication may be sufficient to help the patient tolerate it and realize its therapeutic benefits.

Pregnancy-related host factors are also important to the selection of appropriate antibiotics, because several antibiotics can pass through the placenta and cause harm to the developing fetus. Drugs that cause developmental abnormalities in the fetus are called **teratogens**. Their use by pregnant women can result in birth defects.

Some patients also have certain genetic abnormalities that result in various enzyme deficiencies. These conditions can adversely affect drug actions in the body. Two of the most common examples of such genetic host factors are **glucose-6-phosphate dehydrogenase (G6PD) deficiency** and **slow acetylation**. The administration of antibiotics such as sulfonamides, nitrofurantoin, and dapsone to a person with G6PD deficiency may result in the *hemolysis,* or destruction, of red blood cells. Patients who are slow acetylators have a physiologic makeup that causes certain drugs to be metabolized more slowly than usual in a chemical step known as *acetylation.* This can lead to toxicity from drug accumulation (see Chapter 4).

The anatomic site of the infection is a very important host factor to consider when deciding not only which antibiotic to use but also the dosage, route of administration, and duration of therapy. Some antibiotics do not penetrate into the site of infection, such as the lung or bone or abscesses, which can lead to treatment failures.

Consideration of these host factors helps prescribers to ensure optimal drug selection for each individual patient. Continued patient assessment and proper monitoring of antibiotic therapy increase the likelihood that this therapy will be safe and effective.

ANTIBIOTICS

Antibiotics are classified into broad categories based on their chemical structure. The common categories include sulfonamides, penicillins, cephalosporins, macrolides, quinolones, aminoglycosides, and tetracyclines. In addition to chemical structure, other characteristics that distinguish classes of drugs include antibacterial spectrum, mechanism of action, potency, toxicity, and pharmacokinetic properties. The four most common mechanisms of antibiotic action are: (1) interference with bacterial cell wall synthesis, (2) interference with protein synthesis, (3) interference with replication of nucleic acids (deoxyribonucleic acid [DNA] and ribonucleic acid [RNA]), and (4) antimetabolite action that disrupts critical metabolic reactions inside the bacterial cell. Figure 38-3 portrays these mechanisms in combating bacterial infections and indicates which mechanism is used by several major antibiotic classes.

Perhaps the greatest challenge in understanding antimicrobial therapy is remembering the types and species of microorganisms against which a given drug can act. The list of microorganisms that a given drug has activity against can be quite extensive and can seem daunting to the inexperienced

practitioner. Most antimicrobials have activity against only one type of microbe (e.g., bacteria, viruses, fungi, protozoans). However, a few drugs do have activity against more than one class of organisms.

The field of infectious disease treatment is continually evolving, largely because of the continual emergence of resistant bacterial strains. For this reason, drug indications change frequently, often from year to year, as various bacterial species become resistant to previously effective antiinfective therapy. It is always appropriate to check the most current reference materials or consult with colleagues (e.g., nurses, pharmacists, prescribers) when questions remain. Pharmacists are excellent resources regarding antibiotics. Many hospitals now have pharmacists who are specially trained in the treatment of infectious diseases.

SULFONAMIDES

Sulfonamides were one of the first groups of drugs used as antibiotics. Although there are many compounds in the sulfonamide family, only sulfamethoxazole combined with trimethoprim (a nonsulfonamide antibiotic), known as Bactrim, Septra, or co-trimoxazole and often abbreviated as SMZ-TMP, is used commonly in clinical practice. Sulfisoxazole combined with erythromycin (a macrolide antibiotic) is occasionally used in pediatrics. Sulfasalazine, another sulfonamide, is used to treat ulcerative colitis and rheumatoid arthritis and is not used as an antibiotic.

Mechanism of Action and Drug Effects

Sulfonamides do not actually destroy bacteria but rather inhibit their growth. For this reason, they are considered **bacteriostatic antibiotics.** They inhibit the growth of susceptible bacteria by preventing bacterial synthesis of folic acid. Folic acid is a B-complex vitamin that is required for the proper synthesis of purines, one of the chemical components of nucleic acids (DNA and RNA). Specifically, in a process known as *competitive inhibition,* sulfonamides compete with PABA for the bacterial enzyme tetrahydropteroic acid synthetase, which incorporates PABA into the folic acid molecule. Because sulfonamides are capable of blocking a specific step in a biosynthetic pathway, they are also considered antimetabolites. Microorganisms that require exogenous folic acid (not synthesized by the bacterium itself) are not affected by sulfonamide antibiotics. Therefore, these drugs do not affect folic acid metabolism in human cells. Trimethoprim, although not a sulfonamide, works via a similar mechanism, inhibiting dihydrofolic acid reduction to tetrahydrofolate, which results in inhibition of the enzymes of the folic acid pathway.

Indications

Sulfonamides have a broad spectrum of antibacterial activity, including activity against both gram-positive and gram-negative organisms. These antibiotics achieve very high concentrations in the kidneys, through which they are eliminated. Therefore, sulfamethoxazole/trimethoprim is often used in the treatment of UTIs. The combination of these two drugs allows for

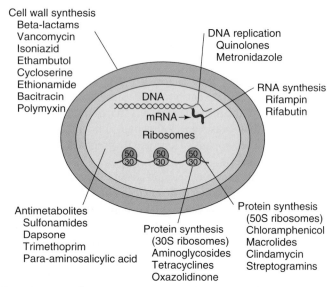

FIGURE 38-3 Basic sites of antibiotic activity. *DNA,* Deoxyribonucleic acid; *mRNA,* messenger ribonucleic acid; *RNA,* ribonucleic acid. (From Murray PR, Rosenthal KS, Pfaller MA: *Medical microbiology,* ed 6, St Louis, 2009, Mosby.)

a synergistic (see Chapter 2) antibacterial effect. Commonly susceptible organisms include strains of *Enterobacter* species (spp.), *Escherichia coli*, *Klebsiella* spp., *Proteus mirabilis*, *Proteus vulgaris*, and *S. aureus*. Unfortunately, however, resistant bacterial strains are a growing problem, as is the case with other antibiotic classes. Results of culture and sensitivity testing help to optimize drug selection in individual cases. Often times a urinary analgesic, phenazopyridine (Pyridium), is given along with an antibiotic to help with the pain associated with a urinary tract infection. Phenazopyridine is available over the counter. Sulfamethoxazole/trimethoprim is also used for respiratory tract infections. However, it is now less effective against streptococci infecting the upper respiratory tract and pharynx. Another specific use for sulfamethoxazole/trimethoprim is prophylaxis and treatment of opportunistic infections in patients with human immunodeficiency virus (HIV) infection, especially infection by *Pneumocystis jirovecii*, a common cause of HIV-associated pneumonia. Sulfamethoxazole/trimethoprim is also a drug of choice for infection caused by the bacterium *Stenotrophomonas maltophilia*. Sulfamethoxazole/trimethoprim has become common treatment for outpatient *Staphylococcus* infections, due to the high rate of community-associated methicillin-resistant *S. aureus* (MRSA) infections. MRSA and other resistant organisms are discussed in Chapter 39.

Contraindications

Use of sulfonamides is contraindicated in cases of known drug allergy to sulfonamides. Chemically related drugs such as the sulfonylureas (used to treat diabetes; see Chapter 32), thiazide and loop diuretics (see Chapter 28), and carbonic anhydrase inhibitors (see Chapter 28) are generally considered relatively safe in a patient who has a sulfonamide allergy. However, the cyclooxygenase-2 inhibitor celecoxib (Celebrex) should not be used (see Chapter 44) in patients with a known sulfonamide allergy. It is important to differentiate between sulfites and sulfonamides. Sulfites are commonly used as preservatives in everything from wine to food to injectable drugs. A person allergic to sulfonamide drugs may or may not also be allergic to sulfite preservatives. The use of sulfonamides is also contraindicated in pregnant women at term and in infants younger than 2 months of age.

Adverse Effects

Sulfonamide drugs are a common cause of allergic reaction. Patients will sometimes refer to this as "sulfa allergy" or even "sulfur allergy." Although immediate reactions can occur, sulfonamides typically cause delayed cutaneous reactions. These reactions frequently begin with fever followed by a rash (morbilliform eruptions, erythema multiforme, or toxic epidermal necrolysis). Photosensitivity reactions are another type of skin reaction that is induced by exposure to sunlight during sulfonamide drug therapy. In some cases, such reactions can result in severe sunburn. Such reactions are also common with the tetracycline class of antibiotics discussed later in this chapter, as well as with various other drug classes and may occur immediately or have a delayed onset. Other reactions to sulfonamides include mucocutaneous, GI, hepatic, renal, and hematologic

TABLE 38-2 Sulfonamides: Reported Adverse Effects

Body System	Adverse Effects
Blood	Agranulocytosis, aplastic anemia, hemolytic anemia, thrombocytopenia
Gastrointestinal	Nausea, vomiting, diarrhea, pancreatitis, hepatotoxicity
Integumentary	Epidermal necrolysis, exfoliative dermatitis, Stevens-Johnson syndrome, photosensitivity
Other	Convulsions, crystalluria, toxic nephrosis, headache, peripheral neuritis, urticaria, cough

complications, all of which may be fatal in severe cases. It is believed that sulfonamide reactions are immune mediated and involve the production of reactive drug metabolites in the body. Reported adverse effects of the sulfonamides are listed in Table 38-2.

Interactions

Sulfonamides can have clinically significant interactions with a number of other medications. Sulfonamides may potentiate the hypoglycemic effects of sulfonylureas in diabetes treatment, the toxic effects of phenytoin, and the anticoagulant effects of warfarin, which can lead to hemorrhage. Sulfonamides may increase the likelihood of cyclosporine-induced nephrotoxicity. Patients receiving any of the above drug combinations may require more frequent monitoring. Sulfonamides, and all antibiotics, may also reduce the efficacy of oral contraceptives. Instruct patients taking these drugs to use additional contraceptive methods.

Dosages

For dosage information on selected sulfonamides, see the table on the next page.

DRUG PROFILE

Sulfonamides work by interfering with the bacterial synthesis of folic acid. Most sulfonamide therapy today uses the combination drug sulfamethoxazole/trimethoprim.

sulfamethoxazole/trimethoprim (co-trimoxazole)

Co-trimoxazole (Bactrim) is a fixed-combination drug product containing a 5:1 ratio of sulfamethoxazole to trimethoprim. It is available in both oral and injectable dosage forms.

Pharmacokinetics: Sulfamethoxazole/Trimethoprim (Co-Trimoxazole)

Route	Onset of Action	Peak Plasma Concentration	Elimination Half-life	Duration of Action
PO	Variable	2-4 hr	7-12 hr	12 hr

BETA-LACTAM ANTIBIOTICS

The beta-lactam antibiotics are very commonly used drugs. They are so named because of the beta-lactam ring that is part of their chemical structure (Figure 38-4). This broad group of

Selected Sulfonamide Combination Drug Products

Drug (Pregnancy Category)	Pharmacologic Class	Usual Adult Dosage Range*	Indications
Sulfamethoxazole/trimethoprim (co-trimoxazole, SMZ-TMP) (Bactrim, Septra) (C)	Sulfonamide and folate antimetabolite	IV/PO: 8-20 mg/kg/day in divided doses (dose is in terms of trimethoprim component) PO: 160 mg TMP/800 mg SMZ twice daily (every 12 hr)	UTI, shigellosis enteritis; higher doses for nocardiosis and *Pneumocystis jirovecii* infection *P. jirovecii* prophylaxis, acute exacerbation of chronic bronchitis

*Dosage ranges are typical but are not necessarily exhaustive due to space limitations. Clinical variations may occur. Check current drug handbook for exact dosages for specific indications.

TABLE 38-3   Classification of Penicillins

Subclass	Generic Drug Names	Description
Natural penicillins	penicillin G, penicillin V	Although many modifications of the original natural (mold-produced) structure have been made, these are the only two in current clinical use. Penicillin G is the injectable form for IV or IM use; penicillin V is a PO dosage form (tablet and liquid).
Penicillinase-resistant drugs	cloxacillin, dicloxacillin, nafcillin, oxacillin	Stable against hydrolysis by most staphylococcal penicillinases (enzymes that normally break down the natural penicillins).
Aminopenicillins	amoxicillin, ampicillin	Have an amino group attached to the basic penicillin structure that enhances their activity against gram-negative bacteria compared with natural penicillins.
Extended-spectrum drugs	piperacillin, ticarcillin, carbenicillin, piperacillin/tazobactam	Have wider spectra of activity than do all other penicillins.

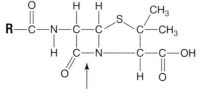

Beta-lactam ring

FIGURE 38-4 Chemical structure of penicillins showing the beta-lactam ring. **R,** Variable portion of drug chemical structure.

drugs includes four major subclasses: penicillins, cephalosporins, carbapenems, and monobactams. They share a common structure and mechanism of action: they inhibit the synthesis of the bacterial peptidoglycan cell wall.

Some bacterial strains produce the enzyme beta-lactamase. This enzyme provides a mechanism for bacterial resistance to these antibiotics. The enzyme can break the chemical bond between the carbon (C) and nitrogen (N) atoms in the structure of the beta-lactam ring. When this happens, all beta-lactam drugs lose their antibacterial efficacy. Because of this, additional drugs known as beta-lactamase inhibitors are added to several of the penicillin antibiotics to make the drug more powerful against beta-lactamase–producing bacterial strains. Each of the four classes of beta-lactam antibiotics is examined in detail in the following sections. The beta-lactams exhibit time-dependent killing (meaning their concentration must be above the minimum inhibitory concentration to kill bacteria). Because of this property, it is not unusual to see them given by

continuous IV infusion. They are also given by intermittent infusion (i.e., every 4 to 6 hours).

PENICILLINS

The penicillins are a very large group of chemically related antibiotics that were first derived from a mold (fungus) often seen on bread or fruit. The penicillins can be divided into four subgroups based on their structure and the spectrum of bacteria they are active against: natural penicillins, penicillinase-resistant penicillins, aminopenicillins, and extended-spectrum penicillins. Examples of penicillin antibiotics in each subgroup and a brief description of their characteristics are given in Table 38-3.

Penicillins are bactericidal antibiotics, meaning they kill a wide variety of gram-positive and some gram-negative bacteria. However, some bacteria have acquired the capacity to produce enzymes capable of destroying penicillins. These enzymes are called *beta-lactamases,* and they can inactivate the penicillin molecules by opening the beta-lactam ring. The beta-lactamases that specifically inactivate penicillin molecules are called *penicillinases.* Bacterial strains that produce these drug-inactivating enzymes were a therapeutic obstacle until drugs were synthesized that inhibit these enzymes. Three of these beta-lactamase inhibitors are clavulanic acid (also called *clavulanate*), tazobactam, and sulbactam. These drugs bind with the beta-lactamase enzyme itself to prevent the enzyme from breaking down the penicillin molecule, although they are not always effective. The following are examples of currently available combinations of a penicillin and a beta-lactamase inhibitor:

- ampicillin/sulbactam (Unasyn)
- amoxicillin/clavulanic acid (Augmentin)
- ticarcillin/clavulanic acid (Timentin)
- piperacillin/tazobactam (Zosyn)

Mechanism of Action and Drug Effects

The mechanism of action of penicillins involves the inhibition of bacterial cell wall synthesis. Once distributed by the patient's bloodstream to infected areas, penicillin molecules slide through bacterial cell walls to get to their site of action. Some penicillins, however, are too large to pass through the openings in the cell walls, and because they cannot get to their site of action they cannot kill the bacteria. Some bacteria make the openings in their cell walls small so that the penicillin cannot get through to kill them. The penicillin molecules that do gain entry into the bacterium must then find the appropriate binding sites. These are known as *penicillin-binding proteins*. By binding to these proteins, the penicillin molecules interfere with normal cell wall synthesis, causing the formation of defective cell walls that are unstable and easily broken down (see Figure 38-3). Bacterial death usually results from lysis (rupture) of the bacterial cells due to this drug-induced disruption of cell wall structure.

Indications

Penicillins are indicated for the prevention and treatment of infections caused by susceptible bacteria. The microorganisms most commonly destroyed by penicillins are gram-positive bacteria, including *Streptococcus* spp., *Enterococcus* spp., and *Staphylococcus* spp. Most natural penicillins have little if any ability to kill gram-negative bacteria. However, the extended-spectrum penicillins (i.e., piperacillin/tazobactam [Zosyn]) have excellent gram-positive, gram-negative, and anaerobic coverage. Because of this, the extended-spectrum penicillins are used to treat many health care–associated infections, including pneumonia, intraabdominal infections, and sepsis.

Contraindications

Penicillins are usually safe and well-tolerated medications. The only usual contraindication is known drug allergy. It is very important to obtain an accurate history regarding the type of reaction that occurs in patients who state they are allergic to penicillins. It is also important to note that often drugs are referred to by their trade names, and these don't always end in "*cillin*" (e.g., Zosyn, Augmentin). Many medication errors have occurred when a penicillin drug called by its trade name is given to a patient with a penicillin allergy (see the Safety and Quality Improvement: Preventing Medication Errors box on this page).

Adverse Effects

Allergic reactions to the penicillins occur in 0.7% to 4% of treatment courses. The most common reactions are urticaria, pruritus, and angioedema. A wide variety of idiosyncratic (unpredictable) drug reactions can occur, such as maculopapular eruptions, eosinophilia, Stevens-Johnson syndrome, and exfoliative dermatitis. Maculopapular rash occurs in about 2% of treatment courses with natural penicillin and 5.2% to 9.5%

⚡ SAFETY AND QUALITY IMPROVEMENT: PREVENTING MEDICATION ERRORS

Do You Know Your Penicillins?

Medication errors have occurred when nurses gave penicillin products to patients who were allergic to penicillin. In these cases, the drugs were referred to by their trade names, which lack the *"cillin"* suffix. Examples of these drugs are Zosyn and Unasyn. Both drugs contain a form of penicillin and a beta-lactamase inhibitor. Zosyn is a combination of piperacillin and tazobactam; Unasyn is a combination of ampicillin and sulbactam. Analysis of these errors revealed that the person administering the drug did not realize that the drug with the non-*"cillin"* name was a penicillin.

These errors illustrate why is it important to use both trade and generic names when ordering medications for patients. It is essential to know what you are administering to your patients! Be sure to check both names of the medications you give, and check the patient's allergies.

---

of those with ampicillin. Anaphylactic reactions are much less common, occurring in 0.004% to 0.015% of patients. Severe reactions are much more common with injected than with orally administered penicillin, as is the case with most drugs. Patients who are allergic to penicillins have an increased risk for allergy to other beta-lactam antibiotics. The incidence of cross-reactivity between cephalosporins and penicillins is reported to be between 1% and 4%. Patients reporting penicillin allergy need to describe their prior allergic reaction. It is very important to document the type of reaction. The decision to treat with cephalosporin therapy in such cases is often a matter of clinical judgment, based on the severity of reported prior reactions to penicillin drugs, the nature of the infection, the drug susceptibility of the infective organism if known, and the availability and patient tolerance of other alternative antibiotics. Generally speaking, only those patients with a history of throat swelling or hives from penicillin should not receive cephalosporins. Some patients may require skin testing and desensitization.

Penicillins are generally well tolerated and associated with very few adverse effects. As with many drugs, the most common adverse effects involve the GI system. The intravenous (IV) formulations of some penicillins contain large amounts of sodium and/or potassium. Doses must be adjusted for patients with renal dysfunction. The most common adverse effects of the penicillins are listed in Table 38-4.

Interactions

Many drugs interact with penicillins; some have positive effects, and others have harmful effects. The most common and clinically significant drug interactions associated with penicillin use are listed in Table 38-5.

Dosages

For dosage information on selected penicillins, see the table on p. 609.

DRUG PROFILES

Penicillins are classified as pregnancy category B drugs. They are very safe antibiotics. Their use is contraindicated in patients

TABLE 38-4 Penicillins: Reported Adverse Effects

Body System	Adverse Effects
Central nervous	Lethargy, anxiety, depression, seizures
Gastrointestinal	Nausea, vomiting, diarrhea, taste alterations, oral candidiasis
Hematologic	Anemia, bone marrow depression, granulocytopenia
Metabolic	Hyperkalemia, hypernatremia, alkalosis
Skin	Pruritus, hives, rash

TABLE 38-5 Penicillins: Drug Interactions

DRUG Interacting with Penicillins	Mechanism	Result
Aminoglycosides (IV) and clavulanic acid	Additivity	More effective killing of bacteria
methotrexate	Decreased renal elimination of methotrexate	Increased methotrexate levels
NSAIDs	Compete for protein binding	More free and active penicillin (may be beneficial)
Oral contraceptives	Uncertain	May decrease efficacy of the contraceptive
probenecid	Competes for elimination	Prolongs the effects of penicillins
rifampin	Inhibition	May inhibit the killing activity of penicillins
warfarin	Reduced vitamin K from gut flora	Enhanced anticoagulant effect of warfarin

with a known hypersensitivity to them, but because of their relatively good adverse effects profile, there are otherwise very few contraindications to their use.

NATURAL PENICILLINS
◆penicillin G and penicillin V potassium

Penicillin G has three salt forms: benzathine, procaine, and potassium. All of these forms are given by injection, either IV or intramuscularly (IM). The benzathine and procaine salts are used as longer-acting IM injections. They are formulated into a thick, white, pastelike material that is designed for prolonged dissolution and absorption from the IM site of injection. Never give these preparations IV, however, because their consistency is too thick for IV administration, and such use can be fatal. The IM formulations can be especially helpful for treating the sexually transmitted disease syphilis, because often only one injection is needed. Penicillin G potassium is formulated for IV use. Penicillin V potassium is available only for oral use.

Pharmacokinetics: Penicillin G

Route	Onset of Action	Peak Plasma Concentration	Elimination Half-life	Duration of Action
PO	Variable	30-60 min	30 min	4-6 hr
IV	Variable	30 min	24-54 min	4-6 hr

PENICILLINASE-RESISTANT PENICILLINS
nafcillin

Nafcillin is one of the four currently available penicillinase-resistant penicillins; the other three are cloxacillin, dicloxacillin, and oxacillin. Methicillin is part of this group but is no longer used clinically. Nafcillin is available only in injectable form, whereas cloxacillin and dicloxacillin are available only in oral form. Oxacillin is available in both oral and injectable forms. The penicillinase-resistant penicillins are able to resist breakdown by the penicillin-destroying enzyme (penicillinase) commonly produced by bacteria such as staphylococci. For this reason, they may also be referred to as *antistaphylococcal penicillins*. The chemical structure of these drugs features a large, bulky side chain near the beta-lactam ring. This side chain serves as a barrier to the penicillinase enzyme, preventing it from breaking the beta-lactam ring, which would inactivate the drug. There are, however, certain strains of staphylococci, specifically *S. aureus,* that are resistant to these drugs. Such bacteria therefore require alternative antibiotic regimens.

Pharmacokinetics: Nafcillin

Route	Onset of Action	Peak Plasma Concentration	Elimination Half-life	Duration of Action
IV	Variable	15-30 min	30-60 min	6 hr

AMINOPENICILLINS

There are two aminopenicillins: amoxicillin and ampicillin. They are so named because of the presence of a free amino group ($-NH^2$) in their chemical structure. This structural feature gives aminopenicillins enhanced activity against gram-negative bacteria against which the natural and penicillinase-resistant penicillins are relatively ineffective. The aminopenicillins are also effective against some gram-positive organisms. Amoxicillin is an analogue of ampicillin.

◆amoxicillin

Amoxicillin is a commonly prescribed aminopenicillin. Amoxicillin is used to treat infections caused by susceptible organisms in the ears, nose, throat, genitourinary tract, skin, and skin structures. Pediatric dosages are sometimes higher than in the past because of the development of increasingly resistant *Streptococcus pneumoniae* organisms. The drug is available only for oral use and can be given with or without food.

Pharmacokinetics: Amoxicillin

Route	Onset of Action	Peak Plasma Concentration	Elimination Half-life	Duration of Action
PO	0.5-1 hr	1-2 hr	1-1.5 hr	6-8 hr

ampicillin

Ampicillin is available in three different salt forms: anhydrous, trihydrate, and sodium. The different salt forms are administered by different routes. Ampicillin anhydrous and trihydrate are both administered orally, whereas ampicillin sodium is given parenterally. This drug is still currently

DOSAGES

Selected Penicillins

Drug (Pregnancy Category)	Pharmacologic Class	Usual Adult Dosage Range	Indications
◆amoxicillin (Amoxil, generics) (B)	Aminopenicillin	PO: 250-500 mg every 8 hr	Otitis media; sinusitis; various susceptible respiratory, skin, and urinary tract infections; dental prophylaxis for bacterial endocarditis; *Helicobacter pylori* infection
ampicillin (generic only) (B)	Aminopenicillin	PO/IV/IM: 1-12 g/day divided every 4-6 hr	Primarily infection with gram-negative organisms such as *Shigella, Salmonella, Escherichia, Haemophilus, Proteus,* and *Neisseria* spp.; infection with some gram-positive organisms
nafcillin (generic only) (B)	Penicillinase-resistant penicillin	IV: 500-2000 mg every 4-6 hr	Infection with penicillinase-producing staphylococci
◆penicillin V potassium (Pen-Vee K) (B)	Natural penicillin	PO: 125-500 mg every 6-8 hr	Primarily infection with gram-positive organisms such as Streptococcus (including *Streptococcus pneumoniae*)

spp., Species.

available, although it is now used less frequently than before because of resistance. The combination product ampicillin and sulbactam (Unasyn) is commonly used. Sulbactam is a beta-lactamase inhibitor that decreases resistance and increases the spectrum of activity.

Pharmacokinetics: Ampicillin

Route	Onset of Action	Peak Plasma Concentration	Elimination Half-life	Duration of Action
PO	Variable	1-2 hr	1-1.5 hr	4-6 hr
IV	Variable	5 min	1-1.8 hr	6-8 hr

EXTENDED-SPECTRUM PENICILLINS

By making a few changes in the basic penicillin structure, drug developers produced another generation of penicillins that have a wider spectrum of activity than that possessed by either of the other two classes of semisynthetic penicillins (penicillinase-resistant penicillins and aminopenicillins) or by the natural penicillins. Currently three extended-spectrum penicillins are available: carbenicillin, piperacillin, and ticarcillin; however, they are rarely used by themselves. Both ticarcillin and piperacillin are available in fixed-combination products that include beta-lactamase inhibitors. The ticarcillin fixed-combination product (Timentin) includes clavulanate potassium. Piperacillin is available in combination with tazobactam (a combination called Zosyn). These beta-lactamase–inhibiting products allow for enhanced multiorganism coverage, especially against anaerobic organisms that are common in intestinal infections and *Pseudomonas* spp., which are common in health care–associated infections. Zosyn is commonly used in hospitalized patients with suspected or documented serious infections. Because of its broad spectrum of activity (gram-positive, gram-negative, and anaerobic), it is often used as empiric therapy. Zosyn and Timentin are available for IV use only.

CEPHALOSPORINS

Cephalosporins are semisynthetic antibiotics widely used in clinical practice. They are structurally and pharmacologically related to the penicillins. Like penicillins, cephalosporins are bactericidal and work by interfering with bacterial cell wall synthesis. They also bind to the same penicillin-binding proteins inside bacteria that were described earlier for the penicillins. Although there are a variety of such proteins, they are collectively referred to as *penicillin binding* regardless of the type of beta-lactam drug involved.

Cephalosporins can destroy a broad spectrum of bacteria, and this ability is directly related to the chemical changes that have been made to their basic cephalosporin structure. Modifications to this chemical structure by pharmaceutical scientists have given rise to five generations of cephalosporins. Depending on the generation, these drugs may be active against gram-positive, gram-negative, or anaerobic bacteria. They are not active against fungi, viruses, or enterococci. The different drugs of each generation have certain chemical similarities, and thus they can kill similar spectra of bacteria. In general, the level of gram-negative coverage increases with each successive generation. The first-generation drugs have the most gram-positive coverage, and the later generations have the most gram-negative coverage. Anaerobic coverage is found only with the second-generation drugs. Cefepime, cefdinir, and cefditoren pivoxil are the oral third-generation cephalosporins. Ceftaroline, the newest cephalosporin, often referred as the fifth generation, has a broad spectrum and covers gram-positive (including MRSA) and gram-negative organisms. The currently available parenteral and oral cephalosporin antibiotics are listed in Table 38-6. As is often the case, injectable drugs produce higher serum concentrations than drugs administered by the oral route and thus are used to treat more serious infections.

The safety profiles, contraindications, and pregnancy ratings of the cephalosporins are very similar to those of the penicillins. The most commonly reported adverse effects are mild diarrhea, abdominal cramps, rash, pruritus, redness, and edema. Because cephalosporins are chemically very similar to penicillins, a person who has had an allergic reaction to penicillin may also have an allergic reaction to a cephalosporin. This is referred to as *cross-sensitivity*. Various investigators have observed that the incidence of cross-sensitivity between penicillins and

TABLE 38-6　**Cephalosporins: Parenteral and Oral Preparations**

FIRST-GENERATION		SECOND-GENERATION		THIRD-GENERATION		FOURTH-GENERATION	FIFTH-GENERATION
IV	PO	IV	PO	IV	PO	IV	IV
cefazolin	cefadroxil	cefoxitin	cefaclor	cefotaxime	cefpodoxime	cefepime	ceftaroline
cephradine	cephalexin	cefuroxime	cefuroxime axetil	ceftizoxime	ceftibuten		
	cephradine	cefotetan	cefprozil	ceftriaxone	cefdinir		
				ceftazidime			

TABLE 38-7　**Cephalosporins: Drug Interactions**

Interacting Drug	Mechanism	Result
Ethanol (alcohol)	Accumulation of acetaldehyde metabolite of ethanol	Acute alcohol intolerance (disulfiram-like reaction) after drinking alcoholic beverages within 72 hr of taking cefotetan. Symptoms include stomach cramps, nausea, vomiting, diaphoresis, pruritus, headache, and hypotension.
Antacids, iron	Decreased absorption of certain oral cephalosporins (cefdinir, cefditoren)	Decreased effectiveness of drug
probenecid	Decreased renal excretion	Increased cephalosporin levels
Oral contraceptives (OCs)	Unknown	Increased risk for unintended pregnancy

cephalosporins is between 1% and 4%. However, only those patients who have had a serious anaphylactic reaction to penicillin must not be given cephalosporins. As a class, the cephalosporins are very safe and effective antibiotics.

Penicillins and cephalosporins are practically identical in their mechanism of action, drug effects, therapeutic effects, and adverse effects. For this reason, this information is not repeated for the cephalosporins, and the reader is referred to the pertinent discussions in the section on the penicillin drugs. Cephalosporins of all generations are very safe drugs that are classified as pregnancy category B drugs. Their use is contraindicated in patients with a known hypersensitivity to them and in patients with a history of life-threatening allergic reaction to penicillins. Drug interactions are listed in Table 38-7.

Dosages

For dosage information on selected cephalosporins, see the table on the next page.

DRUG PROFILES

FIRST-GENERATION CEPHALOSPORINS

First-generation cephalosporins are usually active against gram-positive bacteria and have limited activity against gram-negative bacteria. They are available in both parenteral and oral forms. Currently available first-generation cephalosporins include cefadroxil, cefazolin, cephalexin, and cephradine.

◆ cefazolin

Cefazolin (Ancef) is a prototypical first-generation cephalosporin. As with all first-generation cephalosporins, it provides excellent coverage against gram-positive bacteria but limited

coverage against gram-negative bacteria. It is available only for parenteral use. It is used commonly for surgical prophylaxis and for susceptible staphylococcal infections.

Pharmacokinetics: Cefazolin

Route	Onset of Action	Peak Plasma Concentration	Elimination Half-life	Duration of Action
IV	Variable	5 min	1.2-2.5 hr	8 hr

◆ cephalexin

Cephalexin (Keflex) is a prototypical oral first-generation cephalosporin. It also provides excellent coverage against gram-positive bacteria but limited coverage against gram-negative bacteria. It is available only for oral use. Cephradine is another oral first-generation cephalosporin.

Pharmacokinetics: Cephalexin

Route	Onset of Action	Peak Plasma Concentration	Elimination Half-life	Duration of Action
PO	Variable	1 hr	0.6-2 hr	6-12 hr

SECOND-GENERATION CEPHALOSPORINS

Second-generation cephalosporins have coverage against gram-positive organisms similar to that of the first-generation cephalosporins but have enhanced coverage against gram-negative bacteria. Both parenteral and oral formulations are available. Currently available second-generation cephalosporins include cefaclor, cefoxitin, cefuroxime, cefotetan, and cefprozil. These drugs differ slightly with regard to their antibacterial coverage.

DOSAGES

Selected Cephalosporins

Drug (Pregnancy Category)	Pharmacologic Class	Usual Adult Dosage Range	Indications
◆ cefazolin (Kefzol, Ancef) (B)	First-generation cephalosporin	IV/IM: 500-2000 mg every 8 hr	Infections due to gram-positive organisms, some penicillinase-producing organisms, and some gram-negative organisms; preoperative and postoperative surgical prophylaxis
◆ cefoxitin (Mefoxin) (B)	Second-generation cephalosporin	IV/IM: 3-12 g/day divided every 6-8 hr	Infections; less coverage of gram-positive organisms, greater coverage of gram-negative and anaerobic organisms
cefuroxime* (Zinacef); cefuroxime axetil (Ceftin, tablet form) (B)	Second-generation cephalosporin	PO (tabs): 125-500 mg bid IV/IM: 750-1500 mg every 8 hr	Comparable to those for cefazolin, and provides more coverage of gram-negative organisms
ceftazidime (Fortaz, Tazidime) (B)	Third-generation cephalosporin	IV/IM: 250-2000 mg every 6-12 hr	Infections; more extensive coverage of gram-negative organisms, including *Pseudomonas* spp.
◆ ceftriaxone (Rocephin) (B)	Third-generation cephalosporin	IV/IM: 1-2 g given once daily except for meningitis, for which it is given twice daily (as above)	Comparable to those for ceftazidime, except for *Pseudomonas* spp.
cefepime (Maxipime) (B)	Fourth-generation cephalosporin	IV/IM: 250-2000 mg daily-bid	Infections; provides more extensive coverage of gram-negative organisms and better gram-positive coverage than third generation, including organisms causing intraabdominal infections
Ceftaroline (Teflaro) (B)	Fifth-generation cephalosporin	600 mg every 12 hr	Provides broad-spectrum coverage including MRSA and gram-negative infections (except pseudomonas and acinetobacter)

spp., Species.
*Cefuroxime axetil and cefditoren pivoxil are both prodrugs for PO use that are hydrolyzed into the active ingredient in the fluids of the gastrointestinal tract.

Cefoxitin and cefotetan are often referred to as *cephamycins* and have better coverage against various anaerobic bacteria such as *Bacteroides fragilis*, *Peptostreptococcus* spp., and *Clostridium* spp. than the other drugs in this class.

◆ cefoxitin

Cefoxitin (Mefoxin) is a parenteral second-generation cephalosporin. It provides excellent gram-positive coverage and better gram-negative coverage than the first-generation drugs. Cefoxitin has been used extensively as a prophylactic antibiotic in patients undergoing abdominal surgery because it can effectively kill intestinal bacteria, including anaerobes. Normal intestinal flora include gram-positive, gram-negative, and anaerobic bacteria.

Pharmacokinetics: Cefoxitin

Route	Onset of Action	Peak Plasma Concentration	Elimination Half-life	Duration of Action
IV	Variable	0.5 hr	1 hr	8 hr

cefuroxime

Cefuroxime sodium (Zinacef) is the parenteral form of this second-generation cephalosporin. The oral form is a different salt, cefuroxime axetil (Ceftin). It has more activity against gram-negative bacteria than first-generation cephalosporins

but a narrower spectrum of activity against gram-negative bacteria than third-generation cephalosporins. It differs from the cephamycins such as cefoxitin in that it does not kill anaerobic bacteria. Cefuroxime axetil is a prodrug. It has little antibacterial activity until it is hydrolyzed in the liver to its active cefuroxime form. It is available only for oral use. Cefuroxime sodium is available only in injectable form.

Pharmacokinetics: Cefuroxime

Route	Onset of Action	Peak Plasma Concentration	Elimination Half-life	Duration of Action
PO	Variable	2-3 hr	1.3 hr	6-8 hr
IV	Variable	30 min	1-2 hr	6-8 hr

THIRD-GENERATION CEPHALOSPORINS

The available third-generation cephalosporins include cefotaxime, cefpodoxime, ceftazidime, ceftibuten, cefdinir, ceftizoxime, and ceftriaxone. These are the most potent of the first three generations of cephalosporins in fighting gram-negative bacteria, but they generally have less activity than first- and second-generation drugs against gram-positive organisms.

Because of specific changes in the basic cephalosporin structure, ceftazidime has activity against *Pseudomonas* spp. However, resistance is beginning to limit its usefulness. Cefpodoxime, cefdinir, and ceftibuten are currently the only third-generation cephalosporins available for oral use. All the other third-generation drugs are available only in parenteral forms.

◆ceftriaxone

Ceftriaxone (Rocephin) is an extremely long-acting third-generation drug that can be given only once a day for the treatment of most infections. It also has the unique characteristic of being able to pass easily through the blood-brain barrier. For this reason, it is one of the few cephalosporins that is indicated for the treatment of meningitis, an infection of the meninges of the brain. The spectrum of activity of ceftriaxone is similar to that of the other third-generation drugs cefotaxime and ceftizoxime. It can be given both IV and IM. In some cases of infection, one IM injection can eradicate the infection. Ceftriaxone is 93% to 96% bound to plasma protein, a proportion higher than that of many of the other cephalosporins. This drug is also unique in that it is metabolized in the intestine after biliary excretion. Ceftriaxone is not given to hyperbilirubinemic neonates or to patients with severe liver dysfunction. It should not be administered with calcium infusions. Ceftriaxone is available only for injection.

Pharmacokinetics: Ceftriaxone

Route	Onset of Action	Peak Plasma Concentration	Elimination Half-life	Duration of Action
IV	Variable	1.5-4 hr	4.3-8.7 hr	24 hr

ceftazidime

Ceftazidime (Ceptaz, Fortaz, Tazidime) is a parenterally administered third-generation cephalosporin with activity against difficult-to-treat infections with gram-negative bacteria such as *Pseudomonas* spp. It is the third-generation cephalosporin of choice for many indications because of its excellent spectrum of activity and safety profile; however, resistance is beginning to limit its usefulness, and it is generally given in combination with an aminoglycoside (discussed in Chapter 39). Ceftazidime is available only in injectable form. A recently approved drug, Avycaz (ceftazidime-avibactam), combines ceftazidime with avibactam, which is a new beta-lactamase inhibitor. Avycaz in indicated for intraabdominal infections and complicated urinary tract infections.

Pharmacokinetics: Ceftazidime

Route	Onset of Action	Peak Plasma Concentration	Elimination Half-life	Duration of Action
IV/IM	Variable	1 hr	2 hr	8-12 hr

FOURTH-GENERATION CEPHALOSPORINS
cefepime

Cefepime (Maxipime) is the prototypical fourth-generation cephalosporin. Cefepime is a broad-spectrum cephalosporin that most closely resembles ceftazidime in its spectrum of activity. It differs from ceftazidime in that it has increased activity against many *Enterobacter* spp. (gram-negative) as well as gram-positive organisms. Cefepime is indicated for the treatment of uncomplicated and complicated UTIs, uncomplicated skin and skin structure infections, and pneumonia. It is available only in injectable form.

Pharmacokinetics: Cefepime

Route	Onset of Action	Peak Plasma Concentration	Elimination Half-life	Duration of Action
IV	0.5 hr	0.5-1.5 hr	2 hr	8-12 hr

FIFTH-GENERATION CEPHALOSPORINS
ceftaroline

Ceftaroline (Teflaro) is the newest cephalosporin. It has a broader spectrum of activity than the current cephalosporins. It is effective against a wide variety of organisms, including methicillin-resistant *S. aureus* (MRSA), making it the only cephalosporin that treats MRSA. Ceftaroline is indicated for acute skin and skin structure infections and community-associated pneumonia. The dose needs to be adjusted for decreased renal function. It is available only in injectable form.

Pharmacokinetics: Ceftaroline

Route	Onset of Action	Peak Plasma Concentration	Elimination Half-life	Duration of Action
IV	0.5 hr	1 hr	2.4 hrs	8-12 hr

CARBAPENEMS

Carbapenems have the broadest antibacterial action of any antibiotics to date. They are bactericidal and inhibit cell wall synthesis. Because of this, they are often reserved for complicated body cavity and connective tissue infections in acutely ill hospitalized patients. They are also effective against many gram-positive organisms. One hazard of carbapenem use is drug-induced seizure activity, which occurs in a relatively small percentage of patients. However, the risk for seizures can be reduced by proper dosage adjustment in impaired patients. There is a small risk for cross-allergenicity in patients with penicillin allergies. Only those patients with anaphylactic-type reactions to penicillins must not receive a carbapenem. Currently available carbapenems include imipenem/cilastatin, meropenem, ertapenem, and doripenem. Carbapenems must be infused over 60 minutes.

DRUG PROFILE
◆imipenem/cilastatin

Imipenem/cilastatin (Primaxin) is a fixed combination of imipenem, which is a semisynthetic carbapenem antibiotic similar to beta-lactam antibiotics, and cilastatin, an inhibitor of an enzyme that breaks down imipenem. Imipenem has a wide spectrum of activity against gram-positive and gram-negative aerobic and anaerobic bacteria. Cilastatin is a unique drug in that it inhibits an enzyme in the kidneys called *dehydropeptidase*, which would otherwise quickly break down the imipenem. Cilastatin also blocks the renal tubular secretion of imipenem, which impairs imipenem from being excreted by the kidneys, the primary route of elimination of the drug.

Imipenem/cilastatin exerts its antibacterial effect by binding to penicillin-binding proteins inside bacteria, which in turn inhibits bacterial cell wall synthesis. Unlike many of the penicillins and cephalosporins, imipenem/cilastatin is very resistant to the antibiotic-inhibiting actions of beta-lactamases. Drugs with which it potentially interacts include cyclosporine, ganciclovir, and probenecid, all of which may potentiate the central nervous system (CNS) adverse effects (including seizures) of imipenem. The most serious adverse effect associated with imipenem/cilastatin therapy is seizures, which have been reported in up to 1.5% of patients receiving less than 500 mg every 6 hours. In patients receiving high dosages of the drug (more than 500 mg every 6 hours), however, there is a 10% incidence of seizures. Seizures are more likely in older adults and renally impaired patients. Seizures have been associated with all of the carbapenems, but the data suggest that they are most likely to occur with imipenem/cilastatin.

Imipenem/cilastatin is indicated for the treatment of bone, joint, skin, and soft-tissue infections; bacterial endocarditis caused by *S. aureus;* intraabdominal bacterial infections; pneumonia; UTIs and pelvic infections; and bacterial septicemia caused by susceptible bacterial organisms. The IM form of imipenem/cilastatin contains lidocaine, and its use is therefore contraindicated in patients with a known drug allergy to lidocaine or related local anesthetics. All dosage forms contain the same number of milligrams of both imipenem and cilastatin.

Meropenem (Merrem) is the second drug in the carbapenem class of antibiotics. Compared with imipenem/cilastatin, meropenem appears to be somewhat less active against gram-positive organisms, more active against *Enterobacteriaceae,* and equally active against *P. aeruginosa.* However, meropenem is the only carbapenem currently indicated for treatment of bacterial meningitis. Ertapenem (Invanz) has a spectrum of activity comparable to that of imipenem/cilastatin, although it is not active against *Enterococcal* or *Pseudomonas* spp. It has the advantage of being given once a day. Doripenem (Doribax) is the newest carbapenem. It has less seizure potential than imipenem/cilastatin. It is indicated for intraabdominal infections, pyelonephritis, UTIs, and pneumonia. Recommended dosages of imipenem/cilastatin are given in the table on the next page.

Pharmacokinetics: Imipenem/Cilastatin

Route	Onset of Action	Peak Plasma Concentration	Elimination Half-life	Duration of Action
IV	Variable	2 hr	2-3 hr	6-8 hr

MONOBACTAMS

DRUG PROFILE

aztreonam

Aztreonam (Azactam) is the only monobactam antibiotic to be developed thus far. It is a synthetic beta-lactam antibiotic that is primarily active against aerobic gram-negative bacteria, including *E. coli, Klebsiella* spp., and *Pseudomonas* spp. Aztreonam is a bactericidal antibiotic. It destroys bacteria by inhibiting bacterial cell wall synthesis, which results in lysis. Aztreonam is indicated for the treatment of moderately severe systemic infections and UTIs. It is often combined with other antibiotics for the treatment of intraabdominal and gynecologic infections. Aztreonam is available only in injectable form. Its use is contraindicated in patients with a known drug allergy, although it is believed to have less allergic cross-reactivity with other beta-lactam antibiotics. In fact, it is commonly given to patients who have a penicillin allergy. Common adverse effects include rash, nausea, vomiting, and diarrhea. Recommended dosages for this monobactam are given in the table on the next page.

Pharmacokinetics: Aztreonam

Route	Onset of Action	Peak Plasma Concentration	Elimination Half-life	Duration of Action
IV/IM	Variable	1 hr	1.5-2.1 hr	6-12 hr

MACROLIDES

The macrolides are a large group of antibiotics that first became available in the early 1950s with the introduction of erythromycin. Macrolides are considered bacteriostatic; however, in high enough concentrations they may be bactericidal to some susceptible bacteria. Currently available macrolide antibiotics include: azithromycin, clarithromycin, erythromycin, and fidaxomicin. Azithromycin and clarithromycin are currently the most widely used of the macrolides. Although the spectra of antibacterial activity of both azithromycin and clarithromycin are similar to that of erythromycin, the former have longer durations of action than erythromycin, which allows them to be given less often. They produce fewer and milder GI tract adverse effects than erythromycin, and azithromycin is usually dosed over a shorter length of time than many of the erythromycin products. Azithromycin and clarithromycin also exhibit better efficacy in eradicating various bacteria and are capable of better tissue penetration. Because erythromycin has a bitter taste and is quickly degraded by the acidity of the stomach, several salt forms and many dosage formulations were developed to circumvent these problems. Fidaxomicin (Dificid) is the newest macrolide antibiotic. It is indicated only for the treatment of *Clostridium difficile*–associated diarrhea. The most common adverse effects are nausea, vomiting, and GI bleed. It is classified as a pregnancy category B drug. It has minimal absorption and, as such, there are known drug interactions.

Mechanism of Action and Drug Effects

Macrolide antibiotics are bacteriostatic drugs that inhibit protein synthesis by binding reversibly to the 50S ribosomal subunits of susceptible microorganisms. Macrolides are effective in the treatment of a wide range of infections. These include various infections of the upper and lower respiratory tract, skin, and soft tissue caused by some strains of *Streptococcus* and *Haemophilus;* spirochetal infections such as syphilis and Lyme disease; gonorrhea; and *Chlamydia, Mycoplasma,* and *Corynebacterium* infections. Gonorrheal infections have become increasingly difficult to treat with macrolide monotherapy, so

Selected Carbapenems and Monobactams

Drug (Pregnancy Category)	Pharmacologic Class	Usual Adult Dosage Range	Indications
aztreonam (Azactam) (B)	Monobactam	IV/IM: 500-2000 mg every 6-12 hr	Primarily UTI caused by gram-negative organisms, severe systemic infections
◆ imipenem/cilastatin (Primaxin) (C)	Carbapenem	IV: 250-500 mg every 6-8 hr IM: 500-750 mg every 12 hr	Infection with gram-positive, gram-negative, and aerobic bacteria, including *Pseudomonas aeruginosa*; includes infections of bone, joint, skin, or soft tissue and endocarditis, pneumonia, UTI, intraabdominal, and pelvic infections, and septicemia

these drugs are sometimes used in combination with other antibiotics such as cephalosporins. Macrolides are also somewhat unique among antibiotics in that they are especially effective against several bacterial species that often reproduce inside host cells instead of just in the bloodstream or interstitial spaces. Common examples of such bacteria, some of which were previously listed, are *Listeria, Chlamydia, Legionella* (one species of which causes Legionnaires' disease), *Neisseria* (one species of which causes gonorrhea), and *Campylobacter*.

Indications

Infections caused by *Streptococcus pyogenes* (group A beta-hemolytic streptococci) are inhibited by macrolides, as are mild to moderate upper and lower respiratory tract infections caused by *Haemophilus influenzae*. Spirochetal infections that are treated with erythromycin and other macrolides are syphilis and Lyme disease. Various forms of gonorrhea and *Chlamydia* and Mycoplasma infections are also susceptible to the effects of macrolides.

A therapeutic effect of erythromycin outside its antibiotic actions is its ability to irritate the GI tract, which stimulates smooth muscle and GI motility. This may be of benefit to patients who have decreased GI motility, such as delayed gastric emptying in diabetic patients (known as *diabetic gastroparesis*). It has also been shown to be helpful in facilitating the passage of feeding tubes from the stomach into the small bowel. Azithromycin and clarithromycin are approved for the prevention and treatment of *Mycobacterium avium-intracellulare (MAC)* complex infections. This is a common *opportunistic infection* often associated with HIV infection/acquired immunodeficiency syndrome (AIDS) (see Chapter 40). Clarithromycin also has been approved for use in combination with omeprazole and amoxicillin for the treatment of patients with active ulcer associated with *Helicobacter pylori* infection.

Contraindications

The only usual contraindication to macrolide use is known drug allergy. Macrolides are often used as alternative drugs for patients with allergies to beta-lactam antibiotics.

Adverse Effects

Erythromycin formulations cause many GI-related adverse effects, especially nausea and vomiting. Azithromycin and

TABLE 38-8   Macrolides: Reported Adverse Effects

Body System	Adverse Effects
Cardiovascular	Palpitations, chest pain, QT prolongation
Central nervous	Headache, dizziness, vertigo
Gastrointestinal	Nausea, hepatotoxicity, heartburn, vomiting, diarrhea, flatulence, cholestatic jaundice, anorexia, abnormal taste
Integumentary	Rash, urticaria, phlebitis at intravenous site
Other	Hearing loss, tinnitus

clarithromycin seem to be associated with a lower incidence of these GI tract complications. Reported adverse effects are listed in Table 38-8.

Interactions

There are a number of potential drug interactions with the macrolides. The macrolides possess two properties that can cause drug interactions: they are highly protein bound, and they are metabolized in the liver. For drugs metabolized in the liver, drug interactions arise from competition between the different drugs for metabolic enzymes, specifically the enzymes known as the *cytochrome P-450 complex* (see Chapter 2). Such enzymatic effects generally lead to more pronounced drug interactions than competition for protein binding. The result is a delay in the metabolic clearance of one or more interacting drugs and thus a prolonged and possibly toxic drug effect. Examples of some especially common drugs that compete for hepatic metabolism with the macrolides are carbamazepine, cyclosporine, theophylline, and warfarin. When macrolides are given with these drugs, the results are enhanced effects and possible toxicity of the latter drugs, and patients must be monitored. Macrolides can also reduce the efficacy of oral contraceptives. Clarithromycin and erythromycin are not to be used with moxifloxacin, pimozide, thioridazine, or other drugs that prolong the QT interval, because malignant dysrhythmias can occur. Concurrent use of simvastatin or lovastatin with clarithromycin or erythromycin is not recommended. Azithromycin is not as prone to such interactions as are the other macrolides, because of its minimal effects on the cytochrome P-450 enzymes.

DOSAGES

Selected Macrolides

Drug (Pregnancy Category)	Pharmacologic Class	Usual Adult Dosage Range	Indications
♦ azithromycin (Zithromax) (B)	Semisynthetic macrolide	PO: 500 mg × 1 dose, then 250 mg daily × 4 days IV: 500 mg daily	Comparable to those for erythromycin, but especially GU and respiratory tract infections, including MAC infections
♦ clarithromycin (Biaxin) (C)	Semisynthetic macrolide	PO: 500 mg twice daily	Comparable to those for erythromycin, but especially GU and respiratory tract infections, including MAC infections
♦ erythromycin* (E-mycin, EryPed, Eryc, E.E.S., many others) (B)	Natural macrolide	PO: 250-500 mg qid	Infections of respiratory and GI tracts and skin caused by various gram-positive, gram-negative, and miscellaneous organisms

GU, Genitourinary; MAC, *Mycobacterium avium-intracellulare* complex.
*There are many dosage forms, and dosages may vary from those listed.

Dosages

For dosage information on selected macrolide antibiotics, see the table on this page.

DRUG PROFILES

Macrolide antibiotics are used to treat a variety of infections. Azithromycin and clarithromycin have fewer adverse effects and a better pharmacokinetics profile than erythromycin.

Macrolide use is contraindicated in patients with known drug allergy. Because these drugs are significantly protein bound and are metabolized in the liver, they may interact with other drugs that are also highly protein bound or hepatically metabolized.

♦ erythromycin

Erythromycin, which goes by many product names, was for many years the most commonly prescribed macrolide antibiotic. However, other macrolides are now more commonly used. The drug is available in several different salt and dosage forms for oral use that were developed to circumvent some of the drawbacks it has chemically. An injectable form is also available for IV use. Erythromycin is also available in topical forms for dermatologic use (see Chapter 56) and in ophthalmic dosage forms (see Chapter 57). The absorption of oral erythromycin is enhanced if it is taken on an empty stomach, but because of the high incidence of stomach irritation associated with its use, many of these drugs are taken with a meal or snack. Erythromycin is associated with many drug interactions because it is a strong inhibitor of cytochrome P450 enzymes.

♦ azithromycin and ♦ clarithromycin

Azithromycin (Zithromax) and clarithromycin (Biaxin) are semisynthetic macrolide antibiotics that differ structurally from erythromycin and as a result have advantages over it. These include better adverse-effect profiles, including less GI tract irritation, and more favorable pharmacokinetic properties. Both have very similar spectra of activity that differ only slightly from that of erythromycin. The two drugs are used for the treatment of both upper and lower respiratory tract and skin structure infections. Azithromycin is available in oral and injectable forms, whereas clarithromycin is available only in oral form.

Azithromycin has excellent tissue penetration, so that it can reach high concentrations in infected tissues. It also has a long duration of action, which allows it to be dosed once daily. It is usually given in a regimen of 500 mg on day 1 and then 250 mg/day for 4 days. Taking the drug with food decreases both the rate and extent of GI absorption. The drug is available in oral and injectable forms.

Clarithromycin is given orally twice daily in adults and children older than 6 months of age. It can be given with or without food. The extended-release preparation must not be crushed.

Pharmacokinetics: Azithromycin

Route	Onset of Action	Peak Plasma Concentration	Elimination Half-life	Duration of Action
PO	Variable	2.5-4 hr	60-70 hr	Up to 24 hr

Pharmacokinetics: Clarithromycin

Route	Onset of Action	Peak Plasma Concentration	Elimination Half-life	Duration of Action
PO	Variable	2-4 hr	3-7 hr	Up to 12 hr

KETOLIDES

Telithromycin (Ketek) is currently the only drug in a new class known as ketolides. It is derived from erythromycin A and has better acid stability and better antibacterial coverage than the macrolides. Its mechanism of action is also similar to that of the macrolides. However, telithromycin has been associated with severe liver damage, and its use is very limited.

TETRACYCLINES

The tetracyclines are bacteriostatic drugs that inhibit bacterial protein synthesis by binding to the 30S bacterial ribosome. The three naturally occurring tetracyclines are demeclocycline, oxytetracycline, and tetracycline. The two semisynthetic tetracyclines are doxycycline and minocycline. The newest tetracycline antibiotic is tigecycline (Tygacil). Tigecycline is indicated for skin and soft-tissue infections, intraabdominal infections, and pneumonia. It is effective against many resistant bacteria. The available tetracycline antibiotics are listed in Box 38-1.

Tetracyclines are chemically and pharmacologically similar to one another. The most significant chemical characteristic of these drugs is their ability to bind to (chelate) divalent (Ca^{++}, Mg^{++}) and trivalent (Al^{+++}) metallic ions to form insoluble complexes. Therefore, their coadministration with milk, antacids, or iron salts causes a considerable reduction in the oral absorption of the tetracycline. In addition, their strong affinity for calcium usually precludes their use in pediatric patients younger than 8 years of age, because it can result in significant tooth discoloration. These drugs must be avoided in pregnant women and nursing mothers. The drugs do pass into breast milk, and this can be another route of exposure leading to tooth discoloration in nursing children.

Tetracyclines primarily differ from one another in the following ways:
- *Oral absorption:* All except tigecycline are adequately absorbed, but doxycycline and minocycline have the best absorption.
- *Body tissue penetration:* Doxycycline and minocycline possess the best penetration potential (brain and cerebrospinal fluid).
- *Half-life and resulting dosage schedule:* See the dosages table on this page and pharmacokinetics information in the Drug Profiles section.

Mechanism of Action and Drug Effects

Tetracyclines work by inhibiting protein synthesis in susceptible bacteria. They inhibit the growth of and kill a very wide range

of *Rickettsia*, *Chlamydia*, and *Mycoplasma* organisms, as well as a variety of gram-negative and gram-positive bacteria. They are also useful in the treatment of spirochetal infections, such as syphilis and Lyme disease, and pelvic inflammatory disease. Demeclocycline possesses a unique drug effect in that it inhibits the action of antidiuretic hormone, which makes it useful in the treatment of the syndrome of inappropriate secretion of antidiuretic hormone (SIADH).

Indications

Tetracyclines have a wide range of activity, and all drugs in this class are effective against essentially the same spectrum of microbes. They inhibit the growth of many gram-negative and gram-positive organisms and even of some protozoans. Traditionally used to treat acne in adolescents and adults, they are also considered the drugs of choice for the treatment of the following infections caused by susceptible organisms:
- *Chlamydia:* lymphogranuloma venereum, psittacosis, and nonspecific endocervical, rectal, and urethral infections
- *Mycoplasma: Mycoplasma* pneumonia
- *Rickettsia:* Q fever, rickettsial pox, Rocky Mountain spotted fever, and typhus
- *Other bacteria:* acne, brucellosis, chancroid, cholera, granuloma inguinale, shigellosis, spirochetal relapsing fever, Lyme disease, *H. pylori* infections associated with peptic ulcer disease (used as part of the treatment regimen), syphilis (used as an alternative drug to treat patients with penicillin allergy); tetracyclines are now unreliable in treating gonorrhea due to the development of resistant bacterial strains
- *Protozoa:* balantidiasis

Contraindications

The only usual contraindication is known drug allergy. However, tetracyclines must be avoided in pregnant and nursing women and in children younger than 8 years of age.

Adverse Effects

All tetracyclines cause similar adverse effects. They can cause discoloration of the permanent teeth and tooth enamel hypoplasia in both fetuses and children and possibly retard fetal skeletal development if taken during pregnancy. Other clinically

BOX 38-1 Available Tetracycline Antibiotics

demeclocycline	doxycycline
oxytetracycline	minocycline
tetracycline	tigecycline

DOSAGES

Selected Tetracyclines*

Drug (Pregnancy Category)	Pharmacologic Class	Usual Adult Dosage Range	Indications
demeclocycline (Declomycin) (D)	Tetracycline	PO: 150 mg qid or 300 mg bid	Infections; provides broad antibacterial coverage, including treatment of skin infections and respiratory, GI, and GU tract infections
◆ doxycycline (Vibramycin, others) (D)	Tetracycline	PO: 100 mg bid first day, then 100 mg daily thereafter	Comparable to those for demeclocycline
tigecycline (Tygacil) (D)	Glycylcycline	IV: 100 mg × 1, then 50 mg every 12 hr	Skin and skin structure infections, MRSA infections, intraabdominal infections

MRSA, Methicillin-resistant *Staphylococcus aureus.*
*Use of tetracyclines is contraindicated in children younger than 8 years of age and in pregnant women because of the risk for significant tooth discoloration in children.

significant undesirable effects include photosensitivity, which is most frequent in patients taking demeclocycline; alteration of the intestinal and vaginal flora, which can result in diarrhea or vaginal candidiasis; reversible bulging fontanelles in neonates; thrombocytopenia, possible coagulation irregularities, and hemolytic anemia; and exacerbation of systemic lupus erythematosus. Other effects include gastric upset, enterocolitis, and maculopapular rash.

Interactions

There are several significant drug interactions associated with the use of tetracyclines. When tetracyclines are taken with antacids, antidiarrheal drugs, dairy products, calcium, enteral feedings, or iron preparations, the oral absorption of the tetracycline is reduced. Tetracyclines can potentiate the effects of oral anticoagulants, which necessitates more frequent monitoring of anticoagulant effect and possible dosage adjustment. They can also antagonize the effects of bactericidal antibiotics and oral contraceptives. In addition, depending on the dosage, they can cause increased blood urea nitrogen levels.

Dosages

For dosage information on selected tetracyclines, see the table on this page.

DRUG PROFILES

Tetracyclines were one of the first classes of antibiotic capable of providing coverage against a broad spectrum of microorganisms. Their use is contraindicated in patients with a known hypersensitivity to them. They should be avoided in pregnant and lacting women and children younger than 8 years old. Resistance to one tetracycline implies resistance to all tetracyclines.

demeclocycline

Demeclocycline (Declomycin) is a naturally occurring tetracycline antibiotic that is derived from strains of *Streptomyces*. It is used both for its antibacterial action and for its ability to inhibit the action of antidiuretic hormone in SIADH. Demeclocycline has all the characteristics of this class of tetracyclines. It is available only for oral use.

♦ doxycycline

Doxycycline (Doryx) is a semisynthetic tetracycline antibiotic. It is useful in the treatment of rickettsial infections such as Rocky Mountain spotted fever, chlamydial and mycoplasmal infections, spirochetal infections, and many infections with gram-negative organisms. It can also be used for the prevention and treatment of anthrax and malaria. Doxycycline may also be used in the treatment of acne. It is available in both oral and injectable forms.

Pharmacokinetics: Doxycycline

Route	Onset of Action	Peak Plasma Concentration	Elimination Half-life	Duration of Action
PO	Variable	1.5-4 hr	14-24 hr	Up to 10-12 hr

tigecycline

Tigecycline (Tygacil) is the newest tetracycline, referred to as a *glycylcycline*. It differs from other tetracyclines in that it is effective against many organisms resistant to others in its class. It is indicated for the treatment of complicated skin and skin structure infections caused by susceptible organisms, including MRSA and vancomycin-sensitive *Enterococcus faecalis*, and for the treatment of complicated intraabdominal infections and community-associated pneumonia. Tigecycline is given by injection only. Nausea and vomiting are the most common adverse effects, occurring in 20% to 30% of patients.

Pharmacokinetics: Tigecycline

Route	Onset of Action	Peak Plasma Concentration	Elimination Half-life	Duration of Action
IV	Immediate	Immediate after infusion	27 hr	12 hr

The remaining antibiotic classes are discussed in Chapter 39.

NURSING PROCESS

ASSESSMENT

In general, before the administration of any *antibiotic*, it is crucial to gather data regarding a history of or symptoms indicative of hypersensitivity or allergic reactions (from mild reactions with rash, pruritus, or hives to severe reactions with laryngeal edema, bronchospasm, hypotension, and possible cardiac arrest). Additionally it is important to determine the patient's age, weight, and baseline vital signs with body temperature. Examine the results of any laboratory tests that have been ordered, such as liver function studies (AST and ALT levels), kidney function studies (usually BUN and creatinine levels), cardiac function studies (pertinent laboratory tests, electrocardiogram), ultrasonography (if indicated), culture and sensitivity tests, CBC, and platelet and clotting tests. Obtain specimens for cultures before beginning antibiotic therapy. Assess intake and output measurements, if appropriate (e.g., more than 30 mL/hr or 600 mL/day or 0.5 mL/kg/hr as per institutional protocol). Record baseline neurologic assessment findings because of the possibility of adverse effects impacting the central nervous system by various antibiotics. Assess bowel sounds and bowel patterns/habits because of potential antibiotic-related gastrointestinal tract adverse effects. Further assessment needs include thorough checking for contraindications, cautions, and drug interactions. Obtain a complete list of all the patient's medications, including prescribed and over-the-counter drugs, herbals, and dietary supplements. Cultural assessment is also important because of the well-documented research on variations in response among different racial and ethnic groups as well as some patients' use of folk remedies or alternative therapies to try and alleviate infections. Assess learning preparedness, willingness to learn, and educational level because of the importance of patient education to safe medication administration. Note baseline findings from assessment of the oral mucosa, respiratory tract, gastrointestinal tract, and genitourinary tract because of the risk for superinfection in these areas. Superinfections are often evidenced by fever, lethargy, mouth sores, perineal itching, and other system-related symptoms. Because antibiotic resistance is so prevalent, pose questions about long-term use, overuse, or abuse of antibiotics to the patient or caregiver. Assessment information related to each group of antibiotics is presented in the following paragraphs.

For patients taking *sulfonamides*, perform a careful assessment for drug allergies to sulfa-type drugs and/or sulfites such as the sulfonylurea, oral antidiabetic drugs, and thiazide diuretics (see the pharmacology discussion). Assess for potential drug interactions. Perform a thorough skin assessment before and during drug therapy because of the potential for occurrence of the adverse effect of Stevens-Johnson syndrome (see Table 38-2). Assess complete blood cell count before beginning sulfonamide therapy because of the possibility of drug-related anemias/blood dyscrasias. With frequent or long-term therapy, assess renal function studies such as BUN, creatinine, and urinalysis due to the potential for drug-related crystalluria. Check the patient's medication and medical history for any manifestations of G6PD and slow acetylation (see Chapters 2 and 4).

With *penicillins*, because of the high incidence of hypersensitivity, determine if there are drug allergies before initiation of therapy. Potential drug interactions are presented in Table 38-5. In addition, assess the patient for a history of asthma, sensitivity to multiple allergens, aspirin allergy, and sensitivity to cephalosporins; these factors are associated with a higher risk for penicillin allergy. If *procaine penicillin* is to be given, also assess for procaine hypersensitivity. Note results of culture and sensitivity testing as soon as they are available to confirm the appropriateness of therapy. Because of possible CNS and/or GI adverse effects, complete a thorough neurologic, abdominal, and bowel assessment. Especially important for patients with electrolyte disturbances, cardiac disease, and/or renal disease is assessment of serum sodium and potassium levels, primarily because of the high sodium and potassium ion concentrations in some penicillin preparations. For example, *penicillin G* contains 1.7 mEq of potassium ion per million units and 2 mEq of sodium ion per million units. With these particular preparations, if a patient has heart failure, fluid overload, or cardiac dysrhythmias, a high sodium or potassium level (hypernatremia or hyperkalemia) could lead to exacerbation of these problems. With any dosage form of the penicillins, it is important to patient safety to assess for the possibility of an immediate, accelerated, or delayed allergic reaction. Also, assess the medication order and be aware that many times these drugs are referred to by their trade names and don't always end in *"cillin,"* such as with *Zosyn* and *Augmentin* (see the Safety and Quality Improvement: Preventing Medication Errors box on p. 607).

With *cephalosporins*, conduct a thorough assessment of allergies, including allergy to penicillins, due to the possible cross-sensitivity. Because of the similarity in their mechanism of action to penicillins, assessment data is also similar. Obtain information about the specific drug, and note the generation of cephalosporins to which it belongs. Each of the five drug generations has distinctive adverse effects and/or complications in addition to commonalities with the other groups.

Carbapenems are used when there are complicated connective tissue infections in acutely ill patients who are hospitalized. Assess patients for a history of seizure activity because of the potential seizure-type drug-induced reaction.

With *macrolides*, assessment of baseline cardiac function with documentation of vital signs is important because these drugs may lead to palpitations, chest pain, and ECG changes. Note baseline hearing status because of drug-induced hearing loss and tinnitus. Assess liver function and history of liver disease due to the potential adverse effects of hepatotoxicity. Drug interactions have been discussed previously, but special consideration should be given to concurrent use of a macrolide with warfarin, digoxin, or theophylline, resulting in possible toxicity of the latter drugs. Macrolides also reduce the effectiveness of oral contraceptives.

With *tetracyclines*, carefully assess culture and sensitivity reports as with all antibiotic therapy. There is concern regarding the use of these drugs in patients younger than 8 years of age because of the problem of permanent mottling and discoloration of the teeth. Use of these drugs in pregnancy may also pose problems for the fetus. Assess for any whitish sore patches on the oral mucosa (due to candidiasis or yeast infection) as well as any vaginal itching, pain, and/or cottage cheese–like discharge (due to vaginal candidiasis) for early identification and subsequent prompt treatment of superinfections (see previous discussion). Assess for significant drug interactions, including simultaneous use of antacids, antidiarrheal drugs, dairy products, calcium, enteral feedings, and iron preparations. These medications may lead to reduced absorption of the tetracycline. Tetracyclines may also decrease the effectiveness of oral contraceptives. Assess the patient taking oral anticoagulants more closely due to possible potentiation of bleeding.

Antiseptics and *disinfectants* are also discussed in this chapter. See Box 38-2 for a brief summary of nursing-related considerations for these agents.

NURSING DIAGNOSES

1. Noncompliance with treatment regimen related to lack of information and/or inability to pay for and obtain the necessary medication
2. Deficient knowledge related to lack of information about the disease process and the medication regimen
3. Risk for infection related to the patient's possible development of a compromised immune status (due to use of sulfonamides)

PLANNING: OUTCOME IDENTIFICATION

1. Patient remains compliant with the antibiotic therapy regimen taking drug for the full duration of treatment and as prescribed.
2. Patient demonstrates an increase in knowledge and information about the disease process and related drug therapy with explanation of adverse effects.
3. Patient maintains homeostasis and a healthy immune system and is free of signs and symptoms of infection.

IMPLEMENTATION

Overall nursing interventions that apply to *antibiotics* include the following: (1) Give oral antibiotics within the recommended

BOX 38-2 Brief Summary of Nursing Considerations for Antiseptics and Disinfectants

- Check for allergies to any of the chemicals or compounds contained in the antiseptic or disinfectant before use. These include alcohol, chlorine, and hydrogen peroxide.
- If the agent is iodine based (e.g., povidone-iodine), be sure to ask about any allergies to iodine or seafood. If allergies exist, then the agent must not be used. There is a higher risk for reactions to antiseptics if there have been previous allergic reactions to antibacterial topical drugs. Use of disinfectants may also be associated with allergic reactions.
- Research the product or chemical, and be aware of specific instructions and application technique.
- Always follow Standard Precautions. Dispose of any soiled bandages in a biohazard bag.
- With antiseptics, always research the product and any special application instructions or directions. If the skin is intact, nonsterile gloves are recommended for use unless otherwise indicated. If integrity is broken and the skin is not intact, use sterile gloves and/or sterile technique.
- With antiseptics, cleanse the site of any debris (e.g., pus, drainage) and any residual medication. Use normal saline or lukewarm soap and water for cleansing. Use a tongue blade, cotton-tipped applicator, or gloved finger to apply the antiseptic solution or product. Document any unusual findings at the site of use, such as swelling, redness, or drainage.
- Always follow the instructions related to each specific disinfectant agent.
- Adverse effects of antiseptics may include excessive dryness of the skin, burns to the skin or mucous membranes, blistering, and skin staining.
- Instruct patients to report any increase in redness, drainage, pain, swelling, and/or fever associated with the use of antiseptics, as deemed appropriate.

CASE STUDY

Patient-Centered Care: Antibiotic Therapy

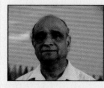

Mr. G. has been a resident of an assisted care facility since experiencing a left-sided stroke 5 years ago. Presently his cardiovascular status and cerebrovascular status are stable. However, he has had a productive cough and a low-grade fever for 2 days. After physical assessment and chest radiographic examination, the prescriber diagnoses pneumonia of the left lower lobe of the lung. The prescriber orders intravenous piperacillin/tazobactam (Zosyn) 2.25 g every 8 hours and oral theophylline (Theo-Dur) 300 mg every 12 hours. Mr. G. also takes warfarin (Coumadin) 2 mg every evening. Maalox 30 mL has been ordered as needed for GI upset, and oral ibuprofen 400 mg can be given as needed for pain. The prescriber also orders blood cultures from 2 different sites, and asks the nurse to start the antibiotic "as soon as possible."

1. Explain the rationale behind the use of tazobactam with piperacillin in Zosyn.
2. Which order will the nurse implement first? Explain your answer.
3. What concerns or drug interactions will the nurse be aware of with the use of Zosyn and the other medications ordered for Mr. G.?
4. What parameters need to be monitored to determine whether the Zosyn is working? Explain your answer.

For answers, see *http://evolve.elsevier.com/Lilley.*

time frames and fluids/foods, as indicated. (2) All medication is to be taken as ordered, for the prescribed length of time and around the clock to maintain effective blood levels unless otherwise instructed by the prescriber. (3) Doses are not to be omitted or doubled up. (4) Oral antibiotics are not to be given at the same time as antacids, calcium supplements, iron products, laxatives containing magnesium, or some of the antilipemic drugs (see pharmacology listing of drug interactions). (5) Herbal products and dietary supplements may be used only if they do not interact with the antibiotic. (6) Continually monitor for hypersensitivity reactions past the initial assessment phase because immediate reactions may not occur for up to 30 minutes, accelerated reactions may occur within 1 to 72 hours, and delayed responses may occur after 72 hours. These are characterized by wheezing; shortness of breath; swelling of the face, tongue, or hands; itching; or rash. (7) If signs of a hypersensitivity reaction occur, the first thing to do is stop the dosage form immediately (if IV, stop the infusion), contact the prescriber, and monitor the patient closely.

Sulfonamides need to be avoided in patients with G6PD and slow acetylation. Encourage an increase in fluids (2000 to 3000 mL/24 hr), preferably water, to prevent drug-related crystalluria. Oral dosage forms are to be taken with food to minimize GI upset. Encourage patients to immediately report the following to the prescriber: worsening abdominal cramps, stomach pain, diarrhea, blood in the urine, severe or worsening rash, shortness of breath, and fever. These may indicate adverse reactions to these drugs; remember that the mucocutaneous, GI, hepatic, and hematologic complications may be fatal in nature.

With *penicillins,* as with other antibiotics, the natural flora in the GI tract may be killed off by the antibiotic. Unaffected GI bacteria such as *C. difficile* may overgrow (see pharmacology discussion for more information). This process may be prevented by the consumption of probiotics, such as products containing *Lactobacillus,* supplements, or cultured dairy products like yogurt, buttermilk, and kefir. Kefir is prepared using milk from sheep, goats, and cows. Soy milk kefirs are now also commercially available. Consider the following important points when giving various penicillin formulations: (1) Advise patients to take oral penicillins with at least 6 ounces of water (not juices); juices are acidic fluids and may nullify the drug's antibacterial action. (2) *Penicillin V, amoxicillin,* and *amoxicillin/clavulanate* are given with water and 1 hour before or 2 hours after meals to maximize absorption; however, because of GI upset, these medications may need to be taken with a snack or meals. (3) *Procaine* and *benzathine salt penicillins* are thick solutions; give them as ordered IM, using at least a 21-gauge needle, and into a large muscle mass, rotating sites as needed. (4) Reconstitute IM *imipenem/cilastin* in sterile saline, with plain lidocaine—as ordered and if the patient has no allergy to it—give into a large muscle mass. (5) With IV *penicillins* (e.g., *ampicillin*), as with any IV therapy, use the proper diluent and infuse the medication over the recommended time. Monitor the IV site frequently for swelling, tenderness, heat, redness, leaking, and pain. Calculate IV rates to deliver the prescribed amount per minute/hour. Change IV sites per institutional protocol. (6) Check for compatibilities of IV fluids and drugs prior to infusion. (7) If the patient experiences an anaphylactic reaction to a *penicillin* (or any drug), give epinephrine and other emergency drugs, as ordered. Have supportive equipment, such as oxygen, available at all times.

Orally administered *cephalosporins* may be given with food to decrease GI upset. Alcohol and alcohol-containing products are to be avoided due to the potentiation of a disulfiram-like reaction (known as *acute alcohol intolerance*) with some of the cephalosporins. This may occur up to 72 hours after taking *cefotetan*. Symptoms that may occur include stomach cramping, nausea, vomiting, headache, diaphoresis, pruritus, and hypotension. With the newer cephalosporins, as with many drug groups, check the drug names carefully to ensure patient safety. Many drug names sound alike, potentially leading to medication errors.

Macrolides need to be administered with the same precautions as used with other antibiotics. Macrolides are *not* to be given with or immediately before or after fruit juices to avoid interaction with the drug. Inform the patient about the many drug interactions (discussed in the pharmacology section), including those with over-the-counter drugs, herbal products, and dietary supplements. Encourage patients to report the following to their prescriber immediately: chest pain, palpitations, dizziness, jaundice, rash, and hearing loss.

Tetracyclines cause photosensitivity, so advise the patient to take precautions to avoid sun exposure and tanning bed use. Encourage the patient to take oral doses with at least 8 ounces of fluids and food to minimize GI upset. However, warn the patient *not* to take tetracyclines with calcium, magnesium, and iron. These chemicals *chelate* or bind with the tetracycline, leading to a significant reduction in the oral absorption, and thus the effectiveness, of this group of antibiotics. Therefore, concurrent use of dairy products, antacids, or iron needs to be avoided. The patient may take these interacting foods and drugs 2 hours before or 3 hours after the *tetracycline* to avoid this interaction. IV *doxycycline* is very irritating to the veins, so check the IV infusion site frequently for patency. Remember that tetracyclines can cause discoloration of the permanent teeth and tooth enamel in fetuses and children. They may also retard fetal skeletal growth if taken during pregnancy. Continually monitor for diarrhea or vaginal yeast infections due to altered intestinal and/or vaginal flora.

▌EVALUATION

Include monitoring of goals, outcome criteria, therapeutic effects, and adverse effects in the evaluation. Therapeutic effects of *antibiotics* include a decrease in the signs and symptoms of the infection; a return to normal vital signs, including temperature; negative results on culture and sensitivity tests; normal results for CBC; and improved appetite, energy level, and sense of well-being. Evaluation for adverse effects includes monitoring for specific drug-related adverse effects (see each drug profile).

▌PATIENT-CENTERED CARE: PATIENT TEACHING

- Provide the patient with a list of foods and beverages that may interact negatively with antibiotics, such as alcohol, acidic fruit juices, and dairy products.

- Advise the patient to report severe adverse effects to the prescriber and to keep any follow-up visits so that the effectiveness of therapy may be monitored. Laboratory tests (e.g., CBC) may also be performed at these visits.

- Foods that may help prevent superinfections (e.g., vaginal yeast infections) include yogurt, buttermilk, and kefir. Probiotic yogurts and/or supplements are available for reestablishing the natural flora of the GI tract while taking antibiotics.

- Educate patients who are taking oral contraceptives for birth control, about the drug interactions between them and certain antibiotics. The effectiveness of oral contraceptives may be decreased with certain antibiotics due to the interaction or from altered metabolism. Reliable backup methods of contraception must be used in addition to the oral contraceptive during antibiotic use.

- Counsel the patient to wear a medical alert bracelet or necklace at all times and to keep a medical card with diagnoses and list of medications and allergies, especially if anaphylactic in nature, on his or her person at all times.

- For *sulfonamides*, the medication is to be taken with plenty of fluids (2000 to 3000 mL/24 hr) and taken with food to decrease GI adverse effects.

- For *penicillins*, medications are to be taken exactly as prescribed and for the full duration indicated, as with all antibiotics. Doses are to be spaced at regularly scheduled intervals. Instruct the patient to take oral dosage forms with water, avoiding the following beverages: caffeine-containing beverages, citrus fruit, cola beverages, fruit juices, and tomato juice (decrease effectiveness of the antibiotic). If the patient must take a penicillin drug four times a day, encourage the patient to set up a reminder system (with cell phone alarms or a watch) so that blood levels remain steady.

- For *cephalosporins*, advise the patient to report unresolved GI upset, such as diarrhea and nausea. Alcohol must be avoided.

- For *tetracyclines*, advise patients to avoid exposure to tanning beds and direct sunlight or to use sunscreen and/or wear protective clothing because of drug-related photosensitivity. These photosensitive effects may be noticed within a few minutes to hours after taking the drug and may last up to several days after the drug has been discontinued.

- For *macrolides*, instruct the patient to take the drug as directed, and check for interactions with other drugs being taken at the same time, especially interactions between erythromycin and other medications. For some drugs in this class (e.g., azithromycin), newer dosage forms are available in 3-day and 1-day dose packs rather than the 5-day dose pack. Always be sure that the patient knows the proper dosage and instructions for the drug the patient is taking.

KEY POINTS

- Antibiotics are either bacteriostatic or bactericidal. Bacteriostatic antibiotics inhibit the growth of bacteria but do not directly kill them. Bactericidal antibiotics directly kill the bacteria.
- Most antibiotics work by inhibiting bacterial cell wall synthesis in some way. Bacteria have survived over the ages because they can adapt to their surroundings. If a bacterium's environment includes an antibiotic, over time it can mutate in such a way that it can survive an attack by the antibiotic. The production of beta-lactamases is one way in which bacteria can fend off the effects of antibiotics.

- Be aware of the most common adverse effects of antibiotics, which include nausea, vomiting, and diarrhea. Inform patients that antibiotics should be taken for the prescribed length of time.
- Each class of antibiotics is associated with specific cautions, contraindications, drug interactions, and adverse effects that must be carefully assessed for and monitored by the nurse.
- Because normally occurring bacteria are killed during antibiotic therapy, superinfections may arise during treatment. These may be manifested by the following signs and symptoms: fever, perineal itching, oral lesions, vaginal irritation and discharge, cough, and lethargy.

NCLEX® EXAMINATION REVIEW QUESTIONS

1. A patient is scheduled for colorectal surgery tomorrow. He does not have sepsis, his WBC count is normal, he has no fever, and he is otherwise in good health. However, there is an order to administer an antibiotic on call before he goes to surgery. The nurse knows that the rationale for this antibiotic order is to
   a. provide empiric therapy.
   b. provide prophylactic therapy.
   c. treat for a superinfection.
   d. reduce the number of resistant organisms.

2. A teenage patient is taking a tetracycline drug as part of treatment for severe acne. When the nurse teaches this patient about drug-related precautions, which is the most important information to convey?
   a. When the acne clears up, the medication may be discontinued.
   b. This medication needs to be taken with antacids to reduce GI upset.
   c. The patient needs to use sunscreen or avoid exposure to sunlight, because this drug may cause photosensitivity.
   d. The teeth should be observed closely for signs of mottling or other color changes.

3. A newly admitted patient reports a penicillin allergy. The prescriber has ordered a second-generation cephalosporin as part of the therapy. Which nursing action is appropriate?
   a. Call the prescriber to clarify the order because of the patient's allergy.
   b. Give the medication, and monitor for adverse effects.
   c. Ask the pharmacy to change the order to a first-generation cephalosporin.
   d. Administer the drug with a nonsteroidal antiinflammatory drug to reduce adverse effects.

4. During patient education regarding an oral macrolide such as erythromycin, the nurse will include which information?
   a. If GI upset occurs, the drug will have to be stopped.
   b. The drug needs to be taken with an antacid to avoid GI problems.
   c. The patient needs to take each dose with a sip of water.
   d. The patient may take the drug with a small snack to reduce GI irritation.

5. A woman who has been taking an antibiotic for a UTI calls the nurse practitioner to complain of severe vaginal itching. She has also noticed a thick, whitish vaginal discharge. The nurse practitioner suspects that
   a. this is an expected response to antibiotic therapy.
   b. the UTI has become worse instead of better.
   c. a superinfection has developed.
   d. the UTI is resistant to the antibiotic.

6. The nurse is reviewing the orders for wound care, which include use of an antiseptic. Which statements best describe the use of antiseptics? (Select all that apply.)
   a. Antiseptics are appropriate for use on living tissue.
   b. Antiseptics work by sterilizing the surface of the wound.
   c. Antiseptics are applied to nonliving objects to kill microorganisms.
   d. The patient's allergies must be assessed before using the antiseptic.
   e. Antiseptics are used to inhibit the growth of microorganisms on the wound surface.

7. The order for a child reads: "Give cefoxitin (Mefoxin) 160 mg/kg/day, IVPB, divided into doses given every 6 hours." The child weighs 55 lb. How much will the patient receive each day? For each dose?

8. The nurse is reviewing the orders for a patient who has been admitted for treatment of pneumonia. The antibiotic orders include an order for doxycycline. However, when the patient is asked about his allergies, he lists "doxycycline" as one of his allergies. What is the nurse's priority action at this time?
   a. Call the prescriber to clarify the order because of the patient's allergy.
   b. Ask the patient to explain what happened when he had the allergic reaction.
   c. Ask the pharmacy to order a different antibiotic.
   d. Administer the drug with an antihistamine to reduce adverse effects.

1. b, 2. c, 3. a, 4. d, 5. c, 6. a, d, e, 7. 4000 mg/day; 1000 mg/dose, 8. b.

CRITICAL THINKING AND PRIORITIZATION QUESTIONS

1. The nurse is reviewing the medications that are due this morning for a patient and notes the following orders:
   doxycycline, 200 mg, PO every morning
   multivitamin with iron, 1 tablet, PO every morning
   Mylanta, 30 mL, PO, twice a day
   What is the nurse's priority action when considering whether these medications can be given together?

2. A 79-year-old patient has been admitted for treatment of osteomyelitis. His orders include IV imipenem/cilastatin, oral lisinopril, oral phenytoin, and a prn order for acetaminophen for a temperature over 101° F (38.3° C) or for pain. The nurse is reviewing the patient's history and new orders. After reviewing the orders, what is the first action the nurse will take?

For answers see *http://evolve.elsevier.com/Lilley.*

Antibiotics Part 2

http://evolve.elsevier.com/Lilley

OBJECTIVES

When you reach the end of this chapter, you will be able to do the following:

1. Review the general principles of antibiotic therapy and all of the antibiotics covered previously in Chapter 38 in preparation for discussion of the following antibiotics or antibiotic classes: aminoglycosides, quinolones, clindamycin, metronidazole, nitrofurantoin, vancomycin, and several other miscellaneous antibiotics.
2. Describe the advantages and disadvantages associated with the use of antibiotics, including overuse and abuse of

antibiotics, development of drug resistance, superinfections, and antibiotic-associated colitis.
3. Discuss the indications, cautions, contraindications, mechanisms of action, adverse effects, toxic effects, routes of administration, and drug interactions for the aminoglycosides, fluoroquinolones, clindamycin, metronidazole, nitrofurantoin, vancomycin, and miscellaneous antibiotics.
4. Develop a nursing care plan that includes all phases of the nursing process for the patient receiving antibiotics.

DRUG PROFILES

amikacin, p. 627
♦ ciprofloxacin, p. 630
♦ clindamycin, p. 630
colistimethate, p. 630
daptomycin, p. 631
♦ gentamicin, p. 627
levofloxacin, p. 630
linezolid, p. 630
♦ metronidazole, p. 632

neomycin, p. 628
nitrofurantoin, p. 632
telavancin, p. 633
tobramycin, p. 628
♦ vancomycin, p. 633

_____

♦ = *Key drug*
! = *High-alert drug*

KEY TERMS

Carbapenem-resistant Enterobacteriaceae (CRE) refers to bacteria that possess an enzyme, carbapenemase, which renders the organism resistant to all carbapenem antibiotics as well as beta-lactam antibiotics and monobactams. Such organisms produce a very serious resistant infection. CRE used to be known as *Klebsiella pneumoniae* carbapenemase (KPC). (p. 624)

Concentration-dependent killing A property of some antibiotics, especially aminoglycosides, whereby achieving high plasma drug concentrations, even if briefly, results in the most effective bacterial kill (compare *time-dependent killing*). (p. 625)

Extended-spectrum beta-lactamases (ESBLs) A group of beta-lactamase enzymes produced by some organisms that makes the organism resistant to all beta-lactam antibiotics (penicillins and cephalosporins) and aztreonam. Patients who are infected by such organisms must be in contact isolation; proper handwashing is key to preventing the spread of these organisms. (p. 624)

Methicillin-resistant *Staphylococcus aureus* (MRSA) A strain of *Staphylococcus aureus* that is resistant to the beta-lactamase penicillin known as *methicillin*. Originally, the abbreviation MRSA referred exclusively to methicillin-resistant *S. aureus*. It is now used more commonly to refer to strains of *S. aureus* that are resistant to several drug classes, and therefore, depending on the context or health care institution, it may also stand for "multidrug-resistant *S. aureus*." (p. 624)

Microgram One millionth of a gram. Be careful not to confuse it with milligram (one thousandth of a gram), which is one thousand times greater than 1 microgram. Confusion of these two units sometimes results in drug dosage errors. (p. 625)

Minimum inhibitory concentration (MIC) A laboratory measure of the lowest concentration of a drug needed to kill a certain standardized amount of bacteria. (p. 625)

Multidrug-resistant organisms Bacteria that are resistant to one or more classes of antimicrobial drugs. These include multidrug-resistant *Staphylococcus aureus,* extended-spectrum beta-lactamase–producing organisms, and carbapenemase-resistant enterobacteriaceae. (p. 624)

Nephrotoxicity Toxicity to the kidneys, often drug induced and manifesting as compromised renal function; usually reversible upon withdrawal of the offending drug. (p. 625)

Ototoxicity Toxicity to the ears, often drug induced and manifesting as varying degrees of hearing loss that is likely to be permanent. (p. 625)

Postantibiotic effect A period of continued bacterial suppression that occurs after brief exposure to certain antibiotic drug classes, especially aminoglycosides (discussed in this chapter) and carbapenems (see Chapter 38). The mechanism of this effect is uncertain. (p. 626)

Pseudomembranous colitis A necrotizing inflammatory bowel condition that is often associated with antibiotic therapy. Some antibiotics (e.g., clindamycin) are more likely to produce it than others. More commonly referred to as *antibiotic-associated colitis* or *Clostridium difficile diarrhea* or *C. difficile infection.* (p. 630)

Synergistic effect Drug interaction in which the bacterial killing effect of two antibiotics given together is greater than the sum of the individual effects of the same drugs given alone. (p. 626)

Therapeutic drug monitoring Ongoing monitoring of plasma drug concentrations and dosage adjustment based on these values as well as other laboratory indicators such as kidney and liver function test results; it is often carried out by a pharmacist in collaboration with medical, nursing, and laboratory staff. (p. 625)

Time-dependent killing A property of most antibiotic classes whereby prolonged high plasma drug concentrations are required for effective bacterial kill (compare *concentration-dependent killing*). (p. 625)

Vancomycin-resistant *Enterococcus* (VRE) *Enterococcus* species that are resistant to beta-lactam antibiotics and vancomycin. Most commonly refers to *Enterococcus faecium.* (p. 624)

OVERVIEW

This chapter is a continuation of Chapter 38 and focuses on additional classes of antibiotics, which are used for more serious and harder-to-treat infections. Most of the drugs discussed in this chapter are given by the *parenteral* (injection) route only, a route generally reserved for treating more clinically serious infections. Also included are miscellaneous drugs that are unique in their class, as well as newer drugs and drug classes. This chapter also focuses on multidrug-resistant organisms, specifically **methicillin-resistant *Staphylococcus aureus* (MRSA)**, **vancomycin-resistant *Enterococcus* (VRE)**, organisms producing **extended-spectrum beta-lactamases (ESBLs)**, and **carbapenem-resistant Enterobacteriaceae (CRE)**.

PATHOPHYSIOLOGY OF RESISTANT INFECTIONS

Organisms that are resistant to one or more classes of antimicrobial drugs are referred to as **multidrug-resistant organisms**. These include MRSA, VRE, ESBL, and CRE. MRSA has been around for many years, and fortunately new antibiotics have been developed to treat MRSA. MRSA is no longer seen just in hospitals; it has spread to the community setting, and over 50% of staphylococcal infections contracted in the community involve MRSA, depending on location. Local community and hospital MRSA strains vary. VRE is usually seen in urinary tract infections. Some newer antibiotics have been developed to successfully treat VRE, as well as MRSA. Unfortunately, ESBL and CRE are the newest players in this saga. Organisms that produce ESBL are resistant to all beta-lactam antibiotics and

aztreonam, and can be treated only with carbapenems or sometimes quinolones. In our noble effort to treat infection with ESBL-producing organisms, the use of carbapenems increased, and unfortunately in response, bacteria created a new means of resistance, namely, the ability to produce the enzyme carbapenemase, which renders all carbapenems ineffective. When patients become infected with CRE, there are only two known antibiotics that can be used, tigecycline and colistimethate. Reports of resistance to these antibiotics have been described, which leaves the patient untreatable. Multidrug-resistant organisms are one of the world's top health problems. When patients become infected with such an organism, they must be placed in contact isolation. Many hospitals are placing all patients infected with CRE in one area, and some hospitals have been shut down due to this organism. Proper handwashing is of the utmost importance. These organisms are spread by contact, so all health care professionals must wash their hands before and after all patient contact. The importance of handwashing cannot be overemphasized. Some research indicates that patterns of antibiotic resistance for a certain class of antibiotics are influenced by the prescription of antibiotics in other, previously-assumed unrelated classes. (For example, quinolone use may influence the emergence of resistance to other antibiotic classes.) Box 39-1 lists the current treatment choices of resistant infections.

AMINOGLYCOSIDES

The aminoglycosides are a group of natural and semisynthetic antibiotics that are classified as bactericidal drugs (see Chapter 38). They are potent antibiotics, which makes aminoglycosides the drugs of choice for the treatment of particularly virulent

BOX 39-1   Selected Resistant Infections and Selected Antibiotic Treatment

Infection	Treatment
MRSA	Vancomycin, daptomycin, linezolid, tedizolid, televancin, ortivancin, dalbavancin, ceftaroline (see Chapter 38)
VRE	Daptomycin, linezolid, tedizolid
ESBL	Carbapenems (see Chapter 38)
CRE	Colistin, tigecycline (see Chapter 38)

MRSA, Methicillin-resistant *Staphylococcus aureus; VRE,* vancomycin-resistant *Enterococcus; ESBL,* extended-spectrum beta-lactamase; *CRE,* carbapenemase-resistant *Enterobacteriaceae.*

TABLE 39-1   Aminoglycoside Antibiotics

Serum Drug Levels	PEAK		TROUGH	
	Multiple Daily Dosing*	Once-Daily Dosing	Multiple Daily Dosing	Once-Daily Dosing
amikacin	15-30 mcg/mL†	Usually not measured	5-10 mcg/mL	Less than 10 mcg/mL
gentamicin and tobramycin	4-10 mcg/mL	Usually not measured	1-2 mcg/mL	Less than 1 mcg/mL

*q8h or q12h.

†*mcg,* **microgram**; note that 1 microgram = 1/1000 (one thousandth) of a milligram or 1/1,000,000 (one millionth) of a gram. Also note that microgram is abbreviated *mcg,* while milligram is abbreviated *mg.*

infections. The commonly used aminoglycoside antibiotics are listed in Table 39-1. These drugs can be given by several different routes, but they are not given orally because of their poor oral absorption. An exception to this is neomycin (see the Drug Profiles section later in the chapter). The three aminoglycosides most commonly used for the treatment of systemic infections are amikacin, gentamicin, and tobramycin. Serum levels of these drugs are routinely monitored in patients' blood samples. Dosages are adjusted to maintain known optimal levels that maximize drug efficacy and minimize the risk for toxicity. This process is known as **therapeutic drug monitoring.** Aminoglycoside therapy is monitored in this way due to the **nephrotoxicity** and **ototoxicity** associated with these drugs. Most commonly, dosing is adjusted to the patient's level of renal function, based on estimates of creatinine clearance calculated from serum creatinine values. This task is often carried out by a hospital pharmacist, consulting for the prescriber. Not only are serum levels measured to prevent toxicity, but it has been shown that for the aminoglycosides to be effective, the serum level needs to be at least eight times higher than the **minimum inhibitory concentration (MIC).** The MIC for any antibiotic is a measure of the lowest concentration of drug needed to kill a certain standard amount of bacteria. This value is determined *in vitro* (in the laboratory) for each drug. It has been shown that other classes of antibiotics, such as beta-lactams, act through **time-dependent killing,** that is, the amount of time

the drug is above the MIC is critical for maximal bacterial kill. However, aminoglycosides work primarily through **concentration-dependent killing;** that is, achieving a drug plasma concentration that is a certain level above the MIC, even for a brief period, results in the most effective bacterial kill. For this reason, although these drugs were originally given in three daily intravenous doses, the current predominant practice is once-daily aminoglycoside dosing. Dosages of 5 to 7 mg/kg/day of gentamicin or tobramycin are used, and doses of 15 mg/kg of amikacin are used. Several clinical studies have shown that once-daily dosing provides a sufficient plasma drug concentration for bacterial kill, along with equal or lower risk for toxicity compared with multiple daily dosing regimens. Use of a once-daily regimen instead of the traditional three-times–daily regimen also reduces the nursing care time required and often allows for outpatient or even home-based aminoglycoside drug therapy.

Peak (highest) drug levels for once-daily regimens are usually not measured, as it is assumed that the peak level for a single daily dose will be short lived and will drop within a reasonable time frame. However, trough (lowest) levels are routinely measured to ensure adequate renal clearance of the drug and avoid toxicity. For dosage information on selected aminoglycosides, see the table on p. 627. Dosage regimens and ranges for serum levels may vary for different health care institutions.

With once-daily dosing, the blood sample for trough measurement is drawn at least 8 to 12 hours after completion of dose administration. The therapeutic goal is a trough concentration at or below 1 mcg/mL (which is considered undetectable for gentamicin and tobramycin). Trough levels above 2 mcg/mL are associated with a greater risk for both *ototoxicity* and *nephrotoxicity.* Ototoxicity (toxicity to the ears) often manifests as some degree of temporary or permanent hearing loss. Nephrotoxicity (toxicity to the kidneys) manifests as varying degrees of reduced renal function. This is generally indicated by laboratory test results such as serum creatinine level. A rising serum creatinine level suggests reduced creatinine clearance by the kidneys and is indicative of declining renal function. Trough levels are normally monitored initially, and then once every 5 to 7 days until drug therapy is discontinued. The patient's serum creatinine level is measured at least every 3 days as an index of renal function, and drug dosages are adjusted as needed for any changes in renal function.

Traditional dosing of aminoglycosides (i.e., three times a day) can still be used. When an aminoglycoside is given in this manner, both peak and trough levels are measured. Samples for measurement of peak levels are drawn 30 minutes after a 30-minute infusion, and samples for measurement of trough levels are drawn just before the next dose. Pharmacists can adjust the dose based on a pharmacokinetic evaluation of these levels. When the drug is given in the traditional manner, the desired peak levels vary depending on the type of organism and the site of infection. Higher levels are needed when treating pneumonia, as opposed to treating a urinary tract infection. Because the aminoglycosides are eliminated by the kidney, the drug concentrates in the urine, so lower dosages can be used to treat urinary tract infections. Regardless of the infection being treated, however, it is desirable to keep gentamicin and tobramycin trough levels below 2 mcg/mL. Table 39-1 lists the traditional desired drug levels for these drugs.

Mechanism of Action and Drug Effects

Aminoglycosides work in a way that is similar to that of the tetracyclines in that they bind to ribosomes, specifically the 30S ribosome, and thereby prevent protein synthesis in bacteria (see Figure 38-3). Aminoglycosides are most often used in combination with other antibiotics such as beta-lactams or vancomycin in the treatment of various infections, because the combined effect of the two antibiotics is greater than the sum of the effects of each drug acting separately. This is known as a synergistic effect. When aminoglycosides are used in combination with beta-lactam antibiotics (i.e., penicillins, cephalosporins, monobactams [see Chapter 38]), the beta-lactam antibiotic is given first. This is because the beta-lactams break down the cell wall of the bacteria and allow the aminoglycoside to gain access to the ribosomes where they work. Aminoglycosides also have a property known as the postantibiotic effect. This is a period of continued bacterial growth suppression that occurs *after* short-term antibiotic exposure, as in once-daily aminoglycoside dosing (see earlier). Carbapenems are another antibiotic class with a postantibiotic effect. The postantibiotic effect is enhanced with higher peak drug concentrations and concurrent use of beta-lactam antibiotics.

As is the case with most antibiotic drug classes, various bacterial mechanisms of resistance to aminoglycosides have emerged among both gram-positive and gram-negative species previously more susceptible to these drugs. The prevalence and strength of such resistance varies for different drugs, organisms, patient populations, disease states, and geographic prescribing patterns. Amikacin is generally reserved for resistant infections.

Indications

The toxicity associated with aminoglycosides limits their use to treatment of serious gram-negative infections and specific conditions involving gram-positive cocci, in which case gentamicin is usually given in combination with a penicillin. Gram-negative infections commonly treated with aminoglycosides include those caused by *Pseudomonas* species (spp.) and several organisms belonging to the Enterobacteriaceae family (facultatively anaerobic gram-negative rods), including *Escherichia coli*, *Proteus* spp., *Klebsiella* spp., *Serratia* spp., and *acinetobacter* spp. Such infections are often treated with a suitable aminoglycoside and an extended-spectrum penicillin, third-generation cephalosporin, or carbapenem. Gram-positive infections treated with aminoglycosides may include infections due to *Enterococcus* spp. and *S. aureus,* and bacterial endocarditis, which is usually streptococcal in origin. A regimen of three daily doses is more common when treating gram-positive infections, because this often enhances synergy with other antibiotics that are used. Aminoglycosides are never used alone to treat gram-positive infections. Aminoglycosides are also used for prophylaxis in procedures involving the gastrointestinal (GI) or genitourinary (GU) tract, because such procedures carry a high risk for

TABLE 39-2 Aminoglycosides: Comparative Spectra of Antimicrobial Activity	
Aminoglycoside	**Spectrum of Activity**
amikacin	*Acinetobacter* spp., *Enterobacter aerogenes*, *Escherichia coli*, *Klebsiella pneumoniae*, *Proteus* spp., *Providencia* spp., *Pseudomonas* spp., *Serratia* spp., Staphylococcus
gentamicin	*E. aerogenes*, *E. coli*, *K. pneumoniae*, *Proteus* spp., *Pseudomonas* spp., *Salmonella* spp., *Serratia* spp. (nonpigmented), *Shigella* spp.
neomycin	Toxicity limits use to gastrointestinal tract (hepatic coma, *E. coli* diarrhea, and antisepsis) and as a topical antibacterial
streptomycin	*Klebsiella granulomatis* (granuloma inguinale), *Yersinia pestis* (plague), *Francisella tularensis* (tularemia), *Mycobacterium tuberculosis* (tuberculosis), *Streptococcus* spp. (nonhemolytic endocarditis)
tobramycin	*Citrobacter* spp., *Enterobacter* spp., *E. coli*, *Klebsiella* spp., *Proteus* spp., *Providencia* spp., *P. aeruginosa*, *Serratia* spp.

spp., Species.

enterococcal bacteremia. They are also commonly given in combination with either ampicillin or vancomycin (for penicillin-allergic patients) to surgical patients with a history of valvular heart disease, because diseased heart valves are also more prone to enterococcal infection.

Aminoglycosides are to be administered with caution in premature and full-term neonates. Because of the renal immaturity of these patients, prolonged actions of the aminoglycosides and a greater risk for toxicities may result. Serious pediatric infections for which aminoglycosides are used include pneumonia, meningitis, and urinary tract infections. Drug selection for both pediatric and adult patients is based on the susceptibility of the causative organism. Refer to Table 39-2 for more information on the antibacterial spectra of specific aminoglycosides. A few aminoglycosides have more specific indications. Streptomycin is active against *Mycobacterium* spp. (see Chapter 41), whereas paromomycin is used to treat amebic dysentery, a protozoal intestinal disease (see Chapter 43). Aminoglycosides are inactive against fungi, viruses, and most anaerobic bacteria.

Contraindications

The only usual contraindication is known drug allergy. The pregnancy categories of these drugs range from C to D. Aminoglycosides have been shown to cross the placenta and cause fetal harm when administered to pregnant women. There have been several case reports of total irreversible bilateral congenital deafness in the children of women receiving aminoglycosides during pregnancy. Therefore, aminoglycosides are used in pregnant women only in the event of life-threatening infections when safer drugs are ineffective. These drugs are also distributed in breast milk. They should not be used by lactating women to avoid the risk for drug toxicity in nursing infants.

Adverse Effects

Aminoglycosides are very potent antibiotics and are capable of potentially serious toxicities, especially to the kidneys (nephrotoxicity) and to the ears (ototoxicity), in which they can affect hearing and balance functions. Duration of drug therapy needs to be as short as possible, based on sound clinical judgment and monitoring of the patient's progress. Nephrotoxicity typically occurs in 5% to 25% of patients and is usually manifested by urinary casts (visible remnants of destroyed renal cells), proteinuria, and increased blood urea nitrogen (BUN) and serum creatinine levels. It is usually reversible, but the patient's renal function test results must be monitored throughout therapy. In contrast, ototoxicity is less common, occurring in 3% to 14% of patients, and often is not reversible. It can result in varying degrees of permanent hearing loss, depending on the dosage and duration of drug therapy. It is believed to result from injury to the eighth cranial nerve (CN VIII, also called the *cochleovestibular nerve* or *auditory nerve*) and involves both cochlear damage (hearing loss) and vestibular damage (disrupted sense of balance). Symptoms include dizziness, tinnitus, a sense of fullness in the ears, and hearing loss. Other less common effects include headache, paresthesia, vertigo, skin rash, fever, overgrowth of nonsusceptible organisms, and neuromuscular paralysis (very rare and reversible). The risk for these toxicities is greatest in patients with preexisting renal impairment, patients already receiving other renally toxic drugs, and patients receiving high-dose or prolonged aminoglycoside therapy.

Interactions

The risk for nephrotoxicity can be increased with concurrent use of other nephrotoxic drugs such as vancomycin, cyclosporine, and amphotericin B. Concurrent use with loop diuretics increases the risk for ototoxicity. In addition, because aminoglycosides, like many other antibiotics, kill intestinal bacterial flora, they also reduce the amount of vitamin K produced by these gut bacteria. These normal flora normally serve to balance the effects of oral anticoagulants such as warfarin (Coumadin). Therefore, aminoglycosides can potentiate warfarin toxicity. Concurrent use with neuromuscular blocking drugs may prolong the duration of action of the neuromuscular blockade.

Dosages

For dosages information on selected aminoglycosides, see the table on this page.

DRUG PROFILES

Historically, the aminoglycoside antibiotics were used primarily to treat gram-negative infections. However, they are now used as a synergistic drug in the treatment of gram-positive infections as well. They are normally given intravenously or intramuscularly, but neomycin is administered only orally, rectally, or topically. Topical dosage forms of both gentamicin and tobramycin are also available for dermatologic (see Chapter 56)

DOSAGES

Selected Aminoglycosides*

Drug (Pregnancy Category)	Usual Adult Dosage Range	Indications/Uses
amikacin (generic only) (D)	IV: 15 mg/kg/day divided 2-3 times daily or 15-20 mg/kg once daily	Primarily infection with gentamicin- and tobramycin-resistant gram-negative organisms along with severe staphylococcal infections
◆ gentamicin (generic only) (C)	IV/IM: 3-5 mg/kg/day (frequency depends on renal function)	Primarily gram-negative infections along with severe staphylococcal infections
neomycin (C)	PO/PR: 4-12 g/day in divided doses	Preoperative bowel cleansing (also used with different dosage regimens for hepatic encephalopathy)
tobramycin (generic, TOBI) (D)	IV/IM: 3-6 mg/kg/day (frequency depends on renal function)	Primarily gram-negative infections along with severe staphylococcal infections

*Dosing and frequency vary depending on the age of the patient.

and ophthalmic (see Chapter 57) use. Currently available aminoglycosides include amikacin, gentamicin, kanamycin, neomycin, streptomycin, and tobramycin. Dosage and other information are given in the table above.

amikacin

Amikacin is a semisynthetic aminoglycoside antibiotic that is often used to treat infections that are resistant to gentamicin or tobramycin. It is available only in injectable form.

Pharmacokinetics: Amikacin

Route	Onset of Action	Peak Plasma Concentration	Elimination Half-life	Duration of Action
IV	Variable	1 hr	2-3 hr	8-12 hr
IM	Variable	30 min-2 hr	2-3 hr	8-12 hr

◆ gentamicin

Gentamicin can be given either intravenously or intramuscularly, and the dosage is the same for both routes. It is indicated for the treatment of infection with several susceptible gram-positive and gram-negative bacteria. Gentamicin is available in several dosage forms, including injections, topical ointments, and ophthalmic drops and ointments.

Pharmacokinetics: Gentamicin

Route	Onset of Action	Peak Plasma Concentration	Elimination Half-life	Duration of Action
IV	Variable	30 min	2-3 hr	Up to 24 hr
IM	Variable	30-90 min	2-3 hr	Up to 24 hr

tobramycin

Tobramycin has dosages, routes of administration, and indications that are comparable to those for gentamicin for generalized infections. In addition, it is commonly used to treat recurrent pulmonary infections in patients with cystic fibrosis by both injectable and inhaled dosing. It is also available in topical and ophthalmic dosage forms.

Pharmacokinetics: Tobramycin

Route	Onset of Action	Peak Plasma Concentration	Elimination Half-life	Duration of Action
IV	Variable	30 min	2-3 hr	Up to 24 hr
IM	Variable	30-90 min	2-3 hr	Up to 24 hr

neomycin

Neomycin is most commonly used for bacterial decontamination of the GI tract before surgical procedures, and it is given both orally and rectally (as an enema) for this purpose. Other uses include topical application for skin infections, bladder irrigation, and treatment of *E. coli* diarrhea, hepatic encephalopathy, and eye infections. In hepatic encephalopathy, the drug helps reduce the number of ammonia-producing bacteria in the GI tract. The subsequent reduced blood ammonia levels sometimes result in improvement of neurologic symptoms of the hepatic illness. This drug is not available in injectable form but instead is available in tablets, solutions, and powders for oral, topical, or irrigation administration.

Pharmacokinetics: Neomycin

Route	Onset of Action	Peak Plasma Concentration	Elimination Half-life	Duration of Action
PO	Variable	1-4 hr	3 hr	Up to 24 hr

QUINOLONES

Quinolones, sometimes referred to as *fluoroquinolones,* are very potent bactericidal broad-spectrum antibiotics. Currently available quinolone antibiotics include norfloxacin, ciprofloxacin, levofloxacin, moxifloxacin, and gemifloxacin. With the exception of norfloxacin, these antibiotics have excellent oral absorption. In most cases, the extent of oral absorption is comparable to that of intravenous injection.

Mechanism of Action and Drug Effects

Quinolone antibiotics destroy bacteria by altering their deoxyribonucleic acid (DNA) (see Figure 38-3). They accomplish this by interfering with the bacterial enzymes DNA gyrase and topoisomerase IV. Quinolones do not inhibit the production of human DNA.

The quinolones kill susceptible strains of mostly gram-negative and some gram-positive organisms. Some quinolones are also believed to diffuse into and concentrate themselves in human neutrophils, killing bacteria such as *S. aureus, Serratia marcescens,* and *Mycobacterium fortuitum* that sometimes accumulate in these cells. Bacterial resistance to quinolone antibiotics has been identified among several bacterial species, including *Pseudomonas aeruginosa, S. aureus, Pneumococcus* spp., *Enterococcus* spp., and the broad Enterobacteriaceae family that includes *E. coli.*

Indications

Quinolones are active against a wide variety of gram-negative and selected gram-positive bacteria, although resistance is becoming common. Most are excreted primarily by the kidneys as unchanged drug. This characteristic, together with the fact that they have extensive gram-negative coverage, makes them suitable for treating complicated urinary tract infections. They are also commonly used to treat respiratory, skin, GI, and bone and joint infections.

Ciprofloxacin (Cipro) was the first quinolone to enjoy widespread use. Resistance was soon seen in *Pseudomonas* and some *Streptococcus* spp. Ciprofloxacin and levofloxacin are available both orally and by injection and are both available in generic form, which means that it costs significantly less than brand name quinolones. Levofloxacin (Levaquin) is somewhat more active than ciprofloxacin against gram-positive organisms such as *Streptococcus pneumoniae,* including penicillin-resistant strains, as well as *Enterococcus* and *S. aureus.* Moxifloxacin is also effective against *S. pneumoniae* as well as some strains of *S. aureus* and enterococci. However, MRSA and VRE are generally also resistant to moxifloxacin. The activity of moxifloxacin against many enteric gram-negative bacteria and *P. aeruginosa* is similar to that of levofloxacin and less than that of ciprofloxacin. Moxifloxacin often has stronger anaerobic bacterial coverage. Norfloxacin has limited oral absorption and is available only in oral form, and its use is limited to GU tract infections. Quinolones are often combined with aminoglycosides to treat *P. aeruginosa* infections. Moxifloxacin also has some *in vitro* activity against anaerobes.

The use of quinolones in prepubescent children is not generally recommended, because these drugs have been shown to affect cartilage development in laboratory animals. However, more recent evidence suggests that judicious use in children might be less of a risk than previously thought, and in fact these drugs are used commonly in children with cystic fibrosis. Box 39-2 lists selected microbes commonly susceptible to quinolone

---

BOX 39-2   Overview of Quinolone-Susceptible Organisms

- Gram-positive: Streptococcus (including *Streptococcus pneumoniae*), Staphylococcus, Enterococcus, *Listeria monocytogenes*
- Gram-negative: *Neisseria gonorrhea, Neisseria meningitidis, Haemophilus influenzae, Haemophilus parainfluenzae,* Enterobacteriaceae (including *Escherichia coli, Enterobacter, Klebsiella, Proteus mirabilis, Salmonella, Shigella*), Acinetobacter, *Pseudomonas aeruginosa**, *Pasteurella multocida, Legionella, Mycoplasma pneumoniae,* Chlamydia
- Anaerobes: *Bacteroides fragilis,* Peptococcus, Peptostreptococcus (moxifloxacin is strongest)
- Other: Rickettsia (ciprofloxacin only)

*Most pseudomonas infections are now resistant to quinolone therapy.

therapy in general, but there is some variation in spectra among drugs. Table 39-3 gives common indications for individual drugs.

Contraindications

The only true contraindication is known drug allergy.

Adverse Effects

Quinolones are capable of causing a variety of adverse effects, the most common of which are listed in Table 39-4. Bacterial overgrowth is another possible complication of quinolone therapy, but this is more commonly associated with long-term use. More worrisome is a cardiac effect that involves prolongation of the QT interval on the electrocardiogram (ECG). Dangerous cardiac dysrhythmias are more likely to occur when quinolones are taken by patients who are also receiving class Ia and class III antidysrhythmic drugs, such as disopyramide and amiodarone. For this reason, such drug combinations are best avoided. The U.S. Food and Drug Administration requires a black box warning for all quinolones because of the increased risk for tendinitis and tendon rupture with use of these drugs. This effect is more common in older adult patients, patients with renal failure, and those receiving concurrent glucocorticoid therapy (e.g., prednisone). Central nervous system stimulation (i.e., seizures) has been reported. Quinolones can also cause peripheral neuropathy, which may be permanent. New evidence suggests that they may also cause liver injury in older adults. Quinolones must be infused over 1 to 1.5 hours.

Interactions

There are several drugs that interact with quinolones. Concurrent use of oral quinolones with antacids, calcium, magnesium, iron, zinc preparations, or sucralfate causes a reduction in the oral absorption of the quinolone. Patients need to take the interacting drugs at least 1 hour before or after taking quinolones. Dairy products also reduce the absorption of quinolones and should be separated as stated previously for interacting drugs. Enteral tube feedings can also reduce the absorption of quinolones. Probenecid can reduce the renal excretion of quinolones. Nitrofurantoin (which is discussed later in the chapter) can antagonize the antibacterial activity of the quinolones, and oral anticoagulants are to be used with

TABLE 39-3 Quinolones: Common Indications for Specific Drugs

Generic Name (Trade Name)	Antibacterial Spectrum	Common Indications
norfloxacin (Noroxin)	Extensive gram-negative and selected gram-positive coverage	Urinary tract infections, prostatitis, STIs
ciprofloxacin (Cipro)	Comparable to that of norfloxacin	Anthrax (inhalational, postexposure); respiratory, skin, urinary tract, prostate, intraabdominal, GI, bone, and joint infections; typhoid fever; selected health care–associated pneumonias
levofloxacin (Levaquin)	Comparable to that of ciprofloxacin with better gram-positive coverage	Respiratory and urinary tract infections; prophylaxis in various transrectal and transurethral prostate surgical procedures
moxifloxacin (Avelox)	Comparable to that of levofloxacin plus anaerobic coverage	Respiratory and skin infections; CAP caused by PRSP; anaerobic infections
gemifloxacin (Factive)	Comparable to ciprofloxacin	CAP, exacerbation of COPD

CAP, Community-associated pneumonia; *COPD*, chronic obstructive pulmonary disease; *PRSP*, penicillin-resistant streptococcal pneumonia; *STI*, sexually transmitted infection.

TABLE 39-4 Quinolones: Reported Adverse Effects

Body System	Adverse Effects
Central nervous	Headache, dizziness, insomnia, depression, restlessness, convulsions, neuropathy
Gastrointestinal	Nausea, constipation, increased AST and ALT levels, flatulence, heartburn, vomiting, diarrhea, oral candidiasis, dysphagia
Integumentary	Rash, pruritus, urticaria, flushing
Other	Ruptured tendons and tendonitis (black box warning added in 2008), fever, chills, blurred vision, tinnitus

ALT, Alanine aminotransferase; *AST*, aspartate aminotransferase.

DOSAGES

Selected Quinolones

Drug	Pharmacologic Class	Usual Adult Dosage Range	Indications
◆ ciprofloxacin* (Cipro) (C)	Fluoroquinolone	IV: 200-400 mg every 8-12 hr PO: 250-750 mg every 12 hr	Broad gram-positive and gram-negative coverage for infections throughout the body
levofloxacin (Levaquin) (C)		IV/PO: 250-750 mg once daily	Various susceptible bacterial infections

*Not normally recommended for children younger than 18 years of age due to finding of adverse musculoskeletal effects in studies of immature animals.

caution in patients receiving quinolones because of the antibiotic-induced alteration of the intestinal flora, which affects vitamin K synthesis.

Dosages

For dosage information on selected quinolones, see the table on the previous page.

DRUG PROFILES

◆ ciprofloxacin

Ciprofloxacin (Cipro) was one of the first of the broad-coverage, potent quinolones to become available. It was first marketed in an oral form but is also available in injectable, ophthalmic (see Chapter 57), and otic (see Chapter 58) formulations. Because of its excellent bioavailability, it can work orally as well as many intravenous antibiotics. It is capable of killing a wide range of gram-negative bacteria and is even effective against traditionally difficult-to-kill gram-negative bacteria. Ciprofloxacin can also kill some anaerobic bacteria as well as atypical organisms such as *Chlamydia*, *Mycoplasma*, and *Mycobacterium*. It is also a drug of choice for the treatment of anthrax (infection with *Bacillus anthracis*).

Pharmacokinetics: Ciprofloxacin

Route	Onset of Action	Peak Plasma Concentration	Elimination Half-life	Duration of Action
IV	30 min	1 hr	3-4.8 hr	Up to 12 hr
PO	Variable	1-2 hr	3-4.8 hr	Up to 12 hr

levofloxacin

Levofloxacin (Levaquin) is one of the most widely used quinolones. It has a broad spectrum of activity similar to that of ciprofloxacin, but it has the advantage of once-daily dosing. The oral form has excellent bioavailability. Levofloxacin is available in both oral and injectable forms.

Pharmacokinetics: Levofloxacin

Route	Onset of Action	Peak Plasma Concentration	Elimination Half-life	Duration of Action
IV	Variable	1-2 hr	6-8 hr	Up to 24 hr
PO	Variable	2 hr	6-8 hr	Up to 24 hr

MISCELLANEOUS ANTIBIOTICS

There are a number of antibiotics that do not fit into any of the previously described broad categories. Most have somewhat unique indications or are especially preferred for a particular type of infection. Although they may not be used as commonly as drugs from the other major classes, they are still of clinical importance. Several of these drugs are described individually in the following drug profiles. Dosage information for these drugs is given in the table on the next page.

DRUG PROFILES

◆ clindamycin

Clindamycin (Cleocin) is a semisynthetic antibiotic. Clindamycin can be either bactericidal or bacteriostatic (see Chapter 38), depending on the concentration of the drug at the site of infection and on the infecting bacteria. It inhibits protein synthesis in bacteria (see Figure 38-3). It is indicated for the treatment of chronic bone infections, GU tract infections, intraabdominal infections, anaerobic pneumonia, septicemia caused by streptococci and staphylococci, and serious skin and soft-tissue infections caused by susceptible bacteria. Most gram-positive bacteria, including staphylococci, streptococci, and pneumococci, are susceptible to clindamycin's actions. It also has the special advantage of being active against several anaerobic organisms and is most often used for this purpose. However, resistant strains of gram-positive, gram-negative, and anaerobic organisms do exist. Also, all *Enterobacteriaceae* are resistant to clindamycin.

Clindamycin is contraindicated in patients with a known hypersensitivity to it, those with ulcerative colitis or enteritis, and infants younger than 1 month of age. GI tract adverse effects are the most common and include nausea, vomiting, abdominal pain, diarrhea, pseudomembranous colitis, and anorexia. **Pseudomembranous colitis** (also known as antibiotic-associated colitis, *C. difficile* diarrhea, or *C. difficile* infection) is a necrotizing inflammatory bowel condition that is often associated with antibiotic therapy, especially clindamycin therapy. Clindamycin is available in oral, injectable, and topical (see Chapter 56) forms.

Clindamycin is also known to have some neuromuscular blocking properties that may enhance the actions of neuromuscular drugs (see Chapter 11). Patients receiving both drugs need to be monitored for excessive neuromuscular blockade and respiratory paralysis, and appropriate ventilatory support provided as needed.

Pharmacokinetics: Clindamycin

Route	Onset of Action	Peak Plasma Concentration	Elimination Half-life	Duration of Action
PO	30 min	45 min	2-3 hr	6 hr
IM/IV	Variable	IM: 3 hr	2-3 hr	IM: 8-12 hr

colistimethate

Colistimethate (Coly-Mycin) is a polypeptide antibiotic that penetrates and disrupts the bacterial membrane of susceptible strains of gram-negative bacteria. It is commonly referred to as *colistin*. It is an old drug that fell out of clinical use when newer, less toxic drugs became available. Unfortunately, due to the emergence of CRE infections it is now being used again, often as one of the only drugs available to treat CRE. Colistin is available for intravenous, intramuscular, and inhalational administration. It has serious adverse effects, including renal failure and neurotoxic effects such as paresthesia, numbness, tingling, vertigo, dizziness, and impairment of speech. It can cause acute respiratory failure when administered by inhalation. Colistin

DOSAGES

Selected Miscellaneous Antibiotics

Drug (Pregnancy Category)	Pharmacologic Class	Usual Adult Dosage Range	Indications
◆ clindamycin (Cleocin) (B)	Lincosamide	PO: 150-450 mg every 6 hr IV: 1.2-2.7 g/day in divided doses	Anaerobic infections; streptococcal and staphylococcal infections of bone, skin, respiratory, and GU tract
colistimethate (Colisitin) (C)	Polypeptide	2.5-5 mg/kg/day in divided doses	Treatment of CRE-producing organisms; renal and neurotoxicity common
daptomycin (Cubicin) (B)	Lipopeptide	IV: 4-6 mg/kg once daily × 7-14 days	Complicated skin and soft-tissue infections
linezolid (Zyvox) (C)	Oxazolidinone	IV/PO: 600 mg every 12 hr	VRE infections; skin and respiratory infections caused by various *Staphylococcus* and *Streptococcus* spp.
◆ metronidazole* (Flagyl) (B)	Nitroimidazole	IV/PO: 250-500 mg every 6-12 hr	Primarily anaerobic and gram-negative infections of abdominal cavity, skin, bone, and respiratory and GU tracts
nitrofurantoin (Macrodantin, Furadantin) (B)	Nitrofuran	PO: 50-100 mg qid	Primarily UTIs caused by gram-negative organisms and *Staphylococcus aureus*
quinupristin/dalfopristin (Synercid) (B)	Streptogramins	IV: 7.5 mg/kg every 8-12 hr	VRE infections; skin infections caused by streptococcal and staphylococcal infections
telavancin (Vibativ) (C)	Lipoglycopeptides	IV: 10 mg/kg/day	Serious gram-positive infections, including MRSA
◆ vancomycin (Vancocin, Vancoled) (B, oral; C injection)	Tricyclic glycopeptide	IV: 15-20 mg/kg/day (frequency dependent on renal function) PO†: 125-500 mg every 6 hr	Severe staphylococcal infections, including MRSA infections; other serious gram-positive infections, including streptococcal infections

CRE, Carbapenemase-resistant *Enterobacteriaceae*; *GU*, genitourinary; *MRSA*, methicillin-resistant *Staphylococcus aureus*; *PO*, oral; *spp.*, species; *UTI*, urinary tract infection; *VRE*, vancomycin-resistant *Enterococcus*.
*Not normally used in children except to treat amebiasis.
†Oral is not absorbed and is used only for *C. difficile* diarrhea.

crosses the placenta and needs to be used with caution in pregnant women. Colistin is infused over 3 to 5 minutes.

Pharmacokinetics: Colistimethate

Route	Onset of Action	Peak Plasma Concentration	Elimination Half-life	Duration of Action
IV	Unknown	10 min	2-3 hr	8-12 hr

daptomycin

Daptomycin (Cubicin) is currently the only drug of the new class known as *lipopeptides*. Its mechanism of action is not completely known, but it binds to gram-positive cells in a calcium-dependent process and disrupts the cell membrane potential. It is used to treat complicated skin and soft-tissue infections caused by susceptible gram-positive bacteria, including MRSA and VRE. It can also be used to treat vancomycin-intermediate or vancomycin-resistant strains of MRSA. This drug is contraindicated in cases of known drug allergy. It is available only in injectable form. Adverse reactions include hypotension or hypertension (low incidence for both), headache, dizziness, rash, GI discomfort, elevated liver enzyme levels, local injection site reaction, renal failure, dyspnea, and fungal infection. The precise mechanisms for these reactions are uncertain, but all occur in a relatively small percentage of patients (fewer than 5%). Major drug interactions have yet to

be identified; however, there is a theoretical risk for increased myopathy when daptomycin is given in conjunction with hydroxymethylglutaryl–coenzyme A (HMG-CoA) reductase inhibitors, commonly referred to as *statins*.

Pharmacokinetics: Daptomycin

Route	Onset of Action	Peak Plasma Concentration	Elimination Half-life	Duration of Action
IV	Unknown	30 min	8-9 hr	Unknown

linezolid

Linezolid (Zyvox) was the first antibacterial drug in a class of antibiotics known as oxazolidinones. This drug works by inhibiting bacterial protein synthesis. Linezolid was originally developed to treat infections associated with vancomycin-resistant *Enterococcus faecium*, more commonly referred to as VRE. VRE infection is notoriously difficult to treat and often occurs as a health care–associated infection (previously known as *nosocomial*). Linezolid is commonly used to treat health care–associated pneumonia; complicated skin and skin structure infections, including cases caused by MRSA; and gram-positive infections in infants and children. MRSA is a virulent organism and stands for "methicillin-resistant *S. aureus*." However, methicillin, a penicillinase-resistant penicillin, has recently been removed from the U.S. market. Nonetheless,

MRSA is still the term used, although oxacillin is now the test drug for this organism. To confuse things even further, oxacillin is rarely used for therapy, and nafcillin is the most commonly used drug for methicillin-susceptible *S. aureus*. MRSA is notorious for causing serious infections, especially in the hospital setting. Linezolid is also approved for treatment of community-associated pneumonia and uncomplicated skin and skin structure infections.

The most commonly reported adverse effects attributed to linezolid are headache, nausea, diarrhea, and vomiting. It has also been shown to decrease platelet count. Linezolid is contraindicated in patients with a known hypersensitivity to it. It is available in oral and injectable forms. It has excellent oral absorption, which allows patients to continue oral therapy at home for serious infections that would otherwise require hospitalization. With regard to drug interactions, linezolid has the potential to strengthen the vasopressor (prohypertensive) effects of various vasopressive drugs (see Chapter 18), such as dopamine, by an unclear mechanism. Also, there have been postmarketing case reports of this drug causing serotonin syndrome when used concurrently with serotonergic drugs such as the selective serotonin reuptake inhibitor (SSRI) antidepressants (see Chapter 16). It is recommended that the SSRI be stopped while the patient is receiving linezolid therapy; however, oftentimes this is not realistic and patients must be watched carefully for signs of serotonin syndrome. Finally, tyramine-containing foods such as aged cheese or wine, soy sauce, smoked meats or fish, and sauerkraut can interact with linezolid to raise blood pressure. A new drug, tedizolid (Sivextro), was approved in 2014. Tedizolid is similar to linezolid, and it is effective against some linezolid-resistant strains. Tedizolid is available in oral and intravenous forms and is dosed once a day.

Pharmacokinetics: Linezolid

Route	Onset of Action	Peak Plasma Concentration	Elimination Half-life	Duration of Action
PO	Variable	1-2 hr	5 hr	12 hr
IV	Variable	Immediate	6-7 hr	8-12 hr

◆ metronidazole

Metronidazole (Flagyl) is an antimicrobial drug of the class nitroimidazole. It has especially good activity against anaerobic organisms and is widely used to treat intraabdominal and gynecologic infections that are caused by such organisms. Examples of the anaerobes against which it is active are *Peptostreptococcus* spp., *Eubacterium* spp., *Bacteroides* spp., and *Clostridium* spp. Metronidazole is also indicated for the treatment of protozoal infections such as amebiasis and trichomoniasis (see Chapter 43). It works by interfering with microbial DNA synthesis, and in this regard is similar to the quinolones (see Figure 38-3). It is used orally to treat antibiotic-associated colitis; however, resistance is being noted. Metronidazole is contraindicated in cases of known drug allergy. It is available in both oral and injectable forms. Metronidazole is classified as a pregnancy category B drug, although it is not recommended for use during the first trimester of pregnancy. Adverse effects include dizziness, headache, GI discomfort, nasal congestion, and reversible neutropenia and thrombocytopenia. Drug interactions include acute alcohol intolerance when it is taken with alcoholic beverages, due to the accumulation of acetaldehyde, the principal alcohol metabolite. Patients must avoid alcohol for 24 hours before initiation of therapy and for at least 36 hours after the last dose of metronidazole. Metronidazole may also increase the toxicity of lithium, benzodiazepines, cyclosporine, calcium channel blockers, various antidepressants (e.g., venlafaxine), warfarin, and other drugs. In contrast, phenytoin and phenobarbital may reduce the effects of metronidazole. These interactions occur because of various enzymatic effects involving the cytochrome P-450 liver enzymes that result in altered drug metabolism when these drugs are taken concurrently with metronidazole.

Pharmacokinetics: Metronidazole

Route	Onset of Action	Peak Plasma Concentration	Elimination Half-life	Duration of Action
PO	Variable	1-2 hr	8 hr	Unknown
IV	Variable	1 hr	8 hr	Unknown

nitrofurantoin

Nitrofurantoin (Macrodantin) is an antibiotic drug of the class nitrofuran. It is indicated primarily for urinary tract infections caused by *E. coli, S. aureus, Klebsiella* spp., and *Enterobacter* spp. It works by interfering with the activity of enzymes that regulate bacterial carbohydrate metabolism and also by disrupting bacterial cell wall formation. It is contraindicated in cases of known drug allergy and also in cases of significant renal function impairment, because the drug concentrates in the urine. The drug is available only for oral use. Adverse effects include GI discomfort, dizziness, headache, skin reactions (mild to severe reported), blood dyscrasias, ECG changes, possibly irreversible peripheral neuropathy, and hepatotoxicity. Although hepatotoxicity is rare, it is often fatal. Interacting drugs are few and include probenecid, which can reduce renal excretion of nitrofurantoin, and antacids, which can reduce the extent of its GI absorption. The dose must be reduced for older adult patients or those with decreased renal function. Another drug that is approved for urinary tract infections is fosfomycin (Monurol). It is given as a one-time dose and maintains high concentrations in the urine for up to 48 hours.

Pharmacokinetics: Nitrofurantoin

Route	Onset of Action	Peak Plasma Concentration	Elimination Half-life	Duration of Action
PO	2.5-4.5 hr	30 min	0.5-1 hr	5-8 hr

quinupristin/dalfopristin

Quinupristin and dalfopristin (Synercid) are two streptogramin antibacterials marketed in a 30:70 fixed combination. The combination drug is approved for intravenous treatment of bacteremia and life-threatening infection caused by VRE and for treatment of complicated skin and skin structure infections caused by *S. pyogenes* and *S. aureus,* including MRSA.

Common adverse effects are arthralgias and myalgias, which may become severe. Adverse effects related to the infusion site, including pain, inflammation, edema, and thrombophlebitis, have developed in approximately 75% of patients treated through a peripheral intravenous line. The drug is contraindicated in patients with a known hypersensitivity to it. It is available only in injectable form. Drug interactions are limited, the most serious being potential increase in levels of cyclosporine. Quinupristin/dalfopristin must be infused with 5% dextrose in water (D₅W) only and cannot be mixed with saline or heparin, including heparinized flushes.

Pharmacokinetics: Quinupristin/Dalfopristin

Route	Onset of Action	Peak Plasma Concentration	Elimination Half-life	Duration of Action
IV	1-2 hr	3-4 hr	1-3 hr	8-12 hr

telavancin

Telavancin (Vibativ) is in the class called the *lipoglycopeptides.* It is indicated for the treatment of skin and skin structure infections and pneumonia caused by susceptible gram-positive organisms. It is effective against MRSA. Telavancin must not be used in pregnant women, and the dose needs to be adjusted for renal dysfunction. The most common adverse effects include renal toxicity, infusion-related reactions, and QT prolongation. Recently two new lipoglycopeptides were approved, dalbavancin (Dalvance) and oritavancin (Orbactiv) They differ from telavancin in that they are indicated only for the treatment of skin and skin structure infections caused by susceptible gram-positive organisms, including MRSA. Both of the newer agents have extremely long half-lives. Dalbavancin is dosed as a 1000 mg single dose followed by a 500 mg single dose 1 week later. Common side effects include nausea, diarrhea, and headache. Hypersensitivity reactions, elevated liver function tests and infusion reactions that resemble "red man syndrome" (see vancomycin entry that follows) can occur. Oritavancin (Orbactiv) is given as a single dose of 1200 mg IV over 3 hours. Common side effects include hypersensitivity reactions, infusion reactions, tachycardia, headache, dizziness and anemia. It is contraindicated with use of unfractionated heparin for 48 hours after oritavancin administration as it can falsely elevate aPTT. Coadministration with warfarin may increase bleed risk.

Pharmacokinetics: Telavancin

Route	Onset of Action	Peak Plasma Concentration	Elimination Half-life	Duration of Action
IV	Variable	1 hr	8-9 hr	Up to 24 hr

♦vancomycin

Vancomycin is a bactericidal antibiotic in the glycopeptide class. It destroys bacteria by binding to the bacterial cell wall, producing immediate inhibition of cell wall synthesis and death (see Figure 38-3). This mechanism differs from that of the beta-lactam antibiotics.

Vancomycin is the antibiotic of choice for the treatment of MRSA infection and infections caused by many other gram-positive bacteria. It is not active against gram-negative bacteria, fungi, or yeast. Oral vancomycin is indicated for the treatment of antibiotic-induced colitis (*Clostridium difficile*) and for the treatment of staphylococcal enterocolitis. Because the oral formulation is poorly absorbed from the GI tract, it is used for its local effects on the surface of the GI tract. The parenteral form is indicated for the treatment of bone and joint infections and bacterial bloodstream infections caused by *Staphylococcus* spp. Resistance to vancomycin has been noted with increasing frequency in patients with infections caused by *Enterococcus* organisms. These strains have been isolated most often from GI tract infections but have also been isolated from skin, soft tissue, and bloodstream infections. Resistance to MRSA has been rarely reported to occur with vancomycin.

Vancomycin is contraindicated in patients with a known hypersensitivity to it. It should be used with caution in those with preexisting renal dysfunction or hearing loss, as well as in older adult patients and neonates. Vancomycin is similar to the aminoglycosides in that there are very specific drug levels in the blood that are safe. If the levels are too low (less than 5 mcg/mL), the dosage may be subtherapeutic with reduced antibacterial efficacy. If the blood levels are too high (over 50 mcg/mL), toxicities may result, the two most severe of which are ototoxicity (hearing loss) and nephrotoxicity (kidney damage). Nephrotoxicity is more likely to occur with concurrent therapy with other nephrotoxic drugs such as aminoglycosides, cyclosporine, and contrast media used for CT scans. Vancomycin can also cause additive neuromuscular blocking effects in patients receiving neuromuscular blockers. Another common adverse effect that is bothersome, but usually not harmful, is known as *red man syndrome.* This syndrome is characterized by flushing and/or itching of the head, face, neck, and upper trunk area. It is most commonly seen when the drug is infused too rapidly. It can usually be alleviated by slowing the rate of infusion of the dose to at least 1 hour. Rapid infusions may also cause hypotension. Optimal blood levels of vancomycin are a peak level of 18 to 50 mcg/mL and a trough level of 10 to 20 mcg/mL. Measurement of peak levels is no longer routinely recommended, and only trough levels are commonly monitored. Blood samples for measurement of trough levels are drawn immediately before administration of the next dose. Because of the increase in resistant organisms, many practitioners use a trough level of 15 to 20 mcg/mL as their goal. Vancomycin must be infused over at least 60 minutes, and longer for higher doses.

Pharmacokinetics: Vancomycin

Route	Onset of Action	Peak Plasma Concentration	Elimination Half-life	Duration of Action
IV	Variable	1 hr	4-6 hr	Up to 24 hr Longer in renal dysfunction

NURSING PROCESS

ASSESSMENT

Many of the antibiotics discussed in this chapter, in contrast to those in Chapter 38, are the types of drugs that are often reserved for treatment of more potent infections and are mainly administered by parenteral routes; thus, they demand more skillful and thorough assessment of the patient and the specific drug. These antibiotics all require a critical assessment for any history of or current symptoms indicative of hypersensitivity or allergic reactions, with symptoms ranging from mild reactions with rash, pruritus, or hives to severe reactions with laryngeal edema, bronchospasm, hypotension, to possible cardiac arrest. Additional assessment includes conducting a nursing physical examination with documentation of age, weight, and baseline vital sign values. Diagnostic and laboratory studies that may be ordered include the following: (1) AST and ALT levels for assessing liver function; (2) urinalysis, BUN, and serum creatinine levels for assessing renal function; (3) ECG, echocardiography, ultrasonography, and/or cardiac enzyme levels for assessing cardiac function; (4) culture and sensitivity of infected tissue or blood samples for assessing sensitivity of the bacteria to the antibiotic; and (5) white blood cell (WBC) count, hemoglobin level, hematocrit, RBC count, platelet count, and clotting values for baseline blood count levels. In the baseline neurologic assessment, note sensory and motor intactness and/or assessment of any alterations in neurologic functioning—for example, altered sensorium and level of consciousness—because of the potential for central nervous system adverse effects. Baseline abdominal and gastrointestinal (GI) assessments are important, with a focus on bowel patterns and bowel sounds because of the possibility of GI adverse effects. Note contraindications, cautions, and drug interactions. Obtain a complete list of the patient's medications, including over-the-counter drugs, herbals, and dietary supplements. Perform a cultural assessment because of the various responses of certain racial and ethnic groups to specific drugs as well as the potential use of alternative healing practices.

With any antibiotic, assess for *superinfection,* or a secondary infection that occurs with the destruction of normal flora during antibiotic therapy (see Chapter 38). Fungal superinfections may be evidenced by fever, lethargy, perineal itching, and other anatomically related symptoms. Assess the patient's immune system status and overall condition because the patient's ability to physically resist infection may be diminished if there is a deficiency (e.g., in patients with cancer, autoimmune disorders such as lupus, acquired immunodeficiency syndrome, and any chronic illness). Antibiotic resistance is a continual concern with antibiotic drug therapy, especially in pediatrics and in large health care institutions and long-term care institutions. You must consider this possibility of resistance to certain antibiotics when assessing patients for symptoms of infection and superinfection. Furthermore, it is important to continually assess for carbapenem-resistant Enterobacteriaceae (CRE) because of the serious, resistant infection that is produced.

With *aminoglycosides,* assess for hypersensitivity and preexisting health conditions or altered neurologic and renal function. Obtain a list of all medications the patient is taking because there are numerous cautions, contraindications, and drug interactions associated with these drugs. The aminoglycosides are known for their ototoxicity and nephrotoxicity; therefore, if deemed appropriate, perform baseline hearing tests and assessment of vestibular function. Nephrotoxicity is an increased risk with the use of other nephrotoxic drugs, such as cyclosporine and the intravenous contrast used for CT scan. For patients requiring a CT scan with contrast who are also on a nephrotoxic medication, alert the prescriber to the situation so that the dose may be adjusted and additional fluids and/or medications ordered. Additionally, perform renal function studies (BUN level, urinalysis, serum and urine creatinine levels), as ordered, and document all results. If renal baseline functioning is decreased the prescriber may need to adjust the dosage amounts because of the risk for nephrotoxicity. Complete a thorough neuromuscular assessment because of the potential for drug-related neurotoxicity and higher risk for complications in those with impaired neurologic functioning. For example, patients with myasthenia gravis or Parkinson's disease may experience worsening of muscle weakness because of the drug's neuromuscular blockade. Neonates (because of the immaturity of the nervous and renal systems) and the older adult (because of decreased neurologic and renal functioning) are also at higher risk for nephrotoxicity, neurotoxicity, and ototoxicity and require careful assessment before and during drug therapy. Assess hydration status. The toxicities of these drugs are greater in patients with preexisting renal impairment, those receiving other renally toxic drugs, and those who are taking the aminoglycoside for a long period or are on high-dose therapy.

Quinolones, such as *ciprofloxacin* and *levofloxacin,* require careful assessment for preexisting central nervous system conditions (e.g., seizure or stroke disorders) that may be exacerbated by the concurrent use of these drugs. Assess for existing neuropathies because the quinolones may precipitate peripheral neuropathy. Assess for a cardiac history, and note if the patient is taking certain antidysrhythmics because of the potential for dangerous cardiac irregularities. Liver injury may occur with quinolones, so assess baseline liver function studies. Significant drug interactions include antacids, iron, zinc preparations, and sucralfate as they affect the absorption of the quinolone. Oral anticoagulants also interact with and alter the antibacterial activity of quinolones (see the pharmacology discussion).

If *clindamycin* is being used, assess for hypersensitivity to the drug or related compounds. Clindamycin is not to be used in patients with ulcerative colitis or in those younger than 1 month of age. Perform a thorough assessment of GI disorders because of the possibility of drug-induced pseudomembranous colitis, vomiting, and diarrhea (see the pharmacology discussion). Assess bowel sounds as well as bowel patterns prior to giving this drug. Preoperatively, or if the patient is in an intensive care setting and receiving clindamycin, assess for the concurrent use of neuromuscular blocking drugs because of clindamycin's excessive blockade of neuromuscular functioning and respiratory paralysis. These patients, if in need of *clindamycin*, would need ventilator support.

Linezolid is used to treat health care–associated infections, pneumonia, and complicated skin infections, including MRSA. Use of methicillin (removed from the market) and oxacillin are no longer options for treatment, so this drug offers another pharmacotherapeutic option. Assess for the concurrent use of serotonergic drugs (e.g., SSRIs [antidepressants]) because of drug-induced serotonin syndrome (see Chapter 17). Additionally, assess for intake of tyramine-containing foods (e.g., aged cheese or wine, soy sauce, and smoked fish or meat) because of the risk for elevated blood pressure.

Assess patients taking *metronidazole* for allergy to the drug and to other nitroimidazole derivatives. As with all medications, assess for contraindications, cautions, and drug interactions (see the pharmacology discussion), and document the findings. It is important for patient safety to review culture and sensitivity reports before therapy is initiated. However, it may be necessary to start the medication regimen (due to clinical presentation) prior to results being obtained and then medications can be changed as dictated by the culture and sensitivity results. Baseline assessments are needed of the neurologic system (noting any dizziness, numbness, tingling, and other sensory and motor abnormalities), GI system (checking bowel sounds, problems, and patterns), and GU system (documenting urinary patterns, color of urine, and intake and output). Inquire about alcohol intake because of the interaction of alcohol with the drug and subsequent acute alcohol intolerance. Assess for potential drug interactions, such as with benzodiazepines, calcium channel blockers, various antidepressants, and warfarin.

Assessment of drug allergies is important with *nitrofurantoin*. Renal and liver functions are also important to assess due to the possibility of hepatotoxic adverse effects and the need for a decrease in dosage amounts in the older adult patient with renal function impairment. Complete a baseline assessment of any sensory or motor problems because of the possible adverse effect of peripheral neuropathy, which may be irreversible. Assess the patient's skin color, turgor, intactness, and presence of rash due to the possibility of drug-related mild to severe skin reactions. With *quinupristin/dalfopristin*, assess vital signs as well as for any muscular aches and pains due to drug-induced arthralgia and myalgia.

With *vancomycin*, ask questions about other medications the patient is taking, especially drugs that are nephrotoxic or ototoxic. Assess the patient for a history of preexisting renal disease or hearing loss due to the possibility of nephrotoxicity or ototoxicity. Note the baseline hearing status because of the risk for hearing loss. Part of the prescriber's order will be to order trough levels of vancomycin. These labs will be drawn immediately before the next dose. Assessment of these levels is important to patient safety. Peak levels are no longer utilized. The color of the patient's skin is important to assess because of the risk for red man syndrome. This syndrome is bothersome but not usually harmful, and is characterized by flushing of the face, head, neck, and upper trunk areas. Red man syndrome is seen when infusions are administered too rapidly (see Implementation section). Assess vital signs with attention to blood pressure because too rapid infusions may precipitate hypotension. Because of multiple drug and diluent incompatibilities, as with several of the other parenteral *antibiotics* mentioned previously in this chapter, always assess for potential fluid and medication interactions.

Daptinomycin is a drug now indicated for complicated cases of skin and soft tissue infections caused by MRSA. Assess vital signs and blood pressure prior to and during infusion of this drug.

With the emergence of multidrug-resistant organisms (e.g., MRSA, VRE, and ESBL- and CRE-producing organisms), ensure that proper handwashing techniques are used by health care providers and caregivers.

Dalbavancin (Dalvance) is a newer antibiotic that is similar to telavacin (see the pharmacology section). Specifically assess the medication order for dosing information because it has a long half-life and is dosed once weekly.

CASE STUDY

Vancomycin

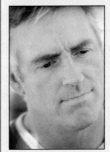

Mr. M., a 45-year-old quadriplegic, is being treated for an infected stage IV sacral pressure ulcer. The wound cultures have indicated the presence of multidrug-resistant Staphylococcus aureus (MRSA). The physician has ordered intravenous vancomycin to be given every 12 hours, application of wet-to-dry dressings (twice a day) as part of the treatment, as well as a referral to the wound care nurse. In addition, Mr. M. is placed on contact precautions because of the MRSA.

1. What will you assess before starting the vancomycin infusion?
2. Two days later, Mr. M. complains of feeling "hot" in his face and neck, and itching in those same areas. His face and neck are flushed. What do you suspect is happening?
3. What can you do to minimize complications during vancomycin infusions?
4. The physician orders measurement of vancomycin blood levels. What is the therapeutic goal when vancomycin levels are monitored?
5. What is the single best action you can take to prevent the spread of Mr. M.'s MRSA infection?

For answers, see *http://evolve.elsevier.com/Lilley*.

NURSING DIAGNOSES

1. Deficient knowledge related to lack of information and experience with the medication regimen
2. Risk for infection related to the patient's compromised immune status before and during treatment
3. Risk for injury (compromised organ function) related to adverse effects of medications (e.g., ototoxicity and nephrotoxicity), weakened physical state from infection, and not completing full therapeutic regimen.

PLANNING: OUTCOME IDENTIFICATION

1. Patient demonstrates adequate knowledge about the rationale for antibiotic therapy and the need to take the full course of antibiotics.
2. Patient remains free from infection without fever, pain, or malaise and has an improved immune status during antibiotic therapy.
3. Patient remains free from injury with minimal to no adverse effects of antibiotic therapy due to adequate dosing of antibiotics with an increase in fluids and eating yogurt and well-balanced meals.

IMPLEMENTATION

Aminoglycosides, as well as any *antibiotics,* need to be given exactly as ordered and with adequate hydration. Encourage fluid intake of up to 3000 mL/day unless contraindicated, especially with oral dosage forms. Parenteral dosage forms are the most commonly used. *Neomycin* is the only oral dosage form available for this class of antibiotic. Oral neomycin is generally used in special situations such as preoperative bowel preparation, treatment of diarrhea caused by *E. coli,* and treatment of hepatic encephalopathy. It is to be given exactly as ordered. Because of the potential for nephrotoxicity and ototoxicity, determine and monitor the patient's renal function during therapy. Dosing is adjusted based on estimates of creatinine clearance calculated from the patient's serum creatinine level. This assists in keeping a close watch on the patient's renal function and thus helps to prevent toxicity. Also monitor BUN levels and glomerular filtration rate (GFR) during therapy. Alteration in auditory, vestibular, or renal function may indicate the need for a possible dosage adjustment or withdrawal of the drug. Consumption of yogurt or buttermilk and/or probiotics may help prevent antibiotic-induced superinfections (see Chapter 38).

With *aminoglycosides,* instruct the patient to report to the prescriber any changes in hearing, ringing in the ears (tinnitus), or a full feeling in the ears. Nausea, vomiting with motion, ataxia, nystagmus, and dizziness should also be reported immediately and may indicate issues with the vestibular nerve. With ophthalmic dosage forms, redness, burning, and itching of the eyes may indicate an adverse reaction to ophthalmic forms, and redness over the skin area may indicate an adverse reaction to topical forms. Check intramuscular administration sites for induration. If noted, report it immediately to the prescriber, and do not reuse the site. Monitor intravenous sites for heat, swelling, redness, pain, or red streaking over the vein (phlebitis), and initiate measures as per institutional protocol or policy. Keep in mind the following special considerations for gentamicin: (1) Intramuscular: Give deeply and slowly into muscle mass (ventrogluteal) to minimize discomfort; and (2) Intravenous: Check for incompatibilities with other drugs, and give only clear or very slightly yellow solutions that have been diluted with either normal saline (NS) or D₅W, infusing at the correct rate.

Quinolones, as with any antibiotics that are self-administered, are to be taken exactly as prescribed and for the full course of treatment. Instruct the patient not to take these medications with antacids, iron, zinc preparations, multivitamins, or sucralfate because the absorption of the antibiotic will be decreased. If the patient needs to take calcium or magnesium, instruct the patient to take it 1 hour before or after the quinolone. Forcing of fluids is recommended, unless contraindicated. See Patient-Centered Care: Patient Teaching later in the chapter for more information.

With *clindamycin,* instruct the patient to take the medication as ordered. Oral dosage forms are to be taken with 8 ounces of water or other fluid. With topical forms, advise patients to avoid the simultaneous use of peeling or abrasive acne products, soaps, or alcohol-containing cosmetics to prevent cumulative effects; however, some products combine clindamycin with anti-acne medications (e.g., Acayna). Topical forms are to be applied in a thin layer to the affected area. Infuse intravenous dosage forms by piggyback technique and as ordered. Most references state *never* to give these drugs via parenteral intravenous push. Dilute doses of the drug, and infuse per manufacturer guidelines. Too rapid an intravenous infusion can lead to severe hypotension and possible cardiac arrest. Give intramuscular dosage forms deep into a large muscle mass (see Chapter 9).

Linezolid is generally given orally or intravenously, which makes it advantageous for those requiring an antibiotic with a spectrum similar to vancomycin for an extended period or on an outpatient basis. Oral doses are to be evenly spaced around the clock, as ordered, and given with food or milk to decrease the possibility of GI upset. Oral suspension forms must be used within 21 days of reconstitution. Protect intravenous doses from light, and infuse over 30 to 120 minutes; do not mix with any other medication. Foods that may increase blood pressure and need to be avoided while taking linezolid include aged cheeses, wine, soy sauce, smoked meats or fish, and sauerkraut due to their tyramine content. *Tedizolid (Sivextra)* is pending FDA approval, similar to linezolid, and is available in once-a-day oral or intravenous dosage forms.

Oral forms of *metronidazole* need to be given with food or meals to help decrease GI upset. Educate patients not to chew extended-release dosage forms. Alcohol is to be avoided with *metronidazole.* Intravaginal doses are recommended to be administered at bedtime. Topical creams, ointments, or lotions are to be applied thinly to the affected area. An applicator should be used for intravaginal dosages. Gloves are worn to protect from undue exposure to the medication and as a part of Standard Precautions. Do not apply topical forms close to the eyes to avoid irritation. Store intravenous dosage forms, which are supplied in a ready-to-use infusion bag, at room temperature.

Nitrofurantoin is available in oral forms and must be given with plenty of fluids, food, or milk to decrease GI upset. Avoid crushing of tablets to help decrease GI upset and prevent staining of teeth. Because of the risk for superinfection, hepatotoxicity, and peripheral neuropathy (which may be irreversible), constantly monitor for signs and symptoms of these adverse effects and document the findings. Be aware that jaundice, itching, rash, and liver enlargement may indicate toxic effects to the liver, whereas numbness and tingling may occur with peripheral neuropathy.

For *quinupristin/dalfopristin*, only intravenous dosage forms are available. Reconstitute the drug using only D_5W. Use a gentle swirling action instead of shaking to mix the drug (to help minimize foaming). A diluted infusion bag of the drug is stable for up to 6 hours, or 54 hours if refrigerated. These characteristics are important to know to help prevent untoward complications. Infusions are generally given over at least 60 minutes. Implement the same measures, as with other antibiotics, to monitor for superinfection.

Vancomycin may be used orally but is poorly absorbed by this route, and is only used to treat microbes in the GI tract (e.g., staphylococcal enterocolitis). Parenteral dosage forms must be used to treat infection outside of the intima of the GI tract. Reconstitute intravenous dosage forms as recommended (e.g., with either D_5W or NS), and infuse over at least 60 minutes. Too rapid an infusion of vancomycin or administration by intravenous push may lead to severe hypotension and red man syndrome. Extravasation may cause local skin irritation and damage, so frequently monitor the infusion, and in particular the intravenous site. Constant monitoring for drug-related neurotoxicity, nephrotoxicity, ototoxicity, and superinfection remain critical to patient safety. In addition, adequate hydration (at least 2 L of fluids every 24 hours unless contraindicated) is important to prevent nephrotoxicity. Trough levels need to be ordered prior to the third or fourth dose; peak levels are no longer used (see the pharmacology discussion for more information).

If the new drug *telavancin* is ordered, use it very carefully and as ordered, especially if the patient has renal dysfunction. When this drug is infused, give it exactly as ordered while also watching for ECG changes, such as changes in the QT segment.

Dalbavancin is given once weekly and is associated with adverse effects of nausea, diarrhea, and headache. It is effective against MRSA.

Because of the significant issue of multidrug-resistant organisms, encourage patients and family members not to abuse or overuse antibiotics and to report immediately to the prescriber any signs and symptoms of an infection that is not resolving or responding to antibiotic therapy. Regardless of drug management, in today's health care settings (acute and long-term

institutions, medical offices, urgent care centers, emergency departments) as well as in the home setting and abroad, teach and demonstrate proper and thorough handwashing technique. Handwashing must be performed often, especially during cold and flu season, before and after preparing food, and after engaging in any of the following activities: going to the bathroom or changing diapers; touching bare human body parts; coughing, sneezing, or using a handkerchief or disposable tissue; eating or drinking; using tobacco; using the telephone; shaking hands; and playing with pets. The Centers for Disease Control and Prevention (CDC) recommend the following as the proper handwashing technique: Wash hands with warm running water and soap; lather well by rubbing hands vigorously for at least 15 to 20 seconds; pay attention to the wrist area, backs of the hands, areas between the fingers, and under the fingernails; and rinse well. Allow the water to run while drying hands with a paper towel and then use a dry paper towel as a barrier between the faucet and clean hands while turning off the water. If soap and water are not available and hands are not visibly soiled, gel hand sanitizers or alcohol-based hand wipes containing at least 60% ethyl alcohol or isopropanol may be used. Once the gel is applied and all surfaces covered, rub hands until gel is dry and do not towel gel off. It is also imperative to educate patients and family members as well as the community at large that taking antibiotics excessively and when not needed may lead to problems of antibiotic resistance!

EVALUATION

Once antibiotic therapy has been initiated, evaluation that is focused on goals, outcome criteria, therapeutic effects, and adverse effects must always be ongoing. Ask patients to report a decrease in symptoms (e.g., infection) as well as absence of injury to self and a decrease in pain. Therapeutic goals include a return to normal of all blood counts and vital signs, negative results on culture and sensitivity testing, and improved appetite, energy level, and sense of well-being. Signs and symptoms of the infection will begin to resolve once therapeutic levels of antibiotics are achieved. Another aspect of evaluation is monitoring for adverse effects of therapy such as superinfections, antibiotic-associated colitis, nephrotoxicity, ototoxicity, neurotoxicity, hepatotoxicity, and other drug-specific adverse effects.

PATIENT-CENTERED CARE: PATIENT TEACHING

Aminoglycosides

- Educate the patient about the drug, its purpose, and its adverse effects, including the risk for hearing loss, which may occur after completion of therapy. Advise the patient to report any change in hearing to the prescriber.
- Increase in fluids up to 3000 mL/day, unless contraindicated, is important with any medication but especially with antibiotics to maximize absorption of oral doses, minimize some of the adverse effects, and ensure adequate hydration.
- Instruct the patient to report to the prescriber any persistent headache, nausea, or vertigo. Educate the patient about the

signs and symptoms of superinfection, such as diarrhea; vaginal discharge; stomatitis; loose and foul-smelling stools; and cough.

Quinolones

- Educate the patient about the incidence of photosensitivity with the use of certain antibiotics. The chemicals in the drug, when taken orally or applied topically, increase the sensitivity of the skin to ultraviolet (UV) light. Photosensitized skin will burn, possibly blister, when exposed to the sun or other UV rays such as with tanning beds/booths. Stress the importance of avoiding exposure to the sun and tanning beds. Recommend the use of sunglasses and sunscreen protection.

- Advise the patient to report to the prescriber any headache, dizziness, restlessness, diarrhea, vomiting, oral candidiasis, flushing of the face, and/or inflammation of the tendons.
- Educate the patient about drug interactions that may occur with the following drugs: calcium, magnesium, probenecid, nitrofurantoin, oral anticoagulants, antacids, iron, sucralfate, and zinc preparations. Instruct the patient to take calcium and magnesium supplements at least 1 hour before or after taking the quinolone. Probenecid may reduce the excretion of the antibiotic and cause toxicity. Since quinolones may alter the intestinal flora and thus vitamin K synthesis, oral anticoagulants must be used with caution in patients taking these antibiotics.
- Instruct the patient to take ciprofloxacin and levofloxacin, both quinolones, exactly as ordered.

Clindamycin

- Instruct the patient not to use topical forms near the eyes or near any abraded areas to avoid tissue irritation.
- When vaginal dosage forms are used, advise the patient not to engage in sexual intercourse for the duration of therapy. The full course of antibiotics are to be taken as ordered to obtain maximal therapeutic benefit.
- If cream dosage forms get into the eyes accidentally, instruct the patient to rinse the eyes immediately with copious amounts of cool tap water.

Linezolid

- Instruct the patient to continue therapy for the full prescribed length of treatment (as with all antibiotics).

- Educate the patient to avoid tyramine-containing foods (e.g., red wine, aged cheeses) while taking the drug.
- Instruct the patient to report to the prescriber immediately any severe abdominal pain, fever, severe diarrhea, and/or worsening of signs and symptoms of infection.

Metronidazole

- Caution the patient to avoid alcohol and any alcohol-containing products (e.g., cough preparations and elixirs) while taking the drug because of the risk for a disulfiram-like reaction (e.g., severe vomiting).
- Educate the patient about the purpose of the drug, such as its use as either an antibacterial or an antifungal medication, because this knowledge is crucial to achieving therapeutic effects and preventing adverse effects.

Nitrofurantoin

- Advise the patient to report to the prescriber any abdominal cramping, dizziness, severe skin reactions, or jaundice.

Vancomycin

- Instruct the patient to report any changes in hearing such as ringing in the ears or a feeling of fullness in the ears. Any nausea, vomiting, unsteady gait, dizziness, generalized tingling (usually after intravenous dosing), chills, fever, rash, and/or hives must also be reported.
- Monitor therapeutic serum levels throughout therapy; this monitoring is key to prevention of toxicity. Trough levels are usually monitored throughout therapy. Stress to the patient that follow-up appointments are important for monitoring serum drug levels and identifying possible toxic effects.

KEY POINTS

- Over the years, bacteria have developed enzymes and mechanisms to interact with antibiotics and render the antibiotic ineffective. Multidrug resistance is a significant health issue, and such resistant organisms include ESBL- and CRE-producing bacteria, MRSA, and VRE.
- The aminoglycosides are a group of natural and semisynthetic antibiotics that are classified as *bactericidal* drugs, are very potent, and are capable of potentially serious toxicities (e.g., nephrotoxicity, ototoxicity).
- Quinolones are very potent, bactericidal, broad-spectrum antibiotics and include norfloxacin, ciprofloxacin, levofloxacin, and moxifloxacin.
- Clindamycin is a semisynthetic derivative of lincomycin, an older antibiotic.
- Linezolid is an antibacterial drug used to treat infections associated with vancomycin-resistant *Enterococcus faecium*, more commonly referred to as VRE. VRE is a difficult infection to treat and often occurs as a health care–associated infection.

- Metronidazole (Flagyl) is an antimicrobial drug of the class nitroimidazole, has good activity against anaerobic organisms, and is widely used for intraabdominal and gynecologic infections; it is also used to treat protozoal infections (e.g., amebiasis, trichomoniasis).
- Nitrofurantoin (Macrodantin) is an antibiotic drug of the class *nitrofuran*. It is indicated primarily for urinary tract infections caused by *E. coli*, *S. aureus*, *Klebsiella* spp., and *Enterobacter* spp.
- Quinupristin and dalfopristin (Synercid) are two streptogramin antibacterials approved for intravenous treatment of bacteremia and life-threatening infection caused by VRE and for treatment of complicated skin and skin structure infections caused by *S. aureus* and *S. pyogenes*.
- Daptomycin (Cubicin) is used to treat complicated skin and soft-tissue infections. Telavancin is a newer drug that is effective against MRSA and is indicated in the treatment of skin and skin structure infections.

- Use of these antibiotics requires a critical assessment for any history or current symptoms indicative of hypersensitivity or allergic reaction (from mild reactions with rash, pruritus, and hives to severe reactions with laryngeal edema, bronchospasm, hypotension, and possible cardiac arrest).
- With use of any antibiotic, it is important to assess for superinfection, or a secondary infection that occurs because of the destruction of normal flora during antibiotic therapy. Superinfections may occur in the mouth, respiratory tract, GI and GU tracts, and on the skin. Fungal infections are evidenced by fever, lethargy, perineal itching, and other anatomically related symptoms.

NCLEX® EXAMINATION REVIEW QUESTIONS

1. While assessing a woman who is receiving quinolone therapy for pneumonia, the nurse notices that the patient has a history of heart problems. The nurse will monitor for which potential cardiac effect of quinolone therapy?
   a. Bradycardia
   b. Dysrhythmias
   c. Tachycardia
   d. Prolonged QT interval

2. A patient has been admitted for treatment of an infected leg ulcer and will be started on intravenous linezolid. The nurse is reviewing the list of the patient's current medications. Which type of medication, if listed, would be of most concern if taken with the linezolid?
   a. Beta blocker
   b. Oral anticoagulant
   c. Selective serotonin reuptake inhibitor antidepressant
   d. Thyroid replacement hormone

3. When administering vancomycin, the nurse knows that which of these is most important to assess before giving the medication?
   a. Renal function
   b. WBC count
   c. Liver function
   d. Platelet count

4. During therapy with an intravenous aminoglycoside, the patient calls the nurse and says, "I'm hearing some odd sounds, like ringing, in my ears." What is the nurse's priority action at this time?
   a. Reassure the patient that these are expected adverse effects.
   b. Reduce the rate of the intravenous infusion.
   c. Increase the rate of the intravenous infusion.
   d. Stop the infusion immediately.

5. When giving intravenous quinolones, the nurse needs to keep in mind that these drugs may have serious interactions with which drugs?
   a. Selective serotonin reuptake inhibitor antidepressants
   b. Nonsteroidal antiinflammatory drugs
   c. Oral anticoagulants
   d. Antihypertensives

6. The nurse is administering an intravenous aminoglycoside to a patient who has had gastrointestinal surgery. Which nursing measures are appropriate? *(Select all that apply.)*
   a. Report a trough drug level of 0.8 mcg/mL, and hold the drug.
   b. Enforce strict fluid restriction.
   c. Monitor serum creatinine levels.
   d. Instruct the patient to report dizziness or a feeling of fullness in the ears.
   e. Warn the patient that the urine may turn darker in color.

7. The order reads: "Give vancomycin, 1250 mg in 250 mL NS, IVPB, every 12 hours. Infuse over 90 minutes." The nurse will set the infusion pump to what setting for mL/hour?

8. A patient has been receiving therapy with the aminoglycoside tobramycin, and the nurse notes that the patient's latest trough drug level is 3 mcg/mL. This drug is given daily, and the next dose is to be administered now. Based on this trough drug level, what is the nurse's priority action?
   a. Administer the drug as ordered.
   b. Hold the drug, and notify the prescriber.
   c. Call the laboratory to have the test repeated and verified.
   d. Hold this dose, but administer the next dose as scheduled.

1. d, 2. c, 3. a, 4. d, 5. c, 6. c, d, 7. 167 mL/hour, 8. b.

CRITICAL THINKING AND PRIORITIZATION QUESTIONS

1. A patient who has been receiving intravenous doses of metronidazole has been discharged and will continue therapy with oral doses of this medication. The patient remarks, "I'm so glad to be going home. Our annual office party is tomorrow night, and I've been looking forward to it all year long." What is the nurse's priority when teaching the patient regarding this drug?

2. A patient has a urinary tract infection caused by *Pseudomonas* spp. Two antibiotics have been ordered, and both are due at 0900:

gentamicin, 300 mg, intravenously, daily (due at 0900), infuse over 60 minutes

ceftazidime, 500 mg intravenously, every 12 hours (due at 0900 and 2100), infuse over 30 minutes

Which antibiotic should the nurse infuse first? Explain your answer.

For answers see *http://evolve.elsevier.com/Lilley*.

EVOLVE WEBSITE

http://evolve.elsevier.com/Lilley

- Animations
- Answer Keys for Textbook Case Studies and Textbook Critical Thinking and Prioritization Questions
- Content Updates
- Key Points
- Review Questions
- Student Case Studies

Antiviral Drugs

http://evolve.elsevier.com/Lilley

OBJECTIVES

When you reach the end of this chapter, you will be able to do the following:

1. Discuss the effects of the immune system with attention to the various types of immunity.
2. Describe the effects of viruses in the human body.
3. List specific drugs categorized as HIV antivirals or antiretrovirals and non–human immunodeficiency virus (HIV) antivirals.
4. Discuss the pathology that occurs with influenza viruses, HSV, VZV, and CMV and hepatitis as well as the process of immunosuppression in patients with viral infections, specifically including HIV infection.
5. Describe the stages of acquired immunodeficiency syndrome (AIDS) and various drugs used to manage the illness.
6. Discuss the mechanism of action, indications, contraindications, cautions, routes, adverse effects, and toxic effects of the various non-HIV antivirals including those for hepatitis B and hepatitis C as well as the HIV antiviral drugs.
7. Develop a nursing care plan that includes all phases of the nursing process for patients receiving non-HIV and HIV antiviral drugs.

DRUG PROFILES

♦ acyclovir, p. 647
amantadine and rimantadine, p. 647
enfuvirtide, p. 653
♦ ganciclovir, p. 647
♦ indinavir, p. 653
♦ nevirapine, p. 654
maraviroc, p. 654
oseltamivir and zanamivir, p. 648
raltegravir, p. 654

ribavirin, p. 648
simeprevir, p. 648
sofosbuvir, p. 648
telbivudine, p. 649
tenofovir, p. 654
♦ zidovudine, p. 654

─────────
♦ = *Key drug*
! = *High-alert drug*

KEY TERMS

Acquired immunodeficiency syndrome (AIDS) Infection caused by the *human immunodeficiency virus (HIV)*, which weakens the host's immune system, giving rise to opportunistic infections. (p. 643)

Antibodies Immunoglobulin molecules that have an antigen-specific amino acid sequence and are produced by the humoral immune system (antibodies produced from B lymphocytes) in response to exposure to a specific antigen, the purpose of which is to attack and destroy molecules of this antigen. (p. 643)

Antigen A substance, usually a protein, that is foreign to a host and causes the formation of an antibody that reacts specifically with that antibody. Examples of antigens include bacterial exotoxins, viruses, and allergens. An allergen (e.g., dust, pollen, mold) is a specific type of antigen that causes allergic reactions (see Chapter 36). (p. 643)

Antiretroviral drugs A specific term for antiviral drugs that work against retroviruses such as HIV. (p. 644)

Antiviral drugs A general term for drugs that destroy viruses, either directly or indirectly by suppressing their replication. (p. 643)

Cell-mediated immunity One of two major parts of the immune system. It consists of nonspecific immune responses mediated primarily by T lymphocytes (T cells) and other immune system cells (e.g., monocytes, macrophages, neutrophils) but not by antibody-producing cells (B lymphocytes). (p. 643)

Deoxyribonucleic acid (DNA) A nucleic acid composed of nucleotide units that transmit genetic information and are found primarily in the nuclei of cells. (Compare with *ribonucleic acid [RNA].*) (p. 642)

Fusion The process by which viruses attach themselves to, or fuse with, the cell membranes of host cells, in preparation for infecting the cell for purposes of viral replication. (p. 642)

Genome The complete set of genetic material of any organism; it may consist of multiple chromosomes (groups of DNA or RNA molecules) in higher organisms; a single chromosome, as in bacteria; or one or two DNA or RNA molecules, as in viruses. (p. 642)

Herpesviruses Several different types of viruses belonging to the family Herpesviridae that cause various forms of herpes infection. (p. 643)

Host Any organism that is infected with a microorganism, such as bacteria or viruses. (p. 642)

Human immunodeficiency virus (HIV) The retrovirus that causes AIDS. (p. 643)

Humoral immunity One of two major parts of the immune system. It consists of specific immune responses in the form of antigen-specific antibodies produced from B lymphocytes. (p. 643)

Immunoglobulins Synonymous with immune globulins. Glycoproteins produced and used by the humoral immune system to attack and kill any substance (antigen) that is foreign to the body. (p. 643)

Influenza viruses The viruses that cause influenza, an acute viral infection of the respiratory tract. (p. 643)

Nucleic acids A general term referring to DNA and RNA. These complex biomolecules contain the genetic material of all living organisms, which is passed to future generations during reproduction. (p. 642)

Nucleoside A structural component of nucleic acid molecules (DNA or RNA) that consists of a purine or pyrimidine base attached to a sugar molecule. (p. 644)

Nucleotide A nucleoside that is attached to a phosphate unit, which makes up the side chain "backbone" of a DNA or an RNA molecule. (p. 644)

Opportunistic infections Infections caused by any type of microorganism that occur in an immunocompromised host but normally would not occur in an immunocompetent host. (p. 643)

Protease An enzyme that breaks down the amino acid structure of protein molecules by chemically cleaving the peptide bonds that link together the individual amino acids. (p. 650)

Replication Any process of duplication or reproduction, such as that involved in the duplication of nucleic acid molecules (DNA or RNA). This term is used most often to describe the entire process of viral reproduction, which occurs only inside the cells of an infected host organism. (p. 642)

Retroviruses Viruses belonging to the family Retroviridae. These viruses contain RNA (as opposed to DNA) as their genome and replicate using the enzyme reverse transcriptase. Currently the most clinically significant retrovirus is HIV. (p. 643)

Reverse transcriptase An RNA-directed DNA polymerase enzyme. It promotes the synthesis of a DNA molecule from an RNA molecule, which is the reverse of the usual process. HIV replicates in this manner. (p. 650)

Ribonucleic acid (RNA) A nucleic acid composed of nucleotide units that transmit genetic information and are found in both the nuclei and cytoplasm of cells. (Compare with *deoxyribonucleic acid [DNA]*.) (p. 642)

Virion A mature virus particle. (p. 642)

Viruses The smallest known class of microorganisms; viruses can only replicate inside host cells. (p. 642)

GENERAL PRINCIPLES OF VIROLOGY

Viruses are not cells, per se, but instead are particles that infect and replicate inside of cells. Viruses can replicate only inside the cells of their **host**. A mature virus particle is known as a **virion**. Virions have a relatively simple structure that consists of the genome, the capsid, and the envelope. The **genome** is the inner core of the virion, which is composed of single- or double-stranded **deoxyribonucleic acid (DNA)** or **ribonucleic acid (RNA)** molecules, but not both. The viral capsid is a protein coat that surrounds and protects the genome. It also plays a role in the process of **fusion** between the virions and the host cells. Fusion occurs when virions attach themselves to host cells in preparation for infecting the cells. The envelope is the outermost layer of the virion and is present in some, but not all, viruses.

Viruses can enter the body through at least four routes: inhalation through the respiratory tract, ingestion via the gastrointestinal (GI) tract, transplacentally via mother to infant, and inoculation via skin or mucous membranes. The inoculation route can take several forms, including sexual contact, blood transfusions, sharing of syringes or needles, organ transplantation, and bites (including human, animal, insect, spider, and others). Once inside the body, the virions begin to attach themselves to the outer membranes of host cells as illustrated in Figure 40-1. The viral genome then passes through the plasma membrane into the cytoplasm of the host cell and enters the nucleus, where the **replication** process begins. In the host cell nucleus, the virus uses the cell's genetic material (the **nucleic acids** RNA and DNA) to construct complete new virions. These new virions exit the infected host cell by budding through the plasma membrane and go on to infect other host cells, where the replication process continues.

Viruses are ubiquitous (widespread) in the environment, and most viral infections may not even be noticed before they are eliminated by the host's immune system. Host immune responses to viral infections are classified as either *nonspecific* or *specific*. Nonspecific immune responses include phagocytosis (eating) of viral particles by leukocytes such as neutrophils, macrophages,

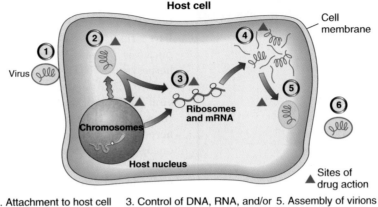

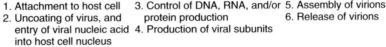

1. Attachment to host cell
2. Uncoating of virus, and entry of viral nucleic acid into host cell nucleus
3. Control of DNA, RNA, and/or protein production
4. Production of viral subunits
5. Assembly of virions
6. Release of virions

FIGURE 40-1 Virus replication. Some viruses integrate into a host chromosome and enter a period of latency. *mRNA,* Messenger RNA. (Modified from Brody TM, Larner J, Minneman KP: *Human pharmacology: Molecular to clinical,* ed 5, St Louis, 2010, Mosby.)

monocytes, and T lymphocytes (T cells). Another nonspecific immune response is the release of cytokines from these leukocytes. Cytokines are biochemical substances (e.g., histamine, tumor necrosis factor) that stimulate other protective immune functions. In addition, these activated immune system cells may also phagocytize infected host cells to curb the growth and spread of infection. These types of immune responses are collectively referred to as cell-mediated immunity. Cell-mediated immunity is nonspecific in the sense that it does not involve antibodies that are specific for a given antigen. This type of immune response is also called humoral immunity. Immune system function is discussed in more detail in Chapters 48 and 49.

OVERVIEW OF VIRAL ILLNESSES AND THEIR TREATMENT

There are at least 6 classes of DNA viruses and at least 14 classes of RNA viruses that are known to infect humans. Some of the more prominent viral illnesses include smallpox (poxviruses), sore throat and conjunctivitis (adenoviruses), warts (papovaviruses), influenza (orthomyxoviruses), respiratory infections (coronaviruses, rhinoviruses), gastroenteritis (rotaviruses, Norwalk-like viruses), human immunodeficiency virus (HIV), which causes acquired immune deficiency syndrome (AIDS) (retroviruses), herpes (herpesviruses), and hepatitis (hepadnaviruses). Effective drug therapy is currently available only for a relatively small number of active viral infections. HIV belongs to the relatively unique viral class known as *retroviruses* and is discussed in more detail in a separate section of this chapter.

Fortunately, many viral illnesses are survivable (e.g., chickenpox). The incidence of some viral illnesses has been reduced by the development of effective vaccines (e.g., vaccines for polio, smallpox, measles, chickenpox, and hepatitis B). However, many other viral illnesses are either fatal or have much more severe long-term outcomes (e.g., hepatitis, HIV infection).

Antiviral drugs can kill or suppress viruses by either destroying virions or inhibiting their ability to replicate. Even the best medications never fully eradicate a virus completely from its

host. However, the body's immune system has a better chance of controlling or eliminating a viral infection when the ability of the virus to replicate is suppressed. Drugs that actually destroy virions include various disinfectants and immunoglobulins. The current antiviral drugs are all synthetic compounds that work indirectly by inhibiting viral replication as opposed to directly by destroying mature virions themselves. Only relatively few of the known viruses can be controlled by current drug therapy. Some of the viruses in this group are the following: cytomegalovirus (CMV), hepatitis viruses, herpes viruses, HIV, influenza viruses, and respiratory syncytial virus (RSV).

Active viral infections are more difficult to eradicate than those caused by bacteria. One reason is that viruses replicate only inside host cells, and antiviral drugs must therefore enter these cells to disrupt viral replication. The HIV/AIDS epidemic that began in the early 1980s strongly boosted antiviral drug research. Many drugs for the treatment of HIV are approved by the U.S. Food and Drug Administration (FDA) via an accelerated process because of the nature of the illness.

Recall that for a virus to replicate, virions must first attach themselves to host cell membranes in a process known as *fusion.* Once inside the cell, the viral genome makes nucleic acids and proteins, which are used to build new viral particles, or virions (see Figure 40-1). Antiviral drugs inhibit replication in various ways. Most antiviral drugs enter the same cells that the viruses enter. Once inside, antiviral drugs interfere with viral nucleic acid synthesis. Other antiviral drugs work by preventing the fusion process itself.

The best responses to antiviral drug therapy are usually seen in patients with competent immune systems. The immune system can work synergistically with the drug to eliminate or suppress viral activity. Patients who are immunocompromised (have weakened immune systems) are at greater risk for opportunistic infections, which are infections caused by organisms that would not normally harm an immunocompetent person (Box 40-1). Such infections often require long-term prophylactic antiinfective drug therapy to control the infection and prevent its recurrence because of compromised host immune functions.

BOX 40-1   Indicator Diseases of AIDS

Opportunistic Infections

Protozoal
- Toxoplasmosis of the brain
- Cryptosporidiosis with diarrhea
- Isosporiasis with diarrhea

Fungal
- Candidiasis of the esophagus, trachea, and lungs
- *Pneumocystis jirovecii* pneumonia
- Cryptococcosis (extrapulmonary)
- Histoplasmosis (disseminated)
- Coccidioidomycosis (disseminated)

Viral
- Cytomegalovirus disease
- Herpes simplex virus infection (persistent or disseminated)
- Progressive multifocal leukoencephalopathy
- Hairy leukoplakia caused by Epstein-Barr virus

Bacterial
- *Mycobacterium avium-intracellulare* complex infection (disseminated)
- Any atypical mycobacterial disease
- Extrapulmonary tuberculosis
- *Salmonella* septicemia (recurrent)
- Pyogenic bacterial infections (multiple or recurrent)

Opportunistic Neoplasias
- Kaposi's sarcoma
- Primary lymphoma of the brain
- Other non-Hodgkin's lymphomas

Others
- HIV wasting syndrome
- HIV encephalopathy
- Lymphoid interstitial pneumonia

AIDS, Acquired immunodeficiency syndrome; *HIV,* human immunodeficiency virus.
Data from Mandell GL, Bennett JE, Dolin R, et al: *Mandell, Douglas, and Bennett's principles and practices of infectious diseases,* ed 7, Philadelphia, 2010, Churchill Livingstone.

Recall that there are two types of nucleic acid found in living organisms: DNA and RNA. A **nucleoside** is a single unit consisting of a base and its attached sugar molecule. A **nucleotide** is a nucleoside plus an attached phosphate molecule. Most antiviral drugs are synthetic purine or pyrimidine nucleoside or nucleotide analogues. **Antiretroviral drugs** are indicated specifically for the treatment of infections caused by HIV. The effectiveness of antiviral drugs varies widely among patients and even over time in the same patient.

HERPES SIMPLEX VIRUS AND VARICELLA-ZOSTER VIRUS INFECTIONS

The family of viruses known as Herpesviridae cause all kinds of herpes infection. Herpes simplex virus type 1 (HSV-1) causes mucocutaneous herpes—usually in the form of perioral blisters ("fever blisters" or "cold sores"). Herpes simplex virus type 2 (HSV-2) causes genital herpes. Human herpesvirus 3 (HHV-3) causes both chickenpox and shingles and is commonly known

as *herpes zoster virus* or *varicella-zoster virus (VZV).* Human herpesvirus 4 (HHV-4), more frequently known as Epstein-Barr virus, is associated with illnesses such as infectious mononucleosis ("mono") and chronic fatigue syndrome. Human herpesvirus 5 (HHV-5) is more commonly known as *cytomegalovirus (CMV)* and is the cause of CMV retinitis (a serious viral infection of the eye) and CMV disease. Human herpesviruses 6 and 7 are not especially clinically significant. Human herpesvirus 8, also known as *Kaposi's sarcoma herpesvirus,* is an oncogenic (cancer-inducing) virus believed to cause Kaposi's sarcoma, an AIDS-associated cancer. Types 3 through 7 normally do not cause diseases that require medication, except in the case of immunocompromised patients. However, the HSVs (types 1 and 2) and VZV (HHV-3) cause illnesses that are now routinely treated with prescription medications.

Herpes Simplex Viruses

Although there can be anatomic overlap between the two types of herpesviruses, HSV-1 infection is most commonly associated with perioral blisters and is therefore often thought of as *oral herpes.* In contrast, HSV-2 infection is most commonly associated with blisters on both male and female genitalia and is therefore commonly referred to as *genital herpes.* Although they usually do not cause serious or life-threatening illness, both infections are highly transmissible through close physical contact. Outbreaks of painful skin lesions occur intermittently, with periods of latency (no sores or other symptoms) occurring between acute outbreaks. Although antiviral medications are *not* curative, they can speed up the process of remission and reduce the duration of painful symptoms. This is especially true if the medications are started early in a given outbreak. Patients may be prescribed an ongoing lower dose of antiviral drug for prophylaxis of outbreaks. HSV infections can become serious, even life-threatening, when the patient is immunocompromised or a newborn infant. Neonatal herpes is often a life-threatening infection. The best strategy to prevent transmission to the newborn infant is usually delivery by cesarean section ("C-section") for any mother with active genital herpes lesions.

Varicella-Zoster Virus

Varicella-zoster virus (VZV) is a type of herpesvirus (HHV-3) that commonly causes chickenpox (varicella) in childhood, remains dormant for many years, and can then reemerge in later adulthood as painful herpes zoster lesions known as *shingles.*

Chickenpox is usually a self-limiting disease of childhood. It is highly contagious and easily spread by direct contact with weeping lesions. Herpes zoster, more commonly known as shingles, is caused by the reactivation of VZV from its dormant state, often decades after a case of childhood chickenpox. It is also referred to simply as *zoster.* Skin lesions that follow nerve tracts, known as *dermatomes,* along the skin surface is the most common clinical manifestation. Zoster lesions are often quite painful, and some patients require opioids for pain control. In addition, postherpetic neuralgias (long-term nerve pain) remain following shingles outbreaks in up to 50% of older adult patients. Early administration (within 72 hours of symptom onset) of antiviral drugs such as acyclovir may speed recovery, but this effect is usually not dramatic. The varicella virus vaccine is now routinely recommended for healthy children older than 1 year of age who have not had chickenpox. A new vaccine, Zostavax, is available for prevention of herpes shingles in patients 50 years of age or older (see Chapter 49).

HEPATITIS

Hepatitis refers to inflammation of the liver that can result in cell damage and liver dysfunction. Hepatitis can be caused by several factors including alcohol abuse, medications, and viruses. Hepatitis can be further characterized as acute or chronic. Acute hepatitis is generally treatable, whereas chronic hepatitis can lead to liver failure. This chapter focuses on chronic hepatitis B and hepatitis C. Hepatitis B is generally milder than hepatitis C; however, it can lead to liver failure and death. Transmission of hepatitis B virus occurs through blood and body fluid exposure. Infants may also develop the disease if they are born to a mother who has the virus. Hepatitis B is preventable by administering a specific vaccine. Antiviral drug therapy for Hepatitis B includes the antiviral drugs lamivudine, tenofovir, and telbivudine, and alfa-interferon, which is discussed in Chapter 47. Hepatitis C is the leading cause of liver failure leading to liver transplantation. Symptoms of hepatitis C are initially mild but progress to chronic liver disease in the majority of patients. Transmission of hepatitis C occurs primarily from contact with infected blood, but can also occur from sexual contact. In addition, people with alcoholic liver disease also tend to develop hepatitis C. Standard drug treatment of Hepatitis C recently changed with the approval of several new drugs, discussed later, and all are considered major breakthrough therapy for hepatitis C.

ANTIVIRALS (NON-HIV)

The drugs discussed in this section include those used to treat non-HIV viral infections such as those caused by influenza viruses, HSV, VZV, CMV, and hepatitis.

Mechanism of Action and Drug Effects

Most of the current antiviral drugs work by blocking the activity of a polymerase enzyme that normally stimulates the synthesis of new viral genomes. The result is impaired viral replication, which allows elimination of the virus by the patient's immune system. If this does not occur, the virus may either enter a dormant state or remain at a low level of replication with continuous drug therapy.

Indications

The antivirals discussed in this section are used to treat HSV, VZV, CMV, and hepatitis B and C infections and are listed in Table 40-1.

Contraindications

Most of the antiviral drugs used to treat non-HIV viral infections are surprisingly well tolerated. The only usual contraindication for most of these drugs is known severe drug allergy. However,

TABLE 40-1 Examples of Antiviral Drugs (Non-HIV)

Drug	Indications
Drugs to Treat Herpesviruses	
acyclovir, valacyclovir	Herpes simplex types 1 and 2, herpes zoster, chickenpox
trifluridine	Herpes simplex keratitis
Drugs to Treat Hepatitis	
simeprevir, sofosbuvir, ledipasvir/sofosubuvir	Hepatitis C
telbivudine, lamivudine, tenofovir	Hepatitis B
Drugs to Treat Influenza Viruses	
amantadine	Influenza A
rimantadine	Influenza A
zanamivir, oseltamivir	Influenza A and B
Miscellaneous Antivirals	
ribavirin	Respiratory syncytial virus infection
cidofovir	Cytomegalovirus infection
foscarnet	Cytomegalovirus infection, herpes simplex infections

HIV, Human immunodeficiency virus.

a small number of contraindications are listed for a few of the antiviral drugs. Amantadine is contraindicated in lactating women, children younger than 12 months of age, and patients with an eczematous rash. Famciclovir is contraindicated in cases of allergy to the drug itself or to a similar drug called *penciclovir,* which is used topically to treat herpes labialis (perioral sores). Ribavirin has a teratogenic potential, therefore it is also contraindicated in pregnant women and even in their male sexual partners. The aerosol form must not be used by pregnant women or by women who may become pregnant during exposure to the drug. This includes health care providers administering the drug in aerosol form, because of the potential for second-hand inhalation on the part of the health care provider.

Adverse Effects

Each antiviral drug has its own specific adverse effect profile. Because viruses reproduce in human cells, selective killing is difficult, and consequently many healthy human cells, in addition to virally infected cells, may be killed in the process, which results in more serious toxicities for these drugs. Adverse effects are listed by drug in Table 40-2.

Interactions

Significant drug interactions that occur with the antiviral drugs arise most often when they are administered via systemic routes. Many of these drugs are also applied topically, and the incidence of drug interactions associated with these routes of administration is much lower. Selected common drug interactions for both antiviral and antiretroviral drugs are listed in Table 40-3.

Dosages

For dosage information on some of the commonly used antiviral drugs, see the table on this page.

TABLE 40-2   Selected Antiviral Drugs: Adverse Effects

Drug	Adverse Effects
acyclovir	Nausea, diarrhea, headache, burning when topically applied
amantadine, rimantadine	Insomnia, nervousness, lightheadedness, anorexia, nausea, anticholinergic effects, orthostatic hypotension, blurred vision
didanosine	Pancreatitis, peripheral neuropathies, seizures
foscarnet	Headache, seizures, electrolyte disturbances, acute renal failure, bone marrow suppression, nausea, vomiting, diarrhea
ganciclovir	Bone marrow toxicity, nausea, vomiting, headache, seizures
indinavir	Nausea; abdominal, back, or flank pain; headache; diarrhea; vomiting; weakness; taste changes; acid regurgitation; nephrolithiasis
nevirapine	Rash, fever, nausea, headache, elevation in liver enzyme levels
ribavirin	Rash, conjunctivitis, anemia, mild bronchospasm
simeprevir	Photosensitivity, rash, pruritus, nausea, myalgia
sofosbuvir	Fatigue, headache
trifluridine	Ophthalmic effects: burning, swelling, stinging, photophobia, pain
telbirudine	Lactic acidosis, fatigue, myopathy, peripheral neuropathy, nausea
vidarabine	Ophthalmic effects: burning, lacrimation, keratitis, foreign body sensation, pain, photophobia, uveitis
zalcitabine	Peripheral neuropathy, rash, ulcers
zidovudine	Bone marrow suppression, nausea, headache

TABLE 40-3   Selected Antiviral Drugs: Interactions

Drug	Interacting Drugs	Interaction
Non-HIV Drugs		
acyclovir	interferon	Additive antiviral effects
	probenecid	Increased acyclovir levels due to decreasing renal clearance
	zidovudine	Increased risk for neurotoxicity
amantadine	Anticholinergic drugs	Increased adverse anticholinergic effects
	CNS stimulants	Additive CNS stimulant effects
ganciclovir	foscarnet	Additive or synergistic effect against CMV and HSV type 2
	imipenem	Increased risk for seizures
	zidovudine	Increased risk for hematologic toxicity (i.e., bone marrow suppression)
ribavirin	Nucleoside reverse transcriptase inhibitors	Increased risk for hepatotoxicity and lactic acidosis
HIV Drugs		
indinavir	Drugs metabolized by the CYP3A4 hepatic microsomal enzyme system (azole antifungals, clarithromycin, doxycycline, erythromycin, isoniazid, nefazodone, nicardipine, protease inhibitors, quinidine, statins, telithromycin, and verapamil)	Competition for metabolism resulting in elevated blood levels and potential toxicity
	rifabutin and ketoconazole	Increased plasma concentrations of rifabutin and ketoconazole
	rifampin	Increased metabolism of indinavir
nevirapine	Drugs metabolized by the CYP3A4 hepatic microsomal enzyme system (see indinavir)	Increased metabolism of these drugs
	Oral contraceptives	Decreased plasma concentrations of oral contraceptives
	Protease inhibitors	Decreased plasma concentrations of protease inhibitors
	rifampin and rifabutin	Decreased serum concentrations of nevirapine
tenofovir	acyclovir, cidofovir, ganciclovir, valacyclovir	May increase serum concentrations of tenofovir
	Protease inhibitors	Increased serum concentrations of tenofovir
maraviroc	CYP3A4 inhibitors (see indinavir)	May increase maraviroc toxicity
	CYP3A4 inducers (phenytoin, carbamazepine, rifampin)	May decrease effects of maraviroc
	St. John's wort	May decrease effects of maraviroc
raltegravir	atazanavir (with or without ritonavir)	May increase effects of raltegravir
	rifampin	May decrease effects of raltegravir
zidovudine	acyclovir	Increased neurotoxicity
	interferon beta	Increased serum levels of zidovudine
	Cytotoxic drugs	Increased risk for hematologic toxicity
	didanosine and zalcitabine	Additive or synergistic effect against HIV
	ganciclovir and ribavirin	Antagonize the antiviral action of zidovudine

DRUG PROFILES

amantadine and rimantadine

Amantadine (Symmetrel), one of the earliest antiviral drugs, is only effective against influenza A viruses. It has been used both prophylactically and therapeutically. However, the most recent guidelines of the Centers for Disease Control and Prevention (CDC) do not recommend the use of amantadine or rimantadine to prevent or treat the flu.

Rimantadine is a structural analogue of amantadine that has the same spectrum of activity, mechanism of action, and clinical indications. However, it differs from amantadine in that it has a longer half-life and causes fewer central nervous system adverse effects such as dizziness and blurred vision. Both medications may be used in children and are available only for oral use.

Pharmacokinetics: Amantadine

Route	Onset of Action	Peak Plasma Concentration	Elimination Half-life	Duration of Action
PO	Within 48 hr	1-4 hr	17 hr	12-24 hr

♦ acyclovir

Acyclovir (Zovirax) is a synthetic nucleoside analogue that is used mainly to suppress the replication of HSV-1, HSV-2, and VZV. Acyclovir is considered the drug of choice for the treatment of both initial and recurrent episodes of these viral infections.

Acyclovir is available in oral, topical, and injectable formulations. Its topical use is discussed in Chapter 56. Other similar antiviral drugs include valacyclovir and famciclovir. However, these latter two drugs are currently available only for oral use and are indicated for the treatment of less serious infections. Note the slight inconsistencies in the spelling of these drug names. Valacyclovir is a prodrug that is metabolized to acyclovir in the body. It has the advantage of greater oral bioavailability and less frequent dosing (three times daily versus five times daily for acyclovir). It may also provide more effective relief of pain from zoster lesions.

Pharmacokinetics (Acyclovir)

Route	Onset of Action	Peak Plasma Concentration	Elimination Half-life	Duration of Action
PO	1.5-2 hr	1.5-2 hr	2-3 hr	10-15 hr
IV	Variable	1 hr	3 hr	8 hr

♦ ganciclovir

Like acyclovir, ganciclovir (Cytovene) is a synthetic nucleoside analogue and is indicated for the treatment of infections caused by CMV. Valganciclovir (Valcyte), foscarnet (Foscavir), and cidofovir (Vistide) are three other antiviral drugs that are used in the treatment of CMV infection. Ganciclovir is most commonly administered intravenously or orally. There is also an ophthalmic form (Vitrasert) for treating active CMV retinitis, which must be surgically inserted. Ganciclovir is also administered to prevent CMV disease (generalized infection) in high-risk patients, such as those receiving organ transplants.

The dose-limiting toxicity of ganciclovir treatment is bone marrow suppression, whereas that of foscarnet and cidofovir is renal toxicity. These toxicities must be kept in mind when

DOSAGES

Antiviral Drugs (Non-HIV)

Drug (Pregnancy Category)	Pharmacologic Class	Usual Dosage Range	Indications
♦ acyclovir (Zovirax) (B)	Antiherpesvirus	**Adult** IV: 5-10 mg/kg every 8 hr for 7-10 days PO: 200-800 mg 5 times daily for 7-10 days	HSV-1 and HSV-2 infection, including genital herpes, mucocutaneous herpes, herpes encephalitis; herpes zoster (shingles); higher-dose therapy for acute episodes; lower-dose therapy for viral suppression
amantadine (Symmetrel) (C)	Antiinfluenza	**Adult** 100-200 mg/day or divided bid	Influenza A
♦ ganciclovir (Cytovene) (C)	Antiviral	**Adult** IV: 5 mg/kg/day divided every 12-24 hr PO: 1000 mg tid	CMV retinitis treatment or maintenance
oseltamivir (Tamiflu) (C)	Antiinfluenza	**Adult** 75 mg twice daily for 5 days	Influenza A or B
ribavirin (Virazole) (X)	Anti-RSV	**Pediatric** Aerosol: 6 g via continuous aerosol 12-18 hr/day for 3-7 days	Severe RSV infection in hospitalized infants and toddlers
zanamivir (Relenza) (C)	Antiinfluenza	**Adult** Inhalation*: 10 mg twice daily	Influenza A or B

HIV, Human immunodeficiency virus; *HSV-1, HSV-2,* herpes simplex virus types 1 and 2; *RSV,* respiratory syncytial virus.
*Use bronchodilator inhaler first if applicable.

deciding which drug is more appropriate in a particular patient. For example, a heart transplant recipient who contracts CMV retinitis is immunocompromised because of immunosuppressant drug therapy and is most likely taking cyclosporine, which is nephrotoxic. Therefore, using foscarnet in this patient may be more dangerous than using ganciclovir. On the other hand, a patient who contracts a CMV infection and is immunocompromised because of a bone marrow transplant might be better treated using foscarnet.

Valganciclovir is a prodrug of ganciclovir, formulated for oral use, that is metabolized to ganciclovir in the body. As in the case described previously for valacyclovir and acyclovir, the prodrug provides greater oral bioavailability and allows less frequent daily dosing. Cidofovir and foscarnet are available only in injectable form.

Pharmacokinetics: Ganciclovir

Route	Onset of Action	Peak Plasma Concentration	Elimination Half-life	Duration of Action
PO	Unknown	24 hr	4.8 hr	Variable

oseltamivir and zanamivir

Oseltamivir (Tamiflu) and zanamivir (Relenza) belong to one of the newest classes of antiviral drugs known as *neuraminidase inhibitors*. The neuraminidase enzyme enables budding virions to escape from infected cells and spread throughout the body. Neuraminidase inhibitors are designed to stop this process in the body, speeding recovery from infection. These drugs are active against influenza virus types A and B. They are indicated for the treatment of uncomplicated acute illness caused by influenza infection in adults. They have been shown to reduce the duration of influenza infection by several days.

The most commonly reported adverse events with oseltamivir are nausea and vomiting; those with zanamivir are diarrhea, nausea, and sinusitis. Oseltamivir is available only for oral use. The drug is indicated for prophylaxis and treatment of influenza infection. Zanamivir is available in dry powder form for inhalation. It is currently indicated only for treatment of active influenza illness. Treatment with oseltamivir and zanamivir needs to begin within 2 days of symptom onset. Peramivir (Rapivab) is the newest agent approved for influenza. It is given as a 600 mg single IV dose.

Pharmacokinetics: Oseltamivir

Route	Onset of Action	Peak Plasma Concentration	Elimination Half-life	Duration of Action
PO	Unknown	1-2 hr	1-3 hr	5-15 hr

Pharmacokinetics: Zanamivir

Route	Onset of Action	Peak Plasma Concentration	Elimination Half-life	Duration of Action
Inhalation	Unknown	1-2 hr	2-5 hr	10-24 hr

ribavirin

Ribavirin (Virazole) is a synthetic nucleoside analogue. It interferes with both RNA and DNA synthesis and as a result inhibits both protein synthesis and viral replication overall. It has a spectrum of antiviral activity that is broader than that of other available antiviral drugs. The inhalational form (Virazole) is used primarily in the treatment of hospitalized infants with severe lower respiratory tract infections caused by respiratory syncytial virus (RSV). This drug was first available only in inhalational form. More recently, oral dosage forms have become available for use in the treatment of hepatitis C. It is classified as a pregnancy category X drug and carries a black box warning. Because of the drug's teratogenic potential, it is contraindicated in pregnant women and their male sexual partners. The aerosol form must not be used by pregnant women or by women who may become pregnant during exposure to the drug. This includes health care providers administering the drug in aerosol form, because of the potential for secondhand inhalation on the part of the health care provider.

Pharmacokinetics: Ribavirin

Route	Onset of Action	Peak Plasma Concentration	Elimination Half-life	Duration of Action
Inhalation	Unknown	End of inhalation	1.4-2.5 hr	Variable
PO	Unknown	2-3 hr	120-170 hr	Unknown

simeprevir

Simeprevir (Olysio) is a protease inhibitor used for the treatment of chronic hepatitis C. It was approved in 2013. It is used in conjunction with standard hepatitis C treatments, interferon and ribavirin. It is not to be used as monotherapy. Simeprevir contains a sulfonamide moiety; however, there is insufficient data to determine if patients with known sulfa allergy will experience adverse effects from simeprevir. Patients of eastern Asian ancestry exhibit higher levels of the drug and more adverse effects. At this time, there are no recommendations to reduce the dose for such patients. Simeprevir alone is a pregnancy category C drug; however, since it is used in conjunction with ribavirin and interferon, it is considered category X. The most common adverse effects include photosensitivity, rash, nausea, and pruritus. Drug interactions include concurrent use with strong CYP3A4 inhibitors and inducers. It is dosed as 150 mg once daily with food.

Pharmacokinetics: Simeprevir

Route	Onset of Action	Peak Plasma Concentration	Elimination Half-life	Duration of Action
PO	Unknown	4-6 hours	10-13 hours	Unknown

sofosbuvir

Sofosbuvir (Solvaldi) is the first-in-class RNA polymerase inhibitor for the treatment of chronic hepatitis C. Sofosbuvir is considered "breakthrough" therapy. It is the first drug treatment for hepatitis C that can be given without interferon. It is, however, used in combination with ribavirin. It is not to be used as monotherapy. It is dosed as 400 mg once daily orally with or without food. Following oral administration, sofosbuvir is rapidly converted to its active metabolite, GS-331007, which accounts for greater than 90% of drug-related activity. The most common adverse effects are fatigue and headache. Drug interactions include strong CYP3A4 inducers, which can lower sofosbuvir concentrations. Rifampin and St. John's wort (both of which are inducers) should be avoided. Because sofosbuvir is given in conjunction with ribavirin, it is considered a pregnancy category X drug. In 2014, the combination of sofosbuvir and ledipasvir (Harvoni) became the first treatment for hepatitis C that does not require the combined use of ribavirin and is a pregnancy category B drug. Serious drug interactions have been reported with Harvoni and Solvadi with amiodrarone. Harvoni is given as a one pill once a day. In late 2014, Viekira Pak (ombitasvir/paritaprevir/ritonavir) also become available. Like Harvoni, it does not require ribavirin in most patients. These drugs can cost up to $100,000 per patient, and thus the payor must make tough decisions as to which patients get treatment. Please refer to the American Association for the Study of Liver Disease (AASLD) for the most current guidelines, as they change rapidly.

Pharmacokinetics: Sofosbuvir

Route	Onset of Action	Peak Plasma Concentration	Elimination Half-life	Duration of Action
PO	Unknown	2-4 hours	27 hours	Unknown

telbivudine

Telbivudine (Tyzeka) is a nucleoside analogue reverse transcriptase inhibitor indicated for chronic hepatitis B. It is excreted by the kidneys and requires dosage adjustments in patients with renal dysfunction. The normal dose is 600 mg orally daily and can be given with or without food. Common adverse effects include fatigue, headache, diarrhea, nausea, arthralgia, myalgia, myopathy, lactic acidosis, and hepatomegaly with steatosis. Severe acute hepatitis B exacerbations have been reported upon discontinuation. Drug interactions include alfa interferons, which can cause severe peripheral neuropathy. Caution should be used with nephrotoxic drugs. Telbivudine is classified as a pregnancy category B drug. Other drugs used to treat hepatitis B include interferon alfa, lamivudine, and tenofovir.

Pharmacokinetics: Telbivudine

Route	Onset of Action	Peak Plasma Concentration	Elimination Half-life	Duration of Action
PO	Unknown	1-4 hours	15 hours	Unknown

HIV INFECTION AND AIDS

HIV infection is a common and devastating viral infection. In 2012, there were 35.3 million people worldwide with HIV infection and over 1.1 million people in the United States. The good news is that new cases of HIV have decreased by 33% since 2001. The most common routes of transmission of HIV are sexual activity, intravenous drug use, and perinatal transfer from mother to child. African-American males and females have a rate of HIV infection seven times higher than that seen in white Americans. No solid evidence to date confirms transmission of HIV by casual contact, including hugging, kissing, coughing, sneezing, swimming in pools, and sharing of food, water, eating utensils, or toilet facilities. HIV also is not transmitted by insect bites, unlike some other viral illnesses. The risk for transmission

to health care workers via percutaneous (needlestick) injuries is currently calculated at approximately 0.3%. Performing hand hygiene and maintaining Standard Precautions to avoid contact with all body fluids during patient care dramatically reduces the risk for caregiver infection (see Table 40-5). The key epidemiologic concepts related to HIV/AIDs are discussed in Box 40-2.

> ### ⚡ SAFETY AND QUALITY IMPROVEMENT: PREVENTING MEDICATION ERRORS   QSEN
> #### *Look-Alike/Sound-Alike Drugs: Zostrix and Zovirax*
>
> An incident was reported that involved the confusion of the two similarly named drugs Zostrix and Zovirax. A provider prescribed Zostrix cream with the directions, "Apply to affected area four times a day." There were no other specific instructions for the medication. The pharmacist mistakenly entered "Zovirax" into the pharmacy computer, and the nursing staff did not catch the error. The next day, the physician saw the tube of Zovirax in the patient's room instead of Zostrix. The sound-alike drug names can be easily confused.
>
> Zostrix is capsaicin, derived from hot chili peppers, and is used topically for the treatment of arthritic pain, muscle strains, and joint sprains. In this case, it was ordered for neuralgic pain. Zovirax 5% ointment is a topical form of acyclovir, an antiviral medication, and is used for the management of initial genital herpes.
>
> This incident illustrates how important it is to clarify the instructions in a medication order (e.g., application to a *specific* site) and how the use of generic names can help to avoid a medication error. In addition, it shows how important it is for nurses to be familiar with the indications of the drugs they are administering.

Modified from *ISMP Medication Safety Alert: NURSE Advise-ERR*, May 2004, Volume 2, Issue 5. Available at *www.ismp.org/newsletters/nursing/issues/nurseadviseerr200405.pdf.* Accessed August 1, 2015.

> ### BOX 40-2 Epidemiology of HIV Infection
>
> **Disease Viral Factors**
> - Developed virus is easily inactivated and must be transmitted in body fluids.
> - Disease has a long prodromal or incubation period.
> - Virus can be shed before development of identifiable symptoms.
>
> **Transmission**
> - Virus is present in blood, semen, and vaginal secretions.
>
> **Groups at Risk**
> - Intravenous drug abusers; sexually active people with many partners (homosexual and heterosexual); prostitutes; newborns of HIV-positive mothers
> - Blood and organ transplant recipients and hemophiliacs: before 1985 (before screening programs)
>
> **Geographic Factors**
> - Continuously expanding epidemic worldwide
> - No particular seasonal pattern of infection (i.e., unlike influenza)
>
> **Modes of Control**
> - Antiviral drugs limit progression of disease.
> - Vaccines for prevention and treatment are in trials.
> - Monogamous sex using safe sexual practices helps limit spread.
> - Sterile injection needles need to be used.
> - Large-scale screening programs have been developed to test blood for transfusions, organs for transplantation, and clotting factors given to hemophiliacs.

Data from U.S. Department of Health and Human Services: AIDSinfo (AIDS information website). Available at *www.aidsinfo.nih.gov.*

HIV is a member of the retrovirus family and was so named upon discovery of a unique feature of its replication process. Retroviruses are all RNA viruses and are unique in their use of the enzyme reverse transcriptase during their replication process. This enzyme promotes the synthesis of complementary (mirror image) DNA molecules from the viral RNA genome. A second enzyme, integrase, promotes the integration of this viral DNA into the host cell DNA. This hybrid DNA complex is known as a *provirus*. It produces new mature HIV virions that infect other host cells. Another important enzyme is protease, which serves to chemically separate the new viral RNA from viral protein molecules. These components are initially synthesized into one large macromolecular strand, and the protease enzyme carefully breaks up this strand into its key components. Figure 40-2 shows the major structural features of the HIV

virion, and Figure 40-3 illustrates the steps in its replication process. Reverse transcriptase is not normally found in host cells—both reverse transcriptase and integrase are carried by the virus itself. "Reversal" of the usual replication processes led to the name *reverse transcriptase* for this enzyme and also to the name *retrovirus* for this family of viruses. Reverse transcriptase has a high rate of errors when stringing together the purine and pyrimidine bases during transcription, which allows frequent genetic mutations among HIV virions and often results in viral strains that are resistant to both medications and the patient's immune system. Such mutations also hamper the development of an effective vaccine against the virus. Drugs used to treat HIV are called *antiretrovirals*.

HIV infection that is untreated or treatment resistant eventually leads to severe immune system failure, with death occurring secondary to opportunistic infections. AIDS often progresses over a period of several years. Various health organizations, including the CDC and the World Health Organization (WHO), have published classification systems describing the various "stages" of this infection. The most recent WHO model lists four stages as follows:

- Stage 1: asymptomatic infection
- Stage 2: early, general symptoms of disease
- Stage 3: moderate symptoms
- Stage 4: severe symptoms, often leading to death

Figure 40-4 illustrates events that roughly correlate with these four stages of HIV infection. This figure shows the hypothetical natural course of the disease through the previously described stages in patients *without* treatment. Patients who are effectively treated with drug therapy usually do not progress through all of these stages, or at least such progression is slowed considerably (by years). In fact, advances in antiretroviral drug

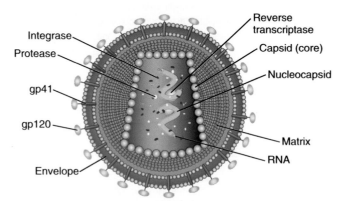

FIGURE 40-2 Human immunodeficiency virus. Within the core capsid, the diploid, single-stranded, positive-sense RNA is complexed to nucleoprotein. *gp,* Glycoprotein. (From *Dorland's illustrated medical dictionary*, ed 32, Philadelphia, 2012, Saunders.)

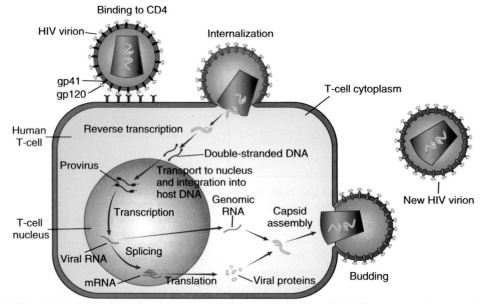

FIGURE 40-3 Life cycle of the human immunodeficiency virus (HIV). The extracellular envelope protein gp120 binds to CD4 on the surface of T lymphocytes or mononuclear phagocytes, while the transmembrane protein gp41 mediates the fusion of the viral envelope with the cell membrane. *gp,* Glycoprotein; *mRNA,* messenger RNA. (From *Dorland's illustrated medical dictionary*, ed 32, Philadelphia, 2012, Saunders.)

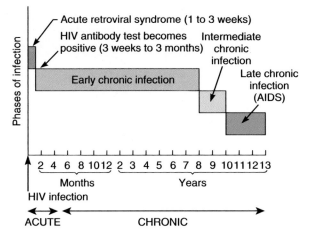

FIGURE 40-4 Timeline for the spectrum of untreated HIV infection. The timeline represents the course of untreated illness from the time of infection to clinical manifestations of disease. (From Lewis SL, Dirksen SR, Heitkemper MM, et al: *Medical-surgical nursing: assessment and management of clinical problems,* ed 8, Philadelphia, 2011, Elsevier.)

therapy have given rise to increasingly greater numbers of long-term survivors of HIV infection. Highly active antiretroviral therapy (HAART) refers to combinations of antiretroviral drugs ("cocktails") that are now standard for treating HIV-infected patients. This combination therapy (HAART) is normally begun immediately upon confirmation of HIV infection. Opportunistic infections are treated with infection-specific antimicrobial drugs as they arise. Prophylactic treatment for opportunistic infections is also common and is most frequently given when a patient's CD4 count falls below 200 cells/mm³. Opportunistic malignancies, such as Kaposi's sarcoma and lymphomas, are also treated with specific antineoplastic medications, which are discussed in Chapters 45 and 46, as well as with radiation and/or surgery as indicated. Long-term survival is defined as living with HIV infection for at least 10 to 15 years after infection. Research attempts to develop an effective anti-HIV vaccine are underway throughout the world. Despite encouraging data regarding potential benefits, the design of an effective HIV vaccine continues to remain elusive.

DRUGS USED TO TREAT HIV INFECTION

The urgency and public awareness of the HIV epidemic stimulated much research in the fields of immunology and pharmacology. This resulted in the development of several effective antiretroviral drugs, as well as of antiviral drugs in general. Although new drug combinations have prolonged lives, these medications often carry significant toxicities. Furthermore, HIV/AIDS is still not considered to be a curable disease. There are currently five classes of antiretroviral drugs, including the reverse transcriptase inhibitors, the protease inhibitors, the fusion inhibitors, and the newest classes, the entry inhibitor–CCR5 coreceptor antagonists and the HIV integrase strand transfer inhibitors. There are currently two subclasses of reverse transcriptase inhibitors: nucleoside reverse transcriptase inhibitors (NRTIs) and nonnucleoside reverse transcriptase inhibitors

TABLE 40-4 Examples of Antiretrovirals Used to Treat HIV	
Generic Name	**Trade Name**
Nucleoside Reverse Transcriptase Inhibitors	
abacavir	Ziagen
abacavir/lamivudine	Epzicom
abacavir/zidovudine/lamivudine	Trizivir
didanosine (enteric coated)	Videx EC
didanosine (dideoxyinosine)	Videx
emtricitabine	Emtriva
lamivudine	Epivir
stavudine (d4t)	Zerit
tenofovir	Viread
tenofovir/emtricitabine	Truvada
zalcitabine	Hivid
zidovudine	Retrovir
Nonnucleoside Reverse Transcriptase Inhibitors	
delavirdine	Rescriptor
efavirenz	Sustiva
etravirine	Intelence
nevirapine	Viramune
Protease Inhibitors	
amprenavir	Agenerase
atazanavir	Reyataz
darunavir	Prezista
fosamprenavir	Lexiva
indinavir	Crixivan
lopinavir/ritonavir	Kaletra
nelfinavir	Viracept
ritonavir	Norvir
saquinavir mesylate	Invirase
tipranavir	Aptivus
Fusion Inhibitor	
enfuvirtide	Fuzeon
Entry Inhibitor–CCR5 Coreceptor Antagonist (Also Known as CCR5 Antagonist)	
maraviroc	Selzentry
HIV Integrase Strand Transfer Inhibitors (Also Known as Integrase Inhibitors)	
dolutegravir	Tivicay
raltegravir	Isentress
Multiclass Combination Products	
efavirenz/emtricitabine/tenofovir	Atripla
abacavir/lamivudine/zidovudine	Trizivir
lamivudine/zidovudine	Combivir
lopinavir/ritonavir	Kaletra
Elvitegravir/cobicistat/emtricitabine/tenofovir	Stribild
Darunavir/cobicistat	Prezcobix

(NNRTIs). Drugs from many of these drug classes are combined into a single drug dosage form for ease of use. Table 40-4 lists these drugs and their respective classes. In 2012, the FDA approved Truvada for the prevention of HIV in high-risk patients. In 2014, cobicistat (Tybost) was approved. Tybost is used as a boosting agent to raise the drug levels of Reyataz (atazanavir) or Prezista (darunavir) in combination with other antiretrovirals (ARVs) to treat HIV. Prezcobix (darunavir and cobicistat) is also available. IV drug therapy is rapidly changing, and the reader is referred to *http://aidsinfo.nih.gov/guidelines* for the most up-to-date treatment recommendations.

Mechanism of Action and Drug Effects

Although HIV/AIDS is a very complex illness, the mechanisms of action of the various drug classes are fortunately straightforward and distinct. The name of each class of medication provides a reminder of its role in suppressing the viral replication process. Thus, reverse transcriptase inhibitors work by blocking activity of the enzyme reverse transcriptase. The protease inhibitors work by inhibiting the protease retroviral enzyme. There is also a combination of protease inhibitors that includes both lopinavir and ritonavir. The ritonavir component also serves to inhibit cytochrome P-450–mediated enzymatic metabolism of the lopinavir component. Fusion inhibitors work by inhibiting viral fusion. The entry inhibitor–CCR5 coreceptor antagonists, or CCR5 antagonists, work by selectively and reversibly binding to the type 5 chemokine coreceptors located on the CD4 cells that are used by the HIV virion to gain entry to the cells. The integrase strand transfer inhibitors, also referred to as *integrase inhibitors,* work by inhibiting the catalytic activity of the enzyme integrase thus preventing integration of the proviral gene into human DNA.

The most effective treatment to date is referred to as highly active antiretroviral therapy (HAART). HAART usually includes at least three medications. Commonly recommended drug combinations include two or three NRTIs; two NRTIs plus one or two protease inhibitors; or a NRTI plus a NNRTI with one or two protease inhibitors. Despite the effectiveness of HAART, prescribers may still need to alter a given patient's drug regimen in cases of major drug intolerance (see Adverse Effects) or drug resistance. A given patient's HIV strain can still evolve and mutate over time, which allows it to become resistant to any drug therapy, especially when that therapy is used for a prolonged period. Evidence of drug resistance includes a falling CD4 count and/or increased viral load.

All antiretroviral drugs have similar therapeutic effects in that they reduce the viral load. A viral load of less than 50 copies/mL is considered to be an undetectable viral load and is a primary goal of antiretroviral therapy. When effective, treatment leads to a significant reduction in mortality and incidence of opportunistic infections, improves patient's physical performance, and significantly increases T-cell counts.

Indications

The only usual indication for all of the current antiretroviral drugs is active HIV infection, although a few are also used to treat hepatitis B. Prophylactic antiretroviral treatment of infected mothers has been shown to reduce infant infection by at least two thirds and is not normally harmful to either the mother or infant. Medication may also be given prophylactically to the newborn infant, typically for the first 6 weeks of life. Infants and children with established HIV infection must

TABLE 40-5 Recommendations for Occupational HIV Exposure Chemoprophylaxis

Type of Exposure	Source	Prophylaxis	Therapy
Any occupational exposure to HIV	Blood; fluid containing visible blood or other potentially infectious fluid or tissue	Recommended	Raltegravir + Truvada (emtricitabine and tenofovir)

NOTE: Recommendations vary and change often, and the reader is referred to the CDC website *(www.cdc.gov)* for updated guidelines.

usually continue taking medication indefinitely. Prophylactic therapy is given to health care workers with a known exposure to HIV (e.g., via needlestick injuries in hospitals [Table 40-5]).

Contraindications

Because of the potentially fatal outcome of HIV infection, the only usual contraindication to a given medication is known severe drug allergy or other intolerable toxicity. Most of the current antiretroviral drug classes have several alternative drugs to choose from if a patient is especially intolerant of a given drug.

Adverse Effects

Common adverse effects of selected antiretroviral drugs are listed in Table 40-2. The need to modify drug therapy because of adverse effects is not uncommon. The goal is to find the regimen that will best control a given patient's infection and that has a tolerable adverse effect profile. Different patients vary widely in their drug tolerance, and their tolerance may change over time. Thus, medication regimens often must be strategically individualized and evolve with the course of the patient's illness.

Approximately 25% of HIV-infected patients in the United States are also infected with hepatitis C virus, and the disease tends to be more severe in HIV patients. HAART is strongly correlated with increased mortality from HCV-induced liver disease, because the anti-HIV drugs produce strain on the liver as these drugs are metabolized via the liver.

A major adverse effect of protease inhibitors is lipid abnormalities, including lipodystrophy, or redistribution of fat stores under the skin. This condition often results in cosmetically undesirable outcomes for the patient, such as a "hump" at the posterior base of the neck and also a skeletonized (bony) appearance of the face. In addition, dyslipidemias such as hypertriglyceridemia can occur, and insulin resistance and type 2 diabetes symptoms can result. It is reported that in these cases, switching a patient from a protease inhibitor to an NNRTI may help to reduce such symptoms without decreasing antiretroviral efficacy. Long-term antiretroviral drug therapy can cause bone demineralization and possible osteoporosis. When this condition occurs, it may require treatment with standard medications for osteoporosis, such as calcium, vitamin D, and bisphosphonates (see Chapter 34).

Interactions

HIV drugs are involved in numerous drug interactions, many of which are severe and necessitate alternative therapy. Common selected drug interactions involving both antiretrovirals and other antivirals are listed in Table 40-3.

Dosages

Because of rapidly changing antiviral drug therapy and the complexity of dosing and the disease state, only selected dosages are listed in this textbook (see the dosages table below). Refer to an up-to-date drug information handbook for specifics on dosing.

DRUG PROFILES

enfuvirtide

Enfuvirtide (Fuzeon) is the only medication in one of the newest classes of antiretroviral drugs, called *fusion inhibitors*. It works by suppressing the fusion process and subsequent viral replication. This mechanism of action serves as yet another example of how antiretroviral drugs are strategically designed to interfere with specific steps of the viral replication process. The use of combinations of drugs that work by different mechanisms improves a patient's chances for continued survival by reducing the likelihood of viral resistance to the drug therapy regimen. Enfuvirtide is indicated for treatment of HIV infection in combination with other antiretroviral drugs. Adult and pediatric patients have shown comparable tolerance of the drug in clinical trials thus far. Use of enfuvirtide in combination with other standard antiretroviral drugs has been associated with markedly reduced viral loads, compared with drug regimens

that did not include this drug. The drug is currently available only in injectable form.

Pharmacokinetics: Enfuvirtide

Route	Onset of Action	Peak Plasma Concentration	Elimination Half-life	Duration of Action
Subcut	Unknown	4-8 hr	4 hr	Unknown

♦ indinavir

Indinavir (Crixivan) belongs to the *protease inhibitor* class of antiretroviral drugs. Others include ritonavir (Norvir), nelfinavir (Viracept), amprenavir (Agenerase), fosamprenavir (Lexiva), atazanavir (Reyataz), tipranavir (Aptivus), ritonavir (Norvir), darunavir (Prezista), and the combination product lopinavir/ritonavir (Kaletra). Indinavir can be taken in combination with other anti-HIV therapies or alone. This drug is best dissolved and absorbed in an acidic gastric environment, and the presence of high-protein and high-fat foods reduces its absorption. Therefore, it is recommended that it be administered in a fasting state. Indinavir therapy produces increases in CD4 cell counts and significant reductions in viral load. Protease inhibitors are commonly given in combination with two reverse transcriptase inhibitors to maximize efficacy and decrease the likelihood of viral drug resistance. Indinavir is relatively well tolerated in most patients. Nephrolithiasis (kidney stones) occurs in approximately 4% of patients. Patients who take indinavir are encouraged to drink at least 48 ounces of liquids every day to maintain hydration and help avoid nephrolithiasis. Indinavir and all other protease inhibitors are available only for oral use.

DOSAGES

HIV/AIDS Drugs

Drug (Pregnancy Category)	Pharmacologic Class	Usual Dosage Range
enfuvirtide (Fuzeon) (B)	Fusion inhibitor	**Adult** Subcut: 90 mg twice daily
♦ indinavir (Crixivan) (C)	Protease inhibitor	**Adult** PO: 800 mg every 8 hr
maraviroc (Selzentry) (B)	CCR5 antagonist	**Adult** PO: 300 mg twice daily
♦ nevirapine (NVP) (Viramune) (C)	Nonnucleoside reverse transcriptase inhibitor	**Adult** PO: 200 mg daily for 14 days, then twice daily
raltegravir (Isentress) (C)	Integrase inhibitor	**Adult** PO: 400 mg twice daily
tenofovir (Viread) (B)	Nucleotide reverse transcriptase inhibitor	**Adult** PO: 300 mg once daily
♦ zidovudine (AZT, ZDV) (Retrovir) (C)	Nucleoside reverse transcriptase inhibitor	**Adult** PO: 300 mg twice daily IV: 1 mg/kg every 4 hr **Pregnant woman** PO: 100 mg 5 times daily during pregnancy until start of labor, then give IV bolus dose of 2 mg/kg over 1 hr followed by an IV infusion of 1 mg/kg/hr until the umbilical cord is clamped

AIDS, Acquired immunodeficiency syndrome; *CCR5,* chemokine receptor 5; *HIV,* human immunodeficiency virus.

Pharmacokinetics: Indinavir

Route	Onset of Action	Peak Plasma Concentration	Elimination Half-life	Duration of Action
PO	2 wk to therapeutic effect	0.5-1 hr	1.5-2.5 hr	6 mo

maraviroc

Maraviroc (Selzentry) is the only drug available in a new class of antiretrovirals called *CCR5 antagonists*. Maraviroc works by selectively and reversibly binding to the chemokine coreceptors located on the CD4 cells. It is used in treatment-experienced patients with evidence of viral replication and HIV-1 strains resistant to multiple antiretroviral therapies. Patients must receive an FDA-approved medication guide before this drug is dispensed. Hepatotoxicity with allergic-type features has been reported. Drug interactions of significance include interactions with cytochrome P-450 3A4 (CYP3A4) inhibitors (azole antifungals, clarithromycin, doxycycline, erythromycin, isoniazid, nefazodone, nicardipine, protease inhibitors, quinidine, telithromycin, and verapamil), which may increase maraviroc toxicity. CYP3A4 inducers, including phenytoin, carbamazepine, nafcillin, and rifampin, may decrease maraviroc's effects. Maraviroc is available only for oral use.

Pharmacokinetics: Maraviroc

Route	Onset of Action	Peak Plasma Concentration	Elimination Half-life	Duration of Action
PO	Unknown	0.5-4 hr	14-18 hr	Unknown

♦ nevirapine

Nevirapine (Viramune) is a nonnucleoside reverse transcriptase inhibitor (NNRTI). Other currently available NNRTIs include delavirdine (Rescriptor), efavirenz (Sustiva), and etravirine (Intelence). These drugs are often used in combination with NRTIs. Nevirapine is well tolerated compared with other therapies for HIV. The most common adverse events associated with nevirapine therapy are rash, fever, nausea, headache, and abnormal liver function test results. Nevirapine and the other NNRTIs are available only for oral use.

Pharmacokinetics: Nevirapine

Route	Onset of Action	Peak Plasma Concentration	Elimination Half-life	Duration of Action
PO	2 hr	2-4 hr	25-30 hr	24 hr

raltegravir

Raltegravir (Isentress) is the only drug in the new class called *integrase inhibitors*. Raltegravir works by inhibiting the activity of the integrase enzyme, thus preventing integration of the proviral gene into human DNA. Raltegravir is used in treatment-experienced patients with virus that shows multidrug resistance and active replication. Myopathy and rhabdomyolysis have been reported, as well as an immune reconstitution syndrome, which may result in an inflammatory response to a residual opportunistic infection. Raltegravir does not interact with CYP3A4 inducers or inhibitors (as do many other AIDS drugs).

Pharmacokinetics: Raltegravir

Route	Onset of Action	Peak Plasma Concentration	Elimination Half-life	Duration of Action
PO	Unknown	3 hr	9 hr	Unknown

tenofovir

Tenofovir (Viread) is one of many nucleoside reverse transcriptase inhibitors (NRTIs). Others in this class include emtricitabine (Emtriva), lamivudine (Epivir), stavudine (Zerit), and abacavir (Ziagen), as well as many combination products. Lactic acidosis and severe hepatomegaly have been reported with this drug and others in its class. Tenofovir is indicated for use against HIV infection in combination with other antiretroviral drugs. It is currently available only for oral use.

Pharmacokinetics: Tenofovir

Route	Onset of Action	Peak Plasma Concentration	Elimination Half-life	Duration of Action
PO	4-8 days for therapeutic effect	1 hr	10-14 hr	7 days

♦ zidovudine

Zidovudine (Retrovir), also known as azidothymidine or AZT, is a synthetic nucleoside analogue of thymidine that has had an enormous impact on the treatment and quality of life of patients who have AIDS. It was the very first and, for a long time, the only anti-HIV medication. Zidovudine, along with various other antiretroviral drugs, is given to HIV-infected pregnant women and even to newborn babies to prevent maternal transmission of the virus to the infant.

The major dose-limiting adverse effect of zidovudine is bone marrow suppression, and this is often the reason a patient with HIV infection must be switched to another anti-HIV drug such as zalcitabine or didanosine. Some patients may receive a combination of two of these drugs, in lower dosages, to maximize their combined actions. This strategy may reduce the likelihood of toxicity. Zidovudine is available in both oral and injectable forms.

Pharmacokinetics: Zidovudine

Route	Onset of Action	Peak Plasma Concentration	Elimination Half-life	Duration of Action
PO	At least 6 mo for therapeutic effect	0.4-1.5 hr	0.8-2 hr	3-5 hr

NURSING PROCESS

ASSESSMENT

Before administering an antiviral drug, perform a thorough head-to-toe physical assessment and take a medical and medication history. Document any known allergies. Assess the patient's nutritional status and baseline vital signs because of the profound effects of viral illnesses on physiologic status, especially if the patient is immunocompromised. Assess for any contraindications, cautions, and drug interactions.

In your assessment related to the use of *non-HIV antivirals*, inquire about the patient's allergy to medications. Ask for a listing of any prescription and over-the-counter drugs, herbals, and dietary supplements. Before initiation of therapy, assess energy levels, any weight loss, vital signs, and the characteristics of any visible lesions. Document the findings for baseline comparison. Age is also important to assess, because amantadine is not to be used in children younger than 12 months of age. *Cidofovir* requires assessment of renal function and is contraindicated in those with renal compromise or with use of other nephrotoxic drugs. *Ribavirin* is contraindicated in pregnant women and in their male sexual partners due to its teratogenic properties; it also carries the contraindication for handling by health care personnel who are or might be pregnant, and there is also potential for secondhand inhalation (on part of the health care provider). With ribavirin, analysis of respiratory secretions via sputum specimen will most likely be ordered for diagnostic purposes prior to initiation of drug therapy. With respiratory illness, assess and document breath sounds, respiratory rate and patterns, cough, sputum production, and vital signs including temperature. A dose-limiting toxicity of *ganciclovir* treatment is bone marrow suppression; thus, perform a close review of the patient's CBC; CBC includes RBCs, WBCs, and platelets. With *foscarnet* and cidofovir, assess renal function because of the potential for renal toxicity.

Before giving *acyclovir*, assess vital signs and take a thorough medication history. Assess pain levels associated with the zoster lesions prior to giving the medication because relief of pain is expected with use of the drug. See Chapter 56 for more information on the topical form of acyclovir. *Famciclovir* also requires assessment of allergies. *Oseltamivir* and *zanamivir*, useful against influenza virus types A and B, must be given as ordered within 2 days of the onset of flu symptoms; therefore, assessment of presenting symptoms and their date of onset is most important to their effective use. Ganciclovir is associated with bone marrow suppression; therefore, assess blood counts prior to and during use.

Simeprevir (Olysio), used for the treatment of chronic hepatitis C in combination with interferon and ribavirin, contains a sulfa-like chemical, thus it is important to assess for a potential drug allergy to sulfonamides. Additionally, it is important to assess racial-ethnicity because it is a known fact that patients of Asian descent exhibit higher levels of the drug and thus have more adverse effects. Assess for interactions with drugs that are strong CYP3A4 inhibitors/inducers. Refer to Table 2-5 in Chapter 2 under the specific enzyme "3A4," and you will find a listing of some of the medications that are considered CYP3A4 inhibitors/inducers. *Sofosbuvir (Solvald)*, also used for treatment of hepatitis C, is another drug to be used in combination therapy. Assess baseline energy levels and any preexisting complaints of headache due to the adverse effects of fatigue and headache. Like simeprevir, there are drug interactions with CYP3A4 inducers and with the herbal product, St. John's wort. *Telbivudine (Tyzeka)*, used in chronic hepatitis B, requires assessment of renal function due to its excretion by the kidneys and does require subsequent dosage adjustments if the patient has altered renal function. Cautious use is needed with the concurrent use with nephrotoxic drugs.

With use of *HIV antivirals* or *antiretrovirals*, closely assess allergies, cautions, contraindications, and drug interactions. Because of the severity of HIV infections and potential for a fatal outcome, the main contraindication includes severe drug allergy and other toxicities. Use of *protease inhibitors* requires assessment of the patient's medical history, vital signs, baseline weight, allergies, medication history, and results of baseline laboratory tests, such as CBC and renal and liver function studies. These laboratory tests are also ordered during the different phases of treatment; monitor and document results appropriately. A major adverse effect of the protease inhibitors is lipid abnormalities with redistribution of fat stores under the skin, leading to undesirable cosmetic outcomes for the patient. Assess emotional status and support systems due to the impact of this adverse effect on body image. Bone demineralization is yet another adverse effect with long-term use, so assessment of calcium and vitamin D levels is crucial to patient safety before, during, and after therapy. *Indinavir (Crixivan)* may precipitate nephrolithiasis, so assess medical history for the occurrence of kidney stones. Assess also the patient's level of hydration.

The *antiretroviral* drug *maraviroc* requires assessment of allergies and liver function as well as a review of the list of medications the patient is taking because of many interacting drugs. *Raltegravir* is associated with myopathies and breakdown of muscle cells; thus, baseline notation of skeletal muscle functioning and pain level is crucial to patient safety. Perform a baseline measurement, and frequently monitor vital signs, including temperature, due to the possibility of opportunistic infections. The prescriber may also order CBCs and other laboratory studies before, during, and after therapy. Avoid *tenofovir* in patients with liver disorders. Bone marrow suppression is a dose-limiting adverse effect of *zidovudine*, so review blood cell counts and results of clotting studies before and during therapy.

With any of the drugs presented in this chapter, especially those used for the management of HIV infection, assessment of the patient's knowledge about the illness and the need for long-term and often lifelong therapy is crucial. In addition, an assessment of the patient's knowledge about the illness as well as his or her educational level, reading level, the way in which he or she learns best, and familiarity with community resources is important in implementing patient education effectively. Be sure to assess mental status and emotional state because of the psychologic impact of chronic illness on the patient, family, and significant others. Value systems, social patterns, hobbies, support systems, and spiritual beliefs also need to be assessed and documented. Perform an assessment of financial status and resources, as well. Many patients need to be referred to social services because of lack of health care insurance and financial resources because many of these drugs are lifelong. For patients with chronic illnesses, the synthesis of the assessment will help ensure the development of a nursing care plan that is complete and holistic.

CASE STUDY

Patient-Centered Care: Antiviral Therapy

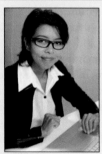

One of your patients, Z.K., a 33-year-old biology professor, has just begun therapy with lamivudine/zidovudine (Combivir) for a human immunodeficiency virus (HIV) infection. She has many questions about this medication therapy, and you are meeting with her to review her questions.

1. Z.K. asks you why there are two drugs in this particular medication. What is your explanation?
2. While she is receiving this drug therapy, Z.K. is continually monitored for what potential major problem?
3. What will be done to monitor for this problem, and how is it manifested?
4. Develop a patient teaching guide for Z.K., emphasizing any specific cautions and symptoms to report to the health care provider.

For answers, see *http://evolve.elsevier.com/Lilley.*

NURSING DIAGNOSES

1. Activity intolerance related to weakness secondary to decreased energy from pathology of viral infections
2. Deficient knowledge related to lack of information about and experience with long-term medication therapy and lack of information about the viral infection, its transmission, and its treatment
3. Risk for injury related to the immunosuppressive effects of viral disease processes and their treatment

PLANNING: OUTCOME IDENTIFICATION

1. Patient experiences improved comfort, energy, and activity level while receiving therapy.
2. Patient demonstrates improved knowledge base about the disease process, its transmission, treatment, and the need for lifelong therapy.
3. Patient remains free from injury and further insults to immune system while taking non-HIV and HIV antiviral medications.

IMPLEMENTATION

Nursing interventions pertinent to patients receiving *non-HIV antivirals* include use of the appropriate technique when applying or administering ointments, aerosol powders, and intravenous or oral forms of medication. Wear gloves and wash hands thoroughly before and after the administration of medication to prevent contamination of the site and spread of infection. It is important to the safety of both the patient and you to always begin by performing hand hygiene and maintain Standard Precautions (see Box 9-1). The use of non-HIV antivirals as well as HIV antivirals or antiretrovirals may lead to superimposed infection or superinfection, so constantly monitor for such infections and implement measures for their prevention (see Chapters 38 and 39).

Instruct the patient to take *oral antivirals* with meals to help minimize GI upset. Advise the patient to store capsules at room temperature and not to crush or break the capsules. *Acyclovir* is available in various dosage forms, and there are slight inconsistencies in the spelling of the drug names, so be sure to double-check the specific drug and dosage form ordered. Topical dosage forms (e.g., acyclovir) must be applied using a finger cot or gloves to prevent autoinoculation. Eye contact must also be avoided. Intravenous acyclovir is stable for 12 hours at room temperature and will often precipitate when refrigerated. Dilute intravenous infusions as recommended (e.g., with 5% dextrose in water or normal saline), and infuse with caution. Infusion over longer than 1 hour is suggested to avoid the renal tubular damage seen with more rapid infusions. Encourage adequate hydration during the infusion and for several hours afterward to prevent drug-related crystalluria. Carefully monitor the intravenous site. Document and report to the prescriber any redness, heat, pain, swelling, or red streaks that may indicate possible phlebitis. Document the characteristics of any lesions. Implement appropriate isolation for individuals with chickenpox or herpes zoster, and give analgesics for comfort, as ordered. Some of the more common adverse effects of acyclovir include nausea, diarrhea, and headache. Comfort measures may need to be implemented.

Amantadine and other *antivirals* need to be taken for the entire course of therapy, and, if a dose is missed, instruct the patient to take the dose as soon as it is remembered or contact the prescriber for further instructions. If dry mouth occurs due to anticholinergic effects, sucking on sugarless candy or chewing gum might be helpful. Encourage daily mouth care, including the use of dental floss, and regular dental preventive visits. Saliva substitutes may be needed, and if dry mouth continues for longer than 2 weeks, contact the prescriber for further instructions. Orthostatic hypotension may occur, so it is important to monitor vital signs with postural blood pressures during therapy. Encourage the patient to change positions slowly and carefully to prevent dizziness and syncope. If given intravenously, dilute ganciclovir with 5% dextrose in water or normal saline to a concentration and in a time frame indicated by the prescriber and authoritative sources. Administration into large veins is recommended to provide the dilution needed to minimize the risk for vein irritation. When handling the solution of ganciclovir, avoid exposure of the eyes, mucous membranes, and skin to the drug, and use latex gloves and safety glasses for handling and preparation. If the drug comes in contact with these areas, flush the eyes with plain water, and thoroughly wash other affected areas with soap and water. Laboratory values including blood counts will most likely be monitored during therapy due to possible bone marrow toxicity. *Ribavirin* may be given by nasal or oral inhalation, but the drug is not to be administered to pregnant women or handled by a health care provider who is (or may be) pregnant. Continually monitor for possible altered breath sounds, as wheezing may occur due to mild bronchospasm. When certain antivirals are given, always check the order closely against the drug being administered, because other drugs are spelled similarly or sound alike. For example, *acyclovir* may be mistaken for *valacyclovir* and *famciclovir*. When the patient is taking oseltamivir and other non-HIV antivirals for influenza, it is important to remember that this medication must be prescribed and is most effective if started within 2 days of the onset of flu symptoms.

Aerosol generators are available from the drug manufacturer. Discard reservoir solutions if levels are low or empty, and change every 24 hours. For patients taking *ribavirin* and similar drugs for treatment of respiratory syncytial virus via a small particle aerosol generator (SPAG) device, provide clear and precise instructions to on how to properly mix and administer the drug. Be sure to reconstitute the drug (e.g., ribavirin powder) as instructed in the manufacturer guidelines. Discard old solutions left in the equipment before adding fresh medication. Drugs administered via SPAG equipment are usually administered 12 to 18 hours daily for up to 7 days, beginning within 3 days of the onset of symptoms. Much controversy exists about the use of this drug in patients on ventilators, and it is to be administered by only health care providers who are specially trained in this drug and its use. Frequently empty any "rain out" in the tubing of the ventilator, and continually monitor breath sounds in patients receiving inhaled forms of this drug, whether they are receiving artificial ventilation or not. *Zanamivir* is administered by inhalation using a Diskhaler device. Be sure that the patient exhales completely first; then, while holding the mouthpiece between the teeth with lips snug around it and tongue down and out of the way, the patient needs to inhale deeply through the mouth and then hold the breath as long as possible before exhaling the drug and the breath. Encourage rinsing of the mouth with water to prevent irritation and dryness, and instruct the patient to never exhale into the Diskhaler.

With use of *simeprevir (Olysio)* and *sofosbuvir (Solvald)*, the drugs for treatment of chronic hepatitis C, remember that they are not to be used as monotherapy. Either drug, when ordered, is to be dosed once daily. Simeprevir is recommended to be taken with food to decrease GI upset. Educate about photosensitivity, and emphasize that it is a skin reaction (rash) precipitated by this medication with exposure to ultraviolet radiation from the sun or an artificial light source. Prevention includes wearing sunscreen and protective clothing or staying out of the sun. Sofosbuvir may be taken with or without food. *Telbivudine (Tyzeka)* may also be taken with or without food.

HIV antivirals, or *antiretrovirals*, include numerous drugs. With regard to dosage forms, there are special administration and handling guidelines for some of these drugs. With *zidovudine*, monitor for the adverse effects of bone marrow suppression by checking RBCs, WBCs, platelets, and other blood counts. If the patient experiences signs and symptoms of an opportunistic infection (e.g., respiratory signs and symptoms, fever, changes in oral mucosa), the prescriber needs to be contacted immediately. The patient may experience headaches; therefore, provide the appropriate form of analgesia, as ordered. See Table 40-2 for a listing of more adverse effects associated with the various antiviral drugs.

With film-coated oral dosage forms, advise the patient not to alter the drugs in any way. Patients may improve the taste of *ritonavir* by mixing it with chocolate milk or a nutritional beverage within 1 hour of its dosing. Emphasize to the patient and family that ritonavir's dosage form needs to be protected from light. Absorption of oral dosage forms of zidovudine is not impeded by taking the drug with food or milk, but instruct the patient to remain upright or with the head of the bed elevated while administering the medication and for up to 30 minutes afterward to prevent esophageal ulceration. Give an intravenous dose only if the solution is clear and does not contain any particulate matter. Be sure to use the appropriate dosage, diluents, and infusion time. Because these drugs often come in oral dosage forms, it is usually recommended that they be given with food. Generally, administer zidovudine and other antiretrovirals at evenly spaced intervals around the clock—as ordered—to ensure steady-state levels. With all oral and parenteral dosage forms of antiretrovirals, observe the patient for nausea and vomiting as well as any changes in weight, anorexia, or changes in bowel activity and patterns. *Indinavir* is best dissolved and absorbed in an acidic GI environment, and its absorption is decreased with high-protein, high-fat foods, so it is recommended to administer this drug in a fasting state. *Maraviroc* and *tenofovir* are available for oral dosing and are to be given as prescribed.

Throughout therapy, always remember that the goal of treatment is to find the regimen that provides the best control of the individual patient's infection with the most tolerable adverse effects possible. Because patients vary greatly in their drug tolerance, carefully individualize medication regimens. Other nursing interventions associated with these drugs include: (1) Continually monitor for adverse effects throughout therapy with a focus on the various organ systems, such as GI, neurologic, renal, and hepatic. (2) *Nevirapine, zidovudine*, and similar drugs may be associated with a rash; however, if the rash is accompanied by blistering, fever, malaise, myalgias, oral lesions, swelling or edema, or conjunctivitis, contact the prescriber immediately. (4) If drug therapy results in worsening of signs and symptoms, notify the prescriber immediately. The drug may be discontinued. (5) Continually monitor laboratory testing (e.g., CBC, renal/liver function studies, HIV RNA levels), and report abnormalities to the prescriber. HIV drug therapy is constantly changing, and an excellent resource is available at *www.fda.gov/ForPatients/Illness/HIVAIDS*. See Patient-Centered Care: Patient Teaching on the next page for more information.

EVALUATION

The therapeutic effects of *non-HIV antivirals* and *HIV antivirals* or *antiretrovirals* include elimination of the virus or a decrease in the symptoms of the viral infection. There may be a delayed progression of HIV infection and AIDS as well as a decrease in flulike symptoms and/or the frequency of herpetic flare-ups and other lesion breakouts. With successful therapy, herpetic lesions will crust over, and the frequency of recurrence will decrease. In addition, constantly evaluate for the occurrence of adverse effects and toxicity associated with specific antiviral and antiretroviral drugs.

These specific adverse effects are listed in Table 40-2. Continually reevaluate the nursing care plan to ensure that the goals and outcome criteria have been met. Remain constantly attentive in reviewing reports from the CDC, other federal and state health care agencies, and public health care organizations regarding new strains of viruses and flu syndromes (see earlier discussion).

PATIENT-CENTERED CARE: PATIENT TEACHING

- Alert the patient to the adverse effect of dizziness, and instruct him or her to use caution while driving or participating in activities requiring alertness while taking antiviral drugs. Advise the patient to take all medications exactly as prescribed and for the full course of therapy.
- Inform the patient of all possible drug interactions including over-the-counter medications.
- Advise immunocompromised patients to avoid crowds and persons with infections.
- Advocate Standard Precautions and safe sex practices for all patients, but especially those with sexually transmitted viral diseases, such as HIV-positive individuals. Condom use is a necessity for prevention of these viral infections and other sexually transmitted diseases. The presence of genital herpes requires sexual abstinence.
- It is generally recommended that female patients with genital herpes undergo a Papanicolaou smear test (Pap test) every 6 months or as ordered by the prescriber to monitor the virus and effectiveness of therapy.
- Instruct the patient taking antivirals to report the following adverse reactions to the prescriber: decreased urinary output, seizure activity, syncope, nervousness, lightheadedness, jaundice, wheezing, abnormal sensations in the hands and feet, anorexia, nausea, vomiting, diarrhea, weakness, changes in taste, acid regurgitation, and abdominal/flank or back pain.
- Provide the patient with adequate demonstrations, teaching aids, and instructions for special application procedures (e.g., instillation of ophthalmic drops, use of finger cots or gloves when applying medication to lesions, use of respiratory inhalation forms). Explain that gloves or finger cots

are needed for medication application and cleansing to prevent the spread of lesions. Instruct the patient to wash hands before and after application of medication.
- Encourage forcing fluids up to 3000 mL/24 hr unless contraindicated.
- Educate the patient about the fact that these drugs suppress but do not cure the viral infection.
- Inform the patient that therapy is to be started as prescribed but at the first sign (as with valacyclovir or other antivirals) of a recurrent episode of genital herpes or herpes zoster. In addition, explain that early treatment within 24 to 48 hours of symptom onset is needed to achieve full therapeutic results.
- Instruct the patient to report to the prescriber immediately any difficulty breathing; drastic changes in blood pressure; bleeding; new symptoms; worsening of infection, fever, or chills; or other unusual problems.
- Emphasize the importance of follow-up appointments with any of the antivirals.
- Ribavirin (Virazole) is associated with teratogenesis and is not to be taken by pregnant women or by women who may become pregnant during exposure to the drug. Educate patients about this concern, and provide education/counseling about appropriate contraceptive measures.
- Educate the patient about the prevention of skin reactions due to photosensitivity associated with the use of simeprevir.
- Telbivudine (Tyzeka) may be taken without regard to food and is associated with common adverse effects of fatigue, headache, diarrhea, nausea, myopathy, and hepatomegaly.

KEY POINTS

- Viruses are difficult to kill and to treat because they live inside human cells, and most antiviral drugs work by inhibiting replication of the virus. In this chapter, antiviral drugs are categorized as either non-HIV antivirals or HIV antivirals (antiretrovirals).
- Non-HIV antivirals include amantadine, rimantadine, acyclovir, ganciclovir, oseltamivir, zanamivir, and ribavirin. HIV antivirals include enfuvirtide, indinavir, maraviroc, nevirapine, raltegravir, tenofovir, and zidovudine.
- Administer antiretroviral drugs only after the prescriber's orders are read and understood and after performing a

thorough nursing assessment that includes a review of the patient's nutritional status, weight, baseline vital signs, and renal and hepatic functioning as well as an assessment of heart sounds, neurologic status, and GI tract functioning.
- Comfort measures and supportive nursing care are to accompany drug therapy. Patients need to drink plenty of fluids and to space medications around the clock, as ordered, to maintain steady blood levels of the drug.

NCLEX® EXAMINATION REVIEW QUESTIONS

1. During treatment with zidovudine, the nurse needs to monitor for which potential adverse effect?
   a. Retinitis
   b. Deep vein thromboses
   c. Kaposi's sarcoma
   d. Bone marrow suppression

2. After giving an injection to a patient with HIV infection, the nurse accidentally receives a needlestick from a too-full needle disposal box. Recommendations for occupational HIV exposure may include the use of which drug(s)?
   a. didanosine
   b. lamivudine and enfuvirtide
   c. emtricitabine and tenofovir
   d. acyclovir

3. When the nurse is teaching a patient who is taking acyclovir for genital herpes, which statement by the nurse is accurate?
   a. "This drug will help the lesions to dry and crust over."
   b. "Acyclovir will eradicate the herpes virus."
   c. "This drug will prevent the spread of this virus to others."
   d. "Be sure to give this drug to your partner, too."

4. A patient who has been newly diagnosed with HIV has many questions about the effectiveness of drug therapy. After a teaching session, which statement by the patient reflects a need for more education?
   a. "I will be monitored for side effects and improvements while I'm taking this medicine."
   b. "These drugs do not eliminate the HIV, but hopefully the amount of virus in my body will be reduced."
   c. "There is no cure for HIV."
   d. "These drugs will eventually eliminate the virus from my body."

5. After surgery for organ transplantation, a patient is receiving ganciclovir, even though he does not have a viral infection. Which statement best explains the rationale for this medication therapy?
   a. Ganciclovir is used to prevent potential exposure to the HIV virus.
   b. This medication is given prophylactically to prevent influenza A infection.
   c. Ganciclovir is given to prevent CMV infection.
   d. The drug works synergistically with antibiotics to prevent superinfections.

6. The nurse is reviewing the use of multidrug therapy for HIV with a patient. Which statements are correct regarding the reason for using multiple drugs to treat HIV? (Select all that apply.)
   a. The combination of drugs has fewer associated toxicities.
   b. The use of multiple drugs is more effective against resistant strains of HIV.
   c. Effective treatment results in reduced T-cell counts.
   d. The goal of this treatment is to reduce the viral load.
   e. This type of therapy reduces the incidence of opportunistic infections.

7. The order for a patient who has a severe case of shingles is for acyclovir (Zovirax) 10 mg/kg IV every 8 hours for 7 days. The patient weighs 165 pounds. How much is each dose?

8. The nurse notes in the patient's medication history that the patient is taking sofosbuvir (Solvaldi) with ribavirin. Based on this finding, the nurse interprets that the patient has which disorder?
   a. Cytomegalovirus
   b. Genital herpes
   c. Chronic hepatitis C
   d. Respiratory syncytial virus infection

1. d, 2. c, 3. a, 4. d, 5. c, 6. b, d, e, 7. 750 mg per dose, 8. c.

CRITICAL THINKING AND PRIORITIZATION QUESTIONS

1. A young adult female patient underwent bone marrow transplantation, and less than 1 year later she contracted a cytomegalovirus (CMV) infection. She is concerned about the medications and asks, "Are these antiviral drugs going to be a problem? What if I get pregnant?" What is the nurse's priority when responding to her questions? Explain your answer.

2. A college student has had symptoms of the flu since Friday, but she does not go to the student health office until the following Tuesday. She tells the nurse that she is "miserable" and that she heard about Tamiflu on the Internet. She wants to take it to "keep the flu from getting worse." What is the nurse's best response to the student's request?

For answers, see *http://evolve.elsevier.com/Lilley*.

EVOLVE WEBSITE

Antitubercular Drugs

http://evolve.elsevier.com/Lilley

OBJECTIVES

When you reach the end of this chapter, you will be able to do the following:

1. Identify the various first-line and second-line drugs indicated for the treatment of tuberculosis.
2. Discuss the mechanisms of action, dosages, adverse effects, routes of administration, special dosing considerations, cautions, contraindications, and drug interactions of the various antitubercular drugs.
3. Develop a nursing care plan that includes all phases of the nursing process for patients receiving antitubercular drugs.
4. Develop a comprehensive teaching guide for patients and families impacted by the diagnosis and treatment of antitubercular drugs.

DRUG PROFILES

ethambutol, p. 664
♦ isoniazid, p. 664
pyrazinamide, p. 665
rifabutin, p. 665
rifampin, p. 665

rifapentine, p. 666
streptomycin, p. 666

_____

♦ = *Key drug*
! = *High-alert drug*

KEY TERMS

Aerobic Requiring oxygen for the maintenance of life. (p. 661)

Antitubercular drugs Drugs used to treat infections caused by *Mycobacterium* bacterial species. (p. 662)

Bacillus A rod-shaped bacterium. (p. 661)

Granulomas Small nodular aggregations of inflammatory cells (e.g., macrophages, lymphocytes) characterized by clearly delimited boundaries, as found in tuberculosis. (p. 660)

Isoniazid The primary and most commonly prescribed tuberculostatic drug. (p. 661)

Multidrug-resistant tuberculosis (MDR-TB) Tuberculosis that demonstrates resistance to two or more drugs. (p. 661)

Slow acetylator An individual with a genetic defect that causes a deficiency in the enzyme needed to metabolize isoniazid, the most widely used tuberculosis drug. (p. 664)

Tubercle The characteristic lesion of tuberculosis; a small round gray translucent granulomatous lesion, usually with a caseated (cheesy) consistency in its interior. (See *granuloma*.) (p. 661)

Tubercle bacilli Another common name for rod-shaped tuberculosis bacteria; essentially synonymous with *Mycobacterium tuberculosis*. (p. 661)

Tuberculosis (TB) Any infectious disease caused by species of *Mycobacterium*, usually *Mycobacterium tuberculosis* (adjectives: *tuberculous, tubercular*). (p. 660)

PATHOPHYSIOLOGY OF TUBERCULOSIS

Tuberculosis (TB) is the medical diagnosis for any infection caused by a bacterial species known as *Mycobacterium*. TB is most commonly characterized by granulomas in the lungs. These are nodular accumulations of inflammatory cells (e.g., macrophages, lymphocytes) that are delimited ("walled off" with clear boundaries) and have a center that has a cheesy or caseated consistency. (*Casein* is the name of a protein that is prevalent in cheese and milk.) There are two mycobacterial species that can cause TB, *Mycobacterium tuberculosis* and *Mycobacterium bovis*. Infections caused by *M. tuberculosis* (abbreviated MTB) are the most common. There are also several other mycobacterial species, including *Mycobacterium leprae*, which causes leprosy, and *Mycobacterium avium-intracellulare* complex (MAC). Infections with these bacteria are much less of a public health problem and hence are not the focus of this chapter.

MTB is an aerobic bacillus, which means that it is a rod-shaped microorganism (bacillus) that requires a large supply of oxygen to grow and flourish (aerobic). This bacterium's need for a highly oxygenated body site explains why *Mycobacterium* infections most commonly affect the lungs. Other common sites of infection are the growing ends of bones and the brain (cerebral cortex). Less common sites of infection include the kidney, liver, and genitourinary tract.

Tubercle bacilli (a common synonym for MTB) are transmitted from one of three sources: humans, cattle (adjective: *bovine,* hence the species name *M. bovis*), or birds (adjective: *avian*), although bovine and avian transmission are much less common than human transmission. Tubercle bacilli are conveyed in droplets expelled by infected people or animals during coughing or sneezing and then inhaled by the new host. After these infectious droplets are inhaled, the infection spreads to the susceptible organ sites by means of the blood and lymphatic system. MTB is a very slow-growing organism, which makes it more difficult to treat than most other bacterial infections. Many of the antibiotics used to treat TB work by inhibiting growth (bacteriostatic) rather than by directly killing the organism. The reason why microorganisms that grow slowly are more difficult to kill is because their cells are not as metabolically active. Most bactericidal (cell-killing) drugs work by disrupting critical cellular metabolic processes in the organism. Therefore, the most drug-susceptible organisms are those with faster (not slower) metabolic activity.

The first infectious episode is considered the primary TB infection; reinfection represents the chronic form of the disease. TB does not develop in all people who are exposed to the bacteria. In some cases, the bacteria become dormant and walled off by calcified or fibrous tissues. These patients may test positive for exposure but are not necessarily infectious because of this dormancy process. In immunocompromised patients, TB can inflict devastating and irreversible damage. The steps for diagnosis of TB are listed in Box 41-1.

TB cases have been reported on a national level in the United States beginning in 1953. Since that time, the TB incidence decreased in most years until about 1985. At that point, the epidemic of human immunodeficiency virus (HIV) infection was growing strongly, and the TB incidence began to rise for the first time in 20 years because of the development of TB in patients coinfected with HIV. In 1992, there was a resurgence peak in the United States, but it has decreased since that time. A rate of 3.2 TB cases per 100,000 persons was reported in 2012,

with a 5.4% and 6.1% decline in cases reported and case rate, respectively. The number of reported TB cases in 2012 was the lowest recorded rate since national reporting began in 1953. The decline is attributed to intensified public health efforts aimed at preventing, diagnosing, and treating TB as well as HIV infection. However, the concern now focuses on the increasing number of multidrug-resistant tuberculosis (MDR-TB) cases.

The prevalence and growth of TB continues to be greater in the larger global community, and TB infects one third of the world's population. It is currently second only to HIV infection in the number of deaths caused by a single infectious organism. MDR-TB is defined as TB that is resistant to both isoniazid and rifampin, according to the World Health Organization. Close contacts of patients with MDR-TB need to be treated as well. Extensively drug-resistant tuberculosis (XDR-TB) is a relatively rare type of MDR-TB. It is resistant to almost all drugs used to treat TB, including the two best first-line drugs, isoniazid and rifampin, as well as to the best second-line medications. Because XDR-TB is resistant to the most powerful first-line and second-line drugs, patients are left with treatment options that are much less effective and often have worse treatment outcomes. XDR-TB is of special concern for patients who have AIDS or are otherwise immunocompromised. Not only are these patients more likely to contract TB, they are also more likely to die from it. Several factors have contributed to this health care crisis, but one very important source of the problem is the increasing numbers of people in groups that are particularly susceptible to the infection—the homeless, undernourished or malnourished individuals, HIV-infected persons, drug abusers, cancer patients, those taking immunosuppressant drugs, and those who live in crowded and poorly sanitized housing facilities. All of these circumstances also favor the acquisition of a drug-resistant infection. Members of racial and ethnic minority groups are at greater risk than white populations and account for two thirds of new cases. Asian and Hispanic immigrants are at particularly high risk, accounting for more than half of all U.S. cases of foreign-acquired TB.

ANTITUBERCULAR DRUGS

The drugs used to treat infections caused by all forms of *Mycobacterium* are called antitubercular drugs. These drugs fall into two categories: primary or first-line drugs and secondary or second-line drugs. As these designations imply, primary drugs are those tried first, whereas secondary drugs are reserved for more complicated cases, such as those resistant to primary drugs. The antimycobacterial activity, efficacy, and potential adverse and toxic effects of the various drugs determine the class to which they belong. Isoniazid is a primary antitubercular drug and is the most widely used. It can be administered either as the sole drug in the prophylaxis of TB or in combination with other antitubercular drugs in the treatment of TB. The various first-line and second-line antibiotic drugs are listed in Box 41-2. There are also two miscellaneous TB-related injections—one diagnostic, the other a vaccine. These are described in Box 41-3. In 2013, the FDA granted accelerated approval for bedaquiline (Sirturo) for the treatment of MDR-TB.

BOX 41-1 Diagnosis of Tuberculosis

Step 1: Tuberculin skin test (Mantoux test)
Step 2: If skin test results are positive, then chest x-ray
Step 3: If chest x-ray shows signs of tuberculosis, then culture of sputum* or stomach secretions

*The acid-fast bacillus smear test is performed on sputum as a quick method of determining whether tuberculosis treatment and precautions are needed until a more definite diagnosis is made.

It inhibits mycobacterial ATP synthase. Bedaquiline is the first drug in 40 years with a new mechanism of action. Side effects include headache, chest pain, nausea, and QT prolongation. It is classified as a pregnancy category B drug. The following should be avoided while taking bedaquiline: alcohol, mifepristone, strong CYP3A4 inhibitors, and drugs with high risk for causing QT prolongation. Administration with food significantly increases bedaquiline absorption and should be given with food to aid in its absorption.

An important consideration during drug selection is the likelihood of drug-resistant organisms and drug toxicity. Other key elements that are important in effective therapy include the following:

- Drug-susceptibility tests are to be performed on the first *Mycobacterium* species that is isolated from a patient specimen (to prevent the development of MDR-TB).
- Before the results of the susceptibility tests are known, the patient is started on a four-drug regimen consisting of isoniazid, rifampin, pyrazinamide (PZA), and ethambutol or streptomycin, which together are 95% effective in combating the infection. The use of multiple medications reduces the possibility of the organism's becoming drug resistant.
- Once drug susceptibility results are available, the regimen is adjusted accordingly.
- Patient adherence to the prescribed drug regimen and any adverse effects of therapy need to be monitored closely,

because the incidence of both patient nonadherence and adverse effects is high.

Mechanism of Action and Drug Effects

The mechanisms of action of the various antitubercular drugs vary depending on the drug. These drugs act by inhibiting protein synthesis, inhibiting cell wall synthesis, or various other mechanisms. The antitubercular drugs are listed in Table 41-1 by their mechanism of action. The major effects of drug therapy include reduction of cough and, therefore, reduction of the infectiousness of the patient. This normally occurs within 2 weeks of the initiation of drug therapy, assuming that the patient's TB strain is drug sensitive. With appropriate antibiotic treatment, most cases of TB can be cured. Successful treatment usually involves taking several antibiotic drugs for at least 6 months and sometimes for as long as 12 months.

Indications

Antitubercular medications are indicated for the treatment of TB infections, including both pulmonary and extrapulmonary TB. Most antitubercular drugs have not been fully tested for their effects in pregnant women. However, the combination of isoniazid and ethambutol has been used to treat pregnant women without teratogenic complications. Rifampin is another drug that is usually safe during pregnancy and is a more likely choice for more advanced disease.

Besides being used for the initial treatment of TB, antitubercular drugs have also proved effective in the management of treatment failures and relapses. Infection with species of *Mycobacterium* other than *M. tuberculosis* and atypical mycobacterial infections have also been successfully treated with these drugs. Nontuberculous *Mycobacteria* may also be susceptible to antitubercular drugs. However, in general, antitubercular drugs are not as effective against other species of *Mycobacterium* as they are against MTB.

In summary, antitubercular drugs are primarily used for the prophylaxis or treatment of TB. The effectiveness of these drugs depends on the type of infection, adequate dosing, sufficient duration of treatment, adherence to the drug regimen, and selection of an effective drug combination. The indications of the different antitubercular drugs are listed in Table 41-2.

Contraindications

Contraindications to the use of various antitubercular drugs include severe drug allergy and major renal or liver dysfunction. However, it must be recognized that the urgency of treating a potentially fatal infection may have to be balanced against any prevailing contraindications. In extreme cases, patients are sometimes given a drug to which they have some degree of allergy with supportive care that enables them at least to tolerate the medication. Examples of such supportive care are treatment with antipyretics (e.g., acetaminophen), antihistamines (e.g., diphenhydramine), or corticosteroids (e.g., prednisone, methylprednisolone).

One relative contraindication to ethambutol is optic neuritis. Chronic alcohol use, especially when associated with major liver damage, may also be a contraindication to therapy with any

TABLE 41-1 Antitubercular Drugs: Mechanisms of Action

Drugs	Description
Inhibit Protein Synthesis	
kanamycin, capreomycin, rifabutin, rifampin, streptomycin	Streptomycin and kanamycin work by interfering with normal protein synthesis and causing the production of faulty proteins. Rifampin and rifabutin inhibit RNA synthesis and may also inhibit DNA synthesis. Human cells are not as sensitive as the mycobacterial cells and are not affected by rifampin except at high drug concentrations. Capreomycin inhibits protein synthesis by preventing translocation on ribosomes.
Inhibit Cell Wall Synthesis	
cycloserine, ethionamide, isoniazid	Cycloserine acts by inhibiting the amino acid (D-alanine) involved in the synthesis of cell walls. Isoniazid and ethionamide also act at least partly to inhibit the synthesis of wall components, but the mechanisms of these two drugs are still not clearly understood.
Other Mechanisms	
ethambutol, ethionamide, isoniazid, para-aminosalicylic acid, pyrazinamide	Isoniazid is taken up by mycobacterial cells and undergoes hydrolysis to isonicotinic acid, which reacts with cofactor NAD to form a defective NAD that is no longer active as a coenzyme for certain life-sustaining reactions in the *Mycobacterium tuberculosis* organism. Ethionamide directly inhibits mycolic acid synthesis, which eventually has the same deleterious effects on the TB organism as isoniazid. Ethambutol affects lipid synthesis, which results in the inhibition of mycolic acid incorporation into the cell wall and thus inhibits protein synthesis. Para-aminosalicylic acid acts as a competitive inhibitor of para-aminobenzoic acid in the synthesis of folate. The mechanism of action of pyrazinamide in the inhibition of TB is unknown. It can be either bacteriostatic or bactericidal, depending on the susceptibility of the particular *Mycobacterium* organism and the concentration of the drug attained at the site of infection.

NAD, Nicotinamide adenine; *TB,* tuberculosis.

TABLE 41-2 Antitubercular Drugs: Clinical Uses

Drug	Clinical Uses
capreomycin	Used with other antitubercular drugs for the treatment of pulmonary TB caused by *Mycobacterium tuberculosis* after first-line drugs fail, drug resistance appears, or drug toxicity occurs.
cycloserine	Used with other antitubercular drugs for treatment of active pulmonary and extrapulmonary TB after failure of first-line drugs.
ethambutol	Indicated as a first-line drug for treatment of TB.
ethionamide	Used with other antitubercular drugs after failure of first-line drugs and for treatment of other types of mycobacterial infections.
isoniazid	Used alone or in combination with other antitubercular drugs in treatment and prevention of clinical TB.
para-aminosalicylic acid	Used in combination with other antitubercular drugs for treatment of pulmonary and extrapulmonary *M. tuberculosis* infection after failure of first-line drugs.
pyrazinamide	Used with other antitubercular drugs in treatment of clinical TB.
rifabutin	Used to prevent or delay development of *Mycobacterium avium-intracellulare* bacteremia and disseminated infections in patients with advanced HIV infection.
rifampin	Used with other antitubercular drugs in treatment of clinical TB.
	Used in treatment of diseases caused by mycobacteria other than *M. tuberculosis*.
	Used for preventive therapy in patients exposed to isoniazid-resistant *M. tuberculosis*.
	Used to eliminate meningococci from the nasopharynx of asymptomatic *Neisseria meningitidis* carriers when risk for meningococcal meningitis is high.
	Used for chemoprophylaxis in contacts of patients with HiB infection.
	Used with at least one other antiinfective drug in the treatment of leprosy.
	Used in the treatment of endocarditis caused by methicillin-resistant staphylococci, chronic staphylococcal prostatitis, and multiple-antiinfective–resistant pneumococci.
rifapentine	Used with other antitubercular drugs in the treatment of clinical TB.
streptomycin	Used in combination with other antitubercular drugs in the treatment of clinical TB and other mycobacterial diseases.

HiB, Haemophilus influenzae type b; *HIV,* human immunodeficiency virus; *TB,* tuberculosis.

antitubercular drug. Other contraindications for specific drugs, if any, can be found in the drug profiles presented later in the chapter.

Adverse Effects

Antitubercular drugs are fairly well tolerated. Isoniazid, one of the mainstays of treatment, is noted for causing pyridoxine deficiency and liver toxicity. For this reason, supplements of pyridoxine (vitamin B_6; see Chapter 53) are often given concurrently with isoniazid. Adverse effects of antitubercular drugs are listed in Table 41-3.

Interactions

There are many drugs that can interact with antitubercular drugs. See Table 41-4 for a listing of selected interactions. Besides these drug interactions, isoniazid can cause false-positive readings on urine glucose tests (e.g., Clinitest) and an

increase in the serum levels of the liver function enzymes alanine aminotransferase and aspartate aminotransferase.

Dosages

For dosage information on selected antitubercular drugs, see the table on the next page.

DRUG PROFILES

ethambutol

Ethambutol (Myambutol) is a first-line bacteriostatic drug used in the treatment of TB. It works by diffusing into the mycobacteria and suppressing ribonucleic acid (RNA) synthesis, which thereby inhibits protein synthesis. Ethambutol is included with isoniazid, streptomycin, and rifampin in many TB combination-drug therapies. It may also be used to treat other mycobacterial diseases. It is contraindicated in patients with known optic neuritis, because it can both exacerbate and cause this condition, which can result in varying degrees of vision loss. Ethambutol is also contraindicated in children younger than 13 years of age. It is available only in oral form.

Pharmacokinetics: Ethambutol

Route	Onset of Action	Peak Plasma Concentration	Elimination Half-life	Duration of Action
PO	Variable	2-4 hr	3.5 hr	24 hr

◆ isoniazid

Isoniazid (also called INH) is the mainstay in the treatment of TB and the most widely used antitubercular drug. It may be given either as a single drug for prophylaxis or in combination with other antitubercular drugs for the treatment of active TB. It is a bactericidal drug that kills the mycobacteria by disrupting cell wall synthesis and essential cellular functions. Isoniazid is metabolized in the liver through a process called *acetylation*, which requires a certain enzymatic pathway to break down the drug. Some people have a genetic deficiency of the liver enzymes needed for this to occur. Such people are called slow acetylators. When isoniazid is taken by slow acetylators, the isoniazid accumulates, because there is not enough of the enzyme to break down the isoniazid. Therefore, the dosages of isoniazid may need to be adjusted downward in these patients.

TABLE 41-3   Antitubercular Drugs: Common Adverse Effects

Drug	Adverse Effects
bedaquiline	Headache, chest pain, nausea, QT prolongation
capreomycin	Ototoxicity, nephrotoxicity
cycloserine	Psychotic behavior, seizures
ethambutol	Retrobulbar neuritis, blindness
ethionamide	GI tract disturbances, hepatotoxicity
isoniazid	Peripheral neuropathy, hepatotoxicity, optic neuritis and visual disturbances, hyperglycemia
para-aminosalicylic acid	GI tract disturbances, hepatotoxicity
pyrazinamide	Hepatotoxicity, hyperuricemia
rifabutin	GI tract disturbances; rash; neutropenia; red-orange-brown discoloration of urine, feces, saliva, sputum, sweat, tears, and skin
rifampin	Hepatitis; hematologic disorders; red-orange-brown discoloration of urine, tears, sweat, and sputum
rifapentine	GI upset; red-orange-brown discoloration of tears, sweat, skin, teeth, tongue, sputum, saliva, urine, feces, and CSF
streptomycin	Ototoxicity, nephrotoxicity, blood dyscrasias

CSF, Cerebrospinal fluid.

TABLE 41-4   Selected Antitubercular Drugs: Drug Interactions

Drug	Interacting Drugs	Mechanism	Results
isoniazid	Antacids	Reduce absorption	Decreased isoniazid levels
	cycloserine, ethionamide, rifampin	Have additive effects	Increased central nervous system and hepatic toxicity
	phenytoin, carbamazepine	Decrease metabolism	Increased phenytoin and carbamazepine effects
streptomycin	Nephrotoxic and neurotoxic drugs	Have additive effects	Increased toxicity
	Oral anticoagulants	Alter intestinal flora	Increased bleeding tendencies
rifampin	Beta blockers, benzodiazepines, cyclosporine, oral anticoagulants, oral antidiabetics, oral contraceptives, phenytoin, quinidine, sirolimus, theophylline	Increase metabolism	Decreased therapeutic effects of these drugs

DOSAGES

Selected Antitubercular Drugs

Drug (Pregnancy Category)	Pharmacologic Class	Usual Adult Dosage Range	Indications
ethambutol (Myambutol) (B)	Synthetic first-line antimycobacterial	PO: 15-25 mg/kg/day; may also be divided into twice/wk and 3 times/wk dosages	
♦ isoniazid (INH), generic only (C)	Synthetic first-line antimycobacterial	PO: 5 mg/kg daily (max 300 mg) or 15 mg/kg 1-3 times/wk (max 900 mg/dose)	
pyrazinamide (generic only) (C)	Synthetic first-line antimycobacterial	PO: 15-30 mg/kg/day (max 2 g)	
rifabutin (Mycobutin) (B)	Semisynthetic first-line antimycobacterial antibiotic	PO: 150 mg bid or 300 mg daily	Active TB
rifampin* (Rifadin, Rimactane) (C)	Semisynthetic first-line antimycobacterial antibiotic	PO/IV: 10 mg/kg up to 600 mg once daily	
rifapentine (Priftin) (C)	Semisynthetic first-line antimycobacterial antibiotic	PO: 600 mg twice/wk for first 2 mo, then once/wk for 4 mo	
streptomycin (generic) (D)	Aminoglycoside antibiotic used in combination with other drugs for TB	Deep IM: 15 mg/kg/day	

*Use of intramuscular and subcutaneous injections is contraindicated due to soft-tissue toxicity.

Isoniazid is most commonly used in oral form, although an injection is available. There is also a combination oral formulation containing both isoniazid and rifampin (Rifamate). Another combination drug product, Rifater, contains rifampin, isoniazid, and pyrazinamide. Isoniazid is contraindicated in those with previous isoniazid-associated hepatic injury or any acute liver disease. Isoniazid is noted for causing pyridoxine deficiency. For this reason, supplements of pyridoxine (vitamin B_6; see Chapter 53) are often given concurrently with isoniazid.

Pharmacokinetics: Isoniazid

Route	Onset of Action	Peak Plasma Concentration	Elimination Half-life	Duration of Action
PO	Variable	1-2 hr	1-4 hr	24 hr

pyrazinamide

Pyrazinamide (also called PZA) is an antitubercular drug that can be either bacteriostatic or bactericidal, depending on its concentration at the site of infection and the particular susceptibility of the mycobacteria. It is commonly used in combination with other antitubercular drugs for the treatment of TB. Its mechanism of action is unknown, but it is believed to work by inhibiting lipid and nucleic acid synthesis in the mycobacteria. Pyrazinamide is available only in generic oral form. It is contraindicated in patients with severe hepatic disease or acute gout. It is also not normally used in pregnant patients in the United States, due to a lack of teratogenicity data, although it is often used in pregnant patients in other countries.

Pharmacokinetics: Pyrazinamide

Route	Onset of Action	Peak Plasma Concentration	Elimination Half-life	Duration of Action
PO	Variable	2 hr	9-10 hr	24 hr

rifabutin

Rifabutin is one of three currently available *rifamycin* antibiotics. Although it is considered a first-line TB drug by some practitioners, it is more commonly used to treat infections caused by *M. avium-intracellulare* complex, which includes several non-TB mycobacterial species. This is also the case with the two other rifamycin-derived drugs, rifampin and rifapentine. A notable adverse effect of rifabutin, as well as rifampin (see later in the chapter), is that it can turn urine, feces, saliva, skin, sputum, sweat, and tears a red-orange-brown color. Rifabutin is currently available only for oral use.

Pharmacokinetics: Rifabutin

Route	Onset of Action	Peak Plasma Concentration	Elimination Half-life	Duration of Action
PO	Variable	2-4 hr	16-69 hr	1 to several days

rifampin

Rifampin (Rifadin) is the first of the rifamycin class of synthetic macrocyclic antibiotics, which also includes rifabutin and rifapentine. The term *macrocyclic* connotes the very large and complex hydrocarbon ring structure included in all three of the rifamycin compounds. Rifampin has activity against many *Mycobacterium* species, as well as against *Meningococcus*, *Haemophilus influenzae* type b, and *M. leprae*. It is a broad-spectrum bactericidal drug that kills the offending organism by inhibiting protein synthesis. Rifampin is used either alone in the prevention of TB or in combination with other antitubercular drugs in its treatment. It is available in both oral and parenteral formulations and in combination with isoniazid (Rifamate). Rifampin is contraindicated in patients with known drug allergy to it or to any other rifamycin (i.e., rifabutin, rifapentine). The drug is a potent enzyme inducer and is associated with many drug interactions (see Table 41-4.) Rifampin may cause urine, saliva, tears, and sweat to be red-orange-brown colored.

Pharmacokinetics: Rifampin

Route	Onset of Action	Peak Plasma Concentration	Elimination Half-life	Duration of Action
PO	Variable	2-4 hr	3.5 hr	Up to 24 hr

rifapentine

Rifapentine (Priftin) is a derivative of rifampin. It offers advantages over rifampin in that it has a much longer duration of action and possibly better efficacy. It has been shown to have greater antimycobacterial efficacy and macrophage penetration. Its accumulation into tissue macrophages allows it to work synergistically against bacterial cells that are ingested by the macrophage during phagocytosis ("cell eating"). Rifapentine is available only for oral use.

Pharmacokinetics: Rifapentine

Route	Onset of Action	Peak Plasma Concentration	Elimination Half-life	Duration of Action
PO	Unknown	5-6 hr	13-17 hr	1 to several days

streptomycin

Streptomycin is an aminoglycoside antibiotic currently available only in generic form. Introduced in 1944, it was the very first drug available that could effectively treat TB. Because of its toxicities, it is used most commonly in combination drug regimens for the treatment of multidrug-resistant TB infections. Streptomycin is currently available only in injectable form. It is classified as a pregnancy category D drug and is usually not given to pregnant patients.

Pharmacokinetics: Streptomycin

Route	Onset of Action	Peak Plasma Concentration	Elimination Half-life	Duration of Action
IM	Variable	1-2 hr	2-3 hr	Up to 24 hr

▌NURSING PROCESS

▌ASSESSMENT

Before administering any of the *antitubercular drugs,* and to ensure the safe and effective use of these medications, obtain a thorough medical history, medication profile, and nursing history. Perform a complete head-to-toe physical assessment. Note any specific history of diagnoses or symptoms of TB. Determine the results of the patient's last purified protein derivative (PPD) or tuberculin skin test and the reaction at the intradermal injection site. Review the most recent chest x-ray and results. Assess the results of liver function studies (e.g., bilirubin level, liver enzyme levels) and kidney function studies (e.g., BUN, creatinine clearance). As noted earlier, major liver and/or renal dysfunction are contraindications. These specific

laboratory values also provide comparative baseline data throughout therapy.

Because some *antituberculin drugs* may lead to peripheral neuropathies, note baseline neurologic functioning prior to therapy. Assess hearing status, especially when *streptomycin* is to be used, because of its drug-related ototoxicity. A gross eye examination is important due to the drug-induced adverse effect of visual disturbances and optic neuritis with *isoniazid, levofloxacin,* and *ofloxacin.* Blindness may occur with the use of *ethambutol.*

Assessment of age is also important because the likelihood of adverse reactions and toxicity is increased in older adult patients due to age-related liver and kidney dysfunction. Additionally, the safety of these drugs in children 13 years of age and younger has not been established. Assess the patient's CBC prior to giving isoniazid, streptomycin, and *rifampin* because of the potential for drug-related hematologic disorders. Renal function studies, such as creatinine clearance and BUN, may be ordered prior to therapy with streptomycin due to the nephrotoxicity associated with its use. Document uric acid baseline levels with use of *pyrazinamide* due to the drug-induced adverse effect of hyperuricemia and symptoms of gout. Analysis of sputum specimens is usually ordered as well, to aid in determining the appropriate drug regimen. Contraindications, cautions, and drug interactions have been discussed previously. Assess for drug interactions with use of *bedaqulinie (Sirturo)* including alcohol, mifepristone, and strong CYP3A4 drugs.

▌NURSING DIAGNOSES

1. Ineffective family health management related to poor compliance with antitubercular drug therapy and lack of knowledge about long-term therapies
2. Deficient knowledge related to the disease process and treatment protocol
3. Risk for injury related to noncompliance with the drug therapy regimen and an overall poor health status

▌PLANNING: OUTCOME IDENTIFICATION

1. Patient experiences improved therapeutic regimen management with compliance to regimen and understanding about method of spread and improved symptomatology.
2. Patient gains increased knowledge about antitubercular medication therapy and takes medication regularly and for the length of time prescribed with reporting of adverse effects and/or relapse in symptoms.
3. Patient remains free from injury related to noncompliance with antitubercular drug regimen.

▌IMPLEMENTATION

Because drug therapy is the mainstay of treatment for TB and often lasts for up to 24 months, patient education is critical, with a special emphasis on adherence to the drug regimen. Provide simple, clear, and concise instructions to the

CASE STUDY

Patient-Centered Care: Antitubercular Drugs

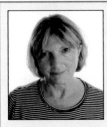

M.C., a 59-year-old homemaker, lives on a farm with her husband, R.C. Recently she has been experiencing weight loss, night sweats, and a chronic cough. When she is given the purified protein derivative (PPD) test, the result is positive, and a chest x-ray indicates areas of consolidation characteristic of tuberculosis. M.C. is hospitalized, and special precautions are initiated to prevent the spread to others.

1. What is the next step in diagnosing the disease?
   The health care provider orders that M.C. be started on a four-drug regimen consisting of isoniazid, rifampin, pyrazinamide, and ethambutol until the final results of testing are back.
2. What is the purpose of the multiple drugs in this order?
3. What needs to be assessed before M.C. begins this medication therapy?
   Two weeks later, M.C. is discharged and given a prescription for Rifamate (combination of rifampin and isoniazid). In addition, she is given instructions to take pyridoxine (vitamin B₆).
4. M.C. asks, "Can't I just take my regular multivitamin? Why do I need this one?" What is the nurse's best response?

For answers, see *http://evolve.elsevier.com/Lilley.*

patient, with appropriate use of audiovisuals and take-home information. All patient teaching must be individualized to the particular patient and in consideration of learning needs (see Chapter 6) and home environment. Include the fact that multiple drugs are often used to improve cure rates. The patient needs to be able to state an understanding of all instructions. Because many of the patients affected by tuberculosis may be from other countries and cultures, it is important to have a translator available.

All *antitubercular drugs* need to be taken exactly as ordered and at the same time every day. Consistent use and dosing around the clock are critical to maintaining steady blood levels and minimizing the chances of resistance to the drug therapy. Always emphasize the need for strict adherence to the therapeutic regimen in the instructions to the patient. Additionally, emphasize that the entire prescription must be finished over the prescribed time and as ordered by the prescriber, even if the patient is feeling better. Successful treatment depends on compliance with drug therapy.

Although many drugs are given without food for maximum absorption, antitubercular drugs may need to be taken with food to minimize gastrointestinal upset. Constantly monitor for any signs and symptoms of liver dysfunction such as fatigue, jaundice, nausea, vomiting, dark urine, and anorexia. If these occur, contact the prescriber immediately. Additionally, monitor kidney function (e.g., BUN, creatinine), and notify the prescriber if levels are altered. If vision changes occur (e.g., altered color perception, changes in visual acuity), in particular with *ethambutol* use, these changes must be reported immediately to the prescriber. Monitor uric acid levels during therapy, and advise the patient to report any symptoms of gout such as hot, painful, or swollen joints of the

big toe, knee, or ankle. In addition, the prescriber must be notified if there are signs and symptoms of peripheral neuropathy (e.g., numbness, burning, and tingling of extremities). Pyridoxine (vitamin B₆) may be beneficial for *isoniazid*-induced peripheral neuropathy. If the prescriber has ordered collection of a sputum specimen to test for acid-fast bacilli, it is best to obtain the sample early in the morning. The most common order is for three consecutive morning specimens and a repeat specimen several weeks later. All drugs are to be taken as ordered and without any omission of doses for maximal therapeutic results. *Bedaqulinie (Sirturo)* is to be taken with food to help with its absorption.

Follow-up visits to the prescriber are important for monitoring therapeutic effects and watching for adverse effects and toxicity. If intravenous dosing of an antitubercular drug is ordered, use the appropriate diluent and infuse over the recommended time. Monitor the intravenous site every hour during the infusion for extravasation with possible tissue inflammation (e.g., redness, heat, and swelling at the intravenous site). See Patient-Centered Care: Patient Teaching on the next page for more information on antitubercular drugs.

Cultural considerations associated with these drugs include the fact that when patients have active TB, thorough patient teaching of all family members is required, and some family members may need prophylactic therapy for up to 1 full year. Because some cultural practices include living in close-knit communities or close living quarters, this teaching is critical to make sure the spread of this highly communicable disease is adequately prevented. All family members or those in close contact with the patient must receive the same thorough instructions about maintaining health while taking their medications appropriately, with emphasis on adherence.

EVALUATION

Always document a patient's response, or lack of, to the therapeutic regimen. A therapeutic response to *antitubercular drugs* is manifested by a decrease in the symptoms of TB, such as cough and fever, and by weight gain. The results of laboratory studies (culture and sensitivity tests) and the chest x-ray findings will aid in the confirmation of resolution of the infection along with improved clinical status. Continually evaluate the meeting of goals and outcome criteria to confirm that the infection is being adequately treated and that the drug therapy is providing therapeutic relief without complications or toxicity and with minimal adverse effects. Also monitor patients for the occurrence of adverse reactions to *antitubercular* drugs, such as hearing loss (ototoxicity); nephrotoxicity; seizure activity; altered vision; blindness; extreme GI upset; fatigue; nausea; vomiting; fever; jaundice; numbness, tingling, or burning of the extremities; abdominal pain; and easy bruising. With the newer drug *bedaqulinie (Sirturo)*, adverse effects include headache, chest pain, nausea, and prolongation of the QT interval. Because of the need for long-term therapy and possible treatment of family or those in close contact, further evaluation of these individuals is important during and after completion of therapy.

PATIENT-CENTERED CARE: PATIENT TEACHING

- Educate the patient to take medications exactly as ordered by the prescriber with attention to long-term therapy and strict adherence to the drug regimen. Emphasize that treatment may be ineffective if drugs are taken intermittently or stopped once the patient begins to feel better.
- Stress the importance of follow-up appointments with the prescriber or health clinic so that the infection and therapeutic effectiveness may be closely monitored.
- Instruct the patient to avoid certain medications while taking antitubercular drugs, such as antacids, phenytoin, carbamazepine, beta blockers, benzodiazepines, oral anticoagulants, oral antidiabetic drugs, oral contraceptives, and theophylline. Inform and provide a listing to the patient of all drug interactions prior to beginning therapy.
- Educate the patient taking isoniazid about the occurrence of adverse effects such as numbness/tingling of extremities, abdominal pain, jaundice, and visual changes. Encourage the patient to promptly report these adverse effects.
- Pyridoxine (vitamin B_6) may be indicated to prevent isoniazid-precipitated peripheral neuropathies and numbness, tingling, or burning of the extremities.
- Advise the patient taking rifampin to report the occurrence of the following adverse effects to the prescriber immediately: fever, nausea, vomiting, loss of appetite, jaundice, and/or unusual bleeding. These may indicate the possible occurrence of the adverse effects of hepatitis and/or various hematologic disorders.
- Encourage the patient to wear sunscreen and protective clothing during therapy to avoid ultraviolet light exposure. Drug-related photosensitivity reactions may be avoided by preventing exposure to the sun.
- Women taking oral contraceptives who are prescribed rifampin must be switched to another form of birth control.

Oral contraceptives become ineffective when given with rifampin.
- During initial periods of the illness, instruct the patient to make every effort to wash hands and cover the mouth when coughing or sneezing. Emphasize methods of proper disposal of secretions. Emphasize and demonstrate proper handwashing technique.
- Emphasize the importance of proper rest, good sleep habits, adequate nutrition, and maintenance of general health. Advise the patient to always keep antitubercular drugs and other medications out of the reach of children.
- Recommend wearing of a medical alert tag or bracelet with a list of allergies, prescription drugs, and medical conditions at all times. Written medical information must also be kept on the patient's person at all times.
- Instruct the patient to contact the prescriber immediately if there is any increase in fatigue, cough and/or sputum production. The prescriber must also be contacted immediately or emergency medical care initiated in the case of bloody sputum, chest pain, unusual bleeding, or yellow skin and/or eyes.
- Patients taking rifampin, rifabutin, or rifapentine may experience red-orange-brown discoloration of the skin, sweat, tears, urine, feces, sputum, saliva, and tongue as an adverse effect of the drug. The discoloration reverses with discontinuation of the drug; however, contact lenses may be permanently stained.
- For patients taking bedaquiline (Sirturo), educate about the need to take this drug with food because it aids in the absorption of the drug. Educate also about significant drug interactions with alcohol, mifepristone, strong CYP3A4 inhibitors, and drugs with high risk for causing a prolongation in the QT interval.

KEY POINTS

- All antitubercular drugs are to be taken exactly as prescribed. Emphasize adherence to the therapeutic regimen and long-term dosing combined with healthy living practices.
- Therapeutic effects include resolution of pulmonary and extrapulmonary MTB infections.
- Vitamin B_6 is needed to combat the peripheral neuropathy associated with isoniazid.
- Counsel women taking oral contraceptive therapy who are prescribed rifampin on other forms of birth control because

of the ineffectiveness of oral contraception when rifampin is taken.
- Educate the patient about the importance of strict adherence to the drug regimen for improvement or cure of the condition. Provide instructions in written and oral forms about drug interactions and the need to avoid alcohol while taking any of these medications.

NCLEX® EXAMINATION REVIEW QUESTIONS

1. The nurse is teaching a patient who is starting antitubercular therapy with rifampin. Which adverse effects would the nurse expect to see?
   a. Headache and neck pain
   b. Gynecomastia
   c. Reddish brown urine
   d. Numbness or tingling of extremities

2. During antitubercular therapy with isoniazid, a patient received another prescription for pyridoxine. Which statement by the nurse best explains the rationale for this second medication?

a. "This vitamin will help to improve your energy levels."

b. "This vitamin helps to prevent neurologic adverse effects."

c. "This vitamin works to protect your heart from toxic effects."

d. "This vitamin helps to reduce gastrointestinal adverse effects."

3. The nurse is counseling a woman who is beginning antitubercular therapy with rifampin. The patient also takes an oral contraceptive. Which statement by the nurse is most accurate regarding potential drug interactions?

a. "You will need to switch to another form of birth control while you are taking the rifampin."

b. "Your birth control pills will remain effective while you are taking the rifampin."

c. "You will need to take a stronger dose of birth control pills while you are on the rifampin."

d. "You will need to abstain from sexual intercourse while on the rifampin to avoid pregnancy."

4. When counseling a patient who has been newly diagnosed with TB, the nurse will make sure that the patient realizes that he or she is contagious

a. during all phases of the illness.

b. any time up to 18 months after therapy begins.

c. during the postictal phase of TB.

d. during the initial period of the illness and its diagnosis.

5. While monitoring a patient, the nurse knows that a therapeutic response to antitubercular drugs would be:

a. The patient states that he or she is feeling much better.

b. The patient's laboratory test results show a lower white blood cell count.

c. The patient reports a decrease in cough and night sweats.

d. There is a decrease in symptoms, along with improved chest x-ray and sputum culture results.

6. The nurse is monitoring for liver toxicity in a patient who has been receiving long-term isoniazid therapy. Manifestations of liver toxicity include: *(Select all that apply.)*

a. Orange discoloration of sweat and tears

b. Darkened urine

c. Dizziness

d. Fatigue

e. Visual disturbances

f. Jaundice

7. The order for isoniazid (INH) reads: "Give 5 mg/kg PO daily." The patient weighs 275 pounds. What is the amount per dose? Is this a safe dose?

8. Bedaquiline (Sirturo) is prescribed for a patient, and the nurse is providing instructions to the patient about the medication. Which statement by the patient indicates a correct understanding of the instructions?

a. "I will take this with food."

b. "I need to take this 1 hour before breakfast."

c. "I can stop this drug if the side effects bother me."

d. "It's okay to have a glass of wine while taking this drug."

1. c, 2. b, 3. a, 4. d, 5. d, 6. b, d, f, 7. 625 mg/dose; no, maximum dose is 300 mg, 8. a.

CRITICAL THINKING AND PRIORITIZATION QUESTIONS

1. A 28-year-old patient has been diagnosed with active TB and will be taking rifampin. She is reviewing her current list of medications with the office nurse and asks, "I use birth control because we really don't want children right now. Can I still use 'the pill'?" What is the nurse's priority when answering the patient's questions?

2. P.T., a 48-year-old businessman, has been taking rifapentine as part of therapy for TB. He has been told that his bodily secretions will turn a reddish orange-brown color, and he asks, "What about my contact lenses? I can still wear them, right?" What is the nurse's best answer?

For answers, see *http://evolve.elsevier.com/Lilley.*

Ⓔ EVOLVE WEBSITE

42

Antifungal Drugs

OBJECTIVES

When you reach the end of this chapter, you will be able to do the following:

1. Identify the various antifungal drugs.
2. Describe the mechanisms of action, indications, contraindications, routes of administration, adverse and
toxic effects, and drug interactions of the various antifungal drugs.
3. Develop a nursing care plan that includes all phases of the nursing process for patients receiving antifungal drugs.

DRUG PROFILES

♦ amphotericin B, p. 673
caspofungin, p. 674
♦ fluconazole, p. 674
nystatin, p. 675
terbinafine, p. 675

voriconazole, p. 675

————
♦ = *Key drug*
! = *High-alert drug*

KEY TERMS

Antimetabolite A drug that is a either a receptor antagonist or that resembles a normal human metabolite and interferes with its function in the body, usually by competing for the metabolite's usual receptors or enzymes. (p. 672)

Dermatophyte One of several fungi that are often found in soil and infect the skin, nails, or hair of humans. (p. 670)

Ergosterol The main sterol in fungal membranes. (p. 672)

Fungi A very large, diverse group of eukaryotic microorganisms; consist of yeasts and molds. (p. 670)

Molds Multicellular fungi characterized by long, branching filaments called *hyphae,* which entwine to form a complex branched structure known as a *mycelium.* (p. 670)

Mycosis The general term for any fungal infection. (p. 670)

Pathologic fungi Fungi that cause mycoses. (p. 670)

Sterols Substances in the cell membranes of fungi to which polyene antifungal drugs bind. (p. 672)

Yeasts Single-celled fungi that reproduce by *budding.* (p. 670)

FUNGAL INFECTIONS

Fungi are a very large and diverse group of microorganisms that include all yeasts and molds. **Yeasts** are single-celled fungi that reproduce by budding (in which a daughter cell forms by pouching out of and breaking off from a mother cell). These organisms have common practical uses in the baking of breads and the preparation of alcoholic beverages. **Molds** are multicellular and are characterized by long, branching filaments. Some fungi are part of the normal flora of the skin, mouth, intestines, and vagina.

An infection caused by a fungus is called a **mycosis.** A variety of fungi can cause clinically significant infections or *mycoses.*

These are called **pathologic fungi,** and the infections they cause range in severity from mild infections with annoying symptoms (e.g., athlete's foot) to systemic mycoses that can become life-threatening. These infections are acquired by various routes: the fungi can be ingested orally; can grow on or in the skin, hair, or nails; and, if the fungal spores are airborne, can be inhaled. There are four general types of mycotic infection: *systemic, cutaneous, subcutaneous,* and *superficial.* The latter three are infections of various layers of the *integumentary* system (skin, hair, or nails). Fungi that cause integumentary infections are known as **dermatophytes,** and such infections are known as *dermatomycoses.* The most severe systemic fungal infections

TABLE 42-1   Mycotic Infections

Mycosis	Fungus	Endemic Location	Reservoir	Transmission	Primary Tissue Affected
Systemic Infections					
Aspergillosis	*Aspergillus* spp.	Universal	Soil	Inhalation	Lungs
Blastomycosis	*Blastomycesdermatitidis*	North America	Soil, animal droppings	Inhalation	Lungs
Candidiasis	*Candida albicans, glabrata, krusei, tropicalisis, parapsilosis*	Universal	Humans	Direct contact, overgrowth in response to treatment with antibiotic to which it is nonsusceptible	Blood, lungs
Coccidioidomycosis	*Coccidioidesimmitis*	Southwestern United States	Soil, dust	Inhalation	Lungs
Cryptococcosis	*Cryptococcus neoformans*	Universal	Soil, bird and chicken droppings	Inhalation	Lungs, meninges of brain
Histoplasmosis	*Histoplasmacapsulatum*	Universal		Inhalation	Lungs
Superficial/Topical Infections					
Candidiasis	*Candida albicans*	Universal	Humans	Direct contact, overgrowth in response to treatment with antibiotic to which it is nonsusceptible	Mucous membrane, skin; disseminated (may be systemic)
Dermatophytosis, tinea	*Epidermophyton* spp. *Microsporum* spp. *Trichophyton* spp.	Universal	Humans	Direct and indirect contact with infected persons	Scalp, skin (e.g., groin, feet)
Tineaversicolor	*Malassezia furfur*	Universal	Humans	Unknown*	Skin

*Malassezia spp. are a usual part of the normal human flora and appear to cause infection in only select individuals.
spp., Species.

generally affect people whose host immune defenses are compromised. Commonly, these are patients who have received organ transplants and are taking immunosuppressive drug therapy, cancer patients who are immunocompromised as a result of their chemotherapy, and patients with acquired immunodeficiency syndrome (AIDS). In addition, the use of antibiotics, antineoplastics, or immunosuppressants such as corticosteroids may result in colonization of *Candida albicans,* followed by the development of a systemic infection. When the infection affects the mouth, it is referred to as oral *candidiasis,* or thrush. It is common in newborns and immunocompromised patients. Vaginal candidiasis, commonly called a *yeast infection,* often affects pregnant women, women with diabetes mellitus, women taking antibiotics, and women taking oral contraceptives. The characteristics of some of the systemic, cutaneous, and superficial mycotic infections are summarized in Table 42-1.

ANTIFUNGAL DRUGS

Drugs used to treat fungal infections are called *antifungal drugs.* Systemic mycotic infections and some cutaneous or subcutaneous mycoses are treated with oral or parenteral drugs. Antifungals are a fairly small group of drugs. There are few such drugs because the fungi that cause these infections have proved to be very difficult to kill, and research into new and improved drugs

has occurred at a slow pace. One difficulty is that often the chemical concentrations required for experimental drugs to be effective cannot be tolerated by humans. The drugs that proved successful in the treatment of systemic mycoses as well as severe dermatomycoses include amphotericin B, caspofungin, fluconazole, flucytosine, griseofulvin, itraconazole, ketoconazole, micafungin, nystatin, terbinafine, anidulafungin, isavuconazonium and voriconazole. These drugs are the focus of this chapter.

Topical antifungal drugs are the most commonly used drugs in this class and are often administered without prescription for the treatment of dermatomycoses as well as oral and vaginal mycoses. Although topical drug therapy is usually sufficient for these conditions, systemic oral medications are sometimes used, especially for more severe or recurrent cases. Antifungal drugs available for topical use are discussed further in Chapter 56. There is also a single antifungal drug (natamycin) for ophthalmic use (see Chapter 57).

Two antifungal drugs, flucytosine and griseofulvin, are individually listed and are not specifically classified according to their chemical structures. The remaining drugs currently include four specific chemical classes: *polyenes* (amphotericin B and nystatin), *imidazoles* (ketoconazole), *triazoles* (fluconazole, itraconazole, voriconazole, posaconazole and isavuconazonium), and the *echinocandins* (caspofungin, micafungin, and anidulafungin). The imidazoles and triazoles are often referred to by the more general term *azole antifungals.*

Mechanism of Action and Drug Effects

The mechanisms of action of the various antifungal drugs differ between drug subclasses. Flucytosine, also known as *5-fluorocytosine (5-FC)*, acts in much the same way as the antiviral drugs. It is an **antimetabolite**, which is a drug that disrupts critical cellular metabolic pathways of the fungal cell. Once inside a susceptible fungal cell, the drug is deaminated by the enzyme *cytosine deaminase* to 5-fluorouracil (5-FU). Because human cells do not have this enzyme, they are not harmed by this antimetabolite. Once the 5-FU is generated inside the fungal cell, it interferes with fungal deoxyribonucleic acid (DNA) synthesis, which results in both inhibition of cell growth and reproduction, and cell death. 5-fluorouracil is also available as an antineoplastic (anticancer) drug and is discussed in more detail in Chapter 45.

Griseofulvin, like flucytosine, is one of the older types of antifungal drugs. It works by preventing susceptible fungi from reproducing. It enters the fungal cell through an energy-dependent transport system and inhibits fungal mitosis (cell division) by binding to key structures known as *microtubules*. It has also been proposed that griseofulvin causes the production of defective DNA, which is then unable to replicate. Although both griseofulvin and flucytosine are still currently available in the U.S. market, their use has been largely replaced by the newer antifungal drug classes.

The polyenes (amphotericin B and nystatin) act by binding to **sterols** in the cell membranes of fungi. Once the polyene drug molecule binds to the **ergosterol**, a channel forms in the fungal cell membrane that allows potassium and magnesium ions to leak out of the fungal cell. This loss of ions causes fungal cellular metabolism to be altered, which leads to death of the cell.

Imidazoles and triazoles (ketoconazole, fluconazole, itraconazole, voriconazole, isavuconazonium and posaconazole) act as either fungistatic or fungicidal drugs, depending on their concentration in the fungus. They are most effective in combating rapidly growing fungi and work by inhibiting fungal cell cytochrome P-450 enzymes that are needed to produce ergosterol. The allylamine terbinafine is believed to act by a similar mechanism. When the production of ergosterol is inhibited, it results in a defect similar to that caused by the polyene antifungals, namely, a leaky cell membrane that allows needed electrolytes to escape. The fungal cells die because they cannot carry on cellular metabolism.

The echinocandins (caspofungin, micafungin, and anidulafungin) act by preventing the synthesis of glucans, essential components of fungal cell walls that are not present in human cells. This also contributes to fungal cell death.

Indications

Indications for the use of the various antifungal drugs are specific to the drug. Amphotericin B is effective against a wide range of fungi. It is sometimes given with flucytosine in the treatment of *Candida* and cryptococcal infections because of the synergy of the two drugs. Amphotericin B is also effective for treating aspergillosis, blastomycosis, candidiasis, coccidioidomycosis, cryptococcosis, fungal endocarditis, histoplasmosis,

zygomycosis, fungal septicemia, and many other systemic fungal infections. The activity of nystatin is similar to that of amphotericin B, but its usefulness is limited because of its toxic effects when given in the dosages required to accomplish the same antifungal actions as amphotericin B. It is also not available in parenteral form. Nystatin is most commonly used to treat oropharyngeal candidiasis, commonly referred to as *thrush,* and is frequently used as a topical powder.

Fluconazole, ketoconazole, itraconazole, voriconazole, isavuconazonium, and posaconazole are synthetic azole antifungals. Fluconazole is indicated for the treatment of esophageal, oropharyngeal, peritoneal, urinary tract, vaginal, and systemic candida infections and cryptococcal meningitis. Ketoconazole use is no longer recommended unless all other therapies fail. Itraconazole is indicated for the treatment of blastomycosis, histoplasmosis, aspergillosis, and oncychomycosis of the toe nail. Voriconazole is indicated for the treatment of invasive aspergillosis, candida infections, and infections caused by *Fusarium spp.* Isavuconazonium is indicated for the treatment of invasive aspergillosis and invasive mucormycosis. Posaconazole is indicated for the prophylaxis of invasive aspergillus and candida infections in severly immunocompromised patients.

Flucytosine is indicated for the treatment of endocarditis and cryptococcal meningoencephalisitis in conjunction with amphotericin B. Griseofulvin is indicated for tinea infections. Terbinafine is a synthetic allylamine derivative used in a systemic oral form for treatment of onychomycoses—fungal infections of the fingernails or toenails. Topical forms of terbinafine are also used for various skin infections (see Chapter 56).

Contraindications

Drug allergy, liver failure, kidney failure, and porphyria (for griseofulvin) are the most common contraindications for antifungal drugs. Itraconazole should not be used to treat onychomycoses in patients with severe cardiac problems. Voriconazole can cause fetal harm in pregnant women.

Adverse Effects

Drug interactions and hepatotoxicity are the primary concerns in patients receiving antifungal drugs. The most common adverse effects of the various antifungal drugs are listed in Table 42-2. Amphotericin B is associated with a multitude of adverse effects, and prescribers commonly order various premedications (including antiemetics, antihistamines, antipyretics, and corticosteroids) to prevent or minimize infusion-related reactions. The likelihood of such reactions can also be reduced by using longer-than-average drug infusion times (i.e., 2 to 6 hours) for this particular drug.

Interactions

There are many important drug interactions associated with antifungal drugs, some of which can be life-threatening. A common underlying source of the problem is that many of the antifungal drugs, as well as other drugs, are metabolized by the *cytochrome P-450 enzyme system.* The result of the coadministration of two drugs that are both broken down by this system is that they compete for the limited amount of enzymes, and

TABLE 42-2   Selected Antifungal Drugs: Common Adverse Effects and Cautions

Body System	Adverse Effects	Cautions
Amphotericin B (Sy)		
Cardiovascular	Cardiac dysrhythmias	Recheck dosage and type of amphotericin B being administered
Central nervous	Neurotoxicity; tinnitus; visual disturbances; hand or feet numbness, tingling, or pain; convulsions	
Renal	Renal toxicity, potassium loss, hypomagnesemia	
Pulmonary	Pulmonary infiltrates	
Other (infusion related)	Fever, chills, headache, malaise, nausea, occasional hypotension, gastrointestinal upset, anemia	
Fluconazole (Sy)		
Gastrointestinal	Nausea, vomiting, diarrhea, stomach pain	Use with caution in patients with renal or hepatic dysfunction
Other	Increased liver enzyme levels, dizziness	
Caspofungin (Sy)		
Central nervous	Fever, chills, headache	Adjust dose for patients with hepatic dysfunction
Cardiovascular	Hypotension, peripheral edema, tachycardia	
Gastrointestinal	Nausea, vomiting, diarrhea, hepatotoxicity	
Hematologic	Decreased hemoglobin and hematocrit, leukopenia, anemia	
Integumentary	Rash, facial edema, itching	
Voriconazole (Sy)		
Central nervous	Hallucinations	
Gastrointestinal	Nausea, vomiting	
Hepatic	Increased liver enzyme levels	
Integumentary	Rash	
Other	Photophobia, hypokalemia	
Nystatin (T)		
Gastrointestinal	Nausea, vomiting, diarrhea, cramps	Local irritation may occur
Integumentary	Rash, urticaria	
Terbinafine (Sy, T)		
Central nervous	Headache, dizziness	Rarely causes irritation
Gastrointestinal	Nausea, vomiting, diarrhea	
Integumentary	Rash, pruritus	
Other	Alopecia, fatigue	

Sy, Systemic; *T*, topical.

one of the drugs ends up accumulating. In addition, itraconazole and posaconazole are inhibitors of gastric P-glycoprotein. Key drug interactions for the systemic antifungal drugs are summarized in Table 42-3.

Dosages

For dosage information on selected antifungal drugs, see the table on the next page.

DRUG PROFILES

♦amphotericin B

Amphotericin B (Fungizone) remains one of the drugs of choice for the treatment of severe systemic mycoses. The main drawback of amphotericin B therapy is that the drug causes many adverse effects. Almost all patients given the drug intravenously experience fever, chills, hypotension, tachycardia, malaise, muscle and joint pain, anorexia, nausea and vomiting, and

headache. For this reason, pretreatment with antipyretics, antihistamines, antiemetics, and corticosteroids is common to decrease the severity of the infusion-related reaction.

Lipid formulations of amphotericin B were developed in an attempt to decrease the incidence of its adverse effects and increase its efficacy. There are currently three lipid preparations of amphotericin B: amphotericin B lipid complex (Abelcet), amphotericin B cholesteryl complex (Amphotec), and liposomal amphotericin B (AmBisome). These lipid dosage forms have a much higher cost than conventional amphotericin B and for this reason are often used only when patients are intolerant of or have an infection refractory to nonlipid amphotericin B.

Amphotericin B is contraindicated in patients who have a known hypersensitivity to it and in those with severe bone marrow suppression or renal impairment. However, patients who have life-threatening fungal infections may still be treated with this drug if culture results indicate that no other drug will kill the causative organism. The drug is available in injectable, oral, and topical preparations. Often a 1-mg test dose is given over 20 to 30 minutes to see if the patient will tolerate the drug. Amphotericin B has been used as a local irrigant (in bladder irrigation) for the treatment of candidal cystitis and has been used intrapleurally and intraperitoneally for the treatment of fungal infections in those body cavities.

Pharmacokinetics: Amphotericin B

Route	Onset of Action	Peak Plasma Concentration	Elimination Half-life	Duration of Action
IV	Variable	1 hr	1-15 days	18-24 hr

caspofungin

Caspofungin (Cancidas) was the first echinocandin antifungal drug. It is used for treatment of severe *Aspergillus* infection (invasive aspergillosis) in patients who are intolerant of or have infections refractory to other drugs. Caspofungin doses need to be reduced in patients with impaired liver function. The drug is available only in injectable form. Other echinocandins include micafungin (Mycamine) and anidulafungin (Eraxis).

Pharmacokinetics: Caspofungin

Route	Onset of Action	Peak Plasma Concentration	Elimination Half-life	Duration of Action
IV	Unknown	1 hr	9-50 hr	Unknown

♦ fluconazole

Fluconazole (Diflucan) has proved to be a significant improvement in the area of antifungal treatment. It has a much better adverse effect profile than that of amphotericin B, and it also has excellent coverage against many fungi. In fact, it is often preferred to amphotericin B because of these qualities. Oral fluconazole has excellent bioavailability, which means that almost the entire dose administered is absorbed into the circulation. Fluconazole is available in both oral and injectable forms. A single oral dose of fluconazole is usually effective for the treatment of vaginal candidiasis infections.

DOSAGES

Selected Antifungal Drugs

Drug (Pregnancy Category)	Pharmacologic Class	Usual Adult Dosage Range	Indications
♦ amphotericin B (Amphocin, Fungizone) (B)	Polyene antifungal	IV: Initial daily dose, 0.25 mg/kg; titrate up to 0.5-1.5 mg/kg/day	Systemic infections with broad spectrum of fungi
amphotericin B lipid complex; dosages vary with product as follows:	Polyene antifungal		
Abelcet (B)		IV: 5 mg/kg once daily	
Amphotec (B)		IV: 3-4 mg/kg/day	Systemic fungal infections
AmBisome (B)		IV: 3-5 mg/kg/day	
caspofungin (Cancidas) (C)	Echinocandin antifungal	IV: 70 mg loading dose on day 1, followed by 50 mg/day thereafter	Invasive aspergillosis in patients who do not tolerate or respond to other drugs
♦ fluconazole (Diflucan) (C)	Synthetic triazole antifungal	PO: 150 mg in a single dose	Vaginal candidiasis
		IV/PO: 100-400 mg/day for 2-5 wk (dose and duration depend on severity of infection)	Oropharyngeal and esophageal candidiasis, systemic candidiasis
		IV/PO: 200-400 mg/day for 10-12 wk after negative CSF culture results	Cryptococcal meningitis
nystatin (Nilstat, Mycostatin, Nystex) (C)	Polyene antifungal	PO: 400,000-600,000 units (4-6 mL) oral suspension in oral cavity 4 times daily	Oral candidiasis
		Topical (cream, lotion, or powder): apply 2-3 times daily	Topical candidiasis
terbinafine (Lamisil) (B)	Synthetic allylamine antifungal	PO: 250 mg/day for 6 wk (fingernail) or for 12 wk (toenail)	Onychomycosis (fungal infection of fingernail or toenail)
		Topical cream or solution: Apply once to twice daily to affected area for 1-4 wk	Athlete's foot *(tineapedis)*, jock itch *(tineacruris)*, or ringworm *(tineacorporis)*
voriconazole (Vfend) (D)	Synthetic triazole antifungal	PO: 200 mg every 12 hr	Invasive aspergillosis; other major fungal infections in patients who do not tolerate or respond to other antifungal drugs
		IV: 6 mg/kg every 12 hr for 2 doses followed by 4 mg/kg every 12 hr	

CSF, Cerebrospinal fluid.

TABLE 42-3 Antifungal Drugs: Drug Interactions

Drug	Possible Effects
Amphotericin B	
Digitalis glycosides	Amphotericin B–induced hypokalemia may increase the potential for digitalis toxicity
Nephrotoxic drugs	Additive nephrotoxicity
Thiazide diuretics	Severe hypokalemia or decreased adrenal cortex response to corticotrophin
Azole Antifungals	
cyclosporine, sirolimus, tacrolimus, calcium channel blockers, benzodiazepines	Increased plasma concentrations of target drugs
Oral anticoagulants	Increased effects of anticoagulants
Oral hypoglycemics, statins	Reduced metabolism of hypoglycemic and statins; increased toxicity
quinidine	Prolongation of QT interval on electrocardiogram
Phenytoin, rifampin, phenobarbital, carbamazepine	Decreased levels of azole antifungals

Pharmacokinetics: Fluconazole

Route	Onset of Action	Peak Plasma Concentration	Elimination Half-life	Duration of Action
PO	1 hr	1-2 hr	22-30 hr	Variable

nystatin

Nystatin (Mycostatin) is a polyene antifungal drug that is often applied topically for the treatment of candidal diaper rash, taken orally as prophylaxis against candidal infections during periods of neutropenia in patients receiving immunosuppressive therapy, and used for the treatment of oral and vaginal candidiasis. It is not available in a parenteral form but does come in several oral and topical formulations.

Pharmacokinetics: Nystatin

Route	Onset of Action	Peak Plasma Concentration	Elimination Half-life	Duration of Action
PO	24 hr	2 hr	Unknown	Unknown

terbinafine

Terbinafine (Lamisil) is classified as an allylamine antifungal drug and is currently the only drug in its class. It is available in a topical cream, gel, and spray for treating superficial dermatologic infections, including *tineapedis* (athlete's foot), *tineacruris* (jock itch), and *tineacorporis* (ringworm). A tablet form is also available for systemic use and is used primarily to treat onychomycoses of the fingernails or toenails.

Pharmacokinetics: Terbinafine

Route	Onset of Action	Peak Plasma Concentration	Elimination Half-life	Duration of Action
PO	Unknown	1-2 hr	22-26 hr	Unknown

voriconazole

Voriconazole (Vfend) is used for treating severe fungal infections caused by *Aspergillus* spp. (invasive aspergillosis). It is also used for a variety of other severe fungal infections, such as those caused by *Scedosporium* and *Fusarium* spp. Voriconazole is contraindicated in patients who have a known drug allergy to it and in patients who are taking certain other drugs metabolized by the cytochrome P-450 enzyme 3A4 (e.g., quinidine) because of the risk for induction of serious cardiac dysrhythmias. It is also the only antifungal drug contraindicated in pregnancy. The drug is available in oral and injectable forms.

Pharmacokinetics: Voriconazole

Route	Onset of Action	Peak Plasma Concentration	Elimination Half-life	Duration of Action
PO	Unknown	1-2 hr	Variable	Unknown

▌NURSING PROCESS

▌ASSESSMENT

Although topical dosage forms are discussed in detail in Chapter 56, it is important to discuss all *antifungal* dosage forms and their related nursing process. Before initiation of therapy with antifungals, assess and document vital signs, weight, hemoglobin (Hgb) level, hematocrit (Hct), red blood cell (RBC) counts, complete blood counts (CBCs) with differential, liver and renal function test results, and culture and sensitivity test results.

Before administering *amphotericin B* (or any other antifungal drug), identify any contraindications, cautions, and drug interactions (see Tables 42-2 and 42-3). Baseline renal function studies are generally ordered as well as hepatic function tests due to adverse effects of nephrotoxicity and hepatotoxicity. Avoid any concurrent administration of nephrotoxic drugs if at all possible. There is a risk for severe adverse reactions (e.g., cardiac dysrhythmias, headache, chills, malaise, nausea, hypotension, anemia, GI upset) with intravenous amphotericin B administration; therefore, assessment and documentation of any issues with cardiovascular and gastrointestinal systems is needed. Perform an assessment of any special pre-medication orders for antiemetics, antihistamines, antipyretics, and/or antiinflammatory drugs prior to giving *amphotericin B*. Bone marrow suppression is another contraindication to the use of this drug.

Caspofungin use requires careful assessment of blood pressure, pulse rate, liver function, RBC counts, and WBC counts due to potential drug-induced adverse effects of hypotension, tachycardia, hepatotoxicity, decreased Hgb and Hct, and leukopenia. *Fluconazole* requires a close assessment of preexisting GI problems and of renal and/or hepatic functioning due to drug-induced adverse effects impacting these systems. *Nystatin* lozenges are generally not used in children younger than 5 years of age. See Tables 42-2 and 42-3 for more information about specific adverse effects and drug interactions for all antifungals.

NURSING DIAGNOSES

1. Acute pain related to symptoms of the infectious process
2. Deficient knowledge related to lack of information and experience with the antifungal drug therapy
3. Risk for injury related to adverse effects of the medication treatment regimen
4. Risk for injury related to possible poor adherence to completion of the treatment regimen.

CASE STUDY

Patient-Centered Care: Amphotericin B

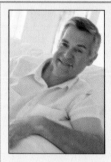

A.B., a 63-year-old retired delivery driver, has been hospitalized for respiratory distress. Since his admission, he has been diagnosed with a severe systemic fungal infection, and an amphotericin B infusion will be started. Before beginning this medication, the nurse assesses the results of his renal and liver function laboratory studies, as well as his complete blood count. The patency of the intravenous line is verified, and the nurse gives A.B. a dose of acetaminophen (Tylenol) as well as an antihistamine before starting the infusion.

1. What is the purpose of the acetaminophen and antihistamine?
2. The nurse stays with A.B. for the first 15 minutes of the infusion and monitors his vital signs. Explain the rationale for these nursing actions.
3. One hour after the infusion is completed, A.B. calls the nurse and says that he feels as if he may vomit and has chills, yet feels hot at the same time. What is the nurse's priority action at this time?
4. A.B. continues to feel "terrible" the rest of the night, and the next morning his physician, Dr. F., changes the order to liposomal amphotericin B (AmBisome). Why did the physician continue an antifungal medication? What is the rationale behind this order change?

For answers, see *http://evolve.elsevier.com/Lilley.*

PLANNING: OUTCOME IDENTIFICATION

1. Patient has minimal to no pain, resolution of fever, and improved well-being after antifungal therapy has been initiated.
2. Patient gains increased knowledge about the antifungal drug, its use, and adverse effects and reports taking medication as prescribed and for the full course of therapy.
3. Patient experiences minimal to no injury to self as related to the adverse effects of antifungal therapy and returns to prescriber for constant monitoring of health status.
4. Patient experiences minimal injury to self as related to completion of full course of therapy.

IMPLEMENTATION

The nursing interventions appropriate for patients receiving *antifungal* drugs vary depending on the particular drug.

When administering intravenous dosage forms, use an in-line filter (see manufacturer guidelines) and monitor the IV site for extravasation. With intravenous *amphotericin B*, do not administer solutions that are cloudy or have precipitates. Use of an intravenous infusion pump is recommended. Once the intravenous infusion has begun, monitor vital signs every 15 minutes, or as needed, to assess for adverse reactions such as cardiac dysrhythmias, visual disturbances, paresthesias (numbness or tingling of the hands or feet), respiratory difficulty, pain, fever, chills, and nausea (see Table 42-2 for a listing of adverse effects). If a severe reaction occurs (e.g., exacerbation of adverse effects and/or a decline in vital signs), discontinue the infusion while continuing to closely monitor the patient. Contact the prescriber immediately. Monitor the intravenous site for signs of phlebitis (e.g., heat, pain, and redness over the vein), as per institutional policy. Monitor intake and output, and report decreasing urinary output of less than 240 mL/8 hrs or less than 0.5 mL/kg per output. Continually monitor all laboratory values during therapy (see earlier discussion). Document weight frequently, as indicated, with long-term or at-home therapy. A gain of 2 pounds or more in a 24-hour period or 5 pounds or more in 1 week may indicate possible medication-induced renal damage and the need for prompt medical attention. Follow manufacturer guidelines and the prescriber's order for specific solutions and rates of intravenous administration. See Patient-Centered Care: Patient Teaching on the next page for further information.

Only use clear solutions of *caspofungin*, and dilute doses with the recommended amount of normal saline. Do not use with dextrose-containing products for diluting, and do not give as a bolus. As with most IV infusions, administer IV fluids at room temperature. Blood is 98.6 degrees, so ideally IV fluids need to be near the same temperature when given to a patient to prevent a drop in body temperature and subsequent adverse effects. Liver toxicity may occur, so monitor liver function tests during therapy as ordered. In addition, constantly monitor the patient for the occurrence of tachycardia, hypotension, fever, hives, rash, increased feeling of warmth, flushing, chills, wheezing, or bleeding. Hemoglobin and hematocrit levels must also be monitored frequently because of the possibility of drug-induced anemias. *Fluconazole* may be given either orally or intravenously, with intravenous dosage forms used if there is a specific indication or if the oral dosage forms are poorly tolerated. Only administer intravenous dosage forms if the solution is clear, and do not add other medications. Protect the IV dosage form from moisture and light. Diluted solutions are only stable for 24 hours. If itching or a rash occurs, stop the infusion, take vital signs, and contact the prescriber immediately. *Nystatin* may be given orally in the form of lozenges or troches, which the patient should slowly and completely dissolve in the mouth for optimal effects; these should not be chewed or swallowed whole. If a suspension is used, instruct the patient to swish the medication solution thoroughly in the mouth for as long as possible before swallowing. *Terbinafine (Lamisil)* oral dosage forms may be taken without regard to food. Granules are to be taken with food, with sprinkling of packet contents on pudding or a nonacidic food item. It is then to be swallowed without chewing. Local skin reactions that need to be reported include blistering, itching, oozing, redness, and swelling. With *voriconazole*, oral doses are to be given 1 hour before or 1 hour after a meal. Intravenous doses may be diluted with 5% dextrose in water or normal saline, with the accurate dose infused over the recommended time. Monitor visual acuity when this drug is given (especially if ordered for longer than 28 days), and report any visual changes to the prescriber.

EVALUATION

The therapeutic effects of *antifungals* include improvement and eventual resolution of the signs and symptoms of the fungal infection if the patient has remained totally adherent to the therapy regimen. Improved energy levels and improvement in overall sense of well-being with a normal temperature and other vital sign values also indicate a therapeutic response. Specific adverse effects for which to monitor in patients receiving these drugs are listed in Table 42-2. Evaluate goals and outcome criteria in the context of the nursing care plan.

PATIENT-CENTERED CARE: PATIENT TEACHING

- Instruct female patients taking antifungal medications for the treatment of vaginal infection to abstain from sexual intercourse until the treatment is completed and the infection is resolved. Advise patients to continue to take the medication even if actively menstruating. Encourage patients to contact their prescriber if symptoms persist once treatment is completed.
- Some patients receiving amphotericin B may need long-term treatment (i.e., 2 weeks to possibly 3 months). If so, possible adverse effects include tinnitus, blurred vision, burning and itching at the infusion site, headache, rash, fever, chills, hypokalemia, gastrointestinal upset, and various anemias. The prescriber is to be notified immediately if there is bleeding, bruising, and/or soft-tissue swelling.
- It is not uncommon to see the following prescribed for symptomatic management of adverse effects: aspirin, acetaminophen and/or ibuprofen, antihistamines, antiemetics, and antispasmotics.
- Instruct patients taking caspofungin to immediately report to the prescriber any problems with shortness of breath, itching, facial swelling, and/or a rash.
- Encourage the patient to practice good hand-washing technique at all times.
- Instruct the patient on the proper dosing instructions for nystatin. For oral solutions, the suspension needs to be shaken thoroughly before measuring out each dose. Each dose is to be taken as directed; for example, for oral suspensions often the dosing instructions are to place half in each

cheek and then swallow and not to mix with food. Other directions may be to swish and swallow. Avoid commercial mouthwashes during therapy. If vaginal troches are prescribed, use the appropriate applicator with a gloved hand, and insert high into the vagina, followed by thorough hand washing (see Chapter 9).
- Encourage the patient to keep affected body areas clean and dry and to wear light and cool clothing. Avoid contact of the topical dosage form with the eyes, mouth, nose, or other mucous membranes.
- With fluconazole, educate patients about the need for an alternative method of contraception while taking this drug. Report any jaundice, nausea, vomiting, clay-colored stools, and/or dark urine.
- With terbinafine (Lamisil), educate about the need for long-term therapy of up to 10 weeks for toenail infection and 4 weeks for fingernail infection. Voriconazole use is often for weeks up to 3 months, depending on the type of infection. It is to be taken 1 hour before or 1 hour after meals. Warn the patient about the adverse effect of photophobia with use of this drug.
- With voriconazole, educate about the reporting to the prescriber any of the following: bleeding, bruising, soft-tissue swelling, dark urine, persistent nausea or diarrhea, rash, or yellow skin/eyes. Caution the patient not to drive at night while on this medication because of vision changes. Women of childbearing age need to use effective contraception due to teratogenic effects.

KEY POINTS

- Fungi are a very large and diverse group of microorganisms and consist of yeasts and molds. Yeasts are single-celled fungi that may be harmful (e.g., causing infections) or helpful (e.g., aiding in baking or brewing beer). Molds are multicellular and are characterized by long, branching filaments called *hyphae*.
- Candidiasis is an opportunistic fungal infection caused by *C. albicans* and occurs in patients taking broad-spectrum antibiotics, antineoplastics, or immunosuppressants, as well as

in immunocompromised persons. When candidiasis occurs in the mouth, it is commonly called *oral candidiasis* or *thrush*. Oral candidiasis is more commonly seen in newborns or immunocompromised persons.
- Vaginal candidiasis is a yeast infection and occurs most commonly in individuals with diabetes mellitus, women taking oral contraceptives, pregnant women, and post–antibiotic therapy.
- Antifungals may be administered either systemically or topically. Some of the most common systemic antifungals are

- amphotericin B and fluconazole; an example of a topical antifungal is nystatin.
- Before administering antifungals, thoroughly assess for allergies as well as interactions with other drugs patients are taking, including prescription drugs, over-the-counter drugs, and herbals.
- Amphotericin B must be properly diluted according to manufacturer guidelines and administered using an intravenous infusion pump. Tissue extravasation of fluconazole at the intravenous infusion site leads to tissue necrosis; therefore, check the site hourly and document the assessment.

▌NCLEX® EXAMINATION REVIEW QUESTIONS

1. The nurse is assessing a patient who is about to receive antifungal drug therapy. Which problem would be of most concern?
   a. Endocrine disease
   b. Hepatic disease
   c. Cardiac disease
   d. Pulmonary disease

2. While monitoring a patient who is receiving intravenous amphotericin B, the nurse expects to see which adverse effect(s)?
   a. Hypertension
   b. Bradycardia
   c. Fever and chills
   d. Diarrhea and stomach cramps

3. When administering antifungal drug therapy, the nurse knows that an issue that contributes to many of the drug interactions with antifungals is the patient's
   a. history of cardiac disease.
   b. history of gallbladder surgery.
   c. ethnic background.
   d. cytochrome P-450 enzyme system.

4. During an infusion of amphotericin B, the nurse knows that which administration technique may be used to minimize infusion-related adverse effects?
   a. Forcing of fluids during the infusion
   b. Infusing the medication quickly
   c. Infusing the medication over a longer period of time
   d. Stopping the infusion for 2 hours after half of the bag has infused, and then resuming 1 hour later

5. When teaching a patient who is taking nystatin lozenges for oral candidiasis, which instruction by the nurse is correct?
   a. "Chew the lozenge carefully before swallowing."
   b. "Dissolve the lozenge slowly and completely in your mouth."
   c. "Dissolve the lozenge until it is half the original size, and then swallow it."
   d. "These lozenges need to be swallowed whole with a glass of water."

6. When monitoring a patient who is receiving caspofungin, the nurse will look for which serious adverse effects? *(Select all that apply.)*
   a. Blood dyscrasias
   b. Hypotension
   c. Pulmonary infiltrates
   d. Tinnitus
   e. Hepatotoxicity

7. The order reads, "Give nystatin (Mycostatin) suspension, 500,000 units by mouth (swish and swallow) 4 times a day for 1 week." The medication is available in a suspension of 100,000 units per mL. How many milliliters will the nurse give per dose?

8. The nurse notes in a patient's medication history that the patient is taking terbinafine (Lamisil). Based on this finding, the nurse interprets that the patient has which disorder?
   a. Vaginal candidiasis
   b. Cryptococcal meningitis
   c. Invasive aspergillosis
   d. Onychomycosis

1. b, 2. c, 3. d, 4. c, 5. b, 6. a, b, e, 7. 5 mL, 8. d.

▌CRITICAL THINKING AND PRIORITIZATION QUESTIONS

1. The nurse is reviewing newly written orders for a patient who has a vaginal yeast infection. One order reads, "Fluconazole, 150 mg, one tablet by mouth now for vaginal yeast infection." When the nurse goes to administer the medication, the patient asks, "Is that a mistake? How can one pill help that problem?" What is the nurse's best answer to this question?

2. When the nurse is administering medications, the patient takes the dosage cup of the oral nystatin suspension and says, "I know how to take this." He then swallows the liquid medication all at once. What is the nurse's priority action at this time?

For answers, see *http://evolve.elsevier.com/Lilley.*

ⓔ EVOLVE WEBSITE

http://evolve.elsevier.com/Lilley
- Animations
- Answer Keys for Textbook Case Studies and Textbook Critical Thinking and Prioritization Questions
- Content Updates
- Key Points
- Review Questions
- Student Case Studies

Antimalarial, Antiprotozoal, and Anthelmintic Drugs

OBJECTIVES

When you reach the end of this chapter, you will be able to do the following:

1. Briefly discuss the infectious process associated with malaria, other protozoal infections, and helminthic infections.
2. Compare the signs and symptoms of malarial, other protozoal, and helminthic infection processes.
3. Identify the more commonly used antimalarial, antiprotozoal, and anthelmintic drugs.
4. Discuss the mechanisms of action, indications, cautions, contraindications, adverse effects, dosages, drug interactions, and routes of administration of the antimalarial, antiprotozoal, and anthelmintic drugs.
5. Develop a nursing care plan that includes all phases of the nursing process for patients receiving antimalarial, antiprotozoal, or anthelmintic drugs.

DRUG PROFILES

atovaquone, p. 686
♦ chloroquine and ♦ hydroxychloroquine, p. 682
♦ mefloquine, p. 683
♦ metronidazole, p. 686
pentamidine, p. 686
praziquantel, p. 689

♦ primaquine, p. 683
pyrantel, p. 689
pyrimethamine, p. 683

_____
♦ = *Key drug*
! = *High-alert drug*

KEY TERMS

Anthelmintic A drug that destroys or prevents the development of parasitic worm (helminthic) infections. Also called *antihelmintic* or *vermicide;* notice that the terms for the drug categories are spelled with only one *h*, which appears in the second syllable of the term, whereas the term for worm infection *(helminthic)* is spelled with two *h*s, appearing in both the first and third syllables of the term. (p. 686)

Antimalarial drugs Drugs that destroy or prevent the development of the malaria parasite *(Plasmodium* sp.) in humans. Antimalarial drugs are a subset of the broader category of antiprotozoal drugs. (p. 680)

Antiprotozoal A drug that destroys or prevents the development of protozoans in humans. (p. 684)

Helminthic infections Parasitic worm infections. (p. 687)

Malaria A widespread protozoal infectious disease caused by four species of the genus *Plasmodium.* (p. 680)

Parasite Any organism that feeds on another living organism (known as a *host*) in a way that results in varying degrees of harm to the host organism. (p. 680)

Parasitic protozoans Harmful protozoans that live on or in humans or animals and cause disease in the process. (p. 679)

Protozoans Single-celled organisms that are the smallest and simplest members of the animal kingdom. (p. 679)

OVERVIEW

There are more than 28,000 known types of **protozoans,** which are single-celled organisms. Those that live on or in humans are called **parasitic protozoans.** Billions of people worldwide are infected with these organisms, and, as a result, these infections are considered a serious public health problem. Some of the more common protozoal infections are malaria, leishmaniasis, trypanosomiasis, amebiasis, giardiasis, and trichomoniasis. They are relatively uncommon in the United States but are becoming increasingly prevalent in immunocompromised individuals, including those with acquired immunodeficiency

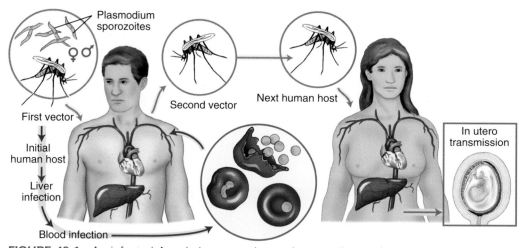

FIGURE 43-1 An infected Anopheles mosquito carries parasites to humans, causing malaria. These parasites mature in the liver before entering the bloodstream and rupturing red blood cells. A pregnant woman infected with malaria may transmit the disease to her unborn child.

syndrome (AIDS). Protozoal diseases are especially prevalent among people living in tropical climates because it is easier for protozoans to survive and be transmitted in environments that are warm and humid year round. Although the population of the United States is relatively free of many of these protozoal infections, international travel and the immigration of people from other countries where such infections are endemic are providing opportunities for increased exposure.

PATHOPHYSIOLOGY OF MALARIA

The most significant protozoal disease in terms of morbidity and mortality is malaria. Worldwide, it is estimated that 350 to 500 million people are infected, with an annual death rate of 1 million to 2 million people. In Africa alone, malaria accounts for more than 1 million infant deaths per year. The geographic areas with the highest prevalence are sub-Saharan Africa, Southeast Asia, and Latin America. Approximately 1200 cases of malaria are reported in the United States annually, seen mostly in people who traveled to malaria-infested countries. Malaria is caused by a particular genus of protozoans called *Plasmodium*. These four species are *Plasmodium vivax, Plasmodium falciparum, Plasmodium malariae,* and *Plasmodium ovale.* Although *P. vivax* is the most widespread of the four, *P. falciparum* is nearly as widespread and causes greater problems with drug resistance. The two remaining species are much less common and more geographically limited in their occurrence, but they can still cause serious malarial infections.

Most commonly, malaria is transmitted by the bite of an infected female anopheline mosquito. This type of mosquito is endemic to many tropical regions of the earth. Malaria can also be transmitted by blood transfusions, congenitally from mother to infant via an infected placenta, or through the use of contaminated needles.

The *Plasmodium* life cycle involves many stages. The organism has two interdependent life cycles: the *sexual cycle,* which takes place inside the mosquito, and the *asexual cycle,* which

occurs in the human host (Figure 43-1). In addition, the asexual cycle of the parasite consists of a phase outside the erythrocyte (primarily in liver tissues) called the *exoerythrocytic phase* (or the *tissue phase*) and a phase inside the erythrocyte called the *erythrocytic phase* (or the *blood phase*).

Malaria signs and symptoms are often described in terms of the *classic malaria paroxysm*. A *paroxysm* is a sudden recurrence or intensification of symptoms. Symptoms include chills and rigors, followed by fever of up to 104° F (40° C) and diaphoresis, frequently leading to extreme fatigue and prolonged sleep. This syndrome often repeats itself periodically in 48- to 72-hour cycles. Other common symptoms include headache, nausea, and joint pain.

ANTIMALARIAL DRUGS

Treatment for malaria is not initiated until the diagnosis has been confirmed by laboratory tests. Once confirmed, appropriate antimalarial treatment must be initiated immediately. Treatment is guided by three main factors: the infecting *Plasmodium* species, the clinical status of the patient, and the drug susceptibility of the infecting parasites as determined by the geographic area where the infection was acquired. Because the resistance patterns are constantly changing, depending on geographic location, the reader is referred to the website of the Centers for Disease Control and Prevention (CDC) at *www.cdc.gov/malaria* for the most up-to-date information. People traveling to different parts of the world may require antimalarial prophylaxis and need to check with their prescribers and/or the CDC website for specific drug therapy.

Antimalarial drugs administered to humans cannot affect the parasite during its sexual cycle when it resides in the mosquito. Instead, these drugs work against the parasite during its asexual cycle, which takes place within the human body. Often these drugs are given in various combinations to achieve an additive or synergistic antimalarial effect. One example is the combination of the two antiprotozoal drugs atovaquone and proguanil (Malarone). The antibiotic combination of pyrimethamine and sulfadoxine (Fansidar) is also commonly used, especially in cases caused by drug-resistant organisms.

Mechanism of Action and Drug Effects

The mechanisms of action of the various antimalarial drugs differ depending on the chemical family to which they belong. The *4-aminoquinoline derivatives* (chloroquine and hydroxychloroquine) work by inhibiting DNA and RNA polymerase, enzymes essential to DNA and RNA synthesis by the parasite cells. Parasite protein synthesis is also disrupted, because protein synthesis is dependent on proper nucleic acid (DNA and RNA) function. These drugs also raise the pH within the parasite, which interferes with the parasite's ability to metabolize and use erythrocyte hemoglobin; this is one reason these drugs are ineffective during the exoerythrocytic (tissue) phase of infection. All of these actions contribute to the destruction of the parasite. Quinine, quinidine, and mefloquine are thought to be similar to the 4-aminoquinoline derivatives in their actions in that all are also believed to raise the pH within the parasite.

The *diaminopyrimidines* (pyrimethamine and trimethoprim [see Chapter 38]) work by inhibiting dihydrofolate reductase, an enzyme that is needed for the production of certain vital substances in malarial parasites. Specifically, inhibiting this enzyme blocks the synthesis of tetrahydrofolate, which is a precursor of purines and pyrimidines (nucleic acid components) and certain amino acids (protein components) that are essential for the growth and survival of plasmodia parasites. These two drugs are effective only during the erythrocytic phase. Pyrimethamine and trimethoprim are often used with a sulfonamide (sulfadoxine or dapsone) because of the resulting synergistic effects exerted by such drug combinations. Tetracyclines such as doxycycline (see Chapter 38) and lincomycins such as clindamycin (see Chapter 39) may also be used in combination with some of the other antimalarial drugs because of the synergistic effects resulting from these drug combinations.

Primaquine, an *8-aminoquinoline* that is structurally similar to the 4-aminoquinolines, has the ability to bind to and alter parasitic DNA. It is one of the few drugs that is effective in the exoerythrocytic phase. Atovaquone/proguanil also works by interference with nucleic acid synthesis.

The drug effects of the antimalarial drugs are mostly limited to their ability to kill parasitic organisms, most of which are *Plasmodium* species (spp.) However, some of these drugs have other effects and therapeutic uses. Hydroxychloroquine also has antiinflammatory effects and is sometimes used in the treatment of rheumatoid arthritis and systemic lupus erythematosus. Quinine and quinidine can also decrease the excitability of both cardiac and skeletal muscles. Quinidine is still used to treat certain types of cardiac dysrhythmias (see Chapter 25).

Indications

Antimalarial drugs are used to kill *Plasmodium* organisms, the parasites that cause malaria. The various antimalarial drugs work during different phases of the parasite's growth inside the human. The antimalarials that exert the greatest effect on all four *Plasmodium* organisms during the erythrocytic or blood

phase are chloroquine, hydroxychloroquine, and pyrimethamine. Other drugs that are known to work during the blood phase are quinine, quinidine, and mefloquine. Because these drugs are ineffective during the exoerythrocytic phase, however, they cannot *prevent* infection. The most effective antimalarial drug for eradicating the parasite during the exoerythrocytic phase is primaquine, which actually works during both phases. Primaquine is indicated specifically for infection with *P. vivax*. Chloroquine and hydroxychloroquine (4-aminoquinolines) are the drugs of choice for the treatment of susceptible strains of malarial parasites. They are highly toxic to all *Plasmodium* spp., except resistant strains of *P. falciparum*.

Quinine is indicated for infection with chloroquine-resistant *P. falciparum*, which can cause a type of malaria that affects the brain. Quinine is commonly given in combination with pyrimethamine, a sulfonamide, or a tetracycline (such as doxycycline). Pyrimethamine is an antimalarial antibiotic that is used in combination with the sulfonamide antibiotic sulfadoxine (Fansidar) for prophylaxis against chloroquine-resistant *P. falciparum* and *P. vivax*. Mefloquine is an antimalarial drug that may also be used for both prophylaxis and treatment of malaria caused by *P. falciparum* or *P. vivax*. The drug combination atovaquone and proguanil (Malarone) is also used for prevention and treatment of *P. falciparum* infection.

Contraindications

Contraindications to various antimalarial drugs include drug allergy, tinnitus (ear ringing), and pregnancy (quinine). Severe renal, hepatic, or hematologic dysfunction may also be a contraindication to the use of antimalarial drugs. Other drug-specific contraindications are noted in the drug profiles that follow.

Adverse Effects

Antimalarial drugs cause diverse adverse effects, and these are listed for each drug in Table 43-1. In 2013, the FDA issued a warning about serious neurologic and psychiatric side effects associated with mefloquine.

Interactions

Some common drug interactions associated with antimalarial drugs are listed in Table 43-2.

Dosages

For dosage information on selected antimalarial drugs, see the table on p. 683.

DRUG PROFILES

The dosing instructions for several of the antimalarial drugs can be confusing, because tablet strengths listed on the medication packaging often indicate the strength of the tablet in terms of the entire salt form of the drug, not just the active ingredient itself, which is referred to as the *base ingredient*. However, dosing guidelines often list recommended dosages in terms of the base ingredient and not the entire salt. For example, as described later in the drug profile for chloroquine, the tablets come in 250-mg and 500-mg strengths of the salt form of the drug, but

TABLE 43-1   Antimalarial Drugs: Common Adverse Effects

Body System	Adverse Effects
Chloroquine and Hydroxychloroquine	
Gastrointestinal	Diarrhea, anorexia, nausea, vomiting
Central nervous	Dizziness, headache, seizures, personality changes
Other	Alopecia, rash, pruritus
Mefloquine	
Central nervous	Headache, fatigue, tinnitus, dizziness, loss of balance, anxiety, depression, hallucinations
Gastrointestinal	Stomach pain, anorexia, nausea, vomiting
Other	Fever, chills, rash, myalgia
Primaquine	
Gastrointestinal	Nausea, vomiting, abdominal distress
Other	Headaches, pruritus, dark discoloration of urine, hemolytic anemia due to G6PD deficiency
Pyrimethamine	
Gastrointestinal	Anorexia; vomiting; taste disturbances; soreness, redness, swelling, or burning of tongue; diarrhea; throat pain; swallowing difficulties; mouth sores and ulcerations; sore throat
Other	Malaise, weakness, rash, abnormal skin pigmentation, hemolytic anemia resulting from G6PD deficiency, hypersensitivity reactions
Quinine	
Central nervous	Visual disturbances, dizziness, headaches, tinnitus
Gastrointestinal	Diarrhea, nausea, vomiting, abdominal pain
Other	Rash, pruritus, hives, photosensitivity, respiratory difficulties

6PD, Glucose-6-phosphate dehydrogenase.

TABLE 43-2   Antimalarial Drugs: Drug Interactions

Drug	Mechanism	Result
Chloroquine		
divalproex, valproic acid, anthelmintics, beta blockers	Decreased serum levels of target drug	Treatment failures of target drugs
digoxin	Increased serum levels of digoxin	Potential toxicity
Mefloquine		
Beta blockers, calcium channel blockers, quinidine, quinine	Unknown	Increased risk for dysrhythmia, cardiac arrest, seizures
Primaquine		
Other hemolytic drugs	Unknown	Increased risk for myelotoxic effects (monitor for muscle weakness)

these tablets actually only have 150 mg and 300 mg, respectively, of the active ingredient or base. Be mindful of these distinctions.

♦chloroquine and ♦hydroxychloroquine

Chloroquine (Aralen) is a synthetic antimalarial drug that is chemically classified as a 4-aminoquinoline derivative. In addition to malaria, it is also indicated for treatment of other parasitic infections, such as amebiasis. Hydroxychloroquine is another synthetic 4-aminoquinoline that differs from chloroquine by only one hydroxyl group (–OH). Its efficacy in treating malaria is comparable to that of quinine. Both medications also possess antiinflammatory actions and have been used to treat rheumatoid arthritis and systemic lupus erythematosus since the 1950s. However, only hydroxychloroquine (Plaquenil) is now used for these indications.

Contraindications include visual field changes, optic neuritis, and psoriasis, but its use may still be warranted in urgent clinical situations, based on sound clinical judgment.

Chloroquine and hydroxychloroquine are available only for oral use. Both drugs are classified as pregnancy category C drugs, but it is recommended that they be used in pregnant women only in truly urgent clinical situations. These drugs are also distributed into breast milk.

Pharmacokinetics: Chloroquine

Route	Onset of Action	Peak Plasma Concentration	Elimination Half-life	Duration of Action
PO	8-10 hr	1-2 hr	3-5 days	Variable

Pharmacokinetics: Hydroxychloroquine

Route	Onset of Action	Peak Plasma Concentration	Elimination Half-life	Duration of Action
PO	4 hr	2-3 hr	32-50 days	Variable

DOSAGES

Selected Antimalarial Drugs

Drug (Pregnancy Category)	Pharmacologic Class	Usual Adult Dosage Range	Indications/Uses
◆ chloroquine (Aralen) (C)	Synthetic antimalarial and antiamebic	PO: 300 mg base weekly, beginning 2 wk before and continuing for 8 wk after visiting endemic area	Malaria prophylaxis
		PO: 600 mg base on day 1, followed by 300 mg 6 hr later and on days 2 and 3	Malaria treatment
◆ hydroxychloroquine (Plaquenil) (C)	Synthetic antimalarial	PO: 400 mg weekly, beginning 1-2 wk before and continuing through 4 wk after visiting endemic area	Malaria prophylaxis
		PO: 800 mg on day 1, followed by 310 mg 6 hr later and once daily on days 2 and 3	Malaria treatment
◆ mefloquine (Lariam) (C)	Synthetic antimalarial	PO: 250 mg weekly beginning 1-2 wk before travel and continuing until 4 wk after visiting endemic area	Malaria prophylaxis
		PO: 1250 mg (5 tabs) in a single dose	Malaria treatment
◆ primaquine (generic only) (C)	Synthetic antimalarial	30 mg PO daily for 1-2 days prior to travel, then continue for 7 days after leaving endemic area; doses vary if dealing with drug-resistant malaria.	Malaria prophylaxis
		PO: 30 mg daily for 14 days	Malaria treatment
pyrimethamine (Daraprim) (C)	Folic acid antagonist, antimalarial, antitoxoplasmotic	PO: 25 mg weekly; continue 10 weeks after exposure	Malaria prophylaxis
		PO: 50 mg daily for 2 days	Malaria treatment

◆ mefloquine

Mefloquine (Lariam) is an analogue of quinine that is indicated for the management of mild to moderate acute malaria and for the prevention and treatment of malaria caused by chloroquine-resistant organisms. It is also used to treat multidrug-resistant strains of *P. falciparum*, which, as already noted, is a very difficult species of *Plasmodium* to kill. The drug is commonly used prophylactically by travelers to prevent malarial infection while visiting malaria-endemic areas. The tetracycline antibiotic doxycycline (see Chapter 38) is also commonly used for this purpose. Mefloquine is available only for oral use.

Pharmacokinetics: Mefloquine

Route	Onset of Action	Peak Plasma Concentration	Elimination Half-life	Duration of Action
PO	Less than 24 hr	7-24 hr	21-22 days	Variable

◆ primaquine

Primaquine is similar in chemical structure and antimalarial activity to the 4-aminoquinolines, but it is classified as an 8-aminoquinoline. It is one of the few antimalarial drugs that can destroy the malarial parasites while they are in their exoerythrocytic phase. Primaquine is indicated for curative therapy in acute cases of *P. vivax, P. ovale,* and to a lesser degree, *P. falciparum* infection.

Primaquine is contraindicated in patients with allergy or any disease states that may cause granulocytopenia (rheumatoid arthritis, systemic lupus erythematosus). Primaquine must be used with caution in patients with methemoglobinemia, porphyria, methemoglobin reductase deficiency, and glucose-6-phosphate dehydrogenase (G6PD) deficiency (see Chapter 2). It is available only for oral use.

Pharmacokinetics: Primaquine

Route	Onset of Action	Peak Plasma Concentration	Elimination Half-life	Duration of Action
PO	2 hr	1-3 hr	4-10 hr	24 hr

pyrimethamine

Pyrimethamine (Daraprim) is a synthetic antimalarial drug that is structurally related to trimethoprim (see Chapter 38). Both drugs are chemically subclassified as *diaminopyrimidines*. Fansidar is a commonly used fixed-combination drug product that contains 500 mg of sulfadoxine and 25 mg of pyrimethamine. Pyrimethamine is contraindicated in patients with megaloblastic anemia caused by folate deficiency. It is available only for oral use.

Pharmacokinetics: Pyrimethamine

Route	Onset of Action	Peak Plasma Concentration	Elimination Half-life	Duration of Action
PO	6 hr	2-6 hr	80-123 hr	Up to 2 wk

OTHER PROTOZOAL INFECTIONS

There are several other common protozoal infections. These include amebiasis (caused by *Entamoebahistolytica*), giardiasis (caused by *Giardia lamblia*), toxoplasmosis (caused by *Toxoplasma gondii*), and trichomoniasis (caused by *Trichomonas vaginalis*). These diseases are more prevalent in tropical regions. Pneumocystosis, which is caused by *Pneumocystis jirovecii* (formerly *Pneumocystis carinii*), used to be classified as a protozoal infection; however, it is now classified as fungal infection. It is a common infection that complicates HIV and AIDS. It is discussed in this chapter as opposed to the antifungal chapter (see Chapter 42) because antifungal drugs are not effective to treat it.

The previously mentioned protozoal infections can be transmitted in a number of ways: from person to person (e.g., via sexual contact), through the ingestion of contaminated water or food, through direct contact with the parasite, or by the bite of an insect (mosquito or tick). These infections can be systemic and occur throughout the body, or they can be localized to a specific region. For example, amebiasis most commonly affects the gastrointestinal tract (e.g., amebic dysentery), whereas pneumocystosis is predominantly a pulmonary infection.

The more common protozoal infections are described briefly in Table 43-3, and the antiprotozoal drugs commonly used in their treatment are listed. Only selected drugs are discussed here. Patients whose immune systems are compromised are at particular risk for acquiring a protozoal infection. Often such infections are fatal in these patients.

ANTIPROTOZOAL DRUGS

Several drugs used to treat malaria are also used to treat nonmalarial protozoal infections, including chloroquine, primaquine, pyrimethamine, and atovaquone. Other antiprotozoal drugs normally used against nonmalarial parasites include iodoquinol, metronidazole, paromomycin, and pentamidine.

Mechanism of Action and Drug Effects

Antiprotozoal drugs work by several different mechanisms. The most commonly used of these drugs, together with brief descriptions of their mechanisms of action, are given in Table 43-4. Pyrimethamine and chloroquine are discussed earlier in this chapter in the section on malaria. The drug effects of antiprotozoal drugs are primarily limited to their ability to kill various forms of protozoal parasites.

Indications

Antiprotozoal drugs are used to treat various protozoal infections, ranging from intestinal amebiasis to pneumocystosis. Indications for selected drugs are summarized in Table 43-5. Atovaquone and pentamidine are used for the treatment of *P. jirovecii* infection. Iodoquinol, metronidazole, and paromomycin are all used to treat intestinal amebiasis. Metronidazole is effective against several forms of bacteria, including anaerobic bacteria (see Chapter 39), as well as against protozoans and helminths (parasitic worms). Worm infection (helminthiasis) is discussed later in the chapter.

Contraindications

Contraindications to the use of antiprotozoal drugs include known drug allergy. Additional contraindications may include serious renal, liver, or other illnesses, with the seriousness of the infection weighed against the patient's overall condition.

Adverse Effects

The adverse effects of antiprotozoal drugs vary greatly depending on the drug and are listed in Table 43-6.

Interactions

The common drug and laboratory test interactions associated with the use of antiprotozoal drugs are listed in Table 43-7.

Dosages

For dosage information for selected antiprotozoal drugs, see the table on p. 686.

TABLE 43-3 Types of Protozoal Infections and Common Drug Therapy

Infection	Description	Antiprotozoal Drug
Amebiasis	Caused by the protozoal parasite *Entamoebahistolytica*. Infection mainly resides in the large intestine but can also migrate to other parts of the body, such as the liver. Usually transmitted in contaminated food or water.	chloroquine, metronidazole, paromomycin, iodoquinol
Giardiasis	Caused by *Giardia lamblia*. The most common intestinal protozoal infection, usually residing in the intestinal mucosa (most commonly the duodenum). May cause diarrhea, bloating, and foul-smelling stools. Transmitted in contaminated food or water or by contact with stool from infected persons.	metronidazole, nitazoxanide, quinacrine, furazolidone, albendazole, paromomycin
Pneumocystosis	Pneumonia caused by *Pneumocystis jirovecii** that occurs exclusively in immunocompromised individuals. Always fatal if left untreated.	trimethoprim/sulfamethoxazole, dapsone, atovaquone, primaquine, pentamidine, clindamycin
Toxoplasmosis	Caused by *Toxoplasma gondii*. Can produce systemic infection Domesticated animals, usually cats, serve as intermediate host for parasites, passing infective oocysts in their feces.	sulfonamides with pyrimethamine, clindamycin, metronidazole
Trichomoniasis	Sexually transmitted disease caused by *Trichomonas vaginalis*.	metronidazole

*Pneumocystis jirovecii is now classified as a fungus.

TABLE 43-4 Selected Antiprotozoal Drugs: Mechanisms of Action

Drug	Mechanism of Action
atovaquone	Atovaquone selectively inhibits mitochondrial electron transport, reducing synthesis of adenosine triphosphate (required for cellular energy). Also inhibits nucleic acid synthesis.
metronidazole	Interferes with DNA, resulting in inhibition of protein synthesis and cell death in susceptible organisms.
pentamidine	Inhibits production of much-needed substances such as DNA and RNA. Can bind to and aggregate ribosomes. Is directly lethal to *Pneumocystis jirovecii** by inhibiting glucose metabolism, protein and RNA synthesis, and intracellular amino acid transport.

*Pneumocystis jirovecii is now classified as a fungus.

TABLE 43-5 Selected Antiprotozoal Drugs: Indications

Drug	Indications
atovaquone	Indicated for treatment of acute mild to moderately severe *Pneumocystis jirovecii* pneumonia in patients who cannot tolerate co-trimoxazole
iodoquinol	Indicated for treatment of intestinal amebiasis in asymptomatic carriers of *Entamoebahistolytica;* also has been used for treatment of *Giardia lamblia* and *Trichomonas vaginalis* infections
metronidazole	Indicated for treatment of bacterial (including anaerobic), protozoal, and helminthic infections
pentamidine	Indicated for treatment of *P. jirovecii** pneumonia

*Pneumocystis jirovecii is now classified as a fungus.

TABLE 43-6 Selected Antiprotozoal Drugs: Adverse Effects

Body System	Adverse Effects
Atovaquone	
Hematologic	Anemia, neutropenia, leukopenia
Integumentary	Pruritus, urticaria, rash
Gastrointestinal	Anorexia, elevated liver enzymes, nausea, constipation
Central nervous	Dizziness, headache, anxiety, fever
Metabolic	Hyperkalemia, hypoglycemia, hyponatremia
Other	Cough
Iodoquinol	
Hematologic	Agranulocytosis
Integumentary	Rash; pruritus; discolored skin, hair, nails
Central nervous	Headache, agitation, peripheral neuropathy
Eyes, ears, nose, and throat	Blurred vision, sore throat, optic neuritis, blindness
Gastrointestinal	Anorexia, gastritis, nausea, vomiting, diarrhea
Metronidazole	
Central nervous	Headache, dizziness, confusion, fatigue, peripheral neuropathy, weakness
Eyes, ears, nose, and throat	Blurred vision, sore throat, dry mouth, metallic taste, glossitis
Gastrointestinal	Anorexia, vomiting, diarrhea, constipation
Genitourinary	Dysuria, cystitis
Hematologic	Neutropenia
Integumentary	Rash, pruritus, urticaria
Paromomycin	
Gastrointestinal	Stomach cramps, nausea, vomiting, diarrhea
Central nervous	Hearing loss, dizziness, tinnitus
Pentamidine	
Cardiovascular	Hypotension, chest pain, dysrhythmias
Hematologic	Leukopenia, thrombocytopenia, neutropenia
Integumentary	Pain at injection site, pruritus, urticaria, rash
Genitourinary	Nephrotoxicity
Gastrointestinal	Increased liver enzyme levels, pancreatitis, metallic taste, nausea, vomiting, diarrhea
Respiratory	Cough, wheezing, dyspnea, pharyngitis
Metabolic	Hypoglycemia followed by hyperglycemia
Other	Fatigue, chills, night sweats

TABLE 43-7 Antiprotozoal Drugs: Drug and Laboratory Test Interactions

Drug	Mechanism	Result
atovaquone	Competition for binding on protein, resulting in free, active atovaquone	Highly protein-bound drugs (e.g., warfarin, phenytoin) may increase atovaquone drug concentrations and risk for adverse reactions.
iodoquinol	Increase in protein-bound serum iodine concentrations, reflecting a decrease in iodine 131 uptake	May interfere with certain thyroid function test results
metronidazole	Decreased absorption of vitamin K from the intestines due to elimination of the bacteria needed to absorb vitamin K, increased plasma acetaldehyde concentration after ingestion of alcohol	Alcohol causes a disulfiram-like reaction; action of warfarin may be increased (increased bleeding risk).
pentamidine	Additive nephrotoxic effects	Use with an aminoglycoside, amphotericin B, colistin, cisplatin, or vancomycin may result in nephrotoxicity.

DOSAGES

Selected Antiprotozoal Drugs

Drug (Pregnancy Category)	Pharmacologic Class	Usual Adult Dosage Range	Indications/Uses
atovaquone* (Mepron) (C)	Synthetic anti-*Pneumocystis* drug	PO: prophylaxis: 1500 mg daily with food; 750 mg bid for 21 days for treatment	Prophylaxis of *Pneumocystis jirovecii* pneumonia; treatment of active *P. jirovecii* pneumonia
◆ metronidazole (Flagyl) (X, first trimester; B, second and third trimesters)	Amebicide, antibacterial, trichomonacide	PO: 750 mg 3 times daily for 7-10 days PO: 250-500 mg 3 times daily for 5-7 days	Amebiasis, including amebic liver abscess Trichomoniasis, giardiasis
pentamidine (NebuPent, Pentam 300) (C)	Synthetic anti-*Pneumocystis*† drug	Inhalation aerosol: 300 mg every 4 wk IV/IM: 4 mg/kg daily for 14-21 days	Prophylaxis of *P. jirovecii* pneumonia; treatment of active *P. jirovecii* pneumonia

*Note: A combination product containing atovaquone and the drug proguanil is also used against malaria.
†*Pneumocystis jirovecii* is now classified as a fungus.

DRUG PROFILES

atovaquone

Atovaquone (Mepron) is a synthetic antiprotozoal drug indicated for the treatment of mild to moderate *P. jirovecii* pneumonia in patients who cannot tolerate co-trimoxazole (trimethoprim/sulfamethoxazole [see Chapter 38]). It is available only for oral use.

Pharmacokinetics: Atovaquone

Route	Onset of Action	Peak Plasma Concentration	Elimination Half-life	Duration of Action
PO	8-24 hr	24-96 hr	2-3 days	Unknown

◆ metronidazole

Metronidazole (Flagyl) is an antiprotozoal drug that also has fairly broad antibacterial activity as well as anthelmintic activity. The therapeutic uses of metronidazole are many and range from the treatment of trichomoniasis, amebiasis, and giardiasis to the treatment of anaerobic bacterial infections and antibiotic-induced pseudomembranous colitis (see Chapters 38 and 39). Metronidazole is believed to directly kill protozoans by causing free-radical reactions that damage their

DNA and other vital biomolecules. Tinidazole (Tindamax) is a newer, similar drug.

Metronidazole is contraindicated during the first trimester of pregnancy. It is available in both oral and injectable forms. Metronidazole interacts with alcohol. Alcohol should be avoided 24 hours before therapy and at least 48 hours after the last dose.

Pharmacokinetics: Metronidazole

Route	Onset of Action	Peak Plasma Concentration	Elimination Half-life	Duration of Action
PO	1 hr	1-2 hr	8 hr	Variable

pentamidine

Pentamidine (NebuPent, Pentam 300) is an antiprotozoal drug that is used for the management of *P. jirovecii* pneumonia, although it is sometimes used to treat various protozoal infections. It works by inhibiting protein and nucleic acid synthesis. It is used for the treatment of active pneumocystosis and for prophylaxis of *P. jirovecii* pneumonia in patients at high risk for initial or recurrent *Pneumocystis* infection, such as patients with HIV infection and AIDS.

The only contraindication to pentamidine is known hypersensitivity to the drug. Hypersensitivity is more common when the drug is administered by inhalation. Due to the seriousness of the *Pneumocystis* infection, an allergic reaction to the inhalational form does not preclude its administration by either the intramuscular or intravenous route. The drug needs to be used with caution in patients with blood dyscrasias, hepatic or renal disease, diabetes mellitus, cardiac disease, hypocalcemia, or hypertension. Pentamidine is available as an oral inhalational solution and also in injectable form.

Pharmacokinetics: Pentamidine

Route	Onset of Action	Peak Plasma Concentration	Elimination Half-life	Duration of Action
Inhalation	0.5-1 hr	Less than 1 hr	6-9 hr	Variable

HELMINTHIC INFECTIONS

Parasitic helminthic infections (worm infections) are a worldwide problem. It has been estimated that one third of the world's population is infected with these parasites. Persons living in undeveloped countries where sanitary conditions are often poor are by far the most common victims. The incidence of worm infection in developed countries where sewage treatment is adequate is much lower. The most prevalent helminthic infection in the United States is enterobiasis, caused by one genus of roundworm, *Enterobius*.

Helminths that are parasitic in humans are classified in the following way:

- Platyhelminthes (flatworms)
- Cestodes (tapeworms)
- Trematodes (flukes)
- Nematodes (roundworms)

The characteristics of a few of the most common of the many helminthic infections are summarized in Table 43-8. These usually first infect the intestines of their host and reside there but can sometimes also migrate to other tissues.

ANTHELMINTIC DRUGS

Unlike protozoans, which are single-celled, helminths are larger and have complex multicellular structures. Anthelmintic drugs (also spelled *antihelmintic*) work to destroy these organisms by disrupting their structures. The currently available anthelmintic drugs are very specific with regard to the worms they can kill. For this reason, the causative worm in an infected host must be accurately identified before treatment is started. This can usually be done by analyzing samples of feces, urine, blood, sputum, or tissue from the infected host for the presence of ova or larvae of the particular parasite.

Several anthelmintics are commercially available in the United States. These include albendazole (Albenza), ivermectin (Stromectol), praziquantel (Biltricide), and pyrantel (Antiminth).

TABLE 43-8	**Helminthic Infections**
Infection	**Organism and Other Facts**
Nematodes (Various Intestinal and Tissue Roundworms)	
Ascariasis	Caused by *Ascaris lumbricoides* (giant roundworm); worm resides in small intestine; treated with pyrantel or albendazole
Enterobiasis	Caused by *Enterobius vermicularis* (pinworm); worm resides in large intestine; treated with pyrantel or albendazole
Platyhelminthes (Intestinal Tapeworms or Flatworms)	
Diphyllobothriasis	Caused by *Diphyllobothrium latum* (fish worm); acquired from fish; treated with paromomycin, praziquantel, or albendazole
Taeniasis	Caused by *Taeniasaginata* (beef tapeworm); acquired from beef; treated with paromomycin, praziquantel, or albendazole

TABLE 43-9	**Anthelmintics: Class of Worms Killed**		
Anthelmintic Drug	**Cestodes**	**Nematodes**	**Trematodes**
albendazole	Yes	Yes	Yes
ivermectin	No	Yes	No
piperazine and pyrantel	No	Yes (giant worm and pinworm)	No
praziquantel	Yes	No	Yes

Other drugs, such as niclosamide and piperazine, may be available either in other countries or by special request from the CDC. Anthelmintics are very specific in their actions. Albendazole can be used to treat both tapeworms and roundworms. Praziquantel is a drug that can kill flukes (trematodes). The most commonly used anthelmintics and the specific class of worms they can effectively kill are summarized in Table 43-9.

Mechanism of Action and Drug Effects

The mechanisms of action of the various anthelmintics vary greatly from drug to drug, although there are some similarities among the drugs used to kill similar types of worms. The various anthelmintic drugs and their respective mechanisms of action are listed in Table 43-10. The drug effects of the anthelmintic drugs are limited to their ability to kill various forms of worms and flukes.

Indications

Anthelmintic drugs are used to treat roundworm, tapeworm, and fluke infections. Specific drugs are used to treat specific helminthic infections.

DOSAGES

Selected Anthelmintic Drugs

Drug (Pregnancy Category)	Pharmacologic Class	Usual Adult Dosage Range	Indications
praziquantel (Biltricide) (B)	Trematode anthelmintic	PO: Approximately 20-25 mg/kg 3 times daily for 1 day	Fluke infections
pyrantel (Pin-X) (C)	Nematode anthelmintic	PO: 11 mg/kg in a single dose (max dose 1 g)	Roundworm infections

PO, Oral.

TABLE 43-10 Anthelmintics: Mechanisms of Action

Drug	Mechanism of Action	Indication
albendazole	Larvae cells are selectively destroyed by degenerating cytoplasmic microtubules. This in turn causes secretory substances to accumulate intracellularly, which leads to impaired cholinesterase secretion and glucose. Glycogen becomes depleted, which leads to decreased ATP production and energy depletion, which immobilizes and kills the worm.	Neurocysticercosis, hydatid disease
ivermectin	Potentiates inhibitory signals in the CNS of nematodes, which leads to their paralysis.	Nondisseminated intestinal infection with *Strongyloides* (threadworms)
praziquantel	Increases permeability of the cell membrane of susceptible worms to calcium, which results in the influx of calcium. This causes the worms to be dislodged from their usual site of residence in the mesenteric veins to the liver; they are then killed by host tissue reactions.	Schistosomiasis, opisthorchiasis (liver fluke infection), clonorchiasis (infection with Chinese or Oriental liver fluke), diphyllobothriasis (fish worm infection), neurocysticercosis
pyrantel	Blocks ACh at the neuromuscular junction, which results in paralysis of the worm. The paralyzed worm is then expelled from the GI tract by normal peristalsis.	Ascariasis, enterobiasis, other helminthic infections
thiabendazole	Inhibits the helminth-specific enzyme fumarate reductase.	Cutaneous larva migrans (creeping eruption), strongyloidiasis, trichinosis

ACh, Acetylcholine; *ATP,* adenosine triphosphate.

Contraindications

The only usual contraindication to a specific anthelmintic drug product is known drug allergy. Pyrantel is contraindicated in patients with liver disease. Praziquantel is also contraindicated in patients with *ocular cysticercosis* (tapeworm infection of the eye).

Adverse Effects

The anthelmintic drugs show a remarkable diversity in their drug-specific adverse effects. Common adverse effects are listed in Table 43-11.

Interactions

The concurrent use of pyrantel with piperazine is not recommended, and pyrantel is used cautiously in patients with hepatic impairment. Pyrantel has also been shown to raise blood levels of theophylline in pediatric patients. Dexamethasone and the anthelmintic praziquantel may raise blood levels of albendazole. Histamine H_2 antagonists (e.g., cimetidine, ranitidine) may also raise blood levels of praziquantel.

Dosages

For dosage information on selected anthelmintic drugs, see the table on this page.

TABLE 43-11 Anthelmintics: Common Adverse Effects

Body System	Adverse Effects
Primaquine	
Gastrointestinal	Nausea, vomiting, abdominal distress
Other	Headaches, pruritus, dark discoloration of urine, hemolytic anemia due to glucose-6-phosphate dehydrogenase deficiency
Pyrantel	
Central nervous system	Headache, dizziness, insomnia
Dermatologic	Skin rash
Gastrointestinal	Anorexia, abdominal cramps, diarrhea, nausea, vomiting
Praziquantel	
Central nervous system	Dizziness, headache, drowsiness
Gastrointestinal	Abdominal pain, nausea
Other	Malaise

DRUG PROFILES

Anthelmintics are available only as oral preparations and, with the exception of pyrantel, all require a prescription. Different drugs are selected to treat infection with different helminthic species.

praziquantel

Praziquantel (Biltricide) is one of the primary anthelmintic drugs used for the treatment of various fluke infections. It is also useful against many species of tapeworm. It is contraindicated in patients with ocular worm infestation (*ocular cysticercosis*). It is available only for oral use.

Pharmacokinetics: Praziquantel

Route	Onset of Action	Peak Plasma Concentration	Elimination Half-life	Duration of Action
PO	1 hr	1-3 hr	4-5 hr	Variable

pyrantel

Pyrantel (Pin-X) is a pyrimidine-derived anthelmintic drug that is indicated for the treatment of infection with intestinal roundworms, including ascariasis, enterobiasis, and other helminthic infections. It is the only anthelmintic available in the United States without a prescription. It is available only for oral use.

Pharmacokinetics: Pyrantel

Route	Onset of Action	Peak Plasma Concentration	Elimination Half-life	Duration of Action
PO	1 hr	1-3 hr	Unknown	Unknown

◼ NURSING PROCESS

◼ ASSESSMENT

Before beginning treatment with an *antimalarial drug*, obtain a thorough medication history, perform a head-to-toe physical assessment, and measure vital signs. Assess and give special attention to assessment findings for any common manifestations of malaria, such as headache, nausea, and joint pain. Other symptoms include chills and rigors followed by fever of up to 104° F (40° C), frequently leading to extreme fatigue and prolonged sleep. Baseline visual acuity tests may be needed due to the contraindications of visual field problems and optic neuritis with *chloroquine, quinine,* and *hydroxychoroquine*. Perform a skin assessment as well, because of the contraindication in individuals with psoriasis. Other drugs, such as *mefloquine, primaquine,* and *pyrimethamine,* require assessment of baseline hearing and of G6PD deficiency due to drug-induced hemolytic anemia. Common drug interactions to assess for are listed in Table 43-2.

Antiprotozoal drugs and their contraindications, cautions, and drug interactions were discussed earlier in the chapter. Assess baseline renal and liver function as well as the patient's overall health status. With *atovaquone,* determine baseline blood counts due to the risk for drug-induced anemia/neutropenia and leukopenia. Assess serum potassium, sodium, and glucose levels as ordered. With *iodoquinol,* it is important to assess blood counts prior to its use as well as baseline vision and neurologic intactness (e.g., presence of normal sensations).

Metronidazole requires assessment for allergy to any of the nitroimidazole derivatives as well as to parabens (for the topical dosage forms). Obtain appropriate specimens for analysis before treatment. Assess blood counts, presence of central nervous system disorders or abnormalities, and bladder function prior to use of metronidazole. This is important because of the adverse effects of dysuria, cystitis, headache, dizziness, confusion, and fatigue (see Table 43-6). *Pentamidine* is associated with serious cardiac, hematologic, skin, renal, GI, and respiratory adverse effects; therefore, documentation of a thorough assessment of each of these systems is critical to patient safety.

With any of the *anthelmintic drugs,* obtain a thorough history of the foods eaten, especially meat and fish, and their means of preparation. Additionally, assess other individuals in the family household for helminth infection. Obtaining stool specimens is usually indicated. Assess the patient's energy level, ability to perform activities of daily living, weight, and appetite. Document the findings. Assess for contraindications, such as liver disease and drug allergy, and any cautions. Drug interactions to assess for include theophylline, antiepileptic drugs, and histamine H_2 antagonists.

◼ NURSING DIAGNOSES

1. Imbalanced nutrition, less than body requirements, related to the disease process and adverse effects of medication
2. Deficient knowledge related to the infection and its drug treatment
3. Ineffective family health management related to poor compliance with treatment and/or lack of knowledge about the infection and its treatment

CASE STUDY

Safety: What Went Wrong? Metronidazole

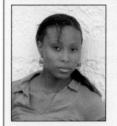

T.J., a 28-year-old graduate student, just returned from an archeology internship in a third-world country. She has had severe diarrhea for several days and has been diagnosed with intestinal amebiasis. She will receive fluids for rehydration and metronidazole (Flagyl) as part of her treatment.

1. What specific laboratory test must be ordered before initiation of the metronidazole therapy? What other laboratory studies will be performed?
2. T.J. is started on the intravenous piggyback infusions, and after 1 day she reports that her diarrhea has decreased and that she feels a little better. During afternoon rounds, T.J. tells the nurse that she feels dizzy and tired, and has some nausea. She asks, "Is this because of my infection?" What is the nurse's best response?
3. T.J. is discharged to home with a prescription to take the metronidazole for 2 more weeks. The nurse reviews several education points about this drug therapy and knows that one serious adverse effect is leukopenia. What symptoms will the nurse tell T.J. to report?
4. One week later, T.J. calls to tell the nurse that she went out to a bar with some friends and became very ill after having a drink. What went wrong?

For answers, see *http://evolve.elsevier.com/Lilley.*

PLANNING: OUTCOME IDENTIFICATION

1. Patient maintains balanced nutrition during drug therapy with balanced nutritional meals with recommended amounts of calorie and protein.
2. Patient, family, and significant others demonstrate adequate knowledge regarding the infection and its treatment, thorough hand washing technique, and symptoms to report to the prescriber such as fever, lethargy, and loss of appetite.
3. Patient, family, and others in the home environment experience improved health management and compliance.

IMPLEMENTATION

With *antimalarials,* encourage adequate dietary and fluid intake while the patient is fighting the infection and taking the medications. Oral doses need to be taken with at least 6 to 8 ounces of water or other fluid. Increase fluids unless contraindicated. Because antimalarials concentrate in the liver first, emphasize to the patient the importance of follow-up visits to the prescriber so that liver function can be monitored during therapy.

Chloroquine and *hydroxychloroquine* are administered orally and are to be taken exactly as prescribed. Follow dosing orders and instructions as prescribed, with specific attention to the loading doses, subsequent doses, and prophylactic dosing. Photosensitivity may occur with *quinine;* provide adequate teaching about the use of sunscreen and sun safety. Sun protection must include coverage against UVA and UVB rays. See Patient-Centered Care: Patient Teaching below for more information.

Most of the *antiprotozoal drugs* (e.g., *atovaquone, metronidazole*) are given with food when taken orally. Infuse intravenous doses of *metronidazole* as ordered. Intravenous (IV) doses are to infuse over 30 to 60 minutes and are never given as an IV bolus. During use of this drug, report to the prescriber any changes in neurologic status (e.g., dizziness, confusion).

All *anthelmintic drugs* are to be administered as ordered and for the prescribed length of time. Warn patients that use of primaquine may lead to dark discoloration of the urine. Perform collection of stool specimens, as ordered. The stool must not be in contact with water, urine, or chemicals because of the risk of destroying the parasitic worms and/or altering the test results. See Patient-Centered Care: Patient Teaching below for more information on these drugs.

EVALUATION

Monitor the patient for therapeutic effects of the *antimalarials, antiprotozoals, and anthelmintics* such as improved energy levels and decrease in and/or eventual resolution of all symptoms. Evaluation of proper hygiene and prevention of the spread of the infestation or infection is also important. With these three groups of drugs, evaluate for the adverse effects associated with each type of drug (see Tables 43-1, 43-6, and 43-11). Some antimalarials and anthelmintics may precipitate hemolysis in patients with G6PD deficiency (mostly African-American patients and those of Mediterranean ancestry); therefore, closely monitor such patients for this complication during the treatment protocol. See Chapter 2 for further discussion of G6PD deficiency.

PATIENT-CENTERED CARE: PATIENT TEACHING

- Antimalarials are known to cause gastrointestinal upset; however, this may be decreased if the medication is taken with food. Encourage the patient to contact the prescriber if there is unresolved nausea, vomiting, profuse diarrhea, or abdominal pain. Patients need to understand the importance of immediately reporting to the prescriber any visual disturbances, dizziness, or respiratory difficulties.
- Educate the patient about the need for prophylactic doses of antimalarials, as prescribed, before visiting malaria-infested countries as well as the need to obtain appropriate treatment upon return.
- Keep antimalarials, like all other medications, out of the reach of children.
- Instruct the patient to take the entire course of medication as directed.

- Oral dosage forms of metronidazole are to be taken with food.
- Inform the patient taking metronidazole for a sexually transmitted disease to avoid sexual intercourse until the prescriber states otherwise.
- When the patient is taking metronidazole for amebiasis, include in your instructions how to check stool samples correctly and safely and how to dispose of samples properly.
- Apply topical forms of the drug with a finger cot or gloved hand and caution the patient to avoid contact of the drug with the eyes.
- Metronidazole may precipitate dizziness. Encourage the patient to be cautious in all activities until a response to the drug is noted and is consistent.
- Anthelmintics are to be taken exactly as prescribed; emphasize the importance of compliance with the drug regimen.

KEY POINTS

- Malaria is caused by *Plasmodium,* a particular genus of protozoans, and is transmitted by the bite of an infected female mosquito. The drug primaquine attacks the parasite when it is outside the exoerythrocytic (tissue) phase.
- Other common protozoal infections are amebiasis, giardiasis, toxoplasmosis, and trichomoniasis. Protozoans are parasites that are transmitted by person-to-person

contact, ingestion of contaminated water or food, direct contact with the parasite, and the bite of an insect (mosquito or tick). Pneumocystosis is now classified as a fungal infection, but it is treated with antiprotozoal drugs.
- Antiprotozoals include atovaquone and pentamidine. Metronidazole is an antibacterial, antiprotozoal, and

anthelmintic. The drugs iodoquinol and paromomycin directly kill protozoans such as *Entamoebahistolytica*.

- Anthelmintics are drugs used to treat parasitic worm infections caused by cestodes (tapeworms), nematodes (roundworms), and trematodes (flukes).

- Nursing considerations with the use of any of the antimalarials, antiprotozoals, and anthelmintics include assessment for contraindications, cautions, and drug interactions.

NCLEX® EXAMINATION REVIEW QUESTIONS

1. The nurse is reviewing the medication history of a patient who is taking hydroxychloroquine. However, the patient's chart does not reveal a history of malaria or travel out of the country. The patient is most likely taking this medication for
   a. *Plasmodium*.
   b. thyroid disorders.
   c. roundworms.
   d. rheumatoid arthritis.

2. Which teaching point would be appropriate to include when the nurse is informing a patient about the adverse effects of antimalarials?
   a. The skin may turn blotchy while these medications are taken.
   b. These medications may cause anorexia and abdominal distress.
   c. These medications may cause increased urinary output.
   d. The patient may experience periods of diaphoresis and chills.

3. When teaching a patient about the potential drug interactions with antiprotozoal drugs, the nurse will include information about
   a. acetaminophen.
   b. warfarin.
   c. decongestants.
   d. antibiotics.

4. Before administering antiprotozoal drugs, the nurse will review which baseline assessment?
   a. Complete blood count
   b. Serum magnesium level
   c. Creatinine clearance
   d. Arterial blood gas concentrations

5. The nurse knows that antimalarial drugs are used to treat patients with infections caused by which microorganism?
   a. *Plasmodium* spp.
   b. Candida albicans
   c. *Pneumocystis jirovecii*
   d. Mycobacterium

6. When giving metronidazole, the nurse implements appropriate administration techniques, including which of these? *(Select all that apply.)*
   a. Giving oral forms with food
   b. Giving oral forms on an empty stomach with a full glass of water
   c. Infusing intravenous doses over 30 to 60 minutes
   d. Administering intravenous doses by bolus over 5 minutes
   e. Obtaining ordered specimens before starting the medication

7. A 5-year-old patient has been diagnosed with malaria after returning from an overseas trip. The patient is to receive one dose of mefloquine (Lariam), 25 mg/kg PO. The child weighs 44 lb. How much mefloquine will this child receive?

8. Praziquantel (Biltricide) is prescribed for a patient with a tapeworm infection. The nurse prepares to administer the medication via which route?
   a. Rectal
   b. Oral
   c. Intravenous
   d. Inhalation

1. d, 2. b, 3. b, 4. a, 5. a, 6. a, c, 7. 500 mg, 8. b.

CRITICAL THINKING AND PRIORITIZATION QUESTIONS

1. You are preparing to give pyrantel (Pin-X) to a patient who has an infection with intestinal roundworms. The patient is very worried about this infection and its treatment, and asks you, "What will this drug do to me? Does it have bad side effects? I'm already sick enough!" What is the nurse's priority when answering the patient's questions?

2. A patient with a history of AIDS has severe *Pneumocystis jirovecii* pneumonia. As you prepare the ordered dose of pentamidine inhalation, the patient asks you, "What are you doing? Why can't you give that to me in a pill?" What is the nurse's priority when answering the patient's questions?

For answers, see *http://evolve.elsevier.com/Lilley*.

ⓔ EVOLVE WEBSITE

Antiinflammatory and Antigout Drugs

http://evolve.elsevier.com/Lilley

KEY TERMS

Chemotaxis The chemical attraction of leukocytes to the site of inflammation, which worsens an inflammatory response. (p. 696)

Done nomogram A standard data graph, originally published in 1960 in the journal *Pediatrics,* for rating the severity of aspirin toxicity following overdose. Serum salicylate levels are plotted against time elapsed since ingestion. (p. 696)

Gout Hyperuricemia (elevated blood uric acid level); the arthritis caused by tissue buildup of uric acid crystals. (p. 699)

Inflammation A localized protective response stimulated by injury to tissues that serves to destroy, dilute, or wall off (sequester) both the injurious agent and the injured tissue. (p. 692)

Nonsteroidal antiinflammatory drugs (NSAIDs) A large and chemically diverse group of drugs that possess analgesic, antiinflammatory, and antipyretic (fever-reducing) activity. (p. 693)

Salicylism The syndrome of salicylate toxicity, including symptoms such as tinnitus (ringing sound in the ears), nausea, and vomiting. (p. 696)

OVERVIEW

Inflammation is defined as a localized protective response stimulated by injury to tissues, which serves to destroy, dilute, or wall off (sequester) both the injurious agent and the injured tissue. Classic signs and symptoms of inflammation include pain, fever, loss of function, redness, and swelling. These symptoms result from arterial, venous, and capillary dilation; enhanced blood flow and vascular permeability; exudation of fluids, including plasma proteins; and leukocyte migration into the inflammatory focus. The inflammatory response is mediated by a host of endogenous compounds, including proteins of the complement system, histamine, serotonin, bradykinin, leukotrienes, and prostaglandins, the latter two being major contributors to the symptoms of inflammation.

Arachidonic acid is released from phospholipids in cell membranes in response to a triggering event (e.g., an injury). It is metabolized in either the prostaglandin pathway or the leukotriene pathway, both of which are branches of the

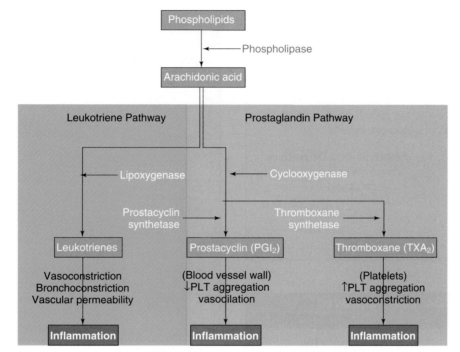

FIGURE 44-1 Arachidonic acid pathway. *PGI2*, Prostaglandin I$_2$; *PLT*, platelet; *TXA$_2$*, thromboxane A$_2$.

arachidonic acid pathway, as shown in Figure 44-1. Both of these pathways lead to inflammation, edema, headache, and other pain characteristic of the body's response to injury or inflammatory illnesses such as arthritis.

In the prostaglandin pathway, arachidonic acid is converted by the enzyme cyclooxygenase into various prostaglandins. Prostaglandins mediate inflammation by inducing vasodilation and enhancing vasopermeability. These effects in turn potentiate the action of proinflammatory substances such as histamine and bradykinin in the production of edema and pain. These symptoms arise as a result of prostaglandin-induced hyperalgesia (excessive sensitivity). In this situation, stimuli that normally would not be painful, such as simply moving a joint through its natural range of motion, become painful because of the inflammatory process at work. Fever occurs when prostaglandin E$_2$ is synthesized in the preoptic hypothalamic region, the area of the brain that regulates temperature.

The leukotriene pathway utilizes lipoxygenases to metabolize the arachidonic acid and convert it into various leukotrienes. Although leukotrienes are more newly discovered than prostaglandins and not as well studied, they are also mediators of inflammation, promoting vasoconstriction, bronchospasm, and increased vascular permeability with resultant edema (see Chapter 37).

NONSTEROIDAL ANTIINFLAMMATORY DRUGS

Nonsteroidal antiinflammatory drugs (NSAIDs) are among the most commonly prescribed drugs. Every year, over 70 million prescriptions are written for these drugs. This represents more than 5% of all prescriptions. Currently more than 23 different NSAIDs are available in the United States. Some of these are used much more commonly than others. A given patient may respond better to one NSAID than to others, in terms of both symptom relief and adverse effects.

NSAIDs comprise a large and chemically diverse group of drugs that possess analgesic, antiinflammatory, and antipyretic (antifever) activity. They are also used for the relief of mild to moderate headaches, myalgia, neuralgia, and arthralgia; alleviation of postoperative pain; relief of the pain associated with arthritic disorders such as rheumatoid arthritis, juvenile arthritis, ankylosing spondylitis, and osteoarthritis; and treatment of gout and hyperuricemia (discussed later in the chapter). Aspirin is used for its effect in inhibiting platelet aggregation, which has been shown to have protective qualities against certain cardiovascular events such as myocardial infarction (MI) and stroke. Aspirin has been shown to reduce cardiac death after an MI and should be administered at the first sign of MI. If not given prior to arriving in the emergency department, aspirin is one of the first drugs given if there are no contraindications. Corticosteroid antiinflammatory drugs (e.g., prednisone, dexamethasone) are also used for similar purposes and are discussed in Chapter 33. NSAIDs have a generally more favorable adverse-effect profile than the corticosteroid antiinflammatory drugs.

In 1899, acetylsalicylic acid (ASA; aspirin) was marketed and rapidly became the most widely used drug in the world. The success of aspirin established the importance of drugs with antipyretic, analgesic, and antiinflammatory properties—the properties that all NSAIDs share. The widespread use of aspirin also yielded evidence of its potential for causing major adverse effects. Gastrointestinal intolerance, bleeding, and renal impairment became major factors limiting its long-term

---

BOX 44-1 **Chemical Categories of NSAIDs**

Salicylates
aspirin
diflunisal (Dolobid)
salsalate (Salistab)
choline salicylate (Arthropan)

Acetic Acid Derivatives
diclofenac sodium (Voltaren)
indomethacin (Indocin)
sulindac (Clinoril)
tolmetin (Tolectin)
etodolac (Lodine)
ketorolac (Toradol)
meclofenamate (generic only)
mefenamic acid (Ponstel)

Cyclooxygenase-2 Inhibitors
celecoxib (Celebrex)

Enolic Acid Derivatives
nabumetone (Relafen)
meloxicam (Mobic)
piroxicam (Feldene)

Propionic Acid Derivatives
fenoprofen (Nalfon)
flurbiprofen (Ansaid)
ibuprofen (Motrin, Advil, others)
ketoprofen (Orudis KT)
naproxen (Naprosyn, Aleve)
oxaprozin (Daypro)

BOX 44-2 **NSAIDs: FDA-Approved Indications**

- Acute gout
- Acute gouty arthritis
- Ankylosing spondylitis
- Bursitis
- Fever
- Juvenile rheumatoid arthritis
- Mild to moderate pain
- Osteoarthritis
- Primary dysmenorrhea
- Rheumatoid arthritis
- Tendinitis
- Various ophthalmic uses

FDA, U.S. Food and Drug Administration.

TABLE 44-1 **Suggested NSAIDs for Patients with Various Medical Conditions**

Medical Condition	Recommended NSAID
Ankylosing spondylitis	indomethacin, diclofenac
Diabetic neuropathy	sulindac
Dysmenorrhea	Fenamates, naproxen, ibuprofen
Gout	indomethacin, naproxen, sulindac
Headaches	aspirin, naproxen, ibuprofen
Hepatotoxicity	tolmetin, naproxen, ibuprofen, piroxicam, fenamates
History of aspirin or NSAID allergy	Avoid if possible; if deemed necessary, consider a nonacetylated salicylate
Hypertension	sulindac, nonacetylated salicylate, ibuprofen, etodolac
Osteoarthritis	diclofenac, oxaprozin, indomethacin
Risk for gastrointestinal toxicity	COX-2 inhibitors (celecoxib), nonacetylated salicylate, enteric-coated aspirin, diclofenac, nabumetone, etodolac, ibuprofen, oxaprozin
Risk for nephrotoxicity	sulindac, nonacetylated salicylate, nabumetone, etodolac, diclofenac, oxaprozin
Warfarin therapy	sulindac, tolmetin, naproxen, ibuprofen, oxaprozin

COX, Cyclooxygenase.

---

administration. As a result, efforts were mounted to develop drugs that did not have the adverse effects of aspirin. This led to the discovery of other NSAIDs, which in general are associated with a lower incidence of and less serious adverse effects and are often better tolerated than aspirin in patients with chronic diseases. If aspirin were to be a newly discovered drug today, it would most likely require a prescription.

As a single class, NSAIDs constitute an exceptional variety of drugs, and they are used for an equally wide range of indications. Box 44-1 categorizes these drugs into a number of distinct chemical classes. The NSAIDs have been approved for a variety of indications and are considered the drug of choice for most of the conditions listed in Box 44-2. Almost all NSAIDs are used for the treatment of rheumatoid arthritis (see Chapter 47) and degenerative joint disease (osteoarthritis). Several of these drugs are available in sustained-release formulations. This allows once- or twice-daily dosing, which is known to improve patients' adherence to prescribed drug therapy regimens.

Mechanism of Action and Drug Effects

The NSAIDs work through inhibition of the leukotriene pathway, the prostaglandin pathway, or both. More specifically, NSAIDs relieve pain, headache, and inflammation by blocking the chemical activity of the enzyme called *cyclooxygenase (COX)*. It is now recognized that there are at least two types of cyclooxygenase. Cyclooxygenase-1 (COX-1) promotes the synthesis of prostaglandins, which have primarily beneficial effects on various bodily functions. One example is their role in maintaining an intact gastrointestinal mucosa. In contrast, cyclooxygenase-2 (COX-2) promotes the synthesis of prostaglandins that are involved in inflammatory processes. In 1998, the newest class of NSAIDs, the COX-2 inhibitors, was approved. These drugs work by specifically inhibiting the COX-2 form of cyclooxygenase and theoretically have limited or no effects on COX-1. Previous NSAIDs nonspecifically inhibited both COX-1 and COX-2 activity. This greater enzyme specificity of the COX-2 inhibitors allows for the beneficial antiinflammatory effects while reducing the prevalence of adverse effects associated with the nonspecific NSAIDs, such as gastrointestinal ulceration. The leukotriene pathway is inhibited by some antiinflammatory drugs, but not by salicylates.

All NSAIDs can be ulcerogenic and induce gastrointestinal bleeding due to their activity against tissue COX-1. One notable effect of aspirin is its inhibition of platelet aggregation, also known as its *antiplatelet activity*. Aspirin has the unique property among NSAIDs of being an irreversible inhibitor of COX-1 receptors within the platelets themselves. This in turn results in reduced formation of thromboxane A_2, a substance that normally promotes platelet aggregation. This antiplatelet action has made aspirin a primary drug in the treatment of acute myocardial infarction and many other thromboembolic disorders. Other NSAIDs lack these antiplatelet effects.

Indications

Some of the therapeutic uses of this broad class of drugs are listed in Table 44-1; however, NSAIDs are primarily used for their analgesic, antiinflammatory, and antipyretic effects, and for platelet inhibition. NSAIDs are also widely used for the treatment of rheumatoid arthritis (see Chapter 47) and osteoarthritis, as well as other inflammatory conditions, rheumatic fever, mild to moderate pain, and acute gout. They also have proved beneficial as adjunctive pain relief medications in patients with chronic pain syndromes, such as pain from bone cancer and chronic back pain. For pain relief, NSAIDs are sometimes combined with an opioid (see Chapter 10). They tend to have an opioid-sparing effect when given together with opioids, because the drugs attack pain using two different mechanisms. This often allows less opioids to be used. Unlike opioids, NSAIDs show a ceiling effect that limits their effectiveness; that is, any further increase in the dosage beyond a certain level increases the risk for adverse effects without a corresponding increase in the therapeutic effect. In contrast, opioid dosages may be titrated almost indefinitely to increasingly higher levels, especially in terminally ill patients with severe pain.

The appropriate selection of an NSAID is a clinical judgment based on consideration of the patient's history, including any previous medical conditions; the intended use of the drug; the patient's previous experience with NSAIDs; the patient's preference; and the cost.

Contraindications

Contraindications to NSAIDs include known drug allergy and conditions that place the patient at risk for bleeding, including vitamin K deficiency and peptic ulcer disease. Patients with documented aspirin allergy must not receive NSAIDs. NSAIDs are generally categorized as pregnancy category C drugs for use during the first two trimesters of pregnancy but are categorized as pregnancy category D (not recommended) for use during the third trimester. This is because NSAID use has been associated with both excessive maternal bleeding and neonatal toxicity during the perinatal period. These drugs also are not recommended for nursing mothers, because they are known to be excreted into human milk. Because of the potential of NSAIDs to increase bleeding, patients undergoing elective surgery need to stop taking NSAIDs at least 1 week prior to surgery.

Adverse Effects

Although NSAIDs are the most widely used class of drugs, and some are available without prescription, their potential for serious adverse events has been underemphasized. Over 100,000 hospitalizations occur each year due to NSAID use, with over 16,000 deaths reported annually. One of the more common and potentially serious adverse effects of the NSAIDs is their effect on the gastrointestinal tract. Symptoms can range from mild symptoms such as heartburn to the most severe gastrointestinal complication, gastrointestinal bleeding. Most fatalities associated with NSAID use are related to gastrointestinal bleeding. In addition, acute renal failure is quite common with NSAID use, especially if the patient is dehydrated. The potential adverse effects of NSAIDs are listed in Table 44-2. Not all of the adverse effects necessarily apply to all drugs, but many do. In 2006, the U.S. Food and Drug Administration (FDA) began requiring a black box warning on all of the NSAIDs (Box 44-3). In 2015, the FDA strengthened the warning of increased chance of heart attack or stroke. Prescription NSAID labels will be revised to reflect the following information: The risk of heart attack or

TABLE 44-2 NSAIDs: Adverse Effects

Body System	Adverse Effects
Cardiovascular	Noncardiogenic pulmonary edema, increased risk for MI and stroke
Gastrointestinal	Dyspepsia, heartburn, epigastric distress, nausea, vomiting, anorexia, abdominal pain, gastrointestinal bleeding, mucosal lesions (erosions or ulcerations)
Hematologic	Altered hemostasis through effects on platelet function
Hepatic	Acute reversible hepatotoxicity
Renal	Reduction in creatinine clearance, acute tubular necrosis with renal failure
Other	Skin eruption, sensitivity reactions, tinnitus, hearing loss

MI, Myocardial infarction.

BOX 44-3 FDA-Required Warnings on All NSAIDs

The following black box warning must now be included in the packaging for all NSAIDs:

Cardiovascular Risk
- NSAIDs may cause an increased risk for serious cardiovascular thrombotic events, myocardial infarction, and stroke, which can be fatal. Patients with cardiovascular disease or risk factors for cardiovascular disease may be at greater risk. The risk of heart attack or stroke can occur as early as the first weeks of using an NSAID. The risk may increase with longer use of the NSAID and with higher doses.
- NSAIDs are contraindicated for the treatment of perioperative pain in the setting of coronary artery bypass graft surgery.

Gastrointestinal Risk
- NSAIDs cause an increased risk for serious gastrointestinal adverse events, including bleeding, ulceration, and perforation of the stomach or intestines, which can be fatal. These events can occur at any time during use and without warning symptoms. Older adult patients are at greater risk for serious gastrointestinal events.
- See Chapter 4 for more information on black box warnings.

FDA, U.S. Food and Drug Administration.

stroke can occur as early as the first weeks. The risk increases with longer use and a higher dose. Patients treated with NSAIDs following a first heart attack are more likely to die in the first year compared with patients who were not treated with an NSAID. There is also an increased risk of heart failure with NSAID use. The most up-to-date information from the FDA can be found at *www.fda.gov/MedWatch*.

Many of the adverse effects of NSAIDs are secondary to their inactivation of protective prostaglandins that help maintain the normal integrity of the stomach lining. The drug misoprostol (Cytotec) (see Chapter 50) has proved successful in preventing gastric ulcers and GI bleeding when given in conjunction with an NSAID. Misoprostol is a synthetic prostaglandin E_1 analogue that inhibits gastric acid secretion and also has a cytoprotective component. This drug also has abortifacient properties, which were discussed in Chapter 34.

TABLE 44-3 Acute or Chronic Salicylate Intoxication: Signs and Symptoms

Body System	Signs and Symptoms
Cardiovascular	Increased heart rate
Central nervous	Tinnitus, hearing loss, dimness of vision, headache, dizziness, mental confusion, lassitude, drowsiness
Gastrointestinal	Nausea, vomiting, diarrhea
Metabolic	Sweating, thirst, hyperventilation, hypoglycemia or hyperglycemia

TABLE 44-4 Acute Salicylate Intoxication: Treatment

Severity	Treatment
Mild	1. Dosage reduction or discontinuation of salicylates
	2. Symptomatic and supportive therapy
Severe	1. Discontinuation of salicylates
	2. Intensive symptomatic and supportive therapy
	3. Dialysis if: high salicylate levels, unresponsive acidosis (pH less than 7.1), impaired renal function or renal failure, pulmonary edema, persistent CNS symptoms (e.g., seizures, coma), progressive deterioration despite appropriate therapy

CNS, Central nervous system.

Renal function depends partly on prostaglandins. Disruption of prostaglandin function by NSAIDs is sometimes strong enough to precipitate acute or chronic renal failure, depending on the patient's current level of renal function. The use of NSAIDs can compromise existing renal function. Renal toxicity can occur in patients who are dehydrated, those with heart failure or liver dysfunction, and those taking diuretics or angiotensin-converting enzyme inhibitors.

All NSAIDS (except aspirin) share a black box warning regarding an increased risk for adverse cardiovascular thrombotic events, including fatal MI and stroke. NSAIDS may counteract the cardioprotective effects of aspirin.

Toxicity and Management of Overdose

Salicylate toxicity, usually from aspirin, is not as common as it once was. Chronic and acute manifestations of salicylate toxicity can occur. Chronic salicylate intoxication is also known as salicylism and results from either short-term administration of high dosages or prolonged therapy with high or even lower dosages. The common signs and symptoms of acute or chronic salicylate intoxication are listed in Table 44-3.

The most common manifestations of chronic salicylate intoxication in adults are tinnitus and hearing loss. Those in children are hyperventilation and central nervous system (CNS) effects such as dizziness, drowsiness, and behavioral changes. Metabolic complications such as metabolic acidosis and respiratory alkalosis often occur to varying degrees in cases of chronic salicylate intoxication. Metabolic acidosis can also occur with acute intoxication, but it is usually less severe than that in patients with chronic intoxication. Hypoglycemia may also arise and can be life-threatening. The treatment of chronic intoxication is based on the presenting symptoms.

The signs and symptoms of acute salicylate toxicity are similar to those of chronic intoxication, but the effects are often more pronounced and occur more quickly. Acute salicylate overdose usually results from the ingestion of a single toxic dose, and its severity can be judged based on the estimated amount ingested (in milligrams per kilogram of body weight), as follows:

- Little or no toxicity: less than 150 mg/kg
- Mild to moderate toxicity: 150 to 300 mg/kg
- Severe toxicity: 300 to 500 mg/kg
- Life-threatening toxicity: over 500 mg/kg

However, doses lower than 150 mg/kg have resulted in fatal toxicity. A serum salicylate concentration measured 6 hours or longer after ingestion may be used in conjunction with the **Done nomogram** to estimate the severity of intoxication and help guide treatment. The Done nomogram is a graphic plot of serum salicylate level as a function of time since salicylate ingestion. It was first published in a 1960 issue of the journal *Pediatrics* and is still used today for gauging salicylate toxicity. This nomogram is intended for estimating only the severity of acute intoxications and not the severity of chronic salicylate intoxication. Table 44-4 describes, in general terms, the treatment for cases of varying severity. Treatment goals include removing salicylate from the gastrointestinal tract and/or preventing its further absorption; correcting fluid, electrolyte, and acid-base disturbances; and implementing measures to enhance salicylate elimination, including hemodialysis.

An acute overdose of nonsalicylate NSAIDs (e.g., ibuprofen) causes effects similar to those of salicylate overdose, but they are generally not as extensive or as dangerous. Symptoms include CNS toxicities such as drowsiness, lethargy, mental confusion, paresthesias (abnormal touch sensations), numbness, aggressive behavior, disorientation, and seizures, and gastrointestinal toxicities such as nausea, vomiting, and gastrointestinal bleeding. Intense headache, dizziness, cerebral edema, cardiac arrest, and death have also been known to occur in extreme cases. Treatment consists of the administration of activated charcoal, with supportive and symptomatic treatment initiated thereafter. Unlike in the case of salicylates, hemodialysis appears to be of no value in enhancing the elimination of nonsalicylate NSAIDs because of their high protein binding.

Interactions

Drug interactions associated with the use of salicylates and other NSAIDs can result in significant complications and morbidity. Some of the more common of these are listed in Table 44-5.

NSAIDs can also interfere with laboratory test results. Specifically, salicylates can cause what are usually minor and transient elevations in the levels of liver enzymes (ALT, AST), but, unlike with acetaminophen (see Chapter 10), cases of severe hepatotoxicity are rare. Hematocrit, hemoglobin level, and RBC count can drop if any drug-induced gastrointestinal bleeding does occur, and bleeding time may be prolonged. NSAID-induced hyperkalemia or hyponatremia can also occur.

TABLE 44-5 Salicylates and Other NSAIDs: Drug Interactions

Interacting Drug	Mechanism	Result
Alcohol	Additive effect	Increased GI bleeding
Anticoagulants	Platelet inhibition, hypoprothrombinemia	Increased bleeding tendencies
Aspirin and other salicylates with other NSAIDs	Reduction of NSAID absorption, additive gastrointestinal toxicities	Increased GI toxicity with no therapeutic advantage
Bisphosphonates	Additive GI toxicities	Increased GI bleeding risk
Corticosteroids and other ulcerogenic drugs	Additive toxicities	Increased ulcerogenic effects
cyclosporine	Inhibition of renal prostaglandin synthesis	Increased nephrotoxic effects of cyclosporine, renal failure
Diuretics and ACE inhibitors	Inhibition of prostaglandin synthesis	Reduced hypotensive and diuretic effects
lithium	Increased lithium absorption	Increased lithium concentrations
Protein-bound drugs	Competition for binding	More pronounced drug actions
Uricosurics	Antagonism	Decreased uric acid excretion
Herbals: feverfew, garlic, ginger, gingko	Interference with platelet function	Increased bleeding risk

ACE, Angiotensin-converting enzyme.

DOSAGES

Most Commonly Used NSAIDs

Drug (Pregnancy Category*)	Pharmacologic Class	Usual Adult Dosage Range	Indications
♦ aspirin (ASA; many product names) (C/D)	Salicylate	PO/PR: 325-650 mg 4-6 times daily (max 4 g/day)	Fever, pain
		PO/PR: 3 g/day divided every 4-6 hr	Arthritis
		PO: 81-325 mg once daily	Thromboprevention
		PO: 325 mg or PR 300 mg at first sign of myocardial infarction	Myocardial infarction
♦ celecoxib (Celebrex) (C/D)	COX-2 inhibitor	PO: 100-200 mg daily or bid	Arthritis, acute pain, primary dysmenorrhea
♦ ibuprofen (Motrin, Advil, others) (C/D)	Propionic acid derivative	1200-3200 mg/day divided 3-4 times daily	Arthritis, fever, pain, dysmenorrhea
♦ indomethacin (Indocin, Indocin SR) (C/D)	Acetic acid derivative	PO/PR: 25-50 mg 2-3 times daily (max 200 mg/day)	Arthritis, including acute gouty arthritis, bursitis, or tendonitis
♦ ketorolac (Toradol) (C/D)	Acetic acid derivative	†PO: 10 mg every 4-6 hr (max 40 mg/day) IV/IM: 15-30 mg every 6-12 hr (max 120 mg/day if younger than 65 yr; max 60 mg/day if 65 yr or older); max combined PO and IV treatment 5 days	Acute painful conditions that would otherwise require opioid-level analgesia

ASA, Acetylsalicylic acid; *COX,* cyclooxygenase.
*Pregnancy category C/D = *C,* first trimester; *D,* third trimester.
†PO form is recommended only when transitioning from injectable form to oral form of ketorolac.

Dosages

For dosage information on selected NSAIDs, see the table on this page.

DRUG PROFILES

SALICYLATES

Aspirin is the most commonly used of all salicylates. Although aspirin is available over the counter, many of the other salicylate drugs do require a prescription. These include diflunisal (Dolobid), choline magnesium trisalicylate (Trilisate), and salsalate (Salsitab). Salicylates are most commonly used in solid oral dosage forms (i.e., tablets, capsules). Other available dosage forms include a topical cream (Aspercreme), rectal suppositories, and oral liquids. Aspirin is also contained in many combination products, including aspirin/acetaminophen/caffeine combinations (e.g., Excedrin) and aspirin/antacid combinations (e.g., Bufferin). Aspirin also is available in special dosage forms, such as enteric-coated aspirin (e.g., Ecotrin), which are designed to protect the stomach mucosa by dissolving in the duodenum.

♦ aspirin

Aspirin is known chemically as acetylsalicylic acid (ASA). It is the prototype salicylate and NSAID and is the most widely used drug in the world. A daily aspirin tablet (81 mg or 325 mg) is now routinely recommended as prophylactic therapy for adults who have strong risk factors for developing coronary artery disease or stroke. It is also effective after a myocardial infarction. The 81-mg strength (which is traditionally thought of as baby or children's aspirin) and the 325-mg strength appear to be equally beneficial for the prevention of thrombotic events. For this reason, the lower strength is often chosen for patients who have any elevated risk for bleeding, such as those with previous stroke history or history of peptic ulcer disease and those taking the anticoagulant warfarin (Coumadin). Aspirin is also often used to treat the pain associated with headache, neuralgia, myalgia, and arthralgia, as well as other pain syndromes resulting from inflammation. These include arthritis, pleurisy, and pericarditis. Patients with systemic lupus erythematosus may also benefit from aspirin therapy because of its antirheumatic effects. Aspirin is also used for its antipyretic action.

Aspirin and other salicylates all have one very specific contraindication. This drug class is contraindicated in children with flulike symptoms, because the use of these drugs has been strongly associated with Reye's syndrome. This is an acute and potentially life-threatening condition involving progressive neurologic deficits that can lead to coma and may also involve liver damage. It is believed to be triggered by viral illnesses such as influenza as well as by salicylate therapy itself, in the presence of a viral illness. Survivors of this condition may or may not suffer permanent neurologic damage. See the Patient-Centered Care: Lifespan Considerations for the Pediatric Patient Box on p. 700.

Pharmacokinetics: Aspirin

Route	Onset of Action	Peak Plasma Concentration	Elimination Half-life	Duration of Action
PO	15-30 min	1-2 hr	5-9 hr	4-6 hr

ACETIC ACID DERIVATIVES

There are several acetic acid derivatives, and they are listed in Table 44-1. Indomethacin and ketorolac are the most commonly used.

◆ indomethacin

Like the other NSAIDs, indomethacin (Indocin) has analgesic, antiinflammatory, antirheumatic, and antipyretic properties. Its therapeutic actions are of particular use in the treatment of rheumatoid arthritis, osteoarthritis, acute bursitis or tendonitis, ankylosing spondylitis, and acute gouty arthritis. The drug is available for both oral and rectal use. An injectable form of the drug is also used intravenously (IV) to promote closure of patent ductus arteriosus, a heart defect that sometimes occurs in premature infants. It is also used for the treatment of preterm labor (see Chapter 34).

Pharmacokinetics: Indomethacin

Route	Onset of Action	Peak Plasma Concentration	Elimination Half-life	Duration of Action
PO	30 min	2 hr	4.5 hr	4-6 hr

◆ ketorolac

Ketorolac (Toradol) is somewhat unique in that, although it does have some antiinflammatory activity, it is used primarily for its powerful analgesic effects. Its analgesic effects are comparable to those of narcotic drugs such as morphine, which can make it a desirable choice for opiate-addicted patients who have acute pain-control needs, because ketorolac lacks the addictive properties of the opioids. Ketorolac is indicated for the treatment of moderate to severe acute pain such as that resulting from orthopedic injuries or surgery. Ketorolac can be given orally or by injection, and there is also a dosage form for ophthalmic use (see Chapter 57). It is available only by prescription. It is indicated for short-term use (up to 5 days) to manage moderate to severe acute pain. It is not indicated for treatment of minor pain or chronic pain. The main adverse effects of ketorolac include renal impairment, edema, gastrointestinal pain, dyspepsia, and nausea. It is important to note that the drug can only be used for 5 days, because of its potential adverse effects on the kidney and gastrointestinal tract.

Pharmacokinetics: Ketorolac

Route	Onset of Action	Peak Plasma Concentration	Elimination Half-life	Duration of Action
IM	30-60 min	2-3 hr	2-6 hr	6-8 hr

PROPIONIC ACID DERIVATIVES

◆ ibuprofen

Ibuprofen (Motrin, Advil) is the prototype NSAID in the propionic acid category, which also includes fenoprofen, flurbiprofen, ketoprofen, naproxen, and oxaprozin. Ibuprofen is the most commonly used of the propionic acid drugs because of the numerous indications for its use and because of its relatively safe adverse-effect profile. It is often used for its analgesic effects in the management of rheumatoid arthritis, osteoarthritis, primary dysmenorrhea, gout, dental pain, and musculoskeletal disorders; in addition, it is used for its antipyretic actions. Naproxen is the second most commonly used NSAID, with a reportedly somewhat better adverse-effect profile than ibuprofen, as well as fewer drug interactions with angiotensin-converting enzyme inhibitors given for hypertension. Both drugs are available for oral use in both over-the-counter and prescription strengths. In 2011, an injectable form of ibuprofen became available.

Pharmacokinetics: Ibuprofen

Route	Onset of Action	Peak Plasma Concentration	Elimination Half-life	Duration of Action
PO	30-60 min (analgesic) 7 days (antiinflammatory)	1-2 hr	2-4 hr	4-6 hr

CYCLOOXYGENASE-2 INHIBITORS

The COX-2 inhibitors were developed primarily to decrease the gastrointestinal adverse effects characteristic of other NSAIDs because of their COX-2 selectivity. However, they are not totally devoid of gastrointestinal toxicity. Gastritis and upper gastrointestinal bleeding have been reported with their use, although much less frequently than with the older NSAIDs. Originally there were three COX-2 inhibitors; however, because the use of rofecoxib (Vioxx) and valdecoxib (Bextra) was found to be associated with an increased risk for adverse cardiovascular events, including myocardial infarction, stroke, and death, they were removed from the U.S. market.

◆ celecoxib

Celecoxib (Celebrex) was the first COX-2 inhibitor and is the only one remaining on the market. It is indicated for the treatment of osteoarthritis, rheumatoid arthritis, acute pain symptoms, ankylosing spondylitis, and primary dysmenorrhea. It is available only for oral use. There is evidence that celecoxib may pose a risk for cardiovascular events similar to that associated with rofecoxib and valdecoxib. However, there is inconsistency in the literature regarding the true potential for these effects. Celecoxib currently remains on the U.S. market, although its use is now being monitored more closely by the FDA. Other adverse effects associated with celecoxib include headache, sinus irritation, diarrhea, fatigue, dizziness, lower extremity edema, and hypertension. COX-2 inhibitors have little effect on platelet function. Celecoxib and sulfa antibiotics share a similar structure; therefore, celecoxib should not be used in patients with known sulfa allergy.

Pharmacokinetics: Celecoxib

Route	Onset of Action	Peak Plasma Concentration	Elimination Half-life	Duration of Action
PO	1 hr	3 hr	11 hr	4-8 hr

ENOLIC ACID DERIVATIVES

The enolic acid derivatives include piroxicam, meloxicam, and nabumetone. Piroxicam and meloxicam are very potent drugs that are commonly used in the treatment of mild to moderate osteoarthritis, rheumatoid arthritis, and gouty arthritis. Both are available only in oral dosage formulations and have contraindications similar to those of the other NSAIDs.

Nabumetone (Relafen) is better tolerated than some of the others in terms of gastrointestinal adverse effects. It is relatively nonacidic compared with most of the other NSAIDs, which may account for its improved gastrointestinal tolerance. Currently it is indicated only for the treatment of osteoarthritis and rheumatoid arthritis.

ANTIGOUT DRUGS

Gout is caused by the overproduction of uric acid or decreased uric acid excretion, or both. This overproduction and/or decreased excretion can often result in hyperuricemia (too much uric acid in the blood). Persons with gout either overproduce or underexcrete uric acid. When the body contains too much uric acid, deposits of uric acid crystals collect in tissues and joints. This causes an inflammatory response and extreme pain, because these crystals are like small needles that jab and stick into sensitive tissues and joints, which is an end product of purine metabolism. Purines are part of the normal dietary intake and are used to make the essential structural units of deoxyribonucleic acid (DNA) and ribonucleic acid (RNA). During purine metabolism, they are converted from hypoxanthine to xanthine and eventually to uric acid. The normal pathway for purine metabolism is depicted in Figure 44-2. This pathway is overactive in patients with gout and is reduced by antigout drug therapy. The goals of gout treatment are to decrease the symptoms of an acute attack and to prevent recurrent attacks.

DRUG PROFILES

Although specific antigout drugs are available, the NSAIDs (described earlier) are considered first-line therapy for most patients with gout. The specific antigout drugs—allopurinol, febuxostat, colchicine, probenecid, and sulfinpyrazone—are targeted at the underlying defect in uric acid metabolism, which causes either overproduction or underexcretion of uric acid (see Figure 44-2). Both of these pathologic processes lead to tissue accumulations of uric acid crystalline deposits (gouty deposits) and symptoms of gout. Not all gouty deposits occur within joints. Gouty arthritis is the condition in which one or more joints are inflamed due to the collection of gouty deposits inside the joint anatomy. This is also called *articular gout*, whereas gout that occurs in tissues outside of the joints is called *abarticular gout*.

◆ allopurinol

The beneficial effect of allopurinol (Zyloprim) in the relief of gout is the inhibition of the enzyme xanthine oxidase, which thereby prevents uric acid production. Allopurinol is indicated for patients whose gout is caused by the excess production of uric acid (hyperuricemia). Oxypurinol, a

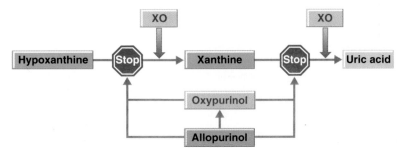

FIGURE 44-2 Uric acid production. *XO,* Xanthine oxidase.

metabolite of allopurinol, also prevents uric acid production. Oxypurinol is available as an orphan drug for patients with hyperuricemia who are intolerant of allopurinol therapy. Allopurinol is also used to prevent acute tumor lysis syndrome (see Chapter 45).

Allopurinol is contraindicated in patients with a known hypersensitivity to it. Significant adverse effects of the drug include agranulocytosis, aplastic anemia, and serious and potentially fatal skin conditions such as exfoliative dermatitis, Stevens-Johnson syndrome, and toxic epidermal necrolysis. Azathioprine and mercaptopurine both significantly interact with allopurinol, and, as a result, their dosages may have to be adjusted. Allopurinol is available only for oral use. The usual recommended adult dosage is 200 to 600 mg/day, and the maximum dosage is 800 mg/day. It is categorized as a pregnancy category C drug.

The new drug febuxostat (Uloric) is non-purine selective inhibitor of xanthine oxidase. It is the first new drug approved for the treatment of gout since the 1960s. It is more selective for xanthine oxidase than allopurinol. Clinical trials suggest that it may pose a greater risk for cardiovascular events than allopurinol, although the mechanism is still being debated. It is not to be given along with theophylline, azathioprine, or mercaptopurine. It is dosed as 40 to 80 mg/day, with a maximum dose of 120 mg/day.

Pharmacokinetics: Allopurinol

Route	Onset of Action	Peak Plasma Concentration	Elimination Half-life	Duration of Action
PO	1-2 wk	30-120 min	18-30 hr	Unknown

QSEN PATIENT-CENTERED CARE: LIFESPAN CONSIDERATIONS FOR THE PEDIATRIC PATIENT

Reye's Syndrome

Reye's syndrome is associated with the administration of aspirin to children and teenagers and is a potentially life-threatening illness. Reye's syndrome is most often seen in children 4 to 12 years of age. Most cases that occur with the chickenpox are in children 5 to 9 years of age. Cases of Reye's syndrome that occur with the flu are usually in those 10 to 14 years of age. Encephalopathy and liver damage are two of the serious complications resulting from Reye's syndrome, which usually occurs after a viral infection such as chickenpox or influenza B, during which time aspirin is often given to decrease fever. To reduce the risk for Reye's syndrome, aspirin or medications that contain aspirin must not be given to children or teenagers to treat viral illnesses or fever. Other names for aspirin include *acetylsalicylic acid, acetylsalicylate, salicylic acid,* and *salicylate*. Other drugs that can be used instead of aspirin to reduce fever and relieve pain include acetaminophen and ibuprofen. Avoid aspirin for several weeks after a child/teenager has received a varicella vaccine. Check the label on any medication that is to be given to a child, because aspirin is contained in many over-the-counter drugs, for example, Alka-Seltzer, some Excedrin products, and Pepto-Bismol. Substances with oil of wintergreen may also contain salicylates.

Signs and Symptoms of Reye's Syndrome
- Altered liver function
- Encephalopathy and fatty degeneration of the viscera, primarily in children and teenagers
- Changes in level of consciousness
- Coma, flaccid paralysis, loss of deep tendon reflexes
- Hypoglycemia
- Seizures
- Vomiting

Suspect Reye's syndrome in an infant with diarrhea; respiratory disturbances such as hyperventilation with apneic episodes; seizures; hypoglycemia; or elevated liver enzymes, such as ALT or AST in the absence of jaundice. Elevation of these liver enzymes is a fairly reliable indication of liver status, with ALT being more specific. Also, suspect Reye's syndrome in a patient presenting with unexpected vomiting after any viral illness, such as a flulike upper respiratory infection or chickenpox, or signs of disturbed brain function characterized by lethargy, stupor, agitated delirium, coma, screaming, and rigidity.

Medical Management
- Provide supportive treatment in intensive care unit
- Maintain life functions, restore metabolic balance, and control cerebral edema; maintain oxygen to brain and other vital organs
- Administer intravenous glucose (10% or higher) for treatment of hypoglycemia
- Monitor blood glucose level; insulin may be needed
- Administer vitamin K for clotting problems
- Give fresh frozen plasma if needed for significant bleeding
- Provide prophylactic antiepileptic drugs
- Monitor intracranial pressure
- Initiate cautious fluid administration
- Administer osmotic diuretics with steroids if needed to treat cerebral edema

Nursing Management
- Critical care setting is often indicated for care of these patients
- Assess neurologic status, vital signs, and arterial and central venous pressures
- Monitor blood gas concentrations and intracranial pressure as ordered
- Control temperature to prevent elevations and increased O_2 demands
- Elevate the head of the bed
- Monitor intake and output
- Initiate hyperventilation (if patient is intubated and if ordered) to reduce intracranial pressure by lowering CO_2 levels and increasing O_2 levels
- Provide a quiet environment
- Handle gently
- Monitor for seizure activity
- Provide family support during critical phase of the illness
- Provide physical and emotional support for the child and family with recovery
- Ensure appropriate spiritual care
- Educate the public about Reye's syndrome and its life-threatening complications

Data from Mayo Foundation for Medical Education and Research: Reye's syndrome, September 17, 2011. Available at *www.mayoclinic.com/health/reyes-syndrome*. Updated August 12, 2014. Accessed May 15, 2015.

colchicine

Colchicine is the oldest available therapy for acute gout and is considered second-line therapy, after the NSAIDs. Colchicine appears to be effective in the treatment of gout by reducing the inflammatory response to the deposits of urate crystals in joint tissue. Its mechanism of action is not clearly defined, but it is thought to inhibit the metabolism, mobility, and *chemotaxis* of polymorphonuclear leukocytes. Chemotaxis is the chemical attraction of leukocytes to the site of inflammation, which worsens an inflammatory response.

Colchicine is a powerful inhibitor of cell mitosis and can cause short-term leukopenia. For this reason, it is generally used for the short-term treatment of acute attacks of gout. However, it may be used for prophylaxis of acute attacks in dosages of 0.6 mg once or twice a day. More severe adverse effects include bleeding into the gastrointestinal or urinary tracts, and the drug needs to be stopped if such effects appear. Colchicine is contraindicated in patients with a known hypersensitivity to it and in those with severe renal, gastrointestinal, hepatic, or cardiac disorders, and blood dyscrasias. There is no specific antidote for colchicine poisoning. The drug is available in oral forms only. Until 2008, it was also available in an injectable form, but at that time the FDA asked that it no longer be manufactured in or shipped to the United States, because of the potential for life-threatening adverse effects. In 2010, the FDA required the withdrawal of all "unapproved" colchicine products that had been used for decades. Currently, there are two FDA-approved colchicine products, Colcrys and Mitigare.

For acute gout, colchicine is given in an initial dose of 0.6 to 1.2 mg, followed by 0.6 mg/hr until pain is relieved, the patient develops severe nausea and diarrhea, or a total of 6 mg has been administered. Some practitioners choose to limit the cumulative dose to 3 mg. When colchicine is used for treatment of acute gout, 3 days must pass before a second course of therapy is initiated. Colchicine dosage must be reduced with renal impairment. It is categorized as a pregnancy category D drug.

Pharmacokinetics: Colchicine

Route	Onset of Action	Peak Plasma Concentration	Elimination Half-life	Duration of Action
PO	12 hr	0.5-2 hr	12-30 min	12 hr

probenecid

Probenecid (generic) inhibits the reabsorption of uric acid in the kidney and thus increases the excretion of uric acid. Drugs that promote uric acid excretion are known as *uricosurics*. In some patients, gout is due to the underexcretion of uric acid. Probenecid works by binding to the special transporter protein in the proximal convoluted renal tubule that takes uric acid from the urine and places it back into the blood. The probenecid is then reabsorbed back into the bloodstream while the uric acid remains in the urine and is excreted. Besides being used to treat the hyperuricemia associated with gout and gouty arthritis, it also has the ability to delay the renal excretion of penicillin, which increases the serum levels of penicillin and prolongs its effect (see Chapter 38). Probenecid is available as a 500-mg

oral tablet. The usual adult dosage is 250 mg twice a day with food, milk, or antacids for 1 week, followed by 500 mg twice daily thereafter. This dosage may be adjusted as needed to maintain desirable serum uric acid levels. Contraindications include peptic ulcer disease and blood dyscrasias. Probenecid is ineffective and is not to be used in patients with renal impairment. It is categorized as a pregnancy category B drug.

Pharmacokinetics: Probenecid

Route	Onset of Action	Peak Plasma Concentration	Elimination Half-life	Duration of Action
PO	1 hr	3 hr	3-17 hr	8 hr

NURSING PROCESS

ASSESSMENT

Prior to giving an *antiinflammatory, antigout,* and/or related drugs, it is critical for patient safety and drug effectiveness to assess drug allergies, contraindications, cautions, and drug interactions associated with each drug in these major groups. Before administering antiinflammatory drugs, perform a thorough head-to-toe physical assessment, measure vital signs, perform a nursing assessment, and take a thorough medication history, noting any prescription, over-the-counter, herbal, and/or alternative drugs that the patient is taking. Analyze results of laboratory tests reflecting hematologic, renal, and hepatic functioning before initiation of therapy as ordered, especially if long-term use is indicated. These tests will most likely include RBC count, hemoglobin level, hematocrit, WBC count, platelet count, BUN level, and liver enzyme levels such as ALP, AST, and LDH. If NSAIDs are used short-term for other conditions (e.g., fever, acute pain), laboratory studies are not usually indicated since these drugs are available over the counter and often self-administered.

With *aspirin, NSAIDs,* other *antiinflammatory* drugs, and *antigout* drugs, assess and document the duration, onset, location, and type of inflammation and/or pain the patient is experiencing as well as any precipitating, exacerbating, or relieving factors. Note any interference of the symptoms with the patient's ability to perform activities of daily living (ADLs). Inspect all joints with attention to deformities, immobility or limitations in mobility, overlying skin condition, and presence of any heat or swelling over the joint. Age is a critical factor to assess because aspirin and many other NSAIDs (because they contain aspirin, also known as *salicylate*) are not to be used in children and teenagers due to the increased risk for Reye's syndrome (see Patient-Centered Care: Lifespan Considerations for the Pediatric Patient on the previous page). These drugs are to be used very cautiously in the older adult patient. Assessing the odor of *aspirin* is also important because a vinegary odor is associated with chemical breakdown of the drug. With aspirin, assess the patient for a history of asthma, wheezing, or other respiratory problems because of the increased incidence of allergic reactions to aspirin in these individuals. With aspirin, identify patients who have been diagnosed with what is called the aspirin triad, which includes asthma, nasal polyps, and rhinitis. These conditions are considered to put the patient at risk for reactions to *aspirin*. Other contraindications, cautions, and drug interactions for aspirin and other *NSAIDs* have been discussed previously. However, in 2015, the FDA strengthened the warning of increased chance of heart attack or stroke when taking NSAIDs (see pharmacology discussion about adverse effects of NSAIDs). Remember that salicylic acid or aspirin and other NSAIDs have antiinflammatory, antipyretic, analgesic, and antiplatelet activity but also carry a risk for ulcerogenic and gastrointestinal bleeding adverse effects. NSAIDs carry the risk for acute reversible hepatotoxicity, renal failure, hearing loss, and noncardiogenic pulmonary edema, so a review of the patient's history of preexisting medical conditions is important.

QSEN 🍃 **SAFETY: HERBAL THERAPIES AND DIETARY SUPPLEMENTS**

Glucosamine and Chondroitin

Overview
Glucosamine is chemically derived from glucose. Its chemical name is 2-amino-2-deoxyglucose sulfate.
 Chondroitin is a protein usually isolated from bovine (cow) cartilage. To date, there are no reports of any type of disease transmission from cows to humans with chondroitin.

Common Uses
These two supplements are often used in combination, and sometimes individually, to treat pain from osteoarthritis. Although they are most commonly taken orally, injectable forms are commercially available (e.g., for administration by naturopathic prescribers).

Adverse Effects
Glucosamine: Usually mild adverse effects that are comparable to those of placebo in clinical studies, including gastrointestinal discomfort, drowsiness, headache, and skin reactions.
 Chondroitin: No major ill effects in studies lasting from 2 months to 6 years. Gastrointestinal discomfort is the most common adverse effect but is usually well tolerated.

Potential Drug Interactions
Both supplements: May enhance the anticoagulant effects of warfarin. The patient's international normalized ratio needs to be measured more frequently during glucosamine/chondroitin therapy, and the warfarin dosage adjusted if indicated.
 Glucosamine: May cause an increase in insulin resistance, necessitating the need for higher dosages of oral hypoglycemics or insulin.

Contraindications
Both supplements: No specific contraindications listed, but avoidance during pregnancy is recommended due to lack of firm safety data.

In addition to patient assessment, the use of *ketorolac* requires assessment of the drug order because it is important to be sure the drug has been ordered for a short term (e.g., no more than 5 days) and for patients experiencing moderate to severe acute pain. Assess the patient for underlying signs of infection before the use of any NSAID or other *antiinflammatory drug*, because these drugs may mask symptoms. With use of celecoxib,

document any cardiovascular disorders or symptoms because use of the drug, as with *rofecoxib* and *valdecoxib*, carries a risk for cardiovascular events.

With *antigout* drugs, perform a thorough assessment of hydration status and baseline serum uric acid levels. Closely assess urinary output prior to and during drug therapy to ensure an output of at least 30 to 60 mL/hr or 0.5 mL/kg/hr (the latter parameter accounts for various patient weights). Determine and assess renal function through monitoring of BUN and serum creatinine as well as liver function through monitoring of liver enzymes, AST and ALT. If receiving *febuxostat (Uloric)*, assess the patient for a history of cardiovascular disease due to risk for adverse effects linked to the cardiac system. Additionally, drug interactions may occur with theophylline, azathiaprine, or mercaptopurine. If the patient is taking *allopurinol*, assess the integrity of the skin due to potentially life-threatening skin adverse effects of exfoliative dermatitis, Stevens-Johnson syndrome, and toxic epidermal necrolysis. Assess blood counts because of the potential for aplastic anemia and agranulocytosis. With *colchicine*, conduct a thorough assessment for a history of gastrointestinal distress; ulcers; or cardiac, renal, or liver disease. When assessing the prescriber's order, remember that there is only one colchicine product available, *Colcrys*, because of FDA recall. Also worthy of mentioning for antigout drugs (e.g., *allopurinol, Colcrys, probenecid*) is that these drugs may be used for either their short-term or long-term effects. Therefore, assess the order and indication for the antigout drug to ensure that the patient is receiving the appropriate treatment. Also assess for all contraindications, cautions, and drug interactions (see earlier discussion).

NURSING DIAGNOSES

1. Acute pain related to the disease process or injury to joints and other disease-affected areas
2. Deficient knowledge related to first-time drug therapy for treatment of a disease process
3. Risk for injury related to the effects of the disease and treatment on mobility and the performance of ADLs

PLANNING: OUTCOME IDENTIFICATION

1. Patient remains pain free or near pain free with adequate drug and nondrug therapy during periods of inflammation, injury, or disease process.
2. Patient demonstrates increased knowledge about disease process, lifestyle changes, and required treatment with NSAID or antigout drug therapy.
3. Patient remains free from injury because of knowledge about drug therapy, its indication, safe dosing, adverse effects, and symptoms to report to health care provider.

Implementation

If *aspirin* is used as an *antigout drug*, the oral dosage forms are given with food, milk, or meals. Advise the patient that sustained-release or enteric-coated tablets are not to be crushed

PATIENT-CENTERED CARE: LIFESPAN CONSIDERATIONS FOR THE OLDER ADULT PATIENT

NSAIDs

The Administration on Aging estimates that by 2030 there will be more than 72.1 million Americans older than 65 years of age, which is approximately double what the population was in 2000. Understanding, preventing, monitoring, and managing adverse events in the older adult patient are difficult tasks. The aging process itself and/or the physiologic changes occurring in this age group poses the older individual at an increased risk for experiencing more adverse events. In the 2011 Drug Abuse Warning Network (DAWN) report, it was estimated, in 2008, that 31% of people 65 years of age and older were hospitalized due to an adverse medication event, and some 51.5% of all hospitalizations were in those patients older than 50 years of age and due to these adverse events. NSAIDS have been a mainstay option for chronic pain management for many years, but side effects impact the gastrointestinal, cardiovascular, renal, and hematologic systems. Additionally, NSAIDS interact with many other medications. It is also anticipated that the use of over-the-counter NSAIDs will be widespread and increasing in this population and require special attention and education to prevent and/or minimize adverse effects. Understanding the physiologic changes of the older adult patient will help ensure safe and effective use of these medications:

- The underlying pharmacokinetic characteristics and physical and biologic changes in older adult patients must be understood. Even if older patients have normal kidney and liver function, they have a reduced rate of drug metabolism and drug elimination compared with younger adults.
- Patients 65 years of age and older do not have to be ill for NSAIDs to adversely affect them because of normal age-related physiologic changes. The presence of chronic or multiple illnesses may result in an increased incidence of adverse reactions.
- Some changes noted in older adult patients that effect drug treatment include changes in renal elimination, protein binding, body composition, drug distribution, drug clearance, and sensitivity to drugs, as well as an increased incidence of adverse reactions to all types of medications (see Chapter 3).
- Older patients who are at risk for renal insufficiency because of natural physiologic changes may experience changes in fluid balance as well as changes in drug reabsorption, excretion, and filtration processes. This may lead to drug toxicity.
- Cardiac output decreases by 25% between 25 and 65 years of age, which results in decreased blood flow to the kidneys and, consequently, reduced glomerular filtration rate. There is also an overall decline in circulating blood volume, which may affect overall pharmacokinetics and lead to decreased drug absorption, distribution, metabolism, and excretion.
- Many individuals older than 65 years of age become slow metabolizers of medications, which affects the way NSAIDs are handled by the liver. In addition, the liver decreases in size and weight with advancing age. Liver blood flow is also decreased. These changes affect drug metabolism, resulting in the need to possibly decrease drug dosages and/or monitor very closely for toxicity.
- Gastrointestinal functioning is impacted by aging, with a more acidic content of gastric juice and decreased gastric motility. This may lead to slower emptying of the stomach and result in decreased intestinal absorption and drug absorption. Serum levels of drugs, including NSAIDs, may be higher due to these changes, and the overall drug dosage may need to be decreased. It has also been documented that these individuals may be at increased risk for developing NSAID-related gastrointestinal problems.

In addition to the physiologic changes, the presence of other disease processes in the older adult patient precipitates the use of therapy with other drugs leading to significant issues with interactions. Some of these drug interactions include antiplatelets, anticoagulants, aspirin/salicylates, thombolytics, antineoplastics, radiation, alcohol, tobacco, corticosteroids, oral antidiabetic drugs, furosemide, herbals such as feverfew, garlic, ginger, ginkgo, and ginseng.

Interventions to help decrease NSAID-related adverse reactions include asking questions, listing all drugs, teaching about all medications, and assessing the patient's gastrointestinal, cardiovascular, and neurologic systems, depending on patient complaints.

Findings from: Substance Abuse and Mental Health Services Administration, Center for Behavioral Health Statistics and Quality. The DAWN Report: Emergency department visits involving adverse reactions to medications among older adults. Rockville, Md. Accessed May 15, 2015.

or broken. Monitor serum levels of aspirin if aspirin therapy is used for its antiarthritic effect; however, this indication is very rare. Because of the high risk for adverse effects that may be severe, aspirin is mainly used in lower doses (e.g., 81 mg) for cardioprotective reasons. If used in higher doses, monitor for clinical presentation as well as serum aspirin levels to help distinguish among mild, moderate, and severe toxicity (see pharmacology discussion). If aspirin is used in higher doses, it is important to be aware of signs and symptoms of toxicity such as gastrointestinal bleeding, other bleeding, and abdominal pain. If these occur, report the findings to the prescriber for immediate treatment. If aspirin is used as an antipyretic, the patient's temperature generally begins to decrease within 1 hour. See Patient-Centered Care: Patient Teaching for more information on the safe use of aspirin.

Non-aspirin NSAIDs or other *antiinflammatory drugs* may also come in enteric-coated or sustained-release preparations; stress to the patient that these are not to be crushed or chewed. Oral dosage forms of these drugs, including *ketorolac*, may be taken with antacids or food to decrease gastrointestinal upset or irritation. Instruct the patient to report to the prescriber

immediately any moderate to severe gastrointestinal upset, dyspepsia with nausea, vomiting, abdominal pain, or blood in the stool or vomitus. Advise the patient to avoid other ulcerogenic substances (e.g., alcohol, prednisone, aspirin-containing products, other NSAIDs) to help minimize the risk for gastrointestinal mucosal breakdown. During therapy with NSAIDs, continuously monitor the patient for bowel patterns, stool consistency, and any occurrence of gastrointestinal symptoms and/or dizziness, and document the findings. Monitor, as indicated, laboratory tests during high-dose or long-term treatment, including CBC, BUN levels, platelet counts, and serum bilirubin, AST, and ALT levels. Emphasize safe ambulation with NSAID use as well as with the use of any other antiinflammatory drugs and/or analgesics. With ketorolac, understand that dosing is not to exceed a 5-day period for either the oral, intramuscular, or IV dosage forms. Administer intramuscular injections slowly into a large muscle mass, and administer IV dosage forms over a period of no less than 15 seconds. Educate the patient to take *celecoxib* only as ordered and, as with the other NSAIDs, to avoid alcohol, aspirin, salicylates, and over-the-counter drugs containing any of these. Celecoxib may be taken without regard to meals; however, taking the drug with food and fluids may decrease gastrointestinal upset. Instruct the patient to report immediately to the prescriber any stomach or abdominal pain, gastrointestinal problems, unusual bleeding, blood in the stool or vomitus, chest pain, edema, and/or palpitations.

The *antigout drugs* are somewhat different from the NSAIDs, with different mechanisms of action and also very different nursing considerations. *Colchicine* needs to be taken on an empty stomach for more complete absorption but is best tolerated if given with food. Educate the patient with gout on the importance of increasing fluid intake of up to 3 L/day, unless contraindicated. Advise the patient to avoid alcohol and any over-the-counter cold relief products that contain alcohol while this medication is being taken. In addition, instruct the patient with gout that adherence to the complete medical regimen—both pharmacologic and nonpharmacologic—is critical to successful treatment. If *allopurinol* is prescribed, it is to be given with meals to minimize the occurrence of gastrointestinal symptoms such as nausea, vomiting, and anorexia. If allopurinol is to be administered in conjunction with chemotherapy (in an attempt to decrease hyperuricemia associated with malignancy and cell death from successful treatment), it is recommended that it be given a few days before the antineoplastic therapy. Patients taking allopurinol must also increase fluid intake to 3 L/day if not contraindicated. Patients need to avoid hazardous activities if dizziness or drowsiness occurs with the medication. Alcohol and caffeine must also be avoided because these drugs will increase uric acid levels and decrease the level of allopurinol.

EVALUATION

Aspirin and *NSAIDs* may vary in their potency and antiinflammatory and analgesic effects. Therapeutic responses to NSAIDs include the following: decrease in acute pain; decrease in swelling, pain, stiffness, and tenderness of a joint or muscle area; improved ability to perform ADLs; improved muscle grip and strength; reduction in fever; return to normal laboratory values for CBC and sedimentation rate; and return to a less inflamed state as evidenced by improved sedimentation rates, radiographic examination, computed tomographic scan, or magnetic

resonance imaging. Monitoring for the occurrence of adverse effects and toxicity is essential to the safe and effective use of *antiinflammatory drugs* (e.g., *aspirin, COX-2 inhibitors, other NSAIDs*) and *antigout drugs* (see Box 44-3 and Tables 44-2 and 44-3).

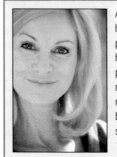
Therapeutic responses to the *antigout* drug colchicine include decreased pain in the affected joints and increased sense of well-being. Monitor the patient closely for any increased pain, blood in the urine, excessive fatigue and lethargy, or chills or fever, and contact the prescriber immediately should these occur. A therapeutic response to *allopurinol*, another antigout drug, includes a decrease in pain in the joints, a decrease in uric acid levels, and a decrease in stone formation in the kidneys.

PATIENT-CENTERED CARE: PATIENT TEACHING

- Instruct the patient that these drugs—if in sustained-release or enteric-coated dosage forms—are not to be crushed or chewed. Instruct the patient to report to the prescriber immediately any ringing in the ears, persistent gastrointestinal or abdominal pain, or easy bruising or bleeding.
- Educate the patient that the full antiinflammatory effect of the drug may not be apparent immediately, depending on the specific drug. For example, onset of full therapeutic antiinflammatory action may take 7 days for ibuprofen or 30 to 60 minutes for its analgesic effects.

- Advise the patient to share a list of all medications with all health care providers/dentists especially if the patient is taking high dosages of aspirin or has been taking aspirin or other NSAIDs for prolonged periods. Aspirin and other NSAIDs are generally discontinued 1 week before any type of surgery, including oral or dental surgery, per the prescriber's or surgeon's orders.
- Always keep aspirin and other drugs out of the reach of children. If a child (or adult) has consumed large or unknown quantities of aspirin or other NSAIDs, contact a poison control center and/or seek emergency medical attention

immediately. Children and teenagers must never take aspirin because of the risk for Reye's syndrome (see Patient-Centered Care: Lifespan Considerations for the Pediatric Patient on p. 700). Acetaminophen in the recommended dosage range is usually preferred.

- Educate the patient about the adverse effects of NSAIDS (including aspirin), such as dyspepsia, heartburn, and gastrointestinal bleeding. (See Table 44-2 for a more complete listing of NSAID-related adverse effects and Box 44-3 for the "black box" warnings on all NSAIDs.) Instruct the patient to immediately report to their prescriber any of the following: black or tarry stools, bleeding around the gums, petechiae (very small red-brown spots), ecchymosis (easy bruising), or purpura (large red spots).
- Encourage the patient to report any signs and symptoms of acute or chronic salicylate toxicity such as tinnitus, hearing loss, increased heart rate, dizziness, mental confusion and diarrhea (review Table 44-3).
- Advise the patient to take NSAIDs with food, milk, or antacids to help minimize gastrointestinal distress.

- Educate the patient about the many drug interactions with aspirin, other NSAIDs, and antigout drugs.
- Alert the patient to look-alike sound-alike drugs, especially Celebrex (celecoxib), which may be confused with Celexa (citalopram) or Cerebyx (fosphenytoin).
- Within the teaching plan, remember that NSAIDS carry FDA black box warnings. The FDA has requested that sponsors of all NSAIDs make labeling changes to their products for both the prescription and over-the-counter (OTC) NSAIDs. All sponsors of marketed prescription NSAIDs, including celecoxib (Celebrex), a cyclooxygenase-2 (COX-2) selective NSAID, have been asked to revise the labeling (package insert) for their products to include a boxed warning, highlighting the potential for increased risk for cardiovascular events and the well-described, serious, potentially life-threatening gastrointestinal bleeding associated with their use. The agency based its advice on a review of the regulatory histories and databases on the various NSAIDs.

KEY POINTS

- Antiinflammatory drugs include aspirin, NSAIDs, and COX-2 inhibitors.
- NSAIDs are one of the most commonly prescribed categories of drugs.
- The first drug in this category to be synthesized was salicylic acid or aspirin. Aspirin is often identified as and included in discussion of antiinflammatory drugs. NSAIDs have analgesic, antiinflammatory, and antipyretic activity; aspirin also has antiplatelet activity. NSAIDs are often used in the treatment of gout, osteoarthritis, juvenile arthritis, rheumatoid arthritis, dysmenorrhea, and musculoskeletal injuries such as strains and sprains.
- The three main adverse effects of NSAIDs are gastrointestinal intolerance, bleeding (often gastrointestinal bleeding), and renal impairment. Misoprostol (Cytotec) may be given to prevent gastrointestinal intolerance and ulcers resulting

from NSAID use. It is classified as a prostaglandin analogue. There are also many contraindications to the use of NSAIDs, such as gastrointestinal tract lesions, peptic ulcers, and bleeding disorders.
- Most oral NSAIDs are better tolerated if taken with food to minimize gastrointestinal upset.
- When NSAIDs are used to decrease joint inflammation in arthritis patients, full therapeutic effects may not be experienced for 1 week or longer.
- Antigout drugs are indicated for either acute or chronic gout or gout prophylaxis. Diarrhea and abdominal pain are common adverse effects. Antigout drugs are often given to patients to avoid goutlike syndromes and pain during cancer chemotherapy that causes cell death.
- Review the black box warnings issued by the FDA (see *www.fda.gov/Drugs/DrugSafety*) for NSAIDS.

NCLEX® EXAMINATION REVIEW QUESTIONS

1. When a patient is receiving long-term NSAID therapy, which drug may be given to prevent the serious gastrointestinal adverse effects of NSAIDs?
   a. misoprostol (Cytotec)
   b. metoprolol (Lopressor)
   c. metoclopramide (Reglan)
   d. magnesium sulfate
2. The nurse recognizes that manifestations of NSAID toxicity include
   a. constipation.
   b. nausea and vomiting.
   c. tremors.
   d. urinary retention.

3. During a teaching session about antigout drugs, the nurse tells the patient that antigout drugs work by which mechanism?
   a. Increasing blood oxygen levels
   b. Decreasing leukocytes and platelets
   c. Increasing protein and rheumatoid factors
   d. Decreasing serum uric acid levels
4. When the nurse is teaching about antigout drugs, which statement by the nurse is accurate?
   a. "Drink only limited amounts of fluids with the drug."
   b. "This drug may cause limited movements of your joints."
   c. "There are very few drug interactions with these medications."
   d. "Colchicine is best taken on an empty stomach."

5. A mother calls the clinic to ask what medication to give her 5-year-old child for a fever during a bout of chickenpox. The nurse's best response would be:
   a. "Your child is 5 years old, so it would be okay to use children's aspirin to treat his fever."
   b. "Start with acetaminophen or ibuprofen, but if these do not work, then you can try aspirin."
   c. "You can use children's dosages of acetaminophen or ibuprofen, but aspirin is not recommended."
   d. "It is best to wait to let the fever break on its own without medication."

6. A 49-year-old patient has been admitted with possible chronic salicylate intoxication after self-treatment for arthritis pain. The nurse will assess for which symptoms of salicylate intoxication? *(Select all that apply).*
   a. Tinnitus
   b. Headache
   c. Constipation
   d. Nausea
   e. Bradycardia

7. An order for a child reads: "Give ibuprofen suspension 30 mg/kg/day, divided into four doses, for pain." The child weighs 33 pounds. How many milligrams will this child receive per dose?

8. The nurse is reviewing a patient's medication list during a preoperative visit. The patient is scheduled for diagnostic laparoscopy in 2 weeks. He asks the nurse, "I hope I can continue the Motrin, because I really ache if I don't take it. It's just minor surgery, right?" What is the nurse's best response?
   a. "You can continue to take it as the laparoscopy is considered minor surgery."
   b. "You will need to take a lower dosage during the preoperative period.
   c. "I'll check with your prescriber, but this drug is usually stopped a week before the surgery because it can cause increased bleeding tendencies."
   d. "You can switch to aspirin before the surgery; both aspirin and Motrin are over-the-counter pain relievers."

1. a, 2. b, 3. d, 4. d, 5. c, 6. a, b, d, 7. 112.5 mg per dose, 8. c.

CRITICAL THINKING AND PRIORITIZATION QUESTIONS

1. P.T., 68 years of age, is instructed to take aspirin, 81 mg every morning with breakfast, as part of treatment after having a myocardial infarction. When discussing the aspirin therapy, he asks the nurse, "Will this also help my arthritis?" What is the nurse's best answer?

2. J.D. has been diagnosed with gout and will be taking colchicine. When reviewing the instructions for the medication, he asks, "I like to take my pills with breakfast." What is the nurse's priority when providing teaching to J.D.?

For answers, see *http://evolve.elsevier.com/Lilley.*

ⓔ EVOLVE WEBSITE

http://evolve.elsevier.com/Lilley
- Animations
- Answer Keys for Textbook Case Studies and Textbook Critical Thinking and Prioritization Questions
- Content Updates
- Key Points
- Review Questions
- Student Case Studies

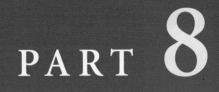
Chemotherapeutic Drugs and Biologic and Immune Modifiers

APPLICATION OF PHARMACOLOGY AND MAKING CONNECTIONS

In Part 7 you were reminded that nursing students are tested not only on knowledge of pharmacology terms and concepts, but also on their ability to apply that knowledge to the nursing process. As you learn about the different classifications of drugs, pay attention to the information in the text boxes, tables, figures, and case studies presented in your chapters. You will discover connections between this information, your previous learning experiences, and the courses you are currently taking including clinical training.

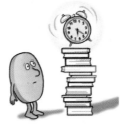

If you are taking anatomy and physiology (AP) concurrently with nursing pharmacology, you will want to make connections between how the different drugs affect the various body systems. You will discover shared terminology and vocabulary between your AP course and the anatomy, physiology, and pathophysiology review at the beginnings of the chapters. Recognizing these commonalities will make learning easier. The review section in Chapter 37 on respiratory drugs examines the function, structure, and physiology of the respiratory tract and lungs. The words printed in blue should already be familiar to you. Box 37-1, *Steps Involved in an Attack of Allergic Asthma,* and Figure 37-1, *Overview of the effects of various antiasthmatic medications,* both provide you with a connection to physiology.

If you are enrolled in beginning nursing courses concurrently with your pharmacology, you will notice that nursing textbooks mention drug therapy when discussing patient care. For example, in most nursing programs, the respiratory system is one of the first systems you will learn. Students learn how to conduct a thorough respiratory assessment. When learning about abnormal respiratory conditions, various medications will be included in the treatment plan. Looking again at Chapter 37, asthma, chronic bronchitis, and emphysema are discussed. The chapter then provides the information on the types of medications that are used in the treatment of these disorders. This is the same information you will encounter in your nursing textbooks. Make the connections. On p. 589, there is a *Case Study* box about *Bronchodilators and Corticosteroids for COPD.* Using this strategy allows you to make the connections between the patient, Ms. B's disease, and her pharmaceutical treatment plan. The questions contained in the scenario allow you to further connect your learning in pharmacology and your nursing instruction. Perhaps you cared for a patient in your clinical rotation with COPD.

This case study allows you to see the similarities and differences between two patients with the same diagnosis. This is an important connection to make.

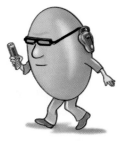

These examples demonstrate that nursing pharmacology is not meant to be learned in isolation. Looking for these types of connections among and between your other courses will assist your learning. Making connections means you are not just memorizing information for your test day, but retaining the conceptual relationships for a deeper understanding. When you become aware of medications and their actions in the human body and their indications as treatment for various diseases, you are applying your knowledge. You can take that application a step further and use it to produce concept maps for patient care, or use the deeper understanding to assist your learning in other courses.

Another connection that you will notice in your textbook is the *Patient-Centered Care: Lifespan Considerations* section that appears at the end of every chapter. In Chapter 3 you were introduced to lifespan considerations. You learned how the pharmacodynamics are altered in both the young patient and the older adult patient. There is a big difference between providing nursing care for children and for the older adult. In your nursing courses, you will learn more about lifespan considerations. You will notice that drug dosages will differ based on a child's weight, and the effects of aging on the human body. The safe dosage for children is much lower and must be calculated based on their weight. The older adult does not metabolize or excrete some medications as readily as younger adults. These are just two examples of lifespan considerations. In the *Patient-Centered Care: Lifespan Considerations for the Pediatric Patient* box on p. 385 in Chapter 24 on heart failure drugs, there is important information about heart failure in the pediatric population. Young children may be taking medications for cardiac issues related to congenital defects. In infants and children, the symptoms of heart failure to observe for include difficulty with feeding. The importance of careful dosage calculation is also emphasized. The *Patient-Centered Care: Lifespan Considerations for the Older Adult Patient* box on p. 590 in Chapter 37 on respiratory drugs provides considerations for the older adult population taking xanthine derivatives. Caution must be used with this drug class because of slower metabolism in older adults. You will need to monitor laboratory results to ensure therapeutic levels and avoid toxicities. The actual drug dosages may also need to be lowered in this patient population. The information in both of these lifespan considerations can be transferred to your patient care in the clinical setting.

As you move through your nursing program, it will become evident that what you are reading and studying in pharmacology will show up again and again. Making these connections early in your nursing program will assist as you in learning more complex disease processes and the required nursing care. When you finish the nursing pharmacology course, do not sell the book; it will become a great reference for you to utilize throughout your nursing program.

Antineoplastic Drugs Part 1: Cancer Overview and Cell Cycle–Specific Drugs

http://evolve.elsevier.com/Lilley

OBJECTIVES

When you reach the end of this chapter, you will be able to do the following:

1. Briefly describe the concepts related to carcinogenesis.
2. Define the different types of malignancy.
3. Discuss the purpose and role of the various treatment modalities in the management of cancer.
4. Define *antineoplastic*.
5. Discuss the role of antineoplastic therapy in the treatment of cancer.
6. Contrast the cell cycle of normal cells and malignant cells with regard to growth, function, and response of the cell to chemotherapeutic drugs and other treatment modalities.
7. Compare the characteristics of highly proliferating normal cells (including cells of the hair follicles, gastrointestinal tract, and bone marrow) with the characteristics of highly proliferating cancerous cells.
8. Briefly describe the specific differences between cell cycle–specific and cell cycle–nonspecific antineoplastic drugs (cell cycle–nonspecific drugs and miscellaneous other antineoplastics are discussed in Chapter 46).
9. Identify the drugs that are categorized as cell cycle–specific, including mitotic inhibitors, topoisomerase inhibitors, and antineoplastic enzymes.
10. Describe the common adverse effects and toxic reactions associated with the various antineoplastic drugs, including the causes for their occurrence and methods of treatment, such as antidotes for toxicity.
11. Discuss the mechanisms of action, indications, dosages, routes of administration, cautions, contraindications, and drug interactions of cell cycle–specific drugs, including mitotic inhibitors, topoisomerase inhibitors, and antineoplastic enzymes.
12. Apply knowledge about the various antineoplastic drugs to the development of a comprehensive nursing care plan for patients receiving cell cycle–specific drugs, including mitotic inhibitors, topoisomerase inhibitors, and antineoplastic enzymes.

DRUG PROFILES

◆ asparaginase, p. 724
capecitabine, p. 721
cladribine, p. 720
◆ cytarabine, p. 721
◆ etoposide, p. 722
fludarabine, p. 720
fluorouracil, p. 721
gemcitabine, p. 721
irinotecan, p. 723

◆ methotrexate, p. 719
◆ paclitaxel, p. 722
pegaspargase, p. 724
topotecan, p. 723
◆ vincristine, p. 722

_____
◆ = *Key drug*
! = *High-alert drug*

KEY TERMS

Analogue A chemical compound with a structure similar to that of another compound but differing from it with respect to some component. (p. 717)

Anaplasia The absence of the cellular differentiation that is part of the normal cellular growth process (see *differentiation*; adjective: *anaplastic*). (p. 714)

Antineoplastic drugs Drugs used to treat cancer. Also called *cancer drugs, anticancer drugs, cancer chemotherapy,* and *chemotherapy.* (p. 714)

Benign Denoting a neoplasm that is noncancerous and therefore not an immediate threat to life. (p. 711)

Cancer A malignant neoplastic disease, the natural course of which is fatal (see *neoplasm*). (p. 710)

Carcinogen Any cancer-producing substance or organism. (p. 713)

Carcinomas Malignant epithelial neoplasms that tend to invade surrounding tissue and metastasize to distant regions of the body. (p. 711)

Cell cycle–nonspecific Denoting antineoplastic drugs that are cytotoxic in any phase of the cellular growth cycle. (p. 715)

Cell cycle–specific Denoting antineoplastic drugs that are cytotoxic during a specific phase of the cellular growth cycle. (p. 715)

Clone A cell or group of cells that is genetically identical to a given parent cell. (p. 711)

Differentiation An important part of normal cellular growth in which immature cells mature into specialized cells. (p. 710)

Dose-limiting adverse effects Adverse effects that prevent an antineoplastic drug from being given in higher dosages, often restricting the effectiveness of the drug. (p. 716)

Emetic potential The potential of a drug to cause nausea and vomiting. (p. 716)

Extravasation The leakage of any intravenously or intraarterially administered medication into the tissue space surrounding the vein or artery; can cause serious tissue injury. (p. 717)

Gene expression How a cell expresses a receptor or gene; the process in which information from a gene is used in the synthesis of a gene product. (p. 712)

Growth fraction The percentage of cells in mitosis at any given time. (p. 713)

Intrathecal A route of drug injection through the theca of the spinal cord and into the subarachnoid space. This route is used to deliver certain chemotherapy medications to kill cancer cells in the central nervous system. (p. 720)

Leukemias Malignant neoplasms of blood-forming tissues characterized by the replacement of normal bone marrow cells with leukemic blasts resulting in abnormal numbers and forms of immature white blood cells in the circulation. (p. 712)

Lymphomas Malignant neoplasms of lymphoid tissue. (p. 712)

Malignant Tending to worsen and cause death; anaplastic, invasive, and metastatic. (p. 711)

Metastasis The process by which a cancer spreads from the original site of growth to a new and remote part of the body (adjective *metastatic*). (p. 711)

Mitosis The process of cell reproduction occurring in somatic (nonsexual) cells and resulting in the formation of two genetically identical daughter cells containing the diploid (complete) number of chromosomes characteristic of the species. (p. 713)

Mitotic index The number of cells per unit (usually 1000 cells) undergoing mitosis during a given time. (p. 713)

Mutagen A chemical or physical agent that induces or increases genetic mutations by causing changes in deoxyribonucleic acid (DNA). (p. 713)

Mutation A permanent change in DNA that is transmissible to future cellular generations. Mutations can transform normal cells into cancer cells. (p. 710)

Myelosuppression Suppression of bone marrow function, which can result in dangerously reduced numbers of red blood cells, white blood cells, and platelets. (p. 717)

Nadir Lowest point in any fluctuating value over time; for example, the lowest white blood cell count measured after the count has been depressed by chemotherapy. (p. 717)

Neoplasm Any new and abnormal growth, specifically growth that is uncontrolled and progressive; a synonym for *tumor*. A malignant neoplasm or tumor is synonymous with *cancer*. (p. 711)

Nucleic acids Molecules of DNA and ribonucleic acid (RNA) in the nucleus of every cell (hence the name *nucleic acid*). Chromosomes are made up of DNA and encode all of the genes necessary for cellular structure and function. (p. 713)

Oncogenic Cancer producing; often applied to tumor-inducing viruses. (p. 713)

Paraneoplastic syndromes Symptom complexes arising in patients with cancer that cannot be explained by local or distant spread of their tumors. (p. 712)

Primary lesion The original site of growth of a tumor. (p. 711)

Sarcomas Malignant neoplasms of the connective tissues arising in bone, fibrous, fatty, muscular, synovial, vascular, or neural tissue, often first presenting as painless swellings. (p. 711)

Tumor A new growth of tissue characterized by a progressive, uncontrolled proliferation of cells. Tumors can be solid (e.g., brain tumor) or circulating (e.g., leukemia or lymphoma), and benign (noncancerous) or malignant (cancerous). Circulating tumors are more precisely called *hematologic tumors* or *hematologic malignancies*. A tumor is also called a *neoplasm*. (p. 711)

Tumor lysis syndrome A common metabolic complication of chemotherapy for rapidly growing tumors. It is characterized by the presence of excessive cellular waste products and electrolytes, including uric acid, phosphate, and potassium, and by reduced serum calcium levels. (p. 718)

OVERVIEW

Cancer is a broad term encompassing a group of diseases that are characterized by cellular transformation (e.g., by genetic mutation), uncontrolled cellular growth, possible invasion into surrounding tissue, and metastasis to other tissues or organs distant from the original body site. This cellular growth differs from normal cellular growth in that cancerous cells do not possess a growth control mechanism. Lack of cellular differentiation or maturation into specialized, productive cells is also a common characteristic of cancer cells. Figure 45-1 illustrates the multiple steps involved in the development of cancer. Cancerous cells will continue to grow and invade adjacent structures. They may break away from the original tumor mass and travel by means of the blood or lymphatic system to establish a new clone of cancer cells and create a metastatic growth

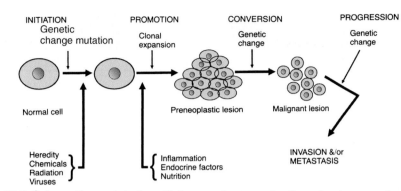

FIGURE 45-1 Schematic model of multistep carcinogenesis. Genetic change refers to events such as the activation of protooncogenes or drug resistance genes or the inactivation of tumor suppressor genes, antimetastasis genes, or apoptosis (normal cell death). Genetic change may be relatively minimal, as with the translocations seen in various leukemias, or it may involve multiple sequential genetic alterations, as exemplified by the development of colon cancer. (From Haskell CM: *Cancer treatment*, ed 5, Philadelphia, 2001, Saunders.)

elsewhere in the body. A **clone** is a cell or group of cells that is genetically identical to a given parent cell. For the remainder of this and the next chapter, the term *cancer* will generally be used to refer to any type of malignant neoplasm.

Metastasis refers to the spreading of a cancer from the original site of growth (**primary lesion**) to a new and remote part of the body (secondary or metastatic lesion). The terms *malignancy, neoplasm,* and *tumor* are often used as synonyms for *cancer.* A **neoplasm** ("new tissue") is a mass of new cells. It is another term for **tumor.** There are two types of tumors: benign and malignant. A **benign** tumor is of a uniform size and shape and displays no invasiveness (in terms of infiltrating other tissues) or metastatic properties. The terms *nonmalignant* and *benign* suggest that tumors may be harmless, which is true in most cases. However, a benign tumor can be lethal if it grows large enough to mechanically interrupt the normal function of a critical tissue or organ. **Malignant** neoplasms consist of cancer cells that invade (infiltrate) surrounding tissues and metastasize to other tissues and organs. Some of the various characteristics of benign and malignant neoplasms are listed in Table 45-1.

Over 100 types of cancer affect humans. Various tumor types based on tissue categories include sarcomas, carcinomas, lymphomas, leukemias, and tumors of nervous tissue origin. Examples of these common types of malignant tumors are presented in Table 45-2. It is important to know the tissue of origin, because this determines the type of treatment, the likely response to therapy, and the prognosis.

Carcinomas arise from epithelial tissue, which is located throughout the body. This tissue covers or lines all body surfaces, both inside and outside the body. Examples are the skin, the mucosal lining of the entire gastrointestinal (GI) tract, and the lining of the bronchial tree (lungs). **Sarcomas** are malignant tumors that arise primarily from connective tissues, but some sarcomas are tumors of epithelial cell origin. Connective tissue is the most abundant and widely distributed of all tissues and includes bone, cartilage, muscle, and lymphatic and vascular structures. Its purpose is to support and protect other tissues.

TABLE 45-1 Tumor Characteristics: Benign and Malignant

Characteristic	Benign	Malignant
Potential to metastasize	No	Yes
Encapsulated	Yes	No
Similar to tissue of origin	Yes	No
Rate of growth	Slow	Unpredictable and unrestrained
Recurrence after surgical removal	Rare	Common

TABLE 45-2 Tumor Classification Based on Specific Tissue of Origin

Tissue of Origin	Malignant Tissue
Epithelial = Carcinomas	
Glands or ducts	Adenocarcinomas
Respiratory tract	Small- and large-cell carcinomas
Kidney	Renal cell carcinoma
Skin	Squamous cell, epidermoid, and basal cell carcinoma; melanoma
Connective = Sarcomas	
Fibrous tissue	Fibrosarcoma
Cartilage	Chondrosarcoma
Bone	Osteogenic sarcoma (Ewing's tumor)
Blood vessels	Kaposi's sarcoma
Synovia	Synoviosarcoma
Mesothelium	Mesothelioma
Lymphatic = Lymphomas	
Lymph tissue	Lymphomas (e.g., Hodgkin's, non-Hodgkin's)
Glia	Glioma
Adrenal medulla nerves	Pheochromocytoma
Blood and Bone Marrow	
White blood cells	Leukemia
Bone marrow	Multiple myeloma

TABLE 45-3   Paraneoplastic Syndromes Associated with Some Cancers

Paraneoplastic Syndrome	Associated Cancer
Hypercalcemia, sensory neuropathies, SIADH	Lung
Disseminated intravascular coagulation	Leukemia
Cushing's syndrome	Lung, thyroid, testes, adrenal
Addison's syndrome	Adrenal, lymphoma

SIADH, Syndrome of inappropriate secretion of antidiuretic hormone.

TABLE 45-4   Cancer: Proposed Etiologic Factors

Risk Factor	Associated Cancer
Environment	
Radiation (ionizing)	Leukemia, breast, thyroid, lung
Radiation (ultraviolet)	Skin, melanoma
Viruses	Leukemia, lymphoma, nasopharyngeal
Food	
Aflatoxin	Liver
Dietary factors	Colon, breast, endometrial, gallbladder
Lifestyle	
Alcohol	Esophageal, liver, stomach, laryngeal, breast
Tobacco	Lung, oral, esophageal, laryngeal, bladder
Medical Drugs	
Diethylstilbestrol (DES)	Vaginal in offspring, breast, testicular, ovarian
Estrogens	Endometrial, breast
Alkylating drugs	Leukemia, bladder
Occupational	
Asbestos	Lung, mesothelioma
Aniline dye	Bladder
Benzene	Leukemia
Vinyl chloride	Liver
Reproductive History	
Late first pregnancy, early menses	Breast
No children	Ovarian
Multiple sexual partners	Cervical, uterine

Lymphomas are cancers within the lymphatic tissues. **Leukemias** arise from the bone marrow and are cancers of blood and bone marrow. Leukemias differ from carcinomas and sarcomas in that the cancerous cells do not form solid tumors but are interspersed throughout the lymphatic or circulatory system and interfere with the normal functioning of these systems. For this reason, they are sometimes referred to as *circulating tumors,* although *hematologic malignancy* is a more precise term. Lymphomas can be quite bulky and are usually classified as solid tumors.

Cancer patients may also experience various groups of symptoms that cannot be directly attributed to the spread of a cancerous tumor. Such symptom complexes are referred to as **paraneoplastic syndromes.** They are estimated to occur in up to 15% of patients with cancer and may even be the first sign of malignancy. *Cachexia* (general ill health and malnutrition) is the most common such symptom complex. Examples of other common paraneoplastic syndromes are given in Table 45-3. These syndromes are believed to result from the effects of biologically or immunologically active substances, such as hormones and antibodies, secreted by the tumor cells. Many patients also exhibit more generalized symptoms, such as anorexia, weight loss, fatigue, and fever.

ETIOLOGY OF CANCER

The etiology of cancer remains a mystery for the most part, and cancer researchers have made slow progress toward identifying possible causes. Certain etiologic factors have been identified, and some of these factors and the cancers with which they are causally associated are listed in Table 45-4. Causative factors that have been identified include age-related and sex-related characteristics; genetic and ethnic factors; oncogenic viruses; environmental and occupational factors; radiation; and immunologic factors.

Age- and Sex-Related Differences

The probability that a neoplastic disease will develop generally increases with advancing age. A number of rare cancers, such as acute lymphocytic leukemia and Wilms tumor, occur predominantly in pediatric patients.

With the exception of cancers affecting the reproductive system, few cancers exhibit a sex-related difference in incidence. Lung and urinary cancers are more common in men than in women, but this may have more to do with exogenous factors such as smoking patterns and occupational exposure to environmental toxins than to sex-related characteristics. The incidence of colon, rectal, pancreatic, and skin cancers are comparable in men and women. A number of hematologic cancers have a slight male predominance.

Genetic and Ethnic Factors

Few cancers have been confirmed to have a hereditary basis (some types of breast, colon, and stomach cancer are exceptions). The understanding of tumor biology has helped guide therapy tremendously. Two such advances are determination of hormone receptor status and identification of specific **gene expression** in various types of tumor cells. For example, some tumor cells express themselves on their cell membrane surfaces, either estrogen receptors or progesterone receptors, and some tumor cells express specific genes such as the *HER2/neu* gene. Because these indicators aid in classification of a patient's tumor, they also help in choosing appropriate drug therapy, predicting response to therapy, and anticipating prognosis. Discovery of the *BRCA1* and *BRCA2* genes has allowed identification of women who are at risk for breast cancer because they have a certain alteration in one of these *BRCA* genes. Many women with a family history of breast cancer choose to be tested for the presence of a *BRCA* gene mutation, which has led some women to undergo prophylactic breast removal. Tumors with identifiable gene expression patterns can show a familial pattern of inheritance. For example, Burkitt's lymphoma is more common in young African children and children of African descent. Another example of an ethnic predisposition is the high incidence of nasopharyngeal cancer in persons of Chinese descent.

Oncogenic Viruses

Extensive research has indicated that there are cancer-causing (oncogenic) viruses that can affect most mammalian species. Examples include human papillomavirus, the various cat leukemia viruses, the Rous sarcoma virus in chickens, and the Shope papillomavirus in rabbits.

The herpesviruses are common examples of oncogenic viruses. Epstein-Barr virus is a type of herpesvirus. It is most commonly recognized as the cause of infectious mononucleosis (commonly referred to as "mono" or the "kissing disease"). However, it is also associated with the development of Burkitt's lymphoma and nasopharyngeal cancer. Infection with human papillomavirus (often abbreviated as HPV) has been linked to both cervical and anal cancer.

Occupational and Environmental Carcinogens

A carcinogen is any substance that can cause cancer. In the nucleus of every cell are found molecules of nucleic acids, namely deoxyribonucleic acid (DNA) and ribonucleic acid (RNA). Genes are transcribed into messenger RNA molecules, which in turn are translated into protein molecules necessary for cellular structure and function. This process is discussed further in the section on alkylating drugs in Chapter 46. A mutagen is any substance or physical agent (e.g., radiation) that induces changes in DNA molecules. Mutations often transform normal cells into cancer cells. Thus, mutagenicity is associated with and often (but not always) leads to carcinogenicity. The U.S. Food and Drug Administration (FDA) mandates that carcinogenic studies be performed before any new drug is approved for use. However, no amount of clinical testing can fully reveal all of a drug's possible carcinogenic effects. Carcinogenic effects may not be observed until the drugs are used in the general population. If patterns of carcinogenicity begin to emerge during this period of postmarketing surveillance (or post-marketing studies), the drug may be recalled from the market.

Radiation

Radiation is a well-known and potent carcinogenic agent. There are two basic types of radiation: (1) ionizing, or high-energy, radiation, and (2) nonionizing, or low-energy, radiation. Both types can be carcinogenic. Ionizing radiation is very potent and can penetrate deeply into the body. It is called *ionizing* because it causes the formation of ions within living cells. This type of radiation (e.g., that used in radiographic studies) is also used to treat (irradiate) cancerous tumors (e.g., radium implants). Nonionizing radiation is much less potent and cannot penetrate deeply into the body. Ultraviolet light is an example of this type of radiation and is the cause of skin cancer. In contrast to chemotherapy, radiation therapy is considered to be a locoregional

and not a systemic cancer treatment. Adverse effects of radiation therapy (e.g., radiation burns; nausea with GI tract irradiation) tend to be more localized to the site of treatment as well.

Immunologic Factors

The immune system plays an important role in terms of cancer surveillance and the elimination of neoplastic cells. Neoplastic cells are believed to develop in everyone; however, a healthy person's immune system recognizes them as abnormal and eliminates them by means of cell-mediated immunity (cytotoxic T lymphocytes; see Chapter 47). It has also been shown that the incidence of cancer is much higher in immunocompromised individuals.

CELL GROWTH CYCLE

Normal cells in the body divide (proliferate) in a controlled and organized fashion, and this growth is regulated by various mechanisms. In contrast, cancer cells lack such regulatory mechanisms and divide uncontrollably. Often the growth of cancer cells is more constant than that of nonmalignant cells. Thus, one important growth index for malignant tumors is the time it takes for the tumor to double in size. This doubling time varies greatly for different types of cancers and is important in determining the prognosis. The time it takes for regrowth to occur depends on the doubling time of the particular cancer. Tumors with shorter doubling times are often difficult to cure due to rapid regrowth.

The cell growth characteristics of normal and neoplastic cells are similar. Both types of cells pass through five distinct gap phases: G_0, the resting phase, in which the cell is considered out of the cell cycle; G_1, the first gap phase; S, the synthesis phase; G_2, the second gap phase; and M, the mitosis phase (Figure 45-2). During mitosis, one cell divides into two identical daughter cells. Mitosis is further subdivided into four distinct subphases related to the time periods before and during the alignment and separation of the chromosomes (DNA strands): prophase, metaphase, anaphase, and telophase. A complete cell cycle from one mitosis to the next is called the *generation time*. It is different for all tumors, ranging from hours to days. The cell growth cycle and the events that occur in the various phases are summarized in Table 45-5. Figure 45-3 shows where in the general phases of the cell cycle the various cell cycle–specific chemotherapeutic drugs show their greatest activity.

The growth activity in a mass of tumor cells has an important bearing on the killing power of chemotherapeutic drugs. The percentage of cells undergoing mitosis at any given time is called the growth fraction of the tumor. The actual number of cells that are in the M phase of the cell cycle is called the mitotic index. Chemotherapy is most effective when used in a rapidly dividing or highly proliferative tumor.

Hematopoietic stem cells are cells in the bone marrow that have the capacity for self-renewal and repopulation of the different types of blood and bone marrow cells. In the bone marrow, the hematopoietic stem cell divides asynchronously, regenerating itself while producing a cell that will go through a series of cell divisions to produce mature blood cells. Tumors

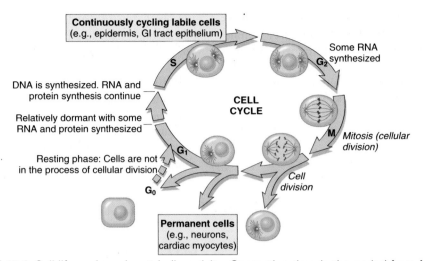

FIGURE 45-2 Cell life cycle and metabolic activity. Generation time is the period from M phase to M phase. Cells not in the cycle but capable of division are in the resting phase (G_0). (From Lewis SL, Dirksen SR, Heitkemper MM, et al: *Medical-surgical nursing: assessment and management of clinical problems,* ed 8, St Louis, 2011, Mosby).

TABLE 45-5	Cell Cycle Phases
Phase	**Description**
G_0: Resting phase	Most normal human cells exist predominantly in this phase. Cancer cells in this phase are not susceptible to the toxic effects of cell cycle–specific drugs.
G_1: First gap phase or postmitotic phase	Enzymes necessary for DNA synthesis are produced.
S: DNA synthesis phase	DNA synthesis takes place, from DNA strand separation to replication of each strand to create duplicate DNA molecules.
G_2: Second gap phase or premitotic phase	RNA and specialized proteins are made.
M: Mitosis phase	Divided into four subphases: prophase, metaphase, anaphase, and telophase; cell divides (reproduces) into two daughter cells.

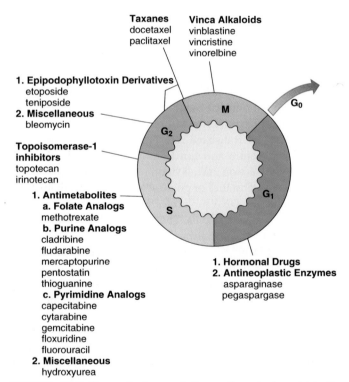

FIGURE 45-3 General phase of the cell cycle in which the various cell cycle–specific chemotherapeutic drugs have their greatest proportionate kill of cancer cells.

in the bone marrow that affect a cell close to the stem cell are unable to mature and are considered poorly differentiated. The level of differentiation within a tumor, whether solid or circulating, becomes especially important in the treatment of neoplasms. This is because more highly differentiated tumors generally have a better therapeutic response (tumor shrinkage) to treatments such as chemotherapy and radiation. In contrast, some cancers, such as leukemia, involve proliferation of immature white blood cells (WBCs) known as *blast cells.* Cancers with a larger proportion of undifferentiated cells are often less responsive to chemotherapy or radiation. Lack of normal cellular differentiation is known as **anaplasia,** and such undifferentiated cells are said to be *anaplastic* cells.

CANCER DRUG NOMENCLATURE

The more technical term for cancer is *malignant neoplasm.* Drugs used to treat cancer are therefore known as **antineoplas-**

tic drugs but are also called *cancer drugs, anticancer drugs,* and, most commonly, *cytotoxic chemotherapy* or just *chemotherapy.* The nomenclature (naming system) of cancer drugs can be somewhat more complex and confusing than that for other drug classes. Cancer treatment is an intensively researched area in health care with many active research protocols. Multiple names are often used for the same drug, depending on its stage of development.

Recall from Chapter 2 that medications have a chemical name, a generic name, and a trade name. This section introduces yet another name for medications, especially cancer drugs: the investigational or protocol name. A drug's chemical name is used by the chemists who first discover and work with the drug. The generic name is frequently first assigned to a chemical compound after a pharmaceutical manufacturer has determined that it is worthy of continued clinical research. It is often at this point that the chemical compound becomes an investigational drug. The trade name is a marketing name used by the manufacturer of a given drug. During the time before marketing and while a given medication is undergoing clinical research, it is frequently referred to by its protocol name. The protocol name is often a code name that consists of a combination of letters and numbers separated by one or more dashes. The following are two typical examples that illustrate these concepts:

Other Name	Generic Name	Trade Name
STI-571 (protocol name)	imatinib	Gleevec
5-fluorouracil* (chemical name)	fluorouracil	Adrucil

*The "5" refers to the position of a fluorine atom in the cyclic ring structure of the uracil molecule.

DRUG THERAPY

Cancer is normally treated using one or more of three major medical approaches: surgery, radiation therapy, and chemotherapy. The term *chemotherapy* refers to the pharmacologic treatment of cancer.

Normal cells in the body divide (proliferate) in a controlled and organized fashion, and this growth is regulated by means of various mechanisms. In contrast, cancer cells lack regulatory mechanisms, and they proliferate uncontrollably. Figure 45-4 shows how various combinations of cancer treatment may succeed, or fail, over time.

Cancer chemotherapy drugs can be subdivided into two main groups based on where in the cell cycle they have their effects. Antineoplastic drugs that are cytotoxic (cell killing) in any phase of the cycle are called cell cycle–nonspecific drugs. Those drugs that are cytotoxic during a specific cell cycle phase are called cell cycle–specific drugs. These are broad categories that describe the activity of a drug with regard to cell cycle. Individual drugs may have actions that fall into both of these categories. Regardless of the cell cycle characteristics of a drug, it is more effective on rapidly growing tumors. This chapter discusses the cell cycle–specific drugs. Chapter 46 focuses on cell cycle–nonspecific drugs as well as various miscellaneous antineoplastic drugs.

The ultimate goal of any anticancer regimen is to kill every neoplastic cell and produce a cure, but this goal is not achieved in most cases. Fortunately, some patients' immune systems may be able to clear the remaining tumor. Factors that affect the chances of cure and the length of patient survival include the cancer stage at time of diagnosis, the type of cancer and its doubling time, the efficacy of the cancer treatment, the development of drug resistance, and the general health of the patient. When total cure is not possible, the primary goal of therapy is

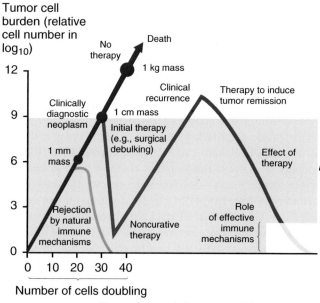
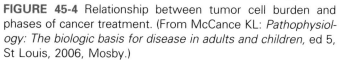

FIGURE 45-4 Relationship between tumor cell burden and phases of cancer treatment. (From McCance KL: *Pathophysiology: The biologic basis for disease in adults and children*, ed 5, St Louis, 2006, Mosby.)

to control the growth of the cancer while maintaining the best quality of life for the patient with the least possible level of discomfort and fewest treatment adverse effects.

It must be emphasized that cancer care and treatment involve many rapidly evolving medical sciences. Cancer is an intensively researched area, with the ultimate goals being to prevent cancer and to prevent premature death. Chemotherapy medications are often dosed as part of complex, specific treatment protocols that are subject to frequent revision by oncology practitioners and researchers. For these reasons, doses of chemotherapeutic agents are not listed in this textbook. When faced with a chemotherapy drug, one must check the dose against standard chemotherapy textbooks and the specific protocol being utilized. Furthermore, the indications that are listed for each specific drug are the primary FDA-approved indications that are current at the time of this writing. These, too, may change unpredictably with time as a given drug is determined to be more (or less) effective for treating certain types of cancer. Also, in clinical practice, patients are often treated with one or more antineoplastic medications in "off-label" uses; that is, the drug is not currently approved for those particular uses by the FDA.

No antineoplastic drug is effective against all types of cancer. Most cancer drugs have a low therapeutic index, which means that a fine line exists between therapeutic and toxic levels. Clinical experience has shown that a combination of drugs is usually more effective than single-drug therapy. Because drug-resistant cells often develop, exposure to multiple drugs with multiple mechanisms and sites of action will destroy more subpopulations of cells. The delayed onset of resistance to a particular antineoplastic drug is one benefit of combination drug therapy.

To be most effective, drugs used in a combination regimen would ideally possess the following characteristics:

- Some efficacy even as single drugs in the treatment of the particular type of cancer
- Different mechanisms of action so that the cytotoxic effect is maximized; this includes differences in cell-cycle specificity
- No or minimal overlapping toxicities

One major drawback to the use of antineoplastic drugs is that nearly all of them cause adverse effects. These toxicities generally stem from the fact that chemotherapy drugs affect rapidly dividing cells—both harmful cancer cells and healthy, normal cells. Three types of rapidly dividing human cells are the cells of hair follicles, GI tract cells, and bone marrow cells. Because most of today's antineoplastic drugs cannot differentiate between cancer cells and healthy cells, the healthy cells are also destroyed, so hair loss, nausea and vomiting, and bone marrow toxicity are the undesirable consequences. Effects on the GI tract and bone marrow are often **dose-limiting adverse effects;** that is, the patient can no longer tolerate an increase in dosage that may be necessary to adequately treat the cancer and achieve good disease response.

Hair follicle cells are rapidly dividing cells. Cancer drugs that affect these cells often cause the adverse effect known as *alopecia,* or hair loss. Many patients, especially women, choose to wear wigs, hats, or scarves to disguise this adverse effect. Some antineoplastic drugs are more harmful to the epithelial cells of the stomach and intestinal tract, which often leads to diarrhea and mucositis, and may also increase the risk for nausea and vomiting. The likelihood that a given drug will produce vomiting is known as its **emetic potential**. Anticancer drugs cause nausea and vomiting by stimulating the cells of the chemoreceptor trigger zone. Several antiemetic drugs are used to prevent these symptoms and are described in Chapter 52. Box 45-1 lists the relative emetic potential of selected chemotherapy drugs.

BOX 45-1   Relative Emetic Potential of Selected Antineoplastic Drugs*

Low (Less Than 10% to 30%)
asparaginase
bleomycin
busulfan
capecitabine
chlorambucil
cladribine
cytarabine (less than 1000 mg/m²)
daunorubicin, liposomal
docetaxel
doxorubicin (less than 20 mg/m²)
doxorubicin, liposomal
estramustine
etoposide
floxuridine
fludarabine
fluorouracil (less than 1000 mg/m²)
gefitinib
gemcitabine
hydroxyurea
imatinib
melphalan
mercaptopurine
methotrexate (less than 250 mg/m²)
mitomycin
paclitaxel
pegaspargase
pentostatin
rituximab
teniposide
thioguanine
thiotepa
topotecan
trastuzumab
tretinoin

vinblastine
vincristine
vinorelbine

Moderate (30% to 60%)
altretamine
cyclophosphamide (less than 750 mg/m²)
dactinomycin
daunorubicin (50 mg/m² or less)
doxorubicin (20 to 60 mg/m²)
epirubicin (less than 90 mg/m²)
idarubicin
ifosfamide (1500 mg/m² or less)
irinotecan
methotrexate (250 to 1000 mg/m²)
mitoxantrone (15 mg/m² or less)
temozolomide

High (60% to More Than 90%)
carboplatin
carmustine
cisplatin
cyclophosphamide (750 to more than 1500 mg/m²)
cytarabine (more than 1000 mg/m²)
dacarbazine
dactinomycin
daunorubicin (more than 50 mg/m²)
doxorubicin (more than 60 mg/m²)
ifosfamide (more than 1500 mg/m²)
lomustine
mechlorethamine
methotrexate (more than 1000 mg/m²)
mitoxantrone (more than 15 mg/m²)
oxaliplatin
procarbazine
streptozocin

*Drugs in this list not covered in this chapter are described in Chapter 46.

Myelosuppression, also known as *bone marrow suppression* or *bone marrow depression,* is another unwanted adverse effect of certain antineoplastics. It commonly results from drug- or radiation-induced destruction of rapidly dividing cells in the bone marrow, primarily the cellular precursors of WBCs, red blood cells (RBCs), and platelets. This can also occur due to the disease processes of the cancer itself. Myelosuppression, in turn, leads to leukopenia, anemia, and thrombocytopenia. The cancer patient is often at greater risk for infection because of leukopenia (reduced WBC count) secondary to chemotherapy. Patients often need antibiotics intravenously (IV), either to prevent or to treat bacterial infections. Such patients are referred to as being *neutropenic.* Drug-induced anemia (reduced RBC count) often leads to hypoxia and fatigue, whereas thrombocytopenia (reduced platelet count) makes the patient more susceptible to bleeding. The lowest level of WBCs in the blood following chemotherapy (or radiation) treatment is called the **nadir.** The time until the nadir is reached in a given patient may become shorter and the recovery time for the bone marrow may become longer with multiple courses of antineoplastic treatment. The nadir normally occurs roughly 10 to 28 days after dosing, depending on the particular drug or combination of drugs that is used. Anticipation of this nadir based on known cancer drug data can be used to guide the timing of prophylactic (preventive) administration of antibiotics and blood stimulants known as *hematopoietic growth factors* (see Chapter 47).

Extravasation—unintended leakage of a chemotherapy drug (with vesicant potential) into the surrounding tissues outside of the IV line is a serious complication with chemotherapy. Specific treatment of extravasations vary depending on the drug and are listed in various tables and boxes throughout this chapter and Chapter 46 (Tables 45-8 and 46-2 and Boxes 46-1 and 46-2).

Because of the often severe toxicity of cancer medications, a current major focus of cancer drug research is the development of targeted drug therapy. Targeted drug therapy utilizes drugs that recognize a specific molecule involved in the growth of cancer cells, while mostly sparing healthy cells. One example of such targeted therapy is the newer class of cancer drugs known as *monoclonal antibodies* (see Chapter 47). There has been a recent expansion of targeted drug therapy. Tyrosine kinase inhibitors are drugs that impede the development of new blood vessels, tumor growth, and cancer progression. Lenvatinib (Lenvina) and sorafenib (Nexavar) are approved for thyroid cancer. Palbociclib (Ibrance) is approved for used in breast cancer. Ceritinib (Zykadia) is approved for non–small cell lung cancer. All of the tyrosine kinase inhibitors are given orally. Because this is an rapidly expanding category, the reader is referred to *www.cancer.gov/cancertopics/treatment/types/targeted-therapies/targeted-therapies-fact-sheet* for the latest developments in targeted therapy.

Pharmacokinetic data for antineoplastic medications is seldom used to guide dosing. Only a few anticancer drugs benefit from therapeutic drug monitoring. For these reasons, pharmacokinetic data are not included with the drug profiles in this chapter.

In spite of their notorious toxicity, given the often fatal outcome of neoplastic diseases, most cancer drugs are rarely considered to be absolutely contraindicated. Even if a patient has a known allergic reaction to an antineoplastic medication, the urgency of treating the patient's cancer necessitates administering the medication and treating any allergic symptoms with premedications such as antihistamines, corticosteroids, and acetaminophen. For these reasons, no specific contraindications are listed for any of the drugs in this chapter.

Common relative contraindications for cancer drugs include very low WBC count, ongoing infectious process, severe compromise in nutritional and hydration status, reduced kidney or liver function, or a decline in organ function in any system that may be further affected by the toxic effect of the drug being administered. These are situations in which chemotherapy treatment is commonly delayed until the patient's status improves. In general, most chemotherapy is held when the patient's absolute neutrophil count (ANC) is less than 500 cells/mm³ (severe neutropenia) (see Chapter 46). Dosages are often reduced for older adult patients or others with significantly compromised organ system function, depending on the drugs used.

Reduction in fertility is a major concern in postpubertal patients. Cancer also complicates 1 in 1000 pregnancies. All chemotherapy drugs are classified as pregnancy category D. The choice to use chemotherapy in a pregnant woman is based on risk versus benefit. Both radiation and chemotherapy treatments can cause significant permanent fetal harm or death. The greatest risk is during the first trimester. Chemotherapy treatment during the second or third trimester is more likely to improve maternal outcome without significant fetal risk. Prepubertal patients are more resilient and can have normal puberty and fertility after receiving chemotherapy.

In the older adult, *frailty* refers to loss of most of the patient's functional reserve and limited ability to tolerate even minimal physiologic stress (e.g., chemotherapy treatment). More robust older adults are better candidates for cancer treatment, although frail patients often benefit as well, especially in terms of palliative (noncurative) symptom control.

CELL CYCLE–SPECIFIC ANTINEOPLASTIC DRUGS

Cell cycle–specific drug classes include antimetabolites, mitotic inhibitors, alkaloid topoisomerase II inhibitors, topoisomerase I inhibitors, and antineoplastic enzymes. These drugs are collectively used to treat a variety of solid and/or circulating tumors, although some drugs have much more specific indications than others.

ANTIMETABOLITES

A compound that is structurally similar to a normal cellular metabolite is known as an **analogue** of that metabolite. Analogues may have agonist or antagonist activity. An antagonist analogue is also known as an *antimetabolite.*

Mechanism of Action and Drug Effects

Antineoplastic antimetabolites are cell cycle–specific analogues that work by antagonizing the actions of key cellular metabolites. More specifically, antimetabolites inhibit cellular growth by interfering with the synthesis or actions of compounds critical to cellular reproduction: the vitamin folic acid, purines, and pyrimidines. Purines and pyrimidines make up the bases contained in nucleic acid molecules (DNA and RNA). Antimetabolites work via two mechanisms: (1) by falsely substituting for purines, pyrimidines, or folic acid; and (2) by inhibiting critical enzymes involved in the synthesis or function of these compounds. Thus, they ultimately inhibit the synthesis of DNA, RNA, and proteins, all of which are necessary for cell survival. Antimetabolites work primarily in the S phase of the cell cycle, during which DNA synthesis is most active. The available antimetabolites are listed below. Although some chemotherapy drugs have abbreviations, it is best to avoid use of abbreviations as they have been associated with medication errors. Best practice is to put the generic and brand name on the label of the finished product to serve as a double check:

Folate antagonists
- methotrexate (MTX)
- pemetrexed
- pralatrexate

Purine antagonists
- cladribine
- fludarabine
- mercaptopurine (6-MP)
- pentostatin
- thioguanine

Pyrimidine antagonists
- capecitabine
- cytarabine (ara-C)
- floxuridine fluorouracil (5-FU)
- gemcitabine

Folic Acid Antagonism

The antimetabolite methotrexate is an analogue of folic acid. It inhibits the action of dihydrofolate reductase, an enzyme responsible for converting folic acid to its active form, folate, which is needed for the synthesis of DNA. The result is that DNA is not produced and the cell dies. In practice, the terms *folic acid* and *folate* are often used interchangeably. Pemetrexed is the name of a newer folate antagonist with a mechanism of action similar to that of methotrexate. Pralatrexate (Folotyn) is the newest dihydrofolate reductase inhibitor, specifically indicated for T-cell lymphoma.

Purine Antagonism

The purine bases present in DNA and RNA are adenine and guanine (see the discussion in Chapter 46), and they are required for the synthesis of the purine nucleotides that are incorporated into the nucleic acid molecules. Mercaptopurine and fludarabine are synthetic analogues of adenine, and thioguanine is a synthetic analogue of guanine. Cladribine is a more general purine antagonist, whereas pentostatin inhibits the action of the critical enzyme adenosine deaminase. Cladribine is unique in that it actually lacks cell-cycle specificity relative to other drugs in its class. It is included in this section because of its similar pharmacology and mechanism of action. All of these drugs work by ultimately interrupting the synthesis of both DNA and RNA.

Although allopurinol is chemically similar to purines, it does not disrupt DNA synthesis. Instead, it inhibits xanthine oxidase, which reduces serum and/or urinary levels of uric acid. Rasburicase is an enzyme that degrades uric acid to more soluble end products. Uric acid is a common waste product that often accumulates in the blood following lysis of tumor cells, part of a condition known as **tumor lysis syndrome** (see Adverse Effects).

Pyrimidine Antagonism

The pyrimidine bases, cytosine and thymine, occur in the structure of DNA molecules, and cytosine and uracil are part of the structure of RNA molecules. These bases are essential for DNA and RNA synthesis. Floxuridine and fluorouracil are synthetic analogues of uracil, and cytarabine is a synthetic analogue of cytosine. Capecitabine is actually a prodrug of fluorouracil and is converted to that drug in the liver and other body tissues. Because of its prodrug form, it can be given orally. Gemcitabine inhibits the action of two essential enzymes, DNA polymerase and ribonucleotide reductase. Overall, these drugs act in a way that is very similar to that of the purine antagonists, incorporating themselves into the metabolic pathway for the synthesis of DNA and RNA and thereby interrupting the synthesis of both of these nucleic acids.

Indications

Antimetabolite antineoplastic drugs are used for the treatment of a variety of solid tumors and some hematologic cancers. They may also be used in combination chemotherapy regimens to enhance the overall cytotoxic effect. Methotrexate is also used to treat severe cases of psoriasis (a skin condition) as well as rheumatoid arthritis (see Chapter 47). Because some of these drugs are available in both oral and topical preparations, they are sometimes used for low-dose maintenance and palliative (noncurative) cancer therapy.

Allopurinol and rasburicase are both indicated for the hyperuricemia associated with tumor lysis syndrome and are usually given in anticipation of this condition during various chemotherapy regimens associated with this syndrome. Allopurinol is also used commonly in oral form to treat gout (see Chapter 44). The commonly used drugs and their common specific therapeutic uses are listed in the table on p. 720.

Adverse Effects

Like most antineoplastic drugs, antimetabolites can cause hair loss, nausea, vomiting, diarrhea, and myelosuppression. The relative emetic potentials for some of these drugs are listed in Box 45-1. In addition, other major types of toxicity including neurologic, cardiovascular, pulmonary, hepatobiliary, GI, genitourinary, dermatologic, ocular, otic, and metabolic toxicity. Common manifestations of these various toxicities are listed in Table 45-6, roughly in order of increasing severity. Note that a

TABLE 45-6	Common Manifestations of Antineoplastic Toxicity
Type of Toxicity	**Common Manifestations**
Neurologic	Fatigue, weakness, depression, agitation, euphoria, insomnia, sedation, headache, reduced libido, confusion, amnesia, hallucinations (visual and auditory), dizziness, loss of taste or altered taste sensations, dysarthria (joint pain), polyneuropathy (e.g., numbness in extremities), neuritis, paresthesia (abnormal touch sensations), facial paralysis, migraine, tremor, hemiplegia, loss of consciousness, seizures, ataxia, stroke, encephalopathy
Cardiovascular	Hot flushes, edema, thrombophlebitis and bleeding (e.g., near infusion site), chest pain, tachycardia, bradycardia, other dysrhythmias, angina, venous or arterial thrombosis, transient ischemic attacks, heart failure, myocardial ischemia, pericarditis, pericardial effusion, pulmonary embolism, aneurysm, cardiomyopathy, myocardial infarction, stroke, cardiac arrest, sudden cardiac death
Pulmonary-respiratory	Cough, rhinorrhea (runny nose), sore throat, sinusitis, bronchitis, pharyngitis, laryngitis, epistaxis (nosebleed), abnormal breath sounds, asthma, bronchospasm, atelectasis, pleural effusion, hemoptysis, hypoxia, respiratory distress, pneumothorax, diffuse interstitial pneumonitis, fibrosis, hemorrhage, anaphylaxis and generalized allergic reactions
Hepatobiliary	Increased bilirubin and liver enzyme levels, jaundice, cholestasis, acalculic cholecystitis (inflamed gallbladder without stones), hepatitis, sclerosis, fibrosis, fatty liver changes, venoocclusive hepatic disease, cirrhosis
Gastrointestinal (GI)	Dyspepsia (heartburn), hiccups, gingivitis (inflamed gums), glossitis (inflamed tongue), abdominal pain, nausea, vomiting, diarrhea, constipation, gastroenteritis, stomatitis (painful mouth sores), oral candidiasis (thrush), ulcers, proctalgia (rectal pain), hematemesis, GI hemorrhage, melena (blood in stool), toxic intestinal dilation, ileus (bowel paralysis), ascites, necrotizing enterocolitis
Genitourinary (GU)	Oliguria, nocturia, dysuria, proteinuria, crystalluria, hematuria, urinary retention, abnormal renal function test results, hemorrhagic cystitis, renal failure
Dermatologic	Rash, erythema, pruritus, ecchymosis, dryness, edema, photosensitivity, sweating, discoloration (pigmentation changes), freckling, petechiae, purpura, numbness, tingling, hypersensitivity, fissuring, scaling, seborrhea, acne, eczema, psoriasis, skin hypertrophy, subcutaneous nodules, alopecia, nail disorder including onycholysis (loss of nails), dermatitis, cellulitis, excoriation, maceration, ulceration, urticaria, abscesses, benign skin neoplasm, hemorrhage (at injection site), palmar-plantar dysesthesia-paresthesia, toxic epidermal necrolysis, Stevens-Johnson syndrome
Ocular	Eye irritation, increased lacrimation, nystagmus, photophobia, visual changes, conjunctivitis, keratitis, dacryostenosis (narrowing of lacrimal duct)
Otic	Hearing loss
Metabolic	Weight loss or gain, anorexia, dehydration, hypokalemia, hypocalcemia, hypomagnesemia, hypertriglyceridemia, hyperglycemia, syndrome of inappropriate secretion of antidiuretic hormone, hypoadrenalism, protein-losing enteropathy, hyperuricemia, tumor lysis syndrome
Musculoskeletal	Back pain, limb pain, bone pain, myalgia, joint stiffness, arthralgia, muscle weakness, fibromyositis

single drug may not cause all of the specific symptoms that are listed for each toxicity category, and actual symptoms may vary widely in severity among patients. The most common general symptoms are fever and malaise. Metabolic toxicity also includes tumor lysis syndrome, a common postchemotherapy condition. This syndrome is often associated with induction (initial) chemotherapy for rapidly growing hematologic malignancies. It may include hyperphosphatemia, hyperkalemia, and hypocalcemia. These electrolyte abnormalities are often treated with diuretics such as mannitol, IV calcium supplementation, oral or rectal potassium exchange resin, and oral aluminum hydroxide. Hyperuricemia can lead to nephropathy, and hemodialysis may be required in severe cases of tumor lysis syndrome.

A severe, but usually reversible, form of dermatologic toxicity is known as *palmar-plantar dysesthesia* or paresthesia (also called *hand-foot syndrome*). It can range from mild symptoms such as painless swelling and erythema to painful blistering of the patient's palms and soles. Other severe, but fortunately uncommon, dermatologic syndromes that can similarly affect the skin in more generalized regions include Stevens-Johnson syndrome and toxic epidermal necrolysis.

Interactions

As is true for cancer drugs in general, the administration of one antimetabolite drug with another that causes similar toxicities may result in additive toxicities. Table 45-7 lists some known common examples of drugs that cause interactions with antimetabolites.

DRUG PROFILES

FOLATE ANTAGONIST

♦ methotrexate

Methotrexate is the prototypical antimetabolite of the folate antagonist group and is currently one of only three antineoplastic folate antagonists used clinically. It has proved useful for the treatment of solid tumors such as breast, head and neck, and lung cancers and for the management of acute lymphocytic leukemia and non-Hodgkin's lymphomas. Methotrexate also has immunosuppressive activity, because it can inhibit lymphocyte multiplication. For this reason, it is useful in the treatment of rheumatoid arthritis (see Chapter 47). Its combined immunosuppressant and antiinflammatory properties also make it useful for the treatment of psoriasis.

High-dose methotrexate is associated with severe bone marrow suppression and is always given in conjunction with the "rescue" drug leucovorin. Leucovorin is an antidote for folic acid antagonists. The body produces active folic acid via metabolic steps utilizing the enzyme dihydrofolate reductase. Because methotrexate inhibits this enzyme, healthy cells die due to lack of folic acid. By giving leucovorin (which is rapidly converted

TABLE 45-7   Selected Antimetabolites: Common Drug Interactions

Antimetabolite	Interacting Drug	Observed and Reported Effects*
capecitabine	warfarin	Altered coagulation test results with potential for fatal bleeding
	phenytoin	Reduced phenytoin clearance and toxicity
cytarabine	digoxin	Reduced absorption likely due to cytarabine-induced damage to intestinal mucosa; elixir form may be better absorbed
fluorouracil	warfarin	Enhanced anticoagulant effects
mercaptopurine (6-MP)	allopurinol	Inhibition of 6-MP metabolism by inhibition of xanthine oxidase enzyme, with possible enhanced 6-MP toxicity; reduce dose to one third to one fourth
	warfarin	6-MP reported to both enhance and inhibit effects of warfarin
	Hepatotoxic drugs	Increased risk for liver toxicity
methotrexate (MTX)	Protein-bound drugs and weak organic acids (e.g., salicylates, sulfonamides, sulfonylureas, phenytoin)	Possible displacement of MTX from protein-binding sites, enhancing its toxicity
	Penicillins, NSAIDs	Possible reduced renal elimination of MTX with potentially fatal hematologic and GI toxicity
	Live virus vaccines	Viral infection (true for any immunosuppressive drug)
	folic acid	Reduced MTX efficacy (theoretical only)
	theophylline	Reduced theophylline clearance
	Hepatotoxic drugs	Increased risk for liver toxicity
pentostatin	fludarabine	Potentially fatal pulmonary toxicity

NSAIDs, Nonsteroidal antiinflammatory drugs.
*Not all mechanisms for these drug interactions have been clearly identified.

INDICATIONS: SELECTED ANTIMETABOLITES

Drug (Pregnancy Category)	Pharmacologic Class	Indications
capecitabine (Xeloda) (D)	Pyrimidine antagonist (analogue)	Metastatic colorectal and breast cancer
cladribine (Leustatin) (D)	Purine antagonist (analogue)	Hairy cell leukemia
◆ cytarabine (Cytosar-U) (D)	Pyrimidine antagonist (analogue)	Leukemias (several varieties), NHL
fludarabine (Fludara) (D)	Purine antagonist (analogue)	Various acute and chronic leukemias, NHL
fluorouracil (Adrucil) (D)	Pyrimidine antagonist (analogue)	Colon, rectal, breast, esophageal, head and neck, cervical, and renal cancer
gemcitabine (Gemzar) (D)	Pyrimidine antagonist (analogue)	Pancreatic, non–small-cell lung, and bladder cancer
◆ methotrexate (Trexall, tablet form; otherwise generic) (X)	Folate antagonist (analogue)	Acute lymphocytic[†] leukemia; gestational choriocarcinoma; breast, head and neck, and many other cancers

NHL, Non-Hodgkin's lymphoma.
[†]The term *lymphocytic* is synonymous in the literature with the term *lymphoblastic.*

to the active form of folic acid), it provides the body with active folic acid, which prevents death of normal cells. Methotrexate is available in both injectable and oral (tablet) form. A preservative-free injectable formulation is required for intrathecal (into the subarachnoid space) administration, used in the treatment of some cancers. Other folate antagonists are pemetrexed and pralatrexate, which have actions similar to that of methotrexate. However, they are used less commonly than methotrexate because they have limited indications: lung cancer and T cell lymphoma, respectively.

PURINE ANTAGONISTS

The currently available purine antagonists are cladribine, fludarabine, mercaptopurine, pentostatin, and thioguanine. Mercaptopurine and thioguanine are administered orally, whereas the other three are available only in injectable form. These drugs are used largely in the treatment of leukemia and lymphoma.

cladribine

Cladribine (Leustatin) is indicated specifically for the treatment of a certain type of leukemia known as *hairy cell leukemia,* so named because of the appearance of its cancerous cells under the microscope.

fludarabine

Fludarabine (Fludara), like cladribine, also has a very specific single indication—in this case, chronic lymphocytic leukemia. It is also commonly used in the treatment of follicular lymphoma and as part of salvage therapy in acute myelogenous leukemia.

PYRIMIDINE ANTAGONISTS

The currently available pyrimidine antagonists are capecitabine, cytarabine, floxuridine, fluorouracil, and gemcitabine. These drugs are used more commonly than the purine antagonists. They are available only in parenteral formulations except for capecitabine, which is currently available only in tablet form.

capecitabine

Capecitabine (Xeloda) is indicated primarily for the treatment of metastatic breast cancer.

♦ cytarabine

Cytarabine (ara-C) (Cytosar) is used primarily for the treatment of leukemias (acute myelocytic and lymphocytic leukemia and meningeal leukemia) and non-Hodgkin's lymphomas. It is available only in injectable form and may be given IV, subcutaneously, or intrathecally. It is also now available in a special encapsulated liposomal form for intrathecal use only in treating meningeal leukemia. Cytarabine has a unique set of adverse reactions, called "cytarabine syndrome." Cytarabine syndrome is characterized by fever, muscle and bone pain, maculopapular rash, conjunctivitis, and malaise. It usually occurs 6 to 12 hours following cytarabine administration. The syndrome may be treated or prevented by the use of corticosteroids.

fluorouracil

Fluorouracil (5-FU) (Efudex, Adrucil) is used in a variety of treatment regimens, including the palliative treatment of cancers of the colon, rectum, stomach, breast, and pancreas. It also is used in the adjuvant setting in the treatment of breast and colorectal cancer.

gemcitabine

Gemcitabine (Gemzar) is an antineoplastic drug structurally related to cytarabine. Gemcitabine is believed to have antitumor activity superior to that of cytarabine. It is used as first-line therapy for locally advanced or metastatic cancer of the pancreas and for the treatment of non–small-cell lung cancer. Gemcitabine is increasingly used to treat other solid tumors, including breast cancer.

MITOTIC INHIBITORS

Mitotic inhibitors include natural products obtained from the periwinkle plant and semisynthetic drugs obtained from the mandrake plant (also known as the "may apple"). The periwinkle plant contains antineoplastic alkaloids. These vinca alkaloids include vinblastine, vincristine, and vinorelbine. Two newer plant-derived drugs are the taxanes. These include paclitaxel, once derived from the bark of the slow-growing Western (Pacific) yew tree, and docetaxel, a semisynthetic taxane produced from the needles of the European yew tree. The current process of isolating the starting material for paclitaxel from the needles has made the drug supply more abundant. Docetaxel is pharmacologically similar to paclitaxel. The newest taxanes are cabazitaxel (Jevtana), which is indicated for prostate cancer, and eribulin (Halaven), which is indicated for breast cancer.

Mechanism of Action and Drug Effects

Depending on the particular drug, these plant-derived compounds can work in various phases of the cell cycle (late S phase, throughout G_2 phase, and M phase), but they all work shortly before or during mitosis and thus retard cell division. Each different subclass inhibits mitosis in a unique way.

The vinca alkaloids (vincristine, vinblastine, and vinorelbine) bind to the protein tubulin during the metaphase of mitosis (M phase). This prevents the assembly of key structures called *microtubules*. This, in turn, results in the dissolution of other important structures known as *mitotic spindles*. Without these mitotic spindles, cells cannot reproduce properly. This results in inhibition of cell division and cell death.

The taxanes (paclitaxel, docetaxel, and cabazitaxel) act in the late G_2 phase and M phase of the cell cycle. They work by causing the formation of nonfunctional microtubules, which halts mitosis during metaphase.

Indications

Mitotic inhibitors are used to treat a variety of solid tumors and some hematologic malignancies. They are often used in combination chemotherapy regimens to enhance the overall cytotoxic effect. Selected drugs and some of their specific therapeutic uses are listed in the Indications table on the next page.

Adverse Effects

Like many of the antineoplastic drugs, mitotic inhibitor antineoplastic drugs can cause hair loss, nausea and vomiting, and myelosuppression (see Table 45-6). The emetic potential of some of these drugs is given in Box 45-1.

Toxicity and Management of Extravasation

Most of the mitotic inhibitor antineoplastics are administered IV, and extravasation of these drugs is potentially serious. Specific antidotes and additional measures to be taken for the treatment of extravasation of the mitotic inhibitors are given in Table 45-8.

Interactions

A variety of drug interactions are possible with most antineoplastic drugs, some more significant than others. A few basic principles apply to all antineoplastic drug classes. Any drug that

TABLE 45-8 Mitotic Inhibitor and Etoposide Extravasation: Listed Specific Antidote

Drug	Antidote Preparation	Method
Etoposide Teniposide Vinblastine vincristine	hyaluronidase (Wydase) 150 units/mL: add 1 mL NaCl (150 units/mL)	1. Inject 1-6 mL into the extravasated site with multiple subcut injections. 2. Repeat subcut dosing over the next few hours. 3. Apply warm compresses.* No total dose established.

subcut, Subcutaneous.

*Important: Administration of corticosteroids and topical cooling appear to worsen toxicity.

TABLE 45-9 Selected Mitotic Inhibitors and Etoposide: Common Drug Interactions

Drug	Interacting Drug	Observed and Reported Effects*
etoposide	warfarin	Enhanced anticoagulation
docetaxel	CYP3A4 inhibitors (e.g., azole antifungals, ciprofloxacin, clarithromycin, imatinib, verapamil, many others)	Enhanced docetaxel effect (possible toxicity)
	CYP3A4 inducers (e.g., carbamazepine, rifampin, phenytoin)	Reduced docetaxel effect
paclitaxel	doxorubicin	Increased cardiotoxicity
	CYP3A4 inhibitors and inducers	Same as for docetaxel
vincristine	phenytoin	Reduced phenytoin concentrations with consequent enhanced seizure risk
	CYP3A4 inhibitors and inducers	Same as for docetaxel

CYP3A4, Cytochrome P-450 liver enzyme 3A4.
*Not all mechanisms for these drug interactions have been clearly identified.

reduces the clearance of an anticancer drug also increases the risk for toxicity, whereas a drug that increases the elimination of an anticancer drug reduces its efficacy. The use of multiple antineoplastic drugs can cause severe neutropenia and infection, due to additive bone marrow suppression. Monitor and treat patients accordingly for hematologic toxicity and infections. Observed drug interactions specific for mitotic inhibitors are summarized in Table 45-9.

ALKALOID TOPOISOMERASE II INHIBITORS

Etoposide and teniposide are derivatives of epipodophyllotoxin. They exert their cytotoxic effects by inhibiting the enzyme topoisomerase II, which causes breaks in DNA strands. These drugs work during the late S phase and the G_2 phase of the cell cycle.

DRUG PROFILES
SELECTED MITOTIC INHIBITORS AND ETOPOSIDE
♦ etoposide
Etoposide (VP-16) (generic) is a topoisomerase II inhibitor. Its structure, mechanism of action, and adverse-effect profile are similar to those of teniposide. It is believed to kill cancer cells in the late S phase and the G_2 phase of the cell cycle. It is indicated for the treatment of small-cell lung cancer and testicular cancer. It is available in both oral and injectable forms. The oral form is poorly absorbed and has fallen out of favor because it produces significant toxicities without therapeutic benefit. The IV drug is formulated in a hydroalcoholic diluent, which can cause toxicity (hypotension) if administered in too high a concentration. A water-soluble form of the drug (Etopophos) can eliminate these administration issues, but it is very expensive compared with the standard preparation.

INDICATIONS: SELECTED MITOTIC INHIBITORS AND ETOPOSIDE

Drug (Pregnancy Category)	Pharmacologic Class	Indications
Epipodophyllotoxin Derivative		
♦ etoposide (Toposar, generics) (D)	Topoisomerase II inhibitor	Testicular and small-cell lung cancer
Taxane		
♦ paclitaxel (Taxol, Onxol) (D)	Mitotic inhibitor	Ovarian, breast, esophageal, bladder, head and neck, cervical cancer; non–small-cell and small-cell lung cancer; Kaposi's sarcoma
Vinca Alkaloid		
♦ vincristine (Vincasar PFS, generics) (D)	Mitotic inhibitor	ALL, AML, HL, NHL, rhabdomyosarcoma, neuroblastoma, Wilms tumor, brain tumors, small-cell lung cancer, Kaposi's sarcoma

ALL, Acute lymphocytic leukemia; *AML,* acute myelocytic leukemia; *HL,* Hodgkin's lymphoma; *NHL,* non-Hodgkin's lymphoma.

♦ paclitaxel
Paclitaxel (Taxol) is a natural mitotic inhibitor that was originally isolated from the bark of the Pacific yew tree. The European yew tree is the source for another mitotic inhibitor known as docetaxel (Taxotere). Paclitaxel is currently approved for the treatment of ovarian cancer, breast cancer, non–small-cell lung cancer, and Kaposi's sarcoma, among other cancers. Paclitaxel is water-insoluble (hydrophobic), and for this reason it is put into a solution containing oil rather than water. The particular oil used is a type of castor oil called Cremophor EL, the same oil with which cyclosporine is formulated. Many patients tolerate it poorly and show hypersensitivity associated with infusion. For this reason, before patients receive paclitaxel they are premedicated with a steroid (dexamethasone), H_1 receptor antagonist (diphenhydramine), and H_2 receptor antagonist (ranitidine). Paclitaxel is available only in injectable form. There is an albumin-bound form of the drug (Abraxane) that is not associated with severe infusion reactions.

♦ vincristine
Vincristine is an alkaloid isolated from the periwinkle plant that is indicated for the treatment of acute lymphocytic leukemia and other cancers. It is available only in injectable form. It is an M phase–specific drug that inhibits mitotic spindle formation. Vincristine is the most significant neurotoxin of the cytotoxic drug class, but it continues to be used in part because of its relative lack of bone marrow suppression. Special care must be taken not to inadvertently give vincristine via the intrathecal route. Several deaths have been reported due to this error. The World Health Organization and the Institute for Safe Medication Practices suggest that vincristine be diluted in

25 to 50 mL of fluid and never dispensed via a syringe to prevent this lethal error from occurring. A special warning is required for all vincristine products dispensed that states "For Intravenous Use Only—Fatal If Given By Other Routes." (See Safety and Quality Improvement: Preventing Medication Errors below.)

QSEN ⚡ SAFETY AND QUALITY IMPROVEMENT: PREVENTING MEDICATION ERRORS

Vincristine: Right Route Is Essential

For several years, the Institute for Safe Medication Practices has recommended changes in procedures to ensure that vincristine and other vinca alkaloids are not given intrathecally (via the spinal route) or by any other route. Administering these drugs through the spinal route is almost always fatal, and the death is slow and excruciating. Mistakes occur when the drug is drawn up in a syringe for intravenous administration and then is inadvertently given via the intrathecal route. These errors are preventable. Pharmacies should prepare vincristine in a diluted volume, such as in a 50-mL minibag of normal saline, to deter practitioners from giving the drug intrathecally. Drugs given intrathecally are not normally dispensed in a minibag. The nurse, who may be assisting the health care practitioner with intrathecal procedures, needs to be aware of the potential fatal error that may occur if vincristine is given via the wrong route.

Data from Institute for Safe Medication Practices. Available at *www.ismp.org/tools/bestpractices/TMSBP-for-Hospitals.pdf*. Accessed August 2, 2015.

TOPOISOMERASE I INHIBITORS

Topoisomerase I inhibitors are a relatively new class of chemotherapy drugs. The two drugs currently available in this class are topotecan and irinotecan. Both are semisynthetic analogues of the compound camptothecin, which was originally isolated in the 1960s from *Camptotheca acuminata*, a Chinese shrub. For this reason, these drugs are also referred to as *camptothecins*.

Mechanism of Action and Drug Effects

The camptothecins inhibit proper DNA function in the S phase by binding to the DNA–topoisomerase I complex. This complex normally allows DNA strands to be temporarily cleaved and then reattached in a critical step known as *religation*. The binding of the camptothecin drugs to this complex retards this religation process, which results in a DNA strand break.

Indications

The two currently available topoisomerase I inhibitors are used primarily to treat ovarian and colorectal cancer. Topotecan has been shown to be effective even in cases of metastatic ovarian cancer that have failed to respond to platinum-containing regimens (e.g., cisplatin, carboplatin) and paclitaxel. Topotecan is also used to treat small-cell lung cancer. Irinotecan is currently approved for the treatment of metastatic colorectal cancer, small-cell lung cancer, and cervical cancer.

Adverse Effects

The main adverse effect of topotecan is bone marrow suppression. Other adverse effects are relatively minor compared with those of the other antineoplastic drug classes. These include mild to moderate nausea, vomiting, and diarrhea; headache; rash; muscle weakness; and cough.

Irinotecan causes more severe adverse effects than topotecan. In addition to producing similar hematologic adverse effects, it has been associated with severe diarrhea known as *cholinergic diarrhea*. It is recommended that this condition be treated with atropine unless use of that drug is strongly contraindicated. Delayed diarrhea may occur 2 to 10 days after infusion of irinotecan. This diarrhea can be severe and even life-threatening and must be treated aggressively with loperamide. There is a moderate risk for nausea and vomiting with irinotecan, which requires appropriate supportive care such as IV rehydration and antiemetic drug therapy.

Interactions

Topotecan has a unique drug interaction involving the granulocyte colony-stimulating factor filgrastim (see Chapter 47). Filgrastim is commonly used to enhance WBC recovery after chemotherapy. When topotecan is given along with filgrastim, myelosuppression has actually been shown to be worsened. It is recommended that filgrastim be administered 24 hours after completion of the topotecan infusion. Laxatives and diuretics are not given with irinotecan, because of the potential to worsen the dehydration resulting from the severe diarrhea that this drug can produce. Severe cardiovascular toxicity, including thrombosis, pulmonary embolism, stroke, and acute fatal myocardial infarction, have been reported when irinotecan is given with fluorouracil and leucovorin. The role of irinotecan in this toxicity syndrome is unclear, because fluorouracil is a well-recognized cause of myocardial ischemia, including myocardial infarction and sudden death. Such drug combinations are given with careful monitoring. Several additional recognized drug interactions occur with irinotecan, which are summarized in Table 45-10.

DRUG PROFILES

irinotecan

Irinotecan (Camptosar) is often given with both fluorouracil and leucovorin. It is available only in injectable form.

topotecan

After initial therapy with other antineoplastics, cancer cells commonly become resistant to their effects. The use of topotecan (Hycamtin) to treat ovarian cancer and small-cell lung cancer has been studied extensively. As noted earlier, it produces therapeutic responses, even in cases in which powerful drugs such as cisplatin and paclitaxel have failed. Topotecan is available only in injectable form.

ANTINEOPLASTIC ENZYMES

Two antineoplastic enzymes are commercially available: asparaginase and pegaspargase. A third, *Erwinia* asparaginase, is available only by special request from the National Cancer Institute for patients who have developed allergic reactions to *Escherichia coli*–based asparaginase. All three drugs are

TABLE 45-10 Irinotecan: Common Drug Interactions

Interacting Drug	Observed and Reported Effects*
CYP2B6 inhibitors (e.g., paroxetine, sertraline)	Increased effects and toxicity of irinotecan
CYP3A4 inhibitors (e.g., azole antifungals, ciprofloxacin, clarithromycin, imatinib, isoniazid, verapamil)	Increased effects and toxicity of irinotecan; concurrent use not recommended
CYP2B6 inducers (e.g., carbamazepine, phenytoin, nevirapine)	Reduced effects of irinotecan
CYP3A4 inducers (e.g., aminoglutethimide, rifampin, nevirapine, phenytoin)	Reduced effects of irinotecan
St. John's wort (CYP3A4 inducer)	Reduced effects of irinotecan; stop St. John's wort 2 wk before initiating irinotecan therapy

CYP2B6, Cytochrome P-450 liver enzyme 2B6; *CYP3A4,* cytochrome P-450 liver enzyme 3A4.
*Note that not all mechanisms for these drug interactions have been clearly identified.

INDICATIONS: SELECTED TOPOISOMERASE I INHIBITORS

Drug (Pregnancy Category)	Pharmacologic Class	Indications
irinotecan (Camptosar) (D)	Synthetic camptothecin	Metastatic colorectal cancer, small-cell lung cancer, cervical cancer
topotecan (Hycamtin) (D)	Semisynthetic camptothecin	Ovarian and small-cell lung cancer

synthesized from cultures of certain bacteria using recombinant DNA technology.

Indications

The antineoplastic enzymes are currently approved exclusively for the treatment of acute lymphocytic leukemia.

Adverse Effects

Of particular note for the antineoplastic enzymes is a fairly unique adverse effect of impaired pancreatic function. This can lead to hyperglycemia and severe or fatal pancreatitis. Other types of adverse effects associated with these drugs are dermatologic, hepatic, genitourinary, neurologic, musculoskeletal, GI, and cardiovascular effects.

Interactions

Commonly reported drug interactions involving the antineoplastic enzymes are summarized in Table 45-11.

DRUG PROFILES

◆ asparaginase

Asparaginase (Elspar) is used for the treatment of acute lymphocytic leukemia. Its mechanism of action is slightly different

TABLE 45-11 Selected Antineoplastic Enzymes: Common Drug Interactions

Enzyme	Interacting Drug	Observed and Reported Effects*
asparaginase	cyclophosphamide, mercaptopurine, vincristine	Interference with efficacy or clearance of asparaginase
	mercaptopurine, methotrexate, prednisone	Enhanced liver toxicity of asparaginase
	methotrexate	Reduced antineoplastic effect when given concurrently, but possibly enhanced antineoplastic effect when given 9 to 10 days before or shortly after methotrexate
	prednisone	Hyperglycemia (give asparaginase after prednisone)
	vincristine	Neuropathy (give asparaginase after vincristine)
	aspirin, NSAIDs, dipyridamole, heparin, warfarin	Use with caution due to possible coagulation abnormalities

NSAIDs, Nonsteroidal antiinflammatory drugs.
*Note that not all mechanisms for these drug interactions have been clearly identified.

from that of traditional antineoplastic drugs in that it is an enzyme that catalyzes the conversion of the amino acid asparagine to aspartic acid and ammonia. Leukemic cells are then unable to synthesize the asparagine required for the synthesis of DNA and proteins needed for cell survival.

The only commercially available asparaginase product in the United States is Elspar. It is derived from the *E. coli* bacterium, and it is common for patients to develop allergic reactions to it. When this happens, one alternative is to switch to a product synthesized from *Erwinia* bacteria. This product is not sold commercially in the United States but is available by special request from the National Cancer Institute. Another treatment alternative is to use the commercially available pegaspargase product described in the following drug profile. All antineoplastic enzymes are available only in injectable form.

pegaspargase

Pegaspargase (Oncaspar) has a mechanism of action, indications, and contraindications similar to those of asparaginase. It is essentially the same enzyme that has been formulated so as to reduce its allergenic potential. This process involves chemical conjugation of the enzyme with units of a relatively inert compound known as monomethoxypolyethylene glycol. Because polyethylene glycol is abbreviated PEG, this process is known as *pegylation.* It is a process that is increasingly used in formulating various drugs, some of which are described in other chapters (e.g., see Chapter 47). These drugs are recognized by the prefix *peg* in their generic names. Pegaspargase is usually prescribed for patients who have developed an allergy to asparaginase—a common occurrence, as mentioned earlier, especially with repeated treatment.

INDICATIONS: SELECTED ANTINEOPLASTIC ENZYMES

Drug (Pregnancy Category)	Pharmacologic Class	Indications
♦ asparaginase (Elspar) (C)	*Escherichia coli*–derived L-asparagine amidohydrolase enzyme	Acute lymphocytic leukemia
pegaspargase (Oncaspar) (C)	Pegylated version of asparaginase	Acute lymphocytic leukemia (usually in patients who have developed an allergy to asparaginase)

NURSING PROCESS

ASSESSMENT

With *antineoplastic therapy*, perform the following components of a thorough physical assessment: nursing assessment including past and present medical history and family history; medication profile with a listing of allergies and all prescription drugs, over-the-counter (OTC) drugs, herbals, and supplements; height and weight; vital signs; and baseline hearing and vision testing (as ordered). Assess bowel and bladder patterns, neurologic status, heart sounds, heart rhythm, breath sounds, and lung function. Examine the skin and mucosa, giving attention to turgor, hydration, color, and temperature. Note any signs and symptoms of fear and anxiety with attention to complaints of insomnia, irritability, shakiness, restlessness, and/or palpitations. Complete a thorough assessment of cultural, emotional, spiritual, sexual, and financial influences, concerns, and issues. Assess the patient's past and present ability to perform activities of daily living and the patient's mobility status, gait, and balance. Perform a pain assessment using objective methods such as an intensity rating scale (e.g., 0 to 10, where 0 = no pain and 10 = worst pain ever). Note the pattern of pain, focusing on the location, quality, onset, duration, and precipitating or alleviating factors. Document any oral, pharyngeal, esophageal, and/or abdominal pain; painful swallowing; epigastric or gastric pain, especially after eating spicy or acidic foods; achiness in joints or lower extremities; or numbness, tingling, burning sensation, or sharp pain in the extremities. Question the patient about past experiences with pain and about any drug, nondrug, or alternative therapies used as well as any previous successes or failures in pain management. Cultural beliefs and background as they relate to pain are important to assess because the individual's culture may affect how pain is perceived, verbalized, and treated (see Chapter 10). Culture and racial ethnicity also impact a patient's perspective on health, illness, as well as treatment of illnesses (see Chapters 2 and 4).

Assess contraindications, cautions, and drug interactions. Thoroughly review and document the findings prior to the use of these drugs. Laboratory tests that are usually ordered, but not limited to, include levels of the following: electrolytes, minerals, vitamins, uric acid, red blood cell and white blood cell count, platelets/clotting and bleeding time, renal function (BUN, creatinine, serum uric acid, urine creatinine clearance), hepatic function (AST, ALT, LDH, bilirubin), and cardiac enzymes (see

BOX 45-2 Effects of Antineoplastic Drugs on Normal Cells and Related Adverse Effects

Antineoplastic drugs are designed to kill rapidly dividing *cancer* cells, but they also kill rapidly dividing *normal* cells. Such normal cells include cells of the oral and gastrointestinal (GI) mucous membranes, hair follicles, reproductive germinal epithelium, and components of bone marrow (e.g., WBCs, RBCs, platelets). The more common adverse effects of normal cell kill are as follows:

- Killing of normal cells of the GI mucous membranes may result in adverse effects such as *altered nutritional status, stomatitis* with inflammation and/or ulceration of the oral mucosa throughout the GI tract, *altered bowel function, poor appetite, nausea, vomiting* (often intractable and requiring aggressive antiemetic treatment), and *diarrhea.*
- Killing of the normal cells of hair follicles leads to *alopecia* (loss of hair).
- Killing of normal cells in the bone marrow results in dangerously low (life-threatening) blood cell counts. Because of the negative impact on these normal cells, the nurse must carefully assess the patient's WBCs levels (leukocytes, neutrophils, and band neutrophils), RBC counts, hemoglobin level, hematocrit, and platelet counts (see Safety: Laboratory Values Related to Drug Therapy on the next page). In addition, monitoring of the patient's absolute neutrophil count (ANC) is needed (ANC = % of neutrophils + % bands × WBC). Monitoring ANC values allows the nurse and other health care providers to identify the nadir—the time of the lowest count when the patient is most vulnerable. An ANC of 500 cells/mm^3 or lower indicates high risk for infection.
- Killing of germinal epithelial cells (also rapidly dividing) leads to *sterility* (irreversible) in males, damage to the ovaries with subsequent *amenorrhea* in females, and *teratogenic* effects with possible fetal death in pregnant women.
- Killing of cells leads to release of waste products, such as uric acid, into the blood, resulting in hyperuricemia.

Safety: Laboratory Values Related to Drug Therapy on the next page). Assays of tumor markers may also be ordered to establish baseline levels and determine the impact of the disease and subsequent therapeutic effectiveness (see Safety: Laboratory Values Related to Drug Therapy on p. 727). For more information about the specific adverse effects associated with the destruction of various populations of normal cells due to chemotherapy, see Box 45-2. Specific areas of assessment related to some of the more common adverse effects of chemotherapy on normal, rapidly dividing cells include the following:

- For *altered nutritional status* and *impaired oral mucosa:* Assess signs and symptoms of altered nutrition with a focus on weight loss, abnormal serum protein-albumin and blood urea nitrogen (BUN) levels (a negative nitrogen status due to low protein levels would be indicated by a decreasing BUN level), weakness, fatigue, lethargy, poor skin turgor, and pale conjunctiva. Assess oral mucosa for any signs and symptoms of stomatitis, such as pain or burning in the mouth, difficulty swallowing, taste changes, viscous saliva, dryness, cracking, and/or fissures with or without bleeding of the mucosa.
- For *effects on the GI mucosa:* Assess bowel sounds (hyperactive or hypoactive versus normoactive). Assess presence of diarrhea, such as frequent, loose stools (more than three stools per day), urgency, and abdominal cramping. Assess for the presence of blood in the stool as well as consistency, color, odor, and amount. Assess for nausea and vomiting, and determine whether symptoms are acute, delayed, or anticipatory (occurring in future); if vomiting occurs,

QSEN ⚡ SAFETY: LABORATORY VALUES RELATED TO DRUG THERAPY

Rationales for Assessment and Monitoring of Blood Cell Counts with Antineoplastics

Antineoplastic drugs kill both normal and abnormal cells that are rapidly dividing, and thus the bone marrow and its rapidly dividing cellular constituents are negatively impacted. Because of this characteristic of chemotherapeutic drugs, RBCs, WBCs, and platelets are suppressed and therefore their levels require frequent monitoring. This box presents information specifically on RBCs and hemoglobin (Hgb) and hematocrit (Hct) levels as well as platelet levels. Chapter 46 presents more information on WBCs with neutrophil counts and nadir levels.

Laboratory Test	Normal Ranges	Rationale for Assessment
RBC count	M: 4.6-6.2 million cells/mm^3 F: 4.2-5.4 million cells/mm^3	Bone marrow suppression from antineoplastics affects RBC values, leading to severe anemia. RBCs carry oxygen—attached to the hemoglobin—from the lungs to the rest of the body. RBCs also help carry carbon dioxide back to the lungs for exhalation. Therefore, if RBC counts are low (e.g., with anemia), the body does not get the oxygen it needs, which leads to lack of energy, fatigue, intolerance of activity, shortness of breath, and hypoxemia. For the cancer patient who may already be experiencing the effects of bone marrow suppression from the disease and then from the treatment, this loss of oxygen saturation will be exacerbated, resulting in a lesser ability to get up and about and perform activities of daily living.
Hct	M: 40%-54% F: 37%-47%	Hct measures the amount of space or volume of RBCs in the blood, so if the RBC value is low the Hct is also low. The impact of this low value is discussed above under RBC count.
Hgb level	M: 14-18 g/dL F: 12-16 g/dL	Hgb is the major substance in RBCs. It carries oxygen and is responsible for the red color of the blood cell. With low levels of Hgb, the consequence to the patient is as noted with RBCs.
Platelet count	150,000-140,000 platelets/mm^3	Platelets are the smallest type of blood cell and play a large role in the process of blood clotting. When bleeding occurs, the platelets swell, clump, and form a plug that helps stop the bleeding. Therefore, if platelet levels are lower than 100,000 platelets/mm^3, the patient is at high risk for uncontrolled bleeding and/or hemorrhage. Some guidelines may use a platelet count of 50,000 platelets/mm^3 and above as the criterion. Seek out further information in policies and procedures, or contact the prescriber.

F, Female; *M*, male.

---

determine the color, amount, consistency, frequency, and odor, and whether blood is present (hematemesis). The severity of nausea and vomiting may be rated using a scale of 1 to 10 (where 10 is the worst symptoms) or using the terms mild, moderate, and severe.

- For *alopecia:* Assess the patient's views, concerns, and emotions about potential hair loss. Assess the patient's need to prepare for hair loss, either by leaving the hair as it is and allowing it to fall out on its own; having the hair cut short; or wearing a scarf, hat, bandana, or hair wrap and/or purchasing a wig before the hair is actually lost. Purchasing a wig prior to chemotherapy will allow for a closer match to a patient's pre-chemotherapy hairstyle.

- For *bone marrow suppression:* Assess for signs and symptoms of anemia or a decrease in RBCs, hemoglobin level, and hematocrit (e.g., pallor of the skin, oral mucous membranes, and conjunctiva; fatigue; lethargy; loss of interest in activities; shortness of breath; and inability to concentrate). Assess for signs and symptoms of leukopenia (decrease in WBCs [see Chapter 46] and/or absolute neutrophil count [ANC; normal range is 1500 cells/mm^3, with severe neutropenia being less than 500 cells/mm^3]), including fever; chills; tachycardia; abnormal breath sounds; productive cough with purulent, green, or rust-colored sputum; change in the color of the urine; lethargy, fatigue; and acute confusion. Assess for signs and symptoms of thrombocytopenia (decrease in thrombocytes [usually less than 100,000] and platelet clotting factors), including indications of unusual bleeding such as petechiae; purpura; ecchymosis; gingival (gum) bleeding; excessive or prolonged bleeding from puncture sites (e.g., intramuscular or IV administration sites or blood draw sites); unusual joint pain; blood in the stool, urine, or vomitus; loss of function in extremities; and a decrease in blood pressure with elevated pulse rate (see Safety: Laboratory Values Related to Drug Therapy above as well as those in Chapters 26 and 27; see also Box 45-2). Always assess for the normal ranges of laboratory values.

- For possible *sterility, teratogenesis,* and damage to ovaries with *amenorrhea:* In adult male patients, assess baseline reproductive history with attention to sexual functioning, fathering of children, and past and current reproductive or sexual problems or concerns. In female adult patients, in addition to the relevant aspects already mentioned, inquire about fertility, menstrual and childbearing history, and age of onset of menses and menopause, if applicable.

With *cell cycle–specific drugs,* document all allergies, cautions, contraindications, and drug interactions. Most *antimetabolite drugs* do not produce severe emesis (i.e., in fewer than 10% of cases). *Pentostatin* and some of the *pyrimidine analogues* have emetic potential, so perform an assessment of baseline GI functioning when giving these drugs. In addition, the folate antagonists are not as likely to cause emesis but may be associated with GI abnormalities, such as ulcers and stomatitis. Because these drugs are generally administered parenterally (IV), assessing peripheral access areas or central venous sites is critical to prevent the risk for damage to surrounding tissue, joints, and

SAFETY: LABORATORY VALUES RELATED TO DRUG THERAPY

Tumor Markers Associated with Cancer Diagnosis, Management, and Monitoring

Tumor markers are substances found in blood, urine, stool, bodily fluids, or tissues of some patients with cancer. They are used to help detect, diagnose, and manage some types of cancer as well as predict a patient's response to certain therapies/treatment and to determine recurrence. Tumor markers are combined with other tests, such as biopsies. They are also used in the staging of cancers. There are over 20 tumor markers that are made by normal cells as well as cancer cells, but higher levels are noted in cancerous conditions. Most tumor markers are proteins, but patterns of gene expression and changes to DNA are now used as tumor markers. Tumor markers are measured periodically during cancer treatment to see if levels are decreased or returned to normal, indicating a response to therapy. If there is no change or an increase in the levels, then the tumor is not responding to treatment. The American Society of Clinical Oncology (ASCO) publishes clinical practice guidelines on tumor markers. Some of the tumor markers being used for a wide range of cancer types that meet standards established by the Clinical Laboratory Improvement Amendments include the following:

Tumor Marker	Type of Malignancy
ALK (anaplastic lymphoma kinase) gene arrangements	Non–small-cell lung cancer Anaplastic large-cell lymphoma
AFP (alpha-fetoprotein)	Liver Germ cell tumors
B2M (beta-2-microglobulin)	Multiple myeloma Chronic lymphocytic leukemia Lymphoma
CA15-3/CA27.29 (cancer antigen 15-3; 27.29)	Breast cancer
CA125 (cancer antigen 125)	Ovarian cancer
Calcitonin	Medullary thyroid cancer
ER/PR (estrogen receptor; progesterone receptor)	Breast cancer
HER2/neu (human epidermal growth factor receptor 2; also called HER-2)	Breast, gastric and esophageal cancer
Immunoglobulins	Multiple myeloma
PSA (prostate-specific antigen)	Prostate cancer
Thyroglobulin	Thyroid cancer

tendons. Assess IV sites every hour for redness, swelling, heat and pain, as needed, or as per institutional protocol. One specific assessment consideration associated with the use of the antimetabolite *cytarabine* is monitoring for the occurrence of cytarabine syndrome. This syndrome usually occurs within 6 to 12 hours after drug administration and is characterized by fever, muscle and bone pain, maculopapular rash, conjunctivitis, and malaise. Assessment and quick identification of this syndrome may lead to its prevention and appropriate treatment.

In patients receiving *mitotic inhibitors* (e.g., *vinblastine, vincristine*) and *alkaloid topoisomerase II inhibitors* (e.g., *etoposide*), perform baseline hepatic and renal function tests, as ordered. Serum uric acid levels are usually ordered because these levels rise with increased cell death from cancer and/or its treatment. The increase in uric acid may precipitate or exacerbate gout, which, if diagnosed accurately, may be managed. Other mitotic inhibitors, *docetaxel* and *paclitaxel*, are associated

with severe neutropenia and a decrease in platelet counts (see Safety: Laboratory Values Related to Drug Therapy on this page as well as in Chapter 47); therefore, CBCs are ordered before, during, and after drug therapy. Constantly assess the patient during and after treatment for severe hypersensitivity reactions characterized by dyspnea, severe hypotension, angioedema, and generalized urticaria. Drops in blood cell counts may even occur before any clinical evidence is present, which is why it is important to monitor these laboratory values. Note baseline neurologic functioning with attention to any confusion as well as changes in level of alertness/consciousness. Assess for the presence of any peripheral neuropathies. Because these drugs have multiple incompatibilities and are irritants (irritating the IV site and vein) or vesicants (causing cell death with extravasation and necrosis with ulcerations), you must become familiar with potential solution and/or drug interactions. Consulting with the prescriber and pharmacist as well as current authoritative resources would be appropriate. Documentation must include initial and frequent follow-up assessments of the IV site.

Topoisomerase I inhibitors are associated with hematologic adverse effects; thus, perform baseline WBC counts as ordered. Bone marrow suppression is predictable, noncumulative, reversible, and manageable; therefore, do not give drugs such as topotecan to patients with baseline neutrophil counts of fewer than 1500 cells/mm³. *Irinotecan* causes more severe adverse effects than *topotecan*; assess related systems and note the findings. The potential for irinotecan-related cholinergic diarrhea requires continual assessment of the gastrointestinal tract. Diarrhea may appear 2 to 10 days after the irinotecan infusion. If severe forms of diarrhea occur, the patient requires further medical treatment. The diarrhea may even be life-threatening. There is only a moderate risk for nausea and vomiting with irinotecan, which requires immediate and appropriate assessment and care. Drug interactions to assess for include the concurrent administration of topotecan with *filgrastim*, which results in a worsening of myelosuppression. Do not give laxatives or diuretics with irinotecan due to the potential for severe diarrhea, volume loss, and subsequent dehydration. When given with *fluorouracil* and *leucovorin*, severe cardiovascular toxicity (including thrombosis), pulmonary embolism, stroke, and acute fatal myocardial infarction may occur. Perform a cautious and skillful assessment of related systems. See Table 45-10 for more drug interactions.

With the use of *natural enzyme* drugs (e.g., *asparaginase, pegaspargase*), assess pancreatic function because of the potential for severe or even fatal pancreatitis. Because of this risk for pancreatitis, assess the patient closely for moderate to severe abdominal pain (upper-left quadrant), nausea, vomiting, and hyperglycemia. Serum alkaline phosphatase and WBC counts, if elevated, may indicate possible pancreatitis if also supported by clinical presentation. Additionally, assessment and documentation of dermatologic, hepatic, genitourinary, neurologic, musculoskeletal, GI, and cardiovascular systems is important due to the drug's impact on these systems.

Genetic considerations are an additional area of importance in the treatment of cancer with *antineoplastics*, as well as with all drug therapy. Assess patients for the presence of the following characteristics before chemotherapy is initiated: (1) genetic markers for oral cancers, (2) genetic determinants of testosterone or estrogen metabolism, and (3) genetically linked enzyme system abnormalities such as those involving specific cytochrome P-450 enzymes that metabolically convert nicotine to a carcinogenic substance. These genetic factors are very complex; nevertheless, be aware of the possible influence of genetic differences and be forward in your critical thinking on the impact of drug research and genetics. See Chapter 8 for more information on genetics as related to drug therapy and the nursing process.

NURSING DIAGNOSES

1. Diarrhea related to the adverse effects of antineoplastic drugs
2. Acute pain related to the disease process and drug-induced joint pain, stomatitis, GI distress, and other discomforts associated with antineoplastic cell cycle–specific therapy
3. Risk for infection related to drug-induced bone marrow suppression with possible leukopenia and neutropenia

PLANNING: OUTCOME IDENTIFICATION

1. Patient regains as near normal as possible bowel elimination patterns with control of diarrhea through dietary restrictions, hydration, and drug therapy during antineoplastic therapy.
2. Patient achieves improved comfort levels with reporting of pain before it is uncontrollable/severe with improved nonpharmacologic and pharmacologic pain control, and symptom and adverse effect management.
3. Patient remains free from infection while under the influence of chemotherapeutic treatment and through thorough hand washing, hydration, balanced diet, mouth care, and avoiding crowds.

(Note that the nursing diagnoses, goals, and outcome criteria presented here are appropriate to treatment with many antineoplastic drugs.)

IMPLEMENTATION

Antineoplastic drugs are some of the most toxic medications given to patients because they cause the death of normal cells along with the death of cancer cells. The high potency of these drugs also places the patient at higher risk for toxicity, serious complications, and adverse effects. The possibility of such adverse effects and toxicities requires skillful nursing care based on cautious and thorough assessment and subsequent critical thinking. General considerations in nursing implementation applicable to most antineoplastic drugs as well as some specific aspects of implementation related to *cell cycle–specific drugs* are presented in the following paragraphs. In the following paragraphs, the specific adverse effect(s) associated with cell cycle–specific drugs will be discussed and are italicized. Other nursing process information related to cell cycle–nonspecific drugs is presented in Chapter 46.

For antineoplastic therapy in general, nursing considerations related to *reducing fear* and *anxiety* include establishing a therapeutic relationship beginning with trust and empathy. Approach the patient in a warm, empathic, and supportive manner while projecting confidence in providing nursing care. Provide individualized explanations and teaching about the patient's illness, care, and treatments that are appropriate to the patient's educational level. Collaborate with all members of the health care team. Encourage patients to consider relaxation techniques such as listening to music, performing meditation, or engaging in guided imagery. It may be necessary to call on all potential sources of support, including social services, counseling services, financial assistance services, Meals On Wheels, and religious-spiritual or belief systems with respect to the patient's needs. Appropriate consults may also be necessary with other practitioners such as a licensed clinical social worker, discharge planner, clinical psychiatrist, mental health nurse, nurse practitioner, and oncology nurse specialist, as well as with support groups for the patient, family, and/or significant others.

A variety of interventions that may be indicated for the management of *stomatitis* or excessive oral mucosa dryness and irritation include the following: (1) Instruct the patient to perform oral hygiene before and after eating or as needed to provide cleanliness and comfort. Advise the patient to avoid lemon, glycerin, undiluted peroxide, or alcohol-containing products because they are drying and irritating to the oral mucosa. (2) Recommend use of a soft-bristle toothbrush or soft-tipped toothette or swab with solutions of diluted warm saline. (3) If dentures are worn, encourage the patient to remove and clean them frequently and, if stomatitis is severe, to insert only at mealtimes. (4) Advise using OTC saliva substitutes, keeping the lips moist, and using sugarless candy or gum to stimulate saliva flow. (5) Stress that spicy, acidic, or hot foods; alcohol; and tobacco must be avoided because they are irritants. (6) Oral antifungal suspensions (e.g., nystatin) may be ordered if white patches are noted on the oral mucosa; use analgesic solutions (e.g., lidocaine swish and swallow), as ordered, to help manage discomfort. Other regimens may be prescribed, as needed.

Nausea and vomiting occur commonly with antineoplastic drugs. Emetic potential varies depending on the drug and treatment protocol (see earlier discussion and Box 45-1). Educate the patient on measures to enhance comfort during times of nausea and vomiting, including restricting oral intake as ordered; removing noxious odors or sights to avoid stimulating the vomiting center; performing oral hygiene as needed; promoting relaxation through slow, deep breathing; consuming small, frequent meals and eating slowly; and consuming clear liquids and a bland diet. Use of IV fluids may be indicated for hydration purposes if nausea and vomiting are severe. Antiemetics are also a vital part of antineoplastic therapy (see Chapter 52 for more specific drug-related information). Premedication with antiemetics 30 to 60 minutes before administration of the antineoplastic(s) is the preferred treatment protocol to help reduce nausea and vomiting, prevent dehydration and malnutrition, and promote comfort. Combination antiemetic drug therapy may be more effective than single-drug therapy. An antiemetic may be given with the chemotherapeutic regimen and prescription medication for at-home use. Ginger ale and ginger-based teas may be helpful. While its exact anti-nausea mechanism is unknown, it is thought that there are chemicals in ginger that influence the nervous system, stomach, and intestines to reduce nausea.

Diarrhea is also a common adverse effect of antineoplastic therapy. Perform the following nursing interventions: (1) Advise the patient to avoid or limit oral intake of irritating, spicy, and gas-producing foods; caffeine; high-fiber foods; alcohol; very hot or cold foods or beverages; and lactose-containing foods and beverages. (2) Consult appropriate personnel, as ordered, to help the patient and family plan meals and arrange ways to meet the patient's dietary and bowel elimination needs. (3) Administer opioids (e.g., paregoric) or synthetic opioids (e.g., loperamide, diphenoxylate hydrochloride) as prescribed, for their antidiarrheal properties. Adsorbents-protectants and anti-secretory drugs may also help reduce GI upset and diarrhea (see Chapter 51).

To address *nutritional concerns,* the following measures may prove beneficial in improving oral intake and nutritional status: (1) Perform a 24-hour recall of food intake, and report the typical week's diet for the patient. (2) Use antiemetic therapy, pain management, mouth care, and hydration, as ordered, to reduce the adverse effects of therapy and improve appetite. (3) To ease taste alterations, advise the patient to consume mild-tasting foods and to use chicken, turkey, cheese, or Greek yogurt for protein sources as tolerated. (4) Provide plastic rather than metal utensils if the patient complains of a metallic taste. (5) Encourage eating foods that are easy to swallow, such as cus-tards; gelatins; puddings; milkshakes; eggnog; commercially prepared high-protein, high-calorie supplemental shakes; mashed white or sweet potatoes; blended drinks with crushed ice, fruit, and yogurt; nutritional supplement drinks and snacks; frozen popsicles; and lactose-free ice cream. (6) Instruct the patient to avoid sticky or dry foods. (7) Encourage the con-sumption of small, frequent meals in an environment that is conducive to eating (e.g., free of odors and excess noise). (8) Appetite stimulants such as megestrol acetate or dronabinol may be helpful. (9) Encourage the patient to practice energy conservation, with frequent rest periods before and after meals.

Alopecia is a common adverse effect of antineoplastics and is very disturbing regardless of age or gender. Warn the patient and family about the possibility of hair loss, and tell them when it will occur (usually 7 to 10 days after treatment begins but dependent upon the specific drug used) and that it is reversible. Inform the patient that new hair growth is often a different color and/or texture from the hair lost. Provide information about the options of acquiring a wig or hairpiece, or wearing scarves or hats, before the actual hair loss. The American Cancer Society may be a resource for items such as wigs, scarves, and hats.

Antineoplastic-induced *bone marrow suppression* leads to *anemias, leukopenia, neutropenia,* and *thrombocytopenia* (see previous discussion and Safety: Laboratory Values Related to

Drug Therapy on pp. 726 and 727 in this chapter and Chapter 46). Anemias result in fatigue and loss of energy and are common adverse effects of therapy and the disease process. *Anemias* may require blood transfusions, peripheral blood stem cell treatment, or treatment with prescribed medications such as iron preparations, folic acid, or erythropoietic growth factors (e.g., epoetin or darbepoetin alfa). These injections may be given at home and may be administered at the first sign of a decrease in RBC counts. Conservation of energy and planning of care is very important in minimizing patient fatigue.

Risk for infection from *leukopenia* or *neutropenia* and/or immunosuppression is one of the more significant adverse effects that requires close attention. Inform the patient and family and/or caregivers that when WBC counts are low, the patient is at high risk for infection and that defenses remain low until the counts recover. Following Standard Precautions and using good handwashing technique are most important in pre-venting transmission of infection in the hospital and home settings. Because fever is a principal early sign of infection, take oral or axillary temperature at least every 4 hours during periods in which the patient is at risk. Avoid taking the temperature rectally to minimize tissue trauma, breaks in skin integrity, and thus loss of the first line of defense and increased risk for infec-tion. Encourage the patient to immediately report to the pre-scriber a temperature elevation of 100.5° F (38.1° C) or higher so that appropriate treatment may be initiated and complica-tions avoided.

If needed, and as ordered, administration of colony-stimulating factors may be beneficial. Filgrastim, pegfilgrastim, and sargramostim are examples of drugs given to accelerate WBC recovery during antineoplastic drug therapy. Use these drugs, as ordered, to minimize neutropenia. These medications act on the bone marrow to enhance neutrophil production and help decrease the incidence, severity, and duration of neutrope-nia. You must administer these drugs within a certain time frame (see Chapter 47). Encourage patients with immune sup-pression to be aware of their environments and persons to avoid, such as individuals who have recently been vaccinated (who may have a subclinical infection) or who have a cold or flu or other symptoms of an infection. Maintaining a "low-microbe" diet by washing fresh fruits and vegetables and making sure foods are well cooked is also recommended. Educate patients on the importance of performing oral care frequently (see discussion of stomatitis) and to turn, cough, and deep breathe to help prevent stasis of respiratory secretions.

Thrombocytopenia is also an adverse effect of antineoplastic therapy and puts the patient at risk for bleeding. Monitor plate-let counts, coagulation studies, RBC counts, hemoglobin levels, and hematocrit values, and report any decreases (see Safety: Laboratory Values Related to Drug Therapy on p. 726). Avoid injections if possible, and utilize alternative routes of adminis-tration. If injections or venipunctures are absolutely necessary, always use the smallest-gauge needle possible and apply gentle, prolonged pressure to the site afterward. Monitor patients undergoing bone marrow aspiration closely after the procedure for bleeding at the aspiration site. Perform blood pressure monitoring as needed. Be efficient and quick and without over-inflating the cuff to avoid bruising. Monitor the patient for bleeding from the mouth, gums, and nose. Check for bleeding after toothbrushing, and report excessive bleeding to the prescriber.

Inform the patient that *antineoplastics* may also have a *negative impact on the reproductive tract,* causing destruction of the germinal epithelium of the testes and damage to the ovaries and to a fetus (teratogenesis). Other problems may include sterility; amenorrhea; premature menopausal symptoms of hot flashes, decreased vaginal secretions, mood changes, or irritability; and decreased libido or sexual dysfunction. Counsel male patients about the risk for sterility, which may be irreversible. Discuss with male patients the option and topic of sperm banking before chemotherapy, if deemed appropriate. Stress that female patients of childbearing age who are sexually active need to protect themselves against pregnancy because of the risk for embryonic death. Encourage contraceptive measures during chemotherapy and for up to 8 weeks after discontinuation of therapy; however, some antineoplastic drugs require use of contraception for up to 2 years after completion of treatment because of the long-term risk for genetic abnormalities.

With *antimetabolites,* always follow the prescriber's orders regarding premedication with antiemetics and/or antianxiety drugs. Follow orders or protocol for the use of other symptom-control medications, as prescribed. GI adverse effects are common with antimetabolites and usually occur on about the fourth day and require preplanning for special pharmacologic interventions (e.g., antiemetics, antispasmodics, analgesics) and nonpharmacologic measures (dietary changes, oral care). Antibiotic therapy may also be ordered prophylactically. See earlier discussion of nursing considerations associated with stomatitis, loss of appetite, diarrhea, nausea, nutrition, hydration, vomiting, and anemias. For further discussion on the handling of antimetabolites and other IV antineoplastic drugs, see Box 46-3.

Use extreme caution in handling and administration of *cytarabine* by the various routes (IV, subcutaneous, or intrathecal). Other major concerns with cytarabine therapy are bone marrow suppression (see earlier discussion) and cytarabine syndrome (see the Assessment section). If high dosages are used, cytarabine may also cause central nervous system, GI, and/or pulmonary toxicity, so closely monitor these systems to ensure patient safety and comfort. For intrathecal administration, the drug may be reconstituted with sodium chloride, or the prescriber may use the patient's spinal fluid. Do not add *fluorouracil* to any other IV infusions; administer the drug by itself in the appropriate diluent. When an infusion port is not used, do not use IV sites over joints, tendons, or small veins, or in extremities that are edematous. Give IV dosages exactly as ordered, and constantly monitor the IV site, infusion port, and/or infusion solution and equipment. If IV infiltration occurs, follow the protocol for management of infiltration and contact the prescriber. Follow all hospital or infusion protocols without exception because treatment of extravasation is handled differently depending on the specific drug. If extravasation of a vesicant occurs, the drug is usually discontinued immediately; leave the IV cannula in place (for possible use of antidotes through

cannula to access affected area), and follow institutional protocol. Antidotes and use of other drugs, as well as use of hot or cold packs, is usually outlined in the protocol for managing extravasation (see Box 46-1). If topical forms of the drug are used, inform the patient that it is important to apply the drug exactly as ordered and to the affected area only. Use gloves or a finger cot to apply the topical dosage form.

Gemcitabine, another *antimetabolite,* is dosed based on absolute granulocyte counts and platelet nadirs and is given if the counts exceed 1500×10^6 cells/L and $100,000 \times 10^6$ platelets/L, respectively. Keep IV solutions at room temperature to avoid crystallization, and use within 24 hours. Give infusions as ordered. Antiemetics and antidiarrheals may be needed. *Mercaptopurine* comes in oral dosage forms; give as ordered. Finally, the antimetabolite *methotrexate* has numerous toxicities and adverse effects that may be minimized by appropriate medical treatment. For example, there may be orders for boosting the immune status and blood cell counts before aggressive therapy is initiated. Cytoprotective drugs are used. Continue to monitor creatinine clearance, as ordered, to detect any nephrotoxicity. Nutritional status may be enhanced by the intake of foods high in folic acid, including bran, dried beans, nuts, fruits, asparagus, and other fresh vegetables, if tolerated. Consumption of these foods is yet another measure to help minimize the possibility of methotrexate toxicity. If GI upset and/or stomatitis occur, the patient may need to decrease any sources of irritation (e.g., high-fiber food). Methotrexate is usually given orally or IV. Wear gloves when giving the drug. If any of the solution comes in contact with the skin, wash the area immediately and thoroughly with soap and water. (See Box 46-3 for discussion of concerns in the handling and administration of vesicant drugs.)

For the *mitotic inhibitors,* specifically the *taxane* family of drugs and *docetaxel* in particular, premedication protocols are usually specified and include administration of oral corticosteroids (e.g., dexamethasone) beginning several days before day 1 of therapy to help decrease the risk for hypersensitivity. Measure vital signs frequently during the infusion, especially in the first hour of the infusion. Closely monitor the patient for the sudden onset of bronchospasm, flushing of the face, and localized skin reactions; these may indicate a hypersensitivity response requiring immediate treatment. Contact the prescriber immediately. These symptoms may occur within just a few minutes of beginning the infusion. In addition, any dyspnea, abdominal distension, crackles in the lungs, or dependent edema during therapy require immediate attention. Cutaneous reactions may also appear during therapy and include rash on the hands and feet; these also need immediate attention and treatment. With *paclitaxel,* the patient may also be premedicated with diphenhydramine, corticosteroids, and H_2 antagonist drugs. Take all measures to minimize tissue trauma (e.g., avoidance of intramuscular injections and rectal temperature taking, if possible) to promote comfort and prevent bleeding and infection.

With the *topoisomerase I inhibitors, irinotecan* and *topotecan,* monitor blood counts closely with every treatment. A drop in blood counts and/or severe diarrhea may cause a temporary postponement of therapy. Treat any extravasation of the solution immediately, and follow protocol. Ensuring that IV sites remain patent is critical to the prevention of tissue damage secondary to extravasation of *antineoplastic drugs* that are considered to be irritants and/or vesicants. Nausea and vomiting may lead to dehydration and electrolyte disturbances. Advise patients and family members to report these symptoms immediately before negative consequences occur (see previous discussion for specific interventions). IV incompatibilities are numerous for both drugs and are of constant concern. With *topotecan*, IV extravasation is usually accompanied by a mild local reaction such as erythema or bruising. If these symptoms are noted, they must be managed immediately to avoid further trauma and/or risk for loss of skin integrity (the first line of defense against infection). Headaches and difficulty breathing may be more common with topotecan; therefore, closely and frequently monitor the patient for these symptoms.

Handle the *enzyme antineoplastics asparaginase* and *pegaspargase* with extreme caution and care. The patient may receive an intradermal test dose of asparaginase before therapy begins or when 1 week or longer has passed between doses. With asparaginase and pegaspargase, if the solution comes in contact with the skin, thoroughly wash or rinse the area with copious amounts of water for a minimum of 15 minutes. During therapy, if there are signs and symptoms of oliguria, anuria (renal failure), or pancreatitis, the drug will most likely be discontinued. The intramuscular route of administration is usually preferred because it carries a lower risk for causing clotting abnormalities, GI disorders, and renal and hepatic toxicity. If solutions are cloudy, do not use them. If more than 2 mL is ordered/required for an intramuscular dosing, use two injections. Pancreatitis is problematic with these drugs and can be serious. Pay close attention to symptoms such as severe abdominal pain with nausea and vomiting. Constantly monitor serum lipase and amylase levels. If any signs or symptoms of pancreatitis occur, the prescriber will usually discontinue the drugs immediately. Use of cytoprotective drugs is briefly discussed in the Pharmacology section earlier in the chapter, with further discussion provided in Chapter 46.

▌EVALUATION

Focus evaluation of nursing care on reviewing whether goals and outcomes are being met as well as monitoring for therapeutic responses and adverse and toxic effects of the *antineoplastic therapy*. Therapeutic responses may manifest as clinical improvement, decrease in tumor size, and decrease in metastatic spread. Evaluation of nursing care, with reference to goals and outcomes, may reveal improvements related to a decrease in adverse effects and a decrease in the impact of cancer on the patient's well-being. There will be increases in comfort, nutrition, hydration, energy levels, and ability to carry out activities of daily living, and improved quality of life with therapeutic effectiveness. Revisit goals and outcomes to identify more specific areas to monitor. In addition, certain laboratory studies including tumor marker levels such as carcinoembryonic antigens, RBC and WBC counts, and platelet counts may be performed to aid in determining how well the treatment protocol has worked and to monitor adverse effects of bone marrow suppression. Also, if absolute neutrophil count (ANC) drops below 500 cells/mm³, the prescriber may discontinue chemotherapy but then reinitiate when the level is above 1000 cells/mm³ or as institutional policy or prescriber dictates. Other blood counts are considered, too. As part of the evaluation, the prescriber may also order additional radiographs, computed tomographic scans, magnetic resonance images, tissue analyses, or other studies appropriate to the diagnosis both during and after antineoplastic therapy has been completed, at time intervals related to the anticipated tumor response.

CASE STUDY

Patient-Centered Care: Facing Chemotherapy

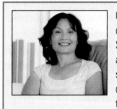 C.D., a 48-year-old married mother of two teenage daughters, has been diagnosed with breast cancer. She has undergone lumpectomy to remove the tumor and is about to start adjuvant chemotherapy. She states that she has "faced the facts" about her disease and the threat to her life but says, "I know this is silly, but I hate the thought of losing my hair to this disease."

1. What measures can be taken to help C.D. deal with her hair loss?
2. Ten days after the chemotherapy, C.D.'s neutrophil count drops to 2000 cells/mm³. She has been hospitalized because she has developed a cough, and several of her friends have come to visit her with a fresh fruit basket. What actions will be taken to protect her from infection?
3. During rounds, the nurse finds C.D. curled up in the bed and sobbing. C.D. says that she feels "so afraid" and is worried about who will care for her family if she dies. What actions will the nurse take at this time?

For answers, see *http://evolve.elsevier.com/Lilley*.

▌PATIENT-CENTERED CARE: PATIENT TEACHING

- Educate patients that GI adverse effects and irritation to the oral and GI mucosa may be decreased by avoiding intake of alcohol, tobacco, spicy and high-fiber foods, citrus fruit juices or foods, and foods that are too hot or cold or have a rough texture.
- Stress that daily mouth care is needed. Instruct the patient to report mouth sores, pain, or white patches to the prescriber immediately. Headache, fatigue, faintness, shortness of breath

(possibly indicative of anemia), bleeding, easy bruising (possibly indicative of a drop in platelet count), sore throat, and fever (possibly indicative of infection) also need to be reported immediately to the appropriate prescriber. Fever and/or chills may be the first sign of an oncoming infection.
- Discuss contraception, sperm banking, and other reproductive issues with male patients and women of childbearing age.

- Emphasize to the patient receiving antineoplastic drugs which OTC medications to avoid (e.g., aspirin, ibuprofen, and any combination products containing these OTC drugs).
- Emphasize pain control measures such as the following: Request and/or self-administer (if at home setting) pain medication prior to the pain becoming severe and uncontrollable. Encourage the use of ranking their pain on a scale of 0 (no pain) to 10 (worst pain ever experienced).
- Review and demonstrate, as appropriate, the use of non-pharmacologic measures of pain control such as relaxation, music therapy, pet therapy, biofeedback, massage, therapeutic touch, and diversion. These may also be used in conjunction with drug therapy to enhance comfort.
- Measures to assist in the support of the patient's immune system and preventing infection include frequent hand washing, deep breathing exercises, increase in fluids/hydration status, consumption of a well-balanced diet, and avoidance of malls/shopping centers or areas/gatherings with large crowds. Avoiding being around those with symptoms of colds, flu, or other communicable illnesses is also important.
- Encourage frequent skin care and enhancement of skin integrity with keeping the skin clean and dry and moisturized.
- Review measures/ways for the patient to minimize oral mucosal breakdown and infection, such as frequent mouth care and dental hygiene measures using mild toothpaste, gentle sponge-type toothettes, and non–alcohol-based mouthwash, as well as taking fluids frequently.
- Emphasize the importance of a daily regimen for increasing urinary health, such as forcing fluids and consuming fluids that minimize urinary infections (e.g., cranberry juice).
- Antineoplastics may cause alopecia (hair loss). Before therapy, provide the patient with the opportunity to discuss options for hair and scalp care. These options may include, but are not limited to, having the hair cut short before treatment; selecting, purchasing, or renting a wig or hairpiece comparable to the patient's existing hair in color, texture, length, and style; or having bandanas, scarves, or hats on hand before the hair is actually lost. Although hair loss is temporary, inform patients that it will occur and that hair

will appear differently upon growing back. The American Cancer Society may be a resource for wigs and hairpieces.
- The following websites are helpful online resources for the patient and significant others: *www.fda.gov, www.cancer.gov, www.nih.gov, www.healthfinder.gov, www.who.int/en/,* and *www.oncolink.org/index.cfm.*
- With *cytarabine,* encourage the patient to increase fluid intake to help decrease the risk for dehydration and/or hyperuricemia.
- With *fluorouracil* and *gemcitabine,* encourage the patient to perform frequent oral hygiene and to report to the prescriber immediately any bleeding, bruising, chest pain, diarrhea, nausea, vomiting, heart palpitations, infection, or changes in vision. Instruct patients to protect themselves from the sun while taking fluorouracil, including avoiding overexposure to sun or ultraviolet light and using protective clothing, sunscreen, and sunglasses.
- With *mercaptopurine,* educate the patient that alcohol must be avoided to help minimize drug toxicity.
- With *methotrexate,* inform the patient to notify the prescriber if nausea and vomiting are problematic or uncontrollable, or if fever, sore throat, muscle aches and pains, or unusual bleeding occurs. Advise the patient to avoid alcohol, salicylates, nonsteroidal antiinflammatory drugs, and exposure to sunlight or ultraviolet light. Instruct both male and female patients to use contraceptive measures for up to 3 months or longer, if appropriate.
- With *taxanes,* specifically paclitaxel, counsel the patient to report to the prescriber immediately any signs or symptoms of neuropathy (e.g., numbness or tingling of the extremities).
- With *etoposide* and *teniposide* as with other antineoplastics, if WBC counts are low, caution the patient to avoid individuals who are ill. Additionally, advise the patient to report to the prescriber immediately any easy bleeding, bruising, difficulty breathing, fever, sore throat, or chills.
- With *asparaginase* and *pegaspargase,* encourage the patient to force fluids and to report any severe nausea or vomiting, bleeding, excessive fatigue, or fever or other signs or symptoms of infection.

KEY POINTS

- Cancers are diseases that are characterized by uncontrolled cellular growth.
- *Malignancy* refers specifically to a neoplasm that is anaplastic, invasive, and metastatic, as opposed to benign.
- Tumors are generally classified by tissue of origin, as follows: epithelial (carcinoma), connective (sarcoma), lymphatic (lymphoma), and leukocytes (leukemia).
- Antineoplastics are drugs that are used to treat malignancies. They may be either cell cycle–specific or cell cycle–nonspecific drugs or may have miscellaneous actions.
- Cell cycle–specific drugs kill cancer cells during specific phases of the cell growth cycle. Cell cycle–nonspecific drugs kill cancer cells during any phase of the cell growth cycle.

- Chemotherapy, or antineoplastic drug therapy, requires very skillful and perceptive nursing care. It is important to act prudently and think critically when making decisions about the nursing care of patients receiving these drugs.
- Cell cycle–specific drug classes include antimetabolites, mitotic inhibitors, alkaloid topoisomerase II inhibitors, topoisomerase I inhibitors, and antineoplastic enzymes.
- Antineoplastic antimetabolites are cell cycle–specific antagonistic analogues that work by inhibiting the actions of key cellular metabolites.
- Two plant-derived antineoplastic drugs are the taxanes paclitaxel, derived from the bark of the slow-growing Western (Pacific) yew tree, and docetaxel, a semisynthetic taxoid

produced from the needles of the European yew tree. Docetaxel is pharmacologically similar to paclitaxel.
• The topoisomerase I inhibitors topotecan and irinotecan compose a relatively new class of chemotherapy drugs.

• Antineoplastic enzymes include asparaginase and pegaspargase.
• Several drugs are available that are classified as cytoprotective and help reduce the toxicity of various antineoplastics.

NCLEX® EXAMINATION REVIEW QUESTIONS

1. A patient is experiencing stomatitis after a round of chemotherapy. Which intervention by the nurse is correct?
   a. Clean the mouth with a soft-bristle toothbrush and warm saline solution.
   b. Rinse the mouth with commercial mouthwash twice a day.
   c. Use lemon-glycerin swabs to keep the mouth moist.
   d. Keep dentures in the mouth between meals.
2. The nurse is caring for a patient who becomes severely nauseated during chemotherapy. Which intervention is most appropriate?
   a. Encourage light activity during chemotherapy as a distraction.
   b. Provide antiemetic medications 30 to 60 minutes before chemotherapy begins.
   c. Provide antiemetic medications only upon the request of the patient.
   d. Hold fluids during chemotherapy to avoid vomiting.
3. The nurse monitors a patient who is experiencing thrombocytopenia from severe bone marrow suppression by looking for
   a. severe weakness and fatigue.
   b. elevated body temperature.
   c. decreased skin turgor.
   d. excessive bleeding and bruising.
4. A patient receiving chemotherapy is experiencing severe bone marrow suppression. Which nursing diagnosis is most appropriate at this time?
   a. Activity intolerance
   b. Risk for infection
   c. Disturbed body image
   d. Impaired physical mobility

5. If extravasation of an antineoplastic medication occurs, which intervention will the nurse perform first?
   a. Apply cold compresses to the site while elevating the arm.
   b. Inject subcutaneous doses of epinephrine around the IV site every 2 hours.
   c. Stop the infusion immediately while leaving the catheter in place.
   d. Inject the appropriate antidote through the IV catheter.
6. The nurse is assessing a patient who has experienced severe neutropenia after chemotherapy and will monitor for which possible signs of infection? *(Select all that apply.)*
   a. Elevated WBC count
   b. Fever
   c. Nausea
   d. Sore throat
   e. Chills
7. The order for chemotherapy reads: "Give asparaginase (Elspar) IV 200 units/kg/day." The patient weighs 297 lb. The pharmacy department will prepare the medication for intravenous infusion. How much drug will be given per dose?
8. The nurse is assessing a patient who has developed anemia after two rounds of chemotherapy. Which of these may be indications of anemia? *(Select all that apply.)*
   a. Hypoxia
   b. Fever
   c. Infection
   d. Bleeding
   e. Fatigue

1. a, 2. b, 3. d, 4. b, 5. c, 6. b, d, e, 7. 27,000 units, 8. a, e.

CRITICAL THINKING AND PRIORITIZATION QUESTIONS

1. A patient is receiving irinotecan as part of his chemotherapy regimen. He will be receiving the dose shortly and then will be sent home. The nurse is providing patient teaching before giving him the medication. What is one of the most important problems for which the patient will need to be ready once he is home? Explain the nurse's priority action.
2. A patient is receiving chemotherapy that includes the antimetabolite cytarabine. Several hours after the treatment, the

patient begins to complain of shortness of breath. The nurse examines the patient and finds that his pulse rate is 118 beats/min, he has slight edema in his lower extremities, and crackles are audible over the bases of the lungs. In addition, his pulse oximetry reading is 89% (previously it was 99%) on room air. What is the nurse's immediate priority action?

For answers, see *http://evolve.elsevier.com/Lilley.*

Ⓔ EVOLVE WEBSITE

http://evolve.elsevier.com/Lilley
• Animations
• Answer Keys for Textbook Case Studies and Textbook Critical Thinking and Prioritization Questions

• Content Updates
• Key Points
• Review Questions
• Student Case Studies

Antineoplastic Drugs Part 2: Cell-Cycle–Nonspecific and Miscellaneous Drugs

ⓔ http://evolve.elsevier.com/Lilley

OBJECTIVES

When you reach the end of this chapter, you will be able to do the following:

1. Review the concepts related to carcinogenesis, the types of malignancies and related terminology, and the different treatment modalities, including the use of cell-cycle–nonspecific and miscellaneous antineoplastic drugs.
2. Identify the various drugs that are classified as cell-cycle nonspecific or hormonal or are considered to be miscellaneous antineoplastic drugs.
3. Discuss the common adverse effects and toxic effects of the cell-cycle–nonspecific and miscellaneous antineoplastic drugs, including the reasons for their occurrence and methods of treatment, such as any antidotes.
4. Describe the mechanisms of action, indications, routes of administration, cautions, contraindications, and drug interactions of the cell-cycle–nonspecific drugs, hormonal drugs, and miscellaneous antineoplastic drugs.
5. Apply knowledge about the cell-cycle–nonspecific, hormonal agonist-antagonist, and other miscellaneous antineoplastic drugs and their characteristics in the development of a comprehensive nursing care plan for patients with cancer who are receiving these drugs.
6. Briefly describe extravasation and other major adverse effects associated with the cell-cycle–nonspecific and miscellaneous antineoplastics, including discussion of protocols and antidotes.

DRUG PROFILES

bevacizumab, p. 739
cisplatin, p. 737
♦ cyclophosphamide, p. 737
♦ doxorubicin, p. 738
hydroxyurea, p. 739
imatinib, p. 740
♦ mechlorethamine, p. 737

mitotane, p. 740
mitoxantrone, p. 738
octreotide, p. 740

_____

♦ = *Key drug*
! = *High-alert drug*

KEY TERMS

Alkylation A chemical reaction in which an alkyl group is transferred from one molecule to another. In chemotherapy, alkylation leads to damage of the cancer cell deoxyribonucleic acid (DNA) and cell death. (p. 735)

Bifunctional Referring to those alkylating drugs composed of molecules that have two reactive alkyl groups and that are therefore able to alkylate at two sites on the DNA molecule. (p. 735)

Extravasation The leakage of any intravenously or intraarterially administered medication into the tissue space surrounding the vein or artery. Such an event can cause serious tissue injury, especially with antineoplastic drugs. (p. 736)

Polyfunctional Referring to the action of alkylating drugs that can engage in several alkylation reactions with cancer cell DNA molecules per single molecule of drug. (p. 735)

OVERVIEW

This chapter is a continuation of Chapter 45 and focuses on additional classes of antineoplastic drugs. Chapter 45 describes the various antineoplastic drugs that are effective against cancer cells during specific phases in the cell growth cycle. In contrast, this chapter focuses on drugs that have antineoplastic activity regardless of the phase of the cell cycle. Also discussed in this chapter are drugs that are classified as miscellaneous antineo-plastics, either because of their lack of clear cell-cycle specificity or their unique or novel (new) mechanisms of action. For a description of the cell growth cycle, see Chapter 45.

CELL-CYCLE–NONSPECIFIC ANTINEOPLASTIC DRUGS

There are currently two broad classes of cell-cycle–nonspecific cancer drugs: alkylating drugs and cytotoxic antibiotics.

ALKYLATING DRUGS

Records of the use of drugs to treat cancer date back several centuries. However, truly successful systemic cancer chemotherapy treatments were not documented until the 1940s. At this time, the first alkylating drugs were developed from mustard gas agents that were used for chemical warfare before and during World War I. The first drug to be developed was mechlorethamine, which is also known as *nitrogen mustard*. It is the prototypical drug of this class and is still used today for cancer treatment. Since its antineoplastic activity was discovered in the mid-twentieth century, many analogues have been synthesized for use in the treatment of cancer, and they are collectively referred to as nitrogen mustards as well.

The alkylating drugs commonly used in clinical practice in the United States today fall into three categories: *classic alkylators* (the nitrogen mustards); *nitrosoureas,* which have a different chemical structure than the nitrogen mustards but also work by **alkylation**; and *miscellaneous alkylators,* which have a different chemical structure than the nitrogen mustards but are known to work at least partially by alkylation. These drugs are used to treat a wide spectrum of malignancies. The drugs in each category are as follows:

Classic alkylators (nitrogen mustards)
- chlorambucil
- cyclophosphamide
- ifosfamide
- mechlorethamine
- melphalan

Nitrosoureas
- carmustine
- lomustine
- streptozocin

Miscellaneous alkylators
- altretamine
- busulfan
- carboplatin
- cisplatin
- dacarbazine
- oxaliplatin
- procarbazine
- temozolomide
- thiotepa

Mechanism of Action and Drug Effects

The alkylating drugs work by preventing cancer cells from reproducing. Specifically, they alter the chemical structure of the cells' deoxyribonucleic acid (DNA). Alkyl groups that are part of the structure of alkylating drugs attach to DNA molecules by forming covalent bonds with the bases. As a result, abnormal chemical bonds form between the adjacent DNA strands, which leads to the formation of defective nucleic acids that are then unable to perform the normal cellular reproductive functions, which leads to cell death. Alkylating drugs can be characterized by the number of alkylation reactions in which they can participate. **Bifunctional** alkylating drugs have two reactive alkyl groups that are able to alkylate two sites on the DNA molecule. **Polyfunctional** alkylating drugs can participate in several alkylation reactions. Figure 46-1 shows the location along the DNA double helix where the alkylating drugs work.

Indications

The most commonly used alkylating drugs today are effective against a wide spectrum of malignancies, including both solid and hematologic tumors. Common examples of the various types of cancer that different alkylating drugs are used to treat are listed in Table 46-1.

Adverse Effects

Alkylating drugs are capable of causing all of the dose-limiting adverse effects described in Chapter 45. Other adverse effects

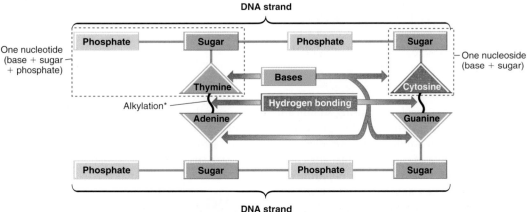

FIGURE 46-1 Organization of deoxyribonucleic acid (DNA) and site of action (*) of alkylating drugs.

TABLE 46-1 Indications: Selected Alkylating Drugs

Drug (Pregnancy Category)	Pharmacologic Subclass	Indications
cisplatin (Platinol-AQ) (D)	Platinum coordination complex	Metastatic testicular, ovarian, and bladder cancer; brain tumors; esophageal, head, neck, lung, and cervical cancer
cyclophosphamide (Cytoxan) (D)	Classic alkylator	HL, NHL, leukemia; breast, ovarian, and testicular cancer; retinoblastoma; almost every solid tumor
mechlorethamine (Mustargen) (D)	Classic alkylator	HL, NHL, leukemia, bronchogenic carcinoma, others

HL, Hodgkin's lymphoma; *NHL,* non-Hodgkin's lymphoma.

TABLE 46-2 Commonly Used Alkylating Drugs: Severe Adverse Effects

Drug	Adverse Effects
busulfan	Pulmonary fibrosis
Carboplatin*	Nephrotoxicity, neurotoxicity, bone marrow suppression
cisplatin	Nephrotoxicity, peripheral neuropathy, ototoxicity
cyclophosphamide	Hemorrhagic cystitis

*Carboplatin has less nephrotoxicity and neurotoxicity but more bone marrow suppression than cisplatin.

are described in Table 46-2. The relative emetic potential of the various alkylating drugs is given in Box 45-1. The adverse effects of these drugs are important because of their severity, but they can often be prevented or minimized by prophylactic measures. For instance, nephrotoxicity from cisplatin can often be prevented by adequately hydrating the patient with intravenous fluids.

Drug **extravasation** (Box 46-1) occurs when an intravenous catheter punctures the vein and medication leaks (infiltrates) into the surrounding tissues. With cancer chemotherapeutic drugs, in particular doxorubicin (a cytotoxic antibiotic), extravasation can cause severe tissue damage and necrosis (tissue death). Extravasation antidotes for selected drugs are listed in Table 46-3.

Interactions

Only a few alkylating drugs are capable of causing significant drug interactions. The most important rule for preventing such drug interactions is to avoid administering an alkylating drug with any other drug capable of causing similar toxicities. For example, a major adverse effect of cisplatin is nephrotoxicity. Therefore, if possible, do not administer it with a drug such as an aminoglycoside antibiotic (gentamicin, tobramycin, or amikacin) because of the resulting additive nephrotoxic effects and hence the increased likelihood of renal failure.

BOX 46-1 Extravasation of Antineoplastics

Extravasation is one of the more devastating complications of antineoplastic therapy and may lead to extensive tissue damage, the need for skin grafting, other problems in the surrounding areas, and even loss of limb. Because many cell-cycle–specific and cell-cycle–nonspecific drugs are given intravenously, there is a constant danger of extravasation of vesicants and subsequent injury, including permanent damage to nerves, tendons, and muscles. Skillful and perceptive nursing care helps to prevent extravasation or to identify it early if it does occur, which may reduce the severity of tissue damage. There are important reasons for the placement of central venous intravenous catheters rather than peripheral catheters when long-term treatment is anticipated. Infiltration may occur with any intravenous catheter; it is the specific drug and its characteristics, such as irritant (irritating the IV site or vein) or vesicant (causing cell death with extravasation and necrosis with ulcerative properties) that poses the concern. Because peripheral veins are small and offer minimal dilution of the intravenous drug with blood, there is a greater risk for severe and irreversible damage if a substance infiltrates and spreads to surrounding areas. If the drug is a vesicant, extravasation may lead to massive tissue injury, whereas extravasation of an irritant results in significantly less damage. Central venous access is needed for administration of vesicants to avoid the problems associated with extravasation. However, extravasation may occur with central lines and PICC lines due to dislodging of the access catheter, venous thrombosis, and catheter breakage. Blood needs to be aspirated prior to administration to check for patency. Extravasation may be suspected if the following occurs at either a central line site, PICC line site, or peripheral IV site: complaints of burning, stinging, pain, or any other acute change of sensation at the site or along the chest wall, neck, or shoulder (central line); or leakage, swelling, or induration at the site. If extravasation of a vesicant is suspected, immediate action must be taken and the antidote, if known, must be given following strict guidelines and procedures. Steps to help manage extravasation of an irritant and/or a vesicant include the following: (1) Stop the infusion immediately and contact the prescriber, leaving the intravenous catheter in place. (2) Next, it is usually recommended to aspirate any residual drug and/or blood from the catheter. (3) Consult institutional policy or guidelines or the pharmacist regarding the use of antidotes, application of hot or cold packs and/or sterile occlusive dressings, and elevation and rest of the affected limb. Document the extravasation incident with attention to all phases of the nursing process related to the problem. Remember to always consult institutional protocol and guidelines.

Data from National Institutes of Health. Available at *www.ncbi.nlm.gov.* Internet resources for additional information: *www.cancer.org, www.oncolink.org/index.cfm,* and *www.acponline.org.* Accessed May 14, 2015.

Mechlorethamine and cyclophosphamide, both of which have significant bone marrow–suppressing effects, are not to be administered with radiation therapy or with other drugs that suppress the bone marrow. In general, you need to work with available pharmacy and oncology staff to proactively anticipate (and avoid, if possible) undesirable drug and treatment interactions.

DRUG PROFILES

The most widely used alkylating drugs, based on standard treatment protocols, are profiled as follows:

TABLE 46-3   Alkylating Drug Extravasation: Specific Antidotes

Drug	Antidote Preparation	Method
carmustine	Mix equal parts 1 mEq/mL sodium bicarbonate (premixed) with sterile NS (1:1 solution); resulting solution is 0.5 mEq/mL.	1. Inject 2-6 mL IV through the existing line along with multiple subcut injections into the extravasated site. 2. Apply cold compresses. 3. Total dose is not to exceed 10 mL of 0.5-mEq/mL solution.
mechlorethamine	Mix 4 mL 10% sodium thiosulfate with 6 mL sterile water for injection.	1. Inject 5-6 mL IV through the existing line with multiple subcut injections into the extravasated site. 2. Repeat subcut injections over the next few hours. 3. Apply cold compresses. 4. No total dose has been established.

♦ cisplatin

Cisplatin (Platinol) is an antineoplastic drug that contains platinum in its chemical structure. It is classified as a probable alkylating drug because it is believed to destroy cancer cells in the same way as the classic alkylating drugs—by forming cross-links with DNA and thereby preventing its replication. It is also considered a bifunctional alkylating drug.

Cisplatin is used for the treatment of many solid tumors, such as bladder, lung, testicular, and ovarian tumors. It is available only in injectable form. Medication errors, resulting in deaths, have occurred when cisplatin was confused for carboplatin. The best practice is to use both trade name and generic name when dealing with chemotherapy drugs.

♦ cyclophosphamide

Cyclophosphamide (Cytoxan) is a nitrogen mustard derivative that was discovered during the course of research to improve mechlorethamine. It is a polyfunctional alkylating drug and is a prodrug requiring *in vivo* activation. It is used in the treatment of cancers of the bone and lymph, as well as other solid tumors. Cyclophosphamide is also used in the treatment of leukemias and multiple myeloma, as well as for noncancer-related illnesses such as prophylaxis for rejection of kidney, heart, liver, and bone marrow transplants and severe rheumatoid disorders. It is available in both oral and injectable dosage forms.

♦ mechlorethamine

Mechlorethamine (nitrogen mustard) (Mustargen) is the prototypical alkylating drug. It is a nitrogen analogue of sulfur mustard (mustard gas) that was used for chemical warfare in World War I. Mechlorethamine was the first alkylating antineoplastic drug discovered. Although its use has declined with the development of newer and better drugs, it continues to be administered in the treatment of Hodgkin's and non-Hodgkin's lymphoma. Mechlorethamine is a bifunctional alkylating drug capable of forming cross-links between two DNA nucleotides, which interferes with RNA transcription and prevents cell division and protein synthesis. It is available in parenteral form only, for administration intravenously or by an intracavitary route, such as intrapleurally or intraperitoneally. It can also be used topically for treatment of cutaneous T-cell lymphoma.

CYTOTOXIC ANTIBIOTICS

The cytotoxic antibiotics consist of natural substances produced by the mold *Streptomyces* as well as semisynthetic substances in which chemical changes are made in the natural molecule. Cytotoxic antibiotics have bone marrow suppression as a common toxicity. The one exception is bleomycin, which instead causes pulmonary toxicity (pulmonary fibrosis and pneumonitis). Other severe toxicities associated with the use of cytotoxic antibiotics are heart failure (daunorubicin) and in rare cases acute left ventricular failure (doxorubicin). The available cytotoxic antibiotics, categorized according to the specific subclass to which they belong, are as follows:

Anthracyclines
- daunorubicin
- doxorubicin
- epirubicin
- idarubicin
- valrubicin

Other cytotoxic antibiotics
- bleomycin (which is actually a cell-cycle–specific drug)
- dactinomycin
- mitomycin
- mitoxantrone
- plicamycin

Mechanism of Action and Drug Effects

Cytotoxic antibiotic antineoplastic drugs are cell-cycle–nonspecific drugs. They interact with DNA through a process called *intercalation*, in which the drug molecule is inserted between the two strands of a DNA molecule, ultimately blocking DNA synthesis. These drugs inhibit the enzyme topoisomerase II, which leads to DNA strand breaks. Many of these drugs are able to generate free radicals, which also leads to DNA strand breaks and programmed cell death.

Indications

Cytotoxic antibiotics are used to treat a variety of solid tumors and some hematologic malignancies as well. Commonly used examples of these drugs and the malignancies they are used to treat are presented in Table 46-4.

TABLE 46-4 Indications: Selected Cytotoxic Antibiotics

Drug (Pregnancy Category)	Pharmacologic Subclass	Indications
Anthracycline Antibiotics		
doxorubicin, conventional (Adriamycin, Rubex) (D)	Anthracycline	Multiple cancers, including breast, bone, and ovarian cancers, leukemia, neuroblastoma, HL, and NHL
doxorubicin, liposomal (Doxil) (D)	Anthracycline	AIDS-related Kaposi's sarcoma when other chemotherapy drugs have failed or patient is intolerant of them; recurrent metastatic ovarian cancer
Anthracenedione Antibiotic		
mitoxantrone (Novantrone) (D)	Anthracenedione	Prostate cancer; acute myelocytic leukemia

HL, Hodgkin's lymphoma; *NHL,* non-Hodgkin's lymphoma.

TABLE 46-5 Cytotoxic Antibiotics: Severe Adverse Effects

Drug	Adverse Effects
bleomycin	Pulmonary fibrosis, pneumonitis
dactinomycin, daunorubicin	Liver toxicity, tissue damage in the event of extravasation, heart failure
doxorubicin, idarubicin	Liver and cardiovascular toxicities
mitomycin	Liver, kidney, and lung toxicities
mitoxantrone	Cardiovascular toxicity
plicamycin	Tissue damage in the event of extravasation

Adverse Effects

As with all of the antineoplastic drugs, cytotoxic antibiotics have the undesirable effects of hair loss, nausea and vomiting, and myelosuppression. The emetic potential of the various drugs in this category is given in Box 45-1. Major adverse effects specific to the cytotoxic antibiotics are listed in Table 46-5.

Toxicity and Management of Overdose

Severe cases of cardiomyopathy are associated with large cumulative doses of doxorubicin. Routine monitoring of cardiac ejection fraction, cumulative dose limitations, and the use of cytoprotective drugs such as dexrazoxane can decrease the incidence of this devastating toxicity. Box 46-2 outlines the management of doxorubicin extravasation.

Interactions

The cytotoxic antibiotics that are used in chemotherapy interact with many drugs. They all tend to produce increased toxicities when used in combination with other chemotherapeutic drugs or with radiation therapy. Some drugs, most notably bleomycin and doxorubicin, have been known to cause serum digoxin levels to increase. Observe patients receiving one of these drugs

BOX 46-2 Treatment of Doxorubicin Extravasation

1. Once detected, contact prescriber, assess, and document. Emergency management is to be started immediately.
2. Stop IV infusion promptly. Know that treatment protocols for severe extravasations may vary from conservative to aggressive management of the acute injury, with additional variations in the management of the wound.
3. If peripheral line infiltration, stop infusion, discontinue drip, leave cannula in place, mark extravasated area, and contact prescriber. Aspirate extravasated drug and attempt to draw blood back from the cannula; if protocol allows, injection of 0.9% sodium chloride may aid in this. Follow individual management protocols regarding heat and cold application. Rest the extremity and elevate as instructed by protocol or as prescribed.
4. If central line, stop infusion, aspirate drug from the line, leave line in place, and inform prescriber. Management from this point often depends on whether the extravasation is in the non-tunneled or tunneled section of the central line.
5. Referral to plastic surgery may be indicated.

Data from Al-Benna A., O'Boyle C., Holley, J. Extravasation injuries in adults. *ISRN Dermatology,* 2013. Available at *www.ncbi.nlm.nih.gov/pmc/articles/PMC3664495.*
Internet resources for additional information: *www.cancer.org, www.oncolink.org/index.cfm, www.hospicenet.org, and www.acponline.org.* Accessed May 17, 2015.

along with digoxin for signs of digoxin toxicity. Dosage reduction or elimination of digoxin therapy may be indicated (see Chapter 24).

DRUG PROFILES

◆ doxorubicin

Doxorubicin (Adriamycin) is used in many combination chemotherapy regimens. The drug is contraindicated in patients with a known hypersensitivity to it, patients with severe myelosuppression, and patients who are at risk for severe cardiotoxicity because they have already received a large cumulative dose of any of the anthracycline antineoplastics. It is available only in injectable form. Doxorubicin is also available in a liposomal drug delivery system (Doxil). In this dosage formulation, the drug is encapsulated in a lipid molecule bilayer called a *liposome.* The advantages of liposomal encapsulation are reduced systemic toxicity and increased duration of action. Liposomal encapsulation extends the biologic half-life of doxorubicin to 50 to 60 hours and increases its affinity for cancer cells. The liposomal dosage formulation is currently indicated for the treatment of ovarian cancer and in combination with bortezomib for the treatment of multiple myeloma.

mitoxantrone

Mitoxantrone (Novantrone) is indicated for the treatment of acute nonlymphocytic leukemia and prostate cancer as well as the neurologic disorder multiple sclerosis. It is available only in injectable form.

MISCELLANEOUS ANTINEOPLASTICS

The miscellaneous antineoplastic drugs are those that, because of their unique structure and mechanism of action, cannot be

⚡ **SAFETY AND QUALITY IMPROVEMENT: PREVENTING MEDICATION ERRORS**

Sound-Alike Drugs: "Rubicins"

> The anthracycline chemotherapy drugs have the same sound-alike suffix and are often nicknamed the "rubicins." These drugs include daunorubicin, doxorubicin, epirubicin, idarubicin, and valrubicin. Even though these drugs are in the same class, their use and drug effects are very different. Medication errors have occurred because one "rubicin" has been mistaken for another. It is important to refer to these drugs by both trade name and generic name rather than as a "rubicin."

classified into the previously described categories. However, some drugs that are originally classified as miscellaneous drugs are later reclassified as more is learned about their mechanisms of action and other characteristics. Drugs currently in the miscellaneous category include bevacizumab, everolimus, hydroxyurea (which is actually cell-cycle–specific), ipilimumab, imatinib, mitotane, ofatumumab, pazopanib, romidepsin, sorafenib, sunitinib, hormonal drugs, and radioactive and related antineoplastic drugs. Selected miscellaneous drugs are profiled in the following sections.

DRUG PROFILES

The various drugs in the miscellaneous category of antineoplastics are used to treat a wide range of neoplasms. Hydroxyurea and imatinib are administered orally. Bevacizumab and mitotane are available only in injectable form. Sipuleucel-T (Provenge) is a new form of treatment for prostate cancer. It is not a chemotherapeutic agent; rather, it is an autologous cellular immunotherapy for the treatment of asymptomatic or minimally symptomatic metastatic hormone-resistant prostate cancer. It uses the patient's own monocytes that are activated and then reinfused into the patient. Infusion-related reactions are common, and patients are to be pretreated with acetaminophen and diphenhydramine. It is restricted to physicians who have undergone extensive training. Certinib (Zykadia) is a new tyrosine kinase inhibitor indicated for ALK-positive lung cancer that is unresponsive to other therapies. It was approved under accelerated approval by the FDA and is considered "breakthrough" therapy. It is administered orally, on an empty stomach, at least 2 hours before or 2 hours after a meal. Serious side effects include bradycardia, severe diarrhea, and nausea and vomiting, and often require dose reduction. Hepatotoxicity, hyperglycemia, QTc prolongation, and life-threatening interstitial lung disease or pneumonitis can also occur. Drug interactions include conivaptan, grapefruit juice, strong CYP3A4 inhibitors, and inducers and drugs that can prolong the QTc interval.

bevacizumab

Bevacizumab (Avastin) was the first antineoplastic drug in a new category—*angiogenesis inhibitors*. *Angiogenesis* is the creation of new blood vessels that supply oxygen and other blood nutrients to growing tissues. In the case of malignant tumors, angiogenesis that occurs within the tumor mass promotes continued tumor growth. Inhibiting this process offers a promising new mechanism for antineoplastic drug action. Bevacizumab is a recombinant "humanized" monoclonal immunoglobulin G_1 antibody derived from mouse antibodies. The scientific name for any compound derived from mouse tissue is *murine*. *Humanization* refers to the use of recombinant DNA techniques to make animal-derived antibody proteins more genetically similar to those of humans. It works by binding to and inhibiting the biologic activity of human vascular endothelial growth factor (VEGF). VEGF is an endogenous protein that normally promotes angiogenesis in the body. Bevacizumab is available only in injectable form. The only recognized contraindication is severe drug allergy or allergy to other murine products. It is approved for the treatment of metastatic colon cancer, rectal cancer in combination with 5-fluorouracil (see Chapter 45), non–small-cell lung cancer, and malignant glioblastoma. Bevacizumab was approved for treatment of breast cancer; however, the FDA revoked the breast cancer indication in 2011.

Adverse reactions include those affecting the cardiovascular system (hypertension or hypotension, deep vein thrombosis), central nervous system (pain, headache, dizziness, asthenia), skin (alopecia, dry skin), metabolism (weight loss, hypokalemia), gastrointestinal (GI) tract (nausea, vomiting, diarrhea, epistaxis, abdominal pain, constipation, GI hemorrhage), kidneys (nephrotoxicity with proteinuria), hematopoietic system (leukopenia), and respiratory tract (infection). More severe effects can occur in any of these systems but are much less common than those listed. Drug interactions reported to date are limited but include potentiation of the cardiotoxic effects of the anthracycline antibiotics such as doxorubicin.

hydroxyurea

Hydroxyurea (Hydrea, Droxia) is an antimetabolite that interferes with the synthesis of DNA by inhibiting the incorporation of thymidine into DNA. More specifically, it inhibits ribonucleotide reductase, which is involved in conversion of ribonucleotides to deoxyribonucleotides. It works primarily in the S and G_1 phases of the cell cycle, which makes it a cell-cycle–specific drug. It is discussed in this chapter because it is included as a miscellaneous drug.

Hydroxyurea is used in the treatment of squamous cell carcinoma in concert with radiation to take advantage of its radiosensitizing activity. It is also used in the treatment of various types of leukemia. The drug is available only in oral form. Adverse reactions include edema, drowsiness, headache, rash, hyperuricemia, nausea, vomiting, dysuria, myelosuppression, elevated liver enzyme levels, muscular weakness, peripheral neuropathy, nephrotoxicity, dyspnea, and pulmonary fibrosis. Hydroxyurea interacts with the anti-HIV drugs zidovudine, zalcitabine, and didanosine (see Chapter 40), all of which can have a synergistic effect with hydroxyurea. Concurrent use with fluorouracil increases the risk for neurotoxic symptoms. Because hydroxyurea can reduce the clearance of cytarabine, dosage reduction of cytarabine is recommended when the two are used concurrently.

imatinib

Imatinib (Gleevec) is the standard of care for the treatment of chronic myeloid leukemia (CML). It works by inhibiting the action of a key enzyme (bcr-abl tyrosine kinase) responsible for causing CML. Although its name sounds similar to those of various monoclonal antibody drugs, imatinib is not a monoclonal antibody but rather a targeted therapy. It is available only in oral form. Common adverse reactions include fatigue, headache, rash, fluid retention, GI and hematologic effects, musculoskeletal pain, cough, and dyspnea. Potential drug interactions are numerous and involve other drugs metabolized by the cytochrome P-450 hepatic enzymes. Examples include amiodarone, verapamil, warfarin, azole antifungals, antidepressants, and antibiotics. A pharmacist may be needed to review the patient's medication regimen and adjust dosages or delete medications accordingly, in collaboration with the patient's prescriber.

mitotane

Mitotane (Lysodren) is an adrenal cytotoxic drug that is indicated specifically for the treatment of inoperable adrenal corticoid carcinoma. It is available only in oral form. Adverse reactions include CNS depression, rash, nausea, vomiting, muscle weakness, and headache. Reported drug interactions include enhanced CNS depressive effects when taken concurrently with other CNS depressants (e.g., benzodiazepines). Mitotane may also increase the clearance of both warfarin and phenytoin, reducing their effects. The potassium-sparing diuretic spironolactone may negate the effects of mitotane.

octreotide

Octreotide (Sandostatin) (see Chapter 30) is a unique medication used for the management of a cancer-related condition called *carcinoid crisis* and treatment of the diarrhea caused by vasoactive intestinal peptide–secreting tumors (VIPomas).

HORMONAL ANTINEOPLASTICS

Hormonal drugs are used in the treatment of a variety of neoplasms. The rationale is that sex hormones act to accelerate the growth of some common types of malignant tumors, especially certain types of breast and prostate cancer. Therefore, therapy may involve administration of hormones with opposing effects (i.e., male versus female hormones) or drugs that block the body's sex hormone receptors. These drugs are used most commonly as palliative and adjuvant therapy. For certain types of cancer, they may be used as drugs of first choice. Some of the more commonly used hormonal drugs for female-specific neoplasms such as breast cancer are the aromatase inhibitors anastrazole and aminoglutethimide, the selective estrogen receptor modulators tamoxifen and toremifene, the progestins megestrol and medroxyprogesterone, the androgens fluoxymesterone and testolactone, and the estrogen receptor antagonist fulvestrant. For male-specific neoplasms such as prostate cancer, the following drugs are used: the antiandrogens bicalutamide, flutamide, and nilutamide; and the antineoplastic hormone estramustine. The most common adverse effects of these drugs used to treat female and male cancers are listed in Table 46-6.

NURSING PROCESS

Antineoplastics are some of the most toxic drugs given to patients (see Chapter 45), and because of these toxicities, serious complications and adverse effects may occur. Nursing care must be based on a thorough knowledge of cancer, its treatment, and the subsequent effects of different treatment modalities. This chapter presents information about cell-cycle–nonspecific, hormonal, and miscellaneous antineoplastic drugs, whereas Chapter 45 covers cell cycle–specific antineoplastic drugs.

ASSESSMENT

Begin the overall assessment of patients taking any of these drugs with a thorough nursing history, medication profile, and past and present medical history. Assess vital signs and weight/height, as both these parameters may be needed to calculate doses. Document the presence of conditions that represent cautions or contraindications as well as potential drug interactions. Perform a head-to-toe physical assessment with specific

TABLE 46-6   Hormonal Antineoplastics: Adverse Effects

Class	Drug	Adverse Effects
Aromatase inhibitors	anastrozole, aminoglutethimide	Vasodilation, hypertension, hot flushes, mood disorders, weakness, arthritis
Selective estrogen receptor modulators	tamoxifen, toremifene	Hypertension, peripheral edema, mood disorders, depression, hot flushes, nausea, weakness
Progestins	megestrol, medroxyprogesterone	Hypertension, chest pain, headache, weight gain, hepatotoxicity, dizziness, abdominal pain
Androgens	fluoxymesterone, testolactone	Menstrual irregularities, virilization of female, gynecomastia, hirsutism, acne, anxiety, headache, nausea
Estrogen receptor antagonists	Fulvestrant	Vasodilation, pain, headache, hot flushes, nausea, vomiting, pharyngitis
Antiandrogens	bicalutamide, flutamide, nilutamide	Peripheral edema, pain, hot flushes, gynecomastia, anemia, nausea, diarrhea
Gonadotropin-releasing hormone agonists	leuprolide, goserelin	Rash, pain on injection, alopecia, body odor
Antineoplastic hormone	Estramustine	Edema, dyspnea, leg cramps, breast tenderness, nausea, anorexia, diarrhea

attention to the following: skin turgor with level of moisture and integrity of the skin and oral mucosa; baseline level of neurologic functioning including motor/sensory intactness, level of consciousness, alertness, deep tendon reflexes, and presence of any abnormal sensations; bowel sounds, bowel patterns, and inquiry into any problems such as diarrhea, constipation, nausea, vomiting, or gastroesophageal reflux; urinary patterns and color, amount, and odor of urine; breath sounds as well as respiratory rate, rhythm, and depth; and heart sounds. Laboratory tests that may be ordered include fluid and electrolyte levels (sodium, potassium, chloride, magnesium, calcium), RBC and WBC counts, hemoglobin, hematocrit, renal and hepatic function tests, and serum protein-albumin levels (see Chapter 45).

For patients receiving *alkylating drugs*, bone marrow suppression *(carboplatin)*, pulmonary fibrosis *(busulfan)*, nephrotoxicity and/or neurotoxicity (more with *cisplatin* than carboplatin), and hemorrhagic cystitis *(cyclophosphamide)* may occur; thus, perform an appropriate and thorough nursing assessment (see Assessment in Chapter 45). Be specific, and assess/document deep tendon reflexes and baseline hearing level. Assess results of any baseline pulmonary function testing, and perform a thorough respiratory assessment. High-dose cyclophosphamide may lead to hemorrhagic cystitis; therefore, document baseline urinary patterns and any abnormal symptoms. Note hydration status before administering cyclophosphamide to avoid hemorrhagic cystitis.

One of the major adverse effects associated with the use of *cytotoxic antibiotics* (e.g., *bleomycin*) is pulmonary fibrosis. A variety of medical testing will be ordered (e.g., radiographs [x-rays], computed tomographic [CT] scans, magnetic resonance imaging [MRI] scans, positron emission tomography [PET] scans, arterial blood gas levels, and partial pressures of CO_2 and O_2), so assess findings. When *dactinomycin* or *daunorubicin* are given intravenously, the drug is generally administered via a central line indwelling catheter device (e.g., Port-A-Cath or MediPort), because if it is given by peripheral intravenous line and extravasation occurs, there is a risk for necrosis with tissue sloughing that may erode through the layers of skin and underlying supportive structures (e.g., muscles, ligaments). See the pharmacology discussion of extravasation as well as Table 46-3 and Box 46-3. In addition, in patients with documented cardiac disease or a history of thoracic irradiation, administer dactinomycin, daunorubicin, and *doxorubicin* with extreme caution due to cardiovascular toxicity. CT scans and ultrasound studies may be needed before and during treatment to assess cardiac ejection fraction because of the risk for cardiotoxicity, which is often associated with cumulative doses.

With use of *hormonal antineoplastic drugs*, obtain a thorough medical, nursing, and medication history. Many of the drugs included in this category are presented in depth in Chapters 34 and 35, which also discuss aspects of the nursing process related to their use. Assessment associated with the use of *estrogen antagonists* such as *fulvestrant, tamoxifen, raloxifene,* and *toremifene* citrates often begins with a review of the results of any tumor estrogen receptor assays, CT scans, x-rays, and other diagnostic testing. Perform a neurologic assessment (see

> **BOX 46-3   Concerns in the Handling and Administration of Vesicant Drugs**
>
> The handling and administration of antineoplastic drugs is of major concern because the nurse mixing and giving the drug may experience negative consequences. The pharmacy department is responsible for mixing these drugs, and preparation must be carried out carefully in an appropriate environment with use of a laminar airflow hood and personal protective equipment (mask, gown, gloves). Many health care institutions recommend taking special precautions during the care of a patient who is receiving chemotherapy, such as double-flushing the patient's bodily secretions in the commode and using special hampers for disposal of all items that come into contact with the patient, including used personal protective equipment. Special spill kits are employed to clean up even the smallest chemotherapy spills. These precautions are necessary to protect the health care provider from the cytotoxic effects of these drugs. In addition, proper and up-to-date knowledge about these drugs is important to safe and appropriate nursing care. All nurses giving these drugs must be certified to administer chemotherapy and must remain current in their level of practice and competencies related to this treatment modality. All equipment and containers must be handled appropriately once the infusion is completed. Hands and any exposed areas must be washed to ensure the safety of the health care provider. The Centers for Disease Control and Prevention and the Oncology Nursing Society offer exceptional resources for individuals involved in the care of patients receiving chemotherapy.

previous discussion and Chapters 34 and 45) with attention to baseline complaints of any pain, abnormal sensations, or headaches. Note any menopausal symptoms upon assessment because of the possible adverse effect of vasodilation and hot flushes. In addition, these drugs may cause nausea and vomiting, so a thorough GI assessment is beneficial.

With the use of *androgens* (e.g., *fluoxymesterone, testosterone*), obtain a thorough gynecologic history of the female patient with attention to any menstrual issues or problems because of the adverse effect of menstrual irregularities. It is also important to assess the patient's body image and feelings of self-esteem because of the possible adverse effects of acne, hirsutism, and virilization in female patients as well as gynecomastia in male patients. See Chapter 35 for more information on the side effects of androgens.

Bicalutamide, flutamide, and *nilutamide* are *antiandrogens* and require thorough assessment of any cardiac diseases due to the potential for peripheral edema. This could exacerbate any preexisting cardiac disorder. Perform a thorough gastrointestinal (GI) and gynecologic assessment because of the possibility for nausea, diarrhea, as well as hot flushes. Documentation of the use of a reliable form of birth control is important because of teratogenic effects. Male sperm production may be affected (see Chapter 45), and a decline in sexual functioning and/or desire may occur because of the antiandrogenic effects.

With use of *gonadotropin-releasing hormone agonists,* such as *leuprolide* and *goserelin,* assess the patient for allergies to the drugs. Contraceptive history is important because women who are taking these drugs must use a nonhormonal contraceptive. Often the prescriber will order laboratory tests for serum testosterone and prostatic acid phosphatase levels for male patients before and during therapy; an increase will be noted during the initial week of therapy, with levels returning to baseline by 4 weeks.

For patients taking *antiadrenal drugs* (e.g., *mitotane*), in addition to performing a basic assessment, inquire about any GI disturbances because of the common adverse effects of nausea and vomiting. With the *miscellaneous antineoplastic drugs*, glucocorticoids and mineralocorticoids may be given to prevent adrenal insufficiency and may also play a part in the therapeutic regimen. An understanding of baseline adrenal functioning through examination of laboratory test results is important to the safe use of these drugs.

With the *miscellaneous* drug *hydroxyurea*, assessment of liver, renal, neurologic, and pulmonary function with baseline blood cell counts are important due to the adverse reactions associated with this drug. With use of *bevacizumab*, an *angiogenesis inhibitor*, assess cardiovascular, central nervous system, GI tract, and renal functioning because of the adverse effects of hypotension or hypertension, headache, pain, dizziness, nausea, vomiting, diarrhea, and nephrotoxicity. *Sipuleucel-T (Provenge)*, a newer drug used with prostate cancer, is not a true chemotherapeutic drug but rather an autologous cellular immunotherapy drug. It is important to understand that sipuleucel-T is associated with infusion reactions, and its use is restricted to those prescribers who have undergone extensive training. With *ceritinib*, assess baseline cardiovascular status with blood pressure, pulse rate, and EKG findings because it is associated with the side effects of bradycardia and changes in QTc interval. Additionally, assess breath sounds, breathing patterns, and pulmonary function testing results due to adverse effects of life-threatening interstitial lung disease or pneumonitis. Drug interactions to assess for include grapefruit juice, strong CYP3A4 inhibitors/inducers, conivaptan, and any drugs that prolong the QTc interval.

CASE STUDY

Safety: What Went Wrong? Chemotherapy with Alkylating Drugs

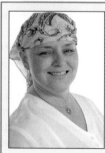

W.S. is receiving cisplatin as part of treatment for ovarian cancer. She is receiving her third treatment today and has just arrived at the cancer treatment center for her outpatient infusion. W.S. says that she felt "okay" during the time between the last treatment and today but is not looking forward to today's treatment because of the side effects.

1. While the nurse prepares to start the infusion, what is important for the nurse to assess before beginning the chemotherapy?
2. What will the nurse do before the infusion to help reduce or prevent adverse effects?
3. During the infusion, W.S. mentions that she is hearing a slight "roaring" sound and that she feels a bit dizzy. What will the nurse do next?
4. After stopping the infusion, the nurse spills some of the chemotherapy solution on her arm and the floor. The nurse wipes up the solution with a paper towel and then notifies the charge nurse. The charge nurse becomes concerned and calls the house supervisor, environmental services department, and the hospital's occupational health nurse. What went wrong?

For answers, see *http://evolve.elsevier.com/Lilley.*

NURSING DIAGNOSES

1. Decreased cardiac output related to the adverse effect of cardiotoxicity associated with cytotoxic antibiotics
2. Diarrhea related to the adverse effects of antineoplastic drugs
3. Imbalanced nutrition, less than body requirements, related to loss of appetite, nausea, and vomiting, as a result of antineoplastic therapy

PLANNING: OUTCOME IDENTIFICATION

1. Patient maintains/regains normal ranges of cardiac output with blood pressure and pulse rates within normal limits (120/80; 60-100 bpm) while implementing daily weights, conserving energy, adequate fluid intake, balanced diet, and reporting of shortness of breath, chest pain, and/or high/low blood pressure/pulse rate.
2. Patient regains normal to near-normal bowel patterns with less diarrhea while avoiding irritating foods/beverages and takes preventive medication (for diarrhea) as prescribed.
3. Patient regains/maintains healthy nutritional patterns with adequate fluid intake, well-balanced diet as tolerated, nutritional supplementation as prescribed, and avoidance of problematic foods/beverages.

IMPLEMENTATION

Before initiating drug therapy with the *cell-cycle–nonspecific drugs, hormonal antineoplastics,* and/or *miscellaneous drugs,* you must be completely knowledgeable about the drug, its use, and impact on all rapidly dividing cells, whether normal or malignant (see Chapters 34, 35, and 45 for additional information).

With *alkylating drugs,* always handle these and all other antineoplastics with caution because of their possible carcinogenic, mutagenic, and teratogenic properties (see Box 46-3). The patient receiving alkylating drugs will more than likely experience problems related to bone marrow suppression, such as anemia, leukopenia, and thrombocytopenia (see Chapter 45 for specific interventions). Most nursing interventions are focused on preventing infection, conserving energy, preventing bleeding and injury, and reducing nausea. Other nursing considerations for these drugs include taking vital signs every 1 to 2 hours or as needed during infusion; increasing fluids; monitoring intake and output; following orders for intravenous therapy for hydration; and monitoring any nausea/vomiting. Contact the prescriber if vomiting is uncontrolled so that appropriate medications can be implemented. Monitor the patient constantly for abnormal peripheral sensations, especially with cisplatin. Report to the prescriber any numbness or tingling of extremities and any ringing or roaring in the ears and/or hearing loss. Encourage the patient experiencing peripheral neuropathies to avoid extremely cold temperatures or the handling of cold objects. *Cisplatin* is particularly nephrotoxic, so closely monitor renal function throughout therapy. Intravenous hydration is often required at a rate of 100 to 200 mL/hr starting before *cisplatin* administration with a total of 2000 to 3000 mL/day, depending on the dose of cisplatin and if not contraindicated. Do not use aluminum needles or administration sets with many of these drugs because aluminum can degrade their platinum compounds; ensure that the proper infusion equipment is used. Because hemorrhagic cystitis is associated with *cyclophosphamide* use, make sure the patient's hydration is maintained to minimize this adverse effect. Pulmonary toxicity may occur with some of the *alkylating drugs*, particularly *busulfan*; therefore, constantly monitor and be alert to cough, shortness of breath, and abnormal breath sounds. Immediately report these adverse effects to the prescriber. Other drugs in this group may be given by various routes, such as intrapericardial, intratumoral, and intravesical. Be sure you perform appropriate interventions per the manufacturer's guidelines or health care institutional policy. Reconstitute the parenteral formulations for any of these drugs according to the manufacturer's guidelines and suggestions. Not all diluents are compatible.

One very important component of nursing care with alkylating drugs and their parenteral administration is monitoring the IV site/infusion continually for signs and symptoms of infiltration. Infiltration could lead to extravasation of the medication into the surrounding tissue. To briefly review, IV infiltration is the leakage of fluids or blood from a dislodged catheter or needle cannula from the intima of the vein and into the surrounding tissue. Signs and symptoms of infiltration include inflammation at or near the insertion site with swollen, taut skin with pain, blanching, and coolness of skin around the IV site; slowed or stopped IV infusion; no backflow of blood into the IV tubing; and/or no blood return obtained. The reason infiltration is of concern with these drugs is that some of them are irritants and others are vesicants with the potential of severe tissue damage. Therefore, if extravasation occurs with some of these drugs, antidotes are required to try and prevent damage from leakage of the drug into the tissue. Specific antidotes for alkylating drugs are presented in Table 46-3. Always follow health care institutional policy when treating extravasation of any medication. With IV infusions of antineoplastics, monitoring of the IV site and infusions is usually more frequent, with many guidelines/policies outlining the standard of care to be hourly assessment with documentation. It is important to note that the vast majority of chemotherapeutic drugs are administered via a central line indwelling catheter device (e.g., Port-A-Cath or MediPort) to minimize the risk for extravasation. Check the device and its patency prior to the drug's administration.

Patients receiving *cytotoxic antibiotics* such as *bleomycin* may require more frequent monitoring of pulmonary function. Baseline chest x-rays may be obtained for comparison with subsequent x-rays if pneumonitis occurs. Monitor results of liver and renal function tests throughout therapy with *dactinomycin*, *daunorubicin*, *doxorubicin*, and *mitomycin*. Heart sounds, daily weights, blood pressure, pulse rate, and monitoring for signs and symptoms of cardiovascular toxicities (e.g., alterations in vital signs, abnormal heart sounds, dyspnea, chest pain) are especially important with doxorubicin, *idarubicin*, and *mitoxantrone*. Additionally, if the patient experiences an increase of 2 pounds or more in 24 hours or 5 pounds or more in 1 week, notify the prescriber, as this may reflect fluid retention related to heart failure. Mitomycin is associated with liver, kidney, and lung toxicities. Close monitoring of these systems during treatment is key to patient safety.

Use of *hormone antagonists* in the treatment of various neoplasms is common, particularly with breast and prostate cancer. Associated nursing interventions and patient education for the use of these drugs are discussed in depth in Chapters 34 and 35. Corticosteroid therapy and related nursing considerations are presented in Chapter 33.

Hydroxyurea is used sparingly but is a component of some treatment protocols. This drug is given orally. Monitor platelet and leukocyte counts before, during, and after treatment due to the adverse effect of bone marrow suppression. If the platelet count falls below 100,000 platelets/mm^3 or leukocyte count falls below 2000 cells/mm^3, therapy may need to be temporarily halted until counts rise toward normal values. See the earlier discussion and Chapter 45 about nursing considerations associated with anemia, fatigue, weakness, bleeding tendencies, and infection. Additionally, hyperuricemia may precipitate gout-related symptoms (e.g., painful, swollen joints); report these to the prescriber so that the appropriate medication may be ordered. Often a drug, such as allopurinol, is prescribed to help control the levels of uric acid caused by cell death from the chemotherapy. The use of *sipuleucel-T* is associated with infusion-related reactions, and those prescribers trained to prescribe/administer the drug will have prescribed a pretreatment protocol with acetaminophen and diphenhydramine. *Ceritinib* is given orally and must be given on an empty stomach or at least 2 hours before or 2 hours after a meal. Closely monitor cardiac and respiratory status during this treatment due to its side effects (see pharmacology discussion).

In addition to the nursing interventions discussed earlier and in Chapter 45, keep epinephrine, antihistamines, and antiinflammatory drugs available in case of an allergic or anaphylactic reaction. Each antineoplastic drug has its own peculiarities and its own set of cautions, contraindications, nursing implementations, and toxicities. *Cytoprotective drugs* are useful in reducing certain toxicities. For example, use of intravenous amifostine may help to reduce the renal toxicity associated with cisplatin. With the occurrence of hyperuricemia (see Table 45-6 and Box 45-2), intravenous or oral allopurinol may be given to reduce uric acid levels. Other major concerns related to the care of patients receiving chemotherapy are the oncologic emergencies that arise because of damage occurring to rapidly dividing normal cells as well as rapidly dividing cancerous cells. Some of the complications that are potential emergencies include infections, infusion reactions and allergy, stomatitis with severe ulceration, bleeding, metabolic aberrations, severe diarrhea, renal failure, liver failure, and cardiotoxicity, including dysrhythmia or heart failure (Box 46-4).

SAFETY: LABORATORY VALUES RELATED TO DRUG THERAPY

Rationales for Assessment and Monitoring of Blood Cell Counts with Antineoplastics

Laboratory Test	Normal Ranges	Rationale for Assessment
Leukocytes (WBCs)	5000 to 10,000 cells/mm^3	WBCs protect against infection, and when an infection develops, the WBCs attack and destroy the causative bacteria, virus, or other organism. In response to the infection, WBCs increase in number dramatically. If WBC levels are decreased from antineoplastic treatment and subsequent bone marrow suppression, and if they decrease to levels less than 2000 cells/mm^3 (leukopenia), there is a high risk for severe infection and immunosuppression.
WBC components: Neutrophils Band neutrophils	47% to 77% or above 1500 cells/mm^3 0% to 3%	The major types of WBCs are neutrophils, lymphocytes, monocytes, eosinophils, and basophils. Immature neutrophils are called *band neutrophils* and their number, along with neutrophil counts, provides a picture of the patient's immune system. If neutrophils are decreased to levels of less than 500 cells/mm^3 (neutropenia), then there is a risk for severe infection. If band neutrophils are included in the WBC differential count, then an abnormally low value reinforces the risk for severe infection (see Chapter 45).
Nadir	See normal range of each blood cell.	*Nadir* refers to the lowest levels of bone marrow cells that are reached. The time to reach this nadir may become shorter and the recovery time longer with successive courses of antineoplastic treatment. A general estimate of the time to nadir is 10 to 28 days. Anticipation of the nadir allows the oncologist and health care team to develop a preventive treatment plan that may include use of biologic response modifiers and antibiotics.

NOTE: Similar information on red blood cell and platelet counts is presented in Chapter 45. Also note that chemotherapy may be discontinued with anemia, leukopenia, neutropenia, and/or thrombocytopenia. Once counts recover (sometimes more quickly with certain drugs), treatment is often reinitiated.

BOX 46-4   Indications of an Oncologic Emergency

Fever and/or chills with a temperature higher than 100.5°F (38.1°C)
New sores or white patches in the mouth or throat
Swollen tongue with or without cracks and bleeding
Bleeding gums
Dry, burning, "scratchy," or "swollen" throat
A cough that is new and persistent
Changes in bladder function or patterns
Blood in the urine
Changes in GI or bowel patterns, including "heartburn" or nausea, vomiting, constipation, or diarrhea lasting longer than 2 or 3 days
Blood in the stools

NOTE: The patient must contact the prescriber immediately if any of the listed signs or symptoms occurs. If the prescriber is not available, the patient must seek medical treatment at the closest emergency department.

EVALUATION

Focus the evaluation of nursing care upon determining whether goals and outcomes have been met, as well as on monitoring for therapeutic responses and adverse and toxic effects of *antineoplastic therapy*. Therapeutic responses may manifest as clinical improvement, decrease in tumor size, and decrease in metastatic spread. Evaluation of nursing care with reference to goals and outcomes may reveal improvements related to a decrease in adverse effects; a decrease in the impact of cancer on the patient's well-being; an increase in comfort, nutrition, and hydration; improved energy levels and ability to carry out activities of daily living; and improved quality of life. The goals and outcomes may be revisited to identify more specific parameters to monitor. In addition, certain laboratory studies such as measurement of tumor markers; levels of carcinoembryonic antigens; and red blood cell, white blood cell, and platelet counts may also be used to determine how well the goals and outcomes have been met. As part of the evaluation, prescribers may also order additional x-rays, CT scans, MRIs, tissue analyses, and other studies appropriate to the diagnosis during and after antineoplastic therapy, at time intervals related to anticipated tumor response.

PATIENT-CENTERED CARE: PATIENT TEACHING

• Advise the patient to avoid aspirin, ibuprofen, and products containing these drugs to help prevent excessive bleeding.
• Be open with discussion about the risk for alopecia (a complete discussion is presented in Chapter 45) as an adverse effect of many of the antineoplastic drugs.
• Encourage the increase of fluids of up to 3000 mL/day, if not contraindicated, to prevent dehydration and further

weakening. In the case of cyclophosphamide therapy, adequate hydration is needed to prevent and/or help manage hemorrhagic cystitis.
• Constipation may be problematic, so educate the patient about ways to help manage this altered bowel status that may be due to the antineoplastic or due to the narcotics used for pain management. To help avoid constipation,

increasing fluids and consumption of a balanced diet are important; however, the oncologist often orders either a stool softener or a mild noncramping laxative to prevent the problem.

- Diarrhea may also be experienced. Advise the patient to avoid spicy, irritating foods; gas-producing foods; caffeine; high-fiber foods; alcohol; and very hot or cold foods and beverages. Preventive medication, such as synthetic opioids (e.g., loperamide) or adsorbents-protectants, may be prescribed to help prevent or treat excess diarrhea.
- Educate the patient about the importance of daily weights and reporting a 2-pound increase in weight over 24 hours or a 5-pound increase in 1 week.
- Demonstrate the proper technique for monitoring blood pressure and pulse rate. Encourage the use of a journal to record daily weights, blood pressure readings, and pulse rate.
- With cytotoxic antibiotics, emphasize the importance of adhering to a daily heart-healthy regimen of conserving energy, planned activities, and seeking/asking for assistance with care and activities of daily living, as needed, to conserve strength and energy. Educate about the importance of reporting the occurrence of hypotension, bradycardia, chest pain, and/or dyspnea.
- The following are helpful online resources for the patient and significant others: *www.fda.gov, www.fda.gov/ForHealth Professionals/default.htm, www.nih.gov, www.healthfinder.gov, www.who.int/en,* and *www.oncolink.org/index.cfm.*

KEY POINTS

- Antineoplastics are drugs that are used to treat malignancies and are classified as cell-cycle–specific drugs, cell-cycle–nonspecific drugs, miscellaneous antineoplastics, and hormonal drugs.
- Cell-cycle–specific drugs kill cancer cells during specific phases of the cell growth cycle, whereas the cell-cycle–nonspecific drugs discussed in this chapter kill cancer cells during any phase of the growth cycle.
- Chemotherapy, or antineoplastic drug therapy, requires very skillful and perceptive care, and you must act prudently and make critical decisions about the nursing care of patients receiving these drugs.
- Knowledge is important to ensure patient and health care provider safety and for protection from the adverse effects of antineoplastics.
- Always exercise extreme caution in the handling and administration of cell-cycle–nonspecific (as well as cell-cycle–specific) drugs.

- Hormonal drugs, both agonists and antagonists, are used to treat a variety of malignancies.
- Extravasation of strong vesicants (e.g., doxorubicin) may lead to severe tissue injury with complications such as permanent damage to muscles, tendons, and ligaments, and possible loss of limb. Constantly monitor the IV site and infusions to prevent this possible complication. Checking the patency of central venous access devices is also important because the majority of chemotherapy drugs are given via this route.
- Oncologic emergencies occur as a consequence of cell death and may be life-threatening. Skillful assessment and immediate intervention may help to decrease the severity of the problem or even reduce the occurrence of such emergencies.

NCLEX® EXAMINATION REVIEW QUESTIONS

1. A patient who is receiving chemotherapy with cisplatin (Platinol) has developed pneumonia. The nurse would be concerned about nephrotoxicity if which type of antibiotic was ordered as treatment for the pneumonia at this time?
   a. Penicillin
   b. Sulfa drug
   c. Fluoroquinolone
   d. Aminoglycoside
2. During treatment with doxorubicin (Adriamycin), the nurse must monitor closely for which potentially life-threatening adverse effect?
   a. Nephrotoxicity
   b. Peripheral neuritis
   c. Cardiomyopathy
   d. Ototoxicity

3. While teaching a patient who is about to receive cyclophosphamide (Cytoxan) chemotherapy, the nurse will instruct the patient to watch for potential adverse effects, such as
   a. cholinergic diarrhea.
   b. hemorrhagic cystitis.
   c. peripheral neuropathy.
   d. ototoxicity.
4. When chemotherapy with alkylating drugs is planned, the nurse expects to implement which intervention to prevent nephrotoxicity?
   a. Hydrating the patient with intravenous fluids before chemotherapy
   b. Limiting fluids before chemotherapy
   c. Monitoring drug levels during chemotherapy
   d. Assessing creatinine clearance during chemotherapy

5. During therapy with the cytotoxic antibiotic bleomycin, the nurse will assess for a potentially serious adverse effect by monitoring
   a. blood urea nitrogen and creatinine levels.
   b. cardiac ejection fraction.
   c. respiratory function.
   d. cranial nerve function.
6. While administering bevacizumab (Avastin), what will the nurse assess to look for drug-related toxicities? *(Select all that apply.)*
   a. Blood pressure
   b. Color of the skin and sclera of the eye (for jaundice)
   c. Blood glucose level
   d. Urine protein level
   e. Hearing
   f. Weight

7. The nurse is preparing to add a dose of bevacizumab (Avastin) to a patient's intravenous infusion. The infusion bag prepared by the pharmacy has 70 mg of bevacizumab in 100 mL of normal saline, and it is to infuse over 90 minutes. The nurse will set the infusion pump to what rate for this dose?
8. The day before a third round of chemotherapy, the nurse reads that a patient's neutrophil count is 1650 cells/mm^3. The nurse expects that the oncologist will follow which course of treatment?
   a. The chemotherapy will be started as scheduled.
   b. The chemotherapy will be given at a lower dosage.
   c. The oncologist will order a neutrophil transfusion to be given first.
   d. The chemotherapy will not be given today.

1. d, 2. c, 3. b, 4. a, 5. c, 6. a, d, f, 7. 67 mL/hour (66.66 rounds to 67), 8. a.

CRITICAL THINKING AND PRIORITIZATION QUESTIONS

1. During an infusion of carmustine, a patient dislodges the intravenous catheter, and infiltration of the medication occurs. What is the nurse's priority action at this time? Explain your answer.
2. A patient has been receiving bleomycin irrigations through a chest tube for 3 days. Today he begins to have an irregular and slow heart rhythm, complains of nausea, and says, "I'm seeing yellow hazy circles around the lights." He thinks the chemotherapy is causing these problems. The nurse reviews the patient's medications and notes that he is taking digoxin (Lanoxin), lisinopril (Zestril), and simvastatin (Zocor). What is the nurse's priority action at this time? Explain your answer.

For answers, see *http://evolve.elsevier.com/Lilley*.

ⓔ EVOLVE WEBSITE

http://evolve.elsevier.com/Lilley
- Animations
- Answer Keys for Textbook Case Studies and Textbook Critical Thinking and Prioritization Questions
- Content Updates
- Key Points
- Review Questions
- Student Case Studies

Biologic Response–Modifying and Antirheumatic Drugs

http://evolve.elsevier.com/Lilley

OBJECTIVES

When you reach the end of this chapter, you will be able to do the following:

1. Describe the basic anatomy, physiology, and functions of the immune system.
2. Compare the two major classes of biologic response–modifying drugs: hematopoietic drugs and immunomodulating drugs.
3. Discuss the mechanisms of action, indications, dosages, routes of administration, adverse effects, cautions, contraindications, and drug interactions of the different biologic response–modifying drugs.
4. Describe the pathology associated with rheumatoid arthritis.
5. Discuss the mechanisms of action, indications, dosages, routes of administration, adverse effects, cautions, contraindications, and drug interactions of the different antirheumatic drugs.
6. Develop a nursing care plan that includes all phases of the nursing process for patients receiving biologic response–modifying drugs and for those receiving antirheumatic drugs.

DRUG PROFILES

abatacept, p. 762
adalimumab, p. 757
♦ aldesleukin, p. 760
alemtuzumab, p. 758
anakinra, p. 760
belimumab, p. 758
bevacizumab, p. 758
certolizumab, p. 758
cetuximab, p. 758
etanercept, p. 762
♦ filgrastim, p. 752
golimumab, p. 758
ibritumomab tiuxetan, p. 758
infliximab, p. 758
♦ interferon alfa-2a, interferon alfa-2b, interferon alfa-n3, peginterferon alfa-2a, and peginterferon alfa-2b, p. 754

♦ interferon beta-1a, interferon beta-1b, p. 755
interferon gamma-1b, p. 755
leflunomide, p. 763
! methotrexate, p. 763
natalizumab, p. 758
♦ oprelvekin, p. 753
♦ rituximab, p. 759
♦ sargramostim, p. 753
ocilizumab, p. 760
tositumomab and iodine I-131 tositumomab, p. 759
rastuzumab, p. 759

_____

♦ = *Key drug*
! = *High-alert drug*

KEY TERMS

Adjuvant A nonspecific *immunostimulant* that enhances overall immune function, rather than stimulating the function of a specific immune system cell. (p. 761)

Antibodies Immunoglobulin molecules (see Chapter 49) that have the ability to bind to and inactivate antigen molecules through formation of an antigen-antibody complex. This process serves to inactivate foreign antigens that enter the body. (p. 750)

Antigen A biologic or chemical substance that is recognized as foreign by the body's immune system. (p. 749)

Arthritis Inflammation of one or more joints. (p. 762)

Autoimmune disorder A disorder that occurs when the body's tissues are attacked by its own immune system. (p. 761)

B lymphocytes (B cells) Leukocytes of the humoral immune system that develop into plasma cells, and then produce the antibodies that bind to and inactivate antigens. B cells are one of the two principal types of lymphocytes; T lymphocytes are the other. (p. 749)

Biologic response–modifying drugs A broad class of drugs that includes hematopoietic drugs and immunomodulating drugs. Often referred to as *biologic response modifiers (BRMs),* they alter the body's response to diseases such as cancer as well as autoimmune, inflammatory, and infectious diseases. Examples are cytokines (e.g., interleukin, interferons), monoclonal antibodies, and vaccines. They are also called *biomodulators* or *immunomodulating drugs.* Biologic response–modifying drugs may be adjuvants, immunostimulants, or immunosuppressants. (p. 749)

Cell-mediated immunity Collective term for all immune responses that are mediated by T lymphocytes (T cells). Also called *cellular immunity.* Cell-mediated immunity acts in collaboration with humoral immunity. (p. 749)

Colony-stimulating factors Cytokines that regulate the growth, differentiation, and function of bone marrow stem cells. (p. 751)

Complement Collective term for about 20 different proteins normally present in plasma that assist other immune system components (e.g., B cells and T cells) in mounting an immune response. (p. 759)

Cytokines The generic term for nonantibody proteins released by specific cell populations (e.g., activated T cells) on contact with antigens. Cytokines act as intercellular mediators of an immune response. (p. 750)

Cytotoxic T cells Differentiated T cells that can recognize and lyse (rupture) target cells that have foreign antigens on their surfaces. These antigens are recognized by the corresponding antigen receptors that are expressed (displayed) on the cytotoxic T-cell surface. Also called *natural killer cells.* (p. 750)

Differentiation The process of cellular development from a simplified into a more specialized cellular structure. In hematopoiesis, it refers to the multistep processes involved in the maturation of blood cells. (p. 751)

Disease-modifying antirheumatic drugs (DMARDs) Medications used in the treatment of rheumatic diseases that have the potential to arrest or slow the actual disease process instead of providing only antiinflammatory and analgesic effects. (p. 762)

Hematopoiesis Collective term for all of the body's processes originating in the bone marrow that result in the formation of various types of blood components (adjective: *hematopoietic*). It includes the three main processes of *differentiation* (see earlier): erythropoiesis (formation of red blood cells, or erythrocytes), leukopoiesis (formation of white blood cells, or leukocytes), and thrombopoiesis (formation of platelets, or thrombocytes). (p. 749)

Humoral immunity Collective term for all immune responses that are mediated by B cells, which ultimately work through the production of antibodies against specific antigens. Humoral immunity acts in collaboration with *cell-mediated immunity.* (p. 749)

Immunoglobulins Complex immune system glycoproteins that bind to and inactivate foreign antigens. The term is synonymous with *immune globulins.* (p. 750)

Immunomodulating drugs Collective term for various subclasses of biologic response–modifying drugs that specifically or nonspecifically enhance or reduce immune responses. The three major types of immunomodulators, based on mechanism of action, are adjuvants, immunostimulants, and immunosuppressants (see Chapter 48). (p. 749)

Immunostimulant A drug that enhances immune response through specific chemical interactions with particular immune system components. An example is interleukin-2. (p. 761)

Immunosuppressant A drug that reduces immune response through specific chemical interactions with particular immune system components. An example is cyclosporine (see Chapter 48). (p. 754)

Interferons One type of cytokine that promotes resistance to viral infection in uninfected cells and can also strengthen the body's immune response to cancer cells. (p. 753)

Leukocytes The collective term for all subtypes of white blood cells. Leukocytes include the granulocytes (neutrophils, eosinophils, and basophils), monocytes, and lymphocytes (B cells and T cells). Some monocytes also develop into tissue macrophages. (p. 750)

Lymphokine-activated killer (LAK) cell *Cytotoxic T cells* that have been activated by interkeukin-2 and therefore have a stronger and more specific response against cancer cells. (p. 759)

Lymphokines Cytokines that are produced by sensitized T lymphocytes on contact with antigen particles. (p. 750)

Memory cells Cells involved in the humoral immune system that remember the exact characteristics of a particular foreign invader or antigen for the purpose of expediting immune response in the event of future exposure to this antigen. (p. 750)

Monoclonal Denoting a group of identical cells or organisms derived from a single cell. (p. 750)

Plasma cells Cells derived from B cells that are found in the bone marrow, connective tissue, and blood. They produce antibodies. (p. 750)

Rheumatism General term for any of several disorders characterized by inflammation, degeneration, or metabolic derangement of connective tissue structures, especially joints and related structures. (p. 761)

T helper cells Cells that promote and direct the actions of various other cells of the immune system. (p. 750)

T lymphocytes (T cells) Leukocytes of the cell-mediated immune system. Unlike B cells, they are not involved in the production of antibodies but instead occur in various cell subtypes (e.g., T helper cells, T suppressor cells, and cytotoxic T cells). They act through direct cell-to-cell contact or through production of cytokines that guide the functions of other immune system components (e.g., B cells, antibodies). (p. 749)

T suppressor cells Cells that regulate and limit the immune response, balancing the effects of T helper cells. (p. 750)

Tumor antigens Chemical compounds expressed on the surfaces of tumor cells. They signal to the immune system that these cells do not belong in the body, labeling the tumor cells as foreign. (p. 749)

OVERVIEW OF IMMUNOMODULATORS

Over the last two decades, medical technology has developed a group of drugs whose primary site of action is the immune system. This has resulted in new additions to the class of drugs known as biologic response–modifying drugs, or biologic response modifiers. These drugs alter the body's response to diseases such as cancer and autoimmune, inflammatory, and infectious diseases. These drugs can enhance or restrict the patient's immune response to disease, can stimulate a patient's hematopoietic (blood-forming) function, and can prevent disease. Hematopoiesis is the collective term for all of the blood component–forming processes of the bone marrow. Two broad classes of biologic response–modifying drugs are hematopoietic drugs and immunomodulating drugs. Subclasses of immunomodulating drugs include interferons, monoclonal antibodies, interleukin receptor agonists and antagonists, and miscellaneous drugs. Disease-modifying antirheumatic drugs are drugs that are used to treat rheumatoid arthritis and are discussed later in the chapter.

Immunomodulating drugs therapeutically alter a patient's immune response. In cancer treatment, they make up the fourth type of cancer therapy, along with surgery, chemotherapy, and radiation. The human immune system is most commonly viewed as the body's natural defense against pathogenic bacteria and viruses. However, it also has effective antitumor capabilities. An intact immune system can identify cells as malignant and destroy them. In contrast to chemotherapeutic drugs, a healthy immune system can distinguish between tumor cells and normal body tissues. Normal cells are recognized as "self" and are not damaged, whereas tumor cells are recognized as "foreign" and are destroyed. People develop cancerous cells in their bodies on a regular basis. Normally the immune system is able to eliminate these cells before they multiply to uncontrollable levels. It is only when the natural immune responses fail to keep pace with these initially microscopic cancer cell growths that a person develops a true "cancer" requiring clinical intervention.

In terms of their activity against cancer cells, biologic response–modifying drugs work by one of three mechanisms: (1) enhancement or restoration of the host's immune system defenses against the tumor; (2) direct toxic effect on the tumor cells, which causes them to lyse, or rupture; or (3) adverse modification of the tumor's biology, which makes it harder for the tumor cells to survive and reproduce.

Some immunomodulating drugs are used to treat autoimmune, inflammatory, and infectious diseases. In these instances, the drug functions either to reduce the patient's inappropriate immune response (in the case of inflammatory and autoimmune diseases such as rheumatoid arthritis) or to strengthen the patient's immune response against microorganisms (especially viruses) and cancer cells. To better understand these complex drugs, a review of immune system physiology is beneficial.

IMMUNE SYSTEM

The immune system is an intricate biologic defense network of cells that are capable of distinguishing an unlimited variety of substances as either foreign ("nonself") or a natural part of the host's body ("self"). When a foreign substance such as a bacteria or virus enters the body, the immune system recognizes it as being foreign and mounts an immune response to eliminate or neutralize the invader. Tumors are not truly foreign substances because they arise from cells of normal tissues whose genetic material (deoxyribonucleic acid [DNA] and ribonucleic acid [RNA]) has somehow mutated. Tumor cells express chemical compounds on their surfaces that signal the immune system that these cells are a threat. These chemical markers are called tumor antigens or *tumor markers,* and they label the tumor cells as abnormal cells. An antigen is any substance that the body's immune system recognizes as foreign. Recognition of antigens varies among individuals, which is why some people are more prone than others to immune-related diseases such as allergies, inflammatory diseases, and cancer.

The two major components of the body's immune system are humoral immunity, which is mediated by B-cell functions (primarily *antibody* production), and cell-mediated immunity, which is mediated by T-cell functions. These two systems work together to recognize and destroy foreign particles and cells in the blood or other body tissues. Communication between these two divisions is important. Attack against tumor cells by antibodies produced by the B lymphocytes (B cells) of the humoral immune system prepares those tumor cells for destruction by the T lymphocytes (T cells) of the cell-mediated immune system.

Humoral Immune System

The functional cells of the humoral immune system are the B lymphocytes. They are also called *B cells* because they originate in the bone marrow. The B cells normally remain dormant until the corresponding antigen is detected. When an antigen binds to receptors located on the B cells, a biochemical signal is sent to the B lymphocytes. These B cells then mature or *differentiate* into **plasma cells,** which in turn produce antibodies. **Antibodies** are **immunoglobulins** that bind to specific antigens, forming an *antigen-antibody complex* that inactivates disease-causing antigens.

The immune system in a healthy individual is genetically preprogrammed to be able to mount an antibody response against literally millions of different antigens. This ability results from the individual's lifetime antigen exposure and is further developed through exposure to new antigens. Antibodies that a single plasma cell makes are all identical and are called **monoclonal** antibodies. Since the 1980s, monoclonal antibodies have also been prepared synthetically using recombinant DNA technology, which has resulted in newer drug therapies.

There are five major types of naturally occurring immunoglobulins in the body: immunoglobulins A, D, E, G, and M. These unique types have different structures and functions and are found in various areas of the body. During an immune response, when B lymphocytes differentiate into plasma cells, some of these B cells become **memory cells.** Memory cells "remember" the exact characteristics of a particular foreign invader or antigen, which allows a stronger and faster immune response in the event of reexposure to the same antigen. The cells of the humoral immune system are shown in Figure 47-1.

Cell-Mediated Immune System

The functional cells of the cell-mediated (as opposed to antibody-mediated) immune system are the T lymphocytes. They are also referred to as *T cells* because they mature in the thymus. There are three distinct populations of T cells: cytotoxic T cells, T helper cells, and T suppressor cells (Figure 47-2). They are distinguished by the different functions that they perform. **Cytotoxic T cells** directly kill their targets by causing cell lysis or rupture. **T helper cells** are considered the master controllers of the immune system. They direct the actions of many other immune components, such as lymphokines and cytotoxic T cells. **Cytokines** are nonantibody proteins that serve as chemical mediators of various physiologic functions. **Lymphokines** are a subset of cytokines. They are released by T lymphocytes upon contact with antigens and serve as chemical mediators of the immune response. **T suppressor cells** have an effect on the immune system that is opposite to that of T helper cells and serve to limit or control the immune response. A

healthy immune system has about twice as many T helper cells as T suppressor cells at any given time.

The cell-mediated immune system (see Figure 47-2) is involved in the destruction of cancer cells. The cancer-killing cells of the cellular immune system are the macrophages (derived from monocytes), natural killer (NK) cells (another type of lymphocyte), and polymorphonuclear **leukocytes** (not lymphocytes), which are also called *neutrophils.* In contrast, T suppressor cells have an important negative influence on antitumor actions of the immune system. Overactive T suppressor cells may be responsible for clinically significant cancers by permitting tumor growth beyond the immune system's control.

PHARMACOLOGY OVERVIEW

Therapy with biologic response–modifying drugs combines the knowledge of several disciplines, including general biology, genetics, immunology, pharmacology, medicine, and nursing. The general therapeutic effects of these drugs are as follows:
- Enhancement of hematopoietic function
- Regulation or enhancement of the immune response, including cytotoxic or cytostatic activity against cancer cells

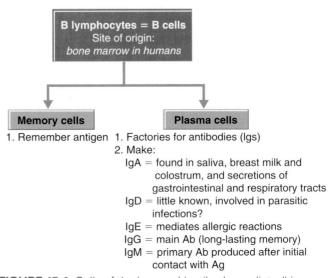

FIGURE 47-1 Cells of the humoral (antibody-mediated) immune system. *Ig,* Immunoglobulin.

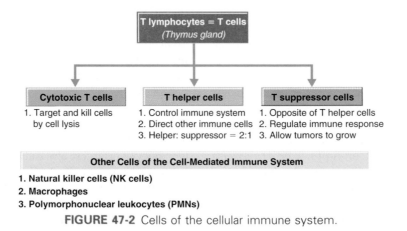

FIGURE 47-2 Cells of the cellular immune system.

BOX 47-1 Selected Biologic Response–Modifying Drugs

Hematopoietic Drugs
Colony-Stimulating Factors
filgrastim (G-CSF)
pegfilgrastim
sargramostim (GM-CSF)

Other
darbepoetin alfa
epoetin alfa
oprelvekin (IL-11)

Immunomodulating Drugs
Interferons
interferon alfa-2a
interferon alfa-2b*
peginterferon alfa-2a
peginterferon alfa-2b
interferon alfa-n3
interferon beta-1a
interferon beta-1b
interferon gamma-1b

Monoclonal Antibodies
adalimumab[†]
alemtuzumab
basiliximab
belimumab
bevacixumab
cetuximab
certolizumab[†]
golimumab[†]
ibritumomab tiuxetan
infliximab[†]

natalizumab
panitumamab
rituximab
secukinumab
trastuzumab

Interleukin Receptor Agonists and Antagonists
Agonist
aldesleukin (IL-2)

Antagonists
anakinra
tocilizumab

Miscellaneous Immunomodulators
Tumor Necrosis Factor Receptor Antagonist
etanercept

Enzymes
Pegademase bovine

Retinoid Receptor Agonists
tretinoin
bexarotene

Adjuvants (Nonspecific Immunostimulants)
Bacille Calmette-Guérin vaccine
leflunomide
levamisole
mitoxantrone
thalidomide
abatacept

G-CSF, Granulocyte colony-stimulating factor; *GM-CSF*, granulocyte-macrophage colony-stimulating factor; *IL*, interleukin.
*Also available in combination with the antiviral drug ribavirin.
[†]Are also considered anti–tumor necrosis factors.

- Inhibition of metastases, prevention of cell division, or inhibition of cell maturation

Box 47-1 lists the currently available biologic response–modifying drugs used in the treatment of cancer and other illnesses that have varying levels of immune system–related pathophysiology. The drugs are classified according to their biologic effects.

HEMATOPOIETIC DRUGS

Hematopoietic drugs include several medications developed over the past 10 to 15 years. Falling into this category are two erythropoietic drugs (epoetin alfa and darbepoetin alfa), three **colony-stimulating factors** (filgrastim, pegfilgrastim, and sargramostim), and two platelet-promoting drugs (oprelvekin, romiplostim). All of these drugs promote the synthesis of various types of major blood components by promoting the growth, **differentiation,** and function of their corresponding precursor cells in the bone marrow.

Mechanism of Action and Drug Effects

Although the hematopoietic drugs are not toxic to cancer cells, they do have beneficial effects in the treatment of cancer. All hematopoietic drugs have the same basic mechanism of action. They decrease the duration of chemotherapy-induced anemia, neutropenia, and thrombocytopenia and enable higher dosages of chemotherapy to be given; decrease bone marrow recovery time after bone marrow transplantation or irradiation; and stimulate other cells in the immune system to destroy or inhibit the growth of cancer cells, as well as virus- or fungus-infected cells. All of these drugs are produced by recombinant DNA technology.

These substances work by binding to receptors on the surfaces of specialized progenitor cells in the bone marrow. Progenitor cells are responsible for the production of three particular cell lines: red blood cells (RBCs), white blood cells (WBCs), and platelets. When a hematopoietic drug binds to a progenitor cell surface, the immature progenitor cell is stimulated to mature, proliferate (reproduce itself), differentiate (transform into its respective type of specialized blood component), and become functionally active. Hematopoietic drugs may enhance certain functions of mature cell lines as well.

Epoetin alfa is a synthetic derivative of the human hormone erythropoietin, which is produced primarily by the kidney. It promotes the synthesis of erythrocytes (RBCs) by stimulating RBC progenitor cells in the bone marrow. Darbepoetin alfa is a longer-acting form of epoetin alfa. These drugs are discussed in detail in Chapter 54. Filgrastim is a colony-stimulating factor that stimulates progenitor cells for the subset of WBCs (leukocytes) known as *granulocytes* (including basophils, eosinophils, and neutrophils). For this reason, it is also commonly called *granulocyte colony-stimulating factor (G-CSF)*. Pegfilgrastim is a longer-acting form of filgrastim. Sargramostim is also a colony-stimulating factor that works by stimulating the bone marrow precursor cells that synthesize both granulocytes and the phagocytic (cell-eating) cells known as *monocytes,* some of which become macrophages. For this reason, it is also called *granulocyte-macrophage colony-stimulating factor (GM-CSF).* Oprelvekin is classified as an *interleukin,* namely, interleukin-11 (IL-11). Other interleukins are discussed later in the chapter. Oprelvekin stimulates the bone marrow cells, specifically megakaryocytes that eventually give rise to platelets. Romiplostim is a colony-stimulating factor used to stimulate platelet production.

Indications

Neutrophils are the most important granulocytes for fighting infection. Infections often appear in patients who have experienced destruction of bone marrow cells as a result of chemotherapy. Colony-stimulating factors stimulate neutrophils to grow and mature and thus directly oppose the detrimental bone marrow actions of chemotherapy. Because these drugs reduce the duration of low neutrophil counts, they reduce the incidence and duration of infections. Colony-stimulating factors also enhance the functioning of mature cells of the immune system, such as macrophages and granulocytes. This increases the ability of the body's immune system to kill cancer cells, as well as virus- and fungus-infected cells. Ultimately these properties allow patients to receive higher dosages of chemotherapy. Similar benefits in RBCs occur with epoetin alfa. Oprelvekin, and romiplostim stimulate the production of platelets. The effect of hematopoietic drugs on the bone marrow cells also reduces the recovery time after bone marrow transplantation and radiation therapy. Dosages of chemotherapy used in bone marrow transplantation are often much higher than those used in conventional chemotherapy. Both the chemotherapy and radiation therapy are toxic to the bone marrow. When one or more colony-stimulating factors are administered as part of the drug therapy for bone marrow transplantation, bone marrow cell counts return to normal in a drastically shortened time. This helps to increase the likelihood of a successful bone marrow transplantation and therefore patient survival. Specific drug indications are listed in the dosages table on this page.

TABLE 47-1 Hematopoietic Drugs: Common Adverse Effects

Body System	Adverse Effects
Cardiovascular	Edema
Gastrointestinal	Anorexia, nausea, vomiting, diarrhea
Integumentary	Alopecia, rash
Respiratory	Cough, dyspnea, sore throat
Other	Fever, blood dyscrasias, headache, bone pain

Contraindications

Contraindications for all these drugs include drug allergy. Use of filgrastim, sargramostim, and pegfilgrastim is contraindicated in the presence of more than 10% myeloid blasts (immature tumor cells in the bone marrow) because colony-stimulating factors may stimulate malignant growth of these myeloid tumor cells.

Adverse Effects

Adverse effects associated with the use of hematopoietic drugs are mild. The most common are fever, muscle aches, bone pain, and flushing. Table 47-1 lists additional adverse effects.

Interactions

Filgrastim and sargramostim have significant drug interactions when these two drugs are given with myelosuppressive (bone marrow suppressant) antineoplastic drugs. Remember that these two drugs are administered to enhance the production of bone marrow cells; therefore, when myelosuppressive antineoplastics are given with them, the drugs directly antagonize each other. Typically filgrastim and sargramostim are not given within 24 hours of administration of myelosuppressive antineoplastics. However, they are given soon after this time to help prevent the WBC nadir from dropping to dangerous levels and also to speed WBC recovery. It is also recommended that these drugs be used with caution or not be given with other medications that can potentiate their myeloproliferative (bone marrow–stimulating) effects, including lithium and corticosteroids.

Dosages

For dosage information on hematopoietic drugs, see the table on this page.

DRUG PROFILES

♦filgrastim

Filgrastim (Neupogen) is a synthetic analogue of human granulocyte colony-stimulating factor and is commonly referred to as *G-CSF.* Filgrastim promotes the proliferation, differentiation, and activation of the cells that make granulocytes. Granulocytes are the body's primary defense against bacterial and fungal infections. Filgrastim has the same pharmacologic effects as endogenous human G-CSF, which is normally secreted by specialized leukocytes known as *monocytes, macrophages,* and *mature neutrophils.* Filgrastim is indicated to prevent or treat febrile neutropenia in patients receiving myelosuppressive

Hematopoietic Drugs

Drug (Pregnancy Category)	Pharmacologic Class	Usual Dosage Range	Indications
♦ filgrastim (Neupogen) (C)	Colony-stimulating factor	IV/subcut: 5-10 mcg/kg/day	Chemotherapy-induced leukopenia
♦ oprelvekin (IL-11) (Neumega) (C)	Synthetic human interleukin analogue	Subcut: 50 mcg/kg/day for up to 21 days	Chemotherapy-induced thrombocytopenia
Romiplostim (NPlate)	Colony-stimulating factor	Subcut: 1 mcg/kg/week	Idiopathic thrombocytopenia purpura
♦ sargramostim (Leukine) (C)	Colony-stimulating factor	IV: 250 mcg/m²/day	Chemotherapy-induced leukopenia

IL, Interleukin.

antineoplastics for nonmyeloid (non–bone marrow) malignancies. It must be given *before* a patient develops an infection, but not within 24 hours before or after myelosuppressive chemotherapeutic drugs. Pegfilgrastim (Neulasta) is a long-acting form of filgrastim that reduces the number of injections required. In 2015, the first biosimilar product was approved in the United States and called filgrastim-sndz (Zarixo). All drugs are available for injection only. These drugs are usually discontinued when a patient's absolute neutrophil count (ANC) rises above 10,000 cells/mm³.

Pharmacokinetics: Filgrastim

Route	Onset of Action	Peak Plasma Concentration	Elimination Half-life	Duration of Action
Subcut or IV	1 hr	2-6 hr	3-5 hr	12-24 hr

♦ sargramostim

Sargramostim (Leukine) is a synthetic analogue of human granulocyte-macrophage colony-stimulating factor and is commonly referred to as *GM-CSF.* There are three major subsets of leukocytes: *granulocytes, monocytes,* and *lymphocytes* (B cells and T cells). Granulocytes are further subdivided into *basophils, eosinophils,* and *neutrophils.* Neutrophils are the most important in fighting infection. Macrophages are tissue-based (as opposed to circulating) cells that are derived from monocytes, which circulate in the blood. Neutrophils, monocytes, and macrophages make up the three main categories of phagocytic (cell-eating) blood cells, and they literally ingest foreign cells and other antigens as part of their immune system function. Sargramostim has the same pharmacologic effects as endogenous human GM-CSF. It stimulates the proliferation, differentiation, and activation of the cells in the bone marrow that eventually become granulocytes, monocytes, and macrophages.

Sargramostim is indicated for promoting bone marrow recovery after autologous (own marrow) or allogenic (donor marrow) bone marrow transplantation in patients with various types of leukemia and lymphoma. This drug is available for injection only.

Pharmacokinetics: Sargramostim

Route	Onset of Action	Peak Plasma Concentration	Elimination Half-life	Duration of Action
Subcut or IV	4 hr	2 hr	2 hr	10 days

♦ oprelvekin

Oprelvekin (Neumega) is both a hematopoietic drug and one of the interleukins. However, its function is similar to that of the colony-stimulating factors (filgrastim and sargramostim) in that it enhances synthesis of a specific blood component—in this case, the platelets. Oprelvekin is indicated for the prevention of chemotherapy-induced severe thrombocytopenia and avoidance of the need for platelet transfusions. Its use is contraindicated in cases of known drug allergy. It is available for injection only. Romiplostim (NPlate) is a colony stimulating factor used specifically for idiopathic thrombocytopenia purpura.

Pharmacokinetics: Oprelvekin

Route	Onset of Action	Peak Plasma Concentration	Elimination Half-life	Duration of Action
Subcut	5-9 days	3 hr	7 hr	14 days

INTERFERONS

Interferons are proteins that have three basic properties: they are antiviral, antitumor, and immunomodulating. There are three different groups of interferon drugs—the alfa, beta, and gamma interferons—each with its own antigenic and biologic activity. Interferons are most commonly used in the treatment of certain viral infections and certain types of cancer.

Mechanism of Action and Drug Effects

Interferons are recombinantly manufactured substances that are identical to the interferon cytokines that are naturally present in the human body. In the body, interferons are produced by activated T cells and by other cells in response to viral infection. Interferons protect human cells from virus attack by enabling the human cells to produce enzymes that stop viral replication and prevent viruses from penetrating into healthy cells. Interferons prevent cancer cells from dividing and replicating and also increase the activity of other cells in the immune system, such as macrophages, neutrophils, and natural killer cells. Their effect on cancer cells is caused by a combination of direct inhibition of DNA and protein synthesis within cancer cells (antitumor effects) and multiple immunomodulatory effects on the host's immune system. Interferons increase the cytotoxic activity of natural killer cells and the phagocytic ability of macrophages. Interferons also increase the expression of cancer cell antigens on the cell surface, which enables the immune system to recognize cancer cells more easily, specifically marking them for destruction.

Overall, interferons have three different effects on the immune system. They can (1) restore its function if it is impaired, (2) augment (amplify) the immune system's ability to function as the body's defense, and (3) inhibit the immune system from working. This latter function may be especially useful when the immune system has become dysfunctional, causing an *autoimmune* disease. This is believed to be the case in multiple sclerosis. Two interferons (interferon beta-1a and interferon beta-1b) are specifically indicated for treatment of multiple sclerosis. Inhibiting the dysfunctional immune system prevents further damage to the body from the disease process.

Indications

The beneficial actions of interferons (antiviral, antineoplastic, and immunomodulatory) make them excellent drugs for the treatment of viral infections, various cancers, and some autoimmune disorders. Currently accepted indications for interferons are listed in the dosages table on this page.

Contraindications

Contraindications to the use of interferons include known drug allergy and may include autoimmune disorders, hepatitis or liver failure, concurrent use of immunosuppressant drugs, and severe liver disease.

Adverse Effects

The most common adverse effects can be described broadly as flulike symptoms: fever, chills, headache, malaise, myalgia, and fatigue. The major dose-limiting adverse effect of interferons is fatigue. Patients taking high dosages become so exhausted that they are often confined to bed. Other adverse effects of interferons are listed in Table 47-2. Interferon alfa-2b has a black box warning related to the potential to cause or aggravate autoimmune disorders and neuropsychiatric symptoms.

Interactions

Drug interactions are seen with both interferon alfa-2a and interferon alfa-2b when they are used with drugs that are metabolized in the liver via the cytochrome P-450 enzyme system. The combination results in decreased metabolism and increased accumulation of these drugs, which leads to drug toxicity. There is also some evidence that using interferons together with antiviral drugs such as zidovudine enhances the activity of both drugs but may lead to toxic levels of zidovudine. Additive toxic effects to the bone marrow can occur when interferon gamma products are used with other myelosuppressive drugs.

Dosages

For dosage information on interferons, see the table on this page.

DRUG PROFILES

The three major classes of interferon drugs are alfa, beta, and gamma, which are sometimes also written using the lowercase Greek letters α, β, and γ, respectively. The "alfa" designation is synonymous with the Greek letter " alpha," but "alfa" is now more commonly used clinically. The interferons vary in their antigenic makeup, biologic actions, and pharmacologic properties. The best known interferon class is interferon alfa. Interferon products are biologic response–modifying drugs that can be broadly classified as cytokines. Cytokines are immune system proteins that serve two essential functions: they direct the actions and communication between the cell-mediated and humoral divisions of the immune system, and they augment or enhance the immune response. Other cytokines include tumor necrosis factor (TNF), interleukins, and colony-stimulating factors.

INTERFERON ALFA PRODUCTS
♦ interferon alfa-2a, interferon alfa-2b, interferon alfa-n3, peginterferon alfa-2a, peginterferon alfa-2b

The most commonly used interferon products are in the alfa class. They are also referred to as *leukocyte interferons* because they are produced from human leukocytes. Two newer types of interferon alfa include peginterferon alfa-2a and peginterferon alfa-2b. The *peg* refers to the attachment of a polymer chain of the hydrocarbon polyethylene glycol (PEG). This "pegylation" process increases the size of the interferon molecule. This increased size delays drug absorption, increases half-life, and decreases plasma clearance rate, which prolongs the drug's therapeutic effects. In addition, pegylation is believed to reduce the immunogenicity of the interferon and thus delay its recognition and destruction by the immune system. Similarly, pegfilgrastim, mentioned previously in this chapter, is a pegylated form of filgrastim and is also longer-acting. The alfa-2a and alfa-2b interferons share the following indications: chronic hepatitis C, hairy cell leukemia, and AIDS-related Kaposi's sarcoma. Interferon alfa-2a (only) is also indicated for the treatment of chronic myelogenous leukemia. Additional indications unique to interferon alfa-2b are chronic hepatitis B, malignant melanoma (an often fatal form of skin cancer), follicular lymphoma (so named because its malignant cells gather in clumps called *follicles*—not to be confused with hair follicles), and condylomata acuminata (virally induced genital or venereal warts).

TABLE 47-2	Interferons: Adverse Effects
Body System	**Adverse Effects**
General	Flulike syndrome, fatigue
Cardiovascular	Tachycardia, cyanosis, ECG changes, orthostatic hypotension
Central nervous	Confusion, somnolence, irritability, seizures, hallucinations
Gastrointestinal	Nausea, diarrhea, vomiting, anorexia, taste alterations, dry mouth
Hematologic	Neutropenia, thrombocytopenia
Renal and hepatic	Increased BUN and creatinine levels, proteinuria, abnormal liver function test

BUN, Blood urea nitrogen; *ECG*, electrocardiogram.

DOSAGES

Interferons

Drug (Pregnancy Category)	Pharmacologic Class	Usual Dosage Range	Indications
◆ interferon alfa-2a (Roferon-A) (C)	Immunomodulator, antiviral, antineoplastic	IM/subcut: 3 million units 3 times/wk, depending on indication	Chronic hepatitis C, hairy cell leukemia, AIDS-related Kaposi's sarcoma, chronic myelogenous leukemia
◆ interferon alfa-2b (Intron-A) (C)	Immunomodulator, antiviral, antineoplastic	IM/subcut: 1-30 million units 3 times/wk*	Hairy cell leukemia, malignant melanoma, follicular lymphoma, condylomata acuminata, Kaposi's sarcoma, chronic hepatitis C, chronic hepatitis B
◆ peginterferon alfa-2a (Pegasys) (C)	Immunomodulator, antiviral	Subcut: 180 mcg once a week for 48 wk	Chronic hepatitis C
◆ peginterferon alfa-2b (PEG-Intron) (C)	Immunomodulator, antiviral	Subcut: 1.5 mcg/kg once a week for 1 yr†	Chronic hepatitis C
◆ interferon alfa-n3 (Alferon-N) (C)	Immunomodulator, antiviral	Intralesional: 250,000 units (0.05 mL) into the base of each wart 2 times/wk for up to 8 wk	Condylomata acuminata
◆ interferon beta-1a (Avonex, Rebif) (C)	Immunomodulator	IM (Avonex): 30 mcg once a week Subcut (Rebif): 44 mcg 3 times/wk	Multiple sclerosis
interferon gamma-1b (Actimmune) (C)	Immunomodulator	**BSA more than 0.5 m²** Subcut: 50 mcg/m² 3 times/wk **BSA less than 0.5 m²** Subcut: 1.5 mcg/kg 3 times/wk	Chronic granulomatous disease, osteopetrosis

BSA, body surface area.
*May also be given by intravenous infusion for melanoma. Route and dose vary depending on indication.
†Dose is 1.5 mcg/kg/wk if given with ribavirin capsules (see Chapter 40).

Peg-interferon alfa-2a and peginterferon alfa-2b are currently indicated only for treatment of chronic hepatitis C.

Interferon alfa-n3 is a polyclonal mixture of all interferon alfa subtypes. It is the product of pooled human leukocytes. Its only current indication is condylomata acuminata.

Interferons are most commonly given by either intramuscular or subcutaneous injection, but intravenous and intraperitoneal routes have been used as well. It is important to note that some interferons are dosed in millions of units. Although it is unacceptable to use the abbreviation MU for "millions of units," you may see it written as such. It is imperative to double-check the dose, because the prescriber's writing of "MU" may be mistaken for "mg" or "mcg." If there is any question about the dose of any medication, double-check with the prescriber, pharmacist, or other experienced colleague before administering the medication to the patient. Although this is true for all medications, it is a special consideration for interferons and other biologic response–modifying drugs, because of both their potency and their dosage variability.

INTERFERON BETA PRODUCTS
◆ interferon beta-1a, interferon beta-1b
Interferon beta-1a and interferon beta-1b are the currently available beta products. They interact with specific cell receptors found on the surfaces of human cells and possess antiviral and immunomodulatory activity. Both are produced by recombinant DNA techniques and are indicated for the treatment of relapsing multiple sclerosis (to slow the progression of physical disability and decrease the frequency of clinical exacer-

bations). The only contraindication is known drug allergy, including allergy to human albumin. Both drugs are available for injection only.

INTERFERON GAMMA PRODUCT
interferon gamma-1b
Interferon gamma-1b (Actimmune) is a synthetic product produced by recombinant DNA technology. It is indicated for the treatment of serious infections associated with chronic granulomatous disease, a genetic immunodeficiency, and osteopetrosis, a genetic bone disease characterized by abnormally dense bone, anemia, and frequent fractures. Interferon gamma-1b is available for injection only.

MONOCLONAL ANTIBODIES

Monoclonal antibodies are quickly becoming standards of therapy in many areas of medicine, including treatment of cancer, rheumatoid arthritis and other inflammatory diseases, multiple sclerosis, and organ transplantation. In cancer treatment, they have advantages over traditional antineoplastics in that they can specifically target cancer cells and have minimal effect on healthy cells. This reduces many of the adverse effects traditionally associated with antineoplastic drugs. There are several commercially available monoclonal antibodies used to treat cancer and rheumatoid arthritis. The most commonly used ones are listed in the dosages table on p. 757. The *mab* suffix in a drug name is usually an abbreviation for

TABLE 47-3	Selected Immunomodulating Drugs: Common Adverse Effects
Drug	**Adverse Effects**
adalimumab	Localized inflammatory reaction at the injection site, upper respiratory tract and urinary tract infections, risk for various malignancies
alemtuzumab	Rash, pruritus, nausea, vomiting, diarrhea, dyspnea, cough, muscle spasms, fever, fatigue, skeletal pain, myelosuppression
belimumab	Nausea, diarrhea, depression, insomnia, fever, infection, anaphylaxis
bevacizumab	Deep vein thrombosis, hypertension, diarrhea, abdominal pain, constipation, vomiting, GI hemorrhage, leukopenia, asthenia, headache, dizziness, dry skin, proteinuria, hypokalemia, epistaxis, weight loss
certolizumab	Arthralgia, respiratory tract infection, cardiac dysrhythmia, rash, bowel obstruction
cetuximab	Headache, insomnia, skin rash, conjunctivitis, GI discomfort, anemia, leukopenia, dehydration, edema, weight loss, dyspnea, asthenia, back pain, fever
golimumab	Hypertension, increased liver function tests, infection
ibritumomab tiuxetan	Nausea, myelosuppression, asthenia, infection, chills
infliximab	Headache, rash, GI discomfort, dyspnea, upper and lower respiratory tract infection
natalizumab	Depression, fatigue, headache, GI discomfort, urinary tract infection, lower respiratory tract infection, joint pain. Of even greater concern are case reports of a rare and potentially fatal brain disorder known as *progressive multifocal leukoencephalopathy.*
rituximab	Fever, chills, headache. Potentially fatal infusion-related events, including severe bronchospasm, dyspnea, hypoxia, pulmonary infiltrates, adult respiratory distress syndrome, hypotension, and angioedema. Tumor lysis syndrome (see Chapter 45) with acute renal failure has also been reported.
tocilizumab	Hypertension, rash, diarrhea, dizziness, anaphylaxis, infection, injection site reaction
tofacitinib	Risk for developing serious infections, GI perforations, anemia, neutropenia, elevated liver enzymes, lipid disturbances, diarrhea
tositumomab and iodine I-131 tositumomab	Headache, rash, GI discomfort, muscle pains, dyspnea, pharyngitis, asthenia, fever, chills, infection
trastuzumab	Fever, chills, headache, infection, nausea, vomiting, diarrhea, dizziness, headache, insomnia, rash, GI discomfort, edema, dyspnea, rhinitis, asthenia, back pain, fever, chills, infection

"monoclonal antibody." Muromonab is used in kidney transplantation and is discussed in Chapter 48.

Mechanism of Action, Drug Effects, and Indications

Because these drugs are so diverse, specific information for each appears in the individual drug profiles provided later in the chapter.

Contraindications

The only clear contraindication to the use of monoclonal antibodies reported thus far is drug allergy to a specific product. Their use is usually contraindicated in patients with known active infectious processes due to their immunosuppressive qualities. Although known drug allergy is a contraindication, depending on the urgency of the clinical situation, a given monoclonal antibody may be the only viable treatment option for a seriously ill patient. In such situations, allergic symptoms may be controlled with supportive medications such as diphenhydramine and acetaminophen. All of the drugs that are TNF antagonists are contraindicated in patients with active tuberculosis or other infections. All TNF-blocking agents have black box warnings regarding the risk for serious infections and lymphoma or other malignancies. Many of the drugs discussed in this chapter carry black box warnings, and the student is referred to the specific drug prescribing information. Infliximab has been shown to worsen severe cases of heart failure. Use of alemtuzumab is also contraindicated in patients with active systemic infections and immunodeficiency conditions, including AIDS.

Adverse Effects

Many, if not most, patients receiving these very potent drugs manifest acute symptoms that are comparable to classic allergy or flulike symptoms, such as fever, dyspnea, and chills. The primary objective is to administer the medication and control such symptoms as well as possible. Because the mechanisms of action of these drugs work through augmentation or inhibition of the human immune response, they can have a variety of adverse effects, some mild, some severe, that affect several body systems. Drug-specific adverse effects with the highest reported incidence (10% to 50% or more) are listed in Table 47-3. The risk for such adverse effects must be weighed against the severity of the patient's underlying illness. Many of these adverse effects may also be associated with the patient's disease process (e.g., infections) and even with life in general (e.g., headache, depression). This is especially true for the milder effects. The risk for acquiring an infection is a serious adverse effect of all of the biologic response–modifying agents, because they alter the normal immune response.

Interactions

Drug interactions associated with monoclonal antibodies are relatively few, and no major food interactions are listed. Administration of adalimumab with the anti–rheumatoid arthritis drug anakinra (an interleukin) may increase the risk for serious infections secondary to neutropenia. The clearance of natalizumab may be reduced by concurrent administration of interferon beta-1a (both used for multiple sclerosis). Coadministration of anti-TNF drugs (e.g., etanercept, anakinra) with infliximab may also increase the risk for neutropenia and infections. Etanercept is not to be given concurrently with varicella-zoster immune globulin (VZIG) because of undesirable drug interactions. However, etanercept may be resumed after completion of VZIG therapy. Bevacizumab is associated with increased risk for severe diarrhea and neutropenia when given concurrently with

DOSAGES

Monoclonal Antibodies

Drug (Pregnancy Category)	Pharmacologic Class	Usual Dosage Range	Indications
adalimumab (Humira) (B)	Anti-TNF monoclonal antibody	Subcut: 40 mg every other week; may advance to 40 mg weekly if indicated	Severe, progressive RA, Crohn's disease, ulcerative colitis
alemtuzumab (Campath) (C)	Anti–glycoprotein CD52	IV: 3-10 mg daily to maximum tolerated dose, then 30 mg 3 times/wk (alternate days) for up to 12 wk	B-cell chronic lymphocytic leukemia
belimumab (Benlysta) (C)	B-lymphocyte stimulator-specific inhibitor	IV: 10 mg/kg ever 2 weeks × 3, then every 4 weeks at 2-week intervals	Systemic lupus erythematosus
certolizumab (Cimzia) (B)	Anti-TNF monoclonal antibody	Subcut: 400 mg at 2-week intervals 3 times, then monthly	RA, Crohn's disease
bevacizumab (Avastin) (C)	Anti–human vascular endothelial growth factor	IV: 5-10 mg/kg every 14 days	Metastatic colorectal cancer
cetuximab (Erbitux) (C)	Anti–human epidermal growth factor	IV: 400 mg/m^2 1 time, then 250 mg/m^2 weekly	Metastatic colorectal cancer
golimumab (Simponi) (B)	Anti-TNF monoclonal antibody	Subcut: 50 mg monthly	RA, ankylosing spondylitis
ibritumomab tiuxetan (Zevalin) (D)	Chelator immunoconjugate	IV: Dose depends on indication	Non-Hodgkin's lymphoma
infliximab (Remicade) (B)	Anti-TNF monoclonal antibody	IV: 3-5 mg/kg at 0, 2, and 6 wk, then every 6-8 wk	Ankylosing spondylitis, Crohn's disease, RA
natalizumab (Tysabri) (C)	Anti–alfa$_4$ integrin subunit MAB	IV: 300 mg every 4 wk	Multiple sclerosis
◆ rituximab (Rituxan) (C)	Anti–CD20 surface antigen	IV: 375 mg/m^2 once a week × 4-8 doses	Non-Hodgkin's lymphoma, RA
tositumomab and iodine I-131 tositumomab (Bexxar) (X)	Radioactive MAB	IV: Complex dosing regimen involving both drug components; follow instructions in package insert as ordered	Non-Hodgkin's lymphoma
trastuzumab (Herceptin) (B)	Anti–HER2 protein MAB	IV: Loading dose, 4 mg/kg IV: Maintenance dose, 2 mg/kg/wk	Breast cancer

MAB, Monoclonal antibody; *RA,* rheumatoid arthritis; *TNF,* tumor necrosis factor.

another anti–colorectal cancer drug, irinotecan (see Chapter 45). Paclitaxel (see Chapter 45) has been shown to reduce the clearance of trastuzumab when the two are administered concurrently to treat breast cancer.

Dosages

For dosage information on the monoclonal antibodies, see the table above.

DRUG PROFILES

All of the monoclonal antibodies are synthesized using recombinant DNA technology. Because of the complexities of this technology, these drugs tend to be much more expensive than most other medications, with prices in the hundreds or thousands of dollars per single dose. Many of the monoclonal antibodies are used to treat various forms of cancer. Their advantage is that they offer greater cell-killing specificity aimed at cancer cells instead of all body cells. Nonetheless, these drugs are associated with significant adverse effects and therefore with risk, which must be weighed against the benefit using expert clinical judgment. Severe allergic inflammatory-type infusion reactions can occur, and patients may therefore be premedicated with acetaminophen or diphenhydramine to reduce the occurrence

of such reactions. If reactions do occur, they may be treated with diphenhydramine and other drugs such as epinephrine and corticosteroids. Conventional pharmacokinetic data are not listed for the majority of these drugs because they do not follow standard pharmacokinetic models owing to their unique behavior in the body. It is known, however, that they may remain in the affected tissues for many weeks or months.

adalimumab

Adalimumab (Humira) works through its specificity for human tumor necrosis factor (TNF). TNF is a naturally occurring cytokine that is involved in normal inflammatory and immune responses. Adalimumab is indicated for the treatment of severe cases of rheumatoid arthritis that have failed to respond to other medications, including methotrexate. It can be used either alone or concurrently with such medications. In patients with rheumatoid arthritis, elevated levels of TNF are found in the synovial fluid in the spaces of affected joints. In addition to preventing TNF molecules from binding to TNF cell surface receptors, adalimumab also modulates the inflammatory biologic responses that are induced or regulated by TNF. Use of adalimumab is contraindicated in patients with any active infectious process, whether localized or systemic, acute or chronic. It is also indicated for Crohn's disease, ulcerative colitis, plaque psoriasis, and psoriatic arthritis.

alemtuzumab

Alemtuzumab (Campath) is approved to treat B cell–mediated chronic lymphocytic leukemia. It is classified as a recombinant humanized antibody that is directed against the CD52 glycoprotein that appears on the surfaces of virtually all B and T lymphocytes. It is used specifically in patients for whom other first-line chemotherapy treatments, including treatment with alkylating drugs and the antimetabolite fludarabine (see Chapter 45), have failed. Its contraindications are known drug allergy, active systemic infection, and documented immunodeficiency disease such as HIV-positive status. The half-life of alemtuzumab is 10 hours to 30 days.

belimumab

Belimumab (Benlysta) is the first drug approved for the treatment of systemic lupus erythematosus in the past 40 years. It is a B-lymphocyte stimulator-specific inhibitor. The most common side effects include nausea, diarrhea, insomnia, bronchitis, migraine, and pain in the extremities. The most serious adverse effects include infection (sometimes fatal), anaphylaxis, and depression. It is given via IV infusion.

bevacizumab

Bevacizumab (Avastin) is approved for the treatment of metastatic colon cancer, rectal cancer in combination with 5-fluorouracil (see Chapter 45), non–small-cell lung cancer, and malignant glioblastoma. It is unique in that it binds to and inhibits vascular endothelial growth factor, a protein that promotes development of new blood vessels in tumors (as well as in normal body tissues). It has no listed contraindications but may complicate surgical wound healing because of its antivascular effects. The half-life of bevacizumab is 11 to 50 days.

certolizumab

Certolizumab (Cimzia) is a tumor necrosis factor (TNF) antagonist. It is indicated for moderate to severe active Crohn's disease that is unresponsive to other therapy and for severe rheumatoid arthritis. The most common adverse effects include headache, nausea, upper respiratory tract infection, hypertension, and infections. A patient medication guide must be dispensed with each prescription, warning patients of potential serious infections and possible lymphoma.

cetuximab

Cetuximab (Erbitux) is approved for the treatment of metastatic colorectal cancer. It is a recombinant monoclonal antibody and is designed for concurrent use with the second-line antineoplastic drug irinotecan (see Chapter 45). It binds to *epidermal growth factor* on the surface of tumor cells, where it hinders cell growth through interference with cell metabolism. Cetuximab is used either in combination with irinotecan or alone in patients who are intolerant of the latter drug. It has no listed contraindications but is known to cause severe infusion

reactions in up to 3% of patients receiving it. The half-life of cetuximab is 97 to 114 hours.

golimumab

Golimumab (Simponi) is a TNF antagonist approved for the treatment of severe rheumatoid arthritis and ankylosing spondylitis. The most common side effects include hypertension, dizziness, increased liver function tests, and infection. It is not to be given with other TNF antagonists. Patients must be monitored for infection, as with all TNF antagonists. Golimumab is given subcutaneously in a dose of 50 mg once a month. It is given in conjunction with methotrexate for RA.

ibritumomab

Ibritumomab (Zevalin) is approved for treating B-cell non-Hodgkin's lymphoma. This drug is an immunoconjugate, consisting of ibritumomab conjugated with the metal chelator tiuxetan. This drug comes in kits that also include one of two radioactive metal isotopes (radioisotopes). The antibody binds to the CD20 antigen that occurs on the surfaces of both normal and malignant B lymphocytes. Once the complex is bound to the cells, the tiuxetan component binds the radioisotope, which is administered as another part of the anticancer therapy. Radioactive beta emission from the bound radioisotope, a unique feature of this drug, induces free radical formation and cell damage in both the cell containing the drug complex and neighboring cells.

infliximab

Infliximab (Remicade) is one of the earliest monoclonal antibodies, approved in 1998. It works through an anti-TNF action, similar to adalimumab. It is approved for the treatment of ankylosing spondylitis, Crohn's disease, ulcerative colitis, plaque psoriasis and rheumatoid arthritis. It has the special contraindication of severe heart failure (class III or IV on the New York Heart Association scale) because it may worsen this condition. It also carries an FDA black box warning reporting cases of fatal tuberculosis and/or fungal infections associated with the use of this drug. It is recommended that patients be tested for latent tuberculosis before it is administered. The half-life of infliximab is 8 to 9 days. A new monoclonal antibody, vedolizumab (Entyvio) was approved in 2014 for the treatment of Crohn's disease and ulcerative colitis. The most common side effects are nausea, nasopharyngitis, upper respiratory tract infection, arthralgia, pyrexia, fatigue, headache, cough, and infusion-related reactions.

natalizumab

Natalizumab (Tysabri) is approved for the treatment of multiple sclerosis. It is a humanized monoclonal antibody derived from murine myeloma cells. Natalizumab works by binding to the $alph_4$ subunits of integrins, proteins found on the surfaces of leukocytes (with the exception of neutrophils). These proteins are implicated in the multiple sclerosis disease process, but its exact mechanism of action has not been determined. However, the drug is known to inhibit the leukocyte adhesion that is mediated by these alpha protein subunits, and this is also believed to be part of the disease process. Natalizumab has no listed contraindications. The half-life is 11 days. Natalizumab was taken off the market only 1 year after it was originally approved in 2004 due to reports of patients developing multifocal leukoencephalopathy, a rare and serious viral infection of the brain. In 2006, the FDA allowed the marketing of natalizumab to resume under a special distribution program. Only patients who are enrolled in the program are allowed to receive the drug. Fingolimod (Gilenya) is a newer oral drug for the treatment of relapsing forms of MS to reduce the frequency of clinical exacerbations and delay disability progression. It is a sphingosine 1-phosphate receptor modulator. It is classified as a pregnancy category C drug. Headache, diarrhea, increased liver function tests, back pain, and flulike symptoms are the most common adverse effects of fingolimod.

♦ rituximab

Rituximab (Rituxan) specifically binds to antigen CD20. This antigen is a protein on the membranes of both normal and malignant B cells found in patients with non-Hodgkin's lymphoma. Antigen CD20 is expressed in more than 90% of B-cell non-Hodgkin's lymphomas. Once rituximab binds to these B cells, a host immune response causes lysis of the cells. Rituximab has become a standard drug for the treatment of patients with follicular low-grade non-Hodgkin's lymphoma for whom previous therapy has failed. It is recommended that patients be premedicated with acetaminophen and diphenhydramine before each infusion of the drug to reduce its well-known infusion-related adverse effects. Rituximab is also indicated for rheumatoid arthritis.

tositumomab and iodine I-131 tositumomab

Tositumomab and iodine (I-131) tositumomab (Bexxar) are approved for the treatment of non-Hodgkin's lymphoma. This drug is a murine monoclonal antibody with a dual radioactive and nonradioactive component. Both components bind to the CD20 antigen, a transmembrane protein that is expressed on the cell membranes of more than 90% of B-cell non-Hodgkin's lymphoma cells. Theoretical mechanisms of action include induction of apoptosis (programmed cell death), *complement-dependent* cytotoxicity, or antibody-dependent cytotoxicity mediated by the drug itself. Complement is a collective term for about 20 different proteins normally present in plasma that aid other immune system components (e.g., B cells and T cells) in mounting an immune response.

trastuzumab

Trastuzumab (Herceptin) kills tumor cells by mediating antibody-dependent cellular cytotoxicity. It accomplishes this by inhibiting proliferation of human tumor cells that overexpress the HER2 protein. The HER2 protein is overexpressed in 25% to 30% of primary malignant breast tumors and has been established as an adverse prognostic factor for early-stage breast cancer. Trastuzumab has a special FDA black box warning reporting cases of ventricular dysfunction and heart failure associated with this drug. Monitor for signs and symptoms of heart failure and ventricular dysfunction before and during

treatment. In addition, fatal hypersensitivity reactions, infusion reactions, and pulmonary events have occurred in association with its use; therefore, careful clinical judgment, risk evaluation, and informed patient consent are called for in its use. The half-life of trastuzumab is 10 to 30 days.

INTERLEUKINS AND RELATED DRUGS

Interleukins are a natural part of the immune system and are classified as *lymphokines.* Lymphokines are soluble proteins that are released from activated lymphocytes such as natural killer cells. There are several known interleukins in the body (IL-2, IL-3, IL-4, IL-5, IL-6,IL-7a and IL-11), and more are being identified as knowledge of the immune system increases.

Mechanism of Action and Drug Effects

Interleukins cause multiple effects in the immune system, one of which is antitumor action. IL-2 is produced by activated T cells in response to macrophage-"processed" antigens and secreted interleukin (IL-1). It was formerly called *T-cell growth factor* because, among other actions, it aids in the growth and differentiation of T lymphocytes. The IL-2 derivative aldesleukin acts indirectly to stimulate or restore immune response. Aldesleukin binds to receptor sites on T cells, which stimulates the T cells to multiply. One type of cell that results from this multiplication is the lymphokine-activated killer (LAK) cell. These LAK cells recognize and destroy only cancer cells and ignore normal cells. Aldesleukin is currently the most widely used of the interleukin drugs. A detailed list of its specific immunomodulating effects appears in Box 47-2.

Anakinra is a recombinant form of the natural human IL-1 receptor antagonist. It competitively inhibits the binding of IL-1 to its corresponding receptor sites, which are expressed in many different tissues and organs. Tocilizumab is a recombinant form of the natural IL-6 receptor antagonist. Secukinumab is an IL-7 antagonist.

Indications

The pharmaceutical interleukin receptor agonists most commonly used are aldesleukin (IL-2) and oprelvekin (IL-11). Aldesleukin was previously indicated only for the treatment of metastatic renal cell carcinoma, a malignancy that originates in

---

BOX 47-2 Interleukin-2: Drug Effects

Modulating Effects
Proliferation of T cells
Synthesis and secretion of cytokines
Increased production of B cells (antibodies)
Proliferation and activation of NK cells
Proliferation and activation of LAK cells

Enhancing Effects
Enhancement of killer T cell activity
Amplification of the effects of cytokines
Enhancement of the cytotoxic actions of NK cells and LAK cells

LAK, Lymphokine-activated killer; *NK,* natural killer.

the kidney tissues. It is now also approved for the treatment of metastatic melanoma. Oprelvekin is used to help patients produce platelets and is discussed with the hematopoietic drugs earlier in the chapter. It has a dual classification as both an interleukin and hematologic drug.

The IL antagonists include secukinumab, tocilizumab, and anakinra. Secukinumab (Cosentyx) was the first IL-7a inhibitor and is indicated for moderate to severe plaque psoriasis. Anakinra (Kineret) is an IL-1 receptor antagonist and tocilizumab (IL-6) antagonist. Both drugs are indicated for rheumatoid arthritis.

Contraindications

Contraindications to the administration of aldesleukin include known drug allergy, organ transplantation, and abnormal results on thallium cardiac stress tests or pulmonary function tests. The only usual contraindication for anakinra, secukinumab, and tocilizumab is known drug allergy.

Adverse Effects

Therapy with aldesleukin is commonly complicated by severe toxicity. A syndrome known as *capillary leak syndrome* is responsible for the severe toxicities of aldesleukin. As the name implies, capillary leak syndrome refers to a condition induced by interleukin therapy in which the capillaries lose their ability to retain vital colloids such as albumin, protein, and other essential components of blood. Because the capillaries are "leaky," these substances migrate into the surrounding tissues. This results in massive fluid retention (20 to 30 pounds), which can lead to the life-threatening problems of respiratory distress, heart failure, dysrhythmias, and myocardial infarction. Fortunately, these are all reversible after discontinuation of the interleukin therapy. Close patient monitoring and vigorous supportive care are essential in the patient receiving aldesleukin therapy. Other adverse effects that may be associated with aldesleukin therapy are fever, chills, rash, fatigue, hepatotoxicity, myalgias, headaches, and eosinophilia.

The most common adverse effects associated withanakinra includes local reactions at the injection site, various respiratory tract infections, and headache. Tocilizumab has a high risk for causing anaphylaxis. Common side effects with secukinumab include nasopharyngitis, diarrhea and upper respiratory infection.

Interactions

Aldesleukin, when given with antihypertensives, can produce additive hypotensive effects. Coadministration of corticosteroids with aldesleukin can reduce its antitumor effectiveness and is to be avoided. Anakinra, secukinumab, and tocilizumab are not to be used (or are to be used cautiously) with other immune modifiers due to increased risk for serious infections.

Dosages

For dosage information on the interleukin agonists and antagonists, see the table on this page.

DRUG PROFILES

The interleukins are a group of naturally occurring cytokines in the body that originally were believed to be produced by and to act primarily on leukocytes (WBCs). They are now recognized as multifunctional cytokines that are produced by a variety of cells but act at least partly within the lymphatic system.

♦ aldesleukin

Aldesleukin (Proleukin) is a human IL-2 derivative that is manufactured using recombinant DNA technology. It is a cytokine that is produced by lymphocytes and is therefore classified as a lymphokine. Aldesleukin is currently approved only for the treatment of metastatic renal cell carcinoma and metastatic melanoma, despite its activity against other cancers. Off-label uses include HIV infection and AIDS, and non-Hodgkin's lymphoma. Aldesleukin is contraindicated in patients with known drug allergy, abnormal thallium stress test or pulmonary function tests (due to potential drug effects on cardiopulmonary function), and organ transplants (due to the immunostimulating qualities of the drug, which may cause organ rejection). Aldesleukin is available only for injection.

anakinra

Anakinra (Kineret) is an IL-1 receptor antagonist that is used to help control the symptoms of rheumatoid arthritis. Its only current contraindication is known drug allergy. Anakinra is available for injection only.

tocilizumab

Tocilizumab (Actemra) is an interleukin-6 antagonist approved for the treatment of severe rheumatoid arthritis. It is approved for patients who have not had an adequate response to other agents. It has a significant risk for anaphylaxis, and premedication must be given. A medication guide must be given to all patients receiving tocilizumab. Serious adverse effects include hepatotoxicity, infections, herpes zoster reactivation, and GI perforation. Tocilizumab is not to be given with other biologic response–modifying agents. It is given as an IV infusion.

DOSAGES

Interleukins and Related Drugs

Drug (Pregnancy Category)	Pharmacologic Class	Usual Dosage Range	Indications
♦ aldesleukin (IL-2) (Proleukin) (C)	Human recombinant IL-2 analogue	IV: 600,000 IU/kg (0.037 mg/kg) every 8 hr (14 doses); hold × 9 days, then repeat cycle × 1	Metastatic renal cell carcinoma or melanoma
anakinra (Kineret) (B)	IL-1 receptor antagonist	Subcut: 100 mg/day	Rheumatoid arthritis
tocilizumab (Actemra)	IL-6 antagonist	IV: 4-8 mg/kg monthly	Rheumatoid arthritis

IL, Interleukin.

TABLE 47-4   Miscellaneous Immunomodulating Drugs

Drug (Trade and Other Names)	Classification	Indications	Mechanism of Action
abatacept (Orencia)	Selective costimulation modulator	RA	Inhibits T-cell activation
bexarotene (Targretin)	Retinoid receptor agonist	Cutaneous T-cell lymphoma	Exact mechanism is unknown; binds to and activates retinoid X receptor subtypes; this regulates the expression of genes that control cellular differentiation
BCG vaccine (Pacis, TICE BCG, TheraCys)	Live virus vaccine, adjuvant	Localized bladder cancer	Promotes local inflammation and immune response in bladder mucosa
etanercept (Enbrel)	TNF receptor antagonist	RA (including juvenile) and psoriatic arthritis	Blocks effects of TNF, a major inflammatory mediator in RA
leflunomide (Arava)	Antimetabolite	RA	Exerts antiinflammatory effects via inhibition of cellular DNA synthesis
levamisole (Ergamisol)	Immunostimulant, adjuvant	Dukes stage C colon cancer (given with fluorouracil)	Exact mechanism is unknown, but may enhance the therapeutic effects of fluorouracil and have its own immunostimulatory effects
mitoxantrone (Novantrone)	Anthracycline antibiotic (also an antineoplastic drug)	MS (secondary chronic type)	Inhibits cellular DNA synthesis, which reduces neurologic disability in MS (exact mechanism is unclear)
pegademase bovine (Adagen)	Immunostimulant	SCID	Modified enzyme that compensates for deficiency of the enzyme adenosine deaminase, which is associated with SCID
thalidomide (Thalomid)	Immunostimulant	Erythremia nodosum*	Exact mechanism is unknown, but may have anti-TNF properties, which counter the disease process
tretinoin (Vesanoid)	Retinoid receptor agonist	Acute promyelocytic leukemia	Induces differentiation and maturation of leukemic cells, reducing proliferation of immature, disease-causing cells

BCG, Bacille Calmette-Guerin; *MS,* multiple sclerosis; *RA,* rheumatoid arthritis; *SCID,* severe combined immunodeficiency disease; *TNF,* tumor necrosis factor.

*An inflammatory reaction in the subcutaneous fat, often following a bacterial infection, or in reaction to drugs such as oral contraceptives or sulfonamides.

MISCELLANEOUS IMMUNOMODULATING DRUGS

In addition to the drugs in the major classes discussed thus far, there are several additional medications that can be broadly classified as miscellaneous immunomodulating drugs. They work by various specific and nonspecific mechanisms. A special term used for **immunostimulant** drugs that work by a nonspecific mechanism is **adjuvant.** These miscellaneous medications, including some that are classified as adjuvants, are listed in Table 47-4.

RHEUMATOID ARTHRITIS

Rheumatism is a general term for any of several disorders characterized by inflammation, degeneration, or metabolic derangement of connective tissue structures, especially joints and related structures such as muscles, tendons, fibrous tissue, and ligaments. Rheumatoid arthritis is a chronic **autoimmune disorder** that commonly causes inflammation and tissue damage in joints. It can also cause anemia and diffuse inflammation in the lungs, eyes, and pericardium of the heart, and subcutaneous nodules under the skin (Figure 47-3). It is a painful and oftentimes disabling disease. It is diagnosed primarily based on symptoms and the results of a blood test for rheumatoid factor. Symptoms include pain, stiffness, and reduced range of motion. Treatment encompasses both pharmacologic and nonpharmacologic modalities, including physical and occupational therapy. There is no known cure for rheumatoid arthritis, and the goal

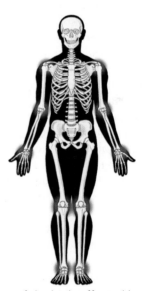

FIGURE 47-3 Areas of the body affected by rheumatoid arthritis. Rheumatoid arthritis is most frequently seen in the shoulders, elbows, wrists, knees, and ankles, and it often affects the joints on both sides of the body equally.

of therapy is to alleviate current symptoms and to prevent further damage of the joints. Rheumatoid arthritis affects over 2 million people in the United States and usually appears between 25 and 50 years of age. Women are two to three times more likely than men to have rheumatoid arthritis. Smokers and those with a family history are also at risk. Osteoarthritis is another type of arthritis that tends to be an age-related degeneration of joint tissues resulting in pain and reduced function. This section focuses on rheumatoid arthritis.

Because rheumatoid arthritis is a disease characterized by inflammation, the nonsteroidal antiinflammatory drugs (NSAIDs) are tried in the early stages of RA (see Chapter 44). Corticosteroids, also potent antiinflammatory drugs (see Chapter 33), are also used to prevent inflammatory symptoms. These drugs, although they are effective in reducing inflammation, do not actually affect the disease itself. Disease-modifying antirheumatic drugs (DMARDs) not only provide antiinflammatory and analgesic effects, but they can arrest or slow the disease processes associated with arthritis.

DISEASE-MODIFYING ANTIRHEUMATIC ARTHRITIS DRUGS (DMARDs)

DMARDs are drugs that modify the disease of rheumatoid arthritis. They exhibit antiinflammatory, antiarthritic, and immunomodulating effects and work by inhibiting the movement of various cells into an inflamed, damaged area, such as a joint. These cells (neutrophils, monocytes, and macrophages) are responsible for causing many of the deleterious effects of chronic rheumatoid arthritis. By preventing the accumulation of these inflammatory cells in the area of the diseased joint, antiarthritic drugs prevent progression of the disease. DMARDs often have a slow onset of action of several weeks, versus minutes to hours for NSAIDs. For this reason, DMARDs are sometimes also referred to as *slow-acting antirheumatic drugs (SAARDs)*. They were previously thought of as second-line drugs for the treatment of arthritis because they can have much more toxic adverse effects than do the NSAIDs. However, the American College of Rheumatology updated its treatment guidelines in 2012 and now recommends the use of DMARDs as first-line therapy in many patients. The guidelines differentiate the DMARDs into nonbiologic and biologic DMARDs. The nonbiologic DMARDs include methotrexate, leflunomide, hydroxychloroquine, and sulfasalazine. The guidelines recommend starting with methotrexate or leflunomide in most patients. Use of the other drugs, including the biologic DMARDs, is generally reserved for those patients who do not respond to methotrexate or leflunomide. The biologic DMARDs include adalimumab, anakinra, certolizumab, etanercept, golimumab, infliximab, adalimumab, abatacept, rituximab, tocilizumab and, most recently, tofacitinib. Box 47-3 lists the DMARDs. Etanercept and abatacept are discussed in this section; the others are discussed in the section on monoclonal antibodies earlier in the chapter. Tofacitinib (Xeljanz) is a Janus kinases inhibitor that was recently approved for adult patients with moderately to severely active RA who have had an inadequate response or intolerance to methotrexate. It is the only DMARD that is given orally. Serious infections—including tuberculosis and bacterial, invasive fungal, viral, and other opportunistic infections—have been reported. Lymphoma and other malignancies have also been observed. The most common side effects include diarrhea, upper respiratory tract infection, headache, hypertension, lipid abnormalities, anemia,

BOX 47-3	Disease-Modifying Antirheumatic Drugs
abatacept	leflunomide
adalimumab	methotrexate
anakinra	rituximab
certolizumab	tocilizumab
etanercept	tofacitinib
golimumab	hydroxychloroquine
infliximab	sulfasalazine

and insomnia. It should not be used in combination with other DMARDS or immunosuppressants.

Mechanism of Action, Indications, and Adverse Effects

The mechanism of action and adverse effects of the different DMARDs vary. The individual drug profiles provide information on mechanism of action and adverse effects. All of these drugs are indicated for the treatment of rheumatoid arthritis, and some have other uses as previously mentioned.

Contraindications

DMARDs are not used in patients with active bacterial infection, active herpes zoster, active or latent tuberculosis, or acute or chronic hepatitis B or C. Etanercept, infliximab, and adalimumab are not to be used in patients with heart failure, lymphoma, or multiple sclerosis. Methotrexate and leflunomide are to be avoided during pregnancy and lactation.

DRUG PROFILES

abatacept

Abatacept (Orencia) is a selective costimulation modulator; it inhibits T-cell activation. Abatacept is indicated for the treatment of rheumatoid arthritis. It is contraindicated in patients with a known hypersensitivity to it or any of its components. Use with caution in patients with a history of recurrent infections or chronic obstructive pulmonary disease. Bring patients up to date with all current immunizations before starting abatacept therapy. Adverse effects include headache, upper respiratory tract infections, and hypertension. Abatacept may increase the risk for infections associated with live vaccines and may decrease the response to dead and/or live vaccines. Abatacept is not to be given with anakinra or TNF-blocking drugs because of the risk for serious infections, or with the herb echinacea, which has immunostimulant properties. Abatacept is dosed according to body weight and is given at 4-week intervals. It is administered intravenously, and a filter must be used. The half-life is 8 to 25 days.

etanercept

Etanercept (Enbrel) is a recombinant DNA–derived TNF-blocking drug. It binds TNF and blocks its interaction with cell surface receptors. It is indicated for the treatment of rheumatoid arthritis (including juvenile rheumatoid arthritis) and moderate to severe chronic plaque psoriasis. It is contraindicated in patients with a known hypersensitivity to it and in those with sepsis and active infections (including chronic or local infections). Use with caution in patients with preexisting demyelinating central nervous system disorders, heart failure, or significant hematologic abnormalities. Some dosage forms may contain latex, so screen patients for latex allergy. Reactivation of hepatitis and tuberculosis have been reported. Live vaccines should not be given with etanercept. Common adverse effects include headache, injection site reaction, upper respiratory tract infection, dizziness, and weakness. The drug is administered subcutaneously. Drugs with which it interacts include anakinra, which may increase the risk for infection, and cyclophosphamide, which may increase the risk for malignancy. Etanercept is classified as a pregnancy category B drug. It is not known if the drug is excreted in breast milk, and its use is not recommended in lactating women. The onset of action is 1 to 2 weeks, and the half-life is 72 to 132 hours.

leflunomide

Leflunomide (Arava) is indicated for the treatment of active rheumatoid arthritis. It modulates or alters the response of the immune system to rheumatoid arthritis. It has antiproliferative, antiinflammatory, and immunosuppressive activity. Most common adverse effects are diarrhea, respiratory tract infection, alopecia, elevated liver enzyme levels, and rash. It is contraindicated in women who are or may become pregnant and is not to be used by nursing mothers or those with a known hypersensitivity to it. It is classified as a pregnancy category X drug. Aspirin, other NSAIDs, and/or low-dose corticosteroids may be continued during leflunomide therapy. Leflunomide is available only for oral use. The half-life is 14 to 15 days.

!methotrexate

Methotrexate is an anticancer drug that is commonly used for treatment of rheumatoid arthritis in much lower dosages than those used for cancer. It is usually started at dosages of 7.5 to 10 mg/wk but can be increased to 25 mg/wk. It is very important to note that the drug is given once per week, not once per day. Serious medication errors, including deaths, have occurred when an order for once weekly is misinterpreted as once daily. It is usually given orally for rheumatoid arthritis, but it can also be given by injection. Bone marrow suppression is the main adverse effect of methotrexate. Most patients are advised to take supplemental folic acid to lessen the likelihood of adverse effects. The onset of antirheumatic action is 3 to 6 weeks. The half-life of the drug is 3 to 10 hours.

NURSING PROCESS

ASSESSMENT

For *hematopoietic* drugs, assess the medication order thoroughly as well as the specific indication for each of the drugs prescribed. Once you understand the indication, specific laboratory value(s) may be easily determined for further assessment (e.g., WBC counts with *sargramostin* and *filgrastim*, platelets with use of *oprelvekin*). After initial assessment and monitoring

of baseline blood counts, measure drug response blood counts against these values. Additionally, prior to administering these medications, assess the following: vital signs, skin turgor/intactness, bowel sounds/bowel patterns, and breath sounds. Assess also for any complaints of pain, and rate accordingly (see discussion in Chapter 10). These areas are all very important to assess when giving hematopoietic drugs because of the adverse effects of edema, nausea, vomiting, diarrhea, rash, cough, dyspnea, sore throat, fever, blood dyscrasias, headache, and bone pain. Additionally, assess potential intravenous and subcutaneous injection sites, as needed. From laboratory values, assess the chemotherapy-induced absolute neutrophil nadir (low point). This is important because timing of the dose is critical in helping to boost blood cell counts. For example, with filgrastim, it is *not* given within 24 hours before or after the chemotherapy drug. Specifically with use of filgrastim, assess for any existing joint or bone pain because of the possible adverse effect of mild to severe bone pain. See Chapter 54 for more information regarding assessment associated with use of epoetin alfa.

With the administration of any of the *biologic response–modifying drugs* (and other drugs included in this chapter), assess your own knowledge about these medications with attention to the drug's action, pharmacokinetic properties, associated cautions, contraindications, drug interactions, adverse effects, and toxicities. Assess the patient for the presence of any conditions and/or medications that represent cautions, contraindications, or interactions. Assess for hypersensitivity to the drug, egg proteins, or immunoglobulin G. Furthermore, assess the following systems: (1) respiratory system with attention to rate, rhythm, and depth as well as breath sounds, listening for any adventitious (abnormal) sounds; (2) cardiac system with attention to vital signs, heart sounds, heart rate and rhythm, and oxygen saturation levels, as well as assessment for edema and/or shortness of breath, presence of cyanotic discoloration around the mouth or nail beds, and any chest pain; (3) central nervous system with a focus on baseline mental status, as well as assessment for any seizure-like activity or central nervous system abnormalities; and (4) immune system, noting any history of chronic illnesses, ability to fight off infections, and history of suppressed immunity. Note nutritional status, height, and weight as well as results of any prescribed laboratory tests, such as CBC and especially hemoglobin and hematocrit levels, serum protein and albumin levels, and immunoglobulin levels (see Nursing Process in Chapters 45 and 46). Also document the presence or absence of underlying diseases, symptoms, and success or failure of past medication regimens. Assess the patient's ability to carry out the activities of daily living, emotional and socioeconomic status, educational level, learning needs, desire and ability to learn, past coping strategies, and support systems.

Before *interferons* (e.g., *interferon alfa-2a or alfa-2b; interferon gamma-1b*) are given, assess the patient's history of drug allergies as well as any history of autoimmune disorders, hepatitis, liver failure, or AIDS. Contraindications include concurrent use of immunosuppressant drugs, liver dysfunction, severe liver disease, and AIDS-related Kaposi's sarcoma. It is important to remember that *interferon alfa-2b* has a black box warning associated with the possible aggravation and/or precipitation of autoimmune disorders and neuropsychiatric symptoms. Determine baseline WBC and platelet counts prior to initiation of therapy due to the potential for drug-induced neutropenia and thrombocytopenia. Monitor other serum laboratory values such as blood urea nitrogen, creatinine levels, and ALP and AST levels before and during treatment due to the risk for problems with renal and liver functioning. It is important to document baseline neurologic functioning, bowel status, heart sounds, pulse rate, and blood pressure (including postural readings). Significant drug interactions to assess for include those drugs that are metabolized via the cytochrome P-450 enzyme system in the liver because of the risk for subsequent drug toxicity. Bone marrow suppression may be exacerbated when the *interferon gamma products* are given with other bone marrow suppressive drugs. *Antiviral drugs* such as *zidovudine* may lead to severe toxicity and myelosuppression.

With the use of *monoclonal antibody drugs* (e.g., *adalimumab, alemtuzumab, bevacizumab, infliximab, natalizumab, trastuzumab, vedolizumab*), assess and document history of allergic reactions. Assess for ranges of responses with these medications including mild to severe reactions (see Table 47-3). Assessment of baseline vital signs and any signs of infection are important because of the risk for acquiring an infection when these drugs are given. Contraindications to their use include any active infectious process and HIV. Assess patient status for possible surgery or presence of wounds because bevacizumab (Avastin) may complicate surgical wound healing. With infliximab (Remicade), assess for a history because it is contraindicated in severe heart failure. Additionally, there is an FDA black box warning stating that fatal tuberculosis and/or fungal infections have been associated with use of this drug, so any infections process needs to be ruled out prior to its use. Testing needs to be completed, as ordered, for latent tuberculosis. Patients with multiple sclerosis may need treatment with natalizumab (Tysabri). It is now only FDA approved in those patients enrolled in a special distribution program because of associated multifocal leukoencephalopathy infections of the brain. Inquire as well as review patient data for the presence of any condition that may weaken the immune system such as an HIV infection or AIDS, leukemia, lymphoma, or organ transplant. These may indeed be contraindications to its use. Additionally, be sure to assess baseline medical conditions as well as a thorough neurologic assessment with attention to thought processes, vision, balance/gait, and bilateral strength in the arms and legs. This is important due to the fact that alterations in the neuroskeletal muscular systems indicate a concern with continuing the treatment. Trastuzumab (Herceptin B) has an FDA black box warning for cases of ventricular dysfunction and heart failure. Fatal hypersensitivity and infusion reactions have occurred with this drug; therefore, prior to administration be very astute in the risk evaluation to enhance subsequent, prudent clinical judgment-making by the prescriber and you. With the administration of vedolizumab (Entyvio), it is important to assess existing pulmonary disease/infection due to the adverse effect of upper respiratory tract infection. Perform close

monitoring and supervision before, during, and after the infusion of these drugs. Table 47-3 provides a listing of common adverse effects associated with these drugs requiring further areas and systems to be assessed.

With *interleukins*, assess for drug allergy as well as the contraindications of organ transplantation, abnormal thallium cardiac stress test, or abnormal pulmonary function tests. Assess vital signs and breath and heart sounds. Document any history of respiratory and/or cardiac disorders due to the severe toxicities of capillary leak syndrome (with *aldesleukin*). As mentioned earlier in the chapter, capillary leak syndrome results in massive fluid retention of 20 to 30 pounds leading to potentially life-threatening problems of respiratory distress and heart failure. These are reversible after discontinuation of the interleukin therapy. Assess liver function studies prior to therapy. Drug interactions of significance include antihypertensives, which produce additive hypotensive effects. Corticosteroid use is contraindicated because of a reduction in antitumor effectiveness. *Tocilizumab* is one interleukin drug that is indicated for severe rheumatoid arthritis and is not to be given with other biologic response modifiers.

With *DMARDs*, perform a close assessment of any past or present medical conditions as well a thorough assessment of allergies. Compile a complete and thorough medication profile, listing prescription drugs, herbals, and over-the-counter drugs. Assess the specific type of DMARD prescribed because there are nonbiologic and biologic DMARDS. *Nonbiologic DMARDs* include *methotrexate, leflunomide, hydroxychoroquine,* and *sulfasalazine.* Biologic DMARDs include several of the monoclonal antibodies such as *adalimumab, infliximab,* and *tocilizumab.* Assess for contraindications to the use of DMARDs such as active bacterial infections, active herpes, active/latent tuberculosis, and acute or chronic hepatitis B or C. Additional contraindications are presented in the pharmacology discussion. Because bone marrow suppression is one of the main adverse effects (e.g., with methotrexate), assess and monitor baseline blood cell and platelet counts before, during, and after therapy. Important to patient safety is the thorough assessment of the medication order. This will help prevent serious medication errors. There is documentation that serious drug errors have occurred when the order for some of these drugs (e.g., methotrexate) has been transcribed incorrectly and the drug given daily instead of in the recommended once-weekly dosing.

Before initiation of therapy with leflunomide, perform a complete assessment of hepatic functioning as well as baseline blood cell counts. Because of the possible adverse effects of diarrhea and respiratory infections, assess respiratory and gastrointestinal functioning including the following: Obtain a history of past and present respiratory disorders and infections, noting breath sounds, presence of sputum, and baseline respiratory rate, rhythm, and depth. Assess bowel patterns, and document the findings. Etanercept is to be avoided in those with sepsis and active infections, so conduct a thorough assessment of WBC counts and for any signs and symptoms of infection or a history of infection. Because some dosage forms may contain latex, it is critical to also assess for latex allergy. The DMARD *abatacept* is given based on weight; thus, there is a need for

TEAMWORK AND COLLABORATION: LEGAL AND ETHICAL PRINCIPLES

The Nurse and Patient Care

Never neglect or deceive a patient, even if a conflict arises with your own cultural, racial-ethnic, spiritual, or personal belief systems. Such a dilemma is often encountered in connection with various treatment modalities for cancer patients or patients needing drugs that alter the body's biologic response. You do have the right to refuse to participate in any treatment or aspect of a patient's care that violates personal ethical principles, but it is important to understand that this refusal of care can in no way involve desertion or neglect of the patient. In these situations, inform the appropriate supervisory personnel about the conflict, and transfer the patient to the safe care of another qualified professional. As detailed in the American Nurses Association *Code of Ethics for Nurses* (2015), nurses are bound by the profession always to remain ethical in the provision of care to patients. This may include participation in the care of a patient who needs the nurse's care but who may be receiving treatment or care that is not "acceptable" by the nurse's own standards or ethics.

an accurate predrug therapy weight. Additionally, assess the patient's immunization record because all immunizations must be current prior to beginning therapy with abatacept. Document the findings of a baseline head-to-toe physical assessment, and note any musculoskeletal changes due to the pathology of arthritis and related changes in activities of daily living and other basic activities before drug therapy is initiated as well as throughout the therapeutic regimen.

NURSING DIAGNOSES

1. Imbalanced nutrition, less than body requirements, related to the adverse effects of biologic response–modifying drugs
2. Impaired skin integrity (rash) related to the adverse effects of biologic response–modifying drugs
3. Risk for infection related to adverse effect of bone marrow suppression related to DMARDs and immunomodulating drugs

PLANNING: OUTCOME IDENTIFICATION

1. Patient regains/maintains predrug healthy nutritional status with a 24-hour recall of food intake; menu planning with use of MyPlate including high-calorie, low-residue, high protein/high-energy foods; and use of antiemetics, as prescribed.
2. Patient's skin integrity remains intact during drug therapy with use of daily bathing, skin care, dental care, and reporting of any redness, irritation, swelling, drainage, or pain.
3. Patient remains free from injury to self with minimizing the risk for infection (proper diet, fluid intake, staying away from crowds) and reports an elevation in temperature of 100.5 to the prescriber for immediate treatment.

IMPLEMENTATION

With *hematopoietic drugs*, it is important to administer the drug as ordered. Determine and rotate subcutaneous and IV sites, as specified by institutional policy. With *filgrastim*, administer the drug before a patient receiving myelosuppressive chemotherapy develops an infection, but not within 24 hours before or after a myelosuppressive chemotherapy drug is given. Once a patient's absolute neutrophil count (ANC) reaches 10,000 cells/mm^3, discontinue the drug, as ordered and as recommended by the manufacturer. Give filgrastim and use D$_5$W to dilute the product. With *sargramostim*, reconstitute the dose with sterile water for injection. Do not use *oprelvekin* if any discoloration or particulate matter is noted in the vial. Treatment may be ordered to begin within 6 to 24 hours after completion of antineoplastic therapy. Daily subcutaneous dosing for 14 days has been found to produce dose-dependent platelet elevations, with counts increasing within 5 to 9 days of starting injections. Once oprelvekin is discontinued, counts remain increased for about 7 days and return to baseline within 14 days. Subcutaneous sites for oprelvekin administration include the thigh, abdomen, hip, and upper arm. When drugs are given subcutaneously, rotate injection sites. See Patient-Centered Care: Patient Teaching on p. 767 for more information.

Administer *biologic response–modifying drugs* exactly as prescribed and in keeping with manufacturer guidelines to minimize adverse effects. It is important to acknowledge that acquiring an infection is a serious adverse effect of these drugs, and so the risk must always be weighed against the severity of the patient's underlying illness. Measure vital signs with special attention to temperature. Premedication with acetaminophen and diphenhydramine is usually the standard of care with use of any of the biologic response–modifying drugs because of the high incidence of drug reactions. With some of the biologic response–modifying drugs, if bone pain and chill are not successfully managed with premedications, then opioids, antihistamines, and/or antiinflammatory drugs may be required. Antiemetics may also be needed for any drug-related nausea or vomiting and may be administered prior to the administration of the biologic response–modifying drug. Antiemetics may need to be dosed around the clock if nausea and vomiting are problematic. Encourage the patient to rest when tired, not to overexert self during therapy, and to contact the prescriber if he or she experiences profound fatigue or loss of appetite. Encourage an increase of fluids to up to 3000 mL/day, unless contraindicated, to promote excretion of the by-products of cellular breakdown and to maintain cellular hydration. Consultation with a dietitian or nutritionist may be helpful to the patient in learning about a nourishing, well-balanced diet to promote health and wellness. Foods high in protein, complex carbohydrates, and necessary minerals and vitamins will be recommended. Discuss menu planning and grocery shopping with attention to patient-specific suggestions. Nowadays, many grocery stores support online food shopping with pickup at the store on the same or next day or home delivery at minimal to no cost. Inform patients about community resources such as Meals On Wheels, respite care organizations within city governments, and support from ones' church or other organization as deemed appropriate and as needed.

When *interferons* are given, be sure to first read the order for correct spelling and be careful not to confuse with any other sound-alike, look-alike drugs. Administer the interferons parenterally by either the subcutaneous, intravenous, or intramuscular route, depending on the specific drug. For example, give *interferon alfa-2a* subcutaneously or intramuscularly. Be sure to rotate sites and use accurate technique (see Chapter 9). With concerns of infection, as with many of the biologic response–modifying drugs, monitor the patient's vital signs with attention to temperature. Monitor also for the occurrence of chills and headache indicative of a fever. An ECG, before and during treatment, is generally prescribed, so monitor the results and report any chest pain, hypotension, hypertension, or dyspnea. Make sure to always check each brand of medication for the dilution directions, as each brand has different directions. Read the package insert prior to giving these drugs. Acetaminophen may be prescribed to help with fever and headache. Encourage increasing of fluids.

With *monoclonals,* serious infections are a major concern. With *belimumab,* the most serious concern is infection, which may sometimes be fatal. Constantly monitor for infection during therapy. *Bevacizumab (Avastin)* is associated with complicating surgical wound healing, so there is a need for documentation of wound assessment. *Certolizumab,* which is used with severe Crohn's disease and severe rheumatoid arthritis, is also associated with the risk for serious infections and possible lymphoma. Discuss all of these concerns and risks with the patient, significant others/family members, and/or caregiver. Complete blood counts will be monitored before, during, and after therapy. Monitor the patient for changes in blood pressure and pulse rate and for chest pain. Contact the prescriber immediately if there are significant changes in baseline parameters. Avoid *infliximab* in patients with severe heart failure. When giving this drug, it is important to monitor heart sounds, blood pressure, pulse rate, pulse oximetry reading, and ECG. If there are signs and symptoms of infection and/or changes in cardiac status, contact the prescriber immediately. This drug carries an FDA black box warning because it may cause fatal tuberculin and/or fungal infections. *Natalizumab (Tysabri),* as with several drugs in this class, has a prolonged half-life and takes days to weeks to be eliminated from the body (see Pharmacology discussion). This pharmacokinetic property may lead to more drug interactions and risk for toxicity. With natalizumab, only patients enrolled in the "Touch" program, a special distribution program mandated by the FDA, can receive the drug. This developed out of the fact that it is associated with multifocal leukoencephalopathy infection of the brain. *Trastuzumab (Herceptin B)* also requires premedication because of the risk for infusion reactions. Additionally, it carries an FDA black box warning for ventricular dysfunction and heart failure.

The interleukin *aldesleukin* is associated with severe toxicity and capillary leak syndrome. When administering this drug, monitor patients very closely for fever, chills, rash, myalgias, headache, and changes in liver function tests and eosinophils, as per institutional protocol and/or through critical decision making.

With the *biologic DMARD methotrexate* a test dose is usually administered to see how the patient reacts to the medication. Be aware of the FDA black box warning about the cautious administration of this drug in those with renal disease,

infection, pulmonary disease, and stomatitis. Be sure that if *methotrexate* is ordered for rheumatoid arthritis, it is administered weekly as ordered. For more information on methotrexate, see Chapter 45. Give *etanercept,* yet another drug with black box warnings (see the pharmacology discussion), subcutaneously into the thigh, abdomen, or upper arm, rotating injection sites. Give *leflunomide* very cautiously while monitoring liver and renal functioning; administer it orally with meals or food to minimize gastrointestinal upset. Monitor daily weights due to possible edema.

CASE STUDY

Patient-Centered Care: Hematopoietic Biologic Response Modifiers

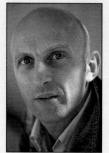

P.S., a 38-year-old surveyor, is receiving a second round of chemotherapy as part of treatment for non-Hodgkin's lymphoma. The oncologist is monitoring for signs of bone marrow suppression of the various blood cell components.

1. What symptoms would the nurse expect to see if P.S. had diminished production of platelets? White blood cells? Explain your answers.
2. One week after this round of chemotherapy, P.S.'s white blood cell count is 0.8 cells/mm³ (pretherapy value was 6200 cells/mm³), and his absolute neutrophil count is 450 cells/mm³ (pretherapy value was 1600 cells/mm³). The oncologist orders strict neutropenic precautions and filgrastrim (Neupogen), 480 mcg, subcut daily. What is the purpose of the order for the filgrastim? The nurse will need to assess P.S. for what conditions before beginning the filgrastim?
3. The nurse notices a woman with an infant about to enter P.S.'s room. The infant is fussy, and the woman is wiping the infant's nose after the baby sneezed. What is the nurse's priority action at this time?
4. P.S. asks the nurse, "How long will I need to take these injections? I hate having to have another shot!" How will the nurse respond to the patient's question?

For answers, see *http://evolve.elsevier.com/Lilley.*

┃EVALUATION

Therapeutic responses to *biologic response–modifying drugs* include a variety of responses, such as a decrease in the growth of the lesion or mass, decreased tumor size, and an easing of symptoms related to the tumor or disease process. Other therapeutic effects are an improvement in WBC and platelet counts and/or a return of blood counts to normal levels, and absence of infection and hemorrhage. Encourage patient journaling, which may help provide health care providers with more data from which to evaluate the patient's response during and after therapy. Possible adverse effects for which to evaluate are presented in Tables 47-1 and 47-2. *DMARDs* are expected to have therapeutic results within a documented time frame (often weeks), with the patient experiencing increased ability to move joints, less discomfort, and an overall increased sense of improvement and well-being. Toxicity of these drugs may be manifested by liver, renal, and respiratory dysfunction and, for methotrexate, bone marrow suppression.

PATIENT-CENTERED CARE: PATIENT TEACHING

- Advise the patient to avoid hazardous tasks because of the central nervous system changes noted with several biologic response–modifying drugs. Fatigue is also a common adverse effect; instruct the patient to report any excessive fatigue.
- Instruct the patient to report to the prescriber immediately any signs of infection, such as sore throat, diarrhea, vomiting, and/or fever of 100.5°F (38.1°C) or higher. Advise the patient also to report excessive fatigue, loss of appetite, edema, or bleeding.
- Pregnancy is discouraged while the patient is taking a biologic response–modifying drug. Educate patients of childbearing age about contraceptive choices and the need to use contraception for up to 2 years after completion of therapy.
- Inform the patient that adverse effects associated with biologic response–modifying drugs usually disappear within 72 to 96 hours after therapy is discontinued.
- Interferons may cause increased fatigue and flulike symptoms. Fatigue may be severe enough to keep the patient in bed, so prepare the patient (and family, caregiver) that this may occur. Interactions occur with any drugs metabolized by the P450 enzyme system. Educate about the various interacting drugs.
- Educate the patient, family, and/or caregiver about the association of capillary leak syndrome (CLS) with interleukins, specifically aldesleukin and interferon. Early signs and symptoms to emphasize include nasal congestion, runny nose, cough progressing to lightheadedness, weakness, fatigue, nausea, and sudden onset of edema (swelling) in the arms, legs, and other parts of the body. The potential to retain up to 30 pounds of fluid progresses rapidly with a drop in blood pressure, respiratory distress, heart failure, dysrhythmias,

and myocardial infarction. Emphasize that CLS is reversible if diagnosed early, the prescriber discontinues the drug, and emergency medical supportive and symptomatic treatment is provided during the onset of early symptoms. CLS may be fatal if not recognized early.

- If anakinra (Kineret), an interleukin, is prescribed, the patient may self-administer (if prescribed), so there is a need to emphasize the specific injection technique and proper disposal of equipment (e.g., needles, syringes). Provide demonstrations, and allow for return demonstration with written instructions for the subcutaneous injection. Encourage the daily keeping of a journal to record the site of injection and an overall rating of how the patient feels.
- Bone pain and flulike symptoms often occur with some of the biologic response–modifying drugs, and the use of nonopioid or, in some cases, opioid analgesics may be required. Some patients may find relief with acetaminophen or ibuprofen.
- Educate patients about the FDA black box warnings for infliximab (Remicade), which include the risk for fatal forms of tuberculosis and/or fungal infections. Trastuzumab (Herceptin B) also has a black box warning because of its ventricular dysfunction and heart failure reactions.
- With DMARDs, the patient will experience improved joint function and decreased pain. Encourage the patient to report any bleeding, excess fatigue, fever, or respiratory symptoms. The newer DMARD, tofacitinib, is the only one that is given orally and used if the patient has an inadequate response or intolerance to methotrexate. However, serious infections including tuberculosis are concerns with use of the drug, and the patient needs to know the signs and symptoms to report to the prescriber.

KEY POINTS

- Over the last two decades, medical technology has developed a group of drugs impacting the immune system, and a new addition to these drugs includes the biologic response-modifying drugs or biologic response modifiers (BRMs).
- These drugs alter the body's response to diseases including cancer, autoimmune, inflammatory, and infectious disease processes. These drugs enhance/restrict the patient's immune response to disease. They can stimulate a patient's hematopoietic function and prevent disease.
- Two broad classes of BRMs include hematopoietic drugs and immunomodulating drugs. Subclasses include interferons, monoclonal antibodies, interleukin receptor agonists/ antagonists, and miscellaneous drugs.
- The two major components of the body's immune system are humoral immunity, mediated by B-cell functions (primarily *antibody* production), and cell-mediated immunity, which is mediated by T-cell functions. These two systems work together to recognize and destroy foreign particles and cells in the blood or other body tissues. The humoral and cellular immune systems act together to recog-

nize and destroy foreign particles and cells. The humoral immune system is composed of lymphocytes that are known as B cells until they are transformed into plasma cells when they come in contact with an antigen (foreign substance). The plasma cells then manufacture antibodies to that antigen.

- Nursing management associated with the administration of biologic response–modifying drugs focuses on the use of careful aseptic technique and other measures to prevent infection; proper nutrition; oral hygiene; monitoring of blood counts; and management of adverse effects, including joint/bone pain and flulike symptoms.
- Monitor the patient for capillary leak syndrome (CLS) if they are taking interleukins. Identification of early symptoms will allow critical, supportive treatment with discontinuation of the interleukin drug.
- Do not administer filgrastim and sargramostim within 24 hours of a myelosuppressive antineoplastic, and follow the timeframe for their use (as prescribed), whether in an inpatient or home setting.

- The recommended therapy with nonbiologic DMARDs usually begins with methotrexate or leflunomide for most patients. Biologic DMARDs are generally reserved for those patients whose disease does not respond to methotrexate or leflunomide. The biologic DMARDs include etanercept, infliximab, adalimumab, abatacept, and rituximab.

NCLEX® EXAMINATION REVIEW QUESTIONS

1. The nurse is conducting a class on drugs for malignant tumors for a group of new oncology staff members. Which best describes the action of interferons in the management of malignant tumors?
   a. Interferons increase the production of specific anticancer enzymes.
   b. Interferons have antiviral and antitumor properties and strengthen the immune system.
   c. Interferons stimulate the production and activation of T lymphocytes and cytotoxic T cells.
   d. Interferons help improve the cell-killing action of T cells because they are retrieved from healthy donors.

2. When planning care for a patient who is receiving interferon therapy, the nurse must keep in mind that the major dose-limiting factor is
   a. fatigue.
   b. bone marrow suppression.
   c. fever.
   d. nausea and vomiting.

3. The nurse is administering methotrexate as part of treatment for a patient with rheumatoid arthritis and will monitor for which sign of bone marrow suppression?
   a. Edema
   b. Tinnitus
   c. Increased bleeding tendencies
   d. Tingling in the extremities

4. In caring for a patient receiving therapy with a myelosuppressive antineoplastic drug, the nurse notes an order to begin filgrastim after the chemotherapy is completed. Which statement correctly describes when the nurse will begin the filgrastim therapy?
   a. It can be started during the chemotherapy.
   b. It will begin immediately after the chemotherapy is completed.
   c. It will be initiated 24 hours after the chemotherapy is completed.
   d. It will not be started until at least 72 hours after the chemotherapy is completed.

5. The nurse is monitoring a patient who has been receiving aldesleukin (IL-2) (Proleukin) for treatment of malignant melanoma. Which adverse effect, if noted on assessment, is of primary concern?
   a. Chills
   b. Fatigue
   c. Headache
   d. Fluid retention

6. The nurse is reviewing the medical history of a patient who is about to receive therapy with etanercept (Enbrel). Which conditions, if present, would be a contraindication or caution for therapy with this drug? *(Select all that apply.)*
   a. Urinary tract infection
   b. Psoriasis
   c. Heart failure
   d. Glaucoma
   e. Latex allergy

7. A patient is to receive filgrastim (Neupogen) after therapy with carmustine and radiation therapy for treatment of a brain tumor. The patient weighs 132 pounds. The protocol that the oncologist has written states that the filgrastim will be dosed at 5 mcg/kg. Filgrastim comes in a 300-mcg/mL vial. What dose will the patient receive? How many milliliters will the patient be given?

8. The nurse notes in the patient's medication history that the patient is taking natalizumab (Tysabri). Based on this finding, the nurse interprets that the patient has which disorder?
   a. Multiple sclerosis
   b. Rheumatoid arthritis
   c. Non-Hodgkin's lymphoma
   d. Crohn's disease

1. b, 2. a, 3. c, 4. c, 5. d, 6. a, c, e, 7. 300 mcg; 1 mL, 8. a.

CRITICAL THINKING AND PRIORITIZATION QUESTIONS

1. A patient who has been receiving an alkylating chemotherapeutic drug is to receive the colony-stimulating factor filgrastim (Neupogen). A new nurse is preparing to start the filgrastim as soon as the chemotherapy is completed, and the charge nurse is reviewing the orders. What is the charge nurse's priority action at this time? Explain your answer.

2. The nurse is monitoring a patient who is receiving the interleukin drug aldesleukin (Proleukin). The patient is experiencing fever, chills, fatigue, dyspnea, slight crackles, ankle edema rated as 2+, and headache. What is the nurse's priority action at this time?

For answers, see *http://evolve.elsevier.com/Lilley*.

EVOLVE WEBSITE

http://evolve.elsevier.com/Lilley
- Animations
- Answer Keys for Textbook Case Studies and Textbook Critical Thinking and Prioritization Questions
- Content Updates
- Key Points
- Review Questions
- Student Case Studies

Immunosuppressant Drugs

⒠ http://evolve.elsevier.com/Lilley

OBJECTIVES

When you reach the end of this chapter, you will be able to do the following:

1. Discuss the role of immunosuppressive therapy in organ transplantation and in the treatment of autoimmune diseases.
2. Discuss the mechanisms of action, contraindications, cautions, adverse effects, routes of administration, drug

interactions, and toxicity of the most commonly used immunosuppressants.

3. Develop a nursing care plan that includes all phases of the nursing process for patients receiving immunosuppressants after organ transplantation or for the treatment of autoimmune disease.

DRUG PROFILES

⬧ **azathioprine, p. 773**
basiliximab, p. 773
⬧ **cyclosporine, p. 773**
glatiramer acetate, p. 775
muromonab-CD3, p. 776

⬧ **mycophenolate mofetil, p. 776**
⬧ **sirolimus and** ⬧ **tacrolimus, p. 776**

⬧ = *Key drug*
! = *High-alert drug*

KEY TERMS

Autoimmune diseases A large group of diseases characterized by the alteration of the function of the immune system so that the immune response is directed against normal tissue(s) of the body, which results in pathologic conditions. (p. 770)

Grafts The term used for transplanted tissues or organs. (p. 773)

Immune-mediated diseases A large group of diseases that result when the cells of the immune system react to a

variety of situations, such as transplanted organ tissue or drug-altered cells. (p. 770)

Immunosuppressants Drugs that decrease or prevent an immune response. (p. 770)

Immunosuppressive therapy A drug treatment used to suppress the immune system. (p. 770)

IMMUNE SYSTEM

The purpose of the *immune system* is to distinguish self from nonself and to protect the body from foreign material (antigens). There are three layers of barriers to protect the body (Figure 48-1). There are two types of immunity: humoral immunity, which is mediated by B lymphocytes, and cellular immunity, which is mediated by T lymphocytes. This chapter focuses on drugs that suppress the T lymphocytes.

The immune system defends the body against invading pathogens, foreign antigens, and its own cells that become cancerous, or neoplastic. Besides performing this beneficial function, it can also attack itself and cause what are known as **autoimmune diseases** or **immune-mediated diseases**. The immune system also participates in hypersensitivity, or anaphylactic, reactions, which can be life-threatening. The rejection of

kidney, liver, and heart (whole organ) transplants is directed by the immune system as well.

Drugs that decrease or prevent an immune response, and hence suppress the immune system, are known as **immunosuppressants**. Treatment with such drugs is referred to as **immunosuppressive therapy**. Immunosuppressants are used for many immune-related disorders, including rheumatoid arthritis, systemic lupus erythematosus, Crohn's disease, multiple sclerosis, myasthenia gravis, psoriasis, and others. Examples of these drugs include cyclophosphamide (see Chapter 46), glatiramer acetate, fingolimod, and many immunomodulators, which are discussed in Chapter 47. This chapter focuses on the drugs used in organ transplantation.

Transplantation is one of the most complex areas of modern medicine. Many different types of transplants are routinely done including, but not limited to, kidney, heart, liver, lung,

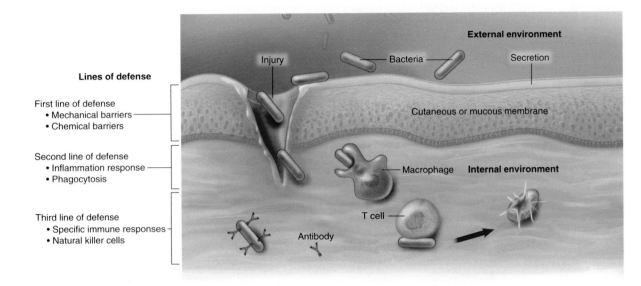

FIGURE 48-1 A simplified depiction of the complicated immune system. (From Patton KT, Thibodeau GA: *Anatomy and physiology*, ed 7, St Louis, 2010, Mosby.)

pancreas, small bowel, bone marrow, and cornea transplantation. The primary concern with transplantation is rejection, which could necessitate the transplanted organ to be removed. Rejection occurs from an immune response targeted against the transplanted organ. Immunosuppressants are used to inhibit the immune system and prevent organ rejection. Transplant patients are on immunosuppressant therapy for the duration of their lifetime. The cost of therapy can average over $2500 per month.

IMMUNOSUPPRESSANT DRUGS

Mechanism of Action and Drug Effects

All immunosuppressants have similar mechanisms of action in that they selectively suppress certain T-lymphocyte cell lines. By suppressing the T-lymphocyte cell lines, they prevent their involvement in the immune response. This results in a pharmacologically immunocompromised state similar to that in a cancer patient or in a patient with acquired immunodeficiency syndrome (AIDS). Each drug differs in the exact way in which it suppresses certain cell lines involved in an immune response. The major classes of immunosuppressant drugs used in preventing organ rejection include glucocorticoids, calcineurin inhibitors, antimetabolites, and biologics. Corticosteroids inhibit all stages of T-cell activation and are used for induction, maintenance immunosuppression, and acute rejection. Corticosteroids are discussed in depth in Chapter 33 and are not discussed further in this chapter. Calcineurin inhibitors (e.g., cyclosporine, tacrolimus, sirolimus) inhibit the phosphate required for interleukin 2 production. Sirolimus does not inhibit calcineurin but instead inhibits mTOR, which ultimately inhibits interleukin 2 communication. Antimetabolites (e.g., azathioprine, mycophenolate) inhibit cell proliferation. Biologics (e.g., muromonab-CD3, basiliximab) inhibit cytotoxic T killer cell function. Table 48-1 gives the mechanisms of action and indications of the available immunosuppressant drugs.

Indications

The therapeutic uses of immunosuppressants vary from drug to drug, as noted in Table 48-1. They are primarily indicated for the prevention of organ rejection. Three of the immunosuppressants are indicated for both prevention of rejection and treatment of organ rejection; they include muromonab-CD3, mycophenolate, and tacrolimus. Fingolimod and glatiramer are immunosuppressants that are indicated for reduction of the frequency of relapses (exacerbations) in a type of multiple sclerosis known as *relapsing-remitting multiple sclerosis.*

Contraindications

The main contraindication for all immunosuppressants is known drug allergy. Relative contraindications, depending on the patient's condition, may include renal or hepatic failure, hypertension, and concurrent radiation therapy. Pregnancy is not necessarily a contraindication to the use of these drugs, but immunosuppressants should be given to pregnant women only in clinically urgent situations. Many of the immunosuppressants have black box warnings, and the student is referred to specific prescribing information for the particular drug.

Adverse Effects

Immunosuppressant drugs have many significant adverse effects, which are listed in Table 48-2. By virtue of their actions, immunosuppressants place patients at increased risk for opportunistic infections. Immunosuppressant drugs may also increase the risk for certain types of cancers, especially skin cancers. Other serious adverse effects are limited to the particular drug. For example, cyclosporine and tacrolimus can cause nephrotoxicity, and corticosteroids, cyclosporine, and tacrolimus can cause posttransplant diabetes mellitus while mycophenolate can cause lymphoma, skin cancers, and progressive multifocal leukoencephalopathy. Patients taking immunosuppressant drugs need to avoid live vaccines.

TABLE 48-1   Available Immunosuppressant Drugs: Mechanisms of Action and Indications

Drug Name	Mechanism of Action	Indications/Uses
azathioprine (Imuran)	Blocks metabolism of purines, inhibiting the synthesis of T-cell DNA, RNA, and proteins and thereby blocking immune response	Prevention of organ rejection in kidney transplantation; treatment of rheumatoid arthritis
basiliximab* (Simulect)	Suppresses T-cell activity by blocking the binding of the cytokine mediator IL-2 to a specific receptor	Prevention of organ rejection in kidney transplantation
cyclosporine (Sandimmune, Neoral, Gengraf)	Inhibits activation of T cells by blocking the production and release of the cytokine mediator IL-2	Prevention of organ rejection in kidney, liver, and heart transplantation; treatment of rheumatoid arthritis and psoriasis. Unlabeled uses* include prevention of rejection in pancreas, bone marrow, and heart/lung transplantation.
fingolimod (Gilenya)	Decreases the amount of lymphocytes available to the central nervous system	Reduction of relapse frequency in patients with RRMS
glatiramer acetate (Copaxone)	Precise mechanism unknown; believed to somehow modify immune system processes that are associated with MS symptoms	Reduction of relapse frequency in patients with RRMS
muromonab-CD3[†] (Orthoclone OKT3)	Binds to CD3 glycoprotein on T-cell receptors, which blocks antigen recognition and reverses graft rejection that is already in progress	Treatment of acute organ rejection in kidney, liver, and heart transplantation
mycophenolate mofetil (CellCept, Myfortic)	Prevents proliferation of T cells by inhibiting intracellular purine synthesis	Prevention of organ rejection in kidney, liver, and heart transplantation
sirolimus (Rapamune)	Inhibits T-cell activation by binding to an intracellular protein known as FKBP-12 that subsequently prevents cellular proliferation	Prevention of organ rejection in kidney transplantation
tacrolimus (Prograf)	Inhibits T-cell activation, possibly by binding to an intracellular protein known as FKBP-12	Prevention of organ rejection in liver, kidney, and heart transplantation. Unlabeled uses[†] include prevention of rejection in bone marrow, pancreas, pancreatic islet cell, and small intestine transplantation; treatment of autoimmune diseases; and severe psoriasis.

FKBP-12, FK-binding protein 12; *IL-2*, interleukin-2; *MS*, multiple sclerosis; *RRMS*, relapsing-remitting multiple sclerosis.
*Non–FDA-approved but under investigation.
[†]Note that "ab" in any drug name usually indicates that it is a monoclonal antibody synthesized using recombinant DNA technology.

Interactions

Because transplant patients are on immunosuppressant drugs for their lifetime and are often on combination therapy, they are at increased risk for drug interactions. Immunosuppressants have narrow therapeutic windows, and drug interactions can be significant. Drugs that cause increased immunosuppressant drug levels can cause toxicity, whereas drugs that reduce immunosuppressant drug levels may lead to organ rejection. The major drug interactions with immunosuppressant drugs are listed in Table 48-3. Many of the immunosuppressant drugs are metabolized by the cytochrome P-450 enzyme system, thus drug interactions are common and can be significant. Grapefruit can inhibit metabolizing enzymes and thus can increase the activity of cyclosporine, tacrolimus, and sirolimus. Grapefruit juice may increase the bioavailability of cyclosporine by 20% to 200% and should be avoided. Foods that are high in potassium, such as bananas and tomatoes, can increase cyclosporine nephrotoxicity. Meals that have a high fat content can increase sirolimus levels.

Because the antibodies basiliximab and muromonab-CD3 are generally given in a relatively short single course of therapy, they have few recognized drug interactions. However, cases of encephalopathy have occurred in patients in whom the antiinflammatory drug indomethacin (see Chapter 44) was used concurrently with muromonab-CD3.

The potential for interactions between immunosuppressant drugs and herbal preparations also should not be overlooked. For example, the enzyme-inducing properties of St. John's wort have been demonstrated to reduce the therapeutic levels of cyclosporine and cause organ rejection. The immunostimulant properties of cat's claw and echinacea may be similarly undesirable in transplant recipients, because they have effects that are opposite those of the immunosuppressants.

Dosages

For dosage information on selected immunosuppressants, see the table on p. 775. Immunosuppressants must be taken exactly as directed and at the exact times and with the exact foods. Adherence to dosing schedules can be very difficult for patients because they are on multiple medications that must be taken at different times throughout the day. Patients should never stop taking their immunosuppressants without being told to do so by their transplant doctor. Cyclosporine and tacrolimus should not be taken at the same time. Sirolimus should be taken 4

TABLE 48-2 Selected Immunosuppressant Drugs: Common Adverse Effects

Body System	Adverse Effects
Azathioprine	
Hematologic	Leukopenia, thrombocytopenia
Hepatic	Hepatotoxicity
Cyclosporine	
Cardiovascular	Moderate hypertension
Central nervous	Neurotoxicity, including tremors
Hepatic	Hepatotoxicity with cholestasis and hyperbilirubinemia
Renal	Nephrotoxicity is common and dose limiting
Other	Posttransplant diabetes mellitus, gingival hyperplasia, and hirsutism
Muromonab-CD3	
Cardiovascular	Chest pain
Central nervous	Pyrexia (fever), chills, tremors
Gastrointestinal	Vomiting, nausea, diarrhea
Respiratory	Dyspnea, wheezing, pulmonary edema
Other	Flulike symptoms, fluid retention
Tacrolimus and Sirolimus	
Cardiovascular	Peripheral edema, hypertension, atrial fibrillation, palpitations, hypotension, tachycardia, thrombosis
Central nervous	Headache, insomnia, pain, anxiety, tremors, confusion, depression, neuropathy, somnolence, hypoesthesia, dizziness, hallucinations
Renal	Albuminuria, dysuria, acute renal failure, renal tubular necrosis
Other	Acne, rash, diabetes mellitus, electrolyte abnormalities, hypertriglyceridemia, hypercholesterolemia, constipation, diarrhea, nausea, urinary tract infection, anemia, thrombocytopenia, arthralgia
Potentially life-threatening reactions	Hepatotoxicity, nephrotic syndrome, anaphylaxis, interstitial lung disease, proteinuria, pulmonary hemorrhage, angioedema, neutropenia, thrombocytopenia, pancreatitis, infections, progressive multifocal leukoencephalopathy, seizures
Antibody Immunosuppressants (basiliximab and muromonab-CD3)	
Multiple body systems	Cytokine release syndrome, which includes such immune-mediated symptoms as fever, dyspnea, tachycardia, sweating, chills, headache, nausea, vomiting, diarrhea, muscle and joint pain, and general malaise

hours after cyclosporine. If a dose is missed, it should be taken as soon as the patient remembers, unless it is close to the time the next dose is due; in this case, the patient must contact the transplant doctor. Because the regimens are complex, this is the perfect opportunity for the nurse to educate the patient. Another important point is to remember that the doses must be taken at the exact times scheduled—the nurse working in a hospital setting must plan medication administration passes accordingly.

DRUG PROFILES

◆azathioprine

Azathioprine (Imuran) is a chemical analogue of the physiologic purines, such as adenine and guanine. It blocks T-cell proliferation by inhibiting purine synthesis, which in turn prevents synthesis of deoxyribonucleic acid (DNA). Azathioprine is used for prophylaxis of organ rejection concurrently with other immunosuppressant drugs, such as cyclosporine and corticosteroids. It is available in both oral and injectable forms. Azathioprine, along with all other immunosuppressants agents, carries a black box warning regarding bone marrow suppression and the development of lymphoma and other malignancies. Azathioprine is also associated with hepatosplenic T-cell lymphoma, a rare white blood cell cancer that is fatal.

Pharmacokinetics: Azathioprine

Route	Onset of Action	Peak Plasma Concentration	Elimination Half-life	Duration of Action
PO	2-4 days*	1-2 hr	5 hr	Unknown

*6-8 weeks for rheumatoid arthritis.

basiliximab

Basiliximab (Simulect) is a monoclonal antibody that works by inhibiting the binding of the cytokine mediator interleukin-2 (IL-2) to the high-affinity IL-2 receptor. It is used to prevent rejection of transplanted kidneys (grafts) and is generally used as part of a multidrug immunosuppressive regimen that includes cyclosporine and corticosteroids. Basiliximab has a tendency to cause the allergy-like reaction known as *cytokine release syndrome*, which can be severe and even involve anaphylaxis. Patients are often premedicated with corticosteroids (e.g., intravenous methylprednisolone) in an effort to avoid or alleviate this problem. Basiliximab is available only in injectable form. Basiliximab has a warning regarding the potential for lymphoproliferative disorders and opportunistic infections, as well as severe hypersensitivity reactions, including anaphylaxis. In addition, it has a black box warning regarding a higher risk for developing new-onset diabetes when used with other immunosuppressants.

Pharmacokinetics: Basiliximab

Route	Onset of Action	Peak Plasma Concentration	Elimination Half-life	Duration of Action
IV	1 day	3-4 days	7-9 days	Unknown

◆cyclosporine

Cyclosporine (Sandimmune) and cyclosporine-modified (Neoral, Gengraf) are immunosuppressant drugs indicated for the prevention of organ rejection. They are classified as calcineurin inhibitors and work by inhibiting the production and release of IL-2. Like azathioprine, they may also be used for the treatment of other immunologic disorders, such as various forms of arthritis, psoriasis, and irritable bowel disease.

Cyclosporine is available in both oral and injectable forms. Neoral and Gengraf are brand names for cyclosporine-modified

TABLE 48-3   Immunosuppressant Drugs: Selected Drug Interactions

Drug	Mechanism	Result
Cyclosporine		
clarithromycin		
fluconazole		
amiodarone		
Estrogens		
verapamil	Inhibit metabolism of cyclosporine	Increased levels of cyclosporine and toxicity
allopurinol		
Protease inhibitors		
HMG-CoA reductase inhibitors		
phenytoin		
phenobarbital		
carbamazepine	Induce metabolism of cyclosporine	Decreased levels of cyclosporine and reduced effect
rifampin		
St. John's wort		
NSAIDs	Inhibit synthesis of renal prostaglandin	Increased nephrotoxic effects of cyclosporine; renal failure
Grapefruit juice	Increases absorption of cyclosporine	Cyclosporine toxicity
Sirolimus		
Cyclosporine	Unknown	Increased concentration of sirolimus
fluconazole		
ketoconazole		
clarithromycin		
erythromycin	Inhibit metabolism of sirolimus	Increased concentration and effect of sirolimus
Protease inhibitors		
verapamil		
Grapefruit juice		
rifampin		
phenytoin		
phenobarbital	Induce metabolism of sirolimus	Decreased concentration and effect of sirolimus
carbamazepine		
St. John's wort		
Tacrolimus		
amphotericin		
gentamicin	Increase nephrotoxicity of tacrolimus	Renal failure
tobramycin		
clarithromycin		
fluconazole		
ketoconazole		
voriconazole		
Protease inhibitors	Inhibit metabolism of tacrolimus	Increased effect of tacrolimus
verapamil		
diltiazem		
Grapefruit juice		
rifampin		
phenytoin		
phenobarbital	Induce metabolism of tacrolimus	Decreased effect of tacrolimus
carbamazepine		
St. John's wort		
Mycophenolate		
Antacids		
Iron	Reduce absorption of mycophenolate	Decreased effect of mycophenolate
cholestyramine		
Oral contraceptives	Mycophenolate decreases progesterone levels	Possible pregnancy
Rifampin	Induces metabolism of mycophenolate	Decreased effect of mycophenolate
Azathioprine		
Allopurinol	Decreases metabolism of azathioprine	Bone marrow suppression
ACE Inhibitors, tacrolimus, ribavirin, sulfamethoxazole/ trimethoprim, roflumilast	Increased azathioprine effects	Bone marrow suppression
Mercaptopurine, live vaccines, leflunomide, natalizumab	Increased effects of drugs listed	Increased toxicity of drugs listed
Warfarin, inactivated vaccines	Decreased effects of drugs listed	Possible clots with warfarin; decreased response to inactivated vaccines

DOSAGES

Selected Immunosuppressant Drugs

Drug (Pregnancy Category)	Pharmacologic Class	Usual Adult Dosage Range	Indications/USES
◆ azathioprine (Imuran) (D)	Antimetabolite	IV/PO: 2-5 mg/kg/day to start, then 1-3 mg/kg/day	Prevention of rejection of kidney transplants
basiliximab (Simulect) (B)	Monoclonal antibody	IV: 20 mg on day of transplant followed by a second dose 4 days posttransplant	Prevention of rejection of kidney and liver transplants
◆ cyclosporine (Sandimmune) (C)	Calcineurin inhibitor	PO: 15 mg/kg 4-12 hr preoperatively; continue same dose daily for 1-2 wk, then reduce by 5%/wk to a maintenance dose of 5-10 mg/kg/day IV: 5-6 mg/kg 4-12 hr preoperatively and continued daily until patient can be switched to oral dosing	Prevention of rejection of kidney, liver, and heart transplants
glatiramer acetate (Copaxone) (B)	Miscellaneous biologic	Subcut: 20 mg once daily	Treatment of RRMS
muromonab-CD3 (Orthoclone OKT3) (C)	Monoclonal antibody	IV: 5 mg/day as a single bolus injection for 10-14 days	Treatment of active rejection of kidney transplants; treatment of active rejection of liver, heart, pancreas, and bone marrow transplants that are resistant to conventional treatment
◆ mycophenolate mofetil (CellCept, Myfortic) (C)	Antimetabolite	IV/PO: 1-1.5 g twice daily	Prevention of rejection of kidney, liver, or heart transplants; treatment of rejection of kidney transplants
◆ sirolimus (Rapamune) (C)	mTOR kinase inhibitor	IV/PO: 6-mg loading dose, followed by 2 mg/day for low-mod risk	Prevention of rejection of kidney transplants
◆ tacrolimus (Prograf) (C)	Calcineurin inhibitor	IV: 0.01-0.05 mg/kg/day as continuous IV infusion; then PO: 0.075-0.2 mg/kg/day divided every 12 hr	Prevention and treatment of rejection of liver, kidney, heart, lung, pancreas, and small bowel transplants

IV, Intravenous; *PO*, oral; *RRMS*, relapsing-remitting multiple sclerosis; *subcut*, subcutaneous.

and were developed to improve absorption over Sandimmune (cyclosporine). Although these three products contain the same active ingredient (cyclosporine), they cannot be used interchangeably. The nurse must double-check the formulation before giving cyclosporine. Neoral, Gengraf, or generic cyclosporine-*modified* refer to interchangeable products; however, if the patient is prescribed the aforementioned, Sandimmune or generic cyclosporine must not be used. If an error occurs in which product is administered, it is extremely important that the prescriber be notified immediately. When a change is made from Neoral or Gengraf to Sandimmune, the starting dose should be a 1:1 mg amount, but dosage adjustments may be necessary to compensate for the greater bioavailability of Neoral and Gengraf. It is recommended that cyclosporine blood concentration be monitored in patients changing from one product to another. Cyclosporine has a narrow therapeutic range, and for this reason laboratory monitoring of drug levels may be used to ensure therapeutic plasma concentrations and to avoid toxicity. Blood levels are to be drawn as a trough (i.e., before the next dose). Cyclosporine has several black box warnings, including renal impairment, which includes structural kidney damage, increased risk for serious and fatal infections, liver injury, seizures, encephalopathy, and skin cancer.

Pharmacokinetics: Cyclosporine

Route	Onset of Action	Peak Plasma Concentration	Elimination Half-life	Duration of Action
PO	1-3 hr	3.5 hr	1-2 hr (parent compound); 10-40 hr (metabolites)	Unknown

glatiramer acetate

Glatiramer acetate (Copaxone) is a mixture of random polymers of four different amino acids. This mixture results in a compound that is antigenically similar to myelin basic protein. This is a protein that is found on the myelin sheaths of nerves. The drug is believed to work by blocking T-cell autoimmune activity against this protein, which reduces the frequency of the neuromuscular exacerbations associated with multiple sclerosis. This drug is mixed in the sugar known as mannitol; therefore, it is contraindicated in patients who are allergic to that component. It is available only in injectable form.

A new drug, fingolimod (Gilenya), which actually failed as an antirejection drug, was approved in 2010 for multiple sclerosis. It is the only oral drug for relapsing forms of multiple sclerosis. It has significant adverse effects, including headache, hepatotoxicity, flulike symptoms, back pain, AV block, bradycardia, hypertension, and macular edema. For these reasons, the FDA requires a patient medication guide for all patients dispensed fingolimod.

muromonab-CD3

Muromonab-CD3 (Orthoclone OKT3) is indicated for the reversal and prevention of graft rejection. It is a monoclonal antibody, synthesized using recombinant DNA technology, and it is very similar to the antibodies produced naturally by the body (immunoglobulins G, M, D, A, and E). It specifically targets the binding sites on the T cells that recognize foreign invaders, such as a transplanted organ. It differs from human antibodies in that it comes from mice. The other monoclonal antibody used for the prevention of organ rejection is basiliximab Muromonab-CD3, often called OKT3, which is contraindicated in patients with hypersensitivity to murine products and in those who are experiencing fluid overload. Muromonab-CD3 can cause cytokine release syndrome, and patients are often pretreated with a corticosteroid as described previously for basiliximab. This drug is available only in injectable form.

Pharmacokinetics: Muromonab-CD3

Route	Onset of Action	Peak Plasma Concentration	Elimination Half-life	Duration of Action
IV	Rapid	3 days	18 hr	Unknown

◆ mycophenolate mofetil

Mycophenolate (CellCept, Myfortic) is an antimetabolite and suppresses T cell proliferation. It is indicated for the prevention of organ rejection as well as the treatment of organ rejection. Mycophenolate has a black box warning from the FDA stating that it is associated with an increased risk for congenital malformations and spontaneous abortions when used during pregnancy, as well as an increased risk for infections and development of lymphoma and skin cancers. Mycophenolate also has a black box warning regarding the potential to develop progressive multifocal leukoencephalopathy. It is available in oral and intravenous forms. Common side effects include hypertension (28% to 77% incidence), hypotension, peripheral edema, tachycardia, pain, headache, hyperglycemia, hyperlipidemia, electrolyte disturbances, abdominal pain, leukopenia, thrombocytopenia, cough, and dyspnea. The different dosage forms, CellCept and Myfortic, should not be used interchangeably due to differences in absorption.

Pharmacokinetics: Mycophenolate

Route	Onset of Action	Peak Plasma Concentration	Elimination Half-life	Duration of Action
PO	4 wk	0.8-1.8 hr	8-16 hr	Unknown

◆ sirolimus and ◆ tacrolimus

Sirolimus (Rapamune) is an immunosuppressant drug, similar in structure to tacrolimus (Prograf). Sirolimus is a macrocyclic immunosuppressive, antifungal, and antitumor drug, and tacrolimus is used to prevent rejection and to treat rejection once it occurs. Sirolimus works by inhibiting T-lymphocyte activation in response to antigenic stimulation and inhibits antibody production, which in turn suppresses cytokine-mediated T-cell proliferation. Sirolimus and tacrolimus are structurally related and act through similar mechanisms. Sirolimus is classified as an mTOR kinase inhibitor, whereas tacrolimus is classified as a calcineurin inhibitor. Sirolimus is available only for oral use, whereas tacrolimus is available in both oral and injectable forms. Sirolimus levels are increased when taken with high-fat meals. Both drugs share black box warnings regarding the potential for developing lymphoma and serious infections, as well as lung dehiscence, hepatic artery thrombosis, and hypersensitivity reactions, including angioedema. The black box warnings also discuss serious drug interactions (see Table 48-3).

Everolimus (Certican) originally was approved for the treatment of advanced renal cell carcinoma and recently has been approved for the prevention of rejection in kidney transplant. It is an analogue of sirolimus.

Pharmacokinetics: Sirolimus

Route	Onset of Action	Peak Plasma Concentration	Elimination Half-life	Duration of Action
PO	Rapid	1-3 hr	60-80 hr	Unknown

Pharmacokinetics: Tacrolimus

Route	Onset of Action	Peak Plasma Concentration	Elimination Half-life	Duration of Action
PO	Variable	0.5-4 hr	21-61 hr	Unknown

NURSING PROCESS

ASSESSMENT

Transplantation is indeed a very complex medical and ethical health care issue. With transplants, the primary concern (as previously discussed) is that of rejection and the possibility of subsequent removal of the transplanted organ. Therefore, *immunosuppressants* are used to inhibit the patient's immune system to help prevent rejection. It also means that patients are on drug therapy for their entire lifetime. Before administering any of the immunosuppressants, perform a thorough patient assessment with baseline measurements of vital signs and weight. Obtain a thorough history of past and present medical conditions, and document findings from the following systems' assessment: (1) preexisting diseases impacting the patient's immune status, such as diabetes, hypertension, and cancer; (2) urinary functioning and patterns; (3) presence of jaundice, edema, and/or ascites; (4) history of cardiac disease and/or dysrhythmias, chest pain, or heart failure; (5) level of central nervous system functioning, with attention to any seizure disorders, alteration of motor or sensory function, paresthesias, or changing levels of consciousness; (6) respiratory status and baseline respiratory functioning, breath sounds, presence of asthma, pulmonary diseases, wheezing, cough, activity intolerance, dyspnea, or sputum production; (7) gastrointestinal (GI) functioning and patterns and bowel disease; (8) musculoskeletal intactness, with attention to ability to perform activities of daily living, range of motion, and appearance of joints and any deformities; and (9) presence and location of any inflammatory reactions as well as any pain, redness, and/or drainage. In addition, the following laboratory and diagnostic tests may be ordered: renal function tests with blood urea nitrogen (BUN) and creatinine levels; hepatic function tests with ALP, AST, ALT, and bilirubin levels; and cardiovascular function with baseline electrocardiogram. See Table 48-2 for information on other systems affected by the *immunosuppressant drugs*. Assess for and document all cautions, contraindications, and drug interactions.

With *azathioprine*, assess for signs of infection such as increased temperature, productive cough with sputum that is not clear in color, and complaints of urinary frequency, urgency and burning. Assess white blood cell and platelet counts, noting any signs and symptoms of infection and bleeding tendencies due to the potential for drug-related leukopenia and thrombocytopenia. This drug has a black box warning for bone marrow suppression, so a thorough assessment for signs and symptoms of infection, anemia, and bleeding is critically important. If leukocytes are less than 3000/mm^3 or platelets less than 100,000/mm^3, the prescriber needs to be contacted because the drug will most likely not be administered. Assess liver function prior to administering this drug due to the risk for hepatotoxicity. Assess for dark urine, jaundice, and increased liver function tests (AST, ALT, bilirubin). Significant drug interactions include ACE inhibitors (leukopenia), cyclosporine (myelosuppression), vaccines (decreased immune response), allopurinol (increased action of azathioprine), and warfarin (decreased action of warfarin).

With *cyclosporine*, thoroughly assess the functional level of all organ systems through laboratory values for liver and renal functioning including alkaline phosphatase, AST, ALT, bilirubin, BUN, and creatinine. Assess also for any underlying cardiovascular and/or central nervous system diseases because of potential drug-related toxicities involving these systems as well as the physiologic impact of the organ transplant process on multiple systems. Perform a baseline oral assessment because of the possible adverse effect of drug-induced gingival hyperplasia. Assess and document baseline blood pressures because as many as 50% of patients on this drug suffer from subsequent moderate hypertension. Baseline assessment of parameters representative of neurologic, renal, and hepatic functioning is also important. Common drug interactions to assess for include estrogens, protease inhibitors, HMG-CoA reductase inhibitors, clarithromycin, phenytoin, phenobarbital, St. John's wort, NSAIDs, and grapefruit juice (see Table 48-3).

Muromonab-DC3 requires assessment for cardiovascular disorders as well as a history of GI and respiratory disorders.

Assess baseline temperature as well as breath sounds and respiratory rate. Assess and document baseline vital signs and weight due to the adverse effect of fluid retention.

With *tacrolimus*, obtain a thorough patient history with attention to medication use. Perform a physical assessment with close attention to renal functioning through monitoring of BUN, serum creatinine, and serum electrolyte levels. With tacrolimus and *sirolimus*, assess baseline vital signs and heart sounds due to adverse effects of hypertension, palpitations, and peripheral edema (see Table 48-2). Due to the potentially life-threatening adverse effects associated with these drugs, assess baseline renal and hepatic laboratory values as well as neurologic and respiratory functioning (Table 48-2). Drug interactions to assess for are listed in Table 48-3.

With *basiliximab* and *muromonab-CD3 (antibody immunosuppressants)*, complete a thorough documentation of baseline vital signs and other presenting complaints because of the possible occurrence of cytokine release syndrome with resultant fever, dyspnea, tachycardia, sweating, chills, vomiting, diarrhea, muscle/joint pain, and general malaise.

With the assessment phase, it is also important to be aware of the difference between *cyclosporine-modified (Neoral, Gengraf)* and *cyclosporine (Sandimmune)*. Neoral and Gengraf were modified to improve absorption over Sandimmune. If cyclosporine-modified drugs are prescribed, they cannot be interchangeably used with Sandimmune. The nurse must always double-check the medication order against the formulation on hand.

NURSING DIAGNOSES

1. Acute pain (e.g., joint and muscle aches and pain and flulike symptoms) related to adverse effects of immunosuppressant medications
2. Risk for injury related to the physiologic effects of the disease, overall weakness, and the adverse effects of immunosuppressants
3. Risk for infection related to altered immune status caused by chronic disease, treatment with immunosuppressants, and/or the transplantation process

PLANNING: OUTCOME IDENTIFICATION

1. Patient experiences maximal comfort during drug therapy with immunosuppressants with the use of drug (acetaminophen) and nondrug therapeutic measures (e.g., biofeedback, imagery, massage).
2. Patient remains free from injury by safe and effective use of the medication and reporting to the prescriber any adverse reactions or unusual symptoms, such as fever, rash, or sore throat.
3. Patient remains free from infection during immunosuppressant therapy with the implementation of improved nutritional intake (increased calorie and protein), reporting of fever/chills/confusion, and minimizing exposure to large crowds or those who are ill.

IMPLEMENTATION

Oral *immunosuppressants* need to be taken with food to minimize GI upset. It is also important, because of the immunosuppressed state of patients receiving immunosuppressants, that oral forms of the drugs be used whenever possible to decrease the risk for infection associated with parenteral injections and subsequent injury to the first line of defense (skin). An oral antifungal medication may be ordered to treat the oral candidiasis that may occur as a consequence of the treatment and the disease process; however, significant drug interactions may occur between the immunosuppressant and the antifungal drug, so always check for drug interactions. It is also important with the use of any of the immunosuppressants to be sure that supportive treatment equipment and related drugs be functional and available in case of an anaphylactic or allergic reaction. Be aware and constantly prepared for the high risk for such a reaction. The use of premedication protocols involving various antihistamines and/or antiinflammatory drugs is also common.

CASE STUDY

Safety: What Went Wrong? Cyclosporine

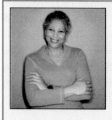 V., a 62-year-old retired orchestra teacher, moved to Florida after her husband died. Over the past few years, she has developed renal problems, and last year she was told that she needed a kidney transplant. After 1 year of waiting and undergoing hemodialysis, V. was told that her niece was a match and was willing to donate a kidney. She has had the transplant, and after 1 week, the transplant seems to be successful so far.

Cyclosporine is one of the immunosuppressant drugs V. will be receiving. She was given her first dose of cyclosporine 12 hours before surgery and is now receiving oral doses. The nurse has provided instructions on how to take the oral doses at home.

1. The next day, when another nurse comes in with V.'s morning medications, V. says, "You can't give me the medicine like that. It's not safe! Don't you know how to mix it?" What do you think the nurse did wrong?
2. What important measures will the nurse take to prevent toxicity?
3. V. tells the nurse that she can't wait to get home and relax by her pool. She is also looking forward to getting her strength back and going shopping with her girlfriends. How will the nurse respond to these statements?
4. After V. gets home, she calls the office to ask about eating grapefruit. "The pill bottle says no grapefruit, but I thought the doctor said I could have a little bit. I have a wonderful grapefruit tree in my backyard, and I love fresh grapefruit juice. What should I do?" What is the nurse's best response to the patient's question?

For answers, see *http://evolve.elsevier.com/Lilley.*

Azathioprine does have a black box warning associated with bone marrow suppression, so always check on blood counts and monitor vital signs during treatment. If leukocytes are less than 3000 cells/mm^3 or platelets are less than 100,000 cells/mm^3, contact the prescriber because the medication will most likely be discontinued. Therapeutic response may take up to 4 months, so educate patients with rheumatoid arthritis about this delay, and advise them to continue with treatment, prescribed exercise, rest, and other medications.

Basiliximab, which comes in an injectable dosage form, is associated with an allergic-like reaction known as cytokine release syndrome. It may be severe and even involve anaphylaxis, so patients are usually premedicated with corticosteroids (e.g., IV methylprednisolone) to try and avoid or alleviate this problem. Continually assess and monitor vital signs and signs and symptoms of a reaction during the administration of these medications.

Cyclosporine is available in both oral and injectable formulations. As noted previously, *Neoral* and *Gengraf* are *cyclosporine-modified* and are not to be used interchangeably with *Sandimmune (cyclosporine)*, which is *unmodified*. If an error occurs, the prescriber must be notified immediately. Do not refrigerate these oral solutions. To safely administer oral liquid dosage forms, use a calibrated liquid measuring device. Oral solutions may be mixed in a glass container with chocolate milk, milk, or orange juice and served at room temperature. Once the solution is mixed, make sure the patient drinks it immediately. Avoid Styrofoam containers or cups because the drug has been found to adhere to the inside wall of such containers. If the prescriber orders a change to be made from Neoral or Gengraf to Sandimmune, there is a dosage adjustment that may be needed (see Pharmacology discussion). With intravenously administered cyclosporine, the dose must be diluted as recommended by the manufacturer and given according to standards of care and institutional policy. Cyclosporine is usually diluted with normal saline or 5% dextrose in water and infused using an intravenous infusion pump. Always infuse over the recommended period. Monitor the patient very closely during the infusion, especially during the first 30 minutes, for any allergic reactions manifested by facial flushing, urticaria, wheezing, dyspnea, and rash. Record vital signs frequently, and document. It is also important to closely monitor the patient's BUN, LDH, AST, and ALT levels during therapy, as ordered, to detect possible renal and hepatic impairment. Oral hygiene may be performed frequently to prevent dry mouth and subsequent infections. The prescriber will also order blood tests to confirm therapeutic serum levels of cyclosporine. These serum drug levels must be closely monitored.

Intravenously administered *muromonab-CD3* is usually infused over 1 minute. When the dose is prepared, withdraw the medication from the ampule through a low protein-binding 0.22-micron filter, detach the filter, and apply a new sterile needle after withdrawing the medication. Follow the premedication protocol to help minimize reactions. *Basiliximab* is administered parenterally. Follow manufacturer guidelines regarding the type and amount of dilutional solution. Closely monitor the intravenous drip, and use an intravenous infusion pump to help ensure that the proper dose is administered.

Sirolimus and *tacrolimus* need to be administered as ordered by either the intravenous or oral route. Sirolimus and tacrolimus are both associated with black box warnings for infection and possible lymphoma, so always be mindful of these concerns when administering the drug. If intravenous tacrolimus is to be discontinued and maintenance dosing needed, oral tacrolimus is usually ordered to be given 8 to 12 hours after the discontinuation of the intravenous drug. Do not store intravenous solution in polyvinyl chloride containers. It must be administered in an appropriately designed container and tubing. Oral doses of *tacrolimus* are given on an empty stomach. As with *cyclosporine*, the oral dosage forms of tacrolimus are not to be put in Styrofoam cups/containers. Inform the patient to avoid the consumption of grapefruit when taking cyclosporine. Both *sirolimus* and tacrolimus have long half-lives, so toxicity is an added concern because of possible cumulative effects.

Because *immunosuppressant therapy* is lifelong, it is important for the patient to receive adequate and appropriate emotional, spiritual, social, and financial support. Additionally, there are other specifics of therapy that must be emphasized with patients, family members, and significant others, such as the need to always have a 1-week supply of medication available so that there is never a risk of running out. There also needs to be discussion about the estimated cost of medication to all involved (see the pharmacology discussion). Drug regimens are expensive and lifelong, and, as such, constant monitoring of drug serum levels is required. Complexity of dosing must be explained clearly and thoroughly.

Ethical dilemmas are also of a complex nature. Organ transplantation raises a number of complex bioethical issues, including definition of death, consents for transplantation, and payment for transplanted organs. Additionally, transplantation tourism and the broader socioeconomic context in which organ harvesting or transplantation may occur are of concern. Organ trafficking is another bioethical issue. More information about the many ethical concerns associated with transplantation is provided by the World Health Organization and the Universal Declaration of Human Rights. Even within developed countries, there is concern that enthusiasm for increasing the supply of organs may adversely and negatively impact the respect for the right to life.

EVALUATION

Continually evaluate and reevaluate patient goals and outcome criteria related to the nursing process and administration of *immunosuppressants*. In addition, evaluate therapeutic responses to immunosuppressants, including acceptance of the transplanted organ or graft and improved symptoms in those with autoimmune disorders. Complete blood count; erythrocyte sedimentation rate; C-reactive protein level; liver, kidney, and cardiac function tests; pulmonary function tests; chest radiography; and analysis of T-lymphocyte surface phenotype are a few of the tests performed to evaluate patients during and after drug therapy. Continually evaluate for drug-specific adverse effects and toxicity (see Table 48-2).

PATIENT-CENTERED CARE: PATIENT TEACHING

- Educate transplant patients on the need for lifelong immunosuppressant therapy with often complex therapeutic regimens.
- Emphasize the importance of avoiding situations that pose an increased risk for exposure to infection, such as being in crowds, malls, or movie theaters.
- Stress the importance of reporting any fever, sore throat, chills, joint pain, or fatigue to the prescriber, as these may indicate infection and require immediate medical attention.
- Educate female patients of childbearing age who are receiving immunosuppressants about the need to use some form of contraception during treatment and for up to 12 weeks after therapy ends.
- Advise patients to take the drug at the same time every day (as with most immunosuppressants) and, if a dose is omitted, to contact the prescriber for further instructions.
- Follow-up appointments are important because of the need to monitor the patient's status through examinations and blood testing.
- Advise the patient to take azathioprine exactly as prescribed and to contact the prescriber if a dose is missed or omitted. Avoid exposure to crowds or those with infection. Treatment with transplant patients is lifelong to avoid transplant rejection. Educate also about reporting to the prescriber any fever, rash, severe diarrhea, sore throat, chills, and any unusual bleeding or bruising.
- Cyclosporine is to be taken the same time of day, every day, with no skipping or doubling-up of doses. Educate also

about not consuming grapefruit/grapefruit juice and not receiving vaccines.
- Instruct patients taking cyclosporine to report the following to their prescriber immediately: fever, chills, increased fatigue, sore throat, bleeding gums, tremors, and/or an increase in blood pressure. A notebook/journal can be helpful in the patient's keeping track of daily treatments, responses to medications, and adverse effects.
- Educate the patient about the black box warning (cyclosporine) of limiting UV exposure (avoiding prolonged exposure, using sunscreen, and wearing protective clothing when outdoors). Inform patients that gel caps are to be stored in a cool, dry environment and must not be exposed to light. The dosage form must be kept in its original packaging. Oral dosage forms may be taken with meals to decrease GI upset. Also, instruct patients about the importance of follow-up appointments.
- With any of the immunosuppressants, encourage patients to inspect the oral cavity frequently for any white patches on the tongue, mucous membranes, and/or oral pharynx. These patches may indicate oral candidiasis and treatment with an oral antifungal is needed.
- With sirolimus, educate the patient to report fever, rash, severe diarrhea, and jaundice and to avoid crowds and those with known infections. Sunscreen and protective clothing is needed when going outside. Grapefruit and vaccines are to be avoided. Encourage follow-up appointments and to take 4 hours after cyclosporine if these medications are both prescribed. Provide patients on tacrolimus with instructions to

report any signs and symptoms of an infection or liver/kidney toxicity. Vaccines, grapefruit, and alcohol are to be avoided.

- Nutritional counseling would be extremely beneficial in understanding food interactions as well as any concerns related to hyperlipidemia and increased triglycerides associated with many of the immunosuppressive drugs.
- All immunosuppressants taken at home are to be taken exactly as ordered and at the same time every day. Educate patients about the adverse effects of the medication. Instruct them to report problems of particular concern,

such as fever, chest pain, dizziness, and headache, problems with urination, rash, and respiratory and/or other infections.

- Provide resources for financial support as well as psychologic/spiritual support for the patient, significant other, and/or family member(s) as needed. One valuable and easily accessible resource is *http://organdonor.gov/about/index.html*. Transplant centers usually have available to the patient a variety of resources, written materials, and videos about the process of becoming an organ donor and also a donor recipient.

KEY POINTS

- Immunosuppressants decrease or prevent the body's immune response.
- Some of the clinical uses for immunosuppressants are suppression of immune-mediated disorders, malignancies, and improvement of short-term and long-term allograft survival.
- Oral antifungals are generally given with immunosuppressant medications to treat the oral candidiasis that occurs as a result of immunosuppression and fungal overgrowth.

- Monitor the results of prescriber-ordered laboratory studies such as hemoglobin level, hematocrit, and red blood cell, white blood cell, and platelet counts. If the values drop below normal ranges, notify the prescriber.
- Because of the lifelong nature of the diseases/disease states being managed with these immunosuppressants, always be aware of the financial, emotional, psychosocial, cultural, and body-image impact to the patient, significant other, and/or family members.

NCLEX® EXAMINATION REVIEW QUESTIONS

1. A patient has a new order for glatiramer acetate. The patient has not had an organ transplant. The nurse knows that the patient is receiving this drug for which condition?
   a. Psoriasis
   b. Rheumatoid arthritis
   c. Irritable bowel syndrome
   d. Relapse-remitting multiple sclerosis
2. While assessing a patient who is to receive muromonab-CD3, the nurse knows that which condition would be a contraindication for this drug?
   a. Acute myalgia
   b. Fluid overload
   c. Polycythemia
   d. Diabetes mellitus
3. During therapy with azathioprine (Imuran), the nurse must monitor for which common adverse effect?
   a. Bradycardia
   b. Diarrhea
   c. Vomiting
   d. Thrombocytopenia
4. During a teaching session for a patient receiving an immunosuppressant drug, the nurse will include which statement?
   a. "It is better to use oral forms of these drugs to prevent the occurrence of thrush."
   b. "You will remain on antibiotics to prevent infections."
   c. "It is important to use some form of contraception during treatment and for up to 12 weeks after the end of therapy."
   d. "Be sure to take your medications with grapefruit juice to increase absorption."

5. During drug therapy with basiliximab, the nurse monitors for signs of cytokine release syndrome, which results in
   a. fever, dyspnea, and general malaise.
   b. neurotoxicity and peripheral neuropathy.
   c. hepatotoxicity with jaundice.
   d. thrombocytopenia with increased bleeding tendencies.
6. When assessing a patient who is to begin therapy with an immunosuppressant drug, the nurse recognizes that such drugs should be used cautiously in patients with which condition(s)? *(Select all that apply.)*
   a. Pregnancy
   b. Glaucoma
   c. Anemia
   d. Myalgia
   e. Renal dysfunction
   f. Hepatic dysfunction
7. The order reads: "Give tacrolimus IV 0.03 mg/kg/day as a continuous IV infusion." The patient weighs 110 lb. How many milligrams per day will this dose provide?
8. The nurse is reviewing cyclosporine and recognizes that this drug works by which mechanism of action?
   a. Suppressing viral replication.
   b. Enhancing the action of macrophages.
   c. Inhibiting activation of T-lymphocyte cells.
   d. Increasing the number of T-lymphocyte cells.

1. d, 2. b, 3. d, 4. c, 5. a, 6. a, e, f, 7. 1.5 mg/day, 8. c.

CRITICAL THINKING AND PRIORITIZATION QUESTIONS

1. A patient is about to receive muromonab-CD3 as part of posttransplant drug therapy. Before administering the muromonab-CD3, what is the nurse's priority action in order to prevent adverse effects? Explain your answer.

2. A patient is on call for lung transplant surgery; she has been told the procedure could occur within 24 hours. The surgeon writes an order that says, "Avoid injections as much as possible." A new nurse questions this order, asking, "What does the surgeon mean by that?" What is the nurse's best response?

For answers, see *http://evolve.elsevier.com/Lilley*.

ⓔ EVOLVE WEBSITE

http://evolve.elsevier.com/Lilley
- Animations
- Answer Keys for Textbook Case Studies and Textbook Critical Thinking and Prioritization Questions

- Content Updates
- Key Points
- Review Questions
- Student Case Studies

Immunizing Drugs

OBJECTIVES

When you reach the end of this chapter, you will be able to do the following:

1. Discuss the importance of immunity as it relates to the various immunizing drugs and their use in patients of all ages.
2. Identify the diseases that are treated or prevented with toxoids or vaccines.
3. Compare the mechanisms of action, indications, cautions, contraindications, adverse effects, toxicity, drug interactions, and routes of administration of various toxoids and vaccines.
4. Develop a nursing care plan that includes all phases of the nursing process related to the administration of immunizing drugs across the lifespan.

DRUG PROFILES

♦ diphtheria and tetanus toxoids and acellular pertussis vaccine tetanus (adsorbed), p. 788
Haemophilus influenzae type b conjugate vaccine, p. 788
♦ hepatitis B immunoglobulin, p. 791
♦ hepatitis B virus vaccine (inactivated), p. 788
herpes zoster vaccine, p. 790
human papillomavirus vaccine, p. 790
♦ immunoglobulin, p. 791
♦ influenza virus vaccine, p. 789
♦ measles, mumps, and rubella virus vaccine (live), p. 789
♦ meningococcal vaccine, p. 789
♦ pneumococcal vaccine, polyvalent and thirteen valent, p. 789

♦ poliovirus vaccine (inactivated), p. 790
rabies immunoglobulin, p. 792
rabies virus vaccine, p. 790
$Rh_0(D)$ immunoglobulin, p. 791
tetanus immunoglobulin, p. 792
♦ varicella virus vaccine, p. 791
varicella-zoster immunoglobulin, p. 792

___
♦ = *Key drug*
! = *High-alert drug*

KEY TERMS

Active immunization A type of immunization that causes development of a complete and long-lasting immunity to a certain infection through exposure of the body to the associated disease antigen; it can be natural active immunization (i.e., having the disease) or artificial active immunization (i.e., receiving a vaccine or toxoid). (p. 784)

Active immunizing drugs Toxoids or vaccines that are administered to a host to stimulate host production of antibodies. (p. 786)

Antibodies Immunoglobulin molecules that have an antigen-specific amino acid sequence and are synthesized by the humoral immune system (B cells) in response to exposure to a specific antigen. Their purpose is to attack and destroy molecules of this antigen. (p. 784)

Antibody titer The amount of an antibody needed to react with and neutralize a given volume or amount of a specific antigen. (p. 786)

Antigens Substances, usually proteins and foreign to a host, that stimulate the production of antibodies and that react

specifically with those antibodies. Examples of antigens include bacterial exotoxins and viruses. An allergen (e.g., dust, pollen, mold) is an antigen that can produce an immediate-type hypersensitivity reaction or allergy. (p. 783)

Antiserum A serum that contains antibodies. It is usually obtained from an animal that has been immunized against a specific antigen. (p. 786)

Antitoxin An antiserum against a toxin (or toxoid). It is most often a purified antiserum obtained from animals (usually horses) by injection of a toxin or toxoid so that antibodies to the toxin (i.e., antitoxin) can be collected from the animals and used to provide artificial passive immunity to humans exposed to a given toxin (e.g., tetanus immunoglobulin). (p. 786)

Antivenin An antiserum against a venom (poison produced by an animal) used to treat humans or other animals that have been envenomed (e.g., by snakebite, spider bite, or scorpion sting). (p. 786)

KEY TERMS—cont'd

Biologic antimicrobial drugs Substances of biologic origin used to prevent, treat, or cure infectious diseases (e.g., vaccines, toxoids, immunoglobulins). These drugs are often simply referred to as *biologics*. However, *biologics* also refers to drugs of bioterrorism (e.g., anthrax spores, smallpox virus), depending on the context. (p. 784)

Booster shot A repeat dose of an antigen, such as a vaccine or toxoid, which is usually administered in an amount smaller than that used in the original immunization. It is given to maintain the immune response of a previously immunized patient at, or return the response to, a clinically effective level. (p. 786)

Cell-mediated immune system The immune response that is mediated by T cells (as opposed to B cells, which produce antibodies). T cells mount their immune response through activities such as the release of cytokines (chemicals that stimulate other protective immune functions) as well as through direct cytotoxicity (e.g., phagocytosis of an antigen). (p. 784)

Herd immunity Resistance to a disease on the part of an entire community or population because a large proportion of its members are immune to the disease. (p. 786)

Immune response A cascade of biochemical events that occurs in response to entry of an antigen (foreign substance) into the body; key processes of the immune response include phagocytosis ("eating of cells") of foreign microorganisms and synthesis of antibodies that react with specific antigens to inactivate them. Immune response centers on the blood but may also involve the lymphatic system and the *reticuloendothelial system* (see later). (p. 783)

Immunization The induction of immunity by administration of a vaccine or toxoid (active immunization) or antiserum (passive immunization). (p. 784)

Immunizing biologics Toxoids, vaccines, or immunoglobulins that are targeted against specific infectious microorganisms or toxins. (p. 784)

Immunoglobulins Glycoproteins synthesized and used by the humoral immune system (B cells) to attack and kill all substances foreign to the body. The term is synonymous with *immune globulins*. (p. 784)

Passive immunization A type of immunization in which immunity to infection occurs by injecting a person with antiserum or concentrated antibodies that directly give the host the means to fight off an invading microorganism (artificial passive immunization). The host's immune system therefore does not have to manufacture these antibodies. This process also occurs when antibodies pass from mother to infant during breastfeeding or through the placenta during pregnancy (natural passive immunization). (p. 784)

Passive immunizing drugs Drugs containing antibodies or antitoxins that can kill or inactivate pathogens by binding to the associated antigens. These are directly injected into a person (host) and provide that person with the means to fend off infection, bypassing the host's own immune system. (p. 786)

Recombinant Relating to or containing a combination of genetic material from two or more organisms. Such genetic recombination is one of the key methods of biotechnology and is often used to manufacture immunizing drugs and various other medications. (p. 786)

Reticuloendothelial system Specialized cells located in the liver, spleen, lymphatics, and bone marrow that remove miscellaneous particles from the circulation, such as aging antibody molecules. (p. 786)

Toxin Any poison produced by a plant, animal, or microorganism that is highly toxic to other living organisms. (p. 784)

Toxoids Bacterial exotoxins that are modified or inactivated (by chemicals or heat) so that they are no longer toxic but can still bind to host B cells to stimulate the formation of antitoxin; toxoids are often used in the same manner as vaccines to promote artificial active immunity in humans. They are one type of active immunizing drug (e.g., tetanus toxoid). (p. 784)

Vaccines Suspensions of live, attenuated, or killed microorganisms that can promote an artificially induced active immunity against a particular microorganism. They are another type of active immunizing drug (e.g., tetanus vaccine). (p. 784)

Venom A poison that is secreted by an animal (e.g., snake, insect, or spider). (p. 786)

IMMUNITY AND IMMUNIZATION

Centuries ago it was noticed that people who contracted certain diseases acquired an immune tolerance to the disease so that, when exposed to it again, they did not experience a second bout of illness. This basic observation prompted scientists to investigate ways of artificially producing this tolerance. Along with this came an understanding of how the normal immune system functions, which is important to an understanding of how immunizing drugs work. Briefly, when the body first comes into contact with antigens (foreign proteins) from an invading organism, specific information is imprinted into a cellular "memory bank" of the immune system. The body can then effectively fight any future invasion by that same organism by mounting an immune response. This cellular memory bank consists of specialized immune cells known as *memory cells*. When an antigen presents itself to a person's humoral immune system (B cells, or B lymphocytes) by binding to B cells, the B cells differentiate into two other types of cells. One type is the memory cells. The second type is plasma cells, which produce

TABLE 49-1   Active versus Passive Immunization

Characteristic	Active	Passive
Artificial		
Type of immunizing drug	Toxoid or vaccine	Immunoglobulin or antitoxin
Mechanism of action	Results from an antigen-antibody response similar to that after antigen exposure in the natural disease process	Results from direct administration of exogenous antibodies; antibody concentration will decrease over time, so if reexposure is expected, it is wise to continue passive immunizations.
Use	To prevent development of active disease in the event of exposure to a given antigen in individuals who have at least a partially functioning immune system	To provide temporary protection against disease in individuals who are immunodeficient, those for whom active immunization is contraindicated, and those who have been exposed to or anticipate exposure to the organism or toxin; an antibody response is not stimulated in the host.
Natural		
Mechanism of action	Production of one's own antibodies during actual infection	Transmission of antibodies from mother to infant through placenta or during breastfeeding

large volumes of antibodies against the antigen in question. Antibodies are immunoglobulin molecules that have antigen-specific amino acid sequences. Immunoglobulins are synthesized by the humoral immune system for the purpose of destroying all substances that the body recognizes as foreign. An immunoglobulin with a specific amino acid sequence is known as an *antibody*. It is because of this process that people rarely suffer twice from certain diseases such as mumps, chickenpox, and measles. Instead they have a complete and long-lasting immunity to those infections.

In contrast to the humoral immune system, which is the focus of this chapter, the cell-mediated immune system is the branch of the immune system that does not synthesize antibodies. Instead, it is driven by T cells (T lymphocytes) and works by the release of cytokines (chemicals that promote other immune system functions, e.g., inflammatory responses, runny nose) and by phagocytosis (engulfing and destruction of the antigens by the T cells). The cell-mediated immune system is discussed in Chapter 48, because it is the target of immunosuppressant drugs. To varying degrees, these two immune system branches work simultaneously or even interdependently.

There are two ways of obtaining immunity to certain infections: active immunization and passive immunization. Each can be an artificial or natural process. In artificial active immunization, the body is clinically exposed to a relatively harmless form of an antigen that does not cause an actual infection. Information about the antigen is then imprinted into the memory of the immune system, and the body's defenses are stimulated to resist any subsequent exposure (by producing antibodies). In contrast, natural active immunization occurs when a person acquires immunity by surviving the disease itself and producing antibodies to the disease-causing organism. Artificial passive immunization involves administration of serum or concentrated immunoglobulins. This directly gives the inoculated person the substance needed to fight off the invading microorganism. This type of immunization bypasses the host's immune system. Finally, natural passive immunization occurs when antibodies are transferred from the mother to her infant in breast milk or through the bloodstream via the

placenta during pregnancy. The major differences between active and passive immunization are summarized in Table 49-1 and are discussed in greater depth in the following sections.

Active Immunization

In general, biologic antimicrobial drugs (also referred to simply as *biologics*) are substances such as antitoxins, antisera, toxoids, and vaccines that are used to prevent, treat, or cure infectious diseases. Toxoids and vaccines are known as immunizing biologics, and they target a particular infectious microorganism.

Toxoids

Toxoids are substances that contain antigens, most often in the form of bacterial exotoxins. These substances have been detoxified or weakened (attenuated), which renders them nontoxic. Nonetheless, they remain highly antigenic and can stimulate an artificial active immune response (production of antitoxin antibodies) when injected into a host patient. These antibodies can then neutralize the same exotoxin upon any future exposure. Toxoids were first developed in 1923 at the Pasteur Institute, and modern versions are effective against diseases such as diphtheria and tetanus caused by toxin-producing bacteria.

Vaccines

Vaccines are suspensions of live, attenuated (weakened), or killed (inactivated) microorganisms that can stimulate production of antibodies against the particular organism. As with toxoids, these slight alterations in the bacteria and viruses prevent the person injected from contracting the disease. They are still able to promote active immunization against the organism, including an antibody response. People vaccinated with live bacteria or viruses (as well as those who recover from an actual infection) enjoy lifelong immunity against that particular disease. However, only partial immunity is conferred on those vaccinated with killed bacteria or viruses, and for this reason they must be given periodic booster shots to maintain immune system protection against infection with the given organism.

Edward Jenner, an English physician born in 1749, noticed that milkmaids who had contracted cowpox infections were rarely victims of smallpox and was the first to study the relationship of cowpox to smallpox immunity. His observation led to the development of the smallpox vaccine. With the help of the modern version of this vaccine, smallpox was considered to be eradicated as of 1980. However, following the terrorist attacks in the United States on September 11, 2001, fears arose of a large-scale bioterrorism attack using the smallpox virus. The Centers for Disease Control and Prevention (CDC) released guidelines recommending routine early detection surveillance activities on the part of all public health agencies. These guidelines also include a plan for rapid vaccination of local populations in the event of a suspected smallpox outbreak and listed several high-priority high-risk groups, including direct health care personnel, who need to be vaccinated first should an outbreak occur.

Today there are more than 20 infectious diseases for which vaccines are available. New vaccines appear periodically but not with the rapidity of other types of drugs, because of the complexities of developing a safe and effective vaccine. Most modern vaccines are produced in a laboratory by genetic engineering methods and contain some extract of the pathogen, or a synthetic extract, rather than the microbe itself. Some vaccines, such as influenza vaccine, may contain actual whole or split virus particles. Most, however, contain a smaller fraction of the organism, such as the bacterial capsular polysaccharides that are used to make pneumococcal vaccine. The attenuating or killing agent is usually a chemical such as formaldehyde or a physical mechanism such as heat. Attenuation may also be accomplished by repeated passage of the microbe through some medium such as a fertile hen egg or a special tissue culture. The search for new and better drugs will never end. Current goals include finding vaccines against human immunodeficiency virus infection/acquired immunodeficiency syndrome (HIV/AIDS) and malaria; the ultimate goal is to develop an effective vaccine against all infectious diseases. The currently available immunizing vaccines are listed in Box 49-1. Note that the drug given to prevent respiratory syncytial virus (RSV) infection is not an immunizing drug per se but is a specialized antiviral drug. It is discussed in Chapter 40. The RSV immunoglobulin is listed in Box 49-1. People who travel to different parts of the world may require specific vaccines. This information can be found on the CDC website at *www.cdc.gov/travel/page/vaccinations.htm.*

The current childhood immunization schedule published by the CDC is available at *www.cdc.gov/vaccines.* This advisory is published annually as a joint effort of the American Academy of Pediatrics, the CDC's Advisory Committee on Immunization Practices, and the American Academy of Family Physicians. The CDC also posts on its website a catch-up schedule for children who may have missed scheduled immunizations. The CDC's current adult immunization schedule can be found online at *www.cdc.gov/vaccines/schedules/index.html.*

Passive Immunization

In passive immunization, the host's immune system is bypassed, and the person is inoculated with serum containing

---

BOX 49-1 Available Immunizing Drugs

Passive Immunizing Drugs

Antivenin, pit viper (Crotalidae), polyvalent
Crotalidae polyvalent immune Fab (for pit viper snakebite; e.g., rattlesnake, water moccasin)
Antivenin, *Latrodectus mactans* (black widow spider)
Antivenin, *Micrurus fulvius* (coral snake)
Botulism immunoglobulin
Cytomegalovirus immunoglobulin (human)
Digoxin immune Fab
Hepatitis B immunoglobulin
Immunoglobulin, intramuscular
Immunoglobulin, intravenous
Lymphocyte immunoglobulin, antithymocyte globulin
Rabies immunoglobulin (human)
Respiratory syncytial virus immunoglobulin, intravenous (human)
$Rh_0(D)$ immunoglobulin
Tetanus immunoglobulin
Vaccinia immunoglobulin
Varicella-zoster immunoglobulin (chickenpox/shingles)

Active Immunizing Drugs

BCG (bacille Calmette-Guérin) vaccine (tuberculosis)
Diphtheria and tetanus toxoids (adsorbed)
Diphtheria and tetanus toxoids, and acellular pertussis vaccine (adsorbed)
Diphtheria and tetanus toxoids, acellular pertussis, and *Haemophilus influenzae* type b conjugate vaccines
Diphtheria and tetanus toxoids, acellular pertussis (adsorbed), hepatitis b (recombinant), and inactivated poliovirus vaccine combined
H. Influenzae type b conjugate vaccine
H. Influenzae type b conjugate vaccine with hepatitis b vaccine
Hepatitis A virus vaccine (inactivated)
Hepatitis B virus vaccine (recombinant)
Hepatitis A virus vaccine (inactivated) and hepatitis b virus vaccine (recombinant)
Herpes zoster virus vaccine (live, attenuated)
Human papillomavirus vaccine (attenuated)
Influenza virus vaccine
Japanese encephalitis virus vaccine
Measles virus* vaccine (live, attenuated)
Measles, mumps, and rubella virus vaccine (live)
Meningococcal bacterial vaccine
Mumps virus vaccine (live)
Pneumococcal bacterial vaccine, polyvalent
Pneumococcal thirteen-valent conjugate vaccine
Poliovirus vaccine (inactivated)
Rabies virus vaccine
Rubella virus vaccine (live)
Rubella and mumps virus vaccine (live)
Rubella, measles, and mumps virus vaccine (live)
Smallpox virus vaccine†
Tetanus toxoid (fluid)
Tetanus toxoid (adsorbed)
Typhoid bacterial vaccine
Varicella virus vaccine
Yellow fever virus vaccine

*Also known as *rubeola* virus.
†Not currently on the U.S. market but according to the Centers for Disease Control and Prevention website may be reintroduced because of current bioterrorism threats.

immunoglobulins obtained from other humans or animals. These substances give the person the means to fight off the invading organism. This is known as *artificially acquired passive immunity,* and it confers temporary immunity against a particular antigen following exposure to the antigen. It differs from active immunization in that it produces a transitory (short-lived) immune state. The antibodies are already prepared for the host—the host's immune system does not have to synthesize its own antibodies. This allows for more rapid prevention or treatment of disease. Important examples include immunization with tetanus immunoglobulin, hepatitis immunoglobulin, rabies immunoglobulin, and snakebite antivenin.

Passive immunization occurs naturally between a mother and the fetus or the nursing infant when the mother passes maternal antibodies directly, either through the placenta to the fetus or through breast milk to the nursing infant. This is called *naturally acquired passive immunity.*

There are specific populations that can benefit from passive immunization but not from active immunization (see Table 49-1). These are people who have been rendered immunodeficient for one reason or another (e.g., by drugs or disease) and who therefore cannot mount an immune response. Passive immunizing drugs are also used in people who already have the given disease, especially those with diseases that are rapidly harmful or fatal, such as rabies, tetanus, and hepatitis. Because these diseases can progress rapidly, the body does not have time to mount an adequate immune defense against them before death occurs. The passive immunization of such individuals confers a temporary protection that is usually sufficient to keep the invading organisms from killing them, even though it does not stimulate an antibody response.

The passive immunizing drugs are divided into three groups: antitoxins, immunoglobulins, and snake and spider antivenins. An antitoxin is a purified antiserum that is usually obtained from horses inoculated with the toxin. An immunoglobulin is a concentrated preparation containing predominantly immunoglobulin G and is harvested from a large pool of blood donors. An antivenin, often referred to as *antivenom,* is an antiserum containing antibodies against a venom, which is a poison secreted by an animal such as a reptile, insect, or other arthropod (e.g., spider). Most antivenins are obtained from animals (usually horses) that have been injected with the particular venom; however, the newer ones are produced by recombinant technology. The serum contains immunoglobulins that can neutralize the toxic effects of the venom.

IMMUNIZING DRUGS

Mechanism of Action and Drug Effects

Active immunizing drugs consist of vaccines and toxoids that may be given either orally or intramuscularly and work by stimulating the humoral immune system. This system synthesizes substances called *immunoglobulins,* of which there are five distinct types, designated as M, G, A, E, and D. These immunoglobulins attack and kill the foreign substances that invade the

body. In this case, these foreign substances are called *antigens,* and the immunoglobulins are called *antibodies.*

Vaccines contain substances that trigger the formation of these antibodies against specific pathogens. They may contain the actual live or attenuated pathogen or a killed pathogen. The antibody titer is a measure of how many antibodies to a given antigen are present in the blood and is used to assess whether enough antibodies are present to protect the body effectively against the particular pathogen. Sometimes the antibody levels decline over time. When this happens, another dose of the vaccine is given to restore the antibody titers to a level that can protect the person against the infection. This repeat dose is referred to as a booster shot. Toxoids are altered forms of bacterial toxins that stimulate the production of antibodies in the same way as vaccines.

Because both toxoids and vaccines rely on the immunized host to mount an immune response, the host's immune system must be intact. Therefore, patients who are immunocompromised (i.e., who cannot mount an immune response) may not benefit from receiving vaccines or toxoids. Instead, their clinical situations may warrant giving them passive immunizing drugs such as immunoglobulins.

Passive immunizing drugs are the actual antibodies (immunoglobulins) that can kill or inactivate the pathogen. The process is called *passive* because the person's immune system does not participate in the synthesis of antibodies; instead, the antibodies are provided by the immunizing drug. Immunity acquired in this way generally lasts for a much shorter time than that produced by active immunization. Passive immunization lasts only until the injected immunoglobulins are removed from the person's immune system by the reticuloendothelial system. The reticuloendothelial system is composed of specialized cells in the liver, spleen, lymphatics, and bone marrow.

Indications

Vaccines and toxoids are active immunizing drugs that have been developed for the prevention of many illnesses caused by bacteria and their toxins, as well as those caused by various viruses. Antivenins, antitoxins, and immunoglobulins are passive immunizing drugs. Such drugs can inactivate spider and snake venom, bacterial toxins (exotoxins), and potentially lethal viruses. Box 49-1 lists the currently available immunizing drugs. The successful immunization of 95% or more of a population confers protection on the entire population. This is called herd immunity.

Antivenins, also known as *antisera,* are used to prevent or minimize the effects of poisoning by the venoms of crotalids (rattlesnakes, copperheads, cottonmouths, water moccasins), black widow spiders, and coral snakes, some of which can be lethal. Most healthy adults do not die from the bites of spiders or snakes if they receive prompt and appropriate treatment (i.e., administration of the appropriate antivenin). However, very young children and older adults with health problems are particularly susceptible to the effects of the venom of some of these animals. In either situation, an antivenin is needed to neutralize the venom.

Contraindications

Contraindications to the administration of immunizing drugs include allergy to the immunization itself or allergy to any of its components, such as eggs or yeast. In the case of a potentially fatal illness such as rabies, the drug may still need to be given and any allergic reaction controlled with other medications. Administration of some immunizing drugs is best deferred until after recovery from a febrile illness or temporary immunocompromised state (e.g., following cancer chemotherapy), if possible. However, this is often a matter of clinical judgment, and the individual patient's condition and risk factors for serious illness may be arguments for or against administration of a given immunizing drug at a given time.

Adverse Effects

The undesirable effects of the various immunizing drugs can range from mild and transient to serious and even life-threatening and are listed in Table 49-2. The overwhelming majority of adverse effects are minor. Minor reactions can be treated with acetaminophen and rest. More severe reactions, such as fever higher than 103°F (39.4°C), can be treated with acetaminophen and sponge baths. Serum sickness sometimes occurs after repeated injections of equine (horse)–derived immunizing drugs. The signs and symptoms consist of edema of the face, tongue, and throat; rash; urticaria; arthritis; adenopathy; fever; flushing; itching; cough; dyspnea; cyanosis; vomiting; and cardiovascular collapse. Serum sickness is best treated with analgesics, antihistamines, epinephrine, and/or corticosteroids. In these cases, hospitalization may be required.

Any serious or unusual reactions to immunizing drugs need to be reported to the Vaccine Adverse Event Reporting System (VAERS). This is a national vaccine safety surveillance program that is cosponsored by the Food and Drug Administration (FDA) and the CDC. A report can be submitted via the toll-free telephone number: 800-822-7967. Alternatively, a reporting form can be printed from either the FDA website (*www.fda.gov*) or the CDC website (*www.cdc.gov*).

In the early 1980s, in response to vaccine-related injuries, many parents became reluctant to immunize their children against common, and even potentially fatal, childhood illnesses. Serious adverse events following vaccination are very uncommon. However, in 1986, the U.S. Congress passed the Childhood Vaccine Injury Act, which in turn established the National Vaccine Injury Compensation Program (VICP). The Vaccine Injury Table published by the Health Resources and Services Administration itemizes serious adverse events reported for vaccines that are covered under the VICP, as well as the expected time frame for such events to occur. For more information, the reader is referred to *www.hrsa.gov/vaccinecompensation/index.html*.

For many years, there was controversy in the national news pertaining to the link between immunizations and autism in children. It was thought that thimerosal (a mercury-containing preservative used in vaccines) may have been a causative link, so since 2001, thimerosal has not been used in the preparation of vaccines. In 2011, the medical community declared that the original study suggesting a link to autism was fraudulent. It is suggested that the original author falsified the medical histories of the patients in his study and that he was "hoping to create a vaccine scare." Although there is absolutely no scientific data to support a link between autism and vaccines, many parents are still reluctant to vaccinate their children.

Interactions

Drug interactions are not generally a problem with the majority of immunizing drugs, because they are normally given in a single dose or a relatively small number of doses. One drug class of note that can potentially reduce the efficacy of immunizing drugs is immunosuppressive drugs, including corticosteroids (see Chapter 33), transplant antirejection drugs (see Chapter 48), and cancer chemotherapy drugs (see Chapters 45 and 46). All of these drugs can, to varying degrees, hinder the generation of the active immunity that would normally occur following vaccine or toxoid administration. The bacille Calmette-Guérin vaccine for tuberculosis (used mostly outside the United States in developing countries) can cause false-positive results on the tuberculin skin test (see Chapter 41).

Some vaccines are not to be given close in time to one other. For example, the meningococcal vaccine, whole-cell pertussis vaccine, and typhoid vaccine together have an undesirably large bacterial endotoxin content and should not be administered simultaneously. The effectiveness of measles, mumps, and rubella vaccines may be reduced by concurrent interferon therapy (see Chapter 47). Influenza vaccine may also theoretically lose efficacy if given while antiviral influenza drugs are being taken (see Chapter 40). Recommendations are to give the influenza vaccine at least 48 hours after stopping such antiviral drug therapy. In general, immunizations requiring intramuscular injection are given with particular caution (and with appropriate monitoring) to patients receiving anticoagulant drugs such as warfarin (see Chapter 26). Review the package insert for any immunizing drugs given to obtain the latest information and identify other specific drug interactions that may occur. Hepatitis B immunoglobulin interacts with live vaccines; defer administration of such vaccines until 3 months after the dose of immunoglobulin is given.

TABLE 49-2	Immunizing Drugs: Minor and Severe Adverse Effects	
Body System	**Adverse Effects**
Minor Effects	
Central nervous	Fever, adenopathy
Integumentary	Minor rash, soreness at injection site, urticaria, arthritis
Severe Effects	
Central nervous	Fever higher than 103° F (39.4° C), encephalitis, convulsions, peripheral neuropathy, anaphylactic reaction, shock
Integumentary	Rash
Respiratory	Dyspnea
Other	Cyanosis

Dosages

For dosage information on selected immunizing drugs, please refer to the following link: *www.immunize.org/catg.d/p3085.pdf.*

DRUG PROFILES

Some of the more commonly used vaccines, toxoids, and immunoglobulins are described in the following sections. The immunizing drugs currently available commercially in the United States, including several combination vaccines for prevention of more than one disease, are listed in Box 49-1. Combination vaccines obviously reduce the number of injections that the patient receives, and thus their use is desirable when possible, especially in children.

ACTIVE IMMUNIZING DRUGS

◆ diphtheria and tetanus toxoids and acellular pertussis vaccine (adsorbed)

The active immunizing drugs include diphtheria and tetanus toxoids and the acellular pertussis vaccine (adsorbed) (Tripedia, Daptacel, Infanrix). *Adsorption* refers to the laboratory techniques used to make most vaccines and toxoids. The biologic materials (i.e., virus or toxin particles) are adsorbed (separated out of solution and dried) onto carrier media such as alum, from which they are later removed for packaging into final dosage forms. Diphtheria, tetanus, and pertussis are very different disorders, but an injection that combines all three vaccines (DTP; also commonly called DPT) was routinely given to children since the 1940s. The vaccine combination called *diphtheria and tetanus toxoids with acellular pertussis vaccine (adsorbed) (DTaP [Daptacel])* was approved for the full childhood immunization series and has replaced DPT. Tdap (Adacel, Boostrix) is also a combination vaccine used for teenagers and adults. DTaP (Daptacel) and Tdap use a different form of the pertussis component, known as *acellular pertussis*. Acellular pertussis consists of only a single weakened toxoid, whereas previous pertussis vaccines contained multiple toxoids; this may reduce the number of adverse effects seen from DTP. Pertussis, also known as *whooping cough,* is highly contagious and is spread through contact with respiratory secretions. Its incidence has increased in several states. Currently DTaP is the preferred preparation for primary and booster immunization against these diseases in children from 6 weeks to 6 years of age, unless use of the pertussis component is contraindicated. Tdap (Adacel) is the recommended vaccine for adolescents and adults. See Safety and Quality Improvement: Preventing Medication Errors on p. 792.

Tetanus, diphtheria, and pertussis are prevalent in the populations of many developing countries throughout the world. Full immunization against these diseases with Tdap or DTaP is recommended for travelers to these areas as well as for their inhabitants. A combination product containing only tetanus and diphtheria toxoids (Td) used to be administered to persons 7 years of age and older who require a primary or booster immunization against tetanus for routine wound management. Booster doses were required approximately every 10 years. However, with the recent increase in pertussis cases, Tdap or DTaP are recommended in place of Td. If persons had received Td in the past, it is recommended that they receive another immunization containing pertussis with Tdap or DTaP.

These toxoids (DTP, DTaP, Tdap, and Td) are available only as parenteral preparations, given as deep intramuscular injections. Their use is contraindicated in persons who have had a prior systemic hypersensitivity reaction or a neurologic reaction to one of the ingredients. Some manufacturers state that use is contraindicated in cases of concurrent acute or active infections but not in cases of minor illness. Although there have been very few studies, if any, documenting the safety of their use in pregnant women, it is generally considered safe to give diphtheria, tetanus, and pertussis toxoids after the first trimester.

Haemophilus Influenzae type b conjugate vaccine

Haemophilus influenzae type b (Hib) (HibTITER, ActHIB, Liquid PedvaxHIB) vaccine is a noninfectious, bacteria-derived vaccine. It is made by extracting *H. influenzae* particles that are antigenic and then chemically attaching these particles to a protein carrier medium for use in injections. The vaccine is given by injection to adults and children considered at high risk for acquiring *H. influenzae* infection. Conditions that may predispose an individual to Hib infection are septicemia, pneumonia, cellulitis, arthritis, osteomyelitis, pericarditis, sickle cell anemia, an immunodeficiency syndrome, and Hodgkin's disease. Before this vaccine was developed, infections caused by Hib were the leading cause of bacterial meningitis in children 3 months to 5 years of age. This form of bacterial meningitis has a mortality rate of 5% to 10%. Of those who survive, 20% to 45% suffer serious morbidity in the form of neurologic deficits. All Hib vaccine products are parenteral formulations that are administered intramuscularly. They are categorized as pregnancy category C drugs.

◆ hepatitis B virus vaccine (inactivated)

Hepatitis B virus vaccine (inactivated) (Recombivax HB, Engerix-B) is a noninfectious viral vaccine containing hepatitis B surface antigen (HBsAg). It is made from viral particles and yeast using recombinant DNA technology. In this technique, DNA from two or more organisms is combined. Yeast cells then produce this viral antigenic substance in mass quantities. The substance is then attached to a carrier medium (alum) and made into a vaccine injection preparation. This antigenic HBsAg is used to promote active immunity to hepatitis B infection in persons considered at high risk for potential exposure to the hepatitis B virus or HBsAg-positive materials (e.g., blood, plasma, serum). Health care workers, for example, are persons considered at high risk, and many hospitals require this vaccination upon employment. It is recommended that all children receive this vaccine, and it is usually started shortly after birth. It is also recommended that adults with diabetes mellitus receive hepatitis B vaccination.

Use of the vaccine is contraindicated in persons who are hypersensitive to yeast. Pregnancy is not considered a contraindication to use (pregnancy category C). The vaccine is administered by intramuscular injection and is given as a series of three injections. There are three main formulations designed for three different populations: a pediatric formulation for neonates, infants, children, and adolescents; an adult formulation for persons older than 20 years of age; and a dialysis formulation for predialysis and dialysis patients and for other immunocompromised individuals.

◆ influenza virus vaccine

The influenza virus vaccine (Fluzone, Fluvirin, FluMist, others) is the vaccine used to prevent influenza. It needs to be given each year before the influenza season begins. Such inoculation is the single most important influenza control measure. FluMist is given intranasally, whereas the others are given intramuscularly. Influenza vaccines are either pregnancy category B or C, depending on the manufacturer.

Each year a new influenza vaccine is developed by virology researchers. It usually contains three different influenza virus strains. These strains are chosen from among the hundreds of influenza virus strains in the environment based on the latest epidemiologic data indicating which influenza viruses will most likely circulate in North America in the upcoming winter. The latest influenza vaccine in the United States also included activity against the H1N1 strain. The vaccine is made from highly purified, egg-grown viruses that have been rendered noninfectious (inactivated).

Influenza is characterized by abrupt onset of fever, myalgia, sore throat, and nonproductive cough. Severe malaise may last several days. More severe illness can occur in certain populations. Older individuals, children, and adults with underlying serious health problems (e.g., HIV infection, asthma, cardiopulmonary disease, cancer, diabetes) are at increased risk for complications from influenza infection. Health care personnel are also considered a high-risk group. Increased mortality results not only from influenza but also from other chronic diseases that can be exacerbated by influenza. More than 90% of the deaths attributed to pneumonia and influenza occur among persons 65 years of age or older. Another fairly unusual but important risk group is children and teenagers who are receiving long-term aspirin therapy (e.g., for juvenile arthritis) and who therefore might be at risk for developing Reye's syndrome after influenza (see Chapter 44).

The effectiveness of influenza vaccine varies. Factors that may alter its effectiveness are the age and immunocompetence of the vaccine recipient and the degree of similarity between the virus strains included in the vaccine and those that actually predominate during a given influenza season. Healthy persons younger than 65 years of age have a 70% chance of avoiding illness caused by influenza virus when there is a good match between the vaccine and the circulating viruses.

Older persons, especially those residing in nursing homes, can avoid severe illness, secondary complications, and death by taking the influenza vaccine. In older adults, the vaccine can prevent hospitalization and pneumonia up to 50% to 60% of the time and death up to 80% of the time. Achieving a high rate of vaccination among nursing home residents can reduce the spread of infection in an institution, thus preventing disease through herd immunity. The CDC now recommends that all people older than 6 months of age receive the influenza vaccine. Two newer formulations of the influenza vaccine are available.

One is the "high dose" Fluzone, which is specifically indicated for older adults. It contains four times more virus antigens, in hopes of helping older adults boost an immune response. Studies have not shown any difference in efficacy, whereas more side effects are produced with the 'high dose' preparation. In 2013, a quadravalent formulation became available. Prior to this, all influenza vaccines were trivalent.

◆ measles, mumps, and rubella virus vaccine (live)

The measles, mumps, and rubella vaccine (M-M-R II) is a virus preparation consisting of live measles, mumps, and rubella viruses that are weakened (attenuated). The vaccine promotes active immunity to these diseases by inducing the production of virus-specific immunoglobulin G and immunoglobulin M antibodies. The antibody response to initial vaccination resembles that caused by primary natural infection.

Administration of the measles vaccine or any of the combination products that includes the measles virus is contraindicated in persons with a history of anaphylactic or anaphylactoid reaction, or some other immediate reaction to egg ingestion. Use of these products is also contraindicated in persons who have had an anaphylactic reaction to topically or systemically administered neomycin, because this antibiotic is used as a preservative in some of the vaccine preparations. These vaccines are not to be administered to pregnant women, and pregnancy needs to be avoided for 3 months after measles virus vaccination and 30 days after vaccination with a rubella-containing (measles-rubella or measles-mumps-rubella [MMR]) measles virus vaccine. This precaution is based on the theoretic risk that the live virus vaccine may cause a fetal infection.

◆ meningococcal vaccine

There are two meningococcal vaccines, Menactra and Menveo. They are indicated for active immunization to prevent invasive meningococcal disease caused by *Neisseria meningitidis*. Menactra is approved for patients 9 months to 55 years of age, and Menveo is approved for persons 11 to 55 years of age. They are classified as pregnancy category B drugs. The powder must be diluted with the included liquid conjugate component. Side effects include a 41% incidence of pain at injection site and a 30% incidence of headache. Other side effects include myalgia, malaise, and nausea. Caution must be used to prevent sound-alike errors with Menactra and Menomune. The most current recommendations indicate that a two-dose series be given for adults with asplenia or those who are immunocompromised. All other patients receive a one-time dose. Two new vaccines were approved in 2014, Trumenba and Bexsero. Both are indicated to prevent invasive disease caused by *Neisseria meningitidis* serogroup B in individuals 10 to 25 years of age. Both are pregnancy category B.

◆ pneumococcal vaccine, polyvalent and thirteen-valent

Two forms of vaccine against pneumococcal pneumonia are available that also protect against any illness caused by *Streptococcus pneumoniae*. *Pneumococcus* is the common name for the bacterium *S. pneumoniae*, the causative organism of this common bacterial infection. The polyvalent type of vaccine (Pneumovax 23) is used primarily in adults. (The term *polyvalent* refers to the fact that the vaccine is designed to be effective against the 23 strains of pneumococcus most commonly implicated in adult cases of pneumonia.) This vaccine also may sometimes be recommended for pediatric patients at higher risk for pneumonia as a result of serious chronic illnesses, especially those who are immunocompromised. However, the thirteen-valent vaccine is the pneumococcal vaccine that is routinely recommended for children. Its official full name is *thirteen-valent conjugate vaccine (PVC13, or Prevnar 13)*. The name *thirteen-valent* refers to the fact that the vaccine is designed to immunize against the top thirteen pneumococcal strains found in pediatric pneumonia cases. In 2008 the CDC recommended that all smokers 19 to 64 years of age receive the pneumococcal vaccine, and in 2014 the CDC recommended that patients 65 years of age receive Prevnar 13 in addition to Pneumovax if they have never received a pneumonia vaccine. Contraindications to the use of either vaccine include known drug allergy to components of the vaccine itself, as well as the presence of current significant febrile illness or immunosuppressed state as a result of drug therapy (e.g., cancer chemotherapy). The vaccine may sometimes still be given in such cases, if it is felt that withholding the vaccine poses an even greater risk to the patient. Prevnar 13 is pregnancy category B, while Prenvar 23 is pregnancy category C.

◆ poliovirus vaccine (inactivated)

The use of live oral polio vaccine (OPV) is no longer routine in the United States. Since 1979, the only indigenous cases of poliomyelitis reported in the United States (44 cases) have been associated with use of the live OPV. Injected doses of inactivated polio vaccine (brand name, IPOL) are instead recommended for routine use. The use of OPV is reserved for the following groups: populations that are the target of mass vaccination campaigns to control outbreaks of paralytic polio, unvaccinated children who will be traveling in fewer than 4 weeks to areas in which polio is endemic, and children of parents who object to the recommended number of IPV injections. It is classified as a pregnancy category C drug.

rabies virus vaccine

Although vaccination against the rabies virus is not normally a routine immunization, situations requiring it occur periodically in many practice settings. Rabies virus vaccine (Imovax, Rab-Avert) is produced using laboratory techniques involving infected human cell cultures and selected antimicrobial drugs. Rabies is a virus that can infect a variety of mammals, including skunks, foxes, raccoons, bats, dogs, and cats. The virus is usually transferred to humans by an animal bite and almost universally causes fatal brain tissue destruction if the patient is not treated with rabies vaccine and immunoglobulin (discussed later). Current recommendations call for a total of five intramuscular injections on days 0, 3, 7, 14, and 28 following an animal bite that raises concern for rabies transmission. This includes a bite by any animal whose rabies immunization status is unknown or which escapes and cannot be observed for signs of rabies. This type of treatment is known as *postexposure prophylaxis*.

Preexposure prophylaxis is recommended for persons at high risk for exposure to the rabies virus (e.g., veterinarians). The preexposure course consists of only three injections on day 0, day 7, and sometime between days 21 and 28. Periodic booster shots are also recommended for such individuals approximately every 2 to 5 years, or based on the levels of the patient's rabies virus antibody titers. Patients who have been previously immunized who have a new bite may need only two booster shots on days 0 and 3. Contraindications to the administration of rabies vaccine include a history of allergic reaction to the vaccine itself or to the drugs neomycin, gentamicin, or amphotericin B. However, given the life-threatening nature of rabies infection, treatment may still be required, with supportive therapy (e.g., epinephrine, diphenhydramine, corticosteroids) provided to minimize allergic reactions. Patients with any kind of febrile illness need to delay occupational preexposure prophylaxis treatment until the illness has subsided. It is classified as a pregnancy category C drug.

human papillomavirus vaccine

Human papillomavirus virus (HPV) is a common cause of genital warts and cervical cancer. Genital HPV is a common virus that is transmitted through genital contact, most often during sex. Most sexually active people will get HPV at some time in their lives, although most will never even know it. It is most common in people in their late teens and early twenties. Every year, about 12,000 women are diagnosed with cervical cancer, and almost 4000 women die from this disease in the United States. The papillomavirus vaccines (Gardasil, Cervarix) are the first and only vaccines known to prevent cancer. Cervarix is a bivalent vaccine, whereas Gardasil is a quadrivalent vaccine. The most current recommendations are that either vaccine is recommended for all girls and boys 11 and 12 years of age and for women 13 to 26 years of age and men up to 21 years of age who have not been vaccinated. The vaccine is also recommended for gay and bisexual men (or any man who has sex with men), and men with compromised immune systems (including those with HIV) through 26 years of age if they were not fully vaccinated when they were younger.

HPV vaccine protects against four types of HPV: two types known to cause 70% of reported cervical cancers and two types known to cause 90% of genital warts. The vaccine is given in three injections—the first dose, and then two more doses 2 months and 6 months later. It is contraindicated in patients who show hypersensitivity to yeast or to their first injection of the vaccine. Although the HPV vaccine is pregnancy category B, it is not recommended for pregnant patients, because appropriate studies have not been completed. Pain on injection is common.

herpes zoster vaccine

Zoster vaccine (Zostavax) is a vaccine for the prevention of herpes zoster. Herpes zoster, also known as *shingles,* is an extremely painful condition caused by the varicella-zoster virus that also causes chickenpox. The vaccine is approved for patients 50 years of age or older to prevent reactivation of the zoster virus that causes shingles. Zostavax is a one-time vaccine. The vaccine does not prevent postherpetic neuralgia.

It can be given to patients who have already had shingles. Herpes zoster virus vaccine is a live attenuated vaccine. Its use is contraindicated in patients with hypersensitivity to neomycin, gelatin, or any component of the vaccine. It is also contraindicated in immunosuppressed patients or those receiving immunosuppressant therapies, as well as in pregnant women. Because it is a live vaccine, there is a risk for transmission of the virus from the person who is vaccinated to other people. The vaccine is not to be used for the prevention of chickenpox and is not given to children. The drug must be stored in a freezer.

◆ varicella virus vaccine

The live attenuated varicella virus vaccine (Varivax) is used to prevent varicella (chickenpox). Varicella primarily occurs in children younger than 8 years of age or in individuals with compromised immune systems, such as older adults and HIV-infected patients. It is estimated that only 10% of children older than 12 years of age are still susceptible to varicella. Only 2% of adults develop varicella-zoster virus infections. However, 50% of the deaths associated with varicella are in adults. Half of these are in immunocompromised patients.

The virus in varicella vaccine is attenuated by the passage of virus particles through human and embryonic guinea pig cell cultures. Varicella vaccine must be stored in a freezer. It is not to be given to immunodeficient patients or to patients who have received high doses of systemic steroids in the previous month. It is also recommended that salicylates be avoided for 6 weeks after administration of varicella vaccine because of the possibility of Reye's syndrome (see Chapter 44). The varicella vaccine is recommended for all children and adults. It should be given at 12 to 15 months of age, and then a second dose given at 4 to 6 years of age. All patients need to receive a second dose. It is classified as a pregnancy category C drug.

PASSIVE IMMUNIZING DRUGS

The currently available antivenins, antitoxins, and immunoglobulins that compose the passive immunizing drugs are listed in Box 49-1. Those that are more commonly used are described in the following profiles.

◆ hepatitis B immunoglobulin

Hepatitis B immunoglobulin (BayHep B, Nabi-HB) is used to provide passive immunity against hepatitis B infection in the postexposure prophylaxis and treatment of persons exposed to hepatitis B virus or HBsAg-positive materials (e.g., blood, plasma, serum). It is prepared from the plasma of human donors with high titers of antibodies to HBsAg. All donors are tested for HIV antibodies to prevent HIV transmission.

Because of the possible devastating consequences of hepatitis B infection, pregnancy is not considered a contraindication to the use of hepatitis B immunoglobulin when there is a clear need for it.

◆ immunoglobulin

Immunoglobulin (BayGam, Octagam) is available in both intramuscular and intravenous dosage forms. It provides passive

BOX 49-2 Current FDA-Approved Indications for Immunoglobulins*
Pediatric HIV infection
B-cell chronic lymphocytic leukemia
Bone marrow transplantation
Hepatitis A
Idiopathic thrombocytopenic purpura
Kawasaki disease
Immunoglobulin deficiencies
Measles
Primary immunodeficiency diseases
Rubella
Varicella

FDA, Food and Drug Administration; *HIV*, human immunodeficiency virus.
*Approved routes of administration are intramuscular and intravenous.

immunity by increasing antibody titer and antigen-antibody reaction potential. Immunoglobulins are given to help prevent certain infectious diseases in susceptible persons or to ameliorate the diseases in those already infected. Immunoglobulins are pooled from the blood of at least 1000 human donors. This plasma is prepared by cold alcohol fractionation and usually washed with a detergent to destroy any harmful viruses, such as hepatitis virus or HIV. There are many FDA-approved and non–FDA-approved uses for immunoglobulins; the approved uses are listed in Box 49-2. In recent years, there has been a shortage of immunoglobulin products. The supply of these drugs is dependent on donors. Because of fluctuations in supply and the unfavorable risk/benefit ratio of using products derived from human donors, product insurers have restricted reimbursement to force practitioners to administer the drugs for FDA-approved indications only. "Off-label" or non–FDA-approved uses have been severely curtailed because of such restrictions as well as because of product shortages

$Rh_0(D)$ immunoglobulin

$Rh_0(D)$ immunoglobulin (RhoGAM, WinRho) is used to suppress the active antibody response and the formation of anti-$Rh_0(D)$ antibodies in an $Rh_0(D)$-negative person exposed to Rh-positive blood. Because an $Rh_0(D)$-negative person reacts to Rh-positive blood as if it were a foreign, "nonself" substance, an immune response develops against it and an antigen-antibody reaction occurs. This reaction can be fatal. The administration of this immunoglobulin helps to prevent the reaction. The most common use of this product is in cases of maternal-fetal Rh incompatibility (postpartum). Only the mother is normally dosed. The objective is to prevent a harmful maternal immune response to a fetus during a future pregnancy if an Rh-negative mother becomes pregnant with an Rh-positive child.

$Rh_0(D)$ immunoglobulin is prepared from the plasma or serum of adults with a high titer of anti-$Rh_0(D)$ antibody to the red blood cell antigen $Rh_0(D)$. Administration of this immunoglobulin is contraindicated in persons who have been previously immunized with this drug and in $Rh_0(D)$-positive/Du-positive patients. It is normally given postpartum but is classified as a pregnancy category C drug.

rabies immunoglobulin

Rabies immunoglobulin (BayRab, Imogam Rabies-HT) is a passive immunizing drug that is administered concurrently with rabies virus vaccine following suspected exposure to the rabies virus. In humans, this usually occurs after an animal bite. Rabies immunoglobulin is derived from human cells that are harvested from persons who have been immunized with rabies vaccine. The only contraindication to its use is known drug allergy, although an allergic patient may still need to be dosed rather than face infection with the almost universally fatal rabies virus. The decision to dose a patient in such a case is based on the probability of rabies infection given the particular circumstances surrounding the animal bite. It is classified as a pregnancy category C drug.

tetanus immunoglobulin

Tetanus immunoglobulin (BayTet) is a passive immunizing drug effective against tetanus. It contains tetanus antitoxin antibodies that neutralize the bacterial exotoxin produced by *Clostridium tetani*, the bacterium that causes tetanus. Tetanus immunoglobulin is prepared from the plasma of adults who are hyperimmunized with the tetanus toxoid and is given as prophylaxis to persons with tetanus-prone wounds. It may also be used to treat active tetanus. It is classified as a pregnancy category C drug.

varicella-zoster immunoglobulin

Varicella-zoster immunoglobulin (VZIG; available only in generic form from the American Red Cross) can be used to modify or prevent chickenpox in susceptible individuals who have had recent significant exposure to the disease. VZIG is best administered within 96 hours of exposure. Candidates for therapy with VZIG are those at high risk for serious disease or complications if they become infected with the varicella-zoster virus. Two examples are newborn children, including premature infants with significant exposure, and immunocompromised adults. If the infection manifests in a pregnant woman within 5 days of delivery, a dose of VZIG is recommended for the infant. It may also be beneficial to both mother and infant when given to the mother during pregnancy, preferably as soon as possible after diagnosis of infection. Healthy adults, including pregnant women, are evaluated on a case-by-case basis. The duration of protection against infection provided by VZIG is at least 3 weeks. VZIG is prepared from the plasma of normal blood donors with high antibody titers to varicella-zoster virus. Pregnancy category has not been established.

NURSING PROCESS

ASSESSMENT

Before administering a *toxoid* or *vaccine*, gather complete information about the patient's health history, including

⚡ SAFETY AND QUALITY IMPROVEMENT: PREVENTING MEDICATION ERRORS   [QSEN]

Tdap and DTaP

The Institute for Safe Medication Practices has reported several errors that involve incorrect use of two vaccines that are used to immunize patients against diphtheria, tetanus, and pertussis (whooping cough). DTaP (Daptacel) and Tdap (Adacel) have similar official names but are used in different situations and for different patients.

DTaP, sold under the trade names Daptacel, Tripedia, and Infanrix, contains toxoids of diphtheria and tetanus as well as the acellular pertussis vaccine. This vaccine is for active immunization of pediatric patients 6 weeks to 6 years of age.

Tdap, sold under the trade names Boostrix and Adacel, contains tetanus toxoid, reduced diphtheria toxoid, and acellular pertussis vaccine. It is used as a booster vaccine for older children, adolescents, and adults.

The lettering gives a clue as to the contents and strengths of the various vaccines contained in each formulation. In the DTaP vaccine, the uppercase letters correspond with higher amounts of antigens of the diphtheria and pertussis components, as compared to the Tdap (where the *d* and *p* are in lowercase letters). The DTaP, with its larger amount of antigens, is indicated for initial immunizations.

If an adult receives the DTaP instead of the Tdap immunization, a higher amount of the antigens is delivered, and the patient usually suffers nothing more than a sore arm at the injection site. However, an infant or child who receives Tdap instead of DTaP receives a lower amount of antigen and may not be sufficiently immunized against diphtheria and pertussis.

The similar names and commonly used abbreviations are the main cause of the confusion between the two vaccines. As a result of these medication mixups, the manufacturers have taken steps to provide the medications with labels that are clearly marked with the vaccines' purpose. Recommendations include encouraging prescribers to order the vaccines by brand names, not by the vaccine abbreviations. In addition, ensure that parents and caregivers are aware of which vaccine is needed through the use of written information sheets.

Data from ISMP: DTaP-Tdap mix-ups now affecting hundreds of patients. *ISMP Medication Safety Alert*, July 2010. Available at *www.ismp.org/Newsletters/acutecare/articles/20100701.asp*.

a list of medications the patient is taking such as prescription medications, over-the-counter medications, herbals, and supplements. Assess also for reactions to drugs in the past, present and past health status, previous allergy test results, use of any immunosuppressants, presence of autoimmune or immunosuppressive diseases or infections, pregnancy and lactation status, and an unusual reaction to any substance. When pediatric patients are to receive a vaccine or toxoid, assess and follow the prescribed immunization schedule and dose. The Department of Health and Human Services, specifically the CDC, provides the latest recommendations for adult and pediatric *immunizations* in the United States. These recommendations along with cautions and contraindications are easily accessible on the Internet at *www.cdc.gov* and are available for referral to gain updated information prior to giving vaccines.

Because *passive immunizing drugs* may precipitate serum sickness, carefully assess patients who have chronic illnesses, are debilitated, or are older adults. This includes measuring vital signs, completing a physical assessment, obtaining a medication history, as well as examining the results of any laboratory testing ordered by the prescriber. Document the patient's general health status with attention to overall well-being and any disease states. See the pharmacology discussion on *passive vaccines* as well as Box 49-1 and Table 49-1 for further information.

For the various *active immunizing drugs,* Tables 49-1 and 49-2 provide more specific insight and information including contraindications, cautions, and drug interactions. It is also important to note that use of these drugs must be considered very carefully in the following group of individuals: pregnant patients; patients with active infections (especially those caused by the same pathogen or organism producing the same toxin); patients with severe febrile illnesses (excluding minor illnesses such as cold, mild infection, ear infection, or low-grade fever); and patients with a history of reactions or serious adverse effects to the specific immunizing drug. In addition, research has shown that patients who are already immunosuppressed (e.g., those with AIDS, neonates, very young and/or older adult patients, those with chronic diseases or cancer) are at increased risk for serious, adverse effects to toxoids or vaccines; therefore, the use of these active immunizing drugs must be done with extreme caution or not at all. Many adults assume that the vaccines they received as children will protect them for a lifetime. This is usually the case. Some adults, however, were never vaccinated as children, or newer vaccines were not available at the time they were vaccinated. In addition, immunity may fade over time, and as an individual ages, he or she may become more susceptible to serious diseases caused by common infections, such as *Pneumococcus* infections.

Tetanus, diphtheria, and pertussis vaccines are to be used in patients 6 weeks to 6 years of age and are contraindicated in those with previous vaccine reactions. In addition, the use of these toxoids is contraindicated in patients with any type of neurologic reaction to the vaccine. Pertussis, or whooping cough, is very contagious, spread through respiratory secretions, and may certainly become a widespread community health problem. With *DTaP,* assess the age of the patient because it is the preferred preparation in children from 6 weeks to 6 years of age unless the pertussis component is contraindicated. In adolescents and adults, *Tdap* is indicated.

The *H. influenzae type b vaccine* is administered to adults and children considered at high risk for acquiring *H. influenzae* infection. This high-risk population includes individuals with septicemia, pneumonia, cellulitis, arthritis, osteomyelitis, pericarditis, sickle cell anemia, immunodeficiency syndrome, or Hodgkin's disease. It is important to note that each year a new *influenza vaccine* is developed (see the pharmacology discussion). The latest one developed in the United States included activity against the H1N1 strain of influenza. Assess whether the patient belongs in a high-risk group for exposure, such as health care personnel. Assessment of age and medical history is important with these vaccines because individuals 65 years of age and older or those with chronic diseases are at risk for increased mortality from the influenza. The influenza virus vaccine is contraindicated in those with a known hypersensitivity to it. *Hepatitis B virus vaccines* are indicated for those at high risk for exposure to the hepatitis B virus or HBsAg-positive materials (e.g., blood, plasma, serum), such as health care workers. This vaccine is contraindicated in those allergic to yeast. Assess the need of the patient receiving the vaccine because there are different formulations for pediatric patients, adults older than 20 years of age, and individuals receiving dialysis or other immunocompromised patients.

The *MMR vaccine* is contraindicated in pregnant women, in persons with a history of anaphylactic reaction or other immediate reaction to egg ingestion, and in those with an anaphylactic reaction to topically or systemically administered neomycin and in cases of active TB. With the *meningococcal vaccine,* gather data about any history of allergies as well as age because Menactra is indicated for patients who are 9 months to 55 years of age, and Menveo is indicated for those who are 11 to 55 years of age. The *pneumococcal vaccine* is contraindicated in those with known allergy to the drug or its components, in patients allergic to latex, and in patients with significant febrile illness or immunosuppressed state as a result of drug therapy (e.g., chemotherapy). It is important to understand that *Pneumovax 23* is primarily for use in adults but may be recommended for pediatric patients at higher risk for pneumonia as a result of a serious chronic illness (see pharmacology discussion). *PVIC13* or *Prevnar 13* is the vaccine routinely recommended for children.

Do not give the *papillomavirus vaccine (Gardasil, Cervarix)* to patients with allergies to yeast or patients who have a documented allergic reaction to the first injection of the vaccine. This vaccine is also contraindicated in pregnancy and in children younger than 9 years of age. The *zoster vaccine (Zostavax)* is for the prevention of herpes zoster. Assessment of age is an important factor in the administration of this vaccine because it is not to be given in children. It is recommended for patients 50 years of age and older to prevent shingles and is not to be given to patients with allergic reactions to neomycin, gelatin, or any component of the vaccine. Assessment of immune status is also important because it is not to be given to those who are pregnant, immunosuppressed, or receiving immunosuppressant therapies. The *varicella vaccine virus, Varivax,* is used to prevent chickenpox, which occurs mainly in those younger than 8 years of age or in those who are immunocompromised. Assess the patient's medical and medication history because it should not be given to individuals who have received high doses of systemic steroids in the previous month. Advise the patient to avoid salicylates for 6 weeks after its administration because of the risk for Reye's syndrome (see Chapter 44). Age of the patient is important because it is given at 12 months of age and then again at 4 to 6 years of age.

NURSING DIAGNOSES

1. Acute pain related to local and/or systemic effects of the injection of a toxoid, vaccine, or passive immunizing drug
2. Deficient knowledge related to the use of toxoids, vaccines, or passive immunizing drugs
3. Risk for injury due to adverse effects associated with toxoids, vaccines, and/or passive immunizing drugs

PLANNING: OUTCOME IDENTIFICATION

1. Patient experiences minimal pain associated with the injection of toxoid, vaccine, or immunizing drug through use of comfort measures, use of analgesics or anti-inflammatory drugs, and rest.
2. Patient demonstrates adequate and updated knowledge regarding the use of toxoids, vaccines, or immunizing drugs including its action and adverse effects.
3. Patient remains free from injury with reporting any of the following symptoms: fever higher than 101°F (38.3°C), infection, wheezing, or other unusual reactions

IMPLEMENTATION

When any *immunizing drug* is administered, always check and then recheck the specific protocols and schedules of administration to ensure patient safety and accuracy. Provide individuals receiving any immunizing drug with the proper instructions and updated written materials about the medication, technique, route of administration, adverse effects, and potential complications. Educate the patient receiving the vaccine that he or she will not "get" the disease in question from receiving the attenuated or dead virus. It is also important to follow the manufacturer's recommendations concerning storage and administration of the drug, routes and site of administration, dosage, precautions pertaining to the drug's use, and contraindications to its use. Always provide the patient with a written record of immunization with the date and a reminder of when a booster is needed, if appropriate. Encourage and teach parents of young children how to maintain an accurate journal of the child's immunization status, including dates of immunization and any reactions if they occur. Prior to giving the vaccine, always inquire again about any previous immunization reaction. Administer all immunizing drugs, as prescribed, using the route specified. The midlateral muscle of the thigh is the preferred site for infants. The deltoid muscle is preferred for older children and adults. If the patient experiences discomfort at the injection site, apply warm compresses to the site, or administer an analgesic, antipyretic, or antiinflammatory medication as ordered. Have epinephrine 1:1000 readily available at the time of injection due to the risk for hypersensitivity reactions. Additionally, if fever (101°F or 38.3°C or higher), convulsions with or without fever, altered consciousness, neurologic symptoms, collapse, or somnolence occur, report them immediately to the prescriber, monitor the patient, and initiate emergency treatment as needed.

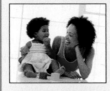
EVALUATION

The therapeutic response in patients receiving *immunizing drugs* is the prevention or amelioration of the specific disease being targeted. Adverse reactions for which to monitor in patients receiving immunizing drugs are specific to the drug, but there may be a localized reaction including swelling, redness, discomfort, and heat at the site of injection or a more serious reaction that must be reported immediately to the prescriber (e.g., high fever, lymphadenopathy, rash, itching, joint pain, severe flulike symptoms, decreased level of consciousness, and/or shortness of breath). For a complete list of expected reactions or adverse effects, including minor and severe, see Table 49-2. As immunizing drugs improve and newer ones are developed, it is hoped that fewer adverse effects will occur and fewer adverse drug events and complications will be seen.

PATIENT-CENTERED CARE: PATIENT TEACHING

- A localized reaction to the injection sometimes occurs when toxoids and vaccines are administered. Inform the patient that the discomfort may be relieved by placing warm compresses on the injection site, resting, and taking acetaminophen and/or diphenhydramine, as directed by the prescriber. Instructions for the care of infants or children experiencing such reactions are generally given by the child's prescriber when the immunizing drug is administered.

- Advise the patient or parent/caregiver to notify the prescriber if high or prolonged fever, rash, itching, or shortness of breath occur after the vaccination.
- Stress that the patient or parent/caregiver always keep a double record (two copies stored in separate places) of all of the medications being taken, especially all vaccinations received.
- Preteens and teens—and everyone else 6 months of age and older—should get the flu vaccine every year as soon as it is

made available in their community. Educate about the two flu vaccines available to preteens and teens: the flu injection that is made from killed flu virus and given usually in the arm (deltoid muscle) and the nasal spray flu vaccine made with live, but weakened, flu virus and is sprayed via the nose. The CDC recommends that preteens and teens with chronic health conditions (e.g., asthma, diabetes, heart disease) do NOT get the nasal spray dosage form of the vaccine. Make sure that parents are aware of the need to inform the doctor, nurse, or whomever is administering the injectable form, of any severe allergy to chicken eggs. It may be helpful to have the patient lie down when getting the shot and up to 15 minutes after to avoid any fainting. The Vaccines for Children program does provide vaccines for children 18 years and younger who are uninsured/underinsured, Medicaid-eligible, Native American, or Alaska Native. Visit *www.cdc.gov* for more information and type VFC in the search box.

- It is important to know that some adults need vaccines: adults who were never vaccinated as children; adults for whom newer vaccines were not available during their childhood; older adults, because immunity may fade over time, and, as aging progresses, individuals become more susceptible to serious disease caused by common infections such as flu and pneumococcus.
- Immunizations that adults need include seasonal influenza (flu); tetanus, diphtheria, and pertussis (whooping cough) (for adults not previously immunized with the Tdap vaccine); shingles (for adults 60 years of age and older), pneumococcal disease (for adults 65 years of age and older and adults with specific health conditions), and hepatitis B infection for adults who have diabetes or are at risk for hepatitis B.
- If patients are not sure which vaccines have been received in the past, there are many ways to find vaccinations records. Visit *www.cdc.gov* for more information.
- A vaccine adverse event reporting system is available through the FDA by calling 800-822-7967.

KEY POINTS

- A foreign substance in the body is termed an *antigen;* the body creates a substance called an *antibody* specifically to bind to it.
- B lymphocytes (B cells), when stimulated by the binding of an antigen molecule, begin to differentiate into memory cells and plasma cells.
- Memory cells remember what that particular antigen looks like in case the body is exposed to the same antigen again in the future. Plasma cells manufacture the antibodies and will mass-produce clones of the antibodies upon reexposure to a particular antigen.
- The two types of immunity are active and passive immunity. Different types of drugs are used to induce each, and these drugs are indicated for different populations, as follows:
  - Active immunization involves administration of a toxoid or a vaccine that exposes the body to a relatively harmless form of the antigen (foreign invader) to imprint cellular memory and stimulate the body's defenses to fight any subsequent exposure. It provides long-lasting or permanent immunity. The recipient must have an active, functioning immune system to benefit.
- Passive immunization involves the administration of immunoglobulins, antitoxins, or antivenins. Serum or concentrated immunoglobulins are obtained from humans or animals and, after screening and testing, are injected into the patient, directly giving the individual the ability to fight off an invading microorganism or inactivate a toxin. Passive immunization provides temporary protection and does not stimulate an antibody response in the host. It is used in patients who are immunocompromised or who have been exposed to, or anticipate exposure to, an organism or toxin.
- Patients who are not to receive immunizing drugs include those with active infections, febrile illnesses, or history of a previous reaction to the drug. Use of these drugs in pregnant women is usually contraindicated.
- Patients who are immunocompromised are at greater risk for experiencing serious adverse effects from immunizing drugs.
- Encourage the updating of all vaccination records.

NCLEX® EXAMINATION REVIEW QUESTIONS

1. When assessing a patient who will be receiving a measles vaccine, the nurse will consider which condition to be a possible contraindication?
   a. Anemia
   b. Pregnancy
   c. Ear infection
   d. Common cold

2. When giving a vaccination to an infant, the nurse will tell the mother to expect which adverse effect?
   a. Fever over 101°F (38.3°C)
   b. Rash
   c. Soreness at the injection site
   d. Chills

3. The nurse is reviewing the Centers for Disease Control (CDC) recommendations for vaccines. The pneumococcal vaccine (Pneumovax 23) is recommended for which group?
   a. Newborn infants
   b. Patients who are immunosuppressed
   c. Patients who are transplant candidates
   d. Smokers between 19 and 64 years of age

4. During a routine checkup, a 72-year-old patient is advised to receive an influenza vaccine injection. He questions this, saying, "I had one last year. Why do I need another one?" What is the nurse's best response?
   a. "The effectiveness of the vaccine wears off after 6 months."
   b. "Each year a new vaccine is developed based on the flu strains that are likely to be in circulation."
   c. "When you reach 65 years of age, you need boosters on an annual basis."
   d. "Taking the flu vaccine each year allows you to build your immunity to a higher level each time."

5. A 28-year-old patient is in the urgent care center after stepping on a rusty tent nail. The nurse evaluates the patient's immunity status and notes that the patient thinks she had her last tetanus booster about 10 years ago, just before starting college. Which immunization would be most appropriate at this time?
   a. Immunoglobulin intravenous (Gammar-P IV)
   b. DTaP (Daptacel) (diphtheria, tetanus, and acellular pertussis)
   c. Tdap (Adacel) (diphtheria, tetanus, and acellular pertussis)
   d. No immunizations are necessary at this time.

6. The nurse is providing teaching after an adult receives a booster immunization. Which adverse reactions will the nurse immediately report to the health care provider? (Select all that apply.)
   a. Swelling and redness at the injection site
   b. Fever of 100°F (37.8°C)
   c. Joint pain
   d. Heat over the injection site
   e. Rash over the arms, back, and chest
   f. Shortness of breath

7. The order for an adult who needs passive hepatitis B prophylaxis reads: "Give hepatitis B immunoglobulin (BayHep B), 0.06 mg/kg IM now, and then again in 30 days." The patient weighs 176 pounds. How many milligrams will this patient receive per dose?

8. An animal control officer was bitten by a stray dog that showed signs of rabies. Which statement by the nurse is correct regarding the treatment for rabies prophylaxis?
   a. "You will receive treatment if you begin to show symptoms of rabies."
   b. "You will receive one oral dose of medication today, and one more in 1 week."
   c. "You will need to receive 3 subcutaneous injections over the next week."
   d. "You will need to receive 5 intramuscular injections over the next 28 days."

1. b, 2. c, 3. d, 4. b, 5. c, 6. c, e, f, 7. 4.8 mg per dose, 8. d.

CRITICAL THINKING AND PRIORITIZATION QUESTIONS

1. R.T. is in the emergency department after receiving a bite from a black widow spider *(Latrodectus mactans).* As you administer the antivenin for the black widow spider bite, he asks you, "Now I will be immune to black widow spiders after this shot, right? That's good, because we have a lot of them around the barn." What is the nurse's best response? Explain your answer.

2. Within 2 hours after a patient receives a tetanus booster vaccination, his wife calls the clinic. "He says that he is feeling weird and a little short of breath. You said to call if he is having a reaction, but it's hard to tell what is happening." What is the first instruction the nurse should give to this patient's wife?

For answers, see *http://evolve.elsevier.com/Lilley.*

ⓔ EVOLVE WEBSITE

PART 9

Drugs Affecting the Gastrointestinal System and Nutrition

Learning Strategies

STUDYING FOR TESTS

Studying for tests or examinations is part of a process. It should never be a cram session. It is best to think in terms of "preparing" for rather than "studying" for a test or examination. If you have been following the learning strategies outlined in the previous chapters, then you have been preparing for the test or examination all along. You have been making connections and forming long-term memory. You have been storing "files" in your brain, as mentioned in Part 7.

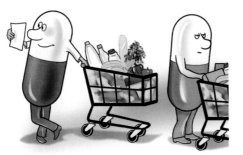

When you sit down to prepare for a test, your success depends on several things. First, remember you are not cramming. Second, you are not rereading all of the corresponding chapters again. Third, you are not writing new notes to "add" to your learning. All of these activities are counterproductive at this point. They add too much information to your existing files. The information that you need for the test or examination is pushed farther down, and too much extra information causes your memory files to overexpand. Too much new information just before a test makes retrieving what you already know much more difficult. So instead of rereading the entire chapter, find the section in the chapter for which you feel you need clarification, and read only that portion. If writing helps you learn, make note cards from your current notes. Extracting new notes from the book introduces too much new information, too late. If you have been making flash cards, composing questions, and quizzing each other in your study group, then you should have a lot of information already stored in your brain (files). The other problem with cramming, rereading, and taking new notes is that it increases your anxiety. You begin to doubt your existing knowledge. You find all sorts of information that you feel you suddenly have to know. Anxiety impedes learning and prevents the free flow of memory.

When preparing for a test or examination, if you are confident in your understanding of a topic, leave it be and move on to something else. Rereading and reviewing material that you have mastered takes time away from reviewing content that you are not so sure of. It is okay; the other information still will be there when you need it. Put the notes and books away early, and get a good night's sleep. In the morning, leave the book and notes alone, unless you absolutely need to look at something. Otherwise you may have the urge to cram.

If your study group likes to meet before the test/examination, decide if that will help or hurt you. If meeting with your group and answering questions confirms that you are ready for the test/examination, then do it. However, if someone mentions a fact you do not know, will that increase your anxiety and cause you to panic and doubt your readiness? If it will, leave the group alone; be confident that you already know what you need to be successful. If listening to music frees your mind and calms your nerves, do that instead and enter the classroom just before the test/examination so your peers will not disturb your calm demeanor. Before you take the test/examination, reassure yourself that you know the material and you will do well. There is power in positive thinking.

TEST-TAKING STRATEGIES

When you take your test or examination, have a system. Will you answer all the questions of a certain type first? It is strongly suggested that, if you do not have an answer within a few minutes, you skip the question and move on. You do not want to increase your anxiety or waste time, as most instructors will set a specific time frame for completion of the test. When you read a multiple choice question, make sure you understand exactly what the question is asking. Many students find highlighting or underlining key words in the *stem* (the question) helps them to quickly decide what it is really asking. If you know that you are looking for an intervention versus a sign or a symptom, it will help you determine which answer to choose.

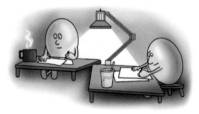

Many students believe the correct answer will be obvious and stand out from the rest. But this is not true, especially when it comes to NCLEX®-style questions, where several answers will seem correct. Your job is to choose the *best* answer. The answer choices are called *distracters*. The wrong answers are there to distract you from choosing the correct answer. Good distracters are very similar to the correct answer, and they allow your instructor to determine whether or not you really understand the concept. A strategy to assist in choosing the best answer is to cover all of the answers as you read the question, which forces you to think critically about the question, recall what you know, and then supply an answer. As you reveal the answers, many times the answer you recalled is one of the options. Choose that answer. Then read the remaining answers to be sure you still like yours. Only change your mind if you are 100% sure that another answer is better. Recheck the stem to make sure your choice indeed answers precisely what the question is asking. This technique works well for the student who has difficulty choosing between two answers. When a student sees all the answers at once and two answers sound correct, it is easy for

doubt to set in. Thinking about the concept and the answer your memory provides before seeing the choices helps avoid this dilemma.

It may also help to make a list next to the question before you reveal the answer. For example, a question is asking about the adverse effects of a medication in the older adult. You recall dizziness, hypotension, diarrhea, and nausea as adverse effects. Write these down. When you reveal the answers, you'll notice "falls" is included in one of your choices. You know this is the correct response since hypotension and dizziness can cause an older adult to fall. If you did not write these down, you may not have made the connection. Instead, you might have been looking for dizziness, hypotension, nausea, and diarrhea in the answer choices, and it may have taken longer to make the connection. This is another example of applying your knowledge. In nursing, most of your test questions will be at this application level, as discussed in Part 7.

Sometimes students circle all the questions they are not sure about then go back and reread them. Many times this causes doubt and changing of answers. You can do this, but studies have shown your first or "gut" response is usually correct. The technique of covering the answers helps with this, as the answer comes to you because you have it stored in your memory where you easily retrieve it. Seeing all the other options at once makes it easy to talk yourself into another choice because you "think" you read it or heard it somewhere.

There will be times when recalling information will not help, or you have no idea where the question is leading. In this case, look at each answer and then look for clues in the stem. Sometimes reading all the answers will alert you to what the answer should be by tugging at your memory. Or you may notice one of the answers is totally wrong. You can start eliminating those that you know are incorrect. If you get down to two answers, you have a 50% chance of being correct, which is better than leaving it blank. So take your best guess.

Be aware of look-alike answers. There may be a subtle difference between the two, so read them carefully. It should then be obvious which one is the distracter. Beware of absolutes like "always," "never," or "must" since very few things in life are absolute. These can be easily eliminated most of the time. In pharmacology, you will often be tested on the terminology or vocabulary involved. You need to be very careful when choosing answers for these types of questions. Again, watch the spelling. You will notice that many terms are similar in spelling and meaning. To know what the question is asking, you may have to also pay attention to the exact spelling of key terms when you make flash cards. Simple words like *hypotension* and *hypertension* may be misread or transposed when you are feeling anxious.

If you have difficulty with a question and you truly do not know what it is asking, seek the assistance of your instructor. There is a 50-50 chance they can help you. The faculty member might either tell you that the query you are posing cannot be answered without giving away the answer, or may rephrase the question in a way that makes it easier for you to understand. If you ask what a term means and the vocabulary word is one that you should know, you will most likely not receive any help. Therefore, again, commit your key terms to memory!

If you are recording your answers on a Scantron or other type of answer sheet, make sure you transfer each one correctly. Correct answers circled on the test usually do not count if they are incorrectly noted on the answer sheet. If you skip one row, the whole answer sheet will be off. When you are taking tests and examinations, remain aware of the time so that you will not have to scramble to complete the last few pages. Not all proctors give a warning when time is almost up.

Once you have finished, turn in the test. Rereading and reviewing your answers invites the temptation to change answers. Be confident that you did your best. When you receive the results, you can complete a performance evaluation to better understand the outcome.

PERFORMANCE EVALUATION

After you have taken your test or examination in pharmacology, it is suggested that you conduct a learning self-evaluation. This evaluation needs to be completed whether or not you performed well on the examination and no matter the score. Some appropriate questions include the following: How well did you actually perform on the examination? Which areas did you struggle with? Which types of answers came effortlessly to you? Which questions or content area did you understand quickly and easily versus a limited or incomplete comprehension? In order to move forward with successful performance on tests, look at your strengths and weaknesses and apply them to acquire greater understanding of the content.

Ask yourself how well you answered questions that reflected understanding of key terms in pharmacology. If this is an area of weakness, it suggests you need to focus more on terminology and vocabulary words when you are studying for the next test. The key terms and vocabulary are the language of pharmacology. As discussed in Part 3, when you learn these key terms you want to be able to apply them and fully understand their connections to nursing and the nursing process.

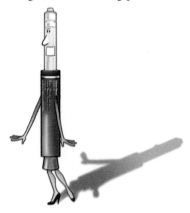

Were there questions that you answered incorrectly because you literally did not know or remember the information? In test taking, there will most likely be questions that assess your knowledge of information or content that you simply do not recall. This forces you to guess at the answer, which is fine. However, if in the self-evaluation process following an examination you notice you answered numerous questions incorrectly because you did not know the information, view this as a red flag warning. Take a look at how you studied, and evaluate your lecture notes and class discussions, as well as your process of taking notes. Are you identifying important key concepts and information from lectures? Are you focusing on the content that your instructor is emphasizing? Do you really comprehend those concepts, or are there blanks or missing parts in your understanding? A major key to taking tests and performing well on them is to identify the most important concepts. Key concepts stressed in course objectives, class, readings, and assignments will be the focus of test questions. If you are not able to determine the rationale for poor performance on a test, or if you lack understanding of lectures, readings, and assignments, do not hesitate to speak with your faculty member, who may be able to identify your problematic areas and is equipped to provide advice for identifying and then focusing on the right content.

It is important that you always focus on your course and lecture objectives. You need to make sure you are connecting complex pharmacologic content with the nursing process and your role as a nurse. Many of the test questions will ask you to apply pharmacologic knowledge to patient care and the nurse's role in assessment, teaching, and evaluating outcomes. This is why active questioning sessions are so important.

If you struggle with multiple choice questions, review the NCLEX® Examination Review Questions and the test-taking strategies. If you run out of time, try to do a better job of self-pacing next time, and do not waste time rereading and reviewing the entire test.

Consider your preparation the night before the test. Did you stay up too late studying? Did you pull an all-nighter? If you did, prepare now to plan ahead. Go back and review your time management, and see if you need to make improvements.

After you have done a thorough self-evaluation, it will be easy to know where you need to change. Reviewing your learning strategies will help ensure your success. Above all, never hesitate to talk with your instructor. It is easier for a faculty member to offer assistance and tutoring to get you back on track early in the term, rather than trying to help when there are only a few points left between you passing and failing the course.

50

Acid-Controlling Drugs

ⓔ http://evolve.elsevier.com/Lilley

OBJECTIVES

When you reach the end of this chapter, you will be able to do the following:

1. Discuss the physiologic influence of various pathologies, such as peptic ulcer disease, gastritis, spastic colon, gastroesophageal reflux disease, and hyperacidic states, on the health of patients and their gastrointestinal tracts.
2. Describe the mechanisms of action, indications, cautions, contraindications, drug interactions, adverse effects,

dosages, and routes of administration for the following classes of acid-controlling drugs: antacids, histamine 2 (H_2)–blocking drugs (H_2 receptor antagonists), proton pump inhibitors, and acid suppressants.
3. Develop a nursing care plan that includes all phases of the nursing process for patients receiving acid-controlling drugs.

DRUG PROFILES

antacids, general, p. 804
⬥ cimetidine, p. 806
⬥ famotidine, p. 806
lansoprazole, p. 808
misoprostol, p. 808
⬥ omeprazole, p. 807
pantoprazole, p. 808

ranitidine, p. 806
simethicone, p. 809
⬥ sucralfate, p. 808

⬥ = *Key drug*
❗ = *High-alert drug*

KEY TERMS

Antacids Basic compounds composed of different combinations of acid-neutralizing ionic salts. (p. 803)

Chief cells Cells in the stomach that secrete the gastric enzyme pepsinogen (a precursor to pepsin). (p. 801)

Gastric glands Secretory glands in the stomach containing the following cell types: parietal, chief, mucous, endocrine, and enterochromaffin. (p. 801)

Gastric hyperacidity The overproduction of stomach acid. (p. 800)

Hydrochloric acid (HCl) An acid secreted by the *parietal cells* in the lining of the stomach that maintains the environment of the stomach at a pH of 1 to 4. (p. 801)

Mucous cells Cells whose function in the stomach is to secrete mucus that serves as a protective mucous coat against the digestive properties of HCl. Also called *surface epithelial cells.* (p. 801)

Parietal cells Cells in the stomach that produce and secrete HCl. These cells are the primary site of action for many of the drugs used to treat acid-related disorders. (p. 801)

Pepsin An enzyme in the stomach that breaks down proteins. (p. 801)

OVERVIEW

One of the conditions of the stomach requiring drug therapy is hyperacidity, or excessive acid production. Left untreated, hyperacidity can lead to serious conditions such as acid reflux, ulcer disease, esophageal damage, and even esophageal cancer. Overproduction of stomach acid is also referred to as gastric hyperacidity.

ACID-RELATED PATHOPHYSIOLOGY

The stomach secretes several substances with various physiologic functions, including the following:

- Hydrochloric acid, an acid that aids digestion and also serves as a barrier to infection
- Bicarbonate, a base that is a natural mechanism to prevent hyperacidity

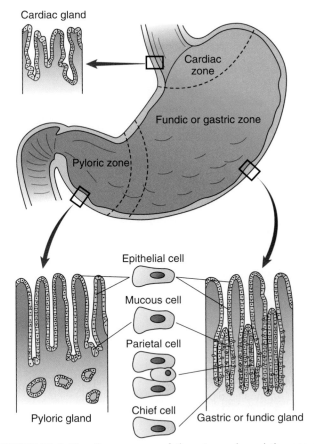

FIGURE 50-1 The three zones of the stomach and the associated glands.

- Pepsinogen, an enzymatic precursor to pepsin, an enzyme that digests dietary proteins
- Intrinsic factor, a glycoprotein that facilitates gastric absorption of vitamin B$_{12}$
- Mucus, which protects the stomach lining from both hydrochloric acid and digestive enzymes
- Prostaglandins, which have a variety of antiinflammatory and protective functions (see Chapter 44)

The stomach, although one structure, can be divided into three functional areas. Each area is associated with specific glands. These glands are composed of different cells, and these cells secrete different substances. Figure 50-1 shows the three functional areas of the stomach and the distribution of the associated types of stomach glands.

The three primary types of glands in the stomach are the cardiac, pyloric, and gastric glands. These glands are named for their positions in the stomach. The cardiac glands are located around the cardiac sphincter (also known as the *gastroesophageal sphincter*); the gastric glands are in the fundus, also known as the *greater part of the body of the stomach;* and the pyloric glands are in the pyloric region and in the transitional area between the pyloric and fundic zones.

The **gastric glands** are highly specialized secretory glands composed of several different types of cells: *parietal, chief, mucous, endocrine,* and *enterochromaffin.* Each cell secretes a specific substance. The three most important cell types are parietal cells, chief cells, and mucous cells. These cells are depicted in Figure 50-1.

Parietal cells produce and secrete **hydrochloric acid (HCl)**. They are the primary site of action for many of the drugs used to treat acid-related disorders. **Chief cells** secrete *pepsinogen.* Pepsinogen is a *proenzyme* (enzyme precursor) that becomes **pepsin** when activated by exposure to acid. Pepsin breaks down proteins and is therefore referred to as a *proteolytic* enzyme. **Mucous cells** are mucus-secreting cells that are also called *surface epithelial cells.* The secreted mucus serves as a protective coating against the digestive action of hydrochloric acid and digestive enzymes.

These three cell types play an important role in the digestive process. When the balance of these cells and their secretions is impaired, acid-related diseases can occur. The most harmful of these involve hypersecretion of acid and include peptic ulcer disease and esophageal cancer. However, the most common condition is mild to moderate hyperacidity. Many lay terms (e.g., *indigestion, sour stomach, heartburn, acid stomach*) have been used to describe this condition of overproduction of hydrochloric acid by the parietal cells. Hyperacidity is often associated with gastroesophageal reflux disease (GERD). This is the tendency of excessive and acidic stomach contents to back up, or reflux, into the lower (and even upper) esophagus. Over time, this condition can lead to more serious disorders such as erosive esophagitis and Barrett esophagus, a precancerous condition. Therefore, to prevent serious disorders from occurring and to promote patient comfort, GERD is aggressively treated with one or more of the medications described in this section.

Hydrochloric acid is secreted by the parietal cells in the lining of the stomach and maintains the environment of the stomach at a pH of 1 to 4. This acidity aids in the proper digestion of food and also serves as one of the body's defenses against microbial infection via the gastrointestinal (GI) tract. Several substances stimulate hydrochloric acid secretion by the parietal cells, such as food, caffeine, chocolate, and alcohol. In moderation, any of these is usually not problematic. However, excessive consumption of large, fatty meals or alcohol, as well as emotional stress, may result in hyperproduction of hydrochloric acid and lead to hypersecretory disorders such as peptic ulcer disease.

The parietal cell is the primary target for many of the most effective drugs for the treatment of acid-related disorders. A closer look at how the parietal cell receives signals to produce and secrete hydrochloric acid will enhance the understanding of the mechanism of action of many of the drugs used to treat acid-related disorders.

The wall of the parietal cell contains three types of receptors: acetylcholine (ACh), histamine, and gastrin. When any one of these is occupied by its corresponding chemical stimulant (ACh, histamine, or gastrin, which can all be considered *first messengers*), the parietal cell will produce and secrete hydrochloric acid. Figure 50-2 shows the parietal cell with its three receptors. Once these receptors have become occupied, a *second messenger* is sent inside the cell. In the case of histamine receptors, occupation results in the production of adenylate cyclase.

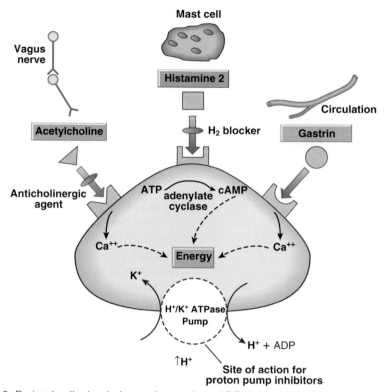

FIGURE 50-2 Parietal cell stimulation and secretion. *ADP,* Adenosine diphosphate; *ATP,* adenosine triphosphate; *ATPase,* adenosine triphosphatase; *cAMP,* cyclic adenosine monophosphate.

Adenylate cyclase converts adenosine triphosphate (ATP) to cyclic adenosine monophosphate (cAMP), which provides energy for the proton pump. The proton pump—or, more precisely, the hydrogen–potassium–adenosine triphosphatase (ATPase) pump—is a pump for the transport of hydrogen ions and is located in the parietal cells. The pump requires energy to work. If energy is present, the proton pump will be activated, and the pump will be able to transport hydrogen ions needed for the production of hydrochloric acid.

In the case of both ACh and gastrin receptors, the second messenger that drives the proton pump is not cAMP but is instead calcium ions. Anticholinergic drugs (see Chapter 21) such as atropine block ACh receptors, which also results in decreased hydrogen ion secretion from the parietal cells. However, these drugs are no longer used for this purpose and have been superseded by other drug classes discussed in this chapter. There is currently no drug to block the binding of the hormone gastrin to its corresponding receptor on the parietal cell surface.

Peptic ulcer disease is a general term for gastric or duodenal ulcers that involve digestion of the GI mucosa by the enzyme pepsin. Pepsin normally breaks down only food proteins and is the activated form of pepsinogen. Pepsinogen is produced by the chief cells of the stomach in response to hydrochloric acid released from the parietal cells. The sight, smell, and taste of food and its presence in the stomach are the primary stimulus for the release of hydrochloric acid from the parietal cells. Because the process of ulceration is driven by the proteolytic

(protein breakdown) actions of pepsin together with the caustic effects of hydrochloric acid, peptic ulcer disease, and related problems are also referred to by the more general term *acid-peptic disorders.*

In 1983, a gram-negative spiral bacterium, *Campylobacter pylori,* was isolated from several patients with gastritis. Over the next few years, this bacterium was studied further, and it became implicated in the pathophysiology of peptic ulcer disease. The official name of the bacterium was changed to *Helicobacter pylori* because it was felt to have more characteristics of the *Helicobacter* genus. The prevalence of *H. pylori* is approximately 40% to 60% for patients older than 60 years of age but only 10% for those younger than 30 years of age. The bacterium is found in the GI tracts of roughly 90% of patients with duodenal ulcers and 70% of those with gastric ulcers. This bacterium is also found in many patients who do not have peptic ulcer disease, and its presence is not associated with acute, perforating ulcers. These latter observations suggest that more than one factor is involved in ulceration. The American College of Gastroenterologists published treatment guidelines, last updated in 2007, for *H. pylori* infections. First-line therapy includes a 10- to 14-day course of a proton pump inhibitor (discussed later in the chapter) and the antibiotics clarithromycin and either amoxicillin or metronidazole (see Chapters 38 and 39) or a combination of a proton pump inhibitor, bismuth subsalicylate (see Chapter 51), and the antibiotics tetracycline and metronidazole (see Chapters 38 and 39). Many different combinations are used, but all incorporate the aforementioned key drugs.

Stress-related mucosal damage is an important issue for critically ill patients. Stress ulcer prophylaxis (or therapy to prevent severe GI damage) is undertaken in almost every critically ill patient in an intensive care unit (ICU) and for many patients on general medical surgical units. GI lesions are a common finding in ICU patients, especially within the first 24 hours after admission. The etiology and pathophysiology of stress-related mucosal damage is multifactorial and is not fully understood. Factors include decreased blood flow, mucosal ischemia, hypoperfusion, and reperfusion injury. Procedures performed commonly in critically ill patients, such as passing nasogastric (NG) tubes, placing patients on ventilators, and others, predispose patients to bleeding of the GI tract. Coagulopathy, a history of peptic ulcer or GI bleed, sepsis, use of steroids, ICU stay of longer than 1 week, and occult bleeding are considered to indicate a high risk for GI lesions. Guidelines suggest that all such patients receive either a histamine receptor–blocking drug or a proton pump inhibitor, both of which are discussed in detail in this chapter. However, data does not support the continued use of stress ulcer prophylaxis once the patient is moved out of the ICU.

ANTACIDS

Antacids are basic compounds used to neutralize stomach acid. Most commonly they are nonprescription salts of aluminum, magnesium, calcium, and/or sodium. They have been used for centuries in the treatment of patients with acid-related disorders. The ancient Greeks used crushed coral (calcium carbonate) in the first century AD to treat patients with dyspepsia. Antacids were the principal antiulcer treatment, along with anticholinergic drugs, until the introduction of the *histamine 2 (H₂) receptor antagonists* in the late 1970s. The use of anticholinergic drugs has fallen out of favor; however, the antacids, especially the over-the-counter (OTC) formulations, are still used extensively. They are available in a variety of dosage forms, some including more than one antacid salt. Many aluminum- and calcium-based formulations also include magnesium, which not only contributes to the acid-neutralizing capacity but also counteracts the constipating effects of aluminum and calcium. However, antacids containing magnesium must be avoided in patients with renal failure. In addition, many antacid preparations also contain the *antiflatulent* (antigas) drug simethicone (see the section on miscellaneous acid-controlling drugs), which reduces gas and bloating.

Mechanism of Action and Drug Effects

Antacids work primarily by neutralizing gastric acidity. They do not prevent the overproduction of acid but instead help to neutralize acid secretions. It is also believed that antacids promote gastric mucosal defensive mechanisms, especially at lower dosages. They do this by stimulating the secretion of mucus, prostaglandins, and bicarbonate from the cells inside the gastric glands. Mucus serves as a protective barrier against the destructive actions of hydrochloric acid. Bicarbonate helps buffer the acidity of hydrochloric acid. Prostaglandins prevent histamine from binding to its corresponding parietal cell receptors, which inhibits the production of adenylate cyclase. Without adenylate cyclase, no cAMP can be formed and no second messenger is available to activate the proton pump (see Figure 50-2).

The primary drug effect of antacids is the reduction of the symptoms associated with various acid-related disorders, such as pain and reflux ("heartburn"). Antacid-associated pain reduction is thought to be a result of base-mediated inhibition of the protein-digesting ability of pepsin, increase in the resistance of the stomach lining to irritation, and increase in the tone of the cardiac sphincter, which reduces reflux from the stomach.

Indications

Antacids are indicated for the acute relief of symptoms associated with peptic ulcer, gastritis, gastric hyperacidity, and heartburn.

Contraindications

The only usual contraindication to antacid use is known allergy to a specific drug product. Other contraindications may include severe renal failure or electrolyte disturbances (because of the potential toxic accumulation of electrolytes in the antacids themselves) and GI obstruction; for example, magnesium antacids may be contraindicated for patients with small bowel obstructions because of the laxative effect.

Adverse Effects

The adverse effects of the antacids are limited. The magnesium preparations, especially milk of magnesia, can cause diarrhea. Both the aluminum- and calcium-containing formulations can result in constipation. Calcium products can also cause kidney stones. Excessive use of any antacid can theoretically result in systemic alkalosis. This is more common with sodium bicarbonate. Another adverse effect that is more common with the calcium-containing products is rebound hyperacidity, or acid rebound, in which the patient experiences hyperacidity when antacid use is discontinued. Chronic use of high-dose calcium-containing antacids or use in renal failure can cause a syndrome known as *milk-alkali syndrome,* which is characterized by headache, nausea, alkalosis, and hypercalcemia. Long-term self-medication with antacids may mask symptoms of serious underlying disease such as bleeding ulcer or malignancy. Patients with ongoing symptoms need to undergo regular medical evaluations, because additional medications or other interventions may be needed. Box 50-1 lists several specific nursing concerns for patients taking antacids.

Interactions

Antacids are capable of causing several interactions when administered with other drugs (see Table 50-1). There are four basic mechanisms by which antacids cause interactions:
- *Adsorption* of other drugs to antacids, which reduces the ability of the other drug to be absorbed into the body
- *Chelation,* which is the chemical inactivation of other drugs that produces insoluble complexes

BOX 50-1 Nursing Concerns for Patients Taking an Antacid

Aluminum, used to reduce gastric acid, binds to phosphate and may lead to hypercalcemia. Early hypercalcemia is characterized by constipation, headache, increased thirst, dry mouth, decreased appetite, irritability, and a metallic taste in the mouth. Later signs and symptoms of hypercalcemia include confusion, drowsiness, increase in blood pressure, irregular heart rate, nausea, vomiting, and increased urination. Use of aluminum-based antacids may also produce hypophosphatemia, which is characterized by loss of appetite, malaise, muscle weakness, and/or bone pain. The use of calcium-containing antacids (e.g., calcium carbonate) may lead to *milk-alkali syndrome*, which is associated with hypercalcemia, headache, nausea, and alkalosis. Use of sodium bicarbonate may lead to metabolic alkalosis if the drug is abused or used over the long term. Alkalosis is manifested by irritability, muscle twitching, numbness and tingling, cyanosis, slow and shallow respirations, headache, thirst, and nausea. Acid rebound occurs with the discontinuation of antacids that have high acid-neutralizing capacity and with overuse or misuse of antacid therapy. If acid neutralization is sudden and high, the result is an immediate elevation in pH to alkalinity and just as rapid a decline in pH to a more acidic state in the gut.

TABLE 50-1 Antacids: Drug Interactions

Interacting Drug	Mechanism	Result
Benzodiazepines Sulfonylureas Sympathomimetics valproic acid	pH effects	Increased effects of interacting drugs
Allopurinol tetracycline Thyroid hormones captopril Corticosteroids digoxin Histamine antagonists Phenytoin isoniazid Ketoconazole Methotrexate Nitrofurantoin Phenothiazines Salicylates Quinolone antibiotics	Decreased GI absorption	Reduced effects of interacting drugs

- *Increased stomach pH,* which increases the absorption of basic drugs and decreases the absorption of acidic drugs
- *Increased urinary pH,* which increases the excretion of acidic drugs and decreases the excretion of basic drugs

Most drugs are either weak acids or weak bases. Therefore, pH conditions in both the GI and urinary tracts will affect the extent to which drug molecules are absorbed. Common examples of drugs whose effects may be chemically enhanced by the presence of antacids (due to pH effects) are benzodiazepines, sulfonylureas (effects may also be reduced, depending on the drugs involved), sympathomimetics, and valproic acid. More commonly, the presence of antacids reduces the efficacy of interacting drugs by interfering with their GI absorption. Such

BOX 50-2 Antacids

Antacids: Salt Content

Magnesium Salts	Aluminum Salts	Calcium Salts	Sodium Salts
Carbonate Hydroxide Oxide Trisilicate	Carbonate Hydroxide	Carbonate	Bicarbonate Citrate

Commonly Available Antacid Products
Magnesium-Containing Antacids
Carbonate salt: Gaviscon Liquid, Gaviscon Extra Strength Relief Formula Tablets
Hydroxide salt: milk of magnesia
Oxide salt: Mag-Ox (included for information only; used primarily as a magnesium supplement)
Trisilicate salt: Gaviscon Tablets

Aluminum-Containing Antacids
Carbonate salt: Basaljel
Hydroxide salt: AlternaGEL, Amphojel
Combination products: Gaviscon, Maalox, Mylanta, Di-Gel

Calcium-Containing Antacids
Carbonate salt: Tums, Maalox Antacid Caplets, Extra Strength Alkets Antacid

Sodium-Containing Antacids
Bicarbonate salt: Alka-Seltzer
Citrate salt: Citra pH

drugs include allopurinol, tetracycline, thyroid hormones, captopril, corticosteroids, digoxin, histamine antagonists, phenytoin, isoniazid, nitrofurantoin, phenothiazines, salicylates, and quinolone antibiotics. Advise patients to dose any interacting drugs at least 1 to 2 hours before or after antacids are taken. Significant patient harm may ensue when the quinolone antibiotics (ciprofloxacin, levofloxacin, moxifloxacin) are given with antacids. These antibiotics are administered orally to treat serious infections. Antacids can reduce their absorption by more than 50%. Thus, antacids must be given either 2 hours before or 2 hours after the dose of a quinolone antibiotic.

Dosages

For dosage information on selected antacid drugs, see the table on the next page.

DRUG PROFILES

antacids, general

Some of the available magnesium, aluminum, calcium, and sodium salts that are used in many of the antacid formulations are listed in Box 50-2. There are far too many individual antacid products on the market to mention all formulations. Briefly, OTC antacid formulations are available as capsules, chewable tablets, effervescent granules and tablets, powders, suspensions, and plain tablets. This allows patients a variety of options for self-medication. Pharmacokinetic parameters are not normally listed for antacids, but these drugs are generally excreted quickly

Selected Antacid Drugs*

Drug (Pregnancy Category)	Pharmacologic Class	Usual Adult Dosage Range	Indications
aluminum hydroxide (Amphojel) (A)	Aluminum-containing antacid	PO: 600-1200 mg 4 times per day	Hyperacidity
aluminum hydroxide and magnesium hydroxide (Maalox, Mylanta) (A)	Combination antacid	PO: 10-20 ml prn	Hyperacidity
calcium carbonate (Tums) (A)	Calcium-containing antacid	PO: 0.5-3 g prn	Hyperacidity
magnesium hydroxide (milk of magnesia) (A)	Magnesium-containing antacid	PO: 400-1200 mg prn, up to 4 times per day	Hyperacidity (more commonly used as a laxative)

*Many more antacid products are available on the market than appear in this table. Dosages given are approximate dosages of active ingredients; there may be variations among different products and different dosage forms of the same product.

through the GI tract and/or the electrolyte homeostatic mechanisms of the kidneys. Antacids are considered safe for use during pregnancy if prolonged administration and high dosages are avoided. It is recommended that pregnant women consult their health care providers before taking an antacid. Aluminum- and sodium-based antacids are often recommended for patients with renal compromise because they are more easily excreted than antacids in other categories. Calcium-containing antacids can be used as an extra source of calcium. Calcium carbonate neutralization will produce gas and possibly belching. For this reason, it may be combined with an antiflatulent drug such as simethicone (see the Miscellaneous Acid-Controlling Drugs section later in the chapter). Magnesium-containing antacids commonly have a laxative effect, and frequent administration of these antacids alone often cannot be tolerated. Both calcium- and magnesium-based antacids are more likely to accumulate to toxic levels in patients with renal disease and are often avoided in this patient group.

H₂ RECEPTOR ANTAGONISTS

H₂ receptor antagonists, commonly abbreviated as H₂RAs and also called *H₂ receptor blockers,* are the prototypical acid-secretion antagonists. These drugs reduce but do not completely abolish acid secretion. They have become the most popular drugs for the treatment of many acid-related disorders, including peptic ulcer disease. This can be attributed to their efficacy, patient acceptance, and excellent safety profile. These drugs include cimetidine, ranitidine, famotidine, and nizatidine. There is little difference among the four available H₂ receptor antagonists from the standpoint of efficacy. All are available OTC.

Mechanism of Action and Drug Effects

H₂ receptor antagonists competitively block the H₂ receptor of acid-producing parietal cells. This makes the parietal cell less responsive not only to histamine but also to the stimulation of ACh and gastrin. This is shown in Figure 50-2. Up to 90% inhibition of vagal- and gastrin-stimulated acid secretion occurs when histamine is blocked. However, complete inhibition has not been shown. The effect of these drugs is reduced hydrogen ion secretion from the parietal cells, which results in an increase in the pH of the stomach and relief of many of the symptoms associated with hyperacidity-related conditions.

Indications

H₂ receptor antagonists have several therapeutic uses, including treatment of GERD, peptic ulcer disease, and erosive esophagitis; adjunct therapy in the control of upper GI tract bleeding; and treatment of pathologic gastric hypersecretory conditions such as Zollinger-Ellison syndrome. The latter is one form of hyperchlorhydria, or excessive gastric acidity. H₂ receptor antagonists are commonly used for stress ulcer prophylaxis in critically ill patients.

Contraindications

The only usual contraindication to the use of H₂ receptor antagonists is known drug allergy. Liver and/or kidney dysfunction are relative contraindications that may warrant dosage adjustment.

Adverse Effects

The H₂ receptor antagonists have a remarkably low incidence of adverse effects (less than 3% of cases). The four available H₂ receptor antagonists are similar in many respects but have some differences in adverse-effect profiles. Table 50-2 lists the adverse effects associated with these drugs. Central nervous system adverse effects occur in less than 1% of patients taking these drugs but are sometimes seen in older adults. These adverse effects include confusion and disorientation. Be alert for mental status changes when giving these drugs, especially if they are new to the patient. Cimetidine may induce impotence and gynecomastia. This is the result of cimetidine's inhibition of estradiol metabolism and displacement of dihydrotestosterone from peripheral androgen-binding sites. All four H₂ receptor antagonists may increase the secretion of prolactin from the anterior pituitary gland. Thrombocytopenia has been reported with ranitidine and famotidine.

Interactions

Cimetidine carries a higher risk for drug interactions than the other three drugs, especially in older adults. These interactions

TABLE 50-2   H₂ Receptor Antagonists: Adverse Effects

Body System	Adverse Effects
Cardiovascular	Hypotension (monitor for this effect with intravenous administration)
Central nervous	Headache, lethargy, confusion, depression, hallucinations, slurred speech, agitation
Endocrine	Increased prolactin secretion, gynecomastia (with cimetidine)
Gastrointestinal	Diarrhea, nausea, abdominal cramps
Genitourinary	Impotence, increased blood urea nitrogen, increased creatinine levels
Hepatobiliary	Elevated liver enzyme levels, jaundice
Hematologic	Agranulocytosis, thrombocytopenia, neutropenia, aplastic anemia
Integumentary	Urticaria, rash, alopecia, sweating, flushing, exfoliative dermatitis

DOSAGES

Selected H₂ Receptor Antagonists

Drug (Pregnancy Category)	Usual Adult Dosage Range	Indications
◆ cimetidine (Tagamet, Tagamet HB) (B)	PO: 200 mg bid	Dyspepsia, heartburn
	PO: 300 mg qid or 400 mg bid or 800 mg at bedtime	Ulcers
	PO: 1600 mg/day divided in 2-4 doses	GERD
	PO/IM/IV: 300-600 mg tid and at bedtime; do not exceed 2400 mg/day	Pathologic hypersecretion
◆ famotidine (Pepcid, Pepcid AC) (B)	PO: 10 mg daily-bid	Dyspepsia, heartburn
	PO: 40 mg daily at bedtime or 20 mg bid	Ulcers
	PO: 20-160 mg every 6 hr	Pathologic hypersecretion
	PO/IV: 20-40 mg bid	GERD
ranitidine (Zantac) (B)	PO: 75 mg bid	Dyspepsia, heartburn
	PO: 150 mg daily or bid or 300 mg at bedtime	Ulcers
	PO: 150 mg qid	Erosive esophagitis

GERD, Gastroesophageal reflux disease.

may be of clinical importance. Cimetidine binds enzymes of the hepatic cytochrome P-450 microsomal oxidase system. By inhibiting the metabolism of drugs metabolized via this pathway, cimetidine may raise the blood concentrations of certain drugs. Ranitidine has only 10% to 20% of the binding action of cimetidine on the P-450 enzyme system, and nizatidine and famotidine have essentially no effect. This interaction has little clinical significance for most drugs; however, significant interactions are more likely to arise with medications having a narrow therapeutic range, such as theophylline, warfarin, lidocaine, and phenytoin. All H₂ receptor antagonists may inhibit the absorption of certain drugs, such as ketoconazole, that require an acidic GI environment for gastric absorption. Smoking has also been shown to decrease the effectiveness of H₂ antagonists. For optimal results, H₂ receptor antagonists are taken 1 to 2 hours before antacids.

Dosages

For dosage information on the H₂ antagonists, see the table on this page.

DRUG PROFILES

H₂ receptor antagonists are the prototypical acid-secretion antagonists. These drugs reduce acid secretion. They are among the most commonly used drugs in the world, due to their efficacy, OTC availability, and overall excellent safety profile. However, this drug class has been partially replaced by proton pump inhibitors (see the next section).

◆ cimetidine

In 1977, cimetidine (Tagamet) became the first drug in this class to be released on the market. It is the prototypical H₂ receptor antagonist and was the first major prescription drug to go OTC. Because of its potential to cause drug interactions, its use has been largely replaced by ranitidine and famotidine. Cimetidine is still used to treat certain allergic reactions.

Pharmacokinetics: Cimetidine

Route	Onset of Action	Peak Plasma Concentration	Elimination Half-life	Duration of Action
PO	15-60 min	1-2 hr	2 hr	4-5 hr

ranitidine

Ranitidine (Zantac) was the second H₂ receptor antagonist introduced. It does not carry the concerns over drug interactions that cimetidine has and has become the most widely used H₂ receptor antagonist. It is available in oral and intravenous forms. Dosing is different for the different forms: oral ranitidine is dosed as 150 mg twice a day or 300 mg at bedtime, whereas the intravenous form is dosed at 50 mg every 8 hours.

Pharmacokinetics: Ranitidine

Route	Onset of Action	Peak Plasma Concentration	Elimination Half-life	Duration of Action
PO	1 hr	2-4 hr	2-3 hr	4-12 hr
IV	Immediate	Less than 15 min	2-3 hr	4-12 hr

◆ famotidine

Famotidine (Pepcid) was the last H₂ receptor antagonist introduced and, like ranitidine, has no drug interaction concerns. It is available in oral and injectable forms. The dosing is the same for both forms.

Pharmacokinetics: Famotidine

Route	Onset of Action	Peak Plasma Concentration	Elimination Half-life	Duration of Action
PO	1.4 hr	3 hr	2.6-4 hr	9-12 hr
IV	Immediate	Less than 15 min	2.6-4 hr	9-12 hr

PROTON PUMP INHIBITORS

The newest drugs introduced for the treatment of acid-related disorders are the proton pump inhibitors (PPIs). These include lansoprazole (Prevacid), omeprazole (Prilosec), rabeprazole (AcipHex), pantoprazole (Protonix), esomeprazole (Nexium), and dexlansoprazole (Dexilant). Zegerid is a combination of omeprazole and sodium bicarbonate. These drugs are even more powerful than the H_2 receptor antagonists. The PPIs bind directly to the hydrogen-potassium-ATPase pump mechanism and irreversibly inhibit the action of this enzyme, which results in a total blockage of hydrogen ion secretion from the parietal cells.

Mechanism of Action and Drug Effects

The action of the hydrogen-potassium-ATPase pump is the final step in the acid-secretory process of the parietal cell (see Figure 50-2). If chemical energy is present to run the pump, the pump will transport hydrogen ions out of the parietal cell, which increases the acid content of the surrounding gastric lumen and lowers the pH. Because hydrogen ions are protons (positively charged atoms), this ion pump is also called the *proton pump*. Proton pump inhibitors (PPIs) bind irreversibly to the proton pump. This inhibition prevents the movement of hydrogen ions out of the parietal cell into the stomach and thereby blocks all gastric acid secretion. The PPIs stop more than 90% of acid secretion over 24 hours, which makes most patients temporarily achlorhydric (without acid). Achlorhydria can cause complications such as bacterial overgrowth, intestinal metaplasia, and hip fracture. However, food absorption is not affected. For acid secretion to return to normal after a PPI has been stopped, the parietal cell must synthesize new hydrogen-potassium-ATPase. Although there are other proton pumps in the body, hydrogen-potassium-ATPase is structurally and mechanically distinct from other hydrogen-transporting enzymes and appears to exist only in the parietal cells. Thus, the action of PPIs is limited to its effects on gastric acid secretion.

Indications

PPIs are currently indicated as first-line therapy for erosive esophagitis, symptomatic GERD that is poorly responsive to other medical treatment such as therapy with H_2 receptor antagonists, short-term treatment of active duodenal ulcers and active benign gastric ulcers, gastric hypersecretory conditions (e.g., Zollinger-Ellison syndrome), nonsteroidal antiinflammatory drug (NSAID)–induced ulcers, and for stress ulcer prophylaxis. Long-term therapeutic uses include maintenance of healing of erosive esophagitis and pathologic hypersecretory conditions, including both GERD and Zollinger-Ellison syndrome. All of the PPIs can be used in combination with antibiotics to treat patients with *H. pylori* infections. The PPIs can be given orally or through an NG or percutaneous enterogastric tube. For example, esomeprazole capsules may be opened, the granules dissolved in 50 mL of water, and the solution given through the tube. Similar tubal administration is also listed by the manufacturer for lansoprazole capsules and omeprazole powder for oral suspension. Consult the drug packaging for drug-specific instructions. Be aware of the particle size of the drug once it is in solution and the tube size being used. For example, pantoprazole granules are to be used with NG tubes that are larger than 16-French, and it may clog the tube if used with small tubes. Several of the PPIs are now also available for intravenous use.

Contraindications

The only usual contraindication to use of the PPIs is known drug allergy.

Adverse Effects

PPIs are generally well tolerated. The frequency of adverse effects has been similar to that for placebo or H_2 receptor antagonists. There are concerns that these drugs may be overprescribed and may predispose patients to GI tract infections because of the reduction of the normal acid-mediated antimicrobial protection. New concerns have arisen over the potential for long-term users of PPIs to develop osteoporosis. This is thought to be due to the inhibition of stomach acid, and it is speculated that PPIs speed up bone mineral loss. The Food and Drug Administration issued a warning in 2010 regarding long-term use of high-dose PPIs, which has been associated with *Clostridium difficile* infections; risk for wrist, hip, and spine fractures; and pneumonia. In 2011, depletion of magnesium was added to the warning.

Interactions

Few drug interactions occur with the PPIs; however, they may increase serum levels of diazepam and phenytoin. There may be an increased chance of bleeding in patients who are taking both a PPI and warfarin. Other possible interactions include interference with the absorption of ketoconazole, ampicillin, iron salts, and digoxin. When given with clopidogrel, there is some concern of an increased risk for death if the patient has acute coronary syndrome; however, recent studies have not substantiated this concern. Sucralfate may delay the absorption of PPIs. Food may decrease the absorption of PPIs, and it is recommended that they be taken on an empty stomach.

Dosages

For dosage information on selected PPIs, see the table on the next page.

DRUG PROFILES

◆ omeprazole

Omeprazole (Prilosec) was the first drug in this breakthrough class of antisecretory drugs. Other PPIs include lansoprazole (Prevacid), esomeprazole (Nexium), rabeprazole (AcipHex), pantoprazole (Protonix), and dexlansoprazole (Dexilant). Zegerid is a combination of omeprazole and sodium bicarbonate. Orally administered PPIs (and H_2 receptor antagonists) often work best when taken 30 to 60 minutes before meals. Many of the PPIs are also available for IV administration.

Pharmacokinetics: Omeprazole

Route	Onset of Action	Peak Plasma Concentration	Elimination Half-life	Duration of Action
PO	2 hr	5 days	0.5-1 hr	1-5 days

lansoprazole

Lansoprazole (Prevacid) is available in a delayed-release capsule, granules for oral suspension, and orally disintegrating tablets (Prevacid SoluTab). The capsules can be opened and mixed (not crushed) with apple juice for administration via NG tube, or the SoluTab can be dissolved in water. Lansoprazole is also available as combination products for the treatment of *H. Pylori* infection.

Pharmacokinetics: Lansoprazole

Route	Onset of Action	Peak Plasma Concentration	Elimination Half-life	Duration of Action
PO	1.7 hr	4 wk	1-2 hr	24 hr

pantoprazole

Pantoprazole (Protonix) was the first PPI available for intravenous use. It was also the first drug to be used as a continuous infusion for the treatment of GI bleeding. It is available as an oral tablet and as delayed-release granules for NG administration. However, the granules are large, and the NG tube must be at least size 16-French, or the granules may clog the tube.

Pharmacokinetics: Pantoprazole

Route	Onset of Action	Peak Plasma Concentration	Elimination Half-life	Duration of Action
PO	2.5 hr	2-2.5 hr	1 hr	7 days
IV	End of infusion	End of infusion	1 hr	7 days

DOSAGES

Selected Proton Pump Inhibitors

Drug (Pregnancy Category)	Usual Adult Dosage Range	Indications
lansoprazole (Prevacid) (B)	PO: 30 mg daily	GERD, ulcer, erosive esophagitis
♦ omeprazole (Prilosec) (C)	PO: 20 mg/day for 4-8 wk	Esophagitis, duodenal ulcer, hypersecretory conditions
	PO: 60 mg PO daily initially, then titrated and given in single or multiple daily doses, with dosage titration up to a maximum of 120 mg PO tid	
pantoprazole (Protonix) (B)	PO/IV: 20-80 mg/day depending on indication	GERD, ulcer, stress ulcer prophylaxis

GERD, Gastroesophageal reflux disease.

MISCELLANEOUS ACID-CONTROLLING DRUGS

There are a few other acid-controlling drugs that are unique in terms of their mechanisms and other features. These include sucralfate, misoprostol, and simethicone. They are profiled individually in the following paragraphs. Other drugs are bismuth subsalicylate (Pepto-Bismol; see Chapter 51) and metoclopramide (see Chapter 52).

DRUG PROFILES

♦ sucralfate

Sucralfate (Carafate) is a drug used as a mucosal protectant in the treatment of active stress ulcerations and in long-term therapy for peptic ulcer disease. Sucralfate acts locally, not systemically, binding directly to the surface of an ulcer. Sucralfate has sucrose as its basic structure. Once sucralfate comes into contact with the acid of the stomach, it begins to dissociate into aluminum hydroxide (an antacid) and sulfate anions. The aluminum salt stimulates secretion of both mucus and bicarbonate base. The sulfated sucrose molecules of sucralfate are attracted to and bind to positively charged tissue proteins at the bases of ulcers and erosions, forming a protective barrier that can be thought of as a liquid bandage. By binding to the exposed proteins of ulcers and erosions, sucralfate also limits the access of pepsin. Pepsin is an enzyme that normally breaks down proteins in food but can have the same effect on GI epithelial tissue, either causing ulcers or making them worse. Sucralfate also binds and concentrates epidermal growth factor, present in the gastric tissues, which promotes ulcer healing. In addition, the drug stimulates the gastric secretion of prostaglandin molecules, which serve a mucoprotective function. Despite its many beneficial actions, sucralfate has fallen out of common use because its effects are transient, and multiple daily dosing (up to four times daily) is therefore needed. It is indicated for stress ulcers, esophageal erosions, and peptic ulcer disease. The only usual contraindication to sucralfate use is known drug allergy. Adverse effects are uncommon but include nausea, constipation, and dry mouth. Only minimal systemic absorption occurs, and the drug is virtually inert. Sucralfate does not display typical pharmacokinetic parameters, and, as such, no pharmacokinetic table is listed. Drug interactions mainly involve physical interference with the absorption of other drugs. This can be alleviated by taking other drugs at least 2 hours ahead of sucralfate. Sucralfate is also best given 1 hour before meals and at bedtime. It is classified as a pregnancy category B drug that is normally dosed at 1 g orally four times daily.

misoprostol

Misoprostol (Cytotec), a prostaglandin E analogue, has been shown to effectively reduce the incidence of gastric ulcers in patients taking NSAIDs (see Chapter 44). Prostaglandins are thought to inhibit gastric acid secretion. They are also believed to protect the gastric mucosa from injury (cytoprotective function), possibly by enhancing the local production of mucus or bicarbonate, by promoting local cell regeneration, and by helping to maintain mucosal blood flow. Use of misoprostol is contraindicated in patients with known drug allergy and in pregnant women (see later in the chapter). Adverse effects include headache, GI distress, and vaginal bleeding. There are no major drug interactions, although antacids may reduce drug absorption.

Although some studies show that synthetic analogues of prostaglandins promote the healing of duodenal ulcers, the drugs must be used in dosages that usually produce disturbing adverse effects, such as abdominal cramps and diarrhea. Thus, they are not believed to be as effective as H_2 receptor antagonists and PPIs for this indication. Misoprostol is also used for its abortifacient properties as discussed in Chapter 34. For this reason, it is classified a pregnancy category X drug. The usual dosage is 200 mcg four times daily with meals for the duration of NSAID therapy in patients at high risk for ulceration.

Pharmacokinetics: Misoprostol

Route	Onset of Action	Peak Plasma Concentration	Elimination Half-life	Duration of Action
PO	30 min	12 min	20-40 min	1-2 days

simethicone

Simethicone (Mylicon) is used to reduce the discomforts of gastric or intestinal gas (flatulence) and aid in its release via the mouth or rectum. It is therefore classified as an antiflatulent drug. Gas commonly appears in the GI tract as a consequence of the swallowing of air as well as normal digestive processes. Gas in the upper GI tract is composed of swallowed air and thus consists largely of nitrogen. It is usually expelled from the body by belching. The composition of flatus, however, is determined largely by the dietary intake of carbohydrates and the metabolic activity of the bacteria in the intestines.

Some foods, including legumes (beans) and cruciferous vegetables (e.g., cauliflower, broccoli), are well known for their gas-producing ability. Gas can also result from disorders such as diverticulitis, dyspepsia (heartburn), peptic ulcers, and spastic or irritable colon; gaseous distention can also occur postoperatively. Simethicone works by altering the elasticity of mucus-coated gas bubbles, which causes them to break into smaller ones. This reduces gas pain and facilitates the expulsion of gas via the mouth or rectum. Simethicone has no listed adverse effects, drug interactions, or pharmacokinetic parameters. It is available only for oral use. The usual simethicone dosage is 1 to 2 tablets four to six times daily as needed. A variety of different simethicone products are available for OTC use.

NURSING PROCESS

ASSESSMENT

Before an *acid-controlling drug* is given, perform a thorough patient assessment with attention to past and present medical history, with special focus on GI tract–related disorders and signs and symptoms of ulcer disease and GERD. Assess current bowel patterns, any change in bowel patterns or GI tract functioning, and GI tract–related pain. Document the findings.

Assess results of any prescribed baseline serum chemistry laboratory tests. Pay special attention to hepatic function (e.g., serum ALP, ALT, AST levels) and renal function (serum creatinine and BUN levels). Assess for contraindications, cautions, and drug interactions. Be aware that acid-controlling drugs have many interactions, so it is critical to patient safety to pay close attention to all medications the patient is taking. This underscores the importance of obtaining a thorough medication history including information about prescription drugs, OTCs, herbals, and supplements. Other components of assessment include performing a physical examination and taking a thorough cardiac history with close attention to a history of heart failure, hypertension, other cardiac diseases, the presence of edema, fluid and electrolyte imbalances, and renal disease. One reason it is important to assess for these conditions is that the high sodium content of various antacids, if used, could lead to exacerbation of cardiac problems, renal dysfunction, and fluid-electrolyte problems.

When *antacids* containing aluminum and/or magnesium are used, identify all other medications the patient is taking. It is important to note that combination products containing both magnesium and aluminum may have fewer adverse effects than either type of antacid by itself. For example, *aluminum-containing antacids* are associated with constipation, whereas *magnesium-containing antacids* may lead to diarrhea. The net effect of a combination of these antacids is a balancing out of both adverse effects and fewer problems with altered bowel patterns. *Calcium-based antacids* may also be used, especially as a source of calcium; however, they carry the risk for rebound hyperacidity, milk-alkali syndrome, and changes in systemic pH, especially if the patient has abnormal renal functioning (see Box 50-1). *Sodium bicarbonate* is generally not recommended as an antacid because of the high risk for systemic electrolyte disturbances and alkalosis. The sodium content of sodium bicarbonate is also high, which is very problematic for patients who have hypertension, heart failure, or renal insufficiency.

For patients using *H_2 receptor antagonist drugs*, assess renal and liver function as well as level of consciousness because of possible drug-related adverse effects. Older adult patients are known to react to these drugs with more disorientation and confusion. Do not administer drugs such as *cimetidine* and *famotidine* simultaneously with antacids. These drugs may be spaced 1 hour apart if both drugs need to be given. In patients taking *nizatidine* or *ranitidine*, assess baseline blood chemistry results with attention to levels of BUN, creatinine, bilirubin, ALP, AST, and ALT to document renal and hepatic functioning before treatment is initiated.

For *PPIs* (e.g., *lansoprazole, omeprazole, pantoprazole*), assess swallowing capacity because of the size of some of the oral capsules. Assess the patient's medical history with an emphasis on any history of GI tract infections due to decreased acid-mediated antimicrobial protection. Since there are documented concerns about the use of PPIs and the development of osteoporosis, thoroughly assess patients for any manifestations and/or history of this disorder. Drug interactions have been discussed previously in the pharmacology section, but important to mention are the interactions with diazepam, phenytoin, warfarin, ampicillin, and iron salts. Always check the patient's medication list before these or any other types of medication are given.

Other GI-related drugs include *sucralfate* and *simethicone*. The use of simethicone (an antiflatulent) and sucralfate (an ulcer adherent) requires assessment of the patient's bowel patterns and bowel sounds. Assess for abdominal distention and rigidity, which may indicate a medical emergency. Treatment of peptic ulcer disease has become focused on the use of antibiotics (to attack the *H. pylori* bacteria) with frequent dosing of other drugs. Inquire also about the presence of any unusual signs and symptoms related to the GI tract.

NURSING DIAGNOSES

1. Constipation related to the adverse effects of aluminum-containing antacids and other drugs used to treat hyperacidity
2. Diarrhea related to the adverse effects of magnesium-containing antacids and other drugs used to treat hyperacidity
3. Deficient knowledge related to lack of information about antacids, H_2 receptor antagonists, or PPIs, including their use and potential adverse effects

PLANNING: OUTCOME IDENTIFICATION

1. Patient experiences minimal to no constipation due to measures taken such as taking only as prescribed and taking aluminum/magnesium combination products, as indicated or prescribed.
2. Patient experiences minimal to no adverse effects of diarrhea through avoiding magnesium-only antacids, especially milk of magnesia, and taking combination aluminum/magnesium products.
3. Patient demonstrates adequate knowledge about the use of acid-controlling medications with stating of the purpose of taking antacids, H_2 receptor antagonists, and PPIs for management of gastric hyperacidity as well as the various adverse effects and when to seek further medical attention.

IMPLEMENTATION

When giving *acid-controlling drugs*, instruct the patient to thoroughly chew the chewable tablets. Liquid forms need to be shaken thoroughly before administered. *Antacids* need to be given with at least 8 ounces of water to enhance absorption of the antacid in the stomach, except for newer dosage forms that are rapidly dissolving drugs. If constipation or diarrhea occurs with single-component drugs, a *combination aluminum- and magnesium-based antacid* may be preferred. Educate the patient about the adverse effects of *aluminum-only* or *magnesium-only products*. It is also recommended that antacids be given as ordered, but not within 1 to 2 hours of other medications because antacids may impair absorption of other oral

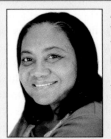
medications. You may safely implement this dosing schedule without interrupting the safe dosing of other medications. The dosing will differ if the prescriber has ordered the drug to be given with antacids. With quinolone antibiotics, there may be serious harm if given with antacids because of a 50% reduction in antibiotic absorption. Serious infections may then go unsuccessfully treated due to altered absorption. Antacid overuse/misuse or the rapid discontinuation of antacids with high acid-neutralizing capacity may lead to acid rebound. Therefore, antacids are only to be used as prescribed and/or as directed.

Because so many *H_2 receptor antagonists* and other acid-controlling drugs are now available OTC, instruct the patient about proper use (see Patient-Centered Care: Patient Teaching on the next page for more information). For example, *cimetidine* is to be taken with meals, and antacids, if also used, need to be taken 1 to 2 hours after the cimetidine. Intravenous dosing and related mixing and infusing for intravenous cimetidine are similar to those described later for intravenous famotidine. *Famotidine* may be given orally in tablet or suspension form and without regard to meals or food. Rapid-release forms of famotidine dissolve quickly under the patient's tongue and can be taken without water. Give *ranitidine* as ordered, and, if administered with antacids, give the antacids 1 hour before or 1 hour after ranitidine. Dilute intravenous forms of famotidine or ranitidine with appropriate solutions, and infuse over the documented time frame. With intravenous H_2 receptor antagonists, hypotension may occur with rapid infusion, so careful monitoring is critical to patient safety. Refer to appropriate sources for information on other specific drugs and their intravenous administration. For all H_2 receptor antagonists, monitor blood pressure readings as needed during intravenous infusion because of the risk for hypotension. Continue to monitor the patient for GI tract bleeding with the diagnosis of ulcers or GI irritation. Report any blood in the stools or the occurrence of black, tarry stools or hematemesis. Listen to bowel sounds, and examine the abdomen to monitor for possible complications.

With *PPIs,* give *lansoprazole* oral dosage forms as ordered. If the patient has difficulty swallowing these capsules, a capsule may be opened and the granules sprinkled over at least a tablespoon of applesauce, which then must be swallowed immediately. Administer *omeprazole* before meals, and educate the patient that the capsule must be taken whole and not crushed, opened, or chewed. Omeprazole may also be given with antacids, if ordered. Always double-check the names and dosages of these drugs to ensure that they are not confused with similarly named drugs. *Pantoprazole* may be given orally without crushing or splitting of the tablet form. Give intravenous dosage forms exactly as ordered using the correct dilutional fluids. Infuse over the recommended time period.

Other GI-related drugs, such as *simethicone,* may also be added to the oral medication protocol with PPIs. Simethicone is usually well tolerated. It is to be taken after meals and at bedtime. Instruct patients to thoroughly chew the tablets or to shake suspensions well before use. *Sucralfate* is usually given 1 hour before meals and at bedtime. Tablets may be crushed or dissolved in water, if needed. Antacids are to be avoided for 30 minutes before or after administration of sucralfate. *Misoprostol* is to be given with food and is usually ordered to be taken with meals and at bedtime. See Patient-Centered Care: Patient Teaching for suggestions on drug-related patient education.

EVALUATION

Therapeutic response to the administration of *antacids, H_2 receptor antagonists, PPIs,* and *other GI-related drugs* includes the relief of symptoms associated with peptic ulcer, gastritis, esophagitis, gastric hyperacidity, or hiatal hernia (i.e., decrease in epigastric pain, fullness, and abdominal swelling). Adverse effects for which to monitor include all of those listed for each of the drug categories and range from constipation or diarrhea to nausea, vomiting, abdominal pain, and hypotension. Milk-alkali syndrome, acid rebound, hypercalcemia, and metabolic alkalosis are known complications associated with the various antacids; evaluate the patient for these adverse effects, and take measures to prevent or resolve them.

PATIENT-CENTERED CARE: PATIENT TEACHING

- Encourage patients to keep a daily journal of precipitating and/or alleviating factors to their symptoms.
- Antacids are to not to be taken within 1 to 2 hours of other medications because of the impaired absorption on oral medications.
- All antacids are to be taken with at least 8 ounces of water to ensure absorption in the stomach, as with all oral medications.
- Advise the patient to contact the prescriber immediately if there is severe or prolonged constipation and/or diarrhea; increase in abdominal pain; abdominal distension; nausea; vomiting; hematemesis; or black, tarry stools (a sign of possible GI tract bleeding).
- If the patient is taking enteric-coated medications, educate about the fact that the use of antacids may promote premature dissolution of the enteric coating. Enteric coatings are used to diminish the stomach upset caused by irritating medications, and if the coating is destroyed early in the stomach, gastric upset may occur.
- Antacids are not to be used for prolonged periods without medical attention. A health care provider should be contacted after 2 weeks of self-prescribed antacid use.
- Encourage the patient to take H_2 receptor antagonists exactly as prescribed. Inform the patient that smoking decreases the drug's effectiveness. Advise the patient taking cimetidine and antacids that the antacid is to be taken either 1 hour before or after the cimetidine.
- Gynecomastia and impotence may occur with cimetidine and are reversible. Encourage patients to report bruising, fatigue, diarrhea, black tarry stools, sore throat, or rash to their prescriber.
- Ranitidine is not to be taken for more than 2 weeks. Once-daily dosing is recommended before bedtime.
- Omeprazole and other PPIs are to be taken before meals. Inform the patient that if lansoprazole is being used, the granules may be sprinkled from the capsule into a tablespoon of applesauce if needed.
- For patients with GERD or hyperacidity, educate about the avoidance of black pepper, caffeine, alcohol, harsh spices, and extremes in food temperature.
- Instruct the patient to follow the manufacturer's directions when taking simethicone. Chewable forms must always be chewed thoroughly; liquid preparations need to be shaken thoroughly before administration. Encourage patients experiencing flatulence to avoid problematic foods (e.g., spicy, gas-producing foods) and carbonated beverages.
- Sucralfate must be taken on an empty stomach, and antacids are to be avoided or, if indicated, taken 30 minutes before or after the use of sucralfate.
- For a patient taking the drug regimen for the treatment of *H. pylori* infection–peptic ulcer disease, it is important to emphasize the need to take each drug, including the antibiotics, exactly as prescribed and without fail to guarantee successful treatment. If treatment protocols are not followed appropriately, the condition may likely recur.

KEY POINTS

- The stomach secretes many substances (hydrochloric acid, pepsinogen, mucus, bicarbonate, intrinsic factor, and prostaglandins).
- The parietal cell is responsible for the production of acid.
- In acid-related disorders, there is an impairment of the balance among the substances secreted by the stomach.
- H_2 receptor antagonists are H_2 blockers that bind to and block histamine receptors located on parietal cells. This blockade renders these cells less responsive to stimuli and thus decreases their acid secretion. Up to 90% inhibition of acid secretion can be achieved with the H_2 receptor antagonists.
- PPIs block the final step in the acid production pathway, the hydrogen-potassium-ATPase pump, and they block all acid secretion.
- Sucralfate is used for the treatment of peptic ulcer disease and stress-related ulcers. It binds to tissue proteins in the eroded area and prevents exposure of the ulcerated area to stomach acid.
- Misoprostol is a synthetic prostaglandin analogue that inhibits gastric acid secretion and is used to prevent NSAID-related ulcers.
- Cautious use of antacids is recommended in patients who have heart failure, hypertension, or other cardiac diseases or who require sodium restriction, especially if the antacid is high in sodium.
- Many drug interactions occur with the acid-controlling drugs due to alteration of oral dosage forms, and so other medications are to be avoided within 1 to 2 hours of taking an antacid.
- Magnesium-aluminum combination antacids are used to prevent the adverse effects of constipation and diarrhea. Some of the more serious concerns with antacids include acid rebound, hypercalcemia, milk-alkali syndrome, and metabolic alkalosis.

NCLEX® EXAMINATION REVIEW QUESTIONS

1. A 30-year-old patient is taking simethicone for excessive flatus associated with diverticulitis. During a patient teaching session, the nurse explains the mechanism of action of simethicone by saying:
   a. "It neutralizes gastric pH, thereby preventing gas."
   b. "It buffers the effects of pepsin on the gastric wall."
   c. "It decreases gastric acid secretion and thereby minimizes flatus."
   d. "It causes mucus-coated gas bubbles to break into smaller ones."

2. When evaluating the medication list of a patient who will be starting therapy with an H_2 receptor antagonist, the nurse is aware that which drug may interact with it?
   a. codeine
   b. penicillin
   c. phenytoin
   d. acetaminophen

3. Which is the correct action when the nurse is administering sucralfate?
   a. Giving the drug with meals
   b. Giving the drug on an empty stomach
   c. Instructing the patient to restrict fluids
   d. Waiting 30 minutes before administering other drugs

4. A patient with a history of renal problems is asking for advice about which antacid he should use. The nurse will make which recommendation?
   a. "Patients with renal problems cannot use antacids."
   b. "Aluminum-based antacids are the best choice for you."
   c. "Calcium-based antacids are the best choice for you."
   d. "Magnesium-based antacids are the best choice for you."

5. A patient who is taking oral tetracycline complains of heartburn and requests an antacid. Which action by the nurse is correct?
   a. Give the tetracycline, but delay the antacid for 1 to 2 hours.
   b. Give the antacid, but delay the tetracycline for at least 4 hours.
   c. Administer both medications together.
   d. Explain that the antacid cannot be given while the patient is taking the tetracycline.

6. When the nurse is administering a proton pump inhibitor (PPI), which actions by the nurse are correct? (Select all that apply.)
   a. Giving the PPI on an empty stomach
   b. Giving the PPI with meals
   c. Making sure the patient does not crush or chew the capsules
   d. Instructing the patient to open the capsule and chew the contents for best absorption
   e. Administering the PPI only when the patient complains of heartburn

7. The order reads: "Give cimetidine (Tagamet) 300 mg in 100 mL normal saline IVPB tid and at bedtime. Infuse over 30 minutes." The infusion pump can only be programmed to deliver over 60 minutes (mL per hour). The nurse will set the pump to deliver how many mL/hour for each IVPB dose?

8. The nurse is preparing to administer the first dose of misoprostol (Cytotec) for a patient who has been diagnosed with a gastric ulcer. What condition would be a contraindication to this medication?
   a. Hypothyroidism
   b. Type 2 diabetes mellitus
   c. Pregnancy
   d. Hypertension

1. d, 2. c, 3. b, 4. b, 5. a, 6. a, c, 7. 200 mL/hour, 8. c.

CRITICAL THINKING AND PRIORITIZATION QUESTIONS

1. A patient with a history of decreased renal function tells the nurse, "I have finally found an antacid that gives me great relief!" The nurse checks the antacid's content and finds that the antacid is a combination of aluminum hydroxide and magnesium hydroxide. What is the nurse's priority action at this time? Explain your answer.

2. A patient tells the nurse, "I like taking antacids because they coat my stomach and protect my ulcer." What is the nurse's priority when answering the patient's question?

For answers, see *http://evolve.elsevier.com/Lilley.*

ⓔ EVOLVE WEBSITE

http://evolve.elsevier.com/Lilley
- Animations
- Answer Keys for Textbook Case Studies and Textbook Critical Thinking and Prioritization Questions

- Content Updates
- Key Points
- Review Questions
- Student Case Studies

Bowel Disorder Drugs

http://evolve.elsevier.com/Lilley

OBJECTIVES

When you reach the end of this chapter, you will be able to do the following:

1. Discuss the anatomy and physiology of the gastrointestinal tract, including the process of peristalsis.
2. Identify the various factors affecting bowel elimination and/or bowel patterns.
3. List the various groups of drugs used to treat alterations in bowel elimination, specifically diarrhea, constipation, and irritable bowel syndrome (IBS).
4. Discuss the mechanisms of action, indications, cautions, contraindications, drug interactions, dosages, routes of administration, and adverse effects of the various antidiarrheals, probiotics, laxatives, and IBS drugs.
5. Develop a nursing care plan that includes all phases of the nursing process for patients taking antidiarrheals, probiotics, laxatives, and IBS drugs.

DRUG PROFILES

belladonna alkaloid combinations, p. 816
bisacodyl, p. 822
bismuth subsalicylate, p. 816
♦ diphenoxylate with atropine, p. 816
♦ docusate salts, p. 821
♦ glycerin, p. 821
♦ *Lactobacillus*, p. 817
♦ lactulose, p. 822
♦ loperamide, p. 816

magnesium salts, p. 822
methylcellulose, p. 820
mineral oil, p. 821
polyethylene glycol 3350, p. 822
♦ psyllium, p. 820
♦ senna, p. 822

─────────
♦ = *Key drug*
! = *High-alert drug*

KEY TERMS

Antidiarrheal drugs Drugs that counter or combat diarrhea. (p. 815)

Constipation A condition of abnormally infrequent and difficult passage of feces through the lower gastrointestinal tract. (p. 818)

Diarrhea The abnormally frequent passage of loose stools. (p. 814)

Irritable bowel syndrome (IBS) A recurring condition of the intestinal tract characterized by bloating, flatulence, and often periods of diarrhea that alternate with periods of constipation. (p. 822)

Laxatives Drugs that promote bowel evacuation, such as by increasing the bulk of the feces, softening the stool, or lubricating the intestinal wall. (p. 818)

OVERVIEW

Diarrhea and the diseases associated with it account for 5 to 8 million deaths per year in infants and small children and are among the leading causes of death and morbidity in underdeveloped nations. The key symptoms of gastrointestinal (GI) disease are abdominal pain, nausea and/or vomiting, and diarrhea. Diarrhea is defined as the passage of stools with abnormally increased frequency, fluidity, and weight, or increased stool water excretion. Acute diarrhea refers to diarrhea of sudden onset in a previously healthy individual. It lasts from 3

days to 2 weeks and is self-limiting. Chronic diarrhea lasts for longer than 3 to 4 weeks and is associated with recurrent passage of diarrheal stools, possible fever, nausea, vomiting, weight reduction, and chronic weakness.

The probable cause of diarrhea needs to be taken into consideration when designing a drug regimen to treat it. Causes of acute diarrhea include drugs, bacteria, viruses, nutritional factors, and protozoa. Causes of chronic diarrhea include tumors, acquired immunodeficiency syndrome (AIDS), diabetes mellitus, hyperthyroidism, Addison's disease, and irritable bowel syndrome (IBS). Treatment is aimed at stopping the stool frequency, alleviating the abdominal cramps, replenishing fluids and electrolytes, and preventing weight loss and nutritional deficits from malabsorption. Often, replacement of fluids is the only treatment needed. Patients with diarrhea associated with a bacterial or parasitic infection must not use antidiarrheal drugs, because this will cause the organism to stay in the body longer and will prolong recovery.

ANTIDIARRHEALS

Drugs used to treat diarrhea are called antidiarrheal drugs. Based on the specific mechanism of action, they are divided into different groups: adsorbents, antimotility drugs (anticholinergics and opiates), and probiotics (also known as *intestinal flora modifiers* and *bacterial replacement drugs*). The specific classes and the drugs in each are listed in Table 51-1. Antidiarrheal and laxative drugs do not have the classic pharmacokinetics of other drugs, and thus pharmacokinetics tables such as those presented throughout the book are not included in this chapter.

Mechanism of Action and Drug Effects

Antidiarrheal drugs have varying mechanisms of action. Adsorbents act by coating the walls of the GI tract. They bind the causative bacteria or toxin to their adsorbent surface for elimination from the body through the stool. Adsorption is similar to absorption but differs in that it involves the chemical binding of substances (e.g., ions, bacterial toxins) onto the surface of an adsorbent. The adsorbent bismuth subsalicylate is a form of aspirin, and therefore it also has many of the same drug effects as aspirin (see Chapter 44). Activated charcoal not only is helpful in coating the walls of the GI tract and adsorbing bacteria but also is useful in cases of overdose because of its drug-binding properties. The antilipemic drugs colestipol and cholestyramine (see Chapter 27) are anion exchange resins that are sometimes prescribed as antidiarrheal adsorbents and lipid-lowering drugs. Besides binding to diarrhea-causing toxins, they have the additional benefit of decreasing cholesterol levels.

Anticholinergic drugs work to slow peristalsis by reducing the rhythmic contractions and smooth muscle tone of the GI tract; they also have a drying effect and reduce gastric secretions. They are used in combination with adsorbents and opiates (see later in the chapter). Anticholinergics are discussed in detail in Chapter 21.

Probiotics are products obtained from bacterial cultures, most commonly *Lactobacillus* organisms, which make up the majority of the body's normal bacterial flora. These organisms are commonly destroyed by antibiotics. Probiotics work by replenishing these bacteria, which helps to restore the balance of normal flora and suppress the growth of diarrhea-causing bacteria.

The primary action of *opiates* (see Chapter 10) in diarrhea treatment is to reduce bowel motility. A secondary effect that makes opiates beneficial in the treatment of diarrhea is reduction of the pain associated with diarrhea by relief of rectal spasms. Because they decrease the transit time of food through the GI tract, they permit longer contact of the intestinal contents with the absorptive surface of the bowel, which increases the absorption of water, electrolytes, and other nutrients from the bowel and reduces stool frequency and net volume.

Indications

Antidiarrheal drugs are indicated for the treatment of diarrhea of various types and levels of severity. Adsorbents are more likely to be used in milder cases, whereas anticholinergics and opiates tend to be used in more severe cases. Probiotics are often helpful in patients with antibiotic-induced diarrhea.

Contraindications

Contraindications to the use of antidiarrheals include known drug allergy and any major acute GI condition, such as intestinal obstruction or colitis, unless the drug is ordered by the patient's prescriber after careful consideration of the specific case.

Adverse Effects

The adverse effects of the antidiarrheals are specific to each drug family. Most of these potential effects are minor and are not life threatening. The major adverse effects of specific drugs in each drug class are listed in Table 51-2. Probiotics do not have any listed adverse effects.

Interactions

Many drugs are absorbed from the intestines into the bloodstream, where they are delivered to their respective sites of action. A number of the antidiarrheals have the potential to

---

TABLE 51-1 Antidiarrheals: Drug Categories and Selected Drugs

Category	Antidiarrheal Drugs
Adsorbents	Activated charcoal, aluminum hydroxide, bismuth subsalicylate, cholestyramine, polycarbophil
Anticholinergics	Atropine, hyoscyamine
Opiates	Opium tincture, paregoric, codeine, diphenoxylate, loperamide
Probiotics and intestinal flora modifiers	*Lactobacillus acidophilus, Lactobacillus GG, Saccharomyces boulardii*

TABLE 51-2 Selected Antidiarrheals: Adverse Effects

Drug	Adverse Effects
bismuth subsalicylate	Increased bleeding time, constipation, dark stools, confusion, tinnitus, metallic taste, blue gums
atropine, hyoscyamine	Urinary retention, impotence, headache, dizziness, anxiety, drowsiness, bradycardia, hypotension, dry skin, flushing, blurred vision
codeine, diphenoxylate	Drowsiness, dizziness, lethargy, nausea, vomiting, constipation, hypotension, urinary retention, flushing, respiratory depression

alter this normal process, by either increasing or decreasing the absorption of these other drugs.

The adsorbents can decrease the effectiveness of many drugs, primarily by decreasing the absorption of certain drugs. Examples include digoxin, quinidine, and hypoglycemic drugs. The oral anticoagulant warfarin (see Chapter 26) is more likely to cause increased bleeding times or bruising when coadministered with adsorbents. This is thought to be because the adsorbents bind to vitamin K, which is needed to make certain clotting factors. Vitamin K is synthesized by the normal bacterial flora in the bowel. The toxic effects of methotrexate are more likely to occur when it is given with adsorbents.

The therapeutic effects of the anticholinergic antidiarrheals can be decreased by coadministration with antacids. Amantadine, tricyclic antidepressants, monoamine oxidase inhibitors, opiates, and antihistamines, when given with anticholinergics, can result in increased anticholinergic effects. The opiate antidiarrheals have additive central nervous system (CNS) depressant effects if they are given with CNS depressants, alcohol, opioids, sedative-hypnotics, antipsychotics, or skeletal muscle relaxants.

Bismuth subsalicylate can lead to increased bleeding times and bruising when administered with warfarin as well as aspirin and other nonsteroidal antiinflammatory drugs. It can also cause confusion in the older adult patient. Cholestyramine, when administered with glipizide, can result in decreased hypoglycemic effects. Cholestyramine also decreases the absorption of any drug that is given within 2 hours of it. It is important not to give any drug within 2 hours before or 2 hours after cholestyramine.

Dosages

For dosage information on the antidiarrheal drugs, see the table on p. 817.

DRUG PROFILES

Drug therapy for diarrhea depends on the specific cause of the diarrhea (if known). All antidiarrheals are orally administered drugs available as suspensions, tablets, or capsules. Some antidiarrheals are over-the-counter (OTC) medications, whereas others require a prescription.

ADSORBENTS
bismuth subsalicylate
Even though it is available OTC, it should be used with caution in children and teenagers who have or are recovering from chickenpox or influenza because of the risk for Reye's syndrome (see Patient-Centered Care: Lifespan Considerations for the Pediatric Patient on the next page). It can also cause all of the adverse effects that are associated with an aspirin-based product (see Chapter 44). Two alarming but harmless adverse effects are temporary darkening of the tongue and the stool. Bismuth subsalicylate is available OTC for oral use.

ANTICHOLINERGICS
The anticholinergics atropine and hyoscyamine are used either alone or in combination with other antidiarrheals because

they slow GI tract motility. These drugs are referred to as *belladonna alkaloids* and are discussed in Chapter 21. Their safety margin is not as wide as that of many of the other antidiarrheals, because they can cause serious adverse effects if used inappropriately. For this reason, they are available only by prescription.

belladonna alkaloid combinations
Belladonna alkaloids can be used to treat many GI disorders, including diarrhea; however, their use is limited. Donnatal is the most commonly used drug in this class. Use of belladonna alkaloid preparations is contraindicated in patients who have a known hypersensitivity to anticholinergics and in patients with narrow-angle glaucoma, GI obstruction, myasthenia gravis, paralytic ileus, and toxic megacolon. Donnatal tablets contain a combination of four different alkaloids: atropine, hyoscyamine, phenobarbital, and scopolamine. Available dosage forms of this combination include elixir, tablets, and extended-release tablets. Donnatal Extentabs contain increased amounts of the aforementioned ingredients. Belladonna alkaloid preparations are classified as pregnancy category C to X drugs, depending on the ingredients of the specific product.

OPIATES
There are five opiate-related antidiarrheal drugs: codeine, diphenoxylate with atropine, loperamide, paregoric, and tincture of opium. The only opiate-related antidiarrheal that is available as an OTC medication is loperamide; all others are prescription-only drugs because of the risk for respiratory depression and dependency associated with opiate use. Numerous medication errors and deaths have been reported with paregoric and tincture of opium. For those reasons, their use is very limited.

♦ diphenoxylate with atropine
Diphenoxylate (Lomotil, Lonox) is a synthetic opiate agonist that is structurally related to meperidine. It acts on smooth muscle of the intestinal tract, inhibiting GI motility and excessive GI propulsion. It has little or no analgesic activity; however, because it is an opioid, abuse and physical dependence may occur. Diphenoxylate is combined with subtherapeutic quantities of atropine to discourage its use as a recreational opiate drug. The amount of atropine present in the combination is too small to interfere with the conjugated diphenoxylate. When taken in large dosages, however, the combination results in extreme anticholinergic effects (e.g., dry mouth, abdominal pain, tachycardia, blurred vision).

Use of the combination of diphenoxylate and atropine is contraindicated in patients experiencing diarrhea associated with pseudomembranous colitis or toxigenic bacteria. It is available only for oral use.

♦ loperamide
Loperamide (Imodium A-D) is a synthetic antidiarrheal that is similar to diphenoxylate. It inhibits both peristalsis in the intestinal wall and intestinal secretion, thereby decreasing the number of stools and their water content. Although the drug

DOSAGES

Selected Antidiarrheal Drugs

Drug (Pregnancy Category)	Pharmacologic Class/Indication	Usual Adult Dosage Range	Onset of Action
belladonna alkaloids/phenobarbital combinations (Donnatal Elixir, Donnatal capsules and tablets) (C to X)	Fixed-combination anticholinergic/diarrhea	PO: Donnatal Elixir, 5-10 mL tid-qid Donnatal capsules and tablets, 1-2 caps or tabs tid-qid	1-2 hr
bismuth subsalicylate (Pepto-Bismol) (D)	Antimicrobial, antidiarrheal/diarrhea	PO: 30 mL or 2 tab Doses repeated every 30-60 min, not to exceed 8 per day	0.5-2 hr
◆ diphenoxylate with atropine (Lomotil) (C)	Opioid with anticholinergic/diarrhea	Initially 5 mg (2 tabs) 3-4 times/day, then reduce to 2.5 mg (1 tab) 3-4 times/day as needed (max of 8 tabs/day)	40-60 min
Lactobacillus acidophilus (Bacid, Lactinex) (A)	Probiotic/dietary supplementation, diarrhea, need for bacterial replacement	PO (Bacid): 2 caps bid-qid PO (Lactinex): 1 packet granules with liquid or food tid-qid; 4 tabs tid-qid with liquid or food	Unknown
◆ loperamide (Imodium A-D) (B)	Opiate antidiarrheal/diarrhea	PO: 4 mg followed by 2 mg after each BM (not to exceed 16 mg/day)	1-3 hr

exhibits many characteristics of the opiate class, physical dependence on loperamide has not been reported. Because of its safety profile, it is the only opiate antidiarrheal drug that is available as an OTC medication. Loperamide use is contraindicated in patients with severe ulcerative colitis, pseudomembranous colitis, and acute diarrhea associated with *Escherichia coli*.

PROBIOTICS

Probiotics suppress the growth of diarrhea-causing bacteria and reestablish the flora that normally resides in the intestine. Most commonly, they are bacterial cultures of *Lactobacillus* organisms. Probiotics are often referred to as *intestinal flora modifiers*. Their mechanism of action is not completely understood, but the general benefits are suppression of growth or invasion by pathogenic bacteria, improvement of intestinal barrier function, modulation of the immune system, and modulation of pain perception.

◆ Lactobacillus

Lactobacillus acidophilus (Bacid) and *Lactobacillus GG* (Culturelle) are acid-producing bacteria prepared in a concentrated, dried culture for oral administration. They are normal inhabitants of the GI tract where, through the fermentation of carbohydrates (which produces lactic acid), they create an unfavorable environment for the overgrowth of harmful fungi and bacteria. *L. acidophilus* has been used for more than 75 years for the treatment of uncomplicated diarrhea, particularly that caused by antibiotic therapy that destroys normal intestinal flora. Another commonly used probiotic is *Saccharomyces boulardii* (Florastor), which is used for *Clostridium difficile* infections.

🎭 PATIENT-CENTERED CARE: LIFESPAN CONSIDERATIONS FOR THE PEDIATRIC PATIENT   [QSEN]

Antidiarrheal Preparations

- If diarrhea is accompanied by fever, malaise, or abdominal pain, contact the prescriber immediately because of the possibility of excessive fluid and electrolyte loss. Dehydration and electrolyte loss occur very rapidly in the pediatric patient because of the patient's size and sensitivity to loss of fluid volume and electrolytes through the stool.
- Always contact the prescriber or pharmacist for the proper dosage of antidiarrheals if the child is 6 years of age or younger or if there is any doubt as to proper dosing. Never hesitate to contact the prescriber with any concern or question regarding any medication recommended for the pediatric patient.
- Bismuth subsalicylate is a salicylate by chemical structure; therefore, it is to be used very cautiously in children and teenagers who have been or are recovering from chickenpox or influenza because of the risk for Reye's syndrome (see Chapter 44).
- Immediately report to the prescriber any abdominal distention, firm abdomen, painful abdomen, or worsening of or lack of improvement in diarrhea 24 to 48 hours after medication administration. Measurement of the amount of diarrhea by the number of soiled diapers or number of stools per day provides important information.
- Antidiarrheal preparations are always to be used very cautiously in the pediatric patient. If symptoms persist or dehydration occurs (e.g., no tears and decreased urine output in the child), contact the prescriber.
- If the patient is sluggish, lethargic, or confused or the diarrhea is bloody, contact the prescriber immediately or go to the closest emergency department.
- Always assess the pediatric patient, including adolescents, for the presence of an eating disorder such as bulimia or anorexia due to the associated use/abuse of laxatives in these conditions.

LAXATIVES

Laxatives are used for the treatment of **constipation**, which is defined as the abnormally infrequent and difficult passage of feces through the lower GI tract. Constipation is a symptom, not a disease; it is a disorder of movement through the colon and/or rectum that can be caused by a variety of diseases or drugs. Some of the more common causes of constipation are listed in Table 51-3.

The GI tract is responsible for the digestive process, which involves (1) ingestion of dietary intake, (2) digestion of dietary intake into basic nutrients, (3) absorption of basic nutrients, and (4) storage and removal of fecal material via defecation (Figure 51-1).

Ingestion → digestion → absorption → storage & removal

The usual time span between ingestion and defecation is 24 to 36 hours. The last segment of the GI tract, the large intestine (colon), is responsible for (1) forming the stool by removing excess water from the fecal material, (2) temporarily storing the stool until defecation, and (3) extracting essential vitamins from the intestinal bacteria (especially vitamin K). The colon is 120 to 150 cm long and is separated from the small intestine by the ileocecal valve. The colon extends into the rectum, which terminates at the anus. The rectum is the temporary storage site for the stool, which is composed of water and unabsorbed and indigestible material. Evacuation of the rectal contents is accomplished by bowel movements.

A bowel movement (defecation) is a reflex act that involves both smooth and skeletal muscles. The entry of feces into the rectum stimulates mass peristaltic movement that results in a bowel movement. However, voluntary initiation or inhibition of defecation is also possible via skeletal muscle pathways.

Treatment of constipation is individualized, with consideration of the patient's age, concerns, and expectations; duration and severity of constipation; and potential contributing factors. Treatment can be either surgical (in extreme cases) or nonsurgical. Nonsurgical treatments can be separated into three broad approaches: dietary (e.g., fiber supplementation), behavioral (e.g., increased physical activity), and pharmacologic. The focus in this chapter is on pharmacologic treatment.

TABLE 51-3   Causes of Constipation

Cause	Examples
Adverse drug effects	Analgesics, anticholinergics, iron supplements, aluminum antacids, calcium antacids, opiates, calcium channel blockers
Lifestyle	Poor bowel movement habits: voluntary refusal to defecate resulting in constipation
	Diet: poor fluid intake and/or low-fiber diet or excessive consumption of dairy products
	Physical inactivity: lack of proper exercise
	Psychologic factors: anxiety, stress, hypochondria
Metabolic and endocrine disorders	Diabetes mellitus, hypothyroidism, pregnancy, hypercalcemia, hypokalemia
Neurogenic disorders	Autonomic neuropathy, intestinal pseudo-obstruction, multiple sclerosis, spinal cord lesions, Parkinson's disease, stroke

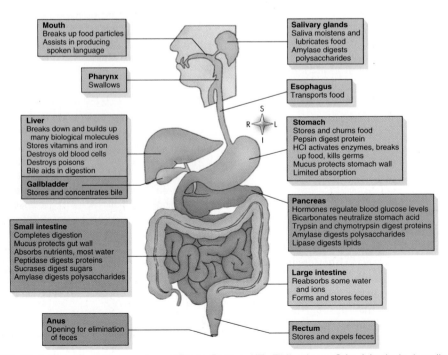

FIGURE 51-1 The digestive system. (From Patton KT, Thibodeau GA: *Mosby's handbook of anatomy and physiology*, St Louis, 2010, Mosby.)

Laxatives are among the most misused OTC medications. Long-term and often inappropriate use of laxatives may result in laxative dependence, produce damage to the bowel, or lead to previously nonexistent intestinal problems. With the exception of the bulk-forming type, laxatives are not to be used for long periods. Based on their mechanisms of action, laxatives are divided into five major groups: bulk-forming, emollient, hyperosmotic, saline, and stimulant laxatives. Table 51-4 lists the currently available laxative drugs categorized by drug family. The onset of action of laxatives is the most important pharmacokinetic feature of these drugs and is listed in the dosages table on p. 821.

Mechanism of Action and Drug Effects

All laxatives promote bowel movements, but each class of laxative has a different mechanism of action. Laxatives may act by (1) affecting fecal consistency, (2) increasing fecal movement through the colon, and/or (3) facilitating defecation through the rectum. Bulk-forming laxatives act in a manner similar to that of the fiber naturally contained in the diet. They absorb water into the intestine, which increases bulk and distends the bowel to initiate reflex bowel activity, thus promoting a bowel movement.

Emollient laxatives are also referred to as *stool softeners* (docusate salts) and *lubricant laxatives* (mineral oil). Fecal softeners work by lowering the surface tension of GI fluids, so that more water and fat are absorbed into the stool and the intestines. The lubricant type of emollient laxative works by lubricating the fecal material and the intestinal wall and preventing absorption of water from the intestines. Instead of being absorbed, this water in the bowel softens and expands the stool. This promotes bowel distention and reflex peristaltic actions, which ultimately lead to defecation.

Hyperosmotic laxatives work by increasing fecal water content, which results in distention, increased peristalsis, and evacuation. Their site of action is limited to the large intestine. Saline laxatives increase osmotic pressure in the small intestine by inhibiting water absorption and increasing both water and electrolyte (salt) secretions from the bowel wall into the bowel lumen. This results in a watery stool. The increased distention promotes peristalsis and evacuation. Rectal enemas of sodium phosphate, a saline laxative, produce defecation 2 to 5 minutes after administration.

As the name implies, stimulant laxatives stimulate the nerves that innervate the intestines, which results in increased peristalsis. They also increase fluid in the colon, which increases bulk and softens the stool. Table 51-5 summarizes the specific drug effects of the different classes of laxatives.

In 2008, a new class of drugs was approved for the treatment of very specific types of constipation related to opioid use and bowel resection surgery. These peripherally acting opioid antagonists include methylnaltrexone (Relistor) and alvimopan (Entereg). These drugs block the entrance of an opioid drug into the bowel cells, thus allowing bowels to function normally, even with continued opioid use. Methylnaltrexone is approved only for terminally ill (hospice) patients who have opioid-induced constipation. It is available as an injection only and is given once a day. Alvimopan is indicated to accelerate GI recovery time following partial large or small bowel resection surgery. Patients must be hospitalized and registered to receive Alvimopan.

Indications

The following are some of the more common uses of laxatives:

- Facilitation of bowel movements in patients with inactive colon or anorectal disorders
- Reduction of ammonia absorption in hepatic encephalopathy (lactulose only)
- Treatment of drug-induced constipation
- Treatment of constipation associated with pregnancy and/or the postobstetric period
- Treatment of constipation caused by reduced physical activity or poor dietary habits
- Removal of toxic substances from the body
- Facilitation of defecation in megacolon
- Preparation for colonic diagnostic procedures or surgery

TABLE 51-4 Laxatives: Drug Categories and Selected Drugs

Category	Laxative Drugs
Bulk-forming	psyllium, methylcellulose
Emollient	docusate salts, mineral oil
Hyperosmotic	polyethylene glycol, lactulose, sorbitol, glycerin
Saline	magnesium hydroxide, magnesium sulfate, magnesium citrate
Stimulant	senna, bisacodyl

TABLE 51-5 Laxatives: Drug Effects

Drug Effect	Bulk	Emollient	Hyperosmotic	Saline	Stimulant
Increases peristalsis	Yes	Yes	Yes	Yes	Yes
Causes increased secretion of water and electrolytes in small bowel	Yes	Yes	No	Yes	Yes
Inhibits absorption of water in small bowel	Yes	Yes	No	Yes	Yes
Increases wall permeability in small bowel	No	Yes	No	No	Yes
Acts only in large bowel	No	No	Yes	No	No
Increases water in fecal mass	Yes	Yes	Yes	Yes	Yes
Softens fecal mass	Yes	Yes	Yes	Yes	Yes

TABLE 51-6   Laxatives: Indications

Category	Indication
Bulk-forming	Acute and chronic constipation, irritable bowel syndrome, diverticulosis
Emollient	Acute and chronic constipation, fecal impaction, anorectal conditions requiring facilitation of bowel movements
Hyperosmotic	Chronic constipation, bowel preparation for diagnostic and surgical procedures
Saline	Constipation, bowel preparation for diagnostic and surgical procedures
Stimulant	Acute constipation, bowel preparation for diagnostic and surgical procedures

TABLE 51-7   Laxatives: Adverse Effects

Category	Adverse Effects
Bulk-forming	Impaction above strictures, fluid disturbances, electrolyte imbalances, gas formation, esophageal blockage, allergic reaction
Emollient	Skin rashes, decreased absorption of vitamins, lipid pneumonia, electrolyte imbalances
Hyperosmotic	Abdominal bloating, rectal irritation, electrolyte imbalances
Saline	Magnesium toxicity (with renal insufficiency), electrolyte imbalances, cramping, diarrhea, increased thirst
Stimulant	Nutrient malabsorption, skin rashes, gastric irritation, electrolyte imbalances, discolored urine, rectal irritation

See Table 51-6 for specific therapeutic indications for each laxative drug class.

Contraindications

All categories of laxatives share the same general contraindications and precautions, including avoidance in cases of drug allergy and the need for cautious use in the presence of the following: acute surgical abdomen; appendicitis symptoms such as abdominal pain, nausea, and vomiting; fecal impaction (mineral oil enemas excepted); intestinal obstruction; and undiagnosed abdominal pain.

Adverse Effects

The adverse effects of the various drugs are specific to the laxative group. Most of the adverse effects from laxatives are confined to the intestine; however, the overuse and misuse of laxatives lead to many unwanted effects that are not expected or designed to occur with appropriate use. The major adverse effects of the laxative drugs are listed in Table 51-7.

Interactions

Laxatives alter intestinal function; therefore, they can interact with other drugs, because many drugs are absorbed in the intestines. Bulk-forming laxatives can decrease the absorption of antibiotics, digoxin, salicylates, tetracyclines, and warfarin.

Mineral oil can decrease the absorption of fat-soluble vitamins (A, D, E, and K). Hyperosmotic laxatives can cause increased CNS depression if they are given with barbiturates, general anesthetics, opioids, or antipsychotics. Oral antibiotics can decrease the effects of lactulose. Stimulant laxatives decrease the absorption of antibiotics, digoxin, nitrofurantoin, salicylates, tetracyclines, and oral anticoagulants.

Dosages

For dosage information on selected laxatives, see the table on the next page.

DRUG PROFILES

Laxatives are used for the treatment of constipation. Such treatment must involve an understanding of the whole patient. Many drugs in the five major groups of laxatives are available as OTC medications, whereas others require a prescription for use. The following profiles describe the prototypical drugs in each of the laxative groups.

BULK-FORMING LAXATIVES

Bulk-forming laxatives are composed of water-retaining (hydrophilic) natural and synthetic cellulose derivatives. Psyllium is an example of a natural bulk-forming laxative, and methylcellulose is an example of a synthetic cellulose derivative. Bulk-forming drugs increase water absorption, which results in greater total volume (bulk) of the intestinal contents. Bulk-forming laxatives tend to produce normal, formed stools. Their action is limited to the GI tract, so there are few, if any, systemic effects. However, they need to be taken with liberal amounts of water to prevent esophageal obstruction and/or fecal impaction. The bulk-forming laxatives are all obtainable OTC, are among the safest laxatives available, and are the only ones that are recommended for long-term use.

methylcellulose

Methylcellulose (Citrucel) is a synthetic bulk-forming laxative that attracts water into the intestine and absorbs excess water into the stool, stimulating the intestines and increasing peristalsis. Specific contraindications include GI obstruction and hepatitis. Methylcellulose is an oral drug available in powdered form that provides approximately 2 g of fiber per heaping tablespoon.

◆psyllium

Psyllium (Metamucil) is a natural bulk-forming laxative obtained from the dried seed of the *Plantago psyllium* plant. It has many of the characteristics of methylcellulose. Psyllium is contraindicated in patients with intestinal obstruction or fecal impaction. Its use is also contraindicated in patients experiencing abdominal pain and/or nausea and vomiting. Psyllium is available for oral use in wafer and powder form.

EMOLLIENT LAXATIVES

Emollient laxatives either directly lubricate the stool and the intestines, as with mineral oil, or act as fecal softeners. By lubricating the fecal material and the intestinal walls, lubricant

DOSAGES

Selected Laxatives

Drug (Pregnancy Category)	Pharmacologic Class	Usual Adult Dosage Range	Onset of Action
bisacodyl (Dulcolax) (C)	Stimulant laxative	5-15 mg oral daily or 10 mg-suppository as a single dose	Oral: 6-12 hr Rectal: 15-60 min
◆ docusate sodium* (Colace, others) (C)	Fecal softener, emollient laxative	PO: 50-300 mg/day divided daily-qid	1-3 days
◆ glycerin (Sani-Supp, Colace, Fleet Babylax) (C)	Hyperosmotic laxative	Rectal only: Insert one suppository PR daily prn; attempt to retain 15-30 min; suppository does not have to melt to induce BM	16-36 min
◆ lactulose† (Enulose, others) (B)	Disaccharide, hyperosmotic laxative	PO: 15-30 ml daily or twice daily	24 hr
magnesium citrate (generic only), magnesium sulfate (Epsom salts by various manufacturers) (B)	Saline laxative	PO: Citrate, 120-300 mL for 1 dose	0.5-3 hr
methylcellulose (Citrucel, others) (B)	Bulk-forming laxative	PO: 1 heaping tbsp in 8 oz cold water daily-tid	12-24 hr
mineral oil (Plain, Fleet Mineral Oil Enema) (B)	Emollient laxative	PO: 15-45 mL oil taken at bedtime PR: Rectal enema, 118 mL one time	6-8 hr
polyethylene glycol (Colyte, GoLYTELY, Half-Lytely, MiraLax) (C)	Hyperosmotic laxative	PO: 4-L solution, usually ending before procedure; patient needs to fast at least 4 hr before drinking solution MiraLax: 17 g once daily	1 hr
◆ psyllium (Metamucil, Fiberall, others) (B)	Bulk-forming laxative	PO: 1 rounded tsp in 8 oz water or juice daily-tid	12-24 hr
◆ senna‡ (Senokot, others) (C)	Stimulant-irritant laxative	PO (tabs): Start with 2 tabs daily (max: 4 tabs bid) PO (liquid): 15 mL daily (max: 30 mL bid)	6-24 hr

BM, Bowel movement; *PR*, per rectum.
*Docusate sodium is available in both capsule and liquid forms. Docusate calcium is available in capsule form only.
†Rectal route is sometimes used to reverse certain types of coma.
‡Many dosage forms; consult product labeling if in doubt. Most common dosage forms are 8.6-mg sennosides in tablet form and 8.8 mg/5 mL of sennosides in liquid form.

emollient laxatives prevent water from moving out of the intestines, which softens and expands the stool. Stool softeners (docusate salts) work by lowering the surface tension of fluids, which allows more water and fat to be absorbed into the stool and the intestines.

◆ docusate salts

Docusate salts (calcium and sodium) (Colace) are stool-softening emollient laxatives that facilitate the passage of water and lipids (fats) into the fecal mass, which softens the stool. These drugs are used to treat constipation, to soften fecal impactions, and to prevent opioid-induced constipation. Docusate does not cause patients to defecate; it simply softens the stool to ease its passage. In addition to the docusate salt formulations, combination products are also available. Docusate use is contraindicated in patients with intestinal obstruction, fecal impaction, or nausea and vomiting.

mineral oil

Mineral oil eases the passage of stool by lubricating the intestines and preventing water from escaping the stool. Mineral oil is the only lubricant laxative in the emollient category. It is a mixture of liquid hydrocarbons derived from petroleum and is most commonly used to treat constipation associated with hard stools or fecal impaction.

Mineral oil use is contraindicated in patients with intestinal obstruction, abdominal pain, or nausea and vomiting. Mineral oil drugs are available as enemas and in products for oral use. There are also combination products that contain mineral oil, such as Haley's M-O, which includes both mineral oil and milk of magnesia (magnesium hydroxide).

HYPEROSMOTIC LAXATIVES

The hyperosmotic laxatives glycerin, lactulose, sorbitol, and polyethylene glycol (PEG) relieve constipation by increasing the water content of the feces, which results in distention, peristalsis, and evacuation. They are most commonly used to treat constipation and to evacuate the bowels before diagnostic and surgical procedures.

◆ glycerin

Glycerin promotes bowel movement by increasing osmotic pressure in the intestine, which draws fluid into the colon. Because it is a very mild laxative, it is often used in children. Glycerin has properties similar to those of sorbitol, another hyperosmotic laxative. Glycerin use is contraindicated in patients who have a known hypersensitivity to it. It is available as a rectal solution and as both adult and pediatric suppositories.

◆ lactulose

Lactulose is a synthetic derivative of the natural sugar lactose, which is not digested in the stomach or absorbed in the small bowel. Instead it passes unchanged into the large intestine, where it is metabolized. Colonic bacteria digest lactulose to produce lactic acid, formic acid, and acetic acid, which creates a hyperosmotic environment that draws water into the colon and produces a laxative effect. This drug-induced acidic environment also reduces blood ammonia levels by converting ammonia to ammonium. Ammonium is a water-soluble cation that is trapped in the intestines and cannot be reabsorbed into the systemic circulation. This effect has proved helpful in reducing serum ammonia levels in patients with hepatic encephalopathy. Lactulose use is contraindicated in patients on a low-lactose diet. It is available as a solution for either oral or rectal use.

polyethylene glycol 3350

PEG-3350 is most commonly given before diagnostic or surgical bowel procedures, because it is a very potent laxative that induces total cleansing of the bowel. The 3350 designation refers to the osmolality of the drug. It is usually available in a powdered dosage form that contains mixtures of electrolytes that also help stimulate bowel evacuation (e.g., Colyte, GoLYTELY, MoviPrep, Half-Lytely). The powder is usually reconstituted in a large volume of fluid (1 gal) that is then gradually drunk by the patient on the afternoon of the day before the procedure. Use of PEG is contraindicated in patients with GI obstruction, gastric retention, bowel perforation, toxic colitis, toxic megacolon, or ileus.

An oral solution of PEG-3350 and electrolytes is available for GI lavage. Diarrhea usually occurs within 30 to 60 minutes after ingestion; complete evacuation and cleansing of the bowel is accomplished within 4 hours. MiraLax is a PEG-3350 product that is available OTC and can be used daily for constipation in much smaller amounts than those used for total bowel cleansing.

SALINE LAXATIVES

Saline laxatives consist of various magnesium or sodium salts. They increase osmotic pressure and draw water into the colon, producing a watery stool, usually within 3 to 6 hours of ingestion. The currently available saline laxatives are listed in Box 51-1. Oral sodium phosphate–containing products used for bowel evacuation, such as Fleet Phospho-Soda, were taken off the market in 2008 because of concerns about acute phosphate nephropathy.

magnesium salts

The magnesium saline laxatives, magnesium citrate (Citroma), and magnesium hydroxide (Phillips Milk of Magnesia) are unpleasant-tasting OTC laxative preparations. They are to be used with caution in patients with renal insufficiency, because

BOX 51-1	Saline Laxatives
Magnesium Laxatives	*Citrate*
Sulfate	Citrate of magnesia
Epsom salts	
	Sodium Laxatives
Hydroxide	Fleet Enema
Milk of magnesia	

they can be absorbed enough to cause hypermagnesemia. They are most commonly used to evacuate the bowel rapidly in preparation for endoscopic examination and to help remove unabsorbed poisons from the GI tract.

Use of magnesium salts is contraindicated in patients with renal disease, abdominal pain, nausea and vomiting, obstruction, acute surgical abdomen, or rectal bleeding. Magnesium hydroxide, more commonly referred to as *milk of magnesia,* is available in oral liquid and tablet form. It is also found in a variety of combination products, such as Haley's M-O (see mineral oil profile). Other magnesium products are listed in the discussion of saline laxatives earlier in the chapter. Note that magnesium *oxide* is used as a supplement, not as a laxative (see Chapter 53).

STIMULANT LAXATIVES

Stimulant laxatives induce intestinal peristalsis. In the past, several different stimulant laxatives were available; however, the U.S. Food and Drug Administration has required that all except bisacodyl (Dulcolax) and senna (Senokot) be removed from the market. Their site of action is the entire GI tract. The action of the stimulant laxatives is proportional to the dose. The stimulant class is the most likely of all laxative classes to cause dependence.

bisacodyl

Bisacodyl (Dulcolax) is the most commonly used stimulant laxative. It is available as an oral tablet and rectal suppository. It is used for constipation or for whole bowel evacuation prior to endoscopic examination. It is available OTC.

◆ senna

Senna (Senokot) is a commonly used OTC stimulant laxative. Senna is obtained from the dried leaves of the *Cassia acutifolia* plant. It may be used for relief of acute constipation or bowel preparation for surgery or examination. Because of its stimulating action on the GI tract, it may cause abdominal pain. It can produce complete bowel evacuation in 6 to 12 hours. Senna is available in a variety of dosages as tablets, syrup, and granules. One product, Senokot-S, includes both senna and the stool softener docusate sodium.

DRUGS FOR IRRITABLE BOWEL SYNDROME

Irritable bowel syndrome (IBS) is a condition of chronic intestinal discomfort characterized by cramps, diarrhea, and/or constipation. Patients usually cope with the symptoms by avoiding irritating foods and/or taking OTC laxatives and antidiarrheal drugs. Women are affected more often than men. There are three drugs specifically indicated for IBS. Lubiprostone (Amitiza) is a chloride channel activator that is indicated for the treatment of chronic idiopathic constipation and IBS with constipation in women 18 years of age and older. The most common adverse effects are nausea, diarrhea, and abdominal pain. It is classified as a pregnancy category C drug. However, lubiprostone was taken off the market in 2012, except for emergencies. Lubiprostone is contraindicated in patients with known or suspected bowel obstruction.

Alosetron (Lotronex) is a selective serotonin 5-HT$_3$ receptor antagonist that is indicated for the treatment of severe, chronic, diarrhea-predominant IBS in women who have failed conventional therapy. If response is inadequate after 4 weeks, the drug is to be discontinued. It must be discontinued immediately if constipation or signs of ischemic colitis occur. Only physicians who have enrolled in the Prometheus Prescribing Program (manufacturer-sponsored) can prescribe alosetron. The FDA has issued a black box warning regarding infrequent but serious GI adverse reactions including ischemic colitis.

Linaclotide (Linzess) is a minimally absorbed peptide guanylate cyclase-C agonist. It is indicated for the treatment of irritable bowel syndrome with constipation and chronic idiopathic constipation. It is contraindicated in patients with GI obstruction and children younger than 17 years of age. The most common side effects include diarrhea, which can be serious, abdominal pain, and flatulence. It is available as an oral capsule, which should be taken on an empty stomach.

NURSING PROCESS

ASSESSMENT

Before giving *antidiarrheal* preparations, obtain a thorough history and perform an assessment of bowel patterns, general state of health, any recent illness, GI complaints, and any dietary changes. Always assess for possible causes of diarrhea such as food intolerance, lactose/wheat/gluten intolerance, fever/infection, and any medications that may be precipitating the changes in bowel patterns. With the abdominal assessment, include auscultation of bowel sounds in all four quadrants of the abdomen *after* inspection *before* percussion and palpation. Performing auscultation and inspection before percussion prevents any possible stimulation of peristalsis or bowel sounds that would not occur otherwise. When the frequency of bowel sounds ranges from 6 to 32 per minute, it is important to describe exactly what is heard and the amount of activity in each of the four quadrants. Terms such as *high-pitched, low-pitched, gurgling,* or *tinkling* may be used to describe the character of the sounds, whereas activity may be described as *hypoactive* (less than 6 sounds per minute), *normoactive* (between 6 and 32 sounds per minute), or *hyperactive* (more than the normal range). Note the presence of tenderness, rigidity, changes in contour, bulges, and obvious peristaltic waves across the abdomen. Assess frequency, consistency, amount, color, and odor (if present) of stools, and

document the findings. In addition, it is critical to patient safety and health to be sure that the possibility of *C. difficile* infection or other infectious diarrhea is ruled out. Assess and document any contraindications, cautions, and drug interactions for all drugs. Report complaints of abdominal pain/distention, bloody stools, confirmation of hypoactive to no bowel sounds, and/or fever to the prescriber immediately. When administering *diphenoxylate* with *atropine,* be wary of overuse because large amounts may result in dry mouth, abdominal pain, tachycardia, and blurred vision. The older adult patient is more susceptible to fluid and electrolyte depletion associated with diarrhea; therefore, closely assess hydration status and age.

Laxative use requires further assessment in addition to the abdominal assessment and bowel pattern history described earlier. For example, focus questions on changes in bowel patterns, long-term use of laxatives (because patients may become laxative dependent), and dietary and fluid intake. Identify if there is an absence of fluids, bulk, or exercise in the patient's lifestyle. Assess vital signs, daily weights, intake and output, and fluid and electrolyte levels, and note the presence of any weakness because of the possibility of hypotension and volume or electrolyte depletion (with long-term laxative use). Assess and document for the presence of rectal bleeding, nausea, and vomiting. Another important area to assess is that of laxative abuse in the older adult patient as well as in pediatric and adolescent patients. Specifically, in pediatric and adolescent patients, assess for eating disorders with concurrent use of laxatives.

The type of laxative and the related mechanism of action dictate specific assessments because of differences in how strongly the patient reacts to the various laxative drugs. The *bulk-forming laxatives* are often used to treat chronic constipation and have few adverse effects, but a basic abdominal and bowel pattern assessment and related history taking are still needed. Always assess and document contraindications, cautions, and drug interactions. Use docusate salts or emollient laxatives cautiously in the older adult patient.

With *hyperosmotic laxatives* (e.g., *polyethylene glycol, lactulose, sorbitol, glycerin*), assess baseline fluid and electrolyte levels to identify any deficits prior to use. All of the previously mentioned assessment measures regarding abdominal examination and bowel patterns are also appropriate for these drugs, with the additional assessment for the presence of abdominal pain, the degree of peristalsis, and any history of recent abdominal surgery, nausea, vomiting, or weight loss. Older adult patients react more adversely to this class of laxatives, so their use is to be avoided.

Saline laxatives (e.g., *magnesium hydroxide, magnesium sulfate, magnesium citrate*) are to be used with caution in older adult patients because of possible dehydration and electrolyte loss. They may also cause magnesium toxicity in those with compromised renal status, thus it is important to assess baseline renal function in those at risk. *Senna* and *bisacodyl* are examples of *stimulant laxatives.* They may also cause electrolyte imbalances, so baseline electrolyte levels are important to assess and monitor.

In patients taking *alosetron (Lotronex)*, a drug for IBS, assess for a history of Crohn's disease, liver disease, GI adhesions/strictures/obstruction/perforation, and ulcerative colitis. Pay close attention to bowel sounds and findings from inspection and palpation of the abdomen.

CASE STUDY

Patient-Centered Care: Long-Term Laxative Use

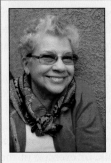 Mrs. M. is a 66-year-old retired schoolteacher. She enjoys good health and exercises three times a week with a senior citizen group in a supervised arthritis swim class at the local recreation center. She arrives at the family practice office with complaints of "constipation" and says that for the past 3 months she has had only one bowel movement every 3 days instead of one every day. In the assessment of this patient, the nurse discovers that Mrs. M. has been taking a stimulant laxative up to twice a day and is also now feeling "weak." Mrs. M. also says that she is experiencing "a lot of tummy cramping."

1. What are at least five questions the nurse should ask Mrs. M.? Provide reasons for each question.
2. What types of problems are generally related to long-term use of laxatives? Explain your answer.
3. What are some nonpharmacologic ways to help prevent constipation?
4. What over-the-counter drug is the best choice to help prevent constipation? Explain your answer.

For answers, see *http://evolve.elsevier.com/Lilley.*

NURSING DIAGNOSES

1. Constipation related to improper and/or inadequate diet
2. Diarrhea related to GI irritation from food, bacteria or viruses, or pathology
3. Deficient fluid volume related to loss of fluids and electrolytes caused by frequent, loose stools

PLANNING: OUTCOME IDENTIFICATION

1. Patient experiences minimal to no constipation by implementing measures to manage/prevent constipation such as forcing fluids; increasing intake of bulk and fiber (unless contraindicated); and increasing physical activity.
2. Patient experiences minimal to no diarrhea through implementation of measures to manage/prevent diarrhea such as increasing bulk; avoiding caffeine and irritating foods and beverages, and taking antidiarrheal as prescribed/instructed.
3. Patient maintains/regains fluid and electrolyte balance with nonpharmacologic and pharmacologic therapies with reporting to the prescriber any signs and symptoms of fluid and electrolyte loss, such as weakness, lethargy, decreased urinary output, and dizziness.

IMPLEMENTATION

With *antidiarrheals,* educate the patient that the drugs must be taken *exactly* as directions indicate, with strict adherence to the recommended dose, frequency, and duration of treatment. Encourage the patient to be aware of fluid intake and any dietary changes that would impact his or her health status or possibly exacerbate present symptoms. Instruct patients to be aware of the factors precipitating the diarrhea and, if symptoms persist, to contact his or her health care provider. Document any changes in bowel patterns, weight, fluid volume, intake and output, as well as in the mucous membranes during and after treatment—whether for constipation or diarrhea. Inform the patient that *bismuth subsalicylate* must be taken as directed and that this medication will turn the stool black or gray. Tablets are available in chewable and non-chewable dosage forms. If the chewable tablets are used, they are to be chewed thoroughly before swallowing and with at least 6 ounces of water. Non-chewable tablets must be taken with at least 6 to 8 ounces of water. Bismuth subsalicylate is a salicylate-based product and is not to be taken with other salicylates to avoid the risk for toxicity. Encourage parents to check with their children's health care provider before giving bismuth subsalicylate to a child or teenager with a viral infection, such as chickenpox or influenza, because of the risk for Reye's syndrome (see Patient-Centered Care: Lifespan Considerations for the Pediatric Patient on p. 817).

Diphenoxylate hydrochloride and *loperamide* may be given without regard to food intake but must be given with adequate fluid. Additionally, advise the patient to follow the specific directions (e.g., the specific number of tablets recommended by the manufacturer after the first loose stool and the total number of tablets to be taken within a 24-hour period). Maximum amounts are not to be exceeded, and if diarrhea continues or other symptoms occur (e.g., fever, abdominal pain, bloody stools), instruct the patient to contact the prescriber immediately. See Patient-Centered Care: Patient Teaching on the next page for more information.

Probiotics may be recommended for a variety of altered bowel elimination patterns, whether diarrhea or constipation. Probiotics are available in foods and dietary supplements and in capsules, tablets, and powder dosage forms. Most of the probiotics are derived from *Lactobacillus* or *Bifidobacterium* bacteria. It is important to educate the patient about probiotics and to emphasize their healthy benefits when administered in the proper amounts. Tell the patient to take probiotics exactly as directed. Foods that contain probiotics include yogurt, fermented milk, miso, tempeh, and some juices and soy beverages.

Bulk-forming laxatives such as *methylcellulose* must be administered as specified by package insert or as ordered. *Methylcellulose* is to be taken with at least 8 ounces or 1 full glass of liquid after the powder form has been thoroughly stirred into it. The fluid must be taken immediately because of a congealing effect that continues to harden with time. To avoid choking or swelling of the product in the throat or esophagus, the patient must swallow or receive the drug immediately upon stirring. The medication must never be taken or administered in its dry form. See Patient-Centered Care: Patient Teaching on the next page for more information.

Docusate is available in a variety of oral dosage forms (e.g., capsules, tablets, syrups, elixir), and it is recommended to take it with at least 6 ounces of water or other fluid. An additional 6 to 8 glasses of water a day is also suggested to help with stool softening. *Bisacodyl*, if ordered, is best taken on an empty stomach for faster action, and whole tablets are not to be chewed or crushed. Advise the patient not to take milk, antacids, or juices with the dose or within 1 hour of taking the medication. Rectal suppositories, if too soft, may be placed in a medicine cup with ice to harden the suppository before insertion. Once the wrapper is removed, apply a water-soluble lubricant to the suppository prior to insertion into the rectum. Use a gloved hand or finger cot for insertion. Encourage the patient to try and keep the suppository in place by lying still on the left side for at least 15 to 30 minutes to allow the drug to dissolve for maximal effectiveness. *Lactulose* may be taken with juice, milk, or water to increase palatability. It is important to note that the normal color of the oral solution is pale yellow. Administer rectal dosage forms as a retention enema with dilution as ordered, and instruct the patient to retain for 30 to 60 minutes. For proper insertion of a retention enema, lubricate the tip of the apparatus well, and insert it carefully with the nozzle pointed toward the umbilicus of the patient, with the patient lying on the left side. Release the fluid gradually, and discontinue administration if the patient experiences severe abdominal pain. If long-term use of the drug is indicated, monitoring serum electrolyte levels is needed.

Magnesium-based laxatives are generally used only in certain situations because they are very potent. Force fluids, and follow other instructions per the prescriber's order or the package instructions. Refrigeration may help increase the palatability of the oral solution. Emphasize the importance that this type of drug is to be taken exactly as prescribed for constipation, with consumption of plenty of fluids and careful attention to adverse effects. Instruct the patient to mix the *PEG-electrolyte solution* with water or a flavored sports drink as directed and to shake well before drinking. Chilled solutions are tolerated better. Rapid drinking of each dose is recommended.

IBS drugs are to be given as ordered. *Alosetron (Lotronex)* is generally given twice daily. Be sure the patient receives the FDA-approved medication guide with each dispensing of alosetron. Encourage the patient to keep a daily journal to help the prescriber identify the effectiveness of therapy.

EVALUATION

Therapeutic responses to any of these medications include an improvement in the GI-related signs and symptoms reported by the patient (e.g., decrease in diarrhea or constipation), return to normal bowel patterns with normal bowel sounds, and absence of abnormal findings on assessment of the abdomen and bowel patterns. Adverse effects for which to monitor patients vary according to the drug. Use goals and outcome criteria as a means to evaluate the nursing care plan related to each problem, whether it is constipation, diarrhea, or both.

PATIENT-CENTERED CARE: PATIENT TEACHING

- Instruct the patient that antidiarrheals are to be taken exactly as prescribed, giving close attention to indicated dosages with warnings of overuse!
- Counsel the patient to take antidiarrheal drugs with caution when performing tasks that require mental alertness or motor skills until it is clear how the drug actually affects him or her. Advise the patient to immediately report to the prescriber any abdominal distention or firm/hard abdomen, abdominal pain, worsening (or no improvement) of symptoms, rectal bleeding, unrelieved constipation or diarrhea, fever, nausea, vomiting or other GI-related signs and symptoms, dizziness, muscle weakness, and muscle cramping.
- Encourage frequent mouth care, fluid intake, or use of sugarless gum or candy to help with the adverse effect of dry mouth.
- Bismuth subsalicylate may turn the stool tarry black, so warn the patient that this may happen. Patients must avoid other drugs containing salicylates while taking bismuth. Always check for cautions and contraindications of this drug, especially for pediatric patients.
- Increasing the intake of fluids, preferably water, as well foods high in fiber and whole grains, green leafy vegetables, and fruits may help to minimize constipation. Exercise is also beneficial.

- Educate the patient that normal bowel patterns for one person may not be normal for another.
- Keep all antidiarrheals and laxatives out of the reach of children.
- For patients taking powder forms of methylcellulose, emphasize the need to have the powder thoroughly mixed with at least 6 ounces of liquid, which is stirred and drunk immediately to avoid esophageal or throat obstruction.
- Probiotics come in various dosages, under different product names, and OTC. Advise the patient to take them exactly as instructed and to be aware that side effects are generally not of concern. Cultured yogurt and cultured milk products provide probiotics.
- Inform the patient taking senna to avoid other medications within 1 hour of taking it and that it often takes 6 to 12 hours for the laxative effect to occur.
- With alosetron, emphasize the importance of reporting to the prescriber immediately any severe constipation, bloody diarrhea, rectal bleeding, or worsening of abdominal pain. Doses are not to be doubled-up if a dose is omitted. Improvement in the patient's condition will take up to 4 weeks, and treatment is only for symptomatic control and not curative.

KEY POINTS

- Diarrhea is a leading cause of morbidity and mortality in underdeveloped countries.
- Drugs used to treat diarrhea include adsorbents, anticholinergics, opiates, and probiotics.
- Most acute diarrhea is self-limiting, subsiding in 3 days to 2 weeks.
- Fluid and electrolyte replacement is vital while a patient is experiencing diarrhea.
- Encourage patients to check and recheck dosage instructions before taking medication and to note any drug-food and drug-drug interactions.
- Anticholinergics work by decreasing GI peristalsis through their parasympathetic blocking effects. Adverse effects include urinary retention, headache, confusion, dry skin, rash, and blurred vision.
- Adsorbents work by coating the walls of the GI tract. They remain in the intestine and bind the causative bacteria or toxin to the adsorbent surface, so that it can be eliminated from the body through the stool. They may increase bleeding and cause constipation, dark stools, and black tongue.

- Probiotics are also used to manage diarrhea and consist of bacterial cultures of *Lactobacillus.* They reestablish normal intestinal flora destroyed by infection or antibiotics and suppress the growth of diarrhea-causing bacteria.
- Opiates are also used as antidiarrheals and help to decrease bowel motility and thus permit longer contact of intestinal contents with the absorptive surface of the bowel. Opiates also help to reduce the pain associated with rectal spasms.
- Laxatives, especially osmotic medications, may cause fluid and electrolyte loss.
- Alert patients to the abuse potential of laxatives and the problems associated with their misuse as well as laxative dependency issues.
- Stool softeners and bulk-forming drugs are often preferred to other drug classes in the treatment of constipation because they are not as problematic with regard to fluid and electrolyte loss.
- Drugs used for treatment of IBS are to be given with extreme caution due to the side effects.

NCLEX® EXAMINATION REVIEW QUESTIONS

1. A patient is being prepared for a colonoscopy. The nurse expects which laxative to be used as preparation for this procedure?
   a. methylcellulose
   b. docusate sodium
   c. PEG-3350
   d. glycerin
2. The nurse is administering oral methylcellulose (Citrucel) and keeps in mind that a major potential concern with this drug is
   a. dehydration.
   b. tarry stools.
   c. renal calculi.
   d. esophageal obstruction.
3. A 45-year-old woman has been diagnosed with irritable bowel syndrome (IBS) and will be taking linaclotide (Linzess). The nurse assesses for conditions that may be contraindications to this drug, such as
   a. constipation.
   b. bowel obstruction.
   c. renal calculi.
   d. anemia.
4. When the nurse teaches a patient about taking bisacodyl tablets, which instruction is correct?
   a. "Take this medication on an empty stomach."
   b. "Chew the tablet for quicker onset of action."
   c. "Take this medication with juice or milk."
   d. "Take this medication with an antacid if it upsets your stomach."

5. A patient has been receiving long-term antibiotic therapy as part of treatment for an infected leg wound. He tells the nurse that he has had "spells of diarrhea" for the last week. Which medication is most appropriate for him at this time?
   a. bismuth subsalicylate
   b. *L. acidophilus*
   c. diphenoxylate with atropine
   d. codeine
6. A parent calls to ask about giving a medication for diarrhea to his child, 15 years of age, who is recovering from the flu. The nurse expects the prescriber to recommend which medication?
   a. bismuth subsalicylate (Pepto-Bismol)
   b. *Lactobacillus GG* (Culturelle)
   c. belladonna alkaloid/phenobarbital combination (Donnatal Elixir)
   d. loperamide (Imodium A-D)
7. A patient has been instructed to use an over-the-counter (OTC) form of the bulk-forming laxative methylcellulose (Citrucel) to prevent constipation. The nurse will advise the patient of potential adverse effects, including (*Select all that apply*)
   a. electrolyte imbalances.
   b. decreased absorption of vitamins.
   c. gas formation.
   d. darkened stools.
   e. discolored urine.

8. A patient has been given a new prescription for alosetron (Lotronex), and the nurse is providing education about this medication. Which statement by the patient indicates a need for further education?
   a. "I will not take a double dose in the afternoon if I forget my morning dose."
   b. "I should be seeing improvement within a few days."
   c. "I will call my doctor if I experience severe constipation or bloody diarrhea."
   d. "This drug will improve symptoms but won't cure my IBS."

1. c, 2. d, 3. b, 4. a, 5. b, 6. d, 7. a, c, 8. b.

CRITICAL THINKING AND PRIORITIZATION QUESTIONS

1. A woman calls the clinic because her 4-month-old daughter has had diarrhea for about 8 hours. What is the nurse's priority action at this time?
2. An 88-year-old patient is undergoing a bowel preparation for colonoscopy. What are the nurse's priorities regarding monitoring the patient during the bowel preparation?

For answers, see *http://evolve.elsevier.com/Lilley.*

ⓔ EVOLVE WEBSITE

http://evolve.elsevier.com/Lilley
- Animations
- Answer Keys for Textbook Case Studies and Textbook Critical Thinking and Prioritization Questions
- Content Updates
- Key Points
- Review Questions
- Student Case Studies

Antiemetic and Antinausea Drugs

http://evolve.elsevier.com/Lilley

OBJECTIVES

When you reach the end of this chapter, you will be able to do the following:

1. Discuss the pathophysiology of nausea and vomiting, including specific precipitating factors and/or diseases.
2. Identify the various antiemetic and antinausea drugs and their drug classification groupings.
3. Describe the mechanisms of action, indications for use, contraindications, cautions, and drug interactions of the various categories of antiemetic and antinausea drugs.
4. Develop a nursing care plan that includes all phases of the nursing process for patients taking antiemetic and antinausea drugs.

DRUG PROFILES

aprepitant, p. 834
dronabinol, p. 834
♦ meclizine, p. 833
♦ metoclopramide, p. 834
♦ ondansetron, p. 834
phosphorated carbohydrate solution, p. 835

♦ prochlorperazine, p. 833
! promethazine, p. 833
scopolamine, p. 833

_____
♦ = *Key drug*
! = *High-alert drug*

KEY TERMS

Antiemetic drugs Drugs given to relieve nausea and vomiting. (p. 829)
Chemoreceptor trigger zone (CTZ) The area of the brain that is involved in the sensation of nausea and the action of vomiting. (p. 828)
Emesis The forcible emptying or expulsion of gastric and, occasionally, intestinal contents through the mouth; also called *vomiting*. (p. 828)

Nausea Sensation often leading to the urge to vomit. (p. 828)
Vomiting center The area of the brain that is involved in stimulating the physiologic events that lead to nausea and vomiting. (p. 828)

NAUSEA AND VOMITING

Nausea and vomiting are two gastrointestinal (GI) disorders that can be extremely unpleasant but also can lead to more serious complications if not treated promptly. **Nausea** is an unpleasant feeling that often precedes vomiting. If it does not subside spontaneously or is not relieved by medication, it can lead to vomiting. Vomiting, which is also called **emesis**, is the forcible emptying or expulsion of gastric and, occasionally, intestinal contents through the mouth. A variety of stimuli can induce nausea and vomiting, including foul odors or tastes, unpleasant sights, irritation of the stomach or intestines, and certain drugs (ipecac or antineoplastic drugs).

The **vomiting center** is an area in the brain that is responsible for initiating the physiologic events that lead to nausea and vomiting. Neurotransmitter signals are sent to the vomiting center from the **chemoreceptor trigger zone (CTZ)**, another area in the brain involved in the induction of nausea and vomiting. These signals alert those areas of the brain to the existence of nauseating substances (noxious stimuli) that need to be expelled from the body. Once the CTZ and vomiting center are stimulated, they initiate the events that trigger the vomiting reflex. The neurotransmitters involved in this process and their respective receptors are listed in Table 52-1. The various pathways and the areas of the body that send the signals to the vomiting center are illustrated in Figure 52-1. Two specific types of nausea and vomiting, chemotherapy-induced and postoperative, produce much more intense symptoms and are treated much more aggressively than general nausea and vomiting.

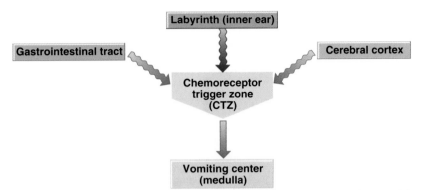

FIGURE 52-1 Various pathways and areas in the body sending signals to the vomiting center.

TABLE 52-1 Neurotransmitters Involved in Nausea and Vomiting

Neurotransmitter (Receptor)	Site in the Vomiting Pathway
Acetylcholine (ACh)	VC in brain; vestibular and labyrinthine pathways in inner ear
Dopamine (D_2)	GI tract and CTZ in brain
Histamine (H_1)	VC in brain; vestibular and labyrinthine pathways in inner ear
Prostaglandins	GI tract
Serotonin (5-HT_3)	GI tract; CTZ and VC in brain
Substance P (Neurokinin 1)	Brainstem

CTZ, Chemoreceptor trigger zone; *ACh,* acetylcholine receptor; *D_2,* dopamine 2 receptor; *H_1,* histamine 1 receptor; *5-HT_3,* 5-hydroxytriptamine 3 receptor; *VC,* vomiting center.

ANTIEMETIC DRUGS

Drugs used to relieve nausea and vomiting are called **antiemetic drugs.** All antiemetic drugs work at some site in the vomiting pathways. There are seven categories of such drugs with varying mechanisms of action. When drugs from different categories are combined, the antiemetic effectiveness is increased because more than one pathway becomes blocked. Some of the more commonly used antiemetics in the various categories are listed in Table 52-2. The sites at which antiemetics work in the vomiting pathway are shown in Figure 52-2. Glucocorticoids (i.e., dexamethasone) are often used for chemotherapy-induced nausea and vomiting and are discussed in Chapter 33.

Mechanism of Action and Drug Effects

Drugs used to prevent or treat nausea and vomiting have many different mechanisms of action. Most work by blocking one of the vomiting pathways, as shown in Figure 52-2. In doing so, they block the neurologic stimulus that induces vomiting. The mechanisms of action of the antiemetic drug categories are summarized in Table 52-3.

Anticholinergic Drugs

Anticholinergics (see Chapter 21) are useful in many different conditions. As antiemetics, they act by binding to and blocking

PATIENT-CENTERED CARE: LIFESPAN CONSIDERATIONS FOR THE PEDIATRIC PATIENT   QSEN

Syrup of Ipecac and Poisoning

- Since November 2003, the American Academy of Pediatrics (AAP) has strongly advised *against* the use of syrup of ipecac as an emetic when children swallow a poisonous substance. In a statement published in the November 2003 issue of *Pediatrics,* the AAP recommended that syrup of ipecac no longer be used as a home treatment for poisoning. Syrup of ipecac is still not recommended for use at this time. See *www.healthychildren.org* for more information.
- If a child has been exposed to a toxic substance, the caregiver must call the national poison control hotline at 800-222-1222. Calls are routed to the local poison control center, or talk to the nearest emergency department.
- Steps to follow to prevent accidental poisoning, as identified by the AAP, include the following: (1) Keep potential poisons out of sight and out of reach. (2) Always check to make sure containers are securely closed and the cabinets where they are stored are securely shut and locked after poisonous substances are used. (3) Never transfer a substance from its original to an alternate container. (4) Safely dispose of all unused and unneeded medications. (5) *Never* refer to medicines as "candy."
- The AAP specifies that the following steps be implemented for the treatment of poisoning in young children: (1) If the poison has been ingested, *first* call the national poison control hotline at 800-222-1222. (2) If the poison has touched the skin or eyes, run tap water over the skin or eyes for 15 to 20 minutes. (3) If the poison has been inhaled, remove the child from the hazardous environment. (4) In *all* cases of poisoning, *if the victim is conscious and alert, call the local poison control center. If the victim has collapsed or stopped breathing, call 911* for emergency transport to a hospital.
- There remains no indication for use of syrup of ipecac in any setting including health care settings.

Modified from American Academy of Pediatrics: Poison treatment in the home, *Pediatrics* 112:1061-1064, 2003; Tips for poison prevention and treatment. Available at *www.healthychildren.org.*

acetylcholine (ACh) receptors in the vestibular nuclei, which are located deep within the brain. When ACh is prevented from binding to these receptors, nausea-inducing signals originating in this area cannot be transmitted to the chemoreceptor trigger zone (CTZ). Anticholinergics also block receptors located in the reticular formation so that nausea-inducing

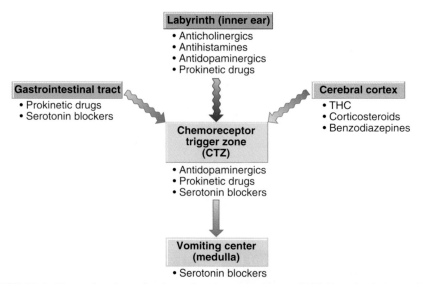

FIGURE 52-2 Sites of action of selected antinausea drugs. *THC,* Tetrahydrocannabinol.

TABLE 52-2 Antiemetic Drugs: Common Drug Categories and Indications

Category	Antiemetic Drugs	Indications
Anticholinergics (acetylcholine blockers)	scopolamine	Motion sickness, secretion reduction before surgery, nausea and vomiting
Antihistamines (H₁ receptor blockers)	dimenhydrinate, diphenhydramine, meclizine	Motion sickness, nonproductive cough, sedation, rhinitis, allergy symptoms, nausea and vomiting
Antidopaminergics	prochlorperazine, promethazine, droperidol	Psychotic disorders (mania, schizophrenia, anxiety), intractable hiccups, nausea and vomiting
Neurokinin antagonists	aprepitant, fosaprepitant	Acute and delayed vomiting associated with chemotherapy
Prokinetics	metoclopramide	Delayed gastric emptying, gastroesophageal reflux, nausea and vomiting
Serotonin blockers	dolasetron, granisetron, ondansetron, palonosetron	Nausea and vomiting associated with chemotherapy, postoperative nausea and vomiting
Tetrahydrocannabinoids	dronabinol	Nausea and vomiting associated with chemotherapy, anorexia associated with weight loss in patients with AIDS and cancer

TABLE 52-3 Antiemetic Drugs: Mechanisms of Action

Category	Mechanism of Action
Anticholinergics	Block ACh receptors in the vestibular nuclei and reticular formation
Antihistamines	Block H₁ receptors, thereby preventing ACh from binding to receptors in the vestibular nuclei
Antidopaminergics	Block dopamine in the CTZ and may also block ACh
Neurokinin receptor antagonists	Inhibit the substance P–neurokinin receptors
Prokinetics	Block dopamine in the CTZ or stimulate ACh receptors in the GI tract
Serotonin blockers	Block serotonin receptors in the GI tract, CTZ, and VC
Tetrahydrocannabinoids	Have inhibitory effects on the reticular formation, thalamus, and cerebral cortex

ACh, Acetylcholine; *CTZ,* chemoreceptor trigger zone; *VC,* vomiting center.

signals originating in this area cannot be transmitted to the vomiting center. Anticholinergics also tend to dry GI secretions and reduce smooth muscle spasms, both of which effects are often helpful in reducing acute GI symptoms, including nausea and vomiting.

Antihistamines

Antihistamines (histamine 1 [H₁] receptor blockers) act by inhibiting vestibular stimulation in a manner that is very similar to that of the anticholinergics. Although they bind primarily to H₁ receptors, they also have potent anticholinergic activity, including antisecretory and antispasmodic effects. Thus, the antihistamines (see Chapter 36) prevent cholinergic stimulation in both the vestibular and reticular systems. Nausea and vomiting occur when these systems are stimulated. Note that these drugs are not to be confused with histamine 2 [H₂] receptor blockers used for gastric acid control (see Chapter 50).

Antidopaminergic Drugs

These drugs are traditionally used for their antipsychotic effects (see Chapter 16), but also prevent nausea and vomiting by blocking dopamine receptors in the CTZ. Many of the antidopaminergics also have anticholinergic actions and calm the central nervous system.

Neurokinin Blockers

Neurokinin receptor antagonists inhibit substance P–neurokinin 1 receptors in the brain stem. Neurokinin blockers are used in conjunction with serotonin blockers and glucocorticoids. Their use augments the serotonin blockers and glucocorticoids to inhibit acute and delayed phases of chemotherapy-induced emesis.

Prokinetic Drugs

Prokinetic drugs, in particular metoclopramide, act as antiemetics by blocking dopamine receptors in the CTZ, which desensitizes the CTZ to impulses it receives from the GI tract. Their primary action, however, is to stimulate peristalsis in the GI tract. This enhances the emptying of stomach contents into the duodenum, as well as intestinal movements.

Serotonin Blockers

Serotonin blockers work by blocking serotonin receptors located in the GI tract, CTZ, and vomiting center. There are many subtypes of serotonin receptors, and they are located throughout the body (CNS, smooth muscle, platelets, and GI tract). The receptor subtype involved in the mediation of nausea and vomiting is the 5-hydroxytryptamine 3 (5-HT_3) receptor. These receptors are the site of action of the serotonin blockers such as ondansetron, granisetron, dolasetron, and palonosetron.

Tetrahydrocannabinoids

Tetrahydrocannabinol (THC), in a drug class by itself, is the major psychoactive substance in marijuana. Nonintoxicating doses in the form of the drug dronabinol are occasionally used as an antiemetic because of the drug's inhibitory effects on the reticular formation, thalamus, and cerebral cortex. These effects cause an alteration in mood and in the body's perception of its surroundings, which may be beneficial in relieving nausea and vomiting. Although this particular category of antiemetics is less commonly prescribed, there are occasionally patients who respond well to THC, including patients being treated for cancer or AIDS who experience nausea and vomiting. In such patients, dronabinol may also stimulate the appetite, and nutritional wasting syndromes are common in both diseases. The drug also demonstrates some benefit in controlling the symptoms of glaucoma.

Indications

The therapeutic uses of the antiemetic drugs vary depending on the drug category. There are several indications for the drugs in each class. These are listed in Table 52-2.

Contraindications

The primary contraindication for all antiemetics is known drug allergy. Other contraindications for various specific drugs are mentioned in the drug profiles.

Adverse Effects

Most of the adverse effects of the antiemetics stem from their nonselective blockade of various receptors. Some of the more common adverse effects associated with the various categories of antinausea drugs are listed in Table 52-4.

Interactions

The drug interactions associated with the antiemetic drugs are specific to the individual drug categories. Anticholinergics

TABLE 52-4 Antinausea Drugs: Adverse Effects	
Body System	**Adverse Effects**
Anticholinergics	
Central nervous	Dizziness, drowsiness, disorientation
Cardiovascular	Tachycardia
Ears, eyes, nose, throat	Blurred vision, dilated pupils, dry mouth
Genitourinary	Difficult urination, constipation
Integumentary	Rash, erythema
Antihistamines	
Central nervous	Dizziness, drowsiness, confusion
Ears, eyes, nose, throat	Blurred vision, dilated pupils, dry mouth
Genitourinary	Urinary retention
Antidopaminergics	
Cardiovascular	Orthostatic hypotension, tachycardia
Central nervous	Extrapyramidal symptoms, tardive dyskinesia, headache
Ears, eyes, nose, throat	Blurred vision, dry eyes
Genitourinary	Urinary retention
Gastrointestinal	Dry mouth, nausea and vomiting, anorexia, constipation
Neurokinin Receptor Antagonists	
Cardiovascular	hypotension, bradycardia
Central nervous	fatigue, dizziness
Gastrointestinal	diarrhea, dyspepsia, abdominal pain, gastritis
Prokinetics	
Cardiovascular	Hypotension, supraventricular tachycardia
Central nervous	Sedation, fatigue, restlessness, headache, dystonia
Gastrointestinal	Dry mouth, nausea and vomiting, diarrhea
Serotonin Blockers	
Central nervous	Headache
Gastrointestinal	Diarrhea
Other	Rash, bronchospasm, prolonged QT interval
Tetrahydrocannabinoids	
Central nervous	Drowsiness, dizziness, anxiety, confusion, euphoria
Ears, eyes, nose, throat	Visual disturbances
Gastrointestinal	Dry mouth

have additive drying effects when given with antihistamines and antidepressants. Increased CNS depressant effects are seen when antihistamine antiemetics are administered with barbiturates, opioids, hypnotics, tricyclic antidepressants, or alcohol. Increased CNS depression also occurs when alcohol or other CNS depressants are given together with antidopaminergic drugs. Combining metoclopramide with alcohol can result in additive CNS depression. Anticholinergics and analgesics can block the motility effects of metoclopramide. Neurokinin antagonists (aprepitant) may induce the metabolism of warfarin, and may reduce the effectiveness of oral contraceptives. Because aprepitant is a major inhibitor of the cytochrome P-450 enzyme system, caution must be used in giving it together with drugs that are primarily metabolized by cytochrome P-450 enzyme 3A4, including azole antifungals, clarithromycin, diltiazem, nicardipine, protease inhibitors, and verapamil. It may increase the bioavailability of corticosteroids, including dexamethasone and methylprednisolone, and dosages of these drugs may need to be adjusted by 25% to 50%. Serotonin blockers and THC have no significant drug interactions.

Dosages

For dosage information on selected antiemetic drugs, see the table on this page.

DRUG PROFILES

Antiemetics are used to treat nausea and vomiting in a variety of clinical situations, including chemotherapy-induced and postoperative nausea and vomiting, both of which can be especially difficult to treat. The ultimate goals of antiemetic therapy

---

DOSAGES

Selected Antiemetic and Antinausea Drugs

Drug (Pregnancy Category)	Pharmacologic Class	Usual Adult Dosage Range	Indications/Uses
Anticholinergics			
scopolamine (Transderm-Scōp) (C)	Anticholinergic, belladonna alkaloid	Apply 1 patch to hairless area behind 1 ear every 3 days (starting at least 4 hr before travel)	Motion sickness prophylaxis
Antihistamines			
◆ meclizine (Antivert, Bonine) (B)	Anticholinergic, antihistamine	PO: 25-50 mg 1 hr before travel and repeated daily during travel	Motion sickness prophylaxis
		PO: 25-100 mg/day, divided 1-4 times daily	Treatment of vertigo
Antidopaminergics			
◆ prochlorperazine (Compazine) (C)	Phenothiazine	PO: 5-10 mg 3-4 times daily IM: 5-10 mg every 3-4 hr (max 40 mg/day) PR: 25 mg twice daily IV: 5-10 mg every 6 hr	Antiemetic
! promethazine (Phenergan) (C)	Phenothiazine	IV, IM, PO, PR: 12.5-25 mg every 4-6 hr	Antiemetic
aprepitant (Emend) (B)	substance P–neurokinin inhibitor	Oral 125 mg on day 1, then 80 mg/day	Chemotherapy antiemetic
Prokinetics			
◆ metoclopramide (Reglan) (B)	Dopamine antagonist	IV: 1-2 mg/kg (30 min before chemotherapy; repeat every 2 hr × 2 doses, then every 3 hr × 3 doses)	Chemotherapy antiemetic
		IM: 10-20 mg × 1 dose near end of surgery; repeat every 4-6 hr as needed	Prevention of postoperative nausea and vomiting
Serotonin Blockers			
◆ ondansetron (Zofran) (B)	Antiserotonergic	PO: 8 mg tid IV: 0.15 mg/kg every 4 hr	Chemotherapy antiemetic
Tetrahydrocannabinoids			
dronabinol (Marinol) (C)	Marijuana-derived antiemetic	PO: Initially, 5 mg/m² 1-3 hr before chemotherapy, then every 2-4 hr after chemotherapy up to 6 times daily for 3 days	Chemotherapy antiemetic

are minimizing or preventing fluid and electrolyte disturbances and minimizing deterioration of the patient's nutritional status. Most of the antiemetics act by blocking receptors in the CNS, but some work directly in the GI tract. There are seven major classes of antiemetic drugs, although there are other drugs that may also be used to treat nausea and vomiting, including corticosteroids such as dexamethasone (see Chapter 33) and anxiolytics such as lorazepam (see Chapter 16). Lorazepam is often used in the treatment and prevention of chemotherapy-induced nausea and vomiting. In addition to an antiemetic effect, it also helps to blunt the memory of the nausea and vomiting experience (especially with cancer chemotherapy). Dexamethasone, lorazepam, and dronabinol are beneficial in preventing nausea and vomiting caused by chemotherapy, especially when used in combination with the serotonin blockers.

ANTICHOLINERGIC
scopolamine

Scopolamine (Transderm-Scōp, Scopace) is the primary anticholinergic drug used as an antiemetic. It has potent effects on the vestibular nuclei, which are located in the area of the brain that controls balance. Scopolamine works by blocking the binding of ACh to the cholinergic receptors in this region and thereby correcting an imbalance between the two neurotransmitters ACh and norepinephrine. These effects make scopolamine one of the most commonly used drugs for the treatment and prevention of the nausea and vomiting associated with motion sickness. Scopolamine is also used to treat postoperative nausea and vomiting. Use of the drug is contraindicated in patients with glaucoma. Scopolamine is available in oral, injectable, transdermal, and even ocular forms (see Chapter 57). The most commonly used formulation for nausea is the 72-hour transdermal patch, which releases a total of 1 mg of the drug.

Pharmacokinetics: Scopolamine (Transderm-Scōp, Scopace)

Route	Onset of Action	Peak Plasma Concentration	Elimination Half-life	Duration of Action
Transdermal	1-2 hr	6-8 hr	8-9.5 hr	72 hr

ANTIHISTAMINES

Antihistamine antiemetics are some of the most commonly used and safest antiemetics. Some of the popular antihistamines are meclizine (Antivert), dimenhydrinate (Dramamine), and diphenhydramine (Benadryl). Many of the antihistamines are available over the counter. Hydroxyzine (Vistaril) is used for antiemetic purposes and is available in oral and intramuscular formulations. Hydroxyzine must never be given by the intravenous route (see Safety and Quality Improvement: Preventing Medication Errors on p. 835).

◆meclizine

Meclizine (Antivert) is commonly used to treat the dizziness, vertigo, and nausea and vomiting associated with motion sickness. Contraindications include shock and lactation. It is available for oral use only.

Pharmacokinetics: Meclizine

Route	Onset of Action	Peak Plasma Concentration	Elimination Half-life	Duration of Action
PO	1 hr	Variable	6 hr	8-24 hr

ANTIDOPAMINERGICS

Prochlorperazine (Compazine) and promethazine (Phenergan) are the most commonly used antiemetics in the antidopaminergic class. These drugs have antidopaminergic as well as antihistaminergic and anticholinergic properties. Droperidol was widely used to treat and prevent postoperative nausea and vomiting for several decades until the U.S. Food and Drug Administration (FDA) called for a black box warning and required continuous electrocardiographic monitoring with its use. These restrictions were in response to concerns over QT widening and possible ventricular dysrhythmias. Some health care institutions still use droperidol, whereas others have banned its use.

◆prochlorperazine

Prochlorperazine (Compazine), especially in the injectable form, is used frequently in the hospital setting. The drug is contraindicated in patients with hypersensitivity to phenothiazines, those in a coma, and those who have seizures, encephalopathy, or bone marrow suppression. It is available for both injection and oral use.

Pharmacokinetics: Prochlorperazine

Route	Onset of Action	Peak Plasma Concentration	Elimination Half-life	Duration of Action
IM	30-40 min	2-4 hr	6-8 hr	3-4 hr

❗promethazine

Promethazine (Phenergan) is commonly used in hospitalized patients as an antiemetic. The preferred route is oral or intramuscular. The intravenous route is not the preferred route but is commonly used. However, extreme care must be taken to avoid accidental intraarterial injection. If promethazine is inadvertently given intraarterially instead of intravenously, severe tissue damage, often requiring amputation, can occur. Promethazine is best diluted in at least 10 mL of fluid (the more dilute the better) and given in a running intravenous line at the port furthest from the patient's vein or through a large-bore vein (not hand or wrist vein). Therapy must be discontinued immediately if burning or pain occurs with administration. Promethazine is contraindicated in children younger than 2 years of age. Sedation is the most common adverse effect and actually may be beneficial. The drug is also available as a rectal suppository. It is not to be given subcutaneously. For more information, see Safety and Quality Improvement: Preventing Medication Errors on p. 835.

Pharmacokinetics: Promethazine

Route	Onset of Action	Peak Plasma Concentration	Elimination Half-life	Duration of Action
IM	20 min	4.4 hr	9-16 hr	2-6 hr

NEUROKININ RECEPTOR ANTAGONISTS
aprepitant

Aprepitant (Emend) is an antagonist of substance P–neurokinin 1 receptors in the brain. In contrast to other antiemetics, this drug has little affinity for 5-HT$_3$ (serotonin) and dopamine receptors. Studies show that aprepitant augments the antiemetic actions of both ondansetron and dexamethasone. This drug is specifically indicated for the prevention of nausea and vomiting associated with highly emetogenic cancer chemotherapy regimens, including high-dose cisplatin, as well as postoperative nausea and vomiting. Common adverse effects include dizziness, headache, insomnia, and GI discomfort, but these are generally no more common than with other standard antiemetic regimens. Aprepitant may induce the metabolism of warfarin, and international normalized ratio (INR) needs to be checked before each cycle of aprepitant. The drug may reduce the effectiveness of oral contraceptives. Aprepitant is a major inhibitor of the cytochrome P-450 enzyme system, thus caution must be used when giving it together with drugs that are primarily metabolized by cytochrome P-450 enzyme 3A4, including azole antifungals, clarithromycin, diltiazem, nicardipine, protease inhibitors, and verapamil. It may increase the bioavailability of corticosteroids. Aprepitant is classified as a pregnancy category B drug. Fosaprepitant is the intravenous form of aprepitant. Akynzeo is a new combination drug that includes a 5-HT3 (palonosetron) and a substance P inhibitor (netupitant); it is indicated for use with highly emetogenic chemotherapy regimens.

Pharmacokinetics: Aprepitant

Route	Onset of Action	Peak Plasma Concentration	Elimination Half-life	Duration of Action
PO	1 hr	3-4 hr	9-13 hr	NA

PROKINETIC

Prokinetic drugs promote the movement of substances through the GI tract and increase GI motility. The only prokinetic drug that is also used to prevent nausea and vomiting is metoclopramide.

◆ metoclopramide

Metoclopramide (Reglan) is available only by prescription because it can cause some severe adverse effects if not used correctly. Metoclopramide is used for the treatment of delayed gastric emptying and gastroesophageal reflux and also as an antiemetic. Its use is contraindicated in patients with seizure disorder, pheochromocytoma, breast cancer, or GI obstruction and also in patients with a known hypersensitivity to it or to procaine or procainamide. Metoclopramide is available in both oral and parenteral formulations. Extrapyramidal adverse effects can occur with its use, especially in young adults. In 2009, the FDA posted a public health advisory regarding the potential for developing tardive dyskinesia with long-term use of metoclopramide.

Pharmacokinetics: Metoclopramide

Route	Onset of Action	Peak Plasma Concentration	Elimination Half-life	Duration of Action
PO	20-60 min	1-2.5 hr	2.5-6 hr	3-4 hr

SEROTONIN BLOCKERS

The serotonin blockers are also called *5-HT3 receptor blockers* because they block the 5-HT$_3$ receptors in the GI tract, the CTZ, and the vomiting center. (The chemical name for serotonin is 5-hydroxytryptamine, or 5-HT.) Drugs in this class have very specific actions, and as a result they have very few adverse effects. No significant drug interactions are known to occur. These drugs are indicated for the prevention of nausea and vomiting associated with cancer chemotherapy and also for the prevention of postoperative or radiation-induced nausea and vomiting. Currently there are four drugs in this category: dolasetron (Anzemet), granisetron (Kytril), ondansetron (Zofran), and palonosetron (Aloxi). This class of drugs revolutionized the treatment of nausea and vomiting, especially in cancer patients and postoperative patients. When used to prevent postoperative nausea and vomiting, a dose is usually given approximately 30 minutes before the end of the surgical procedure. When used to prevent or treat nausea and vomiting associated with cancer treatment, they are given 30 to 60 minutes prior to the start of chemotherapy. All drugs in this class are classified as pregnancy category B drugs. In 2010, the FDA issued a warning regarding dolasetron and the risk for cardiac dysrhythmias. In 2011, the FDA added the same warning for ondansetron. The FDA no longer recommends dolasetron to be used for chemotherapy-induced nausea and vomiting.

◆ ondansetron

Ondansetron (Zofran) is the prototypical drug in this class. Approved in 1992, it represented a major breakthrough in treating chemotherapy-induced nausea and vomiting and, later, postoperative nausea and vomiting. It is also used for the treatment of hyperemesis gravidarum (nausea and vomiting associated with pregnancy). Its only listed contraindication is known drug allergy. It is available in both oral and injectable forms and as orally disintegrating tablets. Doses up to 8 mg can be given by intravenous push over 2 to 5 minutes. Ondansetron was the first of the class to become available as a generic formulation, which significantly increased its use. Granisetron is available as a transdermal patch. Although ondansetron is pregnancy category B, there is concern regarding cleft palate development in the fetus when used in the first trimester.

Pharmacokinetics: Ondansetron

Route	Onset of Action	Peak Plasma Concentration	Elimination Half-life	Duration of Action
IV	15-30 min	1-1.5 hr	3.5-5 hr	6-12 hr

TETRAHYDROCANNABINOID
dronabinol

Dronabinol (Marinol) is the only commercially available tetrahydrocannabinoid. It is a synthetic derivative of THC, the major active substance in marijuana. Dronabinol was approved by the FDA in 1985 for the treatment of nausea and vomiting associated with cancer chemotherapy. It is generally used as a second-line drug after treatment with other antiemetics has failed. It is also used to stimulate appetite and weight gain in patients with AIDS and chemotherapy patients. Its only listed contraindication is known drug allergy. It is available for oral use only.

Pharmacokinetics: Dronabinol

Route	Onset of Action	Peak Plasma Concentration	Elimination Half-life	Duration of Action
PO	30-60 min	1-3 hr	19-36 hr	4-6 hr

MISCELLANEOUS ANTINAUSEA DRUGS
phosphorated carbohydrate solution

Phosphorated carbohydrate solution (Emetrol) is a mint-flavored, pleasant-tasting oral solution used to relieve nausea. It works by direct local action on the walls of the GI tract, where it reduces cramping caused by excessive smooth muscle contraction. It can be used to control mild cases of nausea and vomiting. It does not have a pregnancy category rating, but one of its listed unlabeled (non–FDA-approved) uses is for treatment of morning sickness during pregnancy. Phosphorated carbohydrate solution is not sufficient for treatment of more severe nausea symptoms such as those associated with cancer chemotherapy. Its only contraindication is known drug allergy. It is available for oral use only.

NURSING PROCESS

ASSESSMENT

Before any *antinausea* or *antiemetic drug* is administered, obtain a complete nursing history and perform a thorough physical assessment with attention to the following: history of the symptoms of nausea and vomiting; medical history and current medical status; medication history and drugs currently taken including over-the-counter drugs, herbals, prescription drugs, and social drugs (e.g., cigarettes, alcohol); and use of any alternative therapies. Identify any factors precipitating nausea or vomiting; note any weight loss; measure baseline vital signs; assess intake and output; examine the skin and mucous membranes, noting turgor and color; and assess and document capillary refill time (normal is less than 5 seconds). If laboratory tests are ordered (e.g., serum sodium, potassium, and chloride levels; hemoglobin level and hematocrit; red blood cell and white blood cell counts; urinalysis), assess and document the findings to establish baseline levels. Assess for any contraindications or cautions to the use of these drugs and for drug interactions, as well as any allergies.

Only give the *anticholinergic drug scopolamine* after careful assessment of the patient's health history and medication history. One very important concern to emphasize with scopolamine, which is commonly administered in patch form to prevent motion sickness, is the contraindication to its use in patients with narrow-angle glaucoma. If the patient has a history of this disorder, another antiemetic or antinausea drug

⚡ SAFETY AND QUALITY IMPROVEMENT: PREVENTING MEDICATION ERRORS

Right Route Is Essential

Two commonly used antiemetic drugs may have serious consequences for the patient if they are given via the wrong route.

Hydroxyzine (Vistaril) is an antihistamine-class antiemetic that is only to be given by oral or intramuscular routes. However, when so many other antiemetics are given by the intravenous route, it may be easy to make the mistake of giving hydroxyzine intravenously. It is important to note that intravenous, intraarterial, or subcutaneous administration of hydroxyzine may result in significant tissue damage, thrombosis, and gangrene.

Promethazine (Phenergan) is another commonly used antiemetic. The oral and intramuscular routes are the preferred routes of administration; the intravenous route, while commonly used, is not the preferred route. If this drug is given intraarterially, severe tissue damage, possibly leading to amputation, may occur.

These are just two examples that illustrate the importance of the "right route" with drug administration.

is prescribed. The same concern regarding use in patients with narrow-angle glaucoma applies to *antihistamines* (e.g., *meclizine*). Additionally, antihistamines must be used cautiously in pediatric patients, who may have severe paradoxical reactions. Older adult patients may develop agitation, mental confusion, hypotension, and even psychotic-type reactions in response to these drugs. Other medications need to be considered for patients if these reactions occur. Assess for drug interactions such as other CNS depressants.

Antidopaminergic drugs, such as *promethazine,* are to be used after cautious assessment for signs and symptoms of dehydration and electrolyte imbalance with checking skin turgor and examining the tongue for the presence of longitudinal furrows. Monitor vital signs, especially blood pressure and pulse rate, due to adverse effects of orthostatic hypotension and tachycardia. CNS concerns to assess for include any abnormal movements at baseline functioning because these drugs can lead to adverse effects of extrapyramidal symptoms. Contraindications, cautions, and drug interactions for these drugs are discussed earlier in the chapter. Double-checking the name and mechanism of action is also important (*prochlorperazine* may be confused with *promethazine*) to prevent sound-alike medication errors.

The *neurokinin receptor antagonist, aprepitant,* interacts with several medications such as warfarin, oral contraceptives, antifungals (azoles), clarithromycin, verapamil, and corticosteroids. Assess dosage amount carefully because it usually begins with oral dosage of 125 mg on day 1 of chemotherapy and then is followed with 80 mg/day, as prescribed.

The *prokinetic drug metoclopramide* is often reserved for the treatment of nausea and vomiting associated with antineoplastic drug therapy or radiation therapy and for the treatment of GI motility disturbances. The action of this drug is decreased when it is taken with anticholinergics or opiates; therefore, assess for this interaction as well as for interactions with alcohol. Assess also for contraindications such as individuals with seizure disorders, GI obstruction, and known hypersensitivity to it or to procaine or procainamide. Remember the FDA public health advisory regarding untoward reactions with long-term use of *metoclopramide* (see the pharmacology section).

Only give the *serotonin blocker granisetron* after assessment of baseline vital signs and age; its use has not been established in those younger than 2 years of age. *Ondansetron* use requires assessment for the signs and symptoms of dehydration and electrolyte disturbances. Ondansetron has the warning of its use and the risk for cardiac dysrhythmias. Assess skin turgor, and examine mucous membranes for dryness and/or longitudinal furrows in the tongue.

With the tetrahydrocannabinoid dronabinol, assess patients for signs and symptoms of dehydration, with attention to low urine output, dry mucous membranes, poor skin turgor, and lethargy. Perform a thorough assessment of hydration status because treatment of volume and electrolyte imbalances may be required in addition to treatment with antinausea or antiemetic drugs. Assess motor and cognitive abilities with documentation of baseline findings.

QSEN   ### SAFETY: HERBAL THERAPIES AND DIETARY SUPPLEMENTS

Ginger (Zingiber officinale)

Overview
Ginger (Zingiber officinale) is found naturally in the Asian tropics and is now cultivated in other continents, including part of the United States. Plant parts utilized are the rhizome and root. Active ingredients include gingerols and gingerdione.

Common Uses
It is used as an antioxidant and for relief of varied symptoms such as sore throat, migraine headache, and nausea and vomiting (including that induced by cancer chemotherapy, morning sickness, and motion sickness); There are many other varied uses.

Adverse Effects
Adverse effects include skin reactions, anorexia, nausea, and vomiting.

Potential Drug Interactions
It can increase absorption of all oral medications and may theoretically increase bleeding risk with anticoagulants (e.g., warfarin [Coumadin]) or antiplatelet drugs (e.g., clopidogrel [Plavix])

Contraindications
Ginger is contraindicated in cases of known product allergy. It may worsen cholelithiasis (gallstones). There is anecdotal evidence of abortifacient properties, and some practitioners recommend not using during pregnancy.

NURSING DIAGNOSES

1. Nausea related to disease pathology and adverse effects of specific groups of medications
2. Impaired physical mobility related to adverse effects (e.g., sedation, lethargy, confusion) of antiemetics
3. Risk for injury (falls) related to the adverse effects of antiemetic medications (e.g., sedation and dizziness)

4. Risk for deficient fluid volume related to nausea and vomiting and limited oral intake

PLANNING: OUTCOME IDENTIFICATION

1. Patient remains free from nausea and vomiting with use of pharmacologic and nonpharmacologic therapies such as avoiding irritating, spicy foods/beverages.
2. Patient regains mobility status and/or remains with stable mobility during drug therapy with use of assistance with walking and ADLs as needed.
3. Patient remains free from injury during antiemetic drug therapy with safety measures such as changing positions and rising slowly, taking medications as ordered, and initiating fluids once nausea/vomiting subsides.
4. Patient maintains/regains fluid volume balance while undergoing antiemetic treatment with consumption of fluids beginning with clear liquids

IMPLEMENTATION

Undiluted forms of *diphenhydramine*, an *antihistamine*, must be cautiously administered intravenously at the recommended rate of 25 mg/min as ordered. Administer intramuscular forms into large muscles (e.g., ventral gluteal), and rotate sites if repeated injections are necessary. Frequently monitor blood pressure in patients taking meclizine, especially if they are older adults, due to increased sensitivity to the drug's effects. Be aware of the concern that sedation poses for patient safety, and emphasize the need for cautious movement at all times. Dry mouth, another adverse effect, produced by any of these medications may be alleviated by using sugarless gum or hard candy.

CASE STUDY

Patient-Centered Care: Nausea and Chemotherapy

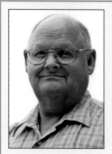

Mr. S., a 68-year-old retired bus driver, has begun outpatient chemotherapy after a recent diagnosis of lung cancer. He has recovered well from a right lung lobectomy, the incisions are well healed, and he is now physically and emotionally ready for a 3-month regimen of chemotherapy. The premedication orders call for a variety of drugs, including granisetron (Kytril). Mr. S. has a prescription for oral ondansetron (Zofran) for use at home.

1. What is the mechanism of action of granisetron that makes it effective in the management of chemotherapy-induced nausea and vomiting?
2. What important patient teaching points should you emphasize to Mr. S. about the ondansetron?
3. After 2 weeks of therapy, the oncologist discontinues the ondansetron because Mr. S. complains that it does nothing to help the nausea and vomiting. Mr. S. receives a prescription for dronabinol but expresses concern, exclaiming, "There's marijuana in that pill!" What would you explain to Mr. S.?

For answers, see *http://evolve.elsevier.com/Lilley*.

Promethazine may be given orally without regard to meals. Suppository forms are available, if needed. Keep suppository dosage forms in their foil covering until use and, once the wrap is removed, the dosage form may be moistened with water or water-soluble lubricating gel before being inserted well into the rectum. For rectal suppository insertion, place the patient on the left side, and keep the patient there for several minutes after insertion (see Chapter 9). Tell the patient to hold in the suppository for as long as possible to increase its absorption. Measure vital signs, and monitor the patient for extrapyramidal symptoms throughout therapy. Encourage the patient to avoid other CNS depressants and alcohol as well as to limit caffeine when using this drug. Instruct the patient to avoid driving and other activities that require mental alertness or motor coordination.

Aprepitant is often used in combination with other medications to prevent nausea and vomiting associated with chemotherapy and may also be given, as ordered, for postoperative nausea and vomiting. The prescriber's orders may indicate other drugs to be administered as well as the timing of the dosage.

Metoclopramide given orally is best taken 30 minutes before meals and at bedtime. Infuse intravenous dosage forms over the recommended time period. In addition, keep solutions for parenteral dosing for only 48 hours, and protect them from light. Do not give metoclopramide in combination with any other medications, such as phenothiazines, that would lead to exacerbation of extrapyramidal reactions. If extrapyramidal reactions occur, they need to be reported to the prescriber immediately. The development of tardive dyskinesia, an involuntary neurologic movement, has been associated with the long-term use of metoclopramide. Monitor for and educate patients about this potential problem.

The *scopolamine* transdermal patch is applied behind the ear as directed. The area behind the ear needs to be cleansed and dried before the patch is applied. If the patch becomes dislodged, the residual drug must be washed off and a fresh patch put in place. Remind the patient to avoid tasks requiring mental clarity or motor skills while taking this medication. The transdermal patch is to be left in place for 72 hours, as ordered.

It is commonly applied to prevent postoperative nausea/vomiting.

Granisetron may be given intravenously or orally. Infuse intravenous doses over the recommended time period, and dilute as appropriate. A transient taste disorder may occur, especially if the drug is taken with antineoplastic medications, but will diminish with continued therapy. Always encourage the use of various relaxation techniques as complementary therapies. *Ondansetron* may be given orally, intramuscularly, or intravenously. Inject intramuscular doses into a large muscle mass. Intravenous push is usually given over 2 to 5 minutes and infusions over 15 minutes as ordered and as per manufacturer guidelines. Oral forms are well tolerated regardless of the relation of dosing to meals. Encourage the patient to avoid alcohol and other CNS depressants during this therapy and to avoid any activities requiring mental alertness or motor skill. If *serotonin blockers* are prescribed to prevent postoperative nausea and vomiting, dosing is usually 30 minutes before the end of the surgical procedure. If used to prevent/treat nausea and vomiting associated with chemotherapy, the drug is usually given 30 to 60 minutes prior to the treatment.

Dronabinol is to be administered 1 to 3 hours before antineoplastic therapy and may be taken at home before the scheduled treatment appointment. Relief of nausea and vomiting usually occurs within approximately 15 minutes of oral drug administration.

EVALUATION

The therapeutic effects of *antiemetic* and *antinausea drugs* include a decrease in or elimination of nausea and vomiting, and avoidance or elimination of complications such as fluid and electrolyte imbalances and weight loss. Monitor the patient for adverse effects such as GI upset, drowsiness, lethargy, weakness, extrapyramidal reactions, and orthostatic hypotension during antiemetic therapy. Laboratory testing (e.g., electrolyte levels, blood urea nitrogen level, urinalysis with specific gravity) may be ordered for evaluation purposes. Defined goals and outcomes may also be used to evaluate therapeutic effectiveness.

PATIENT-CENTERED CARE: PATIENT TEACHING

- Warn the patient using an antiemetic or antinausea drug about the adverse effect of drowsiness. Instruct the patient to use caution while performing hazardous tasks or driving while taking these drugs. Caution the patient about taking antiemetic or antinausea drugs with alcohol and other CNS depressants because of the possible toxicity and exacerbation of CNS depression.
- The antihistamine meclizine is also used for vertigo and motion sickness. It may precipitate sedation and needs to be used with caution.
- Rotate the application sites for transdermal scopolamine patches. Patches are to be applied to nonirritated areas behind the ear. Wash hands thoroughly before and after application.
- Educate the patient about the possible adverse effects of ondansetron, including heart rate irregularities and

headache. Headache may be relieved by taking a simple analgesic such as acetaminophen but avoiding aspirin-containing products. If used during chemotherapy, it is given 30 to 60 minutes prior to the dosing of the antineoplastic drug. The use of an antiemetic generally continues throughout the treatment regimen.
- Remind the patient taking dronabinol to change positions slowly to prevent syncope or dizziness resulting from the hypotensive effects of the drug. Advise the patient to be cautious when engaging in activities that require mental alertness while taking this medication. Phosphorated carbohydrate solution (Emetrol) is given orally to relieve mild cases of nausea, and its use is not sufficient for more severe nausea/vomiting.

KEY POINTS

- Antiemetics help to control vomiting, or emesis, and are also useful in relieving or preventing nausea. Antiemetics are used to prevent motion sickness, reduce secretions before surgery, treat delayed gastric emptying, and prevent postoperative nausea and vomiting. Most of these drugs can cause drowsiness.

- Anticholinergics work by blocking ACh receptors in the vestibular nuclei and reticular formation. This blockade prevents areas in the brain from being activated by nauseous stimuli.

- Antihistamines work by blocking H_1 receptors, which produces the same effect as the anticholinergics. Antidopaminergic antiemetics block dopamine receptors in the CTZ and may also block ACh receptors. Prokinetic drugs also block dopamine receptors in the CTZ.

- The serotonin-blocking drugs (granisetron and ondansetron) may be highly effective antiemetics. They are most commonly used for the prevention of chemotherapy-induced nausea and vomiting.

- Antiemetics are often given 30 to 60 minutes before a chemotherapy drug is administered (time may vary depending on the specific drug) and may also be given during the chemotherapeutic treatment.

- Dronabinol therapy is used to prevent chemotherapy-induced nausea and vomiting and is associated with postural hypotension.

- Caution patients taking antiemetic or antinausea drugs that drowsiness and hypotension may occur and to avoid driving and using heavy machinery while taking these medications.

NCLEX® EXAMINATION REVIEW QUESTIONS

1. The nurse is providing patient teaching regarding scopolamine transdermal patches (Transderm-Scōp) to a patient who is planning an ocean cruise. Which instruction is most appropriate?
   a. "Apply the patch the day before traveling."
   b. "Apply the patch at least 4 hours before traveling."
   c. "Apply the patch to the shoulder area."
   d. "Apply the patch to the temple just above the ear."

2. A middle-aged woman is experiencing severe vertigo. The nurse expects this patient will receive which drug, which is considered the most appropriate drug treatment for vertigo?
   a. meclizine (Antivert)
   b. prochlorperazine (Compazine)
   c. metoclopramide (Reglan)
   d. dronabinol (Marinol)

3. A 33-year-old patient is in the outpatient cancer center for his first round of chemotherapy. The nurse knows that which schedule is the most appropriate timing for the intravenous antiemetic drug?
   a. Four hours before the chemotherapy begins
   b. Thirty to sixty minutes before the chemotherapy begins
   c. At the same time as the chemotherapy drugs are given
   d. At the first sign of nausea

4. When reviewing the various types of antinausea medications, the nurse recognizes that prokinetic drugs are also used for
   a. motion sickness.
   b. vertigo.
   c. delayed gastric emptying.
   d. GI obstruction.

5. A patient who has been receiving chemotherapy tells the nurse that he has been searching the Internet for antinausea remedies and that he found a reference to a product called Emetrol (phosphorated carbohydrate solution). He wants to know if this drug would help him. What is the nurse's best answer?

   a. "This may be a good remedy for you. Let's talk to your prescriber."
   b. "This drug is used only after other drugs have not worked."
   c. "This drug is used only to treat severe nausea and vomiting caused by chemotherapy."
   d. "This drug may not help the more severe nausea symptoms associated with chemotherapy."

6. The nurse is preparing to administer dronabinol (Marinol) to a patient. Which statements about dronabinol therapy are true? *(Select all that apply.)*
   a. It is approved for nausea and vomiting related to cancer chemotherapy.
   b. It is approved for use with hyperemesis gravidarum (nausea and vomiting associated with pregnancy).
   c. It is approved to help stimulate the appetite in patients with nutritional wasting due to cancer or AIDS.
   d. It may cause extrapyramidal symptoms.
   e. It may cause drowsiness or euphoria.

7. The order reads: "Give promethazine (Phenergan) 12.5 mg IM q4h prn nausea/vomiting." The medication is available in 25-mg/mL vials. How many milliliters will the nurse draw up for this dose?

8. The nurse is reviewing the current medications for a patient who has a new prescription for aprepitant (Emend). Which of these medications may have an interaction with aprepitant? *(Select all that apply.)*
   a. digoxin
   b. warfarin
   c. oral contraceptives
   d. nonsteroidal antiinflammatory drugs
   e. corticosteroids

1. b, 2. a, 3. b, 4. c, 5. d, 6. a, c, e, 7. 0.5 mL, 8. b, c, e.

CRITICAL THINKING AND PRIORITIZATION QUESTIONS

1. A patient who has received chemotherapy with a highly emetogenic drug has orders for both ondansetron (Zofran) and prochlorperazine (Compazine). Which drug would be the best choice for the nurse to administer for the patient's nausea and vomiting, and how should it be administered for the best effects? Explain your answer.

2. The nurse has just given an 83-year-old patient a dose of an antinausea drug. Considering this patient's age, what is the nurse's priority action regarding evaluation of the drug's effects?

For answers, see *http://evolve.elsevier.com/Lilley*.

EVOLVE WEBSITE

http://evolve.elsevier.com/Lilley
- Animations
- Answer Keys for Textbook Case Studies and Textbook Critical Thinking and Prioritization Questions

- Content Updates
- Key Points
- Review Questions
- Student Case Studies

53

Vitamins and Minerals

http://evolve.elsevier.com/Lilley

OBJECTIVES

When you reach the end of this chapter, you will be able to do the following:

1. Discuss the importance of the various vitamins and minerals to the normal functioning of the human body.
2. Briefly describe the various acute and chronic disease states and conditions that may lead to various imbalances in vitamin and mineral levels.
3. Discuss the pathologies that result from vitamin and mineral imbalances.
4. Describe the treatment of these vitamin and mineral imbalances.
5. Identify mechanisms of action, indications, cautions, contraindications, drug interactions, dosages, recommended daily allowances, and routes of administration of each of the vitamins and minerals.
6. Develop a nursing care plan related to the use of vitamins and minerals that includes all phases of the nursing process.

DRUG PROFILES

ascorbic acid (vitamin C), p. 853
calcifediol (vitamin D_3), p. 846
calcitriol (vitamin D_3), p. 846
calcium, p. 853
cyanocobalamin (vitamin B_{12}), p. 852
ergocalciferol (vitamin D_2), p. 846
!magnesium, p. 855
niacin (vitamin B_3), p. 850
phosphorus, p. 856

pyridoxine (vitamin B_6), p. 851
riboflavin (vitamin B_2), p. 849
thiamine (vitamin B_1), p. 848
vitamin A, p. 844
vitamin E, p. 847
vitamin K_1, p. 847

_____
♦ = *Key drug*
! = *High-alert drug*

KEY TERMS

Beriberi A disease of the peripheral nerves caused by a dietary deficiency of thiamine (vitamin B_1). Symptoms include fatigue, diarrhea, weight loss, edema, heart failure, and disturbed nerve function. (p. 848)

Coenzyme A nonprotein substance that combines with a protein molecule to form an active enzyme. (p. 841)

Enzymes Specialized proteins that catalyze biochemical reactions. (p. 841)

Fat-soluble vitamins Vitamins that can be dissolved (i.e., are soluble) in fat. (p. 841)

Minerals Inorganic substances that are ingested and attach to enzymes or other organic molecules. (p. 841)

Pellagra A disease resulting from a deficiency of niacin or a metabolic defect that interferes with the conversion of tryptophan to niacin (vitamin B_3). (p. 848)

Rhodopsin The purple pigment in the rods of the retina, formed by a protein, opsin, and a derivative of retinol (vitamin A). (p. 842)

Rickets A condition caused by a deficiency of vitamin D. (p. 845)

Scurvy A condition resulting from a deficiency of ascorbic acid (vitamin C). (p. 852)

Tocopherols Biologically active chemicals that make up vitamin E compounds. (p. 846)

Vitamins Organic compounds essential in small quantities for normal physiologic and metabolic functioning of the body. (p. 841)

Water-soluble vitamins Vitamins that can be dissolved (i.e., are soluble) in water. (p. 841)

OVERVIEW

For the body to grow and maintain itself, it needs the essential building blocks provided by carbohydrates, fats, and proteins. Vitamins and minerals are needed to efficiently utilize these nutrients. Vitamins are organic molecules needed in small quantities for normal metabolism and other biochemical functions, such as growth or repair of tissue. Equally important are minerals, inorganic elements found naturally in the earth. Enzymes are proteins secreted by cells; they act as catalysts to induce chemical changes in other substances. A coenzyme is a substance that enhances or is necessary for the action of enzymes. Many enzymes are useless without the appropriate vitamins and/or minerals that cause them to function properly. Both vitamins and minerals act primarily as coenzymes, binding to enzymes (or other organic molecules) to activate anabolic (tissue-building) processes in the body. For example, coenzyme A is an important carrier molecule associated with the citric acid cycle, one of the body's major energy-producing metabolic reactions. However, it requires pantothenic acid (vitamin B_5) to complete its function in the citric acid cycle.

Vitamins and minerals are essential in our lives. Under most circumstances, daily requirements of vitamins and minerals are met by ingestion of fluids and balanced meals. Ingesting food maintains adequate stores of essential vitamins and minerals, serves to preserve intestinal structure, provides chemicals for hormones and enzymes, and prevents harmful overgrowth of bacteria.

Various illnesses can cause acute or chronic deficiencies of vitamins, minerals, electrolytes, and fluids. These conditions require replacement or supplementation of these nutrients. Common examples include extensive burn injuries and acquired immunodeficiency syndrome (AIDS). Excessive loss of vitamins and minerals may also be the result of poor dietary intake, an inability to swallow after cancer chemotherapy or radiation, or mental disorders such as anorexia nervosa. Poor dietary absorption can also be caused by various gastrointestinal (GI) malabsorption syndromes. In addition, drug and alcohol abuse are frequently associated with inadequate nutritional intake that warrants vitamin and mineral supplementation. Deficiencies in dietary protein, fat, and carbohydrates are also common. These nutrients are discussed in Chapter 55. Because of some of their distinct properties and functions in the body related to blood formation, iron and the vitamin folic acid (vitamin B_9) are discussed separately in Chapter 54.

PHARMACOLOGY OVERVIEW

The human body requires vitamins in specific minimum amounts on a daily basis, and these can be obtained from both plant and animal food sources. In some cases, the body synthesizes some of its own vitamin supply. Supplemental amounts of vitamin B complex and vitamin K are synthesized by normal bacterial flora in the GI tract. Vitamin D can be synthesized by the skin when the skin is exposed to sunlight.

An inadequate diet will cause various nutrition-related vitamin deficiencies. In 1941, the Food and Nutrition Board of

the National Academy of Sciences published its first list of recommended daily allowances (RDAs) of essential nutrients. A newer published standard is the list of dietary reference intakes (DRIs). Whereas the RDAs represented minimum nutrient requirements, the DRIs are designed to represent optimal nutrient amounts for good health. The United States requires that detailed nutritional information be listed on any packaged food product. The values that appear on the labels are the percentage daily values and indicate what percentage of the DRI for a specific nutrient is met by a single serving of the food product. Information regarding DRIs is available from the following sources:

1. Federal Food and Nutrition Information Center: *http://fnic.nal.usda.gov/dietary-guidance/dietary-reference-intakes*
2. Institute of Medicine: Dietary Reference Intakes (DRIs): recommended intakes for individuals, available at *www.iom.edu*

Vitamins are classified as either fat-soluble or water-soluble. Water-soluble vitamins can be dissolved in water and are easily excreted in the urine. Fat-soluble vitamins are dissolvable in fat and tend to be stored longer in the liver and fatty tissues. Because water-soluble vitamins (B-complex group and vitamin C) cannot be stored in the body in large amounts, daily intake is required to prevent the development of deficiencies. Conversely, fat-soluble vitamins (vitamins A, D, E, and K) do not need to be taken daily unless one is deficient, because substantial amounts are stored in the liver and fatty tissues. Deficiencies of these vitamins occur only after prolonged deprivation from an adequate supply or from disorders that prevent their absorption. Table 53-1 lists the fat-soluble and water-soluble vitamins.

One controversial topic related to vitamins is that of nutrient "megadosing" as a strategy both for health promotion and maintenance and for treatment of various illnesses. Some cancer patients elect to use supplemental megadosing of specific nutrients in hopes of strengthening their body's response to more conventional cancer treatments. The American Dietetic Association defines megadosing as "doses of a nutrient that are 10 or more times the recommended amount." A related term was

TABLE 53-1 Fat-Soluble and Water-Soluble Vitamins

FAT-SOLUBLE		WATER-SOLUBLE	
Designation	**Name**	**Designation**	**Name**
vitamin A	retinol	vitamin B_1	thiamine
vitamin D	D_3, cholecalciferol; D_2, ergocalciferol	vitamin B_2	riboflavin
vitamin E	tocopherols	vitamin B_3	niacin
vitamin K	K_1, phytonadione	vitamin B_5	pantothenic acid
	K_2, menaquinone	vitamin B_6	pyridoxine
		vitamin B_9	folic acid
		vitamin B_7	biotin
		vitamin B_{12}	cyanocobalamin
		vitamin C	ascorbic acid

coined in 1968 by the Nobel Prize–winning chemist Linus Pauling. He defined *orthomolecular medicine* to be "the preventive or therapeutic use of high-dose vitamins to treat disease." The best-known claim of Dr. Pauling was that megadoses of vitamin C (at more than 100 times the U.S. RDA) could prevent or cure the common cold and cancer. Many studies since have not substantiated this claim. However, there are some situations in which nutrient megadosing are known to be helpful, including the following:

- When concurrent long-term drug therapy depletes vitamin stores or otherwise interferes with the function of a vitamin. A common clinical example is the use of vitamin B_6 (pyridoxine) supplementation in patients receiving the drug isoniazid for treatment of tuberculosis (see Chapter 41).
- In GI malabsorption syndromes such as those seen in patients with severe colitis and cystic fibrosis (all major nutrient classes, including protein, fat, carbohydrates, vitamins, and minerals).
- For the treatment of pernicious anemia, which results from cyanocobalamin (vitamin B_{12}) deficiency. The GI tract uses a fairly complex mechanism to drive cyanocobalamin absorption. Specifically, a glycoprotein known as *intrinsic factor* is secreted by the parietal cells of the gastric glands (see Chapter 50). Intrinsic factor facilitates absorption of cyanocobalamin in the intestine. When this process is compromised (e.g., by disease), administration of megadoses of cyanocobalamin can bypass this absorption mechanism by allowing a small amount of the vitamin to diffuse on its own through the intestinal mucosa.
- When the vitamin acts as a drug when megadosed. The most common example is niacin (vitamin B_3, also called *nicotinic acid*). At dosages of up to 20 mg daily, it functions as a vitamin, but at dosages 50 to 100 times higher, it reduces blood levels of both triglycerides and low-density lipoprotein cholesterol (see Chapter 27).

In contrast with the aforementioned examples, there are some situations in which nutrient megadosing is known to be harmful. For example, any excess of one or more nutrients can result in deficiencies of other nutrients due to their chemical competition for sites of absorption in the intestinal mucosa. This is likely to be the case with megadosing of minerals, such as calcium, copper, iron, and zinc, and is less likely to result from vitamin megadosing. Vitamin megadosing can lead to toxic accumulations known as *hypervitaminosis*, especially with the fat-soluble vitamins A, D, and K. Vitamin E appears safer, however, even at doses 10 to 20 times the recommended DRI. Hypervitaminosis is less likely to occur with the water-soluble vitamins (B complex and C) because they are readily excreted through the urinary system. Nevertheless, it is known that megadosing with vitamin B_6 (pyridoxine) at 50 to 100 times the DRI can cause nerve damage.

Persons with an illness may be less tolerant of nutrient megadosing, although megadosing regimens are often prescribed for them. For example, megadosing may be more of a strain for a GI tract that is already weakened by illness. Megadosing can even interfere with chemotherapy drugs as well as radiation treatments, because these therapies work to destroy cancer cells

through oxidation processes. Nutritional supplementation with antioxidants may impede such treatment mechanisms. Patients need to tell their health care providers any unusual nutritional regimens that they plan to try, especially if they have a serious illness.

FAT-SOLUBLE VITAMINS

Fat-soluble vitamins are not readily excreted in the urine and are stored in the body. Thus, daily ingestion of these vitamins is not necessary to maintain good health and, in fact, is more likely to result in hypervitaminosis.

The fat-soluble vitamins are A, D, E, and K. As a group, they share the following characteristics:
- They are present in both plant and animal foods.
- They are stored primarily in the liver.
- They exhibit slow metabolism or breakdown.
- They are excreted via the feces.
- They can reach toxic levels (*hypervitaminosis*) if excessive amounts are consumed.

VITAMIN A

Vitamin A (retinol) is derived from animal fats such as those found in dairy products, eggs, meat, liver, and fish liver oils. Vitamin A is also derived from carotenes, which are found in plants (e.g., green and yellow vegetables, yellow fruits). Therefore, vitamin A is an exogenous substance for humans because it must be obtained from either plant or animal foods. There are more than 600 naturally occurring carotenoid compounds in plant-based foods. Of these, 40 to 50 occur commonly in the human diet. Beta carotene is the most prevalent of these, followed by alpha carotene and cryptoxanthin. These are known as *provitamin A carotenoids*, because they are all metabolized to various forms of vitamin A in the body. Table 53-2 lists the food sources for several nutrients.

Mechanism of Action and Drug Effects

Vitamin A is essential for night vision and for normal vision, because it is part of one of the major retinal pigments called **rhodopsin**. Beta carotene is metabolized in the body to retinal (retinaldehyde), and some of this retinal is reduced to *retinol*. The remainder of the retinal may be oxidized to the carboxylic acid compound retinoic acid. Unlike retinal, retinoic acid has no direct role in vision, but it is essential for normal cell growth and differentiation and for the development of the physical shapes of the body's many parts—a process known as *morphogenesis*. It is also involved in the growth and development of bones and teeth and in other body processes, including reproduction, maintenance of the integrity of mucosal and epithelial surfaces, and cholesterol and steroid synthesis.

Indications

Supplements of vitamin A may be used to satisfy normal body requirements or an increased demand, such as in infants and in pregnant and nursing women. A normal diet usually provides adequate amounts of vitamin A, but in cases of excessive need

TABLE 53-2   Food Sources for Selected Nutrients

Vitamins/Minerals	Food Sources
vitamin A	Liver; fish; dairy products; egg yolks; dark green, leafy, yellow-orange vegetables and fruits
vitamin D	Dairy products, fortified cereals and fortified orange juice, liver, fish liver oils, saltwater fish, butter, eggs
vitamin E	Fish, egg yolks, meats, vegetable oils, nuts, fruits, wheat germ, grains, fortified cereals
vitamin K	Cheese, spinach, broccoli, Brussels sprouts, kale, cabbage, turnip greens, soybean oils
vitamin B$_1$ (thiamine)	Yeast, liver, enriched whole-grain products, beans
vitamin B$_2$ (riboflavin)	Meats, liver, dairy products, eggs, legumes, nuts, enriched whole-grain products, green leafy vegetables, yeast
vitamin B$_3$ (niacin)	Liver, turkey, tuna, peanuts, beans, yeast, enriched whole-grain breads and cereals, wheat germ
vitamin B$_6$ (pyridoxine)	Organ meats, meats, poultry, fish, eggs, peanuts, whole grain products, vegetables, nuts, wheat germ, bananas, fortified cereals
vitamin B$_{12}$ (cyanocobalamin)	Liver, kidney, shellfish, poultry, fish, eggs, milk, blue cheese, fortified cereals
vitamin C (ascorbic acid)	Broccoli, green peppers, spinach, Brussels sprouts, citrus fruits, tomatoes, potatoes, strawberries, cabbage, liver
calcium	Dairy products, fortified cereals and calcium-fortified orange juice, sardines, salmon
magnesium	Meats, seafood, milk, cheese, yogurt, green leafy vegetables, bran cereal, nuts
phosphorus	Milk, yogurt, cheese, peas, meat, fish, eggs
zinc	Red meats, liver, oysters, certain seafood, milk products, eggs, beans, nuts, whole grains, fortified cereals

Adapted from USDA: *Dietary guidelines for Americans, 2010.* Available at *http://health.gov/dietaryguidelines.* Accessed March 1, 2015.

TABLE 53-3   Vitamin A: Adverse Effects

Body System	Adverse Effects
Central nervous	Headache, increased intracranial pressure, lethargy, malaise
Gastrointestinal	Nausea, vomiting, anorexia, abdominal pain
Integumentary	Dry skin, pruritus, increased pigmentation, night sweats
Metabolic	Hypomenorrhea, hypercalcemia
Musculoskeletal	Arthralgia, retarded growth

or inadequate dietary intake, vitamin A supplementation is indicated. Symptoms of vitamin A deficiency include night blindness, xerophthalmia, keratomalacia (softening of the cornea), hyperkeratosis of both the stratum corneum (outermost layer) of the skin and the sclera (outermost layer of eyeball), retarded infant growth, generalized weakness, and increased susceptibility of mucous membranes to infection. Vitamin A–related compounds, such as isotretinoin, are also used to treat various skin conditions, including acne, psoriasis, and keratosis follicularis.

Contraindications

Contraindications to vitamin A supplementation include known drug product allergy; known current state of hypervitaminosis; and excessive supplementation beyond recommended guidelines, especially during pregnancy or in oral malabsorption syndromes.

Adverse Effects

There are very few acute adverse effects associated with normal vitamin A ingestion. Only after long-term excessive ingestion of vitamin A do symptoms appear. Adverse effects are usually noticed in bones, mucous membranes, the liver, and the skin. Table 53-3 lists some of the symptoms of long-term excessive ingestion of vitamin A.

Toxicity and Management of Overdose

The major toxic effects of vitamin A result from ingestion of excessive amounts, which occurs most commonly in children. A few hours after administration of an excess dose of vitamin A, irritability, drowsiness, vertigo, delirium, coma, vomiting, and/or diarrhea may occur. In infants, excessive amounts of vitamin A can cause an increase in cranial pressure, resulting in symptoms such as bulging fontanelles, headache, papilledema, exophthalmos (bulging eyeballs), and visual disturbances. Papilledema is the presence of edematous fluid, often including blood, in the optic disc. This is the portion of the eye in the back of the retina, where nerve fibers converge to form the optic nerve. Over several weeks, a generalized peeling of the skin and erythema (skin reddening) may occur. These symptoms seem to disappear a few days after discontinuation of the drug, which is the only treatment necessary in situations of overdose.

Interactions

Vitamin A is absorbed less when used together with lubricant laxatives and cholestyramine. In addition, the concurrent use of isotretinoin and vitamin A supplementation can result in additive effects and possible toxicity.

Dosages

For dosage information on vitamin A, see the table on this page.

DRUG PROFILE

There are three forms of vitamin A: retinol, retinyl palmitate, and retinyl acetate. Medications containing vitamin A may require a prescription, but many over-the-counter (OTC) products, such as vitamin A–containing multivitamins, are also available. All vitamin A products are classified as pregnancy category A.

DOSAGES

Selected Vitamins

Drug	Pharmacologic Class	Usual Adult Dosage Range	Indications/Uses
Vitamin D–Active Compounds			
calcifediol (hydroxyvitamin D₃) (Calderol)	Fat-soluble	PO: 50 mcg once daily	Hypocalcemia in hemodialysis patients
calcitriol (dihydroxyvitamin D₃) (Rocaltrol, Calcijex)	Fat-soluble	PO/IV: 0.25-2 mcg/day	Hypoparathyroidism; hypocalcemia in patients receiving regular hemodialysis
ergocalciferol* (vitamin D₂) (Drisdol, Calciferol)	Fat-soluble	PO: 50,000-200,000 units daily	Rickets, hypoparathyroidism, renal failure
Vitamin B–Active Compounds			
vitamin B₁ (thiamine) (Thiamilate)	Water-soluble, B-complex group	100 mg/day until normal dietary intake is established	Alcohol-induced deficiency
		10-20 mg IM × 2 wk, then 5-30 mg/day for 30 days	Beriberi
vitamin B₂ (riboflavin) (Lactoflavin)	Water-soluble, B-complex group	PO: 5-30 mg/day	Deficiency
vitamin B₃ (niacin, nicotinic acid) (Nicotinex)	Water-soluble, B-complex group	PO: ER: 500-2000 mg/day	Hyperlipidemia
		PO: Up to 500 mg/day	Pellagra (deficiency)
vitamin B₆ (pyridoxine) (Aminoxin, Vitelle)	Water-soluble, B-complex group	PO/IV: 2.5-10 mg/day	Deficiency
		PO/IV: 100-200 mg/day	Drug-induced neuritis (e.g., isoniazid for tuberculosis)
vitamin B₁₂ (cyanocobalamin) (Nascobal)	Water-soluble, B-complex group	IM/subcut: 1000 mcg/month Intranasal gel: 500 mcg/wk	Deficiency; anemia
Vitamins A, C, E, and K			
vitamin A (Aquasol A, others)	Fat-soluble	PO: 100,000 units/day for 3 days, then 50,000 units/day for 14 days	Deficiency
vitamin C (ascorbic acid) (Vita-C, Dull-C, others)	Water-soluble	PO/IV/IM/subcut: 100-250 mg 1-2 times daily	Deficiency; scurvy
vitamin E (d-alpha tocopherol) (Aquavit E, others)	Fat-soluble	PO: 60-75 units/day	Nutritional supplementation
vitamin K (phytonadione) (Mephyton, AquaMEPHYTON)	Fat-soluble	PO: 1.25-10 mg single dose IM/IV: 1-10 mg single dose	Warfarin-induced hypoprothrombinemia

*Dosages are individualized. Higher doses may be required based on response to therapy.

vitamin A

Vitamin A (Aquasol A), also known as *retinol, retinyl palmitate,* and *retinyl acetate,* is available in a variety of oral forms as well as an injectable form. Doses for vitamin A are expressed as *retinol activity equivalents (RAEs).* One RAE is approximately equal to the following:

- 1 mcg of retinol (either dietary or supplemental)
- 2 mcg of supplemental beta carotene
- 12 mcg of dietary beta carotene
- 24 mcg of dietary carotenoids

Pharmacokinetics: Vitamin A

Route	Onset of Action	Peak Plasma Concentration	Elimination Half-life	Duration of Action
PO	N/A	4 hr	50-100 days	Unknown

VITAMIN D

Vitamin D, also called the *sunshine vitamin,* is responsible for the proper utilization of calcium and phosphorus in the body. The two most important members of the vitamin D family are vitamin D$_2$ (ergocalciferol) and vitamin D$_3$ (cholecalciferol). They have different sites of origin but similar functions in the body. Ergocalciferol (vitamin D$_2$) is plant derived and is therefore obtained through dietary sources. The natural form of vitamin D produced in the skin by ultraviolet irradiation (sun) is chemically known as *7-dehydrocholesterol*. It is more commonly referred to as *cholecalciferol* (vitamin D$_3$). This endogenous synthesis of vitamin D$_3$ usually produces sufficient amounts to meet daily requirements. Vitamin D is obtained through both endogenous synthesis and consumption of vitamin D$_2$–containing foods such as fish oils, salmon, sardines, and herring; fortified milk, bread, and cereals; and animal livers, tuna fish, eggs, and butter. Normal serum levels are 12 to 50 ng/mL.

Mechanism of Action and Drug Effects

The basic function of vitamin D is to regulate the absorption and subsequent utilization of calcium and phosphorus. It is also necessary for the normal calcification of bone. Vitamin D in coordination with parathyroid hormone and calcitonin regulates serum calcium levels by increasing calcium absorption from the small intestine and extracting calcium from the bone. Ergocalciferol and cholecalciferol are inactive and require transformation into active metabolites for biologic activity. Both vitamin D$_2$ and vitamin D$_3$ are biotransformed in the liver by the actions of parathyroid hormone. The resulting compound, calcifediol, is then transported to the kidney, where it is converted to calcitriol, which is believed to be the most physiologically active form of vitamin D. Calcitriol promotes the intestinal absorption of calcium and phosphorus and the deposition of calcium and phosphorus into the structure of teeth and bones.

The drug effects of vitamin D are very similar to those of vitamin A and essentially all vitamin and mineral compounds. It is used as a supplement to satisfy normal daily requirements or an increased demand, as in infants and in pregnant and nursing women.

Indications

Vitamin D can be used either to supplement dietary intake or to treat a deficiency of vitamin D. In the case of supplementation, it is given as a prophylactic measure to prevent deficiency-related problems, and it is recommended for breastfed infants. Vitamin D may also be used to treat and correct the result of a long-term deficiency that leads to such conditions as infantile rickets, tetany (involuntary sustained muscular contractions), and osteomalacia (softening of the bones). Rickets is specifically a vitamin D–deficiency state. Symptoms include soft, pliable bones, which causes deformities such as bowlegs and knock knees; nodular enlargement on the ends and sides of the bones; muscle pain; enlarged skull; chest deformities; spinal curvature; enlargement of the liver and spleen; profuse sweating; and general tenderness of the body when touched. Vitamin D can also help promote the absorption of phosphorus and calcium. For this reason, its use is important in preventing osteoporosis. Because of the role of vitamin D in the regulation of calcium and phosphorus, it may be used to correct

deficiencies of these two elements. Other uses include dietary supplementation and treatment of osteodystrophy, hypocalcemia, hypoparathyroidism, pseudohypoparathyroidism, and hypophosphatemia. Many patients have low vitamin D levels, and it is common to see doses of 1000 to 2000 units daily or 50,000 units per week prescribed.

Contraindications

Contraindications to vitamin D products include known drug product allergy to the product, hypercalcemia, renal dysfunction, kidney stones, and hyperphosphatemia.

Adverse Effects

Very few acute adverse effects are associated with normal vitamin D ingestion. Only after long-term excessive ingestion of vitamin D do symptoms appear. Such effects are usually noticed in the GI tract or the central nervous system (CNS) and are listed in Table 53-4.

Toxicity and Management of Overdose

The major toxic effects from ingesting excessive amounts of vitamin D occur most commonly in children. Discontinuation of vitamin D and reduced calcium intake reverse the toxic state. The amount of vitamin D considered to be toxic varies considerably among individuals but is generally thought to be 1.25 to 2.5 mg of ergocalciferol daily in adults and 25 mcg daily in infants and children.

The toxic effects of vitamin D are those associated with hypertension, such as weakness, fatigue, headache, anorexia, dry mouth, metallic taste, nausea, vomiting, abdominal cramps, ataxia, and bone pain.

Interactions

Reduced absorption of vitamin D occurs with the concurrent use of lubricant laxatives and cholestyramine.

Dosages

For dosage information on vitamin D, see the table on the previous page.

DRUG PROFILES

There are three forms of vitamin D: calcifediol, calcitriol, and ergocalciferol. Vitamin D is available in OTC medications,

TABLE 53-4 Vitamin D: Adverse Effects

Body System	Adverse Effects
Cardiovascular	Hypertension, dysrhythmias
Central nervous	Fatigue, weakness, drowsiness, headache
Gastrointestinal	Nausea, vomiting, anorexia, cramps, metallic taste, dry mouth, constipation
Genitourinary	Polyuria, albuminuria
Musculoskeletal	Decreased bone growth, bone and muscle pain

such as multivitamin products, or by prescription. Although various pharmaceutical manufacturers may list their individual vitamin D products as pregnancy category C, these products are generally considered to be category A or B as long as the patient is not dosed at higher levels than recommended.

calcifediol

Calcifediol (Calderol) is the 25-hydroxylated form of cholecalciferol (vitamin D_3). It is a vitamin D analogue used primarily for the management of hypocalcemia in patients with chronic renal failure who are undergoing hemodialysis. Calcifediol is also used for signs of hyperparathyroid disease. It is available only for oral use.

calcitriol

Calcitriol (Rocaltrol) is the 1,25-dihydroxylated form of cholecalciferol (vitamin D_3). It is a vitamin D analogue used for the management of hypocalcemia in patients with chronic renal failure who are undergoing hemodialysis. Calcitriol is also used in the treatment of hypoparathyroidism and pseudohypoparathyroidism, vitamin D–dependent rickets, hypophosphatemia, and hypocalcemia in premature infants. It is available in both oral and injectable forms.

Pharmacokinetics: Calcitriol

Route	Onset of Action	Peak Plasma Concentration	Elimination Half-life	Duration of Action
PO	Less than 3 hr	3-6 hr	3-6 hr	3-5 days

ergocalciferol

Ergocalciferol (Drisdol) is vitamin D_2. It is indicated for use in patients with GI, liver, or biliary disease associated with malabsorption of vitamin D analogues. It is available orally and parenterally.

Pharmacokinetics: Ergocalciferol, Vitamin D_2

Route	Onset of Action	Peak Plasma Concentration	Elimination Half-life	Duration of Action
PO	30 days	Unknown	19 days	Months to years

VITAMIN E

Four biologically active chemicals called **tocopherols** (alpha, beta, gamma, and delta) make up the vitamin E compounds. Alpha tocopherol is the most biologically active natural form of vitamin E and can come from plant and animal sources.

Mechanism of Action and Drug Effects

Vitamin E is a powerful biologic antioxidant and an essential component of the diet. Its exact nutritional function has not been fully demonstrated. The only recognized significant deficiency syndrome for vitamin E occurs in premature infants. In this situation, vitamin E deficiency may result in irritability, edema, thrombosis, and hemolytic anemia.

The drug effects of vitamin E are not as well defined as those of the other fat-soluble vitamins. It is believed to protect polyunsaturated fatty acids, a component of cellular membranes. It has also been shown to hinder the deterioration of substances such as vitamin A and ascorbic acid (vitamin C), two substances that are highly oxygen sensitive and readily oxidized; thus it acts as an antioxidant.

Indications

Vitamin E is most commonly used as a dietary supplement to augment current daily intake or to treat a deficiency. Premature infants are those at greatest risk for complications from vitamin E deficiency. Vitamin E has received much attention as an antioxidant. Preventing the oxidation of various substances prevents the formation of toxic chemicals within the body, some of which are believed to cause cancer. There is a popular but unproved theory that vitamin E has beneficial effects for patients with cancer, heart disease, premenstrual syndrome, and sexual dysfunction. However, the American Heart Association no longer recommends the use of high-dose vitamin E to prevent heart disease. In fact, recent studies have shown no benefit and possible harm.

Contraindications

Contraindications for vitamin E include known allergy to a specific vitamin E product. There are currently no approved injectable forms of this vitamin.

Adverse Effects

Very few acute adverse effects are associated with normal vitamin E ingestion, because it is relatively nontoxic. Adverse effects are usually noticed in the GI tract or CNS and are listed in Table 53-5.

Dosages

For dosage information on vitamin E, see the table on p. 844.

DRUG PROFILE

Vitamin E is available as an OTC medication. It has four forms: alpha, beta, gamma, and delta tocopherol. It is available in many multivitamin preparations and is also available by prescription.

TABLE 53-5   Vitamin E: Adverse Effects

Body System	Adverse Effects
Central nervous	Fatigue, headache, blurred vision
Gastrointestinal	Nausea, diarrhea, flatulence
Genitourinary	Increased blood urea nitrogen level
Musculoskeletal	Weakness

Vitamin E products are usually contraindicated only in cases of known drug allergy.

vitamin E

Vitamin E (Aquasol E) activity is generally expressed in U.S. Pharmacopeia (USP) or international units. It is available for oral and topical use.

VITAMIN K

Vitamin K is the last of the four fat-soluble vitamins (A, D, E, and K). There are three types of vitamin K: phytonadione (vitamin K_1), menaquinone (vitamin K_2), and menadione (vitamin K_3). The body does not store large amounts of vitamin K; however, vitamin K_2 is synthesized by the intestinal flora, which provides an endogenous supply.

Vitamin K is essential for the synthesis of blood coagulation factors, which takes place in the liver. Vitamin K–dependent blood coagulation factors are factors II, VII, IX, and X. Other names for these clotting factors are as follows: factor II (prothrombin); factor VII (proconvertin); factor IX (Christmas factor); and factor X (Stuart-Prower factor). Normal serum levels are 0.1 to 2.2 ng/mL.

Mechanism of Action and Drug Effects

Vitamin K activity is essential for effective blood clotting because, as noted earlier, it facilitates the hepatic biosynthesis of factors II, VII, IX, and X. Vitamin K deficiency results in coagulation disorders caused by hypoprothrombinemia. Coagulation defects affecting these clotting factors can be corrected with administration of vitamin K. Vitamin K deficiency is rare because intestinal flora are normally able to synthesize sufficient amounts. If a deficiency develops, it can be corrected with vitamin K supplementation.

Indications

Vitamin K is indicated for dietary supplementation and for treatment of deficiency states. Although rare, deficiency states can develop with inadequate dietary intake or inhibition of the intestinal flora resulting from the administration of broad-spectrum antibiotics. Deficiency states can also be seen in newborns because of malabsorption attributable to inadequate amounts of bile. For this reason, infants born in hospitals are often given a prophylactic intramuscular dose of vitamin K on arrival to the nursery. Vitamin K deficiency can also result from the administration and pharmacologic action of the oral anticoagulant warfarin (see Chapter 26). Warfarin's anticoagulant effects occur by inhibiting vitamin K–dependent clotting factors II, VII, IX, and X in the liver. Administration of vitamin K overrides the mechanism by which the anticoagulant inhibits production of vitamin K–dependent clotting factors. Thus vitamin K can be used to reverse the effects of warfarin. It is important to note that when vitamin K is used in this manner, the patient becomes unresponsive to warfarin for approximately 1 week after vitamin K administration.

TABLE 53-6 **Vitamin K: Adverse Effects**	
Body System	**Adverse Effects**
Central nervous	Headache, brain damage (large doses)
Gastrointestinal	Nausea, decreased liver enzyme levels
Hematologic	Hemolytic anemia, hemoglobinuria, hyperbilirubinemia
Integumentary	Rash, urticaria

Contraindications

The only usual contraindication to treatment with vitamin K is known drug allergy.

Adverse Effects

Vitamin K is relatively nontoxic and thus causes very few adverse effects. Severe reactions limited to hypersensitivity or anaphylaxis have occurred rarely during or immediately after intravenous administration. Adverse effects are usually related to injection-site reactions and hypersensitivity. See Table 53-6 for a list of such major effects by body system.

Toxicity and Management of Overdose

Toxicity is primarily limited to use in the newborn. Hemolysis of red blood cells (RBCs) can occur, especially in infants with low levels of glucose-6-phosphate dehydrogenase. In severe cases, replacement with blood products may be indicated.

Dosages

For dosage information on vitamin K, see the table on p. 844.

DRUG PROFILE

The most commonly used form of vitamin K is phytonadione (vitamin K_1). Both phytonadione and menadione (vitamin K_3) are available by prescription only in oral and parenteral forms. Menadione is classified as a pregnancy category X drug, whereas phytonadione is a pregnancy category C drug. Both are contraindicated in patients with a known hypersensitivity to them. Their use is also contraindicated in patients who are in the last few weeks of pregnancy and in patients with severe hepatic disease. Vitamin K must be used with caution in patients taking warfarin.

vitamin K_1

Vitamin K_1 (phytonadione) (AquaMEPHYTON) is available in both oral and injectable forms. Because of its potential to cause anaphylaxis (due to the formulation), for intravenous use it is usually diluted and given over 30 to 60 minutes. Vitamin K is given IV or subcutaneously and not intramuscularly when used to reverse warfarin effects.

Pharmacokinetics: Vitamin K_1

Route	Onset of Action	Peak Plasma Concentration	Elimination Half-life	Duration of Action
PO	6-12 hr	24-48 hr	1.2 hr	24 hr
IV	1-2 hr	12-14 hr	1.2 hr	24 hr

WATER-SOLUBLE VITAMINS

The water-soluble vitamins include the vitamin B complex and vitamin C (ascorbic acid). They are present in a variety of plant and animal food sources. The vitamin B complex is a group of 10 vitamins that are often found together in food, although they are chemically dissimilar and have different metabolic functions. Because the B vitamins were originally isolated from the same sources, they were grouped together as B-complex vitamins. Vitamin C (ascorbic acid), the other principal water-soluble vitamin, is concentrated in citrus fruits and is not classified as part of the B complex. The numeric subscripts associated with various B vitamins reflect the order in which they were discovered. In clinical practice, some B vitamins are more often referred to by their common name, whereas others are more often referred to by their numeric designation. For example, "vitamin B_{12}" is used more often in clinical practice than the corresponding common name "cyanocobalamin." However, "folic acid" is rarely referred to as "vitamin B_9." The most commonly used B-complex vitamins, as well as vitamin C, are listed in Box 53-1. Folic acid (vitamin B_9) has a special role in hematopoiesis and therefore is described further in Chapter 54.

Water-soluble vitamins are a chemically diverse group sharing only the characteristic of being dissolvable in water. Like fat-soluble vitamins, they act primarily as coenzymes or oxidation-reduction agents in important metabolic pathways. Unlike fat-soluble vitamins, water-soluble vitamins are not stored in the body in appreciable amounts. Their water-soluble properties promote urinary excretion and reduce their half-life in the body. Therefore, dietary intake must be adequate and regular, or else deficiency states will develop. The body excretes what it does not need, which makes toxic reactions to water-soluble vitamins very rare.

VITAMIN B_1

A deficiency of vitamin B_1 (thiamine) results in the classic disease beriberi or Wernicke's encephalopathy (cerebral beriberi). Common findings in beriberi include brain lesions, polyneuropathy of peripheral nerves, serous effusions (abnormal collections of fluids in body tissues), and cardiac anatomic

changes. Vitamin deficiency can result from poor diet, extended fever, hyperthyroidism, liver disease, alcoholism, malabsorption, and pregnancy and breastfeeding. Normal serum levels are 66 to 200 nmol/L.

Mechanism of Action and Drug Effects

Vitamin B_1 (thiamine) is an essential precursor for the formation of thiamine pyrophosphate. When thiamine combines with adenosine triphosphate (ATP), the result is thiamine pyrophosphate coenzyme. This is required for the citric acid cycle (Krebs cycle), a major part of carbohydrate metabolism, as well as several other metabolic pathways. In addition, thiamine plays a key role in the integrity of the peripheral nervous system, cardiovascular system, and GI tract.

Indications

The essential role of thiamine in many metabolic pathways makes it useful in treating a variety of metabolic disorders. These include subacute necrotizing encephalomyelopathy, maple syrup urine disease, and lactic acidosis associated with pyruvate carboxylase enzyme deficiency and hyper-beta-alaninemia. Some of the deficiency states treated by thiamine are beriberi, Wernicke's encephalopathy, peripheral neuritis associated with pellagra (niacin deficiency), and neuritis of pregnancy. Thiamine is used as a dietary supplement to prevent or treat deficiency in cases of malabsorption such as that induced by alcoholism, cirrhosis, or GI disease. Other situations in which thiamine may have therapeutic value are the management of poor appetite, ulcerative colitis, chronic diarrhea, and cerebellar syndrome or ataxia (impaired muscular coordination). It is also used as an oral insect repellent.

Contraindications

The only usual contraindication to any of the B-complex vitamins is known drug product allergy.

Adverse Effects

Adverse effects are rare but include hypersensitivity reactions, nausea, restlessness, pulmonary edema, pruritus, urticaria, weakness, sweating, angioedema, cyanosis, and cardiovascular collapse. Administration by intramuscular injection can produce local tenderness, and intravenous injections can produce anaphylaxis.

Interactions

Thiamine is incompatible with alkaline- and sulfite-containing solutions.

Dosages

For dosage information on vitamin B_1, see the table on p. 844.

DRUG PROFILE

thiamine

Thiamine is contraindicated only in individuals with a known hypersensitivity to it. Thiamine is available for both oral use and injection. It is classified as a pregnancy category A drug.

BOX 53-1   Water-Soluble Vitamins: Alternate Names

Designation	Alternate Name
vitamin B complex	
vitamin B_1	thiamine
vitamin B_2	riboflavin
vitamin B_3	niacin
vitamin B_5	pantothenic acid
vitamin B_6	pyridoxine
vitamin B_9	folic acid
vitamin B_{12}	cyanocobalamin
vitamin C	ascorbic acid

Pharmacokinetics: Thiamine

Route	Onset of Action	Peak Plasma Concentration	Elimination Half-life	Duration of Action
PO	Unknown	1-2 hr	1.2 hr	24 hr

VITAMIN B₂

A deficiency of vitamin B₂ (riboflavin) results in cutaneous, oral, and corneal changes that include cheilosis (chapped or fissured lips), seborrheic dermatitis, and keratitis.

Mechanism of Action and Drug Effects

Riboflavin serves several important functions in the body. Riboflavin is converted into two coenzymes (flavin mononucleotide and flavin adenine dinucleotide) that are essential for tissue respiration. Riboflavin also plays an important part in carbohydrate catabolism. Another B vitamin, vitamin B₆ (pyridoxine), requires riboflavin for activation. Riboflavin is also needed to convert tryptophan into niacin and to maintain erythrocyte integrity. Deficiency is rare and does not usually occur in healthy people.

Indications

Riboflavin is primarily used as a dietary supplement and for treatment of deficiency states. Patients who may experience riboflavin deficiency include those with long-standing infections, liver disease, alcoholism, or malignancy, and those taking probenecid. Riboflavin supplementation may also be beneficial in the treatment of microcytic anemia; acne; migraine headache; congenital methemoglobinemia (presence in the blood of an abnormal, nonfunctional hemoglobin pigment); muscle cramps; and Grierson-Gopalan syndrome, a symptom of suspected riboflavin (and possibly pantothenic acid [vitamin B₅]) deficiency that involves a sensation of tingling in the extremities (for this reason, it is also called *burning feet syndrome*).

Contraindications

The only usual contraindication to riboflavin is known drug product allergy.

Adverse Effects

Riboflavin is a very safe and effective vitamin; to date, no adverse effects or toxic effects have been reported. In large dosages, riboflavin will discolor urine to a yellow-orange.

Dosages

For dosage information on riboflavin, see the table on p. 844.

DRUG PROFILE

riboflavin

Riboflavin (vitamin B₂) is needed for normal respiratory functions. It is a safe, nontoxic water-soluble vitamin with almost no adverse effects. Riboflavin is available only for oral use. It is classified as a pregnancy category A drug.

Pharmacokinetics: Riboflavin

Route	Onset of Action	Peak Plasma Concentration	Elimination Half-life	Duration of Action
PO	Unknown	Unknown	66-84 min	24 hr

VITAMIN B₃

The body is able to produce a small amount of vitamin B₃ (niacin) from dietary tryptophan, an essential amino acid occurring in dietary proteins and some commercially available nutritional supplements. A dietary deficiency of niacin (vitamin B₃) will produce the classic symptoms known as *pellagra*. Symptoms of pellagra include various psychotic disorders; neurasthenic syndrome; crusting, erythema, and desquamation of the skin; scaly dermatitis; inflammation of the oral, vaginal, and urethral mucosa, including glossitis (inflamed tongue); and diarrhea or bloody diarrhea.

Mechanism of Action and Drug Effects

The metabolic actions of niacin (vitamin B₃) are not due to niacin in the ingested form but rather to its metabolic product, nicotinamide. Nicotinamide is required for numerous metabolic reactions, including those involved in carbohydrate, protein, purine, and lipid metabolism, as well as tissue respiration (Figure 53-1). A key example involves two compounds, nicotinamide adenosine dinucleotide (NAD) and nicotinamide adenosine dinucleotide phosphate (NADP), both of which are necessary for the carbohydrate pathway known as *glycogenolysis* (the breakdown of stored glycogen into usable glucose). The parent compound, niacin itself, also has a pharmacologic role as an antilipemic drug (see Chapter 27). The doses of niacin required for its antilipemic effect are substantially higher than those required for the nutritional and metabolic effects.

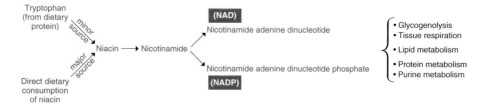

FIGURE 53-1 Niacin, once in the body, is converted to nicotinamide adenosine dinucleotide (NAD) and nicotinamide adenosine dinucleotide (NADP), which are coenzymes needed for many metabolic processes.

TABLE 53-7 Niacin (Vitamin B₃): Adverse Effects

Body System	Adverse Effects
Cardiovascular	Postural hypotension, dysrhythmias
Central nervous	Headache, dizziness, anxiety
Gastrointestinal	Nausea, vomiting, diarrhea, peptic ulcer
Genitourinary	Hyperuricemia
Hepatic	Abnormal liver function test results, hepatitis
Integumentary	Flushing, dry skin, rash, pruritus, keratosis
Metabolic	Decreased glucose tolerance

Indications

Niacin is indicated for the prevention and treatment of pellagra, a condition caused by a deficiency of vitamin B_3 that is most commonly the result of malabsorption. It is also used for management of certain types of hyperlipidemia (see Chapter 27). Niacin also has a beneficial effect in peripheral vascular disease.

Contraindications

Niacin, unlike certain other B-complex vitamins, has additional contraindications besides drug allergy. These include liver disease, severe hypotension, arterial hemorrhage, and active peptic ulcer disease.

Adverse Effects

The most frequent adverse effects associated with the use of niacin are flushing, pruritus, and GI distress. These usually subside with continued use and are most frequently seen when larger doses of niacin are used in the treatment of hyperlipidemia. Table 53-7 lists adverse effects by body system.

Dosages

For dosage information on niacin, see the table on p. 844.

DRUG PROFILE

niacin

Niacin is used to treat pellagra, hyperlipidemias, and peripheral vascular disease. Its use must be monitored closely in patients who have a history of coronary artery disease, gallbladder disease, jaundice, liver disease, or arterial bleeding. Niacin is available only for oral use. It is classified as a pregnancy category A drug.

Pharmacokinetics (Niacin, Vitamin B₃)

Route	Onset of Action	Peak Plasma Concentration	Elimination Half-life	Duration of Action
PO	30-60 min	45 min	45 min	Variable

VITAMIN B₆

Vitamin B_6 (pyridoxine) is composed of three compounds: pyridoxine, pyridoxal, and pyridoxamine. Deficiency of vitamin B_6 can lead to a type of anemia known as *sideroblastic anemia*, neurologic disturbances, seborrheic dermatitis, cheilosis, and xanthurenic aciduria (formation of xanthine crystals or "stones" in urine). It may also result in convulsions, especially in neonates and infants; hypochromic microcytic anemia; and glossitis (inflamed tongue) and stomatitis (inflamed oral mucosa). Pyridoxine deficiency also affects the peripheral nerves, skin, and mucous membranes. Inadequate intake or poor absorption of pyridoxine causes the development of these conditions. Vitamin B_6 deficiency may occur as a result of uremia, alcoholism, cirrhosis, hyperthyroidism, malabsorption syndromes, and heart failure. It may also be induced by various drugs, such as isoniazid and hydralazine.

Mechanism of Action and Drug Effects

Pyridoxine, pyridoxal, and pyridoxamine are all converted in erythrocytes to the active coenzyme forms of vitamin B_6: pyridoxal phosphate and pyridoxamine phosphate. These compounds are necessary for many metabolic functions, such as protein, carbohydrate, and lipid utilization in the body. They also play an important part in the conversion of the amino acid tryptophan to niacin (vitamin B_3) and the neurotransmitter serotonin. They are also essential in the synthesis of gamma-aminobutyric acid, an inhibitory neurotransmitter in the CNS. They are important in the synthesis of heme and the maintenance of the hematopoietic system. In addition, these substances are necessary for the integrity of the peripheral nerves, skin, and mucous membranes.

Indications

Pyridoxine is used to prevent and treat vitamin B_6 deficiency. This includes deficiency that can result from therapy with certain medications, including isoniazid (for tuberculosis) and hydralazine (for hypertension). Although vitamin B_6 deficiency is rare, it can occur in conditions of inadequate intake or poor absorption of pyridoxine. Seizures that are unresponsive to usual therapy, morning sickness during pregnancy, and various metabolic disorders may respond to pyridoxine therapy.

Contraindications

The only usual contraindication to pyridoxine use is known drug product allergy.

Adverse Effects

Adverse effects with pyridoxine use are rare and usually do not occur at normal dosages; high dosages and long-term use may produce the adverse effects listed in Table 53-8. Toxic effects are a result of very large dosages sustained for several months. Neurotoxicity is the most likely result, but this will subside upon discontinuation of the pyridoxine.

Interactions

Pyridoxine will reduce the activity of levodopa; therefore, vitamin formulations containing B_6 must be avoided in patients taking levodopa alone. However, the overwhelming majority of patients with Parkinson's disease take a combination of levodopa and carbidopa, and this interaction does not occur with combination therapy.

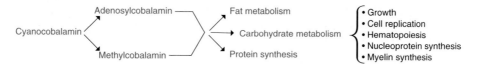

FIGURE 53-2 Cyanocobalamin is a required coenzyme for many body processes.

TABLE 53-8 Pyridoxine (Vitamin B₆): Adverse Effects	
Body System	**Adverse Effects**
Central nervous	Paresthesias, flushing, headache, lethargy
Integumentary	Pain at injection site

Dosages

For dosage information on vitamin B₆, see the table on p. 844.

DRUG PROFILE

pyridoxine

Pyridoxine is a water-soluble B-complex vitamin composed of three components: pyridoxine, pyridoxal, and pyridoxamine. It has several vital roles in the body but is primarily responsible for the integrity of peripheral nerves, skin, mucous membranes, and the hematopoietic system. Pyridoxine is available only for oral use. It is classified as a pregnancy category A drug.

Pharmacokinetics: Pyridoxine

Route	Onset of Action	Peak Plasma Concentration	Elimination Half-life	Duration of Action
PO	Unknown	30-60 min	15-20 days	Unknown

VITAMIN B₁₂

Vitamin B₁₂ (cyanocobalamin) is a water-soluble B-complex vitamin that contains cobalt (hence, its name; and *cyano-* means "blue"). It is synthesized by microorganisms and is present in the body as two different coenzymes: adenosylcobalamin and methylcobalamin. Cyanocobalamin is a required coenzyme for many metabolic pathways, including fat and carbohydrate metabolism and protein synthesis. It is also required for growth, cell replication, hematopoiesis, and nucleoprotein and myelin synthesis (Figure 53-2).

Vitamin B₁₂ deficiency results in GI lesions, neurologic changes that can result in degenerative CNS lesions, and megaloblastic anemia. The major cause of cyanocobalamin deficiency is malabsorption. Other possible but less likely causes are poor diet, chronic alcoholism, chronic hemorrhage, and prolonged use of H₂ blockers or proton pump inhibitors. Normal serum levels are 200 to 900 pg/mL.

Mechanism of Action and Drug Effects

Humans must have an exogenous source of cyanocobalamin, because it is required for nucleoprotein and myelin synthesis, cell reproduction, normal growth, and the maintenance of normal erythropoiesis. The cells that have the greatest require-

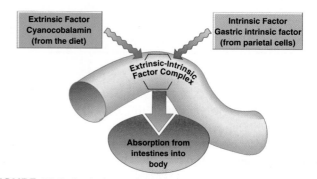

FIGURE 53-3 Oral absorption of cyanocobalamin requires the presence of intrinsic factor, which is secreted by gastric parietal cells.

ment for vitamin B₁₂ are those that divide rapidly, such as epithelial cells, bone marrow, and myeloid cells.

Reduced sulfhydryl (−5H) groups are required to metabolize fats and carbohydrates and to synthesize protein. Cyanocobalamin is involved in maintaining sulfhydryl groups in the reduced form. Cyanocobalamin deficiency can lead to neurologic damage that begins with an inability to produce myelin and is followed by gradual degeneration of the axon and nerve head.

Cyanocobalamin activity is identical to the activity of the anti–pernicious anemia factor present in liver extract called *extrinsic factor* or *Castle factor*. The oral absorption of cyanocobalamin (extrinsic factor) requires the presence of intrinsic factor, which is a glycoprotein secreted by gastric parietal cells. A complex is formed between the two factors, which is then absorbed by the intestines. This is depicted in Figure 53-3.

Indications

Cyanocobalamin is used to treat deficiency states that develop because of an insufficient intake of the vitamin. It is also included in multivitamin formulations that are used as dietary supplements. Deficiency states are most often the result of malabsorption or poor dietary intake, including gastric bypass surgery or consumption of a strict vegetarian diet, because the primary source of cyanocobalamin is foods of animal origin.

The most common manifestation of untreated cyanocobalamin deficiency is pernicious anemia. The use of vitamin B₁₂ to treat pernicious anemia and other megaloblastic anemias results in the rapid conversion of a megaloblastic bone marrow to a normoblastic bone marrow. The preferred route of administration of vitamin B₁₂ in treating megaloblastic anemias is deep intramuscular injection. If not treated, deficiency states can lead to megaloblastic anemia and irreversible neurologic damage. Cyanocobalamin is also useful in the treatment of pernicious anemia caused by an endogenous lack of intrinsic factor.

TABLE 53-9   Cyanocobalamin (Vitamin B₁₂): Adverse Effects

Body System	Adverse Effects
Cardiovascular	Vascular thrombosis, pulmonary edema
Central nervous	Flushing, optic nerve atrophy
Gastrointestinal	Diarrhea
Integumentary	Pruritus, rash, pain at injection site
Metabolic	Hypokalemia

Contraindications

The only usual contraindication to cyanocobalamin (vitamin B₁₂) is known drug product allergy. This may include sensitivity to the chemical element cobalt, which is part of the structure of cyanocobalamin. Another contraindication is hereditary optic nerve atrophy (Leber's disease).

Adverse Effects

Vitamin B₁₂ is nontoxic, and large doses must be ingested to produce adverse effects, which include itching, transitory diarrhea, and fever. Other adverse effects are listed by body system in Table 53-9.

Interactions

Concurrent use with anticonvulsants, aminoglycoside antibiotics, or long-acting potassium preparations decreases the oral absorption of vitamin B₁₂.

Dosages

For dosage information on vitamin B₁₂, see the table on p. 844.

DRUG PROFILE

cyanocobalamin

Cyanocobalamin is a water-soluble B-complex vitamin required for maintenance of body fat and carbohydrate metabolism and protein synthesis. It is also needed for growth, cell replication, blood cell production, and the integrity of normal nerve function. Cyanocobalamin (vitamin B₁₂) is available both as OTC preparations and by prescription. Most of the OTC cyanocobalamin-containing products are oral multivitamin preparations, whereas many of the cyanocobalamin-only products contain large doses for parenteral injection and are available by prescription only. Other available dosage forms are an intranasal gel and a sublingual tablet. It is classified as a pregnancy category A drug.

Pharmacokinetics: Cyanocobalamin, Vitamin B₁₂

Route	Onset of Action	Peak Plasma Concentration	Elimination Half-life	Duration of Action
PO	Unknown	8-12 hr	6 days	Unknown

VITAMIN C

Vitamin C (ascorbic acid) can be used in many therapeutic situations. Prolonged ascorbic acid deficiency results in the nutritional disease *scurvy*, which is characterized by weakness, edema, gingivitis and bleeding gums, loss of teeth, anemia, subcutaneous hemorrhage, bone lesions, delayed healing of soft tissues and bones, and hardening of leg muscles. Scurvy has been recognized for several centuries, especially among sailors. In 1795, the British navy ordered the consumption of limes to prevent the disease.

Mechanism of Action and Drug Effects

Vitamin C is reversibly oxidized to dehydroascorbic acid and acts in oxidation-reduction reactions. It is required for several important metabolic activities, including collagen synthesis and the maintenance of connective tissue; tissue repair; maintenance of bone, teeth, and capillaries; and folic acid metabolism (specifically, the conversion of folic acid into its active metabolite). It is also essential for erythropoiesis. Vitamin C enhances the absorption of iron and is required for the synthesis of lipids, proteins, and steroids. It has also been shown to aid in cellular respiration and resistance to infections.

Indications

Vitamin C is used to treat diseases associated with vitamin C deficiency and as a dietary supplement. It is most beneficial in patients who have larger daily requirements because of pregnancy, lactation, hyperthyroidism, fever, stress, infection, trauma, burns, smoking, and the use of certain drugs (e.g., estrogens, oral contraceptives, barbiturates, tetracyclines, and salicylates). Because vitamin C is an acid, it can also be used as a urinary acidifier. The benefits of other uses of vitamin C are undocumented. For example, taking vitamin C to prevent or treat the common cold is common practice. However, most large controlled studies have shown that ascorbic acid has little or no value as a prophylactic for the common cold.

Contraindications

The only usual contraindication for vitamin C use is known drug product allergy.

Adverse Effects

Vitamin C is usually nontoxic unless excessive dosages are consumed. Megadoses can produce nausea, vomiting, headache, and abdominal cramps and will acidify the urine, which can result in the formation of cystine, oxalate, and urate renal stones. Furthermore, individuals who discontinue taking excessive daily doses of ascorbic acid can experience scurvy-like symptoms.

Interactions

Ascorbic acid has the potential to interact with many classes of drugs. However, clinical experience concerning many interactions is inconclusive. Coadministration with acid-labile drugs such as penicillin G or erythromycin must be avoided. Large doses of vitamin C can acidify the urine and may enhance the excretion of basic drugs and delay the excretion of acidic drugs.

Dosages

For dosage information on vitamin C, see the table on p. 844.

DRUG PROFILE

ascorbic acid

Ascorbic acid is a water-soluble vitamin required for the prevention and treatment of scurvy. It is also required for erythropoiesis and the synthesis of lipids, protein, and steroids. It is available both in OTC preparations such as multivitamin products and by prescription. Ascorbic acid is available in many oral dosage forms as well as an injectable form. It is classified as a pregnancy category A drug.

MINERALS

Minerals are essential nutrients that are classified as inorganic compounds. They act as building blocks for many body structures and thus are necessary for a variety of physiologic functions. They are also needed for intracellular and extracellular body fluid electrolytes. Iron is essential for the production of hemoglobin, which is required for transport of oxygen throughout the body (see Chapter 54). Minerals are necessary for muscle contraction and nerve transmission, and are required components of essential enzymes.

Mineral compounds are composed of various metallic and nonmetallic elements that are chemically combined with ionic bonds. When these compounds are dissolved in water, they separate (dissociate) into positively charged metallic cations and electrolytes or negatively charged nonmetallic anions (Figure 53-4). Ingestion of minerals provides essential elements necessary for vital bodily functions. Elements that are required in larger amounts are called *macrominerals;* those required in smaller amounts are called *microminerals* or *trace elements*. Table 53-10 classifies these nutrient elements as either *macrominerals* or *microminerals* and as *metal* or *nonmetal*.

CALCIUM

Calcium is the most abundant mineral element in the human body, accounting for approximately 2% of the total body weight. The highest concentration of calcium is in bones and teeth. The efficient absorption of calcium requires adequate amounts of vitamin D.

Calcium deficiency results in hypocalcemia and can affect many bodily functions. Causes of calcium deficiency include

inadequate calcium intake and/or insufficient vitamin D to facilitate absorption; hypoparathyroidism; and malabsorption syndrome, especially in older individuals. Calcium deficiency–related disorders include infantile rickets, adult osteomalacia, muscle cramps, osteoporosis (especially in postmenopausal females), hypoparathyroidism, and renal dysfunction. Table 53-11 lists the possible causes of calcium deficiency and the resulting disorders. Normal serum levels are 9 to 10.5 mg/dL.

Mechanism of Action and Drug Effects

Calcium participates in a variety of essential physiologic functions and is a building block for body structures. Specifically, calcium is involved in the proper development and maintenance of teeth and skeletal bones. It is an important catalyst in many of the coagulation pathways in the blood. Calcium acts as a cofactor in clotting reactions involving the intrinsic and extrinsic pathways of thromboplastin. It is also a cofactor in the conversion of prothrombin to thrombin by thromboplastin and the conversion of fibrinogen to fibrin. Calcium is essential for the normal maintenance and function of the nervous, muscular, and skeletal systems and for cell membrane and capillary

TABLE 53-10 Mineral Elements

Element	Symbol	Type	Ionic/Electrolyte Form
Macrominerals			
calcium*	Ca	Metal	Ca^{2+} calcium cation
chlorine	Cl	Nonmetal	Cl^- chloride anion
magnesium*	Mg	Metal	Mg^{2+} magnesium cation
phosphorous*	P	Nonmetal	PO_4^{3-} phosphate anion
potassium	K	Metal	K^+ potassium cation
sodium	Na	Metal	Na^+ sodium cation
sulfur	S	Nonmetal	SO_4^{2-} sulfate anion
Microminerals			
chromium	Cr	Metal	Cr^{3+} chromium cation
cobalt	Co	Metal	Co^{2+} cobalt cation
copper	Cu	Metal	Cu^{2+} copper cation
fluorine	F	Nonmetal	F^+ fluoride anion
iodine*	I	Nonmetal	I^+ iodide anion
iron*	Fe	Metal	Fe^{2+} ferrous cation
manganese	Mn	Metal	Mn^{2+} manganese cation
molybdenum	Mo	Metal	Mo^{6+} molybdenum cation
selenium*	Se	Metal	Se^{2-} selenium cation
zinc*	Zn	Metal	Zn^{2+} zinc cation

*Mineral elements that have a current recommended daily allowance (RDA).

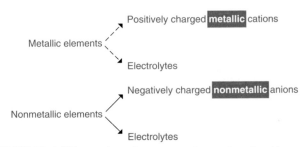

FIGURE 53-4 When mineral compounds are dissolved in water, they separate into positively charged metallic cations or negatively charged nonmetallic anions.

TABLE 53-11 Calcium Deficiency: Causes and Disorders

Cause	Disorder
Inadequate intake	Infantile rickets
Insufficient vitamin D	Adult osteomalacia
Hypoparathyroidism	Muscle cramps
Malabsorption syndrome	Osteoporosis

permeability. It is an important catalyst in many enzymatic reactions, including transmission of nerve impulses; contraction of cardiac, smooth, and skeletal muscles; renal function; respiration; and, as noted earlier, blood coagulation. Calcium also plays a regulatory role in the release and storage of neurotransmitters and hormones, in white blood cell (WBC) and hormone activity, in the uptake and binding of amino acids, and in intestinal absorption of cyanocobalamin (vitamin B_{12}) and gastrin secretion.

Indications

Calcium salts are used for the treatment or prevention of calcium depletion in patients for whom dietary measures are inadequate. Calcium requirements are also high for growing children and for women who are pregnant or breastfeeding. Many conditions may be associated with calcium deficiency, including the following:

- Achlorhydria
- Alkalosis
- Chronic diarrhea
- Hyperphosphatemia
- Hypoparathyroidism
- Menopause
- Pancreatitis
- Pregnancy and lactation
- Premenstrual syndrome
- Renal failure
- Sprue
- Steatorrhea
- Vitamin D deficiency

Calcium is also used to treat various manifestations of established deficiency states, including adult osteomalacia, hypoparathyroidism, infantile rickets or tetany, muscle cramps, osteoporosis, and renal insufficiency. In addition, calcium is used as a dietary supplement for women during pregnancy and lactation.

More than 12 different selected calcium salts are available for treatment or nutritional supplementation. Each calcium salt contains a different amount of elemental calcium per gram of calcium salt. Table 53-12 lists the available salts and their associated calcium content.

Contraindications

Contraindications for administration of exogenous calcium include hypercalcemia, ventricular fibrillation of the heart, and known drug product allergy.

Adverse Effects

Although adverse effects and toxicity are rare, hypercalcemia can occur. Symptoms include anorexia, nausea, vomiting, and constipation. In addition, when calcium salts are administered by intramuscular or subcutaneous injection, mild to severe local reactions, including burning, necrosis and sloughing of tissue, cellulitis, and soft tissue calcification, may occur. Venous irritation may occur with intravenous administration. IV calcium chloride is very caustic to the veins and must be diluted or given via a central line. Taking calcium supplements may increase the

TABLE 53-12 Calcium Salts: Calcium Content

Calcium Salt	Elemental Calcium Content (Per Gram)
phosphate tribasic	400 mg (20 mEq)
carbonate*	400 mg (20 mEq)
phosphate dibasic anhydrous	290 mg (14.5 mEq)
chloride	270 mg (13.5 mEq)
acetate	253 mg (12.7 mEq)
phosphate dibasic dihydrate	230 mg (11.5 mEq)
citrate*	211 mg (10.6 mEq)
glycerophosphate	191 mg (9.6 mEq)
lactate	130 mg (6.5 mEq)
gluconate*	90 mg (4.5 mEq)
gluceptate	82 mg (4.1 mEq)
glubionate	64 mg (3.2 mEq)

*Most commonly used forms for the prevention of osteoporosis.

TABLE 53-13 Calcium Salts: Adverse Effects

Body System	Adverse Effects
Cardiovascular	Hemorrhage, rebound hypertension
Gastrointestinal	Constipation, nausea, vomiting, flatulence
Genitourinary	Renal dysfunction, renal stones, renal failure
Metabolic	Hypercalcemia, metabolic alkalosis

risk for developing kidney stones. Other adverse effects associated with both oral and parenteral use of calcium salts are listed in Table 53-13.

Toxicity and Management of Overdose

Long-term excessive calcium intake can result in severe hypercalcemia, which can cause cardiac irregularities, delirium, and coma. Management of acute hypercalcemia may require hemodialysis, whereas milder cases will respond to discontinuation of calcium intake.

Interactions

Calcium salts will chelate (bind with) tetracyclines and quinolones to produce an insoluble complex. If hypercalcemia is present in patients taking digoxin, serious cardiac dysrhythmias can occur.

Dosages

For dosage information on calcium and other selected minerals, see the table on this page.

DRUG PROFILE

calcium

Calcium salts are primarily used in the treatment or prevention of calcium depletion in patients in whom dietary measures are inadequate. Many calcium salts are available, all with a different content of elemental calcium per gram of salt. Calcium is available in both oral and parenteral forms. Numerous calcium preparations are available that have different names and provide different doses. Consult manufacturer instructions for recommended dosages. The pharmacokinetics of calcium is highly variable and depends on individual patient physiology and the characteristics of the specific drug product used. Medication errors and confusion are common with calcium products, because the amount of the salt is not the same as the amount of elemental calcium. For example, calcium carbonate 1250 mg is equal to 500 mg of elemental calcium. Depending on the institution, the drug may be profiled as 1250 mg, but the tablet is labeled as 500 mg. Additional confusion occurs with the injectable forms, calcium chloride and calcium gluconate. Calcium chloride provides about three times as much elemental calcium as calcium gluconate, but they are both ordered as 1 g or 1 ampule. Calcium chloride can cause severe problems if it infiltrates from the intravenous line. For that reason, it is recommended that it be diluted or given through a central line if it is given by intravenous push. Adding to the confusion is calcium acetate (PhosLo), which is used not for calcium replacement but to bind phosphate in renal patients. Calcium products are classified as pregnancy category C drugs.

MAGNESIUM

Magnesium is one of the principal cations present in the intracellular fluid. It is an essential part of many enzyme systems associated with energy metabolism. Magnesium deficiency (hypomagnesemia) is usually caused by (1) malabsorption, especially in the presence of high calcium intake; (2) alcoholism; (3) long-term intravenous feeding; (4) diuretic use; and (5) metabolic disorders, including hyperthyroidism and diabetic ketoacidosis. Symptoms associated with hypomagnesemia include cardiovascular disturbances, neuromuscular impairment, and mental disturbances. Dietary intake from vegetables and other foods will usually prevent magnesium deficiency. However, magnesium is required in greater amounts in individuals with diets high in protein-rich foods, calcium, and phosphorus. Normal serum levels are 1.7 to 2.2 mg/dL. IV magnesium is considered a high-alert medication; the oral form is not.

DOSAGES

Selected Minerals

Drug	Pharmacologic Class	Usual Dosage Range	Indications/ Uses
calcium carbonate (Tums, others)	Mineral salt	PO: 1000-1500 mg/day	Antacid, nutritional-calcium supplementation, hyperphosphatemia associated with chronic renal failure
magnesium oxide (Max-Ox 400, others)	Mineral salt	PO: 400 mg 1-2 times daily	Magnesium supplementation, hypomagnesemia

SAFETY AND QUALITY IMPROVEMENT: PREVENTING MEDICATION ERRORS

QSEN

All Calcium Forms Are Not the Same!

When calcium is given, it is essential to use the correct form. Calcium chloride has many uses, including treatment of cardiac arrest and hypocalcemic tetany. Both calcium carbonate (Os-Cal, Tums, Caltrate) and calcium citrate (Citracal) are used as antacids and are also used to treat or prevent calcium deficiency and to treat hyperphosphatemia. However, calcium acetate (PhosLo) is not used for calcium replacement. It is used only to control hyperphosphatemia in patients with end-stage renal disease. Be cautious when giving calcium—the different forms are not interchangeable.

Mechanism of Action and Drug Effects

The precise mechanism for the effects of magnesium has not been fully determined. Magnesium is a known cofactor for many enzyme systems. It is required for muscle contraction and nerve function. Magnesium produces an anticonvulsant effect by inhibiting neuromuscular transmission in selected convulsive states.

Indications

Magnesium is used for treatment of magnesium deficiency and as a nutritional supplement in total parenteral nutrition and multivitamin preparations. It is used as an anticonvulsant in magnesium deficiency–induced seizure states; to manage complications of pregnancy, including preeclampsia and eclampsia; as a tocolytic drug for inhibition of uterine contractions in premature labor; for treatment of pediatric acute nephropathy; for management of various cardiac dysrhythmias; and for short-term treatment of constipation.

Contraindications

Contraindications to magnesium administration include known drug product allergy, heart block, renal failure, adrenal gland failure (Addison's disease), and hepatitis.

Adverse Effects

Adverse effects of magnesium are due to hypermagnesemia, which results in tendon reflex loss, difficult bowel movements, CNS depression, respiratory distress and heart block, and hypothermia.

Toxicity and Management of Overdose

Toxic effects are extensions of symptoms caused by hypermagnesemia, a major cause of which is the long-term use of magnesium products (especially antacids in patients with renal dysfunction). Severe hypermagnesemia is treated with intravenous calcium and possibly the diuretic furosemide.

Interactions

The use of magnesium with neuromuscular blocking drugs and CNS depressants produces additive effects.

DRUG PROFILE

‼magnesium

Magnesium is a mineral that has a variety of dosage forms and uses. It is an essential part of many enzyme systems. When it is absent or diminished in the body, cardiovascular, neuromuscular, and mental disturbances can occur. Magnesium sulfate is the most common form of magnesium used as a mineral replacement. It is available in both oral and injectable forms. It is classified as a pregnancy category B drug.

PHOSPHORUS

Phosphorus is widely distributed in foods, and thus a dietary deficiency is rare. Deficiency states are primarily due to malabsorption, extensive diarrhea or vomiting, hyperthyroidism, hepatic disease, and long-term use of aluminum or calcium antacids. Normal serum levels are 2.8 to 4.2 mg/dL.

Mechanism of Action and Drug Effects

Phosphorus in the form of the phosphate group and/or anion (PO_4^{3-}) is a required precursor for the synthesis of essential body chemicals and an important building block for body structures. Phosphorus is required as a structural unit for the synthesis of nucleic acid and the adenosine phosphate compounds (adenosine monophosphate [AMP], adenosine diphosphate [ADP], and adenosine triphosphate [ATP]) responsible for cellular energy transfer. It is also necessary for the development and maintenance of the skeletal system and teeth. The skeletal bones contain up to 85% of the phosphorus content of the body. In addition, phosphorus is required for the proper utilization of many B-complex vitamins, and it is an essential component of physiologic buffering systems.

Indications

Phosphorus is used for treatment of deficiency states and as a dietary supplement in many multivitamin formulations.

Contraindications

Contraindications to phosphorous or phosphate administration include hyperphosphatemia and hypocalcemia.

Adverse Effects

Adverse effects are usually associated with the use of phosphorus replacement products. These effects include diarrhea, nausea, vomiting, and other GI disturbances. Other adverse effects include confusion, weakness, and breathing difficulties.

Toxicity and Management of Overdose

Toxic reactions to phosphorus are extremely rare and usually occur only after ingestion of the pure element.

Interactions

Antacids can reduce the oral absorption of phosphorus.

DRUG PROFILE

phosphorus

Phosphorus is a mineral that is essential to our well-being. It is needed to make energy in the form of ADP and ATP for all bodily processes. Phosphorus is present in a large number of drug formulations and appears as a phosphate salt (PO_4). Phosphorus is to be used with caution in patients with renal impairment. It is available in both oral and parenteral formulations.

ZINC

The metallic element zinc is often taken orally in the form of the sulfate salt as a mineral supplement. Normally a dietary trace element, zinc plays a crucial role in the enzymatic metabolic reactions involving both proteins and carbohydrates. This makes it especially important for normal tissue growth and repair. It therefore also has a major role in wound healing.

NURSING PROCESS

ASSESSMENT

Before administering *vitamins,* assess the patient for nutritional disorders by reviewing the results of various laboratory tests, such as hemoglobin, hematocrit, WBC and RBC counts, serum albumin, and total protein levels. Assess the patient's dietary intake, dietary patterns, menu planning, grocery shopping/food practices and habits, and cultural influences before giving any supplemental therapy. For vitamin A deficiencies, perform a baseline vision assessment, including night vision, and conduct a thorough examination of the skin and mucous membranes, and document the findings. Assess for contraindications to vitamin A such as known drug product allergy as well as a current state of excessive supplementation and/or hypervitaminosis. Additionally, assess for drug interactions with laxatives and cholestyramine leading to possible decreased absorption of the vitamin.

With *vitamin A,* baseline assessment and documentation of level of consciousness, GI functioning and complaints, vision, condition of the skin, and musculoskeletal status is also important due to the adverse effects and signs and symptoms of toxicity associated with overdosage of vitamin A (see the pharmacology discussion and Table 53-3).

For patients who are deficient in *vitamin D,* perform a baseline assessment of skeletal formation with attention to any deformities. Serum vitamin D (12 to 50 ng/mL) and calcium levels are usually ordered as baseline and then during therapy. It is also important to assess for known contraindications such as renal dysfunction and hypercalcemia or hyperphosphatemia. Assess for drug interactions with laxatives and cholestyramine leading to possible decreased absorption of the vitamin. Before *vitamin E* is given, assess patients for hypoprothrombinemia because this condition may occur secondary to vitamin E deficiency. Document any baseline bleeding or hematologic problems, and conduct a thorough skin assessment with attention to skin integrity, presence of edema, muscle weakness, easy bruising, and/or bleeding.

The last of the fat-soluble vitamins, *vitamin K,* is associated with clotting function; therefore, prior to its use, measure and document the patient's prothrombin time, international normalized ratio, and platelet counts. Assess the skin for bruises, petechiae, and erythema. Examine the gums for gingival bleeding. Assess urine and stool for the presence of blood. Additionally, assess vital signs with attention to blood pressure and pulse rate. If intravenous dosage forms are prescribed, baseline assessment must include vital signs because of the risk for anaphylactic reactions. This is particularly important with *vitamin K₁* (*phytonadione* or *AquaMEPHYTON*) because of an associated higher risk for anaphylaxis. Assessment of liver function is also important. It is critical to patient safety to remember that the fat-soluble vitamins are all stored in the body tissue when excessive quantities are consumed and may become toxic if taken in large dosages. Assess and document baseline values of vitamin K; normal ranges are 0.1 to 2.2 ng/mL.

Vitamin B₁ (*thiamine*) hypersensitivity may cause skin rash and wheezing; therefore, document the presence of any allergic reactions to vitamin B compounds. Also, as appropriate, document baseline assessment of vital signs. Because it is rare for a deficiency of only one B-complex vitamin to occur, rule out deficiencies of all the B vitamins before treatment begins. Vitamin B₁ (thiamine) levels range from 66 to 200 nmol/L, and *vitamin B₁₂* (*cyanocobalamin*) levels range from 200 to 900 pg/mL. Urinary thiamine levels may also be ordered (in adults, urinary thiamine levels of less than 27 mcg/dL indicate deficiency). Vitamin B₁ deficiency may result in Wernicke's encephalopathy (see the pharmacology discussion); thus, there is a need for a thorough mental status assessment. Thoroughly assess the medication order for accuracy and for route of administration. Drug interactions include alkaline and sulfite-containing solutions, so be sure to assess for drugs being administered at the same time. *Vitamin B₂* (*riboflavin*) has no major toxic effects or drug interactions, but assessing for any known drug product allergy is important to patient safety. *Vitamin B₃* (*niacin*) has several important indications. Assess for contraindications such as liver disease, severe hypotension, and active peptic ulcer disease. With *vitamin B₆* (*pyridoxine*), perform a thorough neurologic assessment due to associated neurotoxicity with large dosages. Levodopa is a significant drug interaction to assess for with pyridoxine because the vitamin reduces the action of levodopa. *Vitamin B₁₂* (*cyanocobalamin*) requires thorough assessment of the medication order. Note the route of administration because the preferred route is deep IM injection. Drug interactions to assess for include anticonvulsants, aminoglycoside antibiotics, and long-acting potassium supplements because they decrease the oral absorption of vitamin B₁₂.

Vitamin C (*ascorbic acid*) is usually well tolerated; however, assess the patient for any history of nutritional deficits or problems with dietary intake as well as any allergies to a specific vitamin product. Assess for drug interactions that include acid-labile drugs such as penicillin G or erythromycin. Additionally, it is important to note that large doses of vitamin C may increase the excretion of many basic (opposite of acidic) drugs and delay the excretion of acidic drugs.

With the minerals *calcium* and *magnesium*, include allergies, nutritional status, use of medications, medical history, contraindications, cautions, and drug interactions in the baseline assessment. Laboratory studies that may be prescribed include serum calcium (9 to 10.5 mg/dL), magnesium (1.7 to 2.2 mg/dL), hemoglobin, hematocrit, and RBC and WBC counts. Calcium interacts with many medications, as described previously, so a thorough assessment of the patient's medication history is important to patient safety. The specific interaction of calcium is that of chelation or binding with the drug and, in

this case, it is with tetracycline and quinolone antibiotics. The chelation then forms an insoluble complex rendering the antibiotic inactive. Another significant interaction occurs when a patient is hypercalcemic and takes digitalis with the result of serious cardiac dysrhythmias. If there is a history of cardiac disease, a baseline electrocardiogram (ECG) recording may be ordered prior to calcium therapy. Because of the various calcium preparations with different names and doses, always thoroughly assess the medication order and be certain that the right product is being given. Additionally, note that the injectable forms of calcium (e.g., *calcium chloride, calcium gluconate*) may be easily confused, so be cautious to assess the order against your medication preparation. Assess patency of the IV site, if intravenous dosage forms are ordered because infiltrates may lead to severe irritation of the vein and surrounding tissue.

Magnesium is also associated with several drug interactions. Review for potential interactions before drug therapy is initiated, such as with CNS depressants and neuromuscular blocking drugs. Assess the patient's renal, cardiac, and hepatic functioning. Important to document prior to giving magnesium is neurologic functioning and grading of deep tendon reflexes. Hyporeflexia may indicate toxicity. It is also important to assess the prescriber's order for completeness and reason for use so that it is fully understood why the drug is being given (e.g., replacement, antacid, or laxative purposes). In addition, thoroughly assess any order for the use of calcium, magnesium, and/or *zinc* within total parenteral nutritional infusions.

NURSING DIAGNOSES

1. Impaired physical mobility related to poorly developed muscles from vitamin D and/or vitamin E deficiency and/or from fatigue related to poor nutrition and vitamin B deficiency
2. Impaired tissue integrity related to vitamin C deficiency and subsequent decreased healing
3. Risk for injury related to possible night blindness or altered vision due to vitamin A deficiency

PLANNING: OUTCOME IDENTIFICATION

1. Patient regains or maintains normal or near-normal physical mobility and musculoskeletal functioning through a prescribed exercise regimen as well as balanced dietary intake of foods and fluids.
2. Patient maintains intact skin and tissue integrity with frequent mouth care and skin care.
3. Patient remains free from injury with safety measures at home such as minimizing obstacles and adequate lighting at night.

IMPLEMENTATION

Before administering *vitamin A* or any vitamin or supplement, document the patient's dietary intake for the preceding 24 hours. Document any signs and symptoms of hypervitaminosis or hypercarotenemia (excess vitamin A). *Vitamin D* is available

CASE STUDY

Vitamin Supplements

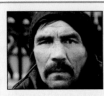

S.C., 49 years of age, was found unconscious in a vacant house and was brought to the emergency department. He had an elevated blood alcohol level and eventually manifested delirium tremens. Now, 1 week later, he is in stable condition on a medical-surgical unit. He is weak and malnourished, and he cannot remember how he got to the hospital. The nurse is reviewing his medication list and notes that several vitamin supplements are ordered.

1. Based on S.C.'s history, what vitamin deficiencies are possible?
2. Which vitamin supplement is especially used to treat complications associated with alcoholism? Explain your answer.
3. S.C. is receiving large doses of several vitamins, and the nurse is concerned about vitamin toxicities. Which type of vitamin, water-soluble or fat-soluble, carries the risk for toxicities? Explain your answer.
4. Because of S.C.'s long-term malnourished state, the prescriber is concerned about the condition of his bones and starts S.C. on phosphorus and calcium supplementation, along with vitamin D. Explain the rationale behind the addition of vitamin D.

For answers, see *http://evolve.elsevier.com/Lilley.*

in oral dosage forms as an OTC product (e.g., multivitamins) or by prescription, but attention to the product prescribed is important to patient safety. For those with GI, liver, biliary, and/or malabsorptive syndromes, intramuscular (IM) dosage forms are available. During therapy, advise the patient to report any palpitations, unresolved nausea, vomiting, constipation, or muscle pain. Instruct the patient to take *vitamin B₁ (thiamine)* as directed. *Vitamin B₂ (riboflavin)* is not associated with any adverse or toxic effects, but it is important to note that in large doses it may turn the urine yellowish-orange. Tell patients to take *vitamin B₃ (niacin)* with milk or food to decrease GI upset. Niacin is often used for hyperlipidemia (see Chapter 27) and in much larger doses. *Vitamin B₆ (pyridoxine)* is more commonly used to treat drug-induced B₆ deficiencies. Two examples of this are with the antituberculin drug isoniazid (INH) and the antihypertensive drug hydralazine. *Vitamin B₁₂ (cyanocobalamin)* is administered orally with meals to increase its absorption. Intranasal gel and sublingual tablets are other dosage forms available. If given for megaloblastic anemia, deep IM injection is the preferred route of administration. Give *vitamin C (ascorbic acid)* orally, and if oral effervescent forms are used, instruct the patient to dissolve it in at least 6 ounces of water or juice. If vitamin C is administered for acidification of urine, it is important to frequently monitor the patient's urinary pH.

Various oral *calcium* products are available and, because of the differences in the amount of elemental calcium they provide (e.g., calcium carbonate 1250 mg is equal to only 500 mg of elemental calcium), medication errors may occur and confusion may arise about the various dosages available OTC. A list of the various calcium salts available is found in Table 53-12. Instruct the patient to take oral dosage forms of calcium 1 to 3 hours after meals. Injectable dosage forms of calcium may also

be confusing. Follow the medication order carefully, and check institutional policy and standards regarding infusions (see previous discussion in the pharmacology section and the Safety and Quality Improvement: Preventing Medication Errors box on p. 855). Because of problems with venous irritation, give intravenous calcium via an intravenous infusion pump and with proper dilution. Giving intravenous calcium too rapidly may precipitate severe hypercalcemia with subsequent cardiac irregularities, delirium, and coma. Administer intravenous calcium slowly, as ordered, and within the manufacturer guidelines (e.g., usually less than 1 mL/min). Patients need to remain recumbent for 15 minutes after the infusion to prevent further problems. Should extravasation of the intravenous calcium solution occur, discontinue the infusion immediately, but leave the intravenous catheter in place for antidote administration. The prescriber may then order an injection of 1% procaine and/or other antidotes or fluids to reduce vasospasm at the site and dilute the irritating effects of calcium on surrounding tissue. However, follow all institutional policies and procedural guidelines and/or manufacturer insert information as is deemed appropriate. In addition, include the appearance of the intravenous site (e.g., erythema, swelling, and drainage) in the documentation.

Administer magnesium according to manufacturer guidelines and as ordered. Always give intravenous *magnesium sulfate* very cautiously; use an infusion pump, and follow manufacturer guidelines for dosage and dilutional concentration. During intravenous magnesium infusion, monitor the patient's ECG and vital signs, and rate patellar or knee-jerk reflexes. Impaired reflexes are used as an indication of drug-related CNS depressant effects. CNS depression may quickly lead to respiratory and/or cardiac depression; thus perform frequent monitoring. Document IV calcium infusion, and record each set of vital sign measurements with ratings of reflexes. If there is a decrease in the strength of reflexes and/or a decrease in respirations to less than 12 breaths/min, contact the prescriber immediately, stop the infusion, and monitor the patient. Other signs that require immediate attention are confusion, irregular heart rhythm, cramping, unusual fatigue, lightheadedness, and dizziness. Calcium gluconate must be readily accessible for use as an antidote to magnesium toxicity. Administer oral dosage forms of magnesium as ordered and in the exact dosage prescribed. See Patient-Centered Care: Patient Teaching on the next page for more information related to the use of vitamins, minerals, and trace elements.

EVALUATION

In the patient's evaluation, always review whether goals and outcome criteria have been met. Monitor for therapeutic responses and adverse effects of each vitamin or mineral. Therapeutic responses to *vitamin A* include restoration of normal vision and intact skin; adverse effects include lethargy, headache, nausea, and vomiting (see Table 53-3). Therapeutic responses to *vitamin D* include improved bone growth and formation and an intact skeleton with decreased or no pain compared with baseline musculoskeletal deformity, weakness, and discomfort; adverse effects include hypertension, dysrhythmias, fatigue, weakness, headache, and decreased bone growth (see Table 53-4). Therapeutic responses to *vitamin E* include improved muscle strength, improved skin integrity, and *alpha tocopherol* levels within normal limits; adverse effects are listed in Table 53-5. Therapeutic responses to *vitamin K* include return to normal clotting; adverse effects include headache, nausea, and hemolytic anemia (see Table 53-6).

Therapeutic responses to *vitamin B₁ (thiamine)* include improved mental status as well as improvement in peripheral neuritis. Monitor for adverse effects such as nausea, itching, weakness, and pulmonary edema. Therapeutic responses to *vitamin B₃ (niacin)* include prevention/improvement in pellagra as well as improvement in certain types of hyperlipidemia and peripheral vascular disease. The most frequent adverse effects of niacin include flushing of the face, itching, and GI upset (see Table 53-7). Therapeutic responses to *vitamin B₆ (pyridoxine)* include improvements in adverse effect linked to certain medications (e.g., the antituberculin drug isoniazid and the antihypertensive drug, hydralazine). *Cyanocobalamin (vitamin B₁₂)* therapy helps to manage pernicious and megoblastic anemia and the related adverse effects include itching, fever, and diarrhea.

Therapeutic responses to *vitamin C* include improvements in capillary intactness, integrity of the skin and mucous membranes, healing, energy level, and mental state. Therapeutic responses to *calcium* include improved deficiency states. Adverse effects are listed in Table 53-13. Therapeutic effects of *magnesium* include bolstering of many enzymatic functions in the body with other uses as an anticonvulsant, treatment of preeclampsia and eclampsia, and management of various dysrhythmias. Adverse effects include loss of deep tendon reflexes, CNS depression, constipation, respiratory distress, and heart block.

PATIENT-CENTERED CARE: PATIENT TEACHING

- Educate the patient about the best dietary sources of both water- and fat-soluble vitamins (vitamins A, B, C, D, E, and K), as well as about the best sources of elements and minerals. See Table 53-2 for the nutrient content of various food items.
- Monitor any patient taking vitamins or minerals closely for therapeutic and adverse effects. Encourage the patient to monitor his or her own progress in how well he or she feels and to note any improvement in the related condition or health status. Encourage intake of fluids with all vitamin and mineral therapy.
- Inform patients who have had a gastrectomy or ileal resection and those with pernicious anemia of the necessity for vitamin B₁₂ injections. Provide written materials on their educational level.
- Educate the patient taking up to 600 mg/day of vitamin C that there may be a slight increase in daily urination and that diarrhea is associated with intake of more than 1 g/day.

- Stress that patients taking calcium and/or magnesium (see Table 53-10) must take the medication as prescribed and with adequate amounts of fluids.
- Educate the patient about calcium therapy and about food items and drugs that will chelate (or bind) with calcium. For example, calcium binds with tetracycline antibiotics and decreases or negates the effect of the antibiotic.
- Encourage an increase in fluids with calcium supplementation to help decrease the risk for kidney stone formation. Most kidney stones are composed of calcium and oxalic acid. If a patient is receiving calcium supplements and has a history of kidney stones, educate about limiting foods high in oxalate such as spinach, rhubarb, and cocoa. Studies also suggest that prolonged use of excessive doses of vitamin D has been known to cause kidney stones. High intake of sodium may also increase the risk for calcium oxalate stones.

KEY POINTS

- OTC use of vitamins and minerals may lead to serious problems and adverse effects and requires careful consideration prior to self-medication. A prescriber may be consulted prior to use if there are any questions or concerns.
- Incorporate the nutritional status of the patient into the nursing care plan to provide comprehensive care during vitamin or mineral therapy.
- Provide information about dietary needs and the body's need for vitamins and minerals as part of the patient's health promotion.

- Focus patient education related to vitamin and mineral replacement on dietary sources of the specific nutrient, drug and food interactions, and adverse effects. Instruct the patient on when it is necessary to contact the prescriber.
- Vitamins and minerals can be dangerous to the patient if given without concern or caution for the patient's overall condition and underlying disease processes.
- Never assume that because the drug is a vitamin or a mineral it does not have adverse reactions or toxicity.

NCLEX® EXAMINATION REVIEW QUESTIONS

1. When giving calcium intravenously, the nurse needs to administer it slowly, keeping in mind that rapid intravenous administration of calcium may cause which problem?
   a. Ototoxicity
   b. Renal damage
   c. Tetany
   d. Cardiac dysrhythmias

2. The nurse will assess which laboratory test results before administration of vitamin K?
   a. Prothrombin time and international normalized ratio
   b. Red blood cell and white blood cell counts
   c. Phosphorous and calcium levels
   d. Total protein and albumin levels

3. A patient has GI malabsorption due to severe intestinal damage from a gastrointestinal infection. The nurse will need to assess for signs of a deficiency of which vitamin?
   a. Vitamin A (retinol)
   b. Vitamin B_{12} (cyanocobalamin)
   c. Vitamin B_6 (pyridoxine)
   d. Vitamin E (tocopherols)

4. The nurse is providing wound care for a patient with a stage IV pressure ulcer and expects that the patient will receive which supplements to assist in wound healing? *(Select all that apply.)*
   a. Vitamin K
   b. Vitamin B_1
   c. Zinc
   d. Calcium
   e. Vitamin C

5. While caring for a newly admitted patient who has a long history of alcoholism, the nurse anticipates that part of the patient's medication regimen will include which vitamin?
   a. Vitamin B_1 (thiamine)
   b. Vitamin B_6 (pyridoxine)
   c. Vitamin C (ascorbic acid)
   d. Vitamin A (retinol)

6. When administering vitamin and mineral supplements, the nurse implements which appropriate interventions? *(Select all that apply.)*
   a. Not administering oral calcium tablets along with oral tetracyclines
   b. Administering intravenous calcium via a rapid intravenous push infusion
   c. Monitoring the heart rhythm (ECG) of a patient receiving an intravenous magnesium infusion
   d. Giving oral niacin with milk or food to decrease gastrointestinal upset
   e. Monitoring for the formation of renal stones in patients taking large doses of vitamin C

7. The order reads: "Give vitamin K (AquaMEPHYTON) 0.5 mg IM within 1 hour of birth." The medication is available in a vial that contains 1 mg/0.5 mL. How many milliliters will the nurse draw up for the injection?

8. The nurse is assessing a patient who has been recently admitted to the hospital after living on the streets for over 1 year. The nurse notes that the patient has severely chapped and fissured lips. This could be a sign of which vitamin deficiency?
   a. Vitamin B_2 (riboflavin)
   b. Vitamin B_6 (pyridoxine)
   c. Vitamin C (ascorbic acid)
   d. Vitamin E (tocopherols)

1. d, 2. a, 3. b, 4. c, e, 5. a, 6. a, c, d, e, 7. 0.25 mL, 8. a.

CRITICAL THINKING AND PRIORITIZATION QUESTIONS

1. The nurse is about to administer calcium supplemental therapy to a patient with a history of cardiac disease. What is the most important assessment that is needed before the nurse gives the drug?

2. A patient receiving a magnesium infusion has developed tendon reflex loss, CNS depression, and some respiratory distress. These problems are a result of what condition? What are the nurse's priority actions at this time?

For answers, see *http://evolve.elsevier.com/Lilley.*

⊜ EVOLVE WEBSITE

http://evolve.elsevier.com/Lilley
• Animations
• Answer Keys for Textbook Case Studies and Textbook Critical Thinking and Prioritization Questions

• Content Updates
• Key Points
• Review Questions
• Student Case Studies

Anemia Drugs

OBJECTIVES

When you reach the end of this chapter, you will be able to do the following:

1. Discuss the importance of iron, vitamin B$_{12}$, and folic acid in the formation of blood cells.
2. Describe the various types of anemia-related drug treatments.
3. Discuss the mechanisms of action, cautions, contraindications, drug interactions, uses, dosages, and special administration techniques of the various drugs used to treat anemia, as well as measures to enhance the effectiveness and decrease the adverse effects of these drugs.
4. Develop a nursing care plan that includes all phases of the nursing process for patients taking drugs used to treat anemia.

DRUG PROFILES

♦ epoetin alfa, p. 863
ferric gluconate, p. 866
ferrous fumarate, p. 866
♦ ferrous sulfate, p. 866
♦ folic acid, p. 866

iron dextran, p. 866
iron sucrose, p. 866

_____

♦ = *Key drug*
! = *High-alert drug*

KEY TERMS

Erythrocytes Another name for red blood cells (RBCs). (p. 861)

Erythropoiesis The process of erythrocyte production. (p. 861)

Globin The protein part of the *hemoglobin* molecule (see later); the four different structural globin chains most often found in adults are the alpha$_1$, alpha$_2$, beta$_1$, and beta$_2$ chains. (p. 862)

Hematopoiesis The normal formation and development of all blood cell types in the bone marrow. (p. 861)

Heme Part of the *hemoglobin* molecule; a nonprotein, iron-containing pigment. (p. 862)

Hemoglobin A complex protein-iron compound in the blood that carries oxygen to the cells from the lungs and carbon dioxide away from the cells to the lungs. (p. 862)

Hemolytic anemias Anemias resulting from excessive destruction of erythrocytes. (p. 863)

Hypochromic Pertaining to less than normal color. The term usually describes an RBC with decreased hemoglobin content and helps further characterize anemias associated with reduced synthesis of hemoglobin. (p. 862)

Microcytic Pertaining to or characterized by smaller than normal cells. (p. 862)

Pernicious anemia A type of megaloblastic anemia usually seen in older adults and caused by impaired intestinal absorption of vitamin B$_{12}$ (cyanocobalamin) due to lack of availability of intrinsic factor. (p. 863)

Reticulocytes An immature erythrocyte characterized by a meshlike pattern of threads and particles at the former site of the nucleus. (p. 862)

Spherocytes Small, globular, completely hemoglobinated erythrocytes without the usual central concavity or pallor. (p. 863)

ERYTHROPOIESIS

The formation of new blood cells is one of the primary functions of bones. This process is known as hematopoiesis, and it includes the production of erythrocytes (red blood cells, or RBCs), as well as leukocytes (white blood cells) and thrombocytes (platelets). This process takes place in the myeloid tissue or bone marrow. This specialized tissue is located primarily in the ends, or *epiphyses,* of certain long bones and also in the flat bones of the skull, pelvis, sternum, scapulae, and ribs.

Erythropoiesis, the process of erythrocyte formation, is the focus of this chapter. This involves the maturation of a nucleated RBC precursor into a hemoglobin-filled, nucleus-free erythrocyte. This process is driven by the hormone erythropoietin, which is produced by the kidneys. Erythropoietin is also produced commercially and is used to treat anemia in certain specific circumstances. It is discussed in detail later in the chapter.

When RBCs are manufactured in the bone marrow by myeloid tissue, they are released into the circulation as immature RBCs called **reticulocytes**. Once in the circulation, reticulocytes undergo a 24- to 36-hour maturation process to become mature, fully functional RBCs. After this, they have a lifespan of about 120 days.

More than one third of an RBC is composed of hemoglobin. **Hemoglobin** (abbreviated *Hgb*) is composed of two parts: heme and globin. **Heme** is a red pigment. Each heme group contains one atom of iron. **Globin** is a protein chain. The four different structural globin chains most often found in adults are the $alpha_1$, $alpha_2$, $beta_1$, and $beta_2$ chains. Together, four heme groups, each linked to one protein chain of globin, make up one hemoglobin molecule (Figure 54-1).

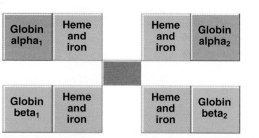

FIGURE 54-1 Schematic structure of a hemoglobin molecule.

TYPES OF ANEMIA

Anemias are classified into four main types based on the underlying causes (Figure 54-2). Anemia of chronic disease is another common type of anemia. Anemias can be caused by maturation defects, or they can be secondary to excessive RBC destruction. Two types of maturation defects lead to anemias, categorized by the location of the defect within the cell: cytoplasmic maturation defects occur in the cell cytoplasm, and nuclear maturation defects occur in the cell nucleus. Factors responsible for excessive RBC destruction can be either intrinsic or extrinsic.

Figure 54-3 summarizes the types of anemias arising from cytoplasmic maturation defects. Major examples include iron-deficiency anemia and genetic disorders such as thalassemia, which result in defective globin synthesis. For each of these anemias, the RBCs appear **hypochromic** (lighter red than normal) and **microcytic** (smaller than normal) on blood smear. Cytoplasmic maturation anemias occur as a result of reduced or abnormal hemoglobin synthesis. Because hemoglobin is synthesized from both iron and globin, a deficiency in either one can lead to a hemoglobin deficiency. Some common causes of iron-deficiency anemia are blood loss, surgery, childbirth, gastrointestinal bleeding (which can be caused by NSAID ingestion; see Chapter 44), menstrual blood loss, and hemorrhoids.

Figure 54-4 summarizes the types of anemias arising from nuclear maturation defects. These occur because of defects in deoxyribonucleic acid (DNA) or protein synthesis. Both DNA and protein synthesis require vitamin B_{12} and folic acid (B_9) to be present in normal amounts for their proper production. If either of these two vitamins is absent or deficient, anemias secondary to nuclear maturation defects may develop. In such

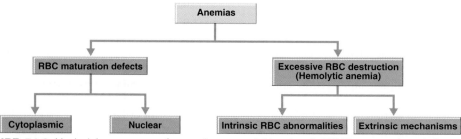

FIGURE 54-2 Underlying causes of anemia are red blood cell (RBC) maturation defects and factors secondary to excessive RBC destruction.

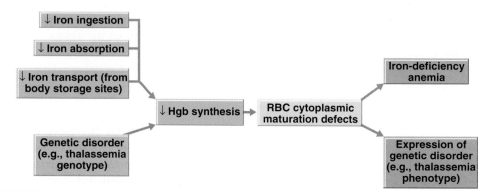

FIGURE 54-3 Schematic showing common causes and results of red blood cell (RBC) cytoplasmic maturation defects. ↓, Decreased.

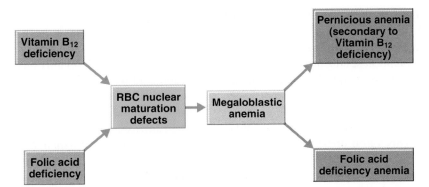

FIGURE 54-4 Schematic showing common causes and results of red blood cell (RBC) nuclear maturation defects.

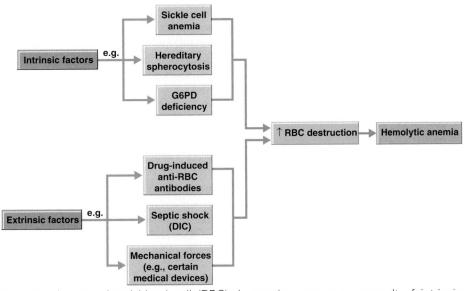

FIGURE 54-5 Increased red blood cell (RBC) destruction occurs as a result of intrinsic and extrinsic factors. ↑, Increased; *DIC,* disseminated intravascular coagulation; *G6PD,* glucose-6-phosphate dehydrogenase.

anemias, RBCs actually appear to be *normochromic* (normal in color) but are commonly *macrocytic* (larger than normal) on blood smear. One example is pernicious anemia. This type of anemia results from deficiency of vitamin B₁₂, which is used in the formation of new RBCs. The usual underlying cause is the failure of the stomach lining to produce intrinsic factor. Intrinsic factor is a gastric glycoprotein that allows vitamin B₁₂ to be absorbed in the intestine (see Chapter 53). Another example is the anemia caused by folic acid deficiency. Both pernicious anemia and folic acid deficiency anemia are also known as types of *megaloblastic* anemia, because they are both characterized by large, immature RBCs. Megaloblastic anemias not caused from a lack of intrinsic factor are usually related to poor dietary intake and are most commonly seen in infancy, childhood, and pregnancy.

Figure 54-5 summarizes the types of anemias arising from excessive RBC destruction, or hemolytic anemias. These can occur because of abnormalities within the RBCs themselves (intrinsic factors) or as a result of factors outside of (extrinsic to) the RBCs. In both cases, the erythrocytes appear on blood

smear as spherocytes. RBC abnormalities caused by intrinsic factors are usually the result of a genetic defect. Examples include sickle cell anemia, hereditary spherocytosis, glucose-6-phosphate dehydrogenase (G6PD) deficiency, and paroxysmal nocturnal hemoglobinuria. Examples of extrinsic mechanisms for excessive RBC destruction include drug-induced antibodies that target and destroy RBCs, septic shock that produces disseminated intravascular coagulation, and mechanical forces such as those created by intraaortic balloon pumps, ventricular assist devices, and continuous veno-venous hemodialysis (CVVHD), commonly used in intensive care units.

ERYTHROPOIESIS-STIMULATING DRUGS

DRUG PROFILES

◆ epoetin alfa

Epoetin alfa (Epogen, Procrit) is a biosynthetic form of the natural hormone erythropoietin, which is normally secreted by the kidneys in response to a decrease in RBCs. It promotes the synthesis of erythrocytes (RBCs) by stimulating RBC progenitor cells in the bone marrow. Epoetin alfa is used to treat anemia that is associated with end-stage renal disease, chemotherapy-induced anemia, and for anemia associated with zidovudine therapy (see Chapter 40). Epoetin causes the progenitor cells in the bone marrow to manufacture large numbers of immature RBCs and to greatly speed up their maturation. This medication is ineffective without adequate body iron stores and bone marrow function. Most patients receiving epoetin alfa need to also receive an oral or intravenous iron preparation. A longer-acting form of epoetin called *darbepoetin (Aranesp)* is available that reduces the required number of injections, although one cost study found that there is no significant difference in overall cost between the two. Both drugs are available for injection only and can be given intravenously or subcutaneously. When the drugs are given by the subcutaneous route, the onset of action is slower, and lower dosages can be used.

Contraindications for erythropoiesis-stimulating drugs (ESAs) include known drug allergy. Use of epoetin and darbepoetin is contraindicated in cases of uncontrolled hypertension and when hemoglobin levels are above 10 g/dL for cancer patients and 11 g/dL for renal patients. Use in patients with head or neck cancers or patients at risk for thrombosis is controversial as these medications increase tumor growth and risk for thrombosis. The most frequent adverse effects include hypertension, fever, headache, pruritus, rash, nausea, vomiting, arthralgia, and injection site reaction.

In 2010, the U.S. Food and Drug Administration (FDA) issued a public health advisory regarding the overzealous use of epoetin. It was found that when hemoglobin levels are above 11 g/dL and the drug is continued, patients experienced serious adverse events, including heart attack, stroke, and death. Based on these findings, the FDA now requires that any patient receiving epoetin for chemotherapy-induced anemia must be registered in a risk mitigation program called ESA Apprise Oncology. Only prescribers and hospitals that are registered in this program may dispense epoetin for cancer patients. The FDA has not yet required the same for its use in chronic kidney disease; however, it is recommended to be dosed to a target hemoglobin level of 11 g/dL for patients on dialysis and 10 g/dL for chronic kidney patients not on dialysis. More information is available at *www.esa-apprise.com/ESAAppriseUI/ESAAppriseUI/default.jsp*. Abuse of erythropoietin by athletes hoping to increase oxygen-carrying capacity and improve performance places the athlete at risk for diseases caused by increased blood viscosity (stroke, myocardial infarction).

Pharmacokinetics: Epoetin Alfa

Route	Onset of Action	Peak Plasma Concentration	Elimination Half-life	Duration of Action
Subcut or IV	7-10 days	5-24 hr	4-13 hr	Variable

IRON

Iron is a mineral that is essential for the proper function of all biologic systems in the body. It is stored in many sites throughout the body (liver, spleen, and bone marrow). Deficiency of this mineral is the principal nutritional deficiency resulting in anemia. Individuals who require the highest amount of iron are women (especially pregnant women) and children, and they are the groups most likely to develop iron-deficiency anemia. For women, this is partly due to ongoing menstrual blood losses. Most vitamin supplements for men contain little or no iron, because men are much less likely to develop iron-deficiency anemia. Nonetheless, dietary iron is usually sufficient for both men and women in developed countries.

Dietary sources of iron include meats and certain vegetables and grains. Oral iron preparations are available as ferrous salts. See Table 54-1 for a list of the currently available oral iron salts and their respective iron content. When a patient cannot tolerate oral iron, intravenous iron may be administered. There are four injectable iron products available: iron dextran (INFeD), iron sucrose (Venofer), ferric gluconate (Ferrlecit, Nulecit), and ferumoxytol (Feraheme).

Mechanism of Action and Drug Effects

Iron is an oxygen carrier in both hemoglobin and *myoglobin* (oxygen-carrying molecule in muscle tissue) and is critical for tissue respiration. Iron is also a required component of a number of enzyme systems in the body and is necessary for energy transfer in the *cytochrome oxidase* and *xanthine oxidase* enzyme systems. Administration of iron corrects iron-deficiency symptoms such as anemia, dysphagia, dystrophy of the nails and skin, and fissuring of the angles of the lips, and also maintains the bodily functions described earlier.

Indications

Supplemental iron contained in multivitamins plus iron or iron supplements alone are indicated for the prevention or treatment of iron-deficiency anemia. In all cases, an underlying cause needs to be identified. After identifying the cause, treatment is aimed at attempting to correct the cause (e.g., chronic blood loss, such as from a peptic or duodenal ulcer, cancerous colon lesion, or Crohn's disease) rather than simply

TABLE 54-1	Ferrous Salts: Iron Content	
Ferrous Salt*	**Iron Content**	**Number of Tablets Taken Per Day (Adults)**
Ferrous fumarate	33% iron or 330 mg/g	6-8 100-mg tablets or 2-3 325-mg tablets
Ferric gluconate	12% iron or 120 mg/g	3-4
Ferrous sulfate	20% iron or 200 mg/g	3-4
Ferrous sulfate (desiccated or dried)	30% iron or 300 mg/g	3-4

*Some patients may tolerate different formulations better; however, the number of tablets that must be consumed may decrease patient adherence.

alleviating the symptoms. Iron supplementation is also used in erythropoietin therapy because it is essential for the production of RBCs.

Contraindications

Contraindications to the use of iron products include known drug allergy, *hemochromatosis* (iron overload), hemolytic anemia, and any other anemia not associated with iron deficiency.

Adverse Effects

The most common adverse effects associated with oral iron preparations are nausea, vomiting, diarrhea, constipation, stomach cramps, and stomach pain. Excess iron intake can lead to accumulation and iron toxicity. See Table 54-2 for a more complete listing of the undesirable effects associated with iron preparations. Older adults tend to respond to lower doses of iron supplementation, and lower doses tend to decrease the rate of adverse effects.

Toxicity and Management of Overdose

Iron overdose is the most common cause of pediatric poisoning deaths reported to U.S. poison control centers. Many iron supplements are enteric coated and resemble candy. Toxicity from iron ingestion results from a combination of the corrosive effects on the gastrointestinal mucosa and the metabolic and hemodynamic effects caused by the presence of excessive elemental iron.

Treatment is based on symptomatic and supportive measures, including suction and maintenance of the airway, correction of acidosis, and control of shock and dehydration with intravenous fluids or blood, oxygen, and vasopressors. Abdominal radiographs may be helpful, because iron preparations are radiopaque and may be visualized on x-ray film. Serum iron concentrations may be helpful in establishing the amount ingested. A serum iron concentration of more than 300 mcg/dL places the patient at serious risk for toxicity. In patients with severe symptoms of iron intoxication, such as coma, shock, or seizures, chelation therapy with deferoxamine is initiated. In 2011, the FDA approved deferiprone, which can also be used for iron overload.

Interactions

The absorption of iron can be enhanced when it is given with ascorbic acid and decreased when it is given with antacids and calcium. Iron preparations can decrease the absorption of certain antibiotics, including tetracyclines and quinolones.

Dosages

For dosage information on iron preparations, see the table on this page.

TABLE 54-2   Iron Preparations: Adverse Effects

Body System	Adverse Effects
Gastrointestinal	Nausea, constipation, epigastric pain, black and tarry stools, vomiting, diarrhea
Integumentary	Temporarily discolored tooth enamel and eyes, pain on injection

DOSAGES

Selected Anemia Drugs

Drug (Pregnancy Category)	Pharmacologic Class	Usual Adult Dosage Range	Indications/Uses
◆ epoetin alfa (Epogen, Procrit) (C)	Human recombinant hormone (erythropoietin) analogue	IV/subcut: 2000-40,000 units 1-3 times per week, depending on weight and indication	Chemotherapy-induced anemia; anemia associated with chronic renal failure
ferric gluconate (Ferrlecit) (B)	Parenteral iron salt	125 mg/dose for 8 doses	Iron deficiency associated with hemodialysis
ferrous fumarate* (Feostat) (A)	Oral iron salt	200-325 mg 3 times daily	Severe iron-deficiency anemia; mild to moderate iron-deficiency anemia; prophylaxis
◆ ferrous sulfate* (A)	Oral iron salt	750-1500 mg/day in divided doses	Iron deficiency
◆ folic acid† (A)	Water-soluble B-complex vitamin	PO/IV/IM/subcut: Normal maintenance dose 400-1000 mcg/day	Folate deficiency; tropical sprue; nutritional supplementation; pregnancy-related supplementation
iron dextran† (INFeD, Dexferrum) (C)	Parenteral iron salt	IM/IV: 25-100 mg/day until total dose reached	Iron deficiency when oral iron therapy is unsatisfactory
iron sucrose (Venofer) (B)	Parenteral iron salt	IV: dialysis: 100 mg 1-3 times weekly to a cumulative dose of 1000 mg; for non-dialysis: 500 mg every 2 wk × 2 doses	Iron deficiency in patients with chronic renal failure

*Doses are expressed in terms of elemental iron, not the salt itself.
†Expressed in milligrams of elemental iron. Dosages are calculated for each patient's weight according to manufacturer's label. Doses are approximate.

DRUG PROFILES

Iron preparations are available by prescription and as over-the-counter (OTC) medications. They are contraindicated in patients with ulcerative colitis and regional enteritis, conditions of excessive body iron stores (e.g., hemosiderosis, hemochromatosis), peptic ulcer disease, hemolytic anemia, cirrhosis, gastritis, and esophagitis. Goals of therapy include maintenance of normal hemoglobin and hematocrit levels, and improved energy level.

ferrous fumarate

The ferrous fumarate iron salts (Femiron) contain the largest amount of iron per gram of salt consumed. Ferrous sulfate and ferric gluconate are two other forms of iron that are commonly used. Ferrous fumarate is 33% elemental iron; therefore, a 325-mg tablet of ferrous fumarate provides 107 mg of elemental iron. Ferrous fumarate is available only for oral use.

Pharmacokinetics: Ferrous Fumarate

Route	Onset of Action	Peak Plasma Concentration	Elimination Half-life	Duration of Action
PO	3-10 days	Unknown	6 hr	Variable

◆ferrous sulfate

Ferrous sulfate is the most frequently used form of oral iron. Ferrous sulfate ($FeSO_4$) is dosed as 300 mg two to three times a day for most adult patients. Confusion arises with ferrous sulfate, because the dose is 300 mg, but many commercially available products are 324 mg. The two doses are used interchangeably. Each tablet contains 65 mg of elemental iron. The adult dose of elemental iron is 50 to 100 mg given two to three times daily. Pediatric dosing is based on elemental iron.

Pharmacokinetics: Ferrous Sulfate

Route	Onset of Action	Peak Plasma Concentration	Elimination Half-life	Duration of Action
PO	1 wk	2 hr	6 hr	Variable

iron dextran

Iron dextran (INFeD, Dexferrum) is a colloidal solution of iron (as ferric hydroxide) and dextran. It is intended for intravenous or intramuscular use for treatment of iron deficiency. Anaphylactic reactions to iron dextran, including major orthostatic hypotension and fatal anaphylaxis, have been reported in 0.3% of patients. Because of this, a test dose of 25 mg of iron dextran is administered before injection of the full dose. Although anaphylactic reactions usually occur within a few minutes after the test dose, it is recommended that a period of at least 1 hour elapse before the remaining portion of the initial dose is given. Because of the potential of iron dextran to cause anaphylaxis, its use has been replaced by the use of newer products, ferric gluconate and iron sucrose. Iron dextran is available only for injection.

Pharmacokinetics: Iron Dextran

Route	Onset of Action	Peak Plasma Concentration	Elimination Half-life	Duration of Action
IM	Unknown	24-48 hr	5-20 hr	3 wk

ferric gluconate

Ferric gluconate (Ferrlecit) is an injectable iron product that is indicated for repletion of total body iron content in patients with iron-deficiency anemia who are undergoing hemodialysis. The risk for anaphylaxis is much less than with iron dextran, and a test dose is not required. Doses higher than 125 mg are associated with increased adverse events, including abdominal pain, dyspnea, cramps, and itching.

Pharmacokinetics: Ferric Gluconate

Route	Onset of Action	Peak Plasma Concentration	Elimination Half-life	Duration of Action
IV	End of infusion	7 min	1 hr	4 days

iron sucrose

Iron sucrose (Venofer) is another injectable iron product indicated for the treatment of iron-deficiency anemia in patients with chronic renal disease. It is also used for patients without kidney disease. Its risk for precipitating anaphylaxis is much less than that of iron dextran, and a test dose is not required. Hypotension is the most common adverse effect and appears to be related to infusion rate. Large doses of iron sucrose are infused over 2.5 to 3.5 hours. Low-weight older adults appear to be at greatest risk for hypotension. The newest injectable iron product is ferumoxytol (Feraheme). It offers the advantage of being given undiluted as IV push in 1 minute.

Pharmacokinetics: Iron Sucrose

Route	Onset of Action	Peak Plasma Concentration	Elimination Half-life	Duration of Action
IV	End of infusion	Unknown	6 hr	Unknown

FOLIC ACID

Folic acid is a water-soluble B-complex vitamin. It is also referred to as *folate*, the name of its anionic form. The human body requires oral intake of folic acid. Dietary sources of folic acid include dried beans, peas, oranges, and green vegetables. Several conditions can lead to folic acid deficiency. However, because folic acid is absorbed in the upper duodenum, malabsorption syndromes are the most common cause of deficiency.

Mechanism of Action and Drug Effects

Folic acid is converted in the body to *tetrahydrofolic acid*, which is used for erythropoiesis and for synthesis of nucleic acids (DNA and ribonucleic acid [RNA]). Dietary ingestion of folate is required for the production of DNA and RNA. It is also essential for normal erythropoiesis. Folic acid is not active in the ingested form. It must first be converted to tetrahydrofolic acid, which is a cofactor for reactions in the biosynthesis of nucleic acids.

Indications

Folic acid is primarily used to prevent and treat folic acid deficiency. Anemias caused by folic acid deficiency can be treated by exogenous supplementation of folic acid. There is also much evidence to support the use of folic acid in the prevention of neural tube defects such as spina bifida, anencephaly, and encephalocele. It is recommended that administration begin at least 1 month before pregnancy and continue through early pregnancy to reduce the risk for fetal neural tube defects. Folic acid is also indicated for the treatment of tropical sprue, a malabsorption syndrome.

Contraindications

Contraindications to the use of folic acid include known drug allergy. Folic acid is not to be used to treat anemias until the underlying cause and type of anemia have been determined. For example, administering folic acid to a patient with pernicious anemia may correct the hematologic changes of anemia (making the CBC normal), while deceptively masking neurologic and other symptoms of pernicious anemia that result from B_{12} deficiency.

Adverse Effects

Adverse effects associated with folic acid use are rare. Allergic reaction or yellow discoloration of urine may occur.

Interactions

No significant drug interactions occur with folic acid. However, oral contraceptives (see Chapter 34), corticosteroids (see Chapter 33), sulfonamides (see Chapter 38), and dihydrofolate reductase inhibitors (including the antineoplastic drug methotrexate [see Chapter 45] and the antibiotic trimethoprim [see Chapter 38]) can all cause signs of folic acid deficiency, but are not affected by folic acid administration.

Dosages

For dosage information on folic acid, see the table on p. 865.

DRUG PROFILE

♦folic acid

Folic acid is a water-soluble B-complex vitamin that is used primarily in the treatment and prevention of folic acid deficiency and anemias caused by folic acid deficiency. Folic acid is available as an OTC medication in multivitamin preparations and by prescription as a single drug. It is contraindicated in patients with uncorrected pernicious anemia. Folic acid is available for both oral and injectable use.

Pharmacokinetics: Folic Acid

Route	Onset of Action	Peak Plasma Concentration	Elimination Half-life	Duration of Action
PO	Unknown	60-90 min	Unknown	Unknown

OTHER ANEMIA DRUGS

Cyanocobalamin (vitamin B_{12}), which is discussed in Chapter 53, is used to treat pernicious anemia and other megaloblastic anemias. It can be given orally or intranasally to treat vitamin B_{12} deficiency but is usually given by deep intramuscular injection to treat pernicious anemia. Once remission of the anemia is seen, cyanocobalamin can be dosed once a month.

NURSING PROCESS

ASSESSMENT

Before any drug is given to treat an anemia, assess the patient's past and present medical history; compile a medication profile, including all prescription, OTC, and herbal medications the patient is taking as well as a listing of any drug allergies. It is important to assess for and document any signs and symptoms of anemia, such as fatigue, changes in nails and skin, and fissuring/cracking of the angles of the lip. Critical to patient safety is the assessment of any allergies, contraindications, cautions, and drug interactions prior to beginning iron supplementation. *Erythropoiesis-stimulating drugs (ESAs) (epoetin alfa* [marketed as *Epogen* and *Procrit*] and *darbepoetin* [marketed as *Aranesp*]) are used to treat anemia associated with end-stage renal disease and/or chemotherapy-induced anemia. Assessment of adequate body iron stores and bone marrow function is needed prior to administration of the drug. Document baseline vital signs because blood pressure may elevate as hematocrit rises; medical intervention may be needed. To ensure patient safety and quality of care, the nurse must be aware of the warnings and recommendations associated with the use of ESAs. See previous discussion of uses and contraindications in the pharmacology section.

TEAMWORK AND COLLABORATION: PHARMACOKINETIC BRIDGE TO NURSING PRACTICE   QSEN

Iron preparations provide a perfect example of how pharmacokinetic properties can impact drug dosing and efficacy. Oral iron is available in a variety of salt forms, such as ferrous fumarate, ferrous sulfate, and ferric gluconate. Although very similar in mechanism of action, the specific salt form is associated with different pharmacokinetic properties and offers varying amounts of elemental iron. The ferrous fumarate iron salts contain some of the largest amount of iron per gram of salt consumed. For example, each 100 mg of ferrous fumarate provides 33 mg of elemental iron, whereas each 324-mg tablet of ferrous sulfate contains 65 mg of elemental iron. Even though the pharmacokinetics of the different oral iron salts are similar, the amount of elemental iron varies significantly per 100 mg. Because of these varying amounts of elemental iron, the iron salts must not be exchanged for one another and must be given with caution to avoid medication errors. Other similar pharmacokinetic properties of oral iron products, such as absorption and excretion, must be understood because unabsorbed iron—though harmless—turns the stool black and may possibly mask melena (blood in the stools). It is recommended to take oral iron with juice (orange juice is preferred) or water but not with milk or antacids because of subsequent decreased drug absorption.

With *iron products,* significant contraindications include hemochromatosis, hemolytic anemia, and any other anemia that is not iron-deficiency related. Drug interactions affecting the absorption of iron preparations include ascorbic acid (increased absorption), antacids (decreased absorption), as well as decreased absorption of other drugs such as tetracyclines and quinolones. Some laboratory studies that may be ordered before, during, and after therapy include RBC count, hemoglobin level, hematocrit, reticulocyte count, bilirubin level, and baseline levels of folate and/or B-complex vitamins. Perform a nutritional assessment with a focus on the amount of iron in the patient's diet. A 24-hour recall of all food intake with serving sizes may prove to be beneficial. A nutritional and dietary consult may also be ordered. In addition, asking questions about the patient's energy levels, ability to carry out activities of daily living, overall immunity to illnesses, and state of health may also provide valuable information.

NURSING DIAGNOSES

1. Activity intolerance related to fatigue and lethargy associated with anemias
2. Imbalanced nutrition, less than body requirements, related to the disease process
3. Constipation related to adverse effects of iron products

PLANNING: OUTCOME IDENTIFICATION

1. Patient maintains/regains normal level of activity, as ordered, with gradual increases and without shortness of breath or intolerance.

2. Patient improves nutrition status through use of nonpharmacologic measures such as dietary intake with use of MyPlate and daily dietary increases of iron including meats and certain vegetables and grains.
3. Patient remains free from or experiences minimal constipation as an adverse effect of iron products through preventive measures such as increased intake of fluids, fiber, fruits, and vegetables and/or use of bulk-forming laxatives.

IMPLEMENTATION

With *erythropoiesis-stimulating drugs,* do not administer with any other product and do not shake the vial. During treatment, always monitor blood pressure and give vitamin B_{12} supplements orally, as prescribed. Instruct the patient to dilute oral liquid dosage forms of *iron products* per manufacturer instructions and to sip through a plastic straw to avoid discoloration of tooth enamel. Other oral forms of iron need to be given with plenty of fluids but not with antacids or milk, and preferably not with meals, because of the risk for decreased absorption of the drug. However, most individuals find that they do need to take oral iron products with meals or food because of the commonly encountered adverse effect of gastrointestinal upset. If antacids or milk products are used, schedule them at least 2 hours before or after the oral dosage of iron. Iron products are generally packaged in a light-resistant, airtight container.

PATIENT-CENTERED CARE: LIFESPAN CONSIDERATIONS FOR THE OLDER ADULT PATIENT   QSEN

Iron Products

- Instructions on how to take oral forms of iron are crucial to safe administration. Implement all types of teaching strategies to reinforce all verbal and/or written instructions. Make sure education is individualized and geared to patients with alterations in sensory perception. Caution patients not to make changes in their medication regimen, such as doubling doses or discontinuing a drug, without the prescriber's order.
- Provide the older adult patient and his or her spouse and/or caregivers with instructions about food sources that are high in iron and how to include these foods in menu planning. Instruct patients to steam vegetables and not to overcook them through excessive boiling. Advise patients that to preserve the content of vitamins and minerals, including iron, it is important to avoid overcooking or boiling vegetables.
- Remind the older adult patient that gastrointestinal upset may occur with many drugs, including vitamins and iron. Iron products are to be taken with food or a snack to help decrease GI upset.
- Always educate older adult patients, as well as spouses, other family members, significant others, and/or caregivers, about appropriate community resources (e.g., Meals On Wheels, senior citizen community centers, public recreation centers). A list of these community resources is often made available through a city web page and/or social services department. Resources are also identified through the following websites: *http://fnic.nal.usda.gov/consumers/ages-stages/seniors, www.nutrition.gov/food-assistance-programs, www.seniorresourcealliance.org/information/food-meals-nutrition/home-delivered-meals-meal-sites/,* and *www.altsa.dshs.wa.gov/pubinfo/services/servicetypes.htm.*

CASE STUDY

Patient-Centered Care: Hematopoietic Biologic Response Modifiers

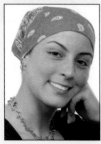

J.T., a 37-year-old homemaker, is receiving a second round of chemotherapy as part of treatment for ovarian cancer. Chemotherapeutic drugs may lead to the adverse effect of bone marrow suppression of various blood cell components.

Two weeks after this round of chemotherapy, J.T.'s hemoglobin level is 7.9 g/dL (pretherapy value was 12 g/dL), and the hematocrit is 28.5% (pretherapy value was 34%). The following orders are received: epoetin alfa (Epogen) 150 units/kg subcutaneously three times a week; ferrous sulfate, 300 mg by mouth daily.

1. What is the purpose of the order for ferrous sulfate?
2. The nurse will assess for what conditions before beginning the epoetin therapy?
3. The nurse needs to monitor J.T. closely. What assessment findings would be of the most concern during this therapy?
4. After 5 weeks, J.T.'s hemoglobin level is 11.6 g/dL and her hematocrit is 33%. The next dose of epoetin is due today. What action will the nurse take?

For answers, see *http://evolve.elsevier.com/Lilley.*

Instruct patients to remain in an upright or sitting position for up to 30 minutes after taking oral dosage forms of *iron, ferrous* products, and related drugs to help minimize esophageal irritation or corrosion. Warn patients that the use of iron products will turn the stools from a normal brown color to a black, tarry color. Patients taking *epoetin alfa* may also be taking oral iron preparations (see the pharmacology discussion for specific information on FDA restrictions). See Patient-Centered Care: Patient Teaching below for more information.

If a patient cannot tolerate oral iron, an intravenous dosage form (e.g., *iron dextran, iron sucrose, ferric gluconate*) may be prescribed. A test dose of iron dextran may be ordered, with the remaining dose given 1 hour later if no adverse reaction occurs. Intramuscularly administered iron must be given deep in a large muscle mass using the Z-track method (see Chapter 9). Intravenous iron dextran must be given after the intravenous line is flushed with 10 mL of normal saline and administered with the recommended amount of diluent and at the recommended drip rate. Premedication with diphenhydramine (Benadryl), acetaminophen, and/or IV hydrocortisone may be prescribed to decrease the risk for a reaction to the intravenous iron. Keep epinephrine and resuscitative equipment available in case of anaphylactic reaction (to iron or any drug that has an increased risk for causing anaphylaxis). In addition, it may be necessary for the patient to remain recumbent for 30 minutes after the intravenous injection to prevent drug-induced orthostatic hypotension. Encourage the patient to move slowly and purposefully during this time.

EVALUATION

Focus the evaluation of therapeutic responses to drugs used for anemia on ensuring that goals and outcome criteria have been met as well as monitoring for therapeutic and adverse effects. Therapeutic responses to *erythropoiesis-stimulating drugs* may take 2 to 6 weeks, so monitor for increased energy, appetite, and sense of well-being. Adverse effects of erythropoiesis-stimulating drugs may include heart attack, stroke, and possible death if used in patients not meeting the criteria presented in the pharmacology section of this chapter. Therapeutic responses to *iron* products include improved nutritional status, increased weight, increased activity tolerance and well-being, and absence of fatigue. Adverse effects of iron products include nausea, constipation, epigastric pain, black and tarry stools, and vomiting. Shock may occur with toxicity and is manifested by hypotension, tachycardia and pallor.

PATIENT-CENTERED CARE: PATIENT TEACHING

- Epoetin alfa (Epogen) is indicated for anemias associated with end-stage renal disease and chemotherapy and requires very careful use. Always check for route of administration with the subcutaneous route having a slower onset of action as compared to the intravenous route.
- Educate the patient about taking oral iron supplements with the erythropoiesis-stimulating drugs. These supplements are often needed to ensure adequate body iron stores, which are needed for the drug therapy to be effective.
- Encourage the patient to take iron products cautiously and to be aware of the potential for poisoning if these drugs are taken in greater than the recommended amounts. Oral iron products need to be taken in their original dosage form and without alteration; for example, without crushing.
- It is recommended that oral dosage forms of iron be taken with at least 4 to 6 ounces of water or other fluid to help minimize gastrointestinal upset and increase absorption.

- Oral dosage forms of iron are not interchangeable, and prescription forms of these products may be very different from one another. Each product contains different forms of the iron salt and also comes in different dose amounts. (One exception is that the 300-mg and 324-mg dosage forms of ferrous sulfate are used interchangeably.)
- Instruct the patient to remain upright for up to 30 minutes after taking an oral iron product to prevent esophageal irritation or corrosion. Remind the patient that iron products may turn the stools a black, tarry color.
- Encourage the patient to maintain a diet high in iron including foods such as meats (mollusks, pork/chicken/turkey/beef liver), certain vegetables (dark leafy greens such as spinach/Swiss chard), and grains (whole grains, fortified cereals, bran).

KEY POINTS

- Erythropoiesis-stimulating drugs are ineffective without adequate body iron stores.
- Iron and folic acid are very important in the treatment of many disorders and diseases (e.g., malignancies) to achieve RBC and hemoglobin formation that is as adequate as possible and to help prevent nutritional deficits that can affect all body systems, especially the immune system.

- Blood-forming drugs are often used in the treatment of pernicious anemia, malabsorption syndromes, hemolytic anemias, hemorrhage, and renal and liver diseases.
- Instruct patients to take iron products exactly as ordered. Parenteral dosage forms may cause anaphylaxis and orthostatic hypotension.

NCLEX® EXAMINATION REVIEW QUESTIONS

1. When administering oral iron tablets, the nurse should keep in mind that the most appropriate substance, other than water, to give with these tablets is
   a. pudding.
   b. an antacid.
   c. milk.
   d. orange juice.

2. The nurse is teaching a patient about oral iron supplements. Which statement is correct?
   a. "You need to take this medication on an empty stomach or else it won't be absorbed."
   b. "It is better absorbed on an empty stomach, but if that causes your stomach to be upset, you can take it with food."
   c. "Take this medication with a sip of water, and then lie down to avoid problems with low blood pressure."
   d. "If you have trouble swallowing the tablet, you may crush it."

3. The nurse is administering an intravenous dose of iron dextran. For which potential adverse effect is it most important for the nurse to monitor at this time?
   a. Anaphylaxis
   b. Gastrointestinal distress
   c. Black, tarry stools
   d. Bradycardia

4. The nurse is assessing a patient who is to receive folic acid supplements. It is important to rule out which condition before giving the folic acid?
   a. Malabsorption syndromes
   b. Pernicious anemia
   c. Tropical sprue
   d. Pregnancy

5. A patient with renal failure has severe anemia, and there is an order for darbepoetin (Aranesp). As the nurse assesses the patient, which condition listed will the nurse consider a contraindication to use of this medication?

   a. Uncontrolled hypertension
   b. Diabetes mellitus
   c. Hypothyroidism
   d. Angina

6. When iron sucrose is administered, which nursing interventions are correct? *(Select all that apply.)*
   a. Administer a test dose before giving the full dose.
   b. Give via deep intramuscular injection into a large muscle mass using the Z-track method.
   c. Administer large doses over 2.5 to 3.5 hours, intravenously.
   d. Monitor the patient for hypertension.
   e. Monitor the patient for hypotension.

7. The order reads: "Give epoetin alfa (Epogen), 3500 units subcut, three times a week." The medication is available in a vial that contains 4000 units/mL. How many milliliters will the nurse draw up for the ordered dose? *(Record your answer using two decimal places.)*

8. A woman who is planning to become pregnant asks the nurse when she should start to take folic acid supplements. What is the nurse's best response?
   a. "There is no evidence to support the use of folic acid during pregnancy."
   b. "You should start taking it at least 1 month before you become pregnant and continue it throughout early pregnancy."
   c. "You need to start it as soon as you discover you are pregnant."
   d. "You should only take it during the last trimester of your pregnancy, and not any earlier."

1. d, 2. b, 3. a, 4. b, 5. a, 6. c, e, 7. 0.88 mL (rounded from 0.875), 8. b.

CRITICAL THINKING AND PRIORITIZATION QUESTIONS

1. The nurse is administering an intravenous dose of iron dextran. A test dose has just been given. What is the nurse's priority action at this time? Explain your answer.

2. A.P. has been receiving epoetin (Epogen), three times a week, during his dialysis treatments for chronic renal failure. This morning, as the nurse prepares to give him a dose, A.P. states,

"I've felt strange today, and last night I had a little chest pain, but it went away after a few minutes so I didn't call the nurse." Will the nurse give the dose of epoetin at this time? Explain your answer. What is the nurse's priority action at this time?

For answers, see *http://evolve.elsevier.com/Lilley.*

ⓔ EVOLVE WEBSITE

http://evolve.elsevier.com/Lilley
- Animations
- Answer Keys for Textbook Case Studies and Textbook Critical Thinking and Prioritization Questions

- Content Updates
- Key Points
- Review Questions
- Student Case Studies

Nutritional Supplements

http://evolve.elsevier.com/Lilley

When you reach the end of this chapter, you will be able to do the following:

1. Describe the various pathophysiologic processes and/or disease states that may lead to nutritional deficiencies and require nutritional supplemental support.
2. Discuss the various enteral and parenteral nutritional supplements used to treat the various deficiencies, including specific ingredients.
3. Describe the nurse's role in the process of initiating and maintaining continuous or intermittent enteral feedings, total parenteral nutrition, and other forms of nutritional supplementation.
4. Compare the various enteral feeding tubes, including specific uses, and detail the special needs of patients requiring this nutritional support.
5. Discuss the mechanisms of action, cautions, contraindications, routes of administration, drug interactions, adverse effects, and complications associated with enteral and parenteral nutritional supplementation.
6. Develop a nursing care plan that includes all phases of the nursing process for patients receiving enteral and parenteral supplemental feedings.
7. Discuss the various laboratory values related to nutritional deficits or altered nutritional status and their impact on monitoring the therapeutic effects of the therapy.

DRUG PROFILES

amino acids, p. 876
carbohydrate formulation, p. 874
carbohydrates, p. 877
fat formulation, p. 874

lipid emulsions, p. 877
protein formulation, p. 874

♦ = *Key drug*
! = *High-alert drug*

KEY TERMS

Anabolism Metabolism characterized by the conversion of simple substances into the more complex compounds; tissue building. (p. 872)

Casein The principal protein of milk and the basis for curd and cheese. (p. 874)

Catabolism A complex metabolic process in which energy is liberated for use in work, energy storage, or heat production by the destruction of complex substances to form simple compounds. (p. 876)

Dumping syndrome A complex reaction to the rapid entry of concentrated nutrients into the jejunum of the small intestine. The patient may experience nausea, weakness, sweating, palpitations, syncope, sensations of warmth, and diarrhea. Most commonly occurs with eating following partial gastrectomy or with enteral feedings that are administered too rapidly into the stomach or jejunum via a feeding tube. (p. 873)

Enteral nutrition The provision of food or nutrients via the gastrointestinal tract, either naturally by eating or through a feeding tube in patients who are unable to eat. (p. 872)

Essential amino acids Those amino acids that cannot be manufactured by the body. (p. 876)

Essential fatty acid deficiency A condition that develops if fatty acids that the body cannot produce are not present in dietary or nutritional supplements. (p. 877)

Hyperalimentation An older term for parenteral nutrition; its use is now discouraged because it may be misinterpreted to mean overfeeding; now referred to as *total parenteral nutrition (TPN)*. (p. 875)

Malnutrition Any disorder of undernutrition. (p. 872)

Multivitamin infusion (MVI) A concentrated solution that contains several water- and fat-soluble vitamins and is used as part of an intravenous (parenteral) nutrition source. (p. 877)

Nonessential amino acids Those amino acids that the body can produce without extracting them from dietary intake. (p. 876)

Nutrients Substances that provide nourishment and affect the nutritive and metabolic processes of the body. (p. 872)

Nutritional supplements Oral, enteral, or intravenous nutritional preparations used to provide optimal nutrients to meet the body's nutritional needs. (p. 872)

Nutritional support The provision of nutrients orally, enterally, or parenterally for therapeutic reasons. (p. 872)

Parenteral nutrition The administration of nutrients by a route other than through the alimentary canal, such as intravenously. (p. 872)

Semiessential amino acids Those amino acids that can be produced by the body but not in sufficient amounts in infants and children. (p. 876)

Total parenteral nutrition (TPN) The intravenous administration of the total nutrient requirements of the patient with gastrointestinal dysfunction, accomplished via peripheral or central venous catheter. (p. 875)

Whey The thin serum of milk remaining after the casein and fat have been removed. It contains proteins, lactose, water-soluble vitamins, and minerals. (p. 874)

OVERVIEW

Nutrients are dietary products that undergo chemical changes when ingested (and metabolized) that cause tissue to be enhanced and energy to be liberated. Nutrients are required for cell growth and division; enzyme activity; protein, carbohydrate, and fat synthesis; muscle contraction; secretion of hormones (e.g., vasopressin, gastrin); wound repair; immune competence; gut integrity; and numerous other essential cellular functions. Providing for these nutritional needs is known as **nutritional support**. Adequate nutritional support is needed to prevent the breakdown of tissue proteins for use as an energy supply to sustain essential organ systems, which is what occurs during starvation. Malnutrition can decrease organ size and impair the function of organ systems (e.g., cardiac, respiratory, gastrointestinal, hepatic, renal). Nutritional supplements are a means of providing adequate nutritional support to meet the body's nutritional needs.

Malnutrition is a condition in which the body's essential need for nutrients is not met by nutrient intake. The purpose of nutritional support is the successful prevention, recognition, and management of malnutrition. **Nutritional supplements** are dietary products used to provide nutritional support. Nutritional supplement products can be administered to patients in a variety of ways. They vary in the amount and chemical complexity of the carbohydrates, proteins, fats, electrolytes, vitamins, and minerals that compose them, as well as in their osmolality. These nutrients may be given in a digested form, a partially digested form, or an undigested form. Nutritional supplements can also be tailored for specific disease states.

Patients' nutrient requirements vary according to age, gender, size or weight, physical activity, preexisting medical conditions, nutritional status, and current medical or surgical treatment. Nutritional supplements are classified according to the method of administration as either enteral or parenteral. **Enteral nutrition** is the provision of food or nutrients via the gastrointestinal tract. Nutritional supplements may also be administered parenterally. **Parenteral nutrition** is the intravenous administration of nutrients. Its purpose is to promote **anabolism** (tissue building), nitrogen balance, and maintenance or improvement of body weight. It is used when the oral or enteral feeding routes cannot be used. The selection of either enteral nutrition or parenteral nutrition and the specific nutritional composition of the product used depend on the specific patient and the clinical situation. Enteral nutrition is used when the patient has a functioning gastrointestinal tract.

Nutritional support
$\nearrow$ enteral nutrition → gastrointestinal tract
$\searrow$ parenteral nutrition → circulation

ENTERAL NUTRITION

Enteral nutrition is the provision of food or nutrients through the gastrointestinal tract. The most common and least invasive route of administration is oral consumption. A feeding tube is used in the other five enteral routes (Figure 55-1). The six routes of enteral nutrition delivery are listed in Table 55-1.

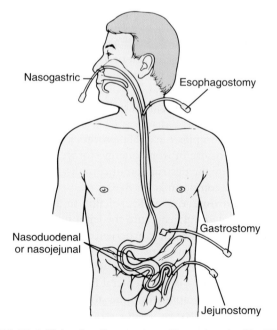

FIGURE 55-1 Tube feeding routes. (From Lewis SL, Dirksen SR, Heitkemper MM, et al: *Medical-surgical nursing: assessment and management of clinical problems*, ed 9, St Louis, 2014, Mosby.)

TABLE 55-1	Routes of Enteral Nutrition Delivery
Route	**Description**
Esophagostomy	Feeding tube surgically inserted into the esophagus
Gastrostomy	Feeding tube surgically inserted directly into the stomach
Jejunostomy	Feeding tube surgically inserted into the jejunum
Nasoduodenal	Feeding tube placed from the nose to the duodenum
Nasojejunal	Feeding tube placed from the nose to the jejunum
Nasogastric	Feeding tube placed from the nose to the stomach
Oral	Nutritional supplements delivered by mouth

Patients who may benefit from feeding tube delivery of nutritional supplements include those with abnormal esophageal or stomach peristalsis, altered anatomy secondary to surgery, depressed consciousness, or impaired digestive capacity. The enteral route is considered to be the superior route of administration of nutritional supplements.

Approximately 100 different enteral supplement formulations are available. The enteral supplements have been divided into groups according to the basic characteristics of the individual formulations. The enteral formulation groups are elemental, polymeric, modular, altered amino acid, and impaired glucose tolerance. These are described in Box 55-1.

Mechanism of Action and Drug Effects

The enteral formula groups provide the basic building blocks for anabolism. Different combinations and amounts of these nutrients are used based on the individual patient's anabolic needs. Enteral nutrition supplies complete dietary needs through the gastrointestinal tract by the normal oral route or by feeding tube.

Indications

Enteral nutrition can be used to supplement an oral diet that is currently insufficient for a patient's nutrient needs or used alone to meet all of the patient's nutrient needs. Box 55-2 lists the main types of enteral nutritional supplements and their indications.

Contraindications

The usual contraindication to nutritional supplements of any kind is known allergy to a specific product or genetic disease that renders a patient unable to metabolize certain types of nutrients.

Adverse Effects

The most common adverse effect of nutritional supplements is gastrointestinal intolerance, manifesting as diarrhea. Infant nutritional formulations are most commonly associated with allergies and digestive intolerance. The other nutritional supplements are commonly associated with osmotic diarrhea. Rapid feeding or bolus doses can result in dumping syndrome,

BOX 55-1   Enteral Formulations

Elemental Formulations

Peptamen	**Contents:** dipeptides, tripeptides, or crystalline amino acids; glucose oligosaccharides; and vegetable oil or medium-chain triglycerides (MCTs)
Vital HN	
Vivonex Plus	
Vivonex TEN	
	Comments: minimal digestion; minimal residue
	Indications: malabsorption, partial bowel obstruction, irritable bowel disease, radiation enteritis, bowel fistula, short bowel syndrome

Polymeric Formulations

Complete	**Contents:** complex nutrients (proteins, carbohydrates, and fat)
Ensure	
Ensure Plus	**Indications:** preferred over elemental formulations for patients with fully functional gastrointestinal tracts and few specialized nutrient requirements
Isocal	
Osmolite	
Portagen	
Jevity	
Sustacal	

Modular Formulations

Carbohydrate	**Contents:** single-nutrient formulas (protein, carbohydrate, or fat)
Moducal	
Polycose	**Indications:** can be added to a monomeric or polymeric formulation to provide a more individualized nutrient formulation
Fat	
MCT Oil	
Microlipid	
Protein	
Casec	
ProMod	
Propac	
Stresstein	

Altered Amino Acid Formulations

Amin-Aid	**Contents:** varying amounts of specific amino acids
Hepatic-Aid	**Indications:** for use in patients with diseases associated with altered metabolic capacities
Travasorb Renal	
Traum-Aid HBC	

Formulation for Impaired Glucose Tolerance

Glucerna	**Contents:** protein, carbohydrate, fat, sodium, potassium
	Indications: for use in patients with impaired glucose tolerance (e.g., diabetic patients)

which produces intestinal disturbances. In addition, tube feeding places the patient at significant risk for aspiration pneumonia. This is especially true in patients in whom mental status, gag reflexes, and general mobility are compromised.

Interactions

Various nutrients can interact with drugs to produce significant food-drug interactions. With some exceptions, food usually delays the absorption of drugs when administered simultaneously. High gastric acid content or prolonged emptying time can result in decreased effects of certain antibiotics (cephalosporins, erythromycin, and penicillins). An increased

BOX 55-2 Enteral Nutritional Supplements: Indications

Complete Nutritional Formulations (i.e., for General Nutritional Deficiencies)
- Inability to consume or digest normal foods
- Accelerated catabolic status
- Undernourishment because of disease

Incomplete Nutritional Formulations (i.e., for Specific Nutritional Deficiencies)
- Genetic metabolic enzyme deficiency
- Hepatic or renal impairment

Infant Nutritional Formulations
- Sole nutritional intake for premature and full-term infants
- Supplemental nutritional intake for older infants receiving solid foods
- Supplemental nutritional intake for breast-fed infants

absorption rate resulting in increased therapeutic effects can be seen when corticosteroids or vitamins A and D are given with nutritional supplements. The antibiotic effects of tetracyclines and quinolones are decreased when they are given with nutritional supplements as a result of chemical inactivation. These drugs must be given at least 2 hours before or after tube feedings.

Tube feedings can also reduce the absorption of phenytoin capsules or tablets, which may result in seizures. It is recommended that tube feedings be held for at least 2 hours before and after the administration of phenytoin. This can be problematic, because the patient may not receive adequate nutrition due to withholding of feedings. This issue is somewhat controversial, and some suggest that the interaction is more theoretical than actual. Thus, some institutions have decided to ignore this possible interaction and to monitor phenytoin levels and patient status, rather than holding the tube feedings, whereas others continue to hold the tube feedings. Often the patient requires intravenous phenytoin when continuous tube feedings are necessary.

Dosages

Because nutrient requirements vary greatly, dosages are individualized according to patient needs.

DRUG PROFILES

Enteral nutrition can be provided by a variety of supplements. Individual patient characteristics determine the appropriate enteral supplement. The four most commonly used enteral formulations are elemental, polymeric, modular, and altered amino acid.

ELEMENTAL FORMULATIONS

Elemental formulations are enteral supplements that contain dipeptides, tripeptides, or crystalline amino acids. Minimal digestion is required with elemental formulations. These supplements are indicated for patients with pancreatitis, partial bowel obstruction, irritable bowel disease, radiation enteritis, bowel fistulas, and short bowel syndrome. They are contraindicated in patients with a known hypersensitivity to them. One of the most commonly used elemental formulations is Vivonex Plus.

POLYMERIC FORMULATIONS

Polymeric formulations are enteral supplements that contain complex nutrients derived from proteins, carbohydrates, and fat. The polymeric formulations are some of the most commonly used enteral formulations because they most closely resemble normal dietary intake. They are preferred over elemental formulations in patients who have fully functional gastrointestinal tracts and have no specialized nutrient needs. Polymeric formulations are less hyperosmolar than elemental formulations and therefore cause fewer gastrointestinal problems. They are contraindicated in patients with a known hypersensitivity to them. They are available without a prescription and have no pregnancy category classification.

The most commonly used enteral supplement in the polymeric formulation category of enteral nutrition products is Ensure. It is lactose free and is also available in a higher-calorie formula called Ensure Plus. Other polymeric formulations are listed in Box 55-1. These drugs contain complex nutrients such as casein and soy protein for protein; corn syrup and maltodextrins for carbohydrates; and vegetable oil or milk fat for fat. They are available in liquid formulations only.

MODULAR FORMULATIONS
carbohydrate formulation

Moducal and Polycose are examples of commonly used enteral supplements in the carbohydrate modular formulation category. Both are carbohydrate supplements that supply carbohydrates only. They are intended to be used in addition to monomeric or polymeric formulations to provide a more individual specialized nutrient mix. They are available in liquid formulations only. These products are obtainable without a prescription, have no pregnancy category classification, and are contraindicated only in patients with a known hypersensitivity to them.

fat formulation

Microlipid and MCT Oil are the formulations available in the fat category. Microlipid is a fat supplement supplying only fats. It is a concentrated source of calories and contains 4.5 kcal/mL. These drugs are given to help individualize nutrient formulations. They may be used in patients with malabsorption and other gastrointestinal disorders and in patients with pancreatitis. They are available in liquid formulations only. These products are obtainable without a prescription, have no pregnancy category classification, and are contraindicated in patients with a known hypersensitivity to them.

protein formulation

Casec, ProMod, and Propac are examples of protein modular formulations. They are used to increase patients' protein intake and provide additional proteins. They are derived from a variety of sources such as whey, casein, egg whites, and amino acids.

All of the available products are dried powders that must be reconstituted with water. They may sometimes be reconstituted by placing them in enteral feedings that are already in liquid form. They are indicated for patients with increased protein needs. They are contraindicated in patients with a known hypersensitivity to them. Protein formulation supplements are available without a prescription and have no pregnancy category classification.

ALTERED AMINO ACID FORMULATIONS

Amin-Aid is one of the many amino acid formulation nutritional supplements available. Many of the nutritional supplements in this category are also listed as modular formulations because they can be used as both single-nutrient formulas and as nutritional formulations for patients with genetic errors of metabolism. Specialized amino acid formulations are used most commonly in patients who have metabolic disorders such as phenylketonuria, homocystinuria, and maple syrup urine disease. They are also used to supply nutritional support to patients with illnesses such as renal impairment, eclampsia, heart failure, or liver failure.

PARENTERAL NUTRITION

Parenteral nutritional supplementation (intravenous administration) is the preferred method for patients who are unable to tolerate and/or maintain adequate enteral or oral intake. Instead of administration of partially digested nutrients into the gastrointestinal tract (as in enteral nutrition), vitamins, minerals, amino acids, dextrose, and lipids are administered intravenously directly into the circulatory system. This effectively bypasses the entire gastrointestinal system, which eliminates the need for absorption, metabolism, and excretion. Parenteral nutrition is also called total parenteral nutrition (TPN) or hyperalimentation.

TPN can supply all of the calories, carbohydrates, amino acids, fats, trace elements, vitamins, and minerals needed for growth, weight gain, wound healing, convalescence, immunocompetence, and other health-sustaining functions.

TPN can be administered through either a peripheral vein (see Table 55-2) or a central vein. Each route of delivery of TPN has specific requirements and limitations. It is generally accepted that TPN is used only when oral or enteral support is impossible or when the gastrointestinal absorptive or functional capacity is not sufficient to meet the nutritional needs of the patient. Some of the factors that must be considered in deciding whether to use peripheral or central TPN for a given patient are listed in Table 55-2.

PERIPHERAL TOTAL PARENTERAL NUTRITION

Peripheral TPN (PPN) is one route of administration of TPN. A peripheral vein is used to deliver nutrients to the patient's circulatory system. PPN is usually a temporary method of administration. The long-term administration of nutritional supplements via a peripheral vein may lead to phlebitis. It is considered a temporary measure to provide adequate nutrients

TABLE 55-2 Peripheral and Central Parenteral Nutrition: Characteristics

Characteristic	Peripheral	Central
Goal of nutritional therapy (total versus supplemental)	Supplemental (total if moderate to low needs)	Total
Length of therapy	Short (fewer than 14 days)	Long (7 days or longer)
Osmolarity	Hyperosmolar (600-900 mOsm/L)	Hyperosmolar (600-900 mOsm/L)
Fluid tolerance	Must be high	Can be fluid restricted
Dextrose	Less than 10%*	10%-35%
Amino acids	Less than 3%	More than 3%-7%
Fats	10%-20%	10%-20%
Calories per day	Less than 2000 kcal/day	More than 2000 kcal/day

*Many institutions use a maximum of 12.5% dextrose.

in patients who have mild deficits or who are restricted from oral intake and have slightly elevated metabolic rates.

PPN is valuable in patients who do not have large nutritional needs, can tolerate moderately large fluid loads, and need nutritional supplements only temporarily. PPN may be used alone or in combination with oral nutritional supplements to provide the necessary fat, carbohydrate, and protein needed by the patient to maintain health.

Mechanism of Action and Drug Effects

PPN provides the basic nutrient building blocks for anabolism. Different combinations and amounts of these nutrients are used based on the individual patient's anabolic needs.

Indications

PPN is used to administer nutrients to patients who need more nutrients than their current oral intake can supply or to provide complete daily nutrition. It is meant only as a temporary means (less than 2 weeks) of delivering TPN.

Circumstances under which patients may benefit from the delivery of PPN are as follows:
- The patient must undergo a procedure that restricts oral feedings.
- The patient has anorexia caused by radiation or cancer chemotherapy.
- The patient has a gastrointestinal illness that prevents oral food ingestion.
- The patient has just undergone surgery of any type.
- The patient's nutritional deficits are minimal, but oral nutrition will not be started for longer than 5 days.

Contraindications

As mentioned previously for the enteral nutritional products, the only usual contraindication to nutritional supplementation of any kind is known drug allergy to a specific product or a genetic disease that renders a patient unable to assimilate certain types of nutrients.

Adverse Effects

The most devastating adverse effect of PPN is phlebitis, which is vein irritation or inflammation of a vein. If phlebitis is severe and is not treated appropriately, it can lead to the loss of a limb, although this is rare. Another potential adverse effect is fluid overload. PPN is limited to solutions with a lower dextrose concentration, generally less than 10%, to avoid sclerosing of the vein. Thus, large volumes are needed to meet a patient's daily nutritional requirements. Some patients, such as those with renal failure or heart failure, cannot tolerate large fluid volumes. In these patients, fluid restrictions may make it impossible to provide adequate calories through PPN.

CENTRAL TOTAL PARENTERAL NUTRITION

In central TPN, a large central vein is used to deliver nutrients directly into the patient's circulation. Usually, the subclavian or internal jugular vein is used. Central TPN is generally indicated for patients who require nutritional supplements for a prolonged period, usually longer than 7 to 10 days. It can also be used in the home care setting. There are a variety of indications for central TPN. The disadvantages of central TPN are the risks associated with venous catheter insertion and the use and maintenance of the central vein. There is a greater potential for infection, more serious catheter-induced trauma and related events, metabolic alterations, and other technical or mechanical problems than with peripheral parenteral nutrition (PPN).

Mechanism of Action and Drug Effects

Central TPN is used to supply nutrients to patients who cannot ingest nutrients by mouth and cannot meet required daily nutritional needs by the enteral or peripheral parenteral routes. Like PPN, central TPN supplies the basic building blocks for anabolism. It provides the necessary fat, carbohydrate, and protein that the patient needs to maintain health.

Indications

TPN delivers total dietary nutrients to patients who require nutritional supplementation. Patients who may benefit from the delivery of TPN include the following:
- Patients who have large nutritional requirements (metabolic stress or hypermetabolism)
- Patients who need nutritional support for prolonged periods (longer than 7 to 10 days)
- Patients who are unable to tolerate large fluid loads

Contraindications

TPN is contraindicated in patients with known hypersensitivity to any of its components. Rarely, a patient who is allergic to eggs may have cross-sensitivity to lipid formulations. TPN is used only when the gastrointestinal tract cannot be used (e.g., in postoperative patients or those who are otherwise unable to eat or digest and absorb nutrients).

Adverse Effects

The most common adverse effects of central TPN are those associated with the use of the central vein for delivery of the

TABLE 55-3 Amino Acids: Recommended Adult Daily Dosage Guidelines	
Healthy	**Malnourished or Trauma/Burn**
0.9 g/kg	Up to 2 g/kg

TPN. The risks associated with insertion of the infusion line, as well as the use and maintenance of the central vein for administration of TPN, can create some complications. There is a greater potential for infection, serious catheter-induced trauma and related events, and other technical or mechanical problems than with PPN. Larger and more concentrated volumes of nutritional supplements are being delivered with central TPN, and therefore there is a greater chance for metabolic complications such as hyperglycemia.

Dosages

Dosage requirements vary from patient to patient. Age, gender, weight, and numerous other factors must be considered for proper administration of TPN. Guidelines for amino acids appear in Table 55-3.

DRUG PROFILES

The individual components of peripheral and central TPN are the same. The difference lies in the concentrations and amounts of the components delivered per volume of nutritional supplement. The basic components of peripheral or central TPN are amino acids, carbohydrates, lipids, trace elements, vitamins, fluids, and electrolytes. Most of the electrolyte components are discussed in Chapter 29.

AMINO ACIDS

Amino acids have many roles in the maintenance of normal nutritional status. The primary role is protein synthesis, or anabolism. Provision of adequate amino acids in nutritional supplements reduces the breakdown of proteins (catabolism) and also helps to promote normal growth and wound healing.

Amino acids are commonly classified as essential or nonessential according to whether they can or cannot be produced by the body. Nonessential amino acids are those that the body produces and therefore need not be present in dietary intake. The body is able to manufacture, from nutritional nitrogen sources, all but eight of the available amino acids. Essential amino acids are those amino acids that cannot be produced by the body. Therefore, they must be included in daily dietary intake. Amino acids are used as building blocks for the protein that is needed for normal growth and development. Two amino acids, histidine and arginine, are not manufactured by the body in large enough quantities during rapid growth periods such as infancy or childhood. Thus, they are referred to as semiessential amino acids. Box 55-3 lists the amino acids according to their categories.

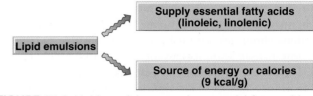

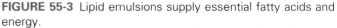

FIGURE 55-3 Lipid emulsions supply essential fatty acids and energy.

BOX 55-3   Amino Acids: Classification

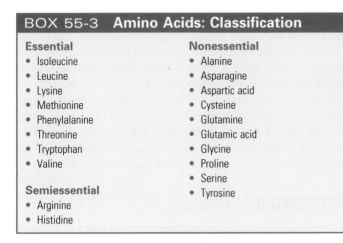

Essential
- Isoleucine
- Leucine
- Lysine
- Methionine
- Phenylalanine
- Threonine
- Tryptophan
- Valine

Semiessential
- Arginine
- Histidine

Nonessential
- Alanine
- Asparagine
- Aspartic acid
- Cysteine
- Glutamine
- Glutamic acid
- Glycine
- Proline
- Serine
- Tyrosine

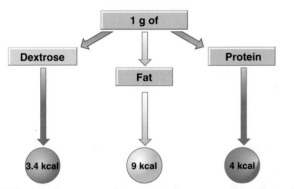

FIGURE 55-2 One gram of dextrose, fat, or protein will provide varying amounts of energy as calories.

amino acids

Amino acid crystalline solutions (Aminosyn 3%, 5%, and 10%, and FreAmine III 8.5% and 10%) can be used in either peripheral or central TPN. Amino acids are a source of both protein and calories. They provide 4 kcal/g. The two currently available brands of amino acid solutions differ only in their respective concentrations. The dosage of these solutions varies depending on the patient's weight and requirements. These drugs have no restrictions regarding pregnancy and have no contraindications to use.

CARBOHYDRATES

In nutritional support, carbohydrates are usually supplied to patients through dextrose. Dextrose is normally the greatest source of calories and provides 3.4 kcal/g. However, protein (amino acids) and lipids are also used as calorie sources (Figure 55-2). The concentration of dextrose in TPN is an important consideration. In PPN, dextrose concentrations are kept below 10% to decrease the possibility of phlebitis. In central TPN, dextrose concentrations can range from 10% to 50%, but they are commonly 25% to 35%. Because dextrose is a sugar, supplemental insulin may be given simultaneously in nutritional supplements. Use of a balanced nutritional supplement that contains dextrose and lipids as caloric sources decreases the need for large amounts of insulin.

FAT

Intravenous fat emulsions serve two functions: they supply essential fatty acids, and they are a source of energy or calories. As with the amino acids, certain fatty acids are essential because the body cannot produce them. Linoleic acid cannot be synthesized by the body. It is needed to produce linolenic and arachidonic acid. If these fatty acids are not present in dietary or nutritional supplements, an **essential fatty acid deficiency** may develop. Clinical signs of essential fatty acid deficiency are hair loss, scaly dermatitis, growth retardation, reduced wound healing, decreased platelet levels, and fatty liver (Figure 55-3).

lipid emulsions

The currently marketed lipid emulsions, Intralipid and Liposyn, are available as 10%, 20%, or 30% emulsions. They differ in fat origin. Liposyn is made from safflower oil, and Intralipid is made from soybean oil.

Lipid emulsions normally deliver 20% to 30% of the total daily calories and must not exceed 60% of daily caloric intake. Fat emulsions are most beneficial when combined with dextrose solutions. The use of fat to meet caloric needs prevents potentially harmful conditions—such as hyperglycemia, hyperinsulinemia, and hyperosmolarity—that can occur when a patient's entire caloric needs are being met solely by dextrose.

TRACE ELEMENTS

Trace elements are available in individual solutions and in many different combinations. The following are considered trace elements:
- Chromium
- Copper
- Iodine
- Manganese
- Molybdenum
- Selenium
- Zinc

Specific dosages and frequencies depend on the individual patient's requirements. Vitamins and other minerals may also be added accordingly. A common multivitamin combination is **multivitamin infusion (MVI)**.

NURSING PROCESS

ASSESSMENT

Perform a thorough nutritional assessment with attention to dietary history, weekly and daily food intake, weight, and height before initiating any *nutritional supplements*. Conduct a thorough nursing history and survey of all systems, including questions about any unusual symptoms, possible nutritional concerns, nausea, vomiting, loss of appetite, and weight gain or loss. Focus other questions on past and present medical and health history; history of any difficulties with nutrition, gastrointestinal absorption, or food intolerance; stressors; and a complete medication profile, including a listing of all prescription drugs, over-the-counter drugs, herbals, and supplements. Consultation with a registered dietitian is crucial to identify the nutrients that are missing in a particular patient's diet. Total body metabolic rate, body mass index, muscle mass, and other variables linked to nutritional status will most likely be assessed and are data that a nutritional consult may provide. Laboratory findings that may need to be assessed include the following: total protein level, albumin level, blood urea nitrogen (BUN) level, red blood cell (RBC) count, white blood cell (WBC) count, serum glucose, vitamin B₁₂ level, hemoglobin level, and hematocrit. Other laboratory studies may include cholesterol level, electrolyte levels, total lymphocyte count, serum transferrin level, iron level, urine creatinine clearance, lipid profile, and urinalysis. All of the objective and subjective data will help the prescriber, nutritionist/dietitian, and other members of the health care team to select the appropriate nutritional supplements for the patient.

Before administering an *enteral nutrition* supplement that is an elemental formulation, determine if the patient has a history of allergic reaction to any of the contents of the solution. Assess for contraindications, cautions, and drug interactions, and document the findings. Of most concern is assessing the patient's cardiac and renal status and ensuring that the ingredients and amount of solution are not too taxing on these systems. In addition, because these solutions are given orally, either by mouth or via tube feedings (see Chapter 9), it is most important to assess ability to swallow, gag reflex, and bowel sounds as well as noting any nausea or vomiting. Remember that protein-based formulations are to be avoided in patients with allergies to egg whites and whey.

With *parenteral nutrition*, assess for allergies to any of the components found within the prescribed intravenous formulation/solution. It is important for patients to also have a solution that considers age as well as individual metabolic needs. There are multiple combinations of products available (see the pharmacology discussion); thus, it is important to assess the patient carefully for allergies to essential proteins, amino acids, carbohydrates, trace elements, minerals, vitamins, lipids, high concentrations of dextrose, and any other ingredients. Assess the patient/family member/caregiver's knowledge about parenteral nutrition and the need for these infusions as well as the possible insertion of a central line, peripherally inserted central line, or peripherally inserted midline catheter. Remain current on the various solutions, methods, and routes of administration. Some complications of parenteral nutrition include pneumothorax, infection, air emboli or emboli related to protein or lipid aggregation (associated with central catheter intravenous lines), septicemia related to the nutrient-rich solutions with invasive intravenous route of administration, and

metabolic imbalances due to the solution ingredients and vomiting (seen with lipid administration in parenteral nutrition). Perform a complete baseline assessment of the following, as deemed appropriate: (1) central line/peripherally inserted line or peripherally inserted midline catheter, with attention to patency and intactness as well as appearance of the site (check for redness, swelling, erythema, drainage, and breaks in integrity of the skin); (2) WBC and RBC counts as well as other laboratory values and parameters (listed earlier), and (3) vital signs.

NURSING DIAGNOSES

1. Nutrition, less than body requirements, related to inability to take in sufficient nutrients
2. Diarrhea related to a decreased tolerance to enteral feedings and their ingredients
3. Risk for infection (sepsis) related to parenteral infusions and use of central venous access line

CASE STUDY

Safety: What Went Wrong? Total Parenteral Nutrition

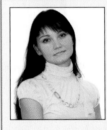

Mrs C., a 28-year-old florist, has been unable to eat due to severe vomiting related to her pregnancy. She is at 13 weeks' gestation and has been admitted to the hospital because of dehydration and inability to eat due to her severe nausea and vomiting. The decision has been made to give her total parenteral nutrition (TPN) for at least 1 week. After 1 week of therapy, her obstetrician will then decide whether to continue or stop the infusion, based on her response. She will be receiving the TPN infusion via a peripheral intravenous catheter with infusion bags that will be changed every 24 hours.

1. Mrs. C. is anxious about this infusion and asks the nurse, "Why is that bag so large? What is in the bag?" What is the nurse's best response?
2. The nurse explains to Mrs. C. that her blood glucose levels will need to be monitored while she is receiving the TPN. Mrs. C. begins to cry, saying, "This morning sickness is bad enough, but now I have diabetes too? How can that be?" What is the nurse's best response?
3. The nurse will monitor for what potential complication that can occur with peripherally administered TPN?
4. The nurse hangs a new bag of TPN to Mrs. C.'s peripheral TPN infusion. After a few hours, Mrs. C. complains of the infusion site hurting her. The nurse checks the infusion site and sees nothing visibly wrong, but the site is tender to the touch. The nurse then checks the TPN bag and notices that one of the contents is listed as 20% dextrose. What do you think went wrong? What is the nurse's priority action at this time? Explain your answer.

For answers, see *http://evolve.elsevier.com/Lilley*.

PLANNING: OUTCOME IDENTIFICATION

1. Patient's nutritional status improves through adequate dietary intake using MyPlate or other prescribed guidelines and/or supplemental feedings or nutrients with improved laboratory values.

2. Patient experienced decreased or no diarrhea as related to enteral supplementation with use of drug and non-drug measures, as prescribed.

3. Patient remains free from infection during parenteral nutritional supplementation and reports to the prescriber any redness, swelling, drainage, abnormal warmth (at site), fever, or chills.

IMPLEMENTATION

A prescriber's order must be complete and dated before *enteral* or *parenteral* (peripheral or central) *nutrition supplementation* is begun. In general, monitoring the status of the patient during and after *enteral feedings* is crucial to safe and prudent nursing care. With nasogastric tube feeding solutions, check for proper placement and/or detect gastric residuals so as to avoid aspiration and other complications. Checking for placement ensures that the tube is within the stomach and has not passed through the larynx into the trachea and down into the bronchi of the lungs. One method of checking tube placement is the aspiration of fluid (from the nasogastric tube) with a syringe and subsequent testing of the pH to determine the acidity of the fluid aspirate. With a pH of 5.5 or lower, the tube is in the correct position (within the stomach). Measure gastric residual volumes, and document before each feeding as well as before administration of each medication. When checking gastric residual volumes, stop the tube feeding and then aspirate stomach contents using a syringe connected to the particular tube. If the volume aspirated is more than the volume delivered over the previous 2 hours (of continuous feeding), return the aspirate, hold the feeding, and contact the prescriber while keeping the head of the patient's bed elevated. For intermittent bolus feedings, if the residual amount is more than 50% of the volume previously infused, it is the standard of care to return the aspirate, withhold the feeding, and contact the prescriber. A reduction in the tube feeding volume will most likely then be ordered. Always check institutional policy or protocol before use of enteral feedings, with attention to procedures involved in checking/managing residuals.

Newer tubes for nasogastric and other enteral feeding have smaller diameters and are thinner (5 French to 10 French) and more pliable for better patient tolerance. However, the smaller-diameter tubes make checking for gastric aspiration more difficult. Confirmation of placement may be through x-ray. To prevent clogging of the feeding tube, it is often helpful to flush the tube with 30 mL of cranberry juice or other designated solution (per institutional policy) followed by 10 mL of water. The juice may help break up the formula residue and unclog certain types of feeding tubes; the water helps to keep the tube clean and free from residue. Percutaneous enteral gastrostomy (PEG) tubes are also commonly used in many situations but do require surgical insertion by a gastroenterologist and are often procedurally done under moderate sedation. Their care includes performing dressing changes during the initial period and then checking for residuals. Placement need not be checked, but if it appears that the tube has come out of the opening and is

longer than previously noted, stop the infusion and contact the prescriber.

Follow prescriber-ordered enteral feeding infusion rates and concentrations carefully. Usually the initial rate is 20 mL/hr, increased at 10 mL/hr every 8 hours as long as it is tolerated, with the goal of 50 mL/hr. If not tolerated, contact the prescriber for further orders/instructions. More rapid feeding increases the risk for hyperglycemia, dumping syndrome, and diarrhea. The prescriber may adjust the infusion rates of enteral feedings as per the patient's tolerance (of the feeding). Tube feeding formulas are to be kept at room temperature and are never to be administered cold or warm. If all the necessary steps to decrease or prevent diarrhea have been taken and failed, antidiarrheal medications may be needed. Lactose-free solutions are available and recommended for patients who are lactose intolerant. Patients with lactose intolerance may present with or complain of abdominal cramping and/or bloating, flatulence, and diarrhea with the ingestion of milk-based enteral feedings.

Monitor parenteral nutrition infusions every hour or per institutional policies and procedures. Document the status of the entire infusion system and equipment as well as the condition of the patient. It is the standard of care to first examine the patient closely and carefully and then follow with checking the insertion site, tubing, infusion pump, and solution. To prevent infection, change the parenteral nutrition tubing every time a new bag is added to the infusion, or as per institutional policy. It is also recommended that tubing changes occur daily with the beginning of each new infusion. A 1.2-micron filter is used to trap bacteria, including *Pseudomonas* species. Document baseline vital signs, and record the patient's temperature every 4 hours, or as prescribed, during the infusion. Report any increase in temperature over 100°F (37.8°C) to the prescriber immediately. Check the patient frequently for signs and symptoms of hyperglycemia such as polydipsia (excessive thirst), polyuria (excessive urination), polyphagia (excessive hunger), headache, dehydration, nausea, vomiting, and weakness. Never accelerate these infusion rates to increase plasma volume because the rapid increase in the amount of dextrose solution may precipitate hyperglycemia and other related complications. Insulin replacement may be needed with the increase in dextrose; therefore, use a glucometer to measure serum glucose levels so that hyperglycemia may be immediately recognized and treated.

Hypoglycemia is manifested by cold, clammy skin; dizziness; tachycardia; and tingling of the extremities. Hypoglycemia associated with parenteral nutrition may be prevented by gradual reduction of the intravenous feeding rate to allow the pancreas time to adapt to the changing blood glucose levels. If parenteral nutrition is discontinued abruptly, rebound hypoglycemia may occur. This can be prevented by providing infusions of 5% to 10% glucose in situations in which parenteral nutrition must be discontinued immediately. Fluid overload may also occur with parenteral nutrition, manifested by weak pulse, hypertension, tachycardia, confusion, decreased urine output, and pitting edema. This may be prevented by maintaining infusion rates as ordered. If signs of fluid overload occur, slow the infusion rate, measure vital signs, contact the prescriber, and remain with the patient until the patient's condition has stabilized. Include auscultation of breath and heart sounds in the patient assessment, especially if additional therapies are administered that may precipitate fluid overload. Measurement of intake and output is usually indicated when *parenteral nutrition* is administered (and with enteral supplementation as well). See Patient-Centered Care: Patient Teaching below for more information on the use of *nutritional supplements*.

EVALUATION

Therapeutic responses to *nutritional supplementation* include improved well-being, energy, strength, and performance of activities of daily living; an increase in weight; and laboratory test results that reflect an improved nutritional status. Specific laboratory values may include some of the following: albumin level, total protein level, hematocrit level, hemoglobin level, RBC and WBC counts, BUN level, electrolyte levels, blood glucose and insulin levels, and iron values. Perform ongoing evaluation for adverse effects associated with all *enteral* and/or *parenteral nutrition* infusions during and after therapy, and complete nutritional reevaluation periodically so that the patient's nutritional needs are met. This may require frequent appointments with the prescriber or monitoring by a home health care nurse. Always refer to goals and outcome criteria to evaluate the effectiveness of therapy.

PATIENT-CENTERED CARE: PATIENT TEACHING

- Because patients are often discharged with the need for various types of tube feedings, provide the patient, family, and/or caregiver with education, instructions, and demonstrations about the daily care of the tube, preparation of tube feedings, and related procedures. Present the education in a way that reflects the learning needs of the patient and/or those involved in the patient's care.

- Instruct the patient, family, and/or caregiver about the need for correct placement of the tube, which should be checked before each tube feeding if a nasogastric tube is used. Incorrect placement of a nasogastric tube would be manifested by coughing, choking, difficulty speaking, cyanosis, and subsequent respiratory distress. The head of the bed must remain elevated during infusions to at least 30 to 45 degrees; this positioning is more critical with nasogastric tube feedings than with gastrostomy tube feedings. Review the need for frequent oral care.

- Provide contact names and phone numbers for the prescriber, home health care nurse, and other resources to the patient, family, and/or caregiver so that therapy can be monitored and problems and complications averted as related to the feeding. A fever, difficulty breathing, sounds of lung congestion, high residual amounts, resistance to the flow of the feeding solution, and resistance in checking for residual are all causes for concern. Appropriate interventions must be implemented, including seeking emergency medical care if needed.

- Patients who are homebound and are receiving parenteral nutrition will need individualized education as well as support from home health care or related health care services. Practice is critical to acquisition of skill by the patient, family, and/or caregiver and must be an integral part of patient education. Before the patient is discharged, explain and demonstrate all procedures for storage, cleansing and care of the site, dressing changes, irrigation of the catheter, pump function and care, and changing of the bag, filters, and tubing, with a return demonstration by the patient. Advise the patient that parenteral nutrition in the home setting requires home health care services—often by a registered nurse—to help prevent the complications of infection at the site, sepsis, fever, and pneumonia.

- Educate the patient about the need to check serum glucose levels at home as ordered by the prescriber if parenteral nutrition or other infused solutions high in dextrose are administered. Thoroughly explain the operation of a glucometer, with specific steps for its use included in a demonstration to the patient, family, and/or caregiver. In addition, include and reinforce instructions in self-administration of insulin, if needed.

- Instruct the patient to report to the prescriber immediately any signs and symptoms of potential complications of parenteral nutrition, including fever, cough, chest pain, dyspnea, and chills (all of which are indicative of adverse reactions to lipid infusions). Restlessness, nervousness, fainting, and tachycardia are associated with hypoglycemia and must also be reported, as must the occurrence of polyuria, polydipsia, polyphagia, nausea, vomiting, dehydration, headache, and/or weakness (indicating hyperglycemia).

KEY POINTS

- A thorough nutritional assessment and possible consultation with a registered dietitian or nutritionist are essential for adequate intervention for the malnourished patient.

- Various enteral feeding formulations with different nutritional content are available, including some that are lactose free.

- Enteral feedings may result in complications such as hyperglycemia, dumping syndrome, and aspiration of the nutritional supplement.

- Parenteral nutrition supplementation (intravenously administered) is total parenteral nutrition (TPN) or hyperalimentation. PN or TPN may be administered through a central vein or through a peripheral vein (PPN).

- TPN is administered through a central venous catheter because of the hyperosmolarity of the substances used and the need for dilution provided by a larger-diameter vein to prevent damage to the vein. Parenteral nutrition given through a peripherally inserted central catheter (PPN) line is another option but uses a solution with a lower concentration of dextrose and other ingredients.

- Parenteral feedings may result in air embolism, fever, infection, fluid volume overload, hyperglycemia, or hypoglycemia. If they are discontinued abruptly, rebound hypoglycemia may result.

- Cautious and skillful nursing care may prevent or decrease the occurrence of complications associated with enteral or parenteral nutritional supplementation.

NCLEX® EXAMINATION REVIEW QUESTIONS

1. The nurse is assessing an enteral feeding that is infusing via a nasogastric feeding tube. Which statement about this tube is accurate?
   a. It is surgically inserted into the stomach.
   b. It is inserted through the nose into the jejunum.
   c. It is surgically inserted directly into the jejunum.
   d. It is inserted through the nose into the stomach.

2. When administering total parenteral nutrition (TPN), the nurse is aware that one purpose of intravenous fat (lipid) emulsions is to provide which nutrient?
   a. Calories
   b. Amino acids
   c. Minerals
   d. Immunoglobulins

3. The nurse is monitoring a patient who is receiving a total parenteral nutrition (TPN) infusion and notes that the patient has cold clammy skin, shows tachycardia, and is complaining of feeling dizzy. What is the nurse's immediate action at this time?
   a. Stop the TPN infusion.
   b. Check the patient's blood glucose level.
   c. Order a stat (immediate) electrocardiogram.
   d. Obtain an order for blood cultures.

4. A patient has new orders for administration of peripheral parenteral nutrition (PPN). The nurse knows that PPN is most appropriate in which situation?
   a. Therapy is expected to last longer than 2 weeks.
   b. Therapy is expected to last fewer than 14 days.
   c. A dextrose concentration of 20% is needed.
   d. Nutritional needs are 3000 kcal/day.

5. During the night shift, a patient's total parenteral nutrition (TPN) infusion runs out, the pharmacy is closed, and a new TPN bag will not be available for about 6 hours. What is the nurse's most appropriate action at this time?
   a. Hang a bottle of lipid solution.
   b. Hang a bag of normal saline.
   c. Hang a bag of 10% dextrose.
   d. Call the prescriber for stat TPN orders.

6. The nurse is assessing a patient who is receiving an enteral tube feeding. Which are possible adverse effects associated with enteral feedings? (Select all that apply.)
   a. Hypoglycemia
   b. Air embolism
   c. Aspiration
   d. Diarrhea
   e. Infection

7. A patient is receiving a tube feeding of Glucerna via percutaneous enteral gastrostomy (PEG) tube at 50 mL/hr. The orders also read to check the residual and flush the tubing every 4 hours with 30 mL of water. Calculate the total intake of fluid at the end of a 12-hour shift.

8. The nurse is assessing a newly admitted patient who had been living his car for several months. Which of these are clinical signs of essential fatty acid deficiency? (Select all that apply.)
   a. Hair loss
   b. Wounds with delayed healing
   c. Increased platelet levels
   d. Scaly dermatitis
   e. Excessive bruising

1. d, 2. a, 3. b, 4. b, 5. c, 6. c, d, 7. 690 mL, 8. a, b, d.

CRITICAL THINKING AND PRIORITIZATION QUESTIONS

1. A patient has been receiving TPN with a 25% glucose content, and the nurse has just discovered that the central intravenous access line is clogged. What is of the most immediate concern, and what is the nurse's priority action at this time? Explain your answer.

2. At the beginning of the morning shift, the nurse is reviewing the medication orders of a patient who is receiving the impaired glucose tolerance formulation Glucerna through a nasogastric feeding tube. The patient has a history of seizures, and a dose of phenytoin (to be given via the tube) is due later in the morning. What is the nurse's priority action at this time?

For answers, see *http://evolve.elsevier.com/Lilley.*

PART 10

Dermatologic, Ophthalmic, and Otic Drugs

Learning Strategies

FUTURE APPLICATION

By this point, you are well aware of just how essential the acquisition of pharmacology knowledge is to the profession of nursing. In the learning strategies introduction, you were told that while the administration of medications is a task that anyone can perform with minimal direction, it takes immense knowledge and understanding of pharmacology to administer medications correctly and safely. One of the features of your pharmacology textbook that has not been discussed in your learning strategies is the safety aspect of medication administration. In Chapter 1, the authors explained QSEN and how quality and safe nursing care are extremely important. Nursing programs are being challenged to begin the inclusion of QSEN in their curriculum. It is the hope that preparing future nurses with the knowledge, skills, and attitudes will enable them to carry those skills into the institutions where they practice and apply them to improve the quality and safety of patient care. Throughout your textbook, you have been learning and applying the QSEN competencies. You have read about Evidence-Based Practice. You have seen examples of Teamwork and Collaboration. Patient-Centered Care has been woven throughout your textbook. It cannot be stressed enough how crucial medication safety is in patient care. As you learn more about medications and the characteristics of the different classifications of drugs, it will become apparent that nurses play a vital role in safe medication delivery and the prevention of medication errors.

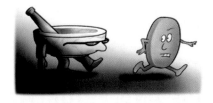

In Chapter 5, you learned about the impact medication errors have on patients and why the prevention and reporting of errors is crucial. As nurses, you will realize that you are the last checkpoint in the chain of safe administration. You cannot fulfill this role if you do not have a strong understanding of the medications and pharmacotherapeutics. As you study your textbook, pay particular attention to these boxes on patient safety. The information is critical to your current lesson and your future nursing practice. To safely administer medications, always use the Nine Rights of medication administration, and watch for high-alert medications and look-alike, sound-alike drugs. Remember also to only use approved abbreviations. In Chapter 5, you also learned how technological advances with computerized order entry and bar coding for medications, while closing the gap on medication errors, is still not foolproof. Technology is only as good as the people using it, so you must still be diligent and careful. Learn to live by the mantra, "When in doubt, check it out." If something does not "feel right," or if your patient questions a medication, that should be your signal to stop and investigate. Never hesitate to call a pharmacist if something does not sound right. Pharmacists and technicians are human, and they have made mistakes. As the final check, nurses and can catch a mistake before it reaches the patient. That is why it is imperative that you have a good understanding of pharmacology so you can easily detect when something is not right. For example, you notice a patient is receiving furosemide (Lasix) 40 mg both intravenous (IV) and orally. You want to make sure the patient is not being double dosed. The 80-mg dose can lead to fluid and electrolyte imbalance much quicker than the 40-mg dose. Ask yourself: Is the IV form only to be given if the patient cannot take the medication orally? Or was it changed from oral to IV and the oral dose not discontinued? Or was the IV dose a one-time-only order? Another example is when a patient is ordered two medications from the same classification. A patient may have several doctors ordering medications. Sometimes they do not realize another prescriber already ordered a drug for the patient. Does the patient need both famotidine (Pepcid) and pantoprazole (Protonix)? Both are used for ulcers, but they differ in classification. Did the second prescriber want to add a different classification to treat the patient's gastrointestinal upset? Or did the doctor not notice the famotidine order and write for pantoprazole because it is his or her preferred drug of choice?

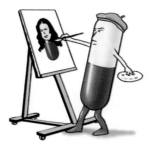

As mentioned earlier, the pharmacology concepts you are learning will reappear in your various nursing courses. The information you learn now will have implications for your future nursing practice, and a certain percentage of pharmacology questions will appear on your NCLEX® examination. New medications are being developed every day. In the future, when you encounter a medication that is brand new or just new to you, you'll want to look it up and learn about it as you do now in your pharmacology course. When you become a nurse, the learning never ends. You never want to be in a situation where your patient asks you a question about his or her medication and you do not know the answer. One way to stay current with pharmacology is to subscribe to nursing journals. Articles may highlight new drugs, or there may be a news section to convey this information. You also can subscribe to various online resources like *Medscape.com*, which provides articles and news briefs on pharmacology. The *FDA.org* website offers a twice-monthly newsletter and e-mail updates on various drug-related topics. Information on medications that have just been approved as well as those on the recall list are also available. Various nursing organizations let their members know about new drugs in their area of expertise. You can have many of these updates sent to you in an e-mail. For example, the Oncology Nursing Society sends out e-mail updates on new chemotherapeutic medications to their members.

There are various drug applications and drug handbooks available for your smart phone or tablet that you can use in your nursing program and future practice. Drug information is readily available on most health care institution computer systems as well. It is also a good idea to become familiar with the pharmacy department at the institution. The pharmacist can provide a wealth of knowledge to assist you with any questions you have about drug administration, adverse effects, or patient teaching. All the knowledge you are gaining in nursing pharmacology will assist you in providing safe, quality nursing care. And this is only the beginning; you will continue to broaden your horizons in nursing pharmacology with increased understanding and application of your knowledge.

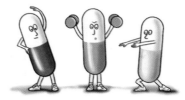

Dermatologic Drugs

http://evolve.elsevier.com/Lilley

OBJECTIVES

When you reach the end of this chapter, you will be able to do the following:

1. Discuss the normal anatomy, physiology, and functions of the skin.
2. Describe the different disorders, infections, and other conditions commonly affecting the skin.
3. Identify the various dermatologic drugs used to treat these disorders, infections, and other conditions, and describe the various classifications of these drugs.
4. Discuss the mechanisms of action, indications, contraindications, cautions, other drug interactions, application techniques, and adverse effects of the various topical dermatologic drugs.
5. Develop a nursing care plan that includes all phases of the nursing process for patients using topical dermatologic drugs.

DRUG PROFILES

anthralin, p. 892
◆ bacitracin, p. 887
◆ benzoyl peroxide, p. 888
calcipotriene, p. 892
clindamycin, p. 888
◆ clotrimazole, p. 889
fluorouracil, p. 894
imiquimod, p. 894
◆ isotretinoin, p. 888
◆ lindane, p. 893
miconazole, p. 890

minoxidil, p. 893
mupirocin, p. 887
neomycin and polymyxin B, p. 887
◆ pimecrolimus, p. 894
◆ silver sulfadiazine, p. 888
tar-containing products, p. 892
tazarotene, p. 892
tretinoin, p. 889

_____
◆ = *Key drug*
! = *High-alert drug*

KEY TERMS

Acne vulgaris A chronic inflammatory disease of the *pilosebaceous* glands of the skin, involving lesions such as *papules* and *pustules* ("pimples" or "comedones"); referred to in this chapter as *acne*. (p. 888)

Actinic keratosis A slowly developing, localized thickening of the outer layers of the skin resulting from long-term, prolonged exposure to the sun; also called *solar keratosis*. (p. 894)

Atopic dermatitis A chronic skin inflammation seen in patients with hereditary susceptibility. (p. 886)

Basal cell carcinoma The most common form of skin cancer; it arises from epidermal cells known as *basal cells* and is rarely metastatic. (p. 886)

Carbuncles Necrotizing infections of skin and subcutaneous tissue caused by multiple furuncles (boils). They are usually caused by the bacterium *Staphylococcus aureus*. (p. 887)

Cellulitis An acute, diffuse, spreading infection involving the skin, subcutaneous tissue, and sometimes muscle as well. It is usually caused by infection of a wound with *Streptococcus* or *Staphylococcus* species. (p. 887)

Dermatitis Any inflammation of the skin. (p. 886)

Dermatophytes Any of the common groups of fungi that infect skin, hair, and nails. These fungi are most commonly from the genera *Microsporum, Epidermophyton,* and *Trichophyton.* (p. 889)

Dermatosis The general term for any abnormal skin condition. (p. 886)

Dermis The layer of the skin just below the epidermis, consisting of papillary and reticular layers and containing blood and lymphatic vessels, nerves and nerve endings, glands, and hair follicles. (p. 885)

Eczema A pruritic, papulovesicular dermatitis occurring as a reaction to many endogenous and exogenous agents, and

KEY TERMS—cont'd

characterized by erythema, edema, and an inflammatory infiltrate of the dermis accompanied by oozing, crusting, and scaling. (p. 886)

Epidermis The superficial, avascular layers of the skin, made up of an outer dead, cornified portion and a deeper living, cellular portion. (p. 885)

Folliculitis Inflammation of a follicle, usually a hair follicle. A follicle is defined as any sac or pouchlike cavity. (p. 887)

Furuncles Painful skin nodules caused by *Staphylococcus* organisms that enter the skin through the hair follicles; also called a *boil.* (p. 887)

Impetigo A pus-generating, contagious superficial skin infection, usually caused by *Staphylococci* or *Streptococci.* It generally occurs on the face and is most commonly seen in children; may be recognized by honey-colored crusts. (p. 887)

Papules Small, circumscribed, superficial, solid elevations of the skin that are usually pink and less than 0.5 to 1 cm in diameter. (p. 887)

Pediculosis An infestation with lice of the family Pediculidae. (p. 892)

Pruritus An unpleasant cutaneous sensation that provokes the desire to rub or scratch the skin to obtain relief. (p. 889)

Psoriasis A common, chronic squamous cell dermatosis with polygenic (multigene) inheritance and a fluctuating pattern of recurrence and remission. (p. 886)

Pustules Visible collections of pus within or beneath the epidermis. (p. 887)

Scabies A contagious disease caused by *Sarcoptes scabiei*, the itch mite, characterized by intense itching of the skin and injury to the skin (excoriation) resulting from scratching. (p. 893)

Tinea A fungal skin disease caused by a dermatophyte and characterized by itching, scaling, and, sometimes, painful lesions. *Tinea* is a general term for an infection with any of various dermatophytes that occur at several sites; also called *ringworm.* (p. 889)

Topical antimicrobials Substances applied to any surface that either kill microorganisms or inhibit their growth or replication. (p. 887)

Vesicles Small sacs containing liquid; also called *cysts.* (p. 887)

OVERVIEW

The skin is the largest organ of the body. It covers the body and serves several functions, including protection, sensation, temperature regulation, excretion, absorption, and metabolism. It acts as a protective barrier for the internal organs. Without skin, harmful external agents such as microorganisms and chemicals would gain access to and damage internal organs. Part of this protection includes the skin's ability to maintain a surface pH of 4.5 to 5.5. This weakly acidic environment discourages the growth of microorganisms that thrive at a more alkaline pH. The skin also has the ability to sense changes in temperature (heat or cold), pressure, or pain—information that is then transmitted along nerve endings. The temperature of the environment changes continually; despite this, the body maintains an almost constant internal temperature due in large part to the skin, which plays a major role in the regulation of body temperature. Heat loss and conservation are regulated in coordination with the blood vessels that supply blood to the skin and by means of perspiration. The skin is also able to excrete fluid and electrolytes through sweat glands. In addition, it stores fat, synthesizes vitamin D, and provides a site for drug absorption.

The skin is made up of two layers: the **dermis** and the **epidermis** (Figure 56-1). The outer skin layer, or epidermis, is itself composed of four layers. From the outermost to innermost, these are the stratum corneum, stratum lucidum, stratum granulosum, and stratum germinativum. The respective functions of these layers are described in Table 56-1.

None of these layers has a direct blood supply of its own. Instead, nourishment is provided through diffusion from the

TABLE 56-1 Epidermal Layers

Layer	Description
Stratum corneum ("horny layer," so named because keratin is the same protein that makes up the horns of animals)	Outermost layer consisting of dead skin cells that are made of a converted water-repellant protein known as *keratin;* it is the protective layer for the entire body. After it is desquamated or shed, it is replaced by new cells from below.
Stratum lucidum ("clear layer")	Layer where keratin is formed; it is translucent and contains flat cells.
Stratum granulosum ("granular layer")	Cells die in this layer; granulated cells are located here, which gives this layer the appearance for which it is named.
Stratum germinativum ("germinative layer")	New skin cells are made in this layer; it contains melanocytes, which produce melanin, the skin color pigment.

dermis below. The dermis lies between the epidermis and subcutaneous fat and differs from the epidermis in many ways. It is approximately 40 times thicker than the epidermis. Traversing the dermis is a rich supply of blood vessels, nerves, lymphatic tissue, elastic tissue, and connective tissue, which provide extra support and nourishment to the skin. Also contained in the dermis are the exocrine glands—the eccrine, apocrine, and sebaceous glands—and the hair follicles. The functions of the various types of exocrine glands are explained in Table 56-2.

Below the dermis is a layer of loose connective tissue called the *hypodermis.* It helps make the skin flexible. It is also here

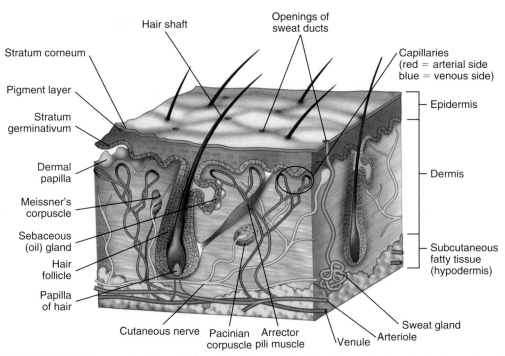

FIGURE 56-1 Microscopic view of the skin. The epidermis, shown in longitudinal section, is raised at one corner to reveal the ridges in the dermis. (Modified from Thibodeau GA, Patton KT: *Anatomy and physiology*, ed 5, St Louis, 2003, Mosby.)

TABLE 56-2	**Exocrine Glands of the Skin**
Gland	**Function**
Sebaceous	Large lipid-containing cells that produce oil or film that covers the epidermis, protects and lubricates the skin, and is water repellent and antiseptic
Eccrine	Sweat glands that are located throughout the skin surface; help regulate body temperature and prevent skin dryness
Apocrine	Mainly in axilla, genital organs, and breast areas; emit an odor; believed to be scent or sex glands

that the subcutaneous fat tissue is located, which provides thermal insulation and cushioning or padding. It is also the source of nutrition for the skin.

Reactions or disorders of the skin are common and numerous. A **dermatosis** is any abnormal skin condition. Dermatoses include a variety of types of **dermatitis** (skin inflammation). Among these are conditions such as **atopic dermatitis**, **eczema**, and **psoriasis**. In addition, there are also a variety of skin cancers, including **basal cell carcinoma**, squamous cell carcinoma, and melanoma.

PHARMACOLOGY OVERVIEW

Drugs that are administered directly to a skin site are called *topical dermatologic drugs*. These drugs are available in a variety of formulations that are suitable for specific indications. Each formulation has certain characteristics that make it beneficial

for certain uses. For example, ointments have an oil base that makes them stickier than creams and better for smaller areas, whereas creams have a water base that makes them better for larger surfaces. Gels tend to enhance penetration of the active ingredient. Lotions are similar to creams but are lighter. More information on the formulations, their characteristics, and examples are provided in Table 56-3. Note that the focus of this chapter is topically administered medications. Because so many topical drugs are available, the scope of this chapter is limited to some of the more commonly used medications. Systemically administered drugs (transdermal) are also used to treat several skin disorders (see Part 7) and are cross-referenced throughout this chapter.

There are many therapeutic categories of dermatologic drugs. Some of the most common ones are the following:

- Antibacterial drugs
- Antifungal drugs
- Antiinflammatory drugs
- Antineoplastic drugs
- Antipruritic drugs (for itching)
- Antiviral drugs
- Burn drugs
- Débriding drugs (promote wound healing)
- Emollients (skin softeners)
- Keratolytics (cause softening and peeling of the stratum corneum)
- Local anesthetics
- Sunscreens
- Topical vasodilators

TABLE 56-3 Dermatologic Formulations: Characteristics and Examples

Formulation	Characteristics	Examples
Aerosol foam	Can cover large area; useful for drug delivery into a body cavity (e.g., vagina, rectum) or hair areas	ProctoFoam, Epifoam, contraceptive foams
Aerosol spray	Spreads thin liquid or powder film; covers large areas; useful when skin is tender to touch (e.g., burns)	Solarcaine, Desenex, Kenalog
Bar	Similar to a bar of soap; useful as a wash with water	PanOxyl (benzoyl peroxide)
Cleanser	Nongreasy; used as an astringent (oil remover) and/or a wash with water	ZoDerm
Cream	Contains water and can be removed with water; not greasy or occlusive; usually white semisolid; good for moist areas	Hydrocortisone cream (Cortaid), Benadryl cream
Gel/jelly	Contains water and possibly alcohol; easily removed and good lubricator; usually clear, semisolid substance; useful when lubricant properties are desirable	K-Y Jelly, Saligel, Surgilube
Lotion	Contains water, alcohol, and solvents; may be a suspension, emulsion, or solution; good for large or hairy areas	Calamine lotion, Lubriderm lotion, Kwell lotion
Oil	Contains very little water, if any; occlusive, liquid; not removable with water	Lubriderm bath oil
Ointment	Contains no water; not removable with water; occlusive, greasy, and semisolid; desirable for dry lesions because of occlusiveness	Vaseline (petrolatum), zinc oxide ointment, A & D ointment
Paste	Similar properties to those of ointments; contains more powder than ointments; excellent protectant properties	Zinc oxide paste (Balmex)
Pledget (pad)	Moistened pad that is applied to or wiped over affected area	EryPads (erythromycin)
Powder	Slight lubricating properties; may be shaken on affected area; promotes drying of area where applied	Tinactin powder, Desenex powder
Shampoo	Soapy liquid for washing hair and/or skin	Nizoral (ketoconazole)
Solution	Nongreasy liquid; dries quickly	Erythromycin topical solution (Eryderm)
Stick	Spreads thin chalky or viscous liquid film; often better for smaller areas	Benadryl Itch Relief
Tape	Most occlusive formulation; consistent topical drug delivery; useful when small, straight areas require drug application	Cordran tape

ANTIMICROBIALS

Topical antimicrobials are antibacterial, antifungal, and antiviral drugs that, as the name implies, are applied topically. Although topical antimicrobials have many of the same properties as the systemic forms, there are differences in terms of their absorption, distribution, toxicities, and adverse effects.

GENERAL ANTIBACTERIAL DRUGS

Common skin disorders caused by various bacteria are folliculitis, impetigo, furuncles, carbuncles, papules, pustules, vesicles, and cellulitis. The bacteria responsible are most commonly *Streptococcus pyogenes* and *Staphylococcus aureus*. Dermatologic antibacterial drugs are used to treat or prevent these skin infections. The most commonly used drugs are bacitracin, polymyxin, and neomycin. Mupirocin is becoming less effective due to increased resistance to methicillin-resistant *S. aureus* (MRSA).

DRUG PROFILES

◆ bacitracin

Bacitracin is a polypeptide antibiotic that is applied topically for the treatment or prevention of local skin infections caused by susceptible aerobic and anaerobic gram-positive organisms such as staphylococci, streptococci, anaerobic cocci, corynebacteria, and clostridia. It works by inhibiting bacterial cell wall synthesis, which leads to cell death. It can be either bactericidal or bacteriostatic, depending on the causative organism.

Its antimicrobial spectrum is broadened in several available combination drug products. Most of these also contain neomycin and/or polymyxin B (see later in the chapter).

Adverse reactions are usually minimal; however, reactions ranging from skin rash to allergic anaphylactoid reactions have occurred. If itching, burning, inflammation, or other signs of sensitivity occur, discontinue bacitracin. This drug is available in ointment form and is usually applied to the affected area one to three times daily. It is also available in systemic and ophthalmic formulations (see Chapter 57).

neomycin and polymyxin B

Neomycin and polymyxin B are two additional broad-spectrum antibiotics that are available as the nonprescription product known as Neosporin. Neosporin cream is a combination of these two drugs alone, whereas Neosporin ointment also contains bacitracin. Several brand name and generic combinations of these three topical antibiotics are available, and all are commonly used as topical antiseptics for minor skin wounds. Although neomycin/polymyxin B is still a very popular over-the-counter (OTC) product, there is evidence that use of the drug can increase the likelihood of future allergic reactions of the skin.

mupirocin

Mupirocin (Bactroban) is an antibacterial product available only by prescription. It is used on the skin for treatment of staphylococcal and streptococcal impetigo. It is used topically and intranasally to treat nasal colonization with MRSA. The drug is applied topically three times daily and intranasally twice daily to treat MRSA colonization. Adverse reactions are usually limited to local burning, itching, or minor pain.

♦ silver sulfadiazine

Silver sulfadiazine (Silvadene) has proved both effective and safe in the prevention and treatment of infections in burns. A major concern for burn victims is infection at the burn site. Because increased systemic absorption of a drug can occur in compromised skin areas, topical burn drugs must not be too potent or toxic to avoid causing dangerous systemic effects. This is especially true when large burned areas must be treated. On the other hand, the blood supply to burned areas is often drastically reduced, so that systemically administered antibiotics either cannot reach the site or do so only in quantities too low to be effective. Therefore, the only way of applying these drugs to ensure that they reach the burn site is to do so topically.

Silver sulfadiazine is a synthetic antimicrobial drug produced when silver nitrate reacts with the chemical sulfadiazine. It appears to act on the cell membrane and cell wall of susceptible bacteria and is used as an adjunct in the prevention and treatment of infection in second- and third-degree burns and less frequently in cellulitic or eczematous extremities. The adverse effects of silver sulfadiazine are similar to those of other topical drugs and include pain, burning, and itching. This drug should not be used in patients who are allergic to sulfonamide drugs. It is available only as a 1% cream and is applied topically to cleansed and débrided burned areas once or twice daily using a sterile-gloved hand.

ANTIACNE DRUGS

Acne vulgaris is the most common skin disorder. Its precise cause is unknown and somewhat controversial. Likely causative factors include heredity, stress, drug reactions, hormones, and bacterial infections. Common bacterial causes include *Staphylococcus* species (spp.) and *Propionibacterium acnes*. Some of the most commonly used antiacne drugs are benzoyl peroxide, clindamycin, erythromycin, tetracycline, isotretinoin, and the vitamin A acid known as *retinoic acid*. Many other drugs are also used in the treatment and prevention of acne, including systemic formulations of the antibiotics minocycline, doxycycline, and tetracycline (see Chapter 38). Some practitioners also prescribe oral contraceptives (see Chapter 34) for female acne patients, because in some controlled studies estrogen has been shown to have beneficial effects against acne, especially hormone-driven acne.

DRUG PROFILES

♦ benzoyl peroxide

The microorganism that most commonly causes acne, *P. acnes*, is an anaerobic bacterium; that is, it needs an environment that is poor in oxygen to grow. Benzoyl peroxide is effective in combating such infection because it slowly and continuously liberates active oxygen in the skin, resulting in antibacterial,

antiseptic, drying, and keratolytic actions. These actions create an environment that is unfavorable for the continued growth of the *P. acnes* bacteria, and they soon die. Drugs such as benzoyl peroxide that soften scales and loosen the outer horny layer of the skin are referred to as *keratolytics*.

Benzoyl peroxide generally produces signs of improvement within 4 to 6 weeks. Adverse effects tend to be related to dose (including overuse) and include peeling skin, red skin, or a sensation of warmth. Blistering or swelling of the skin is generally considered an allergic reaction to the product and is an indication to stop treatment. Overuse of this drug and also of tretinoin is common in teenage patients who are attempting to cure their acne quickly. The result can be painful, reddened skin, which usually resolves on return to use of these medications as prescribed.

Benzoyl peroxide is available in multiple topical dosage forms, including a cleansing bar, liquid, lotion, mask, cream, gel, and cleanser. It is also available in various combination drug products. It is usually applied topically one to four times daily, depending on the dosage form and prescriber's instructions. Benzoyl peroxide is classified as a pregnancy category C drug.

clindamycin

Clindamycin (Cleocin T) is a topical form of the systemic antibiotic described in Chapter 39. Adverse reactions are usually limited to minor local skin reactions, including burning, itching, dryness, oiliness, and peeling. The drug is available in gel, lotion, suspension, foam, and pledgettes (pads saturated with clindamycin solution). Clindamycin is usually applied once or twice daily. It is classified as a pregnancy category B drug.

♦ isotretinoin

Isotretinoin (Amnesteem, Claravis, Sotret) is an oral product indicated for the treatment of severe resistant cystic acne. Isotretinoin inhibits sebaceous gland activity and has antikeratinizing (anti–skin hardening) and antiinflammatory effects. Isotretinoin is one of relatively few medications that are classified as pregnancy category X drugs. This means that it is a proven human *teratogen*, or a chemical that is known to induce birth defects. It is imperative that female patients of childbearing age be counseled and agree not to become pregnant during use of the drug. For these reasons, in 2005, the U.S. Food and Drug Administration (FDA) approved stringent guidelines regarding the prescription and use of this medication. It is now officially required that at least two reliable contraceptive methods be used by sexually active women during therapy with isotretinoin and for 1 month after completion of therapy. A risk management program of unprecedented size and scope has been designed and approved by the FDA especially for this drug. It is known as *iPLEDGE* and was fully implemented as of March 1, 2006. As a result, federal law now requires that any health care provider who prescribes this drug be a registered and active member of this program, and patients must also be qualified and registered. Further information is available at the iPLEDGE call center at 866-495-0654 or online at *www.ipledgeprogram.com*. In addition, there have been case reports of suicide and suicide attempts in patients receiving this medication. It has not been determined if the drug increases the risk for suicide or if psychosocial reactions from severe acne are to blame for increased suicide risk. Educate patients to report any signs of depression immediately to their prescribers. Follow-up treatment may be needed, and simply stopping the drug may be insufficient. Despite these rather strong concerns, this drug does prove to be very helpful in treating severe acne cases. Isotretinoin is available only for oral use.

tretinoin

Tretinoin (retinoic acid, vitamin A acid) (Renova, Retin-A) is a derivative of vitamin A that is used to treat acne and ameliorate the dermatologic changes (e.g., fine wrinkling, mottled hyperpigmentation, roughness) associated with photodamage (sun damage). The drug appears to act as an irritant to the skin, in particular to the follicular epithelium. Specifically, it stimulates the turnover of epidermal cells, which results in skin peeling. While this is occurring, the free fatty acid levels of the skin are reduced, and horny cells of the outer epidermis cannot then adhere to one another. Without fatty acids and horny cells, acne and its comedo, or pimple, cannot exist.

Topically administered tretinoin has been shown to enhance the repair of skin damaged by ultraviolet (UV) radiation, or sunlight. It does this by increasing the formation of fibroblasts and collagen, both of which are needed to rebuild skin. The drug also may reduce collagen degradation by inhibiting the enzyme collagenase that breaks down collagen.

Tretinoin's main adverse effects are local inflammatory reactions, which are reversible when therapy is discontinued. Common adverse effects are excessively red and edematous blisters, crusted skin, and temporary alterations in skin pigmentation. Tretinoin is available in many topical formulations, including creams, gels, and a liquid. Because of its potential to cause severe irritation and peeling, it may initially be applied once every 2 or 3 days, and treatment often starts with a lower-strength product. Severe sunburn can occur with this drug, and patients must use appropriate sunscreens. In addition, waxing procedures are contraindicated in patients using tretinoin.

Retin-A Micro has been approved for the treatment of acne vulgaris. This particular acne product contains tretinoin formulated inside a synthetic polymer called a *Microsponge system*. This system is made of round microscopic particles of synthetic polymer. These microspheres act as reservoirs for tretinoin, allowing the skin to absorb small amounts of the drug over time. Retin-A Micro is currently available only in gel form. All topical forms of tretinoin are classified as pregnancy category C drugs. They are not to be confused with the oral capsule form of tretinoin that is used to treat leukemia, and it is classified as a pregnancy category D drug. Another antiacne retinoid is adapalene, a topical solution.

ANTIFUNGAL DRUGS

A few fungi produce keratinolytic enzymes, which allow them to live on the skin. Topical fungal infections are primarily caused by *Candida* spp. (candidiasis), dermatophytes, and *Malassezia furfur* (tinea versicolor). These fungi are found in moist, warm environments, especially in dark areas such as the feet or groin.

Candidal infections are most commonly caused by *Candida albicans*, a yeastlike opportunistic fungus present in the normal flora of the mouth, vagina, and intestinal tract. Two significant factors that commonly predispose a person to a candidal infection are broad-spectrum antibiotic therapy, which promotes an overgrowth of nonsusceptible organisms in the natural body flora, and immunodeficiency disorders. Because these infections favor warm, moist areas of the skin and mucous membranes, they most commonly occur orally (e.g., thrush in infants), vaginally, and cutaneously in sites such as beneath the breasts and in diapered areas. They may also cause nail infections.

Dermatophytes are a group of three closely related genera consisting of *Epidermophyton* spp., *Microsporum* spp., and *Trichophyton* spp. that use the keratin found on the skin to feed their growth. They produce superficial mycotic (fungal) infections of keratinized tissue (hair, skin, and nails). Infections caused by dermatophytes are called **tinea**, or *ringworm*, infections. The name *ringworm* comes from the fact that the infection sometimes assumes a circular pattern at the site of infection. Tinea infections are further identified by the body location where they occur: tinea pedis (foot), tinea cruris (groin), tinea corporis (body), and tinea capitis (scalp). Tinea infections of the foot are also known as *athlete's foot* and those of the groin as *jock itch*.

Fungi usually invade the stratum corneum, which is the dead layer of desquamated (shed) cells. Inflammation occurs when the fungi invade this layer; sensitivity (e.g., itching) occurs when they penetrate the epidermis and dermis.

Many of the fungi that cause topical infections are very difficult to eradicate. The organisms are very slow growing, and antifungal therapy may be required for periods ranging from several weeks to as long as 1 year. However, many topical antifungal drugs are available for the treatment of both dermatophytic infections and those caused by yeast and yeastlike fungi. Some of these drugs, their dosage forms, and their uses are listed in Table 56-4. Systemically administered antifungal drugs are sometimes used to treat skin conditions as well. These drugs are discussed in Chapter 42.

The most commonly reported adverse effects of topical antifungals are local irritation, **pruritus**, a burning sensation, and scaling. Ciclopirox and clotrimazole are classified as pregnancy category B drugs, and econazole, ketoconazole, and miconazole are classified as pregnancy category C drugs. Efinaconazole (Jublia) and luliconazole (Luzu) are the newest topical antifungals approved in 2014. They are indicated for toenail fungus. Patients using efinaconazole must avoid heat, nail polish, and pedicures. Both drugs are classified as a pregnancy category C drug.

Hypersensitivity is the one contraindication to the use of any of these drugs.

DRUG PROFILES

clotrimazole

Clotrimazole (Lotrimin, Mycelex-G) is available both OTC and by prescription. It is available as a lozenge for the treatment of

TABLE 56-4   Topical Antifungal Drugs

Drug	Trade Name	Dosage Form	Indications	Legal Status
butenafine	Mentax, Lotrimin Ultra	1% cream	Tinea pedis	Rx
butoconazole	Femstat 3	2% vaginal cream	Candidiasis	OTC
ciclopiroxolamine	Loprox	0.77% cream and lotion, 8% solution (for nails)	Candidiasis, dermatophytoses, tinea versicolor	Rx
clotrimazole	Gyne-Lotrimin 3	2% vaginal cream, 100- and 200-mg vaginal tabs	Candidiasis	OTC
	Lotrimin	2% cream, 1% lotion and solution	Candidiasis, tinea versicolor	Rx
	Lotrimin AF	1% cream, lotion, and solution	Dermatophytoses	OTC
	Mycelex	1% cream and solution	Dermatophytoses	Rx
	Mycelex	10-mg troches	Oropharyngeal candidiasis	Rx
	Mycelex-7	1% vaginal cream, 100-mg vaginal tabs	Candidiasis	OTC
ketoconazole	Nizoral	2% cream and shampoo	Candidiasis, dermatophytoses, tinea versicolor	Rx
miconazole	Micatin	2% cream, powder, and spray	Dermatophytoses	OTC
	Monistat-Derm	2% cream	Candidiasis, dermatophytoses, tinea versicolor	Rx
nystatin	Nilstat, Mycostatin	Cream, ointment, powder	Candidiasis	Rx
terbinafine	Lamisil	1% cream and spray	Dermatophytoses	OTC
tolnaftate	Tinactin	1% cream, solution, gel, powder, and spray	Dermatophytoses	OTC
undecylenic acid	Cruex, Desenex	Powder, cream, solution, soap	Dermatophytoses	OTC

OTC, Available over the counter without prescription; *Rx*, currently available by prescription only.

oropharyngeal candidiasis, commonly known as *thrush*. It is also available as a cream, lotion, or solution for the treatment of dermatophytoses (e.g., athlete's foot), superficial mycoses, and cutaneous candidiasis. Similar topical preparations are available for intravaginal administration in the treatment of vulvovaginal candidiasis, commonly called a *yeast infection,* and vaginal trichomoniasis. Clotrimazole is available in many topical formulations: a powder; a 10-mg oral topical lozenge; a 1% cream, lotion, and solution; 1% and 2% vaginal creams; and 100- and 500-mg vaginal tablets. Different dosages and dosage forms are used for the treatment of different fungal infections. Clotrimazole is classified as a pregnancy category B drug.

miconazole

Miconazole (Monistat) is a topical antifungal drug that is available in several OTC and prescription products. It inhibits the growth of several fungi, including dermatophytes and yeast, as well as gram-positive bacteria, and is commonly used to treat dermatophytoses, superficial mycoses, cutaneous candidiasis, and vulvovaginal candidiasis. It is present in many OTC remedies for athlete's foot, jock itch, and yeast infections.

For the treatment of athlete's foot, jock itch, ringworm, and other susceptible fungal infections, miconazole is applied sparingly to the cleansed, dry, infected area twice daily in the morning and evening. For the treatment of yeast infections, one 200-mg suppository is inserted in the vagina once daily at bedtime for 3 consecutive days or 100 mg (one suppository or 5 g of the 2% cream) is administered intravaginally once daily at bedtime for 7 days. The most common adverse effects of topically administered miconazole are vulvovaginal burning and itching, pelvic cramps and rash, urticaria, stinging, and contact dermatitis. Miconazole is available in a variety of topical formulations: as

a 2% aerosol spray and powder, a 2% powder, a 2% cream, a 2% vaginal cream, and a 100- and 200-mg vaginal suppository. It is also available as a 1200-mg vaginal suppository for one-time dosing. It is classified as a pregnancy category C drug.

ANTIVIRAL DRUGS

Topical antivirals are now used less frequently than before, because systemic antiviral drug therapy has generally been shown to be superior for controlling such viral skin conditions. As is the case with systemic drug therapy, these products are best used early in a viral skin lesion outbreak. Topical antivirals are more likely to be used for acute outbreaks, whereas systemic drugs are used for acute outbreaks as well as ongoing prophylaxis against outbreaks. Viral infections are very difficult to treat because they live in the body's own healthy cells and use their cell mechanisms to reproduce. The same holds true for topical viral infections. Infections caused by herpes simplex virus types 1 and 2 and human papillomavirus (which causes anogenital warts) are particularly serious and are becoming more common.

The only topical antiviral drugs currently available to treat such viral infections are acyclovir (Zovirax) and penciclovir (Denavir). They work by comparable mechanisms as described for similar antiviral drugs in Chapter 40. Acyclovir and penciclovir are available as topical ointments (5% and 1%, respectively). Acyclovir is applied every 3 hours, or 6 times daily, for 1 week. Penciclovir is applied every 2 hours while awake for 4 days. A finger cot or rubber glove is to be worn for the application of the ointment to prevent the spread of infection. The most common adverse effects are stinging, itching, and rash. Acyclovir is classified as a pregnancy category C drug and penciclovir as a pregnancy category B drug.

ANESTHETIC, ANTIPRURITIC, AND ANTIPSORIATIC DRUGS

TOPICAL ANESTHETICS

Topical anesthetics are drugs that are used to numb the skin. They accomplish this by inhibiting the conduction of nerve impulses from sensory nerves, thereby reducing or eliminating the pain or pruritus associated with insect bites, sunburn, and allergic reactions to plants such as poison ivy, as well as many other uncomfortable skin disorders. They are also used to numb the skin before a painful injection (e.g., insertion of an intravenous line in a pediatric patient). Topical anesthetics are available as ointments, creams, sprays, liquids, and gels, and are discussed in Chapter 11. A lidocaine/prilocaine combination drug (EMLA) and lidocaine alone (Ela-max) are topical anesthetic drugs that are used frequently, especially in pediatric patients. EMLA is applied 1 hour before the procedure, whereas Ela-max is effective within 30 minutes.

TOPICAL ANTIPRURITICS AND ANTIINFLAMMATORIES

Topical antipruritic (anti-itching) drugs contain antihistamines or corticosteroids. Many exert a combined anesthetic and antipruritic action when applied topically. The antihistamines and their therapeutic effects are covered in Chapter 36. New recommendations for the use of topical antihistamines state that these drugs are not to be used to treat the following conditions because of systemic absorption and subsequent toxicity: chickenpox, widespread poison ivy lesions, and other lesions involving large body surface areas.

The most commonly used topical antiinflammatory drugs are the corticosteroids (see Chapter 33). They are generally indicated for the relief of inflammatory and pruritic dermatoses. When topically administered corticosteroids are used, many of the undesirable systemic adverse effects associated with the use of the systemically administered corticosteroids are avoided. The beneficial drug effects of topically administered corticosteroids are their antiinflammatory, antipruritic, and vasoconstrictive actions.

The many different available dosage forms of the various corticosteroids vary in their relative potency, and this often guides their selection for treating various conditions. For instance, corticosteroids that are fluorinated (which increases the potency) are used for the treatment of dermatologic disorders such as psoriasis. The vehicle in which the corticosteroid is contained also may alter its vasoconstrictive properties and therapeutic efficacy. Ointments are generally the most penetrating, followed next by gels, creams, and lotions. Propylene glycol also enhances the penetration of the corticosteroid and its vasoconstrictive effects. Most corticosteroids are available in many topical formulations, which provide a variety of options. The currently available topical corticosteroids, along with their respective potencies, are listed in Table 56-5.

Adverse effects of these drugs include skin reactions such as acne eruptions, allergic contact dermatitis, burning sensations,

dryness, itching, skin fragility, hypopigmentation, purpura, hirsutism (usually facial), folliculitis, round and swollen face, and alopecia (usually of the scalp). Another adverse effect is the opportunistic overgrowth of bacteria, fungi, or viruses as a result of the immunosuppressive effects of this class of drugs. *Tachyphylaxis* (weakening of drug effect over time) may also occur with these drugs, especially with long-term use or overuse. The usual adult dosage of these drugs is one or two applications daily as a thin layer over the affected area. Less potent topical corticosteroids are used in children, following the same dosing schedule. Corticosteroids are classified as pregnancy category C drugs and are contraindicated in patients with a known hypersensitivity to them. Because many of these products are available orally as well as topically, the potential exists for both to be administered simultaneously. This is not recommended and is potentially harmful. The combined use of topical and oral preparations of the same drug can lead to toxicity.

ANTIPSORIATIC DRUGS

Psoriasis is a common skin condition in which areas of the skin become thick, reddened, and covered with silvery scales. Psoriasis is actually a result of a disordered immune system, although it is generally referred to as a skin condition. It is believed to involve *polygenic* (multigene) inheritance. Psoriasis has fluctuating patterns of recurrence and remission. Flare-ups can be triggered by changes in climate, infection, stress, excessive alcohol intake, or dry skin. Although there are many subtypes, the most classic one is known as *plaque psoriasis* and typically manifests as large, dry, erythematous scaling patches of the skin

Range of Potency*	Corticosteroid
1. Higher potency	Betamethasone dipropionate (cream and ointment), clobetasol propionate, halobetasol propionate, diflorasone diacetate
2. Moderate potency	Amcinonide, betamethasone dipropionate (cream), betamethasone benzoate, betamethasone valerate (0.1% cream, ointment, and lotion), desoximetasone (0.05% cream), desoximetasone, fluocinolone, halcinonide, fluocinolone (cream and ointment), flurandrenolide, mometasone, triamcinolone acetonide (0.5% cream and ointment)
3. Lower potency	Alclometasone, desonide, fluocinolone (0.01% solution), triamcinolone (0.1% cream, lotion), hydrocortisone, dexamethasone

TABLE 56-5 Commonly Used Topical Corticosteroids (in Order of Decreasing Potency)

*Skin penetration and thus potency is enhanced by the vehicle (dosage form) containing the steroid. In decreasing order of effectiveness are ointments, gels, creams, and lotions.

that are often white or silver on top. Commonly affected skin areas include nails, scalp, genitals, and lower back. Treatment usually begins with a topical corticosteroid for mild to moderate cases. When this therapy is not successful, topical antipsoriatic drugs are used. In addition to these topical drugs, there are also newer systemically administered antipsoriatic drugs. A thorough discussion of these drugs is beyond the scope of this chapter on topical medications, but those given by injection include etanercept (Enbrel), which is discussed in Chapter 47 on biologic response modifiers. In addition, the antineoplastic drug methotrexate (see Chapter 45) is also used for its antipsoriatic properties. The newest injectable drug, ustekinumab (Stelara), is an interleukin 12 inhibitor and is indicated for plaque psoriasis. It is given subcutaneously. Patients must receive an FDA-approved patient medication guide when receiving ustekinumab. The most serious side effect is increased risk for infection.

DRUG PROFILES

tazarotene

Tazarotene is a receptor-selective retinoid. It is thought to normalize epidermal differentiation, reducing the influx of inflammatory cells into the skin. Synthetic retinoids are vitamin A analogues and are thought to play a role in skin cell differentiation and proliferation. Tazarotene is available in gel form and is approved for the treatment of stable plaque psoriasis and mild to moderately severe facial acne. Like isotretinoin, tazarotene is classified as a pregnancy category X drug, and a negative pregnancy test 2 weeks before starting therapy is required for female patients.

tar-containing products

Drug products containing coal tar derivatives were among the first medications used to treat psoriasis and are still used today for this purpose. Tar derivatives are known to have antiseptic, antibacterial, and antiseborrheic properties, and they work to soften and loosen scaly or crusty areas of the skin. *Seborrhea* is excessive secretion of *sebum*, a normal skin secretion containing fat and epithelial cell debris. Tar-containing products are available in a variety of shampoo forms (for scalp psoriasis), as well as solution, oil, ointment, cream, lotion, gel, and even soap forms for bathing. These products typically contain 1% to 10% coal tar. Adverse reactions usually include minor skin burning, photosensitivity, and other irritations. These products may be applied from one to four times daily or once or twice weekly as prescribed.

anthralin

Anthralin (Anthra-Derm) is a unique drug that is thought to work by inhibition of deoxyribonucleic acid (DNA) synthesis and mitosis within the epidermis to reduce psoriatic lesions. It is available in ointment and cream form and is usually applied once daily. Adverse reactions are generally limited to minor skin irritation. Anthralin is classified as a pregnancy category C drug.

calcipotriene

Calcipotriene (Dovonex) is a synthetic vitamin D_3 analogue that works by binding to vitamin D_3 receptors in skin cells

known as *keratinocytes*, the abnormal growth of which contributes to psoriatic lesions. Calcipotriene helps to regulate the growth and reproduction of keratinocytes. The most common adverse reaction is minor skin irritation. However, more serious reactions can occur in some cases, including worsening of psoriasis, dermatitis, skin atrophy, and folliculitis. Calcipotriene is usually applied twice daily. It is classified as a pregnancy category C drug. Taclonex is a combination product containing calcipotriene and betamethasone, a topical steroid.

MISCELLANEOUS DERMATOLOGIC DRUGS

There are many other topically applied drugs. Those discussed in this section are the topical ectoparasiticides (scabicides and pediculicides), hair growth drugs, sunscreens, antineoplastics, and immunomodulating drugs. Many of these drugs are available both OTC and by prescription. Aloe vera herbal preparations (see Safety: Herbal Therapies and Dietary Supplements) are also available OTC.

SAFETY: HERBAL THERAPIES AND DIETARY SUPPLEMENTS

Aloe (Aloe vera L.)

Overview
The dried juice of the leaves of the aloe plant contains anthranoids, which give aloe a laxative effect when taken orally. The topical application of the plant juice has been known for years to help aid in wound healing.

Common Uses
Wound healing, constipation

Adverse Effects
Diarrhea, nephritis, abdominal pain, dermatitis when used topically

Potential Drug Interactions
Digoxin, antidysrhythmics, diuretics, corticosteroids

Contraindications
Contraindicated in patients who are menstruating or have renal disease; can increase menstrual blood flow and also cause acute renal failure

DRUG PROFILES

ECTOPARASITICIDAL DRUGS

Ectoparasites are insects that live on the outer surface of the body, and the drugs that are used to kill them are called *ectoparasiticidal drugs*. Lice are transmitted from person to person by close contact with infested individuals, clothing, combs, or towels. A parasitic infestation on the skin with lice is called pediculosis, and such infestations go by one of the following three names, depending on the location of the infestation:

- Pediculosis pubis—pubic louse or "crabs"; infestation by *Phthirus pubis*
- Pediculosis corporis—body louse; infestation by *Pediculus humanus corporis*
- Pediculosis capitis—head louse; infestation by *Pediculus humanus capitis*

Common findings in infested persons include itching; eggs of the lice attached to hair shafts (called *nits*); lice on the skin or clothes; and, in the case of pubic lice, sky blue macules (discolored skin patches) on the inner thighs or lower abdomen. Pediculoses are treated with a class of drugs called *pediculicides*. A second common parasitic skin infection known as scabies is that caused by the itch mite *Sarcoptes scabiei*. Scabies is transmitted from person to person by close contact, such as by sleeping next to an infested person. The scabies mite causes irritation and itching by boring into the horny layers of skin located in cracks and folds. Itching seems to occur most commonly in the evening. The drugs used to treat these infestations are called *scabicides*.

Treatment of these parasitic infestations begins with identification of the source of infestation to prevent re-infestation. Next, the clothing and personal articles of the infested person must be decontaminated. This is best accomplished by washing them in hot, soapy water or by dry cleaning them. All close contacts of the person also need to be treated to prevent re-infestation.

In addition to lindane (see profile), malathion (Ovide) and crotamiton (Eurax) are also ectoparasiticidal drugs. The newest drugs approved for lice treatment are benzyl alcohol 5% (Ulesfia), which works by suffocating the lice, and spinosad (Natroba). Natroba is indicated for children 4 years of age and older and offers the benefit of not requiring nit combing as do the other treatments.

♦ lindane

Lindane (Kwell) is a chlorinated hydrocarbon originally developed as an agricultural insecticide. It is both a scabicide and a pediculicide because it is effective in treating both scabies and pediculosis. High resistance rates to lindane and malathion have limited its use. It is available in two topical formulations: a 1% lotion and a 1% shampoo.

For the treatment of pubic or body lice, the cream or lotion is applied in a sufficient quantity to cover the skin and hair of the infested and surrounding areas. It is left on for 12 hours and then thoroughly washed off. A second application is seldom needed. Head lice can be treated with lindane shampoo, which is worked into the hair and left on for 4 minutes. The hair is then rinsed and dried, after which the nits (eggs) are combed from the hair shafts. The treatment for scabies is similar. It involves the application of lindane over the entire body, from the neck down. It is left on for 8 to 12 hours and then washed off. A similar second application 1 week later is often recommended. The OTC products are applied in similar fashion, although details may vary among individual products. Adverse effects of lindane are an eczematous skin rash and central nervous system toxicity. The latter is more common in young children and in cases of overuse. For many years, lindane was the most widely used pediculicide, but it has been superseded to some degree by permethrin. This is because of case reports of neurotoxicity, including dizziness, seizures, and deaths, caused by lindane. Most of the adverse events occurred due to product misuse (e.g., ingestion) or overuse. Children are at higher risk for neurotoxicity because their skin surface area is larger in relation to body weight. Lindane is still recommended as second-line therapy for lice and scabies after failure of one of the OTC preparations. However, the FDA has recommended that it be sold in smaller containers (1 to 2 ounces) with definitive patient instructions on proper use.

HAIR GROWTH DRUGS

minoxidil

Minoxidil (Rogaine) is a vasodilating drug that is administered systemically to control hypertension (see Chapter 22). Topically it has the same vasodilating effect, but when used in this way it is applied to the scalp to stimulate hair growth. The vasodilation it causes is one possible explanation for how it promotes hair growth. It may also act at the level of the hair follicle, possibly stimulating hair follicle growth directly.

Minoxidil can be used by both men and women who experience baldness or hair thinning. Treatment involves administering the drug to the affected areas (those with balding and anticipated balding) twice daily, usually morning and evening. It generally takes 4 months before results are seen. Systemic absorption of topically applied minoxidil may occur with possible adverse effects, including tachycardia, fluid retention, and weight gain. Local effects may include skin irritation, and the drug is not to be applied to skin that is already irritated, nor used concurrently with other topical medications applied to the same site. Minoxidil is classified as a pregnancy category C drug. Note that the beneficial effects of this drug can be reduced by heat, including the use of a blow dryer.

The systemically administered drug finasteride (Proscar, 5 mg) is used to treat benign prostatic hyperplasia, as discussed in Chapter 35. A lower-strength version known as Propecia (1 mg) is also used to treat male pattern alopecia. Finasteride is classified as a pregnancy category X drug, and women are not to handle this drug without gloves or crush this drug, thereby making it airborne.

SUNSCREENS

Sunscreens are topical products used to protect the skin from damage caused by the UV radiation of sunlight. There are currently nearly 160 specific sunscreen products on the market. None requires a prescription for use. Each is composed of typically three to five various chemical ingredients that work together to provide UV protection and, usually, a moisturizing effect as well. Common examples of these ingredients are titanium dioxide, octyl methoxycinnamate, homosalate, and parabens. Sunscreens are given a sun protection factor (SPF) rating, which is a number ranging from 2 to 50 (and even higher in some newer products) in order of increasing potency of UV protection. In 2011, the FDA stated that only those with an SPF of 15 or greater may state they reduce the risk for skin cancer and early skin aging. Most sunscreens come in lotion, cream, or gel form. A small number of lip balms are also available. It is important for sunscreens to have both UVA and UVB protection. Sunscreen is not to be used on infants.

ANTINEOPLASTIC DRUGS

Skin cancer is the most common form of cancer. There are two types of nonmelanoma skin cancer: basal cell carcinoma and squamous cell carcinoma. Basal cell carcinoma is the most common and is rarely fatal, but it can be highly disfiguring. Squamous cell carcinoma, on the other hand, can be fatal, with 2500 deaths reported annually. The most aggressive skin cancer is melanoma; it accounts for only 3% of all skin cancers but is responsible for 75% of deaths associated with skin cancer. The most common cause of skin cancer is exposure to the sun and tanning beds. Early detection and prevention (with the use of sunscreen) are of the utmost importance.

fluorouracil

Various premalignant skin lesions and basal cell carcinomas may be treated with the topically applied antineoplastic drug fluorouracil (Efudex). As noted in Chapter 45, this drug is an antimetabolite that acts by interfering with key cellular metabolic reactions, destroying rapidly growing cells, such as premalignant and malignant cells. It is also used topically in the treatment of solar or actinic keratosis and superficial basal cell carcinomas of the skin—often in addition to local surgical excision. More aggressive skin cancers (*squamous cell carcinoma* and *malignant melanoma*) are not treated with fluorouracil but are usually treated with more aggressive interventions, such as surgery, radiation therapy, and/or systemic chemotherapy (see Chapters 45 and 46).

The adverse effects associated with the topical use of this antineoplastic drug are generally limited to local inflammatory reactions such as dermatitis, stomatitis, and photosensitivity. More serious effects include swelling, scaling, pain, pruritus, burning, soreness, tenderness, suppuration, scarring, and hyperpigmentation.

Fluorouracil is available in both cream and solution form. It can be applied with a nonmetallic applicator, clean fingertips, or gloved fingers. If the fingers are used, they need to be washed thoroughly immediately after application. Either a 1% or 2% fluorouracil solution is used for the treatment of multiple actinic keratoses of the head and neck. The solution is applied twice daily to the lesions. Superficial basal cell carcinoma may be treated with 5% fluorouracil, administered twice daily for at least 2 to 6 weeks. Another topical drug also used for the treatment of actinic keratoses and basal cell carcinomas is the immunomodulator imiquimod, discussed in the following section.

IMMUNOMODULATORS

◆ pimecrolimus

Pimecrolimus (Elidel) is available in a cream form for use in treating atopic dermatitis. Atopic dermatitis is caused by a hereditary susceptibility to pruritus and is often associated with allergic rhinitis, hay fever, and asthma. This drug works through a mechanism similar to that of the anti–transplant-rejection drug tacrolimus (Prograf), which was discussed in Chapter 48. A topical form of tacrolimus (Protopic) is also used and has similar actions and indications. Adverse reactions to both drugs are usually limited to minor skin irritations.

imiquimod

Imiquimod (Aldara) is an immunomodulating drug that has demonstrated efficacy in treating actinic keratosis, superficial

basal cell carcinoma, and anogenital warts. Its exact mechanism of action is unknown, but it is believed somehow to enhance the body's immune response to these conditions. It is applied two to five times per week, as prescribed, depending on the condition being treated. Adverse reactions include mild skin reactions such as burning, induration (hardness), irritation, pain, and bleeding, which can occur both locally (at the site of medication administration) and at skin areas remote from the site of administration. More severe adverse skin reactions include edema, erosion or ulceration, scaling, scabbing, exudation, and vesicle formation. Systemic reactions, likely related to systemic immunomodulating effects, include cough, upper respiratory tract infection, musculoskeletal reactions (e.g., back pain), and lymphadenopathy. This drug is available only in cream form.

WOUND CARE DRUGS

Although superficial skin wounds usually require minimal interventions, deeper skin wounds often require more definitive care for optimal healing. Such care includes addressing the systemic issues (e.g., body nutritional status) that are critical to tissue repair. Vitamin C (ascorbic acid) and zinc have been shown to improve wound healing when they are given orally. Topical wound care medications are one of the fundamental steps of wound care, referred to in the literature as *preparation of the wound bed*. Wound *débridement* is removal of nonviable tissue and elimination of bacteria by suitable cleansing or surgical intervention. Until 2009, drugs containing papain or papain/urea were commonly used as topical débriding drugs. However, the FDA no longer allows these drugs to be manufactured, because they never received FDA approval. Table 56-6 provides information regarding selected currently available wound care medications.

SKIN PREPARATION DRUGS

The skin must be cleansed before any invasive procedure. Isopropyl alcohol (70%) is most commonly used to prepare the skin before minor procedures such as drawing blood or giving injections. Isopropyl alcohol has been shown to lower the bacterial count for 20 to 40 minutes after application. Other drugs that are used to prepare the skin include povidone-iodine (Betadine), chlorhexidine (Hibiclens), and benzalkonium chloride (Zephiran). Benzalkonium chloride is a surface-active drug that works by denaturing the microorganism or essentially destroying its protein. Chlorhexidine acts by disrupting bacterial membranes and inhibiting cell wall synthesis. It is used primarily as a surgical scrub or hand-washing agent by health care professionals. Povidone-iodine is an antiseptic that kills bacteria, fungi, and viruses. It is used for the prevention or treatment of topical infections associated with surgery, burns, and minor cuts and scrapes, and for relief of minor vaginal infections. It is the most widely used antiseptic, but patients should be screened for iodine or shellfish allergies before using it. It is available in many different dosage forms. See Table 56-7 for more information on selected skin preparation drugs.

TABLE 56-6 Selected Wound Care Products

Product Name	Advantages	Disadvantages	Contraindications
acetic acid (vinegar)	Low cost	Cytotoxic	Allergy
sodium hypochlorite (Dakin's bleach solution, ¼%, ½%, 1%)	Aids débridement; reduces microbial count	Partially toxic and irritating to healing tissue	Clean, noninfected wounds
cadexomer iodine (Iodosorb, others)	Slow release; safe for viable cells; absorbs exudates; promotes wound healing	Partly toxic to fibroblast cells; stains tissue	Iodine allergy
collagenase (Santyl)	Good for patients taking anticoagulants or in whom surgery is contraindicated; selectively removes necrotic tissue; does not harm normal tissue; okay for infected wounds	Requires prescriber's order; not for use with other common wound products such as silver sulfadiazine (Silvadene) or Dakin's solution; expensive	Clean wounds with granulation tissue and signs of healing but with limited areas of necrosis; product allergy
biafine topical emulsion	Can be used for "tunneling" wounds as well as full-thickness wounds and radiation dermatitis	Must not be applied within 4 hr of radiation therapy	Bleeding wounds, skin rashes related to food or drug allergies

TABLE 56-7 Skin Preparation Drugs (Antiseptics)

Drug	Effective Against	Adverse Effects
isopropyl alcohol	Bacteria, fungi, virus	Excessive dryness of skin
chlorhexidine (Hibiclens)	Bacteria, fungi	Central nervous system toxicity in neonates and burn patients
povidone-iodine (Betadine)	Bacteria, fungi, virus	Staining of skin, irritation and pain at wound sites; retards or reverses the granulation process
benzalkonium chloride (Zephiran)	Bacteria, fungi	Chemical burns if left in contact with skin for too long

NURSING PROCESS

ASSESSMENT

Before administering any *dermatologic preparation,* assess the patient for any allergies (including all ingredients), contraindications, cautions, and drug interactions. Topical *antibacterials* are associated with a wide range of reactions because of the generalized sensitivity of patients to antibiotics, even when in a different dosage form; therefore, if a patient is allergic to a systemic antibacterial, he or she will also be allergic to the topical dosage forms. Assess the results of any culture and sensitivity testing that may have been ordered before giving the antibacterial to ensure appropriate drug sensitivity. Before administering any type of topical medication (e.g., *antimicrobial, corticosteroid, antiacne drug*), always consider the concentration of the medication, length of exposure to the skin, condition of the skin, size of the affected area, and hydration of the skin. All of these factors have a significant influence on the action of the medication. Additionally, assess the medication order for the correct drug, dosage/concentration, route, and time/frequency. To inspect the skin or affected area thoroughly, use an adequate light source. Palpate the area with a gloved hand. In dark-skinned patients, an erythematous area may not be visible but may be palpated as an area of warmth. Accompany physical assessment of the skin with an assessment and documentation of surrounding structures, including lymph nodes.

Assess the patient's overall health status and hygiene practices, including whether the patient has experienced any trauma and if there is a history of immunosuppression. Remember that the skin of very young as well as older adult patients is more fragile and permeable to certain topical dermatologic preparations. These characteristics also lead to a higher risk for systemic absorption from the skin. It is also important to note other possible situations that may result in a drug effect that is less than therapeutic, such as the use of topical drugs over an area that is full of pus or debris. The use of herbal products, such as topical aloe vera, also requires thorough assessment and notation of any allergies, contraindications, cautions, and drug interactions (see Safety: Herbal Therapies and Dietary Supplements on p. 892).

With use of *ustekinumab (Stelera),* an *interleukin 12 inhibitor* used for plaque psoriasis, assess the patient's general overall state of health and well-being. Monitor laboratory values, as prescribed, especially WBC counts due to the side effect of increased risk for infection. *Retinoids,* such as *tazarotene,* are used for stable plaque psoriasis and for facial acne, and assessing pregnancy status is needed prior to beginning the drug. Therefore, for tazarotene, as with isotretinoin, a negative pregnancy test 2 weeks before starting therapy is required.

For individuals using *tar-containing products* for seborrhea and/or scalp psoriasis, perform baseline assessment and document the areas to be treated and surrounding scalp/skin areas for intactness, redness, and/or drainage.

With *calcipotriene (Dovonex)* or a synthetic vitamin D_3, baseline assessments of area(s) to be treated and surrounding skin/scalp is needed including notation of any redness, swelling, drainage, and/or pain. If a patient has been prescribed the topical application of *minoxidil,* it is important to assess baseline pulse rate, weight, and the presence of any edema due to the side effects that may occur with potential systemic absorption (see previous pharmacology discussion).

When antineoplastic drugs (e.g., *fluorouracil [Efudex]*) or immunomodulating drugs (e.g., *imiquimod [Aldara]*) are prescribed, assess and document baseline findings of the area to be treated. Because the adverse effects of these drugs are usually limited to local reactions, assess for loss of integrity, redness, discomfort, irritation, and swelling of the application area.

NURSING DIAGNOSES

1. Impaired skin integrity related to specific diseases, reactions, conditions, or breaks in the skin barrier
2. Deficient knowledge related to lack of experience with and exposure to use of topical drugs
3. Noncompliance related to lack of experience taking or applying medication and maintaining frequent dosing

CASE STUDY

Patient-Centered Care: Medications for Wound Care

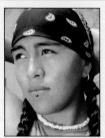 A.T., 16 years of age, was clearing brush with his father when he cut his hand. His mother washed the wound and told him to apply ointment. A.T. checked the family medicine cabinet and applied clotrimazole (Lotrimin) ointment, the only ointment in the cabinet.

Two days later, the wound was not better and was very painful. A.T.'s mother takes him to the clinic to have the wound checked. The physician assistant (PA) finds that the laceration wound is deep but does not have any drainage. The wound is irrigated with normal saline, bacitracin is applied, and the wound is closed with adhesive strips and then covered with a loose gauze dressing. A.T. also receives a tetanus booster vaccine. The nurse gives A.T. instructions on how to care for the wound and tells him that this wound care is to be done twice a day for 1 week. In addition, the PA suggests that A.T. take vitamin C and zinc supplements for the next month and instructs A.T. not to use the clotrimazole ointment on the wound.

1. Why did the PA apply bacitracin instead of clotrimazole? Explain your answer.
2. What is the purpose of the vitamin C and zinc supplements?
3. The next day, A.T. discovers a rash that covers both his arms and legs. The rash is very itchy, and the skin is red with small bumps. He knows that there was poison ivy in the brush and wants something to stop the itching. What will be suggested?
4. The next evening, as he takes off the dressing to clean his wound, A.T. finds that the area is swollen and more inflamed, with tiny red bumps around the wound. There is no drainage. What do you think has happened, and what will be done?

For answers, see *http://evolve.elsevier.com/Lilley*.

PLANNING: OUTCOME IDENTIFICATION

1. Patient's skin integrity remains intact and healed in appearance with less redness, drainage, discomfort, itching, and rash.
2. Patient demonstrates adequate knowledge about the proper dosing, application, and use of the medication.

3. Patient remains compliant as related to the drug regimen while demonstrating safe use of all dosage forms of medication and reporting of side effects.

IMPLEMENTATION

Generally speaking, before any *topical medication* is applied, cleanse the affected area of any debris, drainage, and/or residual medication, taking care to follow any specific directions such as removing water- or alcohol-based topical preparations with soap and water. Always begin (and end) by performing hand hygiene and maintain Standard Precautions (see Box 9-1). Store all dosage forms of medication as recommended. Wear gloves, not only to prevent contamination from secretions/drainage but also to prevent absorption of the medication through your skin. Applying a topical drug using a gloved hand, tongue depressor, or cotton-tipped applicator is recommended. Shake or mix lotions and solutions thoroughly before use, and apply evenly (see Chapter 9). Wash hands before and after application of the medication. Apply any dressings as ordered, paying special attention to directions concerning occlusive, wet, or wet-to-dry dressing changes. It is important to note, however, that most topical dermatologic drugs do not require use of a dressing once the medication is applied. The medication order may also state that any type of dressing or coverage of the affected area is to be avoided. When medications are used for wound care, there is usually a step-by-step protocol for application of a *cleansing agent*, possible *débridement drug*, and *rinsing solution*, as well as final application of an *antibacterial, antifungal, burn, antiseptic,* or other solution that may have been ordered. Provide comprehensive patient education regarding wound care and/or use of topical dermatologic drugs to ensure effective and safe treatment. If home health care is needed after discharge, arrangements need to be in place before the patient leaves the health care institution to return home. Document information about the site of drug application, including drainage (color and amount), swelling, temperature, odor, color, and pain or other sensations, as well as the type of treatment rendered and the response, with each treatment or application, and record a comparative before-and-after assessment.

Follow the manufacturer's guidelines regarding the use of any of the dermatologic preparations because each medication has a different type of base solution. Specific application procedures may be required for different dosage forms. It is also important to follow any instructions or orders regarding other treatments to the affected area, such as the use of an occlusive or wet dressing (see earlier in the chapter). Medicated areas may also need to be protected from exposure to air or sunlight. Strict adherence to the proper method of application and dosage of any dermatologic preparation is important to its effectiveness. Doubling up of a missed dose is not recommended. With *tar*-containing products, various dosage forms include shampoo forms, solutions, oil, gels, creams, and bath soaps. Follow application and dosing instructions as prescribed, which may be from one to four times daily or twice weekly. *Minoxidil* involves application of the drug to the affected areas usually in the morning and evening. Local effects generally include skin irritation, but it is important to emphasize to the patient that it is not to be applied to skin that is already irritated nor is it to be used with other topical medications.

After the medication administration process is complete, dispose of all contaminated dressings, gloves, or equipment properly. Maintain safety, comfort, and privacy of the patient at all times. See Patient-Centered Care: Patient Teaching below for more information. Also see Table 56-6 for information about specific drugs for wound care and their advantages and disadvantages.

EVALUATION

Begin the evaluation by monitoring to ensure that goals and outcome criteria are being met. Therapeutic responses to the various *dermatologic preparations* include improved condition of the skin and healing of lesions or wounds; a decrease in the size of lesions with eventual resolution; and a decrease in swelling, redness, weeping, itching, and burning of the area. Notify the prescriber if a therapeutic response is not observed within an appropriate time (anywhere from 48 to 72 hours or longer, depending on the drug, disorder or skin problem, and acute or chronic nature of the condition) or if signs and symptoms worsen or new ones appear. Adverse effects for which to evaluate include increased severity of symptoms—for example, increased redness, swelling, pain, and drainage; fever; or any other unusual problems at the affected area. Adverse effects may range from slight irritation of the site where the topical drug has been applied to an allergic reaction to toxic systemic effects.

PATIENT-CENTERED CARE: PATIENT TEACHING

- Advise the patient to keep the skin clean and dry or clean and moist as prescribed. Provide instructions to the patient and caregivers about maintaining adequate general hygiene, cleanliness, adequate hydration, and proper nutrition during drug therapy.
- Ensure that the patient has a full understanding on how to prepare the skin for application of the medication and any other instructions.
- Apply dressings to the affected area as directed, if indicated or ordered. Perform dressing application after medication use, and properly dispose of contaminated dressings or equipment. Emphasize the need for thorough hand washing before and after application of medication with a gloved hand, cotton-tipped applicator, or tongue depressor. Demonstrate this to all individuals involved in the care of the patient. Always emphasize the importance of compliance with the drug regimen.
- Encourage the patient to notify the prescriber if any unusual or adverse reactions occur or if the original condition worsens or fails to improve within a designated period.
- Counsel all female patients of childbearing age regarding the birth defect hazards associated with exposure to certain dermatologic drugs. All sexually active women must use contraception during treatment with any teratogenic medication and for at least 1 month after its discontinuation.
- The beneficial effects of minoxidil may be reduced by heat including the use of a blow dryer.
- With finasteride, used for male pattern alopecia, women are not to handle this drug without gloves or crush the drug (which makes it airborne) due to its teratogenic effects.
- Educate the patient about ways to prevent exposure to the sun through the use of sunscreen and protective clothing, and avoidance of overexposure. Tanning beds create the risk

for skin cancer as well, so share with the patient appropriate and accurate information regarding their use and risk. Sunscreen must also be used with tanning beds.
- The most common cause of skin cancer is exposure to the sun and tanning beds, and early detection and prevention including the use of sunscreen are of utmost importance.
- Vitamin D deficiency may be an issue for some sunscreen users and those who live at higher latitudes or are not exposed to sunlight. As adequate oral intake is difficult to achieve without supplementation, many people with minimal exposure to sunlight do not activate vitamin D and are deficient.
- Assess all skin moles or lesions, and monitor for any unusual changes in color, size, texture, and/or shape.
- Educate about the adverse effects of fluorouracil (Efudex) including the more serious effects of swelling, scaling, pain, pruritus, suppuration, scarring, and hyperpigmentation. It is to be applied with a nonmetallic applicator or gloved fingers.
- Patients taking imiquimod (Aldara) need to be aware of the possibility of severe adverse skin reactions such as edema, erosion/ulceration, scabbing, exudation, and vesicle formation. Additionally, educate patients about the possible systemic immunomodulating effects that need to be reported to their prescriber, such as cough, upper respiratory tract infection, back pain, and lymphadenopathy.
- Adverse effects of lindane (for lice) include skin rash and, rarely, central nervous system toxicity. Lindane's use has been surpassed to some degree by perethrin because of case reports of neurotoxicity, including dizziness, seizures, and deaths. Make sure parents or caregivers understand all instructions regarding this drug's use, application, and cautions/concerns.

KEY POINTS

- Drugs administered directly to the skin are called *topical dermatologic drugs* and are available in a variety of formulations with each having specific characteristics that make them beneficial for certain uses.
- Some of the more common therapeutic categories of dermatologic drugs include the following: antibacterial, antifungal, antiinflammatory, antineoplastic, antipruritic, antiviral, keratolytic, and topical vasodilators. Other categories include dermatologic drugs used as emollients, for debriding, as local anesthetics, and for treating burns.
- Corticosteroids are some of the most widely used topical drugs and are indicated for relief of topical inflammatory and pruritic disorders. Beneficial effects of corticosteroids include antiinflammatory, antipruritic, and vasoconstrictive actions.

- Tar derivatives have antiseptic, antibacterial, and antiseborrheic properties.
- Retinoids are used in the treatment of stable plaque psoriasis and mild to moderately severe facial acne.
- Minoxidil (Rogaine) is used topically in men and women for baldness or hair thinning.
- In 2011, the FDA stated that only those sunscreen products with an SPF of 15 or greater may state that they reduce the risk for skin cancer and early skin aging.
- Patient education about the medication, its administration, and its effectiveness are important to ensure compliance with the treatment regimen.

NCLEX® EXAMINATION REVIEW QUESTIONS

1. The nurse is assessing the skin of a teenage patient who has been using a benzoyl peroxide product for 2 weeks as part of treatment for acne. Which assessment findings indicate that the patient is having an allergic reaction and will need to stop treatment?
   a. Reddened skin over the treatment area
   b. Blistering skin over the treatment area
   c. Peeling skin over the treatment area
   d. Sensation of warmth when the product is applied

2. When considering the variety of OTC topical corticosteroid products, the nurse is aware that which type of preparation is generally most penetrating and effective?
   a. Gel
   b. Lotion
   c. Spray
   d. Ointment

3. The nurse is monitoring for an allergic reaction to topical bacitracin, which would be evident by presence of
   a. petechia.
   b. thickened skin.
   c. itching and burning.
   d. purulent drainage.

4. When the nurse is teaching a patient about the mechanism of action of tretinoin, which statement by the nurse is correct?
   a. "This medication acts by killing the bacteria that cause acne."
   b. "This medication actually causes skin peeling."
   c. "This medication acts by protecting your skin from UV sunlight."
   d. "This medication has antiinflammatory actions."

5. When the nurse is providing wound care with Dakin's solution for a patient who has a stage III pressure ulcer, the patient exclaims, "I smell bleach! Why are you putting bleach on me?" What is the nurse's best explanation?
   a. "This is a very dilute solution and acts to reduce the bacteria in the wound so that it can heal."

   b. "This solution is used instead of medication to promote wound healing."
   c. "This solution is used to dissolve the dead tissue in your wound."
   d. "Don't worry; we would never use bleach on a patient!"

6. The nurse is instructing a parent on the use of lindane (Kwell) shampoo for treatment of a child's head lice. Which statement by the parent indicates a need for further education?
   a. "I will wash his hair, and then rinse out the shampoo immediately."
   b. "I will leave the shampoo on his hair for 4 minutes before rinsing."
   c. "After shampooing, I will rinse and dry his hair."
   d. "When the hair is dry, I will comb the hair to remove the nits."

7. The nurse is performing wound care on a burned area using silver sulfadiazine cream in a patient with an arm wound. Which actions by the nurse are correct? (*Select all that apply.*)
   a. Applying the cream over the previous layer to avoid disturbing the wound bed
   b. Gently cleansing the wound to remove the previous layer of cream and wound debris
   c. Using clean gloves to apply the ointment
   d. Using sterile gloves to apply the ointment
   e. Always covering the wound with a dressing after applying the cream
   f. Washing hands before and after the procedure

8. The nurse is reviewing the use of topical anesthetic drugs. Which of these is an appropriate use for the lidocaine/prilocaine combination cream known as EMLA?
   a. To reduce the discomfort of insect bites
   b. To reduce the pain of sunburn
   c. To relieve the itching associated with poison ivy
   d. To reduce pain before a needle insertion

1. b, 2. d, 3. c, 4. b, 5. a, 6. a, 7. b, d, f, 8. d.

CRITICAL THINKING AND PRIORITIZATION QUESTIONS

1. A 22-year-old woman with severe acne is receiving counseling before taking isotretinoin (Amnesteem). She has read the online iPLEDGE information (see *www.ipledgeprogram.com*) and is shocked to see that two negative pregnancy test results are required before therapy is started and that a pregnancy test must be performed monthly during therapy. What is the nurse's best answer to the patient's concerns?

2. The preoperative nurse is about to perform skin preparation with a povidone-iodine (Betadine) preparation kit before a minor surgical procedure. What is the most important thing for the nurse to assess before performing this preparation?

For answers, see *http://evolve.elsevier.com/Lilley*.

EVOLVE WEBSITE

http://evolve.elsevier.com/Lilley
- Animations
- Answer Keys for Textbook Case Studies and Textbook Critical Thinking and Prioritization Questions

- Content Updates
- Key Points
- Review Questions
- Student Case Studies

57

Ophthalmic Drugs

http://evolve.elsevier.com/Lilley

OBJECTIVES

When you reach the end of this chapter, you will be able to do the following:

1. Discuss the anatomy and physiology of the structures of the eye and the impact of glaucoma and other disorders and disease processes on these structures.
2. List the various classifications of ophthalmic drugs, with examples of specific drugs in each class.
3. Discuss the mechanisms of action, indications, dosage forms with application techniques, adverse effects, cautions, contraindications, and drug interactions of the various ophthalmic drugs.
4. Develop a nursing care plan that includes all phases of the nursing process for patients receiving ophthalmic drugs.

DRUG PROFILES

acetylcholine, p. 907
apraclonidine, p. 908
♦ artificial tears, p. 917
♦ atropine sulfate, p. 916
♦ bacitracin, p. 914
♦ betaxolol, p. 909
♦ ciprofloxacin, p. 914
cromolyn, p. 917
cyclopentolate, p. 916
♦ dexamethasone, p. 915
♦ dipivefrin, p. 908
♦ dorzolamide, p. 910
♦ echothiophate, p. 907
♦ erythromycin, p. 913
fluorescein, p. 916
flurbiprofen, p. 915

♦ gentamicin, p. 913
glycerin, p. 911
ketorolac, p. 915
♦ latanoprost, p. 912
mannitol, p. 911
natamycin, p. 914
olopatadine, p. 917
♦ pilocarpine, p. 907
♦ sulfacetamide, p. 914
tetracaine, p. 916
tetrahydrozoline, p. 917
♦ timolol, p. 909
trifluridine, p. 914

♦ = *Key drug*
! = *High-alert drug*

KEY TERMS

Accommodation The adjustment of the lens of the eye for variations in distance. (p. 903)

Angle-closure glaucoma Glaucoma that occurs as a result of a narrowed anatomic angle between the lens and cornea. Also called *closed-angle glaucoma, narrow-angle glaucoma, congestive glaucoma,* and *pupillary closure glaucoma.* (p. 904)

Anterior chamber The bubble-like portion of the front of the eye between the iris and the cornea. (p. 903)

Aqueous humor The clear, watery fluid circulating in the *anterior* and *posterior chambers* of the eye. (p. 903)

Canal of Schlemm A tiny circular vein at the angle of the anterior chamber of the eye through which the aqueous humor is drained and ultimately funneled into the bloodstream. Also called *Schlemm canal.* (p. 903)

Cataract An abnormal progressive condition of the lens of the eye, characterized by loss of transparency with resultant blurred vision. (p. 903)

Ciliary muscle The circular muscle between the anterior and posterior chambers of the eye behind the iris. It is connected to the suspensory ligaments that control the curvature of the lens. (p. 903)

Cones Photoreceptive (light-receiving) cells in the retina of the eye that enable a person to perceive colors and play a large role in central (straight-ahead) vision. (p. 903)

Cornea The convex, transparent anterior part of the eye. (p. 902)

Cycloplegia Paralysis of the ciliary muscles, which prevents the accommodation of the lens for variations in distance. (p. 903)

Cycloplegics Drugs that paralyze the ciliary muscles of the eye. (p. 903)

Dilator muscle A muscle that constricts the iris of the eye but dilates the pupil. Also called *dilator pupillae.* (p. 903)

Glaucoma An abnormal condition of elevated pressure within an eye because of obstruction of the outflow of aqueous humor. (p. 903)

Intraocular pressure The pressure of the fluids of the eye against the tunics (retina, choroid, and sclera). (p. 903)

Iris The round, muscular portion of the eye that gives the eye its color and serves as an aperture controlling the amount of light passing through the pupil. (p. 903)

Lacrimal ducts Small tubes that drain tears from the lacrimal glands into the nasal cavity. (p. 902)

Lacrimal glands Glands located at the medial corners of the eyelids that produce tears. (p. 902)

Lens The transparent, curved structure of the eye that is located directly behind the iris and the pupil and is attached to the ciliary body by ligaments. (p. 903)

Lysozyme An enzyme with antiseptic actions that destroys some foreign organisms. It is normally present in tears, saliva, sweat, and breast milk. (p. 902)

Miotics Drugs that constrict the pupil. (p. 903)

Mydriatics Drugs that dilate the pupil. (p. 903)

Open-angle glaucoma A type of glaucoma that is often bilateral, develops slowly, is genetically determined, and does not involve a narrowing of the angle between the iris and the cornea. (Also called *chronic glaucoma, wide-angle glaucoma,* and *simple glaucoma.*) (p. 904)

Optic nerve A major nerve that connects the posterior end of each eye to the brain, to which it transmits visual signals. (p. 903)

Pupil A circular opening in the iris of the eye, located slightly to the nasal side of the center of the iris. The pupil lies behind the anterior chamber of the eye and the cornea and in front of the lens. (p. 903)

Retina The innermost layer of the eye, containing both rods and cones that receive visual stimuli and transmit them to the optic nerve. (p. 903)

Rods The photoreceptive elements arranged perpendicularly to the surface of the retina. Rods are especially sensitive to low-intensity light and are responsible for black-and-white and peripheral ("off-to-the-side") vision. (p. 903)

Sphincter pupillae A muscle that expands the iris while constricting or narrowing the diameter of the pupil. (p. 903)

Tears Watery saline or alkaline fluid secreted by the lacrimal glands to moisten the conjunctiva (see Figure 57-1). (p. 902)

Uvea The fibrous tunic beneath the sclera that includes the iris, the ciliary body, and the choroid of the eye (see Figure 57-1). Also called *tunica vasculosa bulbi* or *uveal tract.* (p. 903)

Vitreous body A transparent, semigelatinous substance contained in a thin membrane filling the cavity behind the lens. Also called the *corpus vitreum.* (p. 903)

Vitreous humor The fluid component of the vitreous body. (p. 903)

OVERVIEW

The eye is the organ responsible for the sense of sight. The structures of the eye are illustrated in Figure 57-1. Each eyeball is nearly spherical and approximately 1 inch in diameter. Each eye is recessed into a small frontal skull cavity known as an *orbit.* The exposed anterior (front) portion of the eye is covered by three layers: the protective external layer (cornea and sclera), a vascular middle layer known as the *uvea* (includes the choroid, iris, and ciliary body), and the internal layer, known as the *retina.* All of these layers are protected by the eyelid, which serves as an external protective tissue.

Each eye is held in place and moved by six muscles that are controlled by cranial nerves. These muscles include the rectus and oblique muscles. There are four types of rectus muscles: *inferior, superior, medial,* and *lateral.* There are two types of oblique muscles: *inferior* and *superior.* These muscles are shown in Figure 57-2. (The medial rectus muscle is hidden from view in this figure but is directly across from the lateral rectus muscle.) The levator palpebrae superioris muscle opens the eyelid. This muscle rests on top of the superior rectus muscle. There are several other important structures that are either part

of or adjacent to the eye. The structures and the purpose of each are as follows:

- *Eyebrow:* Rows of short hair above (superior to) the upper eyelids. The eyebrow protects the eye from direct light, falling dust or other small particles, and perspiration coming from the forehead.
- *Eyelid:* The layer of muscle and skin lined interiorly by the conjunctiva. The conjunctiva also covers the outer anterior surface of the eye, which includes the cornea. The eyelid is moveable and can open or close. It protects the eye when closed and allows vision when open.
- *Cornea:* The convex (outward-projecting; opposite of concave), transparent, anterior portion of the eye. It can be thought of as a window that sits in front of the lens and allows the passage of light.
- *Eyelashes:* Two or three rows of hairs that are located on the edge (margin) of the eyelids. They help prevent small particles from falling into the eye when it is open.
- *Palpebral fissure:* The space between the upper and lower eyelids when the eyelids are open but relaxed.
- *Sclera:* A tough, white coat of fibrous tissue that surrounds the entire eyeball except for the cornea. It helps maintain the

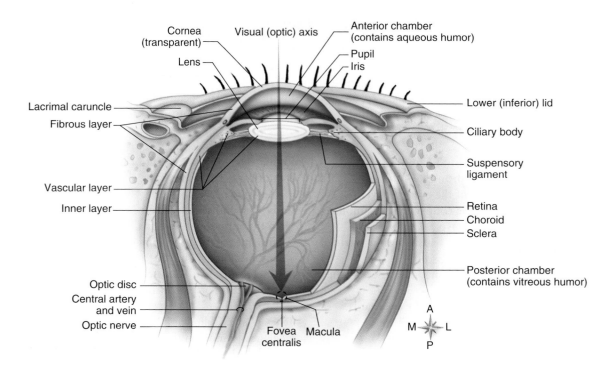

FIGURE 57-1 Horizontal section through the left eyeball, looking from the top down. (Modified from Patton KT, Thibodeau GA: *Anatomy and physiology,* ed 7, St Louis, 2010, Mosby.)

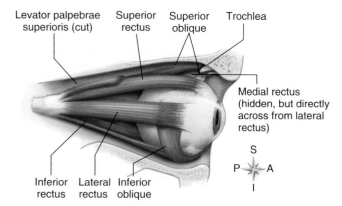

FIGURE 57-2 Extrinsic muscles of the right eye, lateral view. The medial rectus muscle is hidden from view in this figure but is directly across from the lateral rectus muscle. (Modified from Patton KT, Thibodeau GA: *Anatomy and physiology,* ed 7, St Louis, 2010, Mosby.)

shape of the eye. Commonly called the *white* of the eye, the sclera is nonvascular and allows light to pass through it to the lens.

- *Choroid:* One of the middle-layer structures of the eyeball that contains blood vessels that supply the eye; it also absorbs light.
- *Ciliary body:* The structure that supports the ciliary muscles that control the curvature of the lens via attached suspensory ligaments.
- *Conjunctiva:* The mucous membrane that lines the eyelids and also covers the exposed anterior surface of the eyeball.

- *Iris:* The colored (pigmented) muscular apparatus behind the cornea.
- *Pupil:* The variable-sized opening in the center of the iris that allows light to enter into the eyeball when the eyelids are open. The pupil is the rear portion of the window of the eye through which light passes to the lens and the retina (the cornea is the front part of this window).
- *Medial canthus:* The site of union of the upper and lower eyelids near the nose.
- *Lacrimal caruncle:* A small, red, rounded elevation covered by modified skin at the medial angle of the eye; the site of the lacrimal glands (see later in the chapter).
- *Lateral canthus:* The site of union of the upper and lower eyelids away from the nose.

LACRIMAL GLANDS

The eye is kept moist and healthy by an intricate network of connected canals, ducts, and sacs that work together. The lacrimal glands produce tears that bathe and cleanse the exposed anterior portion of the eye. Tears are composed of an isotonic, aqueous solution that contains an enzyme called lysozyme, which acts as an antibacterial to help prevent eye infections. Tears drain into the nasal cavity through the lacrimal ducts.

LAYERS OF THE EYE

Overall, the eye can be thought of as having three separate anatomic layers. The fibrous outer layer of the eye has two parts that are continuous with each other: the sclera and the cornea. The sclera is a tough, fibrous layer that protects and maintains

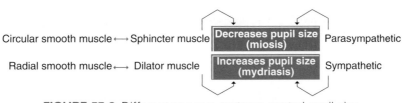

FIGURE 57-3 Different nervous systems control pupil size.

the shape of the eye. The cornea is a nonvascular transparent portion of the outer layer that allows light to enter the eye. It is located at the very front of the eye and is continuous with the sclera. It is pain-sensitive (a protective function) and obtains nutrition from the **aqueous humor**, the clear watery fluid that circulates in the anterior and posterior chambers of the eye.

The vascular middle layer of the eye is composed of the **iris** (to the anterior), ciliary body, and choroid (to the posterior). These three structures are collectively called the **uvea**. The iris gives color to the eye and has an adjustable opening in the center called the **pupil**. The main function of the iris is to regulate the amount of light that enters the eye by causing the size of the pupil to vary. Pupil size is controlled by two smooth muscles. The **sphincter pupillae** muscle is controlled by the parasympathetic nervous system and constricts the diameter of the pupil (called *miosis*) (Figure 57-3). In contrast, the pupil is opened (called *mydriasis*) by a radial smooth muscle called the **dilator muscle**. It is composed of radiating fibers, like spokes of a wheel, which converge from the circumference of the iris toward its center. Sympathetic nervous system impulses control this muscle (see Figure 57-3).

The anterior portions of both the retina and choroid merge to become the ciliary body, which produces aqueous humor. This is the clear, watery fluid that circulates in both the anterior and posterior chambers, not to be confused with tears. Aqueous humor contributes, along with **vitreous humor**, to the **intraocular pressure** of the eye. This is the internal pressure of all fluids against the tunics (retina, choroid, sclera) of the eye. Given the small space of the eye, any change in the volume of aqueous humor present can lead to increased or reduced intraocular pressure. Normally, the aqueous humor is removed from the **anterior chamber** via the **canal of Schlemm** at a rate that balances out its production by the ciliary body. The ciliary body also provides a support for the suspensory ligaments to which the lens is attached. The **lens** is the transparent crystalline structure of the eye, located directly behind the iris and the pupil. It has a biconvex (oval-spherical) shape and is held in place by suspensory ligaments that are attached to the **ciliary muscle**. Contraction of the ciliary muscle changes the shape of the lens. This function is important for visual accommodation as well as the focusing of light (and visual images) onto the retina. The ciliary muscle is controlled by the parasympathetic nervous system through the oculomotor cranial nerve (cranial nerve III). The lens divides the interior of the eyeball into posterior (rear) and anterior (forward) chambers. The larger chamber behind the lens is filled with a jellylike fluid called the **vitreous body**. The lens is transparent to allow light to pass through easily. A loss of lens transparency results in a visual condition

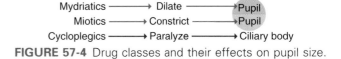

FIGURE 57-4 Drug classes and their effects on pupil size.

called a **cataract**. A cataract is a gray-white opacity that can be seen within the lens. If cataracts are untreated, sight may eventually be completely lost. At the onset of a cataract, vision is blurred and may be further worsened by the glare of bright lights. *Diplopia* or double vision may also develop.

Before light rays reach the retina, they are focused into a sharp image by the lens of the eye. The elasticity of the lens enables it to change its shape and focusing power. This process is called **accommodation** and is facilitated by the ciliary body. Paralysis of accommodation is called **cycloplegia**. **Mydriatics** are drugs that dilate the pupil (e.g., apraclonidine). Drugs that constrict the pupil are called **miotics** (e.g., acetylcholine, pilocarpine). Drugs that paralyze the ciliary body are called **cycloplegics**, but they also have mydriatic properties (e.g., atropine, cyclopentolate) (Figure 57-4). All of these medications are used to facilitate visualization of the inner eye during ophthalmic examinations.

The third and inner layer of the eye is a thin delicate layer known as the **retina**. It contains light-sensitive photoreceptors called **rods** and **cones**. The basic function of the retina is to receive the light image formed by the lens and to convert it via the rods and cones into the neural signals that support vision. Rods produce black-and-white vision, including shades of gray, and are especially sensitive in low light; cones are responsible for color vision (Figure 57-5). In addition, rods are more active in providing peripheral (to-the-side) vision, whereas cones are more active in central (straight-ahead) vision. In the posterior central part of the retina, the nerve fibers of retinal cells join to form the **optic nerve**. The function of this nerve is to connect the retina with the visual center of the brain, located within the occipital lobe that extends above and behind the cerebellum. It is this portion of the brain that interprets incoming visual stimuli.

PATHOPHYSIOLOGY OF GLAUCOMA

Glaucoma is a group of eye disorders that damages the optic nerve. In most cases, this is due to increased intraocular pressure that is caused by abnormally elevated levels of aqueous humor. Glaucoma occurs when the aqueous humor is not drained through the canal of Schlemm as quickly as it is formed by the ciliary body. The accumulated aqueous humor creates a

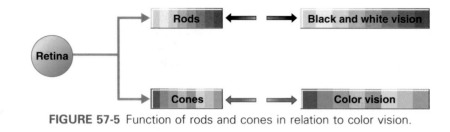

FIGURE 57-5 Function of rods and cones in relation to color vision.

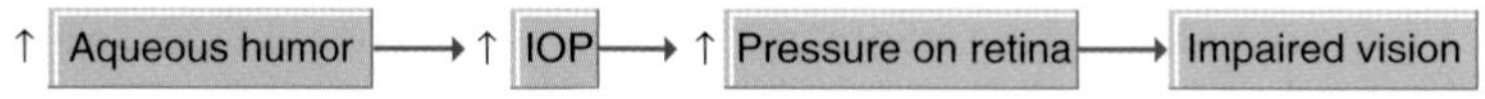

FIGURE 57-6 How increased aqueous humor can result in impaired vision. *IOP*, Intraocular pressure.

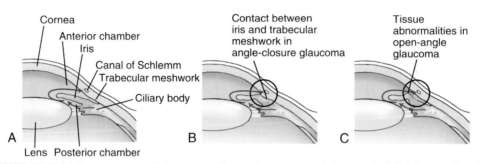

FIGURE 57-7 Main structures of the eye and an enlargement of the canal of Schlemm showing the flow of aqueous humor. **A,** Flow in a normal eye. **B,** In angle-closure glaucoma, the closure of the anterior angle due to contact between the iris and the trabecular meshwork prevents aqueous humor from exiting through the canal of Schlemm, which leads to increased intraocular pressure. **C,** In open-angle glaucoma, the anterior angle remains open, but the canal of Schlemm is obstructed by tissue abnormalities. (Modified from McKenry LM, Tessier E, Hogan MA: *Mosby's pharmacology in nursing,* ed 22, St Louis, 2006, Mosby.)

backward pressure that pushes the vitreous humor against the retina. Continued pressure on the retina destroys its neurons, which leads to impaired vision and eventual blindness (Figure 57-6). Unfortunately, glaucoma is often without early symptoms, and many patients are not diagnosed until some permanent sight loss has occurred.

Two major types of glaucoma are discussed in this chapter: angle-closure glaucoma and open-angle glaucoma. Figure 57-7 shows the pathophysiology of each and provides an enlarged view of the involved eye structures. Table 57-1 lists additional characteristic features of each type. Glaucoma can be a primary illness (occurring on its own), or it can be secondary to another eye condition or injury (e.g., posttraumatic glaucoma). Congenital glaucoma can also occur in infants. The visual and optic nerve changes typical of glaucoma can also occur in the absence of increased intraocular pressure (normotensive glaucoma). There are a few other less common forms of glaucoma (e.g., pigmentary glaucoma, pseudoexfoliative glaucoma) that are beyond the scope of this textbook.

TABLE 57-1	**Glaucoma: Types and Characteristics**	
	Angle-Closure Glaucoma	**Open-Angle Glaucoma**
Synonyms	Closed-angle glaucoma, narrow-angle glaucoma, congestive glaucoma, pupillary closure glaucoma	Chronic glaucoma, wide-angle glaucoma, simple glaucoma
Chronicity	Acute (can cause rapid vision loss)	Chronic
Relative incidence	Less common	More common
Nature of angle	Narrow	Larger
Most common age of onset and race	30 yr or older, white	30 yr or older, African American
Major symptoms	Blurred vision, severe headaches, eye pain	Blurred vision, occasional headaches
Treatment	Topical or systemic drugs, surgery	Topical or systemic drugs, surgery

PHARMACOLOGY OVERVIEW

Medications used to treat disorders of the eye can be divided into several major drug groups: antiglaucoma drugs, antimicrobials, antiinflammatory drugs, topical anesthetics, diagnostic drugs, antiallergic drugs, and lubricants and moisturizers. There are also a variety of combination drug products that include two or more medications from different subclasses. The reader can assume the same therapeutic indications and drug effects for these combination products as for the single-ingredient drug products corresponding to their individual components. The focus of this chapter is on commonly used therapeutic medications. Although rare, systemic adverse effects can occur with eyedrops if given in large quantities. Note that systemic reactions are not discussed in this chapter, unless the frequency is common.

A multitude of various products are also available for use in the care of contact lenses, including contact lens–cleaning enzymes, irrigating solutions, and eye washes. Their use is fairly straightforward, and they carry limited risk. More complicated surgical drugs are beyond the scope of this chapter. The reader is advised to refer to the manufacturer's packaging information for details about any unfamiliar product encountered in clinical practice.

ANTIGLAUCOMA DRUGS

Treatment of glaucoma involves reducing intraocular pressure by either increasing the drainage of aqueous humor or decreasing its production. Some drugs may do both. Drug therapy can delay and possibly even prevent the development of glaucoma. The different classes of eyedrops, including those for glaucoma, are color-coded according to medication class to aid the patient in identification. Eyedrops for glaucoma are listed in Table 57-2. There is a movement by the FDA to eliminate color coding, however it currently exists. It is imperative that nurses never rely merely on color coding. Labels on all medications, including eyedrops, must always be read before administering. Eyedrop labels are particularly bothersome because the print is very small. See Safety and Quality Improvement: Preventing Medication Errors on this page.

Drug classes used to reduce intraocular pressure include the following:

- Direct-acting cholinergics (also called *miotics* and *parasympathomimetic drugs*)
- Indirect-acting cholinergics (also called *miotics, cholinesterase inhibitors,* and *parasympathomimetic drugs*)
- Adrenergics (also called *mydriatics* and *sympathomimetic drugs*)
- Antiadrenergics (beta blockers; also called *sympatholytic drugs*)
- Carbonic anhydrase inhibitors

TABLE 57-2   Antiglaucoma Drugs: Effects on Aqueous Humor

Drug Class	Increased Drainage	Decreased Production
Miotics		
Direct-acting cholinergics	+++	0
Indirect-acting cholinergics (cholinesterase inhibitors)	+++	0
Mydriatics		
Sympathomimetics	++	+++
Others		
Beta blockers	+	+++
Carbonic anhydrase inhibitors	0	+++
Osmotic diuretics	+++	0
Prostaglandin agonists	+++	0

0, No effect; +, minor effect; ++, moderate effect; +++, pronounced effect.

- Osmotic diuretics
- Prostaglandin agonists

See Table 57-2 for a comparison of the effects of these drugs on aqueous humor.

CHOLINERGIC DRUGS (MIOTICS)

There are two categories of ocular parasympathetic drugs, more concisely referred to as *cholinergic drugs:* direct acting and indirect acting. Direct-acting cholinergics include acetylcholine, carbachol, and pilocarpine. Indirect-acting drugs, which are also called *cholinesterase inhibitors,* include echothiophate, currently the only available drug in this class. Because the primary drug effect of these drugs is pupillary constriction, or *miosis* (see later), they are also commonly called *miotics.*

Mechanism of Action and Drug Effects

Acetylcholine is the neurochemical mediator of nerve impulses in the parasympathetic nervous system. It stimulates parasympathetic or cholinergic receptors located in the brain and throughout the body along parasympathetic nerve branches. This results in several effects on the eye: miosis (pupillary constriction), vasodilation of blood vessels in and around the eye, contraction of ciliary muscles, drainage of aqueous humor, and reduced intraocular pressure. Ciliary muscle contraction promotes aqueous humor drainage by widening the space where the drainage occurs. Miosis promotes aqueous humor drainage by causing the iris to stretch, which also serves to widen this space.

Both direct- and indirect-acting miotics have effects similar to those of acetylcholine, but their actions are more prolonged (Figure 57-8). The direct-acting miotics are able to directly stimulate ocular cholinergic receptors and mimic acetylcholine. Indirect-acting miotics work by binding to and inactivating the cholinesterases acetylcholinesterase and pseudocholinesterase, the enzymes that break down acetylcholine. As a result, acetylcholine accumulates and acts longer at the cholinergic receptor sites. This leads to drug effects that include miosis, ciliary muscle contraction, enhanced aqueous humor drainage, and reduced intraocular pressure by an average of 20% to 30% (Figure 57-9). Drug-induced miotic effects may be less pronounced in individuals with dark eyes (e.g., brown or hazel)

⚡ SAFETY AND QUALITY IMPROVEMENT: PREVENTING MEDICATION ERRORS   `QSEN`

Read the Labels! Do Not Rely on Color-Coding

For years, several classes of eye drops for glaucoma have been color-coded so that patients can differentiate the various eye drops that may be prescribed. This practice has long been endorsed by the American Academy of Ophthalmology. However, the practice of relying on bottle cap colors instead of reading the labels or scanning barcodes has led to medication errors. The Institute for Safe Medication Practice (ISMP) has spoken out against this practice because of errors that have occurred when the wrong medication with the same color cap has been administered. The ISMP has also been critical of the small print that manufacturers use on dropper bottles. It is essential to follow the nine rights of medication administration and read all medication labels carefully! For more information, see *www.ismp.org.*

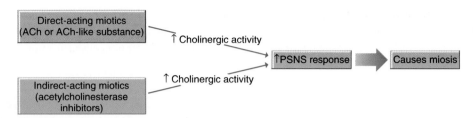

FIGURE 57-8 Cholinergic response of miosis to parasympathomimetic drugs. *ACh*, Acetylcholine; *PSNS*, parasympathetic nervous system.

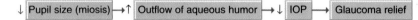

FIGURE 57-9 Therapeutic effects of direct- and indirect-acting miotics on glaucoma. *IOP*, Intraocular pressure.

than in those with lighter eyes (e.g., blue). This is because the pigment of the iris also absorbs the drug (which reduces its therapeutic effects), and dark eyes have more pigment.

Indications

The direct- and indirect-acting miotics are used for treatment of open-angle glaucoma, angle-closure glaucoma, and convergent strabismus (a condition in which one eye points toward the other, or "cross-eye") and in ocular surgery. They are also used to reverse the effect of mydriatic (pupil-dilating) drugs after ophthalmic examination. Specific indications may vary for different drugs, as shown in Table 57-3.

Contraindications

Contraindications to the use of miotics include known drug allergy and any serious active eye disorder in which induction of miosis might be harmful.

Adverse Effects

Most of the adverse effects from the use of cholinergics and cholinergic inhibitors (miotics) are local and limited to the eye. Adverse effects are more likely to occur with indirect-acting miotics because they have longer-lasting effects. Effects include blurred vision, drug-induced myopia (nearsightedness), and accommodative spasms. Such effects are secondary to contraction of the ciliary muscle. Miotic drugs also cause vasodilation of blood vessels supplying the conjunctiva, iris, and ciliary body, which may lead to vascular congestion and ocular inflammation. Other undesirable effects include temporary stinging upon drug instillation, reduced nighttime or low-light vision,

TABLE 57-3   Miotics: Indications

Drug	Indications
acetylcholine	Need for complete and rapid miosis after cataract lens extraction, iridectomy
carbachol	Open-angle glaucoma
echothiophate	Accommodative esotropia, obstructive aqueous humor outflow, open- and angle-closure glaucoma after iridectomy
pilocarpine	Open-angle glaucoma, secondary glaucoma after iridectomy, reversal of cycloplegia

conjunctivitis, lacrimation (tearing), twitching of the eyelids (blepharospasm), and eye or brow pain. Prolonged use can result in iris cysts, lens opacities, and, rarely, retinal detachment.

Interactions

Drug interactions are unlikely because of the local actions of these drugs. When miotic drugs are given with topical adrenergics, antiadrenergics (e.g., beta blockers), or carbonic anhydrase inhibitors, additive lowering effects on intraocular pressure can be seen.

Dosages

For dosage information on selected miotic drugs, see the table on this page.

DRUG PROFILES

Direct-acting ocular cholinergics include acetylcholine (Miochol-E), carbachol (Carboptic), and pilocarpine (Pilocar).

DOSAGES

Selected Miotics

Drug (Pregnancy Category)	Pharmacologic Class	Usual Dosage Range	Indications
acetylcholine (Miochol-E) (C)	Direct-acting cholinergic	0.5 to 2 mL intraocular injection pre-op	Need for surgical miosis
◆ echothiophate (Phospholine Iodide) (C)	Indirect-acting cholinergic	1 drop 1-2 times daily	Early and advanced chronic open-angle glaucoma; glaucoma secondary to cataract surgery; accommodative esotropia
◆ pilocarpine (Pilocar, Isopto Carpine, Akarpine, Pilopine HS) (C)	Direct-acting cholinergic	Solution: 1-2 drops 3-4 times daily Gel: 0.5-inch ribbon into lower conjunctival sac at bedtime (use any other eyedrops at least 5 min before gel)	Chronic open-angle and angle-closure glaucoma; acute angle-closure glaucoma; preoperative and postoperative intraocular hypertension; need for reversal of drug-induced mydriasis

Indirect-acting drugs, which are also called *cholinesterase inhibitors*, include echothiophate (Phospholine Iodide). These drugs are used for management of glaucoma, as adjuncts for ocular surgery, and for treatment of various other ophthalmic conditions.

DIRECT-ACTING MIOTICS
acetylcholine
Acetylcholine (Miochol-E) is a direct-acting cholinergic drug that is used to produce miosis during ophthalmic surgery. It is a pharmaceutical form of the naturally occurring neurotransmitter in the body. It has a very quick onset and may begin to work almost immediately. It is administered directly into the anterior chamber of the eye before and after securing one or more sutures.

Pharmacokinetics: Acetylcholine

Route	Onset of Action	Peak Plasma Concentration	Elimination Half-life	Duration of Action
Ocular	Instant	Instant	3 min	10 min

◆ pilocarpine
Pilocarpine (Pilocar) is a direct-acting cholinergic drug that is used as a miotic in the treatment of glaucoma. Pilocarpine is available in different strengths as an ocular gel and solution. One special formulation is the pilocarpine ocular insert system (Ocusert Pilo-20), which is applied once weekly by the patient.

Pharmacokinetics Pilocarpine

Route	Onset of Action	Peak Plasma Concentration	Elimination Half-life	Duration of Action
Ocular (Immediate Release Formulation)	10-30 min	75 min	Unknown	4-8 hr

INDIRECT-ACTING MIOTIC
◆ echothiophate
Echothiophate (Phospholine Iodide) is an indirect-acting cholinergic that has an organophosphate structure and acts by phosphorylating cholinesterase enzymes. This effect is normally irreversible until new enzymes are synthesized by the body, which may take days or even weeks. For these reasons, this drug is considered to be long acting.

Pharmacokinetics: Echothiophate

Route	Onset of Action	Peak Plasma Concentration	Elimination Half-life	Duration of Action
Ocular	10-30 min	24 hr	Long	7-28 days

SYMPATHOMIMETICS (MYDRIATICS)

Sympathomimetic drugs are used for the treatment of glaucoma and ocular hypertension. These drugs include the alpha receptor agonists brimonidine (Alphagan P) and apraclonidine (Iopidine), as well as the alpha and beta receptor agonists epinephryl (Epinal) and dipivefrin (Propine).

Mechanism of Action and Drug Effects

Sympathomimetic drugs mimic the sympathetic neurotransmitters norepinephrine and epinephrine. They stimulate the dilator muscle to contract by means of alpha and/or beta receptor interaction. This stimulation results in increased pupil size or *mydriasis* (Figure 57-10). Dilation is seen within minutes of instillation of the ophthalmic drops and lasts for several hours, during which time the intraocular pressure is reduced (Figure 57-11). Alpha receptor stimulation reduces intraocular pressure by enhancing aqueous humor outflow through the canal of Schlemm. Production of aqueous humor by the ciliary body is also reduced. Both of these effects appear to be dose dependent.

Indications

Both epinephrine and dipivefrin are used to reduce elevated intraocular pressure in the treatment of chronic open-angle glaucoma, either as initial therapy or as long-term therapy. Increases in intraocular pressure during ophthalmic surgery are usually mediated via increased catecholamine stimulation of the sympathetic nervous system. Apraclonidine stimulates the alpha₂ receptors, which oppose those effects, and thus corrects the surgery-induced elevation in intraocular pressure. Brimonidine also has primarily alpha₂ activity but is used to lower

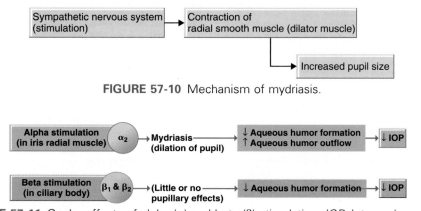

FIGURE 57-10 Mechanism of mydriasis.

FIGURE 57-11 Ocular effects of alpha (α) and beta (β) stimulation. *IOP*, Intraocular pressure.

Selected Ocular Sympathomimetics

Drug (Pregnancy Category)	Pharmacologic Class	Usual Dosage Range	Indications/Uses
apraclonidine (Iopidine) (C)	Direct acting	0.5% solution: 1-2 drops 3 times daily	Short-term adjunctive therapy for glaucoma not controlled by other drugs
◆dipivefrin (Propine) (C)	Direct acting	1 drop every 12 hr	Chronic open-angle glaucoma

intraocular pressure in patients with open-angle glaucoma or ocular hypertension.

Contraindications

Contraindications for the sympathomimetic ophthalmics include known drug allergy.

Adverse Effects

Adverse effects of the sympathomimetic mydriatics are primarily limited to ocular effects and include burning, eye pain, and lacrimation. Such effects are usually temporary and may subside as the patient grows accustomed to the medication. Other ocular effects may include conjunctival hyperemia, localized melanin deposits in the conjunctiva, and release of pigment granules from the iris.

Interactions

With sufficient topical absorption, sympathomimetic mydriatics have the potential to react with other drugs; however, when used in normal doses, drug interactions are not significant.

Dosages

For dosage information on sympathomimetic drugs, see the table on this page.

DRUG PROFILES

Sympathomimetic ophthalmic drugs include dipivefrin (Propine), epinephryl (Epinal), apraclonidine (Iopidine), and brimonidine (Alphagan P). These drugs are used for management of glaucoma and ocular hypertension, and for ocular surgery.

apraclonidine

Apraclonidine (Iopidine) is structurally and pharmacologically related to the alpha$_2$ stimulant clonidine. It reduces intraocular pressure 23% to 39% by stimulating alpha$_2$ and beta$_2$ receptors. It also prevents ocular vasoconstriction, which reduces ocular blood pressure as well as aqueous humor formation. Apraclonidine is primarily used to inhibit perioperative intraocular pressure increases, rather than to treat glaucoma. Brimonidine (Alphagan P) is a similar drug but is used primarily for glaucoma.

Pharmacokinetics: Apraclonidine

Route	Onset of Action	Peak Plasma Concentration	Elimination Half-life	Duration of Action
Ocular	1 hr	3-5 hr	8 hr	12 hr

◆dipivefrin

Dipivefrin (Propine) is a synthetic sympathomimetic miotic drug. It is a prodrug of epinephrine that has little or no pharmacologic activity until hydrolyzed in the eye to two chemically modified forms of epinephrine. These chemical alterations account for the main advantage of this drug over epinephrine: it has enhanced lipophilicity (fat solubility) and can better penetrate into the tissues of the anterior chamber of the eye. This quality also reduces the likelihood of any systemic adverse effects. Dipivefrin typically reduces mean intraocular pressure approximately 15% to 25%. On a weight basis, dipivefrin is 4 to 11 times as potent as epinephrine in reducing intraocular pressure and 5 to 12 times as potent as epinephrine in terms of its mydriatic effects. Epinephryl (Epinal) is a newer drug with similar properties and uses.

Pharmacokinetics: Dipivefrin

Route	Onset of Action	Peak Plasma Concentration	Elimination Half-life	Duration of Action
Ocular	30 min	1 hr	1-3 hr	12 hr

BETA-ADRENERGIC BLOCKERS

The antiglaucoma beta-adrenergic blockers that reduce intraocular pressure include the beta$_1$-selective drugs betaxolol and levobetaxolol.

Mechanism of Action and Drug Effects

The ophthalmic beta blockers reduce both elevated and normal intraocular pressure. They reduce intraocular pressure by reducing aqueous humor formation. In addition, timolol may produce a minimal increase in aqueous outflow.

Indications

Ophthalmic beta blockers are used to reduce elevated intraocular pressure in various conditions, including chronic open-angle glaucoma and ocular hypertension. They may also be used alone or in combination with a topical miotic (e.g., echothiophate iodide, pilocarpine), topical dipivefrin, and/or systemic carbonic anhydrase inhibitors. When used in combination, these drugs may have an additive intraocular pressure-lowering effect. They may also be used to treat some forms of angle-closure glaucoma.

Contraindications

Contraindications for ophthalmic beta blockers include known drug allergy and any ocular condition for which beta-receptor blockade might be harmful.

Adverse Effects

The adverse effects of antiglaucoma beta blockers are primarily limited to ocular effects. The most common ocular effects are transient burning and discomfort. Other effects include blurred vision, pain, photophobia, lacrimation, blepharitis, keratitis (inflammation of the cornea), and decreased corneal sensitivity. Because these drugs are administered topically, few, if any, systemic effects are expected.

Interactions

Drug interactions with systemic drugs are unlikely due to the primarily localized nature of ophthalmically administered drugs.

Dosages

For dosage information on beta-adrenergic blockers, see the table on this page.

DRUG PROFILES

The currently available ophthalmic beta-blocking drugs are betaxolol (Betoptic), carteolol (Ocupress), levobunolol (Betagan), levobetaxolol (Betaxon), metipranolol (OptiPranolol), and timolol (Timoptic). These drugs are used to treat glaucoma and ocular hypertension.

◆ betaxolol

Betaxolol (Betoptic) is a beta$_1$-selective beta blocker. It is one of the most potent and selective beta-blocking drugs. Its ability to decrease aqueous humor formation and reduce intraocular pressure has made it an excellent drug for the treatment of ocular disorders such as open-angle glaucoma and ocular hypertension.

Pharmacokinetics: Betaxolol

Route	Onset of Action	Peak Plasma Concentration	Elimination Half-life	Duration of Action
Ocular	0.5-1 hr	2 hr	Unknown	More than 12 hr

◆ timolol

Timolol (Timoptic) differs slightly from the other ophthalmic beta blockers in that it may increase the outflow of aqueous humor as well as decrease its formation. The drug acts at both beta$_1$ and beta$_2$ receptors and is indicated for the treatment of open-angle glaucoma and ocular hypertension. It is available in various liquid forms, both with and without preservatives. Preservative-free products were developed because of patient allergies to benzalkonium chloride, a commonly used preservative. Timolol is also available in a gel-forming solution (with preservatives). The gel-forming products are longer acting and allow for once-daily dosing, a convenience over the twice-daily dosing that many patients require of the other timolol formulations.

Pharmacokinetics: Timolol

Route	Onset of Action	Peak Plasma Concentration	Elimination Half-life	Duration of Action
Ocular	15-30 min	1-2 hr	Unknown	12-24 hr

CARBONIC ANHYDRASE INHIBITORS

Ophthalmic carbonic anhydrase inhibitors include brinzolamide (Azopt) and dorzolamide (Trusopt). These two drugs are available only in topical ophthalmic form. Systemic carbonic anhydrase inhibitors for oral use are sometimes also used as adjunct drug therapy for glaucoma and are described in Chapter 28. Both drugs are also sulfonamides and are chemically related to the sulfonamide antibiotics (see Chapter 38). They are to be used with caution in patients who are allergic to sulfa antibiotics.

Mechanism of Action and Drug Effects

Carbonic anhydrase inhibitors work by inhibiting the enzyme carbonic anhydrase, which results in decreased intraocular pressure by reduction of aqueous humor formation.

Indications

Ocular carbonic anhydrase inhibitors are used primarily for management of glaucoma, including both open-angle and angle-closure glaucoma; they may also be used preoperatively to control intraocular pressure.

Contraindications

Contraindications include known drug allergy and any ocular condition for which their use might be harmful in the judgment of an ophthalmologist. Allergy to sulfonamide antibiotics is a precaution, not a contraindication; however, patients need to be educated on the possibility of cross-reaction.

Adverse Effects

Systemic absorption of these drugs occurs, although systemic adverse effects are unlikely. The same adverse effects listed for sulfonamide antibiotics in Chapter 38 can theoretically occur with these drugs. Patients with sulfa allergies may develop cross-sensitivities to the carbonic anhydrase inhibitors.

DOSAGES

Selected Ocular Beta Blockers

Drug (Pregnancy Category)	Pharmacologic Class	Usual Dosage Range	Indications
◆ betaxolol (Betoptic, Betoptic S) (C)	Direct acting	1-2 drops twice daily	Chronic open-angle glaucoma; ocular hypertension
◆ timolol (Betimol, Timoptic, Timoptic-XE) (C)	Direct acting	Solution: 1 drop twice daily Gel-forming solution: 1 drop daily	Open-angle glaucoma; ocular hypertension

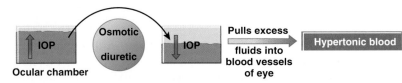

FIGURE 57-12 Mechanism and ocular effects of osmotic diuretics. *IOP,* Intraocular pressure.

DOSAGES
Ocular Carbonic Anhydrase Inhibitor

Drug (Pregnancy Category)	Pharmacologic Class	Usual Dosage Range	Indications
♦ dorzolamide (Trusopt) (C)	Carbonic anhydrase inhibitor	1 drop 3 times daily	Open-angle glaucoma; ocular hypertension

Interactions

Drug interactions with ocular carbonic anhydrase inhibitors are rare.

Dosages

For dosage information on the carbonic anhydrase inhibitor dorzolamide, see the table on this page.

DRUG PROFILE

The two most commonly used ocular carbonic anhydrase inhibitors are brinzolamide (Azopt) and dorzolamide (Trusopt).

♦ dorzolamide

Dorzolamide (Trusopt) is indicated for treatment of elevated intraocular pressure associated with either ocular hypertension or open-angle glaucoma. It is available only as an ophthalmic solution. The other drug in this class, brinzolamide, has comparable indications, dosages, and pharmacokinetics.

Pharmacokinetics: Dorzolamide

Route	Onset of Action	Peak Plasma Concentration	Elimination Half-life	Duration of Action
Ocular	Rapid	Variable	3-4 mo	Variable

OSMOTIC DIURETICS

Osmotic drugs may be administered either intravenously, orally, or topically to reduce intraocular pressure. The osmotic diuretics that are most commonly used for this purpose are glycerin and mannitol.

Mechanism of Action and Drug Effects

Osmotic diuretics reduce ocular hypertension by causing the blood to become hypertonic in relation to both intraocular and spinal fluids. This creates an osmotic gradient that draws water from the aqueous and vitreous humors into the bloodstream,

TABLE 57-4 Osmotic Diuretics: Adverse Effects

Body System	Adverse Effects
Cardiovascular	Edema, thrombophlebitis, hypotension, hypertension, tachycardia, angina-like chest pains, fever, chills
Central nervous	Dizziness, headache, convulsions, rebound increased intracranial pressure, confusion
Electrolytes	Fluid electrolyte imbalances, acidosis, dehydration
Eyes, ears, nose, throat	Loss of hearing, blurred vision, nasal congestion
Gastrointestinal	Nausea, vomiting, dry mouth, diarrhea
Genitourinary	Marked diuresis, urinary retention, thirst

which causes a reduction in the volume of intraocular fluid; the result is a decrease in intraocular pressure (Figure 57-12). Systemic (nonocular) effects of these drugs are discussed in Chapter 28.

Indications

Ocular uses for osmotic diuretics include treatment of acute glaucoma episodes and reduction of intraocular pressure before or after ocular surgery. Typically, glycerin is used first; if the treatment is unsuccessful, mannitol is tried. Isosorbide and urea are two other osmotic drugs that may also be used in similar situations. They are usually administered after glycerin or mannitol has failed.

Contraindications

Osmotic diuretics are contraindicated in patients with known drug allergy, pronounced anuria, acute pulmonary edema, cardiac decompensation, and severe dehydration, because they can worsen all of these conditions.

Adverse Effects

The most frequent reactions to osmotic diuretics are nausea, vomiting, and headache. The most significant adverse effects are fluid and electrolyte imbalances. Other effects are possible irritation and thrombosis at the injection site. Other potential adverse effects are listed in Table 57-4.

Interactions

The only significant drug interaction is increased lithium excretion associated with mannitol and urea.

Dosages

For dosage information on osmotic drugs, see the table on the next page.

DRUG PROFILES

Osmotic diuretics include mannitol, glycerin, urea, and isosorbide. These drugs are normally reserved for acute reduction of intraocular pressure during glaucoma crises and perioperative reduction of intraocular pressure in ophthalmic surgery.

glycerin

Glycerin is an osmotic drug given orally to lower intraocular pressure or topically to reduce superficial corneal edema. Another use is before iridectomy in individuals with acute narrow-angle glaucoma. It is also used preoperatively and/or postoperatively in procedures such as treatment of congenital glaucoma, repair of retinal detachment, cataract extraction, and keratoplasty (corneal transplant). It may also be used in the management of secondary glaucoma.

Pharmacokinetics: Glycerin

Route	Onset of Action	Peak Plasma Concentration	Elimination Half-life	Duration of Action
Ocular	10-30 min	1-1.5 hr	30-45 min	4-5 hr

mannitol

Mannitol (Osmitrol) is administered by intravenous infusion to reduce elevated intraocular pressure when the pressure cannot be lowered by other methods. Mannitol is effective in treating acute episodes of angle-closure, absolute, or secondary glaucoma and in lowering intraocular pressure before intraocular surgery. Mannitol does not penetrate the eye and may be used when irritation is present, unlike some of the other osmotic drugs, such as urea.

Pharmacokinetics: Mannitol

Route	Onset of Action	Peak Plasma Concentration	Elimination Half-life	Duration of Action
IV	30-60 min	1 hr	15-100 min	6-8 hr

PROSTAGLANDIN AGONISTS

The newest class of drugs used to treat glaucoma is the prostaglandin agonists. The three most commonly used drugs in this class include latanoprost (Xalatan), travoprost (Travatan-Z), bimatoprost (Lumigan), and tafluprost (Zioptan).

Mechanism of Action and Drug Effects

Prostaglandins reduce intraocular pressure by increasing the outflow of aqueous humor between the uvea and sclera as well as via the usual exit through the trabecular meshwork (see Figure 57-7). A single dose of a prostaglandin agonist lowers intraocular pressure for 20 to 24 hours, which allows a single daily dosing regimen. The drug effects are primarily limited to these ocular effects.

Indications

Prostaglandin agonists are used in the treatment of glaucoma.

Contraindications

The only usual contraindication is known drug allergy.

Adverse Effects

Prostaglandin agonists are generally well tolerated. Adverse effects include foreign body sensation, punctate epithelial keratopathy (dotted appearance of the cornea), stinging, conjunctival hyperemia ("bloodshot" eyes), blurred vision, itching, and burning. There is one unique adverse effect associated with all prostaglandin agonists: in some people with hazel, green, or bluish-brown eye color, eye color will turn permanently brown, even if the medication is discontinued. This adverse effect appears to be cosmetic only with no known ill effects on the eye.

DOSAGES

Ocular Prostaglandin Agonist

Drug (Pregnancy Category)	Pharmacologic Class	Usual Dosage Range	Indications
◆ latanoprost (Xalatan) (C)	Prostaglandin	1 drop every day in evening	Open-angle glaucoma and ocular hypertension in patients who are intolerant of or whose condition is uncontrolled by other drugs

DOSAGES

Osmotic Diuretics

Drug (Pregnancy Category)	Pharmacologic Class	Usual Dosage Range	Indications/Uses
glycerin (Ophthalgan) (C)	Organic alcohol	1-2 drops before eye examination as a lubricant; more if needed during examination	Gonioscopy of edematous cornea
mannitol (Osmitrol) (C)	Organic alcohol	IV: 1.5-2 g/kg infused over at least 30 min; for preoperative use, give 1-1.5 hr before surgery	Acute reduction of elevated intraocular pressure

Interactions

Concurrent administration of prostaglandin agonists with any other eyedrops containing the preservative thimerosal may result in precipitation. It is recommended that the two medications be administered at least 5 minutes apart.

Dosages

For dosage information on the prostaglandin agonist latanoprost, see the table on the previous page.

DRUG PROFILE

♦ latanoprost

Latanoprost is a prodrug of a naturally occurring prostaglandin known as *prostaglandin F₂-alpha*. When it is administered, it is converted by hydrolysis (with water from ocular fluids) to prostaglandin F_2-alpha, which in turn reduces intraocular pressure. Latanoprost is available only in eyedrop form. About 3% to 10% of patients treated with latanoprost (Xalatan) have shown increased iris pigmentation after 3 to $4\frac{1}{2}$ months of treatment.

Pharmacokinetics: Latanoprost

Route	Onset of Action	Peak Plasma Concentration	Elimination Half-life	Duration of Action
Ocular	30-60 min	2 hr	17 min	24 hr

ANTIMICROBIAL DRUGS

A variety of infections can occur in the eye; many are self-limiting. However, some infections require the use of ocular antimicrobials to be eliminated. Topical antimicrobials used to treat ocular infections include antibacterial, antifungal, and antiviral drugs. All require a prescription. Many of these drugs are also available for systemic administration for treatment of infections elsewhere in the body. The most commonly used antimicrobials from the main antimicrobial drug classes are discussed in this chapter. Some common eye infections may require antibiotic therapy and are listed in Table 57-5. The choice of a particular ophthalmic antimicrobial drug is based on the following:

- Clinical experience
- Sensitivity and characteristics of the organisms most likely to have caused the infection
- Characteristics of the disease itself
- Sensitivity and response of the patient
- Laboratory results (culture and sensitivity testing)

Mechanism of Action and Drug Effects

Topical antimicrobials used to treat infections of the eye work to destroy the invading organism. Their specific antimicrobial actions are similar to those described for systemically administered drugs, which are discussed in Chapters 38, 39, 40, and 42. Some antimicrobials destroy the causative organism, whereas others simply inhibit the organism's growth, allowing the body's immune system to fight the infection.

TABLE 57-5	**Common Ocular Infections**
Infection	**Description**
Blepharitis	Inflammation of the eyelids.
Conjunctivitis	Inflammation of the conjunctiva (the mucous membrane lining the back of the eyelids and the front of the eye except the cornea). It may be bacterial or viral and is often associated with common colds. When caused by *Haemophilus* organisms, it is commonly called *pink eye*. It is highly contagious but usually self-limiting.
Hordeolum (sty)	Acute localized infection of the eyelash follicles and the glands of the anterior lid. It results in the formation of a small abscess or cyst.
Keratitis	Inflammation of the cornea caused by bacterial infection. Herpes simplex keratitis is caused by viral infection.
Uveitis	Infection of the uveal tract or the vascular layer of the eye, which includes the iris, ciliary body, and choroid.
Endophthalmitis	Inflammation of the inner eye structure caused by bacteria.

Indications

The indication for ocular antimicrobials is known or suspected infection with one or more specific microorganisms. Empirical treatment is based on reasonable clinical evaluation of presenting signs and symptoms. Topical use of antimicrobials helps prevent the antimicrobial drug resistance that could arise from unnecessary systemic use. However, systemic antimicrobials may be administered to treat more severe ocular infections.

Contraindications

Contraindications to the use of antimicrobials include known drug allergy or other severe previous adverse drug reaction.

Adverse Effects

The most common adverse effects of ocular antibiotics are local and transient inflammation, burning, stinging, urticaria, dermatitis, angioedema, and drug hypersensitivity. Topical application of antimicrobial drugs may also interfere with growth of the normal bacterial flora of the eye, which may encourage the growth of other, more harmful organisms. If large doses are given, systemic side effects are possible.

Interactions

Systemic drug interactions are unlikely due to the primarily local effects of ocular antimicrobials. One possible interaction involves the concurrent use of antibiotics and corticosteroids (e.g., dexamethasone). Corticosteroids have immunosuppressive effects that may impede the therapeutic effects of ocular antimicrobials.

Dosages

For dosage information on ocular antimicrobials, see the table on the next page.

DRUG PROFILES

AMINOGLYCOSIDES

Aminoglycosides (see Chapter 39) are antimicrobials that destroy bacteria by interfering with protein synthesis in bacterial cells, which leads to bacteria death. Aminoglycosides used to treat ocular infections include gentamicin (Garamycin) and tobramycin (Tobrex). Adverse effects include swollen eyelids, mydriasis, and local erythema. Systemic reactions are rare because of poor topical absorption. Overgrowth of nonsusceptible organisms, which can lead to eye infections that are resistant to treatment, is a possibility.

◆ gentamicin

Gentamicin (Garamycin) is effective against a wide variety of gram-negative and gram-positive organisms. It is particularly useful against *Pseudomonas, Proteus,* and *Klebsiella* organisms. Gram-positive organisms that are effectively destroyed by gentamicin include staphylococci and streptococci that have developed resistance to other antibiotics. Gentamicin is available as an ophthalmic ointment and a solution.

Pharmacokinetics: Gentamicin

Route	Onset of Action	Peak Plasma Concentration	Elimination Half-life	Duration of Action
Ocular	Variable	Immediate	Unknown	6-12 hr

MACROLIDE ANTIBIOTICS

Macrolide antibiotics include erythromycin, azithromycin, and other drugs (see Chapter 38). Erythromycin is the most commonly used macrolide for ophthalmic use.

◆ erythromycin

Erythromycin is a macrolide antibiotic indicated for the treatment of various ophthalmic infections, as well as other infections. It is available in oral and intravenous forms and as an ophthalmic ointment. Erythromycin eye ointment is indicated for the treatment of neonatal conjunctivitis caused by *Chlamydia trachomatis* and for the prevention of eye infections in newborns that may be caused by *Neisseria gonorrhoeae* or other susceptible organisms.

Pharmacokinetics: Erythromycin

Route	Onset of Action	Peak Plasma Concentration	Elimination Half-life	Duration of Action
Ocular	Variable	Immediate	Unknown	Variable

POLYPEPTIDE ANTIBIOTICS

Bacitracin and polymyxin B are polypeptide antibiotics. These drugs are rarely used systemically because of their nephrotoxic effects. They are bactericidal antimicrobials that inhibit protein synthesis in susceptible organisms, which leads to cell death.

DOSAGES

Selected Ocular Antimicrobials

Drug (Pregnancy Category)	Pharmacologic Class	Usual Dosage Range	Indications
Antibacterial Drugs			
◆ bacitracin (AK-Tracin) (C)	Miscellaneous antibiotic	Ointment: 0.5-inch ribbon into lower conjunctival sac 3-4 times daily	
◆ ciprofloxacin (Ciloxan) (C)	Quinolone	Solution: 1-2 drops every 2 hr for 2 days, and then 2 drops every 4 hr	
		Ointment: 0.5-inch ribbon tid for 2 days, then 0.5-inch ribbon twice daily for 5 days	Bacterial ocular infections
◆ erythromycin (Ilotycin) (C)	Macrolide	Ointment: 0.5-inch ribbon 2-6 times/day	
◆ gentamicin (Genoptic, others) (C)	Aminoglycoside	Solution: 1-2 drops every 2-4 hr	
		Ointment: 0.5-inch ribbon 2-3 times/day	
◆ sulfacetamide (Bleph-10, others) (C)	Sulfonamide	Solution: 1-2 drops every 2-3 hr	
		Ointment: Apply 0.5 inch ribbon 4 times a day	
Antifungal Drug			
natamycin (Natacyn) (C)	Antifungal	1 drop into conjunctival sac every 1-2 hr, and then usually reduce after first 3-4 days to 6-8 drops/day; therapy usually continues for 14-21 days	Fungal ocular infections
Antiviral Drug			
trifluridine (Viroptic) (C)	Antiviral	Initially 1 drop every 2 hr while awake (max 9 drops/day and 21 days per episode)	Viral ocular infections: keratitis and keratoconjunctivitis due to HSV types 1 and 2

They are most commonly used in the treatment of superficial infections caused by gram-positive bacteria.

◆bacitracin

Bacitracin (AK-Tracin) is an ophthalmic antimicrobial drug used to treat various eye infections. It is available as a single-ingredient product and as a combination product with polymyxin or neomycin and polymyxin. The combination products have a broader spectrum of activity. Bacitracin is available in ointment form.

Pharmacokinetics: Bacitracin

Route	Onset of Action	Peak Plasma Concentration	Elimination Half-life	Duration of Action
Ocular	Variable	Immediate	Unknown	Variable

QUINOLONE ANTIBIOTICS

Quinolone antibiotics are very effective broad-spectrum antibiotics. They are discussed in detail in Chapter 39. They are bactericidal, destroying a wide spectrum of organisms that are often very difficult to treat. Currently five ophthalmic quinolones are available: ciprofloxacin (Ciloxan), gatifloxacin (Zymar), moxifloxacin (Vigamox), levofloxacin (Quixin), and ofloxacin (Ocuflox).

Significant adverse effects include formation of corneal precipitates during treatment for bacterial keratitis. Other reactions include corneal staining and infiltrates. Systemic reactions are limited because of poor topical absorption. Those that occur are usually taste disorders and nausea. There are no significant drug interactions.

◆ciprofloxacin

Ciprofloxacin (Ciloxan) is a synthetic quinolone antibiotic. It is available in ointment and solution form. Ciprofloxacin is indicated for the treatment of bacterial keratitis and conjunctivitis caused by susceptible gram-positive and gram-negative bacteria. One notable adverse reaction to ophthalmic ciprofloxacin is the appearance of white, crystalline precipitates occurring within any corneal lesions. This has occurred in approximately 17% of patients, and within 1 to 7 days of starting therapy. In all cases to date, the condition has been self-limiting, has not required drug discontinuation, and has not adversely affected clinical outcome.

Pharmacokinetics: Ciprofloxacin

Route	Onset of Action	Peak Plasma Concentration	Elimination Half-life	Duration of Action
Ocular	Variable	Immediate	1-2 hr	Variable

SULFONAMIDES

Sulfonamides are synthetic bacteriostatic antibiotics that work by blocking the synthesis of folic acid in susceptible bacteria. Sulfacetamide sodium (Bleph-10) and sulfisoxazole (Gantrisin) are used to treat conjunctivitis and other ocular infections caused by susceptible bacteria.

The adverse effects are primarily limited to local reactions and include local irritation and stinging. Sulfonamide use can result in the overgrowth of nonsusceptible organisms. No significant topical toxic effects have been reported with the use of ophthalmic sulfonamides.

◆sulfacetamide

Sulfacetamide (Bleph-10) is the most commonly used ophthalmic sulfonamide antibacterial drug. It is available in solution and ointment form.

Pharmacokinetics: Sulfacetamide

Route	Onset of Action	Peak Plasma Concentration	Elimination Half-life	Duration of Action
Ocular	Variable	Immediate	Unknown	Variable

ANTIFUNGAL DRUG

natamycin

Natamycin (Natacyn) is a polyene antifungal drug. It destroys fungi in the eye by binding to sterols in the fungal cell membrane, which disrupts the protective capabilities of the cell and results in cell death. Natamycin is used topically in the treatment of blepharitis, conjunctivitis, and keratitis caused by susceptible fungi (*Candida* and *Aspergillus* species). It is available only in suspension form.

Pharmacokinetics: Natamycin

Route	Onset of Action	Peak Plasma Concentration	Elimination Half-life	Duration of Action
Ocular	Variable	Immediate	Unknown	Variable

ANTIVIRAL DRUGS

Three antiviral ophthalmic drugs are currently available: fomivirsen (Vitravene), ganciclovir (Vitrasert), and trifluridine (Viroptic). Fomivirsen and ganciclovir are used to treat cytomegalovirus infections; they are implanted in the eye by an ophthalmologist and are beyond the scope of this chapter.

trifluridine

Trifluridine (Viroptic, 1% ophthalmic drops) is a pyrimidine nucleoside. It inhibits viral replication by blocking the synthesis of viral deoxyribonucleic acid (DNA) by inhibiting viral DNA polymerase, an enzyme needed for DNA synthesis. It is used for ocular infections (keratitis and keratoconjunctivitis) caused by types 1 and 2 of the herpes simplex virus. Significant adverse effects include secondary glaucoma, corneal punctate defects, uveitis, and stromal edema (edema in the tough, fibrous, transparent portion of the cornea known as the *stroma*). The drugs exhibit no appreciable topical absorption, and no significant drug interactions have been reported.

ANTIINFLAMMATORY DRUGS

Many of the same antiinflammatory drugs used systemically may also be used ophthalmically to treat various ocular

BOX 57-1   Ophthalmic Antiinflammatory Drugs

Nonsteroidal Antiinflammatories
- bromfenac (Xibrom)
- diclofenac (Voltaren)
- flurbiprofen (Ocufen)
- ketorolac (Acular)

Corticosteroids
- dexamethasone (Decadron, others)
- fluocinonide (Retisert)
- fluorometholone (Fluor-Op, others)
- loteprednol (Lotemax, others)
- medrysone (HMS)
- prednisolone (Pred Forte, others)
- rimexolone (Vexol)

inflammatory disorders and ocular surgery-related pain and inflammation. These drugs include both nonsteroidal antiinflammatory drugs (NSAIDs) and corticosteroids and are listed in Box 57-1.

Mechanism of Action and Drug Effects

Corticosteroids and NSAIDs, as discussed in Chapters 33 and 44, respectively, both act to reduce inflammatory responses. When tissues are damaged, the membranes of affected cells release phospholipids, which are broken down by several different enzymes within the arachidonic acid metabolic pathway. Phospholipase is one of the first enzymes involved, and its activity is inhibited by corticosteroids. A second enzyme, cyclooxygenase, is the site of action of the NSAIDs. Both drug actions reduce the production of various inflammatory mediators. This in turn reduces pain, erythema, and other inflammatory processes.

Indications

Corticosteroids and NSAIDs are applied topically for the symptomatic relief of many ophthalmic inflammatory conditions. They may be used to treat corneal, conjunctival, and scleral injuries from chemical, radiation, or thermal burns or from penetration of foreign bodies. They are used during the acute phase of the injury process to prevent fibrosis and scarring, which result in visual impairment. Corticosteroids produce a greater immunosuppressant effect than the NSAIDs. Consequently, NSAIDs are often preferred as initial topical therapy for such injuries. NSAIDs are also used in the symptomatic treatment of seasonal allergic conjunctivitis.

Corticosteroids and NSAIDs are used prophylactically before ocular surgery to prevent or reduce the intraoperative miosis. They are also used prophylactically after ocular surgery, such as cataract extraction, glaucoma surgery, and corneal transplantation, to prevent inflammation and scarring.

Contraindications

These drugs are contraindicated in cases of known drug allergy. In addition, they are not used for minor abrasions or wounds because they may suppress the ability of the eye to resist bacterial, viral, or fungal infections. This is especially true of corticosteroids, which have stronger immunosuppressant effects.

Adverse Effects

The most common adverse effect of corticosteroids is transient burning or stinging on application. The extended use of corticosteroids may result in cataracts, increased intraocular pressure, and optic nerve damage. If large doses are given, systemic absorption is possible. Systemic side effects of corticosteroids and NSAIDs are discussed in Chapters 33 and 44, respectively.

DRUG PROFILES

Corticosteroids and NSAIDs used to treat ophthalmic inflammatory disorders are listed in Box 57-1. The ophthalmic formulations share many of the same characteristics as their systemic drug counterparts. However, the ophthalmic derivatives have limited systemic absorption. Therefore, most therapeutic and toxic effects are restricted to the eye. These drugs are classified as pregnancy category C drugs.

CORTICOSTEROID

♦ dexamethasone

Dexamethasone (Decadron) is a synthetic corticosteroid that is available in many systemic and ophthalmic formulations. It is used to treat inflammation of the eye, eyelids, conjunctiva, and cornea, and it may also be used in the treatment of uveitis, iridocyclitis, allergic conditions, and burns and in the removal of foreign bodies. Dexamethasone is available in ointment, suspension, and solution form.

Pharmacokinetics: Dexamethasone

Route	Onset of Action	Peak Plasma Concentration	Elimination Half-life	Duration of Action
Ocular	Variable	Immediate	Unknown	Variable

NONSTEROIDAL ANTIINFLAMMATORY DRUGS

flurbiprofen

Flurbiprofen (Ocufen) is an NSAID used to treat inflammatory ophthalmic conditions, such as postoperative inflammation after cataract extraction. It is also used to inhibit intraoperative miosis that may be induced by operative trauma and tissue injury. Flurbiprofen is available in solution form.

Pharmacokinetics: Flurbiprofen

Route	Onset of Action	Peak Plasma Concentration	Elimination Half-life	Duration of Action
Ocular	30 min	90 min	Unknown	3 hr

ketorolac

Ketorolac (Acular) is an NSAID that is available in both oral and injectable formulations for systemic use. The ophthalmic formulation is used to reduce ocular inflammation caused by trauma, such as ocular surgery, and inflammation secondary to external agents, such as allergens and bacteria. Ketorolac is contraindicated in patients with known drug allergy. It is available in solution form. It is important to know that this drug may delay eye wound healing and lead to corneal epithelial breakdown; therefore, constantly monitor the eye throughout the duration of therapy.

Pharmacokinetics: Ketorolac

Route	Onset of Action	Peak Plasma Concentration	Elimination Half-life	Duration of Action
Ocular	Rapid	Immediate	Unknown	4-6 hr

TOPICAL ANESTHETICS

Topical anesthetic ophthalmic drugs are local anesthetics that are used to alleviate eye pain. The two currently available topical anesthetics used for ophthalmic purposes are proparacaine and tetracaine.

Mechanism of Action and Drug Effects

As described in Chapter 11, local anesthetics stabilize the membranes of nerves, which results in a decrease in the movement of ions into and out of the nerve endings. When nerves are stabilized in this way, they cannot transmit signals about painful stimuli to the brain. Usually, the application of topical anesthetic drugs to the eye results in local anesthesia in less than 30 seconds.

Indications

Ophthalmic topical anesthetic drugs are used to produce ocular anesthesia for short corneal and conjunctival procedures. They prevent pain during surgical procedures and certain painful ophthalmic examinations, including removal of imbedded foreign objects. They are recommended only for short-term use and are not recommended for self-administration.

Contraindications

Contraindications to local ophthalmic anesthetics include known drug allergy.

Adverse Effects

Adverse effects are rare with ophthalmic anesthetic drugs and are limited to local effects such as stinging, burning, redness, lacrimation, and blurred vision.

Interactions

Because of limited systemic absorption and short duration of action, ophthalmic anesthetic drugs have no significant drug interactions.

DRUG PROFILE

Currently available topical ophthalmic anesthetic drugs are proparacaine (Alcaine) and tetracaine (generic only). They are very similar in their indications and dosing regimens.

tetracaine

Tetracaine is a local anesthetic of the ester type (see Chapter 11). It is applied as an eyedrop to numb the eye for various ophthalmic procedures. Tetracaine begins to work in about 25 seconds and lasts for about 15 to 20 minutes. Additional drops are applied as needed. It is currently available only in solution form. It is classified as a pregnancy category C drug.

Pharmacokinetics: Tetracaine

Route	Onset of Action	Peak Plasma Concentration	Elimination Half-life	Duration of Action
Ocular	Less than 30 sec	1-5 min	Short	15-20 min

DIAGNOSTIC DRUGS

DRUG PROFILES
CYCLOPLEGIC MYDRIATICS
◆ atropine sulfate

Atropine sulfate (Isopto Atropine) solution and ointment are used as mydriatic and cycloplegic drugs. The drug dilates the pupil (mydriasis) and paralyzes the ciliary muscle (cycloplegic refraction), which prevents accommodation. It is used to assist in eye examination or to treat uveal tract inflammatory states. The usual dosage for uveitis (inflammation of the choroid, iris, or ciliary body) in children and adults is 1 to 2 drops of the solution, or 0.3 to 0.5 cm of ointment, 2 to 3 times daily. The dosage for eye examination is 1 drop of solution, ideally 1 hour before the procedure. It is classified as a pregnancy category C drug.

cyclopentolate

Cyclopentolate solution (Cyclogyl) is used primarily as a diagnostic mydriatic and cycloplegic drug. Unlike atropine, it is not used to treat uveitis. The usual adult dose is 1 to 2 drops (0.5%, 1%, or 2%). This is repeated in 5 to 10 minutes if needed. The dose for children is the same as that for adults. The drug effects usually subside within 24 hours. Other cycloplegic mydriatics are scopolamine (Isopto Hyoscine), homatropine (Isopto Homatropine), and tropicamide (Mydriacyl). All three are topical ophthalmic solutions with indications similar to those of atropine and cyclopentolate, except that tropicamide, like cyclopentolate, is generally used for diagnostic purposes only and not for treatment of inflammatory states. It is classified as a pregnancy category C drug.

OPHTHALMIC DYE
fluorescein

Fluorescein (AK-Fluor) is an ophthalmic diagnostic dye used to identify corneal defects and to locate foreign objects in the eye. It is also used in fitting hard contact lenses. After the instillation of fluorescein, various defects are highlighted in either bright green or yellow-orange, and foreign objects have a green halo around them. Fluorescein is available for use as an ophthalmic injection, solution, and diagnostic applicator strips. Dose determination and drug administration are usually carried out by an ophthalmologist. It is classified as a pregnancy category C drug.

ANTIALLERGIC DRUGS

DRUG PROFILES

ANTIHISTAMINES
olopatadine

Olopatadine (Patanol) is an ocular antihistamine used to treat symptoms of allergic conjunctivitis (hay fever), which can be seasonal or nonseasonal. It works by competing at the receptor sites for histamine. Histamine normally produces ocular symptoms such as itching and tearing. Other ocular antihistamines include azelastine (Optivar), emedastine (Emadine), ketotifen (Zaditor), and epinastine (Elestat). These drugs have mechanisms of action, therapeutic and adverse effects, and drug interactions similar to those of the systemic antihistamines described in Chapter 36, although systemic effects are less likely with ophthalmic administration. Recommended dosages for olopatadine are given in the dosages table below. It is classified as a pregnancy category C drug.

MAST CELL STABILIZERS
cromolyn

Cromolyn sodium (Crolom) is an antiallergic drug that inhibits the release of inflammation-producing mediators from sensitized inflammatory cells called *mast cells*. It is used in the treatment of vernal keratoconjunctivitis (springtime inflammation of the cornea and conjunctiva). Other mast cell stabilizers with similar effects are pemirolast (Alamast), nedocromil (Alocril), and lodoxamide (Alomide). Recommended dosages for cromolyn are given in the dosages table below. It is classified as a pregnancy category B drug.

DECONGESTANTS
tetrahydrozoline

Tetrahydrozoline is an ocular decongestant. It works by promoting vasoconstriction of blood vessels in and around the eye. This reduces the edema associated with allergic and inflammatory processes. It is specifically indicated to control redness, burning, and other minor irritations. Other ocular decongestants include phenylephrine (Neo-Synephrine), oxymetazoline (Visine LR), and naphazoline (Clear Eyes). Recommended dosages for tetrahydrozoline are given in the dosages table below. It is classified as a pregnancy category C drug.

LUBRICANTS AND MOISTURIZERS
♦ artificial tears

An array of products is available over the counter to provide lubrication or moisture for the eyes. This is helpful to patients with dry or otherwise irritated eyes. Artificial tears are isotonic and contain buffers to adjust pH. In addition, they contain preservatives for microbial control and may contain viscosity agents for extension of ocular activity. Selected over-the-counter brand names include Moisture Drops, Murine, Nu-Tears, Akwa Tears, and Tears Plus. Many similar products are available on the market both as solutions (eyedrops) and as lubrication ointments. They are often dosed to patient comfort as needed. Restasis is an ophthalmic form of the immunosuppressant drug cyclosporine (see Chapter 48). It is also used to promote tear production in the condition technically known as *keratoconjunctivitis sicca* (dry eyes). It can be used together with artificial tears, if the drugs are given 15 minutes apart. It is classified as a pregnancy category B drug.

NURSING PROCESS

ASSESSMENT

Before administering any *ophthalmic drug* per the prescriber's orders, perform a baseline assessment of the eye and its structures, documenting normal and abnormal findings. It is also important to document any redness, swelling, pain, excessive tearing, eye drainage or discharge, decrease in visual acuity, or other unusual symptoms. Assess the patient for hypersensitivity to any medications or chemicals and for any drug- or disorder-related contraindications, cautions, and drug interactions. Drug interactions are not generally problematic because of the low dosages associated with ophthalmic administered medications. A Snellen visual acuity chart test may need to be performed, if indicated. Note the findings before, during, and after drug treatment. Focus the nursing history on past

DOSAGES

Ocular Antiallergics

Drug (Pregnancy Category)	Pharmacologic Class	Usual Dosage Range	Indications
cromolyn (Crolom) (C)	Mast cell stabilizer	1-2 drops in affected eye(s) 4-6 times daily	Vernal (springtime) conjunctivitis and/or keratitis (corneal inflammation)
olopatadine (Patanol 0.1%) (C)	Antihistamine	1 drop in affected eye(s) 2 times per day at an interval of 6-8 hours	Allergic conjunctivitis
olopatadine (Patanol 0.2%) (C)	Antihistamine	1 drop in affected eye(s) once a day	Allergic conjunctivitis
tetrahydrozoline (Murine Plus, others) (C)	Decongestant	1-2 drops in affected eye(s) up to 4 times daily as needed	Redness, burning, or other minor irritation

or present systemic disease processes and exposure to any chemicals that could be topical irritants to the eye, skin, or mucous membranes, including past or present occupational and environmental exposures.

NURSING DIAGNOSES

1. Acute pain related to the eye disorder, infection, and/or inflammatory eye condition
2. Deficient knowledge related to lack of information about the eye disorder and associated medication therapy
3. Risk for injury (to eye) related to improper use of medication and improper instillation procedures

PLANNING: OUTCOME IDENTIFICATION

1. Patient remains free from eye pain with proper administration of ophthalmic medications and uses non-aspirin analgesics and warm or cold compresses as prescribed.
2. Patient demonstrates adequate knowledge related to the use of the medication, its application, and side effects.
3. Patient remains free from injury (to eye) related to safe, self-administered therapy with implementing of safe environment at home.

CASE STUDY

Safety: What Went Wrong? Medications for Eye Trauma

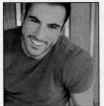 P.L., a construction worker, is being seen in the emergency department because of a possible eye injury. He was working without eye protection, and a gust of wind sprayed metal shavings into his face. The emergency department physician has instilled fluorescein sodium and has noted areas in the eyeball with green halos around them.

1. What is the purpose of the fluorescein sodium, and what is indicated by the green halos?
2. P.L. is sent to an ophthalmologist for further treatment. What eye medication do you expect will be used for the next procedure?
3. After the procedure, P.L. receives a prescription for dexamethasone ocular ointment, to be administered three times a day. What specific patient teaching information will the nurse share with P.L.?
4. How could this accident have been prevented?

For answers, see *http://evolve.elsevier.com/Lilley.*

IMPLEMENTATION

Always inspect the solution, and administer only clear, unexpired products (e.g., drops, ointments, solutions) to the eye. Currently, all classes of eyedrops are color-coded to help the patient in identification. However, the FDA is moving to eliminate all color coding. Imperative to patient safety is to not rely on color coding but to always read the prescriber's order and carry out the Nine Rights of medication administration (see Chapter 1). Shake all solutions, and mix contents thoroughly. Do not use solutions with any particulate matter. One of the most important standards to follow during instillation of drops or ointment is to avoid touching the eye with the tip of the dropper or container to prevent contamination of the product. Remove any excess medication promptly, and apply pressure to the inner canthus for 1 minute (or other specified time frame). Applying pressure to the inner canthus after instillation of medication is needed to prevent or decrease systemic absorption and subsequent systemic adverse effects. Apply ointments and any other ophthalmic topical drug dosage form to the conjunctival sac and never directly onto the eye itself (cornea). To facilitate the instillation of *ophthalmic medication*, tilt the patient's head back and have him or her look up at the ceiling. Several ophthalmic drugs with different actions may be ordered; give each drug exactly as prescribed and within the specified period. This is particularly important when surgical procedures are being performed on the eye because several drugs with different actions may be ordered and must be given at specific times. Ointments may cause a temporary blurring of vision because of the film that bathes the eye. This film will decrease once the drug is absorbed, and vision will then become clearer. Always refer to the medication order, as well as an authoritative drug source for specific instructions and guidelines regarding application technique, length of time to apply pressure to the inner canthus, and any other special directions. See Chapter 9 for ophthalmic drug administration.

Follow directions for the use of *antiviral ophthalmic preparations* closely. Administer *topical anesthetics*, as ordered, for use in removal of a foreign body or treatment of eye injury. Repeated and continuous use is not recommended because of the risk for delayed wound healing, corneal perforation, permanent corneal opacities, and vision loss. When there is an abrasion or other injury to the eye and appropriate medications are ordered, patching of the affected eye is recommended. This helps prevent further injury resulting from loss of the blink reflex due to overuse of topical anesthetic. Include education regarding any change in eye color caused by the medication. For example, *latanoprost* actually changes the eye color permanently from hazel, green, or bluish-brown to brown. See Patient-Centered Care: Patient Teaching on the next page for more information regarding ophthalmic medications.

EVALUATION

Therapeutic responses to *miotics* include decreased aqueous humor of the eye with resultant decreased intraocular pressure and decreased signs, symptoms, and long-term effects associated with glaucoma. *Beta-adrenergic blockers* are therapeutic if there is a resultant decrease in intraocular pressure. Therapeutic responses to *antibiotic, antifungal,* and *antiviral ophthalmic drugs* include elimination of the infection or condition and resolution of symptoms, and prevention of complications. Therapeutic responses to *ophthalmic anesthetics* include prevention/relief of pain associated with the injury. Systemic absorption associated with the specific medication is rare because of the low dosage amount utilized, and so systemic adverse effects are not common. Local reactions may include some discomfort, tearing, and irritation. *Antiinflammatory ophthalmic solutions result* in a decrease in allergic reactions with a decrease in itching, tearing, redness, and eye discharge. Potential complications of these solutions include swelling of the conjunctiva (chemosis). Further monitoring includes reevaluation of goals and outcome criteria.

PATIENT-CENTERED CARE: PATIENT TEACHING

- Educate the patient about correct administration technique. A demonstration with return demonstrations by the patient is a highly recommended teaching strategy.
- Encourage the patient to use only solutions that are clear and unexpired. Keep eyedroppers and solutions in containers for direct application sterile by avoiding touching the tip of the eyedropper or container to the surface of the eye.
- Educate patients that systemic adverse effects are uncommon because of the low dosage amount of the specific drug composed in the ophthalmic solution. With any ophthalmic drug, instruct the patient to report to the prescriber any severe stinging, burning, itching, or redness of the eye; excessive tearing or excessive dryness of the eye; puffiness of the eye/eyelids; discharge from the eye; fever; eye pain; or loss of or change in vision.
- Instill sympatholytic drugs as ordered. Once these drugs (and many other drugs used in the eye) are instilled, instruct the patient to apply pressure to the inner canthus with a tissue or 2-inch by 2-inch gauze pad for 1 full minute or as directed. Application of pressure to the inner canthus helps to minimize absorption and decrease the risk for systemic adverse effects.

- Photosensitivity is an expected adverse effect of mydriatics; therefore, when these drugs are administered, encourage the patient to wear sunglasses to help minimize eye discomfort and/or headaches while in sunlight.
- With topical anesthetics, advise the patient to avoid rubbing or touching the eye while it is numb, because eye damage may result. An eye patch may be worn, if prescribed, to protect the eye because of loss of the blink reflex.
- Instruct the patient to use ophthalmic medications as prescribed and never to overuse. Stress that products with expiration dates that have passed are not to be used and are to be discarded appropriately. Advise the patient never to stop medications without consulting the prescriber first because of the possibility of adverse reactions.
- Inform the patient not to wear contact lenses while ophthalmic drugs are being instilled and for the duration of therapy, because the lenses may lead to further irritation.
- Ophthalmic ketorolac, an antiinflammatory drug, may delay eye wound healing and lead to corneal epithelial breakdown. Instruct the patient to report these problems if present or suspected.

KEY POINTS

- Glaucoma is a disorder of the eye caused by inhibition of the normal flow and drainage of aqueous humor, and treatment helps to reduce intraocular pressure either by increasing the drainage of aqueous humor or decreasing its production.
- Drugs that increase aqueous humor drainage are direct cholinergics, indirect cholinergics, sympathomimetics, and beta blockers.
- A large proportion of the inflammatory diseases of the eye are caused by viruses, and many ocular antimicrobials are available to treat bacterial, viral, and fungal infections of the eye. Common ocular infections include conjunctivitis, hordeolum (sty), keratitis, uveitis, and endophthalmitis.

- Antiinflammatory ophthalmic drugs include corticosteroids and are used to inhibit inflammatory responses to mechanical forces, chemicals, and immunologic reactions.
- Topical anesthetics are used to prevent pain to the eye and are beneficial during surgery, ophthalmic examinations, and removal of foreign bodies.
- Administer all ophthalmic preparations exactly as ordered. Always apply into the conjunctival sac. Safe and accurate application or instillation technique also includes avoiding contact of the eyedropper or tube with the eye to prevent contamination of the drug.
- Advise patients to report to the prescriber immediately any increase in symptoms, such as eye pain or drainage and fever.

NCLEX® EXAMINATION REVIEW QUESTIONS

1. The ophthalmologist has given a patient a dose of ocular atropine drops before an eye examination. Which statement by the nurse accurately explains to the patient the reason for these drops?
   a. "These drops will cause the surface of your eye to become numb so that the doctor can do the examination."

   b. "These drops are used to check for any possible foreign bodies or corneal defects that may be in your eye."
   c. "These drops will reduce your tear production for the eye examination."
   d. "These drops will cause your pupils to dilate, which makes the eye examination easier."

2. When assessing a patient who is receiving a direct-acting cholinergic eyedrop as part of treatment for glaucoma, the nurse anticipates that the drug affects the pupil in which way?
   a. It causes mydriasis, or pupil dilation.
   b. It causes miosis, or pupil constriction.
   c. It changes the color of the pupil.
   d. It causes no change in pupil size.

3. During patient teaching regarding self-administration of ophthalmic drops, which statement by the nurse is correct?
   a. "Hold the eyedrops over the cornea, and squeeze out the drop."
   b. "Apply pressure to the lacrimal duct area for 5 minutes after administration."
   c. "Be sure to place the drop in the conjunctival sac of the lower eyelid."
   d. "Squeeze your eyelid closed tightly after placing the drop into your eye."

4. When the nurse is providing teaching about eye medications for glaucoma, the nurse tells the patient that miotics help glaucoma by which mechanism of action?
   a. Decreasing intracranial pressure
   b. Decreasing intraocular pressure
   c. Increasing tear production
   d. Causing pupillary dilation

5. During the assessment of a glaucoma patient who has newly prescribed carbonic anhydrase inhibitor eyedrops, the nurse would report a history of which condition?
   a. Allergy to sulfa drugs
   b. Decreased renal function
   c. Diabetes mellitus
   d. Hypertension

6. The nurse is preparing to administer ketorolac (Acular) eyedrops. The patient asks, "Why am I getting these eyedrops?" What is the nurse's correct response?
   a. "These drops will reduce the pressure inside your eye as part of treatment for glaucoma."
   b. "These drops are for a bacterial eye infection."
   c. "These drops will relieve your dry eyes."
   d. "These drops work to reduce the inflammation in your eyes."

7. A patient has undergone an eye procedure during which ophthalmic mydriatics and anesthetic drops were used. The nurse gives which instructions to the patient prior to discharge? *(Select all that apply.)*
   a. "Do not rub or touch the numb eye."
   b. "You may reinsert your contact lenses before you leave."
   c. "Be sure to wear sunglasses when you go outside."
   d. "Your pupils will appear very tiny until the medication wears off."
   e. "Report any increase in eye pain or drainage to the ophthalmologist immediately."

8. The nurse is administering sympathomimetic ophthalmic drops. Which therapeutic drug effect will these drops have on the patient's eyes?
   a. Miosis
   b. Reduced intraocular pressure
   c. Reduced inflammation
   d. Increased lubrication.

1. d, 2. b, 3. c, 4. b, 5. a, 6. d, 7. a, c, e, 8. b.

CRITICAL THINKING AND PRIORITIZATION QUESTIONS

1. A patient has a prescription for latanoprost (Xalatan). What is the most important piece of information that the nurse needs to tell the patient *before* the patient starts taking this medication?

2. The nurse is assessing the eyes of a patient who had ocular surgery 1 week earlier. The patient has been receiving ketorolac (Acular) ophthalmic solution. What is the nurse's priority action when assessing the eyes of this patient?

For answers, see *http://evolve.elsevier.com/Lilley*.

ⓔ EVOLVE WEBSITE

http://evolve.elsevier.com/Lilley
- Animations
- Answer Keys for Textbook Case Studies and Textbook Critical Thinking and Prioritization Questions
- Content Updates
- Key Points
- Review Questions
- Student Case Studies

Otic Drugs

OBJECTIVES

When you reach the end of this chapter, you will be able to do the following:

1. Describe the anatomy of the ear including external, middle, and inner ear.
2. Cite the various categories of ear disorders, and describe their causes and signs and symptoms.
3. List the various types of otic preparations and their indications.
4. Discuss the mechanisms of action, dosage, cautions, contraindications, drug interactions, and specific application techniques of each of the otic drugs.
5. Develop a nursing care plan that includes all phases of the nursing process for patients taking otic drugs.

DRUG PROFILES

♦ **carbamide peroxide, p. 923**

♦ = *Key drug*
! = *High-alert drug*

KEY TERMS

Cerumen A yellowish or brownish waxy excretion produced by modified sweat glands in the external ear canal. Also called *earwax.* (p. 923)

Otitis externa Inflammation or infection of the external auditory canal. (p. 922)

Otitis media (OM) Inflammation or infection of the middle ear. (p. 922)

OVERVIEW

The ear is made up of four parts: the external, outer, middle, and inner ears. The external ear is composed of the pinna (outer projecting part of the ear) and the external auditory meatus or opening of the ear canal. Synonyms for the pinna are *auricle* and *ala.* The term *outer ear* refers primarily to the external auditory canal. This is the space between the external auditory meatus and the tympanic membrane (eardrum). The middle ear is composed of the tympanic cavity, which is the space that begins with the tympanic membrane and ends with the oval window. Included in the middle ear are three bony structures of the mastoid bone—the malleus ("hammer"), incus ("anvil"), and stapes ("stirrup")—as well as the auditory or eustachian tube. The inner ear includes the cochlea and semicircular canals. The ear and its associated structures are illustrated in Figure 58-1. Diseases of the inner ear involve highly specialized medical practices that are beyond the scope of this textbook.

Disorders of the ear can be categorized according to the portion of the ear affected. External ear (pinna) disorders are generally the result of physical trauma to the ear and consist of lacerations or scrapes to the skin and localized infection of the hair follicles, which often causes the development of a boil. These disorders also tend to be self-limiting and heal with time. Other examples of external ear disorders are contact dermatitis, seborrhea, and psoriasis, as evidenced by itching, local redness, inflammation, weeping, or drainage. These conditions usually respond to the same topical medications used for any other local skin disorders, as discussed in Chapter 56. However, symptoms such as drainage, pain, and dizziness are sometimes also the first signs of a more serious underlying condition (e.g., head trauma, meningitis) and warrant prompt medical evaluation.

The most common disorders affecting the outer and middle ear are bacterial and fungal infections, inflammation, and earwax accumulation. Such disorders are often self-limiting, and treatments are usually successful. If problems persist or are

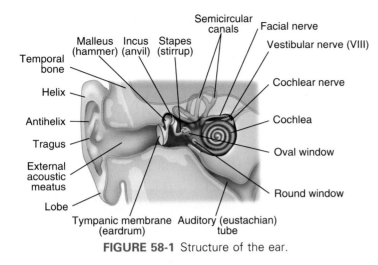

FIGURE 58-1 Structure of the ear.

left untreated, however, more serious problems such as hearing loss may result. Infections affecting the ear canal are known as **otitis externa,** whereas those affecting the middle ear are known as **otitis media (OM).** OM is a common disease of infancy and early childhood. It is often preceded by an upper respiratory tract infection. It may also occur in adults, but it is then generally associated with trauma to the tympanic membrane. Foreign objects and infection or inflammation associated with water sports are the usual sources of such trauma. In adults, the condition is also more likely to manifest as otitis externa, involving the ear canal and/or external tympanic membrane. Common symptoms of both otitis media and otitis externa are pain, fever, malaise, pressure, a sensation of fullness in the ears, and impaired hearing. If the condition is left untreated, tinnitus (ringing in the ears), nausea, vertigo, mastoiditis, and even temporary or permanent hearing deficits may occur.

Otitis media (OM) is the second most common infection in children, accounting for more than 20 million health care provider visits annually. An estimated two thirds of all children in the United States experience at least 1 episode prior to 1 year of age, and an estimated 80% have had at least 1 case of OM by 3 years of age. Medical management of OM is debated among the medical community, primarily due to the increased incidence of antibiotic resistance. Because of these concerns, treatment of OM has significantly changed over the last decade. In 2013, the American Academy of Pediatrics updated their clinical practice guidelines on acute OM. The guidelines highlight more stringent diagnostic criteria. The guidelines recommend antibiotics for severe symptoms with unilateral or bilateral OM and for bilateral nonsevere OM. Patients with nonsevere unilateral OM are either observed or can be placed on antibiotics. They also recommend that a pain assessment and pneumococcal and influenza vaccines be given. They no longer recommend prophylactic antibiotics. If a decision is made to treat with an antibiotic, amoxicillin is the first-line drug for most children. If the patient does not respond, or has received amoxicillin within 30 days, then therapy should be changed to amoxicillin-clavulanic acid (Augmentin). Antibiotics are discussed in Chapters 38 and 39.

TREATMENT OF EAR DISORDERS

Some of the minor ailments that affect the outer or middle ear can be treated with over-the-counter medications, but persistent, painful conditions generally require prescription medications. Drugs used to treat ear conditions are known as *otic drugs,* and most are applied topically to the ear canal. Because of this, they generally are not involved in drug interactions. Adverse effects are uncommon and usually do not extend beyond localized irritation, and otic drugs are normally contraindicated only in cases of known drug allergy. Pertinent classes of otic drugs include the following:

- Antibacterials (antibiotics)
- Antifungals
- Antiinflammatory drugs
- Local analgesics
- Local anesthetics
- Corticosteroids
- Wax emulsifiers

More serious cases of ear disorders may require treatment with systemic drugs such as antimicrobial drugs, analgesics, antiinflammatory drugs, and antihistamines. These medications are discussed in detail in previous chapters dealing with the respective drug classes.

ANTIBACTERIAL AND ANTIFUNGAL OTIC DRUGS

Antibacterial and antifungal otic drugs are often combined with steroids to take advantage of the antiinflammatory, antipruritic, and anti-allergic effects of the steroids. These drugs are used to treat outer and middle ear infections. Because they all work and are dosed very similarly, four products are profiled together here. Systemic antibiotics are also commonly prescribed for these conditions (e.g., amoxicillin; see Chapter 38), either alone or in addition to the otic drugs described in the following sections. Tables 58-1 and 58-2 list several commonly used products and their component amounts. They are classified as pregnancy category C drugs.

DRUG PROFILES
ANTIBACTERIAL PRODUCTS

Cortisporin (and other brands) is a three-drug combination that includes hydrocortisone and two antimicrobials, neomycin (an *aminoglycoside;* see Chapter 39) and polymyxin B. Hydrocortisone is the corticosteroid most commonly used in otic drugs, although there is one preparation (Ciprodex) that contains ciprofloxacin (a *fluoroquinolone;* see Chapter 39) and dexamethasone. In either case, the purpose of the steroid component is to reduce the inflammation and itching associated with ear infections. Ciprofloxacin is also available in combination with hydrocortisone (Cipro HC Otic). Ofloxacin (Floxin Otic) is another fluoroquinolone available only as a single-drug product. All of these products are used for the treatment of bacterial otitis externa or otitis media caused by susceptible bacteria such as *Staphylococcus aureus, Escherichia coli, Klebsiella* species, and others. Neomycin, polymyxin B, and

TABLE 58-1 Common Antibacterial Otic Products

Steroid Component	Antibiotic Component	Trade Name
hydrocortisone (1%)	5 mg of neomycin and 10,000 units of polymyxin B per 10-mL bottle	Cortisporin Otic, others
hydrocortisone (1%)	ciprofloxacin 2 mg/mL	Cipro HT Otic
dexamethasone (0.1%)	ciprofloxacin 3 mg/mL	Ciprodex
None	ofloxacin 3 mg/mL	Floxin Otic

TABLE 58-2 Common Antifungal Otic Products

Ingredients	Trade Name
hydrocortisone, 1%; pramoxine, 1%; chloroxylenol, 0.1%; propylene glycol diacetate, 3%; benzalkonium chloride (amount not specified)	Cortic, Otomar, Aero Otic HC, Mediotic HC
hydrocortisone, 1%; acetic acid, 2%; propylene glycol diacetate, 3%; sodium acetate, 0.015%; benzethonium chloride, 0.02%	Acetasol HC

Neomycin, polymyxin B, and hydrocortisone otic preparations are contraindicated in patients with a perforated eardrum.

hydrocortisone otic preparations are contraindicated in patients with a perforated eardrum; ciprofloxacin and ofloxacin can be used with perforated eardrums. Their usual dosage is 4 drops three to four times daily, except for ofloxacin, which is dosed at 5 to 10 drops twice daily (5-drop dose for children younger than 12 years of age). With some otic drugs, it is recommended to saturate a retrievable cotton or tissue wick and let this wick soak inside the ear canal, as a means of dosing the drug. The wick can be periodically remoistened with additional drug or removed and further eardrops inserted directly into the ear canal. Follow the specific instructions on the drug package or the method recommended by the prescriber or pharmacist.

ANTIFUNGAL PRODUCTS
Fungal infections account for about 4% of ear infections. Antifungal otic drugs are used primarily for otitis externa. These drugs may also have antibacterial and antiviral properties. Two commonly used preparations are Cortic and Acetasol HC, which are composed of hydrocortisone (a steroid), pramoxine (a local anesthetic), chloroxylenol (an antiseptic antifungal), propylene glycol diacetate (an emulsifying drug), and benzalkonium chloride (an antiseptic preservative).

EARWAX EMULSIFIERS

An additional common ear problem is the accumulation and eventual impaction (hardening) of earwax, or cerumen, which can also contribute to or complicate the infectious and inflammatory conditions described earlier. Products that soften and help to eliminate earwax are referred to as *earwax emulsifiers*.

Wax, or cerumen, is a natural product of the ear and is produced by modified sweat glands in the ear canal. However, it can occasionally build up and become impacted, which results in pain and partial temporary deafness. From chemistry, a nonpolar substance is one that is not water-soluble. Such a substance is said to be emulsified when it is chemically and/or physically converted to a more water-soluble form. *Earwax emulsifiers* loosen impacted cerumen, which allows it to be flushed out of the ear canal through irrigation (with water).

DRUG PROFILE

♦ carbamide peroxide
Carbamide peroxide (Debrox) is a commonly used earwax emulsifier. It is combined with other components (e.g., glycerin, a lubricant) that help soften and lubricate cerumen prior to irrigation. Carbamide peroxide slowly releases hydrogen peroxide and oxygen when exposed to moisture. This release of oxygen imparts a weak antibacterial action to this otic drug. In addition, the *effervescence* (foaming) resulting from the release of oxygen has the mechanical effect of emulsifying impacted cerumen to release it from the walls of the ear canal. Earwax emulsifiers are not to be used without health care provider recommendation when ear drainage, tympanic membrane rupture, or significant pain or other irritation is present. After allowing the drug to dissolve the earwax, one can remove it by gentle flushing the ear canal with warm water from a bulb syringe. Some earwax removal products include such a syringe in the package. It is classified as a pregnancy category C drug.

⚡ SAFETY AND QUALITY IMPROVEMENT: PREVENTING MEDICATION ERRORS [QSEN]

Eardrops Do NOT Go into the Eyes!

The Institute for Safe Medication Practices (ISMP) reports that painful medication errors have occurred when eardrops have been mistakenly used in the eyes. The tissues of the eye are more sensitive than ear tissue, and eye medications are specially formulated for ophthalmic use. Patients who receive eardrops in the eyes will immediately complain of burning and stinging; redness and swelling may develop later.

It may seem to be common sense that eardrops should not be used in the eyes, but the ISMP has reported several instances of this occurrence. Some errors are blamed on the similarities between the words "otic" (meaning ear) and "optic" (meaning eye).

The ISMP recommends several actions to reduce the risk for harming patients due to administration of eardrops into the eyes, including:

- Place an extra label on the dropper bottle that specifies "eye" or "ear."
- Keep medications in their original cartons, as these often have drawings of an eye or an ear on the carton, unlike the actual vials.
- In the pharmacy, separate eardrop and eyedrop vials. Storing them together increases the chance of a mixup between medications that have similar names.
- Confirm the medication route with the patient before administering the drops.
- If a patient is receiving both eardrops and eyedrops, administer them on different time schedules if possible.

For more information, see *www.ismp.org/Newsletters/acutecare/ articles/20061019.asp.* Accessed August 9, 2015.

NURSING PROCESS

ASSESSMENT

Before administering any of the *otic preparations,* assess baseline hearing and/or auditory status, if deemed appropriate, and document the findings. Assess the patient's symptoms, past and present medical history, and use of prescription drugs, over-the-counter drugs, and herbals. Document any drug or food allergies. A basic understanding of the anatomy of the ear, especially anatomic variations in patients of different age groups, is needed to ensure proper application technique. Contraindications, cautions, and drug interactions for the otic drugs, chemicals, and/or solutions have been discussed previously in the pharmacology section; always assess the patient for these and document the findings. A perforated eardrum is considered to be a contraindication to the use of otic drugs.

NURSING DIAGNOSES

1. Acute pain related to ear infection or ear disorder
2. Deficient knowledge related to lack of experience with otic drugs and their method of administration
3. Noncompliance related to a lack of motivation and or lack of understanding for the need of frequent eardrop instillation, as ordered

PLANNING: OUTCOME IDENTIFICATION

1. Patient experiences minimal to no ear discomfort with proper use of drug therapy, such as eardrops and analgesics, as well as non-drug therapy with warm compresses.
2. Patient demonstrates adequate knowledge about the treatment regimen, rationale for use, application, adverse effects, and reporting of worsening of symptoms.
3. Patient remains compliant and adheres to medication regimen as prescribed.

IMPLEMENTATION

Instill *otic preparations* only after the ear has been thoroughly cleansed and all cerumen (earwax) has been removed (by irrigation if necessary, or as ordered). Eardrops, solutions, and ointments are to be stored at room temperature before instillation. Administration of solutions that are too cold may cause a vestibular type of reaction with dizziness, "room-spinning" vertigo, and vomiting. If the solution has been refrigerated, allow it to warm to room temperature. Higher temperatures may affect the

potency of these solutions, and storage at room temperature is recommended. When administering eardrops to adults, hold the pinna *up* and back. In children younger than 3 years of age, hold the pinna *down* and back. Allow a period of time for adequate coverage of the ear by the medication. Gentle massage to the tragus area of the ear may also help to increase coverage of the medication after the solution is given. See Patient-Centered Care: Patient Teaching on the next page and also Chapter 9 for more information on eardrop instillation.

CASE STUDY

Patient-Centered Care: Ear Medications

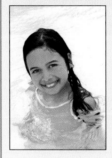 T.E. is 8 years old and loves to swim in the neighborhood pool. Lately she has had a feeling of fullness in her left ear, and today she tells her mother that her ear is hurting and itching and that she feels "awful." Her mother takes her temperature and finds that it is 101° F (38.3° C). She calls the pediatrician's office for an appointment, and T.E. is seen the next morning. After examining T.E., the pediatrician says that T.E. has otitis media in the left ear and some earwax buildup in both ears. The pediatrician removes some of the earwax manually, writes prescriptions for oral antibiotics for T.E., and gives instructions to use an earwax emulsifier. The nurse meets with them to review the instructions.

1. T.E.'s mother asks, "Why is the antibiotic a pill? It seems to me that if she has an ear infection, she should take eardrops!" What is the nurse's best response?
2. T.E.'s mother has another question: "What will happen if this ear infection does not get better?"
3. T.E. complains that her ear "really hurts and itches." What can be given to her for this problem? How will it be given?

For answers, see *http://evolve.elsevier.com/Lilley.*

EVALUATION

The therapeutic effects of *otic drugs,* as with all drugs, are gauged by evaluating whether goals and objectives have been met. Therapeutic effects of otic drugs include less pain, redness, and swelling in the ear; a reduction in fever; and resolution of any other signs and symptoms associated with the ear disorder. Improvement in hearing may also be an anticipated therapeutic effect. Monitor the ear canal for the occurrence of rash and/or any signs of local irritation, such as redness and heat at the site. Evaluate the patient for adverse effects with each application or instillation, and report any unusual appearance of the outer ear and ear canal immediately to the prescriber.

PATIENT-CENTERED CARE: PATIENT TEACHING

- Provide thorough instructions to the patient about the proper use of eardrops or instillation of any medication into the ear. Warn that dizziness may occur after application of the medication, requiring the patient to remain supine or sitting during instillation and for a few minutes thereafter.
- Medication must be at room temperature before administration of eardrops. If needed, this may be achieved by running warm water over the medication bottle, but care must be taken to prevent water from getting into the container, damaging the label so that the directions are unreadable, or making the solution too warm to use. Advise the patient not to heat the medication; for example, a microwave oven

must not be used for warming—because eardrops that are overheated may lose potency. If the pharmacy indicates that the drug should be kept in a refrigerator, instruct the patient to take the drug out of the refrigerator up to 1 hour before it is to be instilled so that it may warm up to room temperature. Most medications for the ear are stored at room temperature.
- Instruct the patient to lie on the side opposite to that of the affected ear for about 5 minutes after instillation of the drug. If the patient prefers, a small cotton ball may be inserted gently into the ear canal to keep the drug in place, but avoid forcing it into the ear or jamming it down into the ear canal.

KEY POINTS

- Otic drugs may include the following ingredients, either by themselves or mixed together (depending on the prescriber's order): steroids, antibacterials, antifungals, antiinflammatories, and wax-emulsifying compounds. Many of the antiinfective drugs are combined with steroids (in solution) to take advantage of the additional antiinflammatory, antipruritic, and antiallergic drug effects of the steroids.
- Some ear infections require additional drug therapy with systemic dosage forms of corticosteroids, antibiotics, antifungals, and antiinflammatory drugs, so remind the patient of oral and other dosage forms.
- Some disorders of the ear are self-limiting to a degree, but appropriate treatment is important to prevent complications

to the ear and/or systemic complications. If left untreated, ear infections or disorders may lead to a decrease in or loss of hearing.
- Wax, or cerumen, is a natural product of the ear and is normally produced by modified sweat glands in the auditory canal; emulsifying otic drugs (such as carbamide peroxide) loosen and help remove this wax.
- Single drugs and combination drug products are used to treat many ear conditions, and it is important to know the indications for and specific information about these drugs to ensure their safe use.

NCLEX® EXAMINATION REVIEW QUESTIONS

1. While teaching a patient about treatment of otitis media, the nurse should mention that untreated otitis media may lead to
   a. mastoiditis.
   b. throat infections.
   c. fungal ear infection.
   d. decreased cerumen production.
2. During a teaching session about eardrops, the patient tells the nurse, "I know why an antibiotic is in this medicine, but why is hydrocortisone in these eardrops?" What is the nurse's best response?
   a. "The hydrocortisone will help to soften the cerumen."
   b. "The hydrocortisone reduces itching and inflammation."
   c. "The hydrocortisone also has antifungal effects."
   d. "This medication helps to anesthetize the area to decrease pain."
3. The nurse is preparing to administer eardrops. Which technique for administering eardrops is correct?
   a. Warm the solution to 100° F (37.7° C) before using.
   b. Position the patient so that the unaffected ear is accessible.
   c. Massage the tragus before administering the eardrops.
   d. Gently insert a cotton ball into the outer ear canal after the drops are given.
4. The nurse is discussing treatment of earwax buildup with a patient. Which statement about earwax emulsifiers is correct?

   a. These drugs are useful for treatment of ear infections.
   b. They loosen impacted cerumen so that it may be removed by irrigation.
   c. They are used to rinse out excessive earwax.
   d. They enhance the secretion of earwax.
5. During an examination, the nurse notes that a patient has a perforated tympanic membrane. There is an order for eardrops. Which is the nurse's most appropriate action at this time?
   a. Give the medication as ordered.
   b. Check the patient's hearing, and then give the drops.
   c. Hold the medication, and check with the prescriber.
   d. Administer the drops with a cotton wick.
6. The nurse is preparing to administer eardrops and finds that the bottle has been stored in the medication room refrigerator. Which is the nurse's best action at this time?
   a. Remove the bottle from the refrigerator, and administer the drops.
   b. Heat the bottle for 5 seconds in the microwave oven before administering the drops.
   c. Let the bottle sit in a cup of hot water for 15 minutes before administering the drops.
   d. Remove the bottle from the refrigerator 1 hour before the drops are due to be given.

7. The nurse is preparing to administer carbamide peroxide (Debrox) to an adult patient with impacted cerumen. Which actions by the nurse are correct? *(Select all that apply.)*
   a. Have the patient lie on his or her side with the affected ear up.
   b. Chill the medication before administering it.
   c. Pull the pinna of the ear down and back.
   d. Pull the pinna of the ear up and back.
   e. Gently irrigate the ear with warm water to remove the softened earwax.

8. A child is in the clinic with a severe case of otitis media. The prescriber has decided to treat it with an antibiotic, and the nurse anticipates that which antibiotic will be prescribed as a first-line drug for this condition?
   a. tetracycline
   b. penicillin
   c. amoxicillin
   d. ciprofloxacin

1. a, 2. b, 3. d, 4. b, 5. c, 6. d, 7. a, e, 8. c.

CRITICAL THINKING AND PRIORITIZATION QUESTIONS

1. When discussing eardrop administration with a patient, the patient says, "I'll keep these in the refrigerator so that they'll be cold when I give them to myself." What is the nurse's best response?

2. The nurse is observing while the mother of an infant administers eardrops for the first time. The mother says, "When I give the drops, I will pull the ear up and back like this, give the drops, and then massage the earlobe." What is the nurse's priority action at this time?

For answers, see *http://evolve.elsevier.com/Lilley.*

ⓔ EVOLVE WEBSITE

http://evolve.elsevier.com/Lilley
- Animations
- Answer Keys for Textbook Case Studies and Textbook Critical Thinking and Prioritization Questions

- Content Updates
- Key Points
- Review Questions
- Student Case Studies

Pharmaceutical Abbreviations

ABBREVIATION	TRANSLATION
Drug Dosage	
cc*†	Cubic centimeter (equivalent to 1 mL)
g or gm	Gram
gr	Grain
gtt	Drop
IU*†	International unit
L	Liter
lb	Pound
mEq	Milliequivalent
min	Minute
ml or mL	Milliliter
no or #	Number
qs†	Quantity sufficient, as much as needed
ss†	One half
oz	Ounce
tbsp	Tablespoon
tsp	Teaspoon
u or U*	Unit
μg*† or mcg	Microgram

Drug Route	
AD†	Right ear
AS†	Left ear
AU†	Both ears
ID	Intradermal
IM	Intramuscular
IV	Intravenous
NG	Nasogastric
OD†	Right eye
OS†	Left eye
OU†	Both eyes
PO	By mouth
SC†, SQ†, subcut	Subcutaneous
SL	Sublingual

Drug Administration	
aa	Of each
ac	Before meals
ad lib	As desired, freely
bid	Twice a day
h or hr	Hour
hs†	Hour of sleep, at bedtime
HS†	Half-strength
noct	Night
NPO	Nothing by mouth
pc	After meals
prn	When needed
qd*†	Every day, once a day
qh	Every hour
qid	Four times a day
qod*†	Every other day
Rx	Prescribe, take
stat	Immediately
tid	Three times a day

*Note: As part of its 2004 National Patient Safety Goals, the Joint Commission announced that all accredited organizations must discontinue using the following abbreviations, acronyms, and symbols: U, IU, qd, qod, MS, MSO_4, and $MgSO_4$. Trailing zeros and lack of leading zeros were also discontinued. In other words, a zero should never appear by itself *after* a decimal point (1 mg instead of 1.0 mg), and a zero should always be used *before* a decimal point (0.1 mg instead of .1 mg). In addition, abbreviations for drug names should not be used because they can be misinterpreted. Other items are being considered for future inclusion on the official "do not use" list, such as the @ sign (write out the word at) and the symbols > and < (write out as *greater than* and *less than*). The abbreviations "cc" and "μg" should also be avoided and are being considered for inclusion on future lists. This National Patient Safety Goal was incorporated into the Information Management standards in 2010.

†These abbreviations are on the *List of Error Prone Abbreviations, Symbols, and Dose Designations* of the Institute for Safe Medication Practices (ISMP). These abbreviations have been reported to the ISMP as being frequently involved in medication errors. The ISMP recommends not ever using these abbreviations when communicating medical information, including medication orders and medication administration records.

Data from Institute for Safe Medication Practices (ISMP): *ISMP's list of error-prone abbreviations, symbols, and dose designations*, 2012. Available at http://www.ismp.org/tools/errorproneabbreviations.pdf. Accessed September 24, 2015.

CASE STUDY PHOTO CREDITS

Chapter 1
© Jose AS Reyes

Chapter 2
© forestpath

Chapter 3
© Katrina Brown

Chapter 4
© Andrew Gentry

Chapter 5
© Oliver Hoffmann

Chapter 6
© Supri Suharjoto

Chapter 7
© David Gilder

Chapter 8
© Felix Mizioznikov

Chapter 10
© Gpalmer

Chapter 11
© Vgstudio

Chapter 12
© Rohit Seth

Chapter 13
© Michael Jung

Chapter 14
© ZanyZeus

Chapter 15
© Jeff Banke

Chapter 16
© Ostill

Chapter 17
© Carme Balcells

Chapter 18
© Andi Berger

Chapter 19
© Sophie Louise Asselin

Chapter 20
© Gina Smith

Chapter 21
© Simone van den Berg

Chapter 22
© Felix Mizioznikov

Chapter 23
© Rohit Seth

Chapter 24
© Steve Carroll

Chapter 25
© YellowCrest Media

Chapter 26
© Martin Allinger

Chapter 27
© William Casey

Chapter 28
© Monkey Business Images

Chapter 29
© Dundanim

Chapter 30
© Junial Enterprises

Chapter 31
© Flashon Studio

Chapter 32
© Rob Marmion

Chapter 33
© Konstantin Sutyagin

Chapter 34
© Martina Ebel

Chapter 35
© Olga OSA

Chapter 36
© Perkus

Chapter 37
© Ragne Kabanova

Chapter 38
© Arvind Balaraman

Chapter 39
© Monkey Business Images

Chapter 40
© William Casey

Chapter 41
© Justin Paget

Chapter 42
© Monkey Business Images

Chapter 43
© Matt Antonino

Chapter 44
© Monkey Business Images

Chapter 45
© Monkey Business Images

Chapter 46
© Lisa F. Young

Chapter 47
© Jacques PALUT

Chapter 48
© Iofoto

Chapter 49
© Monkey Business Images

Chapter 50
© Rob Marmion

Chapter 51
© Layland Masuda

Chapter 52
© Brocreative

Chapter 53
© Wrangler

Chapter 54
© Brian Chase

Chapter 55
© Andry Starostin

Chapter 56
© Mona Makela

Chapter 57
© CURAphotography

Chapter 58
© Juriah Mosin

BIBLIOGRAPHY

GENERAL

American Society of Clinical Oncology website. Available at www.asco.org. Accessed July 5, 2011.

The Joint Commission: *2012 National patient safety goals*. Available at www.jointcommission.org/standards_information/npsgs.aspx. Accessed June 20, 2012.

NANDA International: *Nursing diagnoses—definitions and classification 2012-2014*, Kaukauna, WI, 2012, NANDA International.

National Cancer Institute website. Available at www.nci.hih.gov. Accessed July 5, 2011.

Perry AG, Potter PP: *Clinical skills and nursing techniques*, ed 7, St Louis, MO, 2010, Mosby.

Skidmore-Roth L: *2014 Mosby's nursing drug reference*, ed 27, St Louis, MO, 2014, Mosby.

CHAPTER 1

Bradley D, Benedict B: *The ANA professional nursing development scope and standards, 2009: a continuing education perspective*, Silver Springs, MD, 2010, American Nurses Credentialing Center Accreditation of Continuing Nursing Education.

Bulechek S: *Nursing interventions classification (NIC)*, ed 5, St Louis, MO, 2008, Mosby.

Hill KS: Improving quality and patient safety by retaining nursing expertise, *Online J Issues Nurs* 15(3), 2010.

Cronenwett L, Sherwood G, Barnsteiner J, et al: Quality and safety education for nurses, *Nurs Outlook* 55(3):122–131, 2007.

Dickson GL, Flynn L: Nurses' clinical reasoning: processes and practices of medication safety, *Qual Health Res* 22(1):3–16, 2012.

Institute for Safe Medication Practice: *ISMP's list of error prone abbreviations, symbols and dose designations*. 2013. Available at www.ismp.org. Accessed March 15, 2015.

Institute of Medicine: *Health professions education: A bridge to quality*, Washington DC, 2003, National Academies Press.

The Joint Commission: *Do not use list*, 2004. Available at www.joint commission.org. Accessed November 1, 2015.

Laysa SM, Fabian RJ, Saul MI, et al: Influence of medications and diagnoses on fall risk in psychiatric inpatients, *Am J Health Syst Pharm* 67(15):1274–1280, 2010.

Moorhead SL, Johnson M, Mass ML, et al: *Nursing outcomes classification (NOC)*, ed 4, St Louis, MO, 2008, Mosby.

Mosby's pocket dictionary of medicine, nursing and health professions, ed 6, St Louis, MO, 2010, Mosby.

Ulrich B, Krozek C, Early S, et al: Improving retention, confidence, and competence of new graduate nurses: results from a 10-year longitudinal database, *Nurs Econ* 28(6):363–375, 2010.

Van Cott A, Smith MC: Nursing research: tips and tools to simplify the process, *Dermatol Nurs* 21(3):138–140, 2009.

Weston MJ: Strategies for enhancing autonomy and control over nursing practice, *Online J Issues Nurs* 15(1), 2010. Available at www.nursingworld.org/MainMenuCategories/ANAMarketplace/ANAPeriodicals/OJIN/TableofContents/Vol152010/No1Jan2010/Enhancing-Autonomy-and-Control-and-Practice.html. Accessed November 1, 2015.

CHAPTER 2

Center to Advance Palliative Care: *What is palliative care?* Available at www.getpalliativecare.org/whatis/faq. Accessed September 1, 2011.

Chen JJ, Swope DM, Dashtipour K, et al: Transdermal rotigotine: a clinically innovative dopamine-receptor agonist for the management of Parkinson's disease, *Pharmacotherapy* 29(12):1452–1467, 2009.

Flockhart DA: *Drug interactions: cytochrome P450 drug interaction table, 2009. Indiana University School of Medicine*. Available at http://medicine.iupui.edu/clinpharm/ddis/table.asp. Accessed January 2, 2011.

Lee CA, Cook JA, Reyner EL, et al: P-glycoprotein related drug interactions: clinical importance and a consideration of disease states, *Expert Opin Drug Metabol Toxicol* 6(5):603–619, 2010.

Lucio D, Stevenson J, Hoffman J: Biosimilars: implications for health-system pharmacists, *Am J Health Syst Pharm* 70(15):2004–2017, 2013.

Nolin TD, Naud J, Leblond FA, et al: Emerging evidence of the impact of kidney disease on drug metabolism and transport, *Clin Pharmacol Ther* 83(6):898–903, 2008.

U.S. Food and Drug Administration: *Avoiding drug interactions*. Available at www.fda.gov/forconsumers/consumerupdates/ucm096386.htm. Accessed June 19, 2012.

U.S. Food and Drug Administration: *Drug interactions: what you should know*. Available at www.fda.gov/drugs/resourcesforyou/ucm163354.htm. Accessed June 19, 2012.

CHAPTER 3

Alzheimer's Association: 2010 Alzheimer's disease facts and figures, *Alzheimers Dement* 6:1–66, 2010. Available at: www.alz.org. Accessed September 21, 2012.

The American Geriatric Society Expert Panel: *American Geriatrics Society updated Beers criteria for potentially inappropriate medication use in older adults*. Available at www.americangeriatrics.org/files/documents/beers. Accessed January 15, 2014.

Bernius M, Thibodeau B, Jones A, et al: Prevention of pediatric drug calculation errors by prehospital care providers, *Prehosp Emerg Care* 12(4):486–494, 2008.

Buck ML: Improving pediatric medication safety, part II: evaluating strategies to prevent medication errors, *Pediatr Pharm* 14(12), 2008.

Centers for Disease Control and Prevention: *Health, United States, 2012*. Available at cdc.gov/nchs/data/hus/hus12.pdf#091. Accessed January 15, 2014.

Centers for Disease Control and Prevention: *Life expectancy*. Available at www.cdc.gov/nchs/fastats/lifexpec.htm. Accessed January 15, 2014.

Chang CM, Liu PY, Yang YH, et al: Use of the Beers criteria to predict adverse drug reaction among first-visit elderly outpatients, *Pharmacotherapy* 25(6):831–838, 2005.

DeDea L: The Beers criteria: antibiotic and metoprolol dosing, *JAAPA* 23(10):12, 2010. Available at: www.jaapa.com/the-beers-criteria-antibiotic-and-metoprolol-dosing/article/179953. Accessed June 15, 2015.

Guay D: Geriatric pharmacotherapy updates, *Am J Geri Pharmocother* 8(4):599–609, 2010.

Institute for Safe Medication Practices: Reducing patient harm from opiates. *ISMP Medication Safety Alert! High Alert Medication Feature*, 2007. Available at www.ismp.org/newsletters/acutecare/articles/20070222.asp. Accessed September 21, 2012.

Institute for Safe Medication Practices: Tablet splitting: do it only when you "half" to, and then do it safely. *ISMP Medication Safety Alert! Acute Care*, 2006. Available at www.ismp.org/newsletters/acutecare/articles/20060518.asp. Accessed September 26, 2012.

Jugdutt BI: Heart failure in the elderly: advances and challenges, *Expert Rev Cardiovasc Ther* 8(5):695–715, 2010.

Levy HB, Marcus EL, Christen C: Beyond the Beers criteria: a comparative overview of explicit criteria, *Ann Pharmacother* 44(12):1968–1975, 2010.

Loya AM, Gonzalez-Stuart A, Rivera JO: Prevalence of polypharmacy, polyherbacy, nutritional supplement use and potential product interactions among older adults living on the United States-Mexico border: a descriptive, questionnaire-based study, *Drugs Aging* 26(5):423–436, 2009.

929

MacLeod S: Therapeutic drug monitoring in pediatrics: how do children differ? *Ther Drug Monit* 32(3):253–256, 2010.

Milton JC, Hill-Smith I, Jackson SH: Prescribing for older people, *BMJ* 336:606, 2008.

Molony SL: Beers criteria for potentially inappropriate medication use in the elderly, *J Gerontol Nurs* 29(11):6, 2003.

Stein J: Polypharmacy common in elderly psychiatric inpatients. *Medscape Medical News*. 2010. Available at www.medscape.com/viewarticle/717798. Accessed June 30, 2015.

U.S. Food and Drug Administration: *Drug research and children*. Available at www.fda.gov/Drugs/ResourcesForYou/Consumers/ucm143565.htm. Accessed September 15, 2011.

Wick JY: The Beers criteria: red flags for elders. *Pharmacy Times*, 2006. Available at www.pharmacytimes.com/publications/issue/2006/2006-06/2006-06-5624. Accessed September 21, 2012.

CHAPTER 4

American Nurses Association: *ANA principles for delegation*, Washington, DC, 2005, American Nurses Association.

American Nurses Association: *The American Nurses Association comments on the Wisconsin Department of Justice decision to pursue criminal charges against an RN in Wisconsin*. Available at http://ana.nursingworld.org/FunctionalMenuCategories/MediaResources/PressReleases/2006/CriminalChargesAgainstanRNinWisconsin.aspx. Accessed June 20, 2012.

American Nurses Association: *Code of ethics for nurses with interpretive statements*, Washington, DC, 2001, American Nurses Association.

American Nurses Association: *Nursing: scope and standards of practice*, ed 2, Washington, DC, 2010, American Nurses Association.

American Nurses Association: *Safe nursing staffing poll results*, 2012. Available at www.safestaffingsaveslives.org/WhatisANADoing/PollResults.aspx. Accessed June 20, 2012.

American Nurses Association and National Council of State Boards of Nursing: *Joint statement on delegation*, 2005. Available at www.ncsbn.org/Joint_statement.pdf. Accessed September 21, 2012.

Brooke P: When can you say no?, *Nursing* 39(7):43–47, 2009.

Buppert CT, Klein TA: Dilemmas in mandatory reporting for nurses. *Medscape Top Adv Pract Nurs eJournal*, 2008, 1-17. Available at http://cme.medscape.com/viewprogram/18738. Accessed June 15, 2014.

Colby SL, Ortman JM: *Projections of the size and compostion of the U.S. populations: 2014 to 2060*. U.S. Department of Commerce Economics and Statistics Administration, U.S. Census Bureau, 2015. Available at www.census.gov/content/dam/Census/library/publications/2015/demo/p25-1143.pdf. Accessed July 1, 2015.

Kaldjian L, Jones EW, Wu BJ, et al: Reporting medical errors to improve patient safety, *Arch Intern Med* 168(1):40–46, 2008.

Kalisch B, Landstrom G, Willams R: Missed nursing care: errors of omission, *Nurs Outlook* 57(1):3–9, 2009.

Minor DS, Woford R, Jones DW: Racial and ethnic differences in hypertension, *Curr Atheroscler Rep* 10(2):121–127, 2008.

National Council of State Boards of Nursing (NCSBN): *Working with others; a position paper*, 2005, Chicago, IL. Available at www.ncsbn.org/Working_with_Others.pdf. Accessed June 20, 2012.

National Quality Forum (NQF): *Safe practices for better healthcare—2009 update*, 2009. Executive summary, Washington, DC. Available at www.qualityforum.org/Publications/2009/03/Safe_Practices_for_Better_Healthcare-2009_Update.aspx. Accessed June 20, 2012.

Nguyen TT, Kaufman JS, Whitsel EA, et al: Racial differences in blood pressure response to calcium channel blocker monotherapy: a meta-analysis, *Am J Hypertens* 22(8):911–917, 2009.

Nursing Service Organization (NSO): *CNA Healthpro Nursing Claims Study: an analysis of claims with risk management recommendations 1997-2007*, 2009. Hatboro, PA. Available at www.nso.com/pdfs/db/rnclaimstudy.pdf?fileName=rnclaimstudy.pdf&folder=pdfs/db&isLiveStr=Y&refID=rnclaim. Accessed September 21, 2012.

U.S. Census Bureau: *US Census Bureau news: an older and more diverse nation by mid-century*, 2008. Available at www.census.gov/PressRelease/www/releases/archives/population/012496.html. Accessed July 1, 2015.

U.S. Department of Defense: *Tricare military health plan: Medicare Part D*, 2007. Available at www.tricare.mil/mybenefit/ProfileFilter.do. Accessed July 1, 2015.

U.S. Department of Health and Human Services, Centers for Medicare and Medicaid Services: *Overview of Medicare Part D*. Available at www.cms.hhs.gov/MMAUpdate/01_Overview.asp.

U.S. Department of Health and Human Services, Office of Civil Rights: *Summary of the HIPAA privacy rule*, 2003. Available at www.hhs.gov/OCR/privacysummary.pdf.

U.S. Food and Drug Administration: *Controlled Substances Act*. Available at www.fda.gov/regulatoryinformation/legislation/ucm148726.htm. Accessed January 2, 2011.

U.S. Food and Drug Administration: *The FDA's drug review process: ensuring drugs are safe and effective*. Available at www.fda.gov/drugs/resourcesforyou/consumers/ucm143534.htm. Accessed November 1, 2015.

U.S. Food and Drug Administration: *MedWatch: The FDA Safety Information and Adverse Event Reporting Program*. Available at www.fda.gov/Safety/MedWatch/default.htm. Accessed January 2, 2011.

U.S. Food and Drug Administration: *Timeline: chronology of drug regulation in the United States*. Available at www.fda.gov/cder/about/history/time1.htm.

U.S. Food and Drug Administration, Office of Regulatory Affairs: *Compliance policy guidelines, sec 420.200, compendium revisions and deletions (CPG 7132.02)*. Available at www.fda.gov/ora/compliance_ref/cpg/cpgdrg/cpg420-200.html. Accessed September 26, 2012.

CHAPTER 5

American Medical Association: *Physicians with disruptive behavior*, 2000. Available at www.ama-assn.org/ama/pub/physician-resources/medical-ethics/code-medical-ethics/opinion9045.page. Accessed January 2, 2011.

Barclay L: *Interruptions linked to medication errors by nurses*. Available at www.medscape.com/viewarticle/720803. Accessed January 2, 2011.

Barnsteiner JH: Medication reconciliation, *Am J Nurs* 105(Suppl 3):31–36, 2005.

Clarin OA: Strategies to overcome barriers to effective nurse practitioner and physician collaboration, *J Nurse Pract.* 3(8):538–548, 2007.

Cohen H: Protecting patients from harm: reduce the risks of high-alert drugs, *Nursing* 37(9):49–55, 2007.

Cohen M: Medication errors: reconciling medications, safeguarding transitions, *Nursing* 34(7):14–16, 2005.

Cohen MR: Medication errors, *Nursing* 41(2):11, 2011.

Dennison RD: Creating an organizational culture for medication safety, *Nurs Clin North Am* 40(1):1–23, 2005.

Feldman J: *Magnet nursing and the healthcare team: a physician's view*, 2007. Available at www.medscape.com/viewarticle/562949. Accessed July 5, 2015.

Hughes RE, Edgerton EA: First, do no harm: reducing pediatric medication errors: children are especially at risk for medication errors, *Am J Nurs* 105(5):79–89, 2005.

Hughes RG, Ortiz E: Medication errors: why they happen and how they can be prevented, *Am J Nurs* 105(Suppl 3):14–24, 2005.

Institute for Healthcare Improvement: *Five Million Lives campaign*, 2008. Available at www.ihi.org//IHI/Programs/Campaign. Accessed June 20, 2012.

Institute for Safe Medication Practices: High-reliability organizations (HROs): what they know that we don't (part I), 2005, *ISMP Medication Safety Alert! Acute Care*. Available at www.ismp.org/MSAarticles/20050714.htm. Accessed September 26, 2012.

Institute for Safe Medication Practices: High-reliability organizations (HROs): what they know that we don't (part II). *ISMP Medication Safety Alert!*. *Acute Care*, 2005. Available at www.ismp.org/MSAarticles/20050728.htm. Accessed September 26, 2012.

Institute for Safe Medication Practices: *ISMP's list of error-prone abbreviations, symbols, and dose designations*, 2010. Available at www.ismp.org/Tools/errorproneabbreviations.pdf. Accessed July 5, 2015.

Institute for Safe Medication Practices: *ISMP's list of high-alert medications*, 2010. Available at www.ismp.org/Tools/highalertmedications.pdf. Accessed September 26, 2012.

Institute for Safe Medication Practices: Error-prone conditions that lead to student nurse-related errors, *ISMP Medication Safety Alert! Acute Care*

12(21):1–3, 2007, Available at www.ismp.org/Newsletters/acutecare/articles/20071018.asp. Accessed September 26, 2012.

Intravenous Nurses Society: Medication safety (symposium summary), *J Infus Nurs* 28:42–47, 2005.

The Joint Commission: *Speak Up initiatives*, 2012. Available at www.jointcommission.org/speakup.aspx. Accessed June 20, 2012.

Koppel R, Wtterneck T, Telles JL, et al: Workarounds to barcode medication administration systems: their occurrences, causes and threats to patient safety, *J Am Med Inform Assoc* 15:408–423, 2008.

Lafleur KJ: Tackling med errors with technology, *RN* 67(5):29–34, 2004.

Landrigan C, Parry GJ, Bones CB, et al: Temporal trends in rates of patient harm resulting from medical care, *N Engl J Med* 363:2124–2134, 2010.

Lazoritz S, Carlson PJ: Don't tolerate disruptive physician behavior, *Am Nurse Today* 3(3):2008. Available at: www.americannursetoday.com/article.aspx?id=4882&fid=4860. Accessed September 26, 2012.

Lindeke LL, Sieckert AM: Nurse-physician workplace collaboration, *Online J Issues Nurs* 10(1), 2005.

Manno MS, Hayes DD: Best-practice interventions: how medication reconciliation saves lives, *Nursing* 36(3):63–64, 2006.

Metules TJ, Bauer J: Part 1: JCAHO's patient safety goals: a practical guide, *RN* 69(12):21–27, 2006.

Metules TJ, Bauer J: Part 2: JCAHO's patient safety goals: a practical guide, *RN* 70(1):39–43, 2007.

O'Connell D, et al: Disclosing unanticipated outcomes and medical errors, *J Clin Outcomes Manage.* 10(1):25–29, 2003.

O'Reilly MA: *Change and change again: nurse leaders in the new millennium: highlights of the National Association of Neonatal Nurses' 23rd annual conference*, 2008. Available at www.medscape.com/viewarticle/568013. Accessed January 3, 2014.

Pharm JC, Aswani MS, Rosen M, et al: Reducing medical errors and adverse events, *Annu Rev Med* 63:447–463, 2012.

Richardson WC, et al: *To err is human: building a safer health system*, Washington, DC, 1999, National Academies Press.

Rosenstein AH: Nurse-physician relationships: impact on nurse satisfaction and retention, *Am J Nurs* 102(6):26–34, 2002.

Rosenstein AH, O'Daniel M: Disruptive behavior and clinical outcomes: perceptions of nurses and physicians, *Am J Nurs* 105(1):54–65, 2005.

Schnipper JL, Hamann C, Ndumele CD, et al: Effect of an electronic medication reconciliation application and process redesign on potential adverse drug events: a cluster-randomized trial, *Arch Intern Med* 169:771–780, 2009.

Smith DS, Haig K: Reduction of adverse drug events and medication errors in a community hospital setting, *Nurs Clin North Am* 40(1):25–32, 2005.

Stetina P, Groves M, Pafford L: Managing medication errors—a qualitative study, *Medsurg Nurs* 14(3):174–178, 2005.

Tuohy N, Paparella S: Look-alike and sound-alike drugs: errors waiting to happen, *J Emerg Nurs* 31(6):569–571, 2005.

U.S. Food and Drug Administration: *Medication errors.* Available at www.fda.gov/drugs/drugsafety/medicationerrors/default.htm. Accessed January 2, 2011.

Wager N, Fieldman G, Hussey T, et al: The effects on ambulatory blood pressure of working under favourably and unfavourably perceived supervisors, *Occup Environ Med* 60:468–474, 2003.

CHAPTER 6

Alfaro-Lefevre R: *Critical thinking and clinical judgment: a practical approach to outcome-focused thinking*, ed 4, St Louis, MO, 2009, Saunders.

American Nurses Association: *Nursing: scope and standards of practice*, Silver Spring, MD, 2004, American Nurses Association.

Billings DM: *Teaching in nursing: a guide for faculty*, ed 2, St Louis, MO, 2004, Saunders.

Canobbio MM: *Mosby's handbook of patient teaching*, ed 3, St Louis, MO, 2006, Mosby.

Chang M, Kelly AE: Patient education: addressing cultural diversity and health literacy issues, *Urol Nurs* 27(5):411–417, 2007.

Colby SL, Ortman JM: *Projections of the size and compostion of the U.S. populations: 2014 to 2060*. U.S. Department of Commerce Economics and Statistics Administration, U.S. Census Bureau, 2015. Available at www.census.gov/content/dam/Census/library/publications/2015/demo/p25-1143.pdf. Accessed July 10, 2015.

Hamric AB: *Advanced practice nursing: an integrative approach*, ed 4, St Louis, MO, 2008, Saunders.

Institute of Medicine (IOM): *Health literacy: a prescription to end confusion*, Washington, DC, 2004, The National Academies Press.

The Joint Commission website. Available at www.jointcommission.org. Accessed October 10, 2011.

Leininger MM: *Culture care diversity and universality: a worldwide nursing theory*, ed 2, Boston, MA, 2006, Jones & Bartlett.

Lenahan JL, McCarthy DM, Davis TC, et al: A drug by any other name: Patients ability to identify medication regimens and its association with adherence and health outcomes, *J Health Commun: International Perspectives* 18(1):31–39, 2013.

National Council on Patient Information and Education (NCPIE) website. Available at www.talkaboutrx.org. Accessed February 4, 2011.

Negley DF, Ness S, Fee-Schroeder K, et al: Building a collaborative nursing practice to promote patient education: an inpatient and outpatient partnership, *Oncol Nurs Forum* 36(1):19–23, 2009.

Nies MA: *Community/public health nursing: promoting the health of populations*, ed 4, St Louis, MO, 2006, Saunders.

Redman BK: *Advances in patient education*, New York, NY, 2004, Springer.

Redman BK: *The practice of patient education*, ed 9, St Louis, MO, 2001, Mosby.

U.S. Census Bureau, U.S. Department of Commerce: *U.S. Census Bureau projections show a slower growing, older, more diverse nation a half century from now*, 2012, Available at www.census.gov. Accessed March 6, 2014.

U.S. Department of Commerce: *An older and more diverse nation by midcentury (press release)*, 2008. Available at www.census.gov/newsroom/releases/archives/population/cb08-123.html. Accessed July 10. 2015.

U.S. Department of Health and Human Services: *Healthy People 2010: section 11, health communication*. Available at www.healthypeople.gov/document/html/volume1/11healthcom.htm. Accessed October 10, 2011.

CHAPTER 7

Aschenbrenner DS: The conversion of a prescription drug to OTC status, *Am J Nurs* 107(3):54–57, 2007.

D'Arcy Y: Safety first: what you need to know about NSAIDs, *Nursing Made Incredibly Easy* 5(2):13–15, 2007.

Institute for Safe Medication Practices: *A call to action: protecting U.S. citizens from inappropriate medication use*. Available at www.ismp.org/pressroom/viewpoints/CommunityPharmacy.pdf. Accessed July 20, 2015.

Mennick F: Infant deaths with cold medications, *Am J Nurs* 107(3):22, 2007.

Michna E, Duh MS, Korves C, et al: Removal of opioid/acetaminophen combination prescription pain medications: assessing the evidence for hepatotoxicity and consequences of removal of these medications, *Pain Med* 11(3):369–378, 2010.

Miller S: Drug watch '06: vitamins and minerals, *RN* 69(10):37–43, 2006.

National Center for Complementary and Alternative Medicine website. Available at http://nccam.nih.gov. Accessed February 7, 2011.

Qato DM, Alexander GC, Conti RM, et al: Use of prescription and over the counter and dietary supplements among older adults in the US, *JAMA* 300(24):2867–2878, 2008.

Sand-Jecklin K, Hoggatt B, Badzek L: Know the benefits and risks of using common herbal therapies, *Holist Nurs Pract* 18(4):192–198, 2004.

Shehab N, Schaefer MK, Kegler SR, et al: Adverse events from cough and cold medications after a market withdrawal of products labeled for infants, *Pediatrics* 126:1100–1107, 2010.

Tachjian A, Maria V, Jahangir A: Use of herbal products and potential interactions in patients with cardiovascular diseases, *Am Coll Cardiol.* 55:515–525, 2010.

U.S. Food and Drug Administration: *Acetaminophen and liver injury: Q & A for consumers*. Available at www.fda.gov/forconsumers/consumerupdates/ucm168830.htm. Accessed June 20, 2012.

U.S. Food and Drug Administration: *Consumer update: OTC cough and cold products: not for infants and children under 2 years of age*, 2008. Available at www.fda.gov/consumer/updates/coughcold011708.html. Accessed February 7, 2011.

U.S. Food and Drug Administration: *Dietary supplements*. Available at www.fda.gov/food/dietarysupplements/default.htm. Accessed February 7, 2011.

U.S. Food and Drug Administration: *FDA news: FDA releases recommendations regarding use of over-the-counter cough and cold products*, 2008. Available at www.fda/gov/bbs/topics/NEWS/2008/NEW01778.html. Accessed February 7, 2011.

U.S. Food and Drug Administration: *Now available without a prescription*. Available at www.fda.gov/Drugs/ResourcesForYou/Consumers/ucm143547.htm. Accessed February 7, 2011.

U.S. Food and Drug Administration: *Public health advisory: nonprescription cough and cold medicine use in children*, 2008. Available at www.fda.gov/cder/drug/advisory/cough_cold_2008.htm. Accessed February 11, 2011.

U.S. Food and Drug Administration: *Questions and answers on final rule for labeling changes to over-the-counter pain relievers*. Available at www.fda.gov/Drugs/NewsEvents/ucm144068.htm. Accessed February 7, 2011.

U.S. Food and Drug Administration: *Regulation of nonprescription products*. Available at www.fda.gov/aboutfda/centersoffices/cder/ucm093452.htm. Accessed February 7, 2011.

U.S. Food and Drug Administration, *Office of Nonprescription Products: What we do*. Available at www.fda.gov/cder/Offices/OTC/whatwedo.htm. Accessed February 11, 201.

CHAPTER 8

Daack-Hirsch S, Dieter C, Griffin MT: Integrating genomics into undergraduate nursing education, *J Nurs Sch* 43(3):223–230, 2011.

Gene testing, gene therapy, pharmacogenomics. Human Genome Project Information website. Available at www.ornl.gov/sci/techresources/Human_Genome/home.shtml.

Greco KE: Nursing in the genomic era: nurturing our genetic nature, *Medsurg Nurs* 12(5):307–312, 2003.

Hansson M: Taking the patient's side: the ethics of pharmacogenetics, *Per Med* 7(1):75–85, 2010.

Hoppe R, Brauch H, Kroetz DL, et al: Exploiting the complexity of the genome and trasciptome using pharmcogenomics towards personalized medicine, *Geneome Biol* 12(1):301, 2011.

Janneto P, Bratanow N: Utilization of pharmacogenomics and therapeutic drug monitoring for opioid pain management, *Pharmacogenomics* 10(7):1157–1167, 2009.

Lea DH: Genetic and genomic healthcare: ethical issues of importance to nurses, *Online J Issues Nurs* 13(1):6, 2008.

Lea DH: Look back to move forward: how genetics changes daily practice, *Nurs Manage* 34(11):19–25, 2003.

Lea DH: Tailoring drug therapy with pharmacogenetics, *Nursing* 35(4):22–23, 2005.

Nicol MJ: The variation of response to pharmacotherapy: pharmacogenetics—a new perspective to "the right drug for the right person, *Medsurg Nurs* 12(4):242–249, 2003.

Nussbaum RL, McInnes RR, Willard HE: *Thompson and Thompson genetics in medicine*, ed 6, Philadelphia, PA, 2004, Saunders.

Paice JA: Pharmacokinetics, pharmacodynamics, and pharmacogenomics of opioids, *Pain Manag Nurs* 8(3):82–85, 2007.

Prows CA, Prows DR: Medication selection by genotype, *Am J Nurs* 104(5):60–70, 2004.

Tanzi M: Warfarin pharmacogenomics in clinical practice, *Pharmacy Today* 15(10):35–36, 2009.

Turnpenny P, Ellard S: *Emery's elements of medical genetics*, ed 12, London, UK, 2005, Churchill Livingstone.

Wooten JM: Drug watch 2006: new frontiers, *RN* 69(3):36–41, 2006.

Workman ML: Genetic concepts for medical-surgical nursing. In Ignatavicius DD, Workman ML, editors: *Medical-surgical nursing: critical thinking for collaborative care*, ed 7, St Louis, MO, 2013, Elsevier.

CHAPTER 9

Aschenbrenner DS: Unsafe injection practices put patients at risk, *Am J Nurs* 109(7):45–46, 2009.

Barrons R, Pegram A, Borries A: Inhaler device selection: special considerations in elderly patients with chronic obstructive pulmonary disease, *Am J Health Syst Pharm* 68(13):1221–1232, 2011.

Bower MLM: Is your patient's metered-dose inhaler technique up to snuff?, *Nursing* 35(8):50–51, 2005.

Bradshaw E, Collins B, Williams J: Administering rectal suppositories: preparation, assessment and insertion, *Gastrointestinal Nurs* 7(9):24–28, 2009.

Carter-Templeton H, McCoy T: Are we on the same page? A comparison of intramuscular injection explanations in nursing fundamental texts, *Medsurg Nurs* 17(4):237–240, 2008.

D'Arcy Y: Keeping your patient safe during PCA, *Nursing* 38(1):50–56, 2008.

Hadaway LC: IV rounds: delivering multiple medications via backpriming, *Nursing* 34(3):24–26, 2004.

Hockenberry MJ, Wilson D: *Wong's nursing care of infants and children*, ed 9, St Louis, MO, 2011, Mosby.

Institute for Safe Medication Practices: Hazard alert! Asphyxiation possible with syringe tip caps. *ISMP Medication Safety Alert!*, 2001. Available at www.ismp.org/hazardalerts/Hypodermic.asp. Accessed September 25, 2012.

Institute for Safe Medication Practices: How fast is too fast for IV push medication? *ISMP Medication Safety Alert!*, 2003. Available at www.ismp.org/Newsletters/acutecare/articles/20030515.asp?ptr=y. Accessed September 25, 2012.

Institute for Safe Medication Practices: Oral syringes: A crucial and economical risk reduction strategy that has not been fully utilized, *ISMP Medication Safety Alert! Nurse Advise—ERR* 8(5):1–2, 2010.

Institute for Safe Medication Practices: Preventing errors when administering drugs via an enteral feeding tube. *ISMP Medication Safety Alert! Acute Care*, 2010. Available at www.ismp.org/Newsletters/acutecare/articles/20100506.asp. Accessed September 25, 2012.

Institute for Safe Medication Practices: Smart pumps are not smart on their own. *ISMP Medication Safety Alert!*, 2007. Available at www.ismp.org/Newsletters/acutecare/articles/20070419.asp. Accessed September 25, 2012.

LaDuke S: Playing it safe with barcode medication administration, *Nursing* 39(5):32–34, 2009.

Love GH: Clinical do's and don'ts: administering an intradermal injection, *Nursing* 36(6):20, 2006.

McConnell E: Clinical do's and don'ts: applying nitroglycerin ointment, *Nursing* 31(6):17, 2001.

McErlane K: Keeping track of the patch: transdermal delivery in obese patients, *Am J Nurs* 105(6):36–37, 2005.

Miller D, Miller H: To crush or not to crush?, *Nursing* 30(2):50–52, 2000.

Moureau NL, Dawson RB: Keeping needleless connectors clean, part 1, *Nursing* 40(5):18–19, 2010.

Moureau NL, Dawson RB: Keeping needleless connectors clean, part 2, *Nursing* 40(6):61–63, 2010.

Nicoll LH, Hesby A: Intramuscular injection: an integrative research review and guideline for evidence-based practice, *Appl Nurs Res* 16(2):149–162, 2002.

Prettyman J: Subcutaneous or intramuscular? Confronting a parenteral administration dilemma, *Medsurg Nurs* 14(2):93–99, 2005.

Pruitt W: Teaching your patient to use a peak flowmeter, *Nursing* 35(3):54–55, 2005.

Pullen R: Clinical do's and don'ts: administering medication by the Z-track method, *Nursing* 35(7):24, 2005.

Pullen R: Clinical do's and don'ts: administering an orally disintegrating tablet, *Nursing* 38(1):18, 2008.

Rubin BK: Air and soul: the science and application of aerosol therapy, *Respir Care* 55(7):911–921, 2010.

Rushing J: Clinical do's and don'ts: administering eyedrops, *Nursing* 37(5):18, 2007.

Safety wires: *Nurse Advise ERR* 13(10), 2015. Available at: www.ismp.org/news letters/nursing/issues/NurseAdviseERR201510.pdf. Accessed October 20, 2015.

Schulmeister L: Transdermal drug patches: medicine with muscle, *Nursing* 35(1):48–52, 2005.

Stein HG: Glass ampules and filter needles: an example of implementing the sixth "r" in medication administration, *Medsurg Nurs* 15(5):290–294, 2006.

Walsh L, Brophy K: Most nurses don't follow guidelines on IM injections, *J Adv Nurs* 67(5):1034–1040, 2011.

Williams NT: Medication administration through enteral feeding tubes, *Am J Health Syst Pharm* 65(24):2347–2357, 2008.

CHAPTER 10

Acetadote (acetylcysteine) injection (prescribing information), 2008. *Cumberland Pharmaceuticals, Nashville, TN*. Available at www.acetadote.net. Accessed September 25, 2012.

American Association of Addiction Medicine: *Definitions related to the use of opioids for the treatment of pain*, 2008. Available at www.asam.org/docs/publicy-policy-statements/1opioid-definitions-consensus-2-011.pdf?sfvrsn=0. Accessed July 21, 2015.

Bird A, et al: Competency in managing care in epidural analgesia, *Nurs Times* 109(5):18–20, 2013.

Carlson CL: Use of three evidence-based postoperative pain assessment practices by RN, *Pain Manag Nurs* 10(4):174–187, 2009.

Cohen MR: Acetylcysteine routes: mistakes in the mist?, *Nursing* 35(6):12, 2005.

D'Arcy Y: New pain management options: delivery systems and techniques, *Nursing* 37(2):26–27, 2007.

Drug news: FDA advisory: more deaths linked to methadone, *Nursing* 37(2):31, 2007.

Duragesic (fentanyl) transdermal system (prescribing information), 2009. Ortho-McNeil-Janssen Pharmaceuticals, Titusville, NJ. Available at www.duragesic.com. Accessed July 21, 2015.

Ellis JA, Martelli B, LaMontagne C, et al: Evaluation of a continuous epidural analgesia program for postoperative pain in children, *Pain Manag Nurs* 8(4):146–155, 2007.

Finnerup NB, Otto M, Jensen TS, et al: An evidence-based algorithm for the treatment of neuropathic pain, *Medgenmed* 9(2):36, 2007.

Fontana RJ: Acute liver failure including acetaminophen overdose, *Med Clin North Am* 92:761, 2008.

Ginsburg M, Silver S, Berman H: Prescribing opioids to older adults: a guide to choosing and switching among them, *Geriatrics and Aging* 12(1):48–52, 2009.

Gordon DB, Pellino TA, Higgins GA, et al: Nurses' opinions on appropriate administration of prn range opioid analgesic orders for acute pain, *Pain Manag Nurs* 9(3):131–140, 2008.

Gowing L, Ali R, White JM: Buprenorphine for the management of opioid withdrawal, *Cochrane Database Syst Rev* (3):CD002025, 2009.

Grace PJ: The clinical use of placebos: is it ethical? Not when it involves deceiving patients, *Am J Nurs* 106(2):58–61, 2006.

Jeffrey S: FDA approves tramadol extended-release formulation for chronic pain. *Medscape Medical News*. Available at www.medscape.com/viewarticle/586329. Accessed February 20, 2011.

Joseph EK, Reichling J, Levine D: Shared mechanisms for opioid tolerance and a transition to chronic pain, *J Neurosci* 30(13):4660–4666, 2010.

Lange M, Thom B, Kline NE: Nurses' attitudes toward death and caring for dying patients in a comprehensive cancer center, *Oncol Nurs Forum* 35(6):955–959, 2008.

Lidoderm (lidocaine patch 5%) (prescribing information), 2009, Endo Pharmaceuticals, Chadds Ford, PA. Available at www.lidoderm.com/prescrib.aspx. Accessed September 25, 2012.

Lillefjell M, Krokstad S, Espnes GA: Prediction of function in daily life following multidisciplinary rehabilitation for individuals with chronic musculoskeletal pain: a prospective study, *BMC Musculoskelet Disord*

2007. Available at: www.medscapenursing.com/viewarticle/563476. Accessed July 9, 2013.

McCaffery M, Arnstein P: The debate over placebos in pain management, *Am J Nurs* 106(2):62–65, 2006.

Melvin CS, Oldham L: When to refer patients to palliative care: triggers, traps and timely referrals, *Journal of Hospice and Palliative Nursing* 11(5):291–301, 2009.

National Cancer Institute: *Basic principles of cancer pain management*. Available at www.nci.nih.gov/cancertopics/pdq/supportivecare/pain/Patient/page4. Accessed July 21, 2015.

Nucynta (tapentadol) (prescribing information), 2010, Ortho-McNeil-Janssen Pharmaceuticals, Inc, Raritan, NJ. Available at www.nucynta.com. Accessed November 1, 2015.

Opana and Opana ER: information for health care professionals. Available at www.opana.com. Accessed on July 21, 2015.

Pasero C, Eksterowicz N, Primeau M, et al: Registered nurse management and monitoring of analgesia by catheter techniques: position statement, *Pain Manag Nurs* 8(2):48–54, 2007.

Pasero C, McCaffery M: Authorized and unauthorized use of PCA pumps: clarifying the use of patient-controlled analgesia in light of recent alerts, *AJN* 105(7):30–32, 2005.

Pennington P, Caminiti S, Schein JR, et al: Patients' assessment of the convenience of fentanyl HCL iontophoretic transdermal system (ITS) versus morphine intravenous patient-controlled analgesia (IV PCA) in the management of postoperative pain after major surgery, *Pain Manag Nurs* 10(3):124–133, 2009.

Portenoy RK: Chronic pain. *Merck Manuals Online Medical Library*, 2007. Available at www.merck.com/mmpe/print/sec16/ch209/ch209b.html. Accessed November 1, 2015.

Portenoy RK: Pain: introduction. *Merck Manuals Online Medical Library*, 2007. Available at www.merck.com/mmpe/print/sec16/ch209/ch209a.html. Accessed November 1, 2015.

Reese SM: Doctor, are you telling me the truth? Exclusive ethics survey results. *Medscape Medical Ethics*. Available at www.medscape.com/viewarticle/732693. Accessed February 20, 2011.

Schmader KE, Johnson GR, Saddier P, et al: Effect of a zoster vaccine on herpes zoster-related interference with functional status and health-related quality-of-life measures in older adults, *J Am Geriatr Soc* 58(9):1634–1641, 2010.

Shaw S, Lee A: Student nurses' misconceptions of adults with chronic nonmalignant pain, *Pain Manag Nurs* 11(1):2–14, 2010.

Smith WR, Penberthy LT, Bovbjerg VE, et al: Daily assessment of pain in adults with sickle cell disease, *Ann Intern Med* 148:94, 2008.

Stamer UM, Zhang L, Stuber F: Personalized therapy in pain management: where do we stand?, *Pharmacogenomics* 11(6):843–864, 2010.

Stokowski LA: Adult cancer pain: part 2—the latest guidelines for pain management. *Medscape Hematology-Oncology*. Available at www.medscape.com/viewarticle/733067. Accessed February 20, 2011.

U.S. Food and Drug Administration: *FDA limits acetaminophen in prescription combination products; requires liver toxicity warnings*. Available at www.fda.gov/NewsEvents/Newsroom/PressAnnouncements/ucm239894.htm. Accessed February 6, 2011.

U.S. Food and Drug Administration: *Propoxyphene: withdrawal—risk of cardiac toxicity*, 2010. Available at www.fda.gov/Safety/MedWatch/SafetyInformation/SafetyAlertsforHumanMedicalProducts/ucm234389.htm. Accessed January 2, 2011.

Viscusi ER, Gambling DR, Hughes TL, et al: Pharmacokinetics of extended-release epidural morphine sulfate: pooled analysis of six clinical studies, *Am J Health Syst Pharm* 66(11):1020–1030, 2009.

World Health Organization: *Pain ladder for cancer pain*, 2008. Available at www.who.int/cancer/palliative/painladder/en/print.html. Accessed July 21, 2015.

CHAPTER 11

American Association of Nurse Anesthetists: *Conscious sedation: what patients should expect*. Available at www.aana.com/forpatients/Documents/sedation_brochure03.pdf. Accessed February 25, 2011.

American Society of Anesthesiologists: *Continuum of depth of sedation definition of general anesthesia and levels of sedation/analgesia*, 2004, amended 2009. Available at www.asahq.org/publicationsAndServices/standards/20.pdf. Accessed January 20, 2011.

Bezov D, Ashina S, Lipton R: Post-dural puncture headache: part II—prevention, management, and prognosis, *Headache* 50(9):1482–1498, 2010.

Carter-Templeton H: Malignant hyperthermia, *Nursing* 35(6):88, 2005.

Desai A, Macario A: *Anesthesia, general*. Available at http://emedicine.medscape.com/article/1271543-overview. Accessed January 2, 2011.

Pasero C, McCaffery M: Ketamine: low doses may provide some relief for painful conditions, *Am J Nurs* 105(4):60–64, 2005.

Viscusi ER, Gambling DR, Hughes TL, et al: Pharmacokinetics of extended-release epidural morphine sulfate: pooled analysis of six clinical studies, *Am J Health Syst Pharm* 66(11):1020–1030, 2009.

Yamamoto M, Ishikawa S, Makita K: Medication errors in anesthesia: an 8-year retrospective analysis at an urban university hospital, *J Anesth* 22(3):248–252, 2008.

CHAPTER 12

Barclay L: Medications for insomnia or anxiety linked to 35% increase in mortality risk. *Medscape Medical News.* Available at www.medscape.com/viewarticle/729897. Accessed March 10, 2011.

Barclay L: Sedatives and hypnotics may increase risk for suicide in elderly patients. *Medscape Medical News.* Available at www.medscape.com/viewarticle/703908. Accessed March 10, 2011.

Harsora P, Kessmann J: Nonpharmacologic management of chronic insomnia, *Am Fam Physician* 79(2):125–130, 2009.

Howell HR, McQueeney M, Bostick JR: Prescription sleep aids for the treatment of insomnia. *U.S. Pharmacist.* Available at www.medscape.com/viewarticle/736833. Accessed March 10, 2011.

Marshall G, James R, Landman MP, et al: Pentobarbital coma for refractory intra-cranial hypertension after severe traumatic brain injury: mortality predictions and one-year outcomes in 55 patients, *J Trauma* 69(2):275–283, 2010.

McLarnon ME, Monaghan TL, Stewart SH, et al: Drug misuse and diversion in adults prescribed anxiolytics and sedatives, *Pharmacotherapy* 31(3):262–272, 2011.

Miaskowski C: Pharmacologic management of sleep disturbances in noncancer-related pain. *Pain Management Nursing.* Available at www.medscape.com/viewarticle/736833. Accessed March 10, 2011.

Tariq SH, Pulisetty S: Pharmacotherapy for insomnia, *Clin Geriatr Med* 24:93–105, 2008.

Vgontzas A, Liao D, Bixler E, et al: Insomnia with objective short sleep duration is associated with a high risk for hypertension, *Sleep* 32(4):491–497, 2009.

Wang LH, Lin HC, Lin CC, et al: Increased risk of adverse pregnancy outcomes in women receiving zolpidem during pregnancy, *Clin Pharmacol Ther* 88(3):369–374, 2010.

CHAPTER 13

American Psychiatric Association: *Diagnostic and statistical manual of mental disorders, text revision*, ed 4, Washington, DC, 2000, American Psychiatric Association.

Barclay L: Ibuprofen may help relieve acute migraine headaches. *Medscape Medical News.* Available at www.medscape.com/viewarticle/730343. Accessed March 13, 2011.

Bigal ME, Kurth T, Hu H, et al: Migraine and cardiovascular disease: possible mechanisms of interaction, *Neurology* 72(21):1864–1871, 2009.

Centers for Disease Control and Prevention: *Body mass index*, 2009. Available at www.cdc.gov/healthyweight/assessing/bmi/adult_bmi/index.html. Accessed February 15, 2011.

Centers for Disease Control and Prevention: *Attention deficit hyperactivity disorder*, 2010. Available at www.cdc.gov/ncbddd/adhd/. Accessed February 13, 2011.

Centers for Disease Control and Prevention: *Overweight and obesity*, 2010. Available at www.cdc.gov/obesity/data/trends.html. Accessed February 15, 2011.

Centers for Disease Control and Prevention: *Overweight and obesity: defining overweight and obesity*. Available at www.cdc.gov/nccdphp/dnpa/obesity/defining.htm. Accessed February 13, 2011.

Edvinsson L, Linde M: New drugs in migraine treatment and prophylaxis: telcagepant and topiramate, *Lancet* 376(9741):645–655, 2010.

Faraone S, Mick E: Molecular genetics of attention deficit hyperactivity disorder, *Psychiatr Clin North Amer* 33(1):159–180, 2010.

Kurth T, Schurks M, Logroscino G, et al: Migraine frequency and risk of cardiovascular disease in women, *Neurology* 73(8):581–588, 2009.

CHAPTER 14

Centers for Disease Control and Prevention: *Epilepsy*, 2010. Available at www.cdc.gov/epilepsy/. Accessed February 17, 2011.

Considerations for seniors, Keppra website, 2012. Available at www.keppraxr.com/epilepsy/seniors.aspx. Accessed June 20, 2012.

Epilepsy Foundation: *Discontinuing antiepileptic drugs*. Available at www.epilepsyfoundation.org/about/treatment/medications/discontinuing.cfm. Accessed February 16, 2011.

International League Against Epilepsy: *Seizure types*, 2008. Available at www.ilae-epilepsy.org/Visitors/Centre/ctf/seizure_types.cfm. Accessed February 17, 2011.

Redden L, Pritchett Y, Robieson W, et al: Suicidality and divalproex sodium: analysis of controlled studies in multiple indications, *Ann Gen Psychiatry* 10(1):1–5, 2011.

Stephen LJ, Brodie MJ: Pharmacotherpay of epilepsy: newly approved and developmental agents, *CNS Drugs* 25(2):89–107, 2011.

U.S. Food and Drug Administration: *Antiepileptic drugs*, 2009. Available at www.fda.gov/Safety/MedWatch/SafetyInformation/SafetyAlertsforHumanmedicalProducts/ucm074939.htm. Accessed February 18, 2011.

U.S. Food and Drug Administration: *Consumer update: serious health risks with antiepileptic drugs*, 2008. Available at www.fda.gov/consumer/updates/antiepileptic020508.html. Accessed February 19, 2011.

U.S. Food and Drug Administration: *FDA news: FDA alerts health care providers to risk of suicidal thoughts and behavior with antiepileptic medications*, 2008. Available at www.fda.gov/bbs/topics/NEWS/2008/NEW01786.html. Accessed February 18, 2011.

CHAPTER 15

Barrett MJ: Quality improvement in Parkinson disease. *Medscape Neurology & Neurosrugery.* Available at www.medscape.com/viewarticle/737484. Accessed March 18, 2011.

Brooks M: More evidence of healthcare disparities in Parkinson's disease. *Medscape Medical News.* Available at www.medscape.com/viewarticle/73457. Accessed March 18, 2011.

Clegg A, Young JB: Which medications to avoid in people at risk of delirium: a systematic review, *Age Ageing* 40(1):23–29, 2011.

Forsaa EB, Larsen JP, Wentzel-Larsen T, et al: A 12 year population-based study of pyschosis in Parkinson disease, *Arch Neurol* 67:996–1001, 2010.

Muslimovic D, Post B, Speelman JD, et al: Determinants of disability and quality of life in mild to moderate Parkinson disease, *Neurology* 70:2241–2247, 2008.

National Institutes of Health, National Institute of Neurological Disorders and Stroke: *NINDS Parkinson's disease information page*, 2008. Available at www.ninds.nih.gov/disorders/parkinsons_disease/parkinsons_disease.htm. Accessed February 20, 2011.

National Institute of Neurologic Disease and Stroke: *Parkinson's disease*. Available at www.ninds.nih.gov/disorders/parkinsons_disease/parkinsons_disease.htm. Accessed February 22, 2011.

Parkinson's disease. MedlinePlus website, 2009. Available at www.nlm.nih.gov/medlineplus/parkinsonsdisease.html. Accessed February 18, 2011.

Rabinak CA, Nirenberg MJ: Dopamine agonist withdrawal syndrome in Parkinson disease, *Arch Neurol* 67(9):58–63, 2010.

Zesiesicz TA, Sullivan KL, Arnulf I, et al: Practice parameter: treatment of nonmotor symptoms of Parkinson's disease: report of the Quality Standards Subcommittee of the American Academy of Neurology, *Neurology* 74(11):924–931, 2010.

CHAPTER 16

Barbui C, Cipriani A, Patel V, et al: Efficacy of antidepressants and benzodiazepines in minor depression: systematic review and meta-analysis, *Br J Psychiatry* 198(1; Suppl 1):11–16, 2011.

Belleville G: Mortality hazard associated with anxiolytic and hypnotic drug use in the National Population Health Survey, *Can J Psychiatry* 55(9):558–567, 2010.

Donovan MR, Glue P, Kolluir S, et al: Comparative antidepressants in preventing relapse in anxiety disorders—a meta-analysis, *J Affect Disord* 123(1–3):9–16, 2010.

Fernandez Y, Garcia E, Franks P, et al: Depression treatment preferences of Hispanic individuals: exploring the influence of ethnicity, language and explanatory models, *J Am Board Fam Med* 24(1):39–50, 2010.

Frye MA: Clinical practice. Bipolar disorder—a focus on depression, *N Engl J Med* 364(1):51–59, 2011.

Goldberg JF, Pollack MH, Nierenberg AA: How effective are antidepressants? *Medscape Psychiatry & Mental Health*. Available at http://medscape.com/viewarticle/718270. Accessed March 22, 2011.

Institute for Safe Medication Practices: *ISMP's list of confused drug names*, 2008. Available at www.ismp.org. Accessed February 20, 2011.

Institute for Safe Medication Practices: *ISMP's list of high-alert medications*, 2008. Available at www.ismp.org. Accessed February 20, 2011.

Kessing LV, Thomsen AF, Mogensen UB, et al: Treatment with antipsychotics and the risk of diabetes in clinical practice, *Br J Psychiatry* 197:266–271, 2010.

Lang K, Meyers JL, Korn JR, et al: Medication adherence and hospitalization among patients with schizophrenia treated with antipsychotics, *Psychiatr Serv* 62(12):1239–1247, 2010.

Lowry F: FDA panel gives mixed blessing to duloxetine for chronic pain. *Medscape Medical News*. Available at www.medscape.com/viewarticle/727227. Accessed March 22, 2011.

Mental Health America: *Factsheet: post-traumatic stress disorder*. Available at www.nmha.org. Accessed February 20, 2011.

Meyers BS, Jeste DV: Geriatric psychopharmacology: evolution of a discipline, *J Clin Psychiatry* 71(11):1416–1424, 2010.

National Institute of Mental Health: *What is schizophrenia? (fact sheet)*, 2008. Available at www.nimh.nih.gov/health/publications/schizophrenia/what-is-schizophrenia.shtml. Accessed February 20, 2011.

Owenby RK, Brown LT, Brown JN: Use of risperidone as augmentation treatment of major depressive disorder, *Ann Pharmacother* 45(1):95–100, 2011.

Rubio-Valera M, Serrano-Blanco A, Magdalena-Belío J, et al: Effectiveness of pharmacist care in the improvement of adherence to antidepressants: a systematic review and meta-analysis, *Ann Pharmacother* 45(1):39–48, 2010.

Saad M, Cassagnol M, Ahmed E: The impact of the FDA's warning on the use of antipsychotics in clinical practice: a survey, *Consult Pharm* 25(11):739–744, 2010.

Shim RS, Baltrus P, Ye J, et al: Prevalence, treatment and control of depressive symptoms in the United States: results from the national health and nutrition examination survey (NHANES), 2005-2008, *J Am Board Fam Med* 24(1):33–38, 2011.

U.S. Food and Drug Administration: *Class suicidality labeling language for antidepressants*. Available at www.accessdata.fda.gov/drugsatfda_docs/label/2005/020415s018,021208s009lbl.pdf?utm_campaign. Accessed February 20, 2011.

U.S. Food and Drug Administration Safety Communication: *Antipsychotic drug labels updated on use during pregnancy and risk of abnormal muscle movements and withdrawal symptoms in newborns*. Available at www.fda.gov/Drugs/DrugSafety/ucm243903.htm. Accessed October 14, 2011.

CHAPTER 17

Dube C, Goldstein M, Lewis D, et al, editors: *Project ADEPT: curriculum for primary care physician training, vol. I: core modules*, Providence, RI, 1989, Brown University.

Ewing J: Detecting alcoholism: the CAGE questionnaire, *JAMA* 252:1905–1907, 1984.

Flammer M: *Chantix (varenicline) package insert (safety) update*, 2008. Available at www.chantix.com. Accessed February 20, 2011.

Griffin MR: Teen drug abuse of cough and cold medicine, *WebMD Feature*. In collaboration with Consumer Healthcare Products Association (CHPA). Available at www.webmd.com/parenting/teen-abuse-cough-medicine-9/teens-and-dxm-drug-abuse. Accessed March 25, 2011.

Join Together: *Inhalant use declines among U.S. teens*, 2009. Available at www.jointogether.org/news/headlines/inthenews/2009/inhalant-use-declines-among.html. Accessed March 25, 2011.

National Institute on Drug Abuse: *Commonly abused drugs*. Available at www.nida.nih.gov. Accessed February 20, 2011.

Office of National Drug Control Policy, Executive Office of the President: *Prescription for danger: a report on the troubling trend of prescription and over-the-counter drug abuse among the nation's teens*, 2008. Available at www.theantidrug.com/pdfs/prescription_report.PDF. Accessed September 21, 2012.

The Partnership for a Drug-Free America: *Generation RX: National study reveals new category of substance abuse emerging: teens abusing RX and OTC medications intentionally to get high*. Available at www.drugfree.org/Portal/About/NewsReleases/Generation_Rx_Teens_Abusing_Rx_and_OTC_Medications. Accessed March 25, 2011.

Substance Abuse and Mental Health Services Administration, Office of Applied Studies: *National Survey on Drug Use and Health: misuse of over-the-counter cough and cold medications among persons aged 12 to 25*, 2008. Available at www.oas.samhsa.gov/2k8/cough/cough.htm. Accessed February 20, 2011.

Substance Abuse and Mental Health Services Administration, Office of Applied Studies: *Substance Abuse and Mental Health Data Archive (SAMHDA)*. Available at http://oas.samhsa.gov/SAMHDA.htm. Accessed February 20, 2011.

Sullivan LE, Fiellin DA: Narrative review: buprenorphine for opioid dependent patients in an office practice, *Ann Intern Med* 148(9):662–670, 2008.

Werner E: *Fewer teens sniffing inhalants to get high*, Washington, DC, 2009, Associated Press.

CHAPTER 18

Buddiga P: Use of metered dose inhalers, spaces and nebulizers, *eMedicine*. Available at http://emedicine.medscape.com/article/141336-overview. Accessed March 28, 2011.

DeBacker D, Briston P, Devriendt J, et al: Comparison of dopamine and norepinephrine in the treatment of shock, *N Engl J Med* 362(9):779–783, 2010.

Dellinger RP, Levy MM, Carlet JM, et al: Surviving Sepsis Campaign: international guidelines for management of severe sepsis and septic shock: 2008, *Crit Care Med* 36(1):296–327, 2008.

Kerr M: Asthma patients should not take drug holiday from maintenance therapy. *Medscape Medical News*. Available at www.medscape.com/viewarticle/571616. Accessed March 28, 2011.

Liggett SB: Pharmacogenomics of beta₁-adrenergic receptor polymorphisms in heart failure, *Heart Fail Clin* 6(1):27–33, 2010.

Lowry R: Drug combo reduces need for asthma rescue meds, *Reuters Health Information*. Available at www.medscape.com/viewarticle/732763. Accessed March 28, 2011.

Macon-Bill County Hospital Authority v. Ross, 70785 (176 Ga. App. 221) (335 SE2d 633), 1985. Available at www.lawskills.com/case/ga/id/427/29/index.html. Accessed November 2, 2011.

Russell JA, Walley KR, Singer J, et al: Vasopressin versus norepinephrine infusion in patients with septic shock, *N Engl J Med* 358(9):877–881, 2008.

Skidmore-Roth L: *Mosby's 2014 nursing drug reference*, ed 27, St Louis, MO, 2014, Mosby.

U.S. Food and Drug Administration (FDA): *Questions and answers on final rule of albuterol MDIs*. Available at www.fda.gov/Drugs/DrugSafety/InformationbyDrugClass/ucm080446.htm. Accessed March 28, 2011.

CHAPTER 19

Black HR: Managing hypertension, part II: beta-blockers. *Medscape Cardiology*. Available at www.medscape.com/viewarticle/578378. Accessed March 28, 2011.

Go AS, Yang J, Gurwitz JH, et al: Comparative effectiveness of different beta-adrenergic blocking agents on mortality among adults with heart failure in clinical practice, *Arch Intern Med* 168(22):2415–2421, 2008.

Hunt SA, Abraham WT, Chin MH, et al: 2009 Focused update incorporated into the ACC/AHA 2005 guidelines for the diagnosis and management of heart failure in adults: a report of the American College of Cardiology Foundation/American Heart Association Task Force on Practice Guidelines: developed in collaboration with the International Society for Heart and Lung Transplantation, *Circulation* 119(14):e391–e479, 2009.

van Veldhuisen DJ, Cohen-Solal A, Böhm M, et al: Beta-blockade with nebivolol in elderly heart failure patients with impaired and preserved left ventricular ejection fraction: data from SENIORS (Study of Effects of Nebivolol Intervention on Outcomes and Rehospitalization in Seniors With Heart Failure), *J Am Coll Cardiol* 53(23):2150–2158, 2009.

Waknine Y: FDA approves dutasteride/tamsulosin combo pill for benign prostatic hyperplasia, *Medscape Medical News*. Available at www.medscape.com/viewarticle/723816. Accessed on March 28, 2011.

CHAPTER 20

Folstein MF, Folstein SE, McHugh PR: Mini-mental state: a practical method for grading the cognitive state of patients for the clinician, *J Psychiatr Res* 12(3):189–198, 1975.

National Institute of Neurological Disorders and Stroke: *Myasthenia gravis fact sheet*. Available at www.ninds.nih.gov/disorders/myasthenia_gravis/detail_myasthenia_gravis.htm. Accessed February 11, 2011.

National Institute of Neurological Disorders and Stroke: *Alzheimer's disease information page*. Available at www.ninds.nih.gov/disorders/alzheimersdisease/alzheimersdisease.htm. Accessed February 11, 2011.

Qaseem A, Snow V, Cross JT Jr, et al: Current pharmacologic treatment of dementia: a clinical practice guideline from the American College of Physicians and the American Academy of Family Physicians, *Ann Intern Med* 148(5):370–378, 2008.

Raina P, Santaguida P, Ismaila A, et al: Effectiveness of cholinesterase inhibitors and memantine for the treatment of dementia: evidence review for a clinical practice guideline, *Ann Intern Med* 148(5):379–397, 2008.

Venturelli M, Scarsini R, Schena F: Six-month walking program changes cognitive and ADL performance in patients with Alzheimer, *American Journal of Alzheimer's Disease and Other Dementias* 26(5):381–388, 2011.

Winchester J, Dick MB, Gillen D, et al: Walking stabilizes cognitive functioning in Alzheimer's disease (AD) across one year, *Arch Gerontol Geriatr* 56(1):96–103, 2013.

CHAPTER 21

Gopal M, Haynes K, Bellamy SL, et al: Discontinuation rates of anticholinergic medications used for treatment of lower urinary tract symptoms, *Obstet Gynecol* 112(6):1311–1318, 8a 9a, 2008.

Herschorn S, Stothers L, Carlson K, et al: Tolerability of 5 mg solifenacin once daily versus 5 mg oxybutynin immediate release 3 times daily: results of the VECTOR trial, *J Urol* 183(5):1892–1898, 2010.

Modi A, Weiner M, Craig BA, et al: Concomitant use of anticholinesterase inhibitors and anticholinergics in Medicaid recipients with dementia and residing in nursing homes, *J Am Geriatr Soc* 57(7):1238–1244, 2009.

Shamliyan TA, Kane RL, Wyman J, et al: Systematic review: randomized controlled trials on nonsurgical treatments for urinary incontinence in women, *Ann Intern Med* 148(6):459–473, 2008.

Skidmore-Roth L: *Mosby's 2014 nursing drug reference*, ed 27, St Louis, MO, 2014, Mosby.

Subak LL, Wing R, West DS, et al: Weight loss to treat urinary incontinence in overweight and obese women, *N Engl J Med* 360(5):481–490, 2009.

CHAPTER 22

American Heart Association: *Guidelines for treating resistant hypertension*. Available at www.americanheart.org. Accessed February 18, 2011.

The Antihypertensive and Lipid Lowering Treatment to Prevent Heart Attack Trial website. Available at www.nhlbi.nih.gov/health/allhat/. Accessed February 18, 2011.

Turnbull F, Neal B, et al: Blood Pressure Lowering Treatment Trialists' Collaboration: Effects of different regimens to lower blood pressure on major cardiovascular events in older and younger adults: meta-analysis of randomised trials, *BMJ* 336(7653):1121–1123, 2008.

Cutler JA, Sorlie PD, Wolz M, et al: Trends in hypertension prevalence, awareness, treatment, and control rates in United States adults between 1988-1994 and 1999-2004, *Hypertension* 52(5):818–827, 2008.

Ferdinand KC, Ferdinand DP: Race-based therapy for hypertension: possible benefits and potential pitfalls, *Expert Rev Cardiovasc Ther* 10(6):1357–1366, 2008.

Inspra (prescribing information), 2007, Pfizer, New York. Available at www.pfizer.com/products/rx/rx_product_inspra.jsp. Accessed September 24, 2012.

Law MR, Morris JK, Wald NJ: Use of blood pressure lowering drugs in the prevention of cardiovascular disease: meta-analysis of 147 randomized trials in the context of expectations from prospective epidemiological studies, *BMJ* 336(7653):1121–1123, 2009.

National High Blood Pressure Education Program: *The seventh report of the Joint National Committee on Detection, Evaluation, and Treatment of High Blood Pressure (JNC-7)*, Bethesda, MD, 2004, National Institutes of Health.

National Medical Association (NMA) 2010 Annual Convention and Scientific Assembly: new ARB shows good results in blacks. *Medscape Medical News*. Available at www.medscape.com/viewarticle/726187. Accessed April 10, 2011.

New guidelines for hypertension treatment, *Newsletter No. 1518*, 2008. Available at www.ashp.org. Accessed February 18, 2011.

Remodulin (prescribing information), Research Triangle, 2008, United Therapeutics, Park, NC. Available at www.remodulin.com. Accessed September 24, 2012.

Wang NY, Young JH, Meoni LA, et al: Blood pressure change and risk of hypertension associated with parental hypertension: the Johns Hopkins Precursors Study, *Arch Intern Med* 168(6):643–648, 2008.

CHAPTER 23

Ashkenazi A, Schwedt T: Cluster headache: acute and prophylactic therapy, *Headache* 51(2):272–286, 2011.

Black HR: What about first-line beta blockers? A big issue for JNC 8, *Medscape Cardiology*. Available at www.medscape.com/viewarticle/737001. Accessed April 18, 2011.

Brogden NK, Dunn S: Advances in the treatment of chronic stable angina (continuing education module), *U.S. Pharmacist*, 2008. Available at www.uspharmacist.com. Accessed February 20, 2011.

Fraker TD Jr, Fihn SD, et al: 2002 Chronic Stable Angina Writing Committee: 2007 Chronic angina focused update of the ACC/AHA 2002 guidelines for the management of patients with chronic stable angina: a report of the American College of Cardiology/American Heart Association Task Force on Practice Guidelines Writing Group to develop the focused update of the 2002 guidelines for the management of patients with chronic stable angina, *J Am Coll Cardiol* 50(23):2264–2274, 2007.

Law MR, Morris JK, Wald NJ: Use of blood pressure lowering drugs in the prevention of cardiovascular disease: meta-analysis of 147 randomised trials in the context of expectations from prospective epidemiological studies, *BMJ* 336(7653):1121–1123, 2009.

Morrow DA, Scirica BM, Chaitman BR, et al: Evaluation of the glycometabolic effects of ranolazine in patients with and without diabetes mellitus in the MERLIN-TIMI 36 randomized controlled trial, *Circulation* 119(15):2032–2039, 2009.

Turnbull F, Neal B, et al: Blood Pressure Lowering Treatment Trialists' Collaboration: Effects of different regimens to lower blood pressure on major cardiovascular events in older and younger adults: meta-analysis of randomised trials, *BMJ* 336(7653):1121–1123, 2008.

U.S. Food and Drug Administration: How to dispose of unused medicines. *FDA Consumer Health Information*. 2011. Available at www.fda.gov/ForConsumers/ConsumerUpdates. Accessed on April 18, 2011.

Wilson SR, Scirica BM, Braunwald E, et al: Efficacy of ranolazine in patients with chronic angina observations from the randomized, double-blind, placebo-controlled MERLIN-TIMI (Metabolic Efficiency With Ranolazine for Less Ischemia in Non-ST-Segment Elevation Acute Coronary Syndromes) 36 Trial, *J Am Coll Cardiol* 53(17):1510–1516, 2009.

CHAPTER 24

Beckett NS, Peters R, Fletcher AE, et al: Treatment of hypertension in patients 80 years of age or older, *N Engl J Med* 358(18):1887–1898, 2008.

Fonarow GC, Abraham WT, Albert NM, et al: Influence of beta-blocker continuation or withdrawal on outcomes in patients hospitalized with heart failure: findings from the OPTIMIZE-HF program, *J Am Coll Cardiol* 52(3):190–199, 2008.

Hunt SA, Abraham WT, Chin MH, et al: 2009 focused update incorporated into the ACC/AHA 2005 guidelines for the diagnosis and management of heart failure in adults: a report of the American College of Cardiology Foundation/American Heart Association Task Force on Practice Guidelines. Developed in collaboration with the International Society for Heart and Lung Transplantation, *Circulation* 119(14):e391–e479, 2009.

Maak CA, Taba JA, McClintock DE: Should acute treatment with inhaled beta agonists be withheld from patients with dyspnea who may have heart failure?, *J Emerg Med* 40(2):135–145, 2011.

Massie BM, Carson PE, McMurray JJ, et al: Irbesartan in patients with heart failure and preserved ejection fraction, *N Engl J Med* 359(23):2456–2467, 2008.

Shaddy RE, Webb G: Applying heart failure guidelines to adult congenital heart disease patients, *Expert Rev Cardiovasc Ther* 6(2):165–174, 2008.

Shah RU, Klein L, Lloyd-Jones DM: Heart failure in women: epidemiology, biology and treatment, *Women's Health* 5(5):517–527, 2009.

Task Force for Diagnosis and Treatment of Acute and Chronic Heart Failure 2008 of European Society of Cardiology: ESC guidelines for the diagnosis and treatment of acute and chronic heart failure 2008: the Task Force for the Diagnosis and Treatment of Acute and Chronic Heart Failure 2008 of the European Society of Cardiology. Developed in collaboration with the Heart Failure Association of the ESC (HFA) and endorsed by the European Society of Intensive Care Medicine (ESICM), *Eur Heart J* 29(19):2388–2442, 2008.

Warner C, Bohm M: Is dual blockage most effective for CHF? When to use ARB and ACE inhibitors together, *Geriatrics and Aging* 11(4):224–230, 2008.

CHAPTER 25

Camm AJ, Kirchhof P, Lip GY, et al: Guidelines for the management of atrial fibrillation: The Task Force for the Management of Atrial Fibrillation of the European Society of Cardiology (ESC), *Eur Heart J* 31:2369–2429, 2010.

Fauchier L, Pierre B, de Labriolle A, et al: Antiarrhythmic effect of statin therapy and atrial fibrillation: a meta-analysis of randomized controlled trials, *J Am Coll Cardiol* 51(8):828–835, 2008.

Gaither JB, Tarabar A: *Antidysrhythmic toxicity*. Available at http://emedicicine.medscape.com/article/813046. Accessed April 22, 2011.

Gislason GH, Rasmussen JN, Abildstrom SZ, et al: Increased mortality and cardiovascular morbidity associated with use of nonsteroidal anti-inflammatory drugs in chronic heart failure, *Arch Intern Med* 169(2):141–149, 2009.

Heuzey AL, De Ferrari GM, Radzik D, et al: A short-term, randomized, double-blind, parallel-group study to evaluate the efficacy and safety of dronedarone versus amiodarone in patients with persistent atrial fibrillation: The DIONYSOS study, *J Cardiovasc Electrophysiol* 21(6):606–607, 2010.

Kuber L, Torp-Pedersen C, McMurray JJ, et al: Dronedarone Study Group. Increased mortality after dronedarone therapy for severe heart failure, *N Engl J Med* 358(25):2678–2687, 2008.

Kannankeril PJ: Understanding drug induced torsades de pointes, *Expert Opin Drug Saf* 7(3):231–239, 2008.

Ovetavo OO, Rogers CE, Hoffman PO: Dronedarone: a new antiarrhythmic agent, *Pharmacotherapy* 30(9):904–915, 2010.

Roy D, Talajic M, Nattel S, et al: Rhythm control versus rate control for atrial fibrillation and heart failure, *N Engl J Med* 358:2667–2677, 2008.

U.S. Food and Drug Administration Safety: *Multaq (dronedarone)—drug safety communication: risk of severe liver injury*. Available at www.fda.gov/Safety/MedWatch/SafetyInformation/SafetyAlertsforHumanMedicalProducts/ucm240110.htm. Accessed February 20, 2011.

U.S. Food and Drug Administration Safety: *Multaq (dronedarone)—drug safety communication: increased risk of death or serious cardiovascular events*. Available at www.fda.gov/Safety/MedWatch/SafetyInformation/SafetyAlertsforHumanMedicalProducts/ucm264204.htm. Accessed November 6, 2011.

CHAPTER 26

Becker RC: Next-generation antithrombin therapies, *J Invasive Cardiol* 21(4):179–185, 2009.

Brooks M: Experts mull dabigatran vs. warfarin for stroke prevention in AF. *Medscape Medical News*. Available at www.medscape.com/viewarticle/733652. Accessed April 26, 2011.

Cohen MG, Purdy DA, Rossi JS, et al: First clinical application of an actively reversible direct factor IXa inhibitor as an anticoagulation strategy in patients undergoing percutaneous coronary intervention, *Circulation* 122(6):614–622, 2010.

Edmunds MW, Scudder L: New oral anticoagulants on the horizon. *Medscape Nurses*. Available at www.medscape.com/viewarticle/714692. Accessed April 26, 2011.

Franchini M, Mannucci PM: A new era for anticoagulants, *Eur J Intern Med* 20(6):562–568, 2009.

Garcia D, Libby E, Crowther MA: The new oral anticoagulants, *Blood* 115(1):15–20, 2010.

Gómez-Outes A, Suárez-Gea ML, Lecumberri R, et al: New parenteral anticoagulants in development, *Ther Adv Cardiovasc Dis.* 5(1):33–59, 2011.

Hirsh J, Bauer KA, Donati MB, et al: Parenteral anticoagulants: American College of Chest Physicians evidence-based clinical practice guidelines, edition 8, *Chest* 133(Suppl 6):S141–S159, 2008.

R.E.-M.O.B.I.L.I.Z.E. Writing Committee, Ginsberg JS, Davidson BL, et al: Oral thrombin inhibitor dabigatran etexilate vs North American enoxaparin regimen for prevention of venous thromboembolism after knee arthroplasty surgery, *J Arthroplasty* 24(1):1–9, 2009.

Turpie AG, Lassen MR, Davidson BL, et al: Rivaroxaban versus enoxaparin for thromboprophylaxis after total knee arthroplasty (RECORD4): a randomised trial, *Lancet* 373(9676):1673–1680, 2009.

U.S. Food and Drug Administration: *Safety information: Arixtra (fondaparinux sodium) injection.* Available at www.fda.gov/Safety/MedWatch/SafetyInformation/ucm182229.htm. Accessed March 5, 2011.

van Ryn J, Stangier J, Haertter S, et al: Dabigatran etexilate—a novel, reversible, oral direct thrombin inhibitor: interpretation of coagulation assays and reversal of anticoagulant activity, *Thromb Haemost* 103(6):1116–1127, 2010.

Weitz JI, Hirsh J, Samama MM: New antithrombotic drugs: American College of Chest Physicians evidence-based clinical practice guidelines, edition 8, *Chest* 133(Suppl 6):S234–S256, 2008.

CHAPTER 27

American Heart Association: *Hyperlipidemia.* Available at www.heart.org/HEARTORG/Conditions/Cholesterol/AboutCholesterol/Hyperlipidemia_UCM_434965_Article.jsp. Accessed April 29, 2011.

Barclay L: Overview of lifestyle interventions in the management of hyperlipemia in the primary care setting. *Medscape Medical News.* Available at www.medscape.com/viewarticle/721503. Accessed on April 29, 2011.

Drazen JM, Jarcho JA, Morrissey S, et al: Cholesterol lowering and ezetimibe, *N Engl J Med* 358(14):1507–1508, 2008.

Ford ES, Li C, Zhao G, et al: Hypertriglyceridemia and its pharmacologic treatment among US adults, *Arch Intern Med* 169(6):572–578, 2009.

Ginsberg HN, Elam MB, et al: ACCORD Study Group: Effects of combination lipid therapy in type 2 diabetes mellitus, *N Engl J Med* 362(17):1563–1574, 2010.

The Internet Stroke Center: *Stroke assessment tools: modified Rankin Scale.* Available at www.strokecenter.org/wp-content/uploads/2011/08/modified_rankin.pdf. Accessed April 29, 2011.

Kearney PM, Blackwell L, Cholesterol Treatment Trialists' (CTT) Collaborators, et al: Efficacy of cholesterol-lowering therapy in 18,686 people with diabetes in 14 randomised trials of statins: a meta-analysis, *Lancet* 371(9607):117–125, 2008.

Ní Chróinín D, Callaly EL, Duggan J, et al: Association between acute statin therapy, survival, and improved functional outcome after ischemic stroke: The North Dublin Population Stroke Study, *Stroke* 42(4):1021–1029, 2011.

O'Riordan M: FDA restricts use of simvastatin 80 mg, *Heartwire: Alerts, Approvals, and Safety Changes.* Available at www.medscape.com/viewarticle/744242. Accessed June 13, 2011. 10a 11a.

Pletcher MJ, Lazar L, Bibbins-Domingo K, et al: Comparing impact and cost-effectiveness of primary prevention strategies for lipid lowering, *Ann Intern Med* 150(4):243–254, 2009.

Sarwar N, Sandhu MS, et al: Triglyceride Coronary Disease Genetics Consortium and Emerging Risk Factors Collaboration: Triglyceride-mediated pathways and coronary disease: collaborative analysis of 101 studies, *Lancet* 375(9726):1634–1639, 2010.

Theheart.org: *FDA agrees with SHARP data; vytorin up for expanded use in CKD.* Available at www.theheart.org/condition/lipid-metabolic.do. Accessed November 11, 2011.

CHAPTER 28

Barclay L: Thiazide-like diuretic suitable in patients with hypertension and metabolic syndrome. *Medscape Medical News.* Available at www.medscape.org/viewarticle/570314. Accessed April 30, 2011.

Cross-allergenicity of sulfonamide antibiotics and other drugs: stereochemistry and adverse reactions to sulfonamide antibiotics, 2004. Available at www.medscape.com/viewarticle/482766_4. Accessed February 26, 2011.

Imazio M, Cotroneo A, Gaschino G, et al: Management of heart failure in elderly people, *Int J Clin Pract* 62(2):270–280, 2008.

Jugdutt BI: Heart failure in the elderly: advances and challenges, *Expert Rev Cardiovasc Ther* 8(5):695–715, 2010.

Kaplan NM: The choice of thiazide diuretics: why chlorthalidone may replace hydrochlorothiazide, *Hypertension* 54(5):951–953, 2009.

Khosla N, Kalaitzidis R, Bakris GL: The kidney, hypertension, and remaining challenges, *Med Clin North Am* 93(3):697–715, 2009.

CHAPTER 29

Mount DB: The brain in hyponatremia: both culprit and victim, *Semin Nephrol* 29(3):196–215, 2009.

Palmer BF: A physiologic-based approach to the evaluation of a patient with hyperkalemia, *Am J Kidney Dis* 56(3):387–393, 2010.

Perianayagam A, Sterns RH, Silver SM, et al: DDAVP is effective in preventing and reversing inadvertent overcorrection of hyponatremia, *Clin J Am Soc Nephrol* 3(2):331–336, 2008.

Sterns RH, Hix JK: Overcorrection of hyponatremia is a medical emergency, *Kidney Int* 76(6):587–589, 2009.

Sterns RH, Nigwekar SU, Hix JK: The treatment of hyponatremia, *Semin Nephrol* 29(3):282–299, 2009.

Stiles S: ARB/ACE-inhibitor combo a risk in clinical practice. *Heartwire* 2011. Available at www.medscape.com/viewarticle739632. Accessed May 11, 2011.

Suneja M, Batuman V, Muster HA, et al: Hypocalcemia. *Medscape Reference,* updated October 20, 2011. Available at www.medscape.com/nurses. Accessed November 20, 2011.

CHAPTER 30

Bauer SR, Lam SW: Arginine vasopressin for the treatment of septic shock in adults, *Pharmacotherapy* 30(10):1057–1071, 2010.

Ferguson LA: Growth hormone use in children: necessary or designer therapy?, *J Pediatr Health Care* 25(11):24–30, 2011.

Giavoli C, Bergamaschi S, Ferrante E, et al: Effect of growth hormone deficiency and recombinant hGH replacement on the hypothalamic-pituitary-adrenal axis in children with idiopathic isolation GH deficiency, *Clin Endocrinol* 68(2):247–251, 2008.

Russell JA, Walker KR, Singer J, et al: Vasopressin versus norepinephrine infusion in patients with septic shock, *N Engl J Med* 358(9):877–887, 2008.

Zhang XP, Zhang L, Yang P, et al: Protective effects of baicalin and octreotide on multiple organ injury in severe acute pancreatitis, *Dig Dis Sci* 53(2):581–591, 2008.

CHAPTER 31

Bach-Huynh TG, Nayak B, Loh J, et al: Timing of levothyroxine administration affects serum thyrotropin concentration, *J Clin Endocrinol Metab* 94(10):3905–3912, 2009.

Barclay L: Thyroid drug linked to fracture risk in older adults. *Medscape Medical News.* Available at www.medscape.com/viewarticle/741887. Accessed May 17, 2011.

Benvenga S, Bartolone L, Pappalardo MA, et al: Altered intestinal absorption of L-thyroxine caused by coffee, *Thyroid* 18(3):293–301, 2008.

Brent GA: Clinical practice: Graves' disease, *N Engl J Med* 358(24):2594–2605, 2008.

Flynn RW, Bonellie SR, Jung RT, et al: Serum thyroid-stimulating hormone concentration and morbidity from cardiovascular disease and fractures in patients on long-term thyroxine therapy, *J Clin Endocrinol Metab* 95(1):186–193, 2010.

Jonklaas J: Sex and age differences in levothyroxine dosage requirement, *Endocrin Pract* 16(1):71–79, 2010.

Jonklaas J, Davidson B, Bhagat S, et al: Triiodothyronine levels in athyreotic individuals during levothyroxine therapy, *JAMA* 299(7):769–777, 2008.

CHAPTER 32

The Action to Control Cardiovascular Risk in Diabetes (ACCORD) Study Group: Effects of intensive glucose lowering in type 2 diabetes, *N Engl J Med* 358(24):2545–2569, 2008.

Adamson F: New USDA plate icon: serving it up to your patients. *Medscape Internal Medicine: Medicine Matters.* 2011. Available at www.medscape.com/viewarticle/743918. Accessed June 6, 2011.

American Diabetes Association: Standards of medical care in diabetes—2015, *Diabetes Care* 38(Suppl 1):s1–s93, 2015.

Bergenstal RM: Sensor-augmented insulin pump therapy trumps multiple daily injections in type 1 diabetes, *Medscape Medical News.* Available at www.medscape.com/viewarticle/724427. Accessed June 6, 2011.

Giovannucci E, Harlan DM, Archer MC, et al: Diabetes and cancer: a consensus report, *Diabetes Care* 33(7):1674–1685, 2010.

Kitabchi AE, Umpierrez GE, Murphy MB, et al: Hyperglycemic crises in adult patients with diabetes: a consensus statement from the American Diabetes Association, *Diabetes Care* 29(12):2739–2748, 2006.

Nathan DM, Buse JB, Davidson MB, et al: Medical management of hyperglycemia in type 2 diabetes: a consensus algorithm for the initiation and adjustment of therapy: a consensus statement of the American Diabetes Association and the European Association for the Study of Diabetes, *Diabetes Care* 32(1):193–203, 2009.

Pignone M, Alberts MJ, Colwell JA, et al: Aspirin for primary prevention of cardiovascular events in people with diabetes: a position statement of the American Diabetes Association, a scientific statement of the American Heart Association, and an expert consensus document of the American College of Cardiology Foundation, *Diabetes Care* 33(6):1395–1402, 2010.

Umpierrez GE, Smiley D, Jacobs S, et al: Randomized study of basal-bolus insulin therapy in the inpatient management of patients with type 2 diabetes undergoing general surgery (RABBIT 2 surgery), *Diabetes Care* 34(2):256–261, 2011.

U.S. Food and Drug Administration Safety: *Avandia (rosiglitazone): REMS—risk of cardiovascular events*, 2011. Available at www.fda.gov/safety/medwatch/safetyinformation/safetyalertsforhumanmedicalproducts/ucm226994.htm. Accessed March 11, 2011.

CHAPTER 33

Bornstein SR: Predisposing factors for adrenal insufficiency, *N Engl J Med* 360(22):2328–2339, 2009.

Christiansen CF, Christensen S, Mehnert F, et al: Glucocorticoid use and risk of atrial fibrillation or flutter: a population-based, case-control study, *Arch Intern Med* 169(18):1677–1683, 2009.

Huscher D, Thiele K, Gromnica-Ihle E, et al: Dose-related patterns of glucocorticoid-induced side effects, *Ann Rheum Dis* 68(7):1119–1124, 2009.

Kelly W: Comparison of inhaled corticosteroids: an update, *Annals Pharmacother* 43(3):519–527, 2009.

Panoulas VF, Douglas KM, Stavropoulos-Kalinoglou A, et al: Long-term exposure to medium-dose glucocorticoid therapy associates with hypertension in patients with rheumatoid arthritis, *Rheumatology (Oxford)* 47(1):72–75, 2008.

Schweiger TA, Zdanowicz M: Systemic corticosteroids in the treatment of acute exacerbations of chronic obstructive pulmonary disease, *Am J Health Syst Pharm* 67(13):1061–1069, 2010.

CHAPTER 34

Allard JE, Maxwell GL: Race disparities between black and white women in the incidence, treatment, and prognosis of endometrial cancer, *Cancer Control* 16(1):53–56, 2009.

Cummings SR, San Martin J, McClung MR, et al: Denosumab for prevention of fractures in postmenopausal women with osteoporosis, *N Engl J Med* 361(8):756–765, 2009.

MacLean C, Newberry S, Maglione M, et al: Systematic review: comparative effectiveness of treatments to prevent fractures in men and women with low bone density or osteoporosis, *Ann Intern Med* 148(3):197–213, 2008.

National Osteoporosis Foundation: *Clinician's guide to prevention and treatment of osteoporosis*, 2010. Available at www.nof.org/sites/default/files/pdfs/NOF_ClinicianGuide2009_v7.pdf. Accessed April 21, 2011.

North American Menopause Society: Estrogen and progestogen use in postmenopausal women: 2010 position statement of the North American Menopause Society, *Menopause* 17(2):242–255, 2010.

Ross MG: *Preterm labor*, 2011. Available at http://emedicine.medscape.com/article/260998-overview#aw2aab6b6. Accessed April 21, 2011.

U.S. Food and Drug Administration Drug Safety Communication: *New warnings against use of terbutaline to prevent preterm labor*, 2011. Available at www.fda.gov/Drugs/DrugSafety/ucm243539.htm. Accessed April 21, 2011.

CHAPTER 35

Blanchard N, Abu-Baker A: The treatment of benign prostatic hypertrophy (continuing education module), *U.S. Pharmacist*, 2008. Available at www.uspharmacist.com.

Howlader N, Noone AM, Krapcho M, et al: *SEER cancer statistics review, 1975-2008*, Bethesda, MD., 2011, National Cancer Institute. Available at: http://seer.cancer.gov/csr/1975_2008/. Accessed May 25, 2011.

Jeong YB, Kwon KS, Kim SD, et al: Effect of discontinuation of 5alpha-reductase inhibitors on prostate volume and symptoms in men with BPH: a prospective study, *Urology* 73(4):802–806, 2009.

Marks LS, Gittelman MC, Hill LA, et al: Rapid efficacy of the highly selective alpha1A-adrenoceptor antagonist silodosin in men with signs and symptoms of benign prostatic hyperplasia: pooled results of 2 phase 3 studies, *J Urol* 181(6):2634–2640, 2009.

National Cancer Institute at the National Institutes of Health: *Prostate cancer*, 2011. Available at www.cancer.gov/cancertopics/types/prostate. Accessed May 25, 2011.

Qaseem A, Snow V, Denberg TD, et al: Hormonal testing and pharmacologic treatment of erectile dysfunction: a clinical practice guideline from the American College of Physicians, *Ann Intern Med* 151(9):639–649, 2009.

Tsertsvadze A, Fink HA, Yazdi F, et al: Oral phosphodiesterase-5 inhibitors and hormonal treatments for erectile dysfunction: a systematic review and meta-analysis, *Ann Intern Med* 151(9):650–661, 2009.

Zhu YS, Imperato-McGinley JL: 5alpha-reductase isozymes and androgen actions in the prostate, *Ann N Y Acad Sci* 1155:43–56, 2009.

CHAPTER 36

Bousquet J, Khaltaev N, Cruz N, et al: Allergic Rhinitis and its Impact on Asthma (ARIA) 2008 update (in collaboration with the World Health Organization, GA²LEN and AllerGen), *Allergy* 63(Suppl 86):8–160, 2008.

Dicpinigaitis PV, Gayle YE, Solomon G, et al: Inhibition of cough-reflex sensitivity by benzonatate and guaifenesin in acute viral cough, *Respir Med* 103(6):902–906, 2009.

Driscoll-Maliarakis K: Teen prescription and over-the-counter drug abuse, *Medscape Public Health.* Available at www.medscape.com/viewarticle713306. Accessed May 31, 2011.

Horak F, Zieglmayer P, Zieglmayer R, et al: Placebo-controlled study of the nasal decongestant effect of phenylephrine and pseudoephedrine in the Vienna Challenge Chamber, *Ann Allergy Asthma Immunol* 102(2):116–120, 2009.

Kling J: Acaai 2008: Intranasal steroid outperforms antihistamine in relieving nighttime allergy symptoms, *Medscape Medical News.* Available at www.medscape.com/viewarticle583472. Accessed May 31, 2011.

Shehab N, Schaefer MK, Kegler SR, et al: Adverse events from cough and cold medications after a market withdrawal of products labeled for infants, *Pediatrics* 126(6):1100–1107, 2010.

Wallace DV, Dykewicz MS, Bernstein DI, et al: The diagnosis and management of rhinitis: an updated practice parameter, *J Allergy Clin Immunol* 122(Suppl 2):S1–S84, 2008.

CHAPTER 37

Balkissoon R: Asthma overview, *Prim Car* 35(1):41–60, 2008.

Cyr MC, Beauchesne MF, Lemire C, et al: Effect of theophylline on the rate of moderate to severe exacerbations among patients with chronic obstructive pulmonary disease, *Br J Clin Pharmacol* 65(1):40–50, 2008.

Hurst JR, Vestbo J, Anzueto A, et al: Evaluation of COPD Longitudinally to Identify Predictive Surrogate Endpoints (ECLIPSE) investigators: Susceptibility to exacerbation in chronic obstructive pulmonary disease, *N Engl J Med* 363(12):1128–1138, 2010.

Lindenauer PK, Pekow PS, Lahti MC, et al: Association of corticosteroid dose and route of administration with risk of treatment failure in acute exacerbation of chronic obstructive pulmonary disease, *JAMA* 303(23):2359–2367, 2010.

National Asthma Education and Prevention Program: *Expert panel report 3: guidelines for the diagnosis and management of asthma.* 2007, U.S. Department of Health and Human Services, National Institutes of Health, National Heart, Lung, and Blood Institute, Bethesda, MD, NIH Publication No. 08-5846. Available at www.nhlbi.nih.gov/guidelines/asthma/asthsumm.pdf. Accessed August 1, 2015.

Tamesis GP, Covar RA: Long-term effects of asthma medications in children, *Curr Opin Allergy Clin Immunol* 8(2):163–167, 2008.

U.S. Food and Drug Administration: How to dispose of unused medications. *FDA Consumer Updates.* 2011. Available at www.fda.gov/forconsumers/consumerupdates/ucm101653.htm. Accessed June 8, 2011.

CHAPTER 38

Freifeld AG, Bow EJ, Sepkowitz KA, et al: Clinical practice guideline for the use of antimicrobial agents in neutropenic patients with cancer: 2010 update by the Infectious Diseases Society of America, *Clin Infect Dis* 52(4):e56, 2011.

File TM Jr, Low DE, Eckburg PB, et al: Integrated analysis of FOCUS 1 and FOCUS 2: randomized, doubled-blinded, multicenter phase 3 trials of the efficacy and safety of ceftaroline fosamil versus ceftriaxone in patients with community-acquired pneumonia, *Clin Infect Dis* 51(12):1395, 2010.

Hersh AL, Chambers HF, Maselli JH, et al: National trends in ambulatory visits and antibiotic prescribing for skin and soft-tissue infections, *Arch Intern Med* 168(14):1585, 2008.

Kallen AJ, Mu Y, Bulens S, et al: Health care-associated invasive MRSA infections, 2005-2008, *JAMA* 304(6):641, 2010.

Liu C, Bayer A, Cosgrove SE, et al: Clinical practice guidelines by the Infectious Diseases Society of America for the treatment of methicillin-resistant *Staphylococcus aureus* infections in adults and children, *Clin Infect Dis* 52(3):e18, 2011.

Powers JH, Phoenix JA, Zuckerman DM: Antibiotic uses and challenges—a comprehensive review from NRCWF. *Medscape Family Medicine.* Available at www.medscape.com/viewarticle723457. Accessed June 14, 2011.

Romano A, Gaeta F, Valluzzi RL, et al: Diagnosing hypersensitivity reactions to cephalosporins in children, *Pediatrics* 122(3):521, 2008.

Somech R, Weber EA, Lavi S: Evaluation of immediate allergic reactions to cephalosporins in non-penicillin-allergic patients, *Int Arch Allergy Immunol* 150(3):205, 2009.

Wang JL, Chen SY, Wang JT, et al: Comparison of both clinical features and mortality risk associated with bacteremia due to community-acquired methicillin-resistant *Staphylococcus aureus* and methicillin-susceptible *S. aureus, Clin Infect Dis* 46(6):799, 2008.

CHAPTER 39

Centers for Disease Control and Prevention: Detection of *Enterobacteriaceae* isolates carrying metallo-beta-lactamase—United States, 2010, *MMWR.* 59(24):750, 2010.

Centers for Disease Control and Prevention: *National Antimicrobial Resistance Monitoring System (NARMS)—frequently asked questions (FAQ) about antibiotic resistance,* 2005. Available at www.cdc.gov/narms/faq_antiresis.htm. Accessed December 18, 2011.

Freifeld AG, Bow EJ, Sepkowitz KA, et al: Clinical practice guideline for the use of antimicrobial agents in neutropenic patients with cancer: 2010 update by the Infectious Diseases Society of America, *Clin Infect Dis* 52(4):e56, 2011.

Mainous AG, Everett CJ, Post RE, et al: Availability of antibiotics for purchase without a prescription on the internet, *Ann Fam Med* 7(5):431–435, 2009.

Miller LG: Management of MRSA in the community setting: getting it right the first time, *Medscape CME Infectious Diseases.* Available at www.medscape.org/viewarticle708160. Accessed June 17, 2011.

Nordmann P, Cuzon G, Naas T: The real threat of *Klebsiella pneumoniae* carbapenemase-producing bacteria, *Lancet Infect Dis* 9(4):228, 2009.

Pfaller MA, Mendes RE, Sader HS, et al: Telavancin activity against Gram-positive bacteria isolated from respiratory tract specimens of patients with nosocomial pneumonia, *J Antimicrob Chemother* 65(11):2396, 2010.

Rubinstein E, Lalani T, Corey GR, et al: Telavancin versus vancomycin for hospital-acquired pneumonia due to Gram-positive pathogens, *Clin Infect Dis* 52(1):31, 2011.

Sánchez García M, De la Torre MA, Morales G, et al: Clinical outbreak of linezolid-resistant *Staphylococcus aureus* in an intensive care unit, *JAMA* 303(22):2260, 2010.

CHAPTER 40

Abudalu M, Tyring S, Koltun W, et al: Single-day, patient-initiated famciclovir therapy versus 3-day valacyclovir regimen for recurrent genital herpes: a randomized, double-blind, comparative trial, *Clin Infect Dis* 47(5):651, 2008.

Cernik C, Gallina K, Brodell RT: The treatment of herpes simplex infections: an evidence-based review, *Arch Intern Med* 168(11):1137, 2008.

Cohen MS, Gay CL: Treatment to prevent transmission of HIV-1, *Clin Infect Dis* 50(Suppl 3):S85, 2010.

Dumond JB, Patterson KB, Pecha AL, et al: Maraviroc concentrates in the cervicovaginal fluid and vaginal tissue of HIV-negative women, *J Acquir Immune Defic Syndr* 51(5):546, 2009.

Hoyle B: Valacylovir plus zidovudine may block vertical transmission of HSV-2. *Medscape Medical News.* Available at www.medscape.com/viewarticle/738337. Accessed June 27, 2011.

Mayer KH, Venkatesh KK: Chemoprophylaxis for HIV prevention: new opportunities and new questions, *J Acquir Immune Defic Syndr* 55:S122, 2010.

Phipps W, Saracino M, Magaret A, et al: Persistent genital herpes simplex virus-2 shedding years following the first clinical episode, *J Infect Dis* 203(2):180, 2011.

Smith A, Miles I, Le B, et al: Prevalence and awareness of HIV infection among men who have sex with men—21 cities, United States, 2008, *MMWR.* 59(37):1201–1207, 2010.

Watanabe A, Chang SC, Kim MJ, et al: Long-acting neuraminidase inhibitor laninamivir octanoate versus oseltamivir for treatment of influenza: a double-blind, randomized, noninferiority clinical trial, *Clin Infect Dis* 51(10):1167, 2010.

Wong EY, Hewlett IK: HIV diagnostics: challenges and opportunities, *HIV Therapy* 4(4):399–412, 2010.

CHAPTER 41

Barclay L: Rifampin may be better tolerated than isoniazid for latent tuberculosis. *Medscape Medical News.* Available at www.medscape.com/viewarticle/583731. Accessed June 29, 2011.

Horne DJ, Royce SE, Gooze L, et al: Sputum monitoring during tuberculosis treatment for predicting outcome: systematic review and meta-analysis, *Lancet Infect Dis* 10(6):387–394, 2010.

Johnson JL, Hadad DJ, Dietze R, et al: Shortening treatment in adults with noncavitary tuberculosis and 2-month culture conversion, *Am J Respir Crit Care Med* 180(6):558, 2009.

King J: Aduvant immunotherapy improves tuberculosis outcomes. *Medscape Medical News*. Available at www.medscape.com/viewarticle/731805. Accessed on June 29, 2011.

Sharma SK, Singla R, Sarda P, et al: Safety of 3 different reintroduction regimens of antituberculosis drugs after development of antituberculosis treatment-induced hepatotoxicity, *Clin Infect Dis* 50(6):833, 2010.

World Health Organization: *Treatment of tuberculosis guidelines*, ed 4, Geneva, 2010, World Health Organization. Available at whqlibdoc.who.int/publications/2010/9789241547833_eng.pdf. Accessed April 9, 2011.

CHAPTER 42

Gafter-Gvili A, Vidal L, Goldberg E, et al: Treatment of invasive candidal infections: systematic review and meta-analysis, *Mayo Clin Proc* 83(9):1011, 13a 14a, 2008.

Lyon GM, Karatela S, Sunay S, et al: Antifungal susceptibility testing of *Candida* isolates from the *Candida* surveillance study, *J Clin Microbiol* 48(4):1270–1275, 2010.

Pappas PG, Kauffman CA, Andes D, et al: Clinical practice guidelines for the management of candidiasis: 2009 update by the Infectious Diseases Society of America, *Clin Infect Dis* 48(5):503, 2009.

Thompson GR 3rd, Wiederhold NP, Vallor AC, et al: Development of caspofungin resistance following prolonged therapy for invasive candidiasis secondary to *Candida glabrata* infection, *Antimicrob Agents Chemother* 52(10):3783, 2008.

CHAPTER 43

Centers for Disease Control and Prevention: *Malaria*, 2012. Available at www.cdc.gov/malaria/. Accessed June 20, 2012.

Centers for Disease Control and Prevention: *Malaria travelers*, 2011. Available at www.cdc.gov/malaria/travelers/drugs.html/. Accessed April 18, 2011.

Deen JL, von Seidlein L, Dondorp A: Therapy of uncomplicated malaria in children: a review of treatment principles, essential drugs and current recommendations, *Trop Med Int Health* 13(9):1111, 2008.

Müller IB, Hyde JE: Antimalarial drugs: modes of action and mechanisms of parasite resistance, *Future Microbiol* 5(12):1857–1873, 2010.

CHAPTER 44

Argoff CH: *Optimal pain management in older patients*, 2010. Available at www.medscape.com/viewarticle/730074. Accessed July 2, 2011.

Durrance S: *Older adults and NSAIDs: avoiding adverse reactions*, 2004. Available at www.medscape.com/viewarticle/466796. Accessed July 2, 2011.

Food and Drug Administration: *FDA orders halt to marketing of unapproved single-ingredient oral colchicines*, 2010. Available at www.fda.gov/NewsEvents/Newsroom/PressAnnouncements/ucm227796.htm. Accessed April 21, 2011.

Solomon SD, Wittes J, Finn PV, et al: Cardiovascular risk of celecoxib in 6 randomized placebo-controlled trials: the cross trial safety analysis, *Circulation* 117(16):2104, 2008.

Terkeltaub RA, Furst DE, Bennett K, et al: High versus low dosing of oral colchicine for early acute gout flare: twenty-four-hour outcome of the first multicenter, randomized, double-blind, placebo-controlled, parallel-group, dose-comparison colchicine study, *Arthritis Rheum* 62(4):1060, 2010.

CHAPTER 45

Bang YJ, Van Cutsem E, Feyereislova A, et al: Trastuzumab in combination with chemotherapy versus chemotherapy alone for treatment of HER2-positive advanced gastric or gastro-oesophageal junction cancer (ToGA): a phase 3, open-label, randomised controlled trial, *Lancet* 376(9742):687, 2010.

Nelson R: Chronic pain common in cancer survivors needs to be addressed. *eMedicine Medscape*. 2011. Available at www.medscape.com/viewarticle/736176. Accessed July 5, 2011.

Schore RJ, Coppes MJ: Chemotherapy-induced nausea and vomiting. *eMedicineMedscape*. 2009. Available at http://emedicine.medscape.com. Accessed July 5, 2011.

Scully C, Sonis S, Diz PD: Oral mucositis, *Oral Dis* 12(3):229–241, 2006.

Sonis ST: Pathobiology of oral mucositis: novel insights and opportunities, *J Support Oncol* 5(9; Suppl 4):3–11, 2007.

Treister NS, Elston DM: Chemotherapy-induced oral mucositis. *Medscape Medical News*. 2010. Available at http://emedicine.medscape.com/article/1079570. Accessed July 3, 2011.

Twelves C, Loesch JL, Blum LT, et al: A phase III study (EMBRACE) of eribulin mesylate versus treatment of physician's choice in patients with locally recurrent or metastatic breast cancer previously treated with an anthracycline and a taxane, *J Clin Oncol* 28(Abstr CRA 1004):18s, 2010.

CHAPTER 46

Gahart BL, Nazarena AR: *2011 Intravenous medications*, ed 27, St Louis, MO, 2011, Mosby.

Hamdi T, Latta S, Jallad B, et al: Cisplatin-induced renal salt wasting syndrome, *South Med J* 103(8):793–799, 2010.

Maroto P, Huddart R, Garcia del Muro X, et al: Brief report: phase II multicenter study of temozolomide in patients with cisplatin-Resistant germ cell tumors, *Oncology* 80(3–4):219–222, 2011.

McBride A: Management of chemotherapy extravasations, *US Pharm* 34(9 Oncology Suppl):3–11, 2009.

Sabo B: Reflecting on the concept of compassion fatigue, *Online J Issues Nurs* 16(1):2011. Available at: www.medscape.com/viewarticle/745292. Accessed July 9, 2011.

Wittenberg-Lyles E, Goldsmith J, Ragan S: The shift to early palliative care, *Clin J Oncol Nurs* 15(3):304–310, 2011.

CHAPTER 47

Dall'Era M, Wofsy D: Systemic lupus erythematosus clinical trials—an interim analysis, *Nat Rev Rheumatol* 5(6):348, 2009.

Fleischman R: Don't forget traditional DMARDs: old friends are still useful, *Rheumatology* 50(3):429–430, 2011.

Jolly M: Pitfalls and opportunities in measuring patient outcomes in lupus, *Curr Rheumatol Rep* 12(4):229, 2010.

Saag KG, Teng GG, Patkar NM, et al: American College of Rheumatology 2008 recommendations for the use of nonbiologic and biologic disease-modifying antirheumatic drugs in rheumatoid arthritis, *Arthritis Rheum* 59(6):762, 2008.

Schmajuk G, Trivedi AN, Solomon DH, et al: Receipt of disease-modifying antirheumatic drugs among medicare managed care plans, *JAMA* 305(5):480–486, 2011.

Smolen JS, Landewé R, Breedveld FC, et al: EULAR recommendations for the management of rheumatoid arthritis with synthetic and biological disease-modifying antirheumatic drugs, *Ann Rheum Dis* 69(6):964, 2010.

CHAPTER 48

Armand P, Gannamaneni S, Kim HT, et al: Improved survival in lymphoma patients receiving sirolimus for graft-versus-host disease prophylaxis after allogeneic hematopoietic stem-cell transplantation with reduced-intensity conditioning, *J Clin Oncol* 26(35):5767, 2008.

Gallagher M, Jardine M, Perkovic V, et al: Cyclosporine withdrawal improves long-term graft survival in renal transplantation, *Transplantation* 87(12):1877–1883, 2009.

Gruessner R, Benedetti E: *Living donor organ transplantation*, New York, NY, 2008, McGraw-Hill.

Jain A, Singhal A, Fontes P, et al: One thousand consecutive primary liver transplants under tacrolimus immunosuppression: a 17- to 20-year longitudinal follow-up, *Transplantation* 91(9):1025–1030, 2011.

Levine JE, Paczesny S, Mineishi S, et al: Etanercept plus methylprednisolone as initial therapy for acute graft-versus-host disease, *Blood* 111(4):2470, 14a 15a, 2008.

Mukherjee S, Botha JF, Mukherjee U: Immunosuppression in liver transplantation, *Curr Drug Targets* 10(6):557–574, 2009.

Murphy F: The role of the nurse in pre-renal transplantation, *Br J Nurs* 16(10):582–587, 2007.

CHAPTER 49

Brauser D: *Autism and MMR Vaccine Study an "elaborate fraud", charges BMJ.* Available at www.medscape.com/viewarticle/735354. Accessed May 1, 2011.

Centers for Disease Control and Prevention: *Adult immunization schedule.* Available at www.cdc.gov/vaccines/schedules/hcp/adult.html. Accessed May 1, 2011.

Centers for Disease Control and Prevention: *Child, adolescent, and "catch-up" immunization schedules.* Available at www.cdc.gov/vaccines/schedules/hcp/child-adolescent.html. Accessed May 1, 2011.

Centers for Disease Control and Prevention: *Guide to vaccination contraindications and precautions.* Available at www.cdc.gov/vaccines/recs/vac-admin/contraindications.htm. Accessed May 1, 2011.

Centers for Disease Control and Prevention: *Preventing seasonal flu with vaccination.* Available at www.cdc.gov/flu/protect/vaccine/index.htm. Accessed May 1, 2011.

Centers for Disease Control and Prevention: *Shingles vaccination: what you need to know.* Available at www.cdc.gov/vaccines/vpd-vac/shingles/vac-faqs.htm. Accessed at May 1, 2011.

Centers for Disease Control and Prevention: *Thimerosal.* Available at www.cdc.gov/vaccinesafety/Concerns/thimerosal/. Accessed May 1, 2011.

Centers for Disease Control and Prevention: Updated recommendations for prevention of invasive pneumococcal disease among adults using the 23-valent pneumococcal polysaccharide vaccine (PPSV23), *MMWR.* 59(34):1102–1106, 2010.

Centers for Disease Control and Prevention: Use of hepatitis B vaccination for adults with diabetes mellitus: recommendations of the advisory committee on immunization practices (ACIP), *MMWR.* 60(50):1709–1711, 2011. Available at: www.cdc.gov/mmwr/preview/mmwrhtml/mm6050a4.htm. Accessed January 7, 2012.

Godlee F, Smith J, Marcovitch H, et al: Wakefield's article linking MMR vaccine and autism was fraudulent, *BMJ* 342:c7452, 2011.

Pichichero ME, Gentile A, Giglio N, et al: Mercury levels in newborns and infants after receipt of thimerosal-containing vaccines, *Pediatrics* 121(2):e208, 2008.

Price CS, Thompson WW, Goodson B, et al: Prenatal and infant exposure to thimerosal from vaccines and immunoglobulins and risk of autism, *Pediatrics* 126(4):656, 2010.

U.S. Department of Health and Human Services: *Vaccine adverse event reporting system.* Available at http://vaers.hhs.gov. Accessed May 1, 2011.

U.S. Department of Justice: *Vaccine Injury Compensation Program.* Available at www.justice.gov/civil/common/vicp.html. Accessed May 1, 2011.

U.S. Food and Drug Administration: *Bioterrorism and drug preparedness,* 2011. Available at www.fda.gov/Drugs/EmergencyPreparedness/BioterrorismandDrugPreparedness/default.htm?utm_campaign=Google2&utm_source=fdaSearch&utm_medium=website&utm_term=Drug%20preparedness%20and%20response%20to%20bioterrorism&utm_content=2. Accessed May 1, 2011.

CHAPTER 50

Bhatt D, Cryer B, Contant CF, et al: Clopidogrel with or without omeprazole in coronary artery disease, *N Engl J Med* 363(20):1909–1917, 2010.

Glaser J, Rolita L: Educating the older adult in over-the-counter medication use, *Geriatrics and Aging* 12(2):103–109, 2009.

Leontiadis G, Howden C: The role of proton pump inhibitors in the management of upper gastrointestinal bleeding, *Gastroenterology Clinics* 38(2):199–213, 2009.

Mejia A, Kraft WM: Acid peptic diseases: pharmacological approach to treatment, *Expert Review of Clinical Pharmacology* 2(3):295–314, 2009.

Reimer C, Sondergaard B, Hilsted L, et al: Proton-pump inhibitor therapy induces acid-related symptoms in healthy volunteers after withdrawal of therapy, *Gastroenterology* 137(1):80–87, 2009.

Tsoi KK, Lau JY, Sung JJ: Cost-effectiveness analysis of high-dose omeprazole infusion before endoscopy for patients with upper-GI bleeding, *Gastrointest Endosc* 67(7):1056–1063, 2008.

U.S. Food and Drug Administration: *Possible increased risk of fractures of the hip, wrist, and spine with the use of proton pump inhibitors,* 2011. Available at www.fda.gov/drugs/drugsafety/postmarketdrugsafetyinformationforpatientsandproviders/ucm213206.htm. Accessed October 17, 2011.

U.S. Food and Drug Administration: *Low magnesium levels can be associated with long-term use of Proton Pump Inhibitor drugs (PPIs),* 2011. Available at www.fda.gov/Drugs/DrugSafety/ucm245011.htm. Accessed October 18, 2011.

CHAPTER 51

American College of Gastroenterology Task Force on Irritable Bowel Syndrome, Brandt LJ, Chey WD, et al: An evidence-based position statement on the management of irritable bowel syndrome, *Am J Gastroenterol* 104(Suppl 1):S1, 2009.

Barclay L: Probiotics may shorten acute diarrheal episodes. *Medscape Medical News.* Available at www.medscape.com. Accessed July 24, 2011.

Dalrymple J, Bullock I: Diagnosis and management of irritable bowel syndrome in adults in primary care: summary of NICE guidance, *BMJ* 336(7643):556, 2008.

Ford AC, Talley NJ, Schoenfeld PS, et al: Efficacy of antidepressants and psychological therapies in irritable bowel syndrome: systematic review and meta-analysis, *Gut* 58(3):367, 2009.

Kaptchuk TJ, Kelley JM, Conboy LA, et al: Components of placebo effect: randomised controlled trial in patients with irritable bowel syndrome, *BMJ* 336(7651):999, 2008.

Sherman M: Probiotics and microflora, *US Pharmacist* 34(12):42–44, 2009.

CHAPTER 52

American Society of Health-System Pharmacists: *Guidelines on the prevention of chemotherapy induced nausea and vomiting.* Available at www.ashp.org. Accessed July 26, 2011.

Barclay L: Treatment of acute poisoning from medication ingestion reviewed. *Medscape Medical News.* Available at www.medscape.com/viewarticle/716582. Accessed July 26, 2011.

Hesketh PJ: Chemotherapy induced nausea and vomiting, *N Engl J Med* 258(23):2482–2494, 2008.

U.S. Food and Drug Administration Safety: *Anzemet (dolasetron mesylate): drug safety communication—reports of abnormal heart rhythms,* 2010. Available at www.fda.gov/Safety/MedWatch/SafetyInformation/SafetyAlertsforHumanMedicalProducts/ucm237341.htm. Accessed May 7, 2010.

U.S. Food and Drug Administration Safety: *Zofran (ondansetron): drug safety communication—risk of abnormal heart rhythms,* 2011. Available at www.fda.gov/Safety/MedWatch/SafetyInformation/SafetyAlertsforHumanMedicalProducts/ucm272041.htm. Accessed January 7, 2011.

CHAPTER 53

Allen LH: How common is vitamin B-12 deficiency? *Am J Clin Nutr* 89(2):693S, 2009.

Ebbing M, Bønaa KH, Nygård O, et al: Cancer incidence and mortality after treatment with folic acid and vitamin B₁₂, *JAMA* 302(19):2119, 2009.

Ginde AA, Scragg R, Schwartz RS, et al: Prospective study of serum 25-hydroxyvitamin D level, cardiovascular disease mortality, and all-cause mortality in older U.S. adults, *J Am Geriatr Soc* 57(9):1595, 2009.

Lin J, Cook NR, Albert C, et al: Vitamins C and E and beta carotene supplementation and cancer risk: a randomized controlled trial, *J Natl Cancer Inst* 101(1):14, 2009.

Logan RF, Grainge MJ, Shepherd VC, et al: Aspirin and folic acid for the prevention of recurrent colorectal adenomas, *Gastroenterology* 134(1):29, 2008.

Medline Plus: *Nutritional supplements*. Available at www.nm.nih.gov/medlineplus. Accessed July 29, 2011.

Neuhouser ML, Wassertheil-Smoller S, Thomson C, et al: Multivitamin use and risk of cancer and cardiovascular disease in the Women's Health Initiative cohorts, *Arch Intern Med* 169(3):294, 2009.

CHAPTER 54

Alleyne M, Horne MK, Miller JL: Individualized treatment for iron-deficiency anemia in adults, *Am J Med* 121(11):943, 2008.

Asare K: Anemia of critical illness, *Pharmacotherapy* 28(10):1267–1282, 2008.

Kazory A, Ross EA: Anemia: the point of convergence or divergence for kidney disease and heart failure?, *J Am Coll Cardiol* 53(8):639, 2009.

Kotecha D, Ngo K, Walters JAE, et al: Erythropoietin as a treatment of anemia in heart failure, *Am Heart J* 161(5):822–831, 2011.

Rodgers GM 3rd, Becker PS, Bennett CL, et al: Cancer- and chemotherapy-induced anemia, *J Natl Compr Canc Netw* 6(6):536, 2008.

Silverberg DS, Wexler D, Iaina A, et al: Anemia, chronic renal disease and chronic heart failure: the cardiorenal anemia syndrome, *Transfusion Alternatives in Transfusion Medicine* 10(4):189–196, 2009.

U.S. Food and Drug Administration: *Information on erythropoiesis-stimulating agents (ESA) epoetin alfa (marketed as Procrit, Epogen), darbepoetin alfa (marketed as Aranesp)*, 2010. Available at www.fda.gov/drugs/drugsafety/postmarketdrugsafetyinformationforpatientsandproviders/ucm109375.htm. Accessed May 21, 2011.

CHAPTER 55

DeLegge MH: Enteral feeding, *Gastroenterology* 24(2):184–189, 2008.

Fitzgerald MA: *What do I need to know about drug interactions and enteral feedings? Medscpe Nurses*. Available at www.medscape.com/viewarticle/498270. Accessed August 3, 2011.

Koretz RL: Enteral nutrition: a hard look at some soft evidence, *Nutr Clin Pract* 24(3):316, 2009.

McClave SA, Heyland DK: The physiologic response and associated clinical benefits from provision of early enteral nutrition, *Nutr Clin Pract* 24(3):305, 2009.

McClave SA, Martindale RG, Vanek VW, et al: Guidelines for the provision and assessment of nutrition support therapy in the adult critically ill patient: Society of Critical Care Medicine (SCCM) and American Society for Parenteral and Enteral Nutrition (ASPEN), *J Parenter Enteral Nutr.* 33(3):277, 2009.

CHAPTER 56

American Osteopathic College of Dermatology: *Psoriasis*. Available at www.aocd.org/skin/dermatologic_diseases/psoriasis.html. Accessed May 12, 2011.

Skin Cancer Foundation: *Skin cancer facts*, 2008. Available at www.skincancer.org/Skin-Cancer/2008-Skin-Cancer-Facts.html. Accessed May 15, 2011.

U.S. Food and Drug Administration: *iPLEDGE*, 2010. Available at www.fda.gov/Drugs/DrugSafety/PostmarketDrugSafetyInformationforPatientsandProviders/ucm094307.htm. Accessed May 15, 2011.

U.S. Food and Drug Administration: *Medication guide: Stelara*. Available at www.accessdata.fda.gov/drugsatfda_docs/label/2009/125261mg.pdf. Accessed May 15, 2011.

U.S. Food and Drug Administration: *Questions and answers about FDA's enforcement action regarding unapproved topical drug products containing papain*, 2009. Available at www.fda.gov/Drugs/GuidanceComplianceRegulatoryInformation/EnforcementActivitiesbyFDA/SelectedEnforcementActionsonUnapprovedDrugs/ucm119646.htm. Accessed May 15, 2011.

U.S. Food and Drug Administration: *FDA announces changes to better inform consumers about sunscreen*. Available at www.fda.gov/NewsEvents/Newsroom/PressAnnouncements/ucm258940.htm. Accessed June 17, 2011.

CHAPTER 57

Grus FH, Joachim SC, Wuenschig D, et al: Autoimmunity and glaucoma, *J Glaucoma* 17(1):79–84, 2008.

Kwon YH, Fingert JH, Kuehn MH, et al: Primary open-angle glaucoma, *N Engl J Med* 360(11):1113, 2009.

Realini T: A history of glaucoma pharmacology, *Optom Vis Sci* 88(1):36–38, 2011.

Reeder CE, Franklin M, Bramley TJ: Managed care and the impact of glaucoma, *Am J Manag Care* 14(Suppl 1):S5–S10, 2008.

Susanna R Jr: Unpredictability of glaucoma progression, *Curr Med Res Opin* 25(9):2167, 2009.

CHAPTER 58

American Academy of Pediatrics Subcommittee on Management of Acute Otitis Media: Diagnosis and management of acute otitis media, *Pediatrics* 113(5):1451–1465, 2004.

Benninger MS: Acute bacterial rhinosinusitis and otitis media: changes in pathogenicity following widespread use of pneumococcal conjugate vaccine, *Otolaryngol Head Neck Surg* 138(3):274, 2008.

Broides A, Dagan R, Greenberg D, et al: Acute otitis media caused by *Moraxella catarrhalis*: epidemiologic and clinical characteristics, *Clin Infect Dis* 49(11):1641–1647, 2009.

Chonmaitree T, Revai K, Grady JJ, et al: Viral upper respiratory tract infection and otitis media complication in young children, *Clin Infect Dis* 46(6):815, 2008.

Ely J: Diagnosis of ear pain, *Am Fam Physician* 77(5):621–628, 2009.

Morris P: Acute and chronic otitis, *Ped Clinic North America* 56(6):1383–1399, 2009.

Pages followed by *b*, *t*, or *f* refer to boxes, tables, or figures, respectively. Blue entries indicate disorders. Boldface entries indicate generic drug names.